Eyelid, Conjunctival, and Orbital Tumors

AN ATLAS AND TEXTBOOK

THIRD EDITION

Eyelid, Conjunctival, and Orbital Tumors

AN ATLAS AND TEXTBOOK

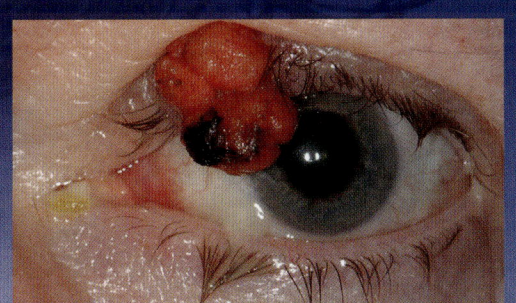
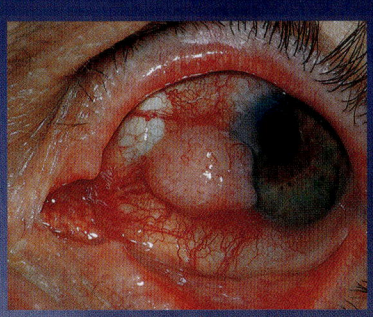
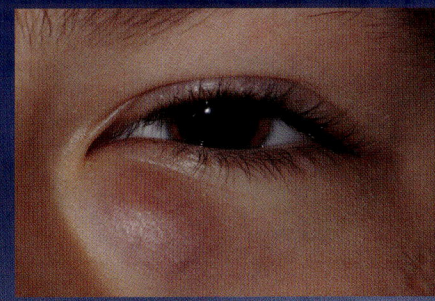

THIRD EDITION

Jerry A. Shields, MD
Director, Ocular Oncology Service
Wills Eye Hospital
Professor of Ophthalmology
Thomas Jefferson University
Philadelphia, Pennsylvania, USA

Carol L. Shields, MD
Co-Director, Ocular Oncology Service
Wills Eye Hospital
Professor of Ophthalmology
Thomas Jefferson University
Philadelphia, Pennsylvania, USA

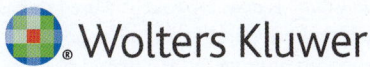

Philadelphia • Baltimore • New York • London
Buenos Aires • Hong Kong • Sydney • Tokyo

Acquisitions Editor: Kel McGowan
Senior Product Development Editor: Emilie Moyer
Marketing Manager: Stephanie Kindlick
Senior Production Project Manager: Alicia Jackson
Design Coordinator: Stephen Druding
Manufacturing Coordinator: Beth Welsh
Prepress Vendor: Aptara, Inc.

Third edition

Copyright © 2016 Wolters Kluwer.

Copyright © 2007 Wolters Kluwer Health | Lippincott Williams & Wilkins. Copyright © 1999 Lippincott Williams & Wilkins, a Wolters Kluwer business. All rights reserved. This book is protected by copyright. No part of this book may be reproduced or transmitted in any form or by any means, including as photocopies or scanned-in or other electronic copies, or utilized by any information storage and retrieval system without written permission from the copyright owner, except for brief quotations embodied in critical articles and reviews. Materials appearing in this book prepared by individuals as part of their official duties as U.S. government employees are not covered by the above-mentioned copyright. To request permission, please contact Wolters Kluwer at Two Commerce Square, 2001 Market Street, Philadelphia, PA 19103, via email at permissions@lww.com, or via our website at lww.com (products and services).

9 8 7 6 5 4 3 2 1

Printed in China

Library of Congress Cataloging-in-Publication Data

Shields, Jerry A., author.
 Eyelid, conjunctival, and orbital tumors : an atlas and textbook / Jerry A. Shields, Carol L. Shields. – Third edition.
   p. ; cm.
 Includes bibliographical references and index.
 ISBN 978-1-4963-2148-0 (alk. paper)
  I. Shields, Carol L., author. II. Title.
  [DNLM: 1. Eyelid Neoplasms–Atlases. 2. Conjunctival Neoplasms–Atlases. 3. Orbital Neoplasms–Atlases. WW 17]
  RC280.E9
  616.99'484–dc23

2015021024

This work is provided "as is," and the publisher disclaims any and all warranties, express or implied, including any warranties as to accuracy, comprehensiveness, or currency of the content of this work.

 This work is no substitute for individual patient assessment based upon healthcare professionals' examination of each patient and consideration of, among other things, age, weight, gender, current or prior medical conditions, medication history, laboratory data and other factors unique to the patient. The publisher does not provide medical advice or guidance and this work is merely a reference tool. Healthcare professionals, and not the publisher, are solely responsible for the use of this work including all medical judgments and for any resulting diagnosis and treatments.

 Given continuous, rapid advances in medical science and health information, independent professional verification of medical diagnoses, indications, appropriate pharmaceutical selections and dosages, and treatment options should be made and healthcare professionals should consult a variety of sources. When prescribing medication, healthcare professionals are advised to consult the product information sheet (the manufacturer's package insert) accompanying each drug to verify, among other things, conditions of use, warnings and side effects and identify any changes in dosage schedule or contraindications, particularly if the medication to be administered is new, infrequently used or has a narrow therapeutic range. To the maximum extent permitted under applicable law, no responsibility is assumed by the publisher for any injury and/or damage to persons or property, as a matter of products liability, negligence law or otherwise, or from any reference to or use by any person of this work.

LWW.com

This book is dedicated to our seven children,

Jerry, Patrick, Bill, Maggie Mae, John, Nellie, and Mary Rose.

They are now in their teens and twenties, and still remain most precious to us.

We wish them satisfaction and success in their home life and careers

and hope that they will flourish as they chase their dreams.

FOREWORD 1

Since Jerry Shields established the Ocular Oncology Service at Wills Eye Hospital in 1974, it has grown into one of the largest and best ocular oncology departments in the world. The ocular oncology team at Wills sees dozens of new patients every week, and performs surgery to treat tumors several days a week. The Service is now headed by Jerry and his wife Carol Shields, two giants in the field. Jerry and Carol and their team have published hundreds of papers in the peer-reviewed ophthalmic literature and lectured extensively throughout the United States and around the world on the diagnosis and management of ocular tumors. I can think of no better doctors to write textbooks dealing with tumors in and around the eye.

The first two editions of the Eyelid, Conjunctival, and Orbital Tumors Atlas and Textbook were superb! This third edition has been updated to include more diagnoses, additional photographs, and cutting edge medical and surgical treatments. The book is divided into three parts which are subdivided into 41 chapters and contains over 2,600 high-quality images. Part 1 deals with tumors of the eyelid. It is composed of 15 chapters on all varieties of eyelid cancers including tumors of the epidermis such as basal cell and squamous cell carcinomas, sebaceous gland tumors, melanocytic tumors, vascular tumors, and numerous conditions simulating neoplasms. The last chapter in this part is on the surgical management of eyelid tumors. Part 2 deals with tumors of the conjunctiva including choristomas such as dermoids, intraepithelial neoplasia and invasive squamous cell carcinoma, vascular tumors, lymphoid tumors, and numerous conditions simulating conjunctival neoplasms. The last chapter in this part is on the surgical management of conjunctival tumors. Part 3 deals with tumors of the orbit including cystic lesions, vascular and hemorrhagic lesions, peripheral and optic nerve tumors, myogenic tumors such as rhabdomyosarcoma, lacrimal gland tumors, lymphoid tumors and leukemias, and numerous inflammatory conditions simulating orbital neoplasms. The last chapter in this part is on the surgical management of orbital tumors.

Each chapter includes discussion of many different tumors or mimicking conditions. For each diagnostic entity, there are general considerations, clinical features, differential diagnosis, pathology, and management. This is followed by numerous superb photos of the clinical entity, imaging studies, pathology, and surgical management. Drs. Jerry and Carol Shields should be congratulated on improving on their already wonderful textbook with this third edition. As clinicians seeing patients with possible ocular and adnexal tumors, we should be extremely thankful to them for putting together such an impressive atlas and textbook!

Christopher J. Rapuano, MD
Chief of the Cornea Service, Co-Chief of the Refractive Surgery Department, Wills Eye Hospital
Professor of Ophthalmology, Sidney Kimmel Medical College at Thomas Jefferson University
Philadelphia, PA

FOREWORD 2

This Third Edition of the 2-volume set on ophthalmic tumors, the second of which is entitled "*Eyelid, Conjunctival and Orbital Tumors: An Atlas and Textbook,*" has been kept to a reasonable length of somewhat more than 800 pages yet embraces many valuable improvements. As an individual with a longstanding interest in orbital and adnexal tumors, I can say without equivocation or reservation that the second volume of the set devoted to the adnexa has no match and should be in every ophthalmologist's and trainee's (along with the first volume) collection of ophthalmic treatises. The accessibility of the knowledge that this volume contains has been facilitated by a highly logical unfolding of topics in the Table of Contents and an excellent Index.

We are well into the era of internet publishing that threatens the very survival of books in both medical and non-medical fields. Today's readers expect to obtain their knowledge in dollops and tweets which means they eschew more considered, in-depth treatments of topics found in textbooks. This is unfortunate. Familiarity with a benchmark source of reasonable length permits one to amble through it so that it becomes like an old friend or companion. While it is not possible to retain everything read in a major textbook, intimacy with it eases a return to it for easily finding the desired information.

Even if books are fast assuming the status of an endangered species, there will always be a role and need for a select few that have passed the test of time. Literary critics refer to such intellectual artifacts that have unarguably transformed into classics as "canonical"—signifying their central and seminal significance among books of their genre. Other examples besides the present enterprise that qualify for this sobriquet are Miller and Newman's revision of the 3-volume *Walsh and Hoyt's Clinical Neuro-Ophthalmology* (Lippincott Williams & Wilkins, 2004), Spencer's 4-volume *Ophthalmic Pathology: An Atlas and Text* (WB Saunders, 1995), and Miller and Albert's 4-volume *Albert and Jakobiec's Principles and Practice of Ophthalmology* (WB Saunders, 2007).

Each section of this volume contains a thoroughly revised, scholarly and comprehensive introductory overview that covers in a succinct and practical fashion what the clinician needs to know about the diagnosis and management of tumors of the eyelids, conjunctiva, and orbit. More than 4,000 carefully chosen and beautiful color illustrations of the relevant clinical and histopathologic features, with a complement of black and white imaging studies, reinforce the points made in the text. The bibliographies for each topic are judiciously selected and up to date. Many new entities have been described since the last edition. Two that appeal to my pedantic side are neurothekeoma (occurring preferentially in the eyelids and exceptionally in the conjunctiva and orbit) and phacomatosis pigmentovascularis of the cesioflammea type. The latter condition combines a nevus flammeus with ipsilateral ocular melanosis, melanocytosis, or melanocytic tumors. The nevus flammeus (but not the melanocytosis) was bilateral in three of seven cases. Choroidal melanoma was observed in three patients and an optic disc melanocytoma in one. (For a more complete description of this recondite subject beyond what is offered in the textbook one should consult Shields et al. *Arch Ophthalmol* 2011; 129:746–750.)

Topical drug treatment for ocular surface tumors as well as plaque brachytherapy are critically assessed and introduced for the first time to the textbook, as is an exploration of the controversial role of sentinel lymph node biopsy and dissection for conjunctival melanoma. Especially helpful for clinicians and pathologists are demystifying descriptions of the clinical and pathologic features, as well as management options, of the challenging entities of primary acquired melanosis, emergent melanoma, and sebaceous carcinoma. Propranolol for promoting regression of eyelid capillary hemangioma is included among the different approaches for this nettlesome problem which can cause amblyopia. An excellent description of the management of malignant lacrimal gland epithelial tumors is offered. Finally, particularly insightful and representative of the contemporary sophistication of the authors is the application of the World Health Organization (WHO) classification of lymphomas for ocular adnexal lesions and the American Joint Commission on Cancer (AJCC) classification of ocular adnexal nonlymphomatous solid tumors.

What makes this textbook a distinctively authoritative resource is the combination of the unrivaled clinical experience of Carol and Jerry Shields as practicing clinical ophthalmic oncologists and their intimate familiarity with the appropriate literature. They have earned the accolade of being the ultimate "power couple" of American ophthalmology and ophthalmic oncology. Their human side, however, has not been adversely affected by their devotion to their professional calling. They have raised a marvelous family with most of their well-adjusted children now launched into adulthood. The Shields are a national, and indeed an international, treasure who have helped untold numbers of patients and who have generously and personally shared their knowledge with colleagues and trainees, and also prodigiously enriched the literature with their high-quality publications based on the codification of their clinical experience. I admire them greatly and am a devoted aficionado of this textbook, to which I frequently refer for digestible summaries of unusual or arcane topics. I wish them many more years of productivity as they persist in their labors to further develop and advance ophthalmic oncology.

Frederick A. Jakobiec, MD, DSc
Henry Willard Williams Professor Emeritus
of Ophthalmology and Pathology
Harvard Medical School
Former Chairman of Ophthalmology
Harvard Medical School
Former Chief of Ophthalmology
Massachusetts Eye and Ear Infirmary
Current Director
David Glendenning Cogan Laboratory of Ophthalmic Pathology
Massachusetts Eye & Ear Infirmary, Boston, Massachusetts

PREFACE

Forty years in the management of eyelid, conjunctival, and orbital tumors

Forty years is a long time. Forty years is beyond the time spent in most careers.

Forty years represents the number of years that we have devoted our medical and surgical practice to the study of eyelid, conjunctival, and orbital tumors. We have focused our career on the topic of periocular tumors, benign or malignant, and the numerous simulating lesions. Every working day, we have traveled from our small farm to the city of Philadelphia and studied and helped patients with periocular tumors, providing diagnoses, treatments, and reconstructions. We have spent precious time exploring new and progressive treatments to maximize patient comfort, safety, and cosmesis. After all is done, then we traveled home in the early evening.

Forty years represents the time that we used to discover, think, design, critique, and perform hours-on-end research that culminated in numerous ocular oncology projects with information pushing the field forward. Slow and steady progress, but looking back, we participated in giant leaps of knowledge.

In 1999, we published our first series of atlases in three volumes, entitled *Atlas of Eyelid and Conjunctival Tumors*, *Atlas of Intraocular Tumors*, and *Atlas of Orbital Tumors*. Following numerous enhancements and updates, we subsequently wrote a second edition in two volumes in 2008 entitled *Intraocular Tumors: An Atlas and Textbook* and *Eyelid, Conjunctival, and Orbital Tumors: An Atlas and Textbook*.

We now provide you with the third edition of our atlases. This volume is embellished with new illustrations, updated references and text, improved imaging modalities, and novel observations. We have carefully planned the layout of this book so that it is reader-friendly with six illustrations per page to tell a story or make a clinical or surgical point. Each diagnostic entity is described in anatomical order based on eyelid then conjunctiva then orbital tissue. Go ahead and flip through to enjoy the full experience.

This book is generously illustrated with numerous images of common lesions, such as chalazion and pinguecula, as well as rare and fascinating conditions like lipoid proteinosis of the eyelid, ligneous conjunctivitis, orbital juvenile xanthogranuloma, and conjunctival hereditary benign intraepithelial dyskeratosis. This atlas is overflowing in clinicopathologic correlations and clinical "pearls" based on our personal experience. Surgical principles are illustrated with high-quality professional drawings and photographs. We hope that this unique textbook and atlas will benefit residents and fellows in ophthalmology, general ophthalmologists, specialists in external disease, oculoplastic surgery, and ophthalmic pathology, as well as other practitioners. We believe the reader will find it useful in clinical practice and enjoyable to read.

Jerry A. Shields, MD
Carol L. Shields, MD

ACKNOWLEDGMENTS

This textbook and atlas represents our lifetime collection of common and rare tumors of the eyelid, conjunctiva, and orbit. This is our work of art, designed to illustrate, describe, categorize, and provide understanding of the sweeping and distinctive spectrum of tumors in the periocular region. This work represents not only our efforts, but it includes the collaborative work of our team and others.

We are grateful to our professors and colleagues for instructing us on the basics of ocular oncology, which stimulated us to explore further. We owe special thanks to our patients for sharing their stories with us and allowing us the honor and trust to care for them.

From the Ocular Oncology Service at Wills Eye Hospital, we would like to thank our first-class team of ophthalmic photographers, Tika Siburt, Tessa Tintle, Jacqueline Hanable, and Sandor Ferenczy for their masterful talents in capturing the distinctive features of ophthalmic tumors. Each photograph was taken with superb skill to provide highest quality imaging of tumor characteristics. We thank Linda Warren for the illustrative surgical drawings. Importantly, we would like to commend the entire staff on the Ocular Oncology Service at Wills Eye Hospital under the direction of David Lashinsky for their devotion and service to our patients. We specifically would like to acknowledge the work of Sandra Dailey in helping with day-to-day matters related to this book. Our staff is the epitome of teamwork and dedication.

We are grateful to the medical staff at Wills Eye Hospital of Thomas Jefferson University, including Julia Haller MD, the Ophthalmologist-in-Chief, and the members of the Pathology, Retina, Uveitis, Cornea, Oculoplastics, Pediatric Ophthalmology, Glaucoma, Neuro-Ophthalmology, and other services for assisting with our patients and sharing ideas. Special thanks to our talented team of oculoplastic surgeons for their cooperative work in repairing surgical defects in challenging cases and providing innovative reconstructions. Special thanks to our corneal colleagues for graciously and expertly consulting on our patients.

We give special thanks to the entire staff at the Department of Neuroradiology at Thomas Jefferson University for their computed tomography and magnetic resonance images. We are particularly appreciative of the many years of assistance from Jack Scully, Director of the Ophthalmic Photography Department at Wills Eye Hospital, who has shown tremendous dedication in the field of ophthalmic imaging and advanced imaging technology.

We would like to credit our physician colleagues on the Ocular Oncology Service at Wills Eye Hospital who have shared in the medical or surgical care of our patients, including Sara Lally, MD, a magnificent surgeon with special interest in eyelid, conjunctival, and orbital tumors. Her innovative and courageous surgical skills are unsurpassed. We thank Arman Masheyekhi, MD, a talented surgeon and pre-eminent scholar, and Emil Say, MD a superb clinician and surgeon in the field of ocular oncology. In addition, there are hundreds of fellows and visitors to the Oncology Service who should be recognized and commended for their dedication to the field of ocular oncology.

We would like to specially recognize the valuable input of our renowned ophthalmic pathologist, Ralph C. Eagle Jr, MD. Throughout the many years that we have worked together, he has provided expert pathologic consultation on ocular tumor cases, some of which were particularly challenging. We are indebted to him for his dedication and unmatched diagnostic insight. Throughout this book, you will note numerous gross and microscopic photographs, courtesy of Dr. Eagle. His unparalleled professional skills in photography are witnessed in the spectacular pathology images.

Finally, we would like to thank our seven children for granting us the time to write this book. They were very young when we generated the first edition, and then they were teenagers during the writing of the second edition. Now they are young adults during this third edition. Their understanding and motivation for this textbook and atlas has provided unending support.

So, now it is time for you to enjoy this third edition of our book. Go ahead and peruse it. Enjoy the dazzling beauty of the 41 chapters. Each chapter boasts splendid new images and updated references with new text and tables. We invite you to savor each page and we hope that this work is useful to you in the care of your patients.

Jerry A. Shields, MD
Carol L. Shields, MD

CONTENTS

PART 1 TUMORS OF THE EYELIDS

Chapter 1 **Benign Tumors of the Eyelid Epidermis** 3

Eyelid Squamous Papilloma 4
Eyelid Seborrheic Keratosis 6
Eyelid Inverted Follicular Keratosis 10
Eyelid Pseudoepitheliomatous Hyperplasia 12
Eyelid Keratoacanthoma and Nonspecific Keratosis 14

Chapter 2 **Premalignant and Malignant Tumors of Eyelid Epidermis** 19

Eyelid Actinic Keratosis 20
Radiation Blepharopathy 24
Eyelid Xeroderma Pigmentosum 26
Sebaceous Nevus 28
Eyelid Basal Cell Carcinoma 30
Eyelid Squamous Cell Carcinoma 43

Chapter 3 **Eyelid Sebaceous Gland Tumors** 49

Eyelid Sebaceous Hyperplasia and Adenoma 50
Eyelid Sebaceous Carcinoma 51

Chapter 4 **Eyelid Sweat Gland Tumors** 67

Eyelid Syringoma 68
Eyelid Eccrine Acrospiroma 70
Eyelid Syringocystadenoma Papilliferum 72
Eyelid Pleomorphic Adenoma (Benign Mixed Tumor) 74
Eyelid Sweat Gland Adenocarcinoma 76

Chapter 5 **Eyelid Hair Follicle Tumors** 81

Eyelid Trichoepithelioma 82
Eyelid Trichofolliculoma and Trichoadenoma 84
Eyelid Trichilemmoma 86
Eyelid Pilomatrixoma 88

| Chapter 6 | **Eyelid Melanocytic Tumors** | 93 |

Eyelid Melanocytic Nevus 94
Oculodermal Melanocytosis (Nevus of Ota) 102
Eyelid Lentigo Maligna (Melanotic Freckle of Hutchinson) 106
Eyelid Blue Nevus 110
Eyelid Primary Malignant Melanoma 114

| Chapter 7 | **Neural Tumors of the Eyelid** | 119 |

Eyelid Neurofibroma 120
Eyelid Schwannoma (Neurilemoma) and Neurothekeoma 124
Eyelid Merkel Cell Carcinoma (Cutaneous Neuroendocrine Carcinoma) 126

| Chapter 8 | **Vascular Tumors of the Eyelids** | 133 |

Eyelid Congenital Capillary Hemangioma (Strawberry Hemangioma) 134
Eyelid Acquired Hemangioma (Cherry Hemangioma) 142
Eyelid Nevus Flammeus (Port Wine Hemangioma) 144
Eyelid Varix 148
Eyelid Lymphangioma 150
Eyelid Glomus Tumor 152
Eyelid Kaposi's Sarcoma 154
Eyelid Angiosarcoma 158

| Chapter 9 | **Eyelid Lymphoid, Plasmacytic, and Metastatic Tumors** | 161 |

Eyelid Lymphoma 162
Eyelid Plasmacytoma 168
Metastatic Neoplasms to the Eyelids 170

| Chapter 10 | **Eyelid Histiocytic, Myxoid, and Fibrous Lesions** | 175 |

Eyelid Xanthelasma and Xanthoma 176
Eyelid Xanthogranuloma 180
Eyelid Necrobiotic Xanthogranuloma with Paraproteinemia 182
Eyelid Angiofibroma 184
Eyelid Nodular Fasciitis 186
Eyelid Miscellaneous Fibrous and Myxomatous Tumors 190

| Chapter 11 | **Eyelid Cystic Lesions Simulating Neoplasms** | 195 |

Eyelid Eccrine Hidrocystoma 196
Eyelid Apocrine Hidrocystoma 198
Eyelid Sebaceous Cyst (Pilar Cyst) 200
Eyelid Epidermal Inclusion Cyst (Epidermoid Cyst) 202
Eyelid Dermoid Cyst 204

| Chapter 12 | **Eyelid Inflammatory Lesions Simulating Neoplasms** | 207 |

Eyelid Molluscum Contagiosum Infection 208
Eyelid Chalazion 210
Miscellaneous Granulomatous Diseases 214
    a. Eyelid Sarcoidosis 214
    b. Eyelid Pseudorheumatoid Nodule (Granuloma Annulare) 215
    c. Eyelid Granulomatosis with Polyangiitis (Wegener's Granulomatosis) 216
Eyelid Mycotic Infections 218
    a. Eyelid Blastomycosis 218
    b. Eyelid Coccidioidomycosis 218
    c. Eyelid Mucormycosis 218

Contents **xiii**

Eyelid Bacterial Infections 220
    a. Eyelid Abscess 220
    b. Necrotizing Fasciitis Involving Eyelid 220

Chapter 13   Eyelid Miscellaneous Conditions Simulating Neoplasms   223

Eyelid Amyloidosis 224
Eyelid Lipoid Proteinosis (Urbach–Wiethe Disease) 226
Miscellaneous Other Pseudoneoplastic Eyelid Lesions 228
    a. Eyelid Granular Cell Tumor 228
    b. Eyelid Malakoplakia 228
    c. Eyelid Subepidermal Calcified Nodule 228
Eyelid Phakomatous Choristoma 230

Chapter 14   Tumors of the Lacrimal Drainage System   233

Lacrimal Drainage System Tumors 234
Lacrimal Sac Squamous Papilloma and Carcinoma 236
Lacrimal Sac Melanoma 238
Lacrimal Sac: Miscellaneous Tumors and Pseudotumors 240

Chapter 15   Surgical Management of Eyelid Tumors   243

Surgical Management of Eyelid Tumors 244

PART 2   TUMORS OF THE CONJUNCTIVA

Chapter 16   Conjunctival and Epibulbar Choristomas   251

Conjunctival Dermoid 252
Conjunctival/Orbital Dermolipoma 256
Epibulbar Osseous Choristoma 260
Lacrimal Gland and Respiratory Choristomas of Conjunctiva 262
Conjunctival Complex Choristoma 264

Chapter 17   Conjunctival Benign Epithelial Tumors   267

Conjunctival Papilloma of Childhood 268
Conjunctival Papilloma of Adulthood 272
Conjunctival Pseudoepitheliomatous Hyperplasia and Keratoacanthoma 276
Conjunctival Hereditary Benign Intraepithelial Dyskeratosis 278
Conjunctival Dacryoadenoma 280

Chapter 18   Premalignant and Malignant Lesions of the Conjunctival Epithelium   283

Conjunctival Keratotic Plaque and Actinic Keratosis 284
Conjunctival Intraepithelial Neoplasia 286
Conjunctival Invasive Squamous Cell Carcinoma 292

Chapter 19   Conjunctival Melanocytic Lesions   307

Conjunctival Melanocytic Nevus 308
Ocular Melanocytosis: Scleral and Episcleral Pigment 320

Complexion-Related Conjunctival Pigmentation (Complexion-Associated
  Melanosis, Racial Melanosis) 322
Conjunctival Primary Acquired Melanosis 324
Conjunctival Malignant Melanoma 332

Chapter 20 Vascular Tumors and Related Lesions of the Conjunctiva — 349

Conjunctival Pyogenic Granuloma 350
Conjunctival Lymphangiectasia and Lymphangioma 354
Miscellaneous Vascular Lesions of the Conjunctiva: Varix, Cavernous Hemangioma,
  Macrovessels, Sentinel Vessels, and Acquired Sessile Hemangioma 358
  a. *Conjunctival Varix* 358
  b. *Cavernous Hemangioma* 358
  c. *Conjunctival Macrovessels and Episcleral Sentinel Vessels* 358
Conjunctival Acquired Sessile Hemangioma and Capillary Hemangioma 360
  a. *Acquired Sessile Hemangioma* 360
  b. *Conjunctival Capillary Hemangioma* 360
Conjunctival Hemangiopericytoma and Glomangioma (Glomus Tumor) 362
  a. *Conjunctival Hemangiopericytoma* 362
  b. *Conjunctival Glomangioma (Glomus Tumor)* 362
Conjunctival Kaposi Sarcoma 364

Chapter 21 Conjunctival Neural, Xanthomatous, Fibrous, Myxomatous, and Lipomatous Tumors — 367

Conjunctival Neuroma and Neurofibroma 368
Conjunctival Schwannoma and Granular Cell Tumor 370
  a. *Conjunctival Schwannoma* 370
  b. *Conjunctival Granular Cell Tumor* 370
Conjunctival Fibrous Histiocytoma 372
Conjunctival Miscellaneous Lesions: Fibroma, Nodular Fasciitis, and
  Juvenile Xanthogranuloma 374
  a. *Conjunctival Fibroma* 374
  b. *Conjunctival Nodular Fasciitis* 374
  c. *Conjunctival Juvenile Xanthogranuloma* 374
Conjunctival Miscellaneous Lesions: Myxoma, Lipoma,
  and Reticulohistiocytoma 376
  a. *Conjunctival Myxoma* 376
  b. *Conjunctival Lipoma* 376
  c. *Conjunctival Reticulohistiocytoma* 376

Chapter 22 Conjunctival Lymphoid, Leukemic, and Metastatic Tumors — 379

Conjunctival Lymphoid and Plasmacytic Tumors 380
Conjunctival Posttransplant Lymphoproliferative Disorder 386
Conjunctival Leukemia 388
Conjunctival Metastatic Tumors 390

Chapter 23 Caruncular Tumors — 393

Caruncular Tumors 394

Chapter 24 Miscellaneous Lesions That Simulate Conjunctival Neoplasms — 403

Conjunctival Epithelial Inclusion Cyst 404
Conjunctival Organizing Hematoma ("Hematic Cyst"; "Hematocele") 406
Conjunctival Foreign Body 408

Episcleritis and Scleritis Simulating Neoplasms   412
Conjunctival Churg–Strauss Allergic Granulomatosis Simulating
Conjunctival Neoplasm   414
Conjunctival Ligneous Conjunctivitis   416
Conjunctival Miscellaneous Infectious Lesions That Simulate Neoplasms   418
Conjunctival Amyloidosis   422
Pinguecula   426
Pterygium   428
Conjunctival and Scleral Miscellaneous Lesions That
Simulate Pigmented Melanoma   430
   a. *Calcified Scleral Plaque*   430
   b. *Staphyloma*   430
   c. *Extraocular Extension of Ciliary Body Melanoma*   430

Chapter 25   Surgical Management of Conjunctival Tumors   433

Surgical Management of Conjunctival Tumors   434

PART 3   TUMORS OF THE ORBIT

Chapter 26   Inflammatory Orbital Lesions That Simulate Neoplasms   443

Thyroid-Related Ophthalmopathy   444
Orbital Cellulitis   448
Orbit: Idiopathic Nongranulomatous Orbital Inflammation (Inflammatory
Pseudotumor, Idiopathic Orbital Inflammatory Syndrome)   450
Immunoglobulin G4–Related Disease (IgG4-RD)   456
Orbital Tuberculosis   457
Orbital Mycotic Infections: Aspergillosis and Mucormycosis   460
Orbital Aspergillosis—Allergic Fungal Sinusitis   461
Orbital Sarcoidosis   464
Orbital Granulomatosis with Polyangiitis (Wegener Granulomatosis)   466
Kimura Disease and Angiolymphoid Hyperplasia with Eosinophilia   468

Chapter 27   Orbital Cystic Lesions   471

Orbital Dermoid Cyst   472
Orbital Simple Primary Cyst of Conjunctival Origin   480
Orbital Teratoma (Teratomatous Cyst)   486
Orbital Congenital Cystic Eye   490
Orbital Colobomatous Cyst (Microphthalmos with Cyst)   492
Orbital Cephalocele   496
Orbital Mucocele   500
Orbital Respiratory Epithelial Cyst   504
Orbital Parasitic Cysts   506

Chapter 28   Orbital Vascular and Hemorrhagic Lesions   509

Orbital Capillary Hemangioma   510
Orbital Cavernous Hemangioma   516
Orbital Hemangiopericytoma   524
Orbital Lymphangioma   528
Orbital Varix   536

Orbital Miscellaneous Vascular Lesions: Intravascular Papillary Endothelial
  Hyperplasia and Glomus Tumor of the Orbit 542
Orbital Angiosarcoma 544
Orbital Hematoma 546

Chapter 29 Orbital Peripheral Nerve Tumors 549

Orbital (Neurilemoma) 550
Orbital Neurofibroma 556
Orbital Paraganglioma (Chemodectoma) 562
Orbital Alveolar Soft Part Sarcoma 564
Miscellaneous Orbital Neural Tumors: Granular Cell Tumor,
  Amputation Neuroma, and Malignant Peripheral Nerve Sheath Tumor 568
  a. Orbital Granular Cell Tumor 568
  b. Orbital Amputation Neuroma 569
  c. Orbital Malignant Peripheral Nerve Sheath Tumor 570

Chapter 30 Optic Nerve, Meningeal, and Other Neural Tumors 573

Optic Nerve Juvenile Pilocytic Astrocytoma (Optic Nerve Glioma) 574
Optic Nerve Malignant Astrocytoma 580
Optic Nerve Sheath Meningioma 582
Orbital Sphenoid Wing Meningioma 588
Orbital Primitive Neuroectodermal Tumor and Primary
  Orbital Neuroblastoma 592

Chapter 31 Orbital Myogenic Tumors 595

Orbital Rhabdomyosarcoma 596
Orbital Malignant Rhabdoid Tumor 606
Orbital Leiomyoma 608
Orbital Leiomyosarcoma 609

Chapter 32 Orbital Fibrous Connective Tissue Tumors 611

Orbital Nodular Fasciitis and Fibroma 612
Orbital Fibromatosis, Myofibromatosis, and Myofibroma 616
Orbital Fibrous Histiocytoma 620
Orbital Solitary Fibrous Tumor 624
Orbital Fibrosarcoma 628

Chapter 33 Orbital Osseous, Fibro-osseous, and Cartilaginous Tumors 631

Orbital Osteoma 632
Orbit Osteosarcoma 636
Orbital Fibrous Dysplasia 638
Orbital Ossifying Fibroma 642
Orbital Giant Cell Reparative Granuloma 646
Orbital Cartilaginous Chondroma 648
Orbital Chondrosarcoma 650

Chapter 34 Orbital Lipomatous and Myxomatous Tumors 653

Orbital Fat Prolapse 654
Orbital/Conjunctival Dermolipoma 658
Orbital Lipoma and Myxoma 662
Orbital Myxoma 666
Orbital Liposarcoma 668

Chapter 35 Orbital Histiocytic Tumors — 671

Orbit Juvenile Xanthogranuloma   672
Orbital Langerhans' Cell Histiocytosis (Eosinophilic Granuloma)   676
Orbital Erdheim-Chester Disease   682
Orbital Rosai-Dorfman Disease (Sinus Histiocytosis with
   Massive Lymphadenopathy)   684
Necrobiotic Xanthogranuloma and Multinucleate Cell Angiohistiocytoma   686

Chapter 36 Orbital Primary Melanocytic Tumors — 689

Orbital Melanoma Arising from Ocular Melanocytosis and Blue Nevus   690
Orbital Melanomas Arising de Novo   692
Orbital Melanocytic Hamartoma and Melanotic Neuroectodermal Tumor   694

Chapter 37 Lacrimal Gland Primary Epithelial Tumors — 697

Introduction: Lacrimal Gland Lesions   698
Lacrimal Gland Ductal Epithelial Cyst (Dacryops)   699
Lacrimal Gland Pleomorphic Adenoma (Benign Mixed Tumor)   702
Lacrimal Gland Pleomorphic Adenocarcinoma   708
Lacrimal Gland Adenoid Cystic Carcinoma   710
Lacrimal Gland Primary Ductal Carcinoma   718
Histopathology of Primary Epithelial Malignancies of Lacrimal Gland   722

Chapter 38 Orbital Metastatic Cancer — 725

Orbital Metastatic Cancer   726

Chapter 39 Orbital Lymphoid Tumors and Leukemias — 743

Orbital Non-Hodgkin Lymphoma   744
Orbital Lymphoma: Atypical Forms   752
Orbital Plasmacytoma and Lymphoplasmacytoid Tumors   754
Orbital Plasmablastic Lymphoma   758
Orbital Burkitt Lymphoma   760
Orbital Post-Transplant Lymphoproliferative Disorder   762
Orbital-Orbital Involvement by Leukemia (Myeloid Sarcoma)   766

Chapter 40 Orbital Secondary Tumors — 771

Orbital Secondary Tumors   772

Chapter 41 Surgical Management of Orbital Tumors — 785

Surgical Management of Orbital Tumors   786

Index   795

PART 1

TUMORS OF THE EYELIDS

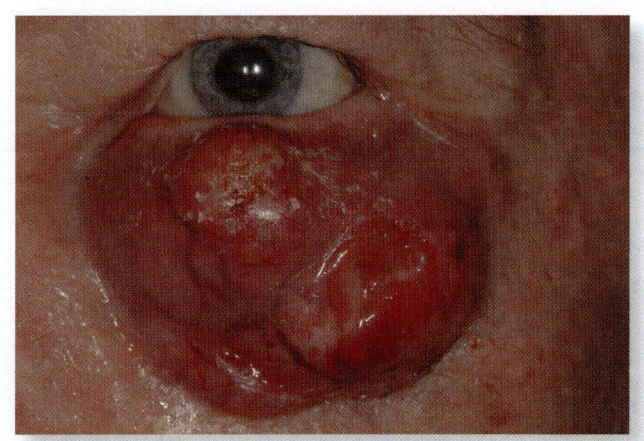

CHAPTER 1

BENIGN TUMORS OF THE EYELID EPIDERMIS

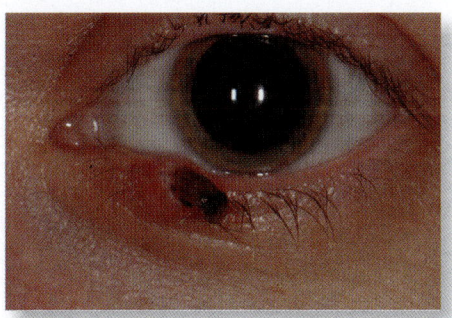

There are many benign tumors and pseudotumors of the epidermis that are discussed in the dermatologic literature (1–3). Many of them can occur on the skin of the eyelid. This section discusses only those that have a tendency to develop on the eyelids and that are better known to ophthalmologists and ophthalmic pathologists.

General Considerations

Squamous papilloma is a nonspecific term used to designate several different conditions characterized clinically by a wart-like lesion and histopathologically by benign hyperplasia of squamous epithelium. Therefore, it is not a specific clinicopathologic entity. However, ophthalmologists and ophthalmic pathologists have come to use the term clinically and histopathologically to characterize the condition described herein. Squamous papilloma is one of the most common eyelid lesions. It usually occurs in middle-aged or elderly individuals and can assume several clinical configurations. This eyelid lesion is quite different from the conjunctival papilloma that is often related to human papilloma virus infection and generally occurs in younger people with a fleshy, pink-red color. It is discussed later, under the topic of conjunctival lesions.

Clinical Features

Clinically, eyelid squamous papilloma can be sessile or pedunculated, solitary or multiple, and is usually of similar color to the adjacent skin; however, it can sometimes be pigmented, particularly in dark-skinned individuals. Sessile papilloma is broad based and slightly elevated and often has a smooth surface. In contrast, pedunculated papilloma is more elevated and generally has a rough, convoluted, cerebriform surface. A rough keratin crust can be palpated on the surface of the lesion (keratotic papilloma or "wart"). Eyelid papilloma tends to have a gradual onset and progress slowly.

Differential Diagnosis

The differential diagnosis includes melanocytic nevus, basal cell carcinoma, seborrheic keratosis (SK), fibroma, and verruca vulgaris. In our experience, a sessile papilloma can be quite similar clinically to amelanotic melanocytic nevus or a nonulcerated basal cell carcinoma.

Pathology

Microscopically, eyelid papilloma is composed of vascularized fibrous connective tissue covered by acanthotic epithelium. The more pedunculated lesions have fingerlike projections of fibrovascular connective tissue lined by epidermis with hyperkeratosis and acanthosis.

Management

Management of eyelid squamous papilloma is usually observation or excision for cosmetic reasons (4–9). Ablative treatment with carbon dioxide laser, argon laser, or photodynamic

EYELID SQUAMOUS PAPILLOMA

therapy has also been reported. More recently, topical or injection of interferon or interferon-related medications like imiquimod can be nonsurgical alternatives. We prefer to remove these lesions by a shaving excision and cautery under local anesthesia.

Prognosis

The prognosis for eyelid papilloma is excellent. Unlike the inverted squamous papilloma that develops in lacrimal drainage system, the eyelid papilloma has little or no malignant potential.

Selected References

Reviews

1. Deprez M, Uffer S. Clinicopathological features of eyelid skin tumors. A retrospective study of 5504 cases and review of literature. *Am J Dermatopathol* 2009;31(3): 256–262.
2. Kersten RC, Ewing-Chow D, Kulwin DR, et al. Accuracy of clinical diagnosis of cutaneous eyelid lesions. *Ophthalmology* 1997;104(3):479–484.
3. Verma V, Shen D, Sieving PC, et al. The role of infectious agents in the etiology of ocular adnexal neoplasia. *Surv Ophthalmol* 2008;53(4):312–331.

Therapy

4. Beckman H, Fuller TA, Boyman R, et al. Carbon dioxide laser surgery of the eye and adnexa. *Ophthalmology* 1980;87:990–1000.
5. Wohlrab TM, Rohrbach JM, Erb C, et al. Argon laser therapy of benign tumors of the eyelid. *Am J Ophthalmol* 1998;125:693–697.
6. Togsverd-Bo K, Haedersdal M, Wulf HC. Photodynamic therapy for tumors on the eyelid margins. *Arch Dermatol* 2009;145(8):944–947.
7. Eshraghi B, Torabi HR, Kasaie A, et al. The use of a radiofrequency unit for excisional biopsy of eyelid papillomas. *Ophthal Plast Reconstr Surg* 2010;26(6): 448–449.
8. Lee BJ, Nelson CC. Intralesional interferon for extensive squamous papilloma of the eyelid margin. *Ophthal Plast Reconstr Surg* 2012;28(2):e47–e48.
9. Ahn HB, Seo JW, Roh MS, et al. Canaliculitis with a papilloma-like mass caused by a temporary punctal plug. *Ophthal Plast Reconstr Surg* 2009;25(5):413–414.

EYELID SQUAMOUS PAPILLOMA

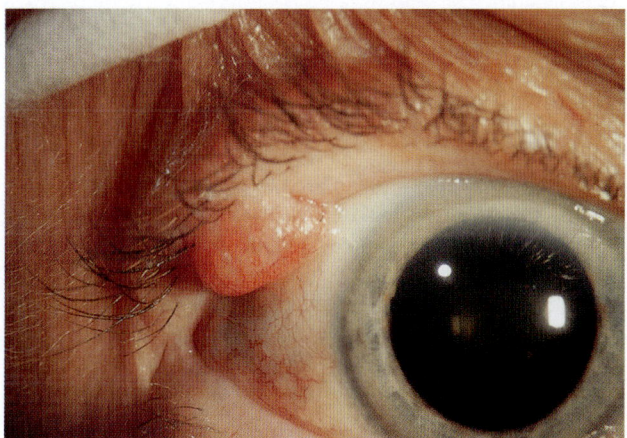

Figure 1.1. Sessile papilloma located on the upper eyelid margin of a 63-year-old woman. It appears as a pink lesion with a smooth surface.

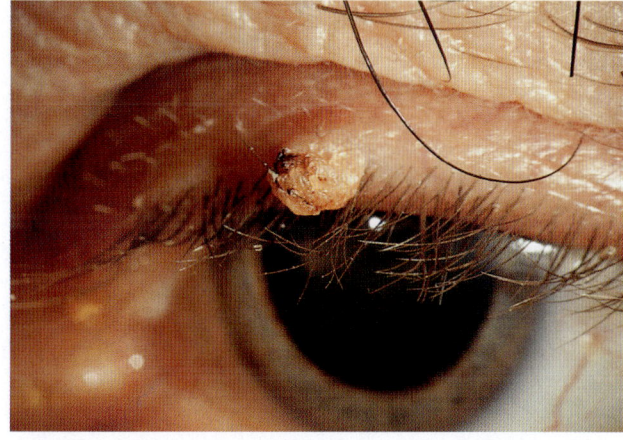

Figure 1.2. Slightly pedunculated papilloma in the upper eyelid of a 72-year-old man. Note the rough, irregular surface of the lesion.

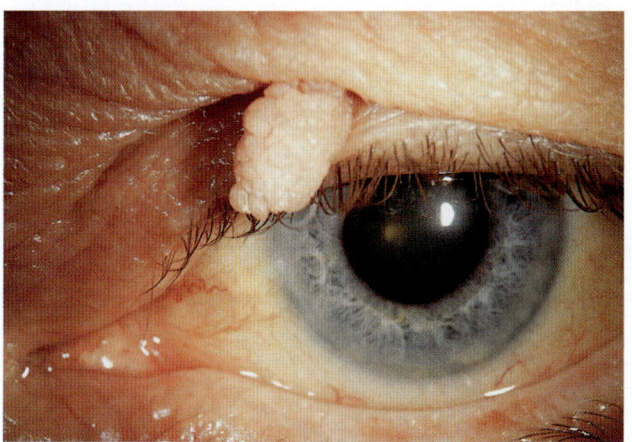

Figure 1.3. Markedly pedunculated papilloma on upper eyelid in a 68-year-old man.

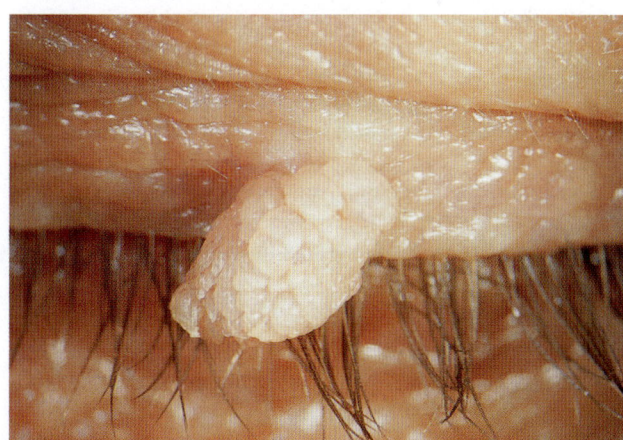

Figure 1.4. Close view of lesion shown in Figure 1.3 depicting the corrugated surface.

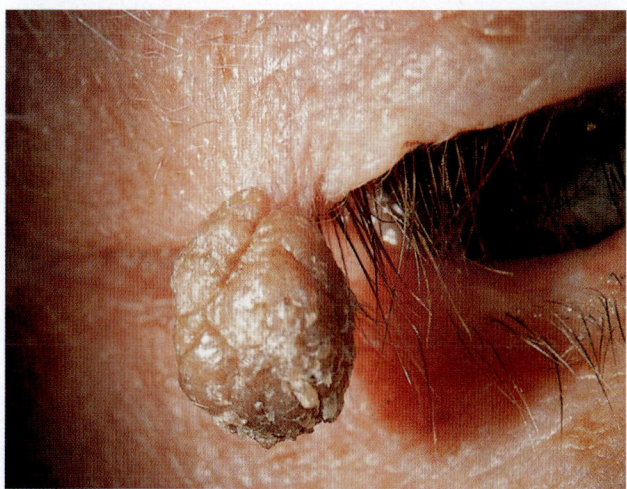

Figure 1.5. Markedly pedunculated papilloma arising from the lateral portion of upper eyelid in an 80-year-old man.

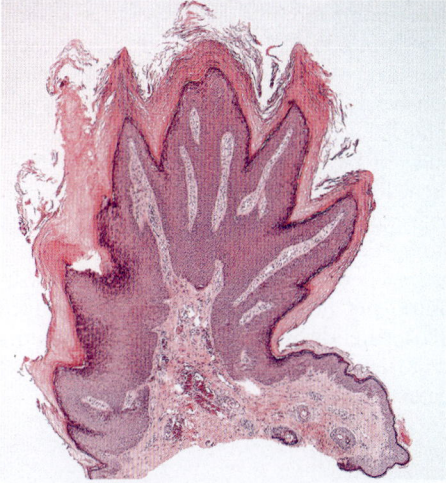

Figure 1.6. Histopathology of eyelid papilloma showing lightly eosinophilic core of fibrovascular tissue, lined by convolutions of acanthotic epithelium with hyperkeratosis and parakeratosis. (Hematoxylin–eosin ×25.)

EYELID SEBORRHEIC KERATOSIS

General Considerations

Seborrheic keratosis (SK; basal cell papilloma; seborrheic wart) is a common, benign, cutaneous lesion that frequently occurs on the chest and back, but is also common on the face and periocular region of older individuals (1–9). This tumor develops in hair-bearing areas of skin and does not occur on the palms, soles, or mucous membranes. It is generally a solitary lesion, but multiple lesions can occur and may have an autosomal-dominant inheritance pattern. The sudden appearance of multiple SKs, or rapid growth of pre-existing SKs, may herald the onset of internal malignancy, particularly gastrointestinal adenocarcinomas. This is called the "sign of Leser–Trélat" (4).

Clinical Features

Clinically, SK first appears as a minimally elevated hyperpigmented, tan to brown plaque. With time, it may become more elevated, and even assume a dome configuration (1). SK can occasionally be more pedunculated and resembles a pedunculated papilloma. Although SK is usually asymptomatic, it can cause pruritus or local irritation, particularly in areas of friction. It usually has a rough surface with irregular fissures. It is usually discrete and movable, and has been compared to a "button stuck on the surface of the skin." A clinical variant of SK, known as dermatosis papulosa nigra, is characterized by multiple, deeply pigmented, elevated papules found in the malar region and periocular area in black individuals (5).

Differential Diagnosis

The clinical differential diagnosis of SK should include any keratotic, pigmented skin lesion, particularly melanoma, melanocytic nevus, and pigmented basal cell carcinoma (1–9).

Pathology and Pathogenesis

Histopathologically, SK is a benign proliferation of basaloid cells. It has been classified into six distinct types and many lesions have combinations of these types. The acanthotic type is the most common. All types of SK are characterized by hyperkeratosis, papillomatosis, and acanthosis, mainly a proliferation of basal cells. A characteristic feature is the presence of intraepithelial keratin cysts (horn cysts or pseudohorn cysts) that should not be confused with the pearl cysts, which are often present in squamous cell carcinoma. These cysts gradually coalesce and migrate superficially, forming a rough surface to the lesion.

The pathogenesis of SK is not clearly established, but age, sun exposure, and hereditary tendency may be predisposing factors. SK apparently arises from the follicular infundibulum and seems to involve an aggregation of immature epidermal keratinocytes.

Management

Treatment of SK is generally observation or excision, depending on the clinical circumstances (6,7). In the eyelid area, a lesion can be removed for cosmetic considerations or because of interference with wearing of glasses. Removal can be accomplished by curettage, shaving excision flush with the skin surface, or standard full-thickness excision of the skin epidermis and dermis down to the subcutaneous tissue, followed by primary closure. The tarsus does not need to be removed. Light freezing with liquid nitrogen has been advocated for smaller flat lesions. There is a slight tendency for local recurrence after excision.

Prognosis

Prognosis for SK is generally excellent. However, it can occasionally occur as multiple eruptive lesions that can herald development of gastrointestinal adenocarcinoma (sign of Leser–Trélat) (6). The cutaneous lesion itself probably has no malignant potential.

EYELID SEBORRHEIC KERATOSIS

Selected References

Reviews

1. Deprez M, Uffer S. Clinicopathological features of eyelid skin tumors. A retrospective study of 5504 cases and review of literature. *Am J Dermatopathol* 2009;31(3):256–262.
2. Kersten RC, Ewing-Chow D, Kulwin DR, et al. Accuracy of clinical diagnosis of cutaneous eyelid lesions. *Ophthalmology* 1997;104(3):479–484.
3. Doxanas MT, Iliff WJ, Iliff NT, et al. Squamous cell carcinoma of the eyelids. *Ophthalmology* 1987;94:538–541.

Clinical Features

4. Ellis DL, Yates RA. Sign of Leser-Trelat. *Clin Dermatol* 1993;11:141–148.
5. Hairston MA Jr, Reed RN, Derbes VJ. Dermatosis papulosa nigra. *Arch Dermatol* 1964;89:655–658.

Therapy

6. Scully J. Treatment of seborrheic keratosis. *JAMA* 1970;213:1498.
7. Beckman H, Fuller TA, Boyman R, et al. Carbon dioxide laser surgery of the eye and adnexa. *Ophthalmology* 1980;87:990–1000.

Case Reports

8. Spott D, Wood M, Healon G. Melanoacanthoma of the eyelid. *Arch Dermatol* 1972;105:898–899.
9. Foley P, Mason G. Keratotic basal cell carcinoma of the upper eyelid. *Aust J Dermatol* 1995;36:95–96.

EYELID SEBORRHEIC KERATOSIS

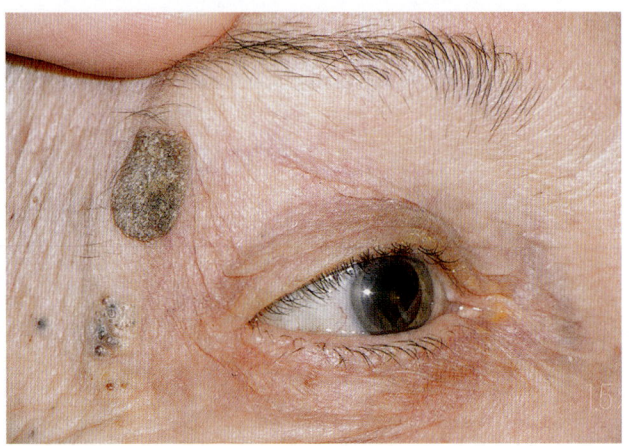

Figure 1.7. SK near the lateral aspect of left upper eyelid in a 74-year-old woman.

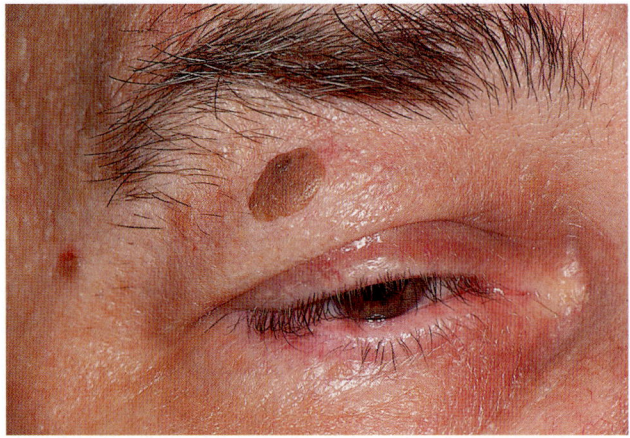

Figure 1.8. SK beneath the right eyebrow in a 62-year-old man.

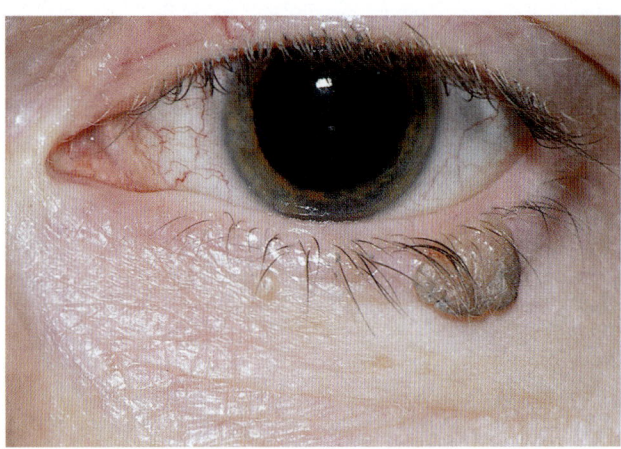

Figure 1.9. Slightly elevated tan SK on left lower eyelid.

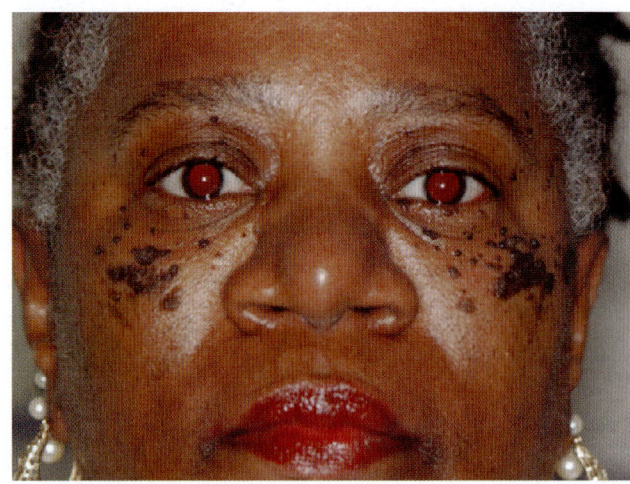

Figure 1.10. Dermatosis papulosa nigra showing SK lesions on face and eyelids of a 62-year-old African-American woman. The lesions are mainly in the periocular and cheek area, and few are present on the neck.

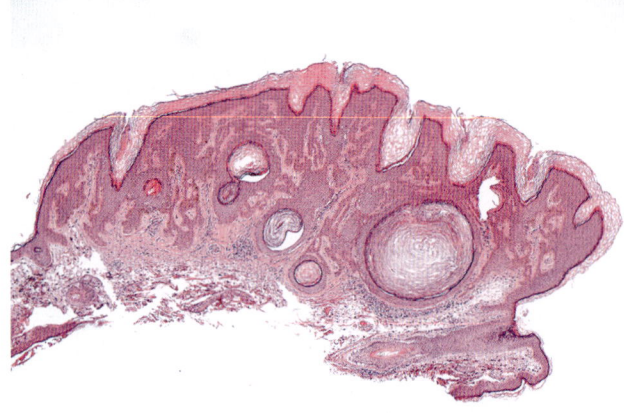

Figure 1.11. Histopathology of hyperkeratotic variant of SK, demonstrating acanthosis, hyperkeratosis, and keratin cysts. (Hematoxylin–eosin ×50.)

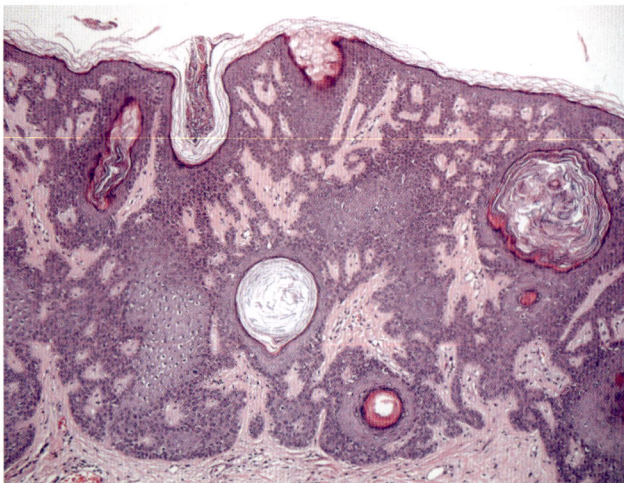

Figure 1.12. Photomicrograph of SK, showing typical keratin cysts within proliferation of basaloid cells. (Hematoxylin–eosin ×100.)

Chapter 1 Benign Tumors of the Eyelid Epidermis

● EYELID SEBORRHEIC KERATOSIS: CLINICAL VARIATIONS

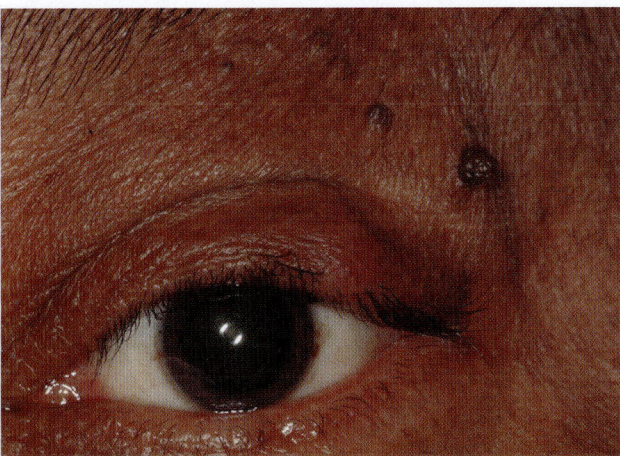

Figure 1.13. Multifocal seborrheic keratosis on left upper eyelid of an African-American man.

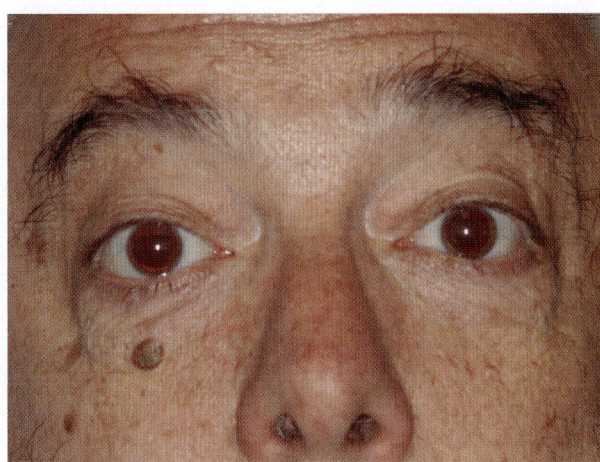

Figure 1.14. Multifocal seborrheic keratosis on right lower eyelid region and right lateral canthus of an elderly Caucasian man.

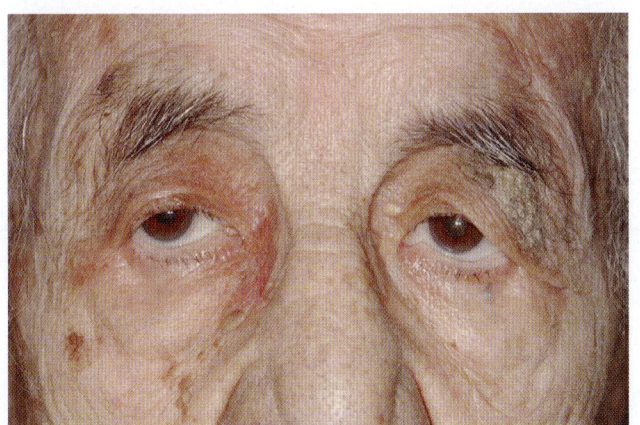

Figure 1.15. Large seborrheic keratosis on the lateral aspect of left upper eyelid in an 82-year-old man.

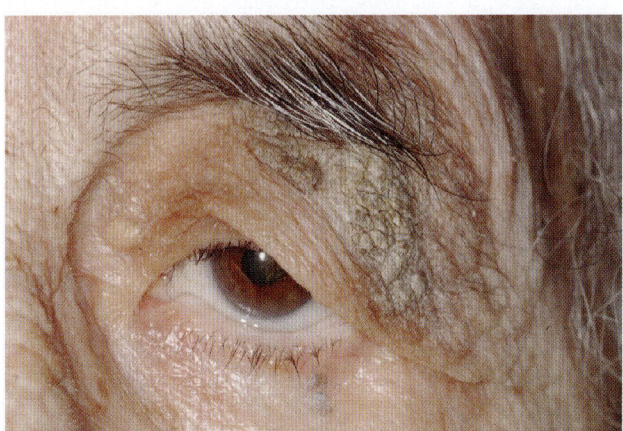

Figure 1.16. Close-up view of seborrheic keratosis in Figure 1.15 showing the "cracked" surface irregularity of the large cutaneous lesion.

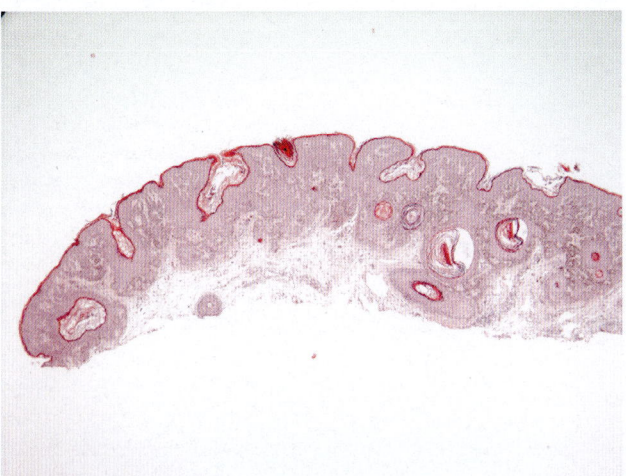

Figure 1.17. Low magnification photomicrograph of seborrheic keratosis exhibiting deeply undulating surface, hyperkeratosis, keratocysts, and acanthosis. (Hematoxylin–eosin ×10.)

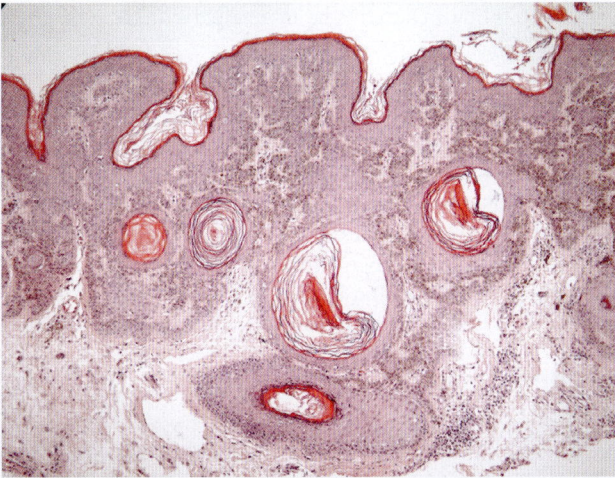

Figure 1.18. Higher magnification of lesion shown in Figure 1.17 demonstrating keratocysts within the acanthotic epithelium. (Hematoxylin–eosin ×40.)

EYELID INVERTED FOLLICULAR KERATOSIS

General Considerations

Inverted follicular keratosis (IFK) is a benign, cutaneous lesion that occurs mainly in middle aged to older adult men and has a wartlike appearance (1–9). The term "inverted follicular keratosis" was introduced by Helwig in 1954 because of his belief that the lesion was of hair follicle origin. However, later reports suggest that it is not of hair follicle origin, but rather a form of "irritated seborrheic keratosis" (9).

Clinical Features

IFK appears clinically as a discrete nodular lesion that may be papillomatous and pigmented, and is often located on or very near the eyelid margin. It may develop rather rapidly over a few months and is believed to have a viral etiology. In the face and eyelid area, the lesion is subject to trauma and may become a scab that causes a burning and itchy sensation. Of the 65 eyelid cases studied by Boniuk and Zimmerman (3), the mean age of the patient at diagnosis was 69 years; 43% occurred at the eyelid margin, and 5 presented as a cutaneous horn. In another series that included all locations, 34 of 40 cases occurred on the face and only 2 were on the eyelids (4).

Differential Diagnosis

The clinical differential diagnosis of IFK is the same as for seborrheic keratosis. It includes any keratotic pigmented skin lesion, particularly melanoma, melanocytic nevus, and pigmented basal cell carcinoma (1).

Pathology

Histopathologically, IFK shows lobular acanthosis with proliferation of both squamous and basal cells (3,9). The epithelium typically shows localized, ill-defined squamous eddies within the acanthotic epithelium. As mentioned, it was once believed to be of hair follicle origin. However, there has been no convincing histopathologic evidence to support that concept and it is now believed to be an inverted irritated seborrheic keratosis (9).

Management

The treatment of IFK is also similar to that of typical seborrheic keratosis. The lesion can be observed or excised depending on the clinical circumstances. In the eyelid area, a lesion can be removed for cosmetic considerations or because of interference with wearing of glasses. Removal can be accomplished by curettage, shaving excision flush with the skin surface, and/or cryotherapy. Recurrence is uncommon after adequate excision.

Prognosis

Prognosis for IFK is generally excellent, but its uncommon association with multiple eruptive lesions with gastrointestinal adenocarcinoma (sign of Leser–Trélat) must be kept in mind. The cutaneous lesion itself probably has no malignant potential.

Selected References

Reviews

1. Deprez M, Uffer S. Clinicopathological features of eyelid skin tumors. A retrospective study of 5504 cases and review of literature. *Am J Dermatopathol* 2009;31(3): 256–262.
2. Doxanas MT, Iliff WJ, Iliff NT, et al. Squamous cell carcinoma of the eyelids. *Ophthalmology* 1987;94:538–541.
3. Boniuk M, Zimmerman LE. Eyelid tumors with reference to lesions confused with squamous cell carcinoma. II: Inverted follicular keratosis. *Arch Ophthalmol* 1963:69: 698–707.
4. Mehregan AH. Inverted follicular keratosis. *Arch Dermatol* 1964;89:229–235.

Therapy

5. Beckman H, Fuller TA, Boyman R, et al. Carbon dioxide laser surgery of the eye and adnexa. *Ophthalmology* 1980;87:990–1000.

Case Reports

6. Sassani JW, Yanoff M. Inverted follicular keratosis. *Am J Ophthalmol* 1979;87:810–813.
7. Scheie HG, Yanoff M, Sassani JW. Inverted follicular keratosis clinically mimicking malignant melanoma. *Ann Ophthalmol* 1977;9:949–952.
8. Schweitzer JG, Yanoff M. Inverted follicular keratosis. A report of two recurrent cases. *Ophthalmology* 1987;94:1465–1468.
9. Lever WF. Inverted follicular keratosis is an irritated seborrheic keratosis. *Am J Dermatopathol* 1983;5:474.

Chapter 1 Benign Tumors of the Eyelid Epidermis

● EYELID INVERTED FOLLICULAR KERATOSIS

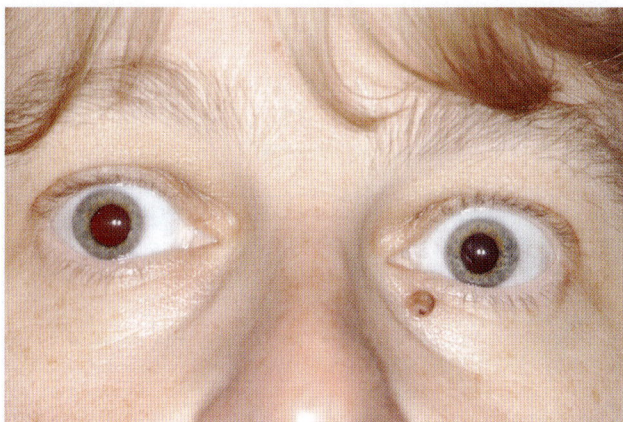

Figure 1.19. Inverted follicular keratosis of the lower eyelid in a 50-year-old woman.

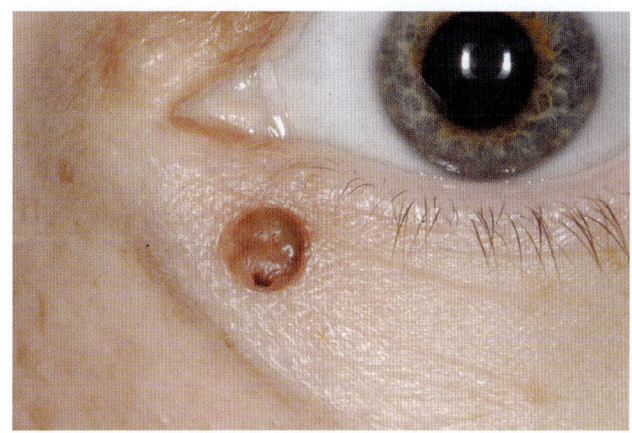

Figure 1.20. Close-up view of lesion shown in Figure 1.19.

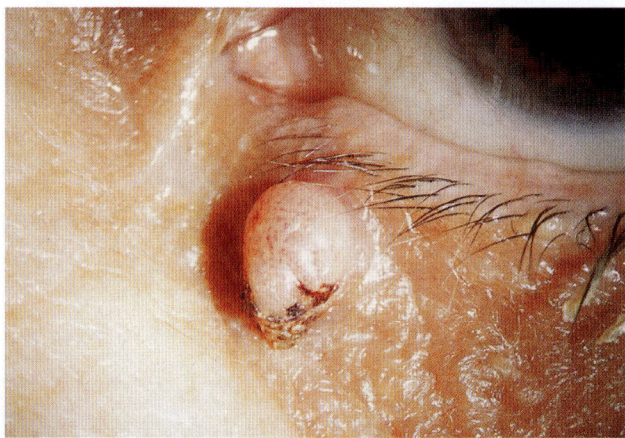

Figure 1.21. Inverted follicular keratosis inferior to the medial canthus in an 80-year-old man.

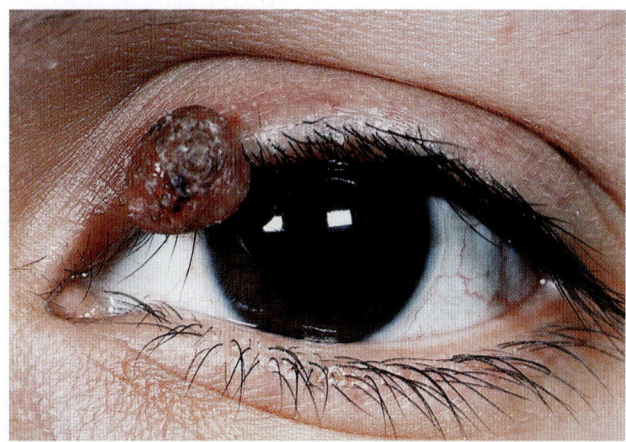

Figure 1.22. Inverted follicular keratosis on upper eyelid in a 24-year-old woman. (Courtesy of James Patrinely, MD.)

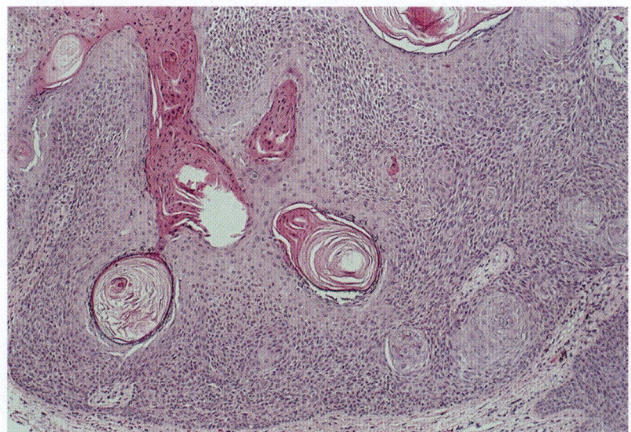

Figure 1.23. Histopathology of inverted follicular keratosis, showing invasive acanthosis and keratin cysts. (Hematoxylin–eosin ×40.)

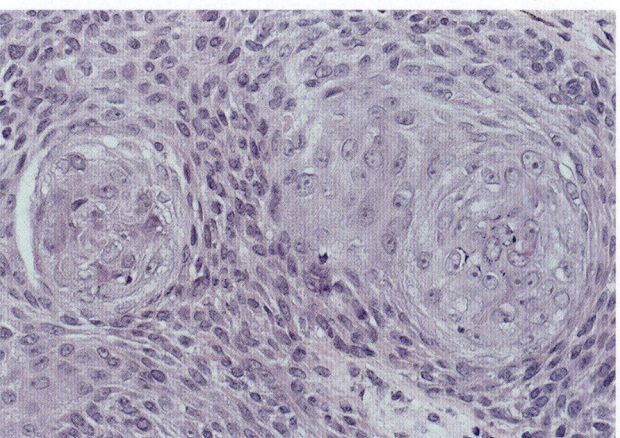

Figure 1.24. Histopathology of inverted follicular keratosis showing squamous eddies in acanthotic epithelium. (Hematoxylin–eosin ×150.)

EYELID PSEUDOEPITHELIOMATOUS HYPERPLASIA

General Considerations
Pseudoepitheliomatous hyperplasia (PEH) is a benign proliferative pseudoneoplastic entity that can attain tumorous proportions (1–6). It often develops rapidly over a few weeks and, if untreated, can gradually regress over a few months. It can simulate basal cell carcinoma clinically and squamous cell carcinoma histopathologically. PEH can be idiopathic or secondary to some mycotic infections, trauma, or certain drugs. It can also occur at the margins of some malignant neoplasms like basal cell carcinoma, squamous cell carcinoma, and metastatic breast cancer.

Clinical Features
PEH can exhibit a variety of clinical manifestations. It is usually nodular, irregular, and crusty, and may eventually ulcerate. An adjacent inflammatory lesion or scar may be present. A well-known, specific variant of PEH, known as "keratoacanthoma," can present as an ulcerated lesion resembling basal cell carcinoma, and is discussed in the next section.

Differential Diagnosis
Several lesions can be clinically similar to PEH. Squamous and basal cell carcinoma are the most frequent lesions that may be difficult to differentiate clinically from PEH (1).

Pathology
Most pathologists agree that it can sometimes be difficult to impossible to differentiate histopathologically PEH from squamous cell carcinoma. PEH is characterized by irregular invasion of the dermis by jagged, often sharply pointed epidermal cell masses, horn cyst formation, and numerous mitotic figures. However, the squamous cells usually are better differentiated and not so invasive as squamous cell carcinoma. Inflammatory cells are frequently present at the base of the lesion and microabscesses are often detectable in the acanthotic epithelium.

The adjacent inflammatory infiltrate should be studied carefully to rule out granulomatous inflammation secondary to tuberculosis, blastomycosis, and other predisposing conditions (4,6). If they are found, then PEH is more likely than squamous cell carcinoma.

Management
PEH is generally managed by surgical excision using preferred methods of treating eyelid malignancies because it so closely resembles squamous cell carcinoma or basal cell carcinoma. If left untreated, however, it is possible that it would eventually regress.

Selected References

Reviews
1. Deprez M, Uffer S. Clinicopathological features of eyelid skin tumors. A retrospective study of 5504 cases and review of literature. *Am J Dermatopathol* 2009;31(3): 256–262.
2. Freeman RG. On the pathogenesis of pseudoepitheliomatous hyperplasia. *J Cutan Pathol* 1974;1:231–237.
3. Stone OJ. Hyperinflammatory proliferative (blastomycosislike) pyodermas. Review, mechanisms, and therapy. *J Dermatol Surg Oncol* 1986;12:271–273.

Case Reports
4. Barr CC, Gamel JW. Blastomycosis of the eyelid. *Arch Ophthalmol* 1986;104:96–97.
5. Kincaid MC, Green WR, Hoover RE, et al. Iododerma of the conjunctiva and skin. *Ophthalmology* 1981;88(12):1216–1220.
6. Ferry AP. Granular cell tumor (myoblastoma) of the palpebral conjunctiva causing pseudoepitheliomatous hyperplasia of the conjunctival epithelium. *Am J Ophthalmol* 1981;91(2):234–238.

EYELID PSEUDOEPITHELIOMATOUS HYPERPLASIA

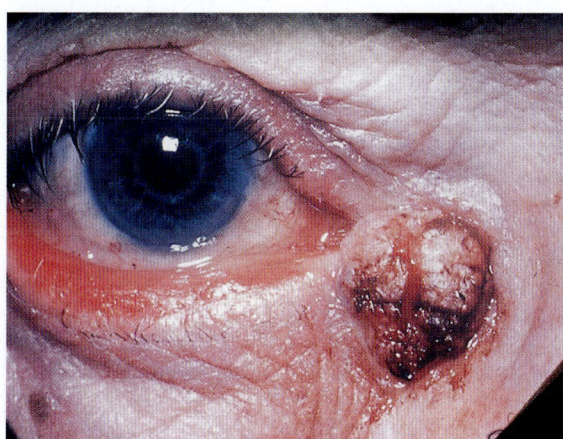

Figure 1.25. Pseudoepitheliomatous hyperplasia near the medial canthus simulating basal cell carcinoma. (Courtesy of Armed Forces Institute of Pathology, Washington, DC.)

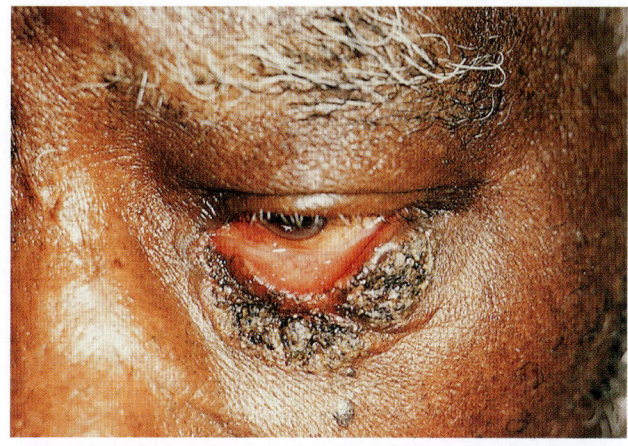

Figure 1.26. Pseudoepitheliomatous hyperplasia secondary to blastomycosis, with secondary ectropion of lower eyelid in an 84-year-old man with history of multiple skin lesions. (Courtesy of Charles Barr, MD.)

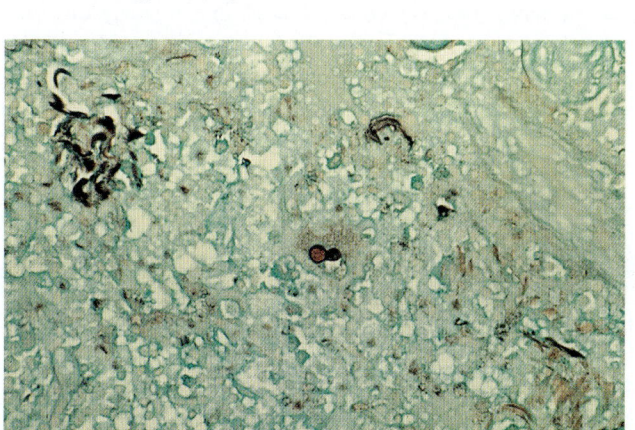

Figure 1.27. Histopathology of lesion shown in Figure 1.26 showing *Blastomyces dermatitidis*. (Gomori methenamine silver stain ×200.) (Courtesy of Charles Barr, MD.)

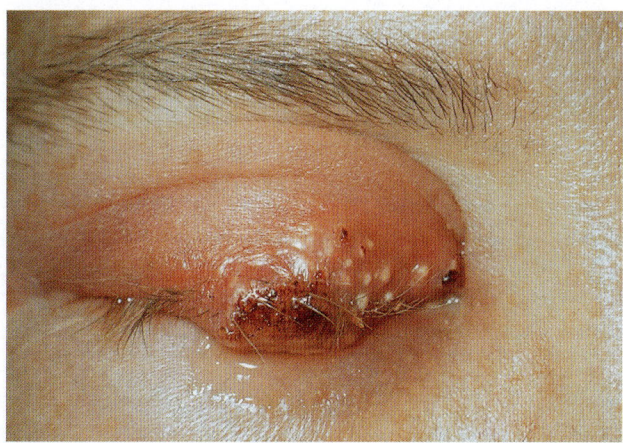

Figure 1.28. Pseudoepitheliomatous hyperplasia of upper eyelid secondary to coccidioidomycosis in an immunosuppressed 37-year-old man who underwent renal transplantation. He previously lived in Arizona where this disease is endemic. (Courtesy of Bruce Johnson, MD.)

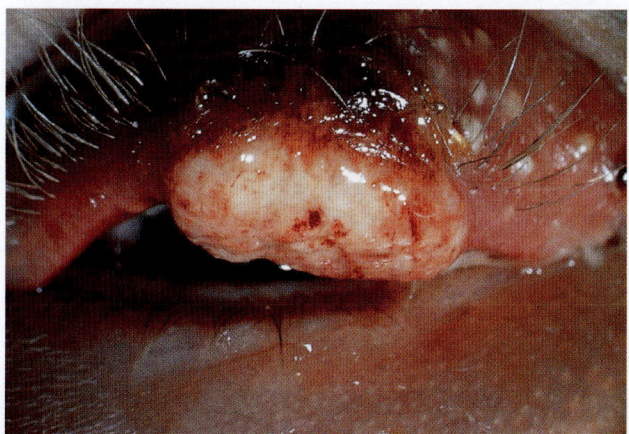

Figure 1.29. Lesion shown in Figure 1.28 with eyelid everted. (Courtesy of Bruce Johnson, MD.)

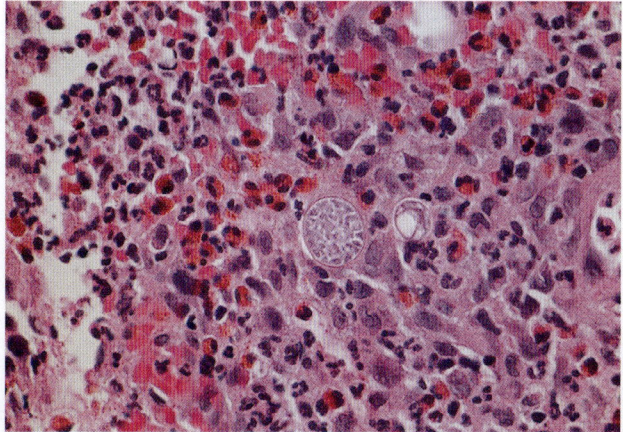

Figure 1.30. Histopathology of lesion shown in Figure 1.28, showing eosinophils, lymphocytes, and spore-containing organisms compatible with *Coccidioides immitis*. (Hematoxylin–eosin ×150.) (Courtesy of Bruce Johnson, MD.)

EYELID KERATOACANTHOMA AND NONSPECIFIC KERATOSIS

General Considerations

Keratoacanthoma (KA) is a specific variant of PEH that deserves separate classification because of its distinctive clinical features (1–11). Although KA is included among benign lesions in this atlas, some authorities now consider it to be a variant of squamous cell carcinoma. About 85% occur on the face with about 5% on the eyelids. In a series of 10 patients (6 men, 4 women) with eyelid KA, patient ages ranged from 27 to 78 years, with a mean of 59 years (1). KA is usually a solitary lesion, but on occasion it can be multiple. The multiple lesions can have several variations and can be associated with cancer family syndromes, including Ferguson–Smith syndrome and Muir–Torre syndrome. Multiple KAs are considered important markers for internal neoplasms that characterize these syndromes (1,2). It has been suggested that all patients with multiple KAs be evaluated for internal cancers. KA is known to occur with greater frequency in immunosuppressed patients, particularly those who have undergone renal transplantation.

Clinical Features

KA characteristically has a rapid onset and growth over a period of ≤2 months, reaches a size of 0.5 to 2 cm and, if untreated, has a tendency to undergo spontaneous regression. If a lesion has a prolonged clinical course, true squamous cell carcinoma is more likely than KA (7,8). The lesion typically develops elevated margins and a central crater, resembling a noduloulcerative basal cell carcinoma. In some cases, KA can be aggressive and assume a large size (9–11). Such cases often prove eventually to be squamous cell carcinoma. A form of "giant KA" (up to 5 cm in diameter) can occasionally involve the periocular skin (10).

Differential Diagnosis

The clinical differential diagnosis of KA mainly includes basal cell carcinoma, squamous cell carcinoma, and other epidermal and adnexal neoplasms.

Pathology and Pathogenesis

Histopathologically, KA is composed of well-differentiated squamous cells with a central, keratin-containing crater (1). Inflammatory cells and microabscesses are often present. As mentioned, it may be almost impossible to differentiate KA from squamous cell carcinoma in some instances. This is particularly true because some presumed KAs are highly aggressive with invasion of dermis, nerve, and muscle (9). Regarding pathogenesis, a viral cause has been postulated, but not unequivocally proven.

Management

Management of KA includes observation for regression or surgical excision with Mohs chemosurgery or frozen section control (1). Most authorities now recommend resection rather than observation, with the assumption that the lesion is potentially squamous cell carcinoma. An incisional biopsy should be done first if the lesion is large and extensive reconstruction is anticipated. It is important that the biopsy includes the solid margin of the lesion and not just the central crater in order to have viable cells for histopathologic study. After meticulous surgical removal, recurrence is unlikely (1). Cryotherapy, corticosteroids, irradiation, chemotherapy, and other methods have been used (1). Local injection of chemotherapeutic agents like 5-fluorouracil (5-FU) (4) or methotrexate (5) have also been used with remarkable success. It is also stated that 5-FU cream three times daily usually results in resolution in 3 to 6 weeks. Imiquimod (Aldara; Graceway Pharmaceuticals, Bristol, TN) may also play a therapeutic role in selected cases (6).

Nonspecific Keratosis

"Nonspecific keratosis" is a term applied to a keratotic lesion that does not meet the specific histopathologic categories mentioned above. In the eyelid, it can assume a variety of forms from a sessile keratotic plaque to a cutaneous horn. It generally occurs in older patients. It can be observed or excised for cosmetic reasons.

Selected References

Reviews
1. Donaldson MJ, Sullivan TJ, Whitehead KJ, et al. Periocular keratoacanthoma: Clinical features, pathology, and management. *Ophthalmology* 2003;110:1403–1407.
2. Reid BJ, Cheesbrough MJ. Multiple keratoacanthomas. A unique case and review of the current classification. *Acta Dermatol Venereol* 1978;58:169–173.
3. Boniuk M, Zimmerman LE. Eyelid tumors with reference to lesions confused with squamous cell carcinoma. III: Keratoacanthoma. *Arch Ophthalmol* 1967;77:29–40.

Therapy
4. Bergin DJ, Lapins NA, Deffer TA. Intralesional 5-fluorouracil for keratoacanthoma of the eyelid. *Ophthal Plast Reconstr Surg* 1986;2:201–204.
5. Melton JL, Nelson BR, Stough DB, et al. Treatment of keratoacanthomas with intralesional methotrexate. *J Am Acad Dermatol* 1991;25:1017–1023.
6. Urosevic M, Dummer R. Role of imiquimod in skin cancer treatment. *Am J Clin Dermatol* 2004;5:453–458.

Case Reports
7. Olver JM, Muhtaseb M, Chauhan D, et al. Well-differentiated squamous cell carcinoma of the eyelid arising during a 20-year period. *Arch Ophthalmol* 2000;118:422–424.
8. Requena L, Romero E, Sanchez M, et al. Aggressive keratoacanthoma of the eyelid: "Malignant" keratoacanthoma or squamous cell carcinoma? *J Dermatol Surg Oncol* 1990;16:564–568.
9. Grossniklaus HE, Wojno TH, Yanoff M, et al. Invasive keratoacanthoma of the eyelid and ocular adnexa. *Ophthalmology* 1996;103:937–941.
10. Reifler DM. Large periocular keratoacanthoma. *Ophthalmic Surg* 1987;18:469–470.
11. Boynton JR, Searl SS, Caldwell EH. Large periocular keratoacanthoma: The case for definitive treatment. *Ophthalmic Surg* 1986;17:565–569.

EYELID KERATOACANTHOMA

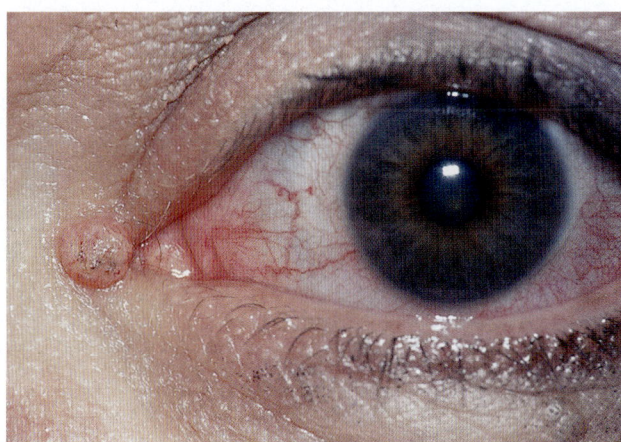

Figure 1.31. Small, minimally ulcerated keratoacanthoma near the medial canthus in a 44-year-old woman. The diagnosis was confirmed histopathologically.

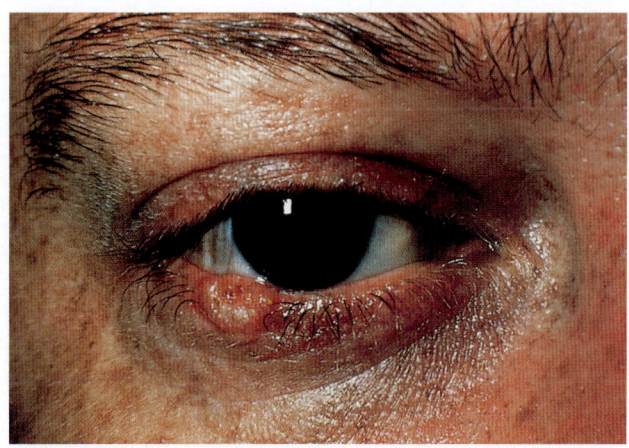

Figure 1.32. Keratoacanthoma of lower eyelid in an immunosuppressed patient who had undergone renal transplantation. (Courtesy of Don Nicholson, MD.)

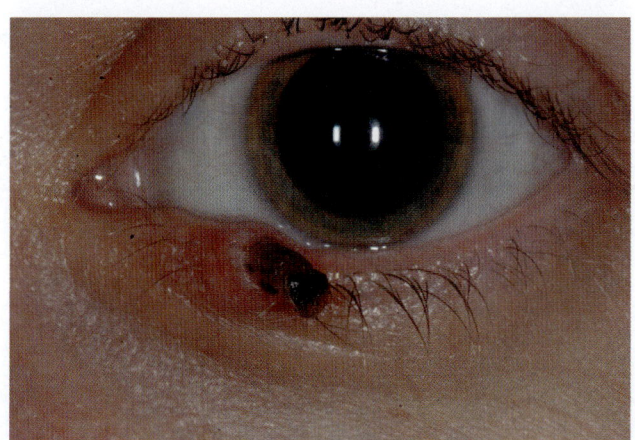

Figure 1.33. Keratoacanthoma with central cutaneous horn in a young female patient.

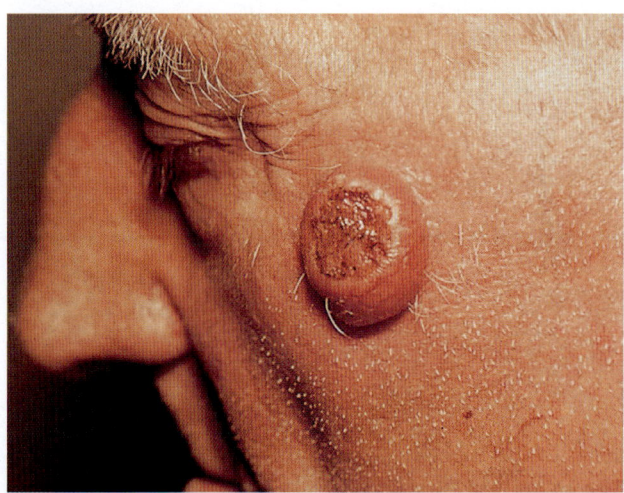

Figure 1.34. Large keratoacanthoma in the malar area. (Courtesy of Margaret Lally, MD.)

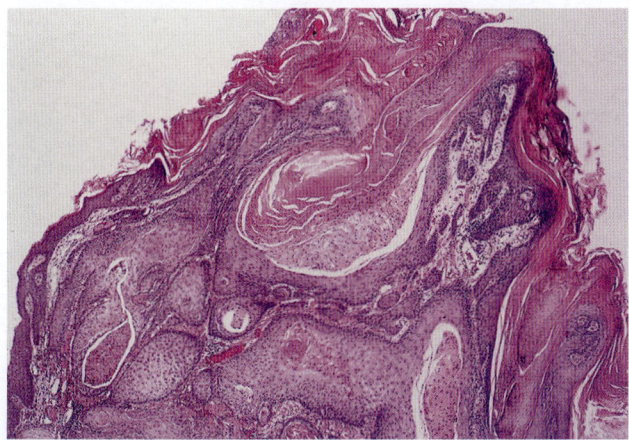

Figure 1.35. Histopathology of lesion shown in Figure 1.32 showing proliferating squamous cells, with acanthosis, hyperkeratosis and a central crater. (Hematoxylin–eosin ×10.) (Courtesy of Don Nicholson, MD.)

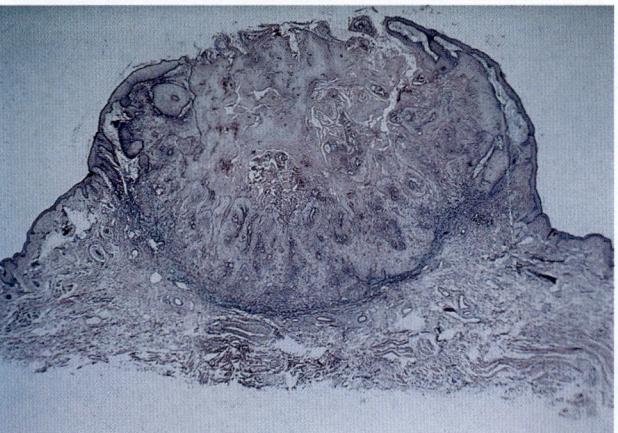

Figure 1.36. Histopathology of another eyelid keratoacanthoma showing well-circumscribed lesion with central keratin-filled crater. (Hematoxylin–eosin ×10.)

EYELID KERATOACANTHOMA: CASE DESCRIPTION AND MANAGEMENT BY EXCISION AND SKIN GRAFT

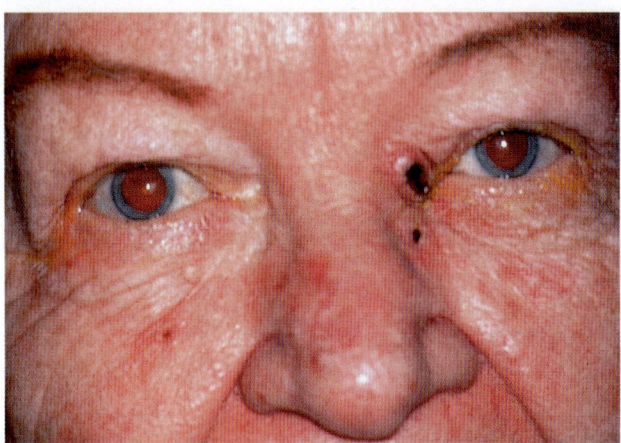

Figure 1.37. Ulcerated KA that evolved over a few weeks near medial canthus in a 75-year-old woman.

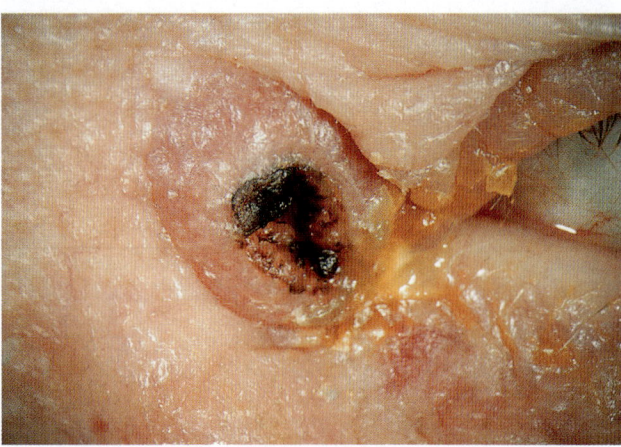

Figure 1.38. Close view of lesion seen in Figure 1.37, showing elevated mass with central crater.

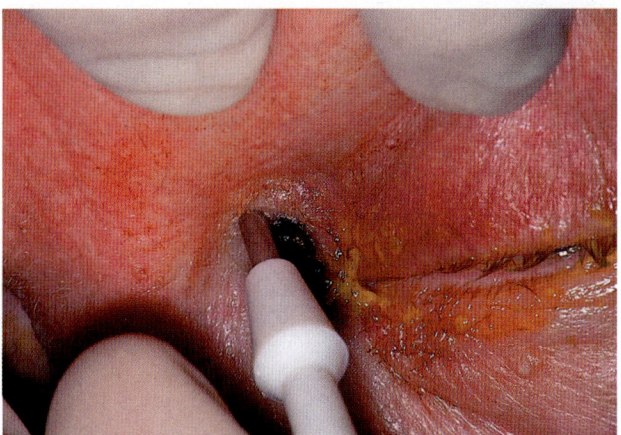

Figure 1.39. A trephine punch biopsy was taken from elevated peripheral margin of the lesion. The biopsy should not be taken from the central crater. The histopathologic findings were compatible with KA.

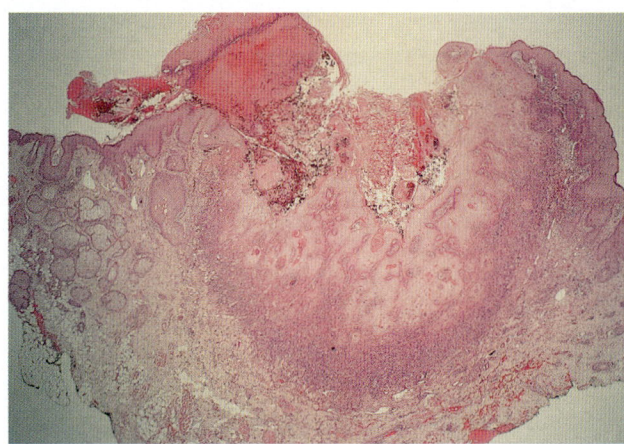

Figure 1.40. Histopathology of KA, showing localized acanthotic lesion with central crater. (Hematoxylin–eosin ×10.)

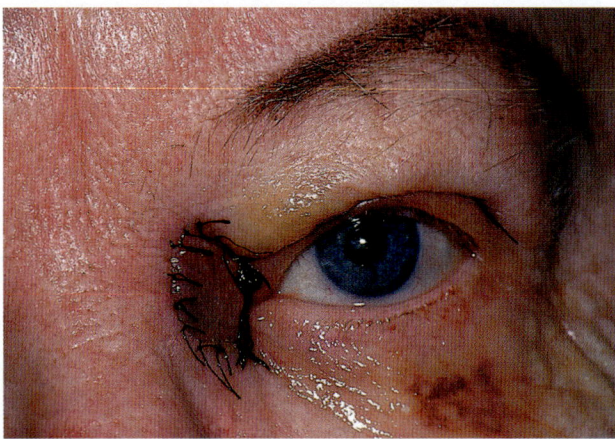

Figure 1.41. Appearance shortly after complete excision of the lesion followed by skin graft.

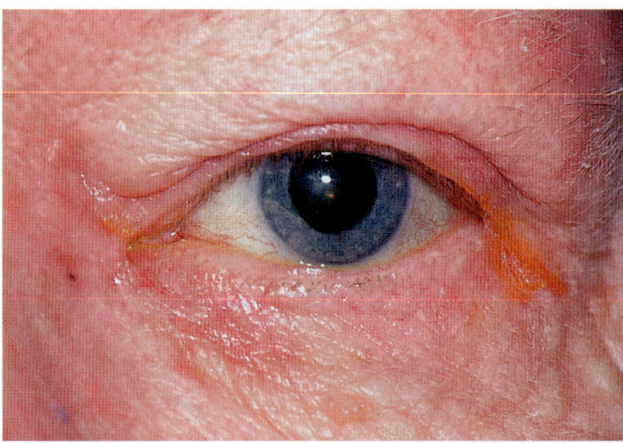

Figure 1.42. Appearance 3 months later showing excellent result.

Chapter 1 Benign Tumors of the Eyelid Epidermis

EYELID KERATOACANTHOMA: CLINICOPATHOLOGIC CORRELATION IN YOUNG AND ELDERLY PATIENTS

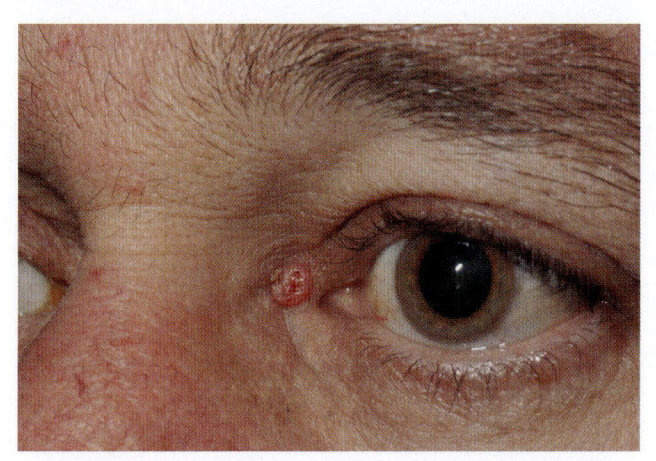

Figure 1.43. Keratoacanthoma in medial canthal region of a young man.

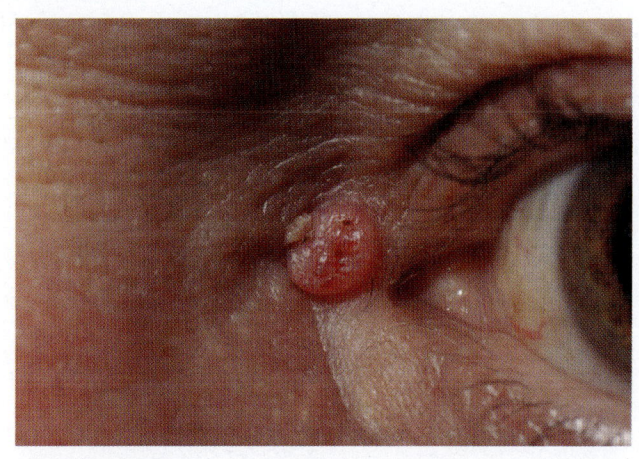

Figure 1.44. Close-up view of lesion shown in Figure 1.43 demonstrating central ulceration.

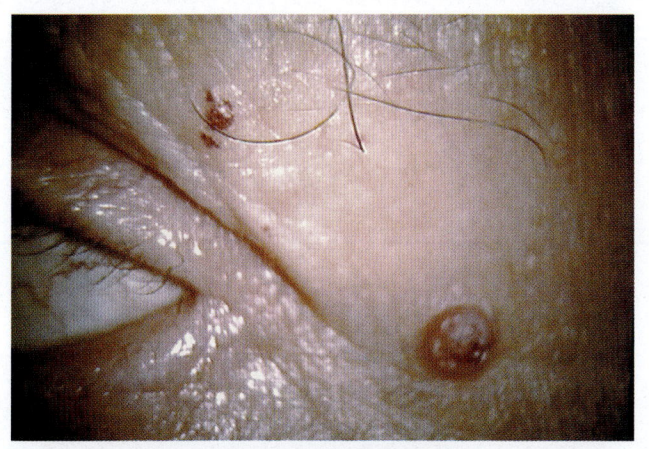

Figure 1.45. Keratoacanthoma near lateral canthus in an elderly man.

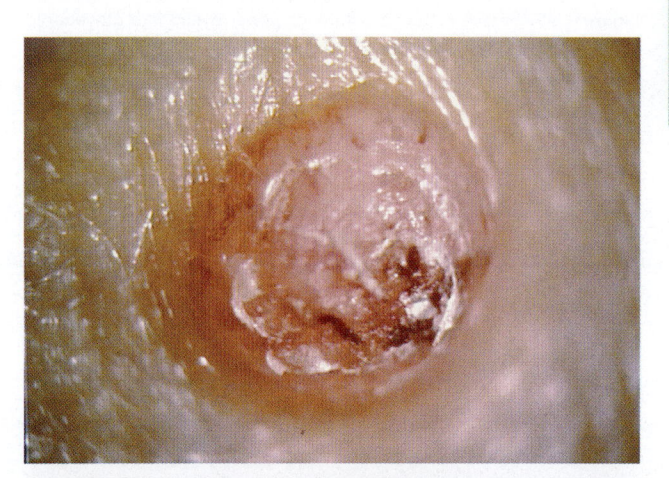

Figure 1.46. Close-up view of lesion shown in Figure 1.45 showing central ulceration.

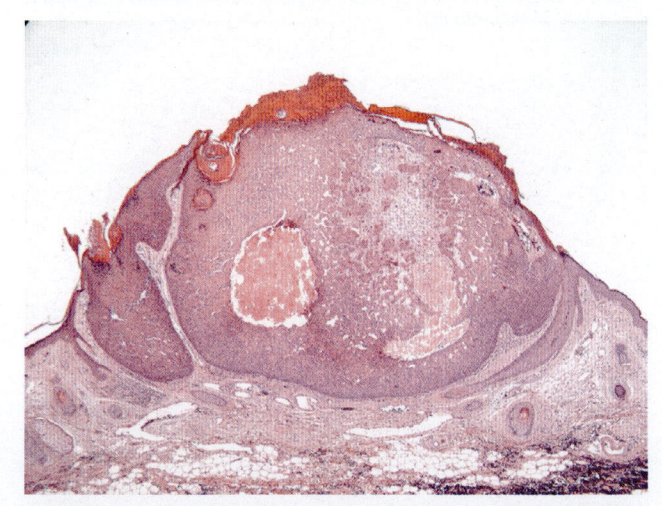

Figure 1.47. Low-magnification photomicrograph showing elevated circumscribed mass with hyperkeratosis and acanthosis. (Hematoxylin–eosin ×10.)

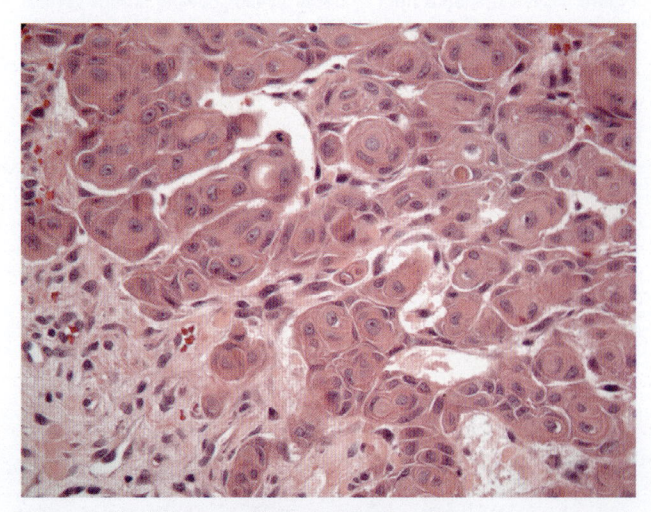

Figure 1.48. Higher-magnification view of proliferating squamous epithelial cells with dyskeratosis. (Hematoxylin–eosin ×100.)

EYELID NONSPECIFIC KERATOSIS

"Nonspecific keratosis" describes a hyperkeratotic lesion that does not fit the clinical description of the aforementioned conditions. It can assume a variety of clinical configurations, including a sessile keratotic plaque or a cutaneous horn.

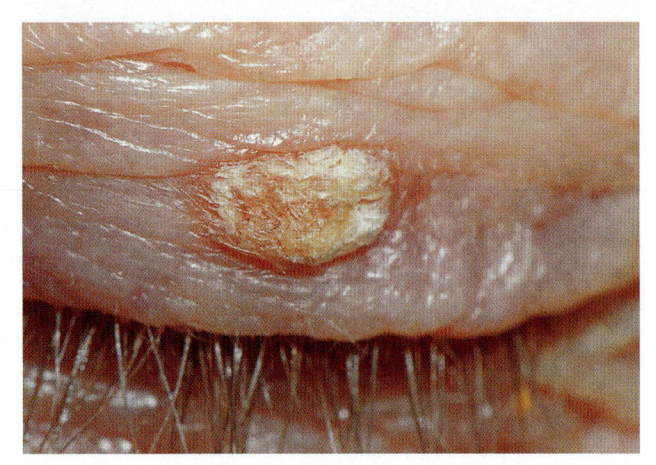

Figure 1.49. Sessile keratotic plaque of upper eyelid in a 65-year-old man.

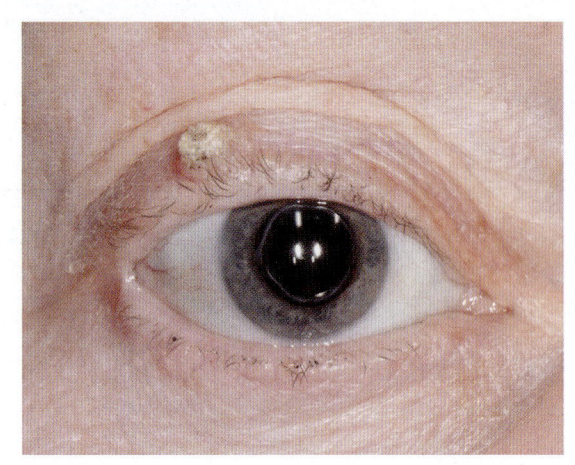

Figure 1.50. Sessile keratotic plaque of upper eyelid in an 82-year-old woman.

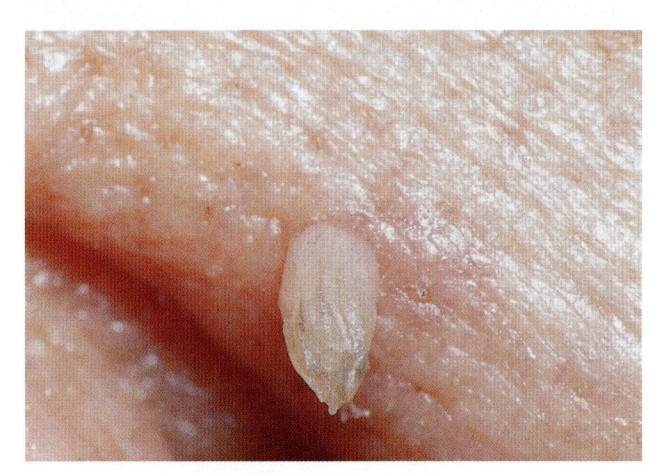

Figure 1.51. Cutaneous horn of upper eyelid showing abrupt vertical configuration in a 65-year-old woman.

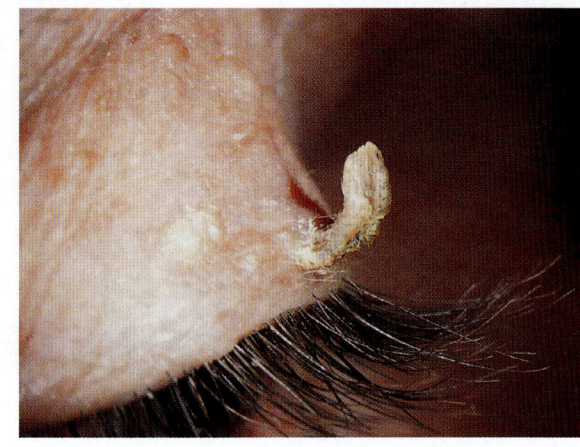

Figure 1.52. Profile view of hyperkeratotic cutaneous horn of upper eyelid in a 55-year-old man.

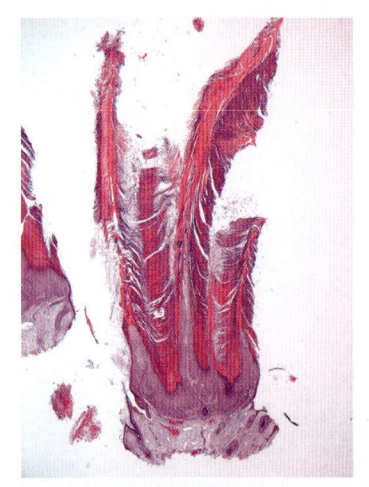

Figure 1.53. Low-power histopathology of cutaneous horn showing marked hyperkeratosis, parakeratosis, acanthosis, and clean base. (Hematoxylin–eosin ×5.)

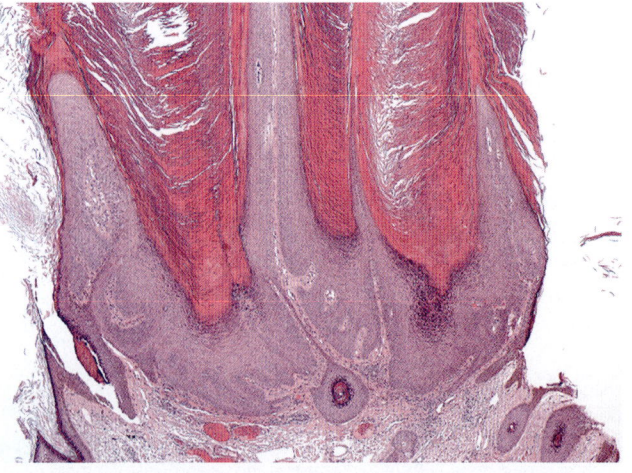

Figure 1.54. High-power histopathology of cutaneous horn showing better visualization o the hyperkeratosis, parakeratosis, and basal acanthosis. (Hematoxylin–eosin ×20.)

CHAPTER 2

PREMALIGNANT AND MALIGNANT TUMORS OF EYELID EPIDERMIS

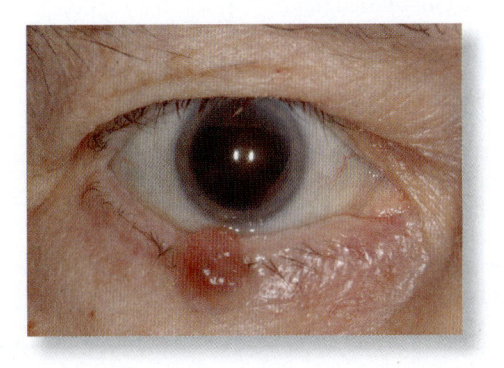

General Considerations
Many aging changes in the skin, including the eyelid, are secondary to gradual damage from lifelong exposure to ultraviolet light. Such damage is particularly prone to occur in light-skinned individuals (1–12). Actinic keratosis (solar keratosis) is a common precancerous cutaneous lesion that affects face, dorsa of the hands, bald areas on the head in men, and commonly the eyelids (1,2). Excessive exposure to sunlight is clearly a predisposing factor. A report from Japan found a mean patient age at diagnosis of 62 years and a slight predilection for females (3). If untreated, approximately 20% are believed to progress to squamous cell carcinoma (SCC).

Clinical Features
Actinic keratosis has several clinical variations, but is usually characterized by multiple, erythematous, excoriated, sessile plaques that may eventually assume a nodular, horny, or wart-like configuration. The lesions range from 1 to 10 mm in diameter and have a pink color. As mentioned, they generally occur on sun-exposed areas of older Caucasians who have had excessive sunlight exposure over a prolonged period of time.

Differential Diagnosis
The differential diagnosis includes most of the benign and malignant epidermal lesions mentioned in this atlas. It differs from seborrheic keratosis in that it has less distinct margins. Some actinic keratoses are pigmented and can simulate lentigo maligna and early melanoma. The presence of multiple actinic lesions in the adjacent skin can facilitate the diagnosis.

Pathology and Pathogenesis
Histopathologically, actinic keratosis is composed of acanthosis, focal hyperkeratosis, dyskeratosis, and mildly atypical keratinocytes with epithelial buds that extend into the papillary dermis (2,3). Clefts often form as a result of dyskeratosis and disruption of intercellular bridges. A characteristic feature is orthokeratosis in the area of the ostea of the pilosebaceous structures. Such sparing of the ostea of these units is unlike true SCC. The dermis shows moderate to severe basophilic collagen degeneration and a moderate lymphoplasmacytic infiltration (2). Several histopathologic variants are described in the literature. Histopathologic study of eyelid SCC generally reveals evidence of actinic keratosis.

EYELID ACTINIC KERATOSIS

Management

There are several ways to manage actinic keratosis and treatment must be individualized depending on the circumstances (1). Small, asymptomatic lesions can be observed. Larger lesions can be selectively resected with a shaving or elliptical approach, or curettage. Liquid nitrogen spray is often helpful for more indurated lesions. Multiple lesions or those that cannot be completely excised can be treated with topical chemotherapeutic agents or cryotherapy. Topical chemotherapy using 5-fluorouracil cream and diclofenac gel has been effective (1,7–11).

There has been recent interest in treatment of actinic keratosis of the face and bald areas of the head with topical imiquimod (Aldara; Graceway Pharmaceuticals, Bristol, TN) cream administered three times weekly (7–9). In a randomized, double-blind, parallel-group, vehicle-controlled trial of 492 patients, complete and partial clearance rates for imiquimod-treated patients (48.3% and 64.0%, respectively) were clinically and statistically significantly higher than for vehicle-treated patients (7.2% and 13.6%, respectively) (9). The median percentage reduction of baseline lesions was 86.6% for the imiquimod-treated group and 14.3% for the vehicle-treated group. It was concluded that 5% imiquimod cream applied three times weekly for 16 weeks is safe and effective for the treatment of actinic keratosis (9). Photodynamic therapy has also been used (10).

Prognosis

SCC that arises from actinic keratosis is low grade and offers an excellent prognosis because local invasiveness is minimal and metastasis occurs in only 1% to 3% of cases (6). In assessing SCC histopathologically, it is important to look for actinic keratosis near the margins. Such a finding imparts a better prognosis and compared with SCC that arises de novo, a condition that is somewhat more likely to metastasize.

EYELID ACTINIC KERATOSIS

Selected References

Reviews

1. Lagler CN, Freitag SK. Management of periocular actinic keratosis: a review of practice patterns among ophthalmic plastic surgeons. *Ophthal Plast Reconstr Surg* 2012;28(4):277–281.
2. López-Tizón E, Mencía-Gutiérrez E, Garrido-Ruíz M, et al. Clinicopathological study of 21 cases of eyelid actinic keratosis. *Int Ophthalmol* 2009;29(5):379–384.
3. Kiyokane K, Sakatani S, Kusakabe H, et al. A statistical study on clinical findings of solar keratosis. *J Med* 1992;23:389–398.
4. Doxanas MT, Iliff WJ, Iliff NT, et al. Squamous cell carcinoma of the eyelids. *Ophthalmology* 1987;94:538–541.
5. Lund HZ. How often does squamous cell carcinoma of the skin metastasize? *Arch Dermatol* 1965;92:635–637.
6. Caya JG, Hidayat AA, Weiner JM. A clinicopathologic study of 21 cases of adenoid squamous cell carcinoma of the eyelid and periorbital region. *Am J Ophthalmol* 1985;99:291–297.

Therapy

7. Urosevic M, Dummer R. Role of imiquimod in skin cancer treatment. *Am J Clin Dermatol* 2004;5:453–458.
8. Ross AH, Kennedy CT, Collins C, et al. The use of imiquimod in the treatment of periocular tumours. *Orbit* 2010;29(2):83–87.
9. Korman N, Moy R, Ling M, et al. Dosing with 5% imiquimod cream 3 times per week for the treatment of actinic keratosis: results of two phase 3, randomized, double-blind, parallel-group, vehicle-controlled trials. *Arch Dermatol* 2005;141:467–473.
10. Toledo-Alberola F, Belinchón-Romero I, Guijarro-Llorca J, et al. Photodynamic therapy as a response to the challenge of treating actinic keratosis in the eyelid area. *Actas Dermosifiliogr* 2012;103(10):938–939.
11. Couch SM, Custer PL. Topical 5-fluorouracil for the treatment of periocular actinic keratosis and low-grade 16. squamous malignancy. *Ophthal Plast Reconstr Surg* 2012;28(3):181–183.
12. Batra R, Sundararajan S, Sandramouli S. Topical diclofenac gel for the management of periocular actinic keratosis. *Ophthal Plast Reconstr Surg* 2012;28(1):1–3.

EYELID ACTINIC KERATOSIS

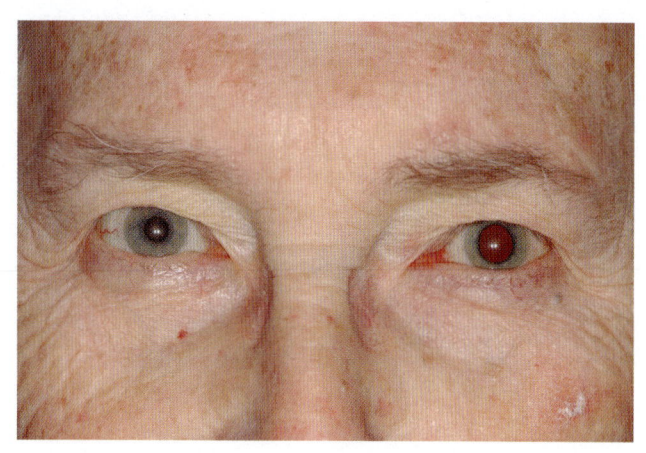

Figure 2.1. Actinic keratosis showing multiple subtle excoriated lesions in the periocular, nasal, cheek, and forehead region of an elderly woman. There is a characteristic actinic keratosis on the left cheek with overlying white hyperkeratosis and surrounding erythema.

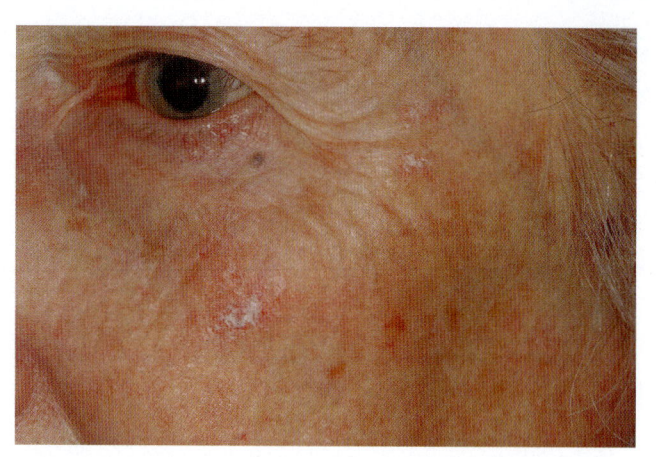

Figure 2.2. Close-up view of Figure 2.1 demonstrating white hyperkeratosis and surrounding erythema of several actinic keratoses.

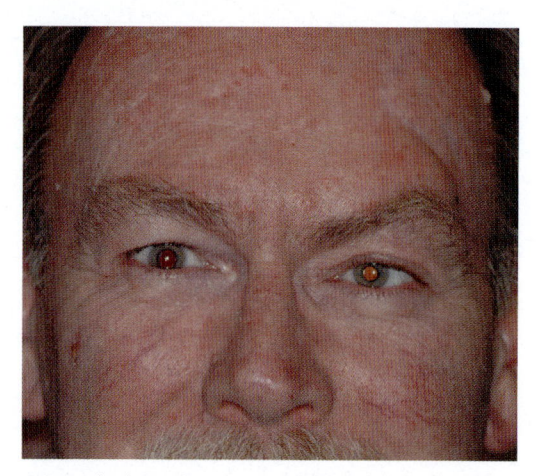

Figure 2.3. Multiple erythematous and flakey facial actinic keratosis on forehead, nasal bridge, suprabrow, and cheek region.

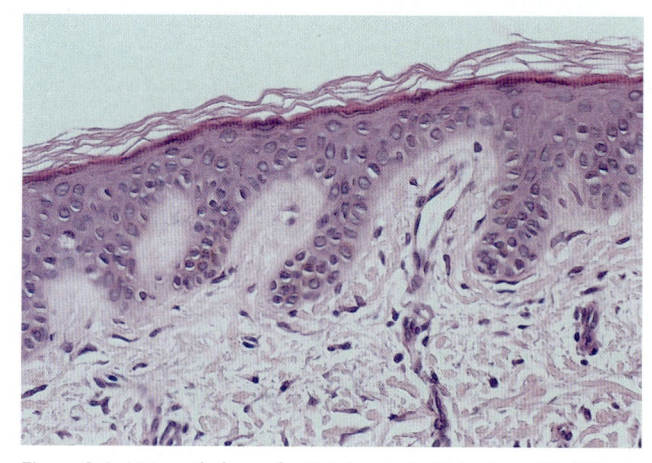

Figure 2.4. Histopathology of actinic keratosis. Note the epithelial buds that extend into the papillary dermis. (Hematoxylin–eosin ×20.)

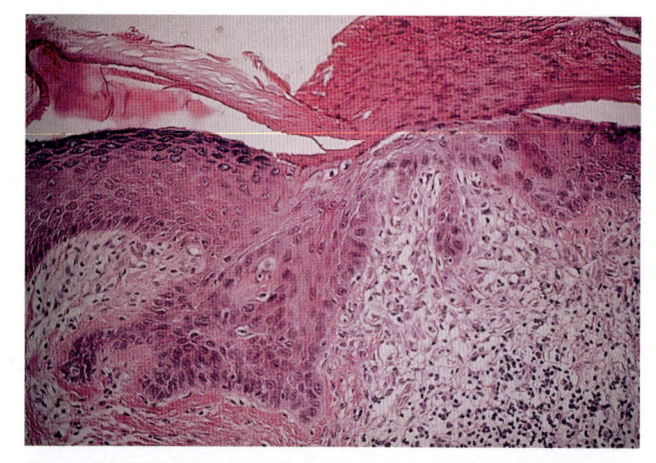

Figure 2.5. Histopathology of more severe actinic keratosis with parakeratosis and dermal inflammation. (Hematoxylin–eosin ×25.)

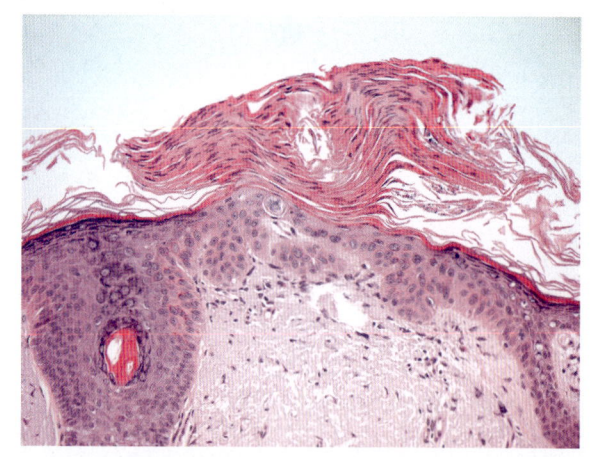

Figure 2.6. High-power histopathology of actinic keratosis with parakeratosis, epithelial buds into dermis, and slightly anaplastic intraepithelial cells. (Hematoxylin–eosin ×50.)

Chapter 2 Premalignant and Malignant Tumors of Eyelid Epidermis

● CUTANEOUS ACTINIC KERATOSIS: ASSOCIATION WITH CONJUNCTIVAL SQUAMOUS CELL CARCINOMA

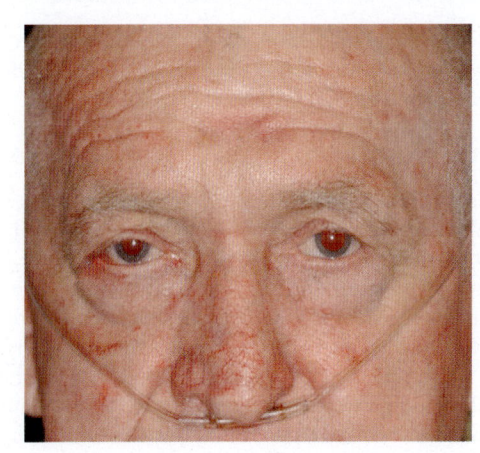

Figure 2.7. Elderly man with rosacea and chronic obstructive lung disease using oxygen. Note the numerous foci of actinic keratosis on face, especially the nose and forehead.

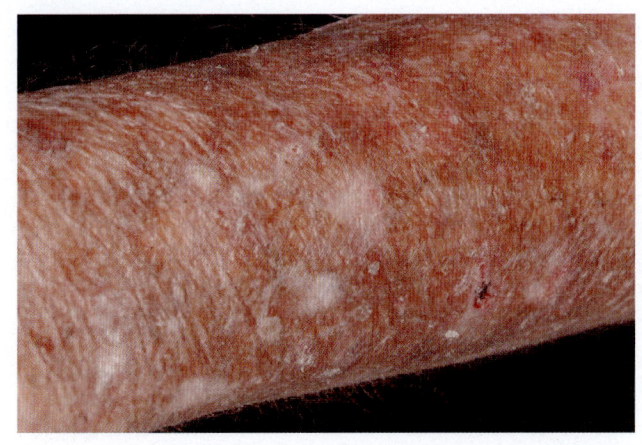

Figure 2.8. Skin involvement on forearm of patient shown in Figure 2.7, showing similar lesions.

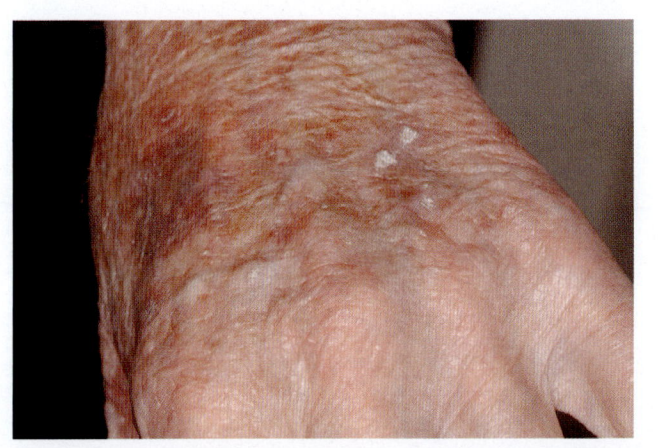

Figure 2.9. Hand of same patient, showing white scales on dorsum of hand.

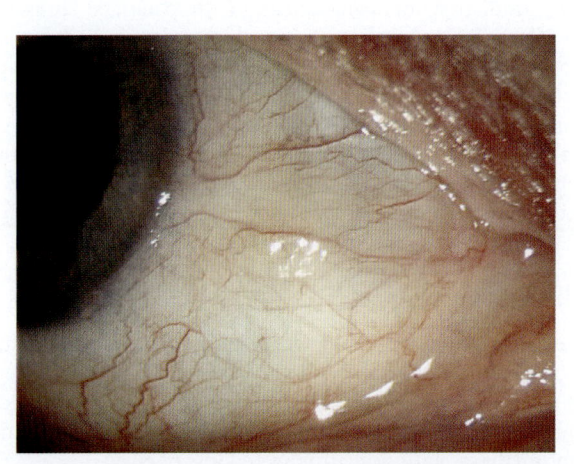

Figure 2.10. Same patient showing actinic keratosis of conjunctiva.

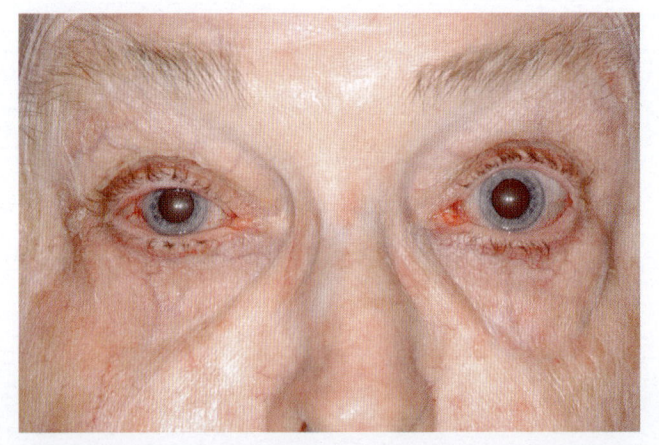

Figure 2.11. Face of another patient showing features of rosacea and actinic keratosis, most pronounced near lateral canthus of right eye.

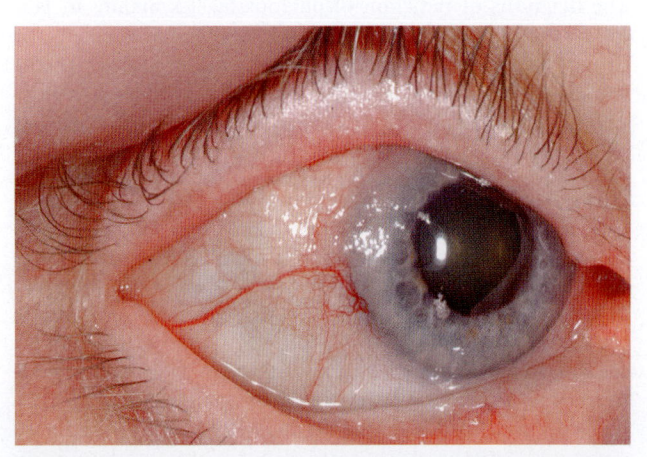

Figure 2.12. Conjunctiva of patient in Figure 2.11 showing SCC of conjunctiva (biopsy proven) on the right eye. Conjunctival SCC has a tendency to occur in patients with actinic keratosis of the skin.

RADIATION BLEPHAROPATHY

General Considerations

In addition to excessive sunlight exposure, there are miscellaneous other insults that can predispose the eyelid to malignant neoplasms. Selected examples include radiation blepharopathy (1–6), xeroderma pigmentosum (XP), and the nevus sebaceous of Jadassohn. In addition, patients who are immunosuppressed for any reason have an increased risk of developing a number of benign and malignant eyelid lesions.

Radiation blepharopathy occurs secondary to therapeutic irradiation to the ocular region for a variety of conditions (1–6). A number of years ago, facial radiation was often used for acne and other benign conditions. This led to acute and chronic changes that predisposed the facial skin to the long-term development of several "radiation-induced" epithelial and glandular neoplasms, as well as soft tissue sarcomas. Ocular irradiation for retinoblastoma, particularly in patients with the germline mutation for that disease, can contribute to a variety of neoplasms, including eyelid tumors (2,4–6). In addition, irradiation for malignancies of the paranasal sinuses or nasopharynx can predispose to radiation blepharopathy and subsequent eyelid malignancies. Sebaceous carcinoma of the eyelid, normally a disease of older individuals, can occur at a young age in children who have undergone irradiation for retinoblastoma (5,6). Many of these neoplasms were more common many years ago when >80 Gy was used in some cases of retinoblastoma. Most radiation today employs a dose of 25 to 40 Gy, depending on the disease being treated.

Clinical Features

The acute stage of radiation blepharopathy develops about a week after initiation of irradiation. It is characterized by eyelid erythema, loss of cilia, and occasional excoriation or ulcer. Chronic radiation blepharopathy can show only minimal abnormalities, with skin atrophy and loss of cilia.

Diagnostic Approaches

The diagnosis of radiation blepharopathy lies mainly in taking a patient history for prior irradiation, combined with the clinical findings mentioned. We have found that some patients who develop eyelid malignancies in middle age may not immediately recall having had irradiation for acne or other reasons when they were young.

Pathology

Acute radiation blepharopathy is characterized by edema and early degenerative changes in the epidermis, and epithelium of sebaceous glands and hair follicles. Late radiation blepharopathy is similar histopathologically to actinic keratosis, with nuclear atypia in the epidermal cells and individual cell keratinization. There may be scattered macrophages in the papillary dermis, fibrosis in the dermis, and atrophy of adnexal structures. Atrophy of sebaceous glands is often profound (3). The blood vessels become telangiectatic and may show individual cell swelling and thrombosis and recanalization. SCC that arises from these changes is generally of spindle cell type with a higher degree of malignancy and a greater tendency to metastasize than ordinary SCC.

Management

Management is directed toward prevention of cutaneous erosion, infection, and long-term cancers. Topical lubrication with antibiotics tends to soothe the site and prevent infection. Avoidance of corticosteroid preparations is advised. The patient should avoid excess exposure to sunlight because actinic stimulation can further increase the chance of malignant transformation. Advanced cases with excoriation or ulceration may require more aggressive management with surgical intervention to restore vascular supply to the site. It is most important to check the patient yearly and to advise the patient to return earlier should there be any suspicious symptoms or signs.

Selected References

Reviews
1. Hsu A, Frank SJ, Ballo MT, et al. Postoperative adjuvant external-beam radiation therapy for cancers of the eyelid and conjunctiva. *Ophthal Plast Reconstr Surg* 2008;24(6):444–449.
2. Abramson DH, Ellsworth RM, Zimmerman LE. Nonocular cancer in retinoblastoma survivors. *Trans Am Acad Ophthalmol* 1976;81:454–456.

Pathology
3. Karp LA, Streeten BW, Cogan DG. Radiation-induced atrophy of the meibomian glands. *Arch Ophthalmol* 1979;97:303–305.

Case Reports
4. Bhatt PR, Al-Nuaimi D, Raines MF. Bilateral basal cell carcinoma of the lower eyelids following radium treatment for blepharitis. *Eye (Lond)* 2008;22(7):980–981.
5. Rundle P, Shields JA, Shields CL, et al. Sebaceous gland carcinoma of the eyelid 16 years after irradiation for retinoblastoma. *Eye* 1999;13:109–110.
6. Kivela T, Asko-Seljavaara S, Pihkala U, et al. Sebaceous carcinoma of the eyelid associated with retinoblastoma. *Ophthalmology* 2001;108:1124–1128.

Chapter 2 Premalignant and Malignant Tumors of Eyelid Epidermis

EYELID RADIATION BLEPHAROPATHY

Radiation blepharopathy can cause acute and chronic changes in the eyelids that can predispose to the development of squamous and sebaceous neoplasms later in life.

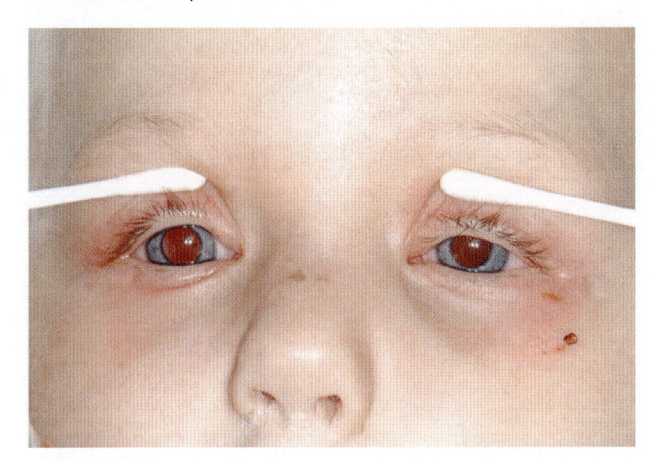

Figure 2.13. Acute radiation blepharitis following external beam irradiation for retinoblastoma.

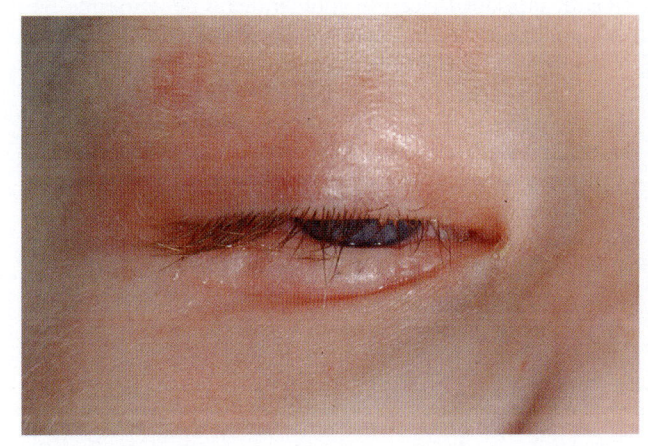

Figure 2.14. Close-up view of patient in Figure 2.13, showing erythema, excoriation, and loss of cilia.

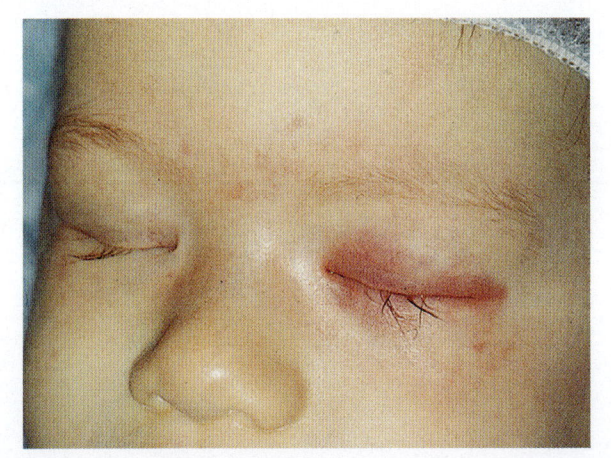

Figure 2.15. Early radiation blepharopathy after irradiation for retinoblastoma in a young child showing eyelid erythema.

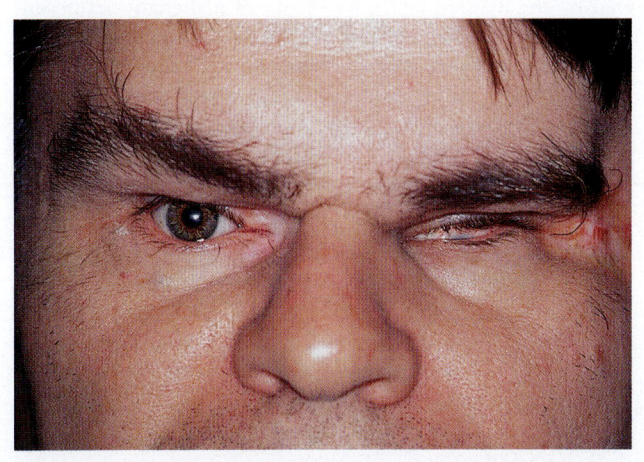

Figure 2.16. Radiation blepharopathy 43 years after treatment for retinoblastoma showing thickening and contraction of eyelid tissues.

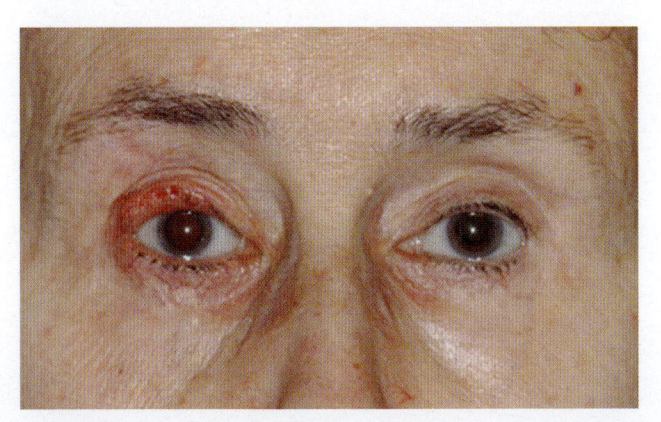

Figure 2.17. Chronic blepharopathy in right eye of a 72-year-old woman who had irradiation for facial acne as a child. Note the thin skin and telangiectasia on nasolabial fold and chin.

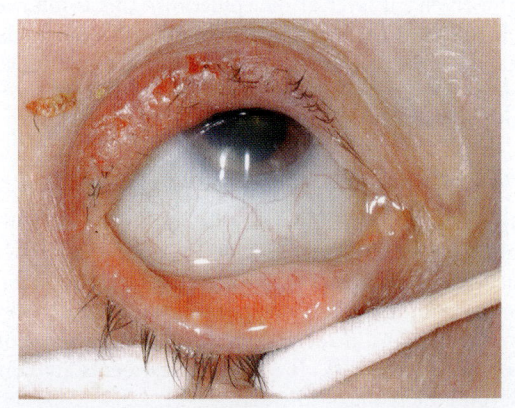

Figure 2.18. Closer view of right eye in patient shown in Figure 2.17. The blepharopathy was worse in the eyelids of right eye and eventual biopsy showed diffuse sebaceous carcinoma.

EYELID XERODERMA PIGMENTOSUM

General Considerations

XP is an autosomal-recessive disorder that is not a specific eyelid lesion like other conditions discussed in this atlas. However, it is appropriate to discuss this disease because affected patients have a marked sensitivity to ultraviolet light that can predispose them to a variety of skin cancers, many of which involve the eyelid and conjunctiva (1–16).

Cultures of skin fibroblasts and blood lymphocytes have demonstrated a deficiency in repair of damaged DNA. Death often occurs by the age of 20 years and, occasionally, by the age of 10 years, usually owing to metastasis from cutaneous SCC or malignant melanoma.

Clinical Features

Six progressive stages of XP are identified, the details of which are beyond the scope of this atlas. In the earlier stages, the exposed skin shows numerous freckles, erythema, and scaling. Later, there is mottled pigmentation with telangiectasia that resembles radiation dermatopathy. The final stage is characterized by the development of a variety of malignant neoplasms often in the second or third decade of life, including SCC, basal cell carcinoma (BCC), malignant melanoma, and some sarcomas (1–3). These multiple benign and malignant tumors can cause bothersome cosmetic problems.

Diagnosis

The diagnosis of XP can generally be made by the classic cutaneous features described, a positive family history, or both. Some patients have associated noncutaneous abnormalities, including mental deficiency, retarded growth, and delayed sexual development. The de Sanctis–Cacchione syndrome is characterized by XP, mental deficiency, microcephaly, dwarfism, hypogonadism, deafness, and ataxia.

Pathology

Histopathologically, the earlier stages are characterized by nonspecific changes, including hyperkeratosis and hyperpigmentation of the basal layer of the epidermis. This is followed by irregular patches of hyperpigmentation with acanthosis and atypical downward proliferation of epidermis similar to actinic keratosis. The final stages are characterized by eruption of the various neoplasms mentioned above (5).

Management

Management of XP mainly includes avoidance of sunlight, topical sunscreens, protective clothing, ultraviolet blocking spectacles, and early removal of premalignant and malignant skin lesions. Some workers have published extensively on treatment of the lesions in the early stages, using a variety of oral and topical agents (2,3). The specific treatments are complex and beyond the scope of this atlas.

Selected References

Reviews

1. Newsome DA, Kraemer KH, Robbins JH. Repair of DNA in xeroderma pigmentosum conjunctiva. *Arch Ophthalmol* 1975;93:660–662.
2. Kraemer KH, DiGiovanna JJ, Moshell AN, et al. Prevention of skin cancer in xeroderma pigmentosum with the use of oral isotretinoin. *N Engl J Med* 1998;318:1633–1637.
3. Kraemer KH, DiGiovanna JJ. Topical enzyme therapy for skin diseases? *J Am Acad Dermatol* 2002;46:463–466.
4. Brooks BP, Thompson AH, Bishop RJ, et al. Ocular manifestations of xeroderma pigmentosum: long-term follow-up highlights the role of DNA repair in protection from sun damage. *Ophthalmology* 2013;120(7):1324–1336.
5. Ramkumar HL, Brooks BP, Cao X, et al. Ophthalmic manifestations and histopathology of xeroderma pigmentosum: two clinicopathological cases and a review of the literature. *Surv Ophthalmol* 2011;56(4):348–361.
6. Alfawaz AM, Al-Hussain HM. Ocular manifestations of xeroderma pigmentosum at a tertiary eye care center in Saudi Arabia. *Ophthal Plast Reconstr Surg* 2011;27(6):401–404.
7. Touzri RA, Mohamed Z, Khalil E, et al. Ocular malignancies of xeroderma pigmentosum: clinical and therapeutic features. *Ann Dermatol Venereol* 2008;135(2):99–104.
8. Dollfus H, Porto F, Caussade P, et al. Ocular manifestations in the inherited DNA repair disorders. *Surv Ophthalmol* 2003;48(1):107–122.
9. Goyal JL, Rao VA, Srinivasan R, et al. Oculocutaneous manifestations in xeroderma pigmentosa. *Br J Ophthalmol* 1994;78(4):295–297.
10. Paridaens AD, McCartney AC, Hungerford JL. Premalignant melanosis of the conjunctiva and the cornea in xeroderma pigmentosum. *Br J Ophthalmol* 1992;76(2):120–122.

Therapy

11. Kheirkhah A, Ghaffari R, Kaghazkanani R, et al. A combined approach of amniotic membrane and oral mucosa transplantation for fornix reconstruction in severe symblepharon. *Cornea* 2013;32(2):155–160.

Case Reports

12. Gaasterland DE, Rodrigues MM, Moshell AN. Ocular involvement in xeroderma pigmentosum. *Ophthalmology* 1982;89:980–986.
13. Kamal S, Bodh SA, Kumar S, et al. Orbital myiasis complicating squamous cell carcinoma in xeroderma pigmentosum. *Orbit* 2012;31(2):137–139.
14. El-Hayek M, Lestringant GG, Frossard PM. Xeroderma pigmentosum in four siblings with three different types of malignancies simultaneously in one. *J Pediatr Hematol Oncol* 2004;26(8):473–475.
15. Calugaru M, Barsu M. Exuberant epibulbar tumor penetrating into the orbit in xeroderma pigmentosum. *Graefes Arch Clin Exp Ophthalmol* 1992;230(4):352–357.
16. Hertle RW, Durso F, Metzler JP, et al. Epibulbar squamous cell carcinomas in brothers with Xeroderma pigmentosa. *J Pediatr Ophthalmol Strabismus* 1991;28(6):350–353.

Chapter 2 Premalignant and Malignant Tumors of Eyelid Epidermis

EYELID XERODERMA PIGMENTOSUM

Like radiation blepharopathy, XP can also predispose the eyelids and conjunctiva to squamous cell carcinoma, basal cell carcinoma, malignant melanoma, and other skin malignancies.

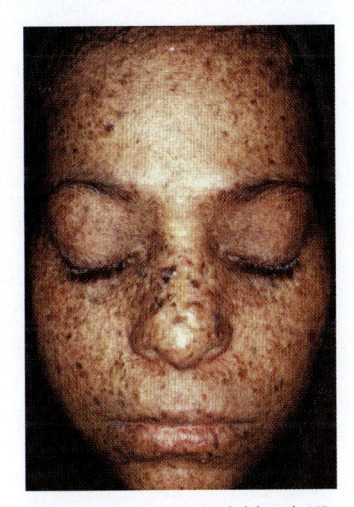

Figure 2.19. Multiple facial lesions in a child with XP.

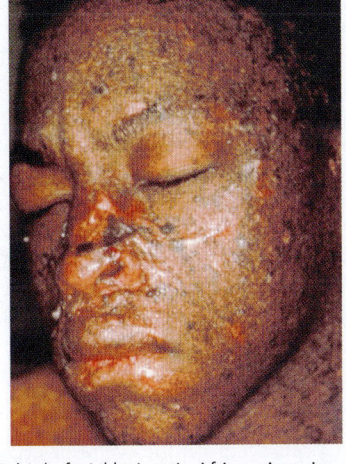

Figure 2.20. Multiple facial lesions in African-American patient with XP.

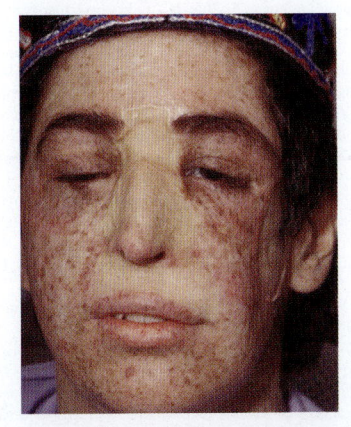

Figure 2.21. A 15-year-old boy with XP showing scars from multiple skin grafts after surgical resections of melanoma and squamous cell carcinoma.

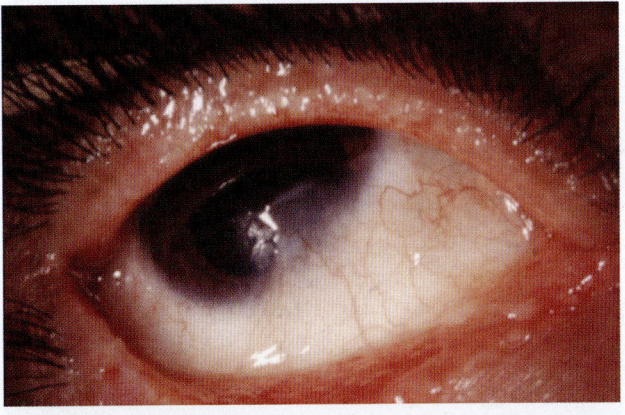

Figure 2.22. Conjunctival fibrosis of patient in Figure 2.21 from previous surgical resection of squamous cell carcinoma.

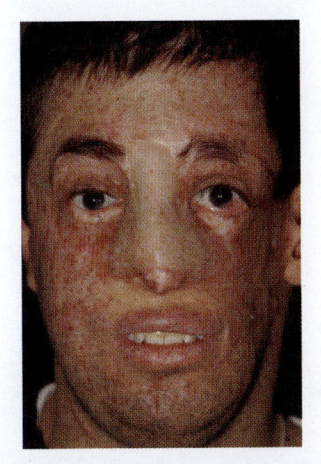

Figure 2.23. At age 24 years, the boy in Figure 2.21 shows continued XP with facial scars.

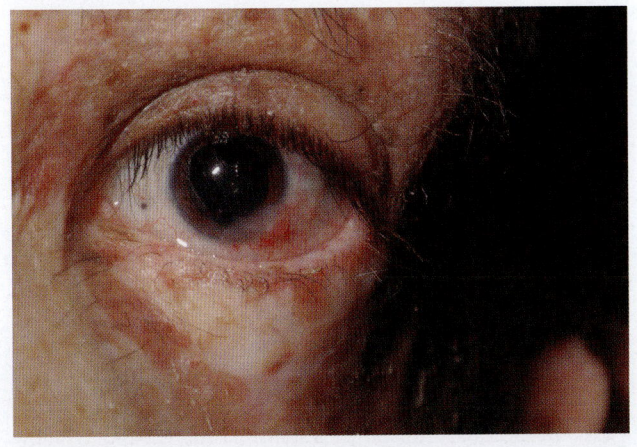

Figure 2.24. Conjunctival fibrosis of patient in Figure 2.23 and the development of a central pink squamous cell carcinoma.

SEBACEOUS NEVUS

General Considerations

Nevus sebaceous of Jadassohn (epidermal nevus syndrome) is an intriguing syndrome that has received attention in the recent literature (1–17). Sebaceous nevus can be an isolated lesion in the eyelid area, or a part of the organoid nevus syndrome. The neurologic aspects of the organoid nevus syndrome include seizures and mental retardation secondary to arachnoid cysts and cerebral atrophy. The best known ocular finding is the epibulbar complex choristoma. The most frequent cutaneous feature of the organoid nevus syndrome is the sebaceous nevus of Jadassohn (1,2). This congenital cutaneous lesion can frequently give rise later in life to BCC and other benign and malignant cutaneous neoplasms. The conjunctival and ocular fundus manifestations of this syndrome are discussed elsewhere in this atlas.

Clinical Features

Sebaceous nevus can occur on the eyelid or eyebrow as a solitary lesion or as a component of a larger geographic lesion that affects the skin of the face, retroauricular area, and scalp, with contiguous involvement of the eyebrow and eyelid. It usually has a pink to brown color and well-defined irregular margins. The component that involves the scalp is usually associated with localized alopecia. The lesions are initially flat but become more elevated about the time of puberty, perhaps owing to sebaceous gland hyperplasia (3–5).

Diagnostic Approaches

The diagnosis can be easily made based on the typical clinical features mentioned. The patient should have a thorough ocular, dermatologic, and neurologic survey to exclude some of the aforementioned systemic findings.

Pathology

Histopathologically, three stages of sebaceous nevus have been proposed. The first (prepubertal) phase consists of epithelial hyperplasia, dense hypercellular stroma, and absence of hair and sebaceous glands in the dermis. The second (adolescent) phase is characterized by acanthosis, papillomatosis, hyperkeratosis, and hyperplasia of sebaceous glands that open directly onto the epidermal surface, and buds of undifferentiated hair structures in the papillary dermis. The third (adult) phase is typified by the development of benign and malignant skin neoplasms, particularly BCC and hidradenoma. About 20% of sebaceous nevi eventually give rise to BCC or other less common adnexal neoplasms. About 75% of all syringocystadenomas arise within a sebaceous nevus.

Management

Small disfiguring lesions in the eyelid area can be removed surgically with primary closure. In some cases, cutaneous flaps or grafts are necessary for larger lesions. Tissue expanders allow enlargement of skin in preparation for cutaneous flaps for extensive lesions. Even though excision is preferred, extensive lesions can be followed conservatively and any small suspicious neoplasms that appear within the lesion should be removed surgically.

Selected References

Reviews

1. Shields JA, Shields CL, Eagle RC Jr, et al. Ophthalmic features of the organoid nevus syndrome. *Trans Am Ophthalmol Soc* 1996;94:65–86.
2. Shields JA, Shields CL, Eagle RC Jr, et al. Ocular manifestations of the organoid nevus syndrome. *Ophthalmology* 1997;104:549–557.
3. Alfonso I, Howard C, Lopez PF, et al. Linear nevus sebaceous syndrome: a review. *J Clin Neuroophthalmol* 1987;7:170–177.
4. Lambert HM, Sipperley JO, Shore JW, et al. Linear nevus sebaceous syndrome. *Ophthalmology* 1987;94:278–282.
5. Solomon LM, Fretzin DF, Dewald RL. The epidermal nevus syndrome. *Arch Dermatol* 1968;97:273–285.
6. Wilkes SR, Campbell RJ, Waller RR. Ocular malformation in association with ipsilateral facial nevus of Jadassohn. *Am J Ophthalmol* 1981;92:344–352.
7. Roth AM, Keltner JL. Linear nevus sebaceous syndrome. *J Clin Neuroophthalmol* 1993;13:44–49.

Case Reports

8. Shields CN, Shields CL, Lin C, et al. Calcified scleral choristoma in organoid nevus syndrome simulating retinoblastoma. *J Pediatr Ophthalmol Strabismus* 2014;51:e1–e3.
9. Kraus JN, Ramasubramanian A, Shields CL, et al. Ocular features of the organoid nevus syndrome. *Retin Cases Brief Rep* 2010;4:385–386.
10. Callahan AB, Jakobiec FA, Zakka FR, et al. Isolated unilateral linear epidermal nevus of the upper eyelid. *Ophthal Plast Reconstr Surg* 2012;28(6):e135–e138.
11. Pushker N, Mehta M, Bajaj MS, et al. Atypical oculo-orbital complex choristoma in organoid nevus syndrome. *J Pediatr Ophthalmol Strabismus* 2006;43(2):119–122.
12. Chiu TY, Fan DS, Chu WC, et al. Ocular manifestations and surgical management of lid coloboma in a Chinese infant with linear nevus sebaceous syndrome. *J Pediatr Ophthalmol Strabismus* 2004;41:312–314.
13. Askar S, Kilinc N, Aytekin S. Syringocystadenoma papilliferum mimicking basal cell carcinoma on the lower eyelid: a case report. *Acta Chir Plast* 2002;44(4):117–119.
14. Mullaney PB, Weatherhead RG. Epidermal nevus syndrome associated with a complex choristoma and a bilateral choroidal osteoma. *Arch Ophthalmol* 1996;114:1292–1293.
15. Pe'er J, Ilsar M. Epibulbar complex choristoma associated with nevus sebaceous. *Arch Ophthalmol* 1995;113:1301–1304.
16. Hayasaka S, Sekimoto M, Setogawa T. Epibulbar complex choristoma involving the bulbar conjunctiva and cornea. *J Pediatr Ophthalmol Strabismus* 1989;26:251–253.
17. Diven DG, Solomon AR, McNeely MC, et al. Nevus sebaceous associated with major ophthalmologic abnormalities. *Arch Dermatol* 1987;123:383–386.

Chapter 2 Premalignant and Malignant Tumors of Eyelid Epidermis   29

EYELID SEBACEOUS NEVUS: ASSOCIATION WITH PERIOCULAR INVOLVEMENT

The cutaneous lesion of nevus sebaceous syndrome, seen best in the medial canthal area, nose, and forehead, has significant malignant potential but the conjunctival lesion (complex choristoma) has not been known to undergo malignant change.

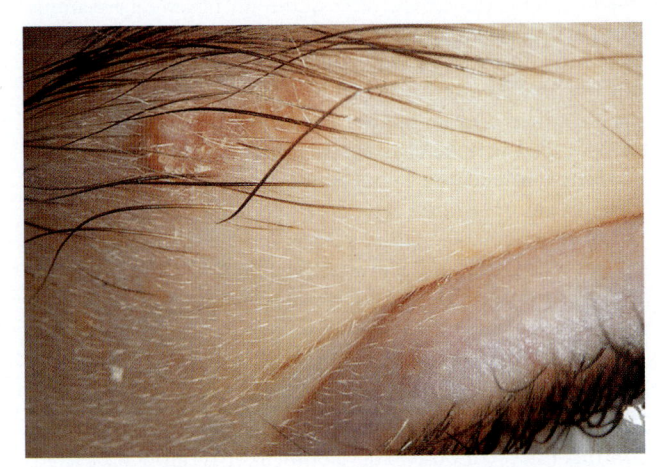

Figure 2.25. Subtle sebaceous nevus localized to lateral aspect of right eyebrow region.

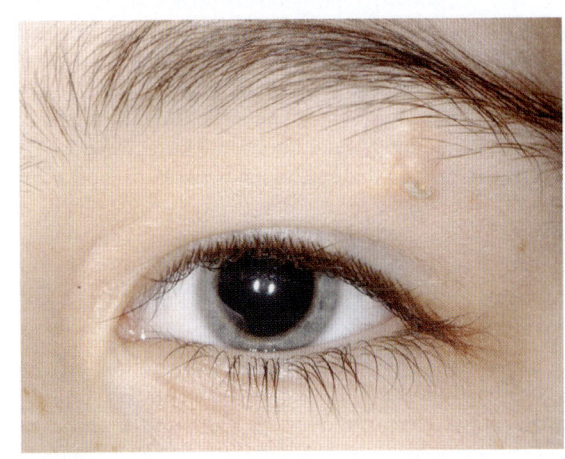

Figure 2.26. Child with subtle sebaceous nevus on left upper eyelid with a more obvious cutaneous horn arising from lesion immediately beneath the eyebrow.

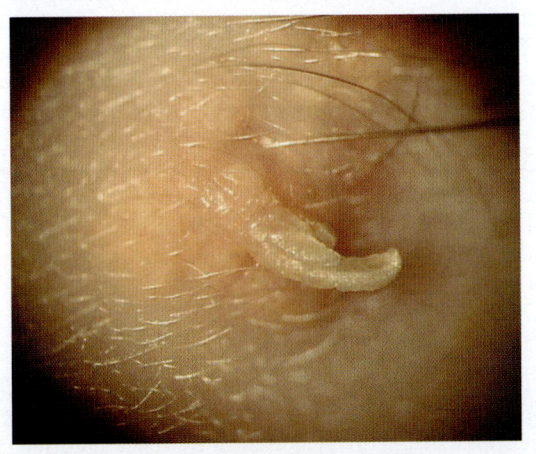

Figure 2.27. Close-up view of lesion shown in Figure 2.26, featuring the cutaneous horn. Note the sessile sebaceous nevus around the base of the horn.

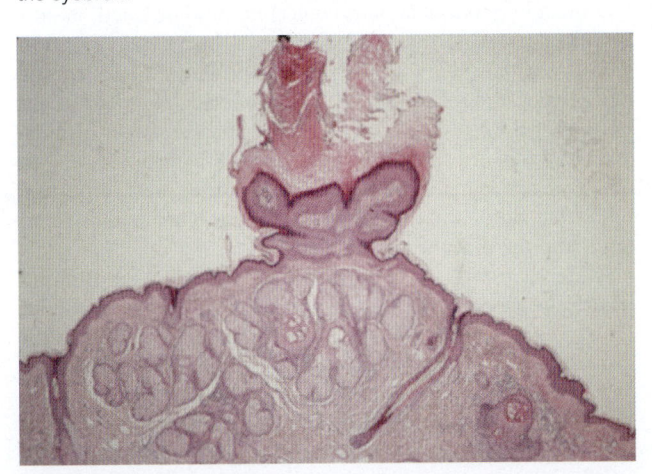

Figure 2.28. Low-magnification photomicrograph of lesion shown in Figure 2.27. Note the irregular, elevated, hyperkeratotic lesion with excess sebaceous glands in dermis. (Hematoxylin–eosin ×5.)

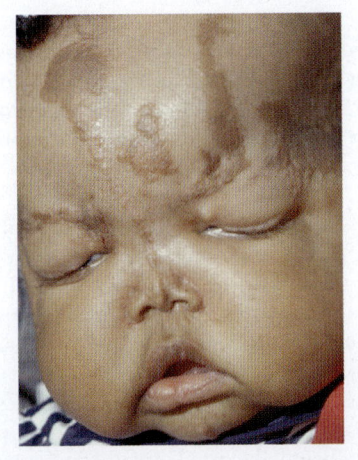

Figure 2.29. Baby with sebaceous nevus in geographic distribution on forehead, eyebrows, eyelids, and nose.

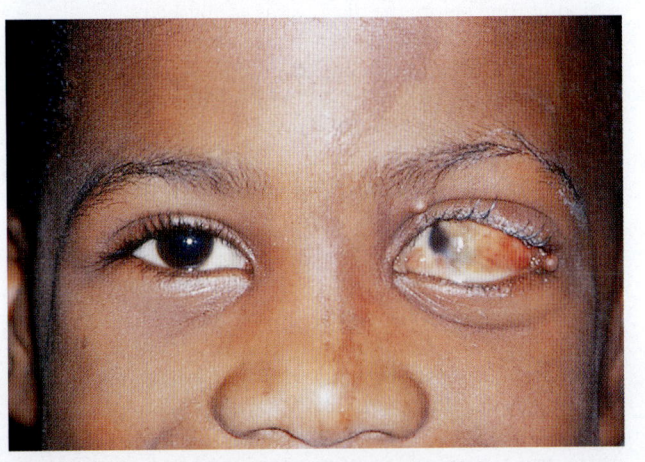

Figure 2.30. Sebaceous nevus of eyelid, nose, and forehead associated with an ipsilateral complex choristoma of the conjunctiva.

EYELID BASAL CELL CARCINOMA

General Considerations

There have been many reports on the diagnosis and management of BCC (1–57). This tumor is the most common malignant lesion of the skin, with >400,000 patients treated yearly in the United States. It occurs mainly in the head and neck region, frequently originates in the eyelids, and accounts for >90% of malignant eyelid tumors in North America. BCC usually occurs in fair-skinned adults between 50 and 80 years of age. BCC can develop in younger patients, especially those who have predisposing lesions like nevoid BCC syndrome, nevus sebaceous of Jadassohn, or XP (9–13).

Clinical Features

Although percents vary from series to series, our experience suggests that eyelid BCC arises on the lower eyelid about 65%, medial canthus 15%, upper eyelid 15%, and lateral canthus 5%. It is usually painless, but more invasive BCCs with perineural spread in the eyelids and orbit can cause pain.

There are several clinical variations that can affect the eyelid, including nodular, noduloulcerative, pigmented, cystic, morpheaform, and superficial varieties. The hallmark of most lesions is the pearly, waxy, or translucent nature of the tumor, best seen on the rolled borders. Telangiectasia, mainly near the borders of the lesion, is a characteristic and consistent finding. When located near the eyelid margin, BCC typically causes loss of cilia over the area of involvement. The three most important types that occur on the eyelid are the nodular, noduloulcerative, and the morpheaform types.

More than 80% of eyelid BCCs are of the nodular or noduloulcerative type (3). It appears initially as a sessile or dome-shaped translucent lesion that gradually enlarges. As it enlarges, the central part of the lesion outstrips its peripheral blood supply, and ulcerates to form the common noduloulcerative variant. The ulcerated lesion may sometimes bleed. Morpheaform or sclerosing BCC is less common, comprising only about 2% of BCCs. This form appears as a pale, relatively flat lesion with clinically ill-defined margins and loss of cilia. Because there is no distinct tumor, it is often misdiagnosed as blepharitis for a period of time before the diagnosis is established.

Neglected or inadequately treated BCC, particularly the morpheaform type, can be highly invasive and extend into the lacrimal drainage system, orbit, and rarely into the cranial cavity. Orbital invasion generally produces diplopia or displacement of the globe, but proptosis is uncommon except in very advanced orbital involvement. Spontaneous regression of BCC is rare (52).

Differential Diagnosis

Most of the lesions discussed in this section can mimic BCC and their clinical features are discussed elsewhere. Keratoacanthoma also shows ulceration but has a more rapid onset and progression. Pigmented BCC must be differentiated from melanocytic nevus, melanoma, and seborrheic keratosis. The cystic type can resemble eccrine or apocrine hydrocystoma.

Pathology

Histopathologically, BCC can assume any of several variations. The circumscribed noduloulcerative lesion typically shows distinct lobules, nests, or cords of well-differentiated basal cells, separated by connective tissue. The tumor cells typically show parallel alignment at the periphery of each lobule, forming the so-called peripheral palisading. The stroma usually shows shrinkage around the lobule, inducing a characteristic clear cleft. The morpheaform type shows ill-defined tumor cells that characteristically lack peripheral palisading and buds or strands of tumor extend for variable distances into the dermis. There is intense stromal fibrous proliferation.

Pathogenesis

Age, light skin, sunlight exposure, arsenic exposure, scars, prior irradiation, and immunosuppression are all believed to be factors that can predispose to development of eyelid BCC. Heredity also plays a role in patients with nevoid BCC syndrome and XP, as mentioned. The relationship to the nevus sebaceous of Jadassohn was also mentioned. Cigarette smoking has been implicated as a predisposing factor in women, but not men (4). One report suggested that chronic infection of the pilosebaceous follicle by the mite *Demodex folliculorum* may also be a pathogenetic triggering factor (5). Demodicidosis is common and more studies are needed to verify those observations.

Cytologically, BCC is believed to arise from pluripotent stem cells that develop throughout life and are associated with basal cells of the epidermis and external root sheath of hair follicles. It is not believed to arise from mature differentiated basal cells.

Management

The goal of management of eyelid BCC should be to achieve complete tumor control, even if treatment compromises cosmetic appearance. For small lesions, complete resection down to the subcutaneous region with frozen section proof of tumor-free margins is performed (17–19). Primary closure or reconstruction with cutaneous flaps and grafts allows for cosmetic rehabilitation. A detailed discussion of reconstruction techniques is beyond the scope of this atlas. In cases where the wound is not readily amenable to primary closure, such as those located in the medial canthal area, the wound can heal spontaneously if left open. This laissez-faire approach can lead to satisfactory cosmetic and functional results in >90% of cases (39).

For larger lesions suspected to be BCC, a small incisional or punch biopsy may provide adequate tissue for histopathologic diagnosis before embarking on wider surgical excision and reconstruction. After confirmation of the diagnosis, wide excision and frozen section control or Mohs chemosurgery offer reliable control rates (38).

In some cases that are not readily amenable to surgical resection, cryotherapy can help to achieve good tumor control (34). Some authors have advocated cryotherapy as the preferred

EYELID BASAL CELL CARCINOMA

primary treatment for small BCCs (40). Radiotherapy is generally reserved as palliative treatment for aggressive recurrent lesions or for patients who are physically unable to undergo surgery (43). If recurrence with orbital extension is suspected, computed tomography (CT) and/or magnetic resonance imaging (MRI) should be performed. If BCC is neglected or not completely excised, it can invade the orbit, nasal cavity, and brain. When eyelid BCC invades these areas, orbital exenteration and/or radiotherapy are often necessary.

We believe that if unresectable orbital tumor is found, orbital exenteration may be the best treatment (49). Orbital exenteration is necessary in only about 1% of eyelid BCCs.

Other methods used to treat extraocular BCC include curettage and electrodessication, photodynamic therapy, interferon, topical neomycin, and local or systemic chemotherapy. These methods have not been widely accepted for BCC. There has been recent interest in the use of topical imiquimod cream to treat selected cases of extraocular and periocular BCCs, with favorable results, particularly useful for nonsurgical elderly patients or those with superficial disease (22–32).

In addition, there has been recent interest in treatment of BCC with vismodegib for BCC (20,21). This oral medication is targeted against the hedgehog pathway which is involved in genetically and somatically related BCC. The treatment can be expensive and intolerable, but patients with multifocal BCCs can have remarkable resolution.

Regional metastasis from BCC is extremely rare (50,51). This tumor rarely exhibits distant metastasis despite the fact that it can invade lymphatic channels. However, incomplete removal can be associated with aggressive recurrence, leading to a poorer cure rate. Neglected or incomplete initial excision can result in orbital invasion and rarely death can ensue due to intracranial invasion via emissaries in the orbital bone. Mortality from eyelid BCC is probably less than 1% (54).

Nevoid Basal Cell Carcinoma Syndrome

The basal cell nevus syndrome, also known as the Gorlin–Goltz syndrome, or Goltz syndrome, deserves special mention. It is a multisystem, autosomal-dominant syndrome involving both ectoderm and mesoderm tissues (10–13). In some cases, it is due to an abnormal *PTCH* (patched) gene on chromosome 9q22.3-q31. It occurs more commonly in males. Typically, the affected patient develops postpubertal onset of multiple BCCs. The associated findings can include odontogenic keratocysts, palmar and plantar pits (which may represent forme frustes of BCC), ectopic calcification of the falx cerebri, and skeletal abnormalities such as bifid ribs and, rarely, other tumors like medulloblastoma and meningioma. Other less common ocular abnormalities include congenital cataracts, uveal and optic nerve coloboma, strabismus, nystagmus, and microphthalmos. It is estimated that 0.7% of patients with BCC have this syndrome.

With nevoid BCC syndrome, patients may manifest only a few to thousands of BCCs. The lesions are often red-brown and vary in size from 1 to 10 mm. They can be pedunculated, pigmented, nodular, erythematous, or ulcerative. There were four cases in our series of 105 patients with eyelid BCC (11). There is a predilection for the BCCs to occur on the face, including the eyelids. Clinically and histopathologically the lesions seen with nevoid BCC syndrome are similar to standard BCCs.

Management of the BCCs associated with nevoid BBC syndrome is similar to that described for other BCCs. It is important to treat BCCs in this syndrome when they are small with surgical excision or other approaches mentioned. There is a report of very successful treatment of diffuse BCCs and basaloid follicular hamartomas in nevoid BCC syndrome by wide-area 5-aminolevulinic acid photodynamic therapy (34). Vismodegib is a specific oral medication for management of nevoid BCC syndrome, causing regression in tumors, but requiring chronic long-term use of a relatively expensive and challenging medication (20,21).

Selected References

Reviews

1. Shinder R, Ivan D, Seigler D, et al. Feasibility of using American Joint Committee on Cancer Classification criteria for staging eyelid carcinomas. *Orbit* 2011;30(5):202–207.
2. Ho SF, Brown L, Bamford M, et al. 5 years review of periocular basal cell carcinoma and proposed follow-up protocol. *Eye (Lond)* 2013;27(1):78–83.
3. Payne JW, Duke JR, Butner R, et al. Basal cell carcinoma of the eyelids: a long-term follow-up study. *Arch Ophthalmol* 1969;81:53–58.
4. Wojno TH. The association between cigarette smoking and basal cell carcinoma of the eyelids in women. *Ophthalmol Plast Reconstr Surg* 1999;15:390–392.
5. Erbagci Z, Erbagci I, Erkilic S. High incidence of demodicidosis in eyelid basal cell carcinomas. *Int J Dermatol* 2003;42:567–571.
6. Leibovitch I, McNab A, Sullivan T, et al. Orbital invasion by periocular basal cell carcinoma. *Ophthalmology* 2005;112:717–723.
7. Allali J, D'Hermies F, Renard G. Basal cell carcinomas of the eyelids. *Ophthalmologica* 2005;219:57–71.
8. Paavilainen V, Tuominen J, Pukkala E, et al. Basal cell carcinoma of the eyelid in Finland during 1953–1997. *Acta Ophthalmol Scand* 2005;83:215–220.
9. Nerad JA, Whitaker DC. Periocular basal cell carcinoma in adults 35 years of age and younger. *Am J Ophthalmol* 1988;106:723–729.

Nevoid Basal Cell Carcinoma Syndrome

10. Gorlin RJ, Goltz RW. Multiple nevoid basal cell epithelioma, jaw cysts and bifid rib. A syndrome. *N Engl J Med* 1960;262:908–912.
11. Honavar SG, Shields JA, Shields CL, et al. Basal cell carcinoma of the eyelids associated with Gorlin-Goltz syndrome. *Ophthalmology* 2001;108:1115–1123.
12. Boonen SE, Stahl D, Kreiborg S, et al. Delineation of an interstitial 9q22 deletion in basal cell nevus syndrome. *Am J Med Genet A* 2005;132:324–328.
13. Lo Muzio L, Nocini P, Bucci P, et al. Early diagnosis of nevoid basal cell carcinoma syndrome. *J Am Dent Assoc* 1999;130:669–674.

Pathology/Genetics

14. Milman T, McCormick SA. The molecular genetics of eyelid tumors: recent advances and future directions. *Graefes Arch Clin Exp Ophthalmol* 2013;251(2):419–433.

Diagnosis

15. Pelosini L, Smith HB, Schofield JB, et al. In vivo optical coherence tomography (OCT) in periocular basal cell carcinoma: correlations between in vivo OCT images and postoperative histology. *Br J Ophthalmol* 2013;97(7):890–894.

Therapy

16. Yin VT, Pfeiffer ML, Esmaeli B. Targeted therapy for orbital and periocular basal cell carcinoma and squamous cell carcinoma. *Ophthal Plast Reconstr Surg* 2013;29(2):87–92.
17. Levin F, Khalil M, McCormick SA, et al. Excision of periocular basal cell carcinoma with stereoscopic microdissection of surgical margins for frozen-section control: report of 200 cases. *Arch Ophthalmol* 2009;127(8):1011–1015.
18. Gayre GS, Hybarger CP, Mannor G, et al. Outcomes of excision of 1750 eyelid and periocular skin basal cell and squamous cell carcinomas by modified en face frozen section margin-controlled technique. *Int Ophthalmol Clin* 2009;49(4):97–110.

19. Bertelmann E, Rieck P. Relapses after surgical treatment of ocular adnexal basal cell carcinomas: 5-year follow-up at the same university centre. *Acta Ophthalmol* 2012;90(2):127–131.
20. Gill HS, Moscato EE, Chang AL, et al. Vismodegib for periocular and orbital basal cell carcinoma. *JAMA Ophthalmol* 2013;31(12):1591–1594.
21. Kahana A, Worden FP, Elner VM. Vismodegib as eye-sparing adjuvant treatment for orbital basal cell carcinoma. *JAMA Ophthalmol* 2013;131(10):1364–1366.
22. Sullivan TJ. Topical therapies for periorbital cutaneous malignancies: indications and treatment regimens. *Curr Opin Ophthalmol* 2012;23(5):439–442.
23. Blasi MA, Giammaria D, Balestrazzi E. Immunotherapy with imiquimod 5% cream for eyelid nodular basal cell carcinoma. *Am J Ophthalmol* 2005;140:1136–1138.
24. Oldfield V, Keating GM, Perry CM. Imiquimod: in superficial basal cell carcinoma. *Am J Clin Dermatol* 2005;6:195–200.
25. Schulze HJ, Cribier B, Requena L, et al. Imiquimod 5% cream for the treatment of superficial basal cell carcinoma: results from a randomized vehicle-controlled phase III study in Europe. *Br J Dermatol* 2005;152:939–947.
26. Peris K, Campione E, Micantonio T, et al. Imiquimod treatment of superficial and nodular basal cell carcinoma: 12-week open-label trial. *Dermatol Surg* 2005;31:318–323.
27. Carneiro RC, de Macedo EM, Matayoshi S. Imiquimod 5% cream for the treatment of periocular Basal cell carcinoma. *Ophthal Plast Reconstr Surg* 2010;26(2):100–102.
28. Ross AH, Kennedy CT, Collins C, et al. The use of imiquimod in the treatment of periocular tumours. *Orbit* 2010;29(2):83–87.
29. Gaitanis G, Kalogeropoulos C, Bassukas ID. Imiquimod can be combined with cryosurgery (immunocryosurgery) for locally advanced periocular basal cell carcinomas. *Br J Ophthalmol* 2011;95(6):890–892.
30. Garcia-Martin E, Gil-Arribas LM, Idoipe M, et al. Comparison of imiquimod 5% cream versus radiotherapy as treatment for eyelid basal cell carcinoma. *Br J Ophthalmol* 2011;95(10):1393–1396.
31. Pakdel F, Kashkouli MB. Re: "Imiquimod 5% cream for the treatment of periocular basal cell carcinoma". *Ophthal Plast Reconstr Surg* 2011;27(4):305; author reply 305–306.
32. Prokosch V, Thanos S, Spaniol K, et al. Long-term outcome after treatment with 5% topical imiquimod cream in patients with basal cell carcinoma of the eyelids. *Graefes Arch Clin Exp Ophthalmol* 2011;249(1):121–125.
33. Jebodhsingh KN, Calafati J, Farrokhyar F, et al. Recurrence rates of basal cell carcinoma of the periocular skin: what to do with patients who have positive margins after resection. *Can J Ophthalmol* 2012;47(2):181–184.
34. Cook BE, Bartley GB. Treatment options and future prospects for the management of eyelid malignancies: an evidence-based update. *Ophthalmology* 2001;108:2088–2098.
35. Doxanas MT, Green WR, Iliff CE. Factors in the successful surgical management of basal cell carcinoma of the eyelids. *Am J Ophthalmol* 1981;91:726–736.
36. Chalfin J, Putterman AM. Frozen section control in the surgery of basal cell carcinoma of the eyelid. *Am J Ophthalmol* 1979;87:802–809.
37. Fraunfelder FT, Zacarian SA, Wingfield DL, et al. Results of cryotherapy for eyelid malignancies. *Am J Ophthalmol* 1984;97:184–188.
38. Conway RM, Themel S, Holbach LM. Surgery for primary basal cell carcinoma including the eyelid margins with intraoperative frozen section control: comparative interventional study with a minimum clinical follow up of 5 years. *Br J Ophthalmol* 2004;88:236–238.
39. Shankar J, Nair RG, Sullivan SC. Management of peri-ocular skin tumours by laissez-faire technique: analysis of functional and cosmetic results. *Eye (Lond)* 2002;16:50–53.
40. Buschmann W. A reappraisal of cryosurgery for eyelid basal cell carcinomas. *Br J Ophthalmol* 2002;86:453–457.
41. Hamada S, Kersey T, Thaller VT. Eyelid basal cell carcinoma: non-Mohs excision, repair, and outcome. *Br J Ophthalmol* 2005;89:992–994.
42. Cuevas P, Arrazola JM. Topical treatment of basal cell carcinoma with neomycin. *Eur J Med Res* 2005;10:202–203.
43. Krema H, Herrmann E, Albert-Green A, et al. Orthovoltage radiotherapy in the management of medial canthal basal cell carcinoma. *Br J Ophthalmol* 2013;97(6):730–734.
44. Apalla Z, Karteridou A, Lallas A, et al. Letter: Immunocryotherapy for difficult-to-treat basal cell carcinoma of the eyelid. *Dermatol Surg* 2013;39(1 Pt 1):146–147.
45. Litwin AS, Rytina E, Ha T, et al. Management of periocular basal cell carcinoma by Mohs micrographic surgery. *J Dermatolog Treat* 2013;24(3):232–234.
46. Lewis CD, Perry JD. Transconjunctival lateral cantholysis for closure of full-thickness eyelid defects. *Ophthal Plast Reconstr Surg* 2009;25(6):469–471.
47. Stafanous S. Five-year cycle of basal cell carcinoma management re-audit. *Orbit* 2009;28(4):264–469.
48. Togsverd-Bo K, Haedersdal M, Wulf HC. Photodynamic therapy for tumors on the eyelid margins. *Arch Dermatol* 2009;145(8):944–947.
49. Shinder R. Risk factors for orbital exenteration in periocular basal cell carcinoma. *Am J Ophthalmol* 2012;154(1):212; author reply 212–213.

Prognosis

50. Von Domarus H, Stevens PJ. Metastatic basal cell carcinoma: report of five cases and review of 170 cases in the literature. *J Am Acad Dermatol* 1984;10:1043.
51. Iuliano A, Strianese D, Uccello G, et al. Risk factors for orbital exenteration in periocular basal cell carcinoma. *Am J Ophthalmol* 2012;153(2):238–241.

Case Reports

52. Gupta M, Puri P, Kamal A, et al. Complete spontaneous regression of a basal cell carcinoma. *Eye (Lond)* 2003;17:262–263.
53. Marty CL, Randle HW, Walsh JS. Eruptive epidermoid cysts resulting from treatment with imiquimod. *Dermatol Surg* 2005;31:780–782.
54. Litwin AS, Shah-Desai SD, Malhotra R. Two new cases of metastatic basal cell carcinoma from the eyelids. *Orbit* 2013;32(4):256–259.
55. Zeitouni NC, Raghu PR, Mansour TN. Orbital invasion by periocular infiltrating Basal cell carcinoma. *Dermatol Surg* 2012;38(12):2025–2027.
56. Kirzhner M, Jakobiec FA. Clinicopathologic and immunohistochemical features of pigmented basal cell carcinomas of the eyelids. *Am J Ophthalmol* 2012;153(2):242–252.
57. Belliveau MJ, Coupal DJ, Brownstein S, et al. Infundibulocystic basal cell carcinoma of the eyelid in basal cell nevus syndrome. *Ophthal Plast Reconstr Surg* 2010;26(3):147–152.

Chapter 2 Premalignant and Malignant Tumors of Eyelid Epidermis

EYELID BASAL CELL CARCINOMA: NODULAR AND NODULOULCERATIVE TYPE

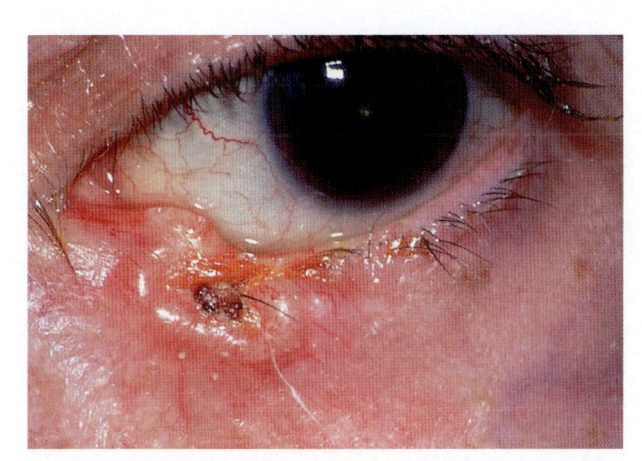

Figure 2.31. Noduloulcerative BCC in lower eyelid in a 71-year-old woman. The lower eyelid is the most common location for periocular BCC.

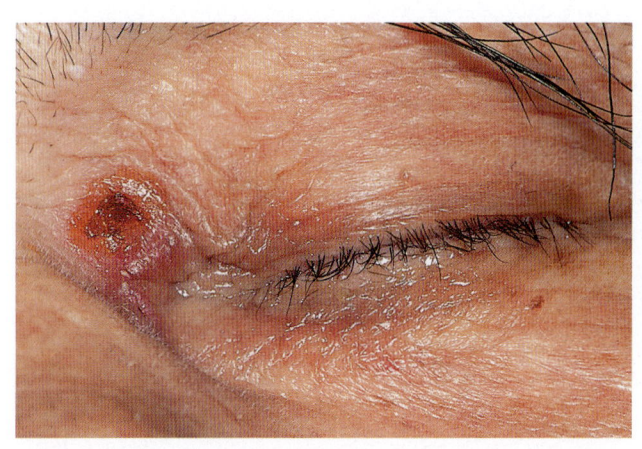

Figure 2.32. Noduloulcerative BCC in medial canthal region in an 85-year-old man. The medial canthal region is the second most common site for periocular BCC.

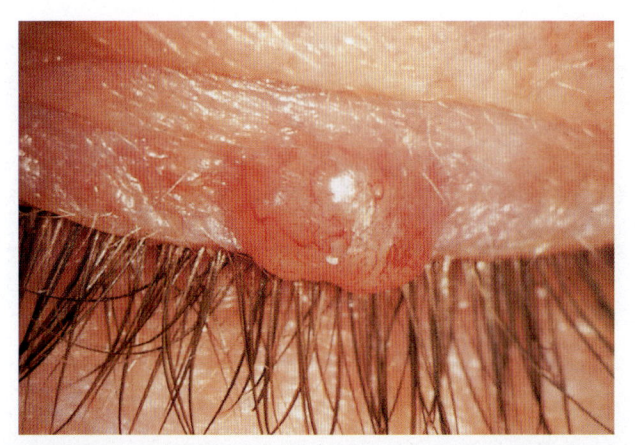

Figure 2.33. Nodular BCC in upper eyelid in a 61-year-old woman. BCC less commonly affects the upper eyelid.

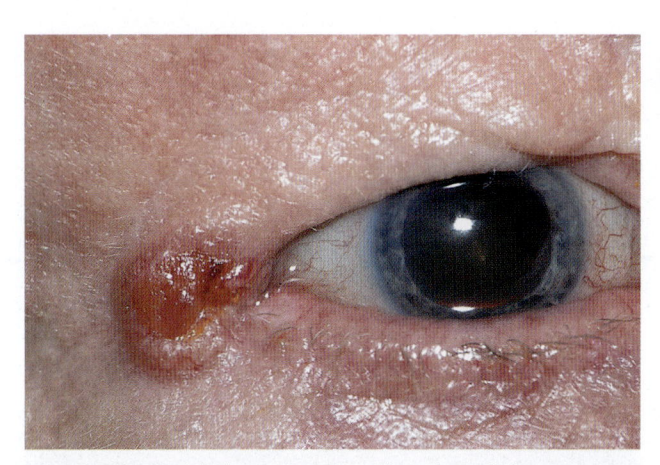

Figure 2.34. Noduloulcerative BCC in lateral canthal region in an 87-year-old man. The lateral canthus is the least common location for eyelid BCC.

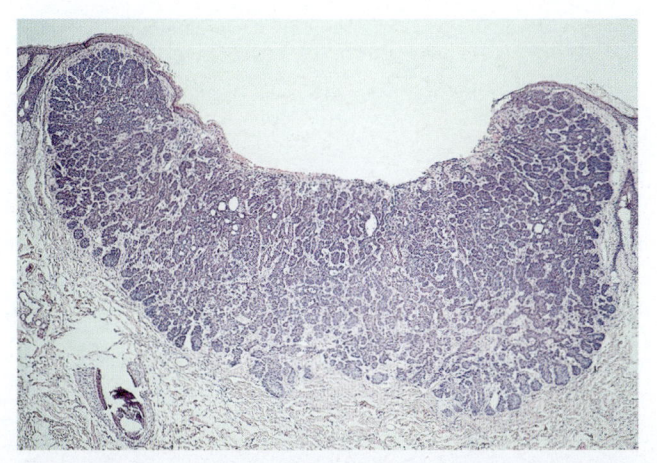

Figure 2.35. Histopathology of noduloulcerative BCC showing closely compact basophilic nuclei and central crater. (Hematoxylin–eosin ×10.)

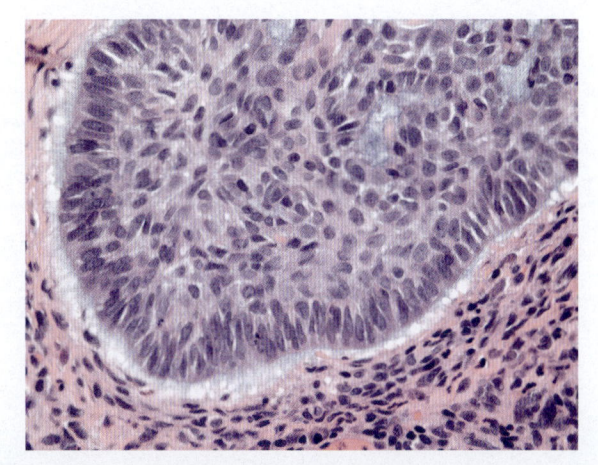

Figure 2.36. Histopathology of noduloulcerative BCC showing well-defined peripheral palisading. (Hematoxylin–eosin ×200.)

EYELID BASAL CELL CARCINOMA: MORPHEAFORM (SCLEROSING) TYPE

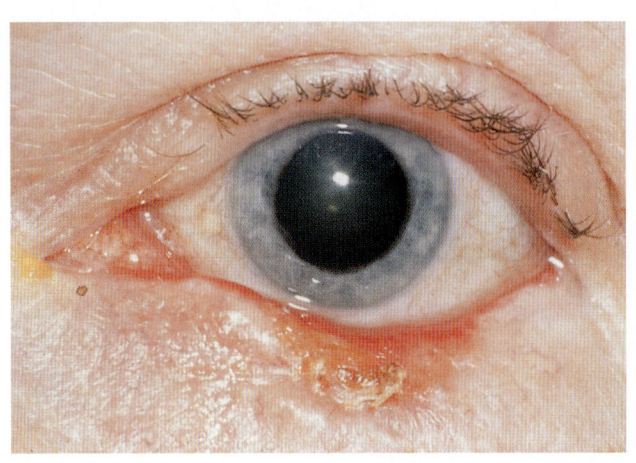

Figure 2.37. Morpheaform BCC involving lower eyelid in a 71-year-old woman. Note the loss of all cilia on lower eyelid and ill-defined margins of the tumor.

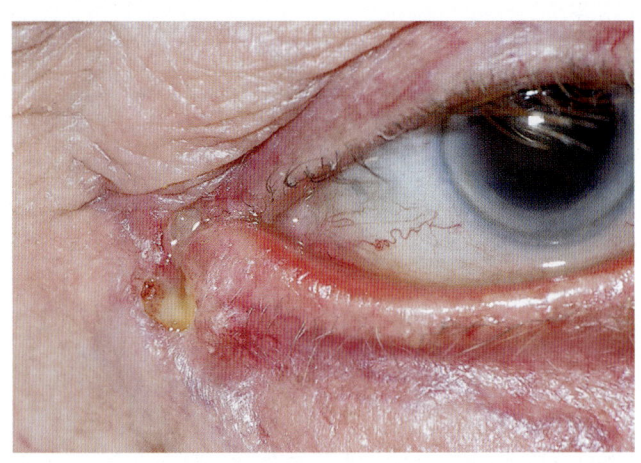

Figure 2.38. Morpheaform BCC in medial canthal region in an 88-year-old man.

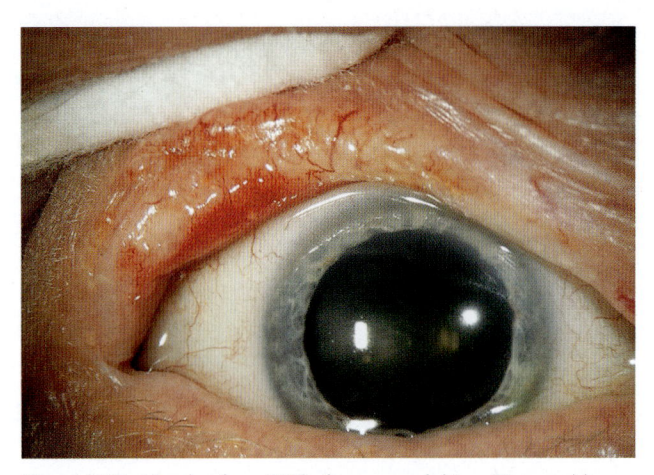

Figure 2.39. Morpheaform BCC of upper eyelid in a 78-year-old man. The diagnosis of sebaceous gland carcinoma was suspected clinically.

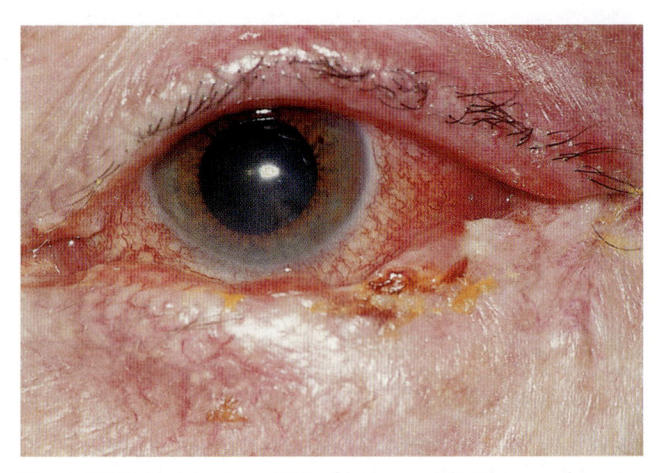

Figure 2.40. Morpheaform BCC of lower eyelid with secondary conjunctival inflammation in a 76-year-old man. Invasive sebaceous carcinoma can have a similar appearance.

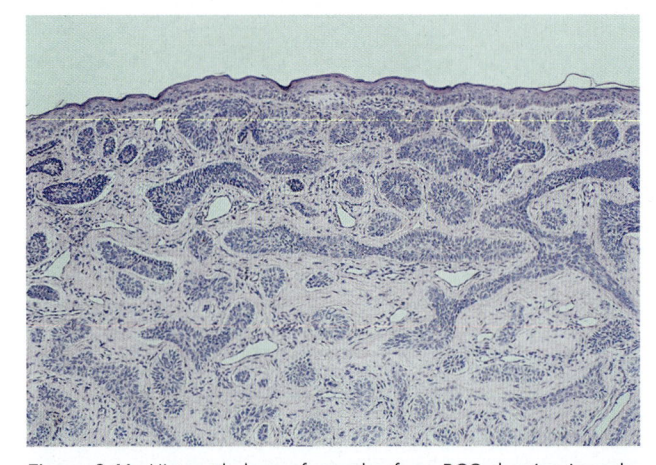

Figure 2.41. Histopathology of morpheaform BCC showing irregular cords of tumor cells interspersed throughout the dermis. The basophilia of the basal cell nuclei give the cellular areas a typical blue color on light microscopy. (Hematoxylin–eosin ×15.)

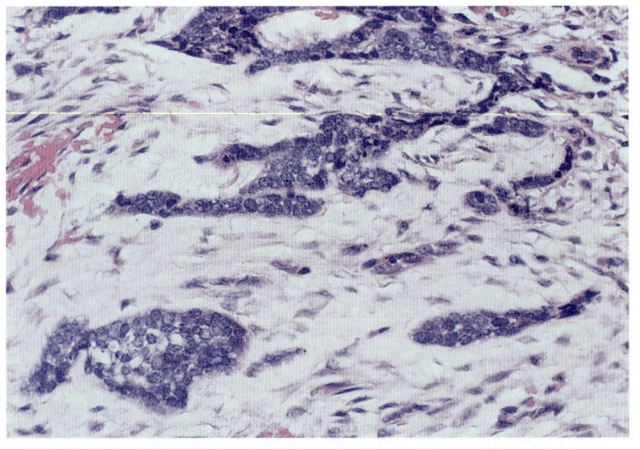

Figure 2.42. Histopathology of morpheaform BCC showing whorls of tumor cells in the dermis. (Hematoxylin–eosin ×100.)

EYELID BASAL CELL CARCINOMA: CLINICAL VARIATIONS

Although most eyelid BCCs have a characteristic nodular, noduloulcerative, or morpheaform growth pattern, the tumor can display many variations.

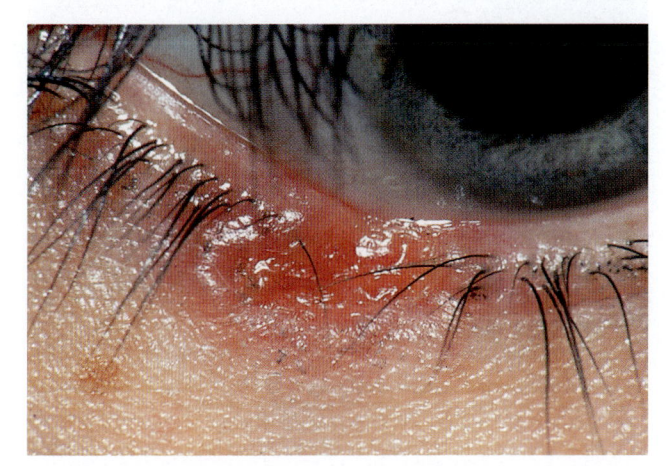

Figure 2.43. Noduloulcerative BCC of lower eyelid in an otherwise healthy 17-year-old girl. This tumor is rare in teenagers.

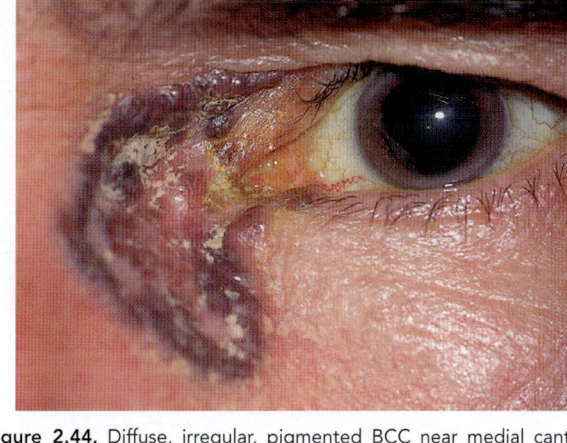

Figure 2.44. Diffuse, irregular, pigmented BCC near medial canthus in an otherwise healthy 52-year-old man. Curiously, the patient had a simultaneous conjunctival malignant melanoma on the opposite eye.

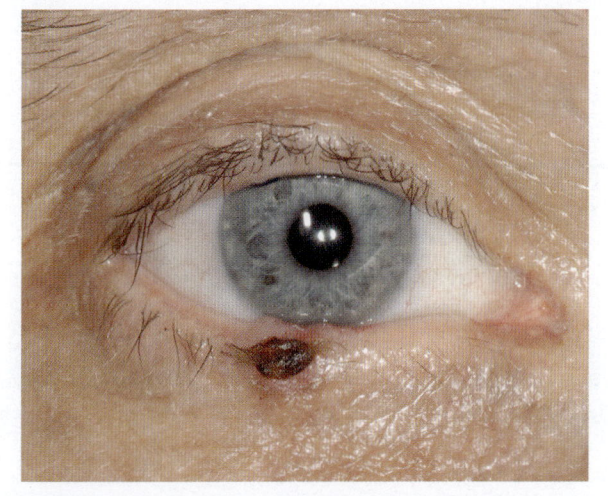

Figure 2.45. Hemorrhagic, ulcerated BCC of lower eyelid.

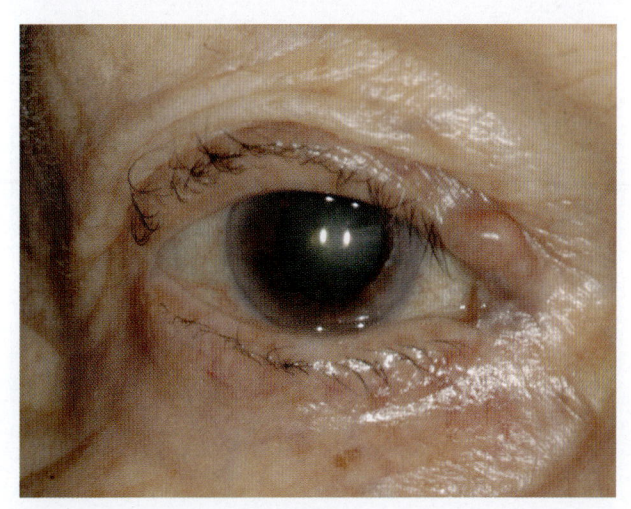

Figure 2.46. Nodular, nonulcerated BCC of upper medial eyelid with notable loss of eyelashes.

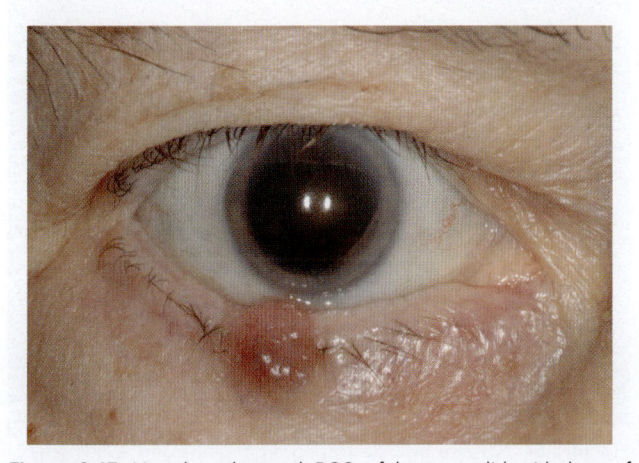

Figure 2.47. Vascular, ulcerated BCC of lower eyelid with loss of eyelashes.

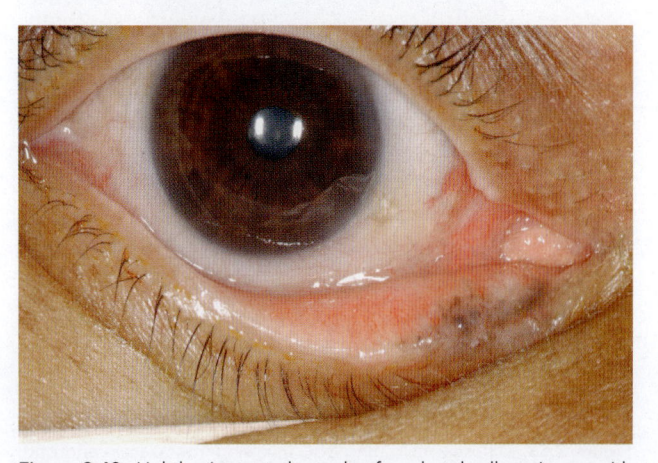

Figure 2.48. Lightly pigmented morpheaform basal cell carcinoma with eyelash loss and conjunctival involvement in an African-American woman.

EYELID BASAL CELL CARCINOMA: ADVANCED CASES

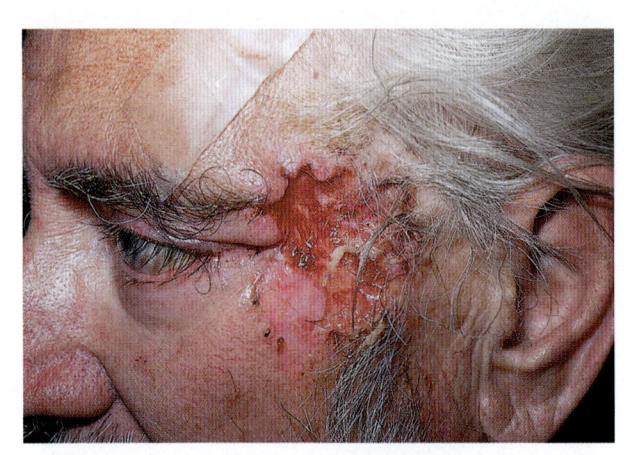

Figure 2.49. Large ulcerated BCC arising from the lateral canthal area and invading skin temporal region in an 80-year-old man.

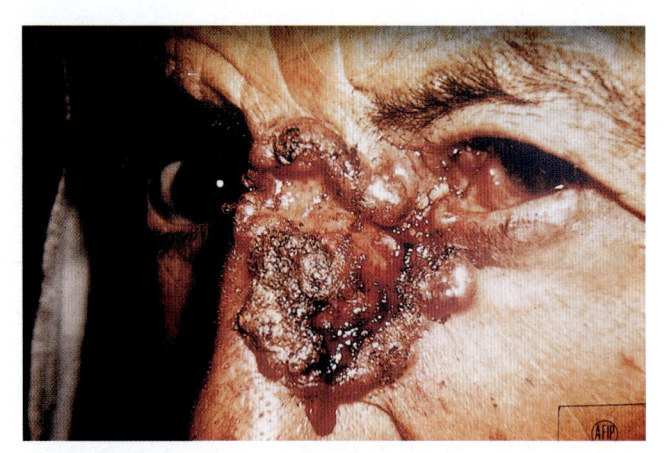

Figure 2.50. Large, ulcerated BCC arising from medial canthal and nasal area with orbital invasion in an 85-year-old man.

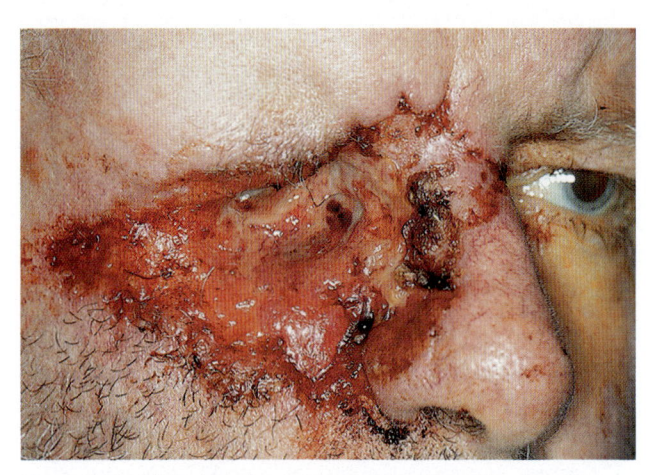

Figure 2.51. BCC arising from lower eyelid and invading the orbit in an elderly man. (Courtesy of Massachusetts Eye and Ear Infirmary.)

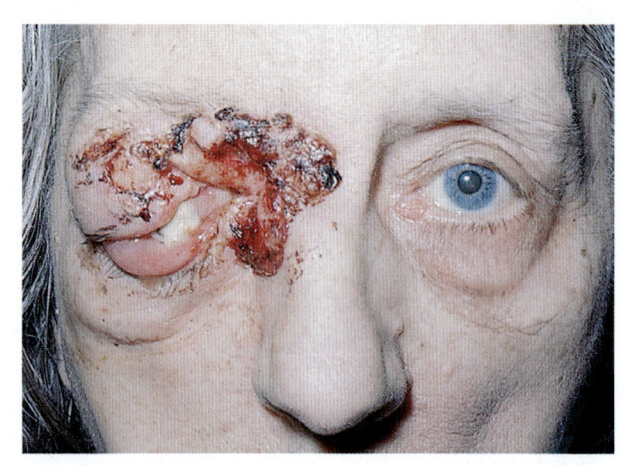

Figure 2.52. BCC with massive diffuse involvement of eyelid and orbit.

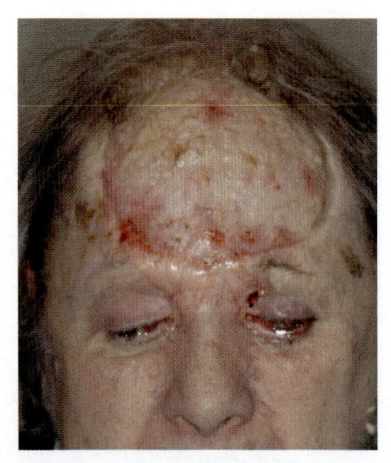

Figure 2.53. Diffusely infiltrating BCC involving frontal scalp and both the left and right orbit.

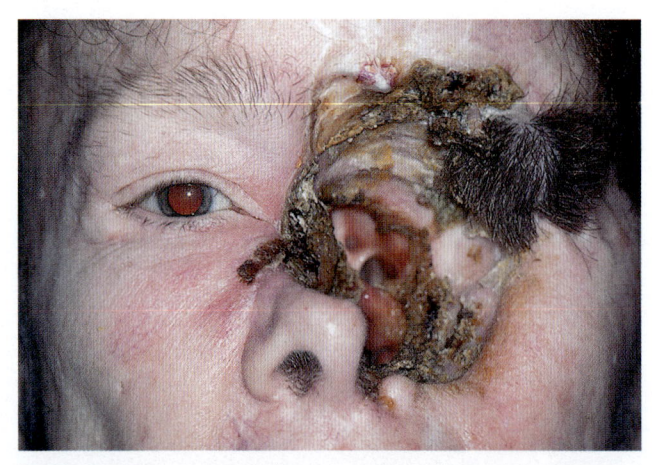

Figure 2.54. Massive BCC destroying orbit, globe and invading nasal tissues in a 67-year-old woman.

Chapter 2 Premalignant and Malignant Tumors of Eyelid Epidermis

EYELID BASAL CELL CARCINOMA: NEVOID BASAL CELL CARCINOMA SYNDROME (GORLIN–GOLTZ SYNDROME)

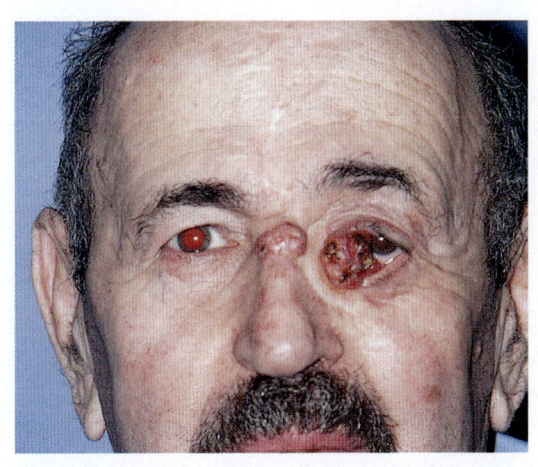

Figure 2.55. Nevoid BCC syndrome with orbital extension of eyelid BCC in a 70-year-old man. His daughter had multiple BCCs.

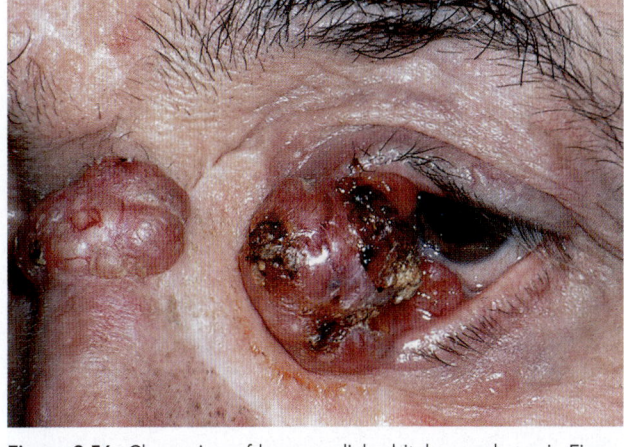

Figure 2.56. Closer view of large medial orbital mass shown in Figure 2.55. Orbital exenteration was performed.

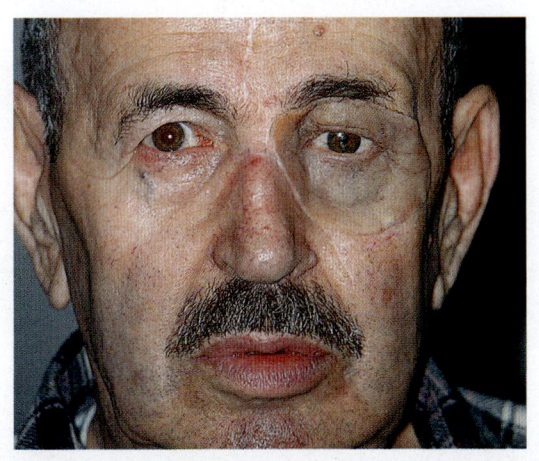

Figure 2.57. Facial appearance of patient shown in Figure 2.55 after orbital exenteration and fitting of a prosthesis.

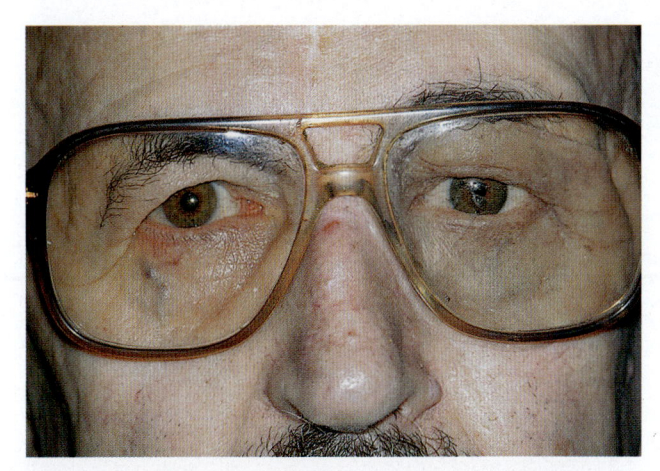

Figure 2.58. Facial appearance of same patient wearing glasses after exenteration and fitting of the prosthesis.

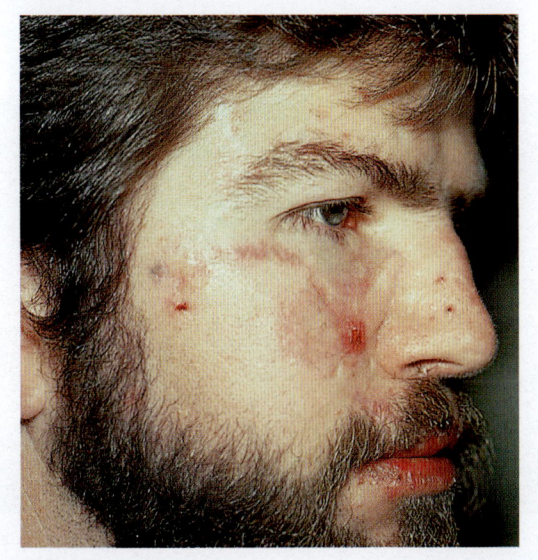

Figure 2.59. Facial lesions in young adult with nevoid BCC syndrome. (Courtesy of Richard Lewis, MD.)

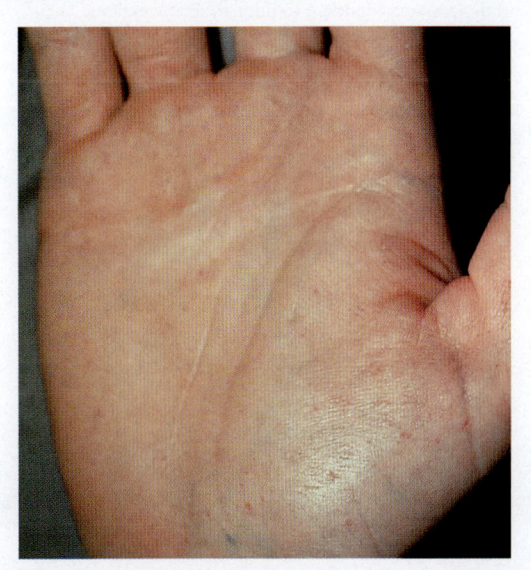

Figure 2.60. Appearance of the palm of the hand in patient shown in Figure 2.59, showing the palmar pits that characterize the nevoid BCC syndrome. (Courtesy of Richard Lewis, MD.)

EYELID BASAL CELL CARCINOMA: NEVOID BASAL CELL CARCINOMA SYNDROME (GORLIN–GOLTZ SYNDROME) WITH MULTIPLE CUTANEOUS MALIGNANCIES

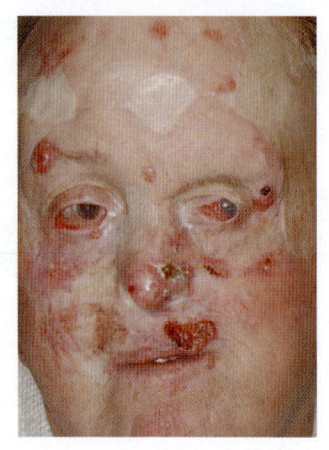

Figure 2.61. Face view of middle-aged man. Note numerous basal cell carcinomas and evidence of several prior skin grafts.

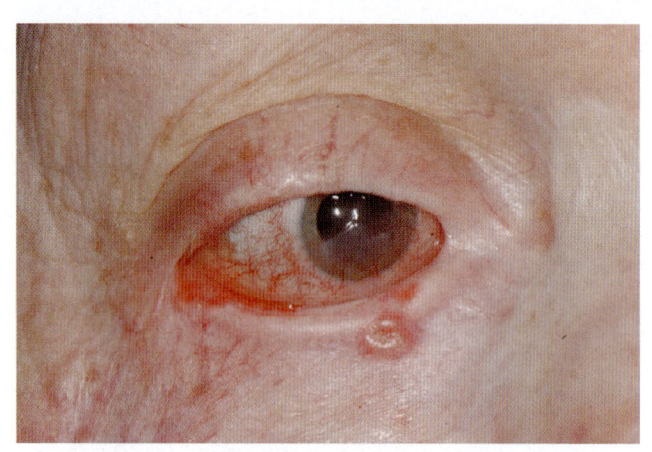

Figure 2.62. Close-up of right lower eyelid, showing noduloulcerative BCC of eyelid and diffuse morpheaform tumor on medial aspect of lower eyelid.

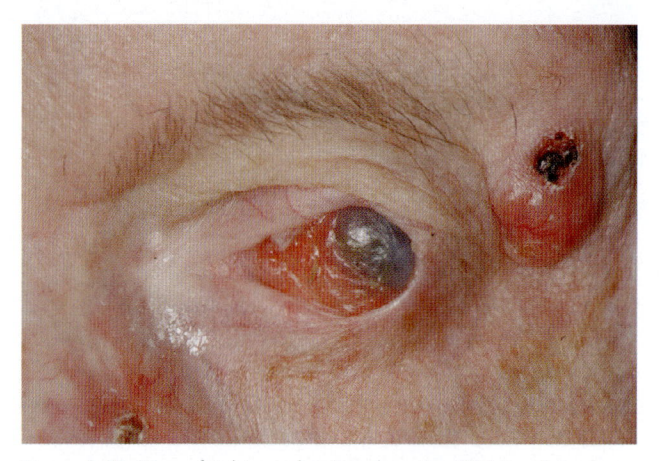

Figure 2.63. View of right eye showing ulcerative BCC near lateral canthus and dry cornea secondary to prior eyelid resections.

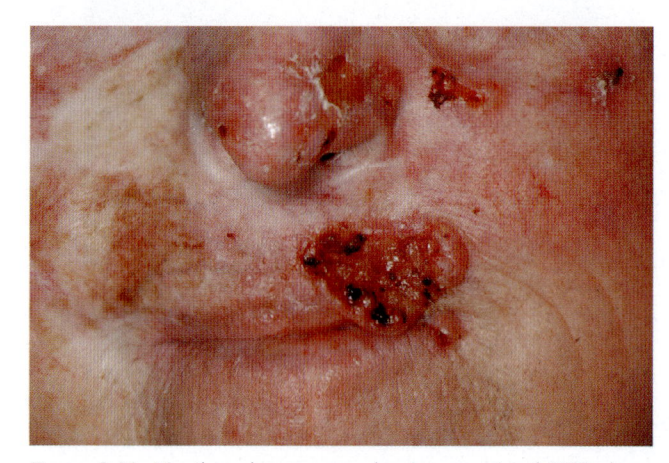

Figure 2.64. Mouth and nose area, showing excoriated BCC above upper lip.

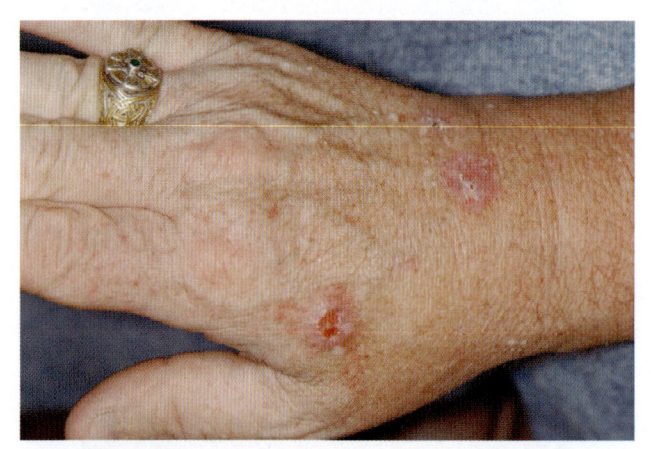

Figure 2.65. Dorsum of hand showing BCC.

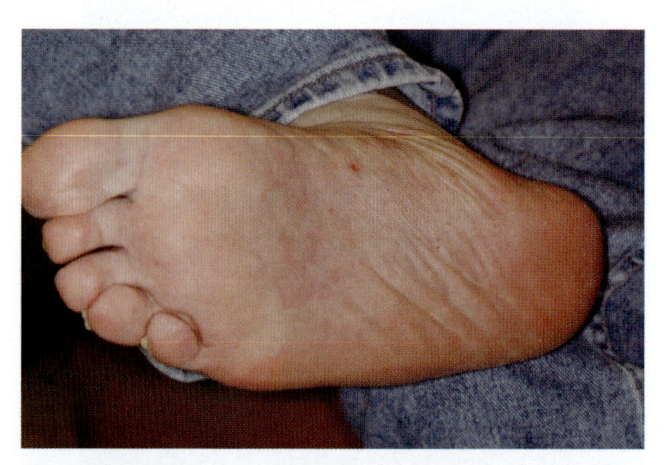

Figure 2.66. Same patient with subtle, plantar pits in arch of the foot.

Chapter 2 Premalignant and Malignant Tumors of Eyelid Epidermis

EYELID BASAL CELL CARCINOMA: NEVOID BASAL CELL CARCINOMA SYNDROME (GORLIN–GOLTZ SYNDROME) WITH ODONTOGENIC KERATOCYST

Nevoid BCC syndrome can be a chronic debilitating condition. Depicted is a patient who has >40-year photographic follow-up.

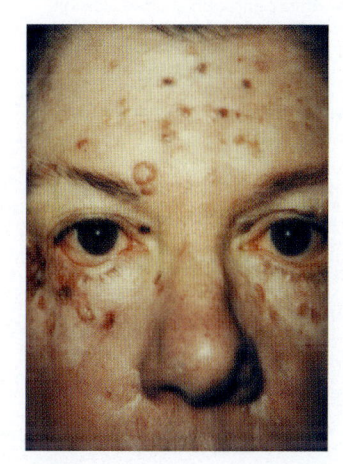

Figure 2.67. Facial appearance of woman at about age 40 years, showing multiple facial basal cell neoplasms.

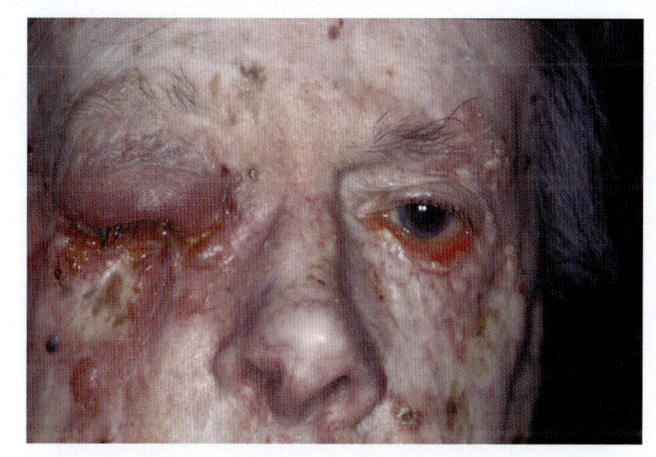

Figure 2.68. Facial appearance of same woman at age 86 years, showing extensive involvement and blepharoptosis. The right globe was immobile secondary to orbital extension of eyelid BCC.

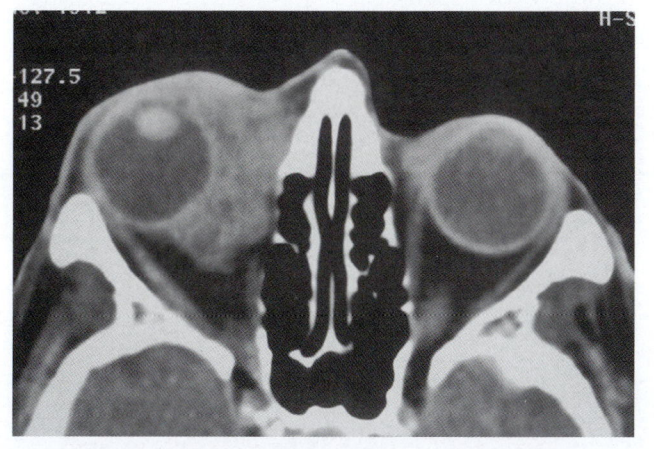

Figure 2.69. Axial CT showing orbital extension of eyelid BCC.

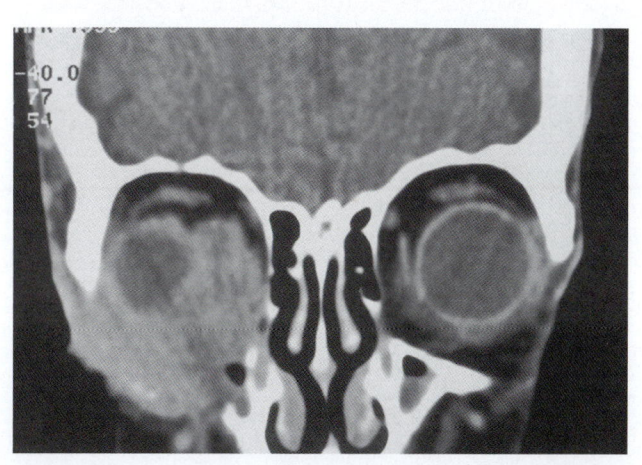

Figure 2.70. Coronal CT showing orbital extension of eyelid BCC.

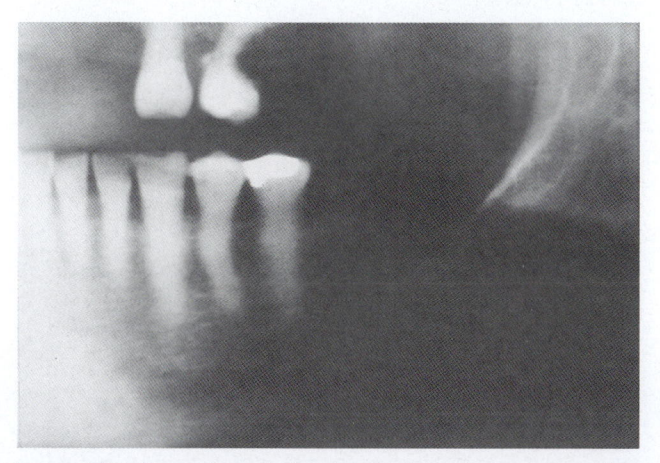

Figure 2.71. X-ray of teeth showing odontogenic keratocyst (clear black area above in area of absence of teeth).

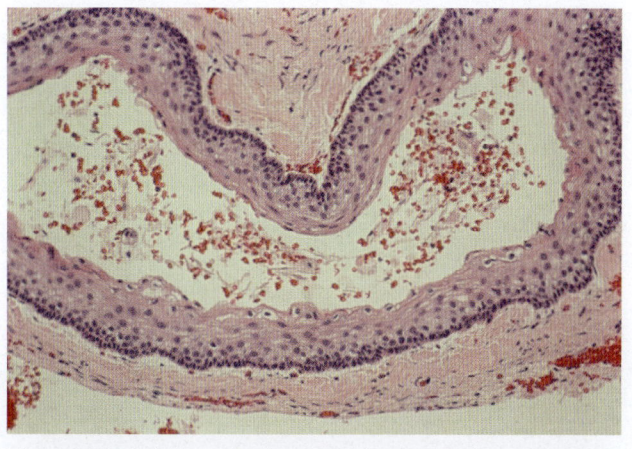

Figure 2.72. Pathology of odontogenic keratocyst, showing keratinizing epithelium and keratin debris in the lumen. (Hematoxylin–eosin ×50.)

EYELID BASAL CELL CARCINOMA: MANAGEMENT WITH PENTAGONAL FULL-THICKNESS EYELID RESECTION AND TOPICAL IMIQUIMOD

Management options for eyelid BCC are discussed in the text. Examples of full-thickness eyelid resection and topical imiquimod are illustrated here. Localized BCC of the eyelid can be removed by full-thickness eyelid resection with a pentagon-shaped incision and frozen section control of the margins. The surgical method is shown briefly below and is illustrated in more detail in Chapter 15. Patients who are very old and poor surgical candidates are treated today with topical imiquimod, an agent that boosts the immune system.

Blasi MA, Giammaria D, Balestrazzi E. Immunotherapy with imiquimod 5% cream for eyelid nodular basal cell carcinoma. *Am J Ophthalmol* 2005;140:1136–1139.

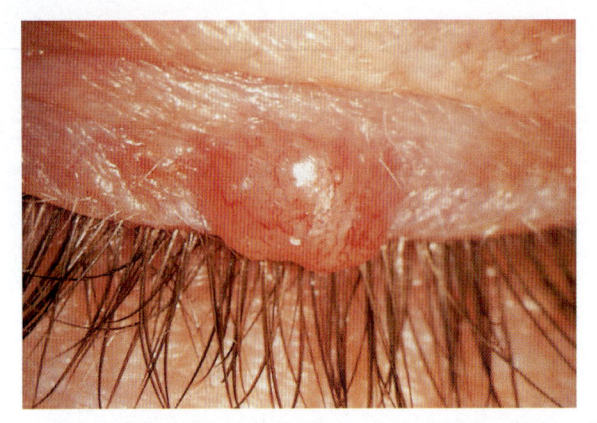

Figure 2.73. Circumscribed BCC of upper eyelid in a 61-year-old woman.

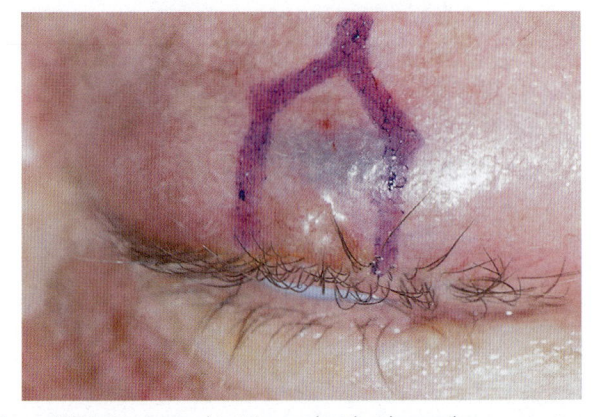

Figure 2.74. Pentagonal incision outlined with pencil.

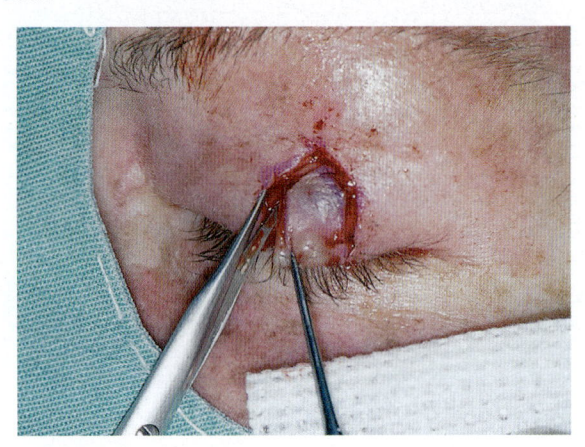

Figure 2.75. Pentagon containing tumor being removed with scalpel and scissors.

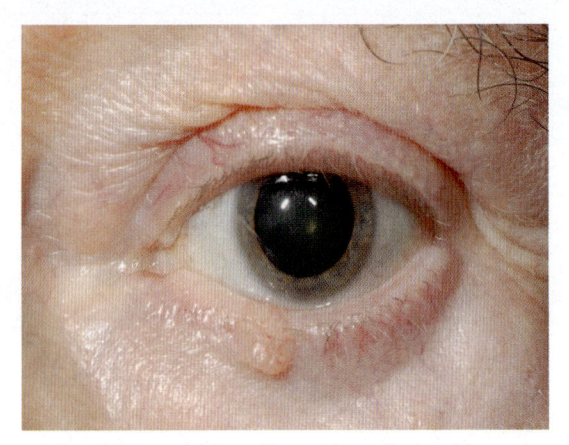

Figure 2.76. BCC in an older patient with medical problems so topical imiquimod was applied.

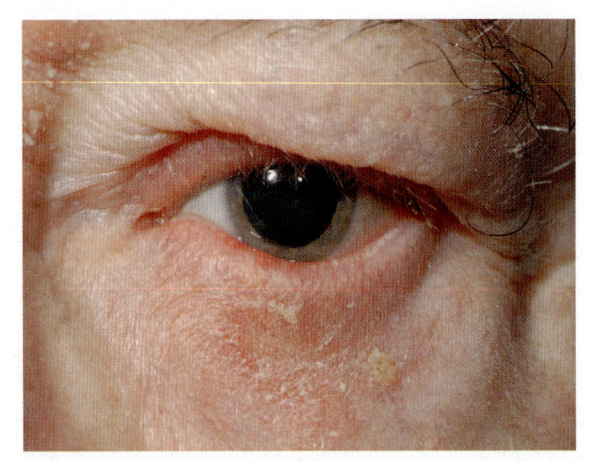

Figure 2.77. Patient in Figure 2.76 following 6 weeks of topical imiquimod, showing cutaneous erythema and scaling and tumor resolution.

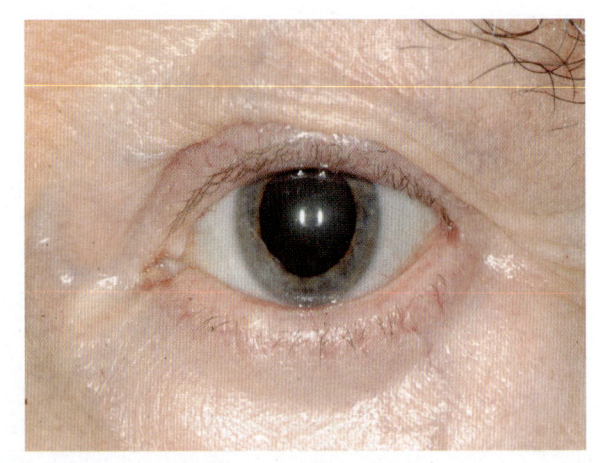

Figure 2.78. Patient in Figure 2.76 at 6 months following topical imiquimod, showing complete tumor regression.

Chapter 2 Premalignant and Malignant Tumors of Eyelid Epidermis

EYELID BASAL CELL CARCINOMA: RESULTS OF SURGICAL MANAGEMENT

The preoperative and postoperative appearance of patients using full-thickness eyelid resection, healing by primary intention, and skin grafting are shown. Drawings depicting these surgical techniques are illustrated in Chapter 15.

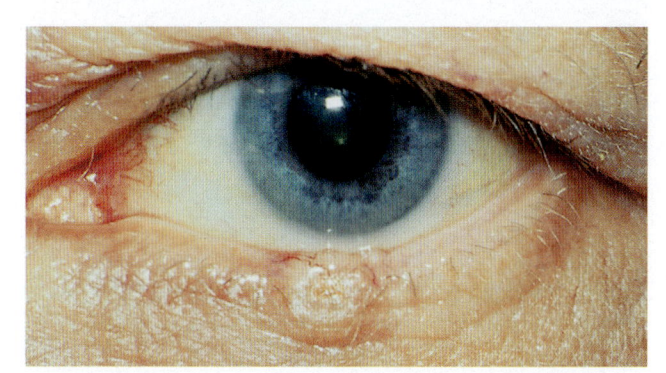

Figure 2.79. Excision of a typical BCC of the lower eyelid of a 60-year-old man by standard pentagonal eyelid incision and primary closure. It was excised with frozen section control and closed by primary closure assisted by a temporal semicircular (Tenzel) flap.

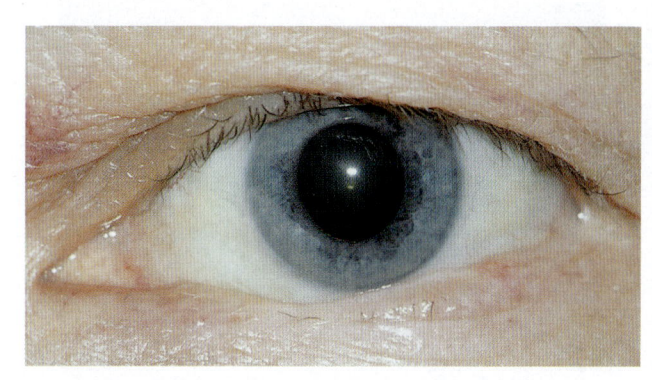

Figure 2.80. Appearance of patient shown in Figure 2.79 several weeks later showing satisfactory result.

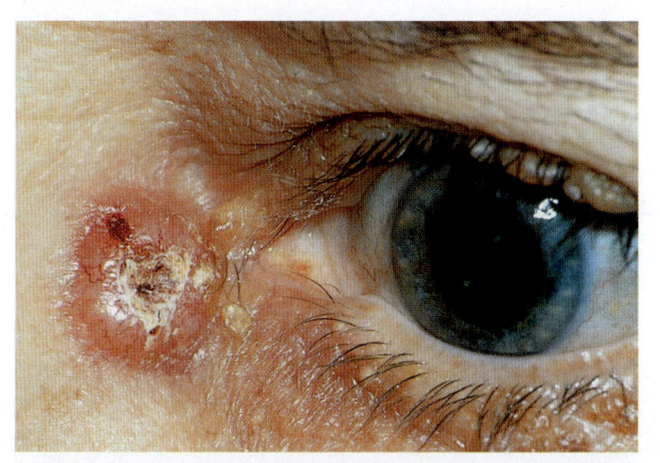

Figure 2.81. Excision with healing by primary intention. Typical BCC near medial canthus in a 70-year-old woman. After circular excision with frozen section control, the large defect and the tight skin made primary closure difficult, so the lesion was allowed to heal by granulation without sutures.

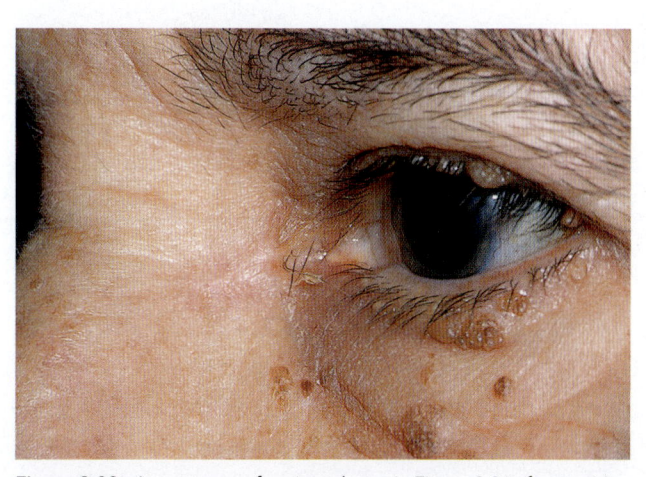

Figure 2.82. Appearance of patient shown in Figure 2.81 after excision and healing by granulation tissue only.

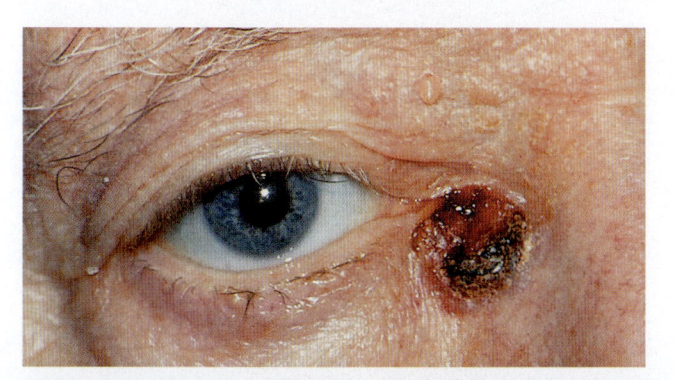

Figure 2.83. Excision and placement of skin graft. Typical BCC near medial canthus. The lesion was removed with frozen section control and a free skin graft from upper eyelid of opposite eye was used to close the defect. Donor skin can also be harvested from the retroauricular area and other sites.

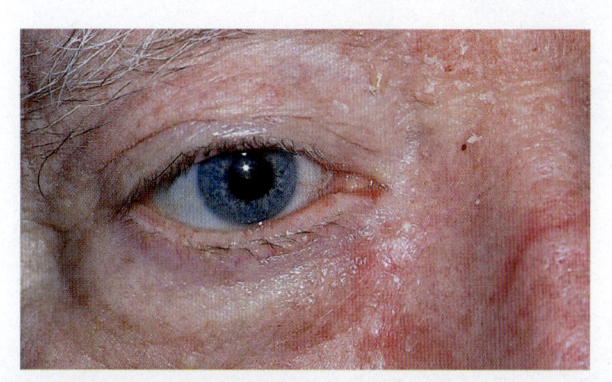

Figure 2.84. Appearance of patient shown in Figure 2.83 after 4 months, showing excellent result.

EYELID BASAL CELL CARCINOMA: ADVANCED, NEGLECTED CASES MANAGED BY ORBITAL EXENTERATION

In advanced cases that have invaded the orbit, orbital exenteration is the preferred treatment.

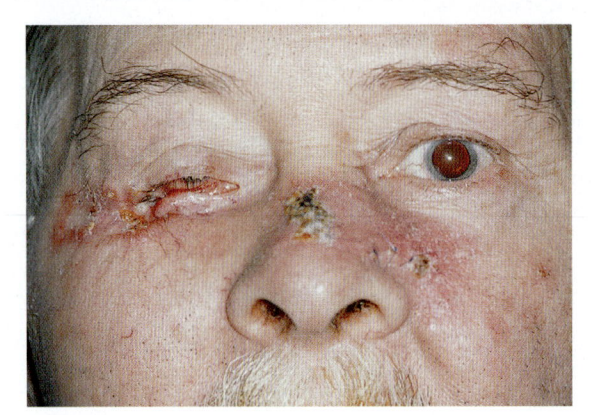

Figure 2.85. Aggressive BCC near lateral canthus that had deeply invaded the orbit in a 63-year-old man.

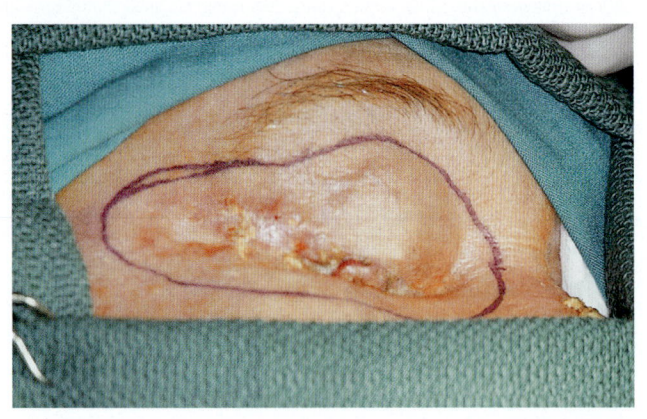

Figure 2.86. Planned incision marked around the tumor shown in Figure 2.85. The eyelids were purposely removed during the surgical procedure.

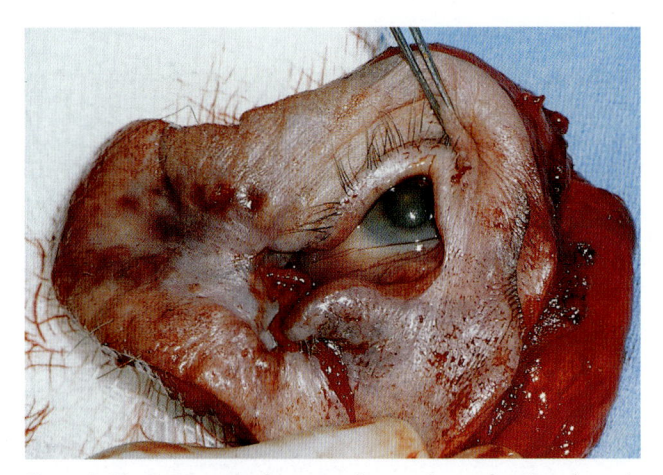

Figure 2.87. Photograph of exenteration specimen of patient shown in Figure 2.85 immediately after surgery.

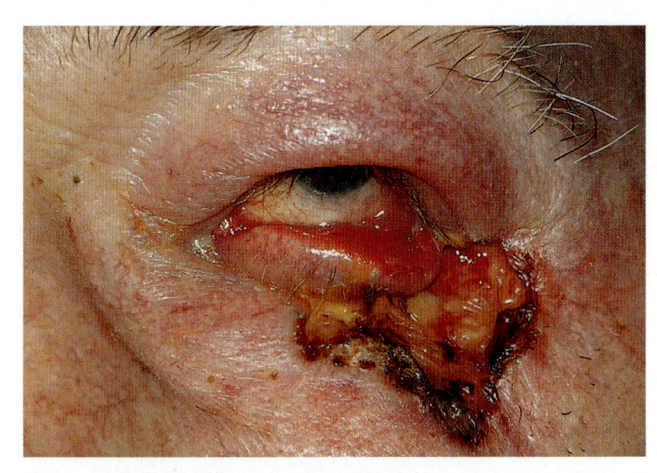

Figure 2.88. BCC of lower eyelid and lateral canthal region that had diffusely invaded the anterior portion of the orbit, causing retraction and superior displacement of the globe in a 69-year-old man.

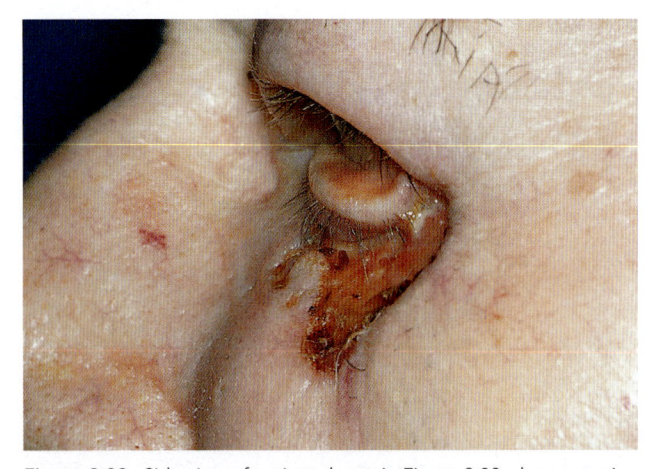

Figure 2.89. Side view of patient shown in Figure 2.88, demonstrating posterior retraction of the inferior eyelid tissues owing to sclerosis and fibrosis of the orbital portion of the tumor. The lesion was a morpheaform (sclerosing) variant of BCC.

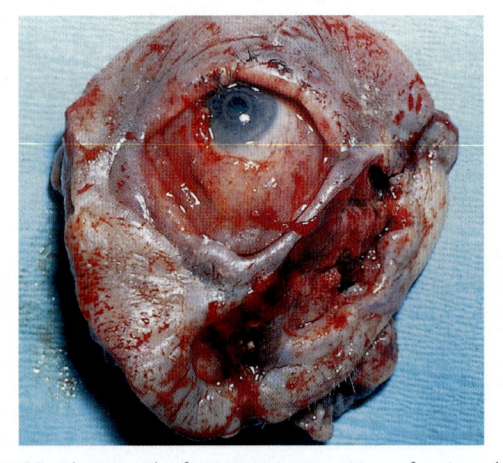

Figure 2.90. Photograph of exenteration specimen of patient shown in Figure 2.88 immediately after surgery.

EYELID SQUAMOUS CELL CARCINOMA

General Considerations

The etiologic factors, clinical features, differential diagnosis, and management of eyelid SCC are fairly similar to those of BCC discussed in the previous section and in other textbooks and articles (1–30). Although opinions vary, it seems preferable to divide eyelid SCC into carcinoma in situ (Bowen's disease) and invasive SCC.

Like BCC, SCC has a marked predilection to occur in fair-skinned individuals who have had extensive exposure to sunlight and other pathogenetic factors mentioned previously. It is also more common in males. It was previously believed that Bowen's disease had a high association with a variety of systemic cancers, including gastrointestinal cancer, but this has become controversial.

Invasive SCC also affects primarily elderly, fair-skinned individuals who have a history of chronic exposure to occupational or recreational sunlight. It can occur at a younger age in patients who are immunosuppressed or who have excess sensitivity to sunlight, particularly albinos. It accounts for about 2% to 10% of eyelid malignancies (1–8). It may arise de novo or from one of the previously mentioned premalignant conditions such as Bowen's disease, actinic keratosis, radiation blepharopathy, or XP, where it may occur at a much younger age.

Clinical Features

Bowen's disease is characterized clinically by an erythematous, crusted, keratotic lesion that occurs on sun-exposed areas in adults. It may be very similar clinically to actinic keratosis (1–8). The average diameter of the lesion is 1.3 cm, which is much larger than typical actinic keratosis.

SCC can have diverse clinical manifestations. In contrast to BCC, it occurs more often on the upper eyelid. It begins as a sessile or papular lesion that is similar to early BCC. It frequently ulcerates centrally, producing the rodent ulcer appearance; it can be irritating and bleed. Occasionally, SCC can assume a papillomatous, cystic, or cutaneous horn configuration. The finding of nearby actinic keratosis may provide a clue to the diagnosis. More advanced eyelid SCC can be highly aggressive and invade the orbit either by soft tissue extension or neural invasion (1). This can lead to numbness, pain, blepharoptosis, diplopia, and displacement of the globe.

Differential Diagnosis

Clinically, SCC of the eyelid area has no pathognomonic features that can differentiate it from the other epidermal lesions described in this section. It can resemble BCC, sebaceous carcinoma, Merkel cell carcinoma, and benign lesions like actinic keratosis, seborrheic keratosis, inverted follicular keratosis, pseudoepitheliomatous hyperplasia, and keratoacanthoma. As mentioned, there is increasing belief that keratoacanthoma is a variant of SCC.

Pathology

Microscopically, Bowen's disease is characterized by plaquelike acanthosis composed of abnormal but well-differentiated epidermal cells that replace the full thickness of the epidermis, but with an intact basement membrane. The squamous cells have eosinophilic cytoplasm, intercellular bridges, and can have keratin pearls. There is cellular atypia and complete loss of maturation of the epithelial cells.

Invasive SCC shows similar features, but is usually more anaplastic and more invasive, with tumor extension beyond the basement membrane into the dermis. Although the tumor foci appear to be discrete microscopically, they actually represent fingerlike extensions passing down from the epidermis. The histopathologic appearance of SCC varies greatly, from well-differentiated cells with obvious keratinization to poorly differentiated anaplastic squamous cells with a sarcomatous appearance. A more poorly differentiated tumor may require immunohistochemistry or electron microscopy to identify the squamous cell origin of the lesion and to rule out other malignant neoplasms.

Pathogenesis

Although some eyelid SCCs can develop de novo, the majority arise from preexisting lesions such as actinic keratosis, Bowen's disease, radiation dermatoses, burn scars, and chronic inflammatory lesions. SCC arises from the prickle-squamous cell layer of the epidermis. Other predisposing factors have been mentioned previously.

Management

The management of SCC of the eyelid is similar to that of BCC and other malignant eyelid tumors (9–17). Most authorities agree that small lesions suspected to be SCC can be managed by primary excisional biopsy. More sizable lesions in which extensive eyelid reconstruction is anticipated should be diagnosed by a shaving or punch biopsy to establish the diagnosis before embarking on definitive surgical management. The lesion should then be surgically excised using Mohs microsurgery or frozen section control. Eyelid reconstruction should be undertaken when the margins are confirmed to be negative for tumor.

As discussed under the subject of BCC, there is a role for radiotherapy, cryotherapy, intralesional chemotherapy, intralesional interferon, and photodynamic therapy in selected cases. Topical imiquimod has been reported to be successful in Bowen's disease of the eyelid (16,17). The indications and techniques of these methods are discussed in more detail elsewhere.

Sentinel lymph node biopsy has been popularized in the overall management of periocular SCC (14,15). Although controversial, it can be helpful in some cases in detecting regional metastasis and in directing further treatment.

Prognosis

The prognosis for eyelid SCC varies with the degree of differentiation, the etiology, tumor size, and tumor depth. Unlike BCC, SCC has a slightly greater tendency to exhibit aggressive local invasion and even metastasis to regional lymph nodes. Reports of regional lymph node metastasis of eyelid SCC have ranged from 2% to 24% (18). It also has a greater tendency toward neurotropism and can extend to the orbit and brain along nerves. Hence, patients with more advanced or recurrent lesions should have imaging studies, preferably orbital MRI and CT, to detect orbital soft tissue and bone invasion. SCC that arises from actinic keratosis appears to have a more favorable prognosis, with a metastatic rate of <2% (4).

Selected References

Reviews

1. Soparkar CN, Patrinely JR. Eyelid cancers. *Curr Opin Ophthalmol* 1998;9:49–53.
2. Doxanas MT, Iliff WJ, Iliff NT, et al. Squamous cell carcinoma of the eyelids. *Ophthalmology* 1987;94:538–541.
3. Kwitko MI, Boniuk M, Zimmerman LE. Eyelid tumors with reference to lesions confused with squamous cell carcinoma. I. Incidence and errors in diagnosis. *Arch Ophthalmol* 1963;69:693–697.
4. Reifler DM, Hornblass A. Squamous cell carcinoma of the eyelid. *Surv Ophthalmol* 1986;30:349–365.
5. Sullivan TJ, Boulton JE, Whitehead KJ. Intraepidermal carcinoma of the eyelid. *Clin Experiment Ophthalmol* 2002;30:23–27.
6. Crawford C, Fernelius C, Young P, et al. Application of the AJCC 7th edition carcinoma of the eyelid staging system: a medical center pathology based, 15-year review. *Clin Ophthalmol* 2011;5:1645–1648.
7. Verma V, Shen D, Sieving PC, et al. The role of infectious agents in the etiology of ocular adnexal neoplasia. *Surv Ophthalmol* 2008;53(4):312–331.
8. Shinder R, Ivan D, Seigler D, et al. Feasibility of using American Joint Committee on Cancer Classification criteria for staging eyelid carcinomas. *Orbit* 2011;30(5):202–207.

Therapy

9. Bowyer JD, Sullivan TJ, Whitehead KJ, et al. The management of perineural spread of squamous cell carcinoma to the ocular adnexae. *Ophthal Plast Reconstr Surg* 2003;19:275–281.
10. Cook BE Jr, Bartley GB. Treatment options and future prospects for the management of eyelid malignancies: an evidence-based update. *Ophthalmology* 2001;108:2088–2098.
11. Rice JC, Zaragoza P, Waheed K, et al. Efficacy of incisional vs punch biopsy in the histological diagnosis of periocular skin tumours. *Eye* 2003;17:478–481.
12. Malhotra R, James CL, Selva D, et al. The Australian Mohs database: periocular squamous intraepidermal carcinoma. *Ophthalmology* 2004;111:1925–1929.
13. Yin VT, Pfeiffer ML, Esmaeli B. Targeted therapy for orbital and periocular basal cell carcinoma and squamous cell carcinoma. *Ophthal Plast Reconstr Surg* 2013;29(2):87–92.
14. Pfeiffer ML, Savar A, Esmaeli B. Sentinel lymph node biopsy for eyelid and conjunctival tumors: what have we learned in the past decade? *Ophthal Plast Reconstr Surg* 2013;29(1):57–62.
15. Vuthaluru S, Pushker N, Lokdarshi G, et al. Sentinel lymph node biopsy in malignant eyelid tumor: hybrid single photon emission computed tomography/computed tomography and dual dye technique. *Am J Ophthalmol* 2013;156(1):43–49.
16. Sullivan TJ. Topical therapies for periorbital cutaneous malignancies: indications and treatment regimens. *Curr Opin Ophthalmol* 2012;23(5):439–442.
17. Couch SM, Custer PL. Topical 5-fluorouracil for the treatment of periocular actinic keratosis and low-grade squamous malignancy. *Ophthal Plast Reconstr Surg* 2012;28(3):181–183.

Prognosis

18. Faustina M, Diba R, Ahmadi MA, et al. Patterns of regional and distant metastasis in patients with eyelid and periocular squamous cell carcinoma. *Ophthalmology* 2004;111:1930–1932.

Case Reports

19. Chak G, Morgan PV, Joseph JM, et al. A positive sentinel lymph node in periocular invasive squamous cell carcinoma: a case series. *Ophthal Plast Reconstr Surg* 2013;29(1):6–10.
20. Trobe JD, Hood I, Parsons JT, et al. Intracranial spread of squamous carcinoma along the trigeminal nerve. *Arch Ophthalmol* 1982;100:608–611.
21. Rossi R, Puccioni M, Mavilia L, et al. Squamous cell carcinoma of the eyelid treated with photodynamic therapy. *J Chemother* 2004;16:306–309.
22. Conill C, Sanchez-Reyes A, Molla M, et al. Brachytherapy with 192Ir as treatment of carcinoma of the tarsal structure of the eyelid. *Int J Radiat Oncol Biol Phys* 2004;59:1326–1329.
23. Brannan PA, Anderson HK, Kersten RC, et al. Bowen disease of the eyelid successfully treated with imiquimod. *Ophthalmol Plast Reconstr Surg* 2005;21:321–322.
24. Martin-Garcia RF. Imiquimod: an effective alternative for the treatment of invasive cutaneous squamous cell carcinoma. *Dermatol Surg* 2005;31:371–374.
25. El-Sawy T, Frank SJ, Hanna E, et al. Multidisciplinary management of lacrimal sac/nasolacrimal duct carcinomas. *Ophthal Plast Reconstr Surg* 2013;29(6):454–457.
26. Inaba K, Ito Y, Suzuki S, et al. Results of radical radiotherapy for squamous cell carcinoma of the eyelid. *J Radiat Res* 2013;54(6):1131–1137.
27. Gill HS, Moscato EE, Chang AL, et al. Vismodegib for periocular and orbital basal cell carcinoma. *JAMA Ophthalmol* 2013;131:1591–1594.
28. Sharkawi E, Hamedani M, Fouladi M. Eyelid squamous cell carcinoma in situ treated with topical 5-fluorouracil. *Clin Experiment Ophthalmol* 2011;39(9):915–916.
29. Ross AH, Kennedy CT, Collins C, et al. The use of imiquimod in the treatment of periocular tumours. *Orbit* 2010;29(2):83–87.
30. Petsuksiri J, Frank SJ, Garden AS, et al. Outcomes after radiotherapy for squamous cell carcinoma of the eyelid. *Cancer* 2008;112(1):111–118.

Chapter 2 Premalignant and Malignant Tumors of Eyelid Epidermis

EYELID SQUAMOUS CELL CARCINOMA

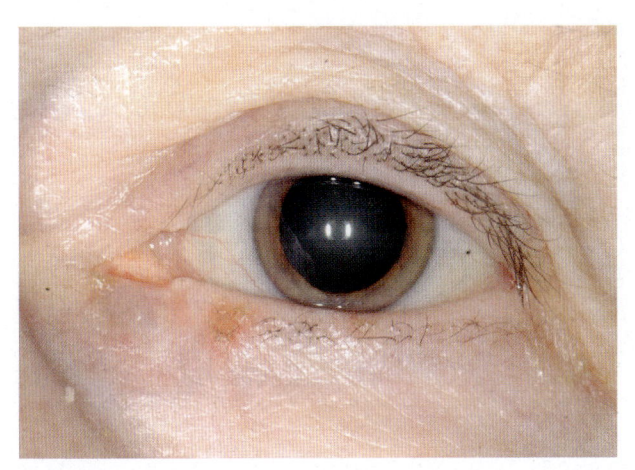

Figure 2.91. Subtle squamous cell carcinoma in situ on lower eyelid demonstrating redness and scaling in a 64-year-old woman.

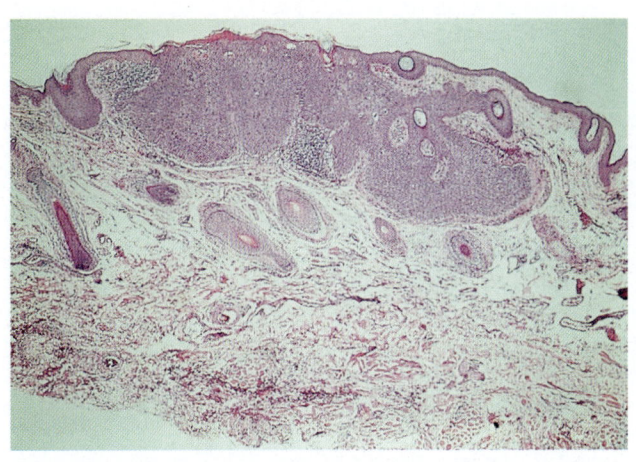

Figure 2.92. Histopathology of squamous cell carcinoma in situ showing thickening of the epidermis due to squamous cell proliferation, with an intact basement membrane. (Hematoxylin–eosin ×15.)

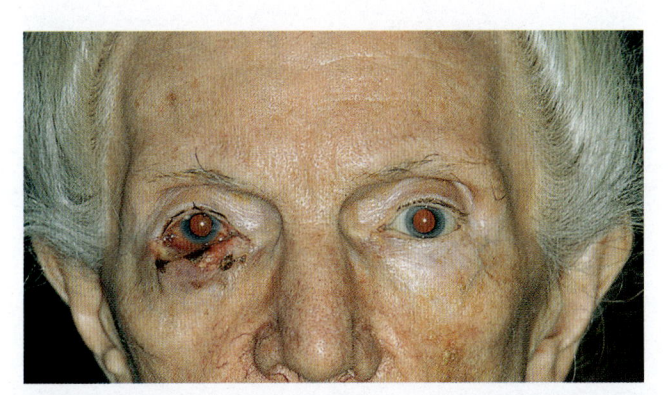

Figure 2.93. Squamous cell carcinoma of right lower eyelid in an 88-year-old woman.

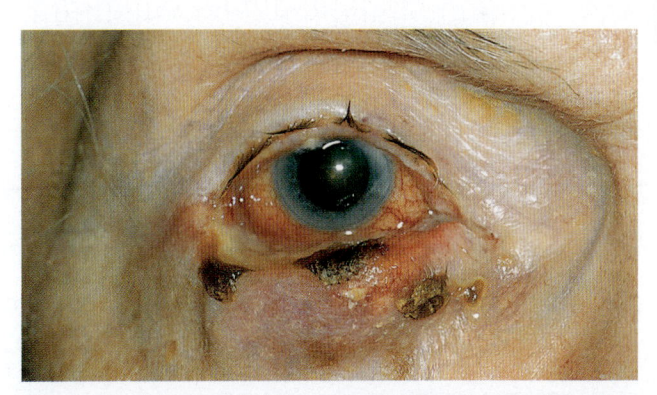

Figure 2.94. Close view of lesion in Figure 2.93, demonstrating diffuse infiltrative tumor with crusting and ectropion of the eyelid.

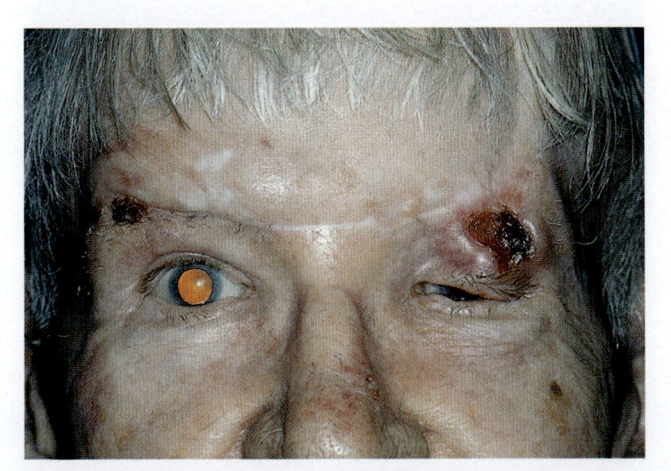

Figure 2.95. Squamous cell carcinoma of upper eyelid in an 87-year-old light-skinned man who had chronic sunlight exposure years earlier as a lifeguard. Note the actinic changes of the skin.

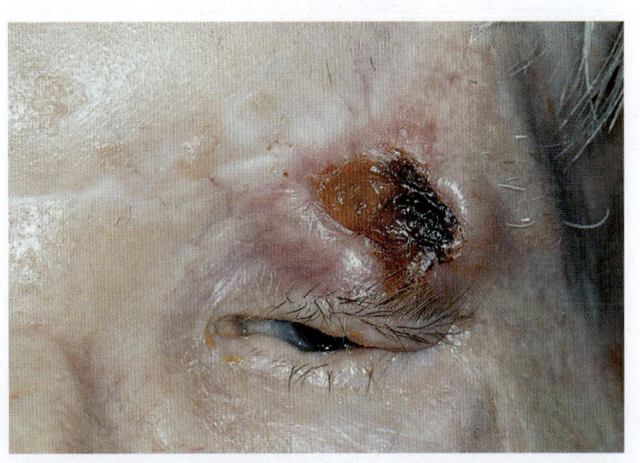

Figure 2.96. Close view of the lesion seen in Figure 2.95, showing the ulcerated lesion on the upper eyelid.

EYELID SQUAMOUS CELL CARCINOMA: DIFFUSE INVOLVEMENT OF UPPER EYELID

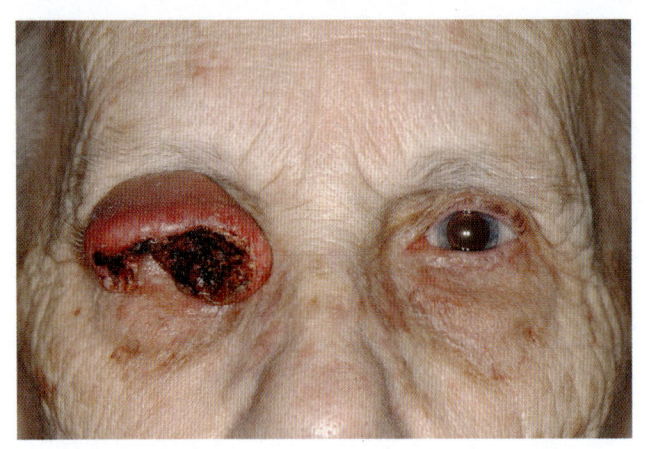

Figure 2.97. Massive squamous cell carcinoma involving entire upper eyelid.

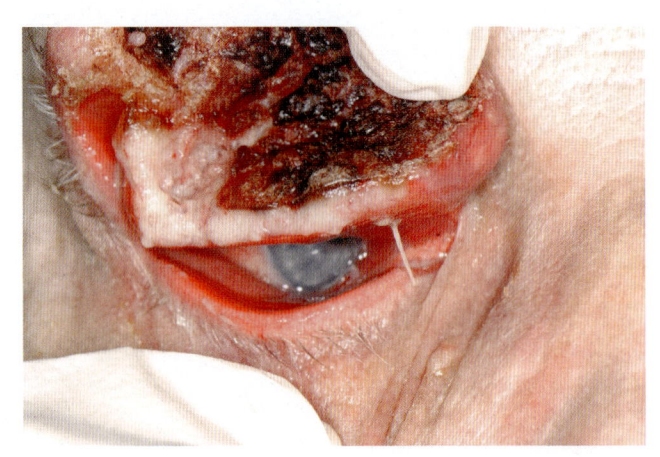

Figure 2.98. The tumor could be retracted to find a normal underlying eye.

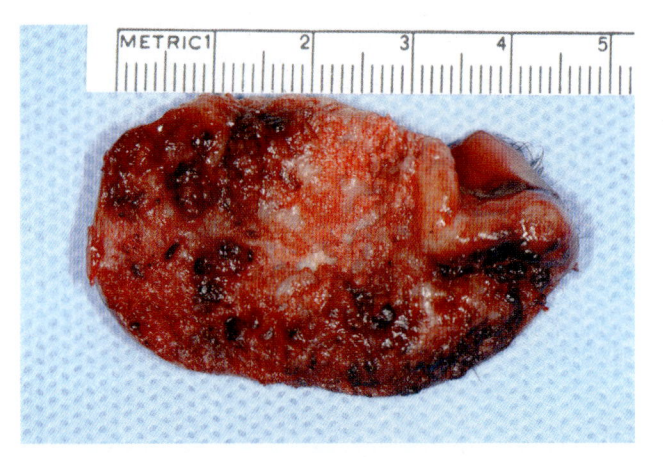

Figure 2.99. The mass was resected completely.

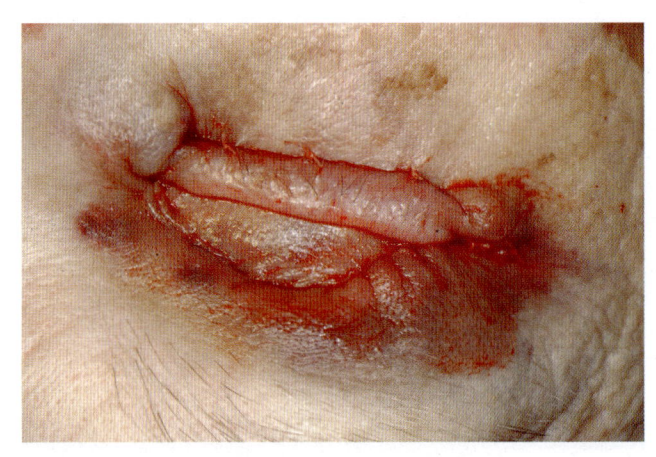

Figure 2.100. A Cutler Beard closure was performed.

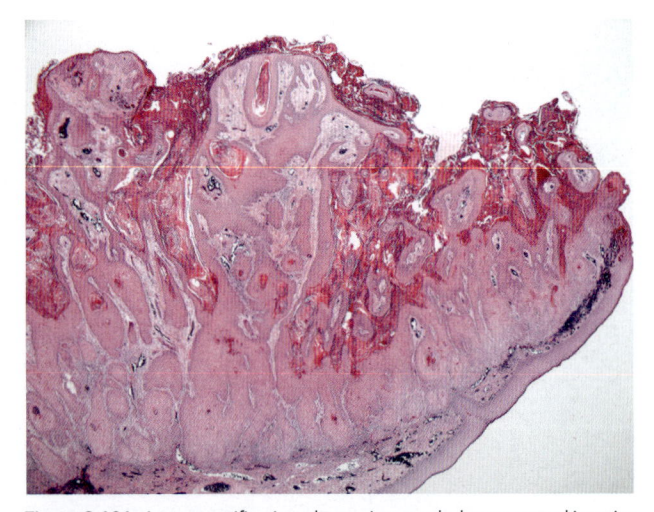

Figure 2.101. Low-magnification photomicrograph demonstrated invasive squamous carcinoma cells with hyperkeratosis. (Hematoxylin–eosin ×50.)

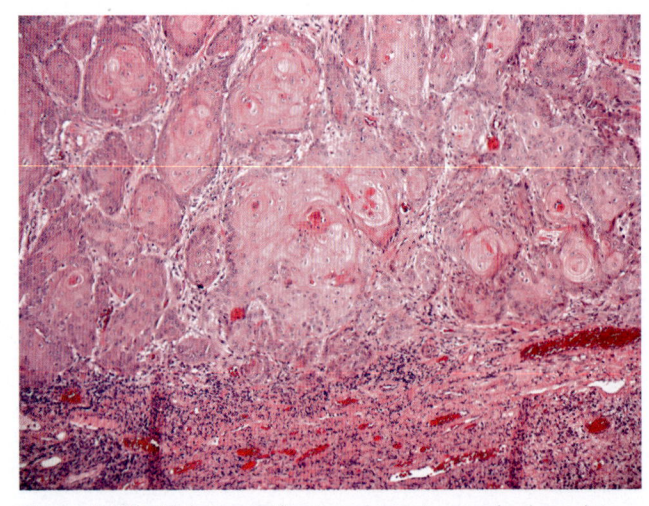

Figure 2.102. Higher-magnification photomicrograph showed invasive anaplastic squamous cell carcinoma with dyskeratosis and marked chronic inflammatory cell infiltration. (Hematoxylin–eosin ×250.)

Chapter 2 Premalignant and Malignant Tumors of Eyelid Epidermis 47

● EYELID SQUAMOUS CELL CARCINOMA: AGGRESSIVE INVASIVE TUMORS

In some instances, SCC can occur in immunosuppressed patients, albinos, or in other predisposed individuals. The tumor can be highly aggressive and can invade the orbit, requiring orbital exenteration.

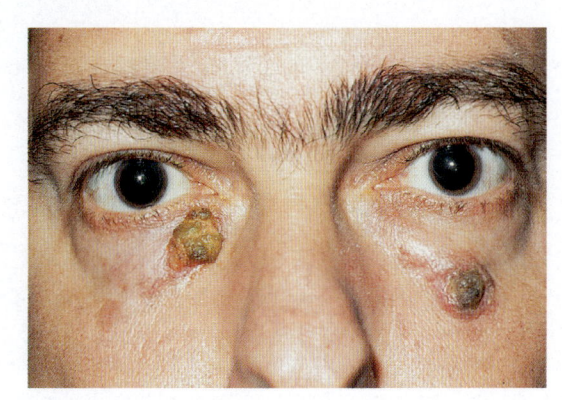

Figure 2.103. Bilateral, crusty, ulcerated SCC of eyelids in a 41-year-old man who was immunosuppressed after renal transplantation. (Courtesy of Narsing Rao, MD.)

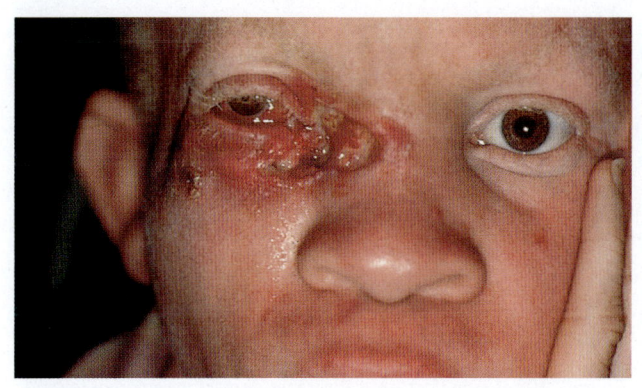

Figure 2.104. Extensive SCC of the eyelid in a young black albino patient from Zaire. Such individuals have a marked predisposition to develop various skin cancers at a young age. (Courtesy of Ralph C. Eagle Jr, MD.)

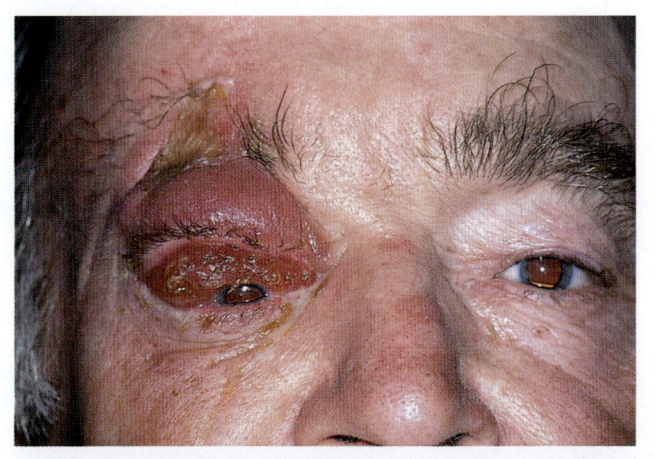

Figure 2.105. Diffuse SCC, presumably originating in upper eyelid, with orbital invasion in a 69-year-old man. Orbital exenteration was necessary.

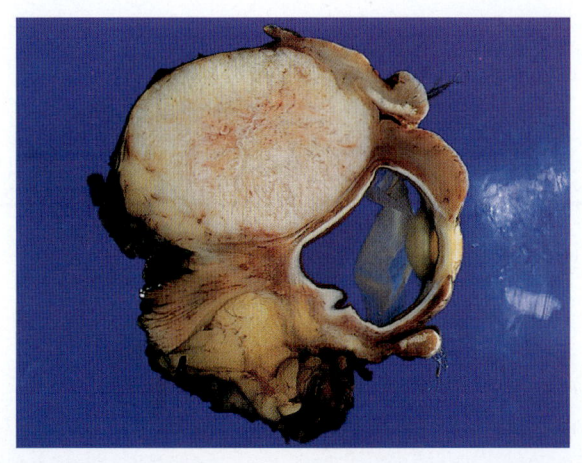

Figure 2.106. Sectioned specimen of the lesion shown in Figure 2.105. Note the large orbital tumor compressing the globe.

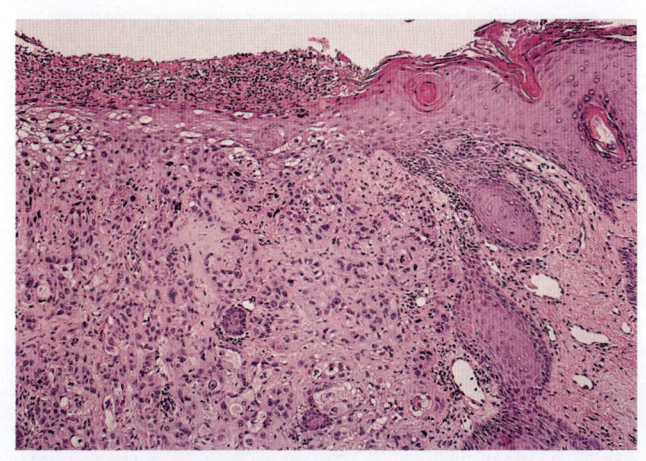

Figure 2.107. Histopathology demonstrating dermal invasion by SCC of the eyelid. (Hematoxylin–eosin ×20.)

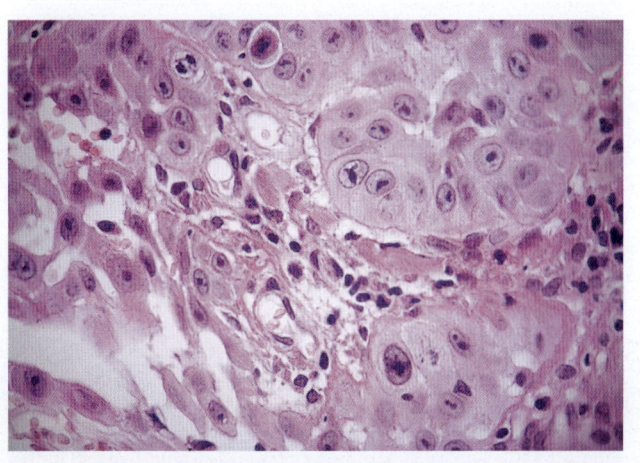

Figure 2.108. Histopathology of eyelid SCC, showing malignant squamous cells. (Hematoxylin–eosin ×200.)

EYELID SQUAMOUS CELL CARCINOMA: DEEP CYSTIC RECURRENT TUMOR

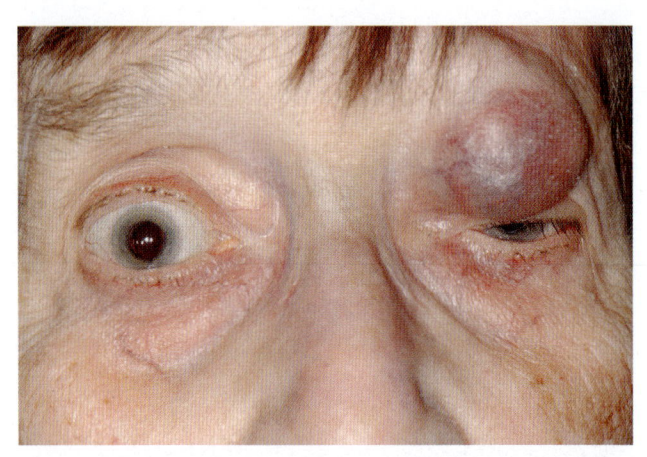

Figure 2.109. Large fluctuant subcutaneous mass in region of left eyebrow of an elderly woman. The patient had been treated elsewhere about 1 year earlier with resection and irradiation of SCC in the same area. The clinical differential diagnosis of this lesion was benign inclusion cyst or cystic recurrence of SCC.

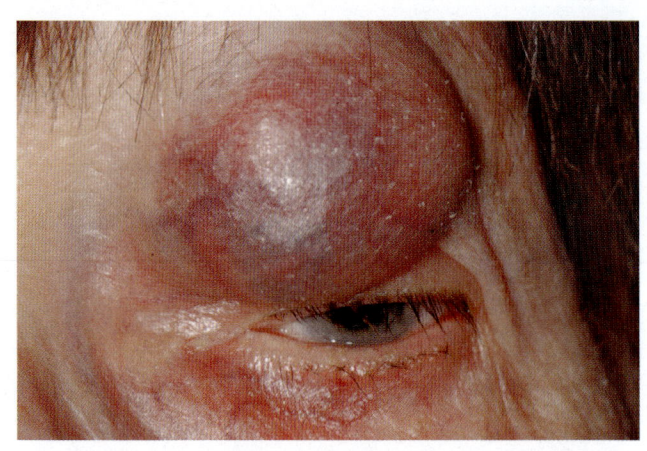

Figure 2.110. Close view of lesion, showing erythematous elevated lesion above left upper eyelid. The lesion was slightly fluctuant to palpation.

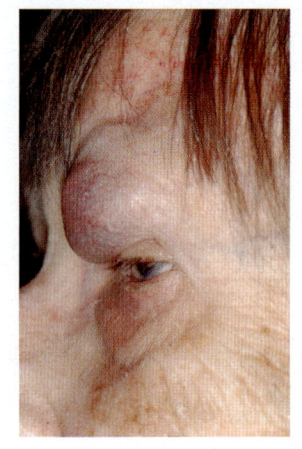

Figure 2.111. Side view of the lesion shown in Figure 2.110.

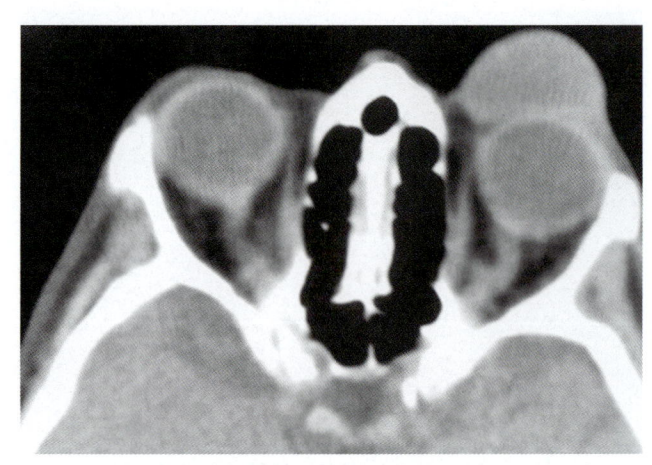

Figure 2.112. Axial CT showing mass anterior to globe.

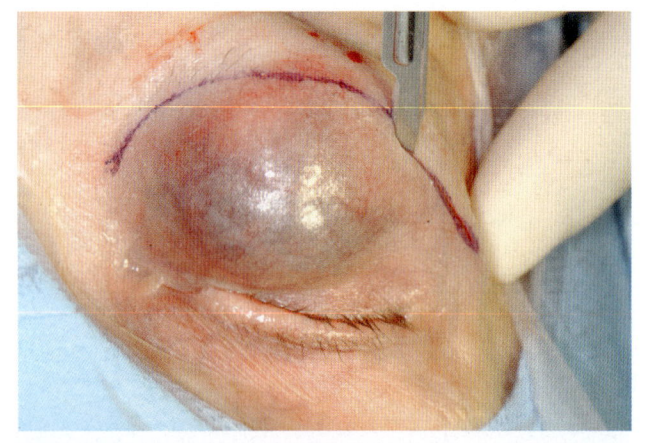

Figure 2.113. Surgical view showing infrabrow incision. She had further recurrences that required irradiation. She died 18 months later of unrelated cardiovascular disease.

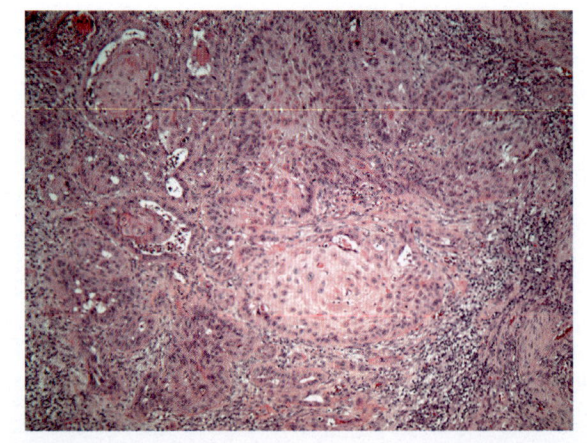

Figure 2.114. Histopathology showing invasive squamous cell carcinoma, showing infiltrating malignant squamous cells. (Hematoxylin–eosin ×150.)

EYELID SEBACEOUS GLAND TUMORS

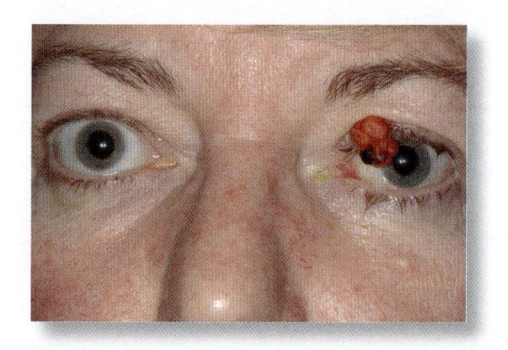

General Considerations

Sebaceous glands of the eyelid area include the meibomian glands of the tarsus, Zeis glands of the cilia, sebaceous glands of the caruncle, and sebaceous glands of the eyebrow. Each can give rise to hyperplasia, adenoma, or adenocarcinoma (sebaceous carcinoma) (1–10). There is an intriguing relationship between sebaceous gland tumors and the Muir–Torre syndrome (MTS) (2–4,6–10).

Muir–Torre Syndrome

MTS is an autosomal-dominant disorder characterized by sebaceous gland adenoma or carcinoma, keratoacanthomas, and gastrointestinal malignancies and other systemic tumors. The number of sebaceous adenomas in MTS can range from 1 to >100 (2–4,6–10).

A patient with one or more cutaneous sebaceous adenomas has a greatly increased chance of developing internal malignancies, particularly gastrointestinal cancers. The internal cancer can become clinically apparent long after the detection of the sebaceous tumor or it can precede it. The associated systemic malignancies can also be multiple. Immunohistochemistry has suggested that lack of expression of the MSH2 mismatch repair gene is an indicator of MTS and may be useful in screening such patients and their family members.

Clinical Features

Eyelid involvement with sebaceous gland hyperplasia is common in middle-aged or older individuals and is apparently unrelated to MTS. It occurs as one or more focal tan-yellow papules or as a diffuse thickening of the eyelids. Sebaceous adenoma, which can be associated with MTS, is clinically similar, but is slightly larger, appearing as a yellow nodule with a smooth surface.

Pathology

Sebaceous hyperplasia is composed of well-demarcated lobules of mature sebaceous glands usually located around a dilated sebaceous duct. In contrast, sebaceous gland adenoma is composed of two types of cells: mature sebaceous cells and poorly differentiated basal cells. The tumor lobules do not usually open into a distinct duct. In some cases, there may be histopathologic overlap between sebaceous hyperplasia and adenoma, making histopathologic classification difficult. The sebaceous tumors seen with MTS often demonstrate typical protrusions of sebaceous tumor cells through the basement membrane into the epidermis (1).

Management

Complete resection is generally the best management. In patients with multiple small lesions, electrodesiccation or cautery and trichloroacetic acid may be effective. As a part of management, any patient with one or more cutaneous sebaceous adenomas should be evaluated for gastrointestinal malignancy or other tumors of the MTS.

EYELID SEBACEOUS HYPERPLASIA AND ADENOMA

Selected References

Reviews/Initial Descriptions

1. Rishi K, Font RL. Sebaceous gland tumors of the eyelids and conjunctiva in the Muir-Torre syndrome: A clinicopathologic study of five cases and literature review. *Ophthal Plast Reconstr Surg* 2004;20:31–36.
2. Muir G, Yates-Bell AJ, Barlow KA. Multiple primary carcinomata of the colon duodenum and larynx associated with keratoacanthoma of the face. *Br J Surg* 1967;54:191–195.
3. Torre D. Multiple sebaceous tumors. *Arch Dermatol* 1968;98:549–551.
4. Rulon DB, Helwig EB. Cutaneous sebaceous neoplasms. *Cancer* 1974;22:82.

Case Reports

5. Bhattacharya AK, Nayak SR, Kirtane MV, et al. Sebaceous adenoma in the region of the medial canthus causing proptosis. *J Postgrad Med* 1995;41:87–88.
6. Tillawi I, Katz R, Pellettiere V. Solitary tumors of meibomian gland origin and Torre's syndrome. *Am J Ophthalmol* 1987;104:179–182.
7. Jakobiec FA. Sebaceous adenoma of the eyelid and visceral malignancy. *Am J Ophthalmol* 1974;78:952–960.
8. Font RL, Rishi K. Sebaceous gland adenoma of the tarsal conjunctiva in a patient with Muir-Torre syndrome. *Ophthalmology* 2003;110:1833–1836.
9. Singh AD, Mudhar HS, Bhola R, et al. Sebaceous adenoma of the eyelid in Muir-Torre syndrome. *Arch Ophthalmol* 2005;123:562–565.
10. Demirci H, Nelson C, Shields CL, et al. Eyelid sebaceous carcinoma associated with Muir-Torre syndrome in two cases. *Ophthal Plast Reconstr Surg* 2007;23:77–79.

EYELID SEBACEOUS CARCINOMA

General Considerations

Sebaceous carcinoma is an important neoplasm that occurs most frequently in the periorbital area, usually the eyelid. It has received a great deal of attention in the ophthalmic literature (1–33). It can exhibit aggressive local behavior and metastasize to regional lymph nodes and distant organs (Table 3.1). Historically, this neoplasm has been notorious for masquerading as other benign and malignant lesions, resulting in delay in diagnosis and higher morbidity and mortality. Hence, it is important for the ophthalmologist to be cognizant of the clinical features and current therapy of periocular sebaceous carcinoma. Recently, greater awareness of this neoplasm has resulted in earlier diagnosis and provided the opportunity for less aggressive therapy (1–5,17,18). Although ophthalmologists have become more familiar with the clinical variations of periorbital sebaceous carcinoma, there remain delays in diagnosis and misdirected therapy (1–3).

Table 3.1 American Joint Committee on Cancer (AJCC) classification of periocular sebaceous gland carcinoma

TNM classification	Definition
Primary tumor (T)	
Tx	Primary tumor cannot be assessed
T0	No evidence of primary tumor
Tis	Sebaceous gland carcinoma in situ
T1	Tumor size <5 mm without involvement of the tarsal plate or eyelid margin
T2a	Tumor size 5–10 mm Or, any tumor <10 mm with involvement of tarsal plate and/or eyelid margin
T2b	Tumor >10 mm to <20 mm Or, any tumor with full thickness involvement of eyelid
T3a	Tumor >20 mm Or, any tumor with involvement of adjacent ocular tissues or orbital structures Or, any tumor with perineural invasion
T3b	Total tumor removal can be achieved only through enucleation, exenteration, or bone resection
T4	Tumor resection is not possible due to invasion of ocular, orbital tissues, craniofacial structures, or brain
Regional lymph node (N)	
Nx	Regional lymph nodes cannot be assessed
cN0	No regional lymph node metastasis based on clinical examination and imaging
pNo	No regional lymph node metastasis, confirmed on biopsy of lymph nodes
N1	Regional lymph node metastasis
Distant metastasis (M)	
M0	No evidence of distant metastasis
M1	Metastasis to distant organs/structures
Staging of sebaceous carcinoma based on TNM classification	
Stage 0	Tis N0 M0
Stage IA	T1 N0 M0
Stage IB	T2a N0 M0
Stage IC	T2b N0 M0
Stage II	T3a N0 M0
Stage IIIA	T3b N0 M0
Stage IIIB	Any T N1 M0
Stage IIIC	T4 Any N M0
Stage IV	Any T Any N M1

From Edge SB, Byrd DR, Compton CC, et al, eds. Carcinoma of the Eyelid. In: *AJCC Cancer Staging Manual.* 7th ed. New York, NY: Springer; 2010:523–530.

Sebaceous carcinoma accounts for 2% to 7% of malignant eyelid tumors in the West. In China and India, where basal cell carcinoma is less common, sebaceous carcinoma accounts for approximately half of all malignant eyelid tumors (18). This aggressive neoplasm can exhibit local recurrence and regional and distant metastases. It generally affects elderly patients, although it has been seen in children and young adults who have undergone irradiation for retinoblastoma or acne (29–31). It has a predilection for elderly females (70%) (1–5). In the periorbital area, it usually arises from the meibomian glands of the upper tarsus, but can originate from the sebaceous glands of the cilia (Zeis glands), caruncle, or eyebrow. Like sebaceous adenoma, sebaceous carcinoma can also be associated with the MTS (11–15).

Clinical Features

The two most common clinical presentations of sebaceous carcinoma are a solitary eyelid nodule and diffuse eyelid thickening. The solitary lesion begins as a firm nodule arising from the tarsus, deep to the epidermis. As it enlarges, it becomes yellow and causes overlying loss of cilia. If the eyelid is everted, the lesion may be more visible in the tarsal conjunctiva. Ulceration is uncommon, but can occur in more advanced cases. The solitary nodular growth pattern is often misdiagnosed in the early stages as a chalazion.

The diffuse growth pattern of sebaceous carcinoma is responsible for its masquerading as chronic blepharoconjunctivitis. Diffuse intraepithelial involvement can extend in a pagetoid pattern across the tarsal conjunctiva, bulbar conjunctiva, and even the cornea and caruncle (1–5). In contrast to most cases of blepharitis, it is unilateral and causes more thickening and induration of the eyelid.

There are other less common presentations of sebaceous carcinoma. When it originates in a Zeis gland, it is located at the eyelid margin rather than deep in the tarsus (27). It can sometimes present as a lacrimal gland mass secondary to deeper invasion of a subtle or subclinical eyelid lesion and can simulate a primary lacrimal gland neoplasm (26). We have also seen it present as a pedunculated mass and as a yellow enlargement of the caruncle.

Classification

The American Joint Commission on Cancer (AJCC) classification of periocular sebaceous gland carcinoma is a staging system for prediction of metastasis and death from this malignancy (16–18). At 10 years, patients with Stage I or II show <5% risk for metastasis whereas those with Stage III or IV show >50% risk for metastasis (18).

Differential Diagnosis

Clinically, sebaceous carcinoma of the eyelid area has no pathognomonic features that differentiate it from the other epidermal lesions described in this section. It should be differentiated from other malignant neoplasms like basal cell carcinoma, squamous cell carcinoma, Merkel cell carcinoma, and from inflammatory lesions like chalazion and blepharoconjunctivitis (1).

Pathology

Sebaceous carcinoma is composed of a malignant proliferation of sebaceous cells with vacuolated cytoplasm owing to the presence of lipid, which is better shown with special fat stains, such as oil red-O stain. In some cases, the exact gland of origin is difficult to identify because of diffuse or multicentric tumor origin.

Although there are several methods of classifying sebaceous carcinoma, most authorities recognize four histopathologic patterns: lobular, comedocarcinoma, papillary, and mixed (9). Histopathologically, sebaceous carcinoma can be further grouped into well-, moderately-, and poorly differentiated varieties. The more common lobular pattern mimics normal sebaceous gland architecture with less differentiated cells situated peripherally, and better differentiated, lipid-producing cells located centrally. In the comedocarcinoma pattern, the lobules show a large necrotic central core surrounded by viable tumor cells. The papillary pattern shows papillary projections and areas of sebaceous differentiation. The mixed pattern can exhibit any combination of the three. When the tumor arises from, and is confined to, the Zeis glands, it appears microscopically to affect the glands near the eyelid margin but spares the tarsus.

A well-known and highly quoted aspect of sebaceous carcinoma is its ability to exhibit intraepithelial (pagetoid) spread into the eyelid epidermis and conjunctival epithelium. This has generally been reported to occur in 44% to 80% of cases (4,9). In an analysis of 25 patients, Chao et al. (4) found that those with pagetoid spread had a significantly higher risk for exenteration.

Management

The best management is wide surgical excision with frozen section or chemosurgery control. If the suspected lesion is large and extensive reconstruction is anticipated, a shaving or punch biopsy can be performed first. For diffuse lesions that affect the bulbar and palpebral conjunctiva, multiple small map biopsies can be done and final surgical planning is based on the extent of the tumors found histopathologically (1–5). Areas that show histopathologic evidence of deep tumor are then surgically resected whereas those that have only intraepithelial pagetoid disease are treated with double freeze-thaw cryotherapy. In advanced diffuse cases with mainly superficial pagetoid involvement of the epithelium, we have used extensive cryotherapy or mitomycin eyedrops for control (23). Deeper tumors of the tarsal region require posterior lamellar resection of the upper eyelid with removal of adjacent conjunctiva, followed by cryotherapy and then reconstruction with buccal mucosal graft or tarsoconjunctival flap.

For patients with sebaceous carcinoma extension into the anterior orbit, orbital exenteration is generally the best approach (1–5). Finally, the role for radiotherapy is not clearly defined. It is probably justified in unresectable tumors because of orbital bone and cranial cavity (24). Systemic chemotherapy can be useful for reduction in tumor size prior to surgical treatment or prevention or treatment of metastatic disease (25).

Prognosis

Although sebaceous carcinoma is a very malignant tumor, the prognosis is improving; clinicians and pathologists have become more familiar with the neoplasm, allowing for earlier recognition and more efficient treatment. Tumors with diffuse or multicentric involvement or with orbital invasion tend to have a worse prognosis. More localized tumors, particularly those that arise from Zeis glands, appear to have a better prognosis, perhaps because they are more apparent and are diagnosed earlier. The AJCC classification is predictive of patient prognosis (16–18).

Selected References

Reviews

1. Shields JA, Demirci H, Marr BP, et al. Sebaceous carcinoma of the ocular region. *Surv Ophthalmol* 2005;50:103–122.
2. Shields JA, Saktanasate J, Lally SL, et al. Sebaceous carcinoma of the eyelids. The 2014 Prof Winifred Mao Lecture. *Asian Pacific J Ophthalmol* 2015; in press.
3. Shields JA, Demirci H, Marr BP, et al. Sebaceous carcinoma of the eyelids. Personal experience with 60 cases. *Ophthalmology* 2004;111:2151–2157.
4. Chao A, Shields CL, Krema H, et al. Outcome of patients with periocular sebaceous gland carcinoma with and without pagetoid conjunctival epithelial invasion. *Ophthalmology* 2001;108:1877–1883.
5. Shields JA, Demirci H, Marr BP, et al. Conjunctival epithelial involvement by sebaceous carcinoma. The 2003 J. Howard Stokes Lecture, part 3. *Ophthal Plast Reconstr Surg* 2005;21:92–96.
6. Doxanas MT, Green WR. Sebaceous gland carcinoma. Review of 40 cases. *Arch Ophthalmol* 1984;103:245–249.
7. DePotter P, Shields CL, Shields JA. Sebaceous gland carcinoma of the eyelids. *Int Ophthalmol Clin* 1993;33:5–9.
8. Kass LG, Hornblass A. Sebaceous carcinoma of the ocular adnexa. *Surv Ophthalmol* 1989;33:477–490.
9. Rao NA, Hidayat AA, McLean IW, et al. Sebaceous gland carcinoma of the ocular adnexa. A clinicopathologic study of 104 cases with five year follow-up data. *Hum Pathol* 1982;13:113–222.
10. Boniuk M, Zimmerman LE. Sebaceous gland carcinoma of the eyelid, eyebrow, caruncle and orbit. *Trans Am Acad Ophthalmol Otolaryngol* 1968;72:619–642.

Muir–Torre Syndrome

11. Muir G, Yates-Bell AJ, Barlow KA. Multiple primary carcinomata of the colon duodenum and larynx associated with keratoacanthoma of the face. *Br J Surg* 1967;54:191–195.
12. Torre D. Multiple sebaceous tumors. *Arch Dermatol* 1968;98:549–551.
13. Rishi K, Font RL. Sebaceous gland tumors of the eyelids and conjunctiva in the Muir-Torre syndrome: A clinicopathologic study of five cases and literature review. *Ophthal Plast Reconstr Surg* 2004;20:31–36.
14. Demirci H, Nelson C, Shields CL, et al. Eyelid sebaceous carcinoma associated with Muir-Torre syndrome in two cases. *Ophthal Plast Reconstr Surg* 2007;23:77–79.
15. Tillawi I, Katz R, Pellettiere V. Solitary tumors of meibomian gland origin and Torre's syndrome. *Am J Ophthalmol* 1987;104:179–182.

Classification

16. Edge SB, Byrd DR, Compton CC, et al, eds. Carcinoma of the eyelid. In: *AJCC Cancer Staging Manual*. 7th ed. New York, NY: Springer; 2010:523–530.
17. Esmaeli B, Nasser QJ, Cruz H, et al. American Joint Committee on Cancer T category for eyelid sebaceous carcinoma correlates with nodal metastasis and survival. *Ophthalmology* 2012;119:1078–1082.
18. Kaliki S, Ayyar A, Nair AG, et al. Neoadjuvant systemic chemotherapy in the management of extensive eyelid sebaceous gland carcinoma: A study of 10 cases. *Ophthal Plast Reconstr Surg* 2015 Feb 11. [Epub ahead of print]

Management

19. Harvey JT, Anderson RL. Management of Meibomian gland carcinoma. *Ophthalmic Surg* 1982;13:56–61.
20. Dzubow LM. Sebaceous carcinoma of the eyelid: Treatment with Mohs surgery. *J Dermatol Surg Oncol* 1985;11:40–44.
21. Putterman AM. Conjunctival map biopsy to determine pagetoid spread. *Am J Ophthalmol* 1986;102:87–90.
22. Lisman RD, Jakobiec FA, Small P. Sebaceous carcinoma of the eyelids. The role of adjunctive cryotherapy in the management of conjunctival pagetoid spread. *Ophthalmology* 1989;96:1021–1026.
23. Shields CL, Naseripour M, Shields JA, et al. Topical mitomycin-C for pagetoid invasion of the conjunctiva by eyelid sebaceous gland carcinoma. *Ophthalmology* 2002;109:2129–2133.
24. Pardo FS, Borodic G. Long-term follow-up of patients undergoing definitive radiation therapy for sebaceous carcinoma of the ocular adnexae. *Int J Radiat Oncol Biol Phys* 1990;34:1189–1190.
25. Murthy R, Honavar SG, Vurman S, et al. Neoadjuvant chemotherapy in the management of sebaceous gland carcinoma of the eyelid with regional lymph node metastasis. *Ophthal Plast Reconstr Surg* 2005;21:301–309.

Case Reports

26. Shields JA, Font RL. Meibomian gland carcinoma presenting as a lacrimal gland tumor. *Arch Ophthalmol* 1974;92:304–308.
27. Shields JA, Shields CL. Sebaceous adenocarcinoma of the glands of Zeis. *Ophthalmol Plastic Reconstr Surg* 1988;4:11–14.
28. Khan JA, Grove AS Jr, Joseph MP, et al. Sebaceous carcinoma. Diuretic use, lacrimal system spread, and surgical margins. *Ophthal Plast Reconstr Surg* 1989;5:227–234.
29. Honavar S, Shields CL, Shields JA, et al. Primary intraepithelial sebaceous gland carcinoma of the palpebral conjunctiva. *Arch Ophthalmol* 2001;119:764–767.
30. Kivela T, Asko-Seljavaara S, Pihkala U, et al. Sebaceous carcinoma of the eyelid associated with retinoblastoma. *Ophthalmology* 2001;108:1124–1128.
31. Rundle P, Shields JA, Shields CL, et al. Sebaceous gland carcinoma of the eyelid seventeen years after irradiation for bilateral retinoblastoma. *Eye* 1999;13:109–110.
32. Howrey RP, Lipham WJ, Schultz WH, et al. Sebaceous gland carcinoma. A subtle second malignancy following radiation therapy in patients with bilateral retinoblastoma. *Cancer* 1998;83:767–771.
33. Khan JA, Doane JF, Grove AS Jr. Sebaceous and meibomian carcinomas of the eyelid. Recognition, diagnosis, and management. *Ophthal Plast Reconstr Surg* 1991;7:61–66.

EYELID SEBACEOUS CARCINOMA: MEIBOMIAN GLAND ORIGIN

The majority of sebaceous carcinomas originate in the meibomian glands of the upper tarsus.

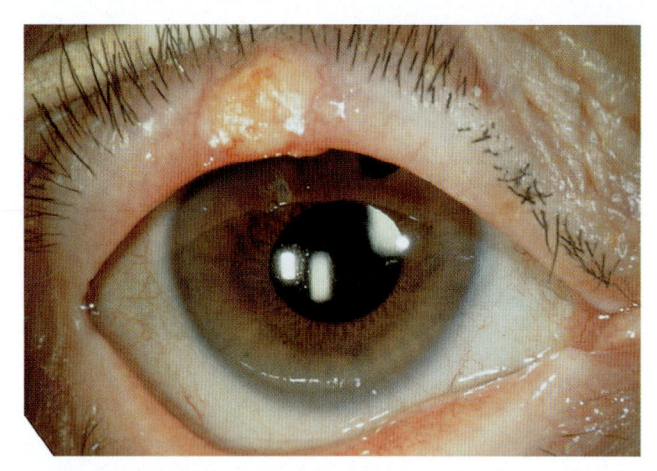

Figure 3.1. Localized sebaceous carcinoma arising from meibomian glands and presenting on cutaneous margin of upper eyelid of a 66-year-old woman.

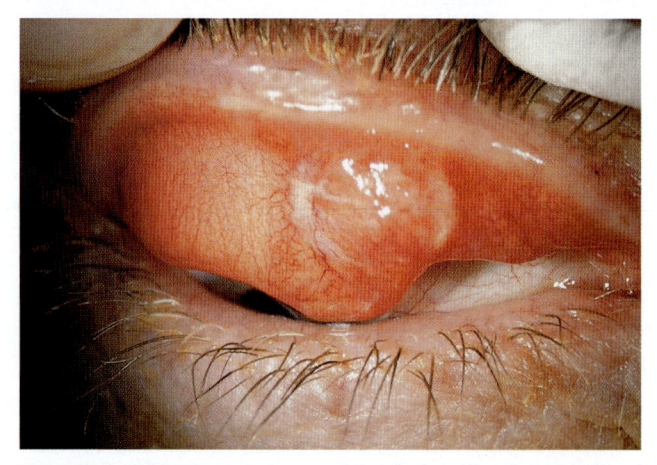

Figure 3.2. Sebaceous carcinoma arising from meibomian glands and presenting on the superior tarsal conjunctiva, seen with the eyelid everted, of a 44-year-old woman.

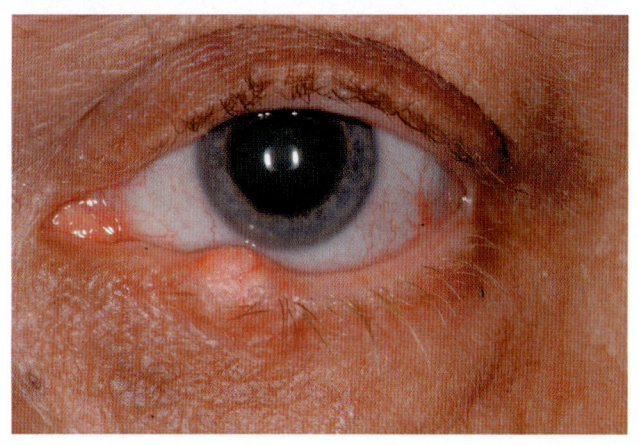

Figure 3.3. Sebaceous carcinoma of lower eyelid simulating a chalazion in a 65-year-old man.

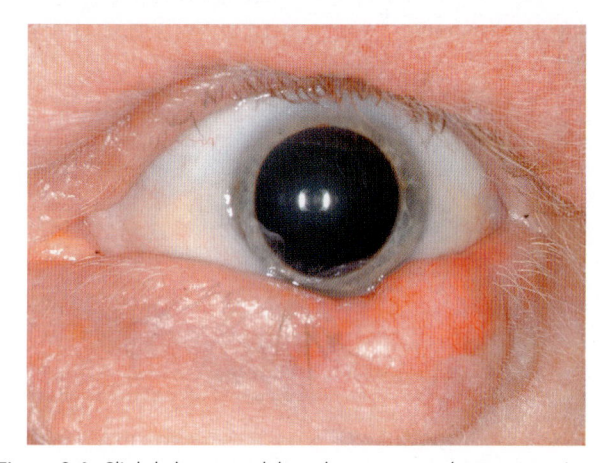

Figure 3.4. Slightly larger nodular subcutaneous sebaceous carcinoma of lower eyelid. Note the typical yellow color and loss of cilia.

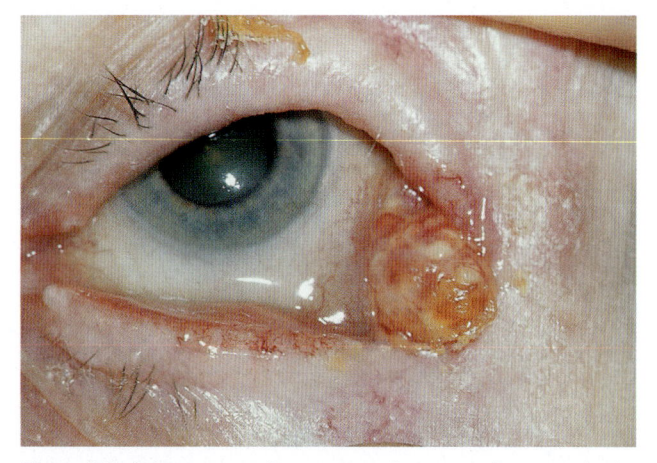

Figure 3.5. Sebaceous carcinoma presenting as a yellow mass in the lateral canthus in a 75-year-old woman.

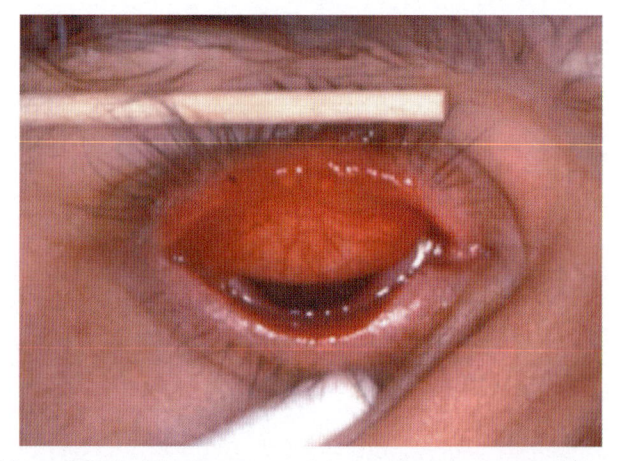

Figure 3.6. Eyelid sebaceous carcinoma arising in a 17-year-old boy, who had undergone ipsilateral ocular irradiation for germ line mutation retinoblastoma. Note the diffuse thickening of the upper eyelid. Prior irradiation for retinoblastoma is one circumstance where sebaceous gland carcinoma can occur in children. It has also occurred in adulthood among patients who had irradiation for acne during childhood.

EYELID SEBACEOUS CARCINOMA: ZEIS GLAND ORIGIN

Sebaceous gland carcinoma that arises from Zeis glands of the cilia tends to occur at the eyelid margin. It is believed to have a better systemic prognosis than sebaceous gland carcinoma that arises from meibomian gland or mixed origin.

Shields JA, Shields CL. Sebaceous adenocarcinoma of the glands of Zeis. *Ophthalmol Plastic Reconstr Surg* 1988;4:11–14.

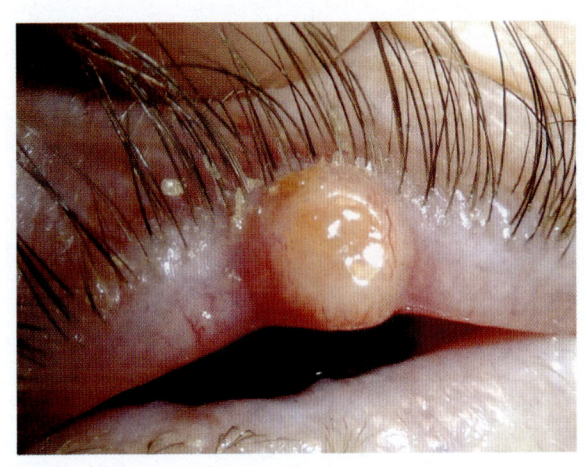

Figure 3.7. Sessile Zeis gland carcinoma on upper eyelid margin in an 80-year-old man.

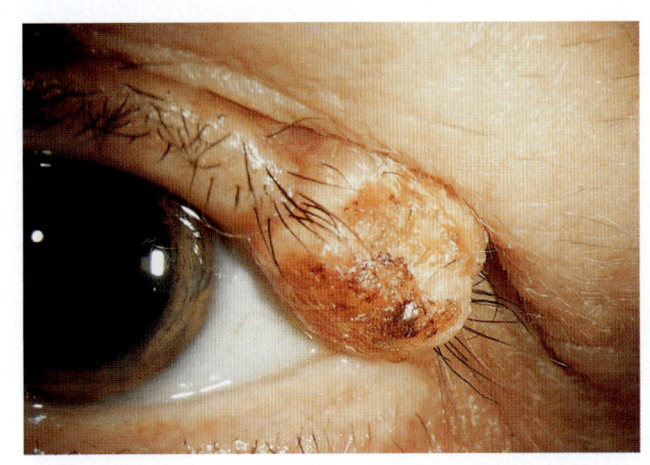

Figure 3.8. Nodular sebaceous carcinoma apparently arising from lateral aspect of tarsus and presenting near lateral aspect of upper eyelid margin in a 64-year-old woman.

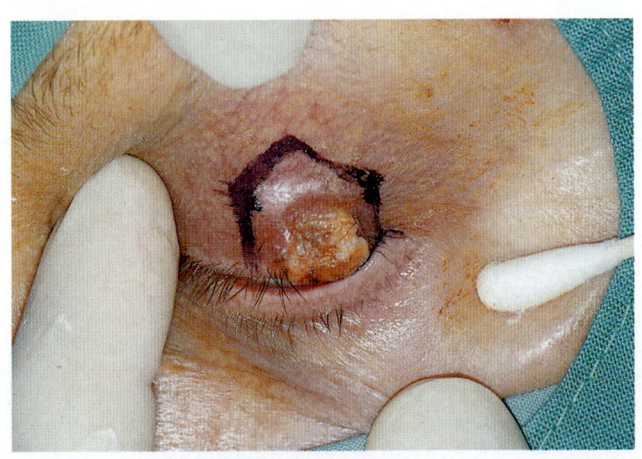

Figure 3.9. Planned pentagonal incision for tumor removal of lesion shown in Figure 3.8. The tumor was removed and the wound was closed primarily.

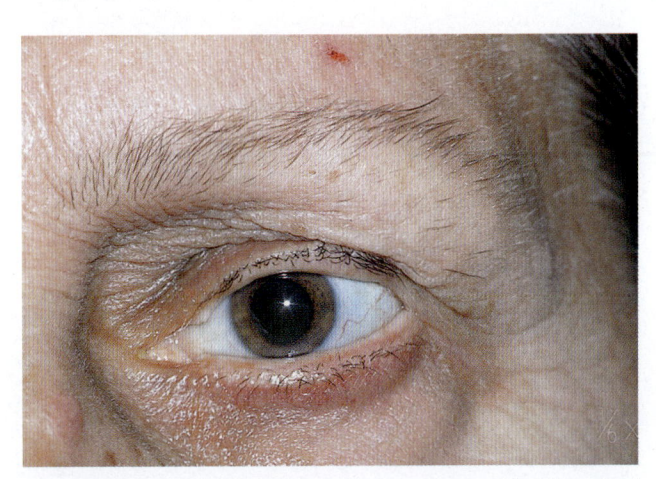

Figure 3.10. Appearance several weeks later, showing that the wound has healed well.

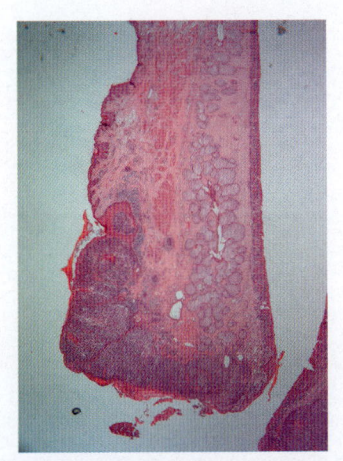

Figure 3.11. Histopathology of lesion shown in Figure 3.8, showing basophilic tumor near eyelid margin. (Hematoxylin-eosin ×5.)

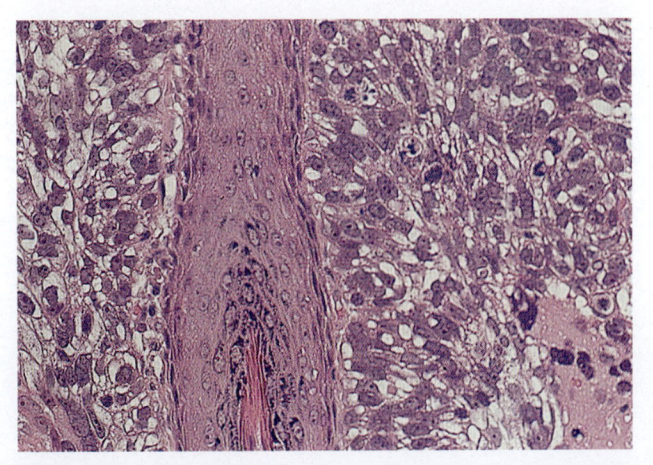

Figure 3.12. Histopathology of same lesion, showing tumor cells around a cilium. (Hematoxylin-eosin ×50.)

EYELID SEBACEOUS CARCINOMA: DIFFUSE NEOPLASM MASQUERADING AS INFLAMMATION

Sebaceous carcinoma can invade the epidermis of the eyelid or the epithelium of the conjunctiva and exhibit diffuse pagetoid spread. This can result in a clinical appearance that simulates an inflammatory process such as blepharoconjunctivitis.

Chao A, Shields CL, Krema H, et al. Outcome of patients with periocular sebaceous gland carcinoma with and without pagetoid conjunctival epithelial invasion. *Ophthalmology* 2001;108:1877–1883.

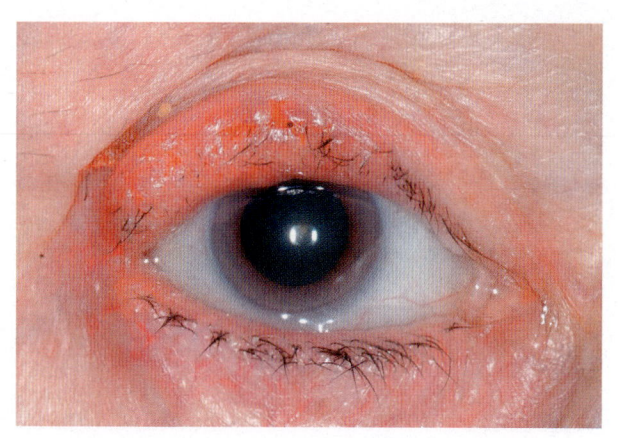

Figure 3.13. Diffuse thickening of upper eyelid due to sebaceous gland carcinoma in a 75-year-old woman. Note the irregular loss of cilia and skin excoriation.

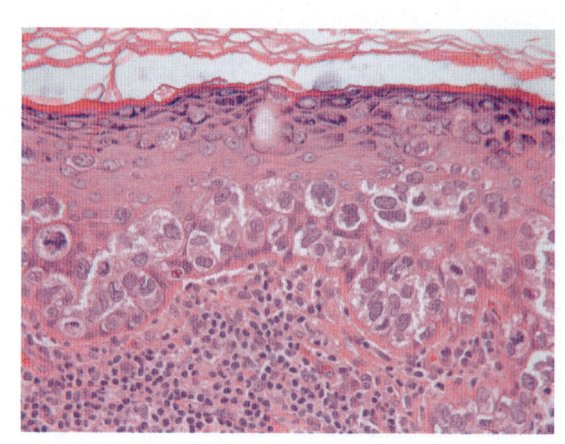

Figure 3.14. Histopathology of diffuse epidermal involvement by sebaceous carcinoma. Note the intact basement membrane and chronic inflammatory cells in the dermis. (Hematoxylin-eosin ×20.)

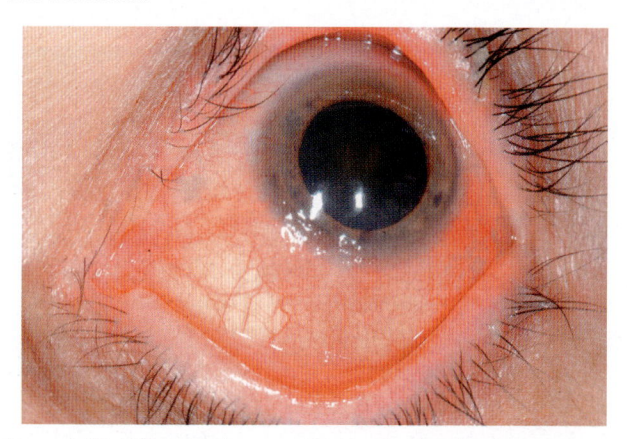

Figure 3.15. Diffuse involvement of conjunctiva by sebaceous carcinoma with early corneal epithelial invasion. Eyelid involvement is minimal.

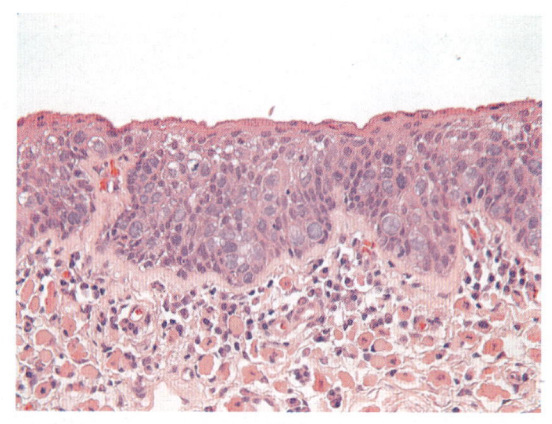

Figure 3.16. Histopathology of diffuse conjunctival epithelial involvement by sebaceous carcinoma. Note the intact basement membrane and chronic inflammatory cells in the conjunctival stroma. (Hematoxylin-eosin ×20.)

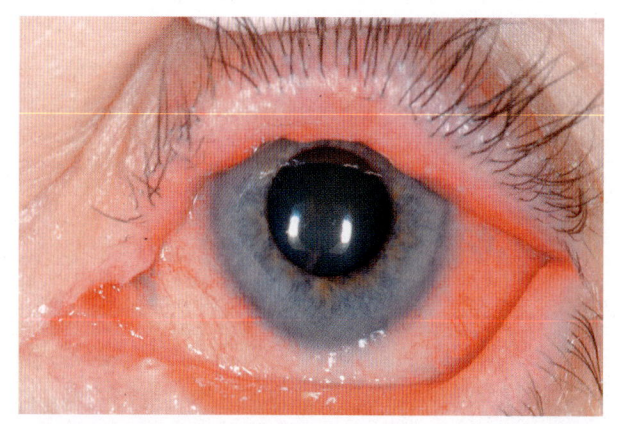

Figure 3.17. Diffuse involvement near eyelid margin, slight eyelid thickening, and diffuse superficial involvement of the conjunctiva secondary to eyelid sebaceous carcinoma.

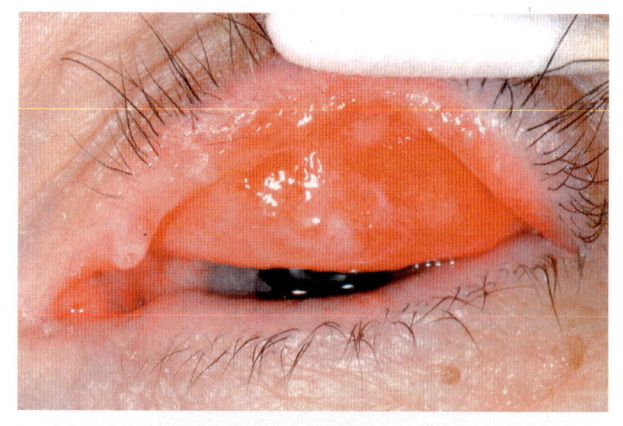

Figure 3.18. Everted eyelid of the patient in Figure 3.17, demonstrating diffuse involvement of the palpebral conjunctiva. It is important to evert the upper eyelid and inspect the palpebral conjunctiva in patients with unexplained blepharoconjunctivitis, because sebaceous carcinoma is a diagnostic consideration. Findings suggestive of sebaceous carcinoma should prompt a biopsy.

Chapter 3 Eyelid Sebaceous Gland Tumors

● EYELID SEBACEOUS CARCINOMA: PEDUNCULATED VARIANT

Shown is a clinicopathologic correlation of a sebaceous carcinoma of tarsus that exhibited a pedunculated growth pattern.

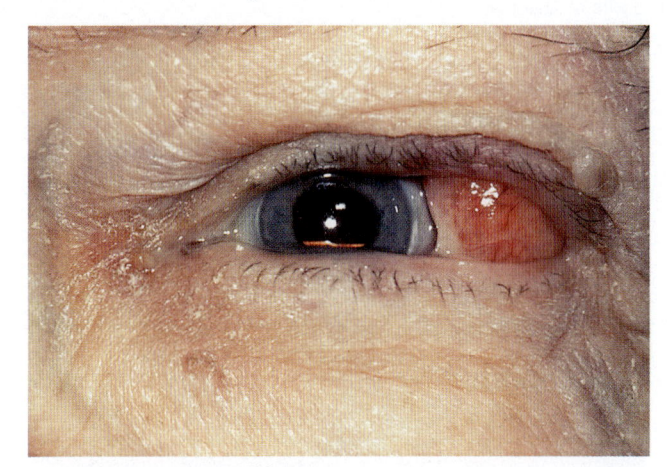

Figure 3.19. Appearance of a lesion near lateral canthus in an 89-year-old woman. She declined treatment.

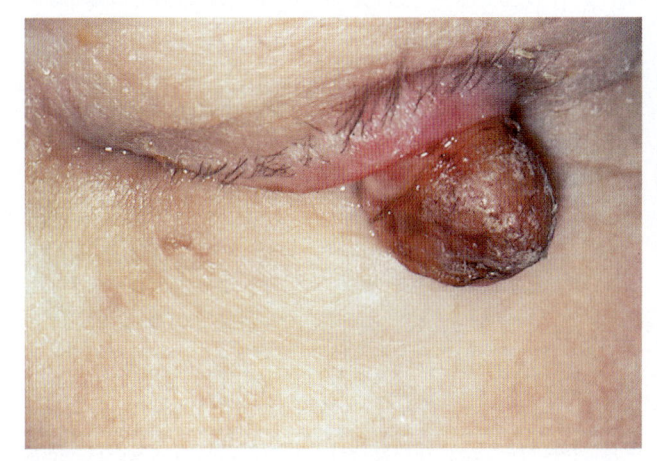

Figure 3.20. Appearance of lesion 1 week later at which time she described rapid progression of the lesion. It is now larger, pedunculated, and crusty.

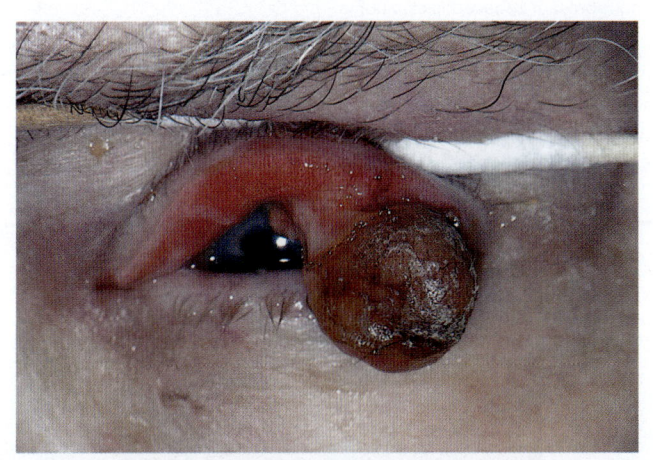

Figure 3.21. Everted upper eyelid showing that pedunculated lesion arose from the tarsal conjunctiva.

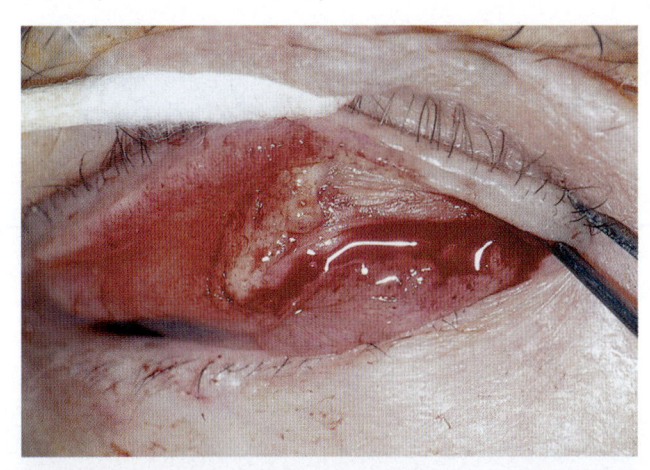

Figure 3.22. Appearance of everted eyelid showing area where lesion was excised by dissection from tarsus. Extensive cryotherapy was applied to tarsal conjunctiva after tumor was removed.

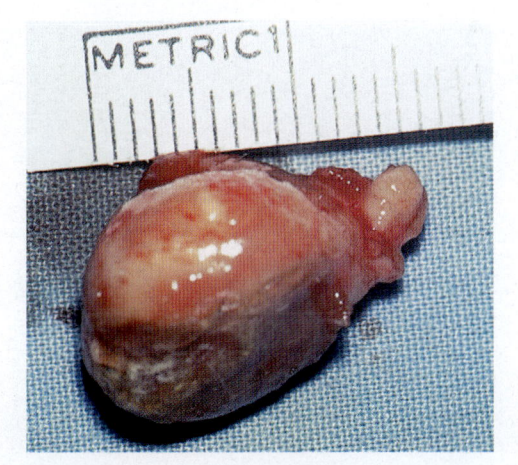

Figure 3.23. Gross photograph of excised lesion.

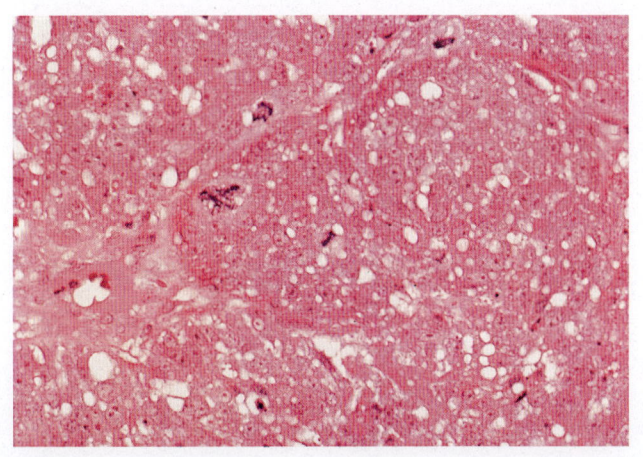

Figure 3.24. Histopathology, showing lobules of malignant sebaceous cells with extensive necrosis. The clear spaces represent dissolved lipid in cytoplasm of cells. (Hematoxylin-eosin ×200.)

TUMORS OF THE EYELIDS

EYELID SEBACEOUS CARCINOMA: CLINICAL VARIATIONS AND HISTOPATHOLOGY

Sebaceous carcinoma is often misdiagnosed histopathologically as squamous cell carcinoma or other lesions. However, most cases can be diagnosed readily by experienced pathologists who have had experience with this neoplasm.

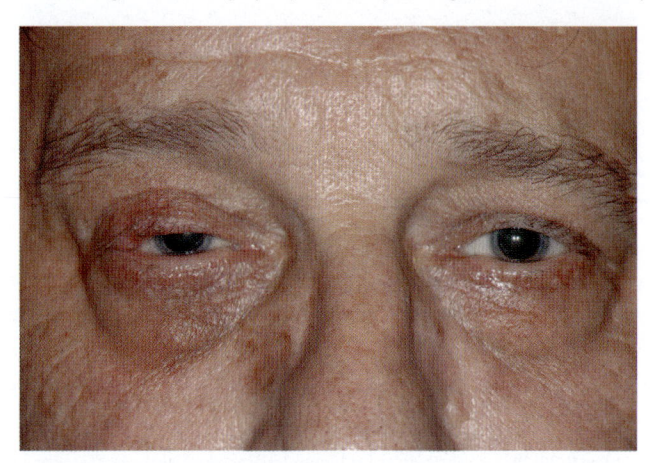

Figure 3.25. Swollen right upper eyelid with ptosis in a 75-year-old man.

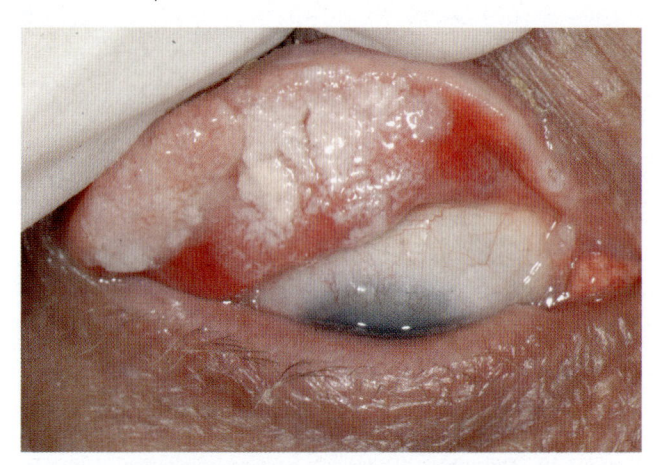

Figure 3.26. Everted eyelid of patient in Figure 3.25 demonstrating extensive white lesion on tarsal conjunctiva that was proven on biopsy to represent sebaceous carcinoma.

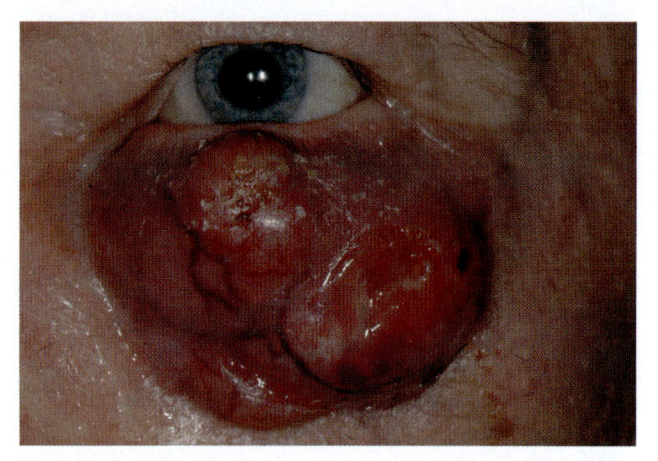

Figure 3.27. Massive left lower eyelid mass in an elderly man, revealing prominent intrinsic vascularity.

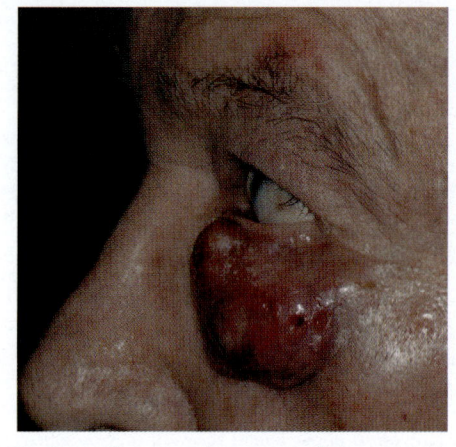

Figure 3.28. On profile view of patient in Figure 3.27, the multilobulated tumor elevation is noted. Histopathology disclosed aggressive sebaceous carcinoma.

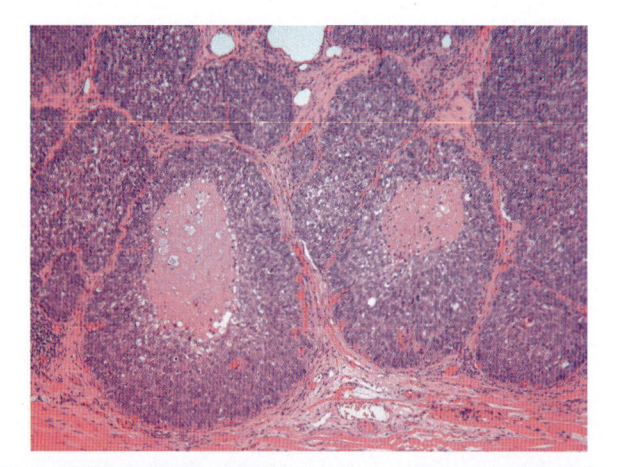

Figure 3.29. Comedo pattern in sebaceous carcinoma, representing areas of central necrosis in center of lobules of viable malignant sebaceous cells. (Hematoxylin-eosin ×50.)

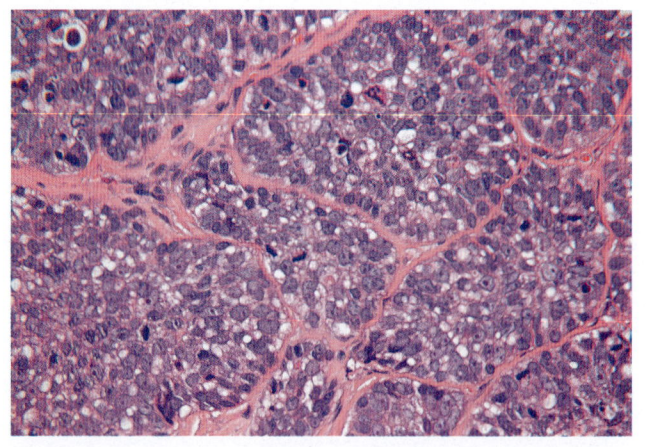

Figure 3.30. Lobules of sebaceous carcinoma, showing cytoplasmic vacuoles and mitotic activity. (Hematoxylin-eosin ×100.)

EYELID SEBACEOUS TUMORS: ASSOCIATION WITH MUIR–TORRE SYNDROME

MTS is an autosomal-dominant disorder characterized by benign or malignant sebaceous neoplasms and malignancies of the gastrointestinal tract, usually colon cancer, as well as other malignancies.

1. Rishi K, Font RL. Sebaceous gland tumors of the eyelids and conjunctiva in the Muir-Torre syndrome: A clinicopathologic study of five cases and literature review. *Ophthal Plast Reconstr Surg* 2004;20:31–36.
2. Demirci H, Nelson C, Shields CL, et al. Eyelid sebaceous carcinoma associated with Muir-Torre syndrome in two cases. *Ophthal Plast Reconstr Surg* 2007;23:77–79.

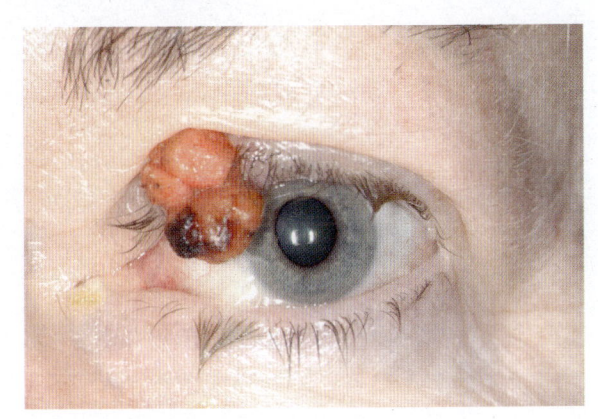

Figure 3.31. Multilobulated sebaceous carcinoma of the upper eyelid in a 60-year-old woman with MTS.

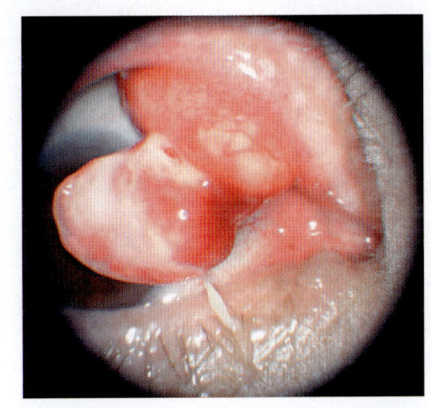

Figure 3.32. Pedunculated sebaceous carcinoma on tarsal eyelid surface with intrinsic vascularization in a 54-year-old man with MTS based on sebaceous carcinoma, colon cancer, and prostate cancer.

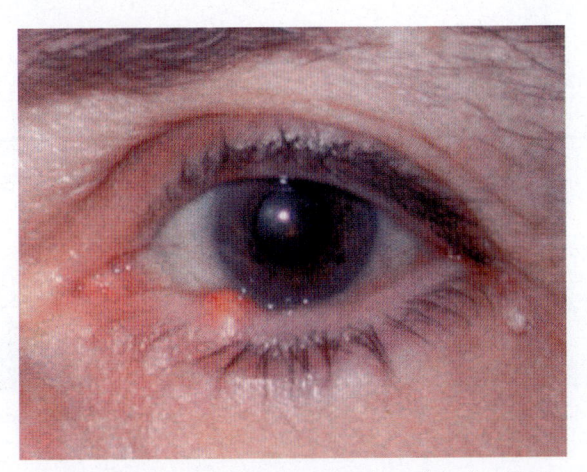

Figure 3.33. Small nodular lesion on lower eyelid of a 79-year-old woman with MTS based on sebaceous carcinoma of the eyelid, colon cancer, and cancers of the uterus, bladder, and kidney.

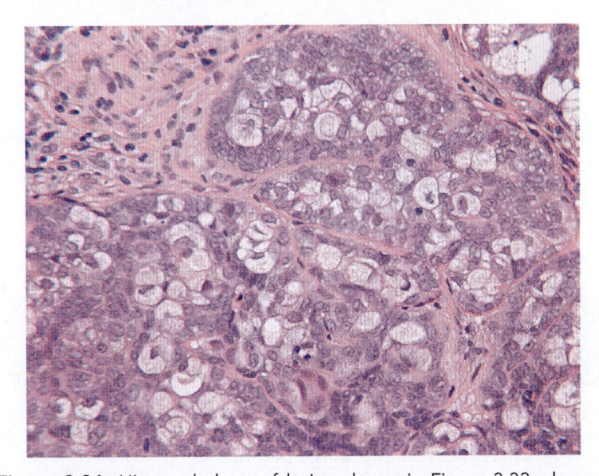

Figure 3.34. Histopathology of lesion shown in Figure 3.33, demonstrating lobules of moderately differentiated sebaceous carcinoma cells. (Hematoxylin-eosin ×200.)

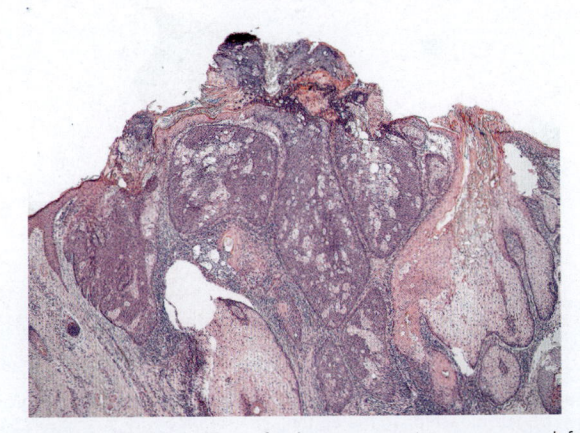

Figure 3.35. Histopathology of sebaceous carcinoma removed from right zygomatic area in a middle-aged man with MTS, showing lobules of tumor with pagetoid invasion of the overlying epithelium and overlying hyperkeratosis. Note the normal sebaceous glands to the right. (Hematoxylin-eosin ×50.)

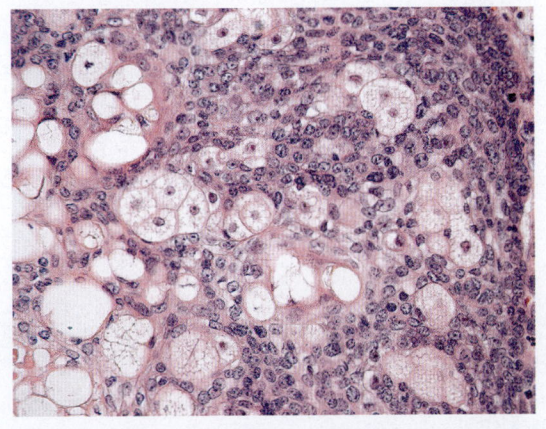

Figure 3.36. Higher magnification view of lesion shown in Figure 3.35 showing typical features of sebaceous carcinoma. (Hematoxylin-eosin ×200.)

EYELID SEBACEOUS CARCINOMA: DIFFUSE NEOPLASM

Sebaceous carcinoma can grow in a pagetoid fashion throughout the eyelid, conjunctiva, and anterior aspect of the orbit. Such cases often require orbital exenteration. A clinicopathologic correlation is presented.

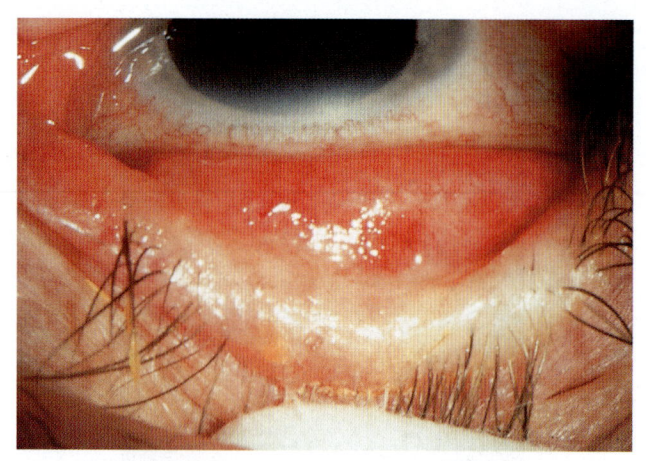

Figure 3.37. Diffuse thickening of the lower tarsal conjunctiva in a 58-year-old woman.

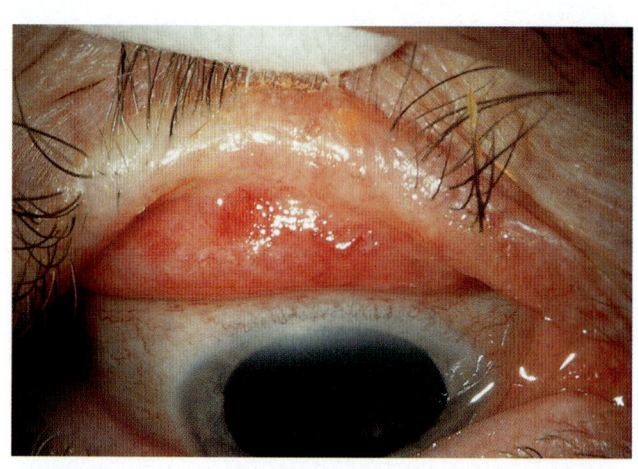

Figure 3.38. Diffuse thickening of the upper tarsal conjunctiva in the same patient.

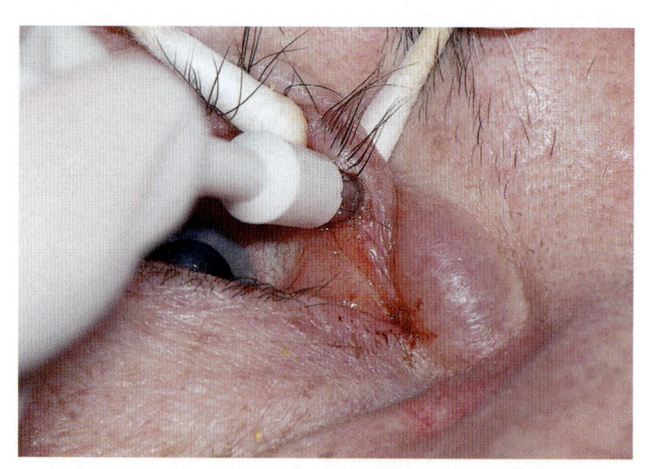

Figure 3.39. Punch biopsy being done in upper tarsus. Biopsies in all areas of upper eyelid, lower eyelid, conjunctiva, and anterior orbit all revealed diffuse sebaceous gland carcinoma.

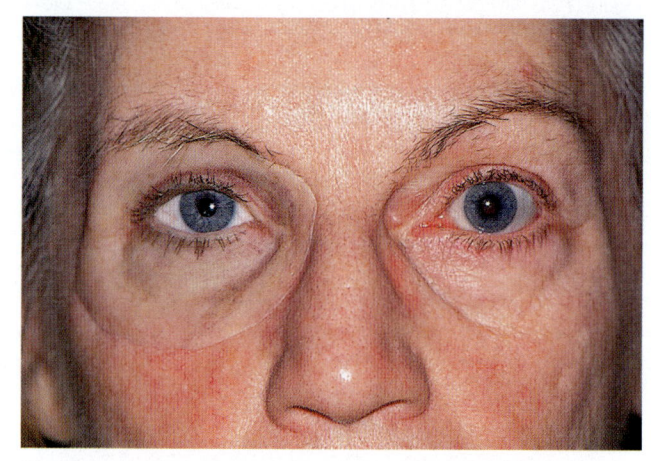

Figure 3.40. Appearance of patient after exenteration of right orbit. Note the glued-on orbital prosthesis.

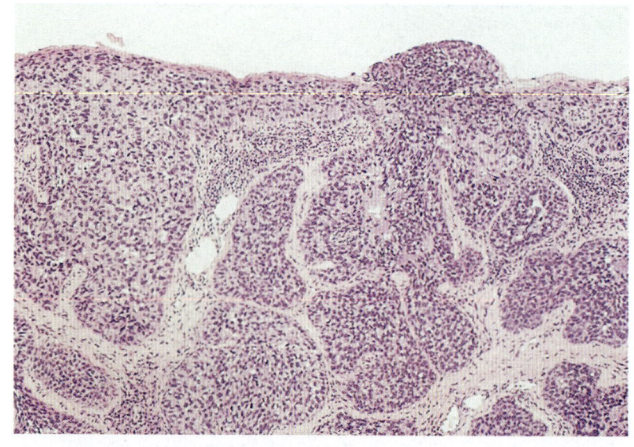

Figure 3.41. Histopathology showing lobules of sebaceous gland carcinoma. (Hematoxylin-eosin ×25.)

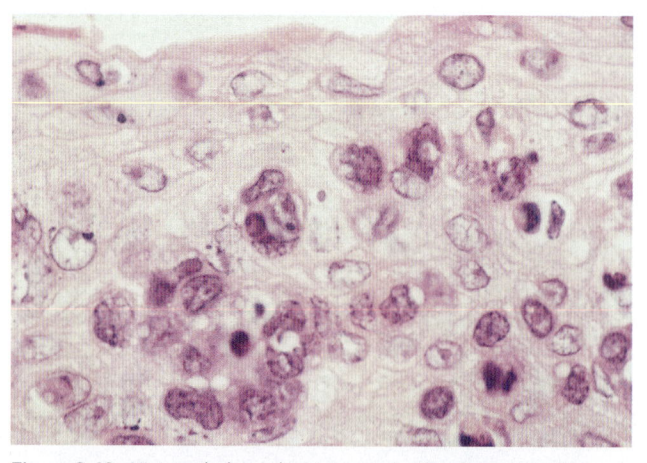

Figure 3.42. Histopathology showing anaplastic sebaceous cells growing in pagetoid fashion in the epithelium. (Hematoxylin-eosin ×200.)

Chapter 3 Eyelid Sebaceous Gland Tumors 61

● EYELID SEBACEOUS CARCINOMA: AGGRESSIVE CLINICAL COURSE

Sebaceous carcinoma can sometimes be locally aggressive and demonstrate regional and systemic metastasis.

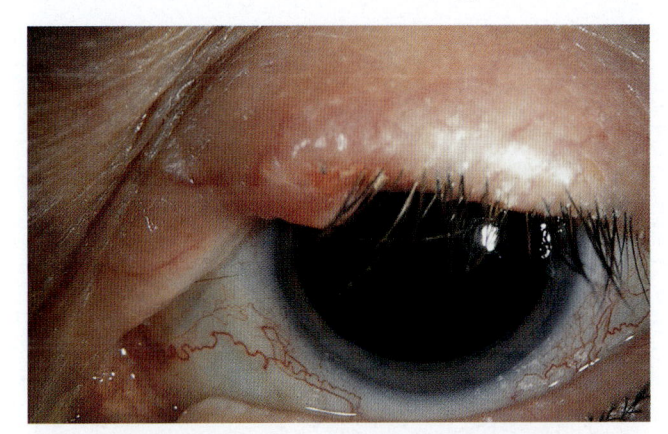

Figure 3.43. Original appearance of upper eyelid lesion in an 84-year-old woman. The clinician diagnosed a chalazion and treated it with curettage. No pathology specimen was submitted. A recurrence 2 years later was biopsied and the diagnosis of sebaceous gland carcinoma was made. The patient was treated with irradiation, but the lesion continued to enlarge.

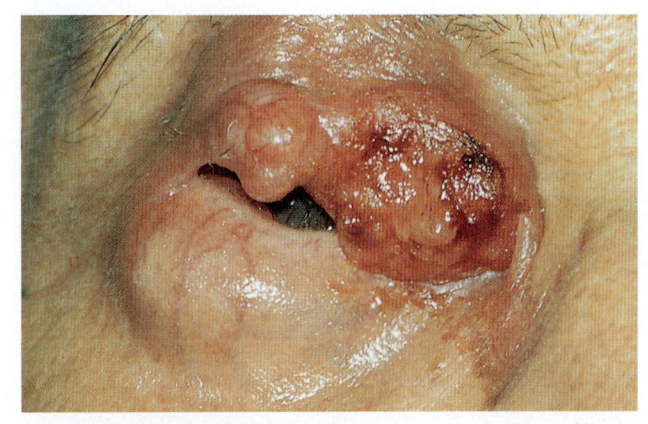

Figure 3.44. Appearance of patient shown in Figure 3.43 when she was referred 2 years later. Note the massive tumor recurrence involving upper and lower eyelids.

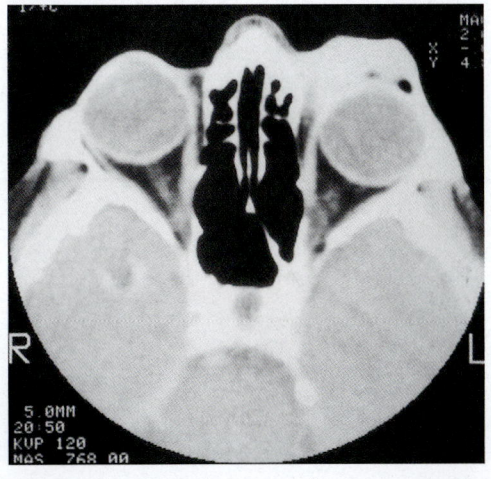

Figure 3.45. Axial computed tomographic image showing tumor encasing anterior portion of orbit.

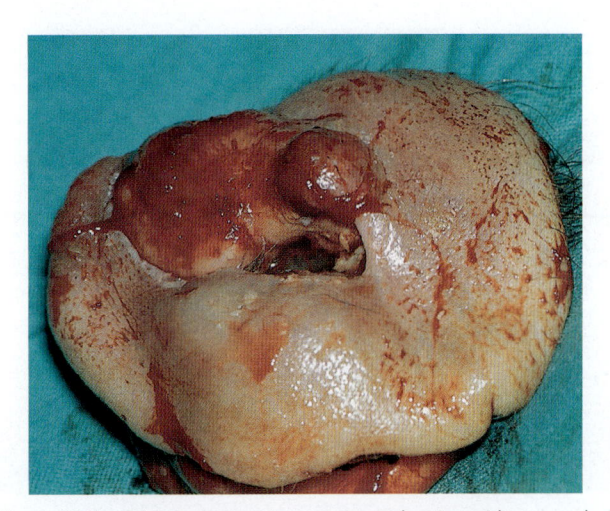

Figure 3.46. Orbital exenteration specimen showing wide removal of eyelid. All margins were free of tumor histopathologically.

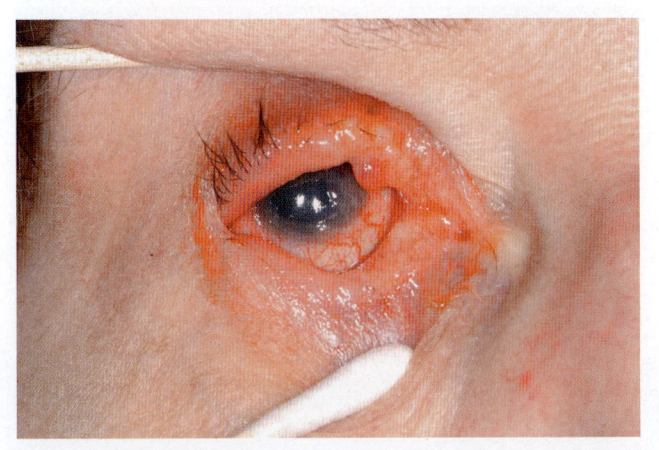

Figure 3.47. Diffuse sebaceous carcinoma involving eyelids of a 51-year-old woman. She had been treated for 2 years for blepharoconjunctivitis with a poor response to treatment and sebaceous carcinoma was eventually suspected.

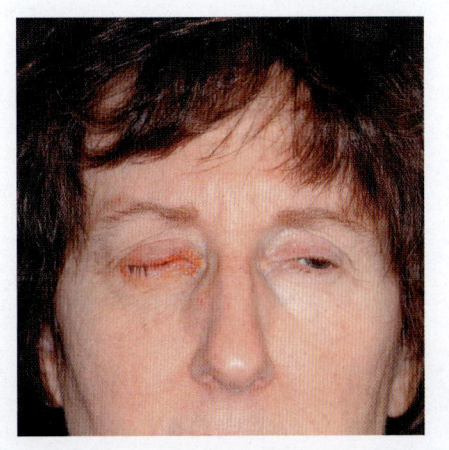

Figure 3.48. The patient seen in Figure 3.47 also had ipsilateral preauricular lymph node metastasis, not well seen in photograph, at the time of referral for the eyelid neoplasm. Preauricular lymph node metastasis developed 2 years later. In spite of lymph node dissection and irradiation, the patient died from tumor dissemination.

EYELID SEBACEOUS CARCINOMA: PENTAGONAL FULL-THICKNESS EYELID RESECTION

Results are shown of a resection of sebaceous carcinoma of the upper eyelid. Details of eyelid resection techniques are shown in Chapter 15.

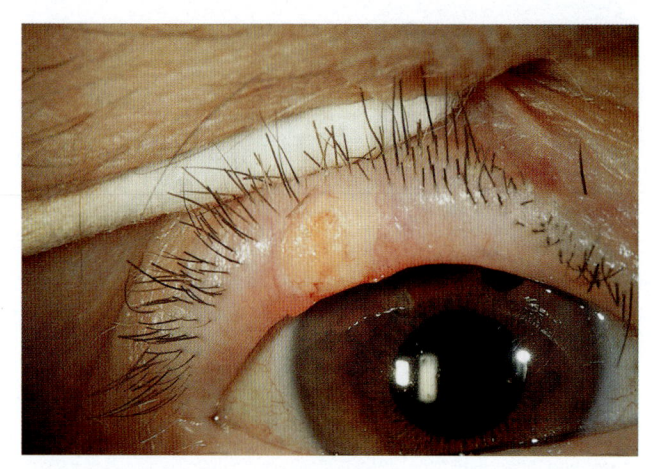

Figure 3.49. Yellow lesion eyelid margin in a 66-year-old woman. Same lesion as shown in Figure 3.1.

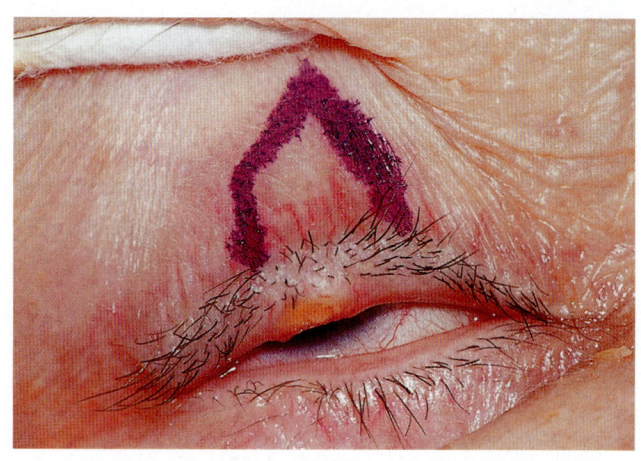

Figure 3.50. Outline of tissue to be removed marked with a sterile pencil.

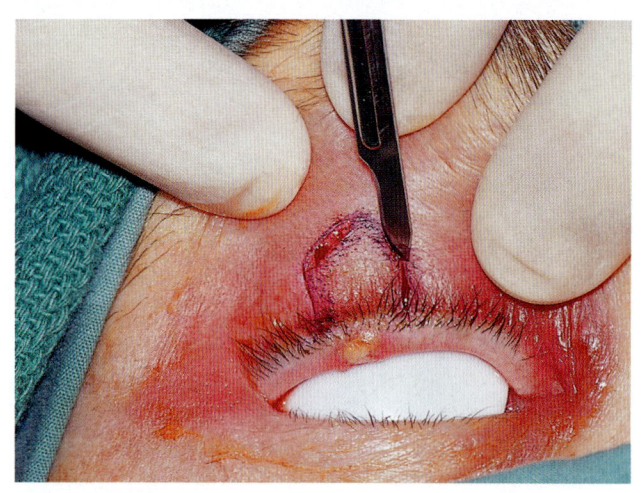

Figure 3.51. Excision of the lesion along line marked with pencil. A plastic shell has been placed to protect the cornea.

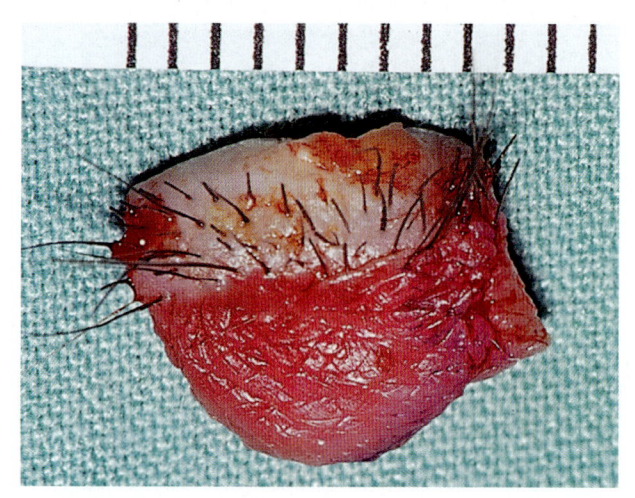

Figure 3.52. Specimen after removal.

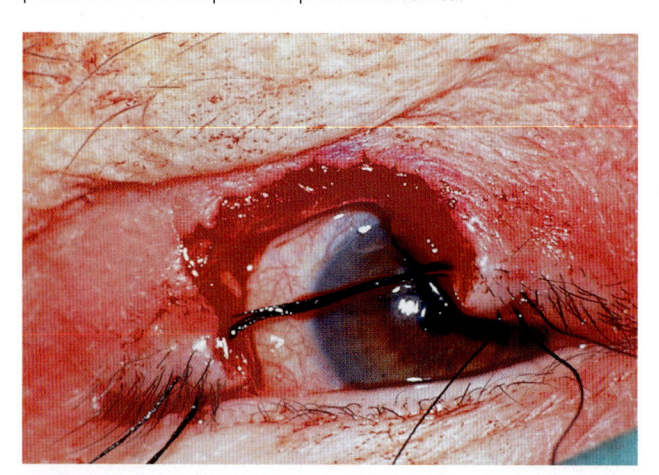

Figure 3.53. Defect after removal. Frozen sections of the margins were negative for tumor. Eyelid margin sutures have been placed. The tarsus was closed with interrupted absorbable sutures.

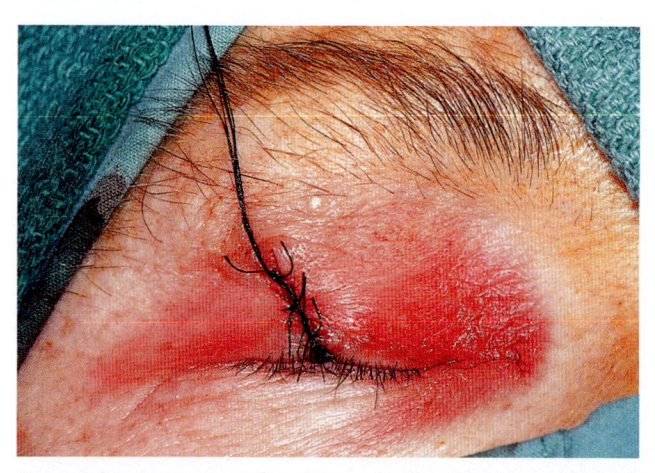

Figure 3.54. Appearance after closure, showing skin sutures. Although the eyelid is tight at the end of the procedure, it resumed its normal position within 2 weeks.

EYELID SEBACEOUS CARCINOMA: PENTAGONAL RESECTION AND SEMICIRCULAR FLAP RECONSTRUCTION

A semicircular flap is used when the eyelid defect cannot be closed primarily. Details of eyelid resection techniques are shown in Chapter 15.

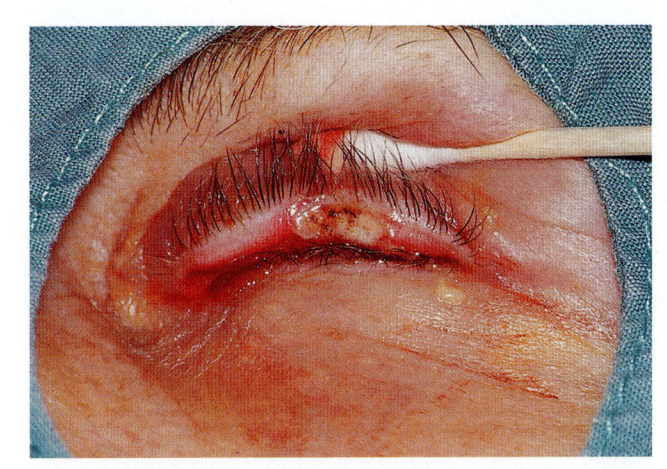

Figure 3.55. Appearance of lesion at eyelid margin in a 72-year-old woman.

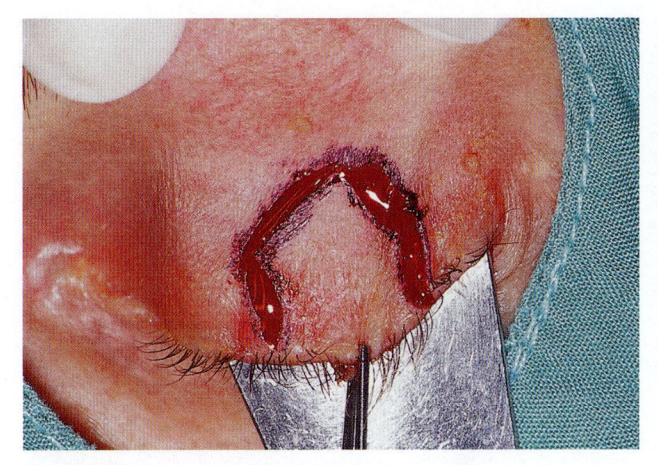

Figure 3.56. Pentagonal skin incision has been made.

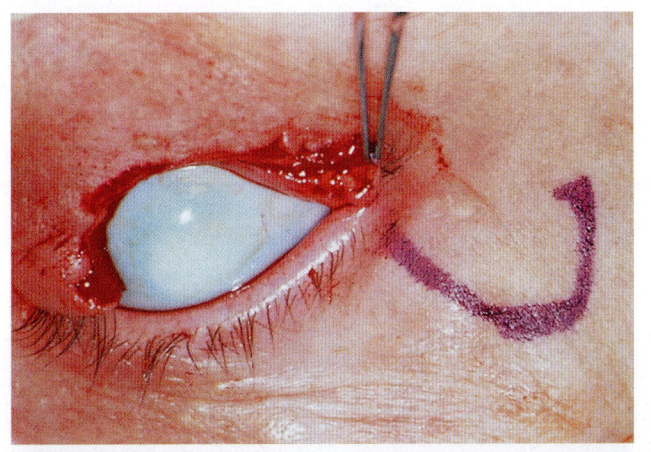

Figure 3.57. The specimen has been removed, leaving a large upper eyelid defect. A plastic shell has been placed temporarily on the cornea for protection. A semicircular flap (Tenzel flap) has been outlined, extending from lateral canthus.

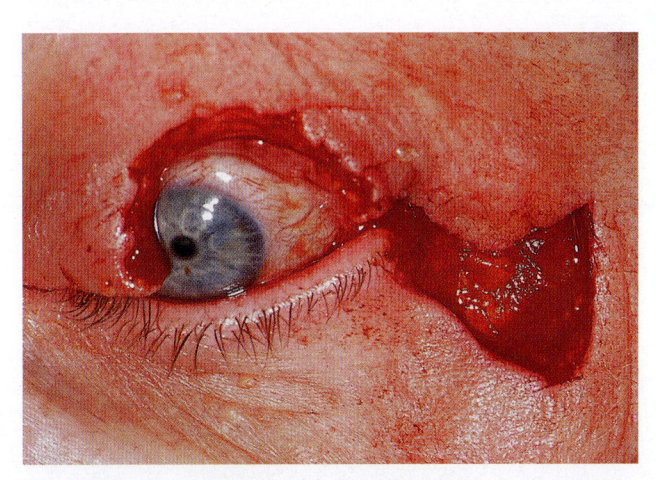

Figure 3.58. Appearance of defect after tumor removal and undermining of the semicircular flap.

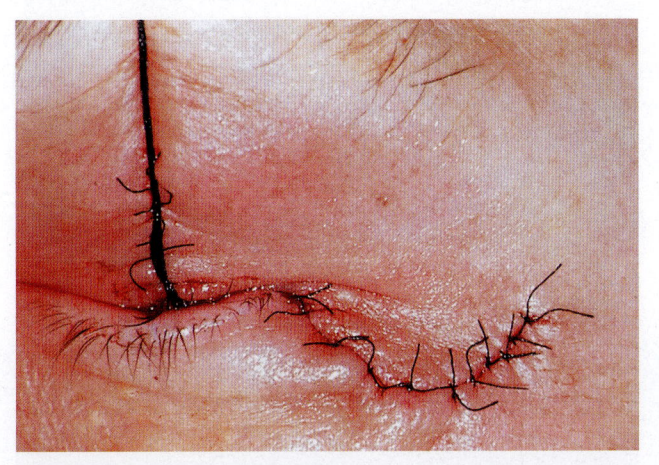

Figure 3.59. Appearance immediately after wound closure.

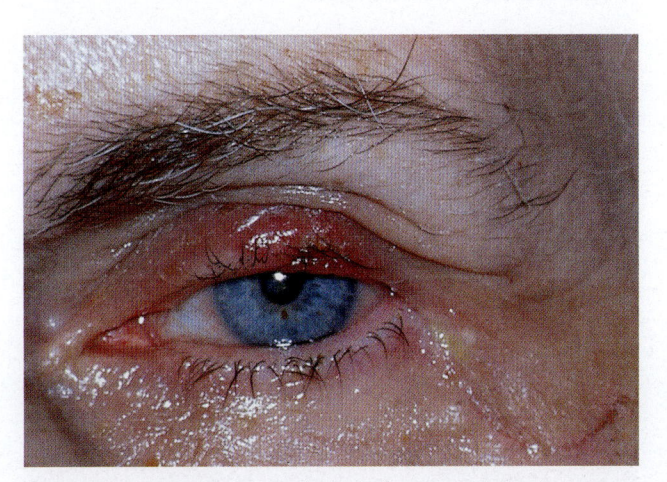

Figure 3.60. Appearance 2 weeks later after suture removal.

EYELID SEBACEOUS CARCINOMA: LARGE TUMOR AND ROTATIONAL FOREHEAD FLAP

After removal of larger tumors near the medial aspect of the eyelid, a rotational forehead flap may be required to achieve satisfactory closure of the wound. A clinicopathologic correlation of a tumor managed by this technique is presented.

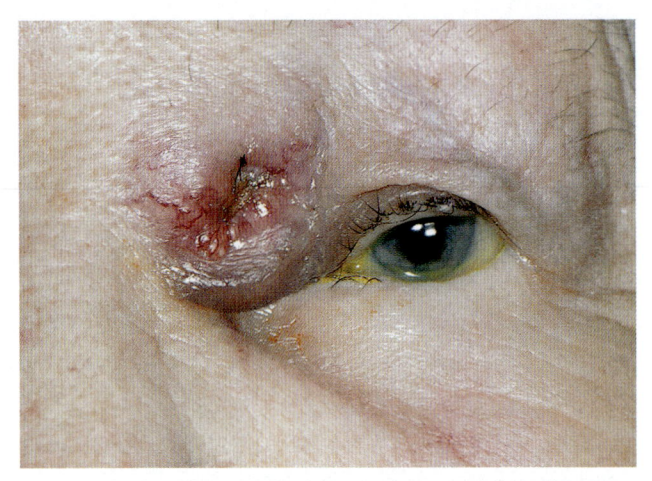

Figure 3.61. Nodular excoriated lesion above medial canthus in an 80-year-old woman. A punch biopsy confirmed the diagnosis of sebaceous carcinoma.

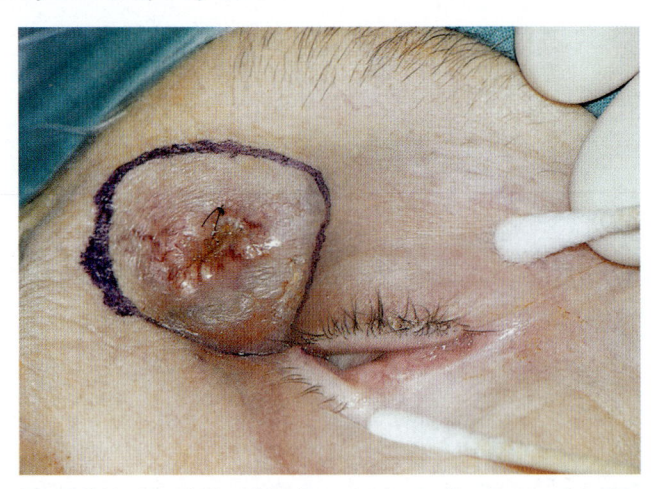

Figure 3.62. A sterile pencil has been used to outline the tumor margins.

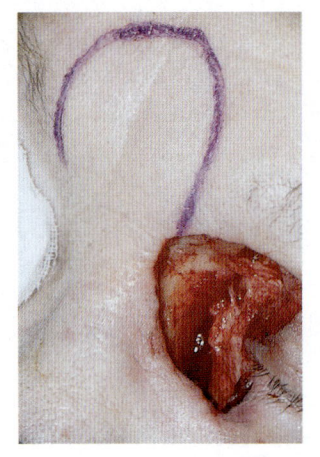

Figure 3.63. The tumor has been removed and frozen section margins are negative. A semicircular incision is outlined to rotate normal skin from the forehead to cover the defect.

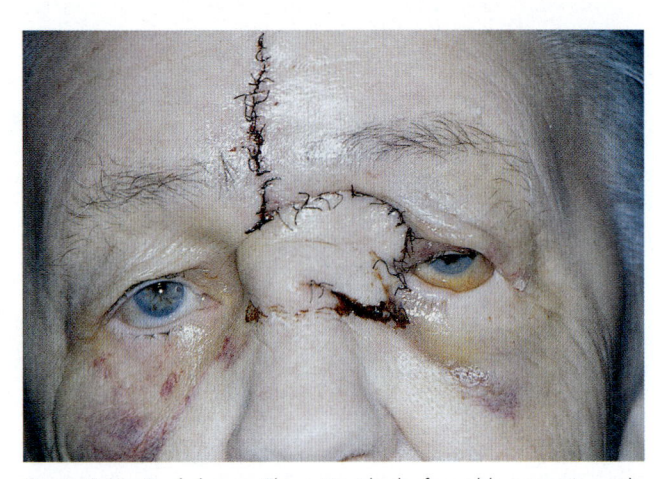

Figure 3.64. Final closure. The patient had a favorable cosmetic result. Posttreatment photographs are not available.

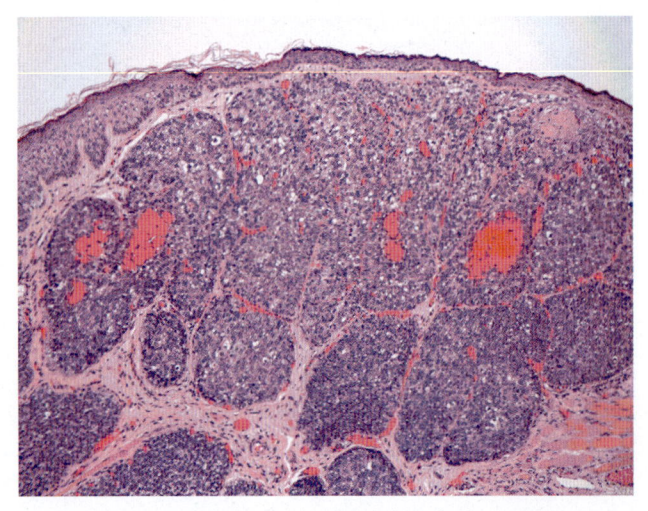

Figure 3.65. Histopathology showing lobules of sebaceous carcinoma with lipid vacuoles and large vessels. (Hematoxylin-eosin ×50.)

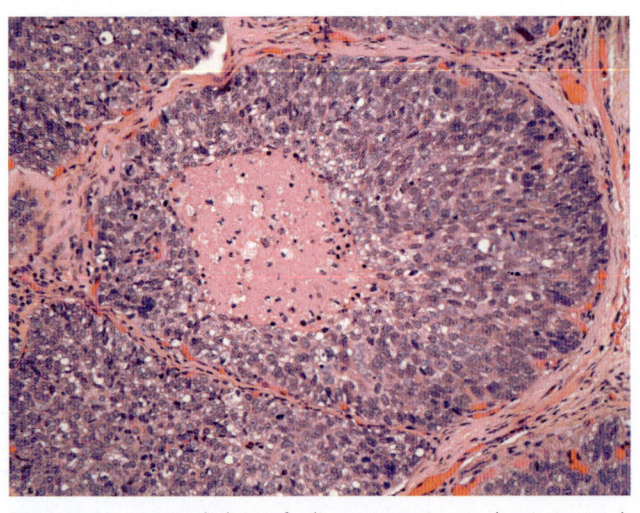

Figure 3.66. Histopathology of sebaceous carcinoma showing comedocarcinoma pattern. (Hematoxylin-eosin ×200.)

Chapter 3 Eyelid Sebaceous Gland Tumors

EYELID SEBACEOUS CARCINOMA: POSTERIOR LAMELLAR EYELID RESECTION AND RECONSTRUCTION

Although surgery is somewhat difficult, posterior lamellar eyelid resection may be a reasonable alternative to orbital exenteration, particularly in older patients who have useful vision in the ipsilateral eye. The technique of map biopsies for diffuse sebaceous carcinoma is shown and can be used for surgical planning.

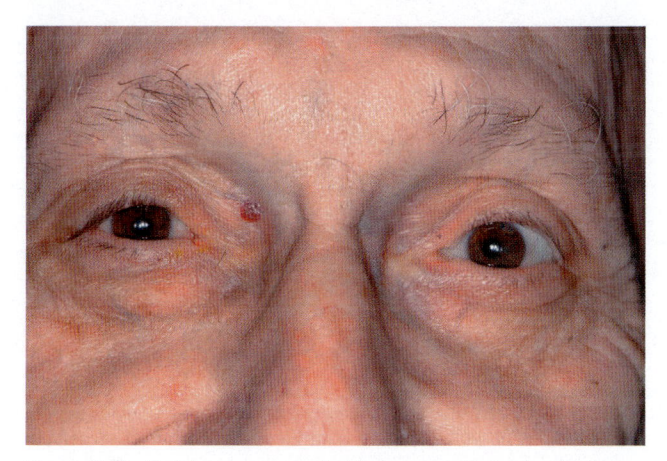

Figure 3.67. Facial appearance of elderly man with foreign body sensation in right eye.

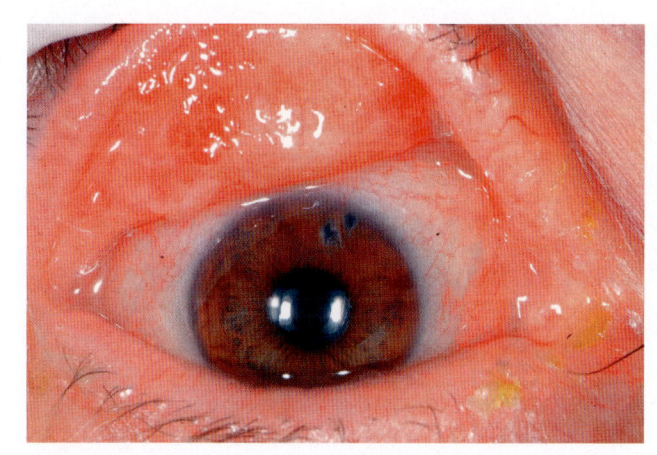

Figure 3.68. Everted eyelid showing diffuse sebaceous carcinoma of entire upper tarsus.

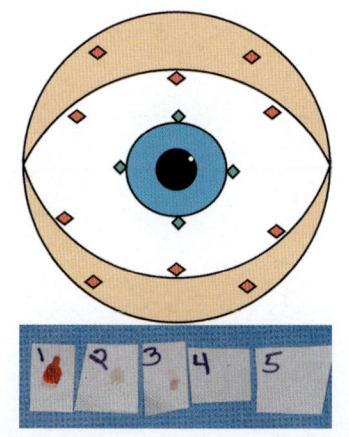

Figure 3.69. Diagram showing technique of map biopsies. Inset shows some of the map biopsy specimens being placed on squares of paper. They are placed separately in fixative and submitted for permanent sections.

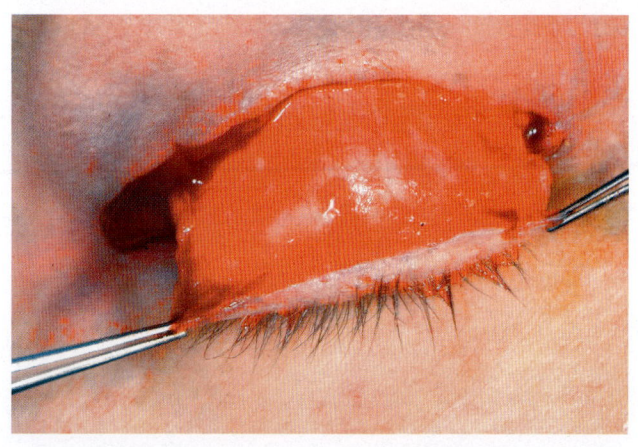

Figure 3.70. Resection of one entire upper eyelid posterior lamella, including conjunctiva and tarsus, but sparing orbicularis muscle and skin.

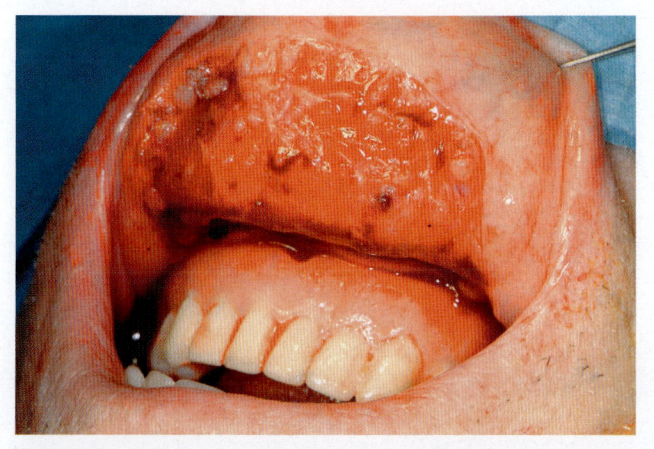

Figure 3.71. Buccal mucosal graft taken from inside mouth.

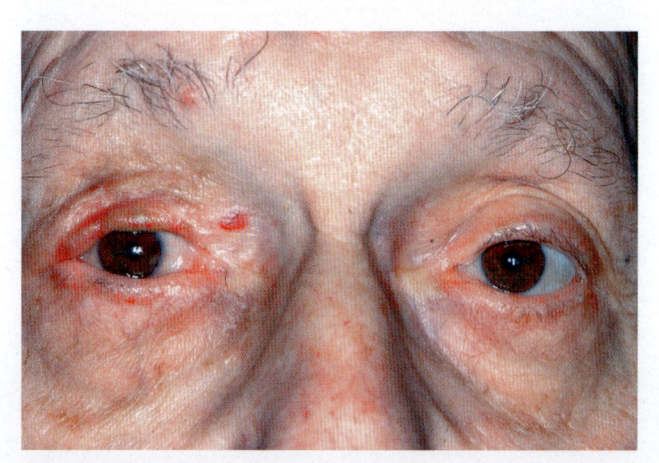

Figure 3.72. Appearance 2 months later. The eyelid has healed and patient is comfortable. There was no evidence of tumor recurrence.

TUMORS OF THE EYELIDS

EYELID SWEAT GLAND TUMORS

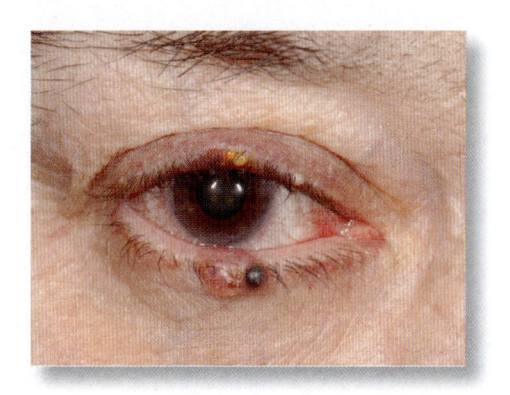

General Considerations

Simple cysts of eccrine or apocrine sweat glands are called eccrine hidrocystoma or apocrine hidrocystoma, respectively (see Chapter 11). Herein, we discuss solid tumors derived from sweat gland epithelium, beginning with syringoma.

Syringoma is a common benign tumor of eccrine sweat gland origin (1–12). About 20% occur on the eyelids (2). It occurs more often in young adult women and has a slight predilection for Asians.

Clinical Features

Syringoma can be solitary or multiple. The multiple variant is more common and is often bilateral, symmetric, and most pronounced on the lower eyelid. They are often subtle and hardly noticed by the patient. Multiple syringomas each ranges from 1 to 3 mm in size and have a yellow-brown color. Multiple syringomas are usually not associated with other conditions. However, some reports indicate that it is more common in patients with Down's syndrome (3,4), Marfan's syndrome, and Ehlers–Danlos syndrome.

Differential Diagnosis

Differential diagnosis includes most of the eyelid lesions discussed in this atlas. Solitary lesions can simulate basal cell carcinoma, sebaceous adenoma, and sebaceous carcinoma. The multiple variety can simulate trichoepithelioma, milium, sarcoidosis, and other conditions.

Pathology

Based on histochemical and electron microscopic findings, syringoma represents an adenoma of eccrine ducts (5). It is composed of cords and nests of solid cells with ducts located within a dense fibrous tissue stroma. The ducts are lined by a double layer of compressed epithelial cells that sometimes assume a comma-shaped or "tadpole" appearance, a feature considered characteristic of this condition. Numerous cystic dilations of the ducts can result in keratin cysts that can suggest the diagnosis of milium, trichoepithelioma, or squamous cell carcinoma. The keratin cysts can rupture and incite a granulomatous inflammatory reaction. Concerning pathogenesis, human papillomavirus types have been detected in solitary eyelid syringoma, suggesting a viral etiology (12).

Management

Management is usually observation. Cosmetics can improve appearance. A larger solitary lesion may require surgical excision to rule out malignancy. Other methods of management include electrodessication and curettage, dermabrasion, and carbon dioxide laser resurfacing (6–11). Some authors have advocated combination of carbon dioxide laser and trichloroacetic acid (10). Although solitary syringoma is cytologically benign, it can recur after incomplete excision and exhibit aggressive behavior.

EYELID SYRINGOMA

Selected References

Reviews
1. Ozdal PC, Callejo SA, Codere F, et al. Benign ocular adnexal tumours of apocrine, eccrine or hair follicle origin. I. 2003;38:357–363.
2. Patrizi A, Neri I, Marzaduri S, et al. Syringoma: a review of twenty-nine cases. *Acta Dermatol Venereol* 1998;78:460–462.
3. Schepis C, Siragusa M, et al. Palpebral syringomas and Down's syndrome. *Dermatology* 1994;189:248–250.
4. Urban CD, Cannon JR, Cole RD. Eruptive syringomas in Down's syndrome. *Arch Dermatol* 1981;117:374.
5. Hashimoto K, Gross BF, Lever WF. Syringoma. *J Invest Dermatol* 1966;46:150–166.

Management
6. Maloney ME. An easy method for removal of syringoma. *J Dermatol Surg Oncol* 1982;8:973–975.
7. Stevenson TR, Swanson NA. Syringoma: removal by electrodessication and curettage. *Ann Plast Surg* 1985;15:151–154.
8. Apfelberg DB, Maser MR, Lash H, et al. Superpulse CO2 laser treatment of facial syringomata. *Lasers Surg Med* 1987;7:533–537.
9. Wang JI, Roenigk HH Jr. Treatment of multiple facial syringomas with the carbon dioxide (CO2) laser. *Dermatol Surg* 1999;25:136–139.
10. Kang WH, Kim NS, Kim YB, et al. A new treatment for syringoma. Combination of carbon dioxide laser and trichloroacetic acid. *Dermatol Surg* 1998;24:1370–1374.
11. Karam P, Benedetto AV. Syringomas: new approach to an old technique. *Int J Dermatol* 1996;35:219–220.

Histopathology
12. Assadoullina A, Bialasiewicz AA, de Villiers EM, et al. Detection of HPV-20, HPV-23, and HPV-DL332 in a solitary eyelid syringoma. *Am J Ophthalmol* 2000;129:99–101.

EYELID SYRINGOMA

Syringoma can be multiple or solitary. Although syringoma is almost always benign, low-grade malignant behavior can rarely occur.

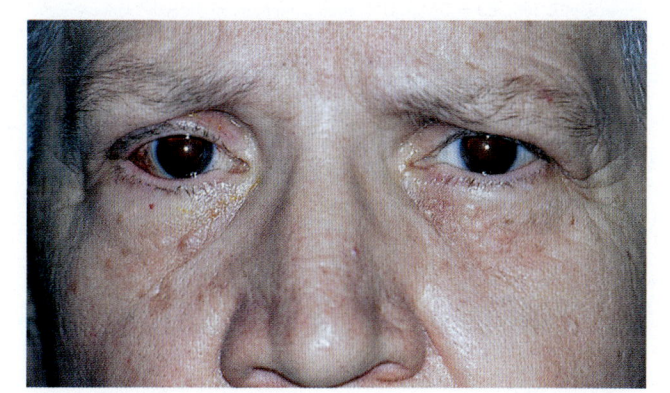

Figure 4.1. Subtle, bilateral syringoma involving the lower eyelids in a 70-year-old woman.

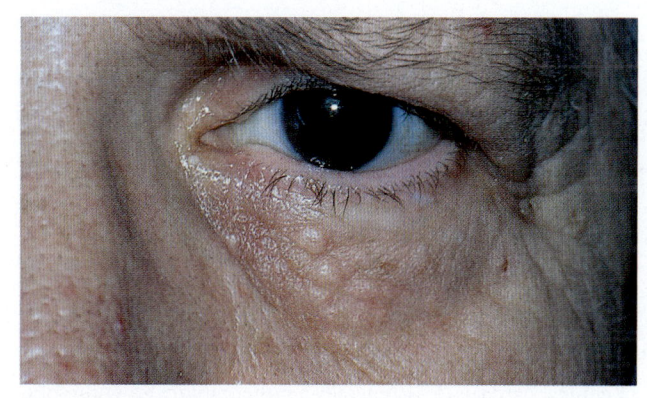

Figure 4.2. Closer view of left eye of patient seen in Figure 4.1, showing elevated tan-colored lesions, similar in color to the adjacent normal skin.

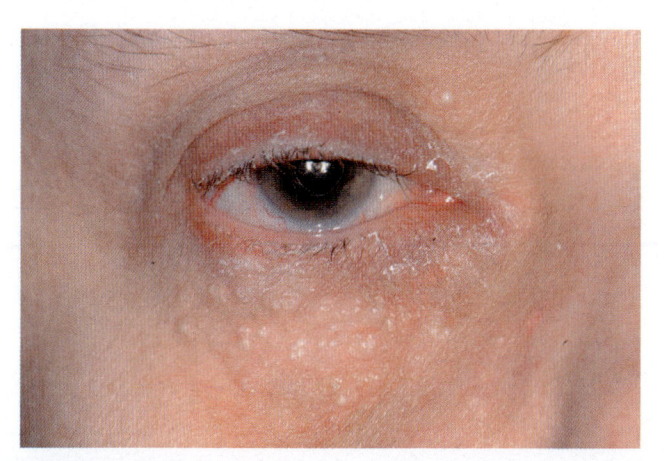

Figure 4.3. Multiple, visible syringomas on lower eyelid and cheek of a 50-year-old woman.

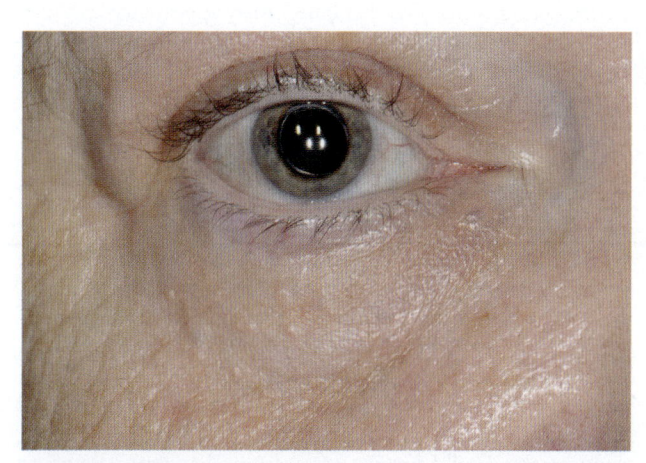

Figure 4.4. Multiple, subtle syringomas on lower eyelid and cheek of a 57-year-old woman.

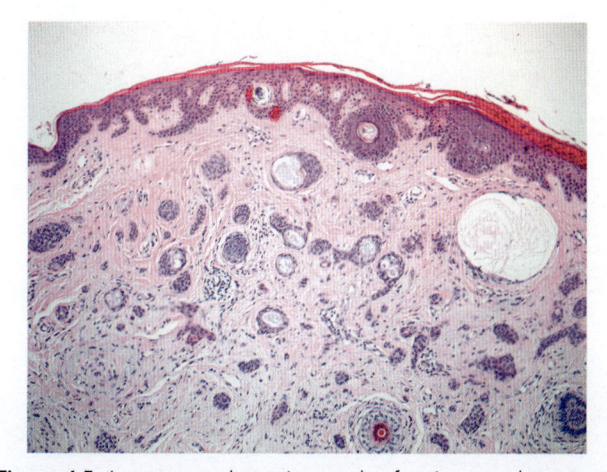

Figure 4.5. Low-power photomicrograph of syringoma demonstrating cords and nests of cells with ducts infiltrating dense fibrous tissue. (Hematoxylin–eosin ×10.)

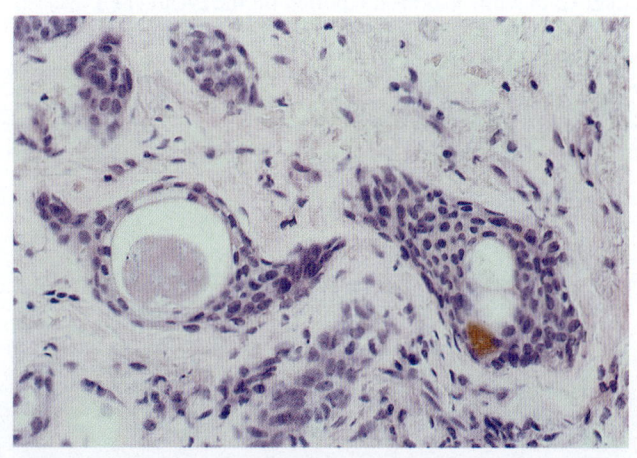

Figure 4.6. High-power photomicrograph of syringoma showing arrangement of ducts and tubules of epithelial cells, with lightly eosinophilic material in lumen. (Hematoxylin–eosin ×200.)

EYELID ECCRINE ACROSPIROMA

General Considerations

Eccrine acrospiroma (also called clear cell hydradenoma, eccrine hydradenoma, and porosyringoma) is a tumor that arises from duct and secretory coil of the eccrine sweat gland (1–15). It is usually solitary and can occur in all parts of the body, with the face and ears being affected in about 10% of cases. It can be nodular, solid, or cystic. Although the majority are benign, a malignant variant has been observed. The terminology regarding this lesion has been the source of some confusion, but "eccrine acrospiroma" seems to be preferred.

Clinical Features

Eccrine acrospiroma of the eyelid can assume any of a variety of clinical patterns. It is generally a rather rapidly growing solid or cystic lesion that may attain a size of 5 to 30 mm (1–3). A smaller lesion may be similar in color to the normal adjacent skin or it may appear as a fleshy subcutaneous mass. A larger eccrine acrospiroma often has blue, crusty appearance and may sometimes become ulcerated. Pain on pressure can be elicited in about 20% of cases. The tumor can occasionally show aggressive growth and invade the conjunctiva and orbit (12).

Pathology

Histopathologically, eccrine acrospiroma has characteristic features (1–6). It is a well-circumscribed lesion deep to the epidermis composed of lobules of epithelial cells that demonstrate a biphasic pattern. One pattern is composed of foci of round to ovoid cells with clear cytoplasm that contain glycogen. The other is composed of closely compact spindle-shaped cells with eosinophilic cytoplasm. In some areas, tumor cells merge with the overlying acanthotic epithelium. Enzyme histochemical and electron microscopic studies have established its eccrine gland origin. Eyelid eccrine acrospiroma has been shown to exhibit oncocytic, apocrine, and sebaceous differentiation, attesting the pluripotentiality of adnexal glandular epithelia (13). Eccrine poroma, a similar tumor that arises from sweat duct epithelium, has been reported on the eyelid (11).

Management

Management of eccrine acrospiroma is complete surgical excision. The diagnosis is not usually suspected clinically and is made on histopathologic evaluation. The prognosis is excellent.

Selected References

Reviews

1. Ozdal PC, Callejo SA, Codere F, et al. Benign ocular adnexal tumours of apocrine, eccrine or hair follicle origin. *Can J Ophthalmol* 2003;38:357–363.
2. Wong TY, Suster S, Cheek RF, et al. Benign cutaneous adnexal tumors with combined folliculosebaceous, apocrine, and eccrine differentiation. Clinicopathologic and immunohistochemical study of eight cases. *Am J Dermatopathol* 1996;18:124–136.
3. Massa MC, Medenica M. Cutaneous adnexal tumors and cysts: a review. Part II – Tumors with apocrine and eccrine glandular differentiation and miscellaneous cutaneous cysts. *Pathol Annu* 1987;22:225–276.

Imaging

4. Furuta M, Shields CL, Danzig CJ, et al. Ultrasound biomicroscopy of eyelid eccrine hidrocystoma. *Can J Ophthalmol* 2007;42(5):750–751.

Histopathology

5. Buchi ER, Peng Y, Eng AM, et al. Eccrine acrospiroma of the eyelid with oncocytic, apocrine and sebaceous differentiation. Further evidence for pluripotentiality of the adnexal epithelia. *Eur J Ophthalmol* 1991;1:187–193.
6. Agarwal S, Agarwal K, Kathuria P, et al. Cytomorphological features of nodular hidradenoma highlighting eccrine differentiation: a case report. *Indian J Pathol Microbiol* 2006;49(3):411–413.

Case Reports

7. Boniuk M, Halpert B. Clear cell hidradenoma or myoepithelioma of the eyelid. *Arch Ophthalmol* 1964;72:59–63.
8. Ferry AP, Haddad HM. Eccrine acrospiroma (porosyringoma) of the eyelid. *Arch Ophthalmol* 1970;83:591–593.
9. Grossniklaus HE, Knight SH. Eccrine acrospiroma (clear cell hidradenoma) of the eyelid. Immunohistochemical and ultrastructural features. *Ophthalmology* 1991;98:347–352.
10. Johnson BL Jr, Helwig EB. Eccrine acrospiroma. A clinicopathologic study. *Cancer* 1969;23:641–657.
11. Vu PP, Whitehead KJ, Sullivan TJ. Eccrine poroma of the eyelid. *Clin Exp Ophthalmol* 2001;29:253–255.
12. Jagannath C, Sandhya CS, Venugopalachari K. Eccrine acrospiroma of eyelid—a case report. *Indian J Ophthalmol* 1990;38:182.
13. Haneveld GT, Hamburg A. Sweat gland tumour of the eyelid with conjunctival involvement. *Ophthalmologica* 1979;179:73–76.
14. Jain R, Prabhakaran VC, Huilgol SC, et al. Eccrine porocarcinoma of the upper eyelid. *Ophthal Plast Reconstr Surg* 2008;24(3):221–223.
15. Boynton JR, Markowitch W Jr. Porocarcinoma of the eyelid. *Ophthalmology* 1997;104(10):1626–1628.

ECCRINE ACROSPIROMA

Unlike a simple eccrine hidrocystoma, eccrine acrospiroma is a solid tumor clinically, although it can sometimes have a cystic component. It can assume a variety of clinical configurations.

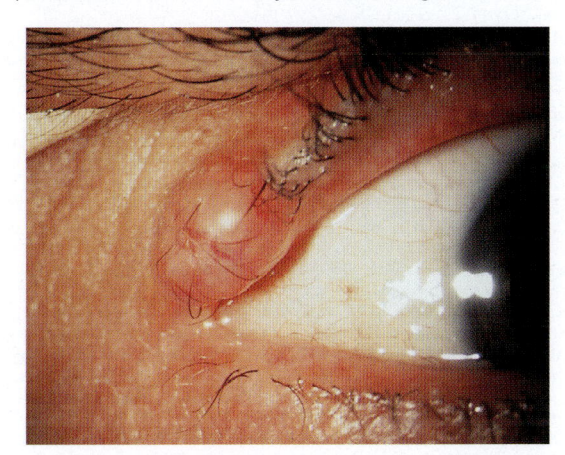

Figure 4.7. Eccrine acrospiroma of upper eyelid of a 75-year-old man. The mass appears as a slightly fleshy nodule deep to the epidermis.

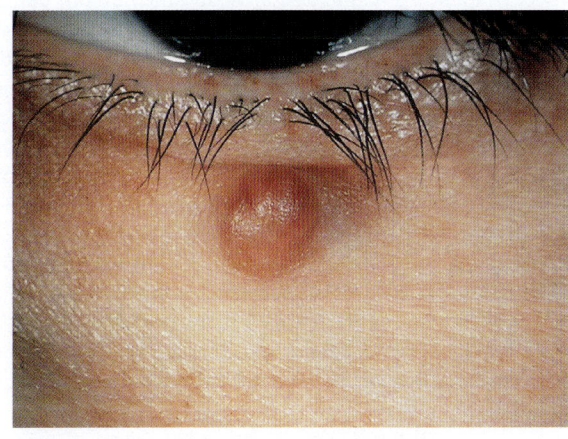

Figure 4.8. Eccrine acrospiroma in lower eyelid. (Courtesy of Ramon Font, MD.)

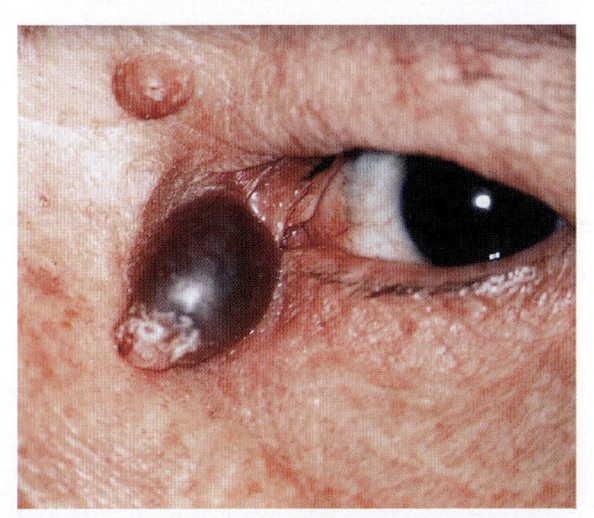

Figure 4.9. Larger, blue-colored eccrine acrospiroma near medial canthus in an elderly person. The lesion had a large cystic component. The smaller solid lesion above is possibly a nevus or papilloma. (Courtesy of Armed Forces Institute of Pathology, Washington, DC.)

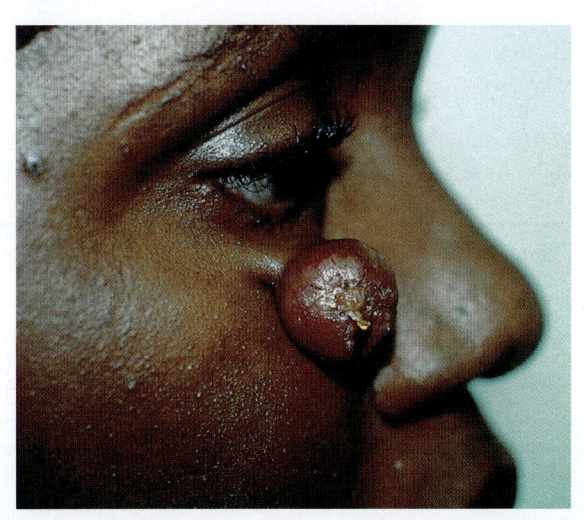

Figure 4.10. Pedunculated eccrine acrospiroma below lower eyelid of a 19-year-old girl. The lesion had been slowly enlarging for 1 year. (Courtesy of Steven Searl, MD.)

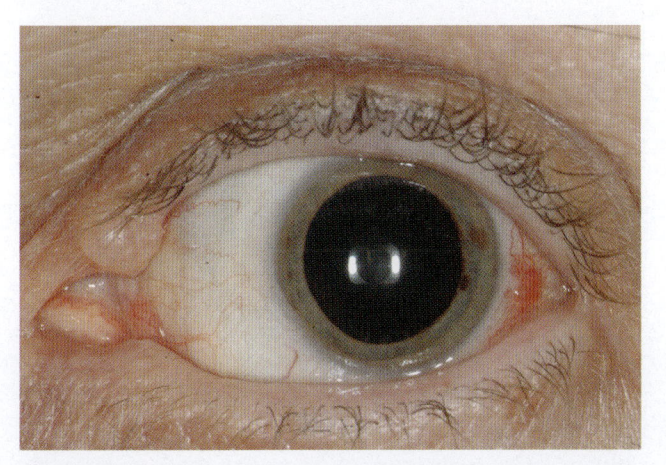

Figure 4.11. Solid eccrine acrospiroma of left upper eyelid in an elderly male.

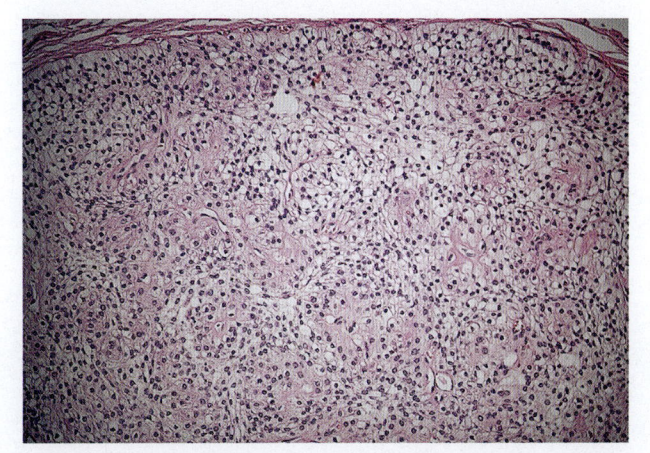

Figure 4.12. Histopathology of eccrine acrospiroma showing biphasic pattern of epithelial cells. Note the intermixing of spindle cells with eosinophilic cytoplasm and more rounded cells with clear cytoplasm. (Hematoxylin–eosin ×75.)

EYELID SYRINGOCYSTADENOMA PAPILLIFERUM

General Considerations

Syringocystadenoma papilliferum is an uncommon benign tumor that arises from apocrine glands (1–17). It occurs most often on the scalp and temple and only occasionally on the eyelid, where it presumably arises from the apocrine glands of Moll. In one series, it accounted for 2% of ocular adnexal tumors of apocrine, eccrine, or hair follicle origin (1). In about 75% of cases, it arises during puberty within a nevus sebaceous of Jadassohn; thus, it may be a component of the organoid nevus syndrome (8,14). When it is confined to the eyelid, it is often a solitary lesion that appears in middle age and is not usually associated with nevus sebaceous of Jadassohn (9). It is believed by some authors that syringocystadenoma papilliferum can evolve into basal cell carcinoma and that it may represent a transition phase between nevus sebaceous of Jadassohn and basal cell carcinoma (13).

Clinical Features

Clinically, syringocystadenoma papilliferum begins as a plaque-like lesion that gradually becomes more elevated and assumes a verrucous or papillomatous configuration. A central ulceration, similar to that seen with basal cell carcinoma, may occur (10). The differential diagnosis includes basal cell carcinoma, squamous cell carcinoma, keratoacanthoma, and other sweat gland and hair follicle neoplasms.

Pathology

Histopathologically, syringocystadenoma papilliferum is a papillomatous lesion with keratinizing epithelial-lined ducts that open on the skin surface. The cells lining the ducts exhibit decapitation secretion, characteristic of apocrine cells, and characteristic papillary projections that extend into the duct-like spaces. Another characteristic feature is infiltration of chronic inflammatory cells, mostly plasma cells, in the connective tissue pores of the papillae. Electron microscopic findings support the apocrine gland origin of this lesion (9).

Management

The management of suspected syringocystadenoma papilliferum is complete surgical resection. The role of supplemental irradiation of other methods of treatment is not clearly established.

Selected References

Reviews

1. Ozdal PC, Callejo SA, Codere F, et al. Benign ocular adnexal tumours of apocrine, eccrine or hair follicle origin. *Can J Ophthalmol* 2003;38:357–363.
2. Wong TY, Suster S, Cheek RF, et al. Benign cutaneous adnexal tumors with combined folliculosebaceous, apocrine, and eccrine differentiation. Clinicopathologic and immunohistochemical study of eight cases. *Am J Dermatopathol* 1996;18:124–136.
3. Massa MC, Medenica M. Cutaneous adnexal tumors and cysts: a review. Part II – Tumors with apocrine and eccrine glandular differentiation and miscellaneous cutaneous cysts. *Pathol Annu* 1987;22:225–276.
4. Al-Faky YH. Epidemiology of benign eyelid lesions in patients presenting to a teaching hospital. *Saudi J Ophthalmol* 2012;26(2):211–216.
5. Rammeh-Rommani S, Fezaa B, Chelbi E, et al. Syringocystadenoma papilliferum: report of 8 cases. *Pathologica* 2006;98(3):178–180.

Histopathology

6. Ni C, Dryja TP, Albert DM. Sweat gland tumor in the eyelids: a clinicopathological analysis of 55 cases. *Int Ophthalmol Clin* 1981;23:1–22.
7. Helmi A, Alaraj AM, Alkatan H. Report of 3 histopathologically documented cases of syringocystadenoma papilliferum involving the eyelid. *Can J Ophthalmol* 2011;46(3):287–289.

Case Reports

8. Helwig EB, Hackney VC. Syringoadenoma papilliferum—lesions with and without naevus sebaceus and basal cell carcinoma. *Arch Dermatol* 1995;71:361–372.
9. Jakobiec FA, Streeten BW, Iwamoto T, et al. Syringocystadenoma papilliferum of the eyelid. *Ophthalmology* 1981;88:1175–1181.
10. Perlman JI, Urban RC, Edward DP, et al. Syringocystadenoma papilliferum of the eyelid. *Am J Ophthalmol* 1994;117:647–650.
11. Johnson BL, Buerger GF Jr. Syringocystadenoma papilliferum of the eyelid. *Am J Ophthalmol* 1994;118:822–823.
12. Rao VA, Kamath GG, Kumar A. An unusual case of syringocystadenoma papilliferum of the eyelid. *Indian J Ophthalmol* 1996;44:168–169.
13. Askar S, Kilinc N, Aytekin S. Syringocystadenoma papilliferum mimicking basal cell carcinoma on the lower eyelid: a case report. *Acta Chir Plast* 2002;44:117–119.
14. Shields JA, Shields CL, Eagle RC Jr, et al. Ocular manifestations of the organoid nevus syndrome. *Ophthalmology* 1997;104:549–557.
15. Shams PN, Hardy TG, El-Bahrawy M, et al. Syringocystadenoma papilliferum of the eyelid in a young girl. *Ophthal Plast Reconstr Surg* 2006;22(1):67–69.
16. Abanmi A, Joshi RK, Atukorala D, et al. Syringocystadenoma papilliferum mimicking basal cell carcinoma. *J Am Acad Dermatol* 1994;30(1):127–128.
17. Fujita M, Kobayashi M. Syringocystadenoma papilliferum associated with poroma folliculare. *J Dermatol* 1986;13(6):480–482.

EYELID SYRINGOCYSTADENOMA PAPILLIFERUM

Perlman JI, Urban RC, Edward DP, et al. Syringocystadenoma papilliferum of the eyelid. *Am J Ophthalmol* 1994;117:647–650.

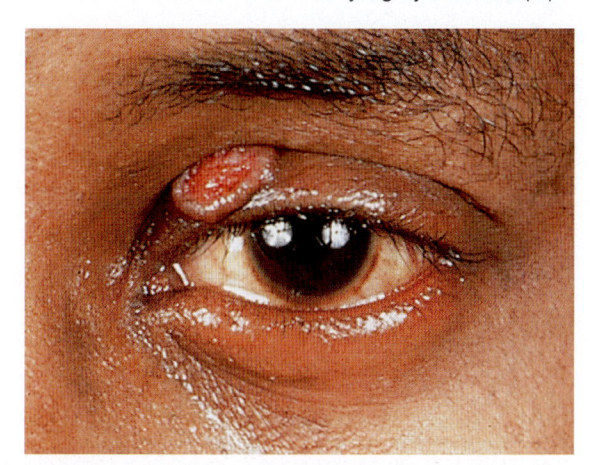

Figure 4.13. Syringocystadenoma papilliferum presenting on the upper eyelid of a 31-year-old man. (Courtesy of Jay Perlman, MD.)

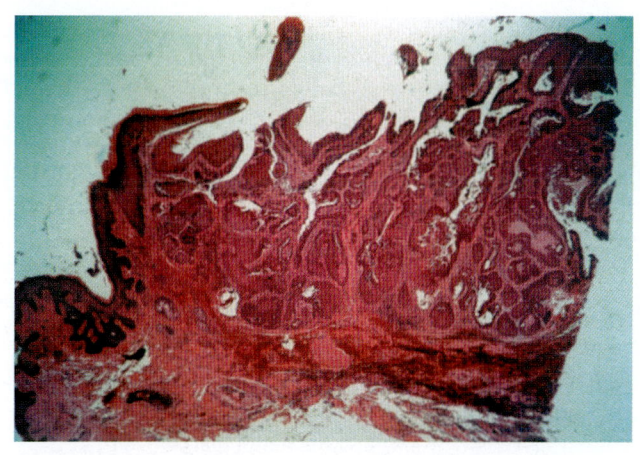

Figure 4.14. Low magnification of lesion shown in Figure 43.1 discloses papillomatous lesion with keratinizing epithelial-lined ducts that open on the skin surface. (Courtesy of Jay Perlman, MD.)

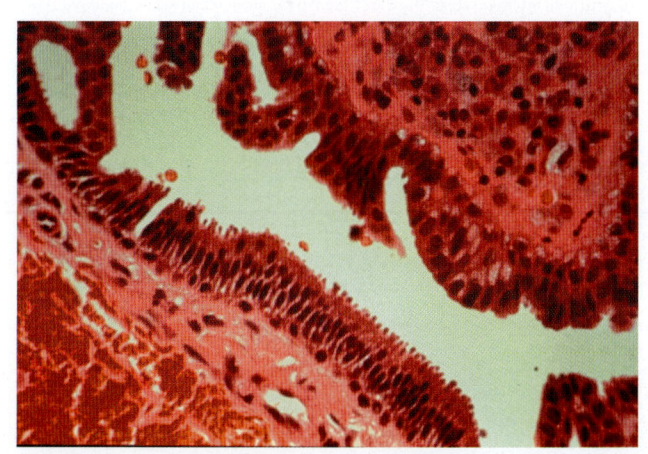

Figure 4.15. Higher magnification of lesion shown in Figure 4.13 showing epithelium lining the ducts that exhibit decapitation secretion, characteristic of apocrine cells. (Courtesy of Jay Perlman, MD.)

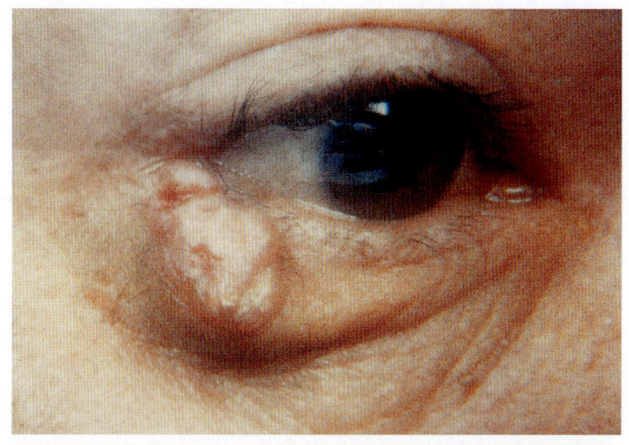

Figure 4.16. Syringocystadenoma papilliferum of lower eyelid of a 46-year-old man.

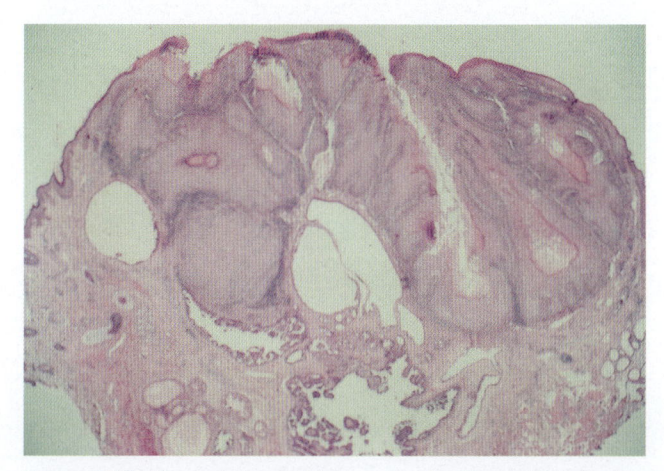

Figure 4.17. Histopathology of lesion seen in Figure 4.16 showing elevated papillomatous lesion with hyperkeratosis and central crater. (Hematoxylin–eosin ×10.)

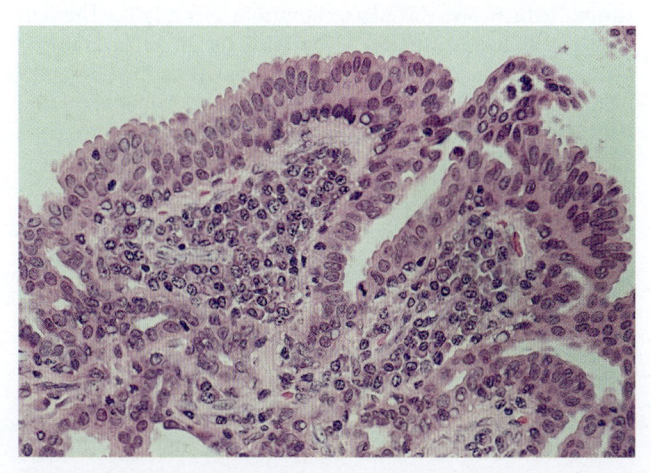

Figure 4.18. Histopathology of lesion shown in Figure 4.16 demonstrating epithelium of apocrine cells with inflammatory infiltrate in the dermis. (Hematoxylin–eosin ×75.)

EYELID PLEOMORPHIC ADENOMA (BENIGN MIXED TUMOR)

General Considerations

Pleomorphic adenoma (benign mixed tumor) is neoplasm that most often occurs in a salivary gland or lacrimal gland (1–12). In some instances, it can arise from either eccrine or apocrine glands of the skin. This tumor was previously called chondroid syringoma based on the terminology by Hirsch and Helwig in 1961, but not all contain cartilage so the preferred term is pleomorphic adenoma (4,12). This tumor can occasionally arise in the eyelid. In a series of 188 tumors, 7 arose in the eyebrow and 1 in the eyelid (4). Like similar tumors of the salivary and lacrimal glands, this tumor can occasionally undergo malignant transformation into pleomorphic adenocarcinoma (malignant mixed tumor) (6). Mandeville et al. (1) reviewed nine cases with eyelid involvement and provided a review of the literature. Palioura et al. described a cystic lesion that arose from an apocrine gland (gland of Moll) at the eyelid margin (12).

Clinical Features

Clinically, eyelid pleomorphic adenoma appears as a slowly enlarging nontender solitary or multilobulated subcutaneous mass that varies in size from 4 to 17 mm at the time of clinical diagnosis. In a collaborative report of nine patients with ocular adnexal lesions, four were at the eyelid margin, three were in the sub-eyebrow area of the upper eyelid, and two in the central eyelids (1). All six cases that did not affect the eyebrow were fixed to the tarsus. None of the lesions was associated with significant changes of the overlying epidermis, although one lesion showed overlying pigmentation. This tumor has no specific clinical features and may be impossible to differentiate clinically from other subcutaneous eyelid lesions.

Pathology

Histopathologically, the eyelid tumor has features identical to pleomorphic adenoma of the lacrimal gland. As the name implies, it has epithelial and mesenchymal components. The glandular epithelial cells form islands or cords in a mucoid stroma, which often displays chondroid metaplasia. The epithelial cells form a double layer, with the inner layer being secretory and the outer layer myoepithelial in nature (12). Like pleomorphic adenoma of the lacrimal gland, areas of malignant transformation can be detected in the eyelid counterpart, although it is less common.

Management

The management of pleomorphic adenoma of the eyelid is complete surgical removal. The diagnosis is rarely suspected clinical and is diagnosed histopathologically after surgical removal. Prognosis is generally excellent (1). Although eyelid lesions rarely undergo malignant change, benign mixed tumors in the extremities or back can metastasize locally and hematogenously (2).

Selected References

Reviews

1. Mandeville JT, Roh JH, Woog JJ, et al. Cutaneous benign mixed tumor (chondroid syringoma) of the eyelid: clinical presentation and management. *Ophthal Plast Reconstr Surg* 2004;20:110–116.
2. Ishimura E, Iwamoto H, Kobushi Y, et al. Malignant chondroid syringoma. Report of a case with widespread metastases and review of pertinent literature. *Cancer* 1983;52:1966–1973.
3. Gündüz K, Demirel S, Heper AO, et al. A rare case of atypical chondroid syringoma of the lower eyelid and review of the literature. *Surv Ophthalmol* 2006;51(3):280–285.
4. Hirsch P, Helwig EB. Chondroid syringoma: mixed tumor of the skin, salivary gland type. *Arch Dermatol* 1961;84:835–847.
5. Kuo YL, Tu TY, Chang CF, et al. Extra-major salivary gland pleomorphic adenoma of the head and neck: a 10-year experience and review of the literature. *Eur Arch Otorhinolaryngol* 2011;268(7):1035–1040.

Case Reports

6. Hilton JMN, Blackwell JB. Metastasizing chondroid syringoma. *J Pathol* 1973;109:167–169.
7. Daicker S, Gafner E. Apocrine mixed tumour of the lid. *Ophthalmologica* 1975:170:548–553.
8. Jordan DR, Nerad JA, Patrinely JR. Chondroid syringoma of the eyelid. *Can J Ophthalmol* 1989;24:24–27.
9. Martorina M, Capoferri C, Dessanti P. Chondroid syringoma of the eyelid. *Int Ophthalmol* 1993;17:285–288.
10. Tyagi N, Abdi U, Tyagi SP, et al. Pleomorphic adenoma of skin (chondroid syringoma) involving the eyelid. *J Postgrad Med* 1996;42:125–126.
11. Mencia-Gutierrez E, Bonales-Daimiel JA, Gutierrez-Diaz E, et al. Chondroid syringomas of the eyelid: two cases. *Eur J Ophthalmol* 2001;11:80–82.
12. Palioura S, Jakobiec FA, Zakka FR, et al. Pleomorphic adenoma (formerly chondroid syringoma) of the eyelid margin with a pseudocystic appearance. *Surv Ophthalmol* 2013;58(5):486–491.

Chapter 4 Eyelid Sweat Gland Tumors

EYELID PLEOMORPHIC ADENOMA (BENIGN MIXED TUMOR)

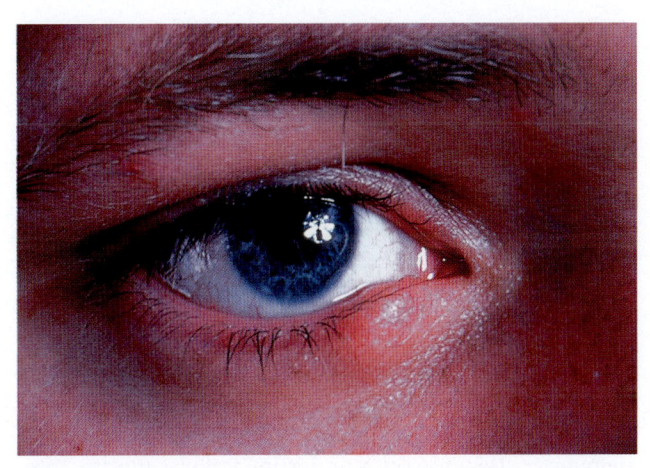

Figure 4.19. Pleomorphic adenoma in the lower eyelid in a young man. (Courtesy of Richard Collin, MD.)

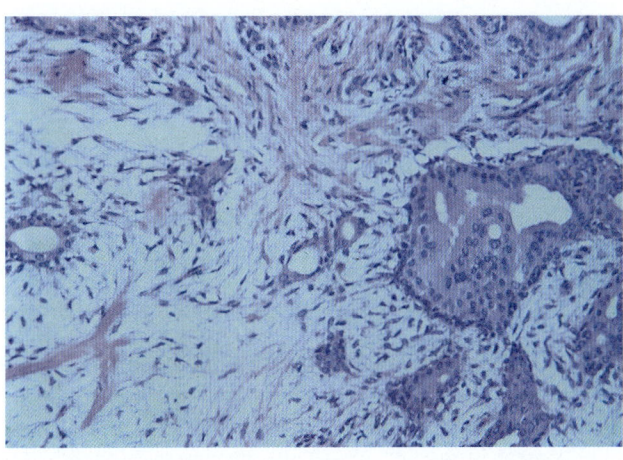

Figure 4.20. Histopathology of lesion shown in Figure 4.19, demonstrating the glandular and mesenchymal elements. (Hematoxylin–eosin ×100.) (Courtesy of Richard Collin, MD.)

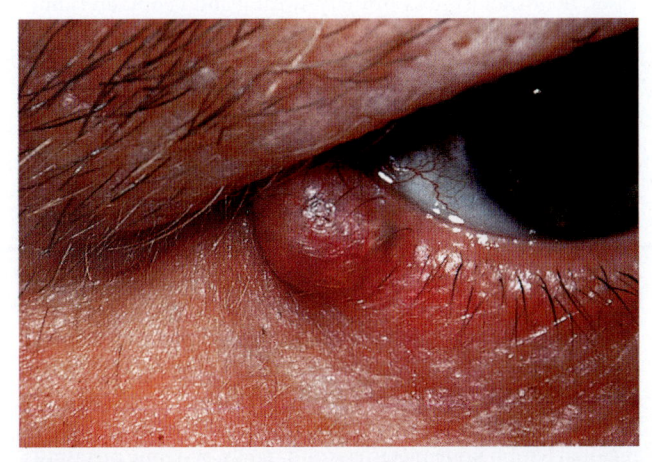

Figure 4.21. Pleomorphic adenoma near lateral aspect of lower eyelid of a 58-year-old man. (Courtesy of Ingolf Wallow, MD.)

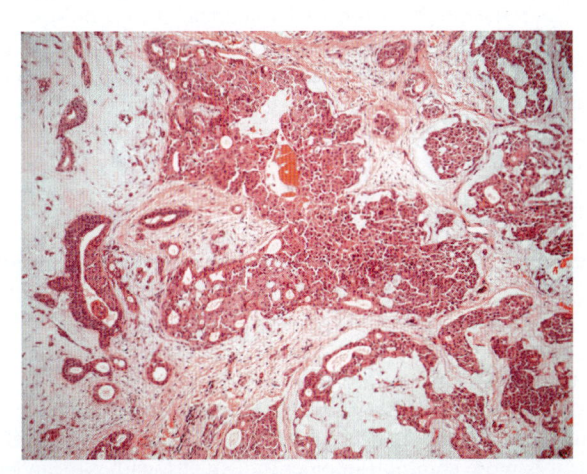

Figure 4.22. Histopathology of pleomorphic adenoma of eyelid, showing glandular, mesenchymal, and chondroid elements. (Hematoxylin–eosin ×100.)

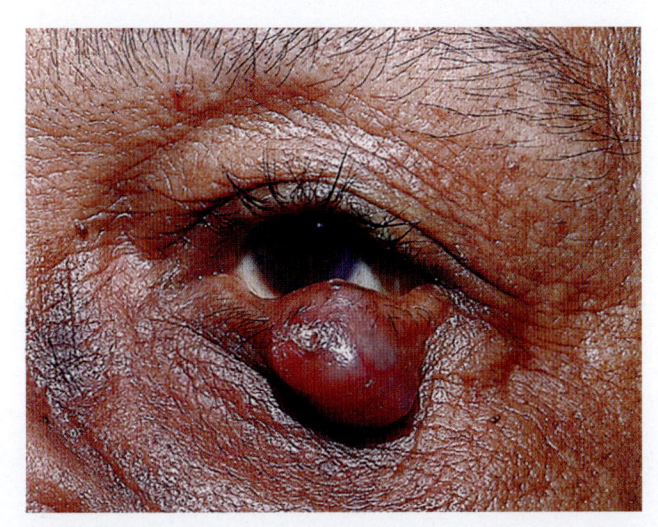

Figure 4.23. Pleomorphic adenoma in lower eyelid. (Courtesy of George Duncan, MD.)

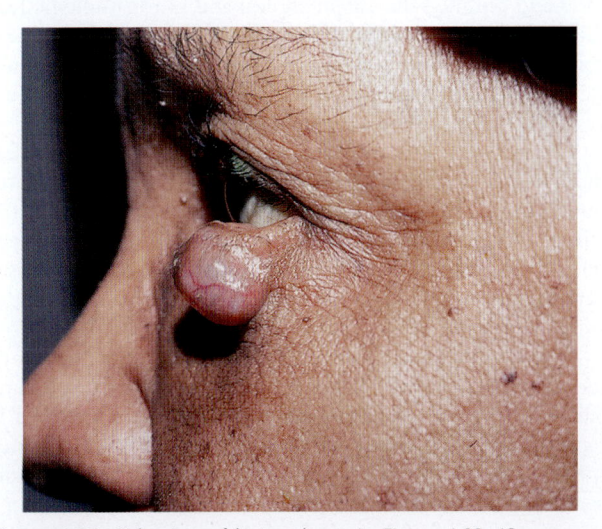

Figure 4.24. Side view of lesion shown in Figure 4.23. (Courtesy of George Duncan, MD.)

EYELID SWEAT GLAND ADENOCARCINOMA

General Considerations

Malignant neoplasms (adenocarcinomas) of sweat gland origin are sufficiently uncommon that, with few exceptions, most reports involve single case descriptions (1–30). The three most often reported malignant eyelid tumors of sweat gland origin are mucinous sweat gland adenocarcinoma, eccrine sweat gland adenocarcinoma, and apocrine adenocarcinoma of the glands of Moll (1–3). Each type has overlapping clinical features, and the diagnosis is often not suspected clinically. Furthermore, they may be difficult to confirm histopathologically, because they may be similar to other primary malignancies and similar to metastatic adenocarcinoma of the eyelid.

Mucinous sweat gland adenocarcinoma arises from the epidermal cells of eccrine sweat glands and is characterized by a high content of mucin (3,7–19,30). Eccrine sweat gland adenocarcinoma (also called "infiltrating signet ring carcinoma") is an unusual variant of adenocarcinoma of sweat gland origin that resembles mammary carcinoma histopathologically (1,22–24). Apocrine adenocarcinoma can occur in areas of the skin where apocrine glands are most dense, such as the perianal region, axilla, and the external auditory canal (ceruminous glands). In the eyelid, it originates in the apocrine glands of Moll (26–29).

Clinical Features

Each type of malignant sweat gland neoplasm begins as a small nodule that grows slowly and, if not controlled locally, has a capacity to recur locally and metastasize to region lymph nodes.

Mucinous sweat gland adenocarcinoma develops in the head and neck region in 75% and in the periorbital area in 40% of cases. It is more common in males with a 2:1 male to female ratio. Patients have ranged in age from 8 to 84 years, but it is more common in older individuals, with a mean age at diagnosis of 63 years (3,15). Although most information is derived from case reports, Wright and Font (3) reported 21 cases and outlined the salient clinical and histopathologic features of mucinous sweat gland adenocarcinoma. It is more common in the lower eyelid and appears as a pink to blue, elevated nodule that may be solid or cystic. It can resemble a cyst, basal cell carcinoma, or keratoacanthoma.

Eccrine sweat gland adenocarcinoma appears as a nodular, indurated subcutaneous mass that has an ill-defined, diffuse, infiltrating margin, and a blue to red color (22–24). When it affects the periocular area, it is most common in the lower eyelid and extends toward the canthal region. Porocarcinoma is a variant of sweat gland carcinoma that arises from the eccrine secretory apparatus (21).

In the eyelid area, apocrine adenocarcinoma develops from the apocrine glands of Moll near the base of the cilia. It is similar to other sweat gland and adnexal tumors, except that it is more likely to be located very near the eyelid margin corresponding to the glands of Moll, can resemble a chalazion, and can ulcerate (26–29).

Pathology

Mucinous sweat gland adenocarcinoma is characterized by lobules and cords of epithelial cells that float in pools of mucin, separated by thin fibrovascular septa (3,7–19,30). Less commonly, the mucin is largely confined to the epithelial cells and not in the extracellular spaces. The epithelial cells can sometimes form ductules or acini, imparting an "adenocystic appearance." Special stains and ultrastructural studies usually confirm the presence of mucin (sialomucin) and the eccrine origin of the tumor cells.

Eccrine sweat gland adenocarcinoma shows cords of atypical epithelial cells (5). The cytoplasm of the cells typically has a foamy or vacuolated appearance. In some cells, a large vacuole displaces the nucleus, producing a characteristic signet ring appearance. The vacuoles stain for intracellular mucin. These cells are said to be indistinguishable from those of the histiocytoid mammary carcinoma metastatic to the eyelid. In such cases, the diagnosis of a primary sweat gland neoplasm cannot be made until breast cancer has been excluded clinically.

Apocrine adenocarcinoma is characterized by a glandular arrangement of large cells with abundant eosinophilic cytoplasm and evidence of decapitation secretion (4). They are identical to the apocrine adenocarcinoma that occurs in the axilla.

Management

The best management of a malignant sweat gland neoplasm is wide surgical excision with frozen section or Mohs surgery to monitor the margins, similar to the management of basal cell carcinoma and other primary malignant eyelid tumors. If that is accomplished, the prognosis is favorable. However, incompletely excised lesions have a tendency toward local recurrence, regional lymph node metastasis and, rarely, systemic metastasis.

EYELID SWEAT GLAND ADENOCARCINOMA

Selected References

Reviews

1. Ni C, Dryja TP, Albert DM. Sweat gland tumors in the eyelids: a clinicopathological analysis of 55 cases. *Int Ophthalmol Clin* 1982;22:1–22.
2. Ni C, Wagoner M, Kieval S, et al. Tumours of the Moll's glands. *Br J Ophthalmol* 1984;68:502–506.
3. Wright JD, Font RL. Mucinous sweat gland adenocarcinoma of eyelid. A clinicopathologic study of 21 cases with histochemical and electron microscopic observations. *Cancer* 1979;44:1757–1768.

Histopathology

4. Thomson SJ, Tanner NS. Carcinoma of the apocrine glands at the base of eyelashes; a case report and discussion of histological diagnostic criteria. *Br J Plast Surg* 1989;42:598–602.
5. Kramer TR, Grossniklaus HE, McLean IW, et al. Histiocytoid variant of eccrine sweat gland carcinoma of the eyelid and orbit: report of five cases. *Ophthalmology* 2002;109:553–559.

Case Reports

6. Grizzard WS, Torczinski E, Edwards WC. Adenocarcinoma of eccrine sweat glands. *Arch Ophthalmol* 1976;94:2119–2120.
7. Rodrigues MM, Lubowitz RM, Shannon GM. Mucinous (adenocystic) carcinoma of the eyelid. *Arch Ophthalmol* 1973;89:493–494.
8. Thomas JW, Fu YS, Levine MR. Primary mucinous sweat gland carcinoma of the eyelid simulating metastatic carcinoma. *Am J Ophthalmol* 1979;87:29–33.
9. Cohen KL, Peiffer RL, Lipper S. Mucinous sweat gland adenocarcinoma of the eyelid. *Am J Ophthalmol* 1981;92:183–188.
10. Gardner TW, O'Grady RB. Mucinous adenocarcinoma of the eyelid. *Arch Ophthalmol* 1984;102:912.
11. Boi S, De Concini M, Detassis C. Mucinous sweat-gland adenocarcinoma of the inner canthus: a case report. *Ann Ophthalmol* 1988;20:189–190.
12. Liszauer AD, Brownstein S, Codere F. Mucinous eccrine sweat gland adenocarcinoma of the eyelid. *Can J Ophthalmol* 1988;23:17–21.
13. Sanke RF. Primary mucinous adenocarcinoma of the eyelid. *Ophthalmic Surg* 1989;20:668–671.
14. Shuster AR, Maskin SL, Leone CR Jr. Primary mucinous sweat gland carcinoma of the eyelid. *Ophthalmic Surg* 1989;20:808–810.
15. Snow SN, Reizner GT. Mucinous eccrine carcinoma of the eyelid. *Cancer* 1992;70:2099–2104.
16. Fox SB, Benson MT, Mody CH, et al. Mucinous sweat-gland adenocarcinoma of the eyelid. *Ger J Ophthalmol* 1992;1:371–373.
17. Werner MS, Hornblass A, Sassoon J, et al. Mucinous eccrine carcinoma of the eyelid. *Ophthal Plast Reconstr Surg* 1996;12:58–60.
18. Boynton JR, Markowitch W Jr. Mucinous eccrine carcinoma of the eyelid. *Arch Ophthalmol* 1998;116:1130–1131.
19. Sudesh R, Siddique S, Pace L. Primary eyelid mucinous adenocarcinoma of eccrine origin. *Ophthalmic Surg Lasers* 1999;30:394–395.
20. Krishnakumar S, Mohan ER, Babu K, et al. Eccrine duct carcinoma of the eyelid mimicking meibomian carcinoma: clinicopathological study of a case. *Surv Ophthalmol* 2003;48:439–446.
21. Boynton JR, Markowitch W Jr. Porocarcinoma of the eyelid. *Ophthalmology* 1997;104:1626–1628.
22. Jakobiec FA, Austin P, Iwamoto T, et al. Primary infiltrating signet ring carcinoma of the eyelids. *Ophthalmology* 1983;90:291–299.
23. Wollensak G, Witschel H, Bohm N. Signet ring cell carcinoma of the eccrine sweat glands in the eyelid. *Ophthalmology* 1996;103:1788–1793.
24. Auw-Haedrich C, Boehm N, Weissenberger C. Signet ring carcinoma of the eccrine sweat gland in the eyelid, treated by radiotherapy alone. *Br J Ophthalmol* 2001;85:112–113.
25. Kodama T, Tane N, Ohira A, et al. Sclerosing sweat duct carcinoma of the eyelid. *Jpn J Ophthalmol* 2004;48:7–11.
26. Aurora AL, Luxenberg MN. Case report of adenocarcinoma of glands of Moll. *Am J Ophthalmol* 1970;70:984–986.
27. Seregard S. Apocrine adenocarcinoma arising in Moll gland cystadenoma. *Ophthalmology* 1993;100:1716–1719.
28. Paridaens D, Mooy CM. Apocrine sweat gland carcinoma. *Eye* 2001;15:253–254.
29. Shintaku M, Tsuta K, Yoshida H, et al. Apocrine adenocarcinoma of the eyelid with aggressive biological behavior: report of a case. *Pathol Int* 2002;52:169–173.
30. Bindra M, Keegan DJ, Guenther T, et al. Primary cutaneous mucinous carcinoma of the eyelid in a young male. *Orbit* 2005;24:211–214.

EYELID MUCINOUS SWEAT GLAND ADENOCARCINOMA

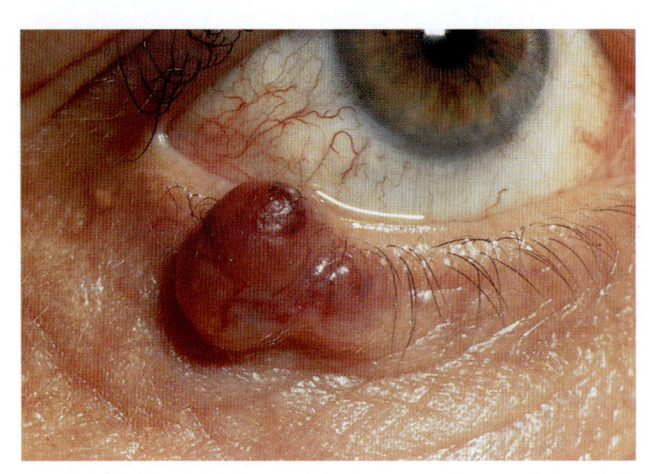

Figure 4.25. Mucin-secreting adenocarcinoma of eccrine origin. Multinodular reddish-blue lesion of lower eyelid. (Courtesy of Richard O'Grady, MD.)

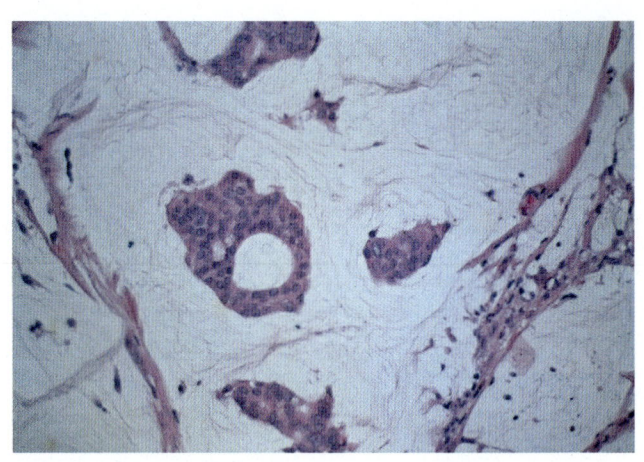

Figure 4.26. Histopathology of lesion shown in Figure 4.27, showing mucin between the cords of epithelial cells. (Hematoxylin–eosin ×100.) (Courtesy of Narsing Rao, MD.)

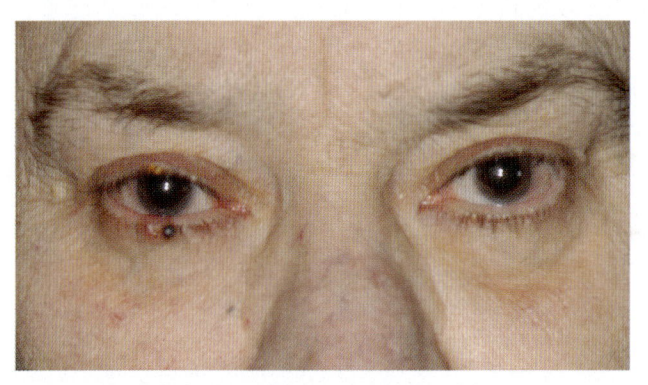

Figure 4.27. Right lower eyelid mass in a 76-year-old woman.

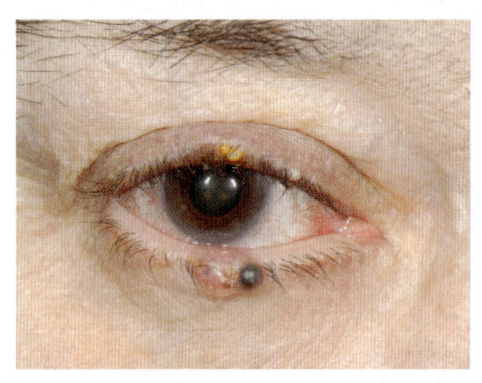

Figure 4.28. Closer view of patient in Figure 4.27 demonstrating the solid pink and cystic purple erosive mass with eyelash loss.

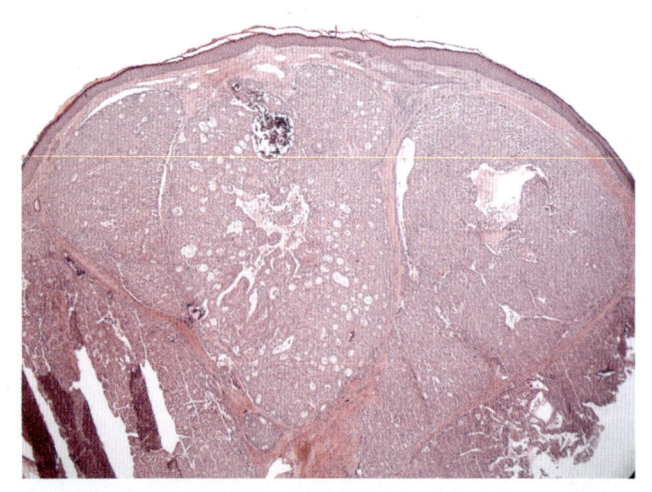

Figure 4.29. Low-power histopathology of mass in Figure 4.28 revealing lobules and cords of tumor separated by fibrous septae. (Hematoxylin–eosin ×10.)

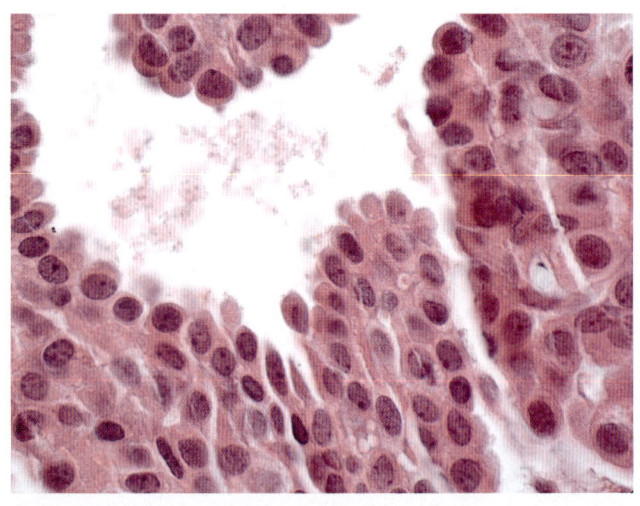

Figure 4.30. High-power histopathology of mass in Figure 4.28 revealing a duct lined by malignant epithelial cells with apical "snouting" and foamy cytoplasm. (Hematoxylin–eosin ×200.)

● EYELID SWEAT GLAND CARCINOMA

Sweat gland adenocarcinoma can occur as a pedunculated lesion or a diffuse infiltrating lesion with a tendency to invade the orbit.

1. Ni C, Dryja TP, Albert DM. Sweat gland tumor in the eyelids: a clinicopathological analysis of 55 cases. *Int Ophthalmol Clin* 1981;23:1–22.
2. Boynton JR, Markowitch W Jr. Porocarcinoma of the eyelid. *Ophthalmology* 1997;104:1626–1828.

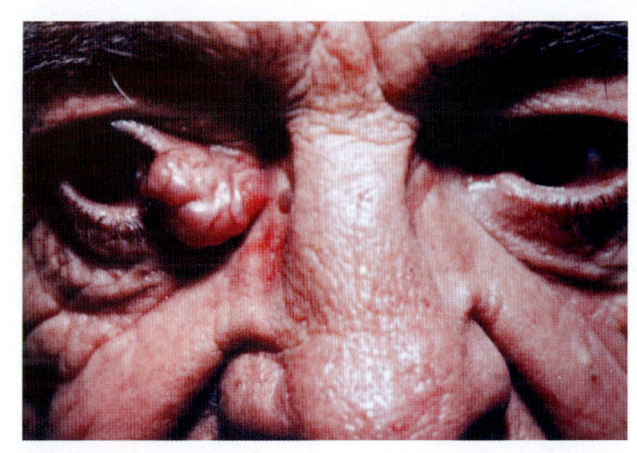

Figure 4.31. Pedunculated apocrine adenocarcinoma near medial canthus in an elderly man.

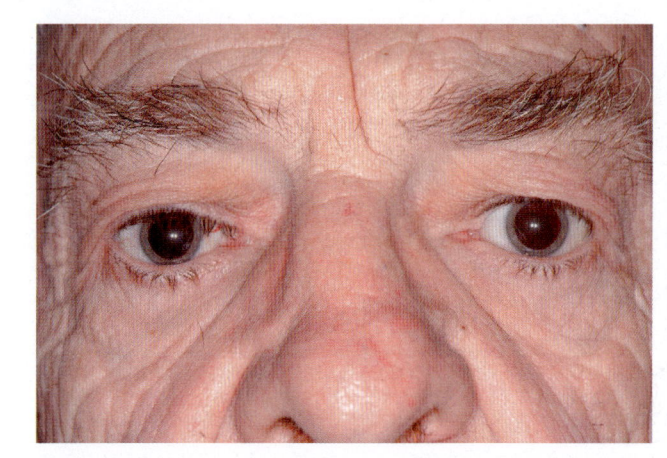

Figure 4.32. Postoperative appearance of lesion shown in Figure 4.31 after resection.

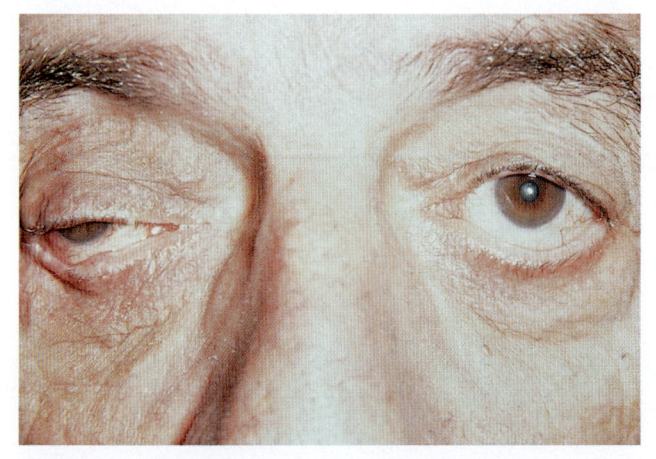

Figure 4.33. Adenocarcinoma of apocrine glands. Blepharoptosis of upper eyelid secondary to a diffuse mass. (Courtesy of Thaddeus Dryja, MD.)

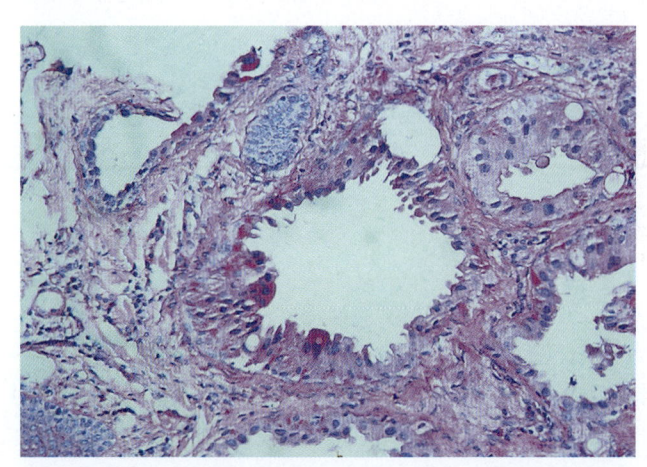

Figure 4.34. Histopathology of case shown in Figure 4.33, revealing a ductule lined by malignant apocrine gland cells. Note the characteristic apical projections of the cells lining the lumen (periodic acid-Schiff; original magnification, ×50.) (Courtesy of Thaddeus Dryja, MD.)

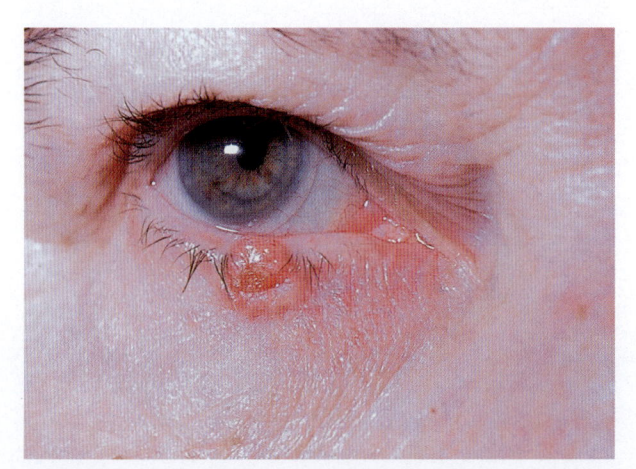

Figure 4.35. Porocarcinoma (carcinoma arising from eccrine secretory apparatus of the eyelid). Nodular lesion of right lower eyelid in a 68-year-old woman. (Courtesy of James Boynton, MD.)

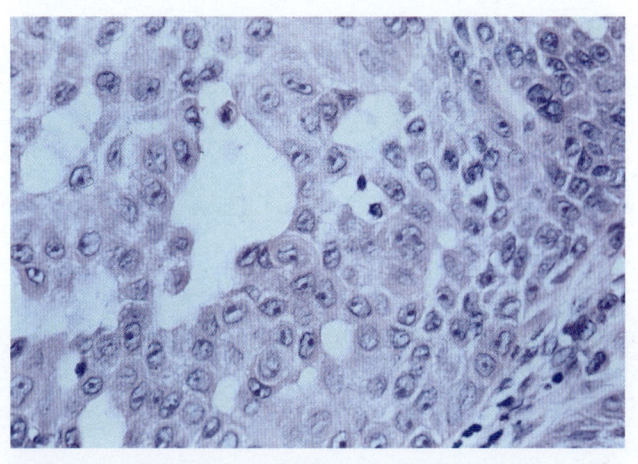

Figure 4.36. Histopathology of lesion shown in Figure 4.35, revealing pleomorphic neoplastic cells. (Courtesy of James Boynton, MD.)

CHAPTER 5

EYELID HAIR FOLLICLE TUMORS

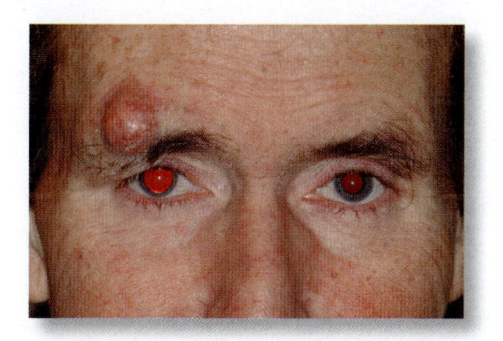

General Considerations

Trichoepithelioma is a benign tumor that can be solitary or multifocal (1–16). Solitary trichoepithelioma is generally unassociated with genetic or systemic abnormalities. It can occur anywhere on the body, but has a predilection for the face and eyelids. The multifocal variant (Brooke's tumor) is transmitted by an autosomal-dominant mode of inheritance (7). Trichoepithelioma accounts for about 1% to 2% of biopsied sweat gland or hair follicle tumors (1,2).

Clinical Features

Solitary trichoepithelioma generally has its onset in early adulthood as a skin-colored, dome-shaped papule that may remain stable or gradually enlarge and become crusty (8,9). Larger trichoepithelioma may have telangiectatic blood vessels and resemble basal cell carcinoma. However, unlike basal cell carcinoma, it is relatively stationary and rarely ulcerates (6).

The autosomal-dominant multiple trichoepithelioma (also called Brooke's tumor and adenoid cystic epithelioma) has its onset in the second decade of life and the lesions slowly increase in number (10–13). It begins as multiple, skin-colored, firm papules usually between 2 and 8 mm in diameter, located mainly in the nasolabial folds, facial skin, and sometimes the eyelids. Ulceration and transformation into basal cell carcinoma are rare. The clinical appearance may be similar to nevoid basal cell carcinoma syndrome, facial angiofibromas of tuberous sclerosis, sarcoidosis, or syringoma. Multiple trichoepitheliomas have also been observed in association with multiple cylindromas, a condition that also has autosomal-dominant inheritance (12,13). The gene for multiple trichoepitheliomas maps to chromosome 9p21 (7).

Pathology

Histopathologically, trichoepithelioma is characterized by irregular lobules of proliferating basal cells with distinct keratin cysts (horn cysts), that represent immature hair structures. The keratin cysts can resemble those seen with seborrheic keratosis or keratotic basal cell carcinoma and the tumor may be difficult to differentiate from basal cell carcinoma or squamous cell carcinoma in many instances. The keratin cysts can occasionally incite a foreign body giant cell reaction. Electron microscopy and immunohistochemical studies suggest that the tumor arises from hair matrix cells and the horn cysts represent attempts at hair shaft formation (1–6).

Management

Management is surgical excision. If an incisional biopsy confirms trichoepithelioma, definitive surgical removal can be done with less generous margins than for basal cell carcinoma, thus facilitating surgical reconstruction (4,5). The carbon dioxide laser has been used for multiple lesions (4). Multiple trichoepitheliomas are managed similarly; management varies with the clinical findings.

EYELID TRICHOEPITHELIOMA

Selected References

Reviews

1. Massa MC, Medenica M. Cutaneous adnexal tumors and cysts: a review. Part I – Tumors with hair follicular and sebaceous glandular differentiation and cysts related to different parts of the hair follicle. *Pathol Annu* 1985;20:189–233.
2. Ozdal PC, Callejo SA, Codere F, et al. Benign ocular adnexal tumours of apocrine, eccrine or hair follicle origin. *Can J Ophthalmol* 2003;38:357–363.
3. Kersten RC, Ewing-Chow D, Kulwin DR, et al. Accuracy of clinical diagnosis of cutaneous eyelid lesions. *Ophthalmology* 1997;104(3):479–484.

Management

4. Wheeland RG, Bailin PL, Kroanberg E. Carbon dioxide (CO2) laser vaporization for the treatment of multiple trichoepitheliomas. *J Dermatol Surg Oncol* 1984;10:470–475.
5. Votruba M, Collins CM, Harrad RA. The management of solitary trichoepithelioma versus basal cell carcinoma. *Eye* 1998;12:43–46.

Histopathology/Genetics

6. Simpson W, Garner A, Collin JRO. Benign hair-follicle derived tumours in the differential diagnosis of basal cell carcinoma of the eyelids: a clinicopathological comparison. *Br J Ophthalmol* 1989;37:347–353.
7. Harada H, Hashimoto K, Ko MS. The gene for multiple familial trichoepithelioma maps to chromosome 9p21. *J Invest Dermatol* 1996;107:41–43.

Case Reports

8. Bishop DW. Trichoepithelioma. *Arch Ophthalmol* 1965;74:4–8.
9. Gray HR, Helwig EB. Epithelioma adenoides cysticum and solitary trichoepithelioma. *Arch Dermatol* 1963;87:102–114.
10. Wolken SH, Spivey BE, Blodi F. Hereditary adenoid cystic epithelioma (Brooke's tumor). *Am J Ophthalmol* 1968;68:26–34.
11. Gaul LE. Heredity of multiple benign cystic epithelioma. *Arch Dermatol* 1953;68:517–519.
12. Parsier RJ. Multiple hereditary trichoepitheliomas and basal cell carcinomas. *J Cutan Pathol* 1986;13:111–117.
13. Sternberg I, Buckman G, Levine MR, et al. Hereditary trichoepithelioma with basal cell carcinoma. *Ophthalmology* 1986;93:531–533.
14. Kirzhner M, Jakobiec FA, Borodic G. Desmoplastic trichoepithelioma: report of a unique periocular case. *Ophthal Plast Reconstr Surg* 2012;28(5):e121–e123.
15. Aurora AL. Solitary trichoepithelioma of the eyelid. *Indian J Ophthalmol* 1974;22:32–33.
16. Kuo DS, Nyong'o OL. Congenital solitary eyelid trichoepithelioma. *J AAPOS* 2010;14(3):277–279.

EYELID AND FACIAL TRICHOEPITHELIOMA

Trichoepithelioma can be solitary or multiple. In some instances, this benign tumor can spawn basal cell carcinoma.

Sternberg I, Buckman G, Levine MR, et al. Hereditary trichoepithelioma with basal cell carcinoma. *Ophthalmology* 1986;93:531–533.

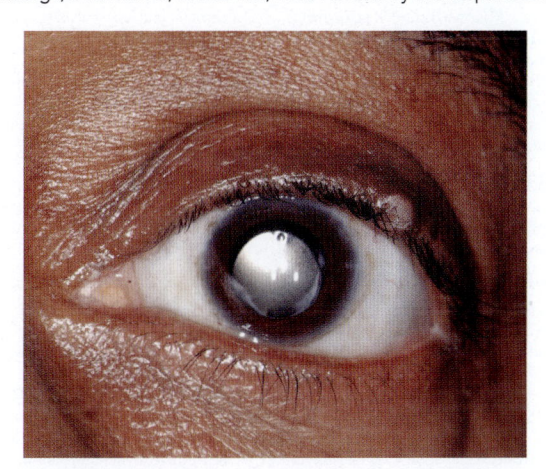

Figure 5.1. Grey-white lesion on eyelid margin with eyelash loss in a middle-aged African-American woman.

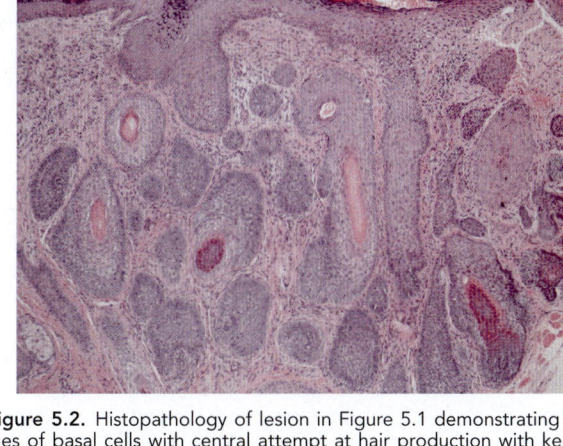

Figure 5.2. Histopathology of lesion in Figure 5.1 demonstrating lobules of basal cells with central attempt at hair production with keratin cyst or lumen. (Hematoxylin–eosin ×150.)

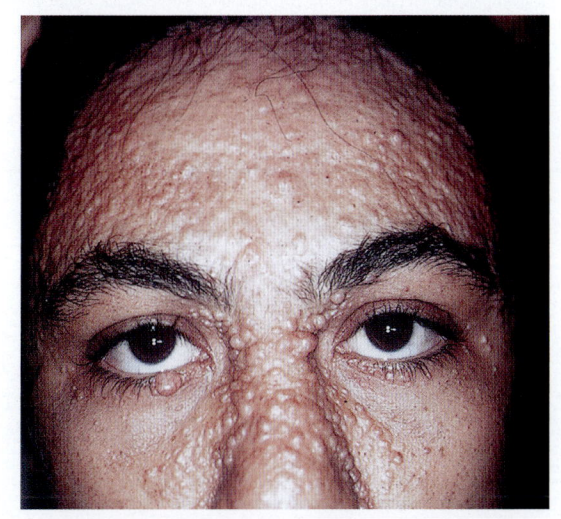

Figure 5.3. Young woman with multiple facial trichoepitheliomas (Brooke's tumor). Three of her nine siblings had similar findings. (Courtesy of the Armed Forces Institute of Pathology, Washington, DC.)

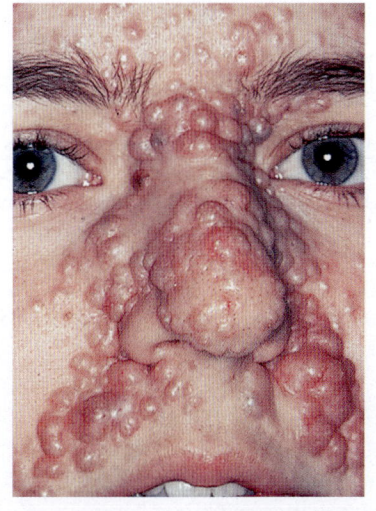

Figure 5.4. Young woman with multiple facial trichoepitheliomas (Brooke's tumor). (Courtesy of Mark Levine, MD.)

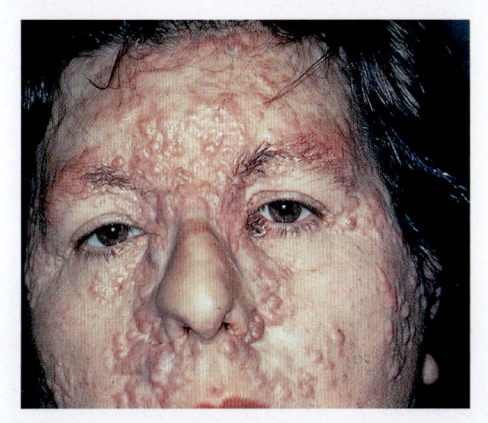

Figure 5.5. Photograph of the mother of the patient shown in Figure 5.4 showing similar lesions and a larger crusted tumor in the left medial canthus. This was excised and proved to be basal cell carcinoma arising in a patient with familial multiple trichoepithelioma. (Courtesy of Mark Levine, MD.)

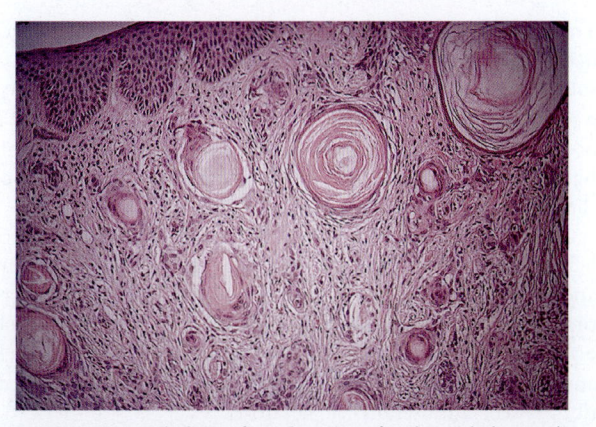

Figure 5.6. Histopathology of another case of trichoepithelioma, showing the well-defined keratin cysts. (Courtesy of the Armed Forces Institute of Pathology, Washington, DC.)

EYELID TRICHOFOLLICULOMA AND TRICHOADENOMA

General Considerations

Trichofolliculoma and trichoadenoma are similar hair follicle tumors that rarely affect the eyelids. Trichofolliculoma, a more common lesion than trichoadenoma, represents a benign, slow-growing tumor of hair follicle origin that occurs most often in the head and neck region and can involve the eyelid (1–10). It accounts for about 1% to 2% of biopsied sweat gland or hair follicle tumors (1–3).

Clinical Features

Trichofolliculoma presents as a dome-shaped, skin-colored nodule with a characteristic central pore through which typical cotton-like fine hairs, sometimes white lanugo hairs, protrude. This is a highly diagnostic feature (1–10). In the ocular region, it has a predilection for the eyelid margin. Sebum-like material can intermittently drain from the pore. Clinically, it may be confused with sebaceous cysts, nevus, or basal cell carcinoma. Trichofolliculoma does not appear to have any systemic associations.

Pathology

Microscopically, trichofolliculoma consists of a dilated hair follicle orifice that contains hair and keratin. It has a duct lined by keratinized stratified squamous epithelium that is continuous with the epidermis, an indication that it represents an enlarged, distorted hair follicle (4). It is a highly differentiated lesion with branching strands of basaloid cells extending from the dilated follicle into the adjacent connective tissue. Fragments of birefringent hair shafts are often present. Glycogen is present in the walls of the hair follicles. Some authorities consider it to be a hamartomatous lesion, representing the most differentiated form of pilar tumor (2).

Management

Trichofolliculoma is generally best managed by complete surgical excision, similar to other benign adnexal tumors. It can recur if incompletely excised.

Trichoadenoma

Trichoadenoma is a rare, benign cutaneous tumor of hair follicle differentiation. It generally occurs on the face and has a solitary, nodular configuration, often with superficial, telangiectatic vessels (11–13). It has only recently been recognized to occur on the eyelid. It usually resembles a basal cell carcinoma, but can have a verrucous configuration and resemble seborrheic keratosis.

Histopathologically, trichoadenoma is a lesion of hair follicle differentiation that is less mature than trichofolliculoma and more mature than trichoepithelioma (11–13). It has keratin cysts that bear a striking resemblance to those seen in seborrheic keratosis, but they are surrounded by eosinophilic cells and are not situated within a solid basaloid cellular proliferation, as seen with seborrheic keratosis.

Selected References

Reviews

1. Massa MC, Medenica M. Cutaneous adnexal tumors and cysts: a review. Part I – Tumors with hair follicular and sebaceous glandular differentiation and cysts related to different parts of the hair follicle. *Pathol Annu* 1985;20:189–233.
2. Ozdal PC, Callejo SA, Codere F, et al. Benign ocular adnexal tumours of apocrine, eccrine or hair follicle origin. *Can J Ophthalmol* 2003;38:357–363.
3. Kersten RC, Ewing-Chow D, Kulwin DR, et al. Accuracy of clinical diagnosis of cutaneous eyelid lesions. *Ophthalmology* 1997;104(3):479–484.

Histopathology

4. Simpson W, Garner A, Collin JRO. Benign hair-follicle derived tumours in the differential diagnosis of basal cell carcinoma of the eyelids: a clinicopathological comparison. *Br J Ophthalmol* 1989;37:347–353.

Case Reports

5. Gray HR, Helwig EB. Trichofolliculoma. *Arch Dermatol* 1962;86:619–625.
6. Pinkus H, Sutton R. Trichofolliculoma. *Arch Dermatol* 1965;91:46–50.
7. Carreras B Jr, Lopez-Marin I Jr, Mellado VG, et al. Trichofolliculoma of the eyelid. *Br J Ophthalmol* 1981;65:214–215.
8. Steffen C, Leaming DV. Trichofolliculoma of the upper eyelid. *Cutis* 1982;30:343–345.
9. Taniguchi S, Hamada T. Trichofolliculoma of the eyelid. *Eye* 1996;10:751–752.
10. Morton AD, Nelson CC, Headington JT, et al. Recurrent trichofolliculoma of the upper eyelid margin. *Ophthal Plast Reconstr Surg* 1997;13:287–288.
11. Rahbari H, Mehregan A, Pinkus H. Trichoadenoma of Nikolowski. *J Cutan Pathol* 1977;4:90–98.
12. Shields JA, Shields CL, Eagle RC Jr. Trichoadenoma of the eyelid. *Am J Ophthalmol* 1998;126:846–848.
13. Lever JF, Servat JJ, Nesi-Eloff F, et al. Trichoadenoma of an eyelid in an adult mimicking sebaceous cell carcinoma. *Ophthal Plast Reconstr Surg* 2012;28(4):e101–e102.

EYELID TRICHOFOLLICULOMA AND TRICHOADENOMA

Shields JA, Shields CL, Eagle RC Jr. Trichoadenoma of the eyelid. *Am J Ophthalmol* 1998;126:846–848.

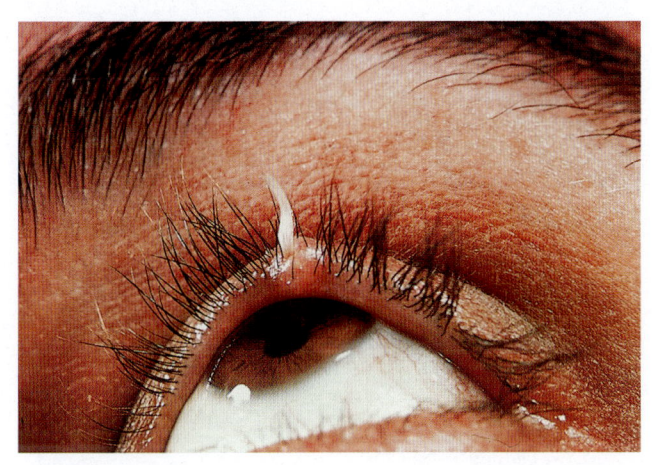

Figure 5.7. Trichofolliculoma of upper eyelid. Note the white hair protruding from the lesion. (Courtesy of Norman Charles, MD.)

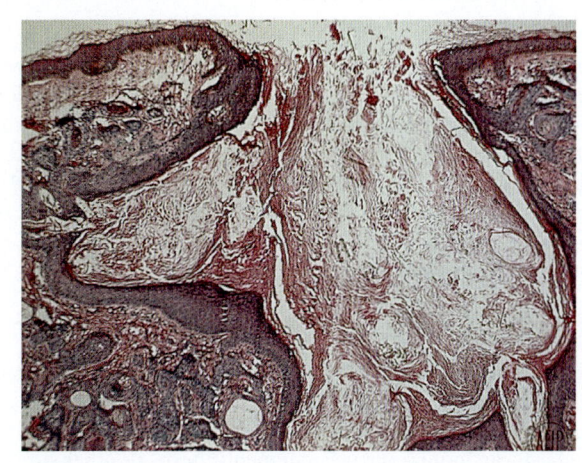

Figure 5.8. Histopathology of trichofolliculoma showing craterlike opening through which keratin and hair are protruding. (Hematoxylin–eosin ×75.) (Courtesy of Armed Forces Institute of Pathology, Washington, DC.)

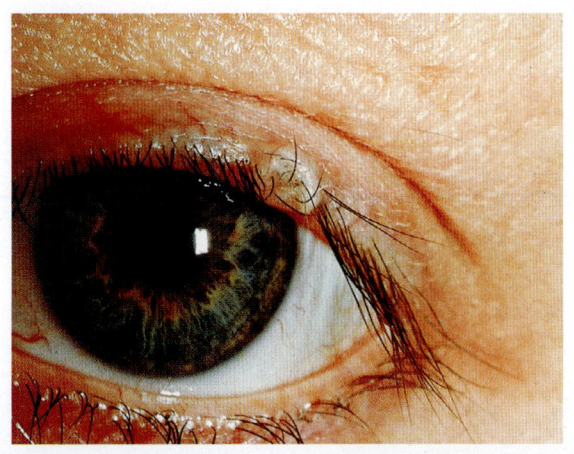

Figure 5.9. Trichofolliculoma on upper eyelid of a 33-year-old woman. Note the dark hair protruding from the lesion. (Courtesy of Victor Elner, MD.)

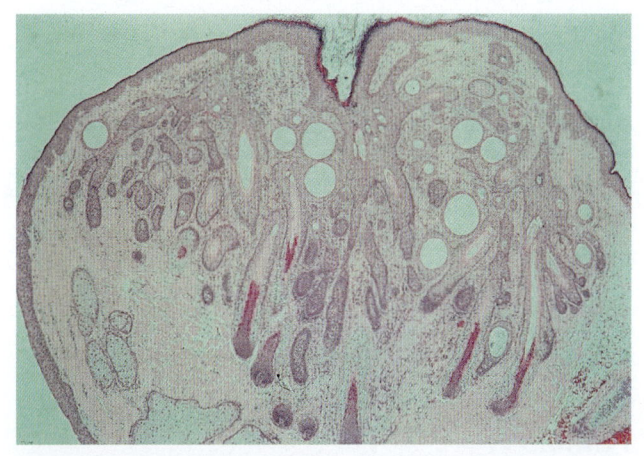

Figure 5.10. Histopathology of lesion shown in Figure 5.9 showing central crater above and dilated abortive hair follicles. (Hematoxylin–eosin ×20.) (Courtesy of Victor Elner, MD.)

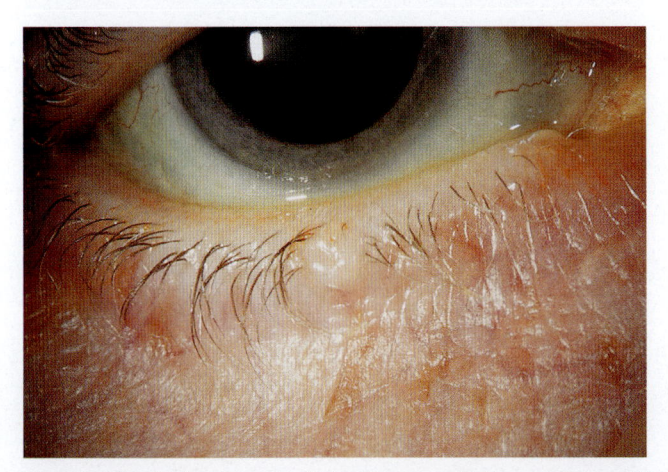

Figure 5.11. Trichoadenoma of the lower eyelid in an 80-year-old woman. Note the loss of cilia and the similarity of the lesion to basal cell carcinoma.

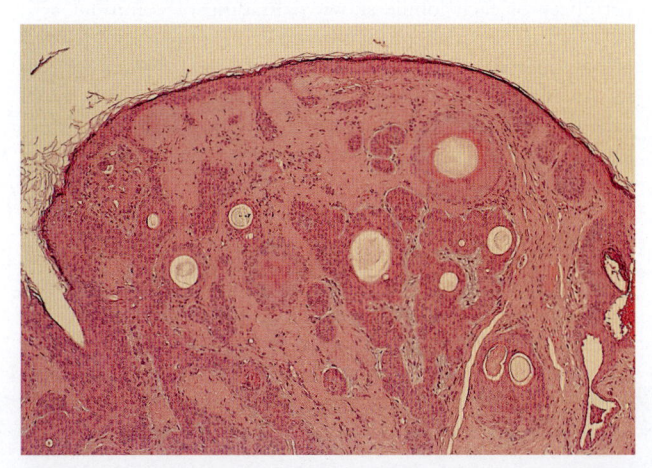

Figure 5.12. Histopathology of lesion shown in Figure 5.11 revealing keratin cysts surrounded by eosinophilic cells in the dermis. Note that the lesion is deep to the epidermis, unlike basal cell carcinoma and seborrheic keratosis. (Hematoxylin–eosin ×40.)

EYELID TRICHILEMMOMA

General Considerations

Trichilemmoma is a benign tumor that arises from the trichilemma, a glycogen-rich zone of clear cells that surrounds the hair shaft. It almost always occurs in the head and neck region (1–14). It has a slight predilection for males (1). It is one of the adnexal tumors that can arise from nevus sebaceous of Jadassohn. In a series of 31 trichilemmomas involving the ocular area, patient ages ranged from 22 to 88 years, with a mean of 56 years (1). The eyelid is the second most common site of involvement after the nose (1).

Clinical Features

Trichilemmoma has no distinctive features. It generally appears as a small, verrucous, or papillomatous nodule. The diagnosis is rarely made clinically and most cases are initially diagnosed as basal cell carcinoma, verruca, cutaneous horn, or other similar lesions.

Cowden's Disease

Multiple facial trichilemmomas can be a marker for an autosomal-dominant condition known as Cowden's disease (multiple hamartoma syndrome) (5–8). Affected patients should be evaluated for other tumors associated with this disease, particularly breast and thyroid cancers. Other benign tumors of Cowden's syndrome include oral mucosal papules, acral keratotic papules, thyroid nodules, lipomas, intestinal polyps, and fibrocystic breast disease. The trichilemmomas can precede breast cancer diagnosis, enabling earlier diagnosis of the malignant breast cancer in such cases. The association of multiple trichilemmomas and Cowden's disease with cerebellar hamartomas is called Lhermitte–Duclos disease (7).

Pathology

Histopathologically, trichilemmoma is characterized by lobular acanthosis composed mainly of glycogen-rich cells. The periphery of each lobule shows palisading of columnar cells with a distinct basement membrane (1). It may resemble basal cell carcinoma, squamous cell carcinoma, or seborrheic keratosis. A variant is the desmoplastic trichilemmoma, which shows irregular extensions of cells of the outer root sheath that project into sclerotic collagen bundles, mimicking invasive basal cell carcinoma (10–12).

Management

Like many other tumors in this section, the management of trichilemmoma is complete surgical excision (2). In some cases, curettage or topical 5-fluorouracil have been used. There are rare reports of trichilemmal carcinoma of the eyelid (13,14). It is not certain whether trichilemmal carcinoma arises de novo or from benign trichilemmoma.

Selected References

Reviews

1. Hidayat AA, Font RL. Trichilemmoma of eyelid and eyebrow. A clinicopathologic study of 31 cases. *Arch Ophthalmol* 1980;98:844–884.
2. Simpson W, Garner A, Collin JRO. Benign hair-follicle derived tumours in the differential diagnosis of basal cell carcinoma of the eyelids: a clinicopathological comparison. *Br J Ophthalmol* 1989;37:347–353.
3. Massa MC, Medenica M. Cutaneous adnexal tumors and cysts: a review. Part I – Tumors with hair follicular and sebaceous glandular differentiation and cysts related to different parts of the hair follicle. *Pathol Annu* 1985;20:189–233.
4. Ozdal PC, Callejo SA, Codère F, et al. Benign ocular adnexal tumours of apocrine, eccrine or hair follicle origin. *Can J Ophthalmol* 2003;38(5):357–363.

Cowden's Disease

5. Brownstein MH, Mehregan AH, Bikowski JB. Trichilemmomas in Cowden's disease. *JAMA* 1977;238:26.
6. Bardenstein DS, McLean IW, Nerney J, et al. Cowden's disease. *Ophthalmology* 1988;95:1038–1041.
7. Padberg GW, Schot JD, Vielvoye GJ, et al. Lhermitte-Duclos disease and Cowden's disease. A single phakomatosis. *Ann Neurol* 1991;29:517–523.
8. Thyresson HN, Doyle JA. Cowden's disease (multiple hamartoma syndrome). *Mayo Clin Proc* 1981;56:179–184.

Case Reports

9. Reifler DM, Ballitch HA, Kessler DL, et al. Trichilemmoma of the eyelid. *Ophthalmology* 1987;94:1272–1275.
10. Boulton JE, Sullivan TJ, Whitehead KJ. The eyelid is a site of occurrence of desmoplastic trichilemmoma. *Eye* 2001;15:257.
11. Topping NC, Chakrabarty A, Edrich C, et al. Desmoplastic trichilemmoma of the upper eyelid. *Eye* 1999;13:593–594.
12. Keskinbora KH, Buyukbabani N, Terzi N. Desmoplastic trichilemmoma: a rare tumor of the eyelid. *Eur J Ophthalmol* 2004;14(6):562–564.
13. Dailey JR, Helm KF, Goldberg SH. Trichilemmal carcinoma of the eyelid. *Am J Ophthalmol* 1993;115:118–119.
14. Lai TF, Huilgol SC, James CL, et al. Trichilemmal carcinoma of the upper eyelid. *Acta Ophthalmol Scand* 2003;81:536–538.

EYELID TRICHILEMMOMA, TRICHILEMMAL CARCINOMA, AND COWDEN'S SYNDROME

Trichilemmoma can occur as a solitary lesion or as multiple lesions in association with Cowden's disease (multiple hamartoma syndrome). About half of facial lesions seen with Cowden's disease are trichilemmomas. On occasion, a trichilemmoma can have malignant changes histopathologically (trichilemmal carcinoma).

Dailey JR, Helm KF, Goldberg SH. Trichilemmal carcinoma of the eyelid. *Am J Ophthalmol* 1993;115:118–119.

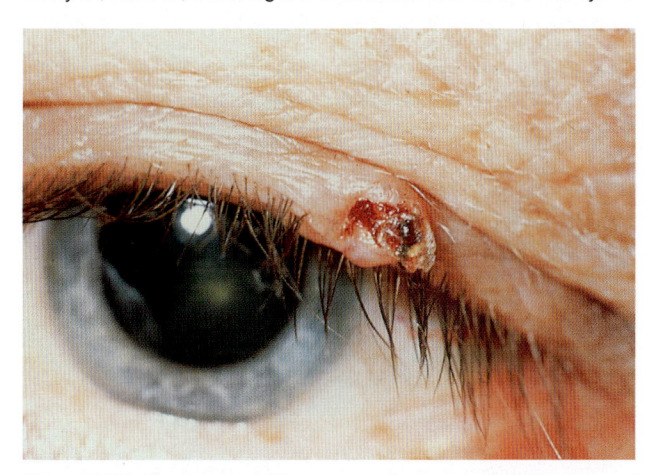

Figure 5.13. Excoriated trichilemmoma of upper eyelid. (Courtesy of Ralph C. Eagle Jr, MD.)

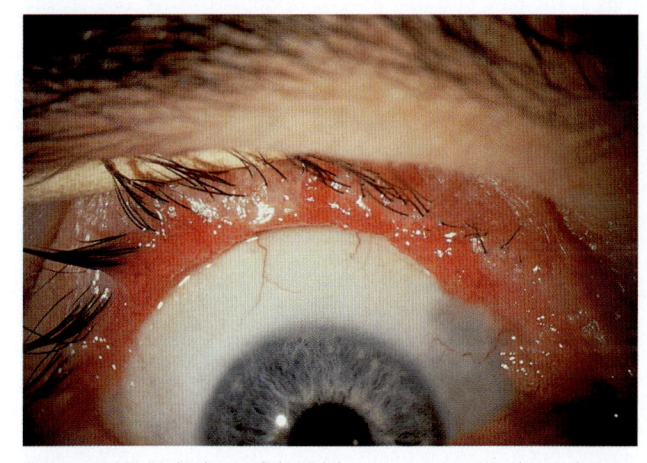

Figure 5.14. Multiple eyelid trichilemmomas in Cowden's disease. (Courtesy of Richard Lewis, MD.)

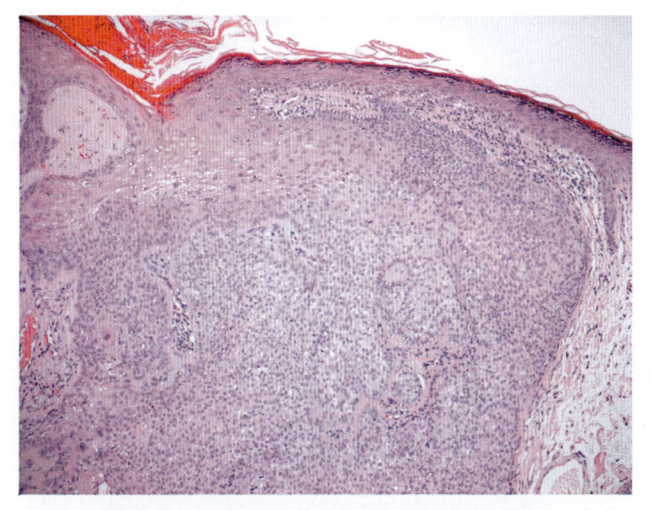

Figure 5.15. Histopathology of trichilemma showing well-defined, glycogen-rich cells continuous with epidermis. (Hematoxylin–eosin ×50.)

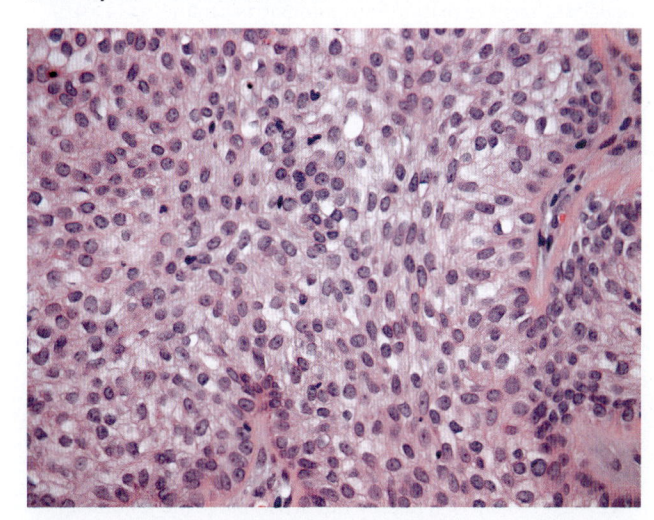

Figure 5.16. Higher magnification view of lesion shown in Figure 5.15, demonstrating clear cells with uniform nuclei.

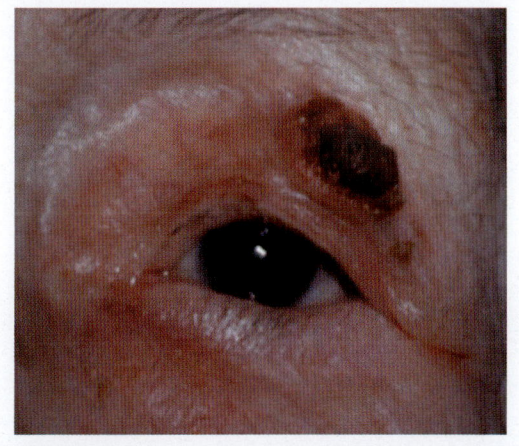

Figure 5.17. Trichilemmal carcinoma. Excoriated lesion of upper eyelid of an elderly woman.

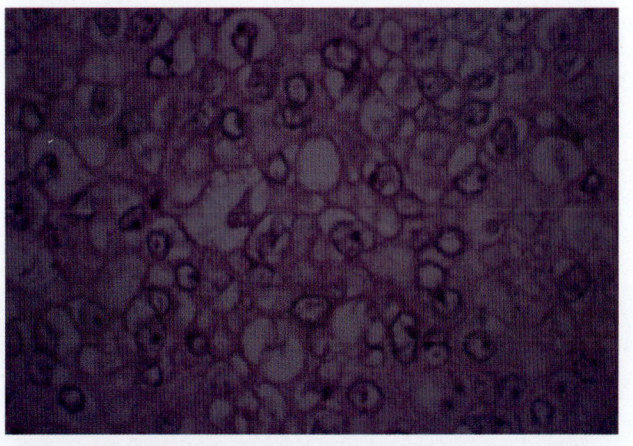

Figure 5.18. Histopathology of lesion shown in Figure 5.17, demonstrating clear cytoplasm in malignant cells.

EYELID PILOMATRIXOMA

General Considerations

Pilomatrixoma ("benign calcifying epithelioma of Malherbe"; pilomatricoma) is a benign neoplasm that arises from the matrix cells at the base of a hair (1–22). "Pilomatrixoma" depicts the lesion's origin in the hair matrix cells. Pilomatrixoma is usually solitary, has a tendency to affect young individuals, and involves the periorbital region in 17% of cases. It is multifocal in about 5% of cases. About 40% develop in the first decade of life and an additional 20% in the second decade (1–8). Pilomatrixoma has a predisposition to occur in the upper eyelid and eyebrow.

Clinical Features

Pilomatrixoma generally presents as a subcutaneous red to blue mass that is fairly well-circumscribed, freely movable, and firm or gritty to palpation (1). Its characteristic location near the lateral aspect of the eyebrow frequently suggests the clinical diagnosis of dermoid cyst. In rare instances, it has presented on the back of the eyelid from the tarsal conjunctiva. It generally grows slowly, but can occasionally exhibit more rapid growth and resemble a keratoacanthoma. Pilomatrixoma can rarely undergo malignant transformation into pilomatrix carcinoma (15,16).

Pathology

Histopathologically, pilomatrixoma is composed of a proliferation of viable basaloid cells, shadow cells, and foci of calcification and occasionally ossification (1–8). The shadow cells represent areas of necrosis of the previously viable basal cells. Foci of calcification gradually develop in the necrotic areas and are present in most cases. About 15% to 20% show areas of ossification but this is uncommon in eyelid lesions.

Management

If the diagnosis of pilomatrixoma is suspected because of the typical clinical features, the lesion should be managed by complete surgical excision. Because this tumor is often confined to the soft tissues, an attempt should be made to remove it intact. Incisional biopsy is generally not advisable if the lesion can be removed completely.

Selected References

Reviews

1. Ni C, Kimball GP, Craft FL, et al. Calcifying epithelioma: a clinicopathological analysis of 67 cases with ultrastructural studies of 2 cases. *Int Ophthalmol Clin* 1982;22:63–86.
2. Orlando RG, Rogers GL, Bremer DL. Pilomatricoma in a pediatric hospital. *Arch Ophthalmol* 1983;101:1209–1210.
3. Duflo S, Nicollas R, Roman S, et al. Pilomatrixoma of the head and neck in children: a study of 38 cases and a review of the literature. *Arch Otolaryngol Head Neck Surg* 1998;124:1239–1242.
4. Yap EY, Hohberger GG, Bartley GB. Pilomatrixoma of the eyelids and eyebrows in children and adolescents. *Ophthal Plast Reconstr Surg* 1999;15:185–189.
5. Mencia-Gutierrez E, Gutierrez-Diaz E, Garcia-Suarez E, et al. Eyelid pilomatricomas in young adults: a report of 8 cases. *Cutis* 2002;69:23–26.
6. Levy J, Ilsar M, Deckel Y, et al. Eyelid pilomatrixoma: a description of 16 cases and a review of the literature. *Surv Ophthalmol* 2008;53(5):526–35.
7. Ozdal PC, Callejo SA, Codere F, et al. Benign ocular adnexal tumours of apocrine, eccrine or hair follicle origin. *Can J Ophthalmol* 2003;38:357–363.
8. Massa MC, Medenica M. Cutaneous adnexal tumors and cysts: a review. Part I – Tumors with hair follicular and sebaceous glandular differentiation and cysts related to different parts of the hair follicle. *Pathol Annu* 1985;20:189–233.

Case Reports

9. Forbis R Jr, Helwig EB. Pilomatrixoma (calcifying epithelioma). *Arch Dermatol* 1961;83:606–618.
10. Boniuk M, Zimmerman LE. Pilomatrixoma (benign calcifying epithelioma) of the eyelid and eyebrow. *Arch Ophthalmol* 1963;70:399–406.
11. Perez RC, Nicholson DH. Malherbe's calcifying epithelioma (pilomatrixoma) of the eyelid. *Arch Ophthalmol* 1979;97:314–315.
12. O'Grady RB, Spoerl G. Pilomatrixoma (benign calcifying epithelioma of Malherbe). *Ophthalmology* 1981;88:1196–1197.
13. Shields JA, Shields CL, Eagle RC Jr, et al. Pilomatrixoma of the eyelid. *J Pediatr Ophthalmol Strabismus* 1995;32:260–261.
14. Katowitz WR, Shields CL, Shields JA, et al. Pilomatrixoma of the eyelid simulating a chalazion. *J Pediatr Ophthalmol Strabismus* 2003;40:247–248.
15. Martelli G, Giardini R. Pilomatrix carcinoma: a case report and review of the literature. *Eur J Surg Oncol* 1994;20:703–704.
16. Cahill MT, Moriarty PM, Mooney DJ, et al. Pilomatrix carcinoma of the eyelid. *Am J Ophthalmol* 1999;127:463–464.
17. Mathen LC, Olver JM, Cree IA. A large rapidly growing pilomatrixoma on a lower eyelid. *Br J Ophthalmol* 2000;84:1203–1204.
18. Kang HY, Kang WH. Guess what! Perforating pilomatricoma resembling keratoacanthoma. *Eur J Dermatol* 2000;10:63–64.
19. Gündüz K, Ecel M, Erden E. Multiple pilomatrixomas affecting the eyelid and face. *J Pediatr Ophthalmol Strabismus* 2008;45(2):122–124.
20. Abalo-Lojo JM, Cameselle-Teijeiro J, Gonzalez F. Pilomatrixoma: late onset in two periocular cases. *Ophthal Plast Reconstr Surg* 2008;24(1):60–62.
21. Huerva V, Sanchez MC, Asenjo J. Large, rapidly growing pilomatrixoma of the upper eyelid. *Ophthal Plast Reconstr Surg* 2006;22(5):401–403.
22. Niitsuma K, Kuwahara M, Yurugi S, et al. Perforating pilomatricoma on the upper eyelid. *J Craniofac Surg* 2006;17(2):372–373.

EYELID PILOMATRIXOMA IN ADULTS

1. O'Grady RB, Spoerl G. Pilomatrixoma (benign calcifying epithelioma of Malherbe). *Ophthalmology* 1981;88:1196–1197.
2. Perez RC, Nicholson DH. Malherbe's calcifying epithelioma (pilomatrixoma) of the eyelid. *Arch Ophthalmol* 1979;97:314–315.

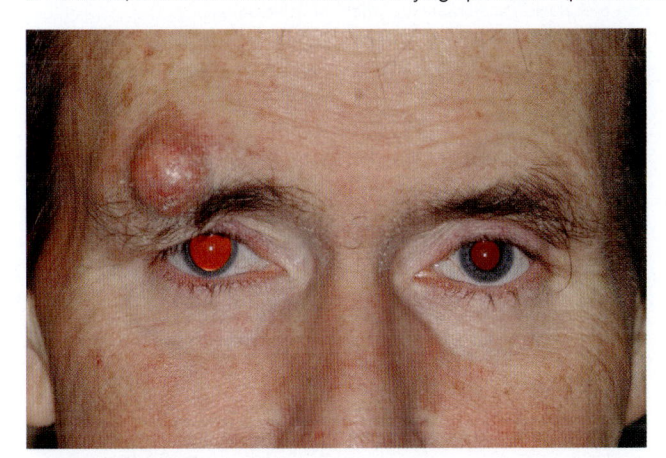

Figure 5.19. Rapidly growing suprabrow lesion in a 75-year-old man.

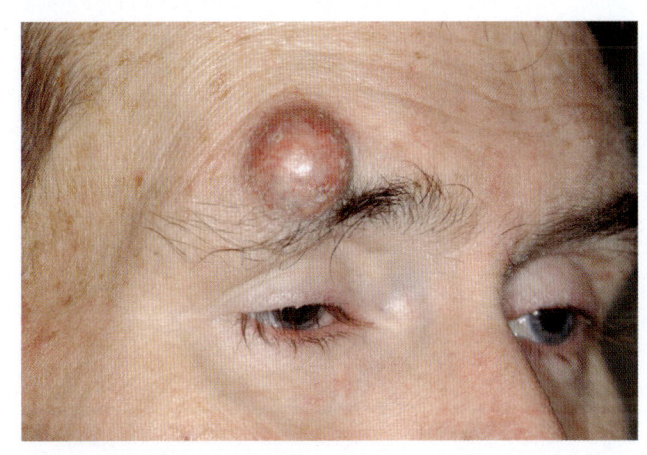

Figure 5.20. Close-up of patient in Figure 5.19 showing the smooth surface and intrinsic vascularity of the slightly pink mass.

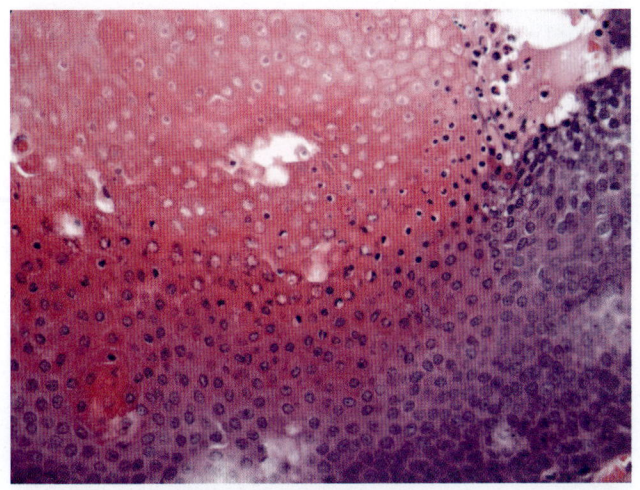

Figure 5.21. Histopathology of mass in Figure 5.20 demonstrating the blue viable cells and pink necrotic "shadow" cells of pilomatrixoma. (Hematoxylin–eosin ×50.)

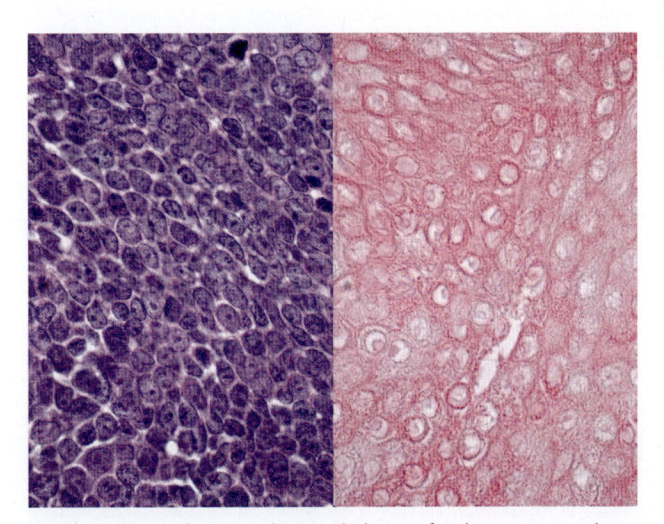

Figure 5.22. High-power histopathology of pilomatrixoma shown above demonstrating the contrast between viable cells (blue) and necrotic shadow cells (pink).

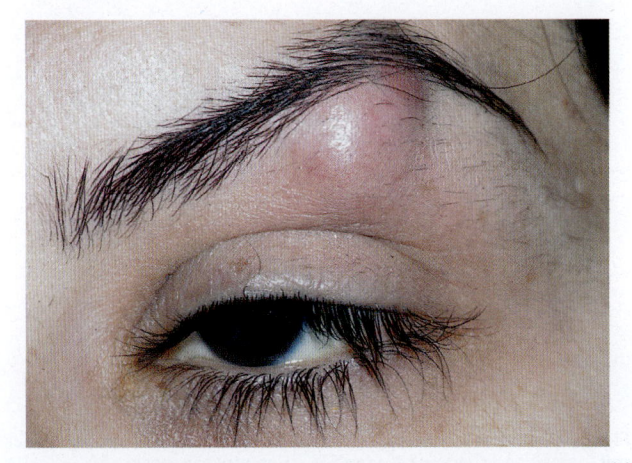

Figure 5.23. Reddish lesion in eyelid beneath eyebrow in a 39-year-old woman.

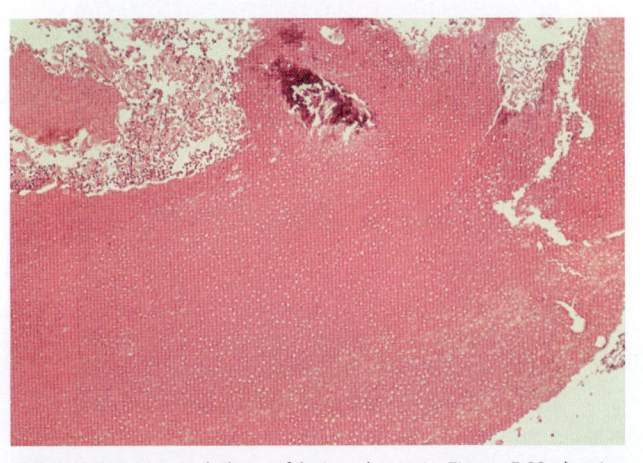

Figure 5.24. Histopathology of lesion shown in Figure 5.23 showing necrotic shadow cells with focus of calcification. (Hematoxylin–eosin ×25.)

EYELID PILOMATRIXOMA IN CHILDREN: SURGICAL EXCISION

Pilomatrixoma of the ocular region should generally be managed by complete excision. A case example is cited.

Katowitz WR, Shields CL, Shields JA, et al. Pilomatrixoma of the eyelid simulating a chalazion. *J Pediatr Ophthalmol Strabismus* 2003;40:247–248.

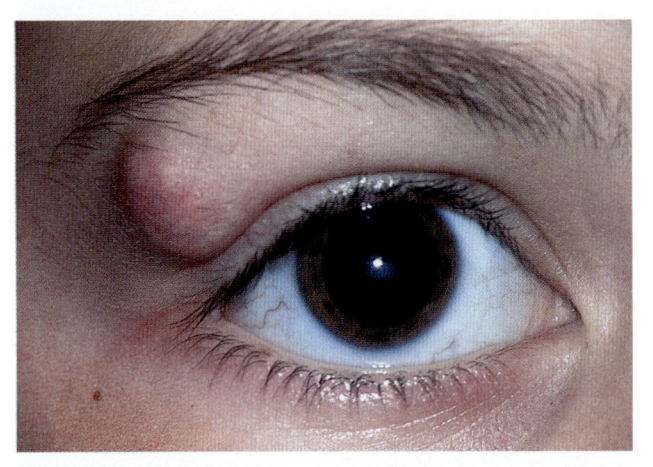

Figure 5.25. Pilomatrixoma in upper eyelid in a 7-year-old girl. It is located deep to the epidermis and has a gritty feeling to palpation.

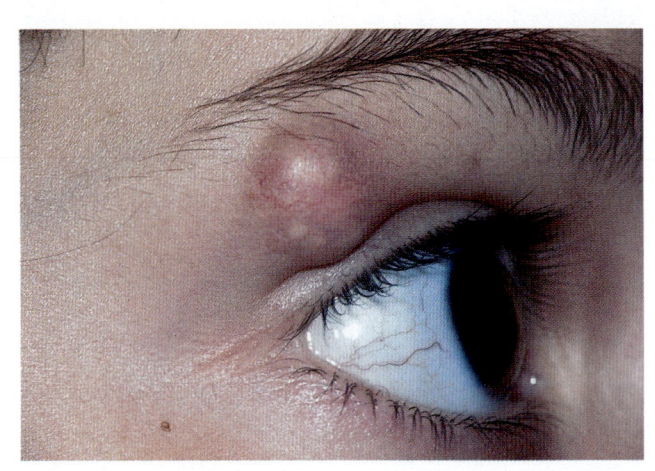

Figure 5.26. Side view of lesion.

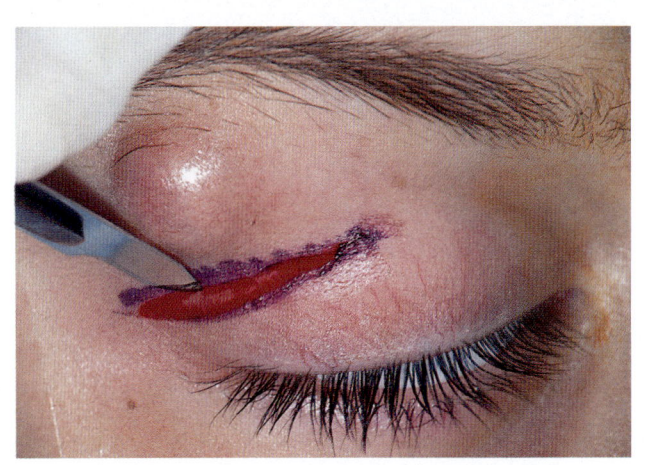

Figure 5.27. Eyelid crease incision inferior to the lesion.

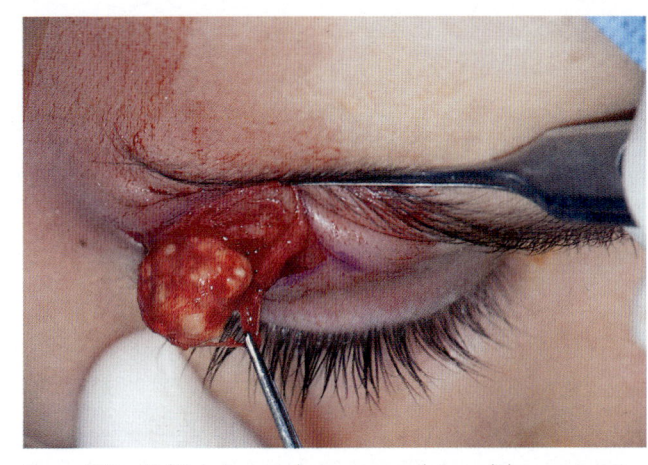

Figure 5.28. Multilobular mass being removed via eyelid crease incision.

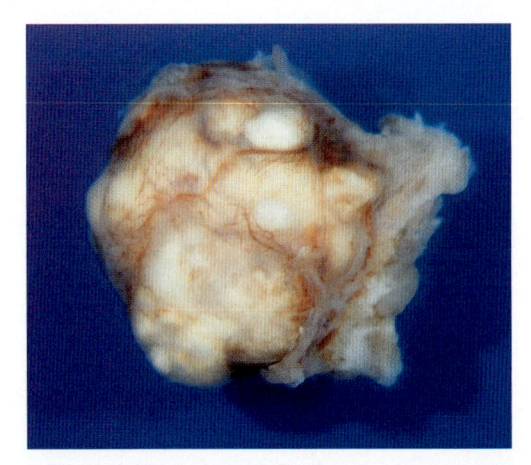

Figure 5.29. Sectioned specimen after fixation showing multinodular mass.

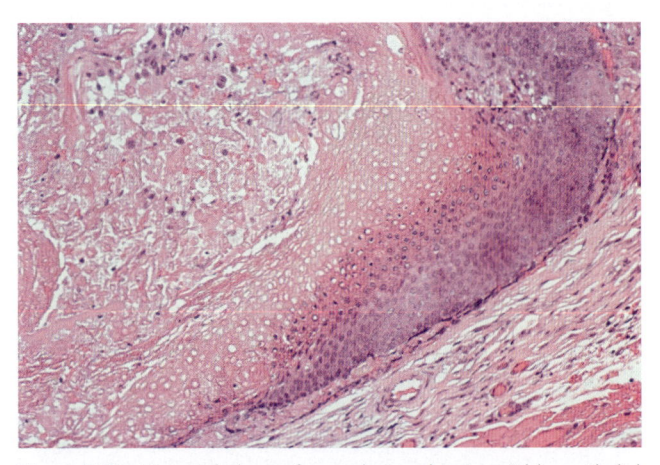

Figure 5.30. Histopathology of same lesion showing viable epithelial cell (below) and shadow cells (above). (Hematoxylin–eosin ×5.)

EYELID PILOMATRIXOMA: SURGICAL EXCISION AND HISTOPATHOLOGY

Pilomatrixoma has a tendency to occur in the eyebrow region of young patients. A clinicopathologic correlation is shown.

Shields JA, Shields CL, Eagle RC Jr, et al. Pilomatrixoma of the eyelid. *J Pediatr Ophthalmol Strabismus* 1995;32:260–261.

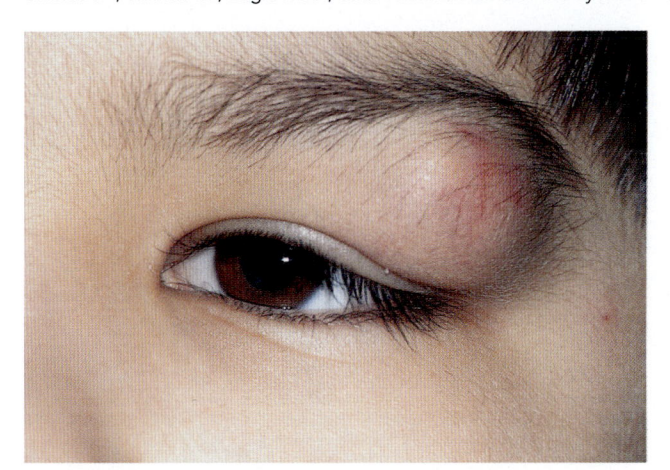

Figure 5.31. Subcutaneous mass beneath the eyebrow superotemporally resembling a dermoid cyst in an 8-year-old boy.

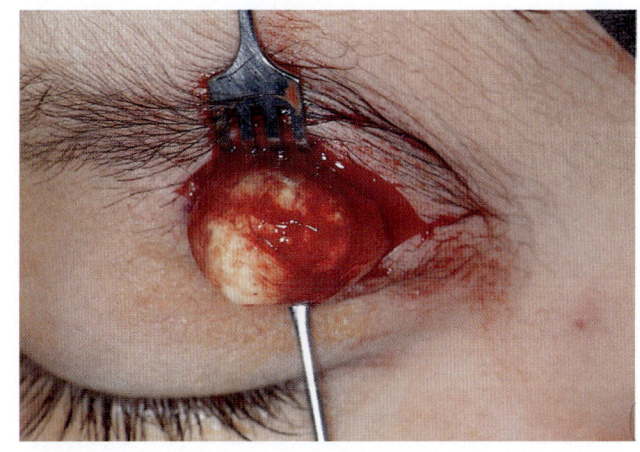

Figure 5.32. Lesion being removed via infrabrow eyelid crease incision.

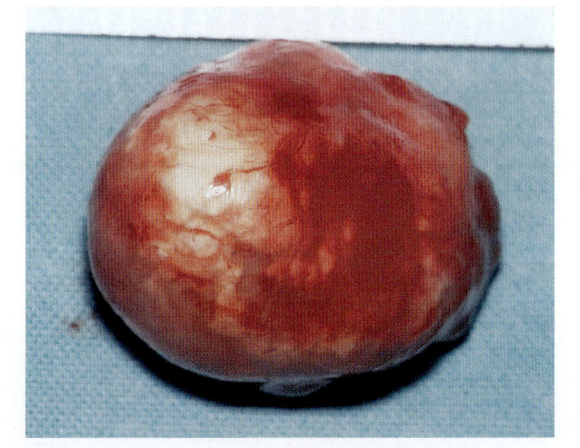

Figure 5.33. Appearance of smooth mass following excision.

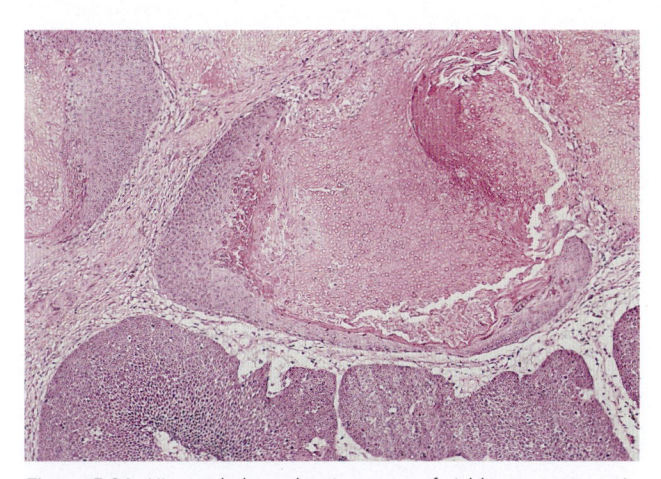

Figure 5.34. Histopathology showing areas of viable tumor, necrosis, and early calcification. (Hematoxylin–eosin ×50.)

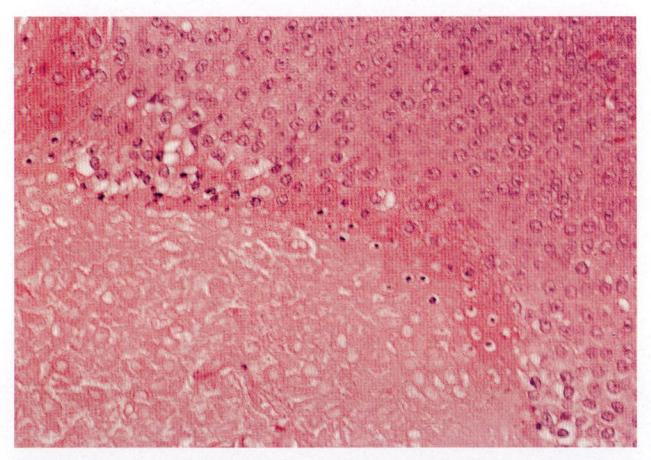

Figure 5.35. Histopathology, showing junction between viable tumor cells (basophilic) and necrotic tumor cells (eosinophilic). (Hematoxylin–eosin ×150.)

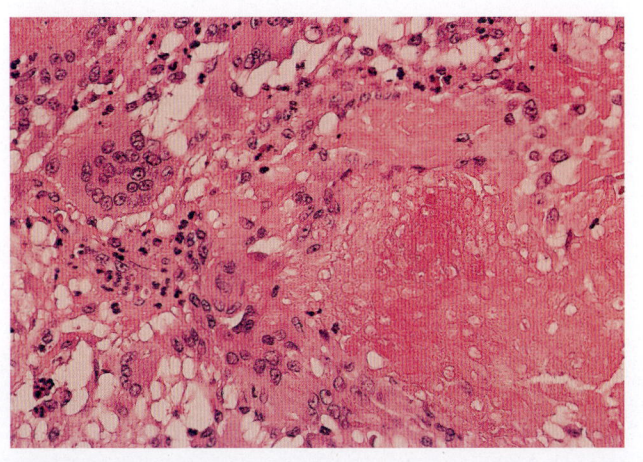

Figure 5.36. Histopathology showing giant cell reaction near the necrotic areas). (Hematoxylin–eosin ×150.)

CHAPTER 6

EYELID MELANOCYTIC TUMORS

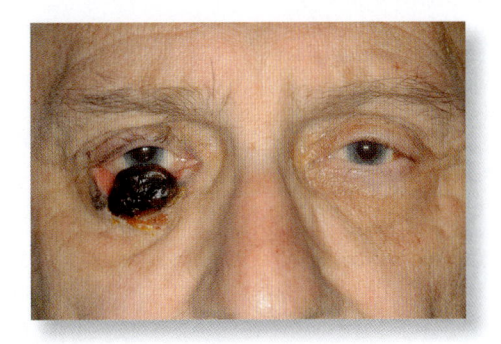

General Considerations

Melanocytic nevus (1–12) consists of melanocytes derived from the neural crest that migrate to the skin during embryonic development. An eyelid nevus can be acquired or congenital. The acquired type becomes clinically apparent in childhood in the basal epithelium (junctional nevus), gradually migrates deeper into the dermis in young adults (compound nevus), and later in life resides entirely in the dermis (dermal nevus). The average young adult has about 15 cutaneous nevi and the eyelid is occasionally affected. Multiple nevi should raise suspicion of the dysplastic nevus syndrome, in which there is a familial tendency toward development of cutaneous melanoma.

Clinical Features

The clinical features vary with patient age and stage of the disease. It usually appears between ages 5 and 15 years as a small macule that gradually evolves through the stages listed above. Eyelid nevus can range from deeply pigmented (melanotic) to completely nonpigmented (amelanotic). An eyelid margin nevus can extend onto the palpebral conjunctiva so it may be necessary to evert the eyelid to visualize the entire lesion. This lesion can surround the lacrimal punctum (peripunctal nevus) (2). The nevus surface can be smooth or verrucous (2,3) and does not generally produce loss of cilia. There is a variant of congenital nevus that is deeply pigmented and larger than an acquired nevus, slightly elevated, and frequently with excessive hairs. As opposed to the junctional nevus, this lesion has a greater chance of malignant transformation, perhaps as high as 5% (5,11,12). Another variant of congenital nevus is the divided nevus of the upper and lower eyelids ("kissing nevus") that develops before embryologic separation of the eyelid and divides when the eyelids separate in utero (10–12).

Pathology

Melanocytic nevi are divided into junctional, compound, and intradermal types. These are not entirely separate categories, but rather represent stages in the "life cycle" of nevus, as discussed above.

The diagnosis of nevus is often made by the arrangement of its cells in nests rather than by cellular characteristics. A junctional nevus has well-circumscribed nests of cells at the basal level of the epidermis. A compound nevus possesses features of both a junctional and an intradermal nevus. It can occasionally have considerable fibrous tissue and may resemble a neurofibroma or other neural tumors.

There are other variants of melanocytic nevus such as balloon cell nevus and epithelioid cell nevus that rarely involve the eyelid. Epithelioid cell nevus (Spitz nevus), a lesion that closely resembles melanoma, has been seen on the eyelid of young children.

EYELID MELANOCYTIC NEVUS

Management

Cutaneous nevi on the trunk and extremities are frequently excised because of their malignant potential. There has been a greater tendency to observe those on the eyelid until growth is documented, partly because of cosmetic considerations. Management is generally periodic observation, with excision of more suspicious lesions. If the lesion is superficial, an elliptical resection is recommended. If it is present on the eyelid margin only, it can be microscopically shaved parallel to the eyelid margin, using an anatomic thin shaving technique. More extensive tumors require anterior lamellar or full-thickness eyelid resection (1). It has recently been found that congenital nevi can be successfully treat immediately after birth using a technique of dermoabrasion.

Some congenital nevi can occasionally involve most of the eyelid area and their management is more difficult. In such cases, the clinician must weigh the chances of malignant transformation with the consequences of radical removal and cosmetic surgery.

Selected References

Reviews

1. Margo CE, Rabinowicz IM, Hagal MB. Periocular congenital melanocytic nevi. *J Pediatr Ophthalmol Strabismus* 1986;23:222–226.
2. Scott KR, Jakobiec FA, Font RL. Peripunctal melanocytic nevi. Distinctive clinical findings and differential diagnosis. *Ophthalmology* 1989;96:994–998.
3. Putterman AM. Intradermal nevi of the eyelid. *Ophthalmic Surg* 1980;11:584–587.
4. McDonnell PJ, Mayou BJ. Congenital divided naevus of the eyelids. *Br J Ophthalmol* 1988;72:198–201.
5. Lorentzen M, Pers M, Bretteville-Jenssen G. The incidence of malignant transformation in giant pigmented nevi. *Scand J Plast Reconstr Surg* 1977;11:163–167.

Histopathology

6. Margo CE, Habal MB. Large congenital melanocytic nevus. Light and electron microscopic findings. *Ophthalmology* 1987;94:9760–9765.
7. Jia R, Zhu H, Lin M, et al. Clinicopathological characteristics and surgical outcomes of divided nevus of the eyelids: a decade's experience on 73 cases. *Ann Plast Surg* 2012;68(2):166–170.
8. Deprez M, Uffer S. Clinicopathological features of eyelid skin tumors. A retrospective study of 5504 cases and review of literature. *Am J Dermatopathol* 2009;31(3):256–162.

Case Reports

9. Kirzhner M, Jakobiec FA, Kim N. Focal blue nevus of the eyelid margin (mucocutaneous junction): a report of a unique case with a review of the literature. *Ophthal Plast Reconstr Surg* 2011;27(5):338–342.
10. Alfano C, Chiummariello S, De Gado F, et al. Divided nevus of the eyelids: three case studies. *In Vivo* 2007;21(1):137–139.
11. Wu-Chen WY, Bernardino CR, Rubin PA. The clinical evolution of a kissing naevus after incomplete excision. *Br J Ophthalmol* 2004;88(6):848–849.
12. Betharia SM, Kumar S. Lid reconstruction for kissing naevus. *Indian J Ophthalmol* 1988;36(1):32–33.

Chapter 6 Eyelid Melanocytic Tumors

● EYELID MELANOCYTIC NEVUS: PIGMENTED TYPES

Many acquired nevi become clinically apparent in childhood and remain relatively dormant for the remainder of the patient's life. Examples are shown of flat and minimally elevated lesions on eyelid margin.

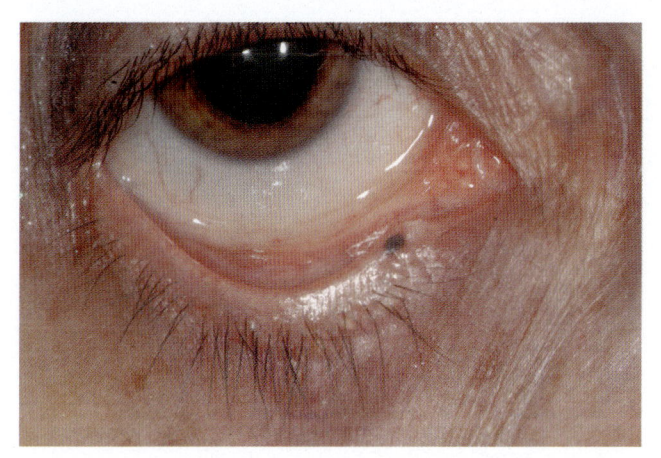

Figure 6.1. Small pigmented melanocytic nevus of left lower eyelid. Note that this benign lesion has not caused loss of cilia.

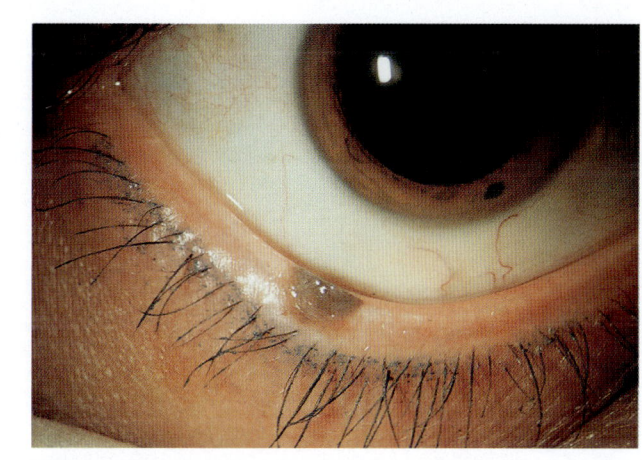

Figure 6.2. Pigmented melanocytic nevus on margin of lower eyelid of a 46-year-old woman.

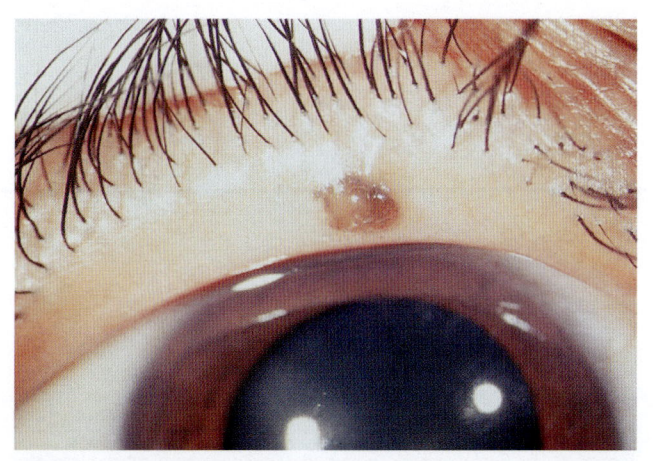

Figure 6.3. Brown melanocytic nevus on margin of upper eyelid of a 40-year-old woman.

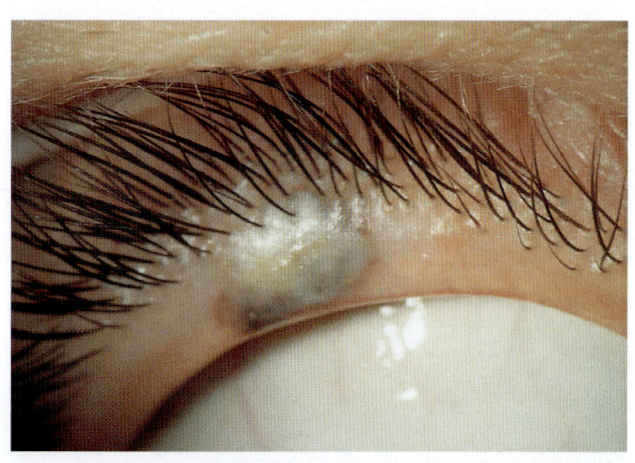

Figure 6.4. Gray melanocytic nevus on margin of upper eyelid in a 44-year-old woman.

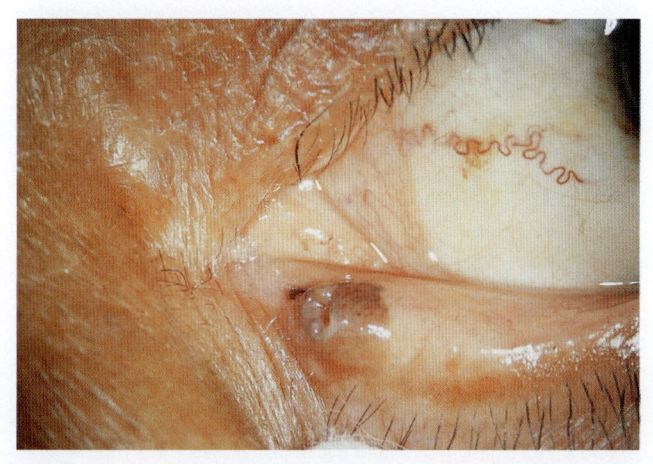

Figure 6.5. Small peripunctal eyelid nevus in a 50-year-old man.

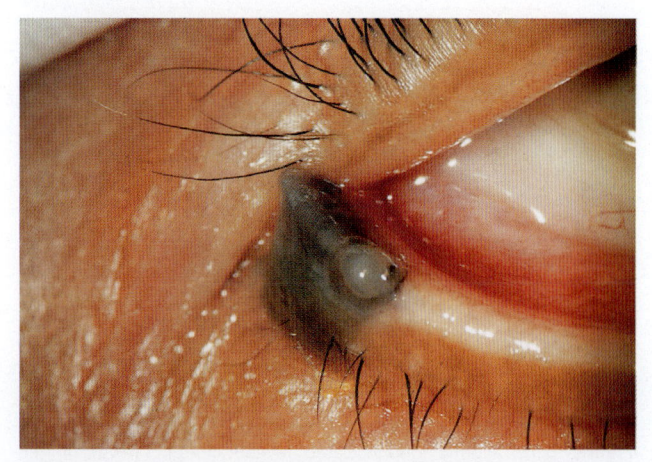

Figure 6.6. Slightly larger peripunctal eyelid nevus in a 90-year-old man. It had been present since childhood and had shown no change.

EYELID MELANOCYTIC NEVUS: AGE AND RACE VARIATIONS

Although it is classically found in Caucasians in the first decade of life, eyelid nevus can be initially diagnosed at any age and in patients of any race.

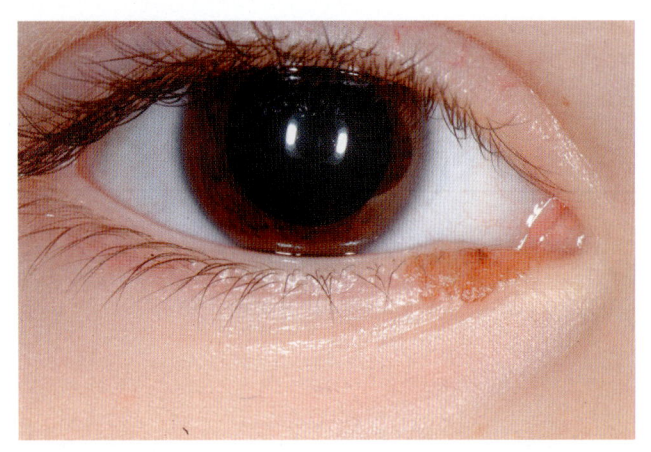

Figure 6.7. Lightly pigmented congenital nevus on right lower eyelid in a young child.

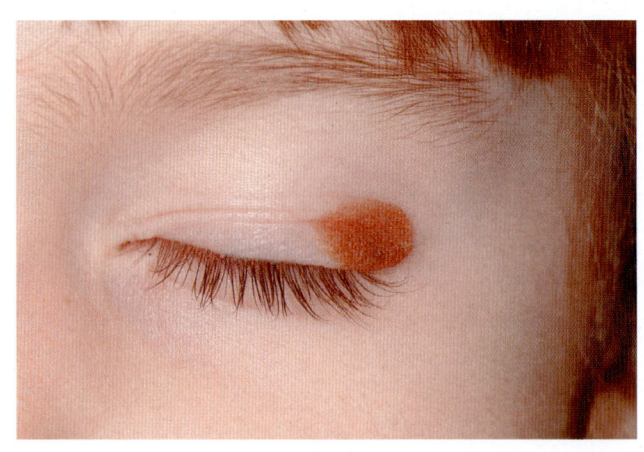

Figure 6.8. Moderately pigmented congenital nevus of upper eyelid in an 8-year-old child.

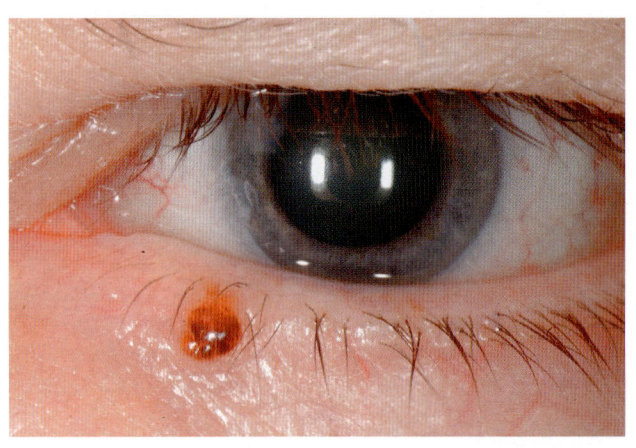

Figure 6.9. Lower eyelid nevus in a Caucasian.

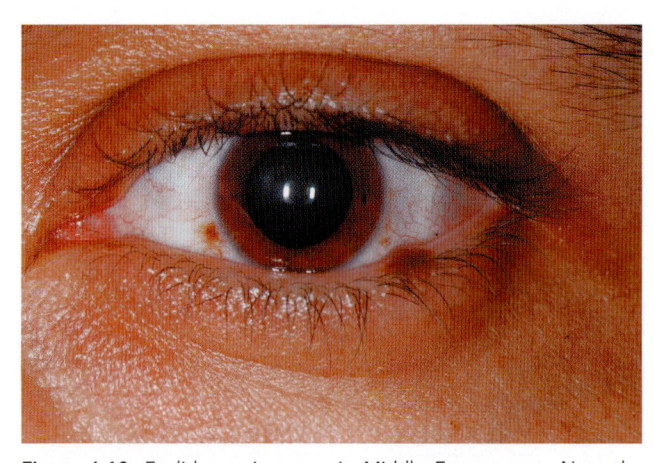

Figure 6.10. Eyelid margin nevus in Middle Eastern man. Note the complexion-related melanosis of conjunctiva, best seen near the limbus.

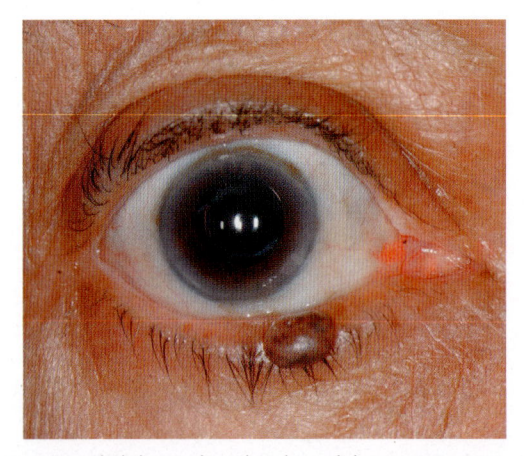

Figure 6.11. Slightly pedunculated eyelid margin nevus in an African-American man. Note again the complexion-related melanosis of the conjunctiva.

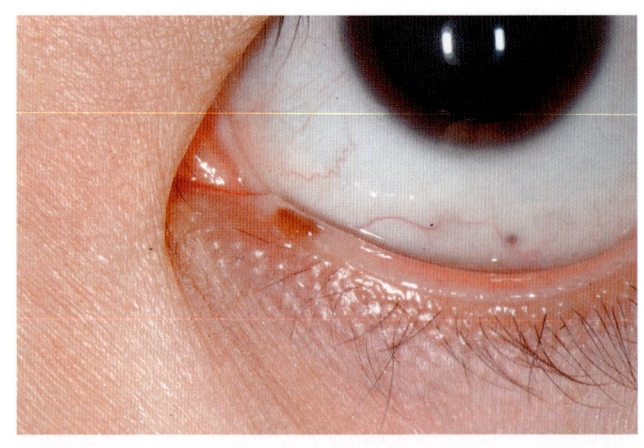

Figure 6.12. Lightly pigmented eyelid margin nevus in a middle-aged Asian woman.

Chapter 6 Eyelid Melanocytic Tumors

● EYELID MELANOCYTIC NEVUS: NONPIGMENTED TYPES

An eyelid nevus can be nonpigmented, thus resembling a papilloma, basal cell carcinoma, or other amelanotic lesion.

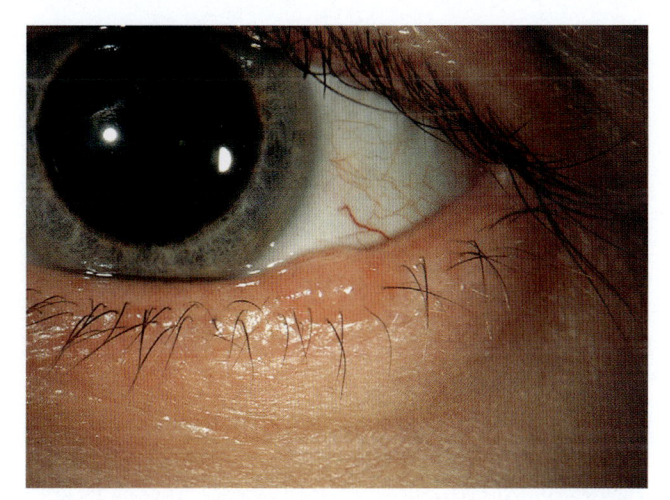

Figure 6.13. Very subtle nonpigmented melanocytic nevus of lower eyelid of a 43-year-old man.

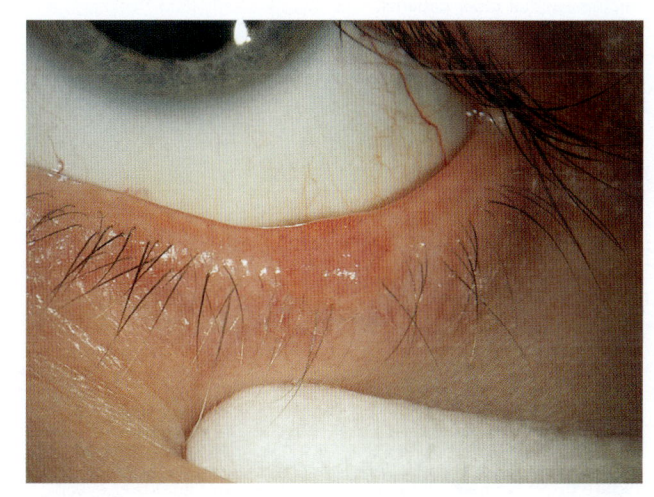

Figure 6.14. Lesion seen in Figure 6.13, with slight eversion of the eyelid, showing that it extends around the eyelid margin to the palpebral conjunctiva.

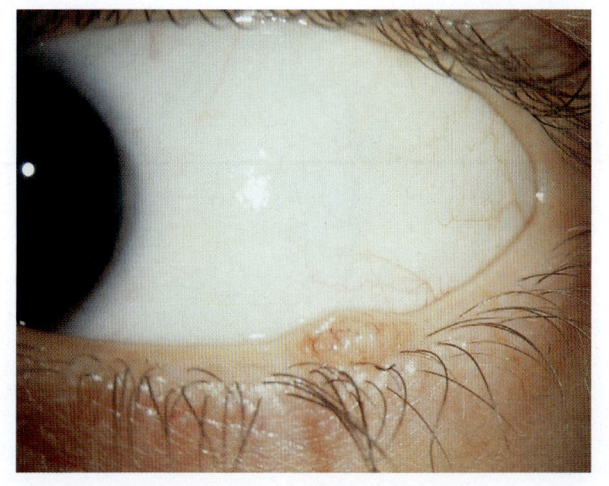

Figure 6.15. Slightly vascular nonpigmented melanocytic nevus of lower eyelid. Such a lesion may be difficult to differentiate clinically from sessile papilloma or nodular basal cell carcinoma.

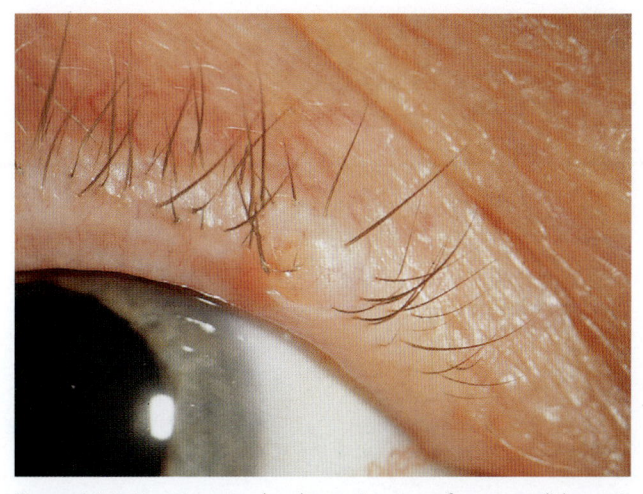

Figure 6.16. Nonpigmented melanocytic nevus of upper eyelid associated with slight loss of cilia in a 59-year-old woman. Such a lesion can resemble basal cell carcinoma.

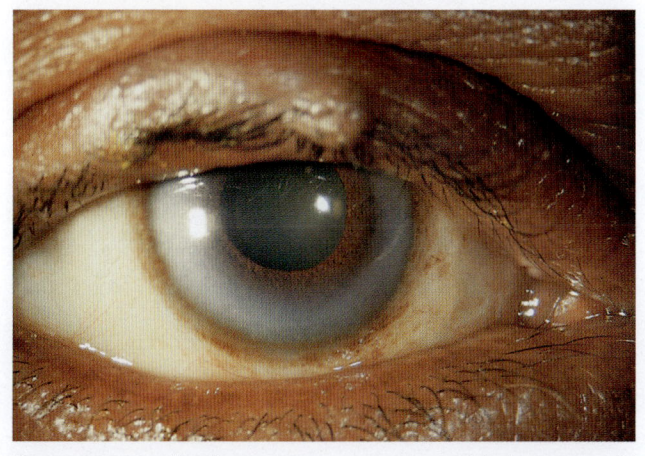

Figure 6.17. Small melanocytic nevus in upper eyelid of a 74-year-old African-American man with slight loss of cilia. Such a lesion can be confused with basal cell carcinoma or many other adnexal tumors.

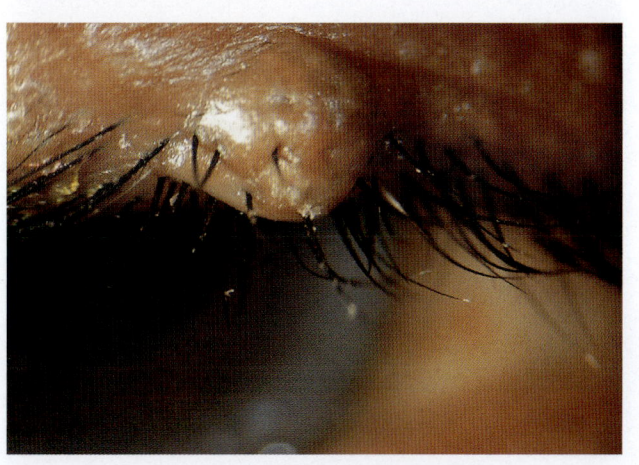

Figure 6.18. Closer view of lesion shown in Figure 6.17.

EYELID MELANOCYTIC NEVUS: CLINICAL VARIATIONS OF NONPIGMENTED TYPE

In some instances, typical eyelid margin nevus can be associated with loss of cilia. It can sometimes be first recognized in middle-aged or older patients.

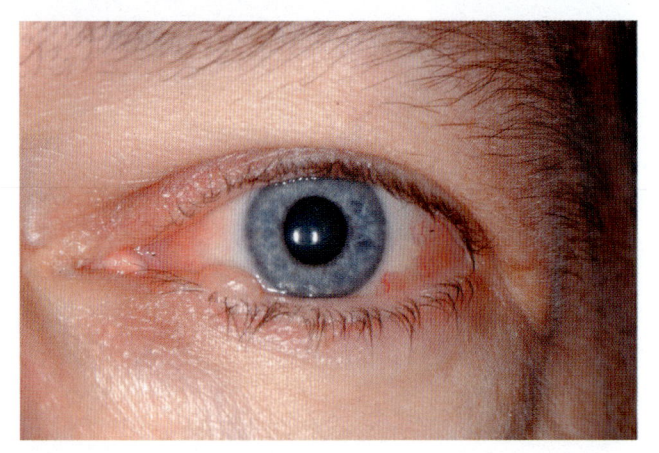

Figure 6.19. Dome-shaped eyelid margin nevus of left lower eyelid.

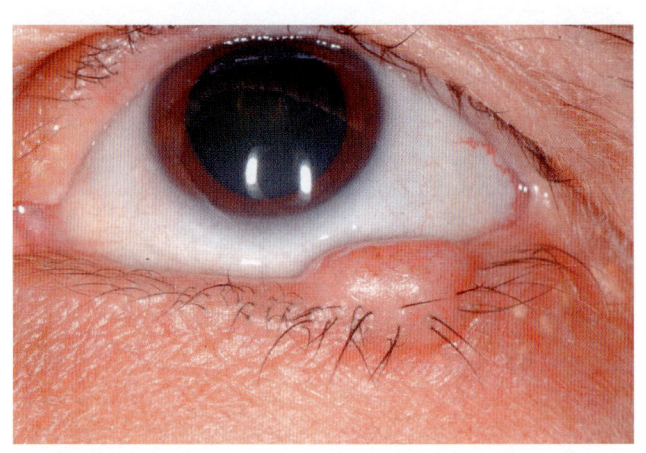

Figure 6.20. Minimally pigmented, slightly vascular lesion on left lower eyelid. Note the sparsity of cilia near the base of the lesion.

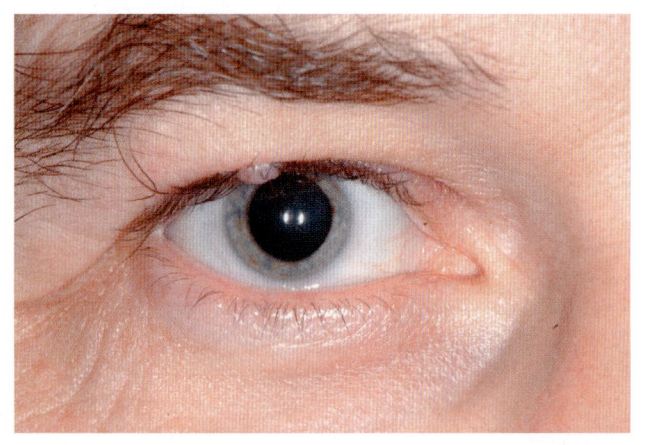

Figure 6.21. Nevus of right upper eyelid margin in adult man. As in the other cases, there is sparsity of cilia in the lesion.

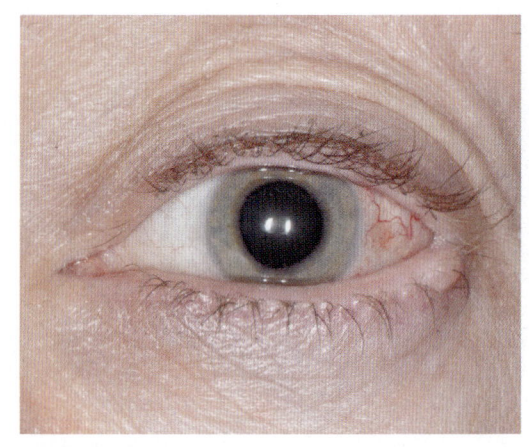

Figure 6.22. Nevus of the left lower eyelid with preservation of eyelashes in adult woman.

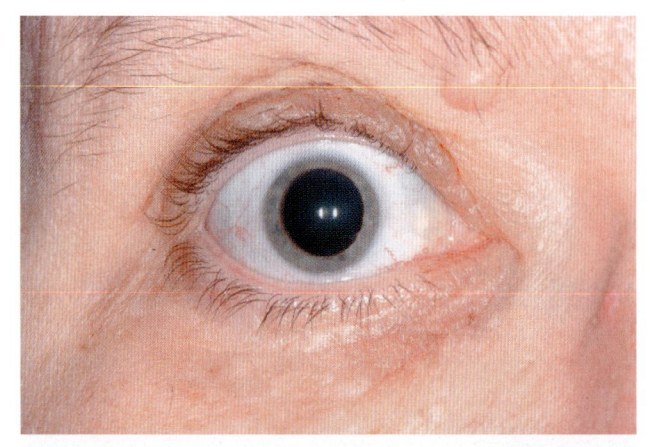

Figure 6.23. Infrabrow nevus in a middle-aged woman. Note the single hair protruding from the lesion.

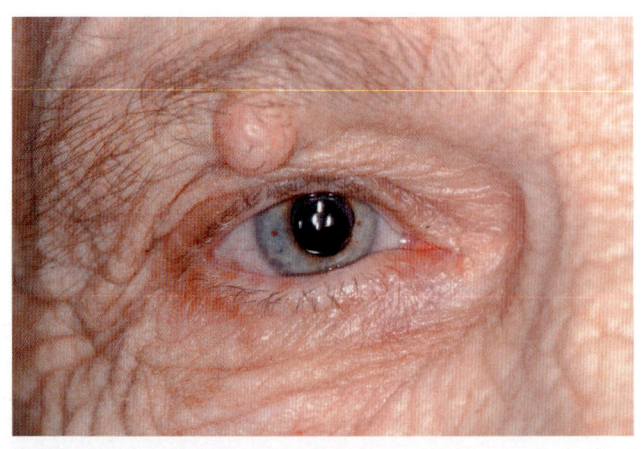

Figure 6.24. Infrabrow nevus in an elderly woman.

Chapter 6 Eyelid Melanocytic Tumors

EYELID MELANOCYTIC NEVUS: EXCISION TECHNIQUE AND PATHOLOGY OF SMALL LESIONS

Suspicious or growing lesions near the eyelid margin can be removed by an elliptical or shaving technique. These methods are illustrated in Chapter 15.

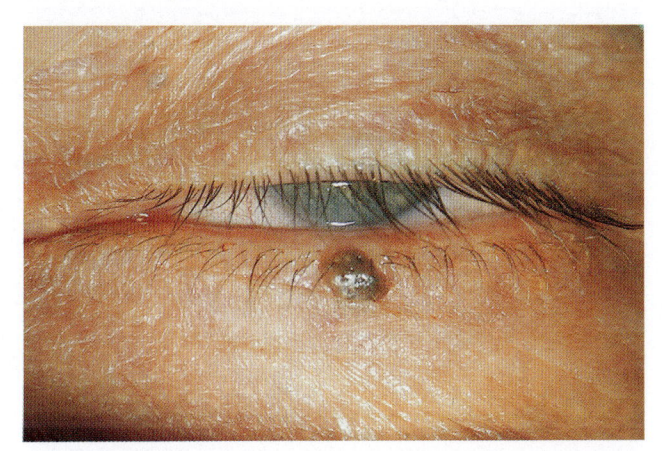

Figure 6.25. Melanocytic nevus of skin of lower eyelid of a 69-year-old man. The lesion had slowly enlarged.

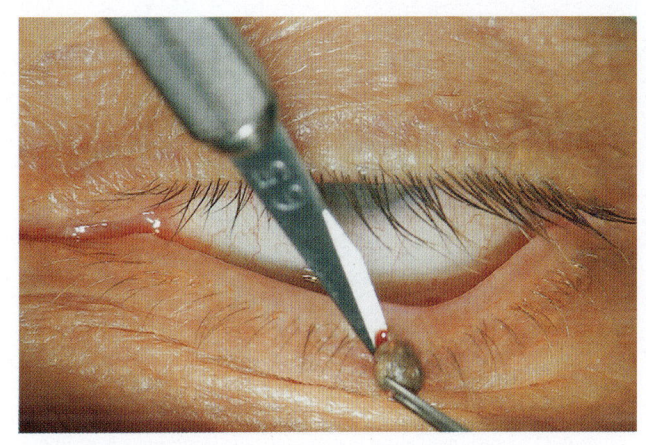

Figure 6.26. Removal of lesion in Figure 6.25 by shaving elliptical excision. The wound was closed with two vertical interrupted skin sutures.

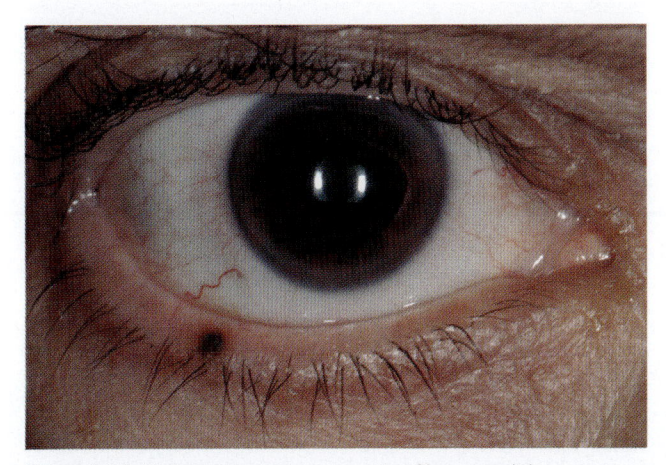

Figure 6.27. Melanocytic nevus on margin of lower eyelid.

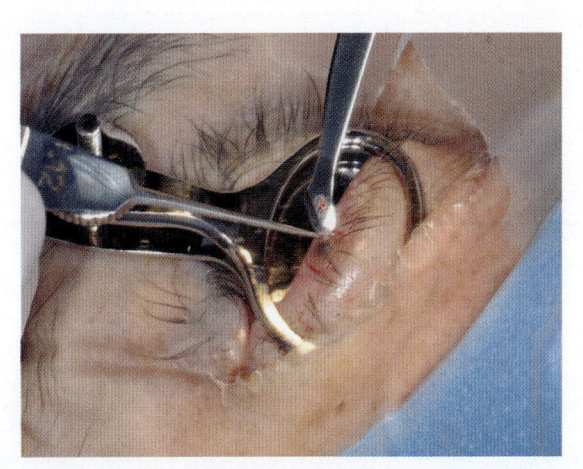

Figure 6.28. Removal of lesion in Figure 6.27 by anatomic shave excision with preservation of tarsus and lid margin using chalazion clamp. Only epithelium is removed from posterior, margin, and anterior eyelid surface. There are no sutures.

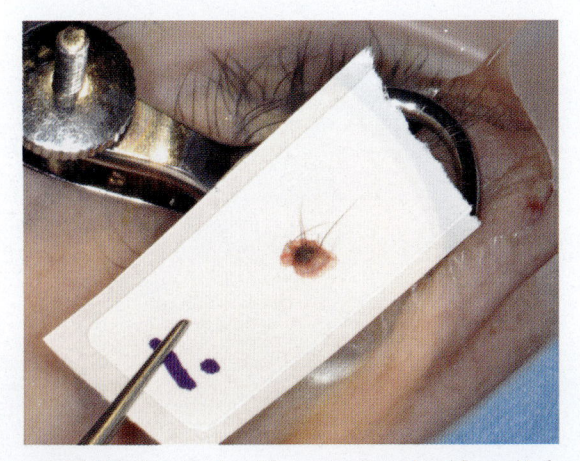

Figure 6.29. Specimen is placed flat on cardboard and floated in formalin for pathology processing.

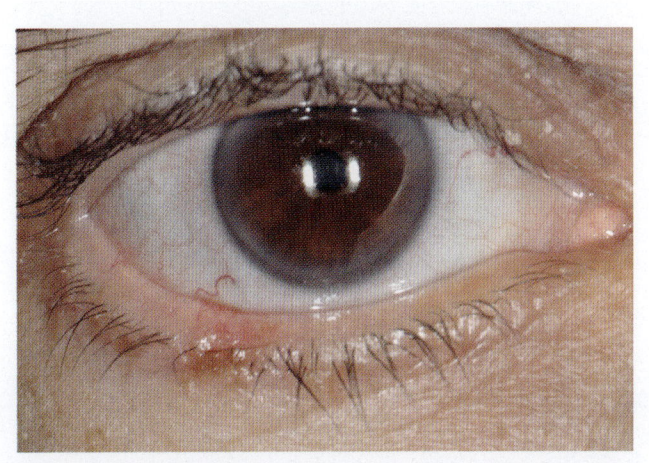

Figure 6.30. At 2-week follow-up of patient in Figure 6.27, the wound has healed with minimal defect.

Part 1 Tumors of the Eyelids

EYELID MELANOCYTIC NEVUS: CONGENITAL DIVIDED ("KISSING") NEVUS

Divided nevus of the eyelid can assume any of several configurations.

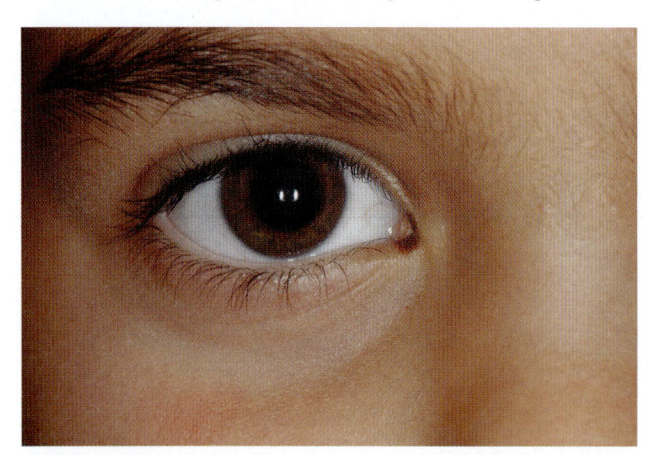

Figure 6.31. Small, medial canthal melanocytic kissing nevus of upper and lower eyelid.

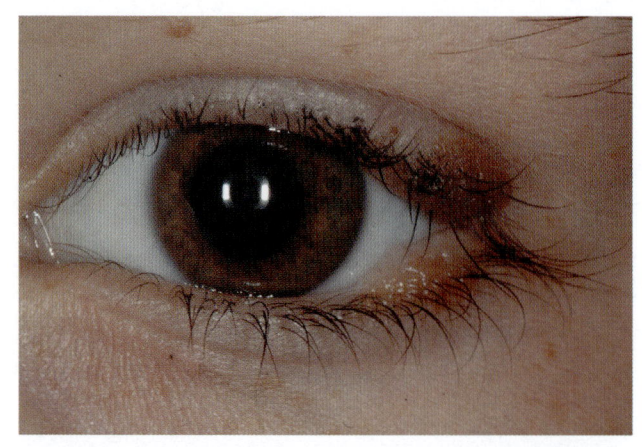

Figure 6.32. Lightly pigmented kissing nevus of upper and lower eyelids with micronodular surface.

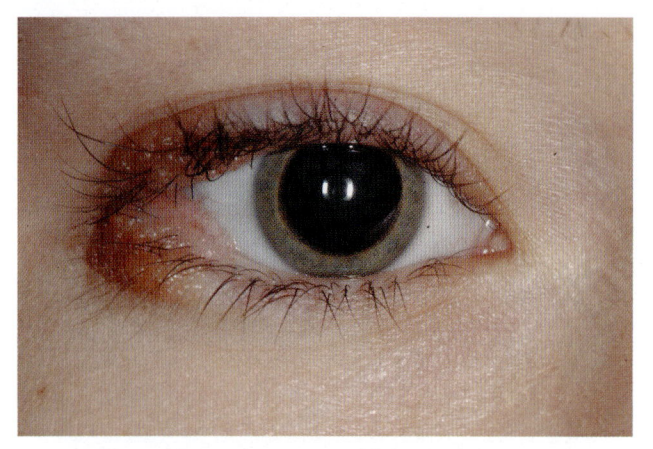

Figure 6.33. Amelanotic kissing nevus of upper and lower eyelids with micronodular surface.

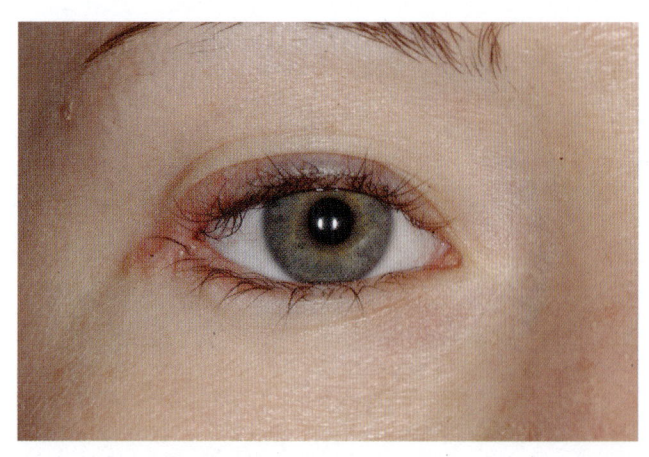

Figure 6.34. Following anatomic shave excision of eyelid nevus in Figure 6.33, the cosmetic appearance has improved, eyelid configuration preserved, and eyelashes intact.

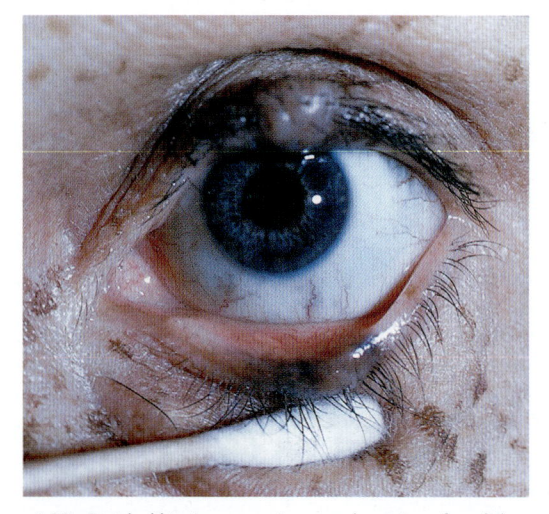

Figure 6.35. Divided kissing nevus in central portion of eyelids.

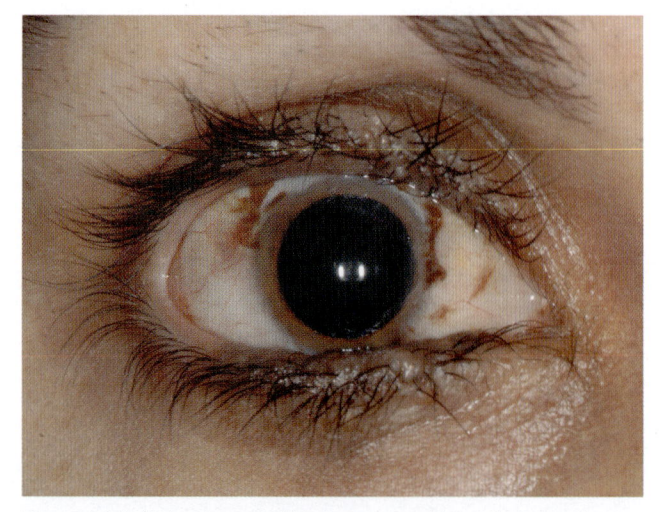

Figure 6.36. Light pigmented kissing nevus with involvement of upper and lower eyelids as well as conjunctiva in between.

● EYELID MELANOCYTIC NEVUS: LARGE CONGENITAL PERIOCULAR TYPE

In some instances, congenital periocular nevus can be very extensive, raising difficult management problems.

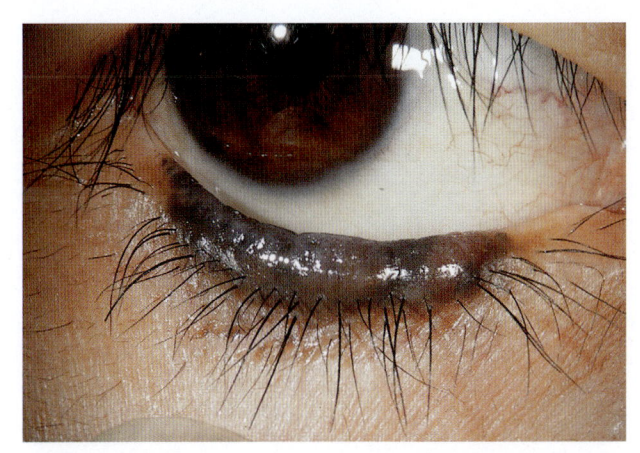

Figure 6.37. Diffuse congenital nevus of lower eyelid in a 30-year-old Asian woman.

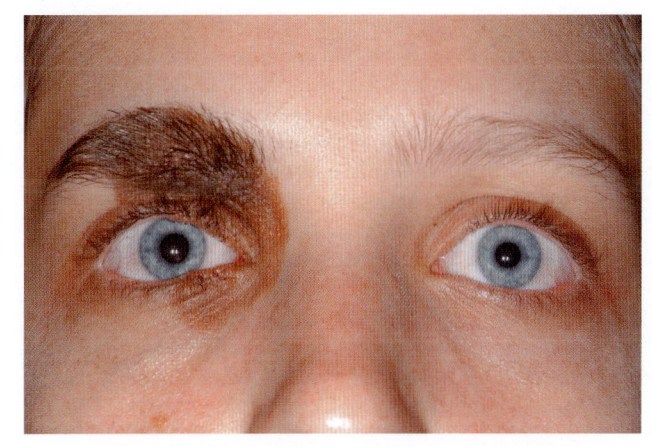

Figure 6.38. Diffuse congenital nevus involving eyelids of right eye.

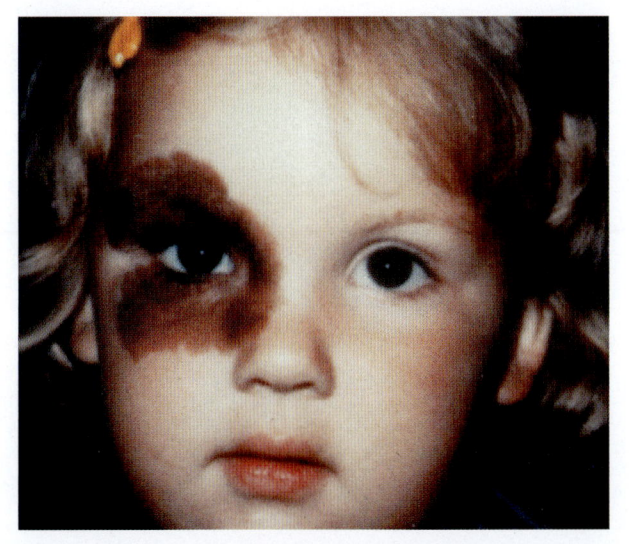

Figure 6.39. Large congenital nevus affecting eyelids and surrounding skin.

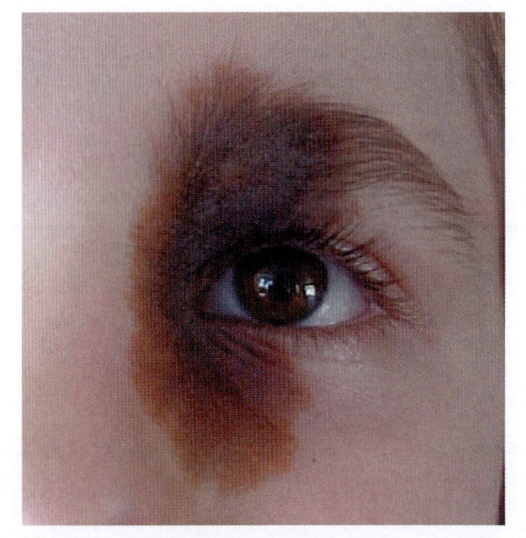

Figure 6.40. Large congenital nevus affecting both eyelids, medial canthal skin, and eyebrow. The indurated lesion was covered with hair. (Courtesy of Curtis Margo, MD.)

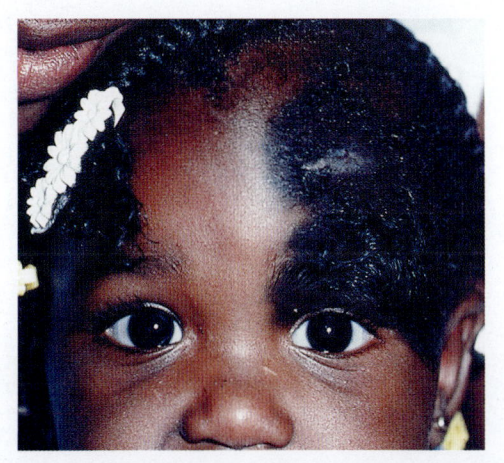

Figure 6.41. Large congenital nevus affects eyelids and scalp. The indurated lesion was covered with hair. (Courtesy of Curtis Margo, MD.)

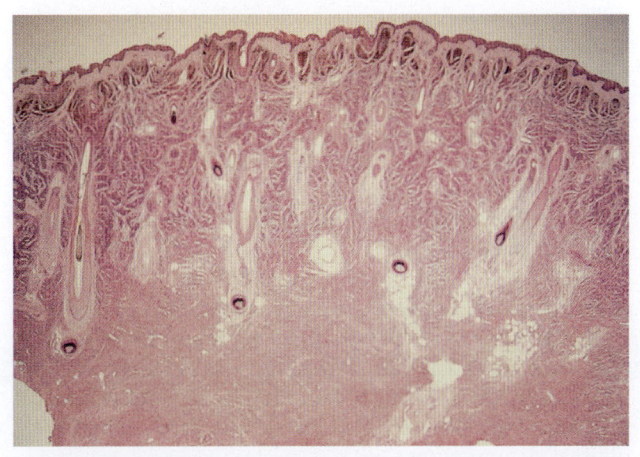

Figure 6.42. Histopathology of biopsy taken from lesion in Figure 6.41, showing heavily pigmented nests of nevus cells in the dermis. (Courtesy of Curtis Margo, MD.)

OCULODERMAL MELANOCYTOSIS (NEVUS OF OTA)

General Considerations

Oculodermal melanocytosis is a congenital pigmentation of periocular skin, uveal tract, and sometimes the orbit, ipsilateral brain meninges, and ipsilateral hard palate (1–18). This condition can occur in Caucasians, Asians, African-American, and other races. The excess melanocytes can spawn malignant melanoma of the uvea, orbit, and brain. Malignant transformation of the eyelid component into cutaneous melanoma is rare. Although oculodermal melanocytosis is generally diagnosed in Caucasians, it can occur in other races, in whom it is also associated with a higher incidence of uveal melanoma (1). This section on eyelid lesions considers mainly the periocular cutaneous lesion as part of the spectrum of oculodermal melanocytosis. The associated uveal melanoma is discussed in the Intraocular Tumors: A Textbook and Atlas.

Clinical Features

Clinically, the cutaneous lesion is a flat, tan-to-gray pigmentation and affects the facial and periocular skin, including the eyelids. Although it may be somewhat irregular, it tends to follow the distribution of the first and second divisions of the trigeminal nerves. It is bilateral in about 10% of cases. Interesting variations include involvement of the temporal skin, hard palate in the roof of the mouth, and eardrum. Another association is iris mammillations, which are often irregular, confluent, dome-shaped elevations on the iris surface. This can be the predominant feature when the episcleral and posterior uveal pigmentation are subtle or absent. Oculodermal melanocytosis can rarely occur in association with other phakomatoses, such as Sturge–Weber syndrome and phakomatosis pigmentovascularis IIa (7,14).

Pathology

Histopathologically, nevus of Ota is characterized by excessive scattered dendritic melanocytes in the dermis. It is not as cellular as a true blue nevus.

Management

A patient with these clinical findings should be evaluated for evidence of ocular melanocytosis and undergo periodic fundus examination to detect early malignant melanoma of the uveal tract (1–3). Uveal melanoma usually occurs in adult Caucasians, but has been recognized in children and African-American patients with congenital melanocytosis, underscoring the need to follow affected patients who would otherwise be at low risk to develop uveal melanoma. The incidence of uveal melanoma in patients with ocular or oculodermal melanocytosis is estimated to be 1:400 cases (1).

Management is generally periodic observation. In cases of cosmetically unacceptable cutaneous lesions, cosmetics may be employed to cover the defect. Laser photocoagulation has also been used and a large series in China has described successful results with Q-switched Alexandrite laser. Surgical removal is generally not advisable, but can be considered in extremely unusual circumstances.

OCULODERMAL MELANOCYTOSIS (NEVUS OF OTA)

Selected References

Reviews

1. Singh AD, De Potter P, Fijal BA, et al. Lifetime prevalence of uveal melanoma in Caucasian patients with ocular (dermal) melanocytosis. *Ophthalmology* 1998;105:195–198.
2. Shields CL, Kaliki S, Livesey M, et al. Association of ocular and oculodermal melanocytosis with the rate of uveal melanoma metastasis: analysis of 7872 consecutive eyes. *JAMA Ophthalmol* 2013;131(8):993–1003.
3. Mashayekhi A, Kaliki S, Walker B, et al. Metastasis from uveal melanoma associated with congenital ocular melanocytosis: a matched study. *Ophthalmology* 2013;120:1465–1468.
4. Lu Z, Fang L, Jiao S, et al. Treatment of 522 patients with nevus of Ota with Q-switched Alexandrite laser. *Chin Med J* 2003;116:226–230.
5. Kopf AW, Bart RS. Malignant blue (Ota's) nevus. *J Dermatol Surg Oncol* 1982;8:442–445.
6. Dorsey CS, Montgomery H. Blue nevus and its distinction from Mongolian spot and the nevus of Ota. *J Invest Dermatol* 1954;22:225–230.
7. Shields CL, Kligman BE, Surianoi MM, et al. Pigmentovascularis of cesioflammea type in 7 cases. Combination of ocular pigmentation (melanocytosis or melanosis) and nevus flammeus with risk for melanoma. *Arch Ophthalmol* 2011;129(6)746–750.

Case Reports

8. Patel BC, Egan CA, Lucius RW, et al. Cutaneous malignant melanoma and oculodermal melanocytosis (nevus of Ota): report of a case and review of the literature. *J Am Acad Dermatol* 1998;38(5 Pt 2):862–865.
9. Gonder JR, Ezell PC, Shields JA, et al. Ocular melanocytosis. A study to determine the prevalence rate of ocular melanocytosis. *Ophthalmology* 1982;89:950–952.
10. Gunduz K, Shields JA, Shields CL, et al. Choroidal melanoma in a 14-year-old patient with ocular melanocytosis. *Arch Ophthalmol* 1998;116:1112–1114.
11. Shields JA, Shields CL, Naseripour M, et al. Choroidal melanoma in a black patient with oculodermal melanocytosis. *Retina* 2002;22:126–128.
12. Honavar SG, Shields CL, Singh AD, et al. Two discrete choroidal melanomas in an eye with ocular melanocytosis. *Ophthalmology* 2002;47:36–41.
13. Gunduz K, Shields CL, Shields JA, et al. Iris mammillations as the only sign of ocular melanocytosis in a child with choroidal melanoma. *Arch Ophthalmol* 2000;118:716–717.
14. Tran HV, Zografos L. Primary choroidal melanoma in phakomatosis pigmentovascularis IIa. *Ophthalmology* 2005;112:1232–1235.
15. Kim JY, Hong JT, Lee SH, et al. Surgical reduction of ocular pigmentation in patients with oculodermal melanocytosis. *Cornea* 2012;31(5):520–524.
16. Dompmartin A, Leroy D, Labbé D, et al. Dermal malignant melanoma developing from a nevus of Ota. *Int J Dermatol* 1989;28(8):535–536.
17. Haim T, Meyer E, Kerner H, et al. Oculodermal melanocytosis (nevus of Ota) and orbital malignant melanoma. *Ann Ophthalmol* 1982;14(12):1132–1136.
18. Croxatto JO, Charles DE, Malbran ES. Neurofibromatosis associated with nevus of Ota and choroidal melanoma. *Am J Ophthalmol* 1981;92(4):578–580.

OCULAR MELANOCYTOSIS: CLINICAL FEATURES

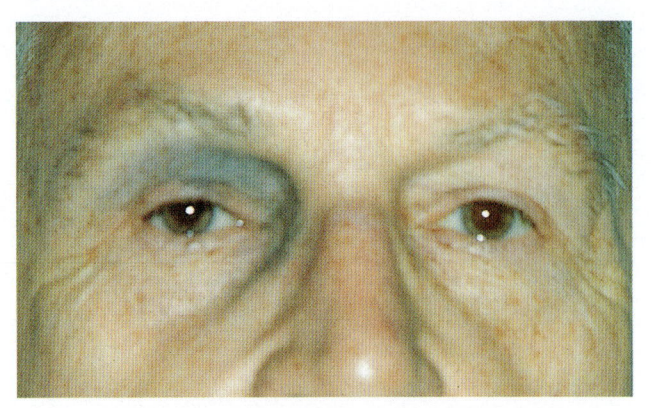

Figure 6.43. Periocular cutaneous pigmentation in a 74-year-old man. This patient did not have scleral or uveal involvement.

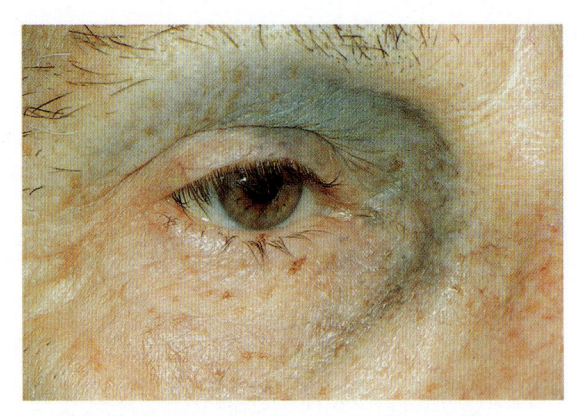

Figure 6.44. Closer view of patient seen in Figure 6.43, showing flat, gray pigmentation involving upper eyelid.

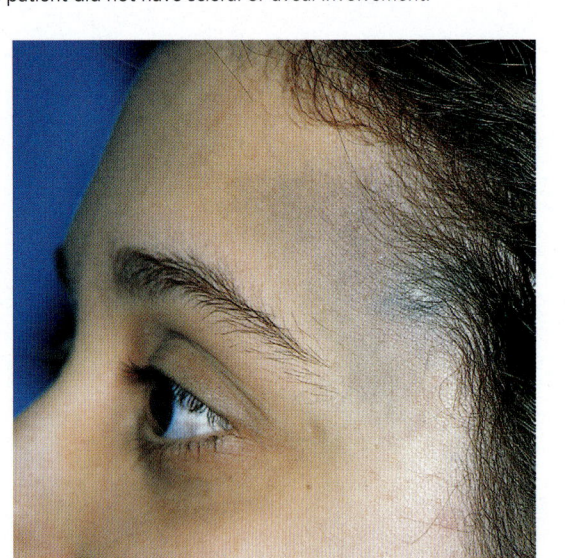

Figure 6.45. Typical patch of pigmentation in temporal region in a patient with ipsilateral oculodermal melanocytosis.

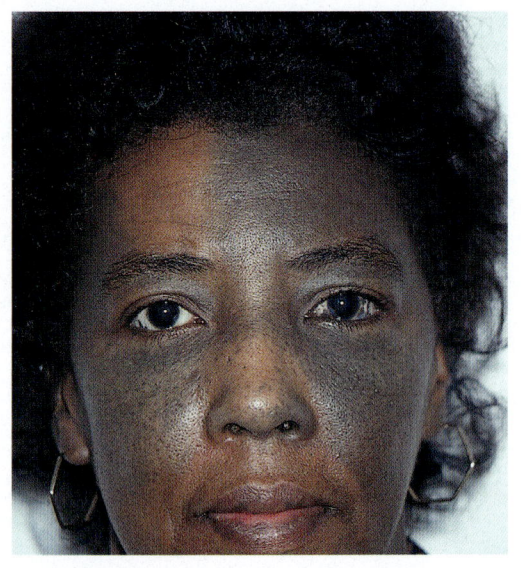

Figure 6.46. Bilateral oculodermal melanocytosis in an African-American patient.

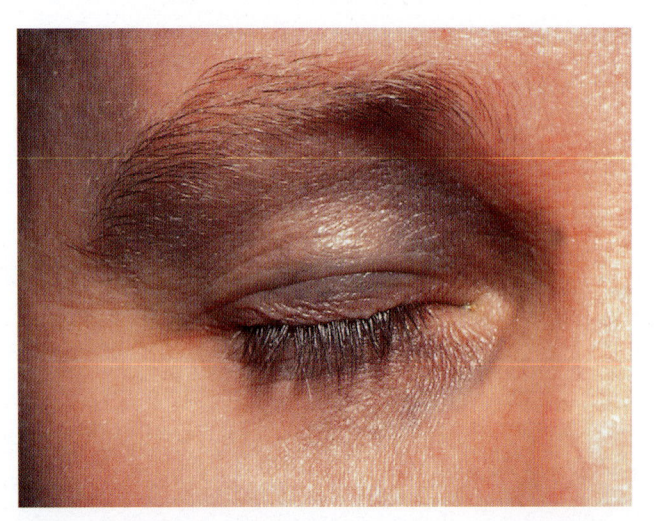

Figure 6.47. Gray pigmentation of right upper and lower eyelids in patient with oculodermal melanocytosis. The patient had a large choroidal melanoma that metastasized to liver despite enucleation.

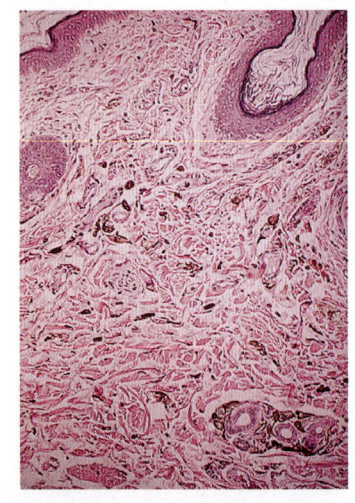

Figure 6.48. Histopathology of eyelid lesion in oculodermal melanocytosis, showing the scattered dendritic melanocytes in the dermis. (Hematoxylin–eosin ×30.)

Chapter 6 Eyelid Melanocytic Tumors

CONGENITAL OCULODERMAL MELANOCYTOSIS: SPECTRUM OF PIGMENTATION

Eyelid changes are often rather subtle, whereas scleral pigmentation is usually more evident. In rare cases, there may be overlap of oculodermal melanocytosis with other systemic hamartoma syndromes, such as nevus flammeus associated with Sturge–Weber syndrome.

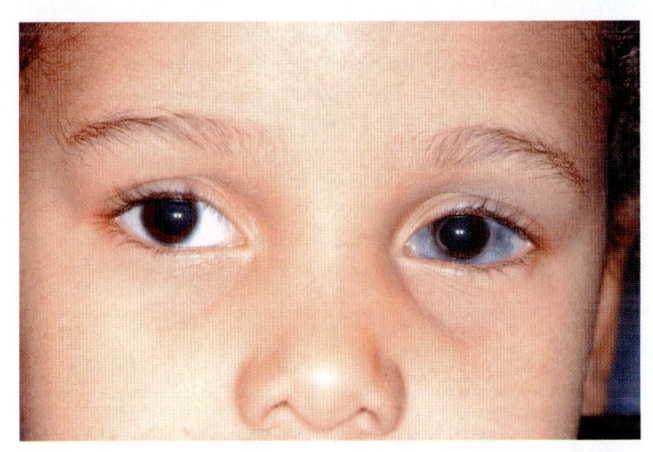

Figure 6.49. Subtle cutaneous pigmentation of upper and lower eyelids in a child. Note the more obvious episcleral pigmentation.

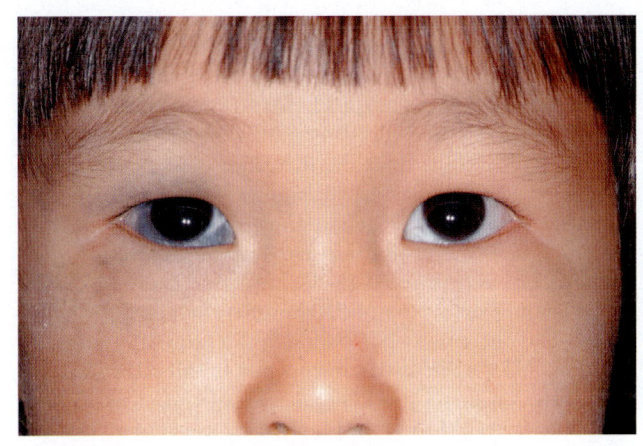

Figure 6.50. Asian child with subtle periocular skin pigmentation. Note again the more obvious episcleral pigmentation.

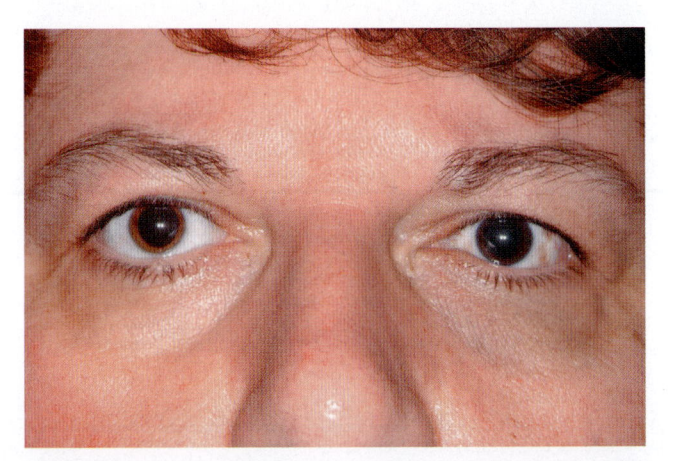

Figure 6.51. Subtle cutaneous pigmentation around left eye in adult Caucasian woman. Note the heterochromia and episcleral pigmentation.

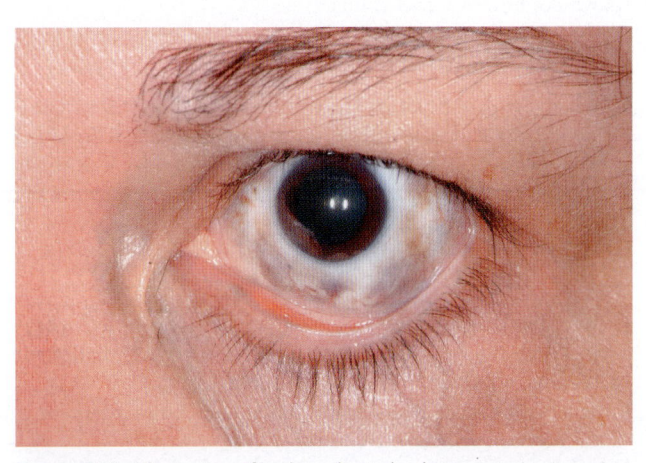

Figure 6.52. Closer view of ipsilateral episcleral pigmentation in patient shown in Figure 6.51.

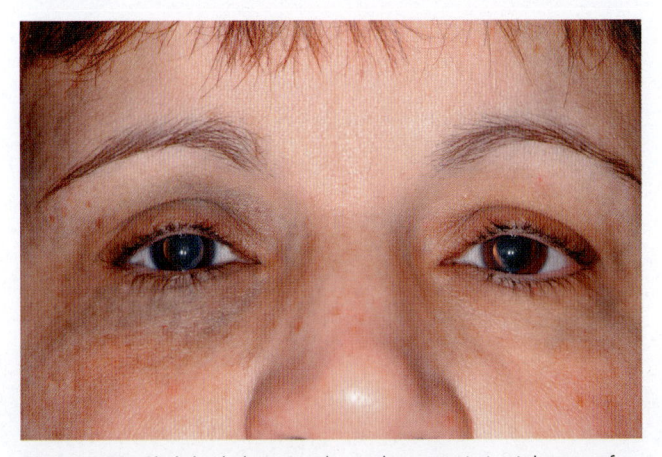

Figure 6.53. Slightly dark periocular melanocytosis in right eye of an adult Caucasian woman. Note the heterochromia with the ipsilateral right iris being darker.

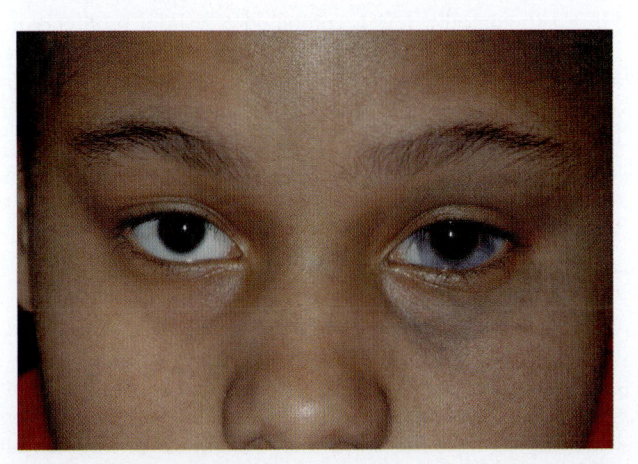

Figure 6.54. Young African-American girl with periocular cutaneous and scleral melanocytosis.

EYELID LENTIGO MALIGNA (MELANOTIC FRECKLE OF HUTCHINSON)

General Considerations

Lentigo maligna (LM; melanotic freckle of Hutchinson) is an acquired pigmentation that usually occurs on sun-exposed areas like the forehead and malar region. It can occasionally involve the eyelid either as a small, localized lesion or as extension from the adjacent skin (1–12). This condition occurs almost exclusively in Caucasians and its prevalence may be as high as 1 in 300 persons. The incidence of evolution into a melanoma (lentigo maligna melanoma [LMM]) varies from report to report (1–12). It is estimated that about 30% of untreated cases will evolve into LMM, usually 10 to 15 years after the LM is first noted (1–5). LMM is believed to be an eyelid counterpart of conjunctival primary acquired melanosis (PAM) and the eyelid and conjunctival lesions are often seen together. PAM is discussed subsequently in this atlas.

Reports on eyelid melanoma have suggested that 19% to 61% arise from LM (3,4). LM is often associated with PAM of the conjunctiva (discussed in conjunctival section), which may represent the mucous membrane counterpart of LM and can spawn conjunctival melanoma.

Clinical Features

Clinically, LM appears in older adults as a flat, well-circumscribed, irregular, tan-to-brown macule (1–12). It enlarges slowly over years. A melanoma secondary to LM is initially flat or minimally elevated (melanoma in situ), but eventually becomes more elevated.

Differential Diagnosis

Differential diagnosis of LM includes lentigo senilis, seborrheic keratosis, acquired melanocytic nevus, and malignant melanoma. Concerning acquired nevus, the age of onset is important, because LM usually has a later onset than junctional melanocytic nevus.

Pathology

Histopathologically, LM is composed of a mild proliferation of intraepidermal melanocytes, usually without distinct nests as seen with junctional nevus (1–12). There may be cellular atypia, prompting some pathologists to equate it with malignant melanoma in situ, although this continues to be controversial. With time LM can slowly evolve into true melanoma and the management depends on the clinical findings as mentioned below.

Management

Older or physically ill patients with mild LM can be followed without immediate treatment. If there appears to be evolution into melanoma (LMM), various treatments have been employed. Ideally, progressive LM should be managed by wide surgical resection, which may be difficult or impractical in the eyelid region. Mohs microsurgery and frozen section control have been used to remove LM and LMM. Alternative treatments include cryotherapy, topical 5-fluorouracil, dermabrasion, and electrodessication and curettage. Intralesional injection of interferon has been advocated to treat recurrent LM of the eyelid. There has been recent interest in the use of topical imiquimod (Aldara; Graceway Pharmaceuticals, Bristol, TN) cream to treat LM in selected cases (8–10).

Some believe that LMM has a better prognosis than superficial spreading or nodular melanoma, with metastasis reported to occur in 10% of cases. However, this is controversial; others have reported that, after adjustment for tumor thickness and other factors, the prognosis for patients with LMM is the same as for other forms of melanoma.

Selected References

Reviews

1. Clark WH Jr, Mihm MC Jr. Lentigo maligna and lentigo maligna melanoma. *Am J Pathol* 1969;55:39–46.
2. Blodi FC, Widner RR. The melanotic freckle (Hutchinson) of the eyelid. *Surv Ophthalmol* 1968;13:23–30.
3. Vaziri M, Buffam FV, Martinka M, et al. Clinicopathologic features and behavior of cutaneous eyelid melanoma. *Ophthalmology* 2002;109:901–909.
4. Naidoff MA, Bernardino VB, Clark WH. Melanocytic lesions of the eyelid skin. *Am J Ophthalmol* 1976;82:371–382.
5. Koh HK, Michalik E, Sober AJ, et al. Lentigo maligna melanoma has no better prognosis than other types of melanoma. *J Clin Oncol* 1984;2:994–1001.

Management

6. Malhotra R, Chen C, Huilgol SC, et al. Mapped serial excision for periocular lentigo maligna and lentigo maligna melanoma. *Ophthalmology* 2003;110:2011–2018.
7. Graham GF, Stewart R. Cryosurgery for unusual cutaneous neoplasms. *J Oncol* 1977;3:437–442.
8. Carucci JA, Leffell DJ. Intralesional interferon alfa for treatment of recurrent lentigo maligna of the eyelid in a patient with primary acquired melanosis. *Arch Dermatol* 2000;136:1415–1416.
9. Demirci H, Shields CL, Bianciotto CG, Shields JA. Topical imiquimod for periocular lentigo maligna. *Ophthalmology* 2010;117(12):2424–2429.
10. Wolf IH, Cerroni L, Kodama K, et al. Treatment of lentigo maligna (melanoma in situ) with the immune response modifier imiquimod. *Arch Dermatol* 2005;141:510–514.

Histopathology

11. Grossniklaus HE, McLean IW. Cutaneous melanoma of the eyelid. Clinicopathologic features. *Ophthalmology* 1991;98:1867–1873.
12. Grossniklaus HE. Correspondence re: A. B. Ackerman, R. Sood, and M. Koenig, Primary acquired melanosis of the conjunctiva is melanoma in situ. *Mod Pathol* 1991;4:253.

Chapter 6 Eyelid Melanocytic Tumors

EYELID LENTIGO MALIGNA (MELANOTIC FRECKLE OF HUTCHINSON)

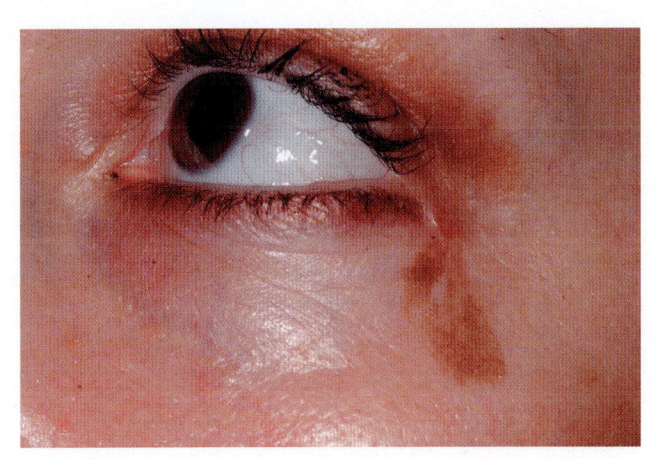

Figure 6.55. Lentigo maligna around the area of lateral canthus of an elderly woman.

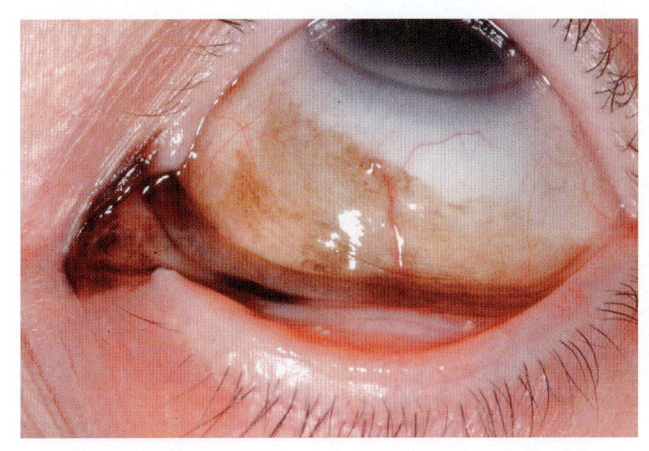

Figure 6.56. Lentigo maligna of eyelid skin with contiguous conjunctival component (primary acquired melanosis).

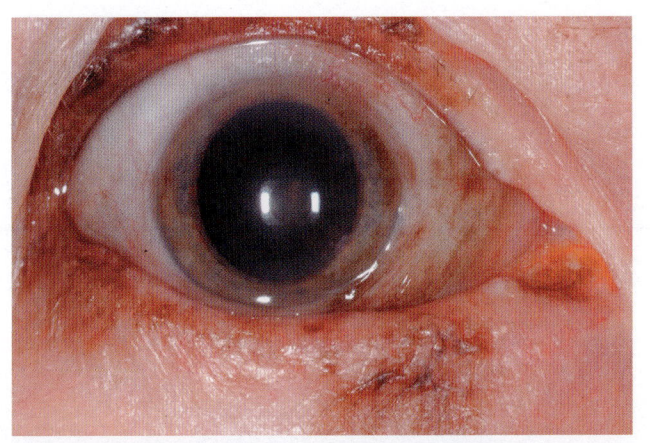

Figure 6.57. Diffuse lentigo maligna on lower eyelid margin in an elderly woman. Note again the associated conjunctival primary acquired melanosis.

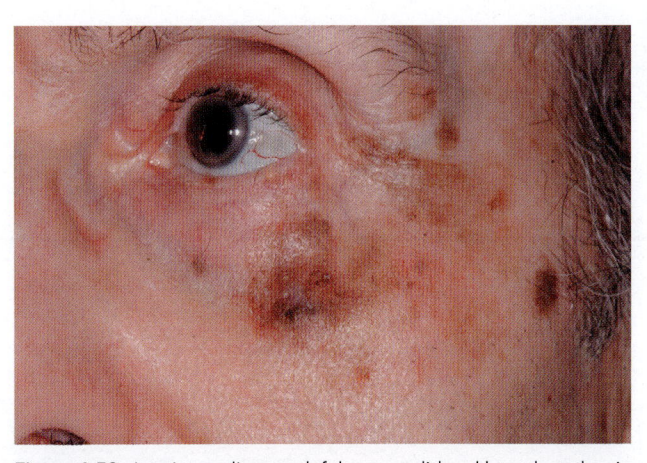

Figure 6.58. Lentigo maligna on left lower eyelid and lateral canthus in a 91-year-old man.

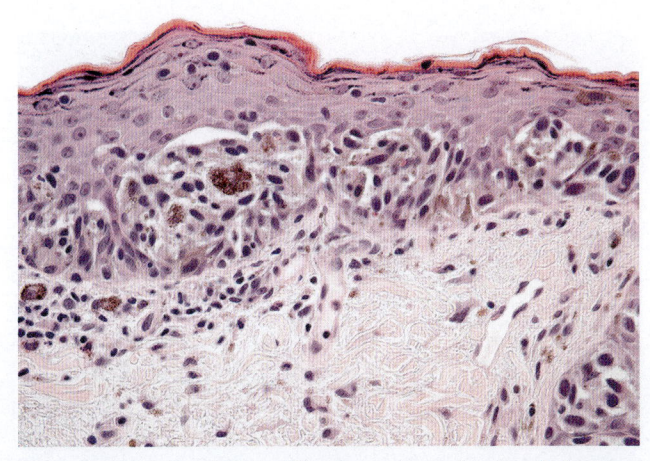

Figure 6.59. Histopathology of lentigo maligna, showing the intraepithelial atypical melanocytes in the epidermis. (Hematoxylin–eosin ×100.)

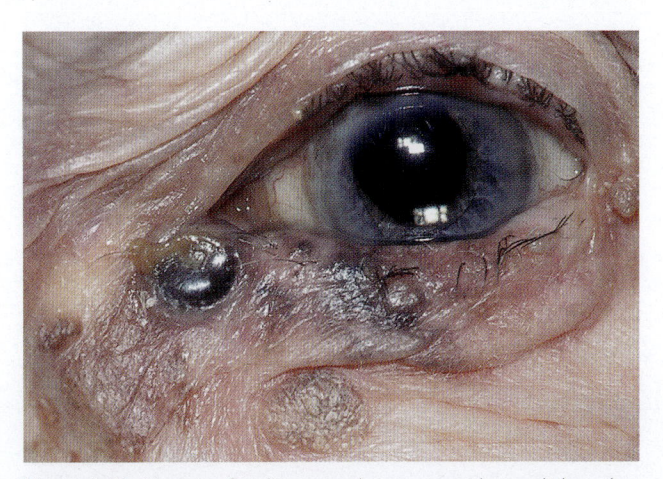

Figure 6.60. Nodule of malignant melanoma near the medial canthus arising from lentigo maligna melanoma in an 88-year-old woman.

EYELID LENTIGO MALIGNA: SURGICAL EXCISION

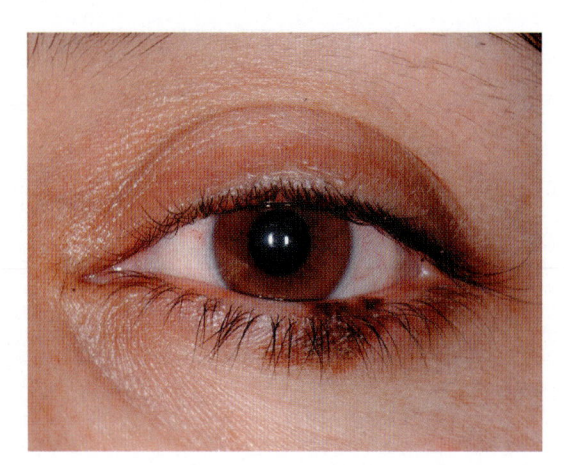

Figure 6.61. Lentigo maligna involving left lower eyelid in a middle-aged woman.

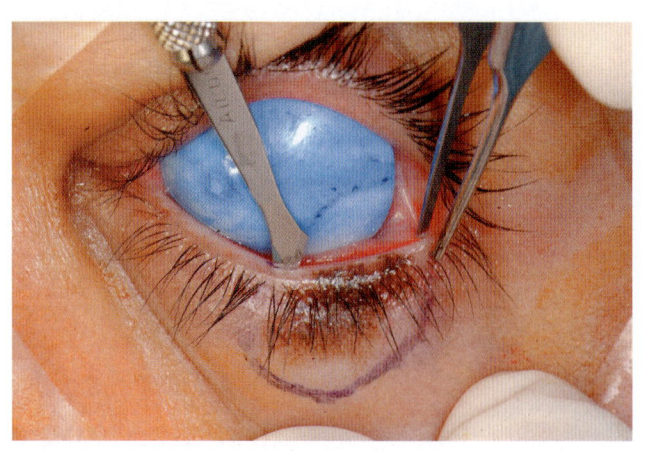

Figure 6.62. Outline of anticipated surgical excision has been marked with a sterile pen and the anterior lamella of the eyelid is divided from the posterior lamella at the eyelid margin. A plastic shell has been inserted to protect the cornea.

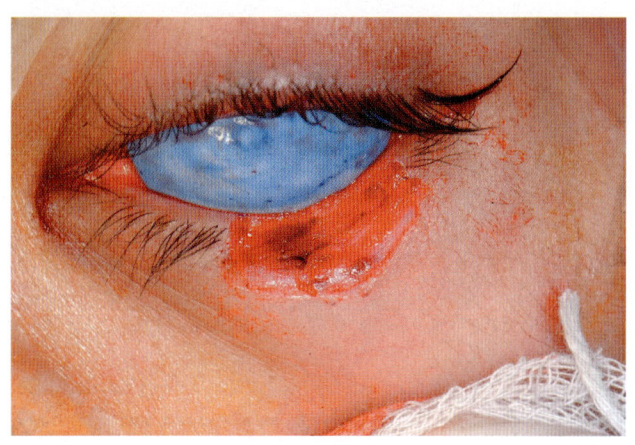

Figure 6.63. The anterior lamella with the pigmented lesion has been removed, exposing the orbicularis muscle.

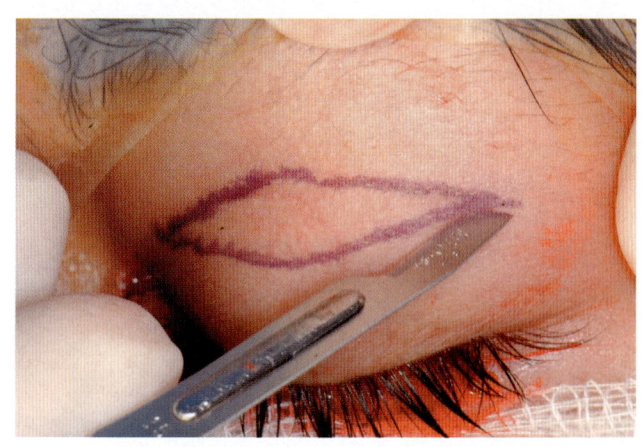

Figure 6.64. Skin is harvested from upper eyelid for grafting to lower eyelid.

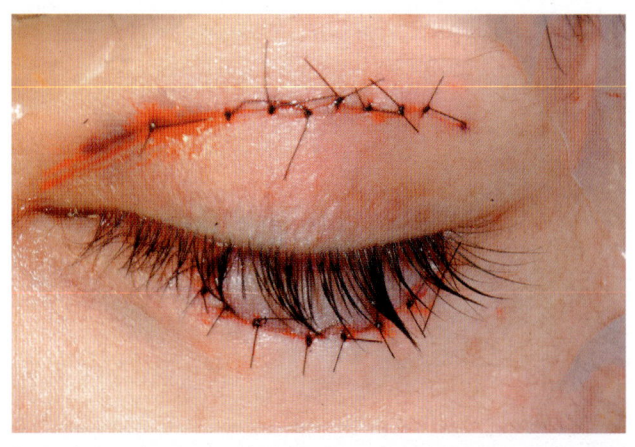

Figure 6.65. The recipient and donor sites have been closed with nylon sutures.

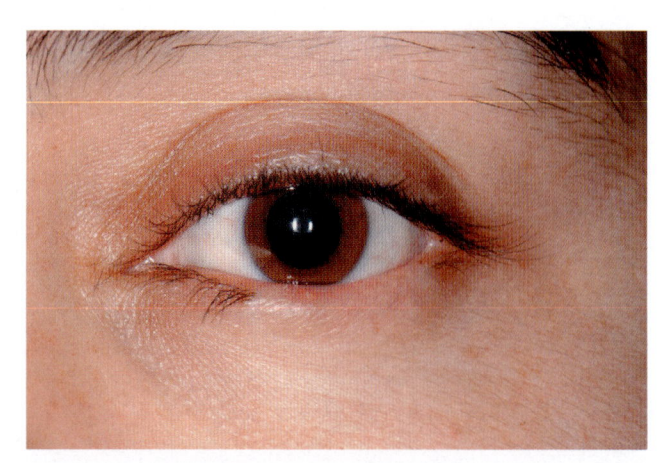

Figure 6.66. Appearance 3 months after surgery. The lower lid has healed and cilia are absent at the upper margin of the skin graft.

Chapter 6 Eyelid Melanocytic Tumors

EYELID LENTIGO MALIGNA: MELANOMA

In this case, the aggressive tumor required orbital exenteration.

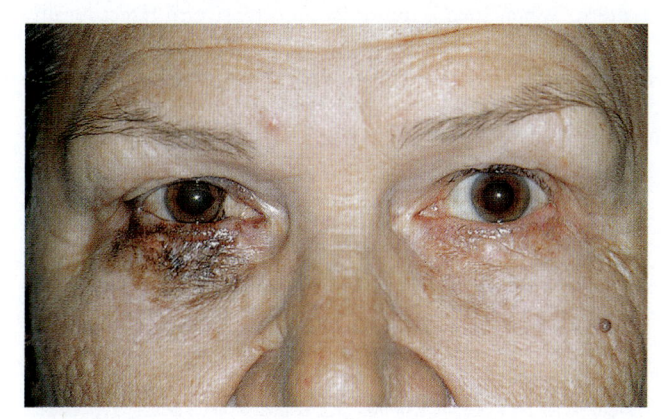

Figure 6.67. Unilateral pigmentation of lower eyelid in a 68-year-old woman. She subsequently developed recurrent eyelid and conjunctival melanoma that were managed by multiple local excisions over 12 years.

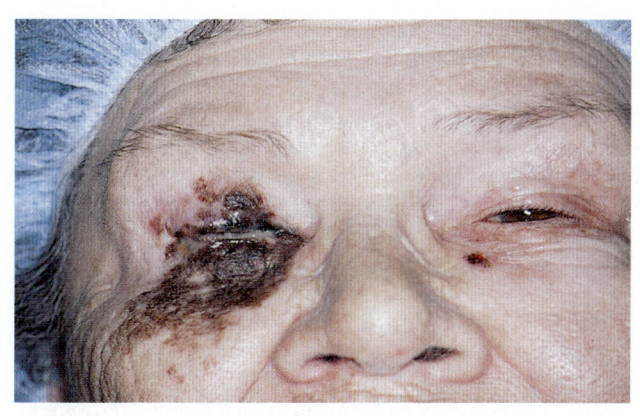

Figure 6.68. Appearance of same patient 11 years later at age 79, showing extensive eyelid recurrence. Biopsies showed lentigo maligna melanoma of skin, conjunctiva, and anterior orbit.

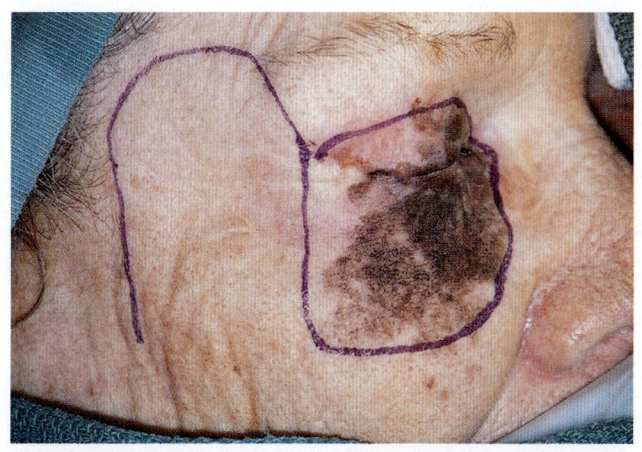

Figure 6.69. Outline of tumor excision from lower and upper eyelids, combined with orbital exenteration. A rotational flap is designed to cover the defect and permit primary closure of the skin over the defect.

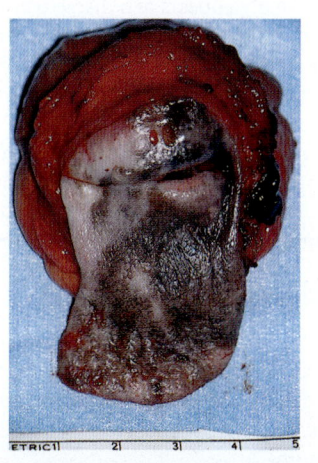

Figure 6.70. Gross appearance of surgical specimen including the eyelids and orbital contents including the globe.

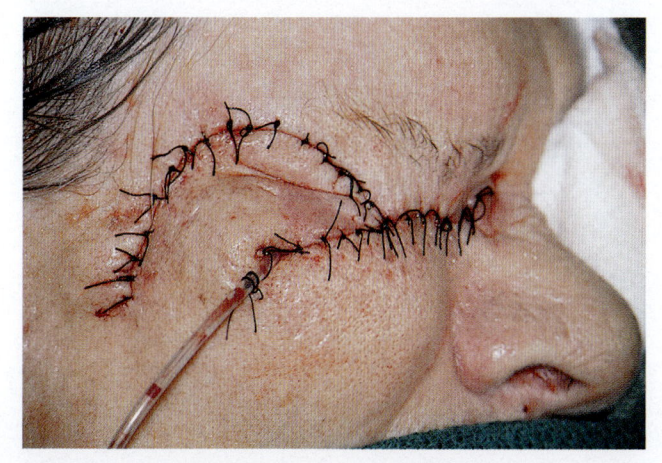

Figure 6.71. Appearance immediately after surgery showing successful closure. A surgical drain has been placed temporally.

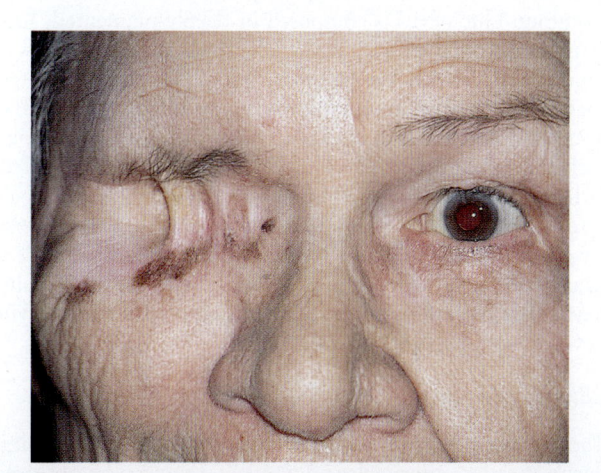

Figure 6.72. Appearance >1 year later. Note that there is mild recurrence of lentigo maligna melanoma. The patient was alive and well 12 years after initial referral. The patient declined an orbital prosthesis. She was lost to follow-up, but reportedly died of an unrelated cause.

EYELID BLUE NEVUS

General Considerations

Blue nevus is a congenital or acquired cutaneous lesion that can take the form of either common blue nevus or cellular blue nevus (1–7). The common blue nevus generally occurs on the dorsa of the hands or feet, but can be found anywhere on the skin. The cellular blue nevus is generally larger and usually occurs in the region of the buttocks or sacrococcygeal region. Blue nevi are so named because of their blue color that results from the reflection of shorter blue wavelengths of light by dermal melanin. The common blue nevus has no known potential to evolve into melanoma, whereas the cellular blue nevus has a low potential to undergo malignant transformation. Both types can uncommonly occur in the eyelid, periocular skin, and orbit. In rare instances, blue nevi are associated with lentigines and cutaneous and atrial myxomas (Lamb syndrome).

Clinical Features

The blue nevus usually appears as a discrete blue-to-black nodule on the eyelid. It is similar to melanocytic nevus described in the previous section, but is deep to the epidermis and has a characteristic blue-gray color. Cellular blue nevus is similar to oculodermal melanocytosis, but it tends to be less distinct, thicker, and more irregular and is not associated with episcleral or uveal pigmentation or with uveal melanoma. The pigmented process can even involve the palate, orbit, and brain, and can spawn melanoma in any of those tissues (3,4).

Differential Diagnosis

Lesions that can resemble common blue nevus include melanoma, seborrheic keratosis, varix, apocrine hidrocystoma, and pigmented basal cell carcinoma. The diffuse periocular cellular blue nevus must be differentiated from oculodermal melanocytosis and melanoma.

Pathology

Common blue nevus is composed of deeply pigmented, fusiform melanocytes that are almost identical to those of nevus of Ota except that they are somewhat more concentrated. Interspersed with the melanocytes are nonpigmented cells that may have a neuroid appearance. The cellular blue nevus has similar melanocytes, but also has cellular islands of closely aggregated, rather large spindle-shaped cells with ovoid nuclei and pale cytoplasm often containing little or no melanin. The cells may have a neuroid appearance (1–7). The overlying epidermis is usually normal. There is a hybrid variant with features of blue nevus and features of junctional or compound melanocytic nevus (combined nevus).

Management

The management of a suspected common blue nevus is similar to that for other melanocytic nevi. They can be observed or removed for cosmetic reasons, but true malignant transformation is uncommon. Periocular cellular blue nevus can be difficult to manage because it may have a more diffuse growth pattern. When such a tumor is too extensive to resect locally, the clinician often must resort to debulking procedures or orbital exenteration if histopathology shows malignant change. Two of our patients with extensive periocular cellular blue nevus developed extensive orbital and brain melanoma that proved to be fatal (4).

Selected References

Reviews

1. Rodriguez HA, Ackerman LV. Cellular blue nevus. Clinical pathologic study of 45 cases. *Cancer* 1968;21:393–405.
2. Wang Q, Prieto V, Esmaeli B, et al. Cellular blue nevi of the eyelid: a possible diagnostic pitfall. *J Am Acad Dermatol* 2008;58(2):257–260.

Case Reports

3. Silverberg GD, Kadin ME, Dorfman RF, et al. Invasion of the brain by a cellular blue nevus of the scalp. A case report with light and electron microscopic studies. *Cancer* 1971;27:349–355.
4. Gunduz K, Shields JA, Shields CL, et al. Periorbital cellular blue nevus leading to orbitopalpebral and intracranial melanoma. *Ophthalmology* 1998;105:2046–2050.
5. Sokol JA, Clark JD, Lee HB, et al. Pigmented epithelioid melanocytoid tumor of the ocular adnexa. *J Pediatr Ophthalmol Strabismus* 2010;21;47 Online:e1–e4.
6. Jakobiec FA, Stacy RC, Thakker MM. Blue nevus of the tarsus as the predominant component of a combined nevus of the eyelid. *Ophthal Plast Reconstr Surg* 2011;27(4):e94–e96.
7. Kirzhner M, Jakobiec FA, Kim N. Focal blue nevus of the eyelid margin (mucocutaneous junction): a report of a unique case with a review of the literature. *Ophthal Plast Reconstr Surg* 2011;27(5):338–342.

Chapter 6 Eyelid Melanocytic Tumors

EYELID CELLULAR BLUE NEVUS: GIVING RISE TO ORBITAL MELANOMA

A clinicopathologic correlation is shown of a deep eyelid and anterior orbital cellular blue nevus that gave rise to melanoma.

Gunduz K, Shields JA, Shields CL, et al. Periorbital cellular blue nevus leading to orbitopalpebral and intracranial melanoma. *Ophthalmology* 1998;105:2046–2050.

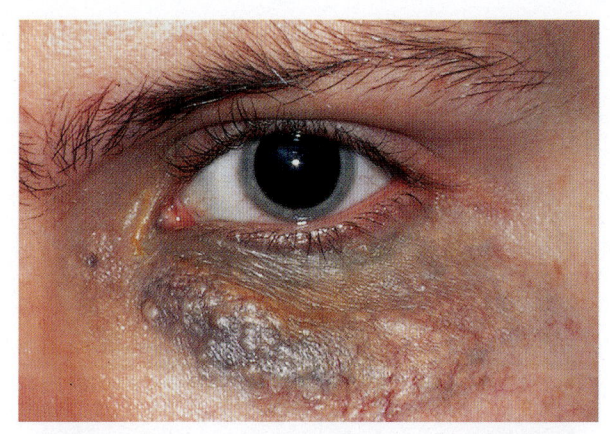

Figure 6.73. Appearance of pigmented thickened eyelid lesion in a 29-year-old man. The thickened lesion was managed by surgical debulking and it proved to be a low-grade melanoma arising from a cellular blue nevus. The patient's opposite eye was amblyopic and the patient declined more extensive surgery.

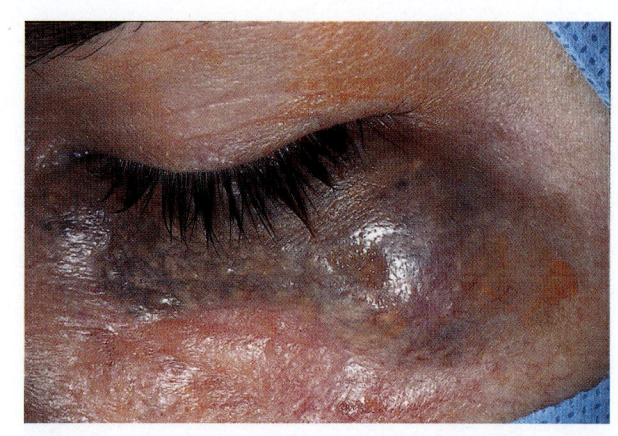

Figure 6.74. Appearance of lesion 10 years later, showing large nodular recurrence.

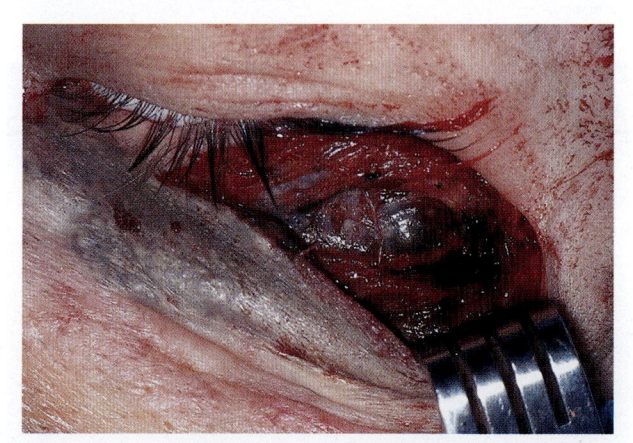

Figure 6.75. Surgically exposed lesion shown in Figure 6.74 after a skin incision was made. A large, well-circumscribed mass was removed.

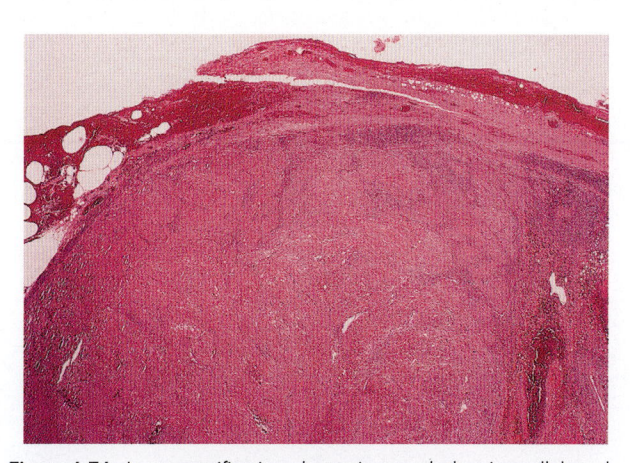

Figure 6.76. Low-magnification photomicrograph showing cellular subcutaneous nodule. (Hematoxylin–eosin ×15.)

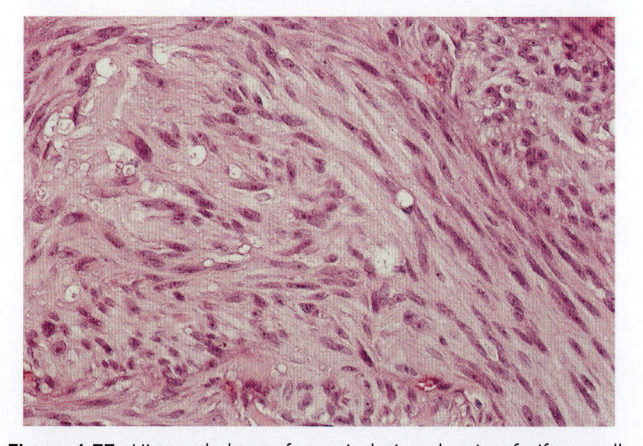

Figure 6.77. Histopathology of area in lesion showing fusiform cells compatible with a cellular blue nevus. (Hematoxylin–eosin ×200.)

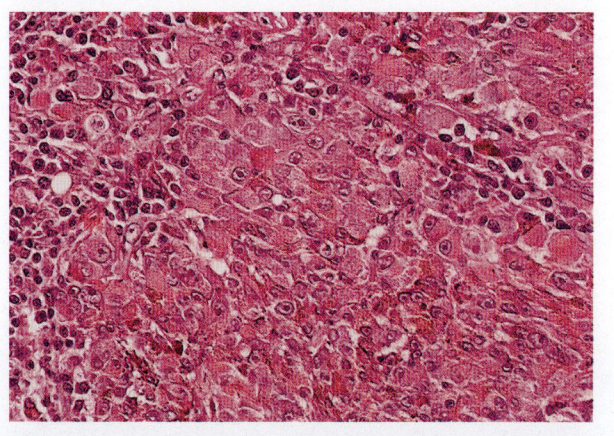

Figure 6.78. Histopathology of another area in lesion showing more anaplastic cells compatible with malignant melanoma. The patient eventually died from orbital recurrence and metastatic melanoma. (Hematoxylin–eosin ×200.)

EYELID CELLULAR BLUE NEVUS: ASSOCIATION WITH ORBITAL AND BRAIN MELANOMA

Extensive orbitopalpebral cellular blue nevus can demonstrate progression, recurrence, and brain involvement. A case is illustrated.

Gunduz K, Shields JA, Shields CL, et al. Periorbital cellular blue nevus leading to orbitopalpebral and intracranial melanoma. *Ophthalmology* 1998;105:2046–2050.

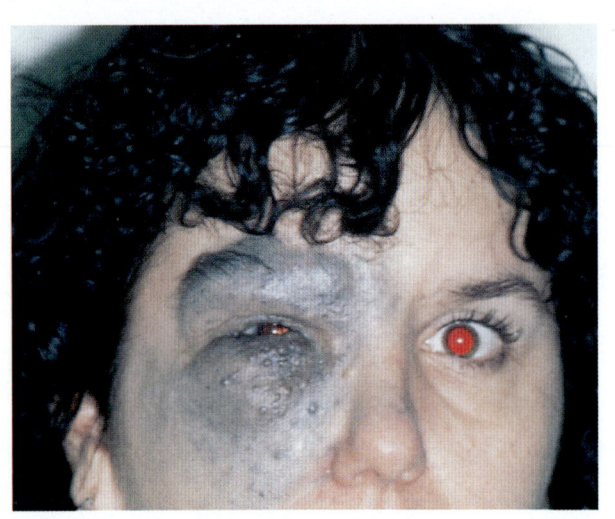

Figure 6.79. Facial photograph of a 31-year-old woman showing a congenital periocular cellular blue nevus affecting both upper and lower eyelids and adjacent skin.

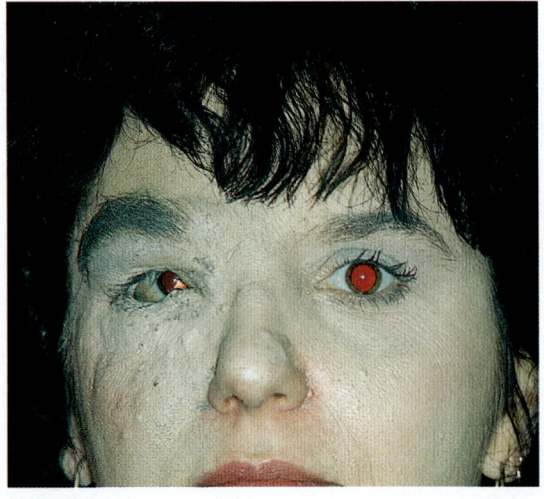

Figure 6.80. Facial appearance of same lesion after application of makeup.

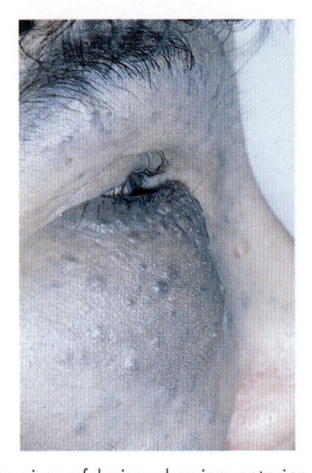

Figure 6.81. Side view of lesion showing anterior bulging of lower eyelid secondary to the subcutaneous mass. Note the small pigmented nodules in the main lesion.

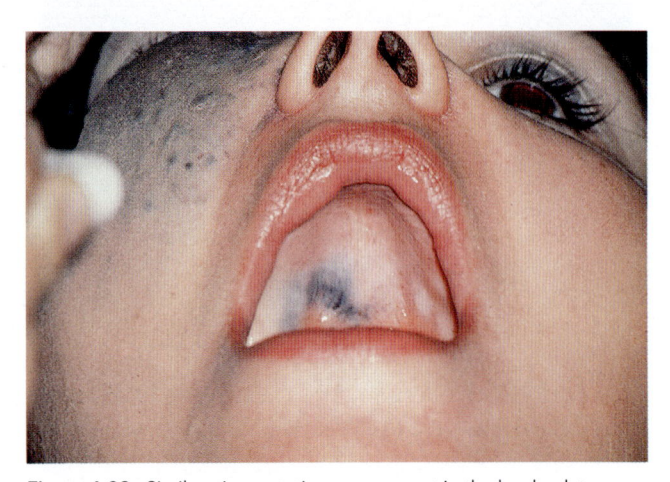

Figure 6.82. Similar pigmentation was present in the hard palate.

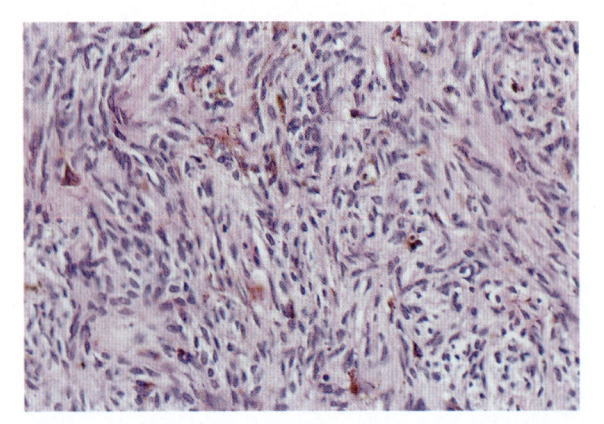

Figure 6.83. Histopathology of biopsy of eyelid lesion showing findings compatible with a cellular blue nevus. (Hematoxylin–eosin ×200.)

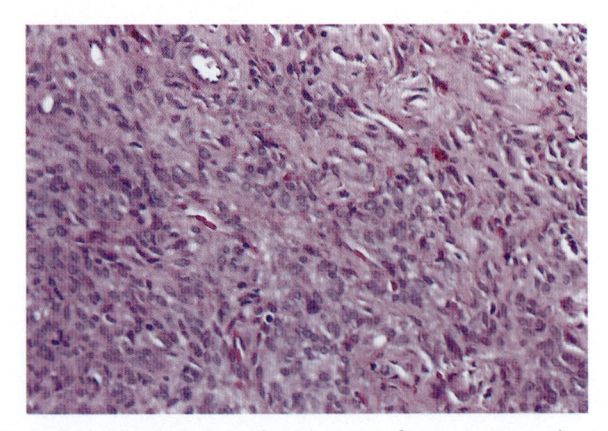

Figure 6.84. Histopathology of another area of same specimen, showing findings compatible with a malignant melanoma. (Hematoxylin–eosin ×200.)

Chapter 6 Eyelid Melanocytic Tumors 113

● EYELID CELLULAR BLUE NEVUS: ASSOCIATION WITH ORBITAL AND BRAIN MELANOMA

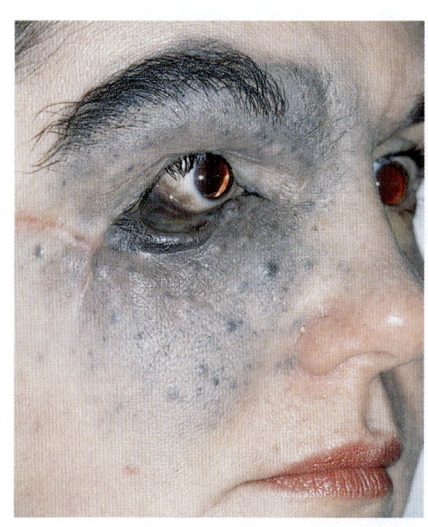

Figure 6.85. Appearance of lesion in patient shown in Figure 6.79 when she was 32 years old, showing ectropion of lower eyelid secondary to prior surgery.

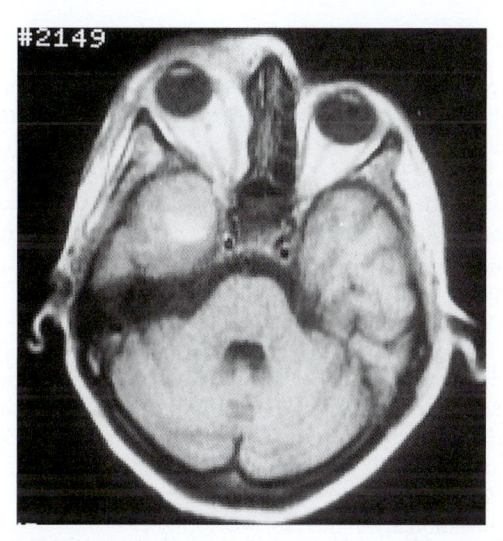

Figure 6.86. T1-weighted axial magnetic resonance image showing expansion of the orbit and a large mass in the brain.

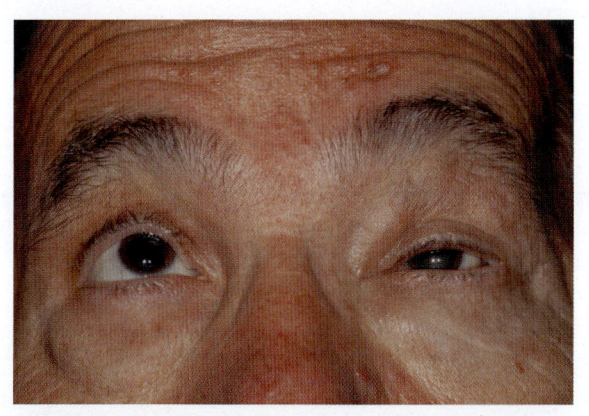

Figure 6.87. Left blepharoptosis was noted in an elderly male.

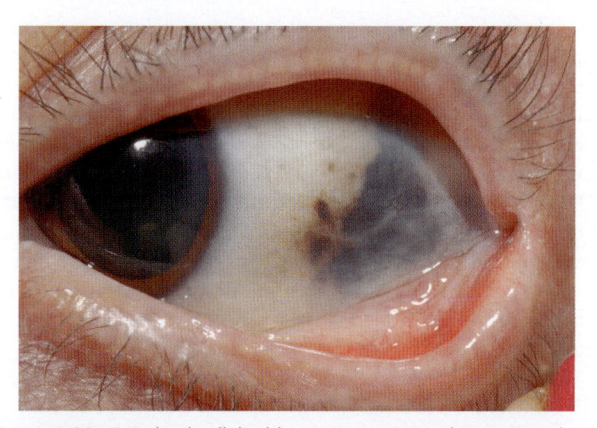

Figure 6.88. Episcleral cellular blue nevus was noted in patient shown in Figure 6.87.

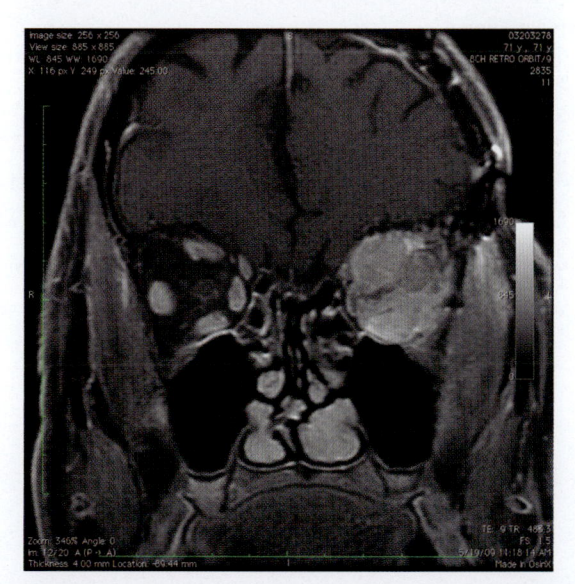

Figure 6.89. T1-weighted coronal magnetic resonance image of patient in Figure 6.87 showing posterior orbit with extensive tumor that proved to be melanoma arising from cellular blue nevus and with brain invasion.

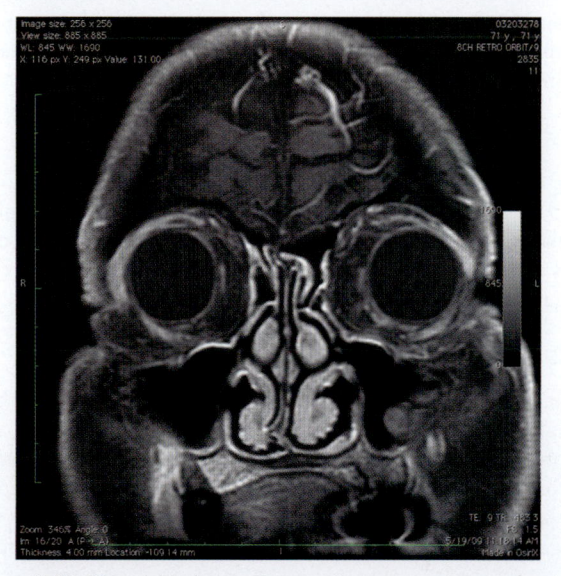

Figure 6.90. T1-weighted coronal magnetic resonance image of patient in Figure 6.87 showing anterior orbit with normal globes.

EYELID PRIMARY MALIGNANT MELANOMA

General Considerations

Cutaneous melanoma generally develops on sun-exposed areas of adult Caucasians who have had excess exposure to ultraviolet light. It can occur in the eyelid as a primary lesion, metastasis from a distant primary melanoma, or extension of a conjunctival melanoma. The clinical features, pathology, and management of eyelid melanoma parallel those of the skin melanomas elsewhere (1–14). There are four types of primary cutaneous melanoma: lentigo maligna melanoma, superficial spreading melanoma, nodular melanoma, and acral lentiginous melanoma. The first three can occur in the eyelids.

Melanoma accounts for about 1% of malignant tumors of the eyelid, being much less common than basal cell carcinoma. It occurs almost exclusively in Caucasians and it is estimated that 1 out of every 75 persons in the United States will develop a cutaneous melanoma. One must assume that the incidence of eyelid melanoma will increase accordingly.

Clinical Features

The many clinical variations of cutaneous melanoma (including eyelid melanoma) are discussed in detail in other textbooks. Clinically, eyelid melanoma appears as a variably pigmented mass that can bleed or ulcerate. In a report of 32 cases, 66% occurred on the lower eyelid; 59% were nodular, 22% superficial spreading, and 19% were lentigo maligna melanoma (1). Melanoma that develops on the eyelid margin may have a worse prognosis (1,2,10). Like other cutaneous melanomas, eyelid melanoma can recur and extend into the orbit by neural invasion (12,13). These neurotropic desmoplastic melanomas can be amelanotic and can simulate fibrous histiocytoma or other spindle cell tumors histopathologically (12,13).

Differential Diagnosis

The differential diagnosis of eyelid melanoma includes melanocytic nevus, pigmented basal cell carcinoma, seborrheic keratosis, apocrine hidrocystoma, and varix. In addition, most nonpigmented lesions discussed in this atlas can sometimes be quite similar to amelanotic eyelid melanoma.

Pathology and Pathogenesis

The histopathologic findings vary with type of melanoma (1,9). Each type is characterized by a proliferation of atypical melanocytes that have a tendency toward invasion of the dermis and lymphogenous metastasis. There is often evidence that the melanoma arose from a preexisting nevus.

Management

The management of primary eyelid melanoma can be challenging. The patient should be checked for preauricular and submandibular lymphadenopathy. Surgical excision and eyelid reconstruction are generally considered the treatment of choice for small lesions suspected to be melanoma. If the lesion is too large for primary wound closure, a biopsy can be taken through the thickest portion and the diagnosis confirmed. Wider surgical excision and repair can then be planned, including orbital exenteration for melanoma with orbital invasion. The role of irradiation, cryotherapy, chemotherapy, and immunotherapy is not clearly established. There has been recent interest in sentinel lymph node biopsy as a tool for staging of eyelid melanoma (6–8). We have employed sentinel lymph node biopsy for several years for malignancies, especially melanoma, of both the eyelid and conjunctiva, but long-term value of this procedure remains controversial.

Prognosis

The prognosis of eyelid melanoma seems to correlate with depth of invasion and type of melanoma. More deeply invasive and nodular melanomas carry a worse prognosis. Because melanoma can metastasize after many years, long-term follow-up is mandatory.

Selected References

Reviews

1. Grossniklaus HE, McLean IW. Cutaneous melanoma of the eyelid. *Ophthalmology* 1991;98:1867–1873.
2. Tahery DP, Goldberg R, Moy RL. Malignant melanoma of the eyelid: a report of eight cases and review of the literature. *J Am Acad Dermatol* 1992;27:17–21.
3. Bianciotto C, Demirci H, Shields CL, Eagle RC Jr, Shields JA. Metastatic tumors to the eyelid: report of 20 cases and review of the literature. *Arch Ophthalmol* 2009;127(8):999–1005.

Management

4. Becerra EM, Blanco G, Saornil MA, et al. Hughes technique, amniotic membrane allograft, and topical chemotherapy in conjunctival melanoma with eyelid involvement. *Ophthal Plast Reconstr Surg* 2005;21(3):238–240.
5. Demirci H, Shields CL, Bianciotto CG, et al. Topical imiquimod for periocular lentigo maligna. *Ophthalmology* 2010;117(12):2424–2429.
6. Pfeiffer ML, Savar A, Esmaeli B. Sentinel lymph node biopsy for eyelid and conjunctival tumors: what have we learned in the past decade? *Ophthal Plast Reconstr Surg* 2013;29(1):57–62.
7. Savar A, Ross MI, Prieto VG, et al. Sentinel lymph node biopsy for ocular adnexal melanoma: experience in 30 patients. *Ophthalmology* 2009;116(11):2217–2223.
8. Turell ME, Char DH. Eyelid melanoma with negative sentinel lymph node biopsy and perineural spread. *Arch Ophthalmol* 2007;125(7):983–984.

Histopathology

9. Garner A, Koornneef L, Levine A, et al. Malignant melanoma of the eyelid skin: histopathology and behaviour. *Br J Ophthalmol* 1983;69:180–186.

Case Reports

10. Zoltie N, O'Neill TJ. Malignant melanoma of the eyelid skin. *Plast Reconstr Surg* 1989;83:994–996.
11. Naidoff MA, Bernardino VB, Clark WH. Melanocytic lesions of the eyelid skin. *Am J Ophthalmol* 1976;82:371–382.
12. Shields JA, Elder D, Arbizo V, et al. Orbital involvement with desmoplastic melanoma. *Br J Ophthalmol* 1987;71:279–285.
13. Dithmar S, Meldrum ML, Murray DR, et al. Desmoplastic spindle-cell melanoma of the eyelid with orbital invasion. *Ophthal Plast Reconstr Surg* 1999;15:134–136.
14. Sanchez R, Ivan D, Esmaeli B. Eyelid and periorbital cutaneous malignant melanoma. *Int Ophthalmol Clin* 2009;49(4):25–43.

Chapter 6 Eyelid Melanocytic Tumors

PRIMARY MALIGNANT MELANOMA OF EYELID

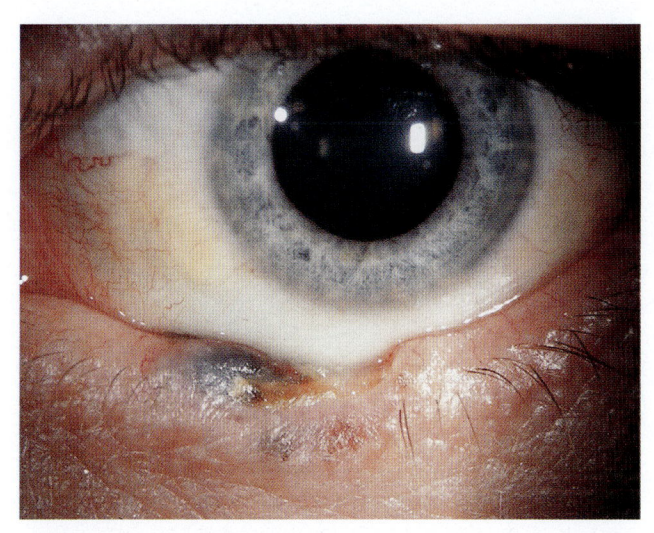

Figure 6.91. Sessile melanoma of lower eyelid showing with ulceration of eyelid margin in a 43-year-old man.

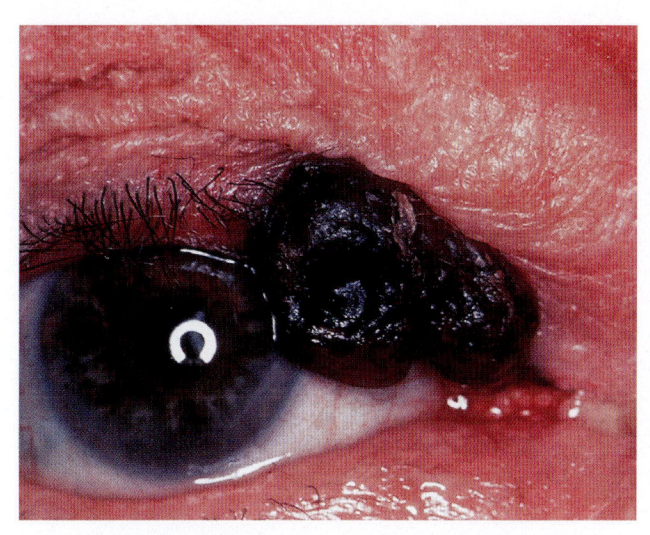

Figure 6.92. Pedunculated melanoma of upper eyelid. (Courtesy of Michael Patipa, MD.)

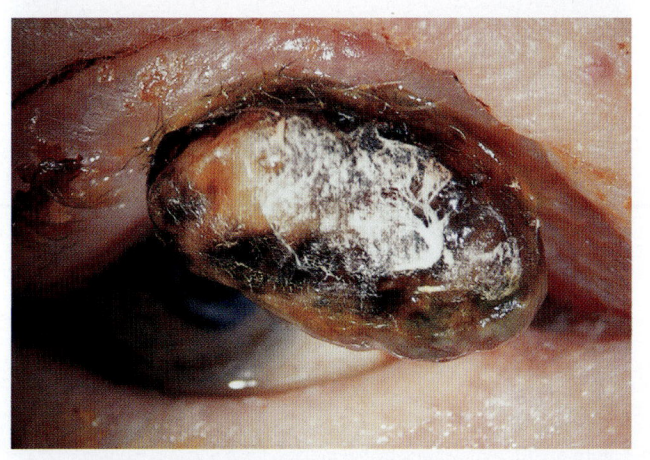

Figure 6.93. Pedunculated melanoma of upper eyelid margin in a 76-year-old man.

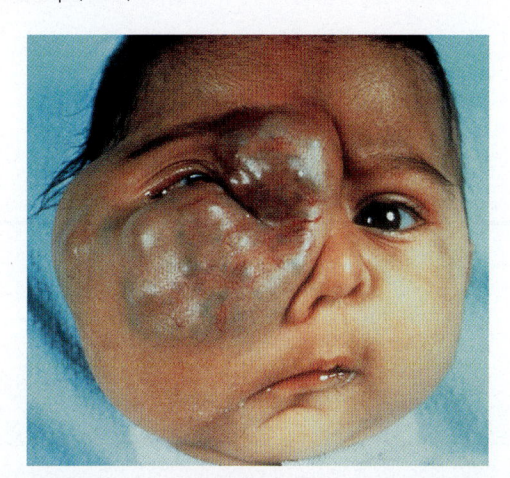

Figure 6.94. Bizarre, congenital melanoma of eyelid and periocular area in a baby. This unusual lesion also massively involved the uveal tract. (Courtesy of Ahmed Hidayat, MD.)

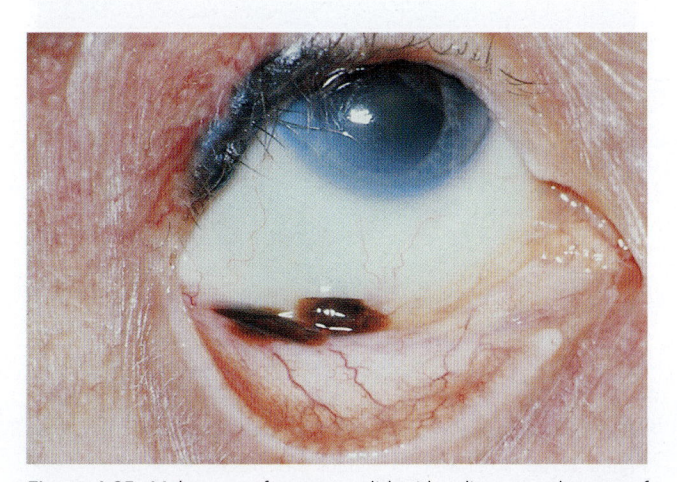

Figure 6.95. Melanoma of upper eyelid with adjacent melanoma of inferior forniceal conjunctiva. It is speculated that the conjunctival melanoma developed from seeding by direct contact from the eyelid lesion during eye closure.

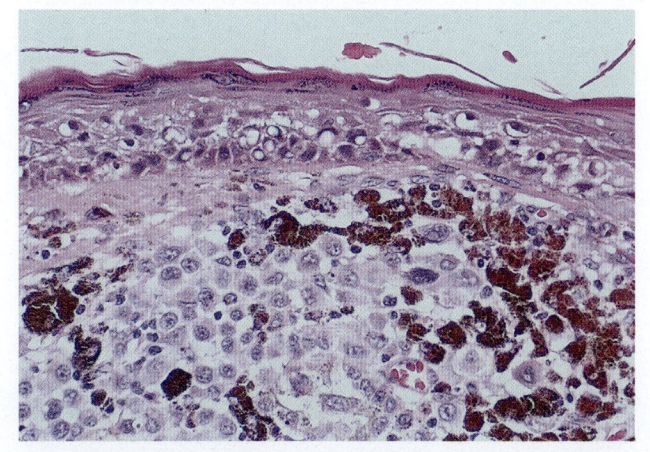

Figure 6.96. Histopathology of eyelid lesion in Figure 6.95, showing malignant melanocytes in the epidermis and dermis. It was necessary to remove the periocular skin and nose before extensive reconstruction was undertaken. (Hematoxylin–eosin ×200.)

PRIMARY EYELID MELANOMA: PIGMENTED AND NONPIGMENTED VARIETIES

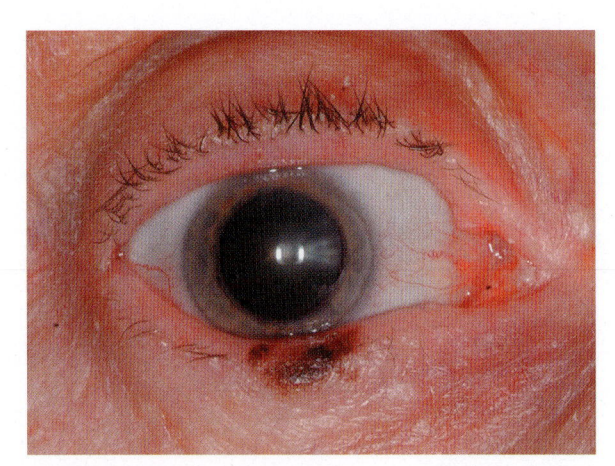

Figure 6.97. Pigmented superficial spreading melanoma of right lower eyelid in an elderly man.

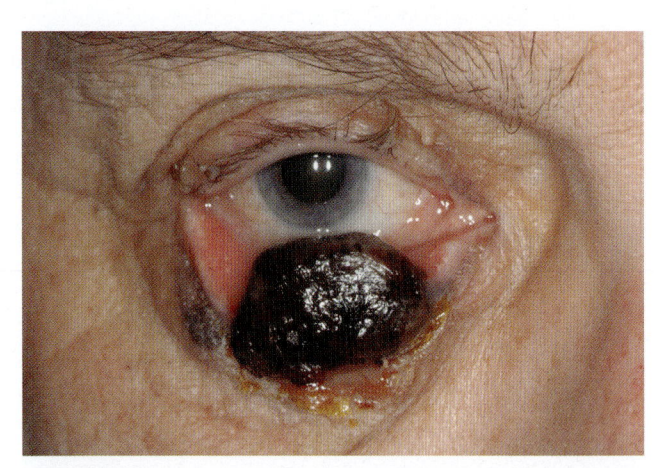

Figure 6.98. Large neglected and pedunculated pigmented melanoma arising along lower eyelid in older man.

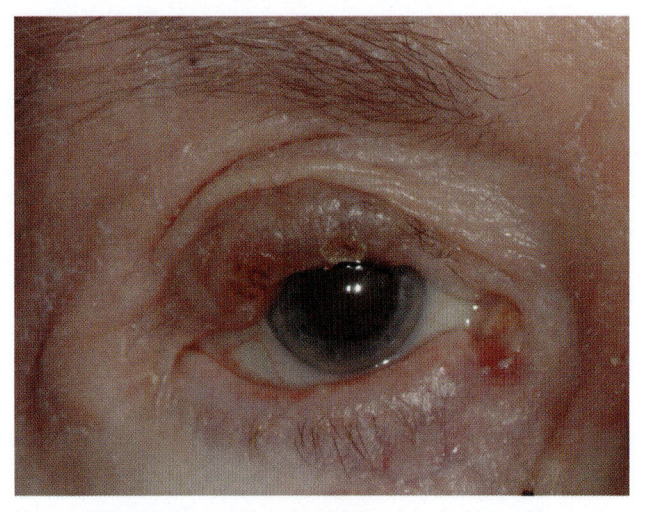

Figure 6.99. Nodular amelanotic eyelid melanoma in an older woman with numerous previous skin cancers.

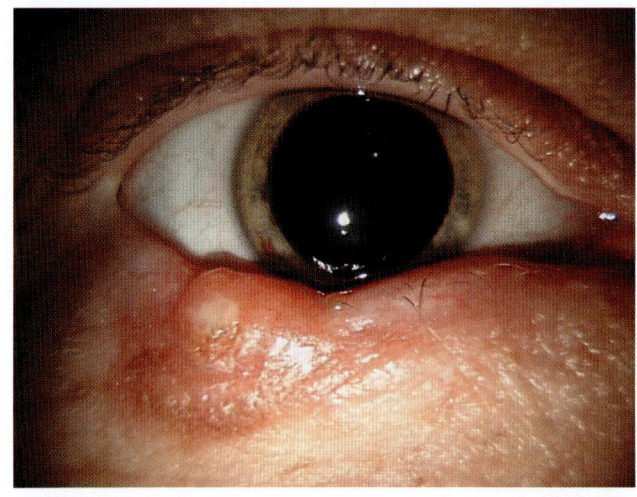

Figure 6.100. Amelanotic eyelid melanoma in a young woman.

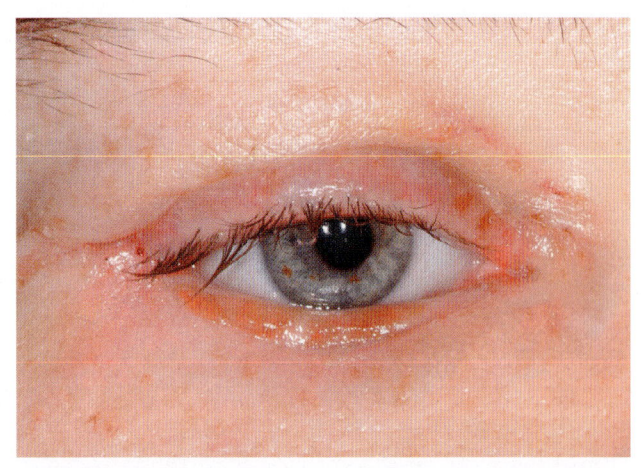

Figure 6.101. Appearance 2 months after excision of entire right lower eyelid of patient shown in Figure 6.100. Note the absence of cilia on lower eyelid. Histopathology suggested that the tumor was completely excised.

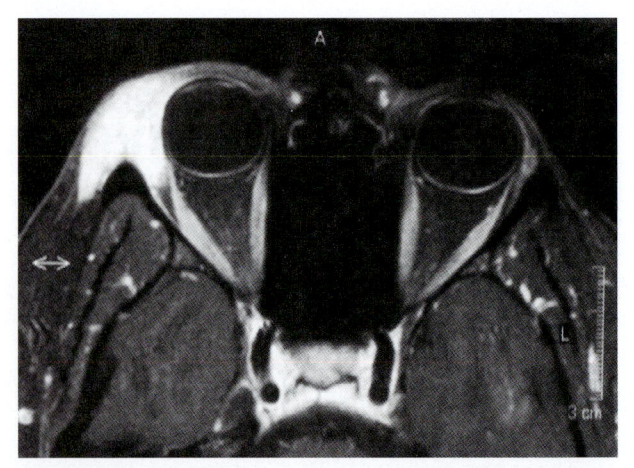

Figure 6.102. Axial MRI 10 months after resection of lesion shown in Figure 6.100, showing orbital recurrence secondary to neurotropic invasion. Patient underwent orbital exenteration but later developed systemic metastasis.

PRIMARY EYELID MELANOMA: SURGICAL EXCISION

Figure 6.103. Variably pigmented superficial spreading melanoma of eyelid margin with loss of cilia in an elderly man.

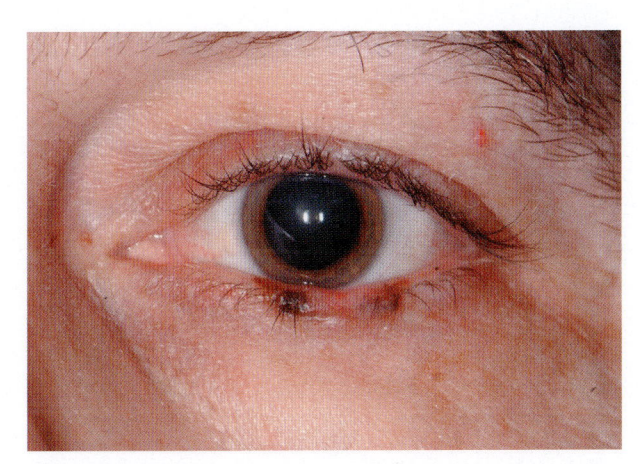

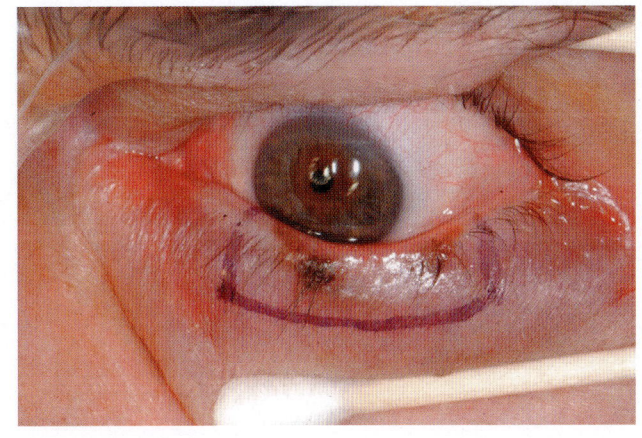

Figure 6.104. Outline of surgical approach designed to obtain surgical margins as wide as possible.

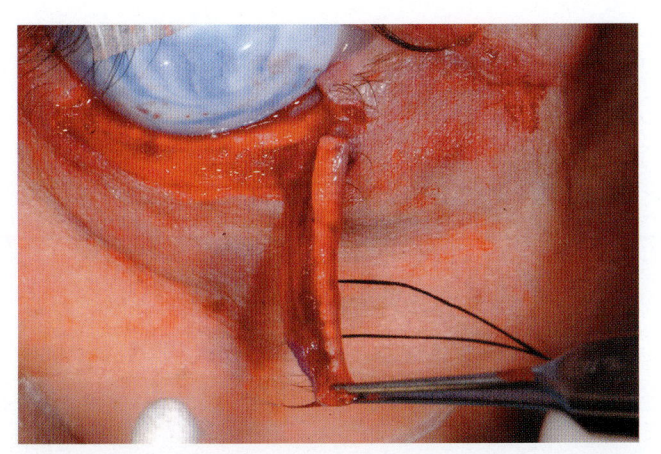

Figure 6.105. The anterior lamella of the lower eyelid was resected, exposing the tarsus. Frozen sections indicated that there was no residual tumor and this was later confirmed with permanent sections.

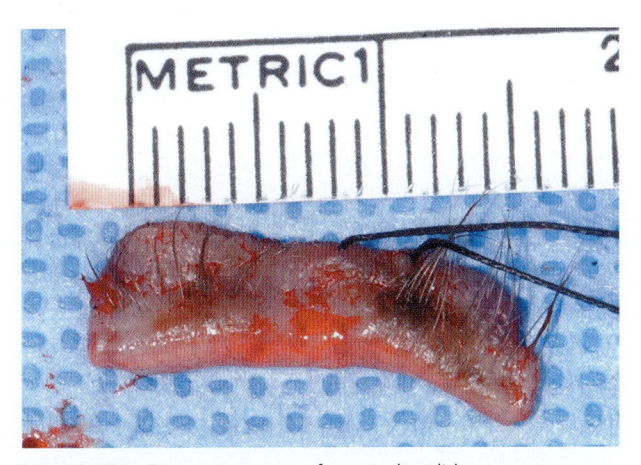

Figure 6.106. Gross appearance of resected eyelid.

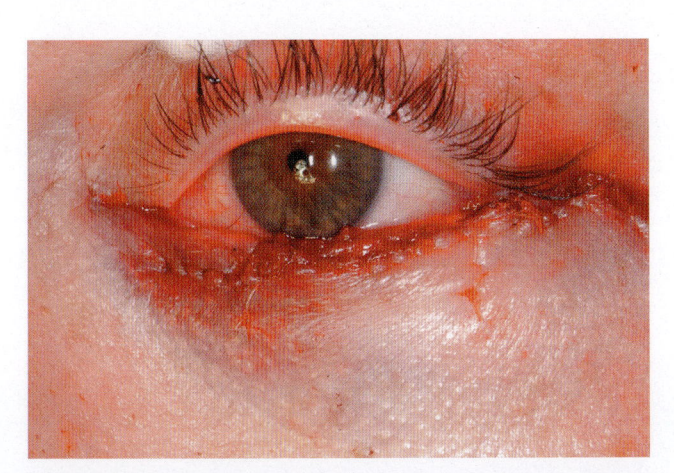

Figure 6.107. Appearance at time of surgical closure by reconstruction with sliding anterior lamellar flap.

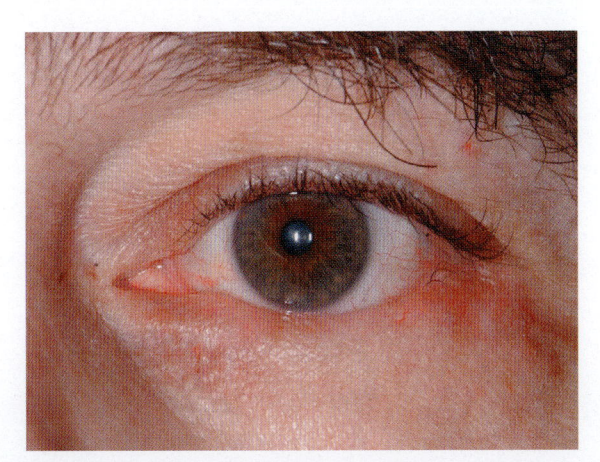

Figure 6.108. Appearance 2 months later showing an absence of cilia. There was no recurrence of the tumor.

CHAPTER 7

NEURAL TUMORS OF THE EYELID

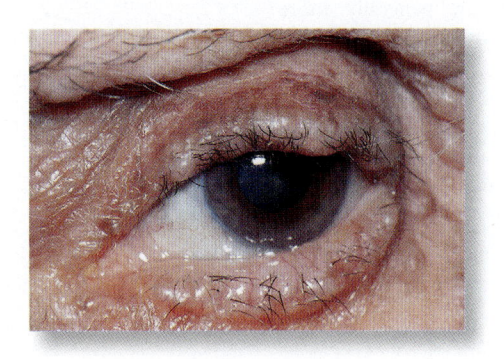

General Considerations

Neurofibroma is an important neural tumor that can affect skin in all parts of the body. It can develop as a solitary lesion unassociated with systemic disease or as multifocal or diffuse lesions associated with type 1 neurofibromatosis. The eyelid and orbit can be involved by neurofibroma in three different ways: solitary neurofibroma, multiple localized neurofibromas, and plexiform neurofibroma (1–9). Plexiform neurofibroma of the eyelid characteristically extends for some distance into the orbit.

Clinical Features

Solitary neurofibroma, also called fibroma molluscum, is a circumscribed subcutaneous nodular lesion of variable size. This tumor can sometimes be painful, reflecting its peripheral nerve origin. Solitary neurofibroma can occur on the eyelid in patients who have no apparent neurofibromatosis. Such a lesion can initially resemble a chalazion or malignant eyelid tumor.

Multiple neurofibromas that affect the skin in patients with type 1 neurofibromatosis can also simultaneously occur on the eyelids. They appear as multiple, discrete, subcutaneous nodules on the eyelid and adjacent skin. They tend to be stable, but can sometimes gradually enlarge. Like the similar neurofibromas on the extraocular skin, they probably have a low potential to undergo malignant transformation; malignant peripheral nerve sheath tumors in the eyelid are quite rare.

Plexiform neurofibroma is considered pathognomonic of type 1 neurofibromatosis (von Recklinghausen's disease). Eyelid involvement is usually associated with contiguous involvement of the deeper tissues in the orbit (1). This tumor develops in young children as a thickening of the entire eyelid that initially causes an S-shaped curve to the margin of the upper eyelid. This lesion can show gradual progressive enlargement and extend into the malar area of the eyebrow and conjunctiva.

Pathology

In contrast to schwannoma (discussed in the next section), which is a tumor composed almost exclusively of Schwann cells, neurofibroma is composed of a combination of Schwann cells, peripheral nerve axons, endoneural fibroblasts, and perineural cells. There are several variations of cutaneous neurofibromas. In brief, each tumor type is composed of bundles of enlarged peripheral nerves. Bodian stain and immunohistochemical stains can help to delineate the axons and additional special stains can assist in the diagnosis.

EYELID NEUROFIBROMA

Management

A small, asymptomatic solitary neurofibroma of the eyelid can be followed conservatively or removed surgically in a patient with NF1. If surgery is performed, the lesion can usually be removed completely by way of an eyelid crease incision with wide undermined margins, sparing the cutaneous surface. If the overlying skin is spared, primary closure without a flap or graft is possible. The multiple small cutaneous neurofibromas associated with neurofibromatosis are usually asymptomatic and can be followed without active treatment. Larger lesions can be individually resected.

Diffuse or plexiform neurofibromas are generally more difficult to manage. The lesion is often ill-defined and bleeds profusely at the time of surgical resection (5–7). When such a lesion becomes cosmetically unacceptable, surgical debulking can be attempted (4). The carbon dioxide laser is reported to be of assistance in such cases (5,6). Because of the extent of many plexiform neurofibromas, a multidisciplinary approach with ophthalmologists, otolaryngologists, and neurosurgeons is often necessary.

EYELID NEUROFIBROMA

Selected References

Reviews

1. Brownstein S, Little JM. Ocular neurofibromatosis. *Ophthalmology* 1983;90:1595–1599.
2. Lewis RA, Riccardi VM. von Recklinghausen neurofibromatosis. *Ophthalmology* 1981;88:348–354.
3. Farris SR, Grove AS Jr. Orbital and eyelid manifestations of neurofibromatosis: a clinical study and literature review. *Ophthal Plast Reconstr Surg* 1996;12:245–259.

Management

4. Lee V, Ragge NK, Collin JR. Orbitotemporal neurofibromatosis. Clinical features and surgical management. *Ophthalmology* 2004;111:382–388.
5. Lapid-Gortzak R, Lapid O, Monos T, et al. CO2 laser in the removal of a plexiform neurofibroma for the eyelid. *Ophthalmic Surg Lasers* 2000;31:432–434.
6. Dailey RA, Sullivan SA, Wobig JL. Surgical debulking of eyelid and anterior orbital plexiform neurofibromas by means of the carbon dioxide laser. *Am J Ophthalmol* 2000;130:117–119.
7. Marchac D, Britto JA. Remodeling the upper eyelid in the management of orbitopalpebral neurofibromatosis. *Br J Plast Surg* 2005;58:944–956.
8. Madill KE, Brammar R, Leatherbarrow B. A novel approach to the management of severe facial disfigurement in neurofibromatosis type 1. *Ophthal Plast Reconstr Surg* 2007;23(3):227–228.

Case Reports

9. Shibata N, Kitagawa K, Noda M, et al. Solitary neurofibroma without neurofibromatosis in the superior tarsal plate simulating a chalazion. *Graefes Arch Clin Exp Ophthalmol* 2012;250(2):309-310.

EYELID NEUROFIBROMA: LOCALIZED AND PLEXIFORM TYPES

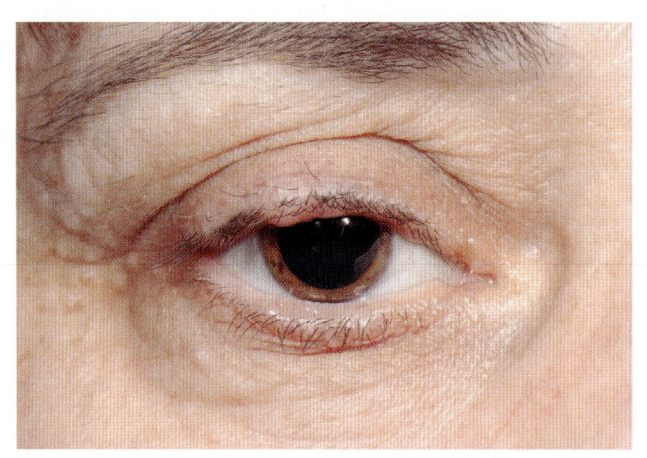

Figure 7.1. Multifocal small neurofibromas along the right upper and lower eyelids in a patient with neurofibromatosis type 1.

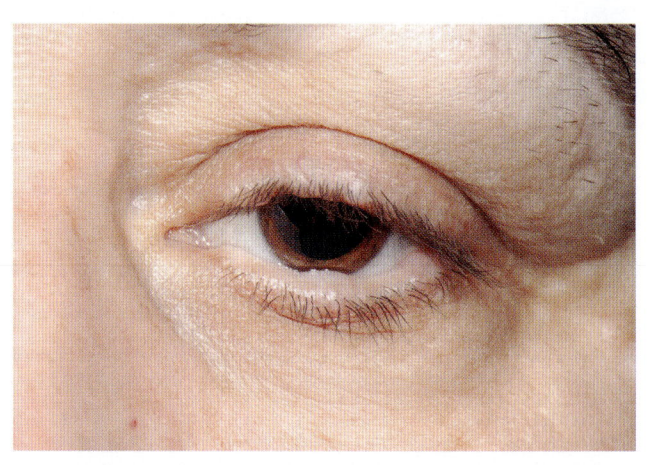

Figure 7.2. Same patient as in Figure 7.1 demonstrating multifocal small neurofibromas along the left upper and lower eyelids.

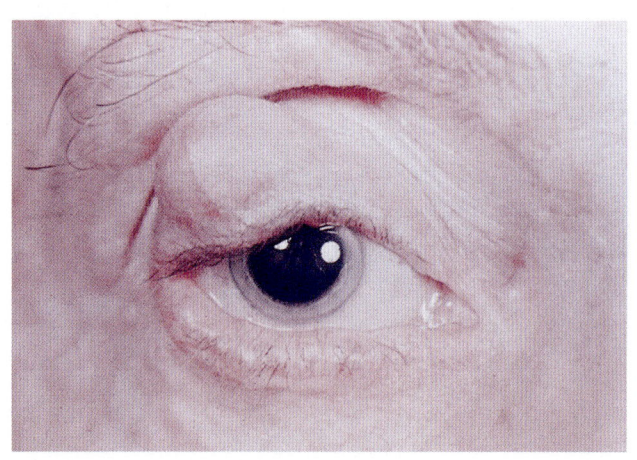

Figure 7.3. Solitary neurofibroma (fibroma molluscum) of the upper eyelid in a patient without neurofibromatosis.

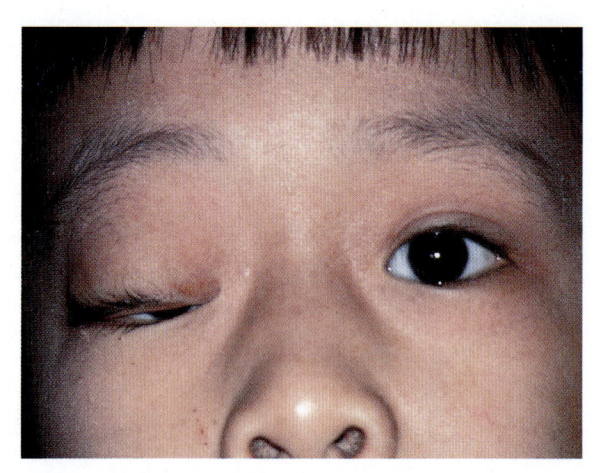

Figure 7.4. Plexiform neurofibroma of upper eyelid and anterior orbit in a 6-year-old boy with von Recklinghausen's neurofibromatosis. Note the eyelid thickening and secondary blepharoptosis.

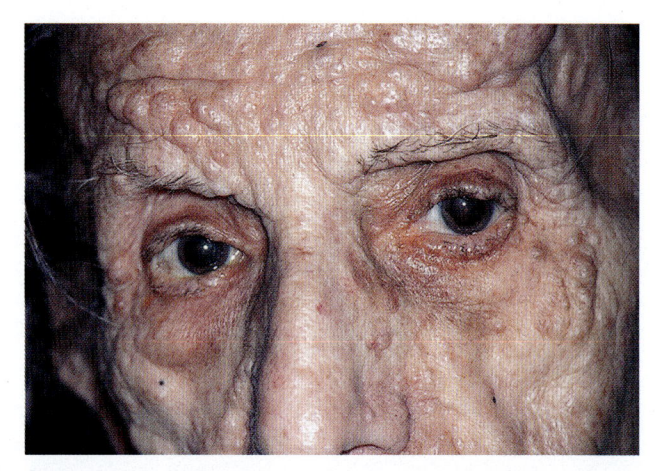

Figure 7.5. Facial appearance of multiple peripheral nerve sheath tumors (neurofibromas) in an 81-year-old woman with von Recklinghausen's neurofibromatosis.

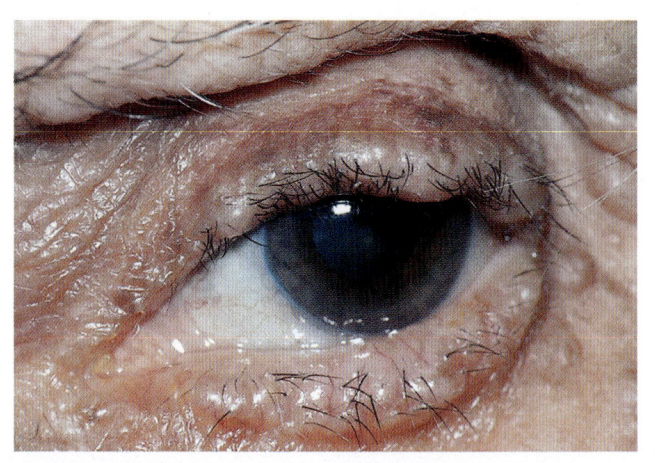

Figure 7.6. Closer view of eyelid margin of patient shown in Figure 7.5, demonstrating the multiple eyelid nodules.

EYELID NEUROFIBROMA: PLEXIFORM TYPE

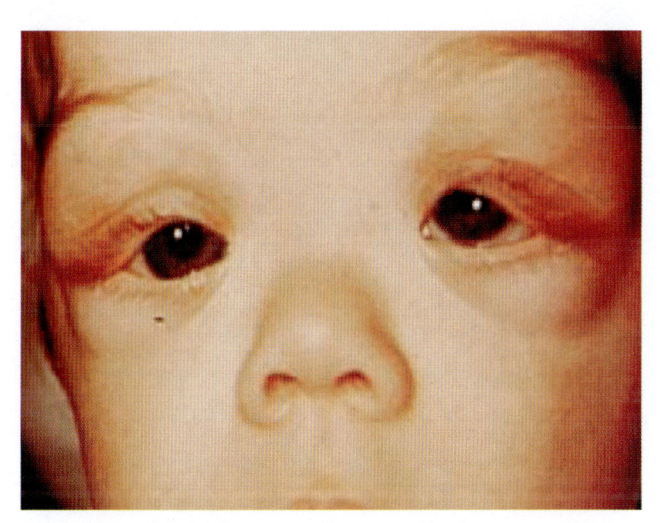

Figure 7.7. Mild plexiform neurofibromas of both upper eyelids in a young girl.

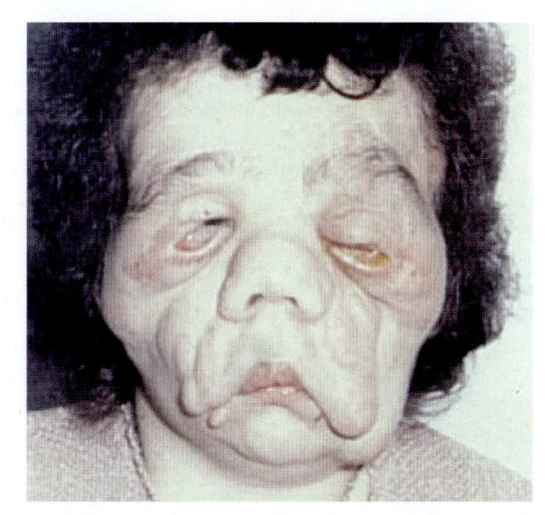

Figure 7.8. Massive enlargement of plexiform neurofibromas of eyelids and face of patient depicted in Figure 7.7, when the patient was a teenager.

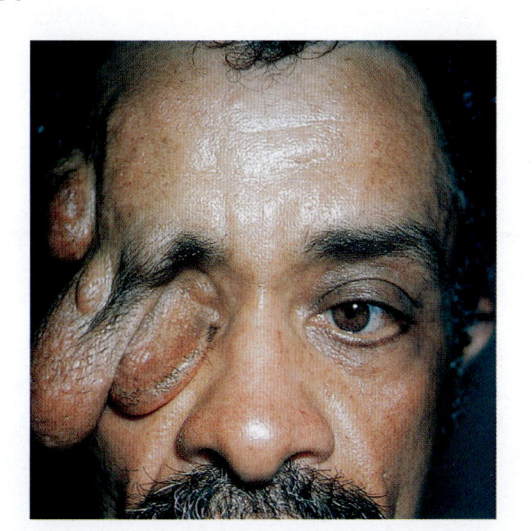

Figure 7.9. Massive plexiform neurofibroma of upper eyelid in a patient with neurofibromatosis. (Courtesy of Charles Lee, MD.)

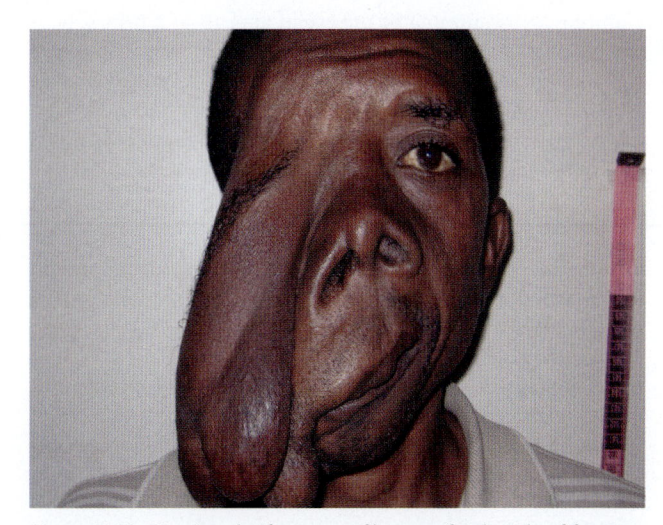

Figure 7.10. Massive plexiform neurofibroma of right side of face in a patient with neurofibromatosis. (Courtesy of Maria Manquez, MD.)

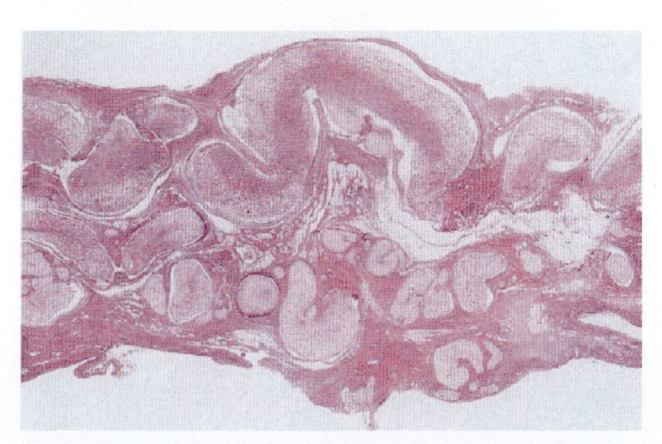

Figure 7.11. Low-power photomicrograph showing intertwining enlarged nerves typical of plexiform neurofibroma. (Hematoxylin–eosin ×5.)

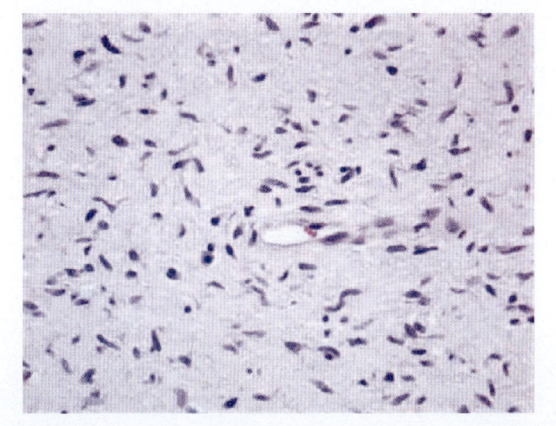

Figure 7.12. Photomicrograph of cutaneous neurofibroma showing randomly arranged spindle cells with mucinous cytoplasm. (Hematoxylin–eosin ×25.)

EYELID SCHWANNOMA (NEURILEMOMA) AND NEUROTHEKEOMA

General Considerations

Schwannoma (neurilemoma) is a benign peripheral nerve sheath tumor that is composed almost exclusively of a proliferation of Schwann cells (1–5). Multiple schwannomas can occur in patients with neurofibromatosis, but solitary schwannoma is usually unassociated with that entity. Schwannoma is known to arise in the orbit, and, occasionally, it can occur in the uveal tract, conjunctiva, caruncle, or eyelid. Only a few cases confined to the eyelid have been reported (1–5). Eyelid cases can occur in elderly patients and young children.

Neurothekeoma is a benign, circumscribed nerve sheath tumor that generally occurs in children or young adults, without systemic associations, and occurs as either a myxomatous nerve sheath tumor or a cellular variant (6–9). This tumor can occur occasionally on the eyelid. The pathogenesis is not clearly defined.

Clinical Features

Clinically, schwannoma of the eyelid appears as a firm subcutaneous mass that can simulate a chalazion. However, it generally is nonpainful, lacks inflammation, and grows very slowly. Neurothekeoma can occur as a solitary lesion on the eyelid that has no typical features and may resemble basal cell carcinoma or other eyelid tumor.

Pathology

Histopathologically, schwannoma is an encapsulated lesion that is composed of closely compact spindle cells (Antoni A pattern) and larger, more round clear cells (Antoni B pattern). Most tumors display a combination of the two patterns. Neurothekeoma is a tumor manifesting a collection of spindle cells in a myxomatous background with immunohistochemical staining for NK1/C3, neuron-specific enolase, and alcian blue (7).

Management

The management of schwannoma and neurothekeoma is complete excision to prevent recurrence. Incomplete removal can be associated with eventual recurrence and more aggressive behavior.

Selected References

Case Reports

1. Baijal GC, Garg SK, Kanhere S, et al. Schwannoma of the eyelid. *Indian J Ophthalmol* 1980;28:155–156.
2. Shields JA, Guibor P. Schwannoma of the eyelid. *Arch Ophthalmol* 1984;102:1650.
3. Shields JA, Kiratli H, Shields CL, et al. Schwannoma of the eyelid in a child. *J Pediatr Ophthalmol Strabismus* 1994;31:332–333.
4. Butt Z, Ironside JW. Superficial epithelioid schwannoma presenting as a subcutaneous upper eyelid mass. *Br J Ophthalmol* 1994;78:586–588.
5. Siddiqui MR, Leslie T, Scott C, et al. Eyelid schwannoma in a male adult. *Clin Experiment Ophthalmol* 2005;33:412–413.
6. Papalas JA, Proia AD, Hitchcock M, Gandhi P, Cummings TJ. Neurothekeoma palpebrae: a report of 3 cases. *Am J Dermatopathol* 2010;32(4):374–379.
7. You TT, Kaiser PK, Netland TP, Jakobiec FA. Neurothekeoma palpebrae: a rare nerve sheath tumor arising in the eyelid. *Ophthal Plast Reconstr Surg* 1999;15(6):448–449.
8. Lefebvre DR, Robinson-Bostom L, Migliori ME. Cellular neurothekeoma of the eyelid: a unique internal palpebral presentation. *Ophthal Plast Reconstr Surg* 2014;30(4):e91–92.
9. Shields JA, Lally SL, Shields CL, et al. Neurothekeoma of the eyelid in a young woman. Submitted for publication (2015).

EYELID SCHWANNOMA AND NEUROTHEKEOMA

1. Shields JA, Guibor P. Neurilemoma of the eyelid. *Arch Ophthalmol* 1984;102:1650.
2. Shields JA, Kiratli H, Shields CL, et al. Schwannoma of the eyelid in a child. *J Pediatr Ophthalmol Strabismus* 1994;31:332–333.

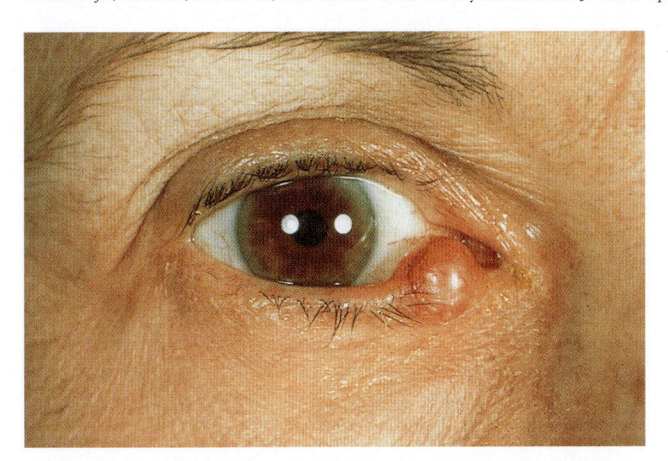

Figure 7.13. Schwannoma near medial aspect of lower eyelid in a 63-year-old woman. This lesion was previously managed elsewhere by curettage with the presumed diagnosis of chalazion, but it subsequently recurred.

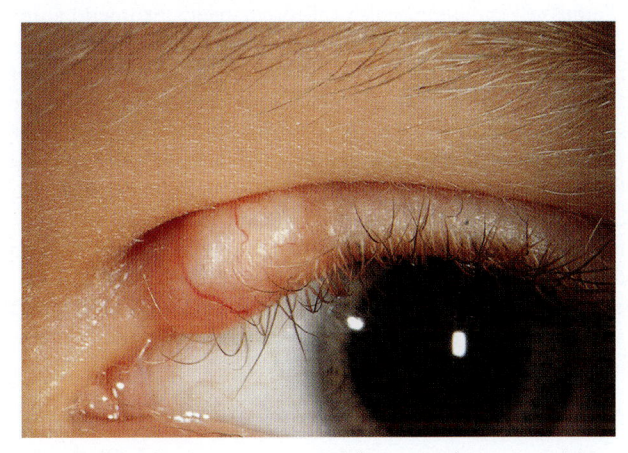

Figure 7.14. Schwannoma near medial aspect of upper eyelid in a 10-year-old boy. This lesion was also previously managed elsewhere by curettage with the presumed diagnosis of chalazion; however, it recurred in the same location.

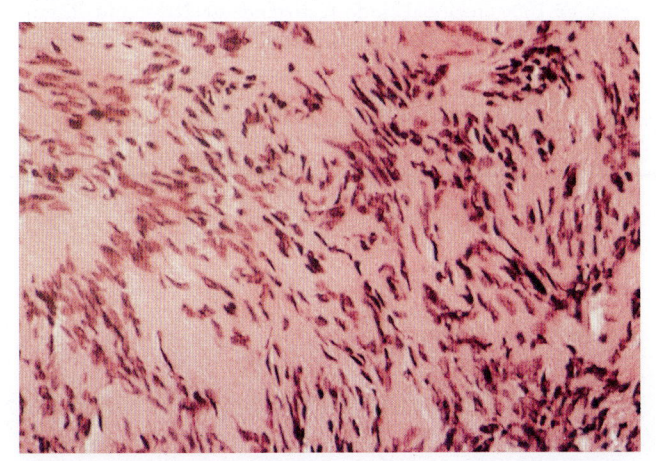

Figure 7.15. Histopathology of lesion in Figure 7.14, showing Antoni A pattern of the tumor. (Hematoxylin–eosin ×75.)

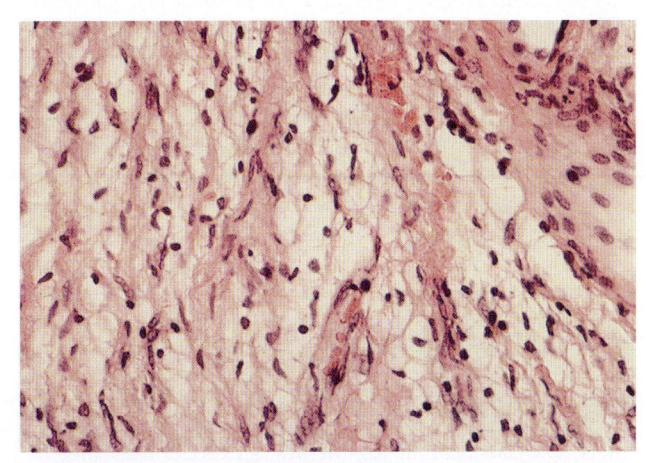

Figure 7.16. Histopathology of lesion in Figure 7.15, showing Antoni B pattern of the tumor. (Hematoxylin–eosin ×75.)

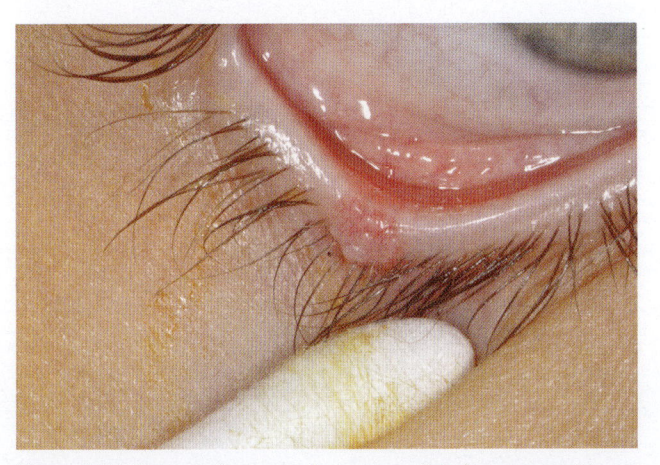

Figure 7.17. Neurothekeoma in the lower eyelid of a teenage girl.

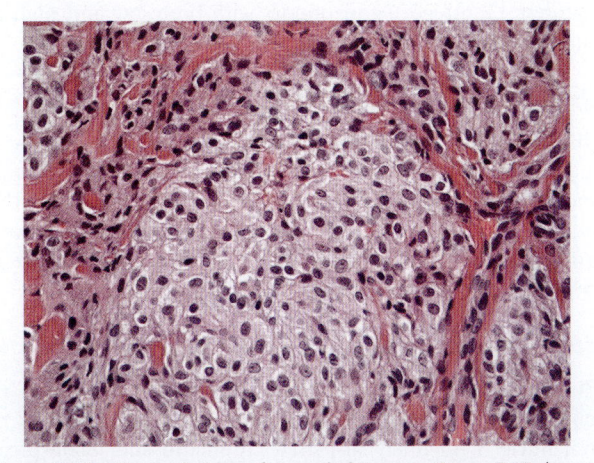

Figure 7.18. Histopathology of neurothekeoma in Figure 7.17 demonstrating whorls of benign nerve sheath cells. (Hematoxylin–eosin ×100.)

EYELID MERKEL CELL CARCINOMA (CUTANEOUS NEUROENDOCRINE CARCINOMA)

General Considerations

Merkel cell carcinoma (also called cutaneous neuroendocrine carcinoma and other terms) is an unusual and intriguing cutaneous neoplasm that can affect the eyelids (1–34). This tumor arises from specialized neuroendocrine receptor cells of the skin and mucous membranes, known as Merkel cells. These cells mediate touch sensation and are thought to be derived from the neural crest. It is an aggressive malignant tumor that can exhibit local recurrence and distant metastasis. Although figures vary, about 10% to 50% of patients are believed to develop regional or distant metastasis (1,2). Merkel cell carcinoma can occur on the trunk, extremities, and face. There are several recent reports and reviews of eyelid and eyebrow involvement (1–34).

Clinical Features

Approximately 10% of all cases of Merkel cell carcinoma affect the eyelid and periocular skin (4). Of those, the upper eyelid is involved in 64%, lower eyelid in 13%, canthi in 11%, and unspecified eyelid sites in 13% of cases (1). Clinically, eyelid Merkel cell carcinoma usually occurs as a painless progressive, red or violaceous, reddish-blue nodule near the eyelid margin. Telangiectasis is frequently present near the surface of the lesion. It has a predilection for elderly women but has been recognized in a 22-year-old woman (18). Like sebaceous carcinoma, Merkel cell carcinoma can masquerade as a chalazion, resulting in serious delay in diagnosis (9,15). Fine needle aspiration biopsy (FNAB) has been employed to make the diagnosis cytopathologically (28), although we do not usually advocate it as a primary diagnosis. However, FNAB has also been used to diagnose parotid metastasis from a biopsy-proven Merkel cell carcinoma of the eyelid (24,25).

Classification

There is a classification for Merkel cell carcinoma using the American Joint Committee on Cancer (AJCC) classification (edge) (34). According to this classification, most patients manifest T2 category and tumors with both low and high T category can develop metastatic disease (1).

Differential Diagnosis

Differential diagnosis includes lymphoma, plasmacytoma, leukemic infiltration, sebaceous carcinoma, squamous cell carcinoma, basal cell carcinoma, and amelanotic melanoma. The reddish-blue color and lack of ulceration of this tumor should arouse suspicion of the diagnosis and to help differentiate it from most other lesions.

Pathology

Histopathologically, Merkel cell carcinoma is composed of lobules of poorly differentiated malignant cells with round to oval nuclei with finely dispersed chromatin and inconspicuous nucleoli (8–13). Mitotic figures are usually abundant. The tumor cells usually involve the dermis and generally spare the epidermis. Electron microscopy and immunohistochemistry may be helpful in confirming the diagnosis. Electron microscopy demonstrates neurosecretory granules in the cytoplasm. Immunohistochemistry can assist in the diagnosis, showing positive reactions to neuron-specific enolase, cytokeratins, and neurosecretory granules (10,11). Diagnosis of Merkel cell carcinoma can be made by fine needle biopsy using cytopathology (12,13).

Management

Management is wide surgical excision with frozen section or Mohs chemosurgery control, similar to that for basal cell carcinoma (1,6). Regional lymph noted dissection, irradiation, and chemotherapy are believed to improve the prognosis, but opinions vary (1).

Concerning prognosis, Merkel cell carcinoma often exhibits early regional lymph node metastasis and distant metastasis. Herbert et al. analyzed 21 patients from five referral centers and found the risk for eyelid Merkel cell carcinoma local recurrence at 10%, regional node recurrence at 10%, and distant metastasis at 19%. They advised sentinel lymph node biopsy for all patients and warned that metastasis can occur, even with relatively small tumors (1).

EYELID MERKEL CELL CARCINOMA (CUTANEOUS NEUROENDOCRINE CARCINOMA)

Selected References

Reviews

1. Herbert HM, Sun MT, Selva D, et al. Merkel cell carcinoma of the eyelid: management and prognosis. *JAMA Ophthalmol* 2014;132:197–204.
2. Kivela T, Tarkkanen A. The Merkel cell associated neoplasms in the eyelids and periocular region. *Surv Ophthalmol* 1990;35:171–187.
3. Rubsamen PE, Tanenbaum M, Grove AS, et al. Merkel cell carcinoma of the eyelid and periocular tissues. *Am J Ophthalmol* 1992;113:674–680.
4. Missotten GS, de Wolff-Rouendaal D, de Keizer RJ. Merkel cell carcinoma of the eyelid review of the literature and report of patients with Merkel cell carcinoma showing spontaneous regression. *Ophthalmology* 2008;115(1):195–201.
5. Singh AD, Eagle RC, Shields CL, et al. Merkel cell carcinoma of the eyelids. In: Shields JA, ed. *Update on Malignant Ocular Tumors (Intl Ophthalmol Clin).* Boston, MA: Little, Brown and Company, 1993:11–17.

Management

6. Peters GB 3rd, Meyer DR, Shields JA, et al. Management and prognosis of Merkel cell carcinoma of the eyelid. *Ophthalmology* 2001;108:1575–1579.
7. Tsukada A, Fujimura T, Hashimoto A, et al. Successful local control of cutaneous Merkel cell carcinoma on the eyelid with CyberKnife radiosurgery eyelid with CyberKnife radiosurgery. *Eur J Dermatol* 2013;23(5):725–726.

Histopathology/Cytopathology

8. Colombo F, Holbach LM, Junemann AG, et al. Merkel cell carcinoma: clinicopathologic correlation, management, and follow-up in five patients. *Ophthal Plast Reconstr Surg* 2000;16:453–458.
9. Furuno K, Wakakura M, Shimizu K, et al. Immunohistochemical studies of Merkel cell carcinoma of the eyelid. *Jpn J Ophthalmol* 1992;36:348–355.
10. Metz KA, Jacob M, Schmidt U, et al. Merkel cell carcinoma of the eyelid: histological and immunohistochemical features with special respect to differential diagnosis. *Graefes Arch Clin Exp Ophthalmol* 1998;236:561–566.
11. Proenca R, Santos MF, Cunha-Vaz JG. Primary neuroendocrine carcinoma of the eyelid, immunohistochemical and ultrastructural study. *Int Ophthalmol* 1990;14:251–258.
12. Gherardi G, Marveggio C, Stiglich F. Parotid metastasis of Merkel cell carcinoma in a young patient with ectodermal dysplasia. Diagnosis by fine needle aspiration cytology and immunocytochemistry. *Acta Cytol* 1990;34:831–836.
13. Gattuso P, Castelli MJ, Shah PA, et al. Fine needle aspiration cytologic diagnosis of metastatic Merkel cell carcinoma in the parotid gland. *Acta Cytol* 1988;32:576–578.

Case Reports

14. Searl SS, Boynton JR, Markowitch W, et al. Malignant Merkel cell neoplasm of the eyelid. *Arch Ophthalmol* 1984;102:907–911.
15. Beyer CK, Goodman M, Dickersin R, et al. Merkel cell tumor of the eyelid. *Arch Ophthalmol* 1983;101:1098–1101.
16. Lamping K, Fischer MJ, Vareska G, et al. A Merkel cell tumor of the eyelid. *Ophthalmology* 1983;90:1399–1402.
17. Mamalis N, Medlock RD, Holds JB, et al. Merkel cell tumor of the eyelid: a review and report of an unusual case. *Ophthalmic Surg* 1989;20:410–414.
18. Saadi AK, Danks JJ, Cree IA, et al. Merkel cell tumour: case reports and review. *Orbit* 1999;18:45–52.
19. Giacomin AL, di Pietro R, Steindler P. Merkel cell carcinoma: a distinct lesion of the eyelid. *Orbit* 1999;18:295–303.
20. Di Maria A, Carnevali L, Redaelli C, et al. Primary neuroendocrine carcinoma ("Merkel cell tumor") of the eyelid: a report of two cases. *Orbit* 2000;19:171–177.
21. Collaco L, Silva JP, Goncalves M, et al. Merkel cell carcinoma of the eyelid: a case report. *Eur J Ophthalmol* 2000;10:173–176.
22. Hocht S, Wiegel T. Primary radiotherapy of recurrent Merkel cell carcinoma of the eyelid. Case report and review of the literature. *Strahlenther Onkol* 1998;174:311–314.
23. Li S, Brownstein S, Addison DJ, et al. Merkel cell carcinoma of the eyelid. *Can J Ophthalmol* 1997;32:455–461.
24. Dini M, Lo Russo G. Merkel cell carcinoma of the eyelid. *Eur J Ophthalmol* 1997;7:108–112.
25. Rubsamen PE, Tanenbaum M, Grove AS, et al. Merkel cell carcinoma of the eyelid and periocular tissues. *Am J Ophthalmol* 1992;113:674–680.
26. Soltau JB, Smith ME, Custer PL. Merkel cell carcinoma of the eyelid. *Am J Ophthalmol* 1996;121:331–332.
27. Hamilton J, Levine MR, Lash R, et al. Merkel cell carcinoma of the eyelid. *Ophthalmic Surg* 1993;24:764–769.
28. Onesti MG, Mazzocchi M, Scuderi N. Merkel cell carcinoma in the orbitopalpebral region. *Scand J Plast Reconstr Surg Hand Surg* 2005;39:48–52.
29. Nicoletti AG, Matayoshi S, Santo RM, et al. Eyelid Merkel cell carcinoma: report of three cases. *Ophthal Plast Reconstr Surg* 2004;20:117–121.
30. Sinclair N, Mireskandari K, Forbes J, et al. Merkel cell carcinoma of the eyelid in association with chronic lymphocytic leukaemia. *Br J Ophthalmol* 2003;87:240.
31. Esmaeli B, Naderi A, Hidaji L, et al. Merkel cell carcinoma of the eyelid with a positive sentinel node. *Arch Ophthalmol* 2002;120:646–648.
32. Silkiss RZ, Green JE, Shetlar DJ. Small cell neuroendocrine carcinoma of the eyelid. *Ophthal Plast Reconstr Surg* 2008;24(4):319–321.
33. Rawlings NG, Brownstein S, Jordan DR. Merkel cell carcinoma masquerading as a chalazion. *Can J Ophthalmol* 2007;42(3):469–470.

Classification

34. Edge SB, Byrd DR, Compton CC, et al., eds. Carcinoma of the eyelid. In: *AJCC Cancer Staging Manual.* 7th ed. New York: Springer, 2010.

EYELID MERKEL CELL CARCINOMA (CUTANEOUS NEUROENDOCRINE CARCINOMA)

Searl SS, Boynton JR, Markowitch W, di Sant'Agnese PA. Malignant Merkel cell neoplasm of the eyelid. *Arch Ophthalmol* 1984;102:907–911.

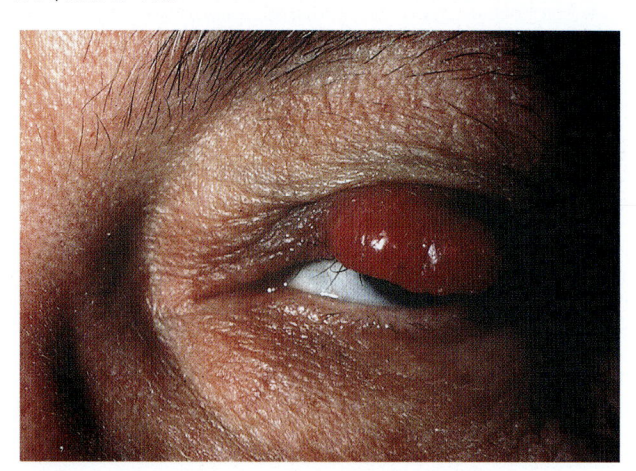

Figure 7.19. Typical Merkel cell carcinoma of the upper eyelid showing reddish, sausage-shaped mass. (Courtesy of Steven S. Searl, MD.)

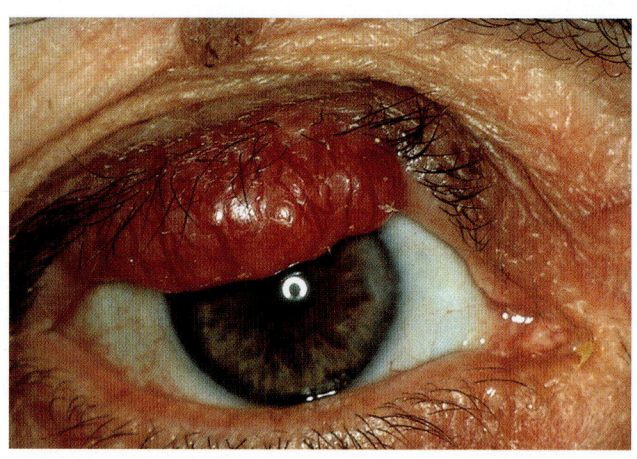

Figure 7.20. Typical Merkel cell carcinoma of the upper eyelid showing reddish, sausage-shaped mass. (Courtesy of Seymour Brownstein, MD.)

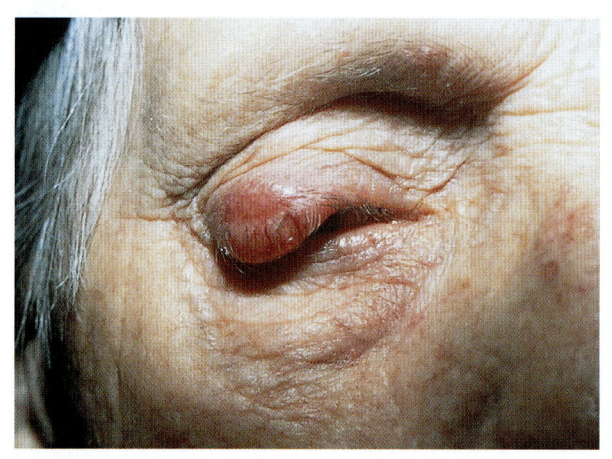

Figure 7.21. Merkel cell carcinoma involving lateral aspect of upper eyelid. (Courtesy of Bruce Johnson, MD.)

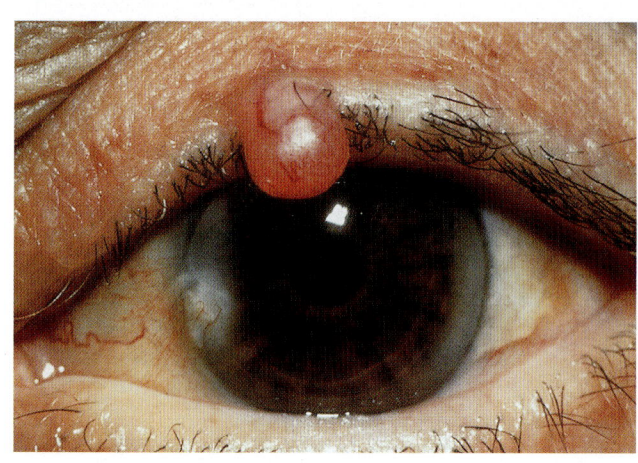

Figure 7.22. Pedunculated Merkel cell carcinoma of upper eyelid. (Courtesy of John Finlay, MD.)

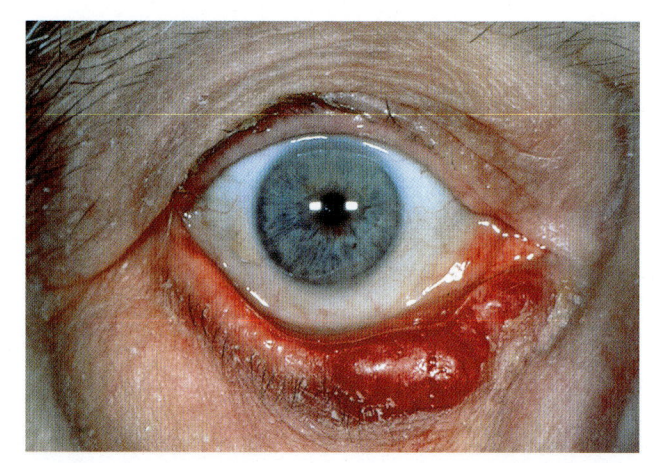

Figure 7.23. Fusiform Merkel cell carcinoma of lower eyelid. (Courtesy of David Addison, MD.)

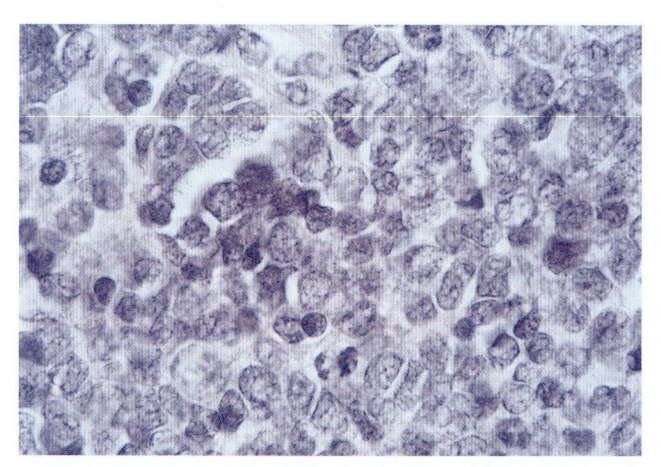

Figure 7.24. Histopathology of Merkel cell carcinoma shown in Figure 7.23 demonstrating poorly differentiated malignant cells with round to oval nuclei with finely dispersed chromatin and inconspicuous nucleoli. (Hematoxylin–eosin ×200.)

Chapter 7 Neural Tumors of the Eyelid

EYELID MERKEL CELL CARCINOMA: MANAGEMENT AND CLINICOPATHOLOGIC CORRELATION

The most appropriate management of Merkel cell carcinoma of the eyelid is surgical resection and eyelid reconstruction, similar to the management of other primary malignant eyelid tumors.

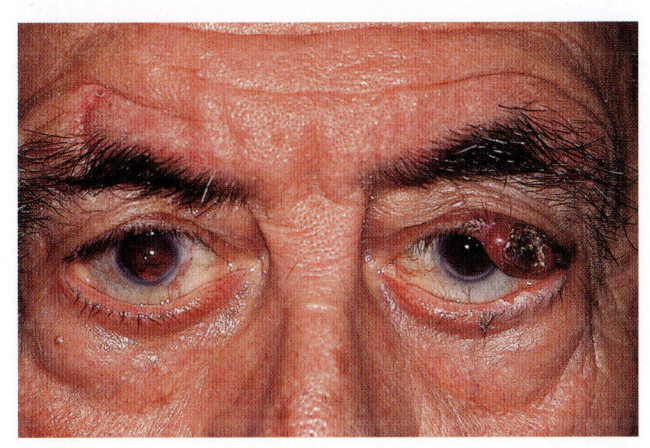

Figure 7.25. Merkel cell carcinoma of upper eyelid in an 80-year-old man.

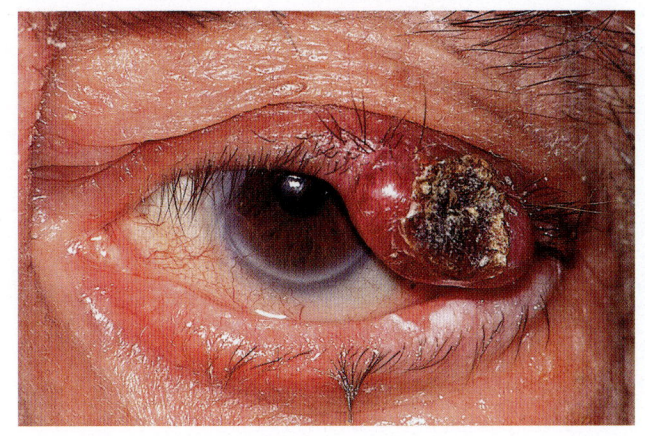

Figure 7.26. Closer view of the lesion shown in Figure 7.25. The crusted surface was secondary to a prior biopsy done elsewhere.

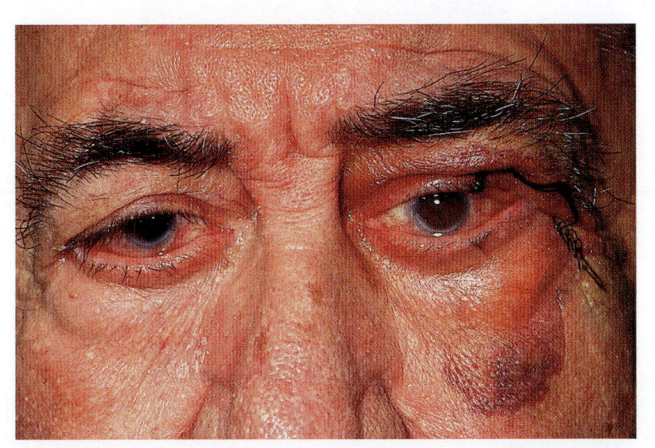

Figure 7.27. Close view 2 days after surgical removal by eyelid resection.

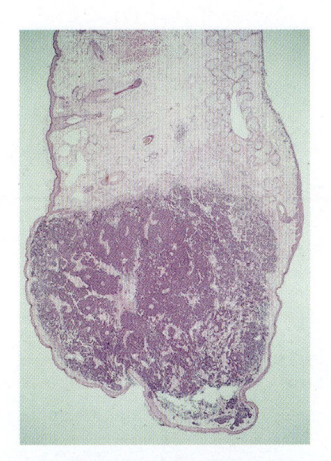

Figure 7.28. Low-magnification photomicrograph of eyelid showing basophilic tumor located near eyelid margin. (Hematoxylin–eosin ×10.)

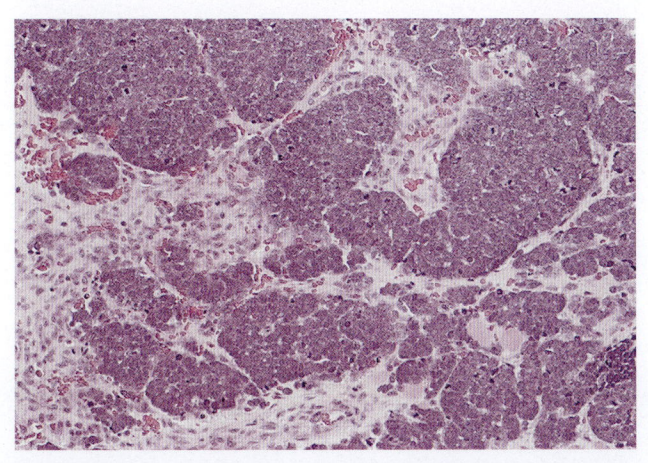

Figure 7.29. Low-magnification photomicrograph showing lobules of basophilic tumor cells. (Hematoxylin–eosin ×100.)

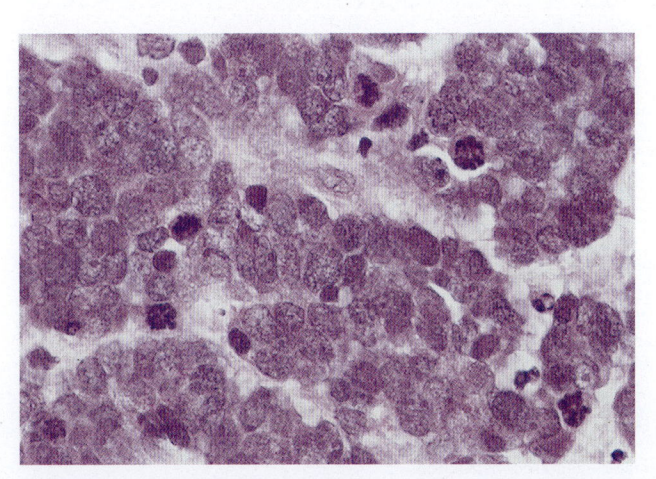

Figure 7.30. Photomicrograph showing anaplastic tumor cells with mitotic activity. (Hematoxylin–eosin ×300.)

EYELID MERKEL CELL CARCINOMA: CLINICAL APPEARANCE AND SURGICAL TECHNIQUE

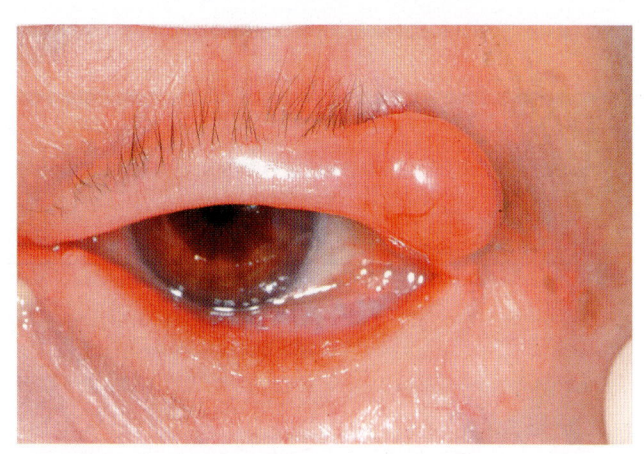

Figure 7.31. Merkel cell carcinoma of upper eyelid in a 76-year-old man.

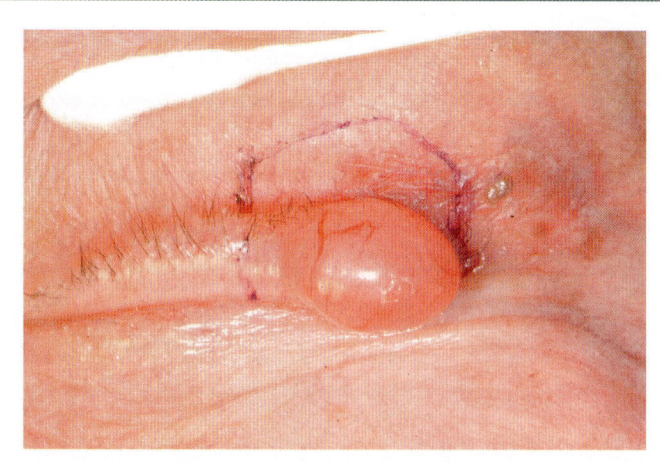

Figure 7.32. Pentagonal resection outlined outside the tumor margins.

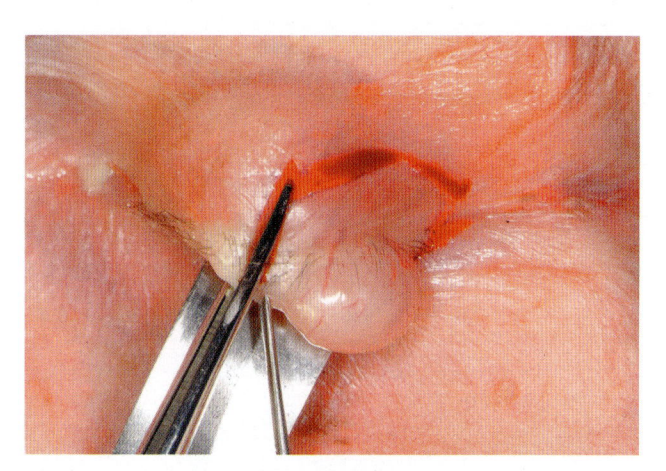

Figure 7.33. Tumor being removed with retractor to protect globe.

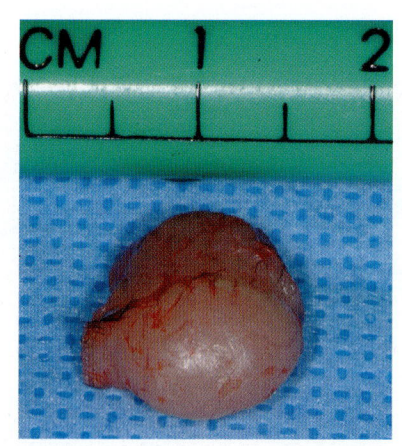

Figure 7.34. Gross appearance of resected mass with surrounding free margins.

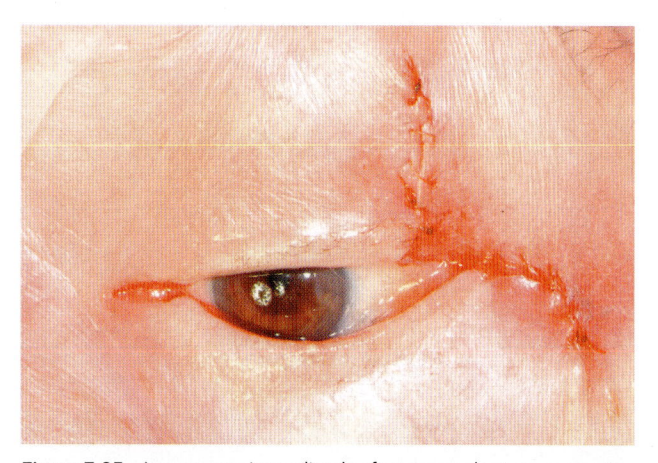

Figure 7.35. Appearance immediately after surgery by tumor resection and eyelid reconstruction.

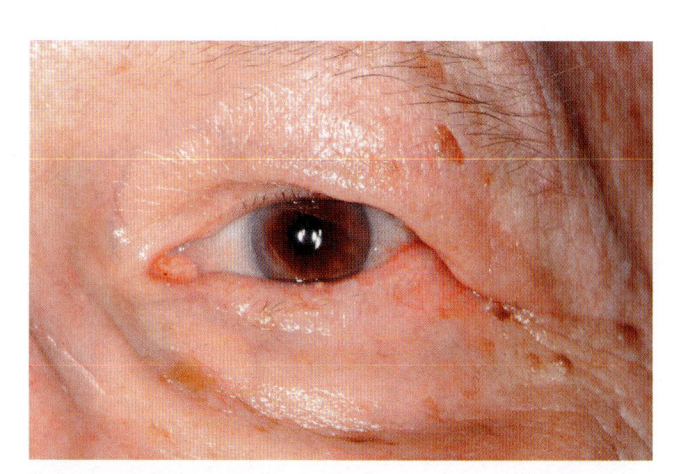

Figure 7.36. Appearance 2 months later.

EYELID MERKEL CELL CARCINOMA: PATHOLOGY

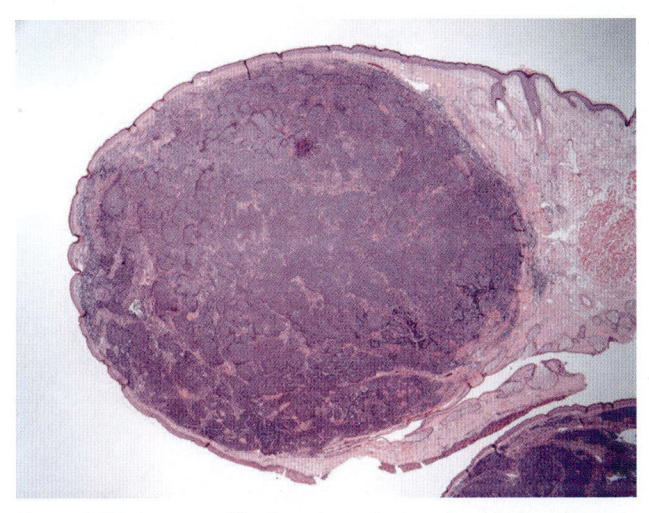

Figure 7.37. Low-magnification photomicrograph of lesion shown in Figures 7.31 to 7.36, demonstrating full-thickness eyelid with basophilic mass near the eyelid margin. (Hematoxylin–eosin ×10.)

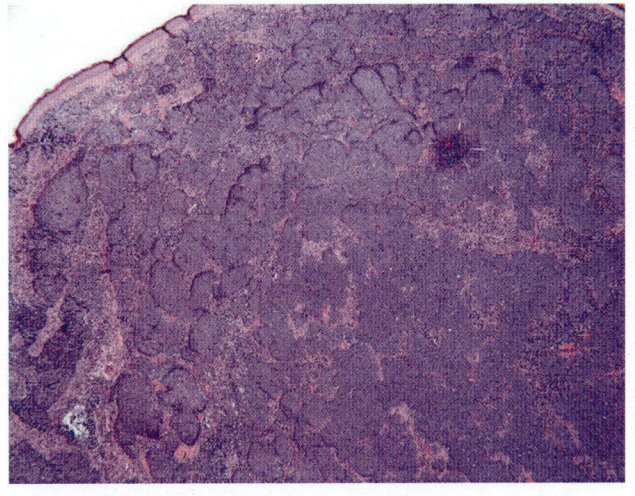

Figure 7.38. Medium-power photomicrograph view showing lobules of basophilic tumor cells. (Hematoxylin–eosin ×25.)

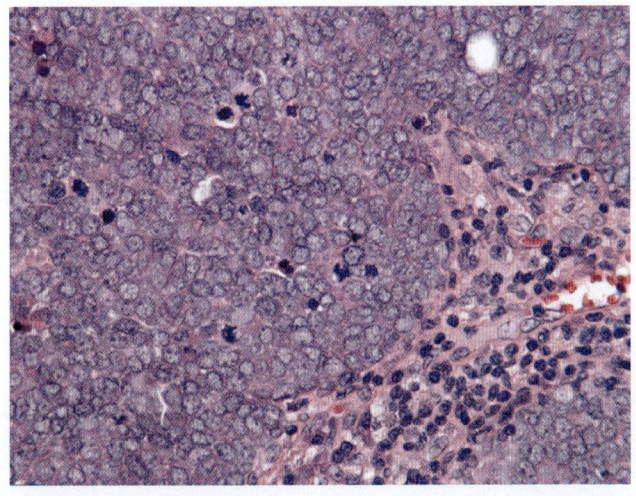

Figure 7.39. Higher-power photomicrograph showing malignant tumor cells. (Hematoxylin–eosin ×100.)

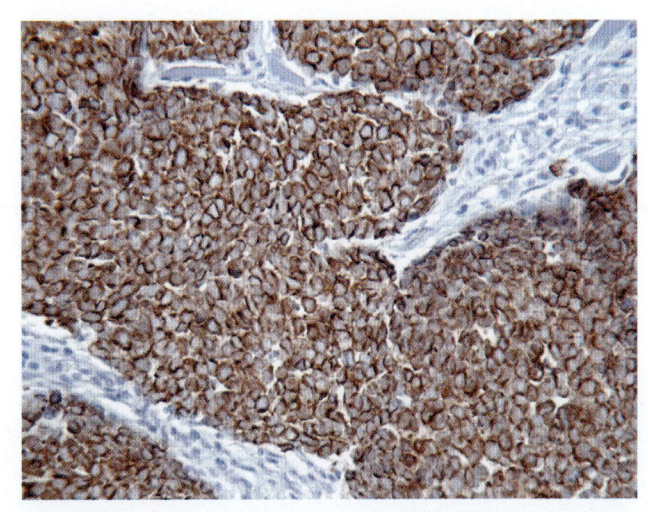

Figure 7.40. Immunohistochemistry showing positive reaction to epithelial marker CAM. (×50.)

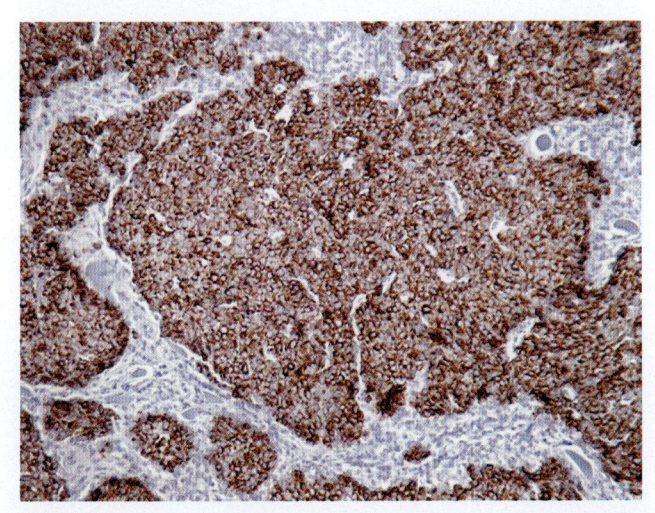

Figure 7.41. Immunohistochemistry showing positive reaction to cytokeratin marker CK20. (×50.)

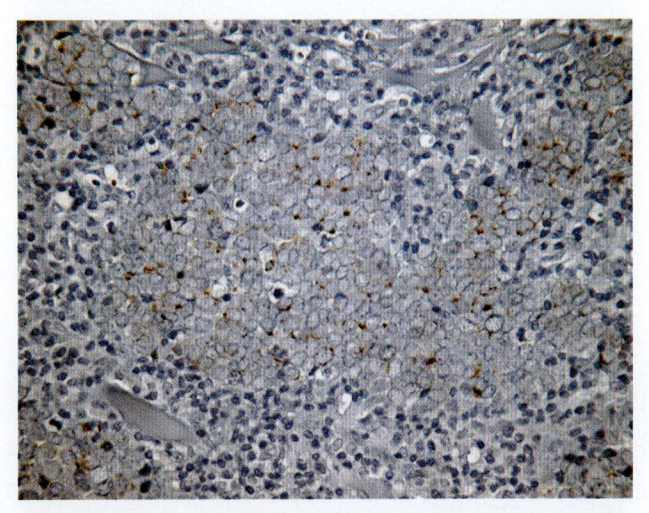

Figure 7.42. Immunohistochemistry showing positive reaction to chromogranin A. (×50.)

CHAPTER 8

VASCULAR TUMORS OF THE EYELIDS

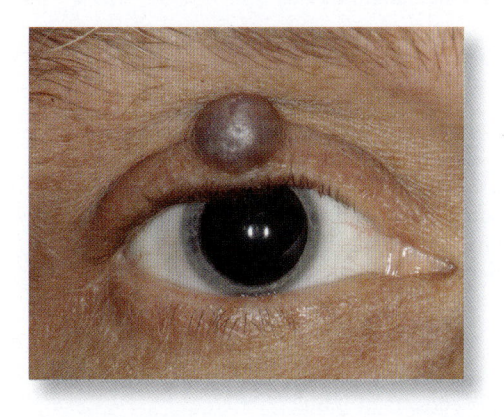

General Considerations

There are a number of vascular tumors and pseudotumors that can affect the eyelid and adjacent tissues (1–39). Congenital cutaneous capillary hemangioma (infantile hemangioma, benign hemangioendothelioma, strawberry nevus) is the most common. This tumor is a benign vascular mass that is either apparent at birth or develops a few weeks after birth. This is one of the most common tumors of infancy (1). Cutaneous capillary hemangioma of infancy can be located superficially, deep, or both. There is a tendency for this lesion to occur in siblings and affected triplets have been described (38). Rarely, cutaneous capillary hemangioma can be associated with extensive hemangiomatosis that can involve the viscera and other organs. Large visceral tumors can trap platelets within their vascular channels, leading to thrombocytopenia and secondary coagulopathy, a condition termed the Kasabach–Merritt syndrome, which can be fatal (1,3). Another important syndrome associated with a large (>5 cm) facial hemangioma is the PHACE syndrome. Major and minor criteria have been established and include anatomic abnormalities of the cerebrovascular, structural brain, cardiovascular, and ocular tissues as well as ventral or midline defects (5).

Clinical Features

The superficial eyelid and periocular capillary hemangioma (strawberry hemangioma) appears initially as a red vascular macule that progressively enlarges and becomes more elevated for 3 to 6 months after diagnosis. It usually becomes stable by age 12 to 18 months and then slowly involutes. It has been estimated that about 30% of cutaneous capillary hemangiomas regress completely by age 3 years and 75% to 90% by age 7 years. Nearly complete regression is achieved by age 5 years. Although this tumor may have a bothersome cosmetic appearance early in its course, the eventual regression can be dramatic, leaving little cosmetic defect or thinned skin.

In contrast to the superficial form, the deep capillary hemangioma lies in the subcutaneous tissues with little or no involvement of the epidermis. It is blue-gray in color, soft to palpation, and becomes more prominent with crying or straining. A tumor that extends deeper in the orbit can produce proptosis and displacement of the globe, and is important in the differential diagnosis of infantile orbital tumors. Both superficial and deep capillary hemangioma can occur together. The natural course of deep hemangioma is similar to the superficial

EYELID CONGENITAL CAPILLARY HEMANGIOMA (STRAWBERRY HEMANGIOMA)

variant, with fairly rapid growth followed by slow regression over several years. This deep capillary hemangioma is discussed later in this atlas under the topic of orbital tumors.

Complications

The main complications of periocular capillary hemangioma are strabismus and amblyopia. The strabismus is either secondary to tumor impingement on the rectus muscles or secondary to amblyopia. The amblyopia can be a result of the tumor obstructing the pupil or a result of the anisometropia induced by the compression of the globe by the tumor. The refractive error often persists even after the hemangioma has regressed (4).

Differential Diagnosis

When the eyelid skin is involved by the typical red lesion, the diagnosis is generally quite evident. The differential diagnosis of deeper capillary hemangioma includes several other childhood anterior orbital neoplasms, including lymphangioma, rhabdomyosarcoma, and myeloid sarcoma (leukemia). These are discussed further in later chapters under the topic of orbital tumors.

Pathology

Histopathologically, capillary hemangioma consists of lobules of capillaries that are separated by fibrous tissue septa. The proliferating endothelial cells may obliterate the capillaries. As a capillary hemangioma undergoes regression, it becomes less cellular and less vascular, and is replaced by fibrous tissue.

Pathogenesis

The pathogenesis of cutaneous capillary hemangioma, previously unknown, has been the subject of recent interest. It has been recognized that placenta and cutaneous capillary hemangiomas share unique immunohistochemical similarities. This has led to speculation that infantile hemangiomas could be of placental origin. Two theories have been proposed to explain this hemangioma–placental connection. First, angioblasts may proliferate toward placental tissue in the site where the hemangioma develops. A second intriguing theory is that cells of placental origin could embolize to the target areas and proliferate into the tumor ("metastatic placenta") (36,37).

Management

Because most infantile capillary hemangiomas regress spontaneously, it is generally appropriate to follow the tumor with observation rather than surgical resection. However, it is important to check visual acuity and do a refraction. Any amblyopia or potential amblyopia should be treated with patching the opposite eye. Most authorities also use local or systemic corticosteroids to hasten resolution.

EYELID CONGENITAL CAPILLARY HEMANGIOMA (STRAWBERRY HEMANGIOMA)

There was previous enthusiasm for the use of systemic corticosteroids or intralesional injection of corticosteroids to hasten regression of capillary hemangioma of the ocular region that have amblyopic potential (6–18). Most patients treated in that manner demonstrated favorable response with minimal complications. However, occasional complications of intralesional corticosteroids include central retinal artery obstruction, linear perilymphatic subcutaneous fat atrophy, eyelid depigmentation, eyelid necrosis, and adrenal gland suppression (9–17). As an alternative, topical corticosteroids have been occasionally used (19–21). Intralesional interferon α-2a and -2b have also been used for capillary hemangioma that is unresponsive to corticosteroids (19). Laser therapy has been advocated for some cutaneous hemangiomas (22,23).

Surgical removal has historically been discouraged for capillary hemangioma due to the potential for rapid blood loss in an infant and possible cosmetic scarring. However, there is a valid argument for selected surgical resection of some cases (34–37). One indication for surgical resection is circumscribed subcutaneous hemangioma that is enlarging in a young infant with risk for amblyopia and globe compression. Such a tumor could become large before it regresses and early surgical removal could avoid more difficult management of a larger tumor. An eyelid crease incision, with removal of the mass intact if possible, and closure of the skin with fine absorbable sutures can achieve a very satisfactory outcome (34). However, surgical resection should generally be avoided for larger superficial lesions that have extensive involvement of the epidermis.

In 2008, Léauté-Labrèze et al. (25) coincidently discovered the benefit of oral propranolol in the management of infants with large cutaneous capillary hemangioma. Currently, propranolol is considered standard of care for this condition with hastening of tumor regression and few side effects (26,29). For deep lesions, oral propranolol is used and for superficial lesions, topical propranolol can be effective (26–31).

Selected References

Reviews
1. Drolet BA, Esterly NB, Frieden IJ. Hemangiomas in children. *N Engl J Med* 1999;341:173–181.
2. Haik BG, Jakobiec FA, Ellsworth RM, et al. Capillary hemangioma of the lids and orbit: an analysis of the clinical features and therapeutic results in 101 cases. *Ophthalmology* 1979;86:760–789.
3. Haik BG, Karcioglu ZA, Gordon RA, et al. Capillary hemangioma (infantile periocular hemangioma). *Surv Ophthalmol* 1994;38:399–426.
4. Robb RM. Refractive errors associated with hemangiomas of the eyelids and orbit in infancy. *Am J Ophthalmol* 1977;83:52–58.
5. Metry D, Heyer G, Hess C, et al. Consensus statement on diagnostic criteria for PHACE syndrome. *Pediatrics* 2009;124:1447–1456.

Management/Corticosteroids
6. Brown BZ, Huffaker G. Local injection of steroids for juvenile hemangiomas which disturb the visual axis. *Ophthalmic Surg* 1982;13:630–633.
7. Zak TA, Morin JD. Early local steroid therapy of infantile eyelid hemangiomas. *J Pediatr Ophthalmol Strabismus* 1981;18:25–27.
8. Kushner BJ. Intralesional corticosteroid injection for infantile adnexal hemangioma. *Am J Ophthalmol* 1982;93:496–506.
9. O'Keefe M, Lanigan B, Byrne SA. Capillary haemangioma of the eyelids and orbit: a clinical review of the safety and efficacy of intralesional steroid. *Acta Ophthalmol Scand* 2003;81:294–298.
10. Ruttum MS, Abrams GW, Harris GJ, et al. Bilateral retinal embolization associated with intralesional corticosteroid injection for capillary hemangioma of infancy. *J Pediatr Ophthalmol Strabismus* 1993;30:4–7.
11. Egbert JE, Schwartz GS, Walsh AW. Diagnosis and treatment of an ophthalmic artery occlusion during an intralesional injection of corticosteroid into an eyelid capillary hemangioma. *Am J Ophthalmol* 1996;121:638–642.
12. Droste PJ, Ellis FD, Sondhi N, et al. Linear subcutaneous fat atrophy after corticosteroid injection of periocular hemangiomas. *Am J Ophthalmol* 1988;105:65–69.
13. Ford MD, Codere F. Perilymphatic subcutaneous atrophy in adnexal hemangioma: a complication of intralesional corticosteroid injection. *Ophthalmic Surg* 1990;21:215–217.
14. Cogen MS, Elsas FJ. Eyelid depigmentation following corticosteroid injection for infantile ocular adnexal hemangioma. *J Pediatr Ophthalmol Strabismus* 1989;26:35–38.
15. Sutula FC, Glover AT. Eyelid necrosis following intralesional corticosteroid injection for capillary hemangioma. *Ophthalmic Surg* 1987;18:103–105.
16. Weiss AH. Adrenal suppression after corticosteroid injection of periocular hemangiomas. *Am J Ophthalmol* 1989;107:518–522.
17. Goyal R, Watts P, Lane CM, et al. Adrenal suppression and failure to thrive after steroid injections for periocular hemangioma. *Ophthalmology* 2004;111:389–395.
18. Elsas JF, Lewis AR. Topical treatment of periocular capillary hemangioma. *J Pediatr Ophthalmol Strabismus* 1994;31:153–156.

Interferon
19. Rosenthal G, Snir M, Biedner B. Corticosteroid resistant orbital hemangioma with proptosis treated with interferon alfa-2-a and partial tarsorrhaphy. *J Pediatr Ophthalmol Strabismus* 1995;32:50–51.
20. Hastings MM, Milot J, Barsoum-Homsy M, et al. Recombinant interferon alfa-2b in the treatment of vision-threatening capillary hemangiomas in childhood. *J AAPOS* 1997;1:226–230.
21. Fledelius HC, Illum N, Jensen H, et al. Interferon-alfa treatment of facial infantile haemangiomas: with emphasis on the sight-threatening varieties. A clinical series. *Acta Ophthalmol Scand* 2001;79:370–372.

Laser
22. Gladstone GJ, Beckman H. Argon laser treatment of an eyelid margin capillary hemangioma. *Ophthalmic Surg* 1983;14:944–946.
23. Chopdar A. Carbon-dioxide laser treatment of eyelid lesions. *Trans Ophthalmol Soc UK* 1985;104:176–180.
24. Shorr N, Goldberg RA, David LM. Laser treatment of juvenile hemangioma. *Ophthalmic Plast Reconstr Surg* 1988;4:131–141.

Propranolol
25. Léauté-Labrèze C, Dumas de la Roque E, Hubiche T, et al. Propranolol for severe hemangiomas of infancy. *N Engl J Med* 2008;358:2649–2651.
26. Vassallo P, Forte R, Di Mezza A, et al. Treatment of infantile capillary hemangioma of the eyelid with systemic propranolol. *Am J Ophthalmol* 2013;155(1):165–170.e2.
27. Rizvi SA, Yusuf F, Sharma R, et al. Management of superficial infantile capillary hemangiomas with topical timolol maleate solution. *Semin Ophthalmol* 2013;30(1):62–64.
28. Xue K, Hildebrand GD. Topical timolol maleate 0.5% for infantile capillary haemangioma of the eyelid. *Br J Ophthalmol* 2012;96(12):1536–1537.
29. Ni N, Guo S, Langer P. Current concepts in the management of periocular infantile (capillary) hemangioma. *Curr Opin Ophthalmol* 2011;22(5):419–425.
30. Ni N, Langer P, Wagner R, et al. Topical timolol for periocular hemangioma: report of further study. *Arch Ophthalmol* 2011;129(3):377–379.
31. Guo S, Ni N. Topical treatment for capillary hemangioma of the eyelid using beta-blocker solution. *Arch Ophthalmol* 2010;128(2):255–256.

Surgical Resection
32. Slaughter K, Sullivan T, Boulton J, et al. Early surgical intervention as definitive treatment for ocular adnexal capillary haemangioma. *Clin Exp Ophthalmol* 2003;31:418–423.
33. Deans RM, Harris GJ, Kivlin JD. Surgical dissection of capillary hemangiomas. An alternative to intralesional corticosteroids. *Arch Ophthalmol* 1992;110:1743–1747.
34. Aldave AJ, Shields CL, Shields JA. Surgical excision of selected amblyogenic periorbital capillary hemangiomas. *Ophthalmic Surg Lasers* 1999;30:754–757.

Other
35. Cruz OA, Zarnegar SR, Myers SE. Treatment of periocular capillary hemangioma with topical clobetasol propionate. *Ophthalmology* 1995;102:2012–2015.

Histopathology
36. North PE, Waner M, Mizeracki A, et al. A unique microvascular phenotype shared by juvenile hemangiomas and human placenta. *Arch Dermatol* 2001;137:559–570.
37. North PE, Waner M, Brodsky MC. Are infantile hemangiomas of placental origin? *Ophthalmology* 2002;109:633–634.

Case Reports
38. Shields CL, Shields JA, Minzter R, et al. Cutaneous capillary hemangiomas of the eyelid, scalp, and digits in premature triplets. *Am J Ophthalmol* 2000;129:528–531.
39. Plager DA, Snyder SK. Resolution of astigmatism after surgical resection of capillary hemangiomas in infants. *Ophthalmology* 1997;104:1102–1106.

Chapter 8 Vascular Tumors of the Eyelids

EYELID CONGENITAL CAPILLARY HEMANGIOMA: SUPERFICIAL TYPE

The superficial type of capillary hemangioma (strawberry hemangioma) has typical clinical features and can show dramatic spontaneous regression.

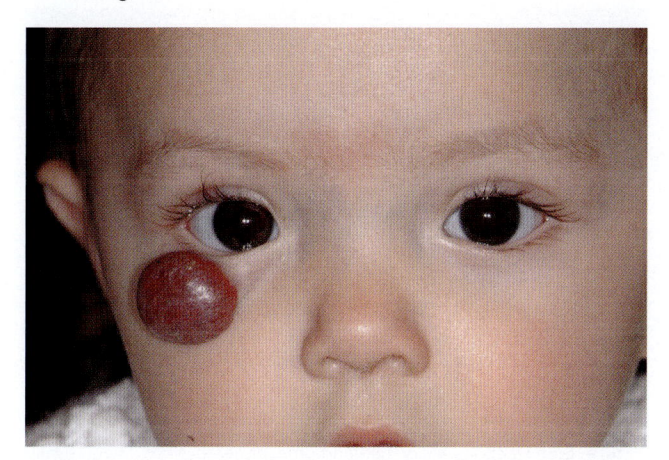

Figure 8.1. Superficial capillary hemangioma on right lower eyelid.

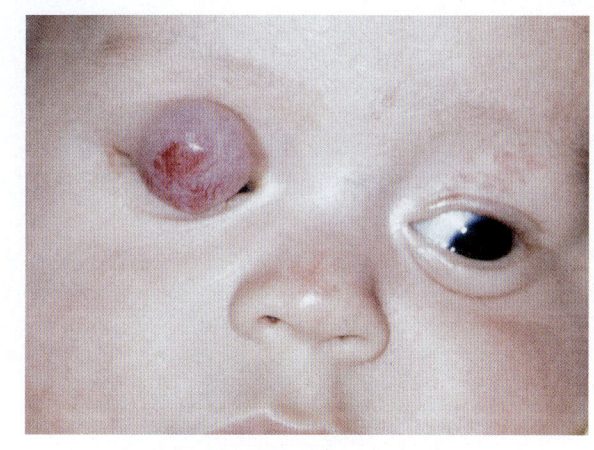

Figure 8.2. Superficial capillary hemangioma on right upper eyelid.

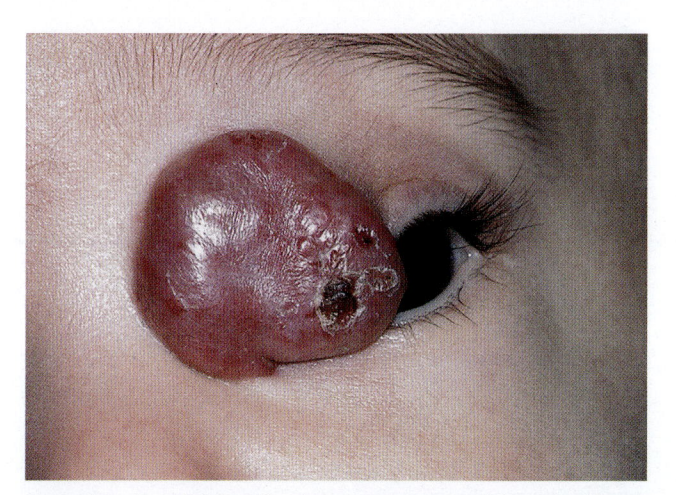

Figure 8.3. Superficial capillary hemangioma on medial aspect of upper eyelid.

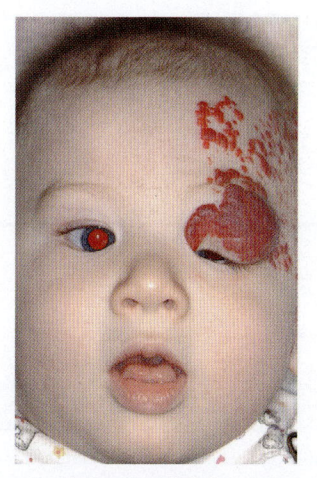

Figure 8.4. Extensive multifocal capillary hemangioma involving upper eyelid, forehead, and temporal scalp.

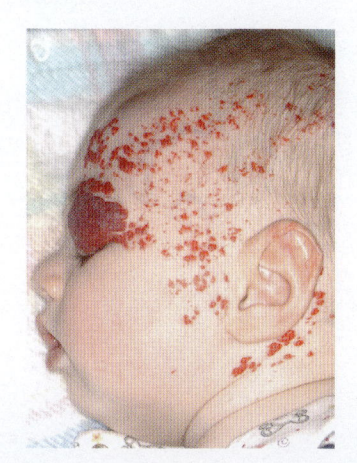

Figure 8.5. Side view of patient shown in Figure 8.4 demonstrating multifocal capillary hemangioma of face, scalp, and neck.

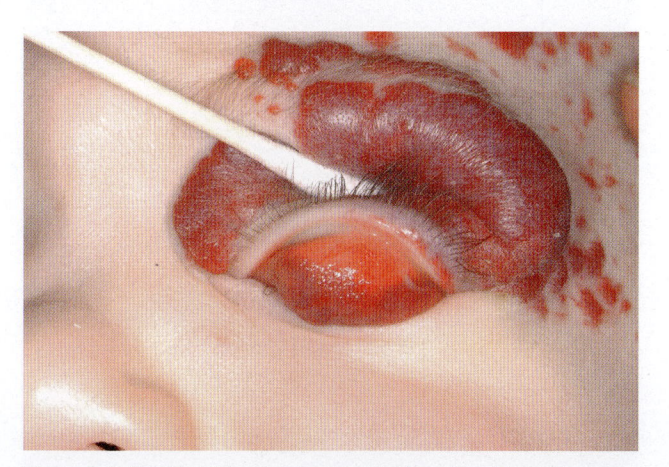

Figure 8.6. Eyelid capillary hemangioma with conjunctival involvement. The upper eyelid is being everted showing diffuse involvement of involved tarsal conjunctiva. It is necessary to evert the eyelid in such cases to determine the full extent of the lesion.

EYELID CONGENITAL CAPILLARY HEMANGIOMA: DEEP TYPE

The deep type of capillary hemangioma does not affect the epidermis and appears as a soft blue or pink subcutaneous mass.

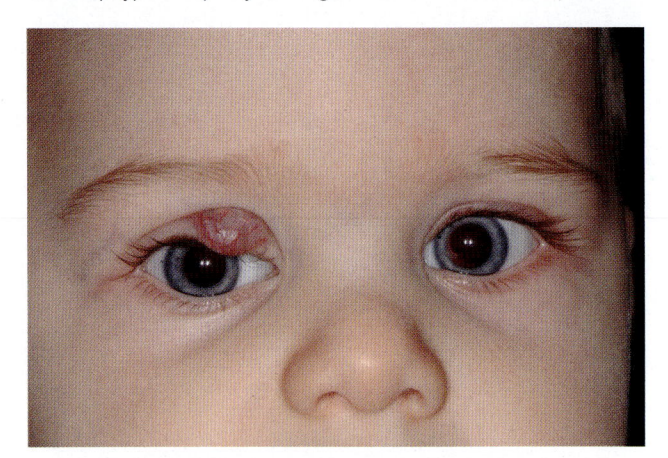

Figure 8.7. Deep capillary hemangioma of upper eyelid with overlying prominent blood vessels.

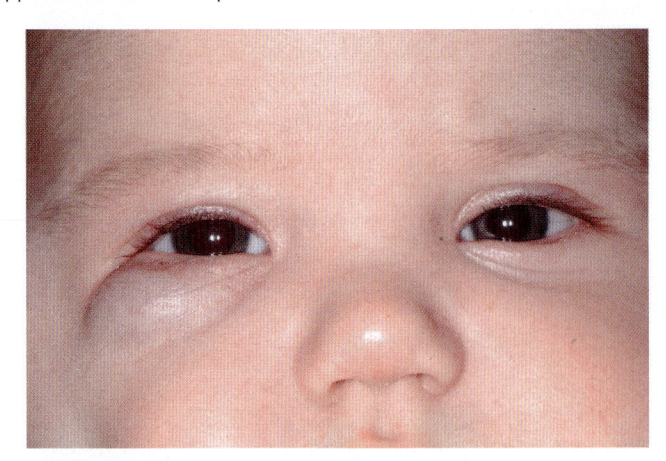

Figure 8.8. Deep capillary hemangioma beneath right lower eyelid imparting blue color to skin.

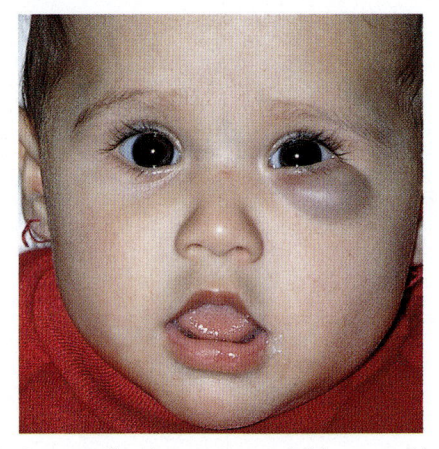

Figure 8.9. Deep capillary hemangioma in left lower eyelid.

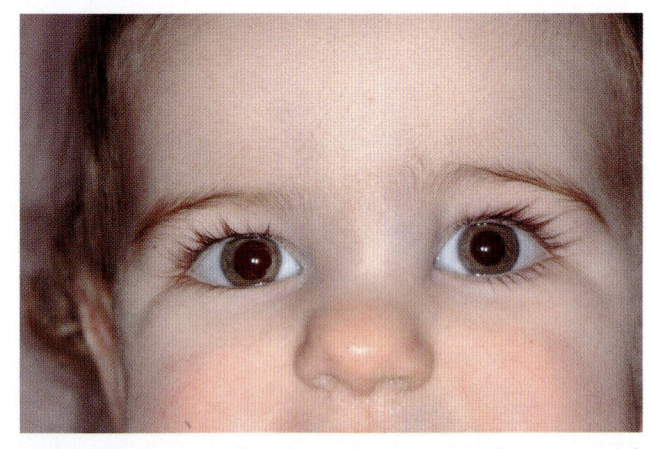

Figure 8.10. Deep capillary hemangioma on side of nose near left medial canthus.

Figure 8.11. Deep capillary hemangioma beneath medial aspect of left upper eyelid.

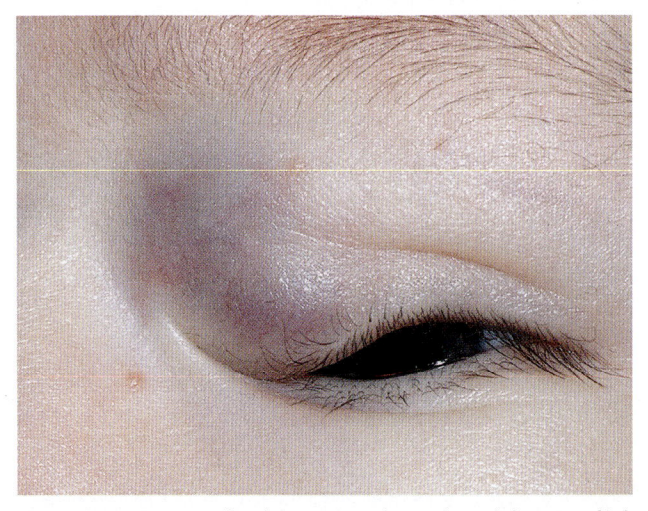

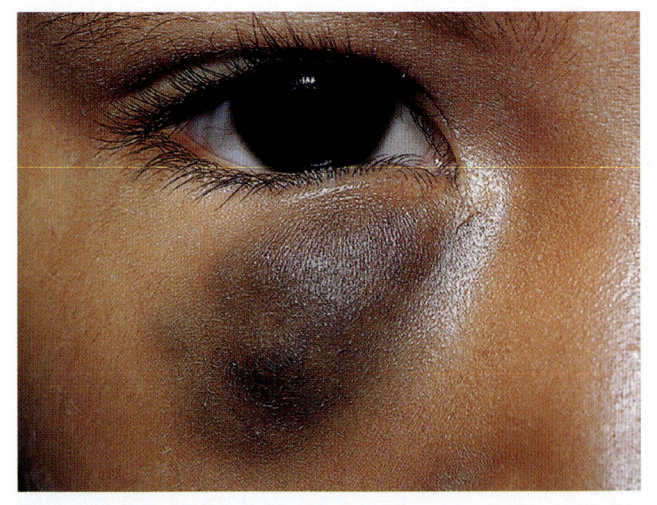

Figure 8.12. Blue-colored deep capillary hemangioma of lower eyelid. This can look similar to hemorrhage into a lymphangioma, but the lesion had slowly regressed and had no acute bleeding episodes.

EYELID CONGENITAL CAPILLARY HEMANGIOMA: REGRESSION OF SUPERFICIAL TYPE

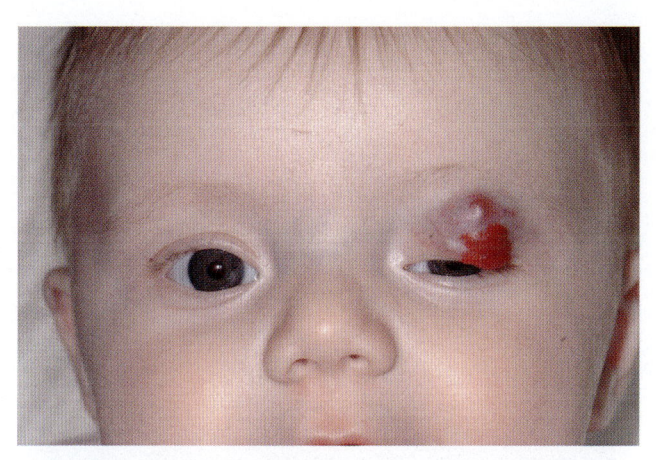

Figure 8.13. Combined superficial and deep capillary hemangioma in 3-month-old child. The child was treated with oral corticosteroids.

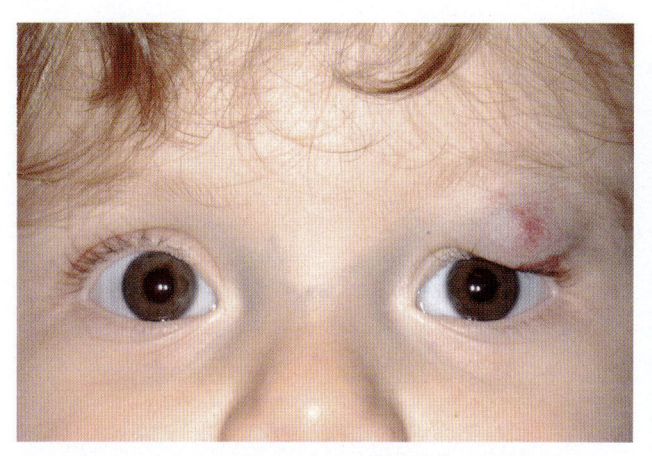

Figure 8.14. Same child 10 months later showing regression of tumor, less blepharoptosis, and more exposure of pupil.

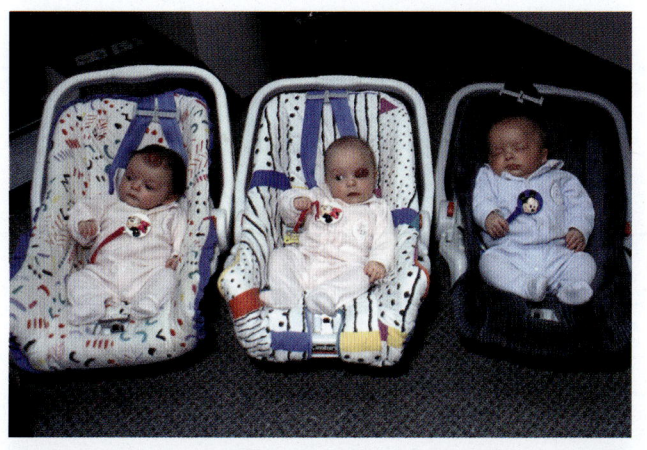

Figure 8.15. Premature triplets, each of whom had multiple cutaneous capillary hemangiomas. The triplet on left shows forehead involvement, the middle one showed involvement of left upper eyelid, and the right one has finger hemangiomas that are not seen.

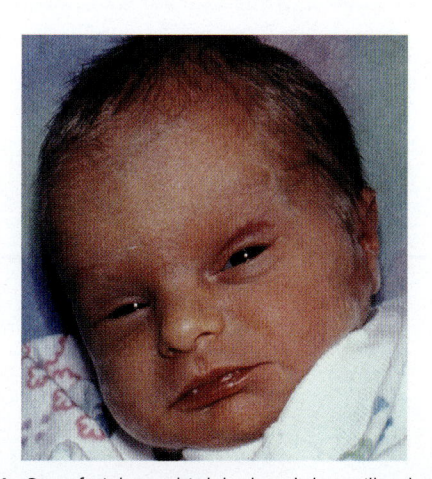

Figure 8.16. One of triplets at birth had a subtle capillary hemangioma of left upper eyelid.

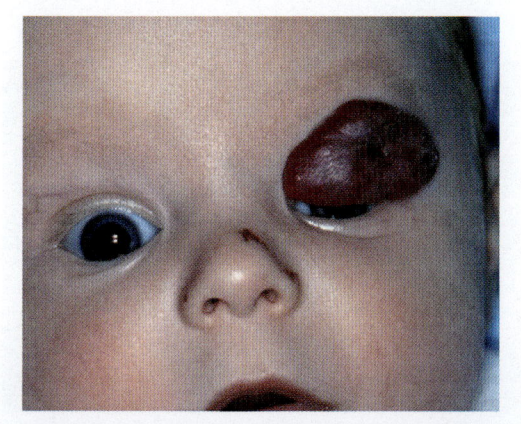

Figure 8.17. Same child shown in Figure 8.16, 2 months later showing larger capillary hemangioma that rapidly developed on left upper eyelid. The child was treated with oral corticosteroids.

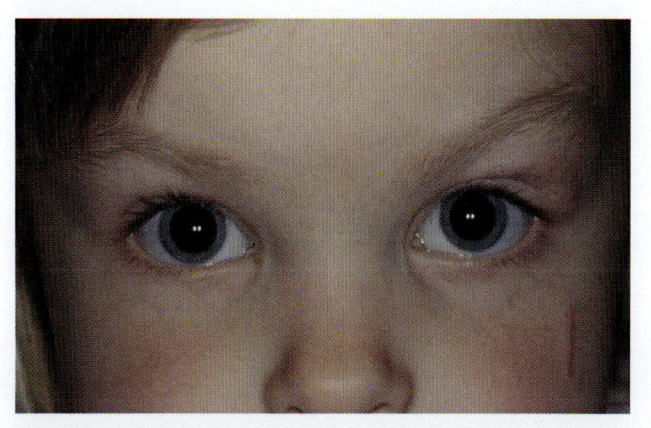

Figure 8.18. Same child at age 3 years, showing complete resolution of the lesion. The resolution was rapid after the oral corticosteroids were initiated.

EYELID CONGENITAL CAPILLARY HEMANGIOMA: REGRESSION OF DEEP TYPE

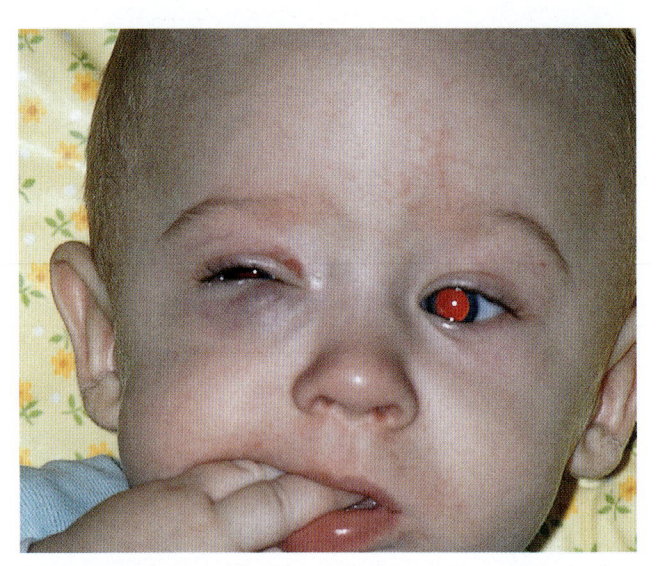

Figure 8.19. Deep capillary hemangioma in lower eyelid of infant. Observation was advised.

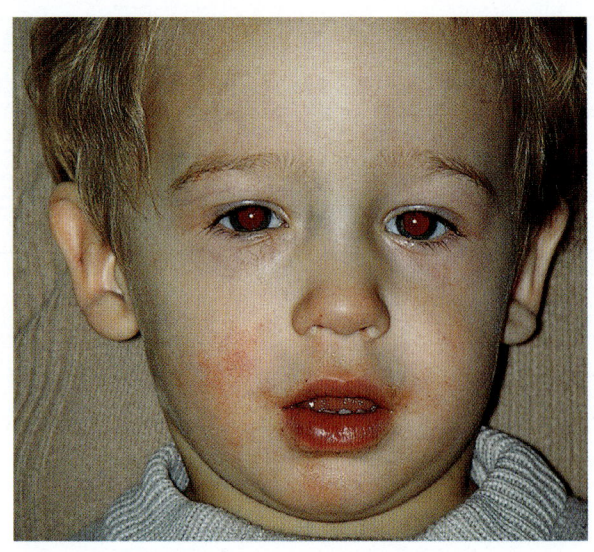

Figure 8.20. Same lesion showing tumor regression 2 years later.

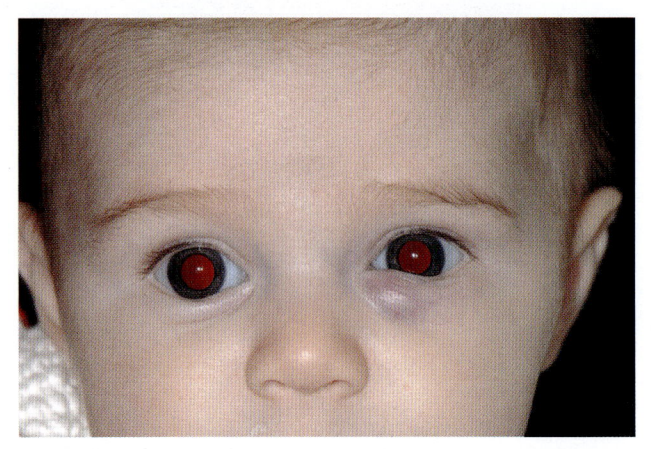

Figure 8.21. Deep capillary hemangioma in lower eyelid of infant.

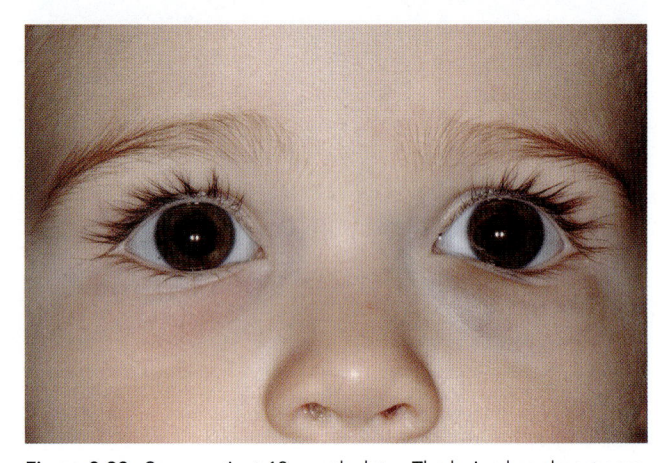

Figure 8.22. Same patient 13 months later. The lesion has almost completely resolved.

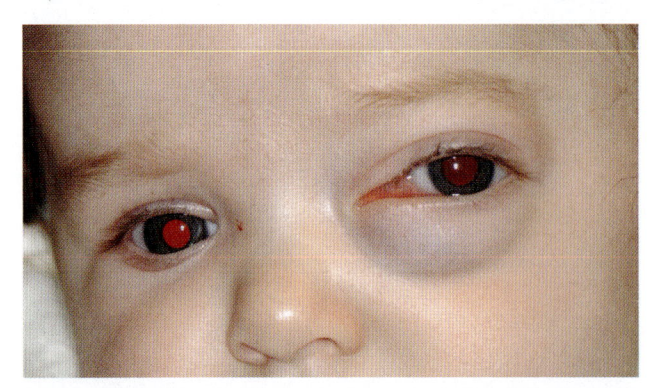

Figure 8.23. Deep capillary hemangioma in medial canthal region causing proptosis in an infant. Such a lesion can simulate an ethmoidal encephalocele.

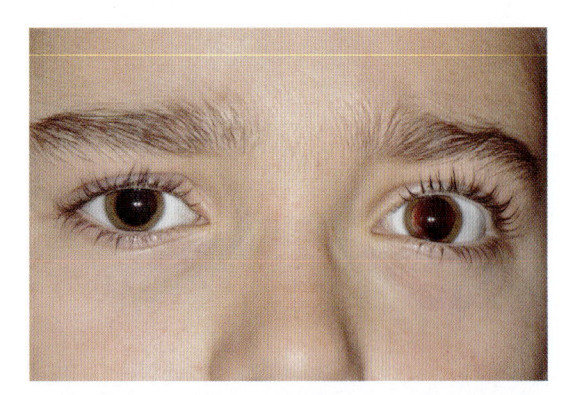

Figure 8.24. Nine years later, the lesion has completely resolved.

Chapter 8 Vascular Tumors of the Eyelids

● EYELID CONGENITAL CAPILLARY HEMANGIOMA: SURGICAL REMOVAL

Sometimes a capillary hemangioma can be resected entirely with a good result without waiting for it to grow to a large size.

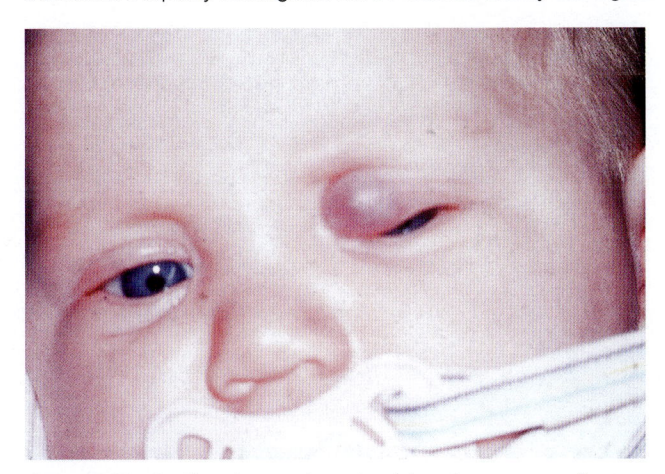

Figure 8.25. Capillary hemangioma involving deep aspect of upper eyelid nasally in an infant. The lesion was removed intact by eyelid crease incision.

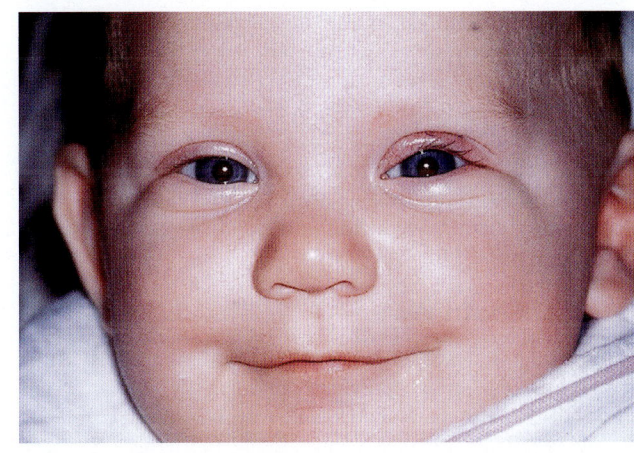

Figure 8.26. Facial appearance of child after surgery, showing good cosmetic result.

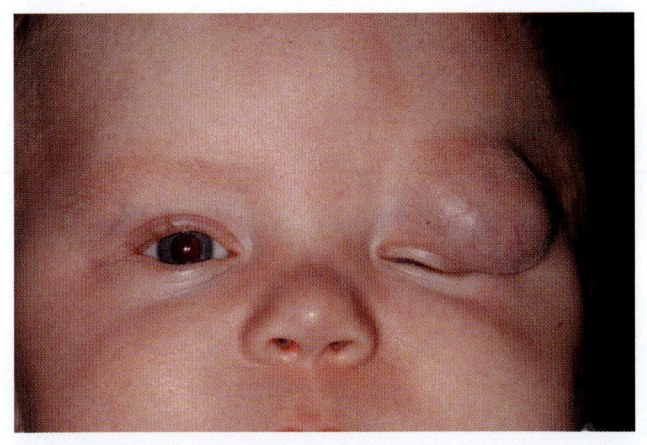

Figure 8.27. Large deep upper eyelid capillary hemangioma in an infant showing complete blepharoptosis.

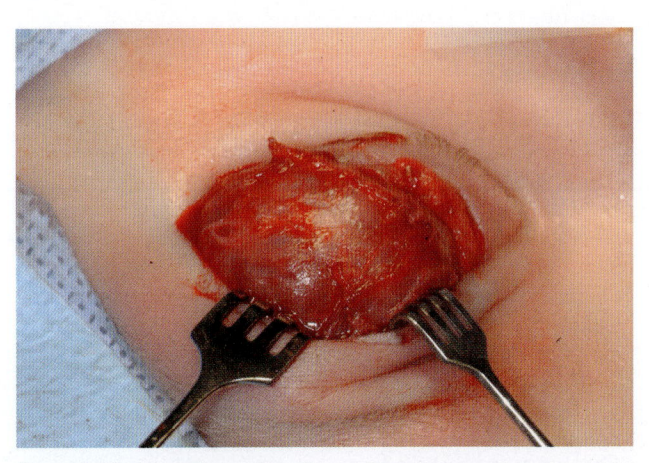

Figure 8.28. Surgical resection of tumor in patient shown in Figure 8.27 using an eyelid crease approach.

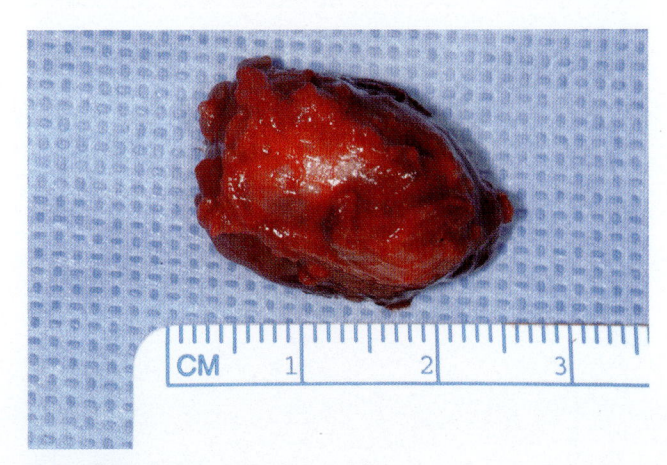

Figure 8.29. Gross specimen removed intact.

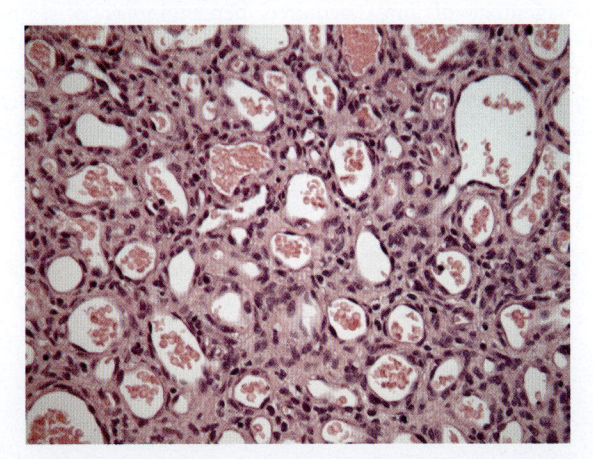

Figure 8.30. Histopathology of eyelid capillary hemangioma shown in Figure 8.29, showing fine vascular channels and proliferating endothelial cells. (Hematoxylin–eosin ×75.)

EYELID ACQUIRED HEMANGIOMA (CHERRY HEMANGIOMA)

General Considerations

Acquired hemangioma (cherry hemangioma; senile hemangioma) is a common cutaneous lesion in middle-aged and older adults (1–5). It occurs in varying numbers in virtually all adults, but the lesions are small and often ignored. The number varies from 1 to 2 in children to hundreds in some elderly individuals. This tumor occurs most commonly on the trunk and extremities, but can occasionally affect the eyelids and periocular region. It can range in size from barely visible to a dome-shaped red mass (1).

Clinical Features

Solitary acquired hemangioma of the eyelid appears as a distinct red to red-blue papule that may range from 0.5 to 5 mm in size (3–5). It is generally movable with skin and it can bleed following trauma. Smaller lesions are red and larger ones have a blue hue. Clinically, the lesion may be very similar to angiosarcoma or pyogenic granuloma. Eyelid acquired hemangioma has been observed to develop and rapidly enlarge during pregnancy (4).

Pathology

In its early stages, acquired hemangioma is very similar histopathologically to the congenital capillary hemangioma of infancy, having numerous newly formed capillaries with narrow lumina and prominent endothelial cells arranged in a lobular fashion in the subpapillary region (1,2). In a fully matured lesion, the vascular lumina become dilated, the endothelial cells more flattened, and the stroma becomes edematous and hyalinized. Some authorities consider the acquired hemangioma to be closely related to pyogenic granuloma, but it generally shows less endothelial proliferation than the latter (2). The term "capillary hemangioma of the pyogenic granuloma type" has been applied to this particular lesion (1).

Management

Management of most acquired hemangiomas is simple periodic observation, because they are generally small and have no malignant potential. When a larger one poses a cosmetic problem, or is suspicious for malignancy, complete excision is appropriate management. Some clinicians used diathermy, electrodessication, and curettage. The prognosis is excellent.

Selected References

Reviews

1. Calonje E, Wilson-Jones E. Vascular tumors. Cherry hemangioma. In: Elder D, Elenitsas R, Jaworsky C, et al., eds. *Lever's Histopathology of the Skin.* 8th ed. Philadelphia, PA: Lippincott-Raven; 1997:899–932.
2. Enzinger FM, Weiss SW. Benign tumors and tumorlike lesions of blood vessels. In: Weiss SW, Goldblum SR, eds. *Enzinger and Weiss's Soft Tissue Tumors.* 4th ed. St. Louis, MO: CV Mosby; 2001:837–890.

Case Reports

3. Murphy BA, Dawood GS, Margo CE. Acquired capillary hemangioma of the eyelid in an adult. *Am J Ophthalmol* 1997;124:403–404.
4. Pushker N, Bajaj MS, Kashyap S, et al. Acquired capillary haemangioma of the eyelid during pregnancy. *Clin Exp Ophthalmol* 2003;31:368–369.
5. Brannan S, Reuser TQ, Crocker J. Acquired capillary haemangioma of the eyelid in an adult treated with cutting diathermy. *Br J Ophthalmol* 2000;84:1322.

EYELID ACQUIRED CAPILLARY HEMANGIOMA

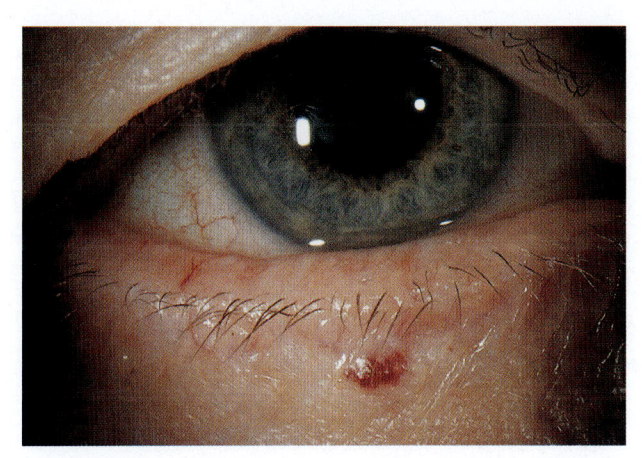

Figure 8.31. Acquired hemangioma in midportion of lower eyelid in a 74-year-old man.

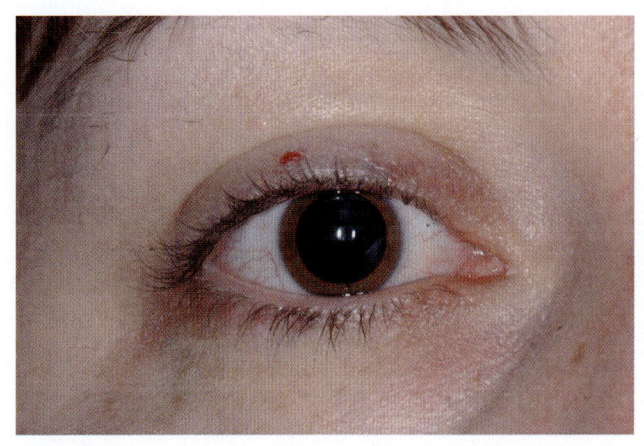

Figure 8.32. Acquired hemangioma in mid portion of right upper eyelid. Another tiny red lesion is present at the eyelid margin nasal to the larger lesion.

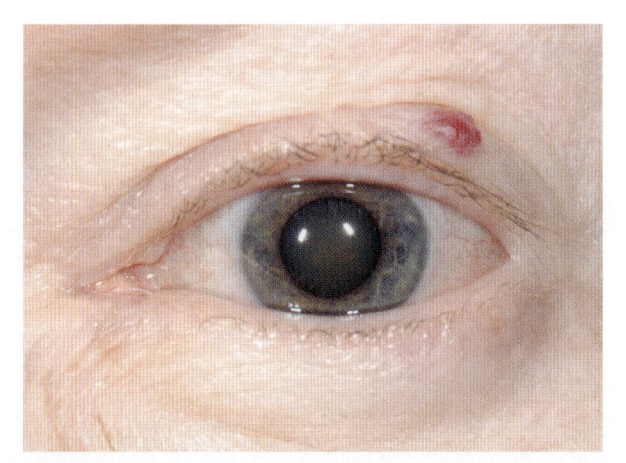

Figure 8.33. Acquired hemangioma in lateral left upper eyelid in older woman.

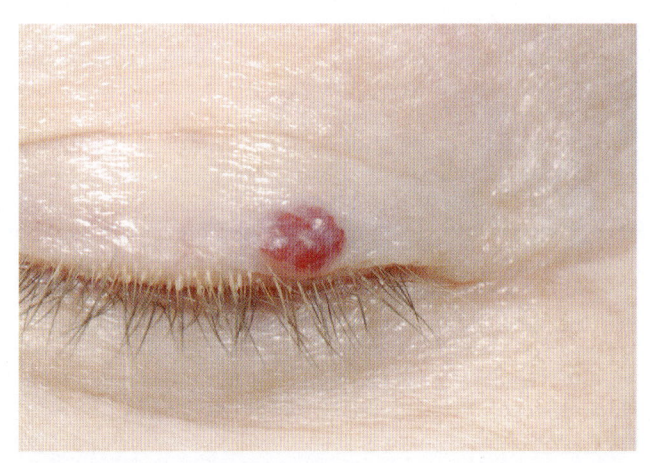

Figure 8.34. Close-up view of patient in Figure 8.33 showing the slightly multilobulated vascular mass.

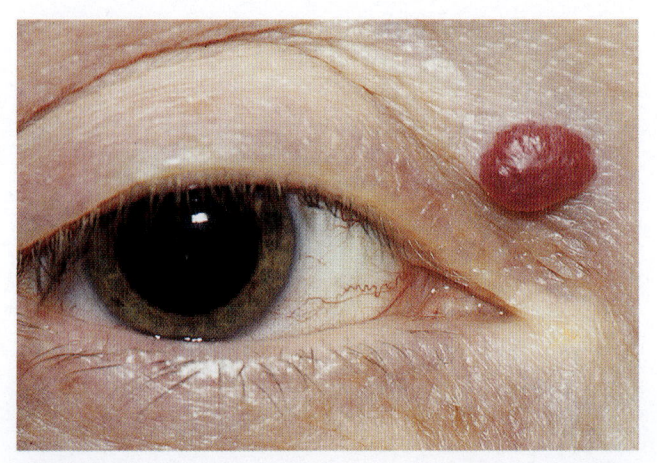

Figure 8.35. Acquired hemangioma of upper eyelid in a 58-year-old woman.

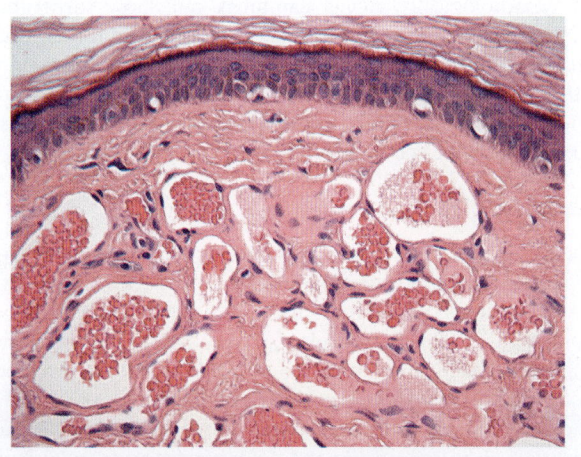

Figure 8.36. Histopathology of lesion shown in Figure 8.35. Note the dilated vascular channels with thin endothelial cells and erythrocytes in the lumen. (Hematoxylin–eosin ×50.)

EYELID NEVUS FLAMMEUS (PORT WINE HEMANGIOMA)

General Considerations

Nevus flammeus ("port wine stain") is a congenital vascular malformation that can affect the eyelids and periorbital region (1–9). Facial nevus flammeus is sometimes seen in patients with no other abnormalities, but it is often associated with variations of the Sturge–Weber syndrome and occasionally the Klippel–Trenaunay–Weber syndrome. The Sturge–Weber syndrome consists of facial nevus flammeus, and ipsilateral epibulbar telangiectasia, congenital glaucoma, diffuse choroidal hemangioma, leptomeningeal hemangiomatosis with calcification, and seizures (1–3). Klippel–Trenaunay–Weber syndrome consists of nevus flammeus and hypertrophy of soft tissues and bone in the extremities, presumably related to arteriovenous fistulas. Although it classically occurs in the cutaneous distribution of cranial nerve V (trigeminal nerve), this condition can have several variations.

Clinical Features

Clinically, nevus flammeus is a congenital, red to purple lesion that can occur in various areas of the skin. When it corresponds to the facial cutaneous distribution of the trigeminal nerve and is associated with neurologic and ocular changes mentioned above, it comprises the Sturge–Weber syndrome (1–3). Trigeminal nerve involvement can range from minor involvement of the first division of the nerve to massive involvement of all three divisions (1). Sometimes the nevus flammeus crosses the midline in an irregular pattern and it is occasionally bilateral. The lesion is present at birth and its slow growth parallels the normal growth of the affected child, appearing flat at birth, and irregular, hypertrophied, and nodular with age (3). In contrast with the capillary hemangioma of infancy, the nevus flammeus does not regress. Upper eyelid involvement is often associated with congenital or juvenile glaucoma, particularly in patients with Sturge–Weber syndrome (1).

Pathology

Histopathologically, nevus flammeus can show surprisingly little abnormality in the early stages, except for minimal capillary dilation in the dermis. In specimens from children under 10 years of age, the dermis shows capillary dilation without endothelial proliferation. There is increased collagenous tissue surrounding the ectatic blood vessels.

Cytogenetics

Recent genetic analysis of nevus flammeus in 97 samples from 50 patients with Sturge–Weber syndrome disclosed a nonsynonymous single-nucleotide variant in GNAQ in 88% of cases compared to 0% in controls (5). The authors speculate that this somatic activating mutation in GNAQ is the cause for port wine stain. We suspect that this mutation could be related to the development of phakomatosis pigmentovascularis, a combination of Sturge–Weber and ocular melanocytosis with risk for uveal melanoma (4).

Management

Management of nevus flammeus consists of cosmetics to conceal the abnormality or laser photocoagulation to reduce the vascular dilation. Treatment with various lasers, mainly carbon dioxide and argon laser, and pulsed dye laser have been effective in permanently closing the dilated blood vessels and improving the cosmetic appearance (6). The glaucoma, choroidal hemangioma, and seizures associated with the Sturge–Weber syndrome require specialized treatment, which is discussed elsewhere (1,2).

Selected References

Reviews
1. Shields JA, Shields CL. The systemic hamartomatoses ("phakomatoses"). In: Shields JA, Shields CL, eds. *Intraocular Tumors: A Text and Atlas*. Philadelphia, PA: WB Saunders; 1991:46–50.
2. Comi AM. Update on Sturge-Weber syndrome: diagnosis, treatment, quantitative measures, and controversies. *Lymphat Res Biol* 2007;5:257–264.
3. Nathan N, Thaller SR. Sturge-Weber syndrome and associated congenital vascular disorders: a review. *J Craniofac Surg* 2006;17:724–728.
4. Shields CL, Kligman BE, Suriano M, et al. Phacomatosis pigmentovascularis of cesioflammea type in 7 cases: combination of ocular pigmentation (melanocytosis, melanosis) and nevus flammeus with risk for melanoma. *Ophthalmology* 2011;129: 746–750.

Cytogenetics
5. Shirley MD, Tang H, Gallione CJ, et al. Sturge-Weber syndrome and Port-wine stains caused by somatic mutation in GNAQ. *N Engl J Med* 2013;368:1971–1979.

Management
6. Quan SY, Comi AM, Parsa CF, et al. Effect of a single application of pulsed dye laser treatment of port-wine birthmarks on intraocular pressure. *Arch Dermatol* 2010;146(9):1015–1018.

Case Reports
7. Lindsey PS, Shields JA, Goldberg RE, et al. Bilateral choroidal hemangiomas and facial nevus flammeus. *Retina* 1981;1:88–95.
8. Shields JA, Shields CL, Oberkircher OR, et al. Unusual retinal and renal vascular lesions in the Klippel-Trenaunay-Weber syndrome. *Retina* 1992;12:355–358.
9. Manquez ME, Shields CL, Demirci H, et al. Choroidal melanoma in a teenager with Klippel Trenaunay syndrome. *J Pediatr Ophthalmol Strabismus* 2006;43:197–198.

Chapter 8 Vascular Tumors of the Eyelids

EYELID NEVUS FLAMMEUS (PORT WINE HEMANGIOMA)

The nevus flammeus is present at birth and typically persists into adulthood without regression.

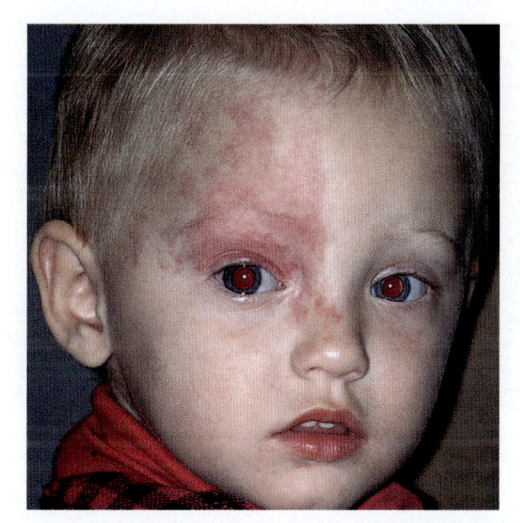

Figure 8.37. Nevus flammeus involving the upper eyelid and forehead of a 2-year-old boy. Note how the lesion respects the midline in the forehead.

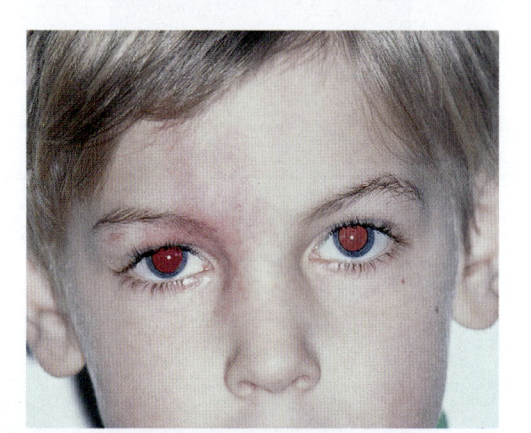

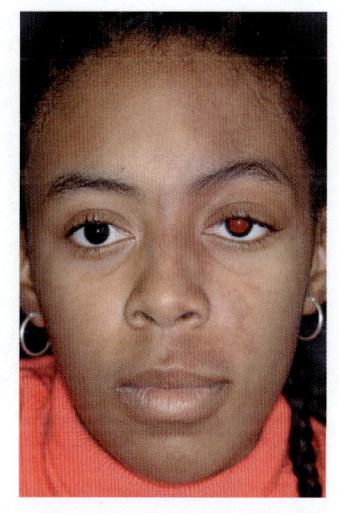

Figure 8.38. Nevus flammeus affecting the left side of the face of an African-American woman.

Figure 8.39. Subtle, irregular nevus flammeus involving the upper eyelid and forehead in a 7-year-old boy.

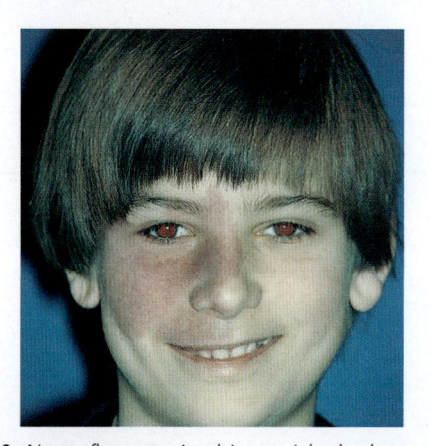

Figure 8.40. Nevus flammeus involving mainly the lower eyelid and cheek of an 11-year-old boy.

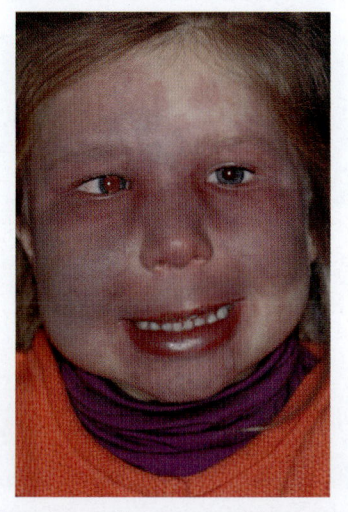

Figure 8.41. Bilateral nevus flammeus involving the forehead, eyelids, cheek, and chin of a 3-year-old girl.

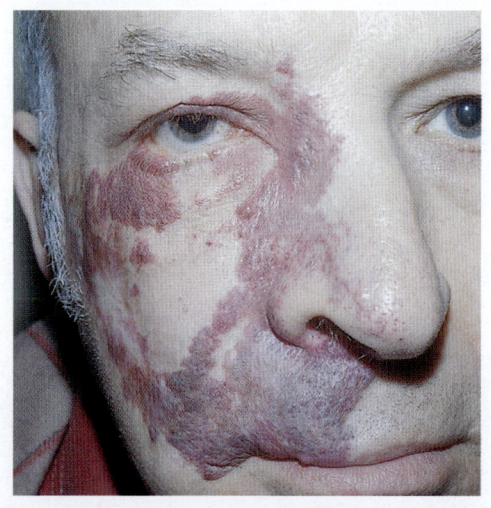

Figure 8.42. Irregular hypertrophied nevus flammeus involving mainly the lower eyelid and cheek of a 70-year-old man. It had been present since birth.

EYELID NEVUS FLAMMEUS: CLINICAL VARIATIONS AND FOLLOW-UP

Nevus flammeus can be bilateral and asymmetric. Cosmetics can be used to improve the appearance.

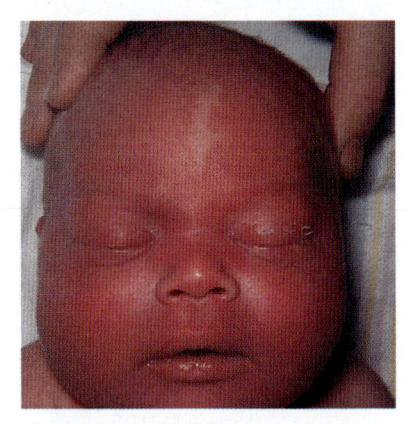

Figure 8.43. Infant with severe bilateral nevus flammeus. Note that only a small area in the middle of the forehead is spared. (Courtesy of Joseph Calhoun, MD.)

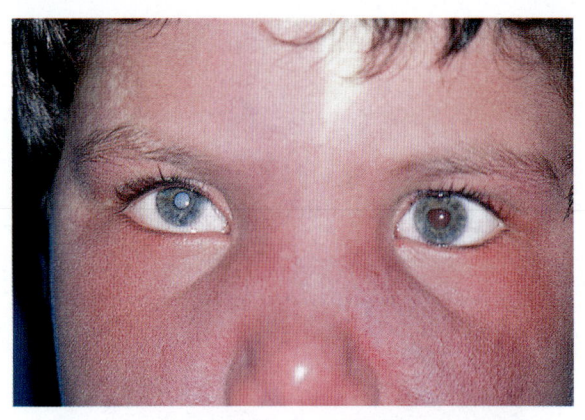

Figure 8.44. Seven-year-old girl with severe bilateral nevus flammeus. The lesion is often less apparent in dark-skinned individuals. Note the subtle involvement of the upper eyelid and forehead. The patient had Sturge–Weber syndrome with bilateral glaucoma, choroidal hemangioma, retinal detachment, and secondary cataracts.

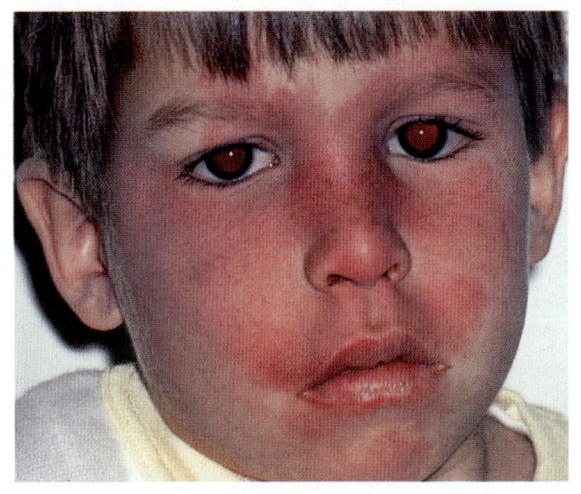

Figure 8.45. Bilateral nevus flammeus sparing most of left upper eyelid in a 6-year-old child.

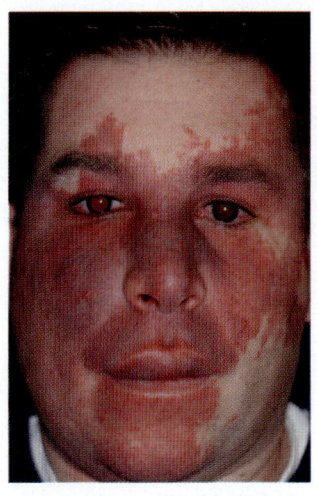

Figure 8.46. Appearance 25 years later of lesion shown in Figure 8.45. The distribution of the vascular lesion has not changed.

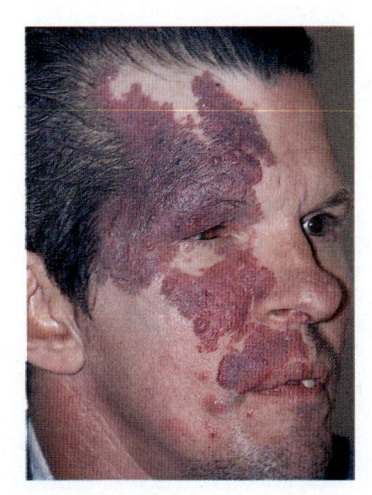

Figure 8.47. Irregular nevus flammeus involving right side of face in a 35-year-old man.

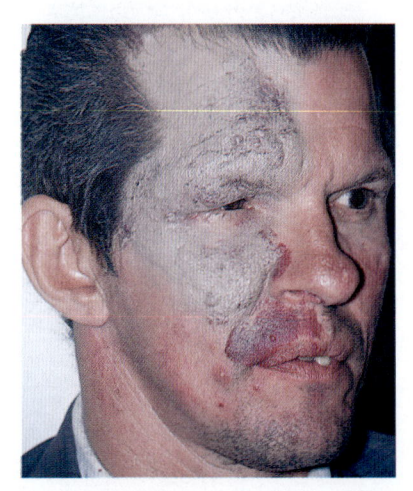

Figure 8.48. Same patient shown in Figure 8.47 after application of cosmetics in an effort to conceal the lesion.

Chapter 8 Vascular Tumors of the Eyelids

EYELID NEVUS FLAMMEUS: ASSOCIATION WITH STURGE–WEBER SYNDROME

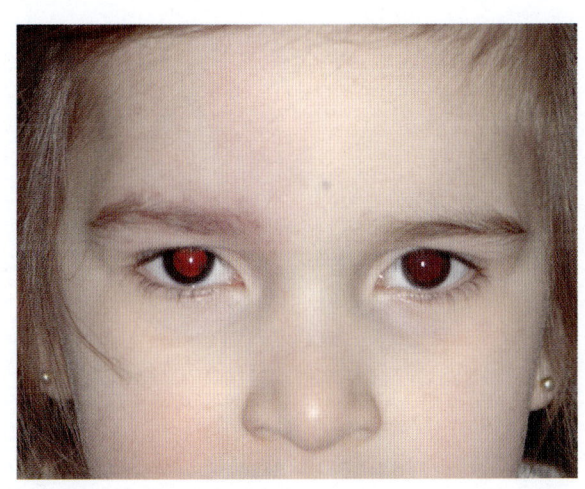

Figure 8.49. Light nevus flammeus on the right side of face, following treatment with tunable dye laser.

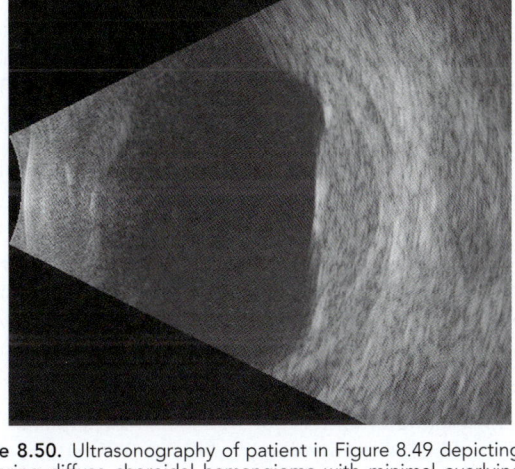

Figure 8.50. Ultrasonography of patient in Figure 8.49 depicting solid appearing diffuse choroidal hemangioma with minimal overlying subretinal fluid.

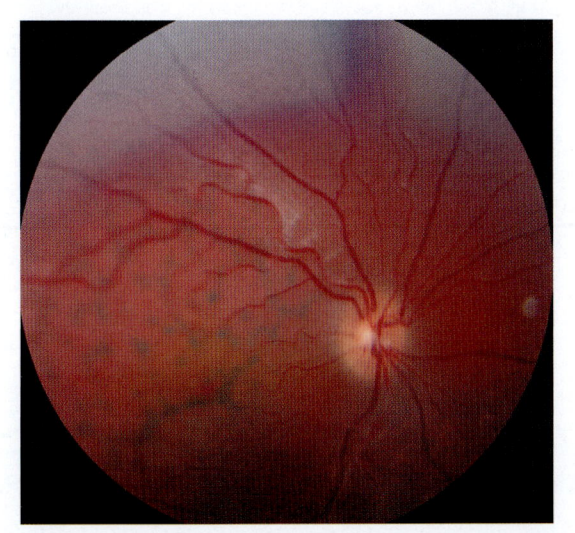

Figure 8.51. Right fundus of patient in Figure 8.49 discloses bright red "tomato catsup" appearance of diffuse hemangioma, with additional overlying retinal pigment epithelial hyperplasia and shallow subretinal fluid.

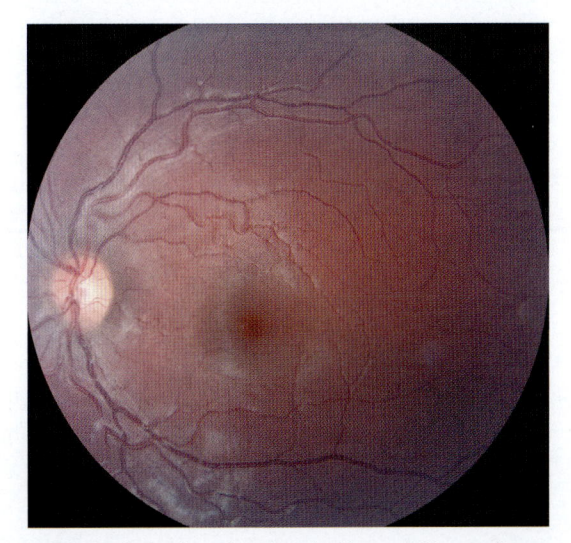

Figure 8.52. Left fundus of patient in Figure 8.49 revealing normal findings.

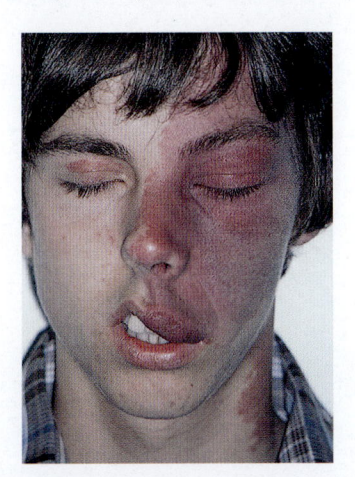

Figure 8.53. Extensive nevus flammeus affecting the left side of the face and neck in a 19-year-old man.

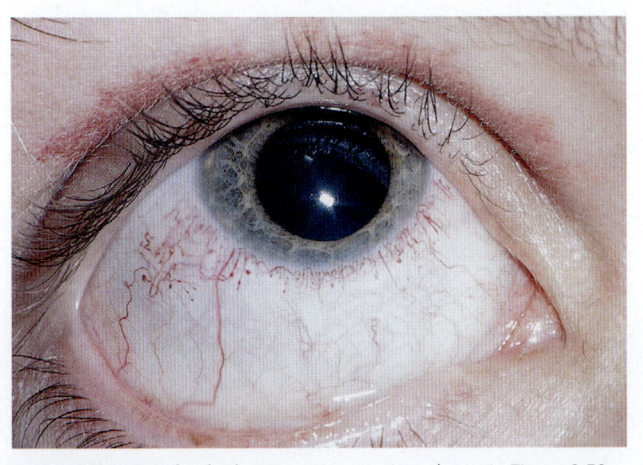

Figure 8.54. Episcleral telangiectasia in patient shown in Figure 8.53.

EYELID VARIX

General Considerations

Miscellaneous benign vascular tumors and related conditions that can affect the orbital and eyelid area include varix, lymphangioma, and glomus tumor. Lymphangioma and varix are more commonly recognized in the orbit than on the eyelid. Many eyelid cases represent an anterior extension of orbital involvement (1–9). Varix and lymphangioma may be difficult to differentiate clinically and histopathologically, and some authorities believe that they represent variations of the same entity (1). Although there is limited information on eyelid varix (5–7), we believe that they share many features with those in the orbit (1,4,8).

Clinical Features

In the eyelid, a varix varies from a small, compressible, cystlike vermiform lesion to a large complex of channels causing thickening and distortion of the eyelid (varices). Extensive involvement may cause an appearance of elephantiasis as seen with neurofibromatosis. A varix that has undergone thrombosis is more firm to palpation.

Pathology

Histopathologically, varix is not a true tumor, but is composed of a thickened wall of a vein with adventitial fibrosis. The lumen contains erythrocytes, scattered mononuclear cells, and a fibrin clot. The lumen may be partially obliterated by an organizing thrombus, with deposition of hemosiderin and foci of dystrophic calcification.

Management

Eyelid varix can be observed or surgically excised, depending on symptoms and cosmetic appearance. Those that are larger can be managed with percutaneous drainage and ablation (2,3).

Selected References

Reviews
1. Wright JE, Sullivan TJ, Garner A, et al. Orbital venous anomalies. *Ophthalmology* 1997;104:905–913.

Management
2. Yue H, Qian J, Elner VM, et al. Treatment of orbital vascular malformations with intralesional injection of pingyangmycin. *Br J Ophthalmol* 2013;97(6):739–745.
3. Hill RH, Shiels WE, Foster JA. Percutaneous drainage and ablation as first line therapy for macrocystic and microcystic orbital lymphatic malformations. *Ophthal Plast Reconstr Surg* 2012;28:119–125.

Case Reports
4. Shields JA, Dolinskas C, Augsburger JJ, et al. Demonstration of orbital varix with computed tomography and valsalva maneuver. *Am J Ophthalmol* 1984;97:108–119.
5. Morikawa M, Rothman MI, Numaguchi Y. Varix of the eyelid: a unique CT finding. *AJR Am J Roentgenol* 1994;162:1505–1506.
6. Mudgil AV, Meyer DR, Dipillo MA. Varix of the angular vein manifesting as a medial canthal mass. *Am J Ophthalmol* 1993;116:245–246.
7. Halasa AH, Matta CS. Varicose veins of the eyelids. Report of a case. *Arch Ophthalmol* 1964;71:176–179.
8. Shields JA, Eagle RC Jr, Shields CL, et al. Orbital varix presenting as a subconjunctival mass. *Ophthal Plast Reconstr Surg* 1995;11(1):37–38.
9. Zakka FR, Jakobiec FA, Thakker MM. Eyelid varix with phlebolith formation, thrombus recanalization, and early intravascular papillary endothelial hyperplasia. *Ophthal Plast Reconstr Surg* 2011;27(1):e8–e11.

Chapter 8 Vascular Tumors of the Eyelids   149

EYELID VARIX

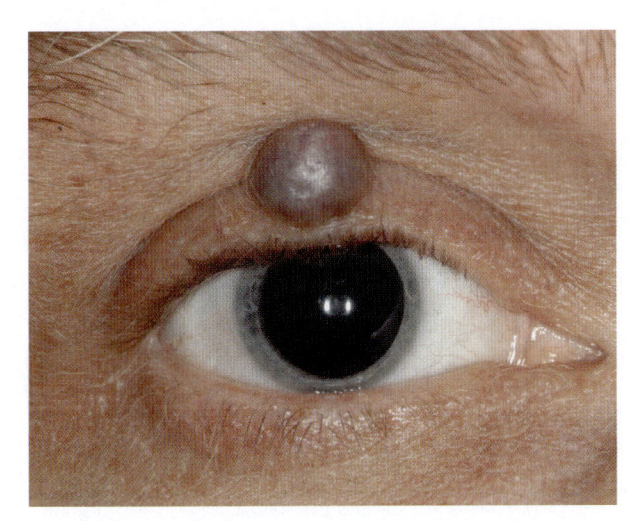

Figure 8.55. Abruptly elevated eyelid varix in a 40-year-old male.

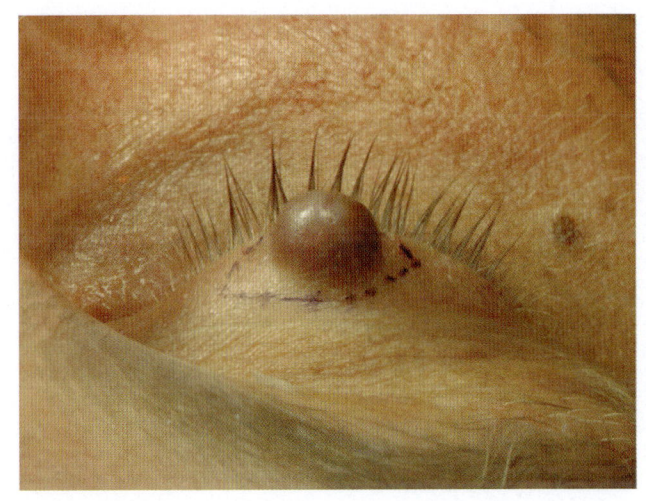

Figure 8.56. Birds-eye-view showing the vascular nodule of patient in Figure 8.55.

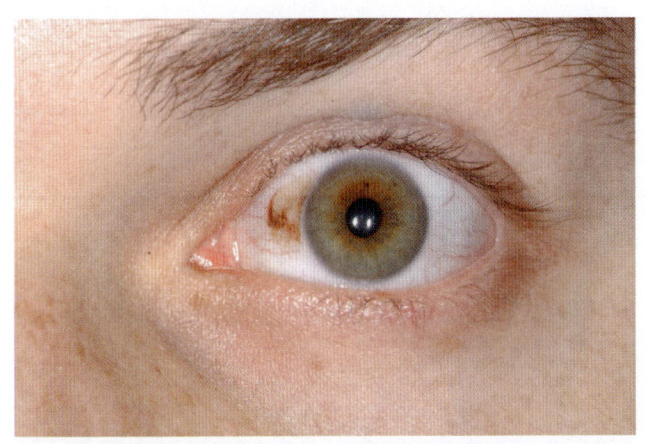

Figure 8.57. Small, subtle blue varix in center of eyelid crease of upper eyelid. There is an unrelated conjunctiva nevus.

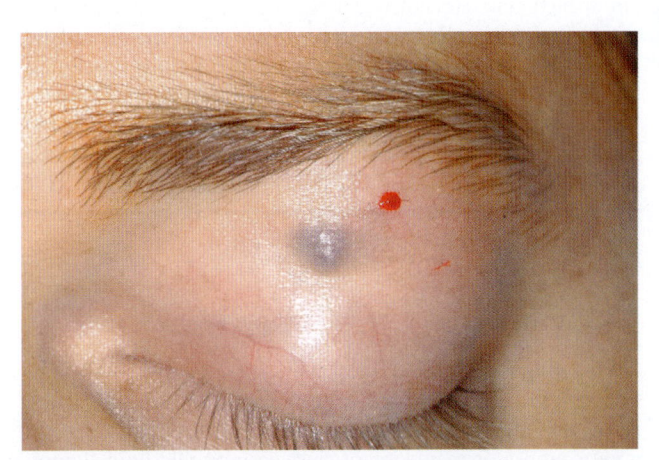

Figure 8.58. Appearance of lesion shown in Figure 8.57 at time of surgery after injection of local anesthetic.

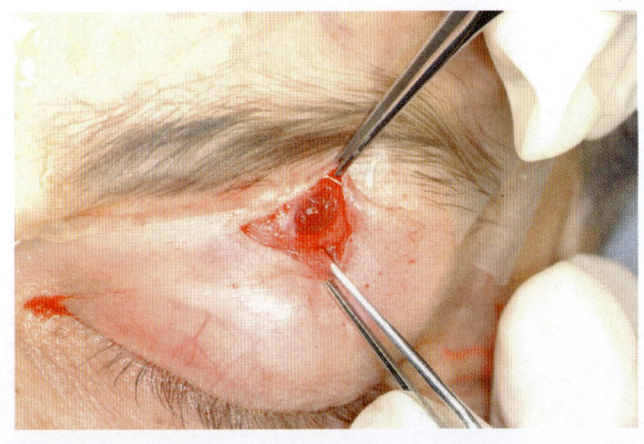

Figure 8.59. Appearance of same lesion exposed at surgery after eyelid incision.

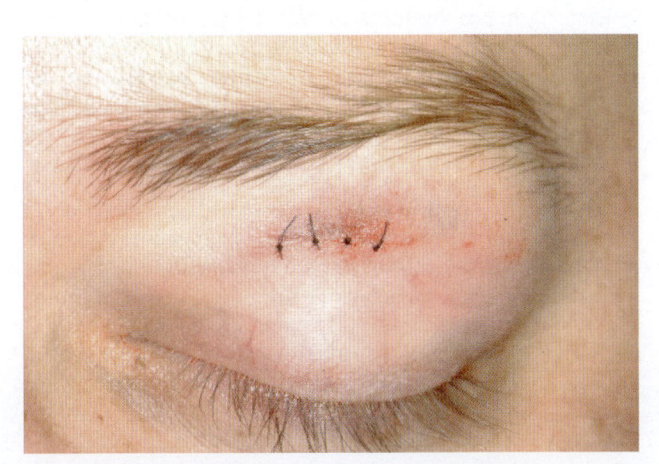

Figure 8.60. Closure of wound with sutures after excision.

EYELID LYMPHANGIOMA

General Considerations
Lymphangioma is a hamartomatous growth of lymph channels that can occur in various parts of the body, including the ocular region (1–17). More than 50% are evident at birth and 90% may become clinically apparent by the second year of life. The main sites of involvement are the head, neck, and axillae. This lesion can involve the conjunctiva and orbit, either individually or combined with eyelid lesions. The majority of eyelid lymphangiomas represent anterior extension of orbital lesions or eyelid extension of facial lesions and lymphangioma confined to the eyelid is exceptionally uncommon. In a series of 62 lymphangiomas of the ocular adnexae, 11 involved the eyelid and 8 of these were present at birth (4). Conjunctival and orbital lymphangiomas are discussed in those sections.

Clinical Features
In the eyelid, lymphangioma usually occurs deep to the epidermis as a dark blue, soft, fluctuant mass. It is generally present at birth and can slowly enlarge. In many instances, it may not become clinically apparent until late in the first or second decade of life, when bleeding into a preexisting subclinical lymphangioma prompts an ophthalmic evaluation. Spontaneous or posttraumatic bleeding into the lymph channels can produce blood-filled cavitary pseudocysts ("chocolate cysts") that can partially or completely resolve into a fibrotic scar. True regression, as seen with capillary hemangioma, does not occur with lymphangioma. On the eyelid, it may be clinically similar to a varix or varices.

Pathology
Histopathologically, most lymphangiomas that involve the eyelid are of the cavernous type. This tumor is composed of dilated vascular channels lined by thin endothelium. The lumen can appear empty or may contain clear eosinophilic fluid (lymph fluid). When hemorrhage has occurred within the spaces, the lesion can be confused histopathologically with a cavernous hemangioma. However, the endothelial cells of hemangioma generally stain positive for factor VIII-related antigen, whereas those of lymphangioma are usually negative with factor 8 but are positive for D2–40 antigen (10). Valves can sometimes be seen in the lymphatic channels as thin-walled protrusions into the lumen.

Management
Management of eyelid lymphangioma, like the more common orbital lymphangioma, is observation or resection for circumscribed tumors, surgical debulking for more diffuse, symptomatic tumors, and percutaneous drainage and ablation using sclerosing agents for extensive lesions (6–9). Management is discussed in more detail in the section on orbital tumors.

Selected References

Reviews
1. Wright JF, Sullivan TJ, Garner A, et al. Orbital venous anomalies. *Ophthalmology* 1997;104:905–913.
2. Rootman J, Hay E, Graeb D, et al. Orbital-adnexal lymphangiomas. A spectrum of hemodynamically isolated vascular hamartomas. *Ophthalmology* 1986;93:1558–1570.
3. Harris GJ, Sakol PJ, Bonavolonta G, et al. An analysis of thirty cases of orbital lymphangioma. Pathophysiologic considerations and management recommendations. *Ophthalmology* 1990;97:1583–1592.
4. Jones IS. Lymphangiomas of the ocular adnexa: an analysis of 62 cases. *Trans Am Ophthalmol Soc* 1959;57:602–665.

Imaging
5. Horgan N, Shields CL, Minzter R, et al. Ultrasound biomicroscopy of eyelid lymphangioma in a child. *J Pediatr Ophthalmol Strabismus* 2008;45(1):55–56.

Management
6. Wesley RE, Bond JB. Carbon dioxide laser in ophthalmic plastic and orbital surgery. *Ophthalmic Surg* 1985;16(10):631–633.
7. Wojno TH. Sotradecol (sodium tetradecyl sulfate) injection of orbital lymphangioma. *Ophthal Plast Reconstr Surg* 1999;15(6):432–437.
8. Yoon JS, Choi JB, Kim SJ, et al. Intralesional injection of OK-432 for vision-threatening orbital lymphangioma. *Graefes Arch Clin Exp Ophthalmol* 2007;245(7):1031–1035.
9. Hill RH, Shiels WE, Foster JA. Percutaneous drainage and ablation as first line therapy for macrocystic and microcystic orbital lymphatic malformations. *Ophthal Plast Reconstr Surg* 2012;28:119–125.

Histopathology
10. Fogt F, Zimmerman RL, Daly T, et al. Observation of lymphatic vessels in orbital fat of patients with inflammatory conditions: a form fruste of lymphangiogenesis? *Int J Mol Med* 2004;13:681–683.

Case Reports
11. Goble RR, Frangoulis MA. Lymphangioma circumscriptum of the eyelids and conjunctiva. *Br J Ophthalmol* 1990;74(9):574–575.
12. Williams CP, Marsh CS, Hodgkins PR. Persistent fetal vasculature associated with orbital lymphangioma. *J AAPOS* 2006;10(3):285–286.
13. Dryden RM, Wulc AE, Day D. Eyelid ecchymosis and proptosis in lymphangioma. *Am J Ophthalmol* 1985;100(3):486–487.
14. Pang P, Jakobiec FA, Iwamoto T, et al. Small lymphangiomas of the eyelids. *Ophthalmology* 1984;91(10):1278–1284.
15. Mortada A. Unilateral lymphangioma of orbit and lids associated with lymphangioma of palate and nose. *Bull Ophthalmol Soc Egypt* 1967;60(64):379–384.
16. Donders PC. Haemorrhagic lymphangiectasia of the conjunctiva. *Ophthalmologica* 1968;155(4):308–312.
17. Quezada AA, Shields CL, Wagner RS, et al. Lymphangioma of the conjunctiva and nasal cavity in a child presenting with diffuse subconjunctival hemorrhage and nosebleeds. *J Ped Ophthalmol Strabism* 2007;44:180–182.

EYELID LYMPHANGIOMA

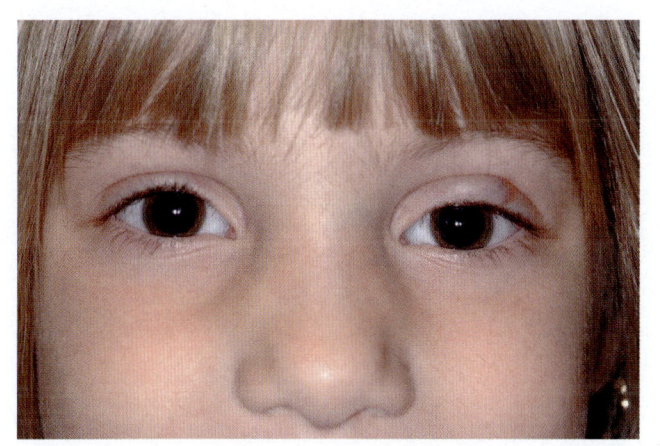

Figure 8.61. Localized lymphangioma in left upper eyelid in a young girl.

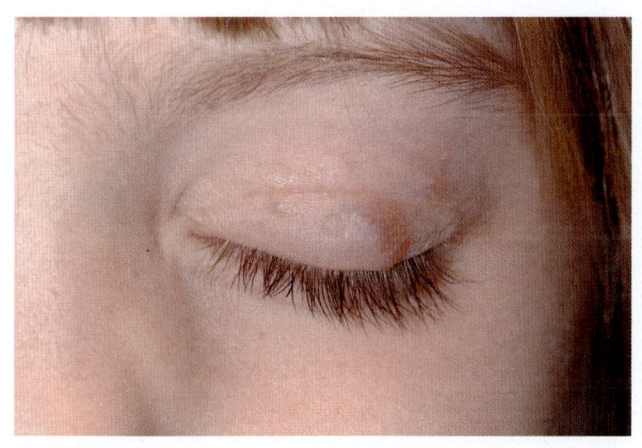

Figure 8.62. Patient shown in Figure 8.61 on down gaze, showing irregular surface of lesion.

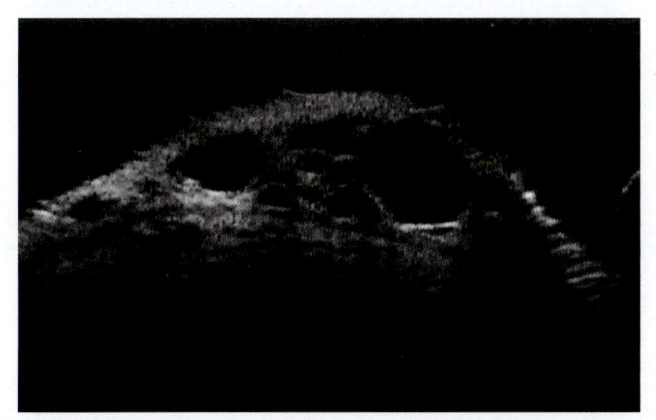

Figure 8.63. Ultrasound biomicroscopy of lesion shown in Figures 8.61 and 8.62. Note the multiple cysts in the subepithelial mass.

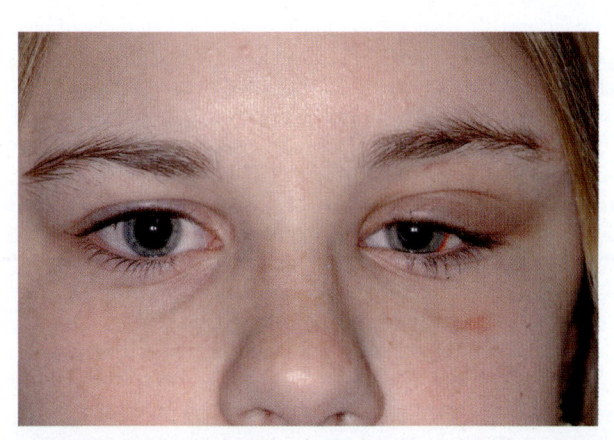

Figure 8.64. Diffuse lymphangioma of left upper eyelid. There is eyelid thickening with slight erythema and conjunctival hemorrhage near the limbus temporally, possibly related to subtle conjunctival involvement.

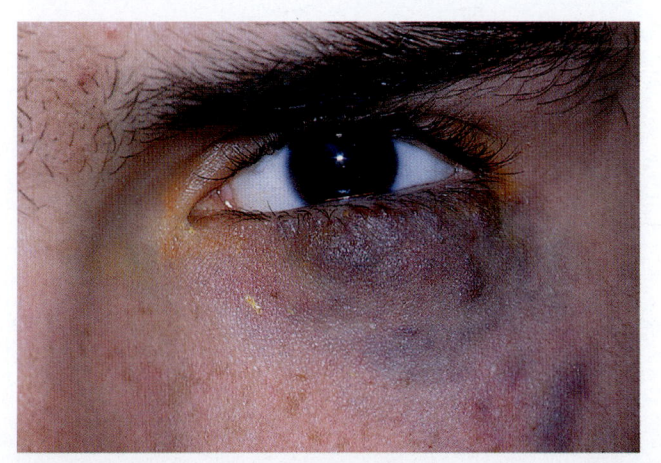

Figure 8.65. Diffuse lymphangioma involving lower eyelid in an 18-year-old man.

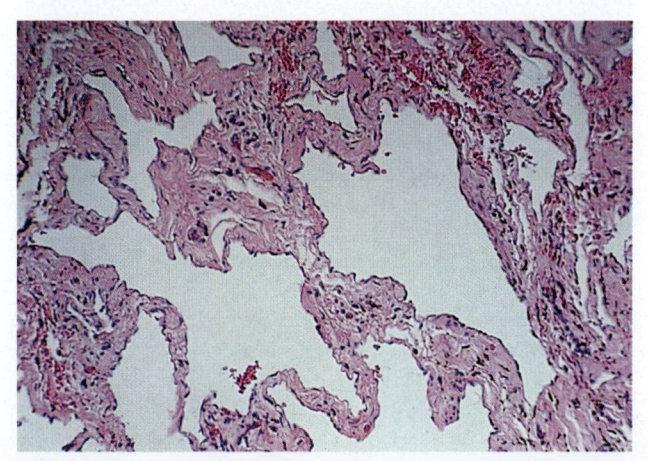

Figure 8.66. Histopathology of lymphangioma showing ectatic bloodless vascular channels. (Hematoxylin–eosin ×25.)

EYELID GLOMUS TUMOR

General Considerations

Glomus tumor (glomangioma) is a relatively common benign vascular lesion that arises from the glomus body, a specialized thermoregulatory structure. It usually develops in young adults between the third and fourth decades of life. The hand is the most frequently affected site, followed by the foot, forearm, ears, and tip of the nose. Subungual glomus tumors tend to be exquisitely tender. Occasionally, a glomus cell tumor can appear in areas where glomus cells are not ordinarily present, including the eyelid, conjunctiva, and facial skin (1–10). BRAF and KRAS mutations have been identified in sporadic glomus tumors (8).

Clinical Features

Glomus tumor in the eyelid and periocular area appears as a reddish-blue, subcutaneous mass that may be indistinguishable from other deep vascular lesions (1). In adulthood, it can be solitary, usually with no hereditary tendency. In a series of seven cases in the face, four involved the lower eyelid (2). Cases that affect the eyelid can extend to affect the orbit and palate (4).

In children, eyelid glomus tumor can occur as a solitary lesion or as multiple lesions with an autosomal-dominant mode of transmission. The term glomangiomatosis has been recommended to designate this multifocal variant. The lesion is sometimes associated with paroxysmal pain that can be elicited by changes in temperature.

Eyelid lesions may simulate lymphangioma, pyogenic granuloma, blue nevus, melanoma, leiomyoma, intravascular papillary endothelial hyperplasia, and angiosarcoma. The diagnosis is not usually made clinically and the nature of the lesion is established histopathologically after surgical removal.

Pathology

Glomus tumor is characterized by varying proportions of glomus cells, convoluted venous channels, and smooth muscle. It can resemble cavernous hemangioma, but the vascular channels are surrounded by a narrow rim of one to three layers of glomus cells (2). This tumor has been subclassified into solid glomus tumor, glomangioma, and glomangiomyoma depending on the histopathologic components. There are sheets of uniform cells with pale or eosinophilic cytoplasm, well-defined cell margins, and round or ovoid nuclei. Rarely, a glomus tumor can have atypical features suggesting malignancy (glomangiosarcoma). However, metastasis is uncommon (1). Multiple glomus tumors must be differentiated from the hemangiomas associated with the blue rubber bleb nevus syndrome. The presence of typical glomus cells in all glomus tumors helps to make that differentiation.

Immunohistochemistry of glomus tumor reveals that the endothelial cell markers (CD34, factor VIII, and *Ulex europaeus*) are consistently nonreactive. The glomus cells stain for antibodies against muscle-specific actin and vimentin, suggesting that the glomus cell is probably of mesenchymal origin and may represent a specialized vascular smooth muscle cell.

Management

Glomus tumor can be surgically excised or simply observed. In the eyelid, this tumor may be larger than suspected clinically (1).

Selected References

Reviews
1. Folpe AL, Fanburg-Smith JC, Miettinen M, et al. Atypical and malignant glomus tumors: analysis of 52 cases, with a proposal for the reclassification of glomus tumors. *Am J Surg Pathol* 2001;25:1–12.
2. Mounayer C, Wassef M, Enjolras O, et al. Facial "glomangiomas": large facial venous malformations with glomus cells. *J Am Acad Dermatol* 2001;45:239–245.

Case Reports
3. Jensen OA. Glomus tumor (glomangioma of the eyelid). *Arch Ophthalmol* 1965;74;511–513.
4. Charles NC. Multiple glomus tumors of the face and eyelid. *Arch Ophthalmol* 1976;94: 1283–1285.
5. Saxe SJ, Grossniklaus HE, Wojno TH, et al. Glomus cell tumor of the eyelid. *Ophthalmology* 1993;100:139–143.
6. Shields JA, Eagle RC Jr, Shields CL, et al. Orbital-conjunctival glomangiomas involving two ocular rectus muscles. *Am J Ophthalmol* 2006;142:511–513.
7. Lai T, James CL, Huilgol SC, et al. Glomus tumour of the eyelid. *Jpn J Ophthalmol* 2004;48(4):418–419.
8. Chakrapani A, Warrick A, Nelson D, et al. BRAF and KRAS mutations in sporadic glomus tumors. *Am J Dermatopathol* 2012;34(5):533–535.
9. Mortada A. Glomangioma of the eyelid. *Br J Ophthalmol* 1963;47:697–699.
10. Kirby DB. Neuromyoarterial glomus tumor in the eyelid. *Trans Am Ophthalmol Soc* 1940;38:80–87.

Chapter 8 Vascular Tumors of the Eyelids

● EYELID GLOMUS TUMOR

1. Saxe SJ, Grossniklaus HE, Wojno TH, et al. Glomus cell tumor of the eyelid. *Ophthalmology* 1993;100:139–143.
2. Charles NC. Multiple glomus tumors of the face and eyelid. *Arch Ophthalmol* 1976;94:1283–1285.

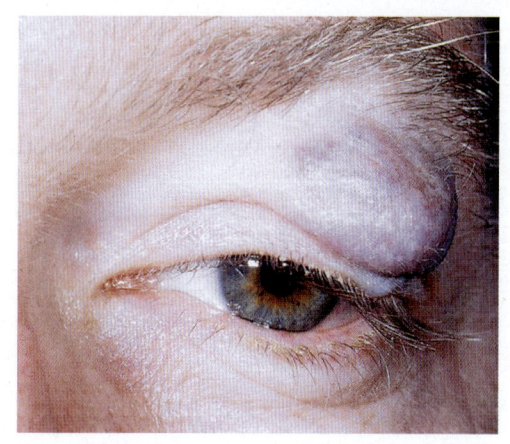

Figure 8.67. Glomus tumor of eyelid in a 39-year-old man. (Courtesy of Hans Grossniklaus, MD.)

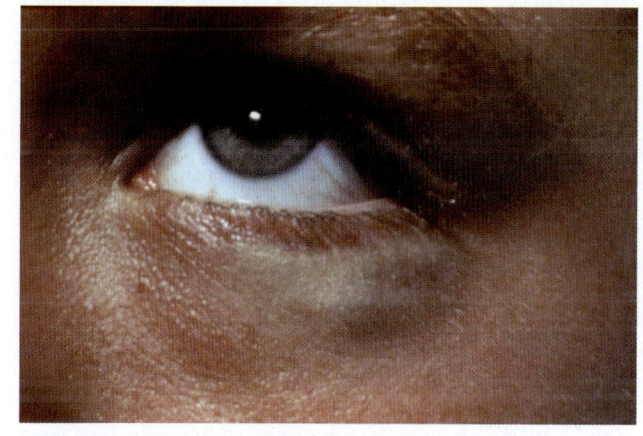

Figure 8.68. Subcutaneous blue glomus tumor of left lower eyelid. (Courtesy of Hans Grossniklaus, MD.)

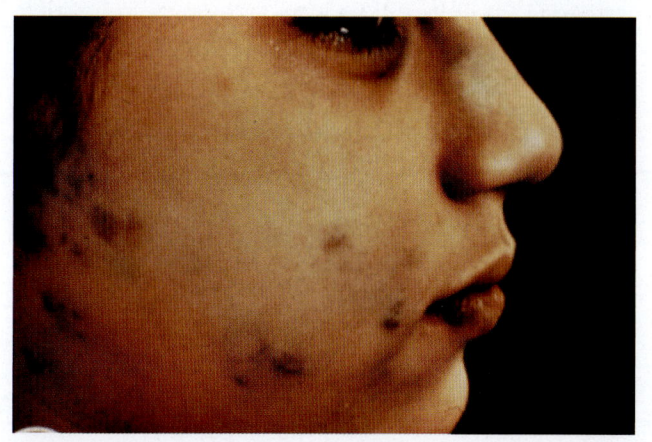

Figure 8.69. Multiple glomus tumors on right lower eyelid and side of face. (Courtesy of Norman Charles, MD.)

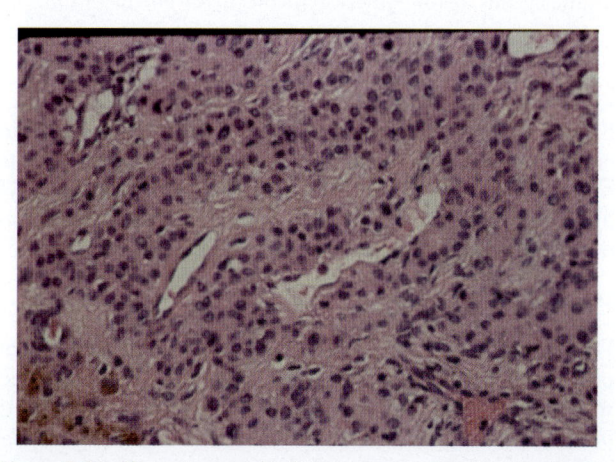

Figure 8.70. Photomicrograph of glomus tumor showing closely compact tumor cells and slitlike vascular spaces. (Hematoxylin–eosin ×50.)

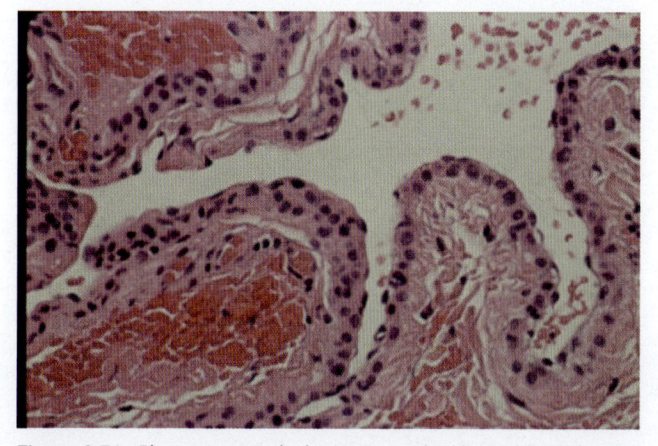

Figure 8.71. Photomicrograph showing vascular channel lined by glomus cells.

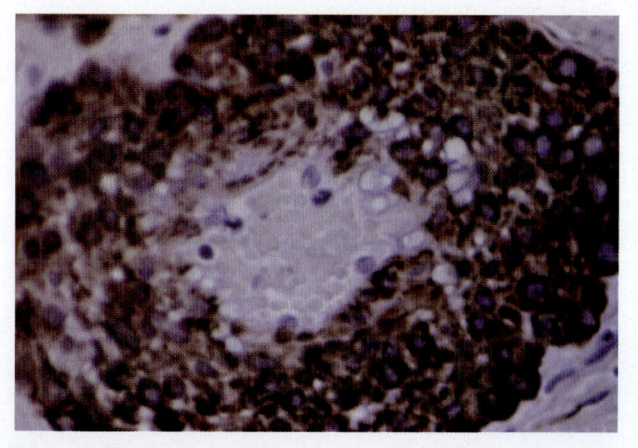

Figure 8.72. Immunohistochemistry showing positive reaction to smooth muscle-specific actin. (×75.)

EYELID KAPOSI'S SARCOMA

General Considerations

Kaposi's sarcoma is a malignant vascular tumor that was first reported by Kaposi in 1872 (1). He described five cases of an unusual neoplasm that occurred primarily in elderly patients. The multiple lesions generally began in the lower extremities and spread to other parts of the skin and eventually the viscera. The demographics and natural history of Kaposi's sarcoma have changed dramatically since recognition of the acquired immunodeficiency syndrome (AIDS).

With the advent of AIDS, Kaposi's sarcoma was observed to occur most often in younger, immunosuppressed adults and was recognized more often in the ocular region (2–15). Like lymphoma and opportunistic infections, this tumor is recognized more often in patients with iatrogenic immunosuppression, particularly after renal transplantation. With the recent decline in severe AIDS cases, it has become less common. Kaposi's sarcoma of the eyelid is generally associated with AIDS and is frequently seen in conjunction with multiple cutaneous tumors. Occasionally, however, it may develop only on the eyelids, before other cutaneous involvement (3,12).

Clinical Features

Eyelid Kaposi's sarcoma appears as a red, purple, brown, or blue flat subcutaneous lesion. It can be circumscribed, diffuse, nodular, or pedunculated. It initially has a smooth surface, but can become rough and crusty. The clinical differential diagnosis includes pyogenic granuloma, cavernous hemangioma, amelanotic melanoma, lymphoma, metastatic carcinoma, and chalazion.

Pathology

Histopathologically, Kaposi's sarcoma appears as a network of proliferating endothelial cells that form slitlike, blood-filled spaces. Positive immunohistochemistry staining for factor VIII in some cases suggests that Kaposi's sarcoma is a form of angiosarcoma.

Management

Management consists of chemotherapy if the lesions are extensive. Low-dose radiotherapy (15 to 20 Gy) in fractionated doses is effective for control of lesions confined to the eyelids or conjunctiva (3–8). Some authors have recommended a single dose of 800 cGy (4). Alpha interferon has also been employed (10,11). Current management of this tumor is focused on treatment of the underlying immune suppression with highly active antiretroviral therapy (HAART) for patients with AIDS or reducing the medical immune suppression in those with transplant-related tumors. Improvement of immune status will cause the Kaposi sarcoma to involute in most cases.

Selected References

Reviews
1. Kaposi M. Idiopatisches multiples Pigmentsarkom der Haut. *Arch Dermatol Syph* 1872;4:265.
2. Brun SC, Jakobiec FA. Kaposi's sarcoma of the ocular adnexa. *Int Ophthalmol Clin* 1997;37(4):25–38.

Management
3. Shields JA, De Potter P, Shields CL, et al. Kaposi's sarcoma of the eyelids: response to radiotherapy. *Arch Ophthalmol* 1992;110:1689.
4. Ghabrial R, Quivey JM, Dunn JP Jr, et al. Radiation therapy of acquired immunodeficiency syndrome-related Kaposi's sarcoma of the eyelids and conjunctiva. *Arch Ophthalmol* 1992;110:1423–1426.
5. Piedbois P, Frikha H, Martin L, et al. Radiotherapy in the management of epidemic Kaposi's sarcoma. *Int J Radiat Oncol Biol Phys* 1994;30:1207–1211.
6. Kirova YM, Belembaogo E, Frikha H, et al. Radiotherapy in the management of epidemic Kaposi's sarcoma: a retrospective study of 643 cases. *Radiother Oncol* 1998;46:19–22.
7. Le Bourgeois JP, Frikha H, Piedbois P, et al. Radiotherapy in the management of epidemic Kaposi's sarcoma of the oral cavity, the eyelid and the genitals. *Radiother Oncol* 1994;30(3):263–266.
8. Ghabrial R, Quivey JM, Dunn JP Jr, et al. Radiation therapy of acquired immunodeficiency syndrome-related Kaposi's sarcoma of the eyelids and conjunctiva. *Arch Ophthalmol* 1992;110(10):1423–1426.
9. Brunetti AE, Guarini A, Lorusso V, et al. Complete response to second line Paclitaxel every 2 weeks of eyelid Kaposi sarcoma: a case report. *Ophthal Plast Reconstr Surg* 2013;29(5):e114–e115.
10. Hummer J, Gass JD, Huang AJ. Conjunctival Kaposi's sarcoma treated with interferon alpha-2a. *Am J Ophthalmol* 1993;116(4):502–503.
11. Qureshi YA, Karp CL, Dubovy SR. Intralesional interferon alpha-2b therapy for adnexal Kaposi sarcoma. *Cornea* 2009;28(8):941–943.

Case Reports
12. Soll DB, Redovan EG. Kaposi's sarcoma of the eyelid as the initial manifestation of AIDS. *Ophthalmic Plast Reconstr Surg* 1989;5:49–51.
13. Shuler JD, Holland GN, Miles SA, et al. Kaposi sarcoma of the conjunctiva and eyelids associated with the acquired immunodeficiency syndrome. *Arch Ophthalmol* 1989;107:858–862.
14. Tunc M, Simmons ML, Char DH, et al. Non-Hodgkin lymphoma and Kaposi sarcoma in an eyelid of a patient with acquired immunodeficiency syndrome. Multiple viruses in pathogenesis. *Arch Ophthalmol* 1997;115(11):1464–1466.
15. Dammacco R, Lapenna L, Giancipoli G, et al. Solitary eyelid Kaposi sarcoma in an HIV-negative patient. *Cornea* 2006;25(4):490–492.

Chapter 8 Vascular Tumors of the Eyelids   155

EYELID KAPOSI'S SARCOMA IN A NONIMMUNOSUPPRESSED PATIENT

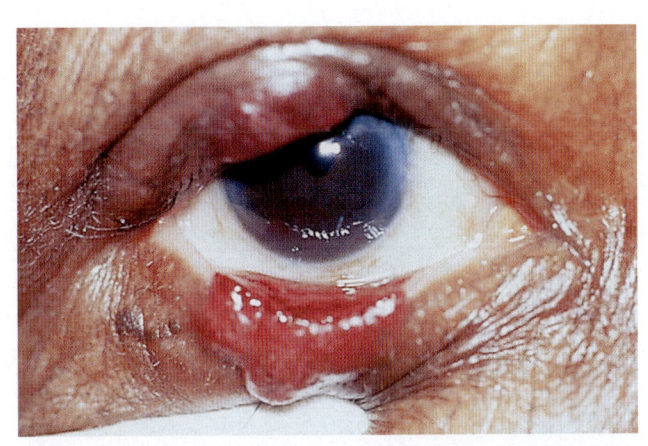

Figure 8.73. Lesions of upper and lower eyelid in a 92-year-old African-American patient. No treatment was given because patient was hospitalized with complications of intestinal Kaposi's sarcomas. (Courtesy of David Apple, MD.)

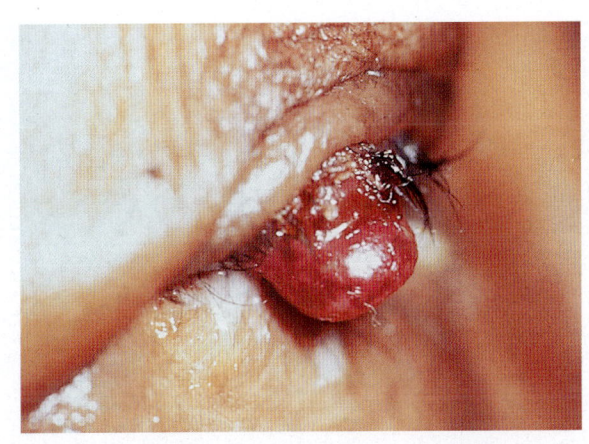

Figure 8.74. Patient seen in Figure 8.73 returned 6 months later with a larger, pedunculated lesion arising near upper eyelid margin.

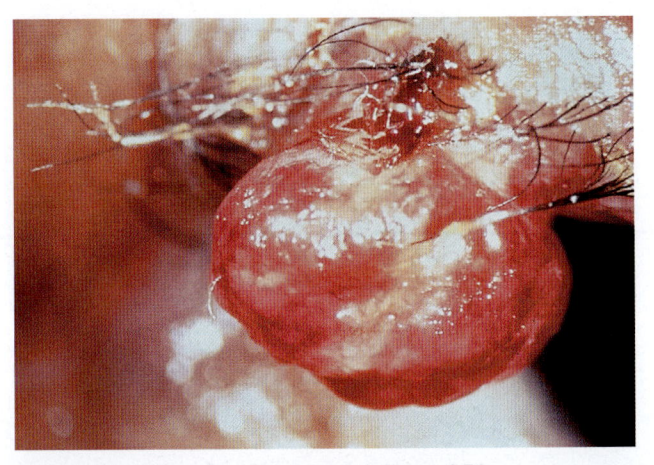

Figure 8.75. Closer view of lesion seen in Figure 8.74.

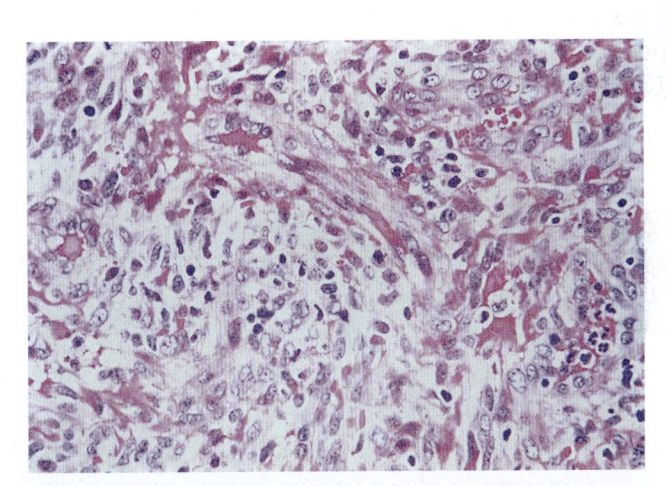

Figure 8.76. Histopathology of lesion shown in Figure 8.74, showing typical features of Kaposi's sarcoma. (Hematoxylin–eosin ×100.) (Courtesy of David Apple, MD.)

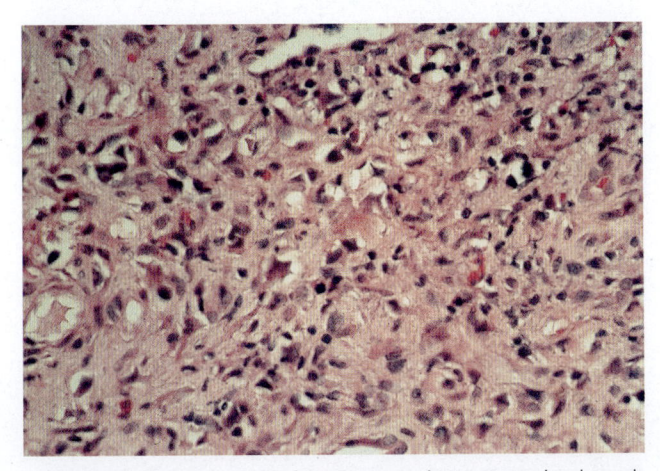

Figure 8.77. Histopathology of another case showing vascular channels and spindle-shaped cells. (Hematoxylin–eosin ×150.) (Courtesy of Anne Huntington, MD.)

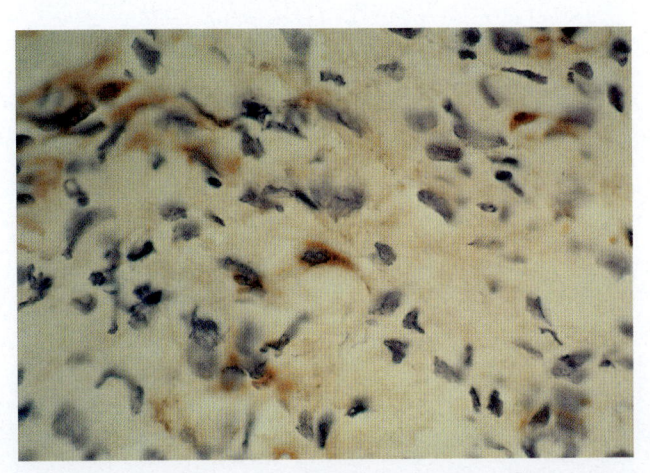

Figure 8.78. Positive immunoreactivity to factor VIII, confirming vascular origin of the lesion shown in Figure 8.77. (×150.) (Courtesy of Anne Huntington, MD.)

EYELID KAPOSI'S SARCOMA IN IMMUNOSUPPRESSED PATIENTS

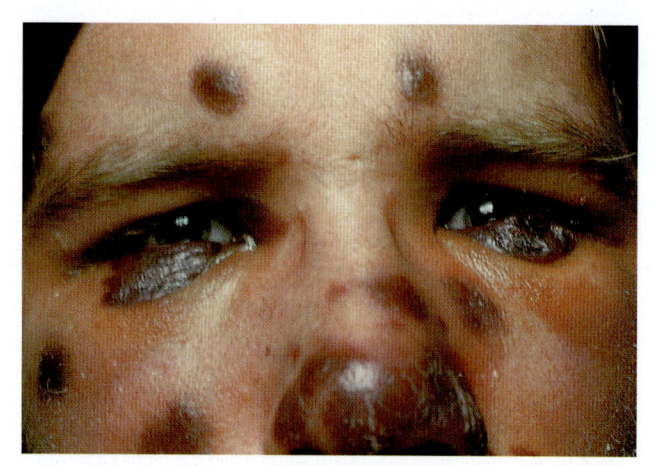

Figure 8.79. Patient with AIDS and multiple Kaposi's sarcomas on face and eyelids. (Courtesy of Wolfgang Lieb, MD.)

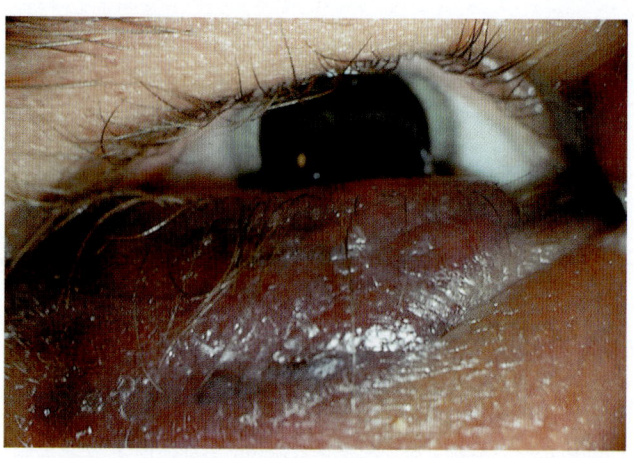

Figure 8.80. Close view of Kaposi's sarcoma of lower eyelid in patient shown in Figure 8.79. (Courtesy of Wolfgang Lieb, MD.)

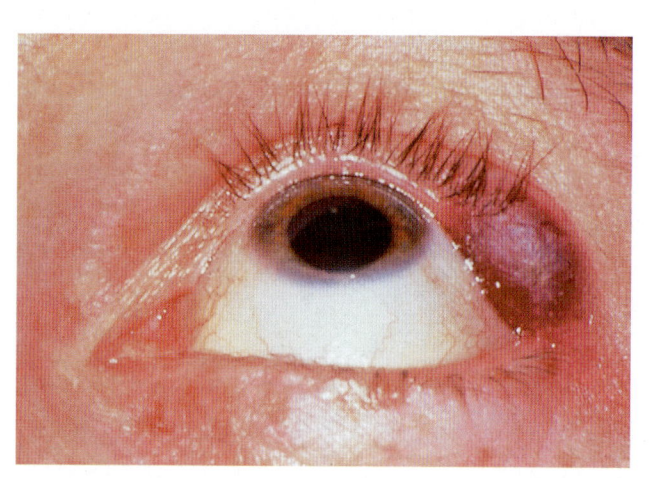

Figure 8.81. Localized Kaposi's sarcoma on upper eyelid margin of a 38-year-old man.

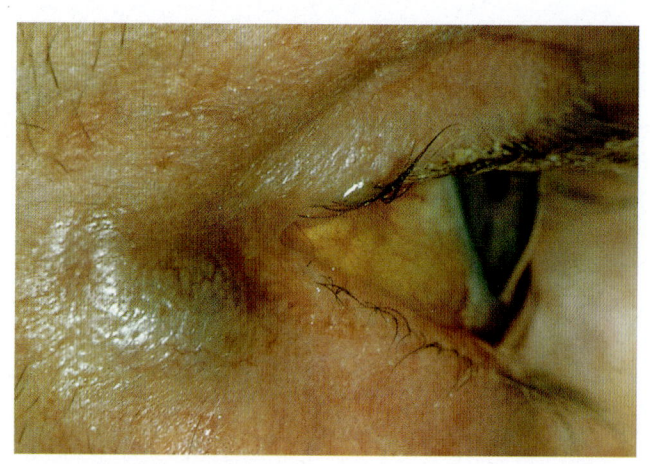

Figure 8.82. Localized Kaposi's sarcoma near lateral canthus. (Courtesy of Peter Savino, MD.)

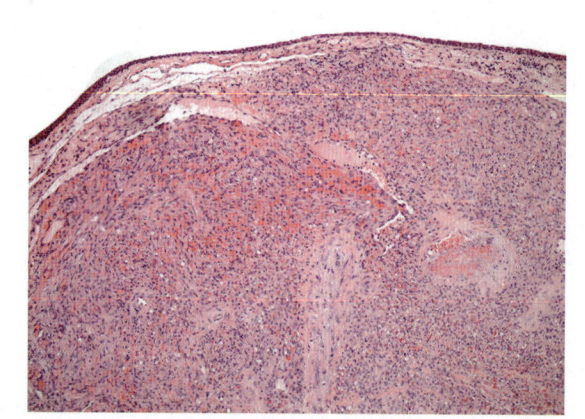

Figure 8.83. Histopathology of Kaposi's sarcoma demonstrating closely compact spindle and ovoid cells with slitlike spaces containing erythrocytes. (Hematoxylin–eosin ×75.)

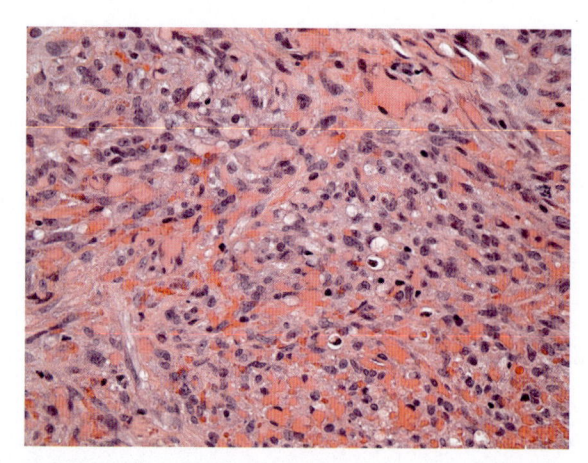

Figure 8.84. Higher magnification view of lesion shown in Figure 8.83. (Hematoxylin–eosin ×200.)

EYELID KAPOSI'S SARCOMA: TREATMENT WITH RADIOTHERAPY

Kaposi's sarcoma of the eyelid is sensitive to irradiation and chemotherapy. A patient treated with radiotherapy is illustrated.

Shields JA, De Potter P, Shields CL, et al. Kaposi's sarcoma of the eyelids: response to radiotherapy. *Arch Ophthalmol* 1992;110:1689.

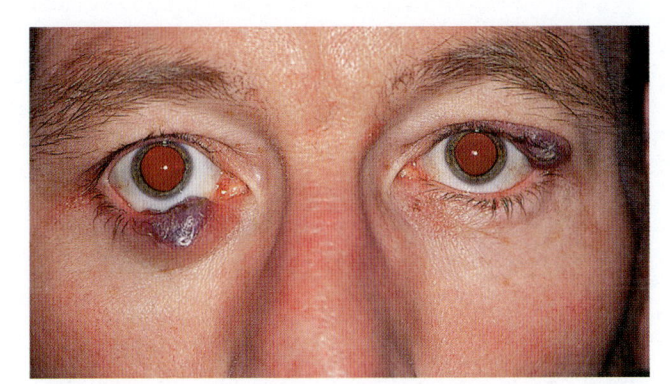

Figure 8.85. Facial view showing Kaposi's sarcoma of right lower eyelid and left upper eyelid.

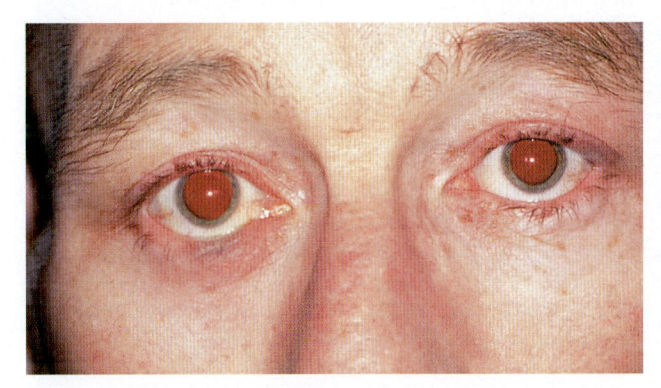

Figure 8.86. Same facial view after 2400 cGy of radiotherapy, showing complete resolution of both tumors.

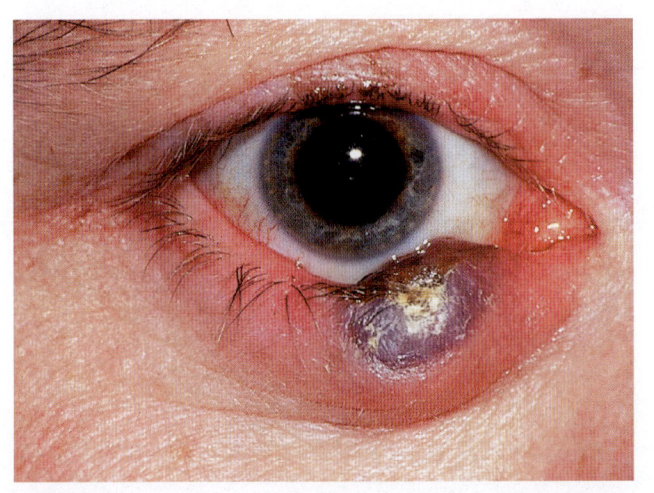

Figure 8.87. Kaposi's sarcoma of right lower eyelid in patient shown in Figure 8.85.

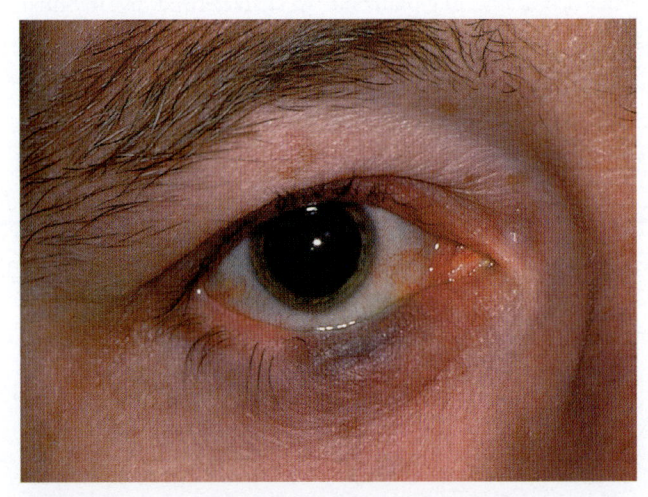

Figure 8.88. Lesion of right lower eyelid after radiotherapy.

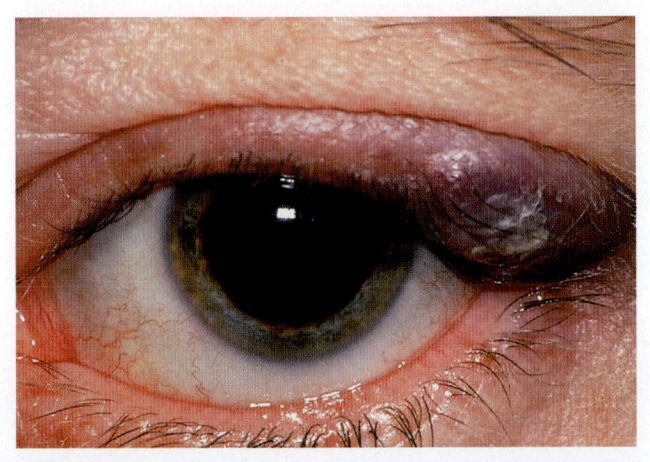

Figure 8.89. Kaposi's sarcoma of left upper eyelid in same patient shown in Figure 8.85.

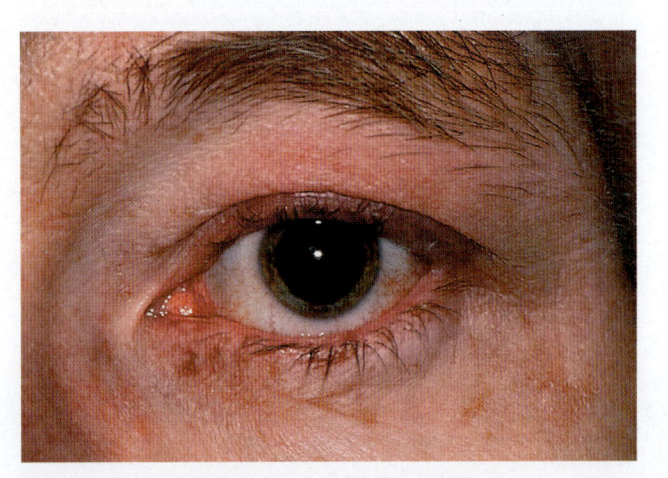

Figure 8.90. Lesion of left upper eyelid after radiotherapy.

EYELID ANGIOSARCOMA

General Considerations
Cutaneous angiosarcoma is a malignant vascular tumor that has a tendency to involve the scalp and face (1–9). Angiosarcoma can be solitary, but 50% of lesions are multifocal. It has a tendency to be more common in elderly men and generally has a poor prognosis.

Clinical Features
Eyelid angiosarcoma can be solitary or diffuse. The diffuse variant can sometimes develop from coalescence of multiple smaller lesions. The tumor typically is reddish-blue and subcutaneous. It may ulcerate and bleed spontaneously. Cutaneous angiosarcoma most often arises spontaneously, but it can develop from a prior benign vascular tumor, including nevus flammeus and an irradiated lymphangioma (1).

Pathology
Microscopically, angiosarcoma is characterized by irregular anastomosing vascular channels lined by atypical endothelial cells with hyperchromatic nuclei (1). Some tumors are very poorly differentiated and special stains and immunohistochemistry may help to elucidate the vascular nature of the lesion. There is some debate as to whether this neoplasm originates from vascular endothelial cells or lymphatic endothelial cells.

Management
The management of cutaneous angiosarcoma involving the eyelids is particularly difficult. Localized lesions may be excised, but more extensive ones may be unresectable and may require radical surgery and radiotherapy, which is generally not effective in achieving tumor control. The mortality rate is approximately 40%, with regional local recurrence and distant metastasis, often to lung and liver.

Selected References

Histopathology
1. Rosai J, Sumner HW, Kostianovsky M, et al. Angiosarcoma of the skin. A clinicopathologic and fine ultrastructural study. *Hum Pathol* 1976;7:83–109.

Management
2. Hiemstra CA, Mooy C, Paridaens D. Excisional surgery of periocular angiosarcoma. *Eye* 2004;18:738–739.

Case Reports
3. Girard C, Johnson WC, Graham JH. Cutaneous angiosarcoma. *Cancer* 1970;26:868–883.
4. Gunduz K, Shields JA, Shields CL, et al. Cutaneous angiosarcoma with eyelid involvement. *Am J Ophthalmol* 1998;125:870–871.
5. Conway RM, Hammer T, Viestenz A, et al. Cutaneous angiosarcoma of the eyelids. *Br J Ophthalmol* 2003;87:514–515.
6. Tay YK, Ong BH. Cutaneous angiosarcoma presenting as recurrent angio-oedema of the face. *Br J Dermatol* 2000;143:1346–1348.
7. Murphy BA, Dawood GS, Margo CE. Acquired capillary hemangioma of the eyelid in an adult. *Am J Ophthalmol* 1997;124:403–404.
8. Lapidus CS, Sutula FC, Stadecker MJ, et al. Angiosarcoma of the eyelid: yellow plaques causing ptosis. *J Am Acad Dermatol* 1996;34:308–310.
9. Bray LC, Sullivan TJ, Whitehead K. Angiosarcoma of the eyelid. *Aust N Z J Ophthalmol* 1995;23:69–72.

EYELID ANGIOSARCOMA: CLINICAL VARIATIONS

Gunduz K, Shields JA, Shields CL, et al. Cutaneous angiosarcoma with eyelid involvement. *Am J Ophthalmol* 1998;125:870–871.

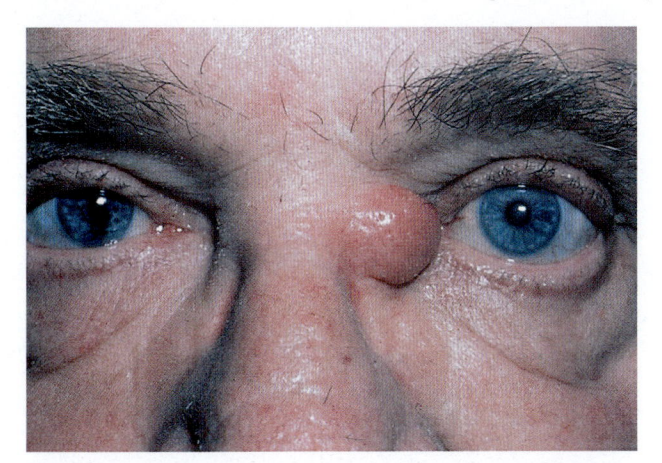

Figure 8.91. Localized nodular angiosarcoma near the medial canthus in a 76-year-old man. (Courtesy of Steven Searl, MD and Robert Kennedy, MD.)

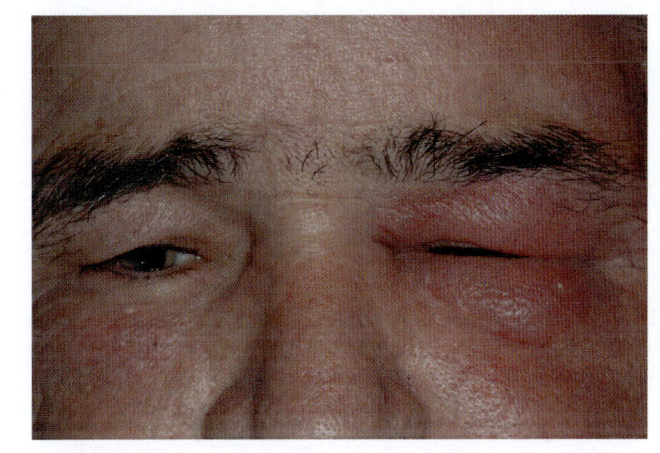

Figure 8.92. Diffuse angiosarcoma involving eyelids and cheek region, leading to mechanical blepharoptosis.

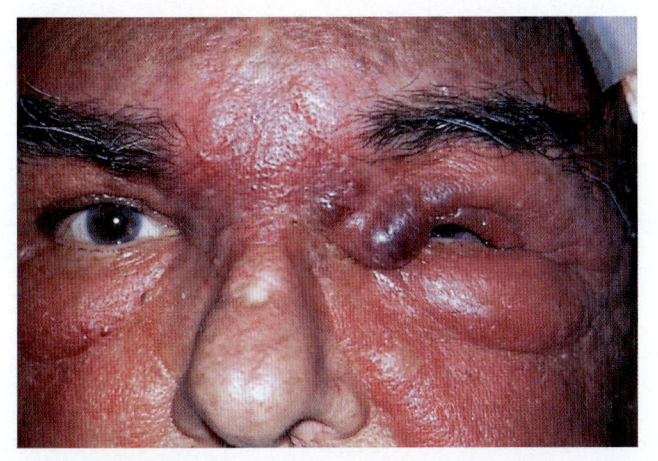

Figure 8.93. Diffuse angiosarcoma involving eyelids and imparting cutaneous erythema in an 83-year-old man.

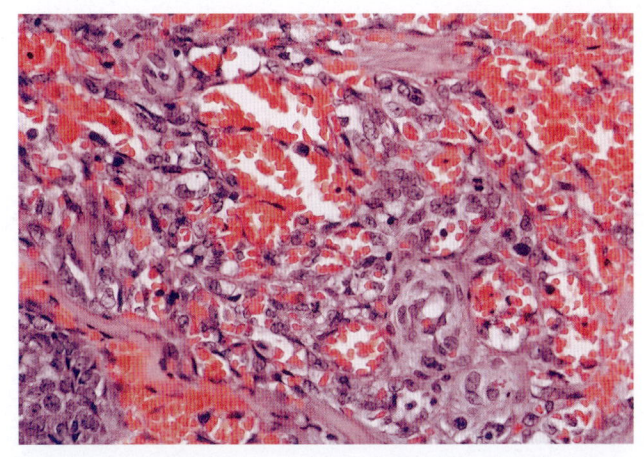

Figure 8.94. Histopathology of lesion shown in Figure 8.93 showing spindle-shaped tumor cells and abundant blood vessels. (Hematoxylin–eosin ×150.)

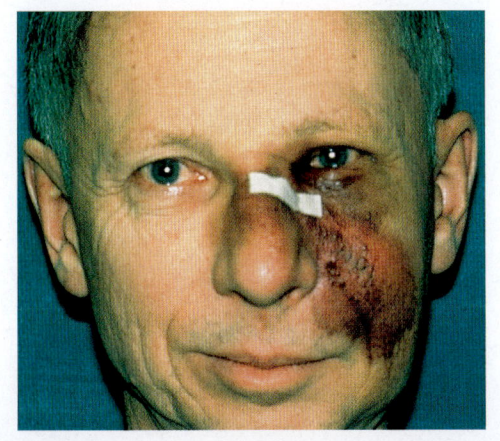

Figure 8.95. Large, diffuse angiosarcoma involving eyelids and lower half of face in a 60-year-old man. The lesion was managed by extensive surgical resection. (Courtesy of Elise Torczynski, MD.)

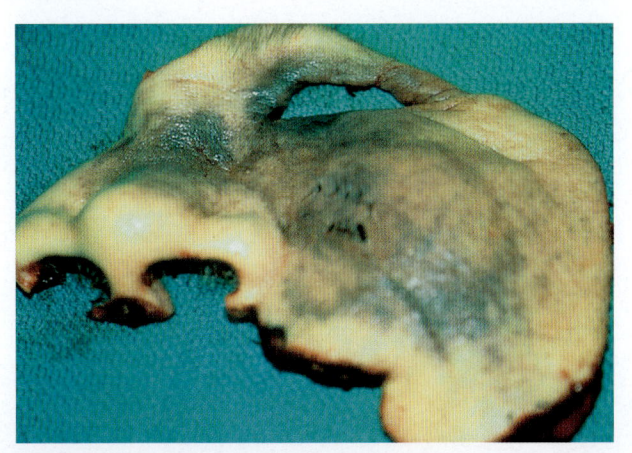

Figure 8.96. Gross appearance of resected specimen from patient seen in Figure 8.95. Note that it was necessary to remove the affected tissues of periocular skin and nose before extensive reconstruction. (Courtesy of Elise Torczynski, MD.)

CHAPTER 9

EYELID LYMPHOID, PLASMACYTIC, AND METASTATIC TUMORS

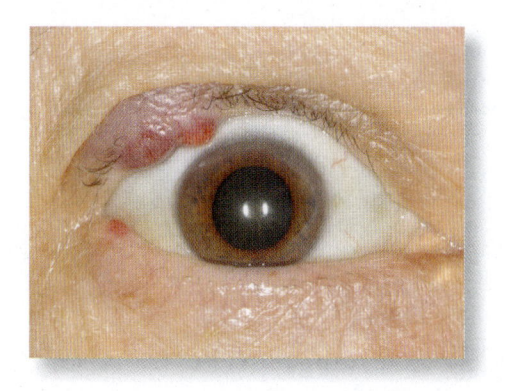

General Considerations

The eyelids, as well as most other ocular structures, can be involved with benign and malignant lymphoid tumors (1–22). There have been several classifications for extranodal lymphoid tumors in the ocular region. The Revised European American Lymphoma classification was the most popular in the past (4,5,11). Ophthalmic pathologists have traditionally classified lymphoid tumors into benign (lymphoid hyperplasia), intermediate, and malignant forms. Clinical differentiation of these forms is often not possible, and biopsy and histopathologic assessment are necessary to make a specific diagnosis. Lymphoma can also be divided into Hodgkin's and non-Hodgkin's types and B-cell or T-cell types (cutaneous lymphoma; mycosis fungoides) depending on the type of lymphocyte that comprises most of the lesion. Currently, the American Joint Committee on Cancer (AJCC) has provided a classification using the tumor, node, metastasis (TNM) system for ocular adnexal lymphoma to unify classification regarding these neoplasms.

Sézary syndrome is a variant of T-cell lymphoma that consists of a triad of erythroderma, leukemia, and large peripheral lymph nodes. It generally affects elderly men and is characterized by a more fulminating course. It often shows atypical mononuclear cells in the blood (Sézary cells). The skin lesions are identical clinically and histopathologically to typical mycosis fungoides and they can rarely involve the eyelids.

Eyelid lymphoid tumors tend to parallel those of the orbit in their degree of malignancy and their clinical behavior. Orbital lymphoid tumors are more common and are discussed in more detail in other chapters. Lymphoma can be confined to the eyelid, but is more often associated with systemic lymphoma. It is generally a disease of elderly patients, but it can occur in younger individuals, particularly those with AIDS or immune suppression. In contrast with conjunctival lymphoma, eyelid lymphoma tends to have a greater association with systemic lymphoma, particularly if it is bilateral (8).

Clinical Features

B-cell lymphoma of the eyelid generally occurs as a smooth, rather firm subcutaneous mass. Ulceration of eyelid B-cell lymphoma is rare (10). Although it may be confined to the eyelid, it is more often continuous with anterior orbital disease.

In contrast, the less common T-cell lymphoma has a tendency to affect the skin more superficially and to exhibit papules, plaques, or ulceration (mycosis fungoides). The lesions can be solitary or multiple. It can often masquerade as other conditions before the diagnosis is realized (12). A severe form of this condition, called adult T-cell leukemia/lymphoma, has recently been recognized to exhibit simultaneous involvement of the eyelid, orbit, and uveal tract (13).

EYELID LYMPHOMA

Pathology

Lymphoma of the eyelids is identical histopathologically to lymphoma in other parts of the body. It is composed of abnormal lymphocytes that range from low grade to intermediate to clearly malignant. Immunohistochemical techniques and flow cytometry are necessary to categorize the specific type of lymphoma (1–4,10). Most eyelid lymphomas are of B-cell lineage.

Management

When either B-cell or T-cell lymphoma are suspected in the eyelid, the affected patient should usually undergo a biopsy of the lesion and study of the cells with immunohistochemistry and flow cytometry to accurately categorize the lesion. It is important that the clinician communicate with the pathologist ahead of time to ensure that the tissue is handled properly. It is often wise to send the fresh material immediately to the pathologist rather than placing it in formaldehyde. If systemic evaluation reveals more widespread lymphoma, then chemotherapy is generally given to control the systemic disease and the eyelid lesion can be followed for regression. If the disease seems to be confined to the eyelid area, then radiotherapy can be considered. The dose of irradiation can vary from 2000 cGy for benign lymphoma to 4000 cGy for malignant lymphoma. The prognosis varies widely with the severity of the disease. A recent collaborative study on follicular subtype of orbital adnexal lymphoma has shown that external beam radiotherapy offered a more favorable prognosis.

EYELID LYMPHOMA

Selected References

Reviews

1. Coupland SE, Krause L, Delecluse HJ, et al. Lymphoproliferative lesions of the ocular adnexa. Analysis of 112 cases. *Ophthalmology* 1998;105:1430–1441.
2. Coupland SE, White VA, Rootman J, et al. A TNM-based clinical staging system of ocular adnexal lymphomas. *Arch Pathol Lab Med* 2009;133(8):1262–1267.
3. Rasmussen PK, Coupland SE, Finger PT, et al. Ocular adnexal follicular lymphoma: a multicenter international study. *JAMA Ophthalmol* 2014;132(7):851–858.
4. Jakobiec FA, Knowles DM. An overview of ocular adnexal lymphoid tumors. *Trans Am Ophthalmol Soc* 1989;87:420–444.
5. Sullivan TJ, Whitehead K, Williamson R, et al. Lymphoproliferative disease of the ocular adnexa: a clinical and pathologic study with statistical analysis of 69 patients. *Ophthal Plast Reconstr Surg* 2005;21:177–188.
6. Lauer SA. Ocular adnexal lymphoid tumors. *Curr Opin Ophthalmol* 2000;11:361–366.
7. McKelvie PA, McNab A, Francis IC, et al. Ocular adnexal lymphoproliferative disease: a series of 73 cases. *Clin Exp Ophthalmol* 2001;29:387–393.
8. Jenkins C, Rose GE, Bunce C, et al. Clinical features associated with survival of patients with lymphoma of the ocular adnexa. *Eye* 2003;17:809–820.
9. Plaza JA, Garrity JA, Dogan A, et al. Orbital inflammation with IgG4-positive plasma cells: manifestation of IgG4 systemic disease. *Arch Ophthalmol* 2011;129(4):421–428.

Histopathology

10. Sharara N, Holden JT, Wojno TH, et al. Ocular adnexal lymphoid proliferations: clinical, histologic, flow cytometric, and molecular analysis of forty-three cases. *Ophthalmology* 2003;110:1245–1254.
11. Go H, Kim JE, Kim YA, et al. Ocular adnexal IgG4-related disease: comparative analysis with mucosa-associated lymphoid tissue lymphoma and other chronic inflammatory conditions. *Histopathology* 2012;60(2):296–312.

Case Reports

12. Game JA, Davies R. Mycosis fungoides causing severe lower eyelid ulceration. *Clin Exp Ophthalmol* 2002;30:369–371.
13. Mori A, Deguchi HE, Mishima K, et al. A case of uveal, palpebral, and orbital invasions in adult T-Cell leukemia. *Jpn J Ophthalmol* 2003;47:599–602.
14. Huerva V, Canto LM, Marti M. Primary diffuse large B-cell lymphoma of the lower eyelid. *Ophthal Plast Reconstr Surg* 2003;19:160–161.
15. Ostler HB, Maibach HI, Hoke AW, et al. Hematological disorders. In: *Diseases of the Skin and the Eye*. Philadelphia, PA: Lippincott Williams & Wilkins, 2004:211.
16. Lugassy G, Rozenbaum D, Lifshitz L, et al. Primary lymphoplasmacytoma of the conjunctiva. *Eye* 1992;6:326–327.
17. Onesti MG, Mazzocchi M, De Leo A, et al. T-cell lymphoma presenting as a rapidly enlarging tumor on the lower eyelid. *Acta Chir Plast* 2005;47:65–66.
18. Ing E, Hsieh E, Macdonald D. Cutaneous T-cell lymphoma with bilateral full thickness eyelid ulceration. *Can J Ophthalmol* 2005;40:467–468.
19. Cloke A, Lim LT, Kumarasamy M, et al. Lymphomatoid papulosis of the eyelid. *Semin Ophthalmol* 2013;28(1):1–3.
20. Shunmugam M, Chan E, O'Brart D, et al. Cutaneous γδ T-cell lymphoma with bilateral ocular and adnexal involvement. *Arch Ophthalmol* 2011;129(10):1379–1381.
21. Raja MS, Gupta D, Ball RY, et al. Systemic T-cell lymphoma presenting as an acute nonresolving eyelid mass. *Ophthal Plast Reconstr Surg* 2010;26(3):212–214.
22. Koestinger A, McKelvie P, McNab A. Primary cutaneous anaplastic large-cell lymphoma of the eyelid. *Ophthal Plast Reconstr Surg* 2012;28(1):e19–e21.

EYELID INVOLVEMENT: B-CELL LYMPHOMA

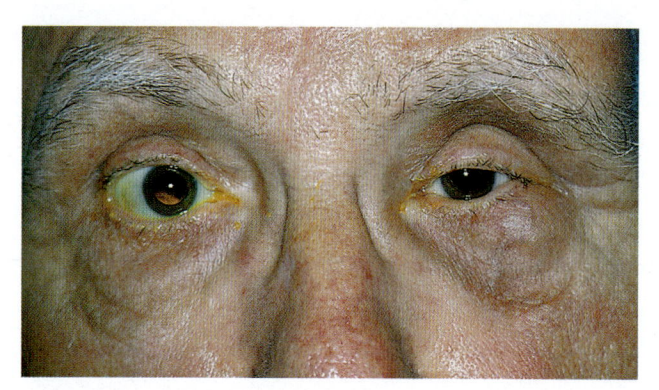

Figure 9.1. B-cell lymphoma involving the left lower eyelid in an 80-year-old man.

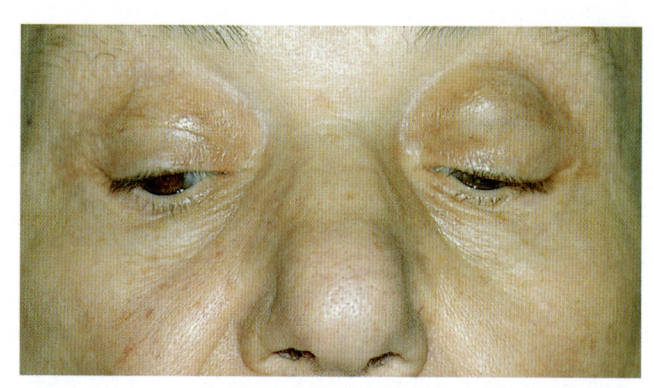

Figure 9.2. B-cell lymphoma involving the left upper eyelid in a 76-year-old man.

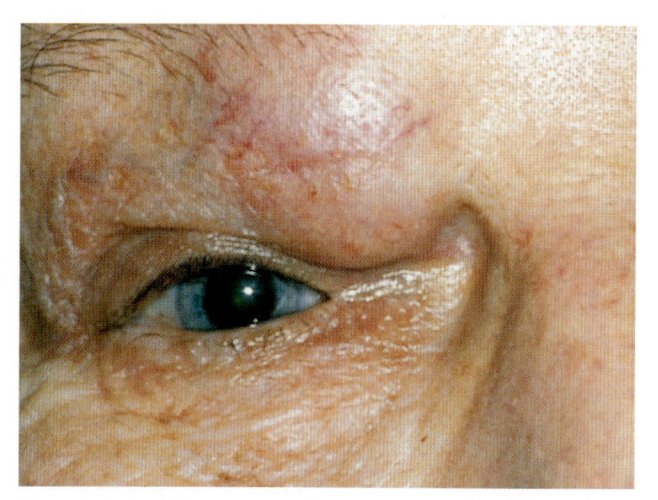

Figure 9.3. B-cell lymphoma of the medial aspect of right upper eyelid in a 71-year-old woman.

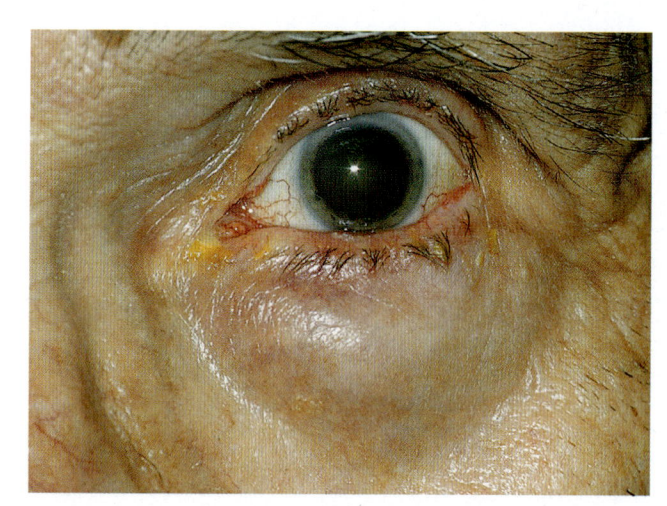

Figure 9.4. B-cell lymphoma of lower eyelid in an 83-year-old man.

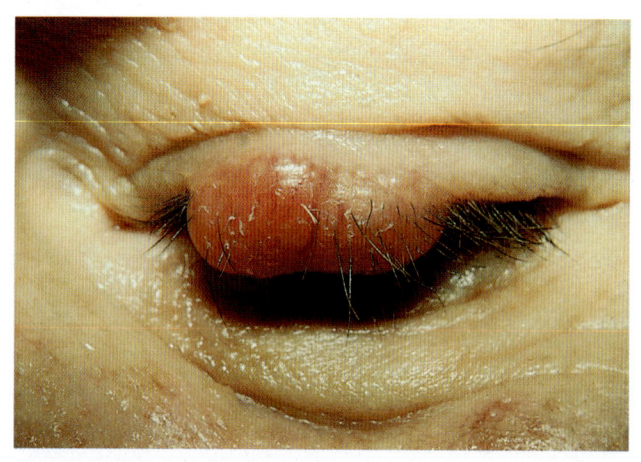

Figure 9.5. B-cell lymphoma of eyelid margin in 62-year-old man. (Courtesy of Zeynel Karcioglu, MD.)

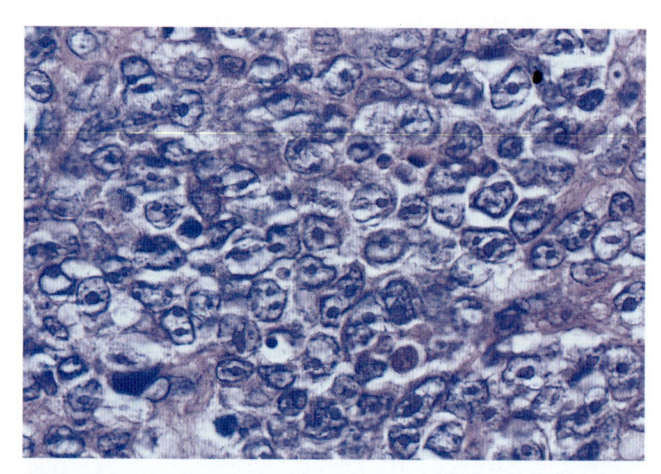

Figure 9.6. Histopathology of lesion shown in Figure 9.5. Note the large malignant lymphocytes. (Hematoxylin–eosin ×200.) (Courtesy of Zeynel Karcioglu, MD.)

Chapter 9 Eyelid Lymphoid, Plasmacytic, and Metastatic Tumors 165

● EYELID INVOLVEMENT: B-CELL LYMPHOMA

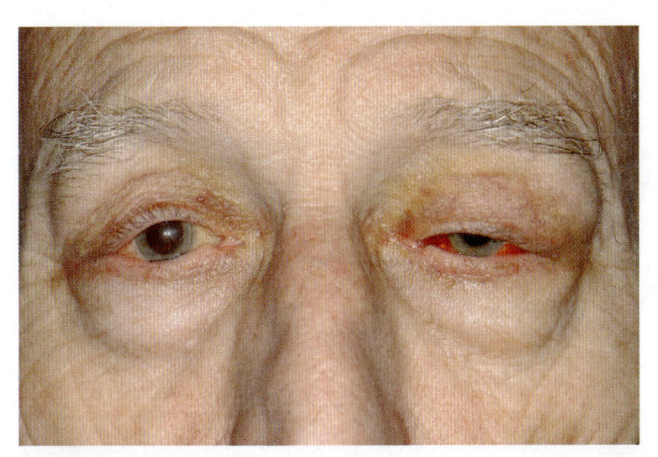

Figure 9.7. Blepharoptosis of left upper eyelid owing to deep eyelid involvement by lymphoma. The hemorrhage was due to prior biopsy to confirm the diagnosis.

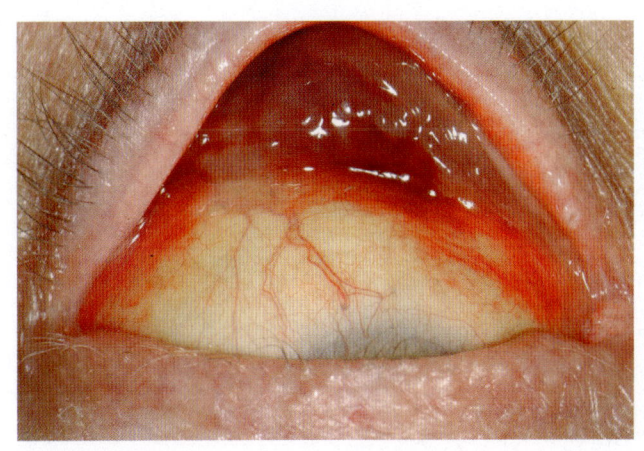

Figure 9.8. Elevation of eyelid in patient shown in Figure 9.7 reveals infiltration of palpebral conjunctiva by the neoplasm.

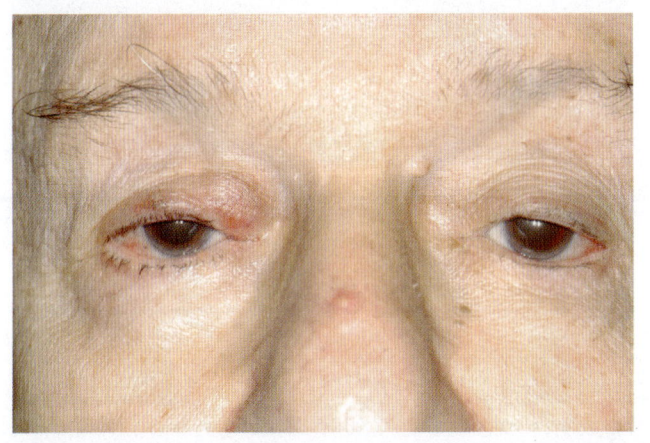

Figure 9.9. Subtle superonasal thickening over right eye from subcutaneous eyelid lymphoma.

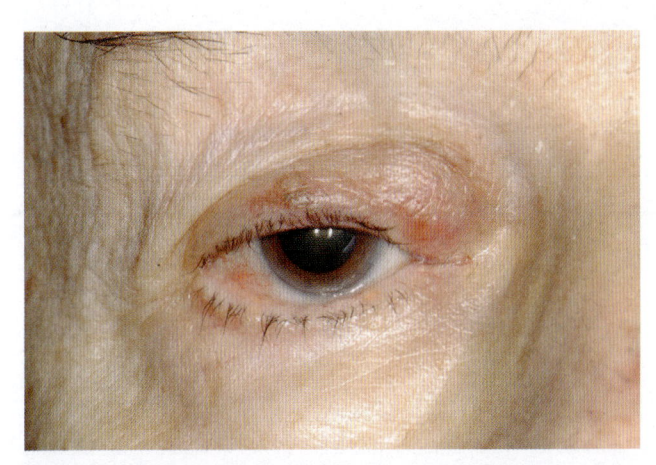

Figure 9.10. Close-up view of lesion shown in Figure 9.9.

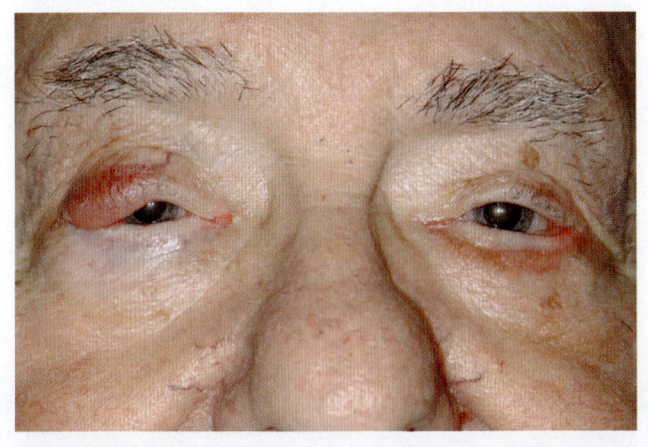

Figure 9.11. More superficial eyelid lymphoma above right eye with surface vascularity.

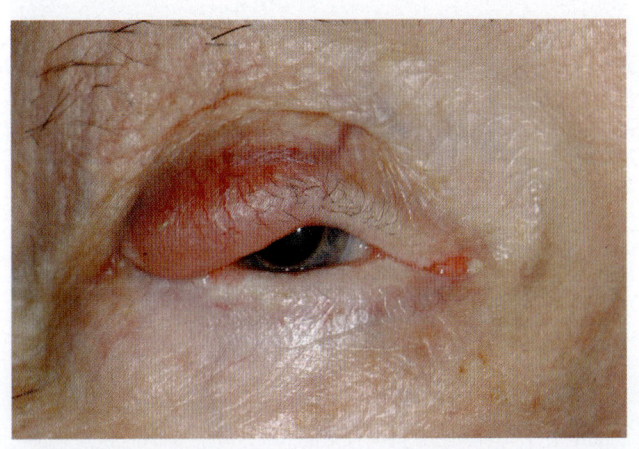

Figure 9.12. Close-up view of lesion shown in Figure 9.11.

EYELID INVOLVEMENT BY LYMPHOMA: ADVANCED CASES

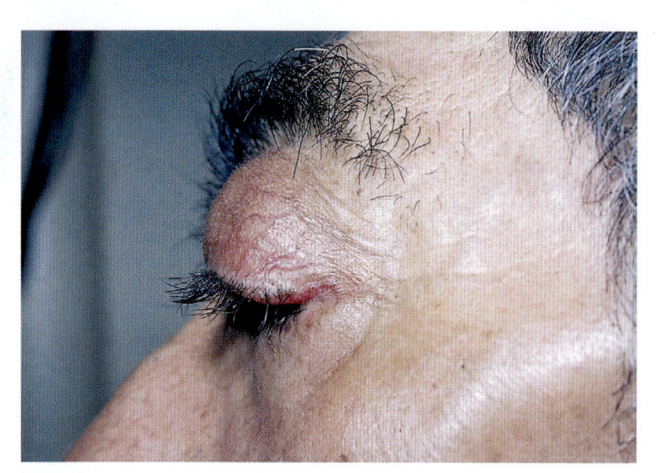

Figure 9.13. Side view of B-cell lymphoma of upper eyelid in a 60-year-old man.

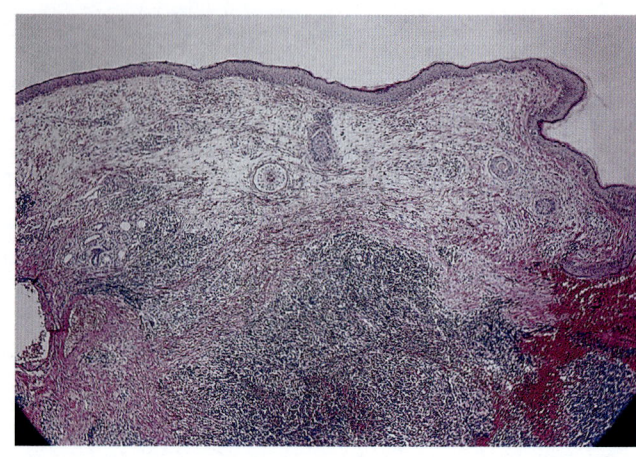

Figure 9.14. Histopathology of lesion shown in Figure 9.13, showing tumor cells in dermis. (Hematoxylin–eosin ×15.)

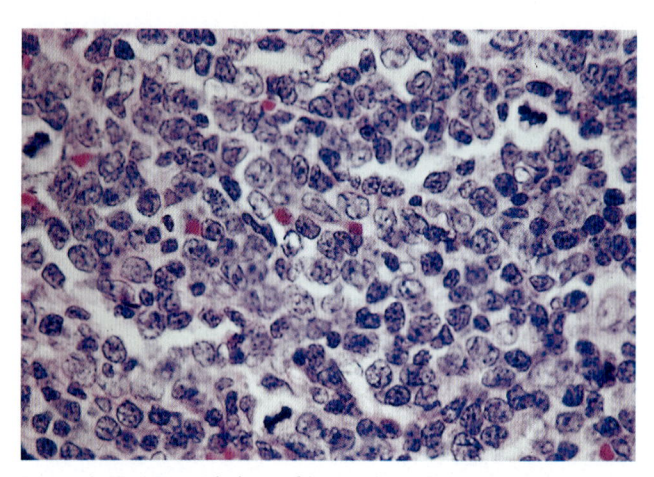

Figure 9.15. Histopathology of lesion shown in Figure 9.13, showing poorly differentiated lymphocytes. (Hematoxylin–eosin ×250.)

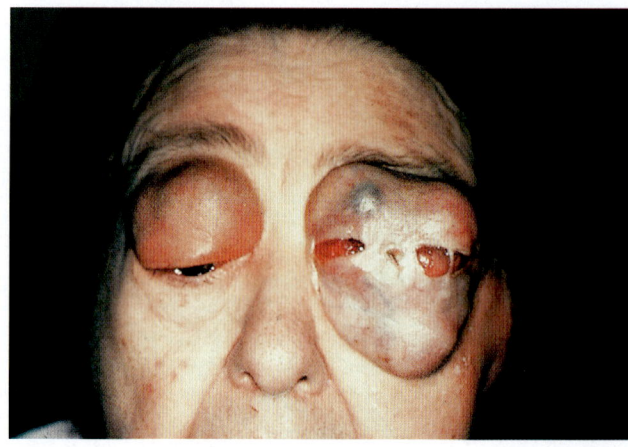

Figure 9.16. Massive bilateral B-cell lymphoma of the eyelids in a patient who also had thyroid ophthalmopathy. (Courtesy of Andrew Ferry, MD.)

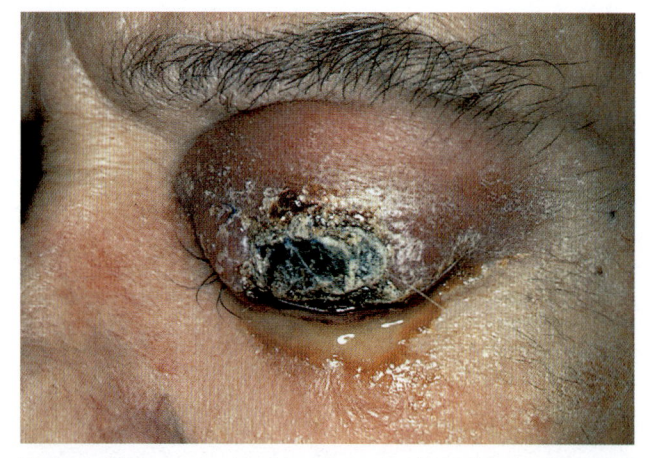

Figure 9.17. Cutaneous T-cell lymphoma involving skin of upper eyelid. Note the ulcerated, crusty appearance of the lesion. (Courtesy of Guy Allaire, MD.)

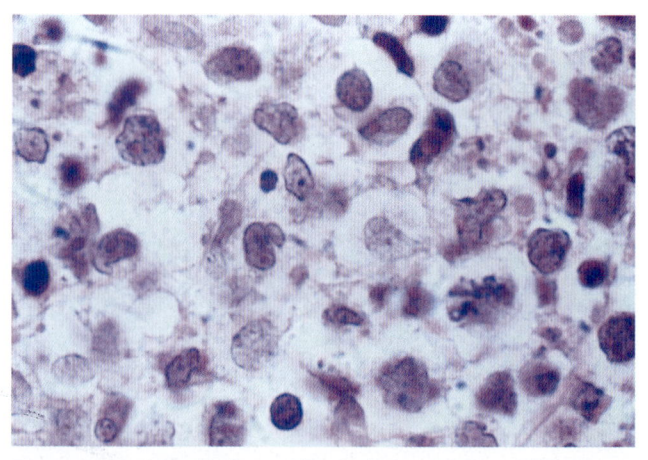

Figure 9.18. Histopathology of lesion shown in Figure 9.17, showing malignant T lymphocytes. (Hematoxylin–eosin ×250.) (Courtesy of Guy Allaire, MD.)

Chapter 9 Eyelid Lymphoid, Plasmacytic, and Metastatic Tumors

● EYELID INVOLVEMENT: T-CELL LYMPHOMA

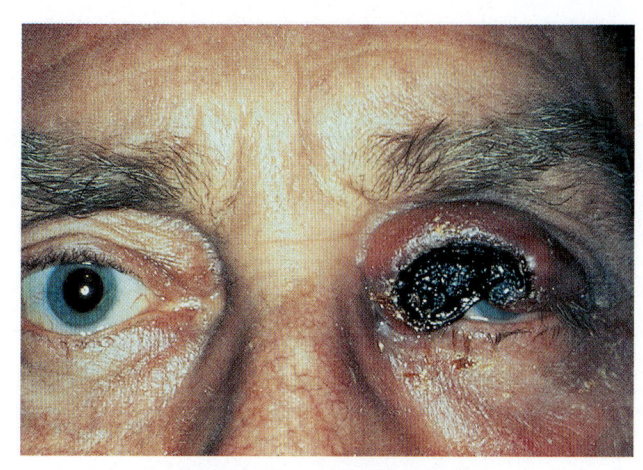

Figure 9.19. Cutaneous T-cell lymphoma involving the skin of upper eyelid in a 59-year-old man. (Courtesy of Seymour Brownstein, MD.)

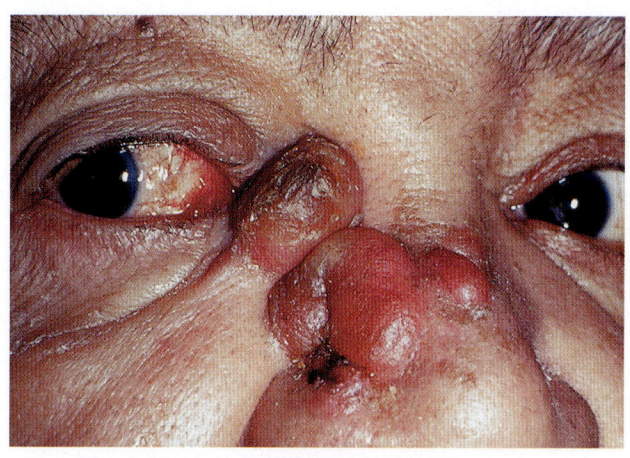

Figure 9.20. Cutaneous T-cell lymphoma involving medial canthus and side of nose. (Courtesy of Bradley Schwartz, MD.)

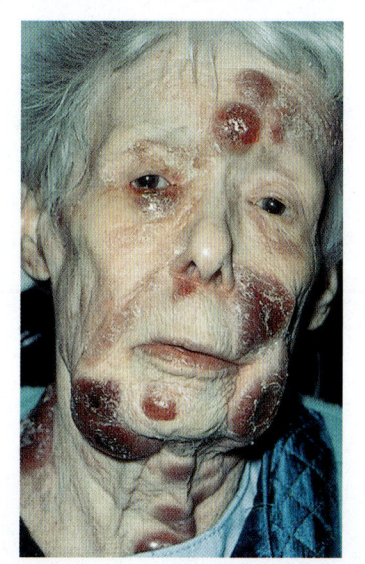

Figure 9.21. Cutaneous T-cell lymphoma affecting right lower eyelid with multiple lesions on face. (Courtesy of Geoffrey Heathcote, MD.)

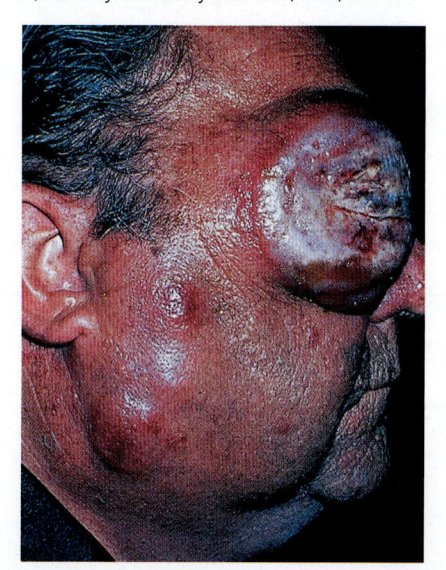

Figure 9.22. Massive cutaneous T-cell lymphoma involving both eyelids and orbit, with subcutaneous lymph node involvement. (Courtesy of Alan Proia, MD.)

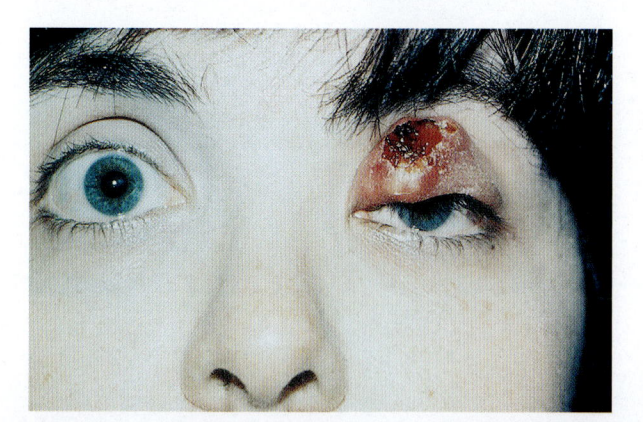

Figure 9.23. Cutaneous T-cell lymphoma in a 33-year-old woman. The patient had no evidence of systemic lymphoma. She declined radiotherapy and was treated with systemic chemotherapy. (Courtesy of Richard O'Grady, MD.)

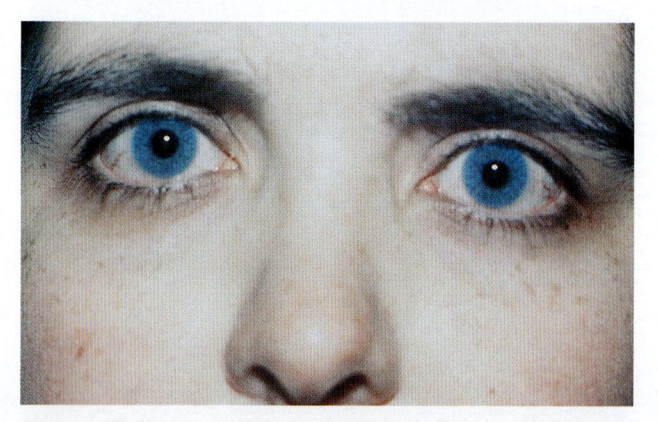

Figure 9.24. Same patient shown in Figure 9.23, 4 years after chemotherapy. There was no recurrence and no evidence of systemic lymphoma at that time. (Courtesy of Richard O'Grady, MD.)

EYELID PLASMACYTOMA

General Considerations

Plasmacytoma is a localized collection of monoclonal plasma cells (1–10). It can occur as a solitary lesion or as a component of multiple myeloma. Solitary extramedullary plasmacytoma is a primary lesion that tends to be locally invasive, but does not often metastasize. Secondary plasmacytoma, on the other hand, is a manifestation of multiple myeloma, which is a malignant systemic plasma cell neoplasm, affecting primarily bones. Multiple myeloma is a more aggressive neoplasm and tends to exhibit systemic metastasis. Both the primary plasmacytoma and multiple myeloma can rarely occur in the choroid, orbit, or eyelid (1–10).

Clinical Features

Plasmacytoma of the eyelid appears as a smooth, circumscribed, violaceous mass involving the dermis and sometimes the epidermis. It may be indistinguishable clinically from lymphoma or other subcutaneous tumors.

Pathology

Cutaneous plasmacytoma is a densely cellular nodule composed of a monomorphous infiltrate or plasma cells that can range from benign to malignant. Its variations are discussed in the literature (3).

Management

Management is excisional biopsy when the lesion is localized and amenable to resection. The tumor is sensitive to irradiation and chemotherapy and these modalities are used for unresectable lesions or those associated with multiple myeloma. Patients with multiple myeloma have a less favorable prognosis.

Selected References

Reviews
1. Adkins JW, Shields JA, Shields CL, et al. Plasmacytoma of the eye and orbit. *Int Ophthalmol* 1997;20:339–343.
2. de Smet MD, Rootman J. Orbital manifestations of plasmacytic lymphoproliferations. *Ophthalmology* 1987;94:995–1003.
3. LeBoit PE, McCalmont TH. Cutaneous lymphomas and leukemias. In: Elder D, Elenitsas R, Jaworsky C, et al., eds. *Lever's Histopathology of the Skin*. Philadelphia, PA: Lippincott-Raven, 1997:814–816.

Case Reports
4. Rodman HJ, Font RL. Orbital involvement in multiple myeloma. *Arch Ophthalmol* 1972;87:30–35.
5. Kremer I, Flex D, Manor R. Solitary conjunctival extramedullary plasmacytoma. *Ann Ophthalmol* 1990;22:126–130.
6. Lugassy G, Rozenbaum D, Lifshitz L, et al. Primary lymphoplasmacytoma of the conjunctiva. *Eye* 1992;6:326–327.
7. Olivieri L, Ianni MD, Giansanti M, et al. Primary eyelid plasmacytoma. *Med Oncol* 2000;17:74–75.
8. Ahamed E, Samuel LM, Tighe JE. Extramedullary plasmacytoma of the eyelid. *Br J Ophthalmol* 2003;87:244–245.
9. Honavar SG, Shields CL, Shields JA, et al. Extramedullary plasmacytoma confined to the choroid. *Am J Ophthalmol* 2001;131:277–278.
10. Morgan AE, Shields CL, Shields JA, et al. Presumed malignant plasmacytoma of the choroid as the first manifestation of multiple myeloma. *Retina* 2003;23:867–868.

Chapter 9 Eyelid Lymphoid, Plasmacytic, and Metastatic Tumors

EYELID PLASMACYTOMA

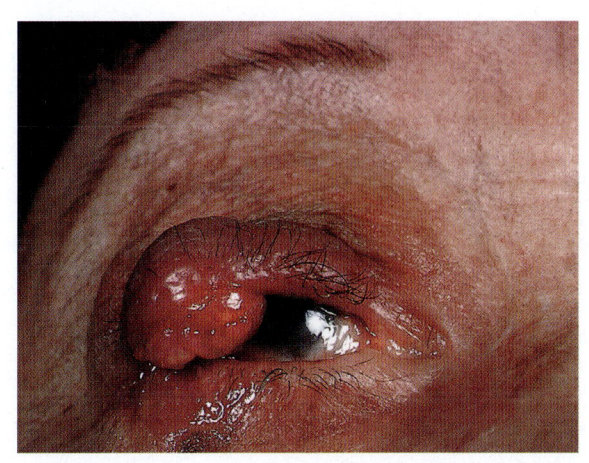

Figure 9.25. Solitary benign plasmacytoma of the upper eyelid in a 60-year-old woman. (Courtesy of Norman Charles, MD.)

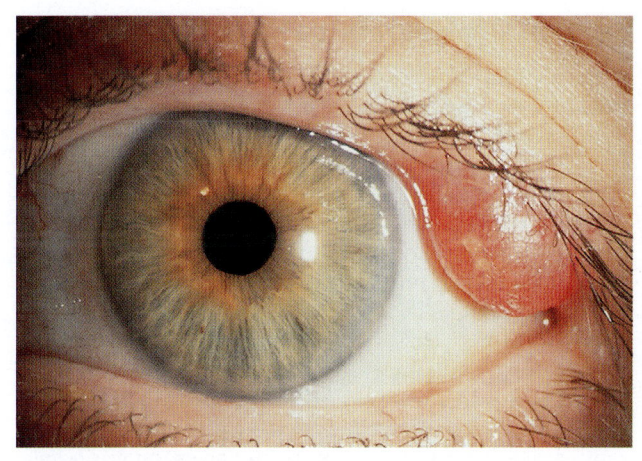

Figure 9.26. Eyelid plasmacytoma as the presenting sign of multiple myeloma in a 49-year-old woman. The lesion was originally suspected to be a chalazion. (Courtesy of Henry Perry, MD.)

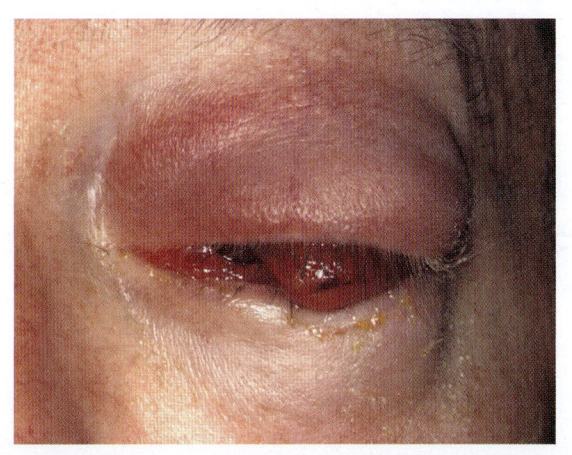

Figure 9.27. Diffuse eyelid and conjunctival involvement by plasmacytoma in a 52-year-old man with multiple myeloma. The lesion extended into the anterior aspect of the orbit.

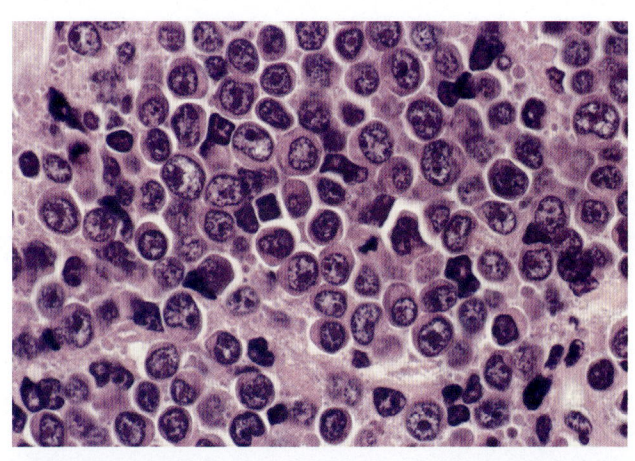

Figure 9.28. Histopathology of lesion shown in Figure 9.27 demonstrating malignant plasma cells in the dermis. (Hematoxylin–eosin ×250.)

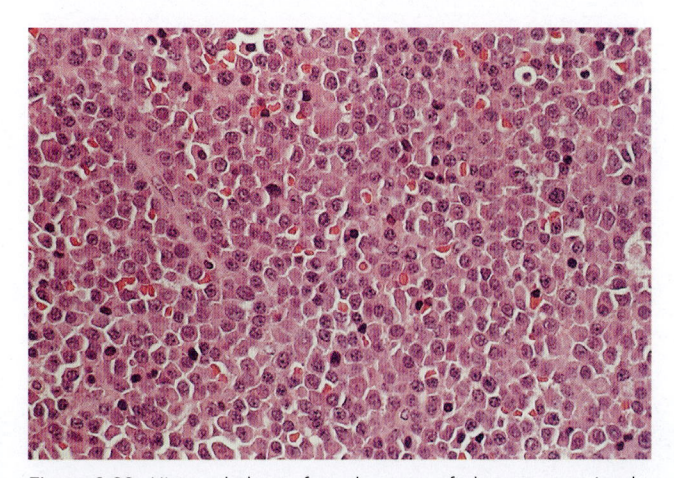

Figure 9.29. Histopathology of another case of plasmacytoma involving orbit and eyelid area. (Hematoxylin–eosin ×100.)

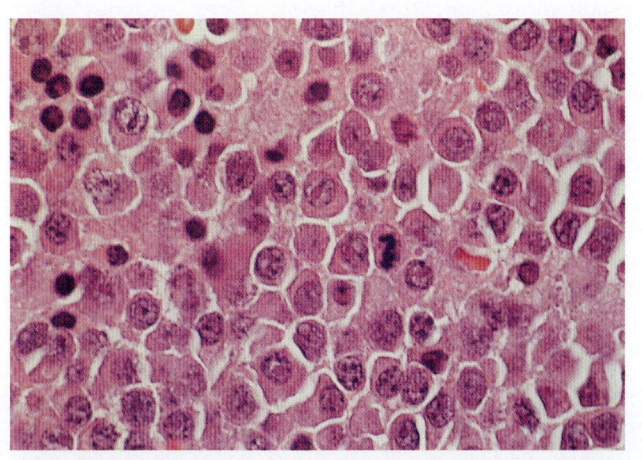

Figure 9.30. Higher-magnification photomicrograph of plasmacytoma shown in Figure 9.29 demonstrating closely compact malignant plasma cells. Note the mitotic figures. (Hematoxylin–eosin ×250.)

METASTATIC NEOPLASMS TO THE EYELIDS

General Considerations

Metastatic cancer to the eyelid is uncommon (1–14). In one series of 240 malignant eyelid tumors, metastasis accounted for three cases (2). In a review of 30 cases of eyelid metastasis, the primary location was breast in 10 cases, cutaneous melanoma in 7 cases, lung in 5 cases, and stomach in 1 case, with individual examples from colon, thyroid, parotid, and trachea (3). A more recent series of 20 cases of eyelid metastasis disclosed tumor origin from cutaneous melanoma (20%), uveal melanoma (20%), breast carcinoma (15%), conjunctival melanoma (15%), renal cell carcinoma (10%), and thyroid, prostate, lung, and salivary gland carcinomas (5% each) (1). Rarely, other primary tumors, such as esophageal leiomyosarcoma (11) and neuroendocrine carcinoma (13) can metastasize to the eyelid. In a few cases, the primary neoplasm was occult. As is the case for uveal metastasis, eyelid metastasis is probably more common than believed, but many are not noted clinically because they occur in patients with extensive metastases.

Clinical Features

Clinically, eyelid metastasis usually presents as a solitary subcutaneous nodule that simulates a chalazion. In contrast to chalazion, however, it usually has fewer inflammatory signs and shows more progressive enlargement and eventual ulceration. In addition, most patients have a history of prior cancer and many have known metastatic disease when they develop the eyelid mass. Metastatic breast cancer to the eyelid, in particular, can often be diffuse and ill-defined, suggesting an inflammatory process such as blepharitis (9). Metastatic melanoma to the eyelid often appears as a deep blue to black nodule. We have seen patients in whom an eyelid metastasis was the first sign of dissemination of choroidal melanoma (5).

Pathology

The histopathologic findings with eyelid metastasis vary with the primary tumor and the degree of differentiation of the metastatic focus. Some lesions, like melanoma (5), breast cancer (6), or renal cell carcinoma (4,7) have characteristic features. Breast cancer metastasis can sometimes have a histiocytoid appearance, thus making the diagnosis difficult (6,9,10). Primary mucinous carcinoma of sweat gland origin can have an almost identical histopathologic appearance. In some instances, the eyelid metastasis is so poorly differentiated that the primary neoplasm cannot be determined based on microscopic appearance alone.

Management

In addition to management of the primary neoplasm, the eyelid metastasis may need specific management. A small progressively enlarging lesion can be removed by local excision. Larger lesions may require a punch biopsy or shaving biopsy to confirm the diagnosis. Needle biopsy can be performed, but it generally yields less tissue, making diagnosis more difficult. If the patient is receiving specific chemotherapy for the primary malignancy, an eyelid metastasis can be observed to assess the response to chemotherapy. Radiotherapy can be employed for cases that are not easily resectable and that are not responding to chemotherapy or other systemic treatment.

Selected References

Reviews

1. Bianciotto C, Demirci H, Shields CL, et al. Metastatic tumors to the eyelid: report of 20 cases and review of the literature. *Arch Ophthalmol* 2009;127(8):999–1005.
2. Aurora AL, Blodi FC. Lesions of the eyelids. A clinicopathologic study. *Surv Ophthalmol* 1970;15:94–104.
3. Riley FC. Metastatic tumors of the eyelids. *Am J Ophthalmol* 1970;69:259–264.
4. Shah SU, Say EA, Chandana D, et al. Renal cell carcinoma metastasis to the eye and ocular adnexa in 38 patients. 2015; in press. [Presented as a poster at the American Academy of Ophthalmology. November, 2014, Chicago IL.]

Case Reports

5. Shields JA, Shields CL, Augsburger JJ, et al. Solitary metastasis of choroidal melanoma to contralateral eyelid. *Ophthal Plast Reconstr Surg* 1987;3:9–12.
6. Hood CI, Font RL, Zimmerman LE. Metastatic mammary carcinoma in the eyelid with histiocytoid appearance. *Cancer* 1973;31:793–800.
7. Kindermann WR, Shields JA, Eiferman RA, et al. Metastatic renal cell carcinoma to the eye and adnexae. A report of 3 cases and review of the literature. *Ophthalmology* 1981;88:1347–1350.
8. Mansour AM, Hidayat AA. Metastatic eyelid disease. *Ophthalmology* 1987;94:667–670.
9. Mottow-Lippa L, Jakobiec FA, Iwamoto T. Pseudoinflammatory metastatic breast carcinoma of the orbits and eyelids. *Ophthalmology* 1981;88:575–580.
10. Tomasini C, Soro E, Pippione M. Eyelid swelling: think of metastasis of histiocytoid breast carcinoma. *Dermatology* 2002;205:63–66.
11. Esmaeli B, Cleary KL, Ho L, et al. Leiomyosarcoma of the esophagus metastatic to the eyelid: a clinicopathologic report. *Ophthal Plast Reconstr Surg* 2002;18:159–161.
12. Benson JR, Querci della Rovere G, Nasiri N. Eyelid metastasis. *Lancet* 2001;20:1370–1371.
13. Bachmeyer C, Henni AM, Cazier A, et al. Eyelid metastases indicating neuroendocrine carcinoma of unknown origin. *Eye* 2004;18:94–95.
14. Kaden IH, Shields JA, Shields CL, et al. Occult prostatic carcinoma metastatic to the medial canthal area. Diagnosis by immunohistochemistry. *Ophthal Plastic Reconstr Surg* 1987;3:21–24.

EYELID METASTATIC TUMORS

Figures 9.35 and 9.36 from Kaden IH, Shields JA, Shields CL, et al. Occult prostatic carcinoma metastatic to the medial canthal area. Diagnosis by immunohistochemistry. *Ophthal Plast Reconstr Surg* 1987;3:21–24.

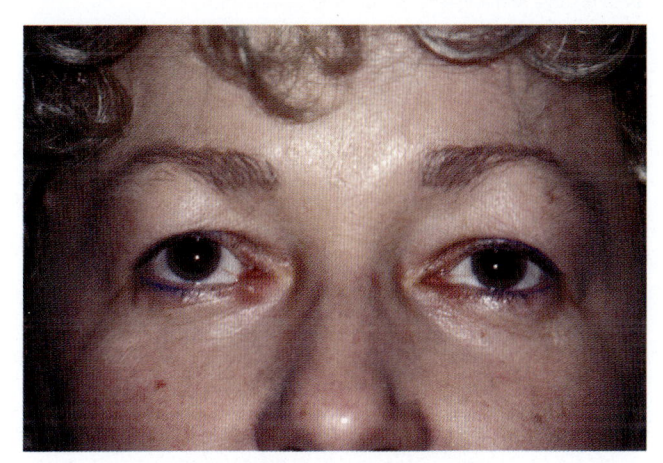

Figure 9.31. Nodular, somewhat discrete metastatic breast cancer to medial aspect of right lower eyelid in a 52-year-old woman. Note the overlying epidermis is not involved.

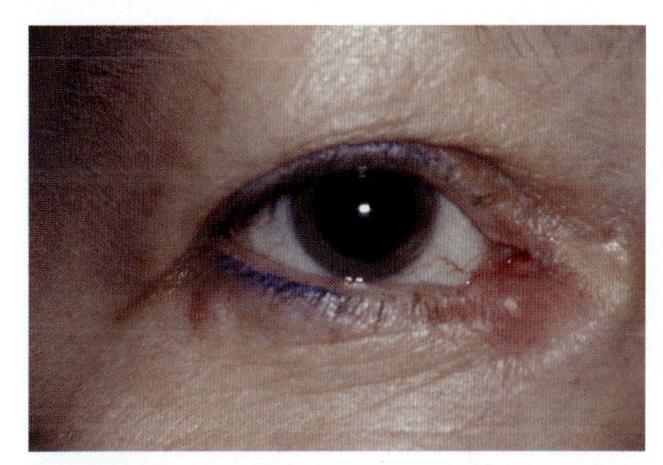

Figure 9.32. Closer view of lesion shown in Figure 9.31.

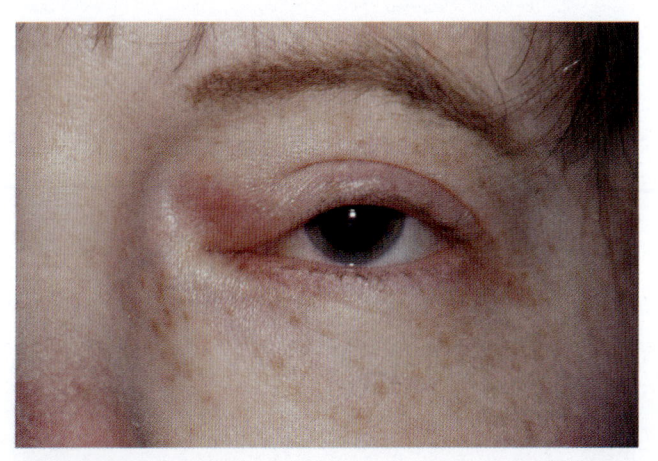

Figure 9.33. Subcutaneous metastatic breast cancer to medial aspect of upper eyelid.

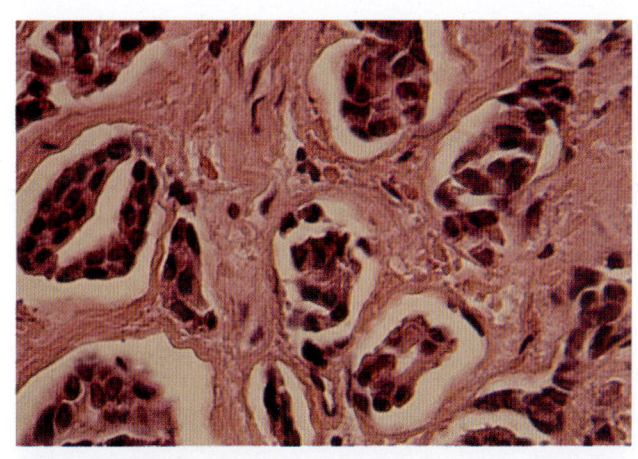

Figure 9.34. Histopathology of metastatic breast cancer, showing acini and cords of malignant tumor cells within dense fibrous tissue stroma. (Hematoxylin–eosin ×100.)

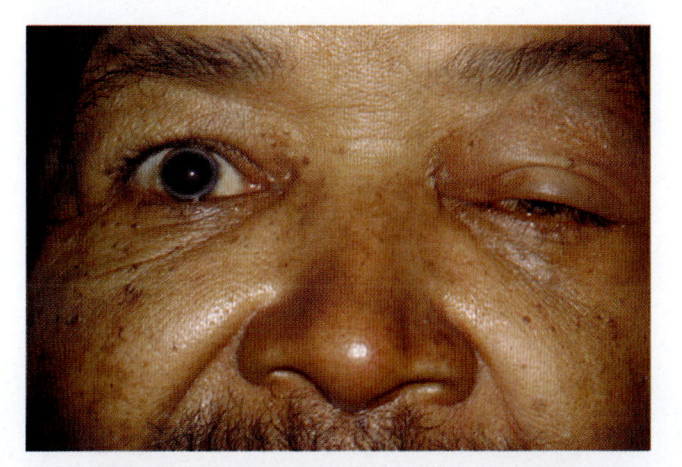

Figure 9.35. Blepharoptosis and thickening of upper eyelid owing to metastatic prostate cancer. The tumor extended posteriorly to involve the frontal bone and orbital soft tissue.

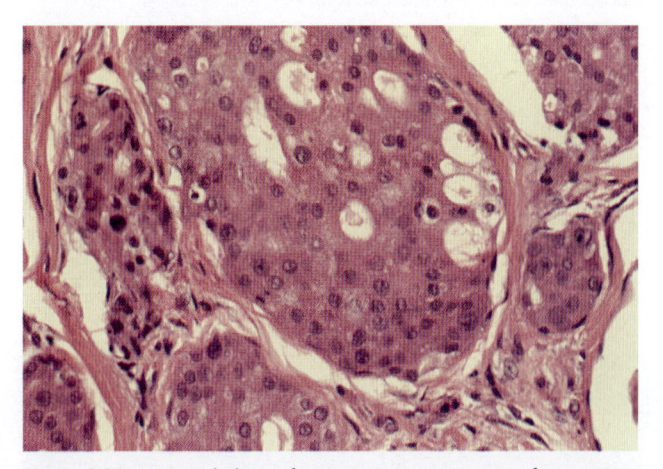

Figure 9.36. Histopathology of metastatic prostate cancer from patient shown in Figure 9.35, showing lobules of malignant tumor cells. The cells showed positive immunohistochemical reaction to prostate-specific antigen. (Hematoxylin–eosin ×100.)

EYELID METASTATIC TUMORS

1. Shields JA, Shields CL, Augsburger JJ, et al. Solitary metastasis of choroidal melanoma to contralateral eyelid. *Ophthal Plast Reconstr Surg* 1987;3:9–12.
2. Kindermann WR, Shields JA, Eiferman RA, et al. Metastatic renal cell carcinoma to the eye and adnexae. A report of 3 cases and review of the literature. *Ophthalmology.* 1981;88:1347–1350.

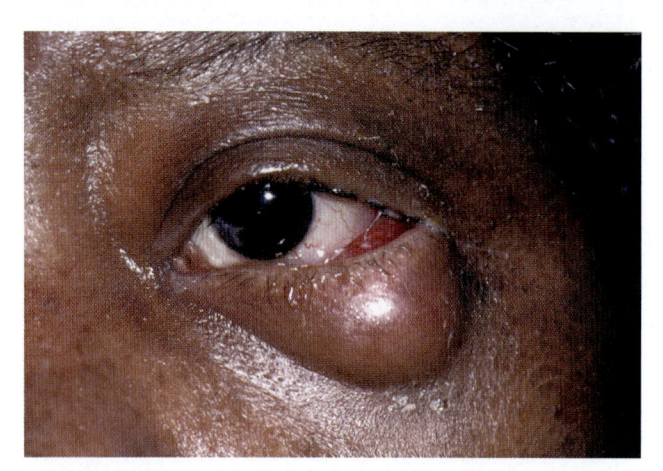

Figure 9.37. Metastatic bronchogenic carcinoma to lower eyelid. There was also metastasis to the ipsilateral temporal fossa.

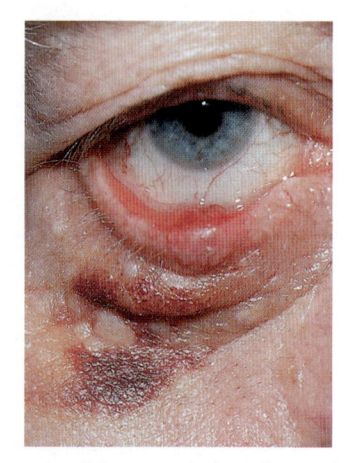

Figure 9.38. Lower eyelid metastasis from ileocecal carcinoid tumor. (Courtesy of Walter Stafford, MD.)

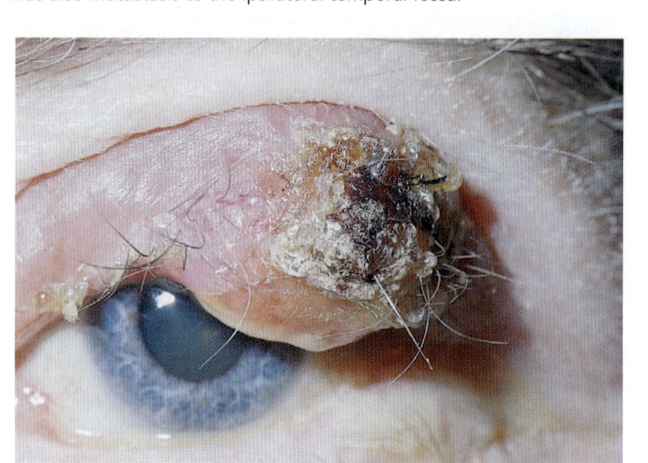

Figure 9.39. Metastatic renal cell carcinoma to the upper eyelid in a 62-year-old man. Biopsy of the eyelid tumor led to the diagnosis and subsequent evaluation disclosed an occult renal neoplasm.

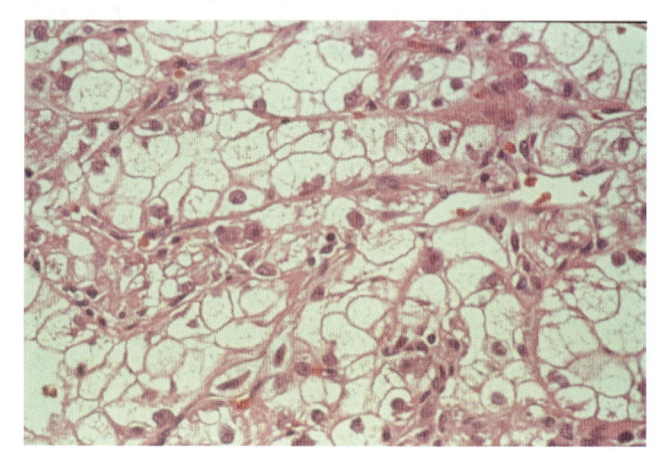

Figure 9.40. Histopathology of lesion shown in Figure 9.39 showing malignant cells with clear cytoplasm, characteristic of renal cell carcinoma.

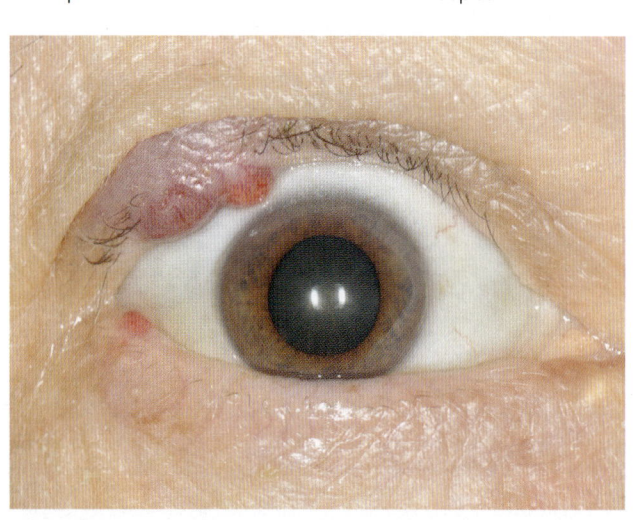

Figure 9.41. Metastatic renal cell carcinoma to the right upper and lower eyelids in an older male.

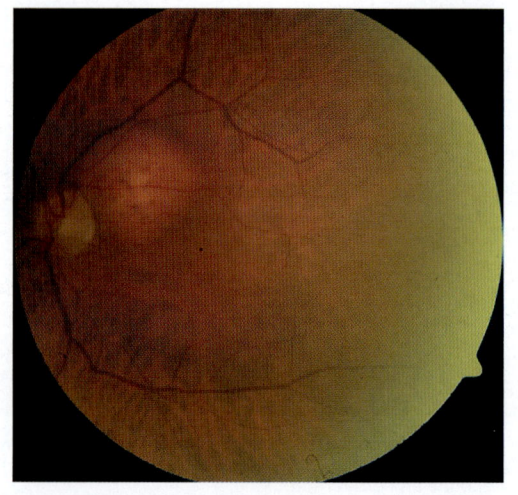

Figure 9.42. Fundus photography of patient in Figure 9.41 demonstrating choroidal metastasis from renal cell carcinoma near the optic disc.

Chapter 9 Eyelid Lymphoid, Plasmacytic, and Metastatic Tumors

EYELID METASTATIC TUMORS FROM CHOROIDAL MELANOMA

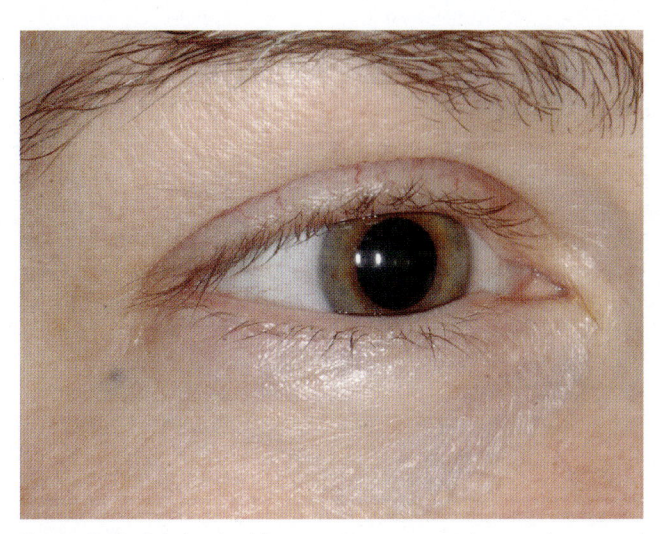

Figure 9.43. Subtle, tiny blue cutaneous metastasis occurring several years after treatment of contralateral choroidal melanoma.

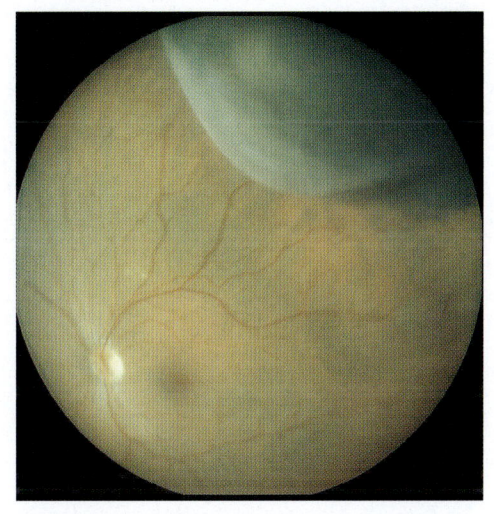

Figure 9.44. Large choroidal melanoma in the opposite eye of patient in Figure 9.43 showing pigmented mass and shallow subretinal fluid prior to treatment.

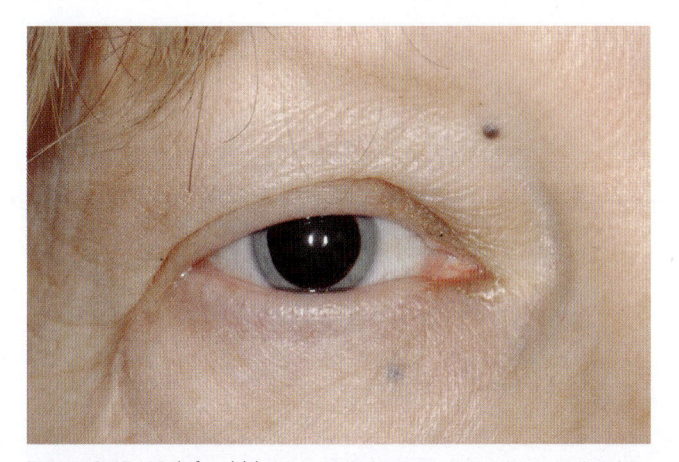

Figure 9.45. Multifocal blue-gray cutaneous metastasis occurring in a patient with no history of choroidal melanoma.

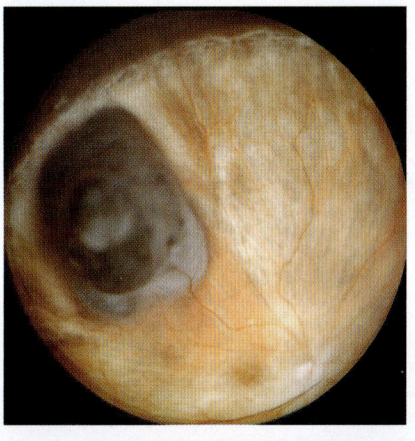

Figure 9.46. Fundus photography of patient in Figure 9.45 illustrating the newly diagnosed mushroom-shaped, retinal invasive melanoma in her right eye. This was treated with plaque radiotherapy.

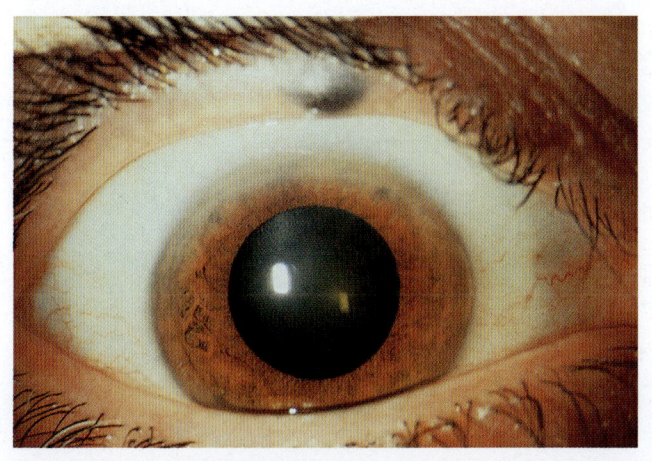

Figure 9.47. Metastatic choroidal melanoma to the upper eyelid in a 51-year-old woman, representing the only sign of systemic metastasis.

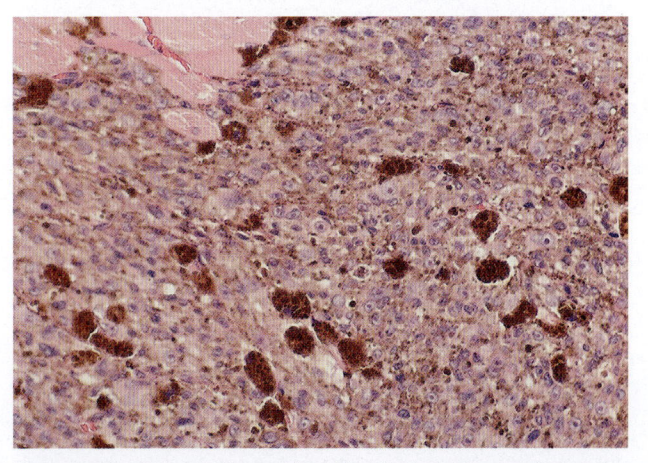

Figure 9.48. Histopathology of the lesion shown in Figure 9.47 showing spindle and epithelioid melanoma cells. (Hematoxylin–eosin ×100.)

CHAPTER 10

EYELID HISTIOCYTIC, MYXOID, AND FIBROUS LESIONS

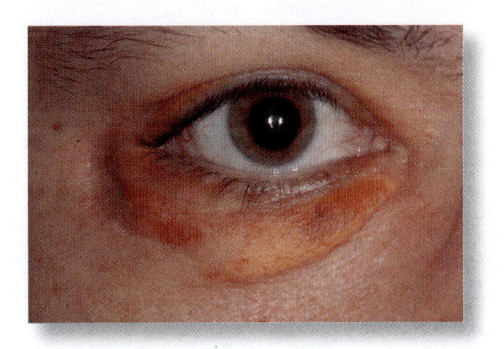

General Considerations

Xanthelasma is an extremely common, benign subcutaneous eyelid lesion that has characteristic clinical and histopathologic features (1–27). When it is larger and nodular, assuming tumorous proportions, it is called a xanthoma. Xanthelasma tends to be bilateral and more common in the elderly. It occurs in 1% to 3% of individuals and is slightly more common in women. Although some patients with xanthelasma are normolipemic, about 50% of them have essential hyperlipidemia (usually type II) or secondary hyperlipidemia owing to conditions like diabetes mellitus or biliary cirrhosis.

Tuberous xanthoma appears as solitary or multiple, placoid, or papular lesions that have a predilection for buttocks, elbows, knees, and fingers. It is more likely to be associated with hyperlipidemia types II and III. It may be a result from hyperlipemic genetic defects in lipid metabolism, and is most often transmitted as an autosomal-dominant trait. It consists of one or more elevated nodules that are usually located in the extremities, but can be found on the eyelids (20–24). In some instances, large bilateral eyelid tumors can be misinterpreted as fibrous histiocytomas, but histopathologically proven to be tuberous xanthomas (see Fig. 10.10).

Multiple eruptive xanthomas can sometimes occur in patients who experience a rapid rise in serum triglyceride levels. In some cases, these lesions can become very large and aggressive despite being benign, and even invade through the orbital septum into the orbital fat. Interestingly, these large xanthomatous lesions have been known to extensively involve all four eyelids in patients with normal serum lipid levels (21–24).

Affected patients are believed to be at higher risk of death from cardiovascular disease. Xanthelasma is also seen with greater frequency in patients with the Erdheim–Chester disease, an idiopathic condition characterized by lipid deposition in bones, heart, retroperitoneum, and orbit (25–27).

Clinical Features

Clinically, xanthelasma appears as one or more, flat or minimally elevated, yellow, placoid lesions that affect the loose skin of the eyelids, more commonly on the medial aspect of the eyelids. It generally occurs in middle-aged or older adults and is more common in women. It is often bilateral and symmetrical, and can sometimes slowly enlarge and coalesce to form large, raised, plaquelike, or nodular lesions. When a xanthelasma becomes elevated and nodular, it is more properly called a tuberous xanthoma (20–24).

Pathology

Microscopically, xanthelasma and xanthoma are forms of lipoma that consist of an infiltration of the superficial reticular dermis by foamy histiocytes. The cells tend to be more concentrated around blood vessels. Touton giant cells are occasionally present. There is generally an absence of fibrosis.

EYELID XANTHELASMA AND XANTHOMA

Management

There are several approaches to management of xanthelasma and xanthoma, depending on the clinical circumstances (2–18). Management should include evaluation of the affected patient for various hyperlipidemias and Erdheim–Chester disease. The eyelid lesions can generally be observed. Surgical excision should be considered for larger or cosmetically unacceptable lesions. The wound can be closed with sutures or allowed to heal by secondary intention (3–6). An intriguing technique has been reported in which the xanthelasma is raised with a skin flap and resected from the back side of the skin and then the skin flap without the tumor is sutured into its original position (4). Others have modified that technique to treat the xanthelasma on the back side of the flap with erbium:yttrium-aluminum-garnet (YAG) laser and then suturing the flap into position (12). Topical application of bichloroacetic acid or trichloroacetic acid can also be effective (13–15). Positive results have also been obtained by using a carbon dioxide laser to vaporize the lesions (7,11). More recently, the erbium:YAG laser has also been reported to be effective (12). The treatment options have recently been reviewed in detail (1–18). In addition, affected patients should be treated medically for elevated serum lipids. Sometimes such medical treatment alone brings about resolution of xanthelasma (18). The larger, tuberous xanthomas generally require surgical excision.

EYELID XANTHELASMA AND XANTHOMA

Selected References

Reviews
1. Rohrich RJ, Janis JE, Pownell PH. Xanthelasma palpebrarum: a review and current management principles. *Plast Reconstr Surg* 2002;110:1310–1314.

Management
2. Cartwright MJ. Xanthelasma procedures. *Plast Reconstr Surg* 1999;104:878.

Surgical Resection
3. Lee HY, Jin US, Minn KW, et al. Outcomes of surgical management of xanthelasma palpebrarum. *Arch Plast Surg* 2013;40(4):380–386.
4. Doi H, Ogawa Y. A new operative method for treatment of xanthelasma or xanthoma palpebrarum: microsurgical inverted peeling. *Plast Reconstr Surg* 1998;102:1171–1174.
5. Eedy DJ. Treatment of xanthelasma by excision with secondary intention healing. *Clin Exp Dermatol* 1996;21:273–275.
6. Levy JL, Trelles MA. New operative technique for treatment of xanthelasma palpebrarum: laser-inverted resurfacing: preliminary report. *Ann Plast Surg* 2003;50:339–343.

Laser Therapy
7. Ullmann Y, Har-Shai Y, Peled IJ. The use of CO_2 laser for the treatment of xanthelasma palpebrarum. *Ann Plast Surg* 1993;31:504–507.
8. Sampath R, Parmar D, Cree IA, et al. Histology of xanthelasma lesion treated by argon laser photocoagulation. *Eye* 1998;12:479–480.
9. Park EJ, Youn SH, Cho EB, et al. Xanthelasma palpebrarum treatment with a 1,450-nm-diode laser. *Dermatol Surg* 2011;37(6):791–796.
10. Karsai S, Czarnecka A, Raulin C. Treatment of xanthelasma palpebrarum using a pulsed dye laser: a prospective clinical trial in 38 cases. *Dermatol Surg* 2010;36(5):610–617.
11. Raulin C, Schoenermark MP, Werner S, et al. Xanthelasma palpebrarum: treatment with the ultrapulsed CO_2 laser. *Lasers Surg Med* 1999;24:122–127.
12. Borelli C, Kaudewitz P. Xanthelasma palpebrarum: treatment with the erbium:YAG laser. *Lasers Surg Med* 2001;29:260–264.

Others
13. Haygood LJ, Bennett JD, Brodell RT. Treatment of xanthelasma palpebrarum with bichloracetic acid. *Dermatol Surg* 1998;24:1027–1031.
14. Cannon PS, Ajit R, Leatherbarrow B. Efficacy of trichloroacetic acid (95%) in the management of xanthelasma palpebrarum. *Clin Exp Dermatol* 2010;35(8):845–848.
15. Nahas TR, Marques JC, Nicoletti A, et al. Treatment of eyelid xanthelasma with 70% trichloroacetic acid. *Ophthal Plast Reconstr Surg* 2009;25(4):280–283.
16. Dincer D, Koc E, Erbil AH, et al. Effectiveness of low-voltage radiofrequency in the treatment of xanthelasma palpebrarum: a pilot study of 15 cases. *Dermatol Surg* 2010;36(12):1973–1978.
17. Hawk JL. Cryotherapy may be effective for eyelid xanthelasma. *Clin Exp Dermatol* 2000;25:351.
18. Shields CL, Mashayekhi A, Racciato P, et al. Disappearance of eyelid xanthelasma following oral simvastatin (Zocor™). *Br J Ophthalmol* 2005;89:639.

Case Reports
19. Pinto X, Ribera M, Fiol C. Dyslipoproteinemia in patients with xanthelasma. *Arch Dermatol* 1989;125:1281–1282.
20. Shukla Y, Ratnawat PS. Tuberous xanthoma of upper eyelid (a case report). *Indian J Ophthalmol* 1982;30:3.
21. Rose EH, Vistnes LM. Unilateral invasive xanthelasma palpebrarum. *Ophthal Plast Reconstr Surg* 1987;3:91–94.
22. Tosti A, Varotti C, Tosti G, et al. Bilateral extensive xanthelasma palpebrarum. *Cutis* 1988;41:113–114.
23. Depot MJ, Jakobiec FA, Dodick JM, et al. Bilateral and extensive xanthelasma palpebrarum in a young man. *Ophthalmology* 1984;91:522–527.
24. Ohta M, Suzuki Y, Sawada M. Bilateral tumor-like invasive xanthelasma palpebrarum in the superior palpebra. *Ophthal Plast Reconstr Surg* 1996;12:196–198.

Erdheim–Chester Disease
25. Alper MG, Zimmerman LE, LaPiana FG. Orbital manifestations of Erdheim-Chester disease. *Trans Am Ophthalmol Soc* 1983;81:64–85.
26. Shields JA, Karcioglu Z, Shields CL, et al. Orbital and eyelid involvement with Erdheim-Chester disease. *Arch Ophthalmol* 1991;109:850–854.
27. Opie KM, Kaye J, Vinciullo C. Erdheim-Chester disease. *Australas J Dermatol* 2003;44:194–198.

EYELID XANTHELASMA

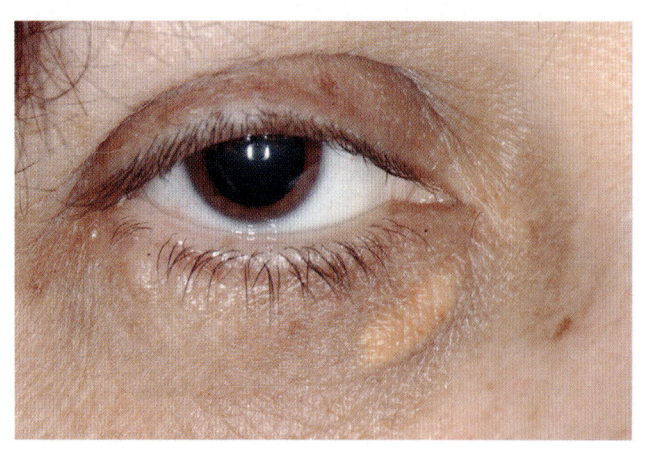

Figure 10.1. Typical xanthelasma appearing as a yellow, slightly elevated placoid lesion in the medial aspect of lower eyelid.

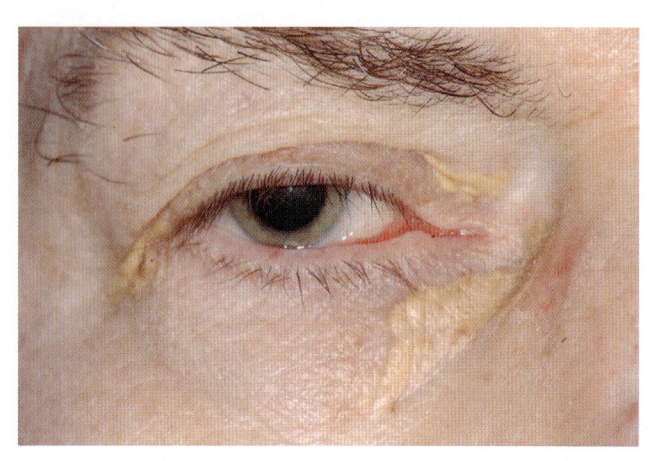

Figure 10.2. Xanthelasmas of upper and lower eyelids at lateral and medial canthus in an elderly man.

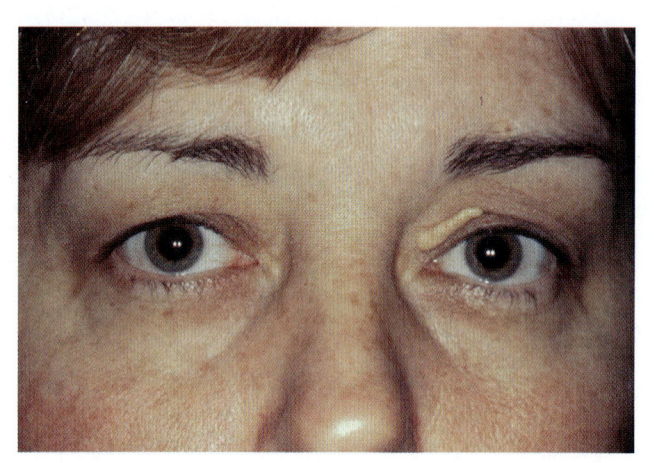

Figure 10.3. Xanthelasma in medial aspect of left upper eyelid in a middle-aged woman.

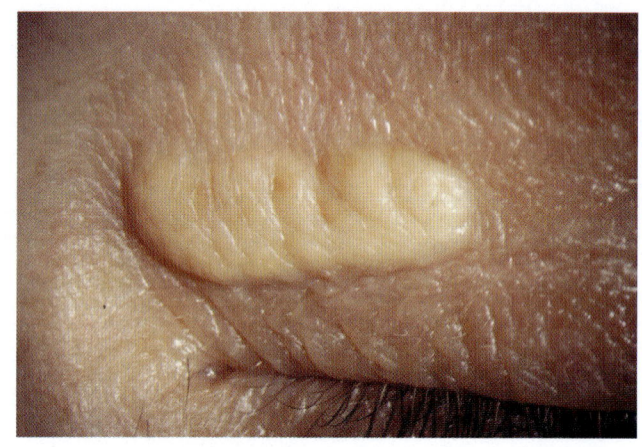

Figure 10.4. Close-up view of lesion shown in Figure 10.3, showing yellow color and preservation of skin creases.

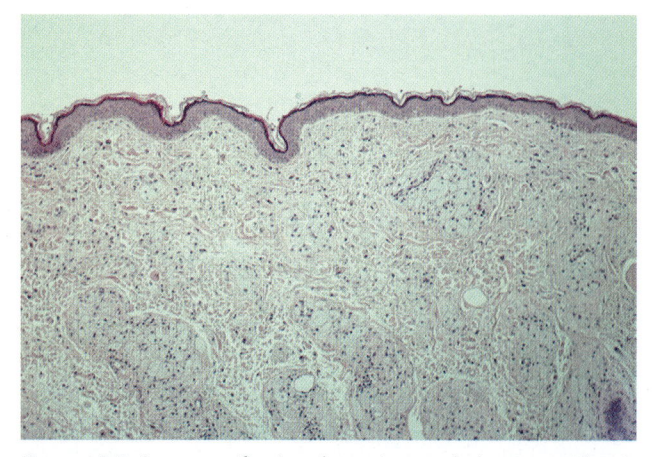

Figure 10.5. Low-magnification photomicrograph showing epidermis and appearance of lipid-containing cells in dermis. (Hematoxylin–eosin ×10.)

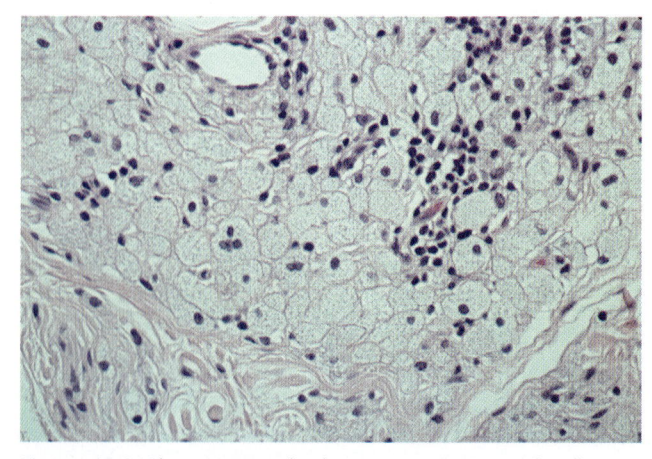

Figure 10.6. Photomicrograph showing compact round cells containing lipid. There is a mild infiltration of chronic inflammatory cells. (Hematoxylin–eosin ×50.)

Chapter 10 Eyelid Histiocytic, Myxoid, and Fibrous Lesions

● EYELID XANTHELASMA: ASSOCIATION WITH SYSTEMIC CONDITIONS

1. Shields CL, Mashayekhi A, Racciato P, et al. Disappearance of eyelid xanthelasma following oral simvastatin (Zocor). *Br J Ophthalmol* 2005;89:639.
2. Shields JA, Karcioglu Z, Shields CL, et al. Orbital and eyelid involvement with Erdheim–Chester disease. *Arch Ophthalmol* 1991;109:850–854.

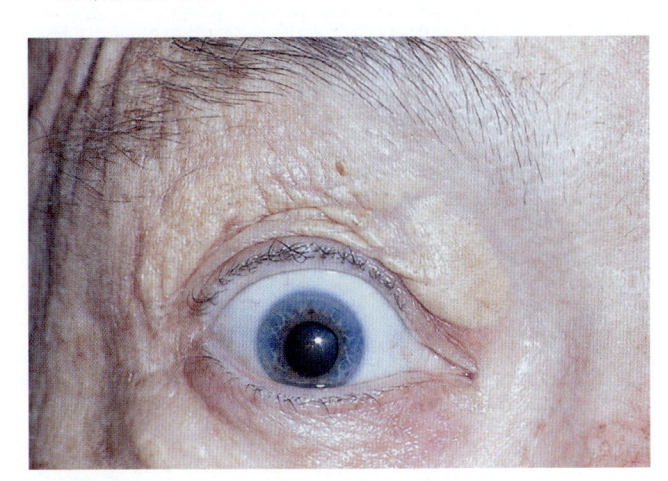

Figure 10.7. Xanthelasma in a patient with Erdheim–Chester disease. This patient also had massive bilateral orbital involvement (shown later in section on orbital diseases).

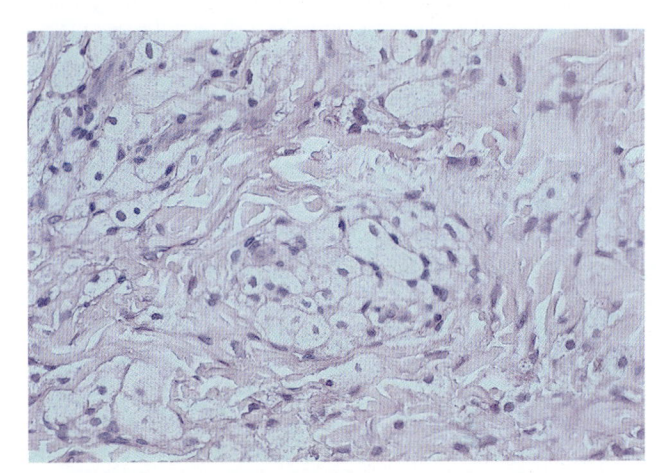

Figure 10.8. Histopathology of lesion shown in Figure 10.7 showing large, round lipid-containing cells in the dermis. The xanthoma cells seem to be most concentrated around blood vessels. (Hematoxylin–eosin ×150.)

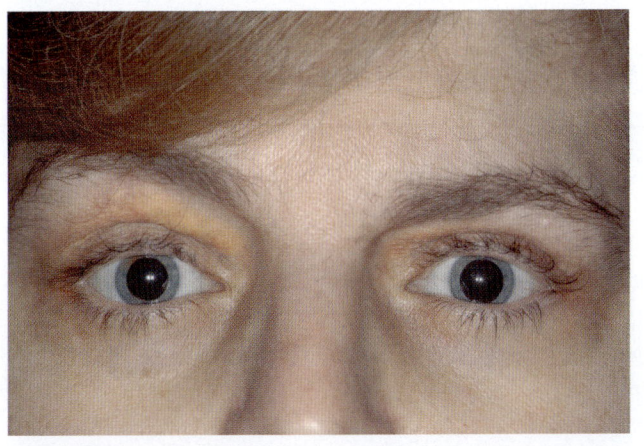

Figure 10.9. Xanthelasma in a patient with adult onset orbital xanthogranuloma with asthma.

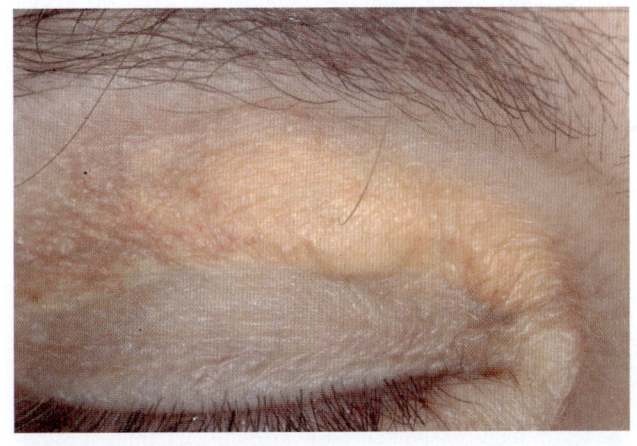

Figure 10.10. Close up showing flat, extensive upper eyelid xanthelasma of patient in Figure 10.9.

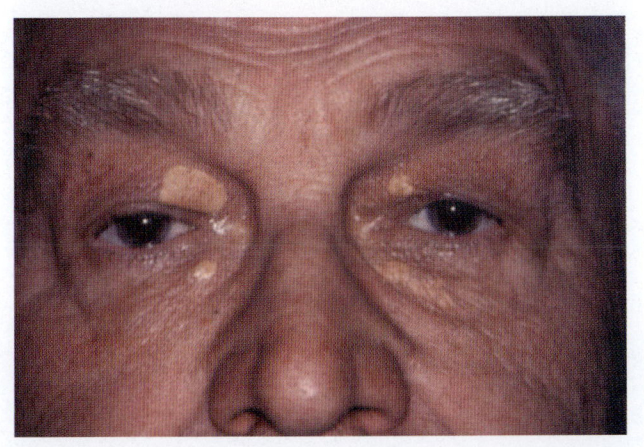

Figure 10.11. Bilateral xanthelasma associated with hyperlipidemia. Patient started taking simvastatin for hyperlipidemia.

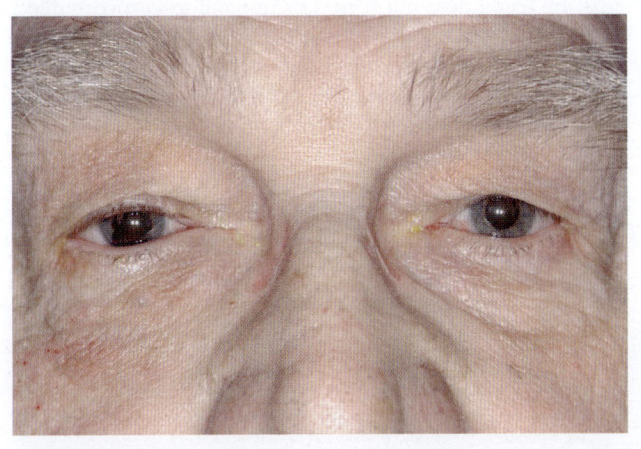

Figure 10.12. Same patient 10 years later, showing disappearance of the xanthelasma after long-term use of simvastatin.

EYELID XANTHOGRANULOMA

General Considerations

Juvenile xanthogranuloma (JXG) is an idiopathic granulomatous inflammation that usually affects the skin of infants, but can occur in ocular tissues of adults as well as children (1–14). Hence, the word "juvenile" may not be always accurate. We use "JXG" here because of its widespread usage, but we briefly mention adult xanthogranuloma as well. In a series of 53 cases of ocular JXG, the eyelid was involved in 13 (25%) (1).

Lesions on the eyelid, conjunctiva, or orbit are usually solitary (3–9). The best-known ocular involvement is an iris lesion that can cause spontaneous hyphema (6–8). Iris JXG is discussed in the *Atlas and Textbook of Intraocular Tumors*.

Clinical Features

Eyelid JXG usually is solitary and tends to occur in older children or young adults (1,2), but in some cases it is present at birth (4,5). This tumor appears as a fleshy tan or orange nodule that can rarely ulcerate. It is generally self-limited and gradually resolves, leaving a small atrophic scar. Sometimes, a large congenital macronodular form of JXG can simulate a malignancy clinically and histopathologically (4,5).

The adult form of xanthogranuloma can occur as a solitary lesion often in patients with asthma (10,11,13). In these instances, it may be similar clinically and histopathologically to the eyelid xanthelasmas seen with Erdheim–Chester disease (14).

Pathology

Early JXG is characterized by a monomorphous infiltration of histiocytes, lymphocytes, mononuclear cells, scattered eosinophils, and Touton giant cells (1). JXG can be similar to fibrous histiocytoma (dermatofibroma), reticulohistiocytoma (13), and other granulomatous inflammations.

Management

Management of eyelid JXG is generally observation, because the lesion tends to spontaneously involute. Systemic or intralesional corticosteroids can be employed in recalcitrant cases. Surgical excision may be considered if malignancy is suspected or if the lesion does not regress or respond to corticosteroids. Irradiation is rarely a therapeutic consideration today. Little is known about the best management of the adult form associated with bronchial asthma, but treatment with asthma medications and systemic corticosteroids should be considered.

Selected References

Reviews
1. Zimmerman LE. Ocular lesions of juvenile xanthogranuloma. *Trans Am Acad Ophthalmol Otolaryngol* 1965;63:412–442.

Case Reports/Juvenile Xanthogranuloma
2. DeStafeno JJ, Carlson JA, Meyer DR. Solitary spindle-cell xanthogranuloma of the eyelid. *Ophthalmology* 2002;109:258–261.
3. Chalfin S, Lloyd WC 3rd. Juvenile xanthogranuloma of the eyelid in an adult. *Arch Ophthalmol* 1998;116:1546–1547.
4. Schwartz TL, Carter KD, Judisch GF, et al. Congenital macronodular juvenile xanthogranuloma of the eyelid. *Ophthalmology* 1991;98:1230–1233.
5. Shields CL, Thaler AS, Lally SE, et al. Massive macronodular juvenile xanthogranuloma of the eyelid in a newborn. *J AAPOS* 2014;18(2):195–197.
6. Manjandavida FP, Arepalli S, Tarlan B, et al. Optical coherence tomography characteristics of epi-iridic membrane in a child with recurrent hyphema and presumed juvenile xanthogranuloma. *J AAPOS* 2014;18:93–95.
7. Danzig C, Shields CL, Mashayekhi A, et al. Fluorescein angiography of iris juvenile xanthogranuloma. *J Ped Ophthalmol Strabism* 2008;45(2):110–112.
8. Shields JA, Eagle RC, Shields CL, et al. Iris juvenile xanthogranuloma studied by immunohistochemistry and flow cytometry. *Ophthal Surg Lasers* 1997;98:40–44.
9. Shields CL, Shields JA, Buchanon H. Solitary orbital involvement with juvenile xanthogranuloma. *Arch Ophthalmol* 1990;108:1587–1589.

Adult Onset Xanthogranuloma
10. Nasr AM, Johnson T, Hidayat A. Adult onset primary bilateral orbital xanthogranuloma: clinical, diagnostic, and histopathologic correlations. *Orbit* 1991;10:13–17.
11. Rose GE, Patel BC, Garner A, et al. Orbital xanthogranuloma in adults. *Br J Ophthalmol* 1991;75:681–686.
12. Bakri SJ, Carlson JA, Meyer DR. Recurrent solitary reticulohistiocytoma of the eyelid. *Ophthal Plast Reconstr Surg* 2003;19:162–164.
13. Jakobiec FA, Mills MD, Hidayat AA, et al. Periocular xanthogranulomas associated with severe adult-onset asthma. *Trans Am Ophthalmol Soc* 1993;91:99–129.
14. Shields JA, Karcioglu Z, Shields CL, et al. Orbital and eyelid involvement with Erdheim-Chester disease. *Arch Ophthalmol* 1991;109:850–854.

Chapter 10 Eyelid Histiocytic, Myxoid, and Fibrous Lesions

● EYELID JUVENILE XANTHOGRANULOMA

1. Shields CL, Thaler AS, Lally SE, et al. Massive macronodular juvenile xanthogranuloma of the eyelid in a newborn. *J AAPOS* 2014;18(2):195–197.
2. Shields CL, Shields JA, Buchanon H. Solitary orbital involvement with juvenile xanthogranuloma. *Arch Ophthalmol* 1990;108:1587–1589.

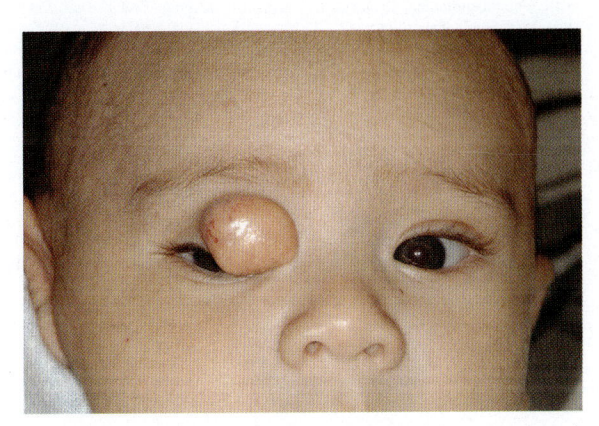

Figure 10.13. Large eyelid juvenile xanthogranuloma present at birth and then enlarged rapidly in this 6-week-old child.

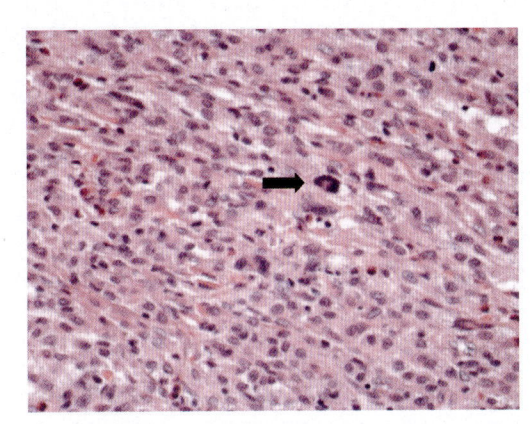

Figure 10.14. Following surgical resection of mass in patient in Figure 10.13, the cellular tumor was confirmed as juvenile xanthogranuloma with rare Touton giant cell (*arrow*). (Hematoxylin–eosin ×200.)

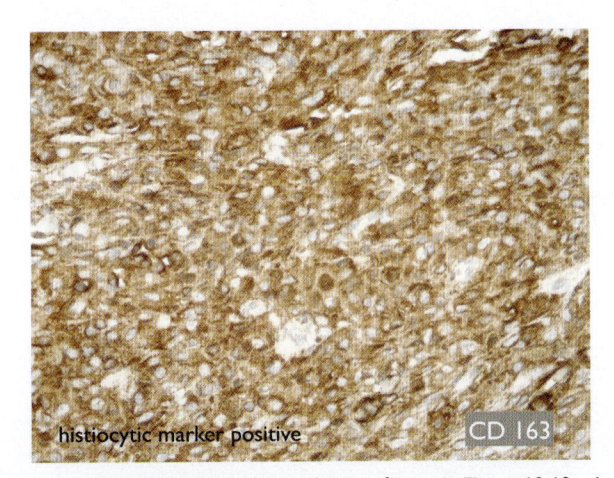

Figure 10.15. Immunohistochemical stain of mass in Figure 10.13 using CD 163, macrophage marker, is positive. (CD 163 ×200.)

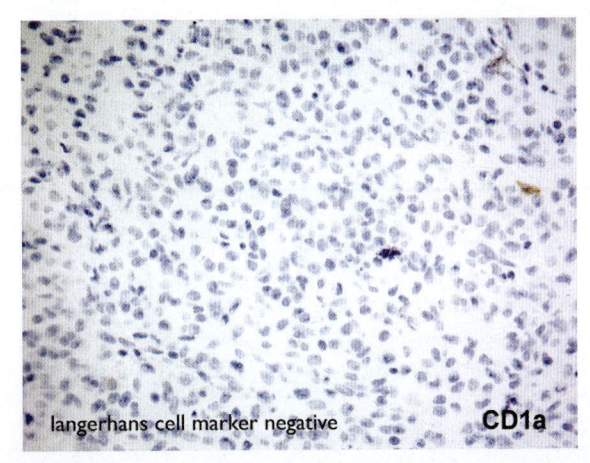

Figure 10.16. Immunohistochemical stain of mass in Figure 10.13 using CD1a, Langerhans marker, is negative. (CD1a ×200.)

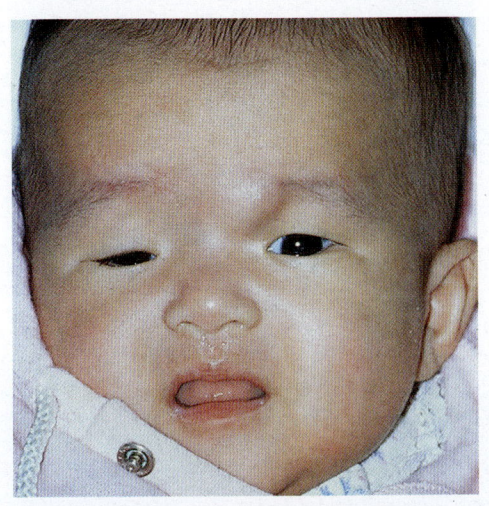

Figure 10.17. Deep eyelid involvement with juvenile xanthogranuloma. Note the subcutaneous mass at nasal aspect of left eyebrow. The lesion extended posteriorly into the medial portion of the orbit.

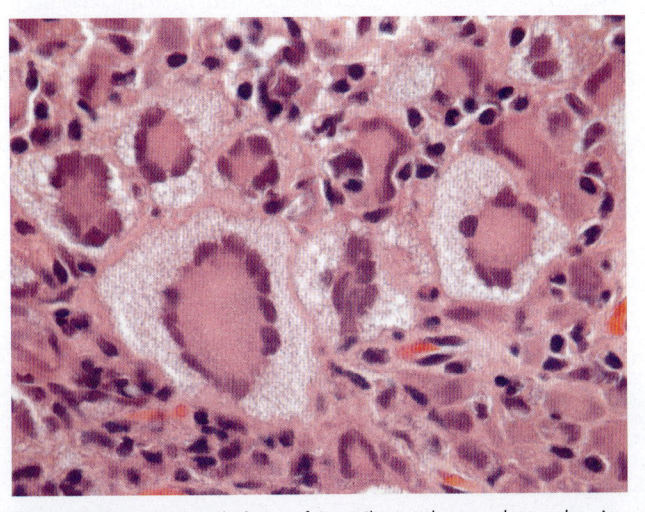

Figure 10.18. Histopathology of juvenile xanthogranuloma showing histiocytes and several Touton giant cells. (Hematoxylin–eosin ×250.)

EYELID NECROBIOTIC XANTHOGRANULOMA WITH PARAPROTEINEMIA

General Considerations

Necrobiotic xanthogranuloma with paraproteinemia is an uncommon histiocytic disorder characterized by multiple yellow xanthomatous skin lesions in patients with dysproteinemias (1–13). This condition has a predilection for the periorbital area, face, and trunk with a mean age of onset of about 55 years. The periorbital region, including the eyelids, is the most common site of involvement. The dysproteinemia is frequently due to a monoclonal immunoglobulin G paraprotein (1).

Clinical Features

Eyelid involvement by necrobiotic xanthogranuloma is characterized by multiple, painless, yellow nodules or plaques on the eyelid skin. Although the eyelid lesions may resemble xanthelasmas, they are more diffuse, indurated, and may extend deeper into the orbit. The condition usually has a progressive clinical course, sometimes with development of multiple myeloma or other cancers. Patients can occasionally develop an associated iritis and disc edema.

Pathology

Histopathologically, necrobiotic xanthogranuloma is composed of a diffuse replacement of the subcutaneous tissue and dermis by a polymorphic infiltrate of foamy histiocytes, multinucleated giant cells of the Touton type, and lymphocytes. The most striking feature is widespread areas of necrobiosis of collagen, a finding which is absent in JXG and Erdheim–Chester disease (1,3). There may be cholesterol clefts within the infiltrate. Immunohistochemically, these lipid-containing cells show a positive reaction for monocyte and macrophage markers but negative for S-100 protein, which differentiates it from Langerhans cell histiocytosis and sinus histiocytosis of Rosai–Dorfman.

Management

Management is difficult and focuses on the treatment of the paraproteinemia. Corticosteroids and chemotherapy have been employed with some success. More recently, injection of corticosteroids has been beneficial in reducing the subcutaneous deposits (13). Radiotherapy may sometimes be effective (9).

Selected References

Reviews

1. Kossard S, Winkelmann RK. Necrobiotic xanthogranuloma with paraproteinemia. *J Am Acad Dermatol* 1980;3:257–270.

Case Reports

2. Codere F, Lee RD, Anderson RL. Necrobiotic xanthogranuloma of the eyelid. *Arch Ophthalmol* 1983;101:60–63.
3. Robertson DM, Winkelmann RK. Ophthalmic features of necrobiotic xanthogranuloma with paraproteinemia. *Am J Ophthalmol* 1984;97:178–183.
4. Bullock JD, Bartley GB, Campbell RJ, et al. Necrobiotic xanthogranuloma with paraproteinemia. Case report and a pathogenetic theory. *Ophthalmology* 1986;93:1233–1236.
5. Cornblath WT, Dotan SA, Trobe JD, et al. Varied clinical spectrum of necrobiotic xanthogranuloma. *Ophthalmology* 1992;99:103–107.
6. Scupham RK, Fretzin DF. Necrobiotic xanthogranuloma with paraproteinemia. *Arch Pathol Lab Med* 1989;113:1389–1391.
7. Plotnick H, Taniguchi Y, Hashimoto K, et al. Periorbital necrobiotic xanthogranuloma and stage I multiple myeloma. Ultrastructure and response to pulsed dexamethasone documented by magnetic resonance imaging. *J Am Acad Dermatol* 1991;25:373–377.
8. Valentine EA, Friedman HD, Zamkoff KW, et al. Necrobiotic xanthogranuloma with IgA multiple myeloma: a case report and literature review. *Am J Hematol* 1990;35:283–285.
9. Char DH, LeBoit PE, Ljung BE, et al. Radiation therapy for ocular necrobiotic xanthogranuloma. *Arch Ophthalmol* 1987;105:174–175.
10. Lam K, Brownstein S, Jordan DR, et al. Bilateral necrobiotic xanthogranuloma of the eyelids followed by a diagnosis of multiple myeloma 20 years later. *Ophthal Plast Reconstr Surg* 2013;29(5):e119–e120.
11. Rayner SA, Duncombe AS, Keefe M, et al. Necrobiotic xanthogranuloma occurring in an eyelid scar. *Orbit* 2008;27(3):191–194.
12. Schaudig U, Al-Samir K. Upper and lower eyelid reconstruction for severe disfiguring necrobiotic xanthogranuloma. *Orbit* 2004;23(1):65–76.
13. Elner VM, Mintz R, Demirci H, et al. Local corticosteroid treatment of eyelid and orbital xanthogranuloma. *Ophthal Plast Reconstr Surg* 2006;22:36–40.

Chapter 10 Eyelid Histiocytic, Myxoid, and Fibrous Lesions

EYELID NECROBIOTIC XANTHOGRANULOMA WITH PARAPROTEINEMIA

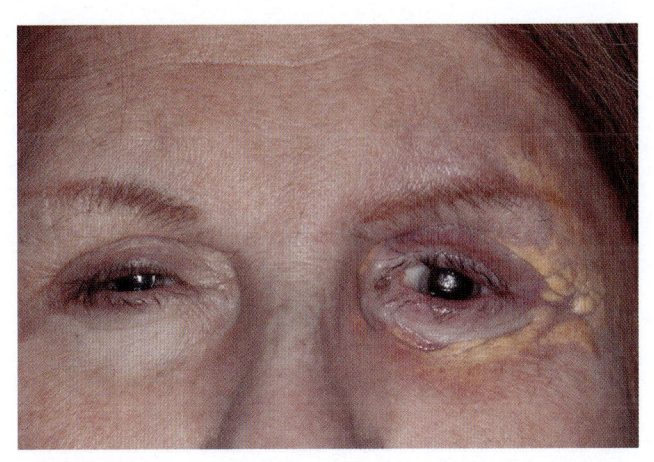

Figure 10.19. Extensive eyelid xanthelasmas with dry irritated eye in a middle-aged woman with necrobiotic xanthogranuloma and monoclonal gammopathy.

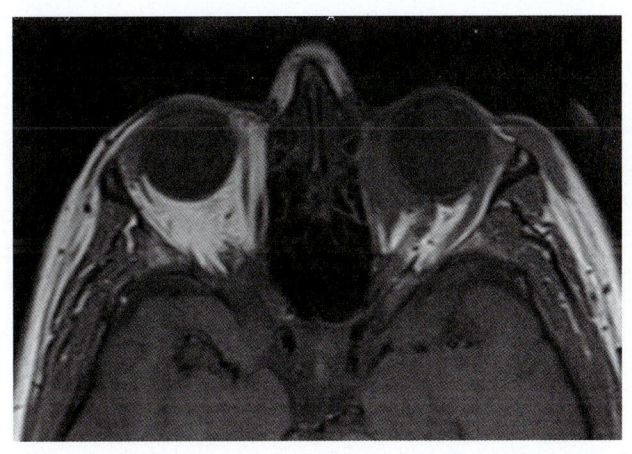

Figure 10.20. Magnetic resonance imaging reveals orbital invasion of necrobiotic xanthogranuloma in patient in Figure 10.19.

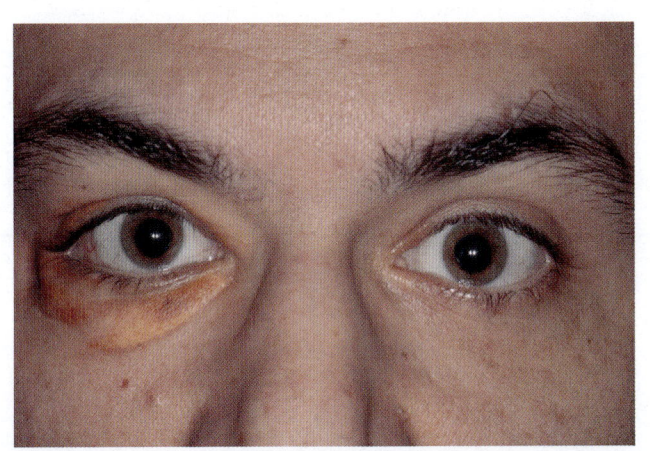

Figure 10.21. Eyelid xanthelasma in a young male that progressed over 2 years and was eventually discovered to have necrobiotic xanthogranuloma of the orbit and later monoclonal gammopathy.

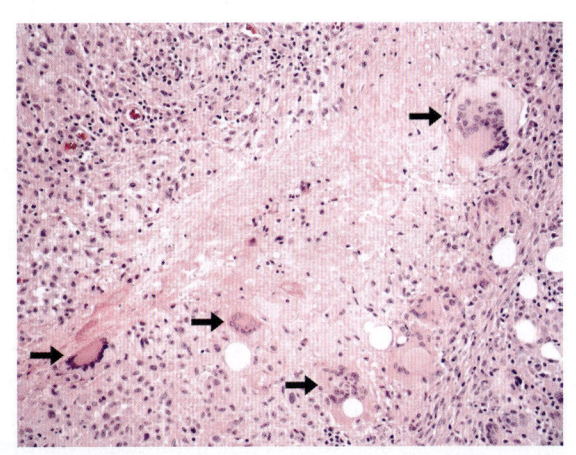

Figure 10.22. Photomicrograph of necrobiotic xanthogranuloma of patient in Figure 10.21 showing granulomatous inflammation with central necrobiosis and Touton giant cells (*arrows*). (Hematoxylin–eosin ×150.)

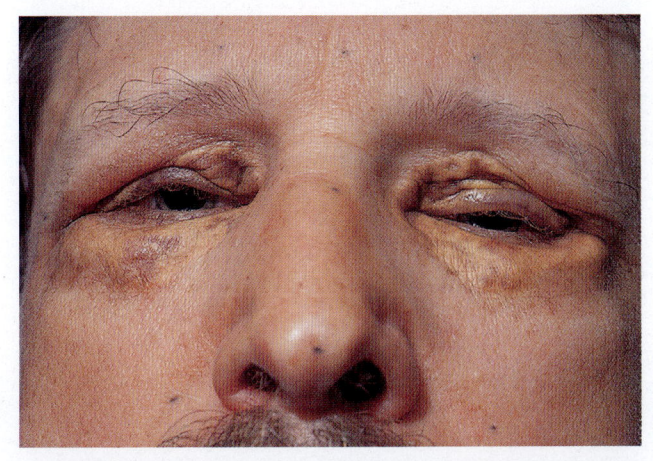

Figure 10.23. Bilateral eyelid involvement with necrobiotic xanthogranuloma in a 53-year-old man with a monoclonal gammopathy.

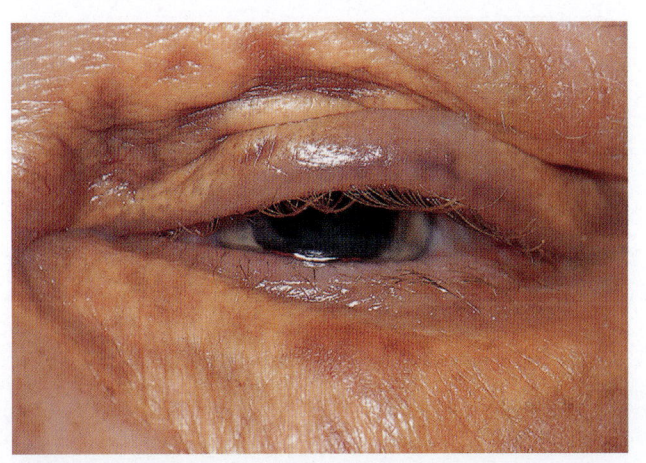

Figure 10.24. Closer view of left eyelid area in the patient shown in Figure 10.23 demonstrating the yellow color of the eyelid skin.

EYELID ANGIOFIBROMA

General Considerations

Angiofibroma often occurs in the first decade of life, and is usually seen in children with tuberous sclerosis complex (TSC) (1–6). TSC has an autosomal-dominant mode of inheritance. It can result from mutations of two separate genes: *TSC1* located at 9q34 and *TSC2* located at 16p13. These encode for the tumor suppressor proteins hamartin and tuberin, respectively. Some of the cutaneous manifestations of TSC include angiofibroma, white macules ("ash leaf sign"), shagreen patches, skin tags, and subungual and periungual angiofibromas. These findings are discussed extensively (1). The main cutaneous manifestation to affect the eyelid area is angiofibroma, which for years has been called "adenoma sebaceum." This is a misnomer, because the tumor is not a neoplasm of sebaceous gland, but rather an angiofibroma with normal or slightly hyperplastic sebaceous glands. The best-known intraocular lesion is the astrocytic hamartoma, which is discussed in the *Atlas and Textbook of Intraocular Tumors*. This section covers angiofibroma of the eyelid area and other common cutaneous features of TSC.

Clinical Features

Angiofibroma of TSC appears as multiple red-brown papules on the skin, often in a butterfly distribution in the ocular area. They are slightly soft to palpation and movable with manipulation. They generally become clinically apparent during early childhood and are rarely identified at birth. The affected patient should be evaluated for retinal astrocytic hamartomas and for systemic findings of TSC, including depigmented cutaneous macules ("ash leaf sign"), calcified cerebral astrocytoma, cardiac rhabdomyoma, and renal angiomyolipoma.

Pathology

Histopathologically, angiofibroma is a fibrovascular hamartomatous proliferation composed of dermal fibrous tissue and dilated capillaries. The sebaceous glands may be atrophic or hyperplastic. The secondary sebaceous gland hyperplasia that is frequently present has led to the erroneous designation of "adenoma sebaceum."

Management

Smaller angiofibromas of the eyelids can be observed but larger lesions may require excision by standard techniques.

Selected References

Reviews

1. Shields JA, Shields CL. The systemic hamartomatoses ("Phakomatoses"). In: Shields JA, Shields CL. *Intraocular Tumors. A Text and Atlas*. Philadelphia, PA: WB Saunders; 1992:516–518.
2. Rowley SA, O'Callaghan FJ, Osborne JP. Ophthalmic manifestations of tuberous sclerosis: a population based study. *Br J Ophthalmol* 2001;85(4):420–423.

Case Reports

3. Hayashi N, Borodic G, Karesh JW, et al. Giant cell angiofibroma of the orbit and eyelid. *Ophthalmology* 1999;106:1223–1229.
4. Mawn LA, Jordan DR, Nerad J, et al. Giant cell angiofibroma of the eyelids: an unusual presentation of tuberous sclerosis. *Ophthalmic Surg Lasers* 1999;30:320–322.
5. Zolli C, Rodrigues MM, Shannon GM. Unusual eyelid involvement in tuberous sclerosis. *J Pediatr Ophthalmol* 1976;13:156–151.
6. Lopez JP, Ossandón D, Miller P, et al. Unilateral eyelid angiofibroma with complete blepharoptosis as the presenting sign of tuberous sclerosis. *J AAPOS* 2009;13(4):413–414.

EYELID AND FACIAL ANGIOFIBROMA WITH TUBEROUS SCLEROSIS COMPLEX

Cutaneous angiofibroma can be isolated but is more often associated with TSC. Illustrated is the typical eyelid angiofibroma and some other associated cutaneous findings of TSC. The fundus and brain manifestations of TSC are further discussed in the *Atlas of Intraocular Tumors*.

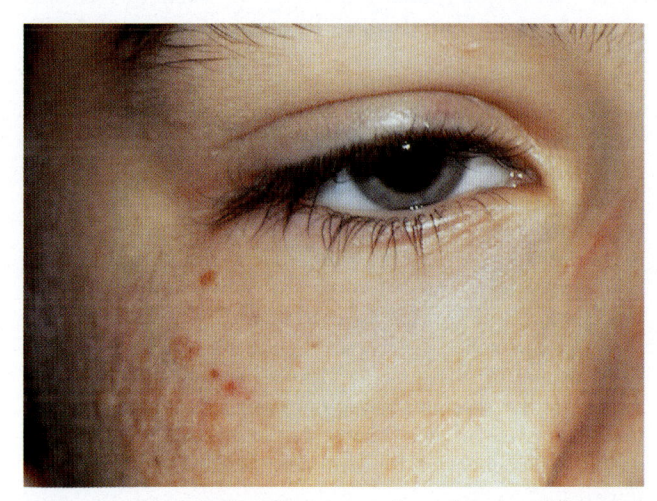

Figure 10.25. Subtle angiofibromas on face of 9-year-old boy with tuberous sclerosis complex.

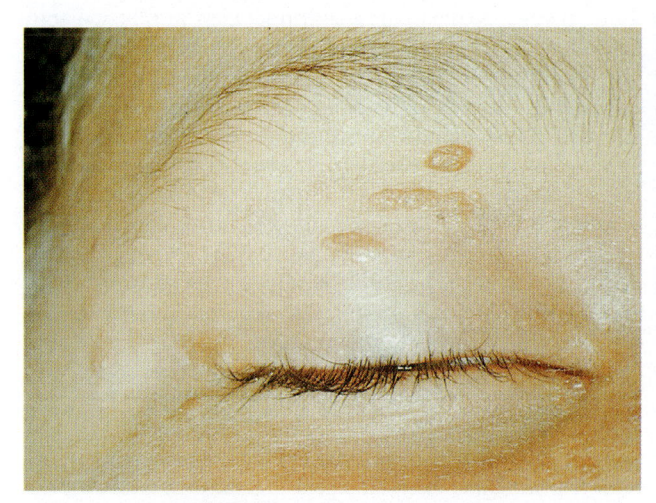

Figure 10.26. Angiofibromas on upper eyelid of a 10-year-old girl with tuberous sclerosis complex.

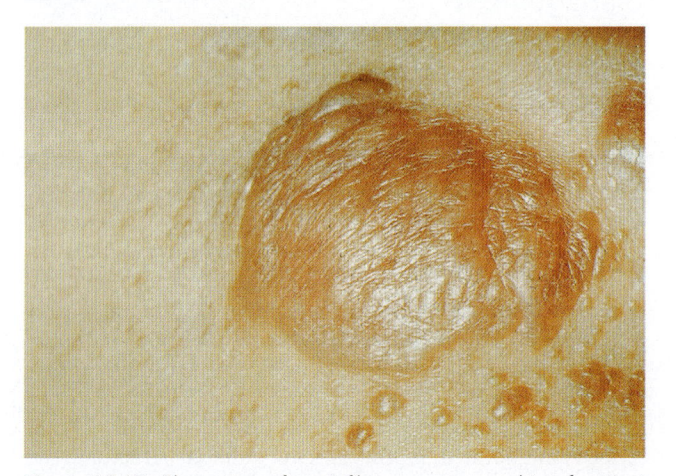

Figure 10.27. Close view of angiofibroma seen on chin of patient shown in Figure 10.26 showing typical appearance of a lesion.

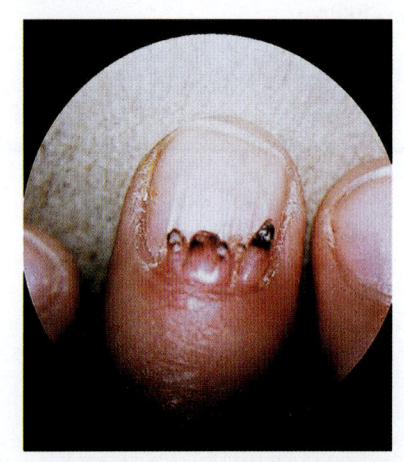

Figure 10.28. Presumed angiofibroma adjacent to fingernail in a patient with tuberous sclerosis complex. (Courtesy of Joseph Calhoun, MD.)

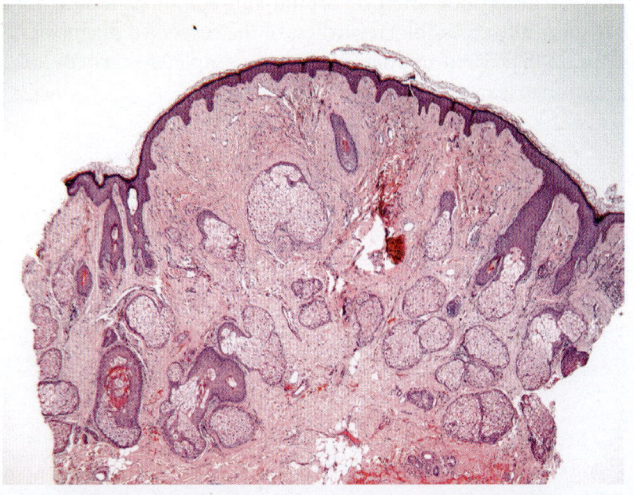

Figure 10.29. Histopathology of angiofibroma showing dermal fibrous tissue and sebaceous gland hyperplasia. (Hematoxylin–eosin ×50.)

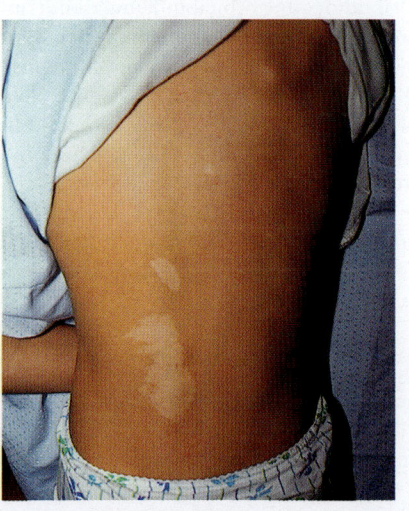

Figure 10.30. Cutaneous hypopigmented macule in patient with tuberous sclerosis complex ("ash leaf sign").

EYELID NODULAR FASCIITIS

General Considerations

Nodular fasciitis is a benign, reactive, pseudoneoplastic condition that generally occurs as a distinct mass in subcutaneous tissues of the trunk and upper extremities in adults (1–18). The etiology is unknown and it appears to have no systemic associations. Because of its rapid onset and progression, nodular fasciitis can simulate a malignant neoplasm clinically. In 1955, Konwaler et al. elucidated the benign nature of nodular fasciitis and stressed that it was a reactive condition rather than a malignancy (3). Subsequently, other reported series have substantiated the benign nature of this condition. Nodular fasciitis usually occurs in the head and neck region of children.

In 1966, Font and Zimmerman reported the occurrence of nodular fasciitis in the ocular region in a series of 10 cases (1). Their report was primarily a histopathologic study with limited clinical correlation. Since the initial series of Font and Zimmerman, there have been several additional reports of nodular fasciitis occurring in the ocular region (4–18). The reported cases have been tabulated in a detailed review of the subject (4). Although most cases of nodular fasciitis in the ocular region have occurred in adults, it has also been seen frequently in children.

Clinical Features

Most affected patients present with a fairly rapid onset of a visible or palpable subcutaneous mass without proptosis or displacement of the globe. Pain may be minimal or absent; severe pain is exceptional. Nodular fasciitis tends to occur in anterior periocular structures and it only rarely arises in the deep orbit (9). Several cases have been reported to develop on the epibulbar surface, presumably arising from Tenon's fascia (1). Those on the epibulbar surface have most often occurred near the insertion of a rectus muscle, although it can rarely develop at the corneoscleral limbus and rarely exhibit intraocular extension (1,4,10).

The clinical differential diagnosis of nodular fasciitis includes many tumors of adulthood and childhood. The rather rapid onset and progression of the mass may suggest a ruptured dermoid cyst, idiopathic orbital inflammation ("inflammatory pseudotumor"), eosinophilic granuloma, rhabdomyosarcoma, metastatic neuroblastoma, or myeloid sarcoma (leukemia, chloroma). Imaging studies such as computed tomography and magnetic resonance imaging may be helpful in excluding some of these conditions. Eosinophilic granuloma and metastatic neuroblastoma tend to arise within bone and to produce distinctive osseous changes. However, it can be difficult with imaging studies to differentiate nodular fasciitis from malignant tumors of soft tissue, such as rhabdomyosarcoma and myeloid sarcoma.

Pathology

Histopathologically, nodular fasciitis closely resembles a malignant spindle cell tumor, including rhabdomyosarcoma and fibrosarcoma. Hence, it is sometimes called "pseudosarcomatous fasciitis" (1–4). The histopathologic diagnosis of nodular fasciitis can be challenging. Abundant spindle cells, often with mitotic activity, can raise the possibility of rhabdomyosarcoma or another soft tissue sarcoma. Pathologists experienced with soft tissue tumors usually can make the diagnosis based on characteristic light microscopic features. Plump, mitotically active stellate or spindle-shaped fibroblasts are often arranged in parallel bundles and extend in all directions, resembling cells in a tissue culture. There are variable amounts of myxoid ground substance intermixed with the fibroblasts. The cells are much larger than mature fibroblasts and their nuclei are far more active in appearance. Numerous newly formed parallel capillaries often ramify through the lesion, forming slitlike spaces reminiscent of those seen in Kaposi's sarcoma.

Immunohistochemistry and electron microscopy can assist in the diagnosis. With immunohistochemistry, nodular fasciitis shows positive reactions for smooth muscle actin and vimentin. With electron microscopy, one sees parallel bundles of actinlike filaments with fusiform densities as seen with smooth muscle tumors (2).

Management

Even though nodular fasciitis is a benign self-limited disorder, the mass is usually excised because of suspected malignancy. It can sometimes recur locally. Reported cases of nodular fasciitis in the ocular area have been managed by surgical excision. Consequently, the natural course of this condition is not well established. Because it represents a reactive process, one may speculate that it would respond to corticosteroids or undergo spontaneous regression. A recently reported case of nodular fasciitis in the arm showed a favorable response following intralesional steroids (15). However, because it may be impossible to differentiate from rhabdomyosarcoma clinically and radiographically, surgical excision is generally the most appropriate management.

Because ocular nodular fasciitis usually is well circumscribed and located in the anterior adnexal structures, we recommend complete surgical removal, rather than a partial diagnostic biopsy. This principle should generally apply to all well-circumscribed anterior orbital and epibulbar lesions that are surgically accessible, regardless of the suspected diagnosis. It appears that when nodular fasciitis is completely excised, local recurrence is extremely rare or nonexistent.

EYELID NODULAR FASCIITIS

Selected References

Reviews
1. Font RL, Zimmerman LE. Nodular fasciitis of the eye and adnexa. *Arch Ophthalmol* 1967;75:475–481.

Histopathology
2. Sakamoto T, Ishibashi T, Ohnishi Y, et al. Immunohistological and electron microscopical study of nodular fasciitis of the orbit. *Br J Ophthalmol* 1991;75:636–638.

Case Reports
3. Konwaler BE, Keasbey L, Kaplan L. Subcutaneous pseudosarcomatous fibromatosis (fasciitis). *Am J Clin Pathol* 1955;25:241–252.
4. Shields JA, Shields CL, Christian C, et al. Orbital nodular fasciitis simulating a dermoid cyst in an eight-month-old infant. *Ophthal Plast Reconstr Surg* 2001;17:144–148.
5. Tolls RE, Mohr S, Spencer WH. Benign nodular fasciitis originating in Tenon's capsule. *Arch Ophthalmol* 1966;75:482–483.
6. Levitt JM, deVeer JA, Ogushan C. Orbital nodular fasciitis. *Arch Ophthalmol* 1969;81:235–237.
7. Meacham CT. Pseudosarcomatous fasciitis. *Am J Ophthalmol* 1974;77:747–749.
8. Ferry AP, Sherman SE. Nodular fasciitis of the conjunctiva apparently originating in the fascia bulbi (Tenon's capsule). *Am J Ophthalmol* 1974;78:514–517.
9. Perry RH, Ramani PS, McAllister SR, et al. Nodular fasciitis causing unilateral proptosis. *Br J Ophthalmol* 1975;59:404–408.
10. Holds FB, Mamalis N, Anderson RL. Nodular fasciitis presenting as rapidly enlarging episcleral mass in a 3-year-old. *J Pediatr Ophthalmol Strabismus* 1990;27:157–160.
11. Vestal KP, Bauer TW, Berlin AJ. Nodular fasciitis presenting as an eyelid mass. *Ophthalmol Plast Reconstr Surg* 1990;6:130–132.
12. Reccia FM, Buckley EG, Townshend LM, et al. Nodular fasciitis of the orbital rim in a pediatric patient. *J Pediatr Ophthalmol Strabismus* 1997;34:316–318.
13. Hymas D, Mamalis N, Pratt DV, et al. Nodular fasciitis of the lower eyelid in a pediatric patient. *Ophthal Plast Reconstr Surg* 1999;15:139–142.
14. Graham BS, Barrett TL, Goltz RW. Nodular fasciitis: response to intralesional corticosteroids. *J Am Acad Dermatol* 1999;40:490–492.
15. Husain A, Cummings T, Richard MJ, et al. Nodular fasciitis presenting in an adult woman. *Ophthal Plast Reconstr Surg* 2011;27(6):e168–e170.
16. de Paula SA, Cruz AA, de Alencar VM, et al. Nodular fasciitis presenting as a large mass in the upper eyelid. *Ophthal Plast Reconstr Surg* 2006;22(6):494–495.
17. Stone DU, Chodosh J. Epibulbar nodular fasciitis associated with floppy eyelids. *Cornea* 2005;24(3):361–362.
18. Meffert JJ, Kennard CD, Davis TL, et al. Intradermal nodular fasciitis presenting as an eyelid mass. *Int J Dermatol* 1996;35(8):548–552.

EYELID NODULAR FASCIITIS

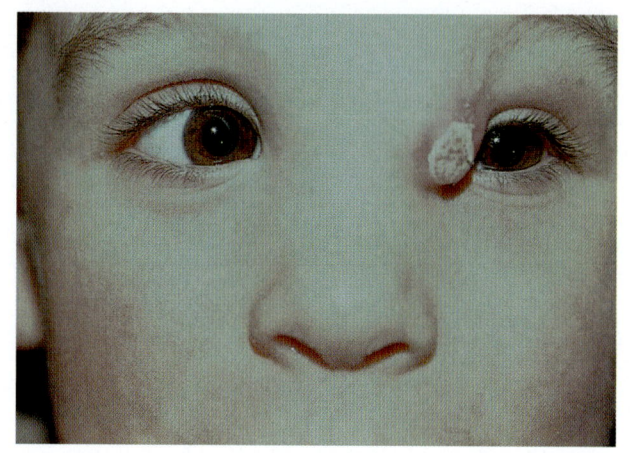

Figure 10.31. Lesion near medial canthus in a 3-year-old boy. The lesion appeared as a painless, rapidly progressive lesion that did not recur after incomplete excision. (Courtesy of Russell Manthey, MD.)

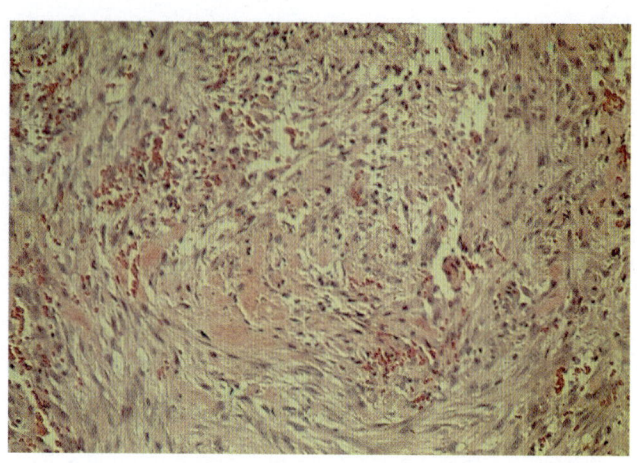

Figure 10.32. Histopathology of case shown in Figure 10.31 showing whorls of closely compact spindle cells. (Hematoxylin–eosin ×150.) (Courtesy of Russell Manthey, MD.)

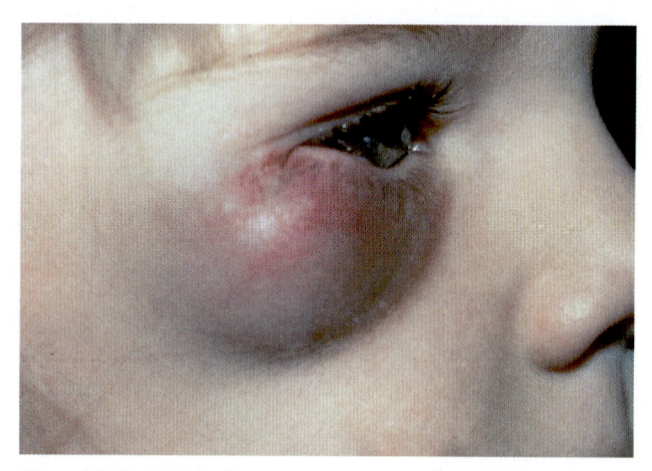

Figure 10.33. Nodular fasciitis occurring as a rapidly enlarging subcutaneous mass in lateral portion of the eyelid in a 2-year-old girl. (Courtesy of Mark Ost, MD.)

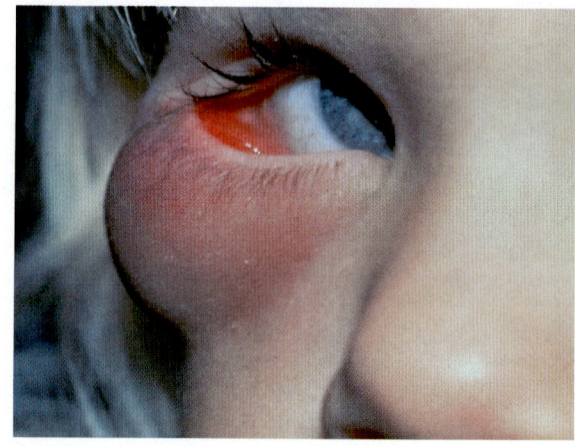

Figure 10.34. Another view of lesion shown in Figure 10.33, showing adjacent involvement of conjunctiva. (Courtesy of Mark Ost, MD.)

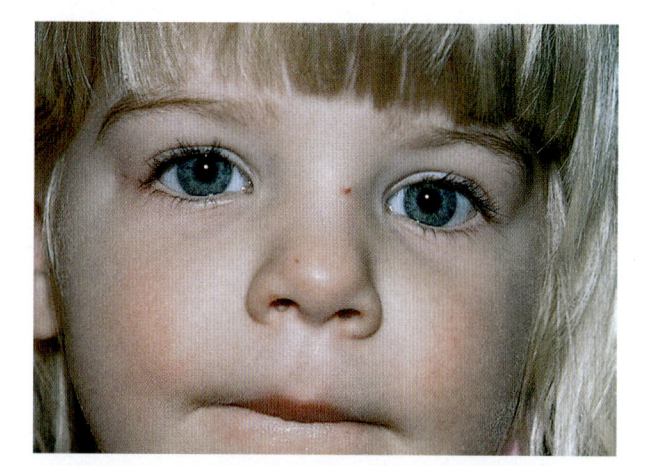

Figure 10.35. Appearance of patient shown in Figure 10.33 showing good result after excision of the lesion. (Courtesy of Mark Ost, MD.)

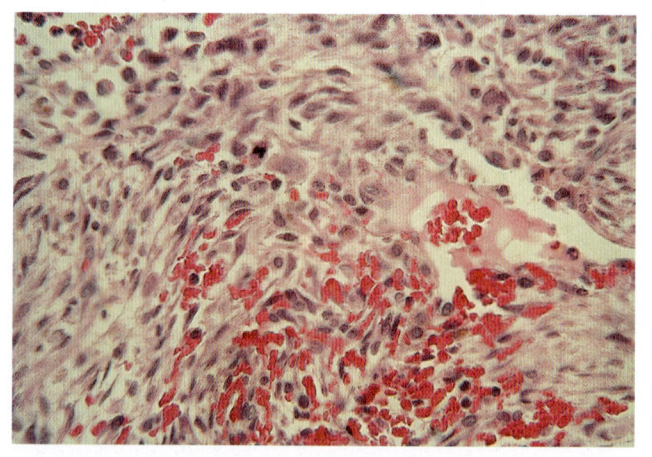

Figure 10.36. Histopathology of lesion shown in Figure 10.33 showing closely compact spindle cells and operative hemorrhage. (Hematoxylin–eosin ×150.) (Courtesy of Mark Ost, MD.)

Chapter 10 Eyelid Histiocytic, Myxoid, and Fibrous Lesions

EYELID NODULAR FASCIITIS: CLINICOPATHOLOGIC CORRELATION

Depicted is a case of nodular fasciitis that resembled clinically a dermoid cyst.

Shields JA, Shields CL, Christian C, et al. Orbital nodular fasciitis simulating a dermoid cyst in an 8-month-old infant. *Ophthal Plast Reconstr Surg* 2001;17:144–148.

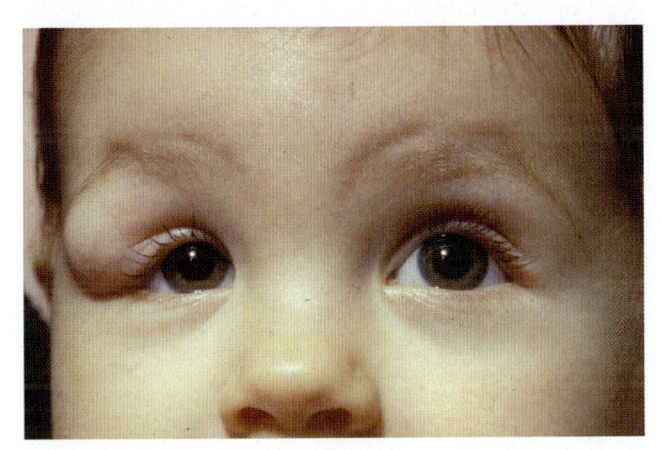

Figure 10.37. Subcutaneous mass superotemporal to the right eye in an 8-month-old boy, resembling a dermoid cyst.

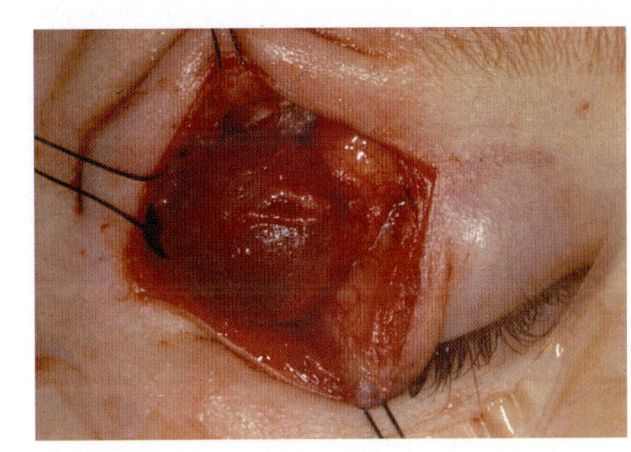

Figure 10.38. Appearance of lesion at surgery, showing exposure of circumscribed mass.

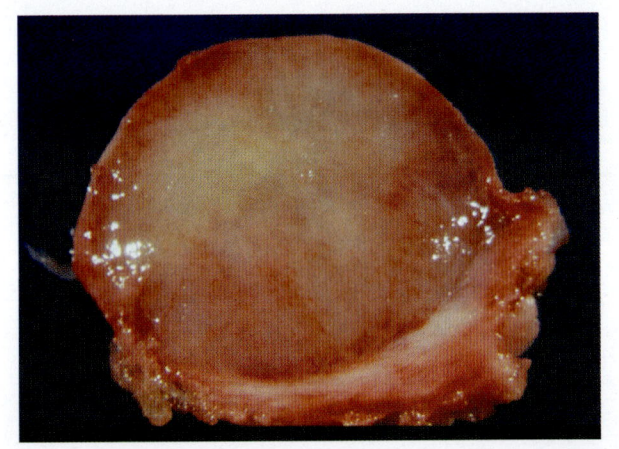

Figure 10.39. Gross appearance of sectioned tumor after removal.

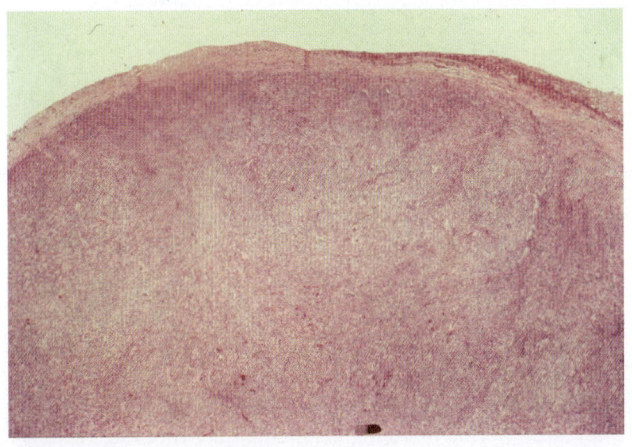

Figure 10.40. Low-magnification photomicrograph showing compact spindle cells. (Hematoxylin–eosin ×10.)

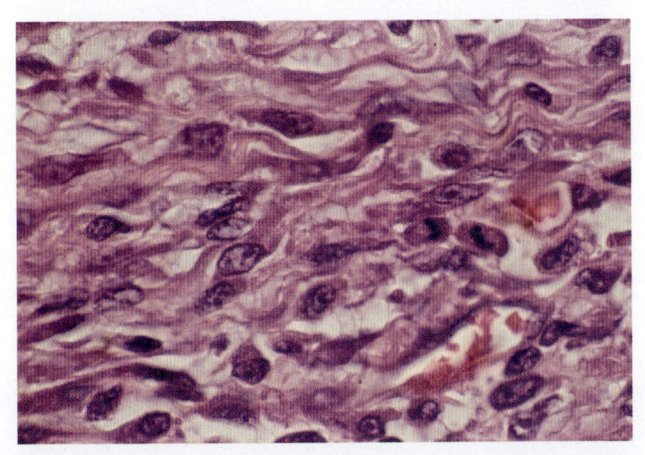

Figure 10.41. Higher-magnification photomicrograph showing intertwining spindle cells and mitotic activity. The lesion superficially resembles a sarcoma. (Hematoxylin–eosin ×150.)

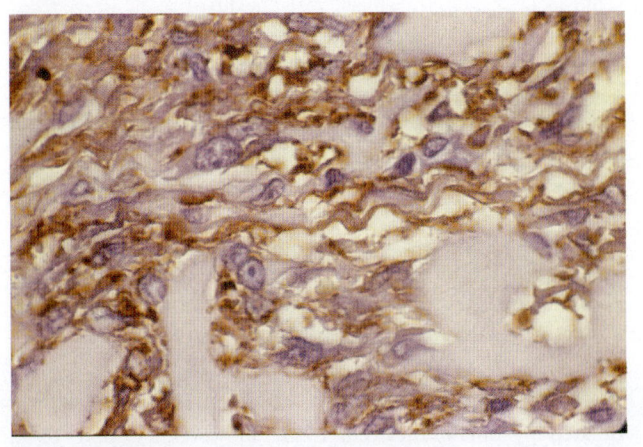

Figure 10.42. Immunohistochemistry shows positive reaction to muscle-specific actin. (×150.)

EYELID MISCELLANEOUS FIBROUS AND MYXOMATOUS TUMORS

There are several other fibrous and myxomatous tumors that can rarely affect the eyelids, they are mentioned for completeness. Selected examples include juvenile fibromatosis, fibrous histiocytoma, fibrosarcoma, myxoma, and multicentric reticulohistiocytosis (1–24). Some of these conditions may overlap clinically and histopathology and a precise classification is difficult. Spindle cell tumors, like nodular fasciitis, fibromatosis, fibrous histiocytoma, and fibrosarcoma, may require knowledge of the clinical history and the assistance of an excellent pathologist to make the definitive diagnosis. Some of these lesions are more likely to occur in the orbit and are discussed in more detail in the section on orbital tumors.

Juvenile Fibromatosis

Juvenile fibromatosis is a benign, fibrous tissue proliferation that can occasionally affect the eyelid area of young children as a diffuse, nonencapsulated subcutaneous growth (1–9). It has a tendency to affect the lower eyelid and inferior orbit. The mean age at diagnosis is 8 years. The differential diagnosis includes leiomyoma, neurofibroma, and well-differentiated fibrosarcoma. Local excision may be difficult and recurrence is common.

Fibrous Histiocytoma

Fibrous histiocytoma is a soft tissue tumor composed of a proliferation of fibroblasts and histiocytes. Although it is better known to occur in the orbital tissues, it can occasionally affect the eyelid as a subcutaneous mass (10,11). It is more common in young adults. Although fibrous histiocytoma of the eyelid is a benign tumor, some orbital fibrous histiocytomas are malignant.

Fibrosarcoma

Fibrosarcoma is a malignant neoplasm that can develop spontaneously or can occur in the eyelid and orbital region following irradiation for the hereditary form of retinoblastoma. The primary form occurs in young children with a mean age at diagnosis of 4 years. Clinically, this tumor is poorly circumscribed and grows rather rapidly (12–15). It is composed histopathologically of immature spindle-shaped fibroblastic cells in a classic herringbone pattern or in interlacing fascicles. Mitotic figures are often abundant. The best management is wide surgical excision when necessary, which may necessitate orbital exenteration in some cases, particularly if the tumor is incompletely removed or recurs (4). Supplemental chemotherapy or irradiation may be necessary depending on the clinical circumstances. Although the tumor can recur locally after incomplete excision, metastasis is uncommon and the systemic prognosis for the primary type is favorable. The prognosis for a patient with radiation-induced fibrosarcoma is less favorable because of risk for additional new cancers associated with the hereditary form of retinoblastoma.

Myxoma

Isolated myxoma of the eyelid is rare. However, it appears to be more common in patients with Carney's complex, a syndrome that includes cardiac myxoma, cutaneous myxoma, myxoid fibroadenoma of the breast, spotty mucocutaneous pigmentation, testicular tumors, adrenal hyperplasia, melanotic schwannoma, and other benign and malignant neoplasms (16–20). A patient with an eyelid myxoma should be evaluated for the various components of Carney's complex (16–20,23,24). Histopathology shows scattered benign spindle cells in a loose, myxoid stroma.

Multicentric Reticulohistiocytosis

Multicentric reticulohistiocytosis is a rare systemic disorder characterized by an idiopathic proliferation of histiocytes (21,22). The affected patient typically has multiple cutaneous nodules. The lesions can occasionally affect the eyelids. Periosteal and bone involvement can lead to destructive arthritis.

EYELID MISCELLANEOUS FIBROUS AND MYXOMATOUS TUMORS

Selected References

Juvenile Fibromatosis
1. Hidayat AA, Font RL. Juvenile fibromatosis of the periorbital region and eyelid: a clinicopathologic study of 6 cases. *Arch Ophthalmol* 1980;98:280–285.
2. Andrew N, Dodd T, Selva D, et al. Tendon sheath fibroma of the medial canthal tendon. *Ophthal Plast Reconstr Surg* 2013;29(1):e1–e2.
3. Mencía-Gutiérrez E, Gutiérrez-Díaz E, Ricoy JR, et al. Re: "trichoblastic fibroma of the eyelid." *Ophthal Plast Reconstr Surg* 2012;28(1):77.
4. Wladis EJ, Linos K, Carlson JA. Trichoblastic fibroma of the eyelid. *Ophthal Plast Reconstr Surg* 2012;28(3):e62–e64.
5. Joung Lee M, Khwarg S. Fibroma of the medial canthal area: a case report. *Ophthal Plast Reconstr Surg* 2011;27(1):e21–e23.
6. Kohl SK, Persidsky I, Gigantelli JW. Tendon sheath fibroma of the medial canthus. *Ophthal Plast Reconstr Surg* 2007;23(4):341–342.
7. Clinch TJ, Kostick DA, Menke DM. Tarsal fibroma. *Am J Ophthalmol* 2000;129(5):691–693.
8. Sandinha T, Lee WR, Reid R. Pleomorphic fibroma of the eyelid. *Graefes Arch Clin Exp Ophthalmol* 1998;236(5):333–338.
9. Boynton JR, Markowitch W Jr, Searl SS. Atypical fibroxanthoma of the eyelid. *Ophthalmology* 1989;96(10):1480–1484.

Fibrous Histiocytoma
10. Font RL, Hidayat AA. Fibrous histiocytoma of the orbit. A clinicopathologic study of 150 cases. *Hum Pathol* 1982;13:199–209.
11. Jakobiec FA, DeVoe AG, Boyd J. Fibrous histiocytoma of the tarsus. *Am J Ophthalmol* 1977;84(6):794–797.

Fibrosarcoma
12. Weiner JM, Hidayat AA. Juvenile fibrosarcoma of the orbit and eyelid. A study of five cases. *Arch Ophthalmol* 1983;101;253–259.
13. Chawla B, Pushker N, Sen S, et al. Recurrent bilateral dermatofibrosarcoma protuberans of eyelids. *Ophthal Plast Reconstr Surg* 2011;27(6):e167–e168.
14. Brazzo BG, Saffra N. Dermatofibrosarcoma protuberans of the brow and eyelid. *Ophthal Plast Reconstr Surg* 2004;20(4):332–334.
15. Li J, Ge X, Ma JM, et al. Dermatofibrosarcoma protuberans. *Ophthalmology* 2012;119(1):197.e1–e3.

Carney's Complex
16. Kennedy RH, Waller RR, Carney JA. Ocular pigmented spots and eyelid myxomas. *Am J Ophthalmol* 1987;104:533–538.
17. Grossniklaus HE, McLean IW, Gillespie JJ. Bilateral eyelid myxomas in Carney's complex. *Br J Ophthalmol* 1991;75:251–252.
18. Kennedy RH, Flanagan JC, Eagle RC, et al. The Carney complex with ocular signs suggestive of cardiac myxoma. *Am J Ophthalmol* 1991;11:699–702.
19. Hartstein ME, Thomas SM, Ellis LS. Orbital desmoid tumor in a pediatric patient. *Ophthal Plast Reconstr Surg* 2006;22(2):139–141.
20. Tsilou ET, Chan CC, Sandrini F, et al. Eyelid myxoma in Carney complex without PRKAR1A allelic loss. *Am J Med Genet A* 2004;130A(4):395–397.

Multicentric Reticulohistiocytosis
21. Eagle RC Jr, Penne RA, Hneleski IS Jr. Eyelid involvement in multicentric reticulohistiocytosis. *Ophthalmology* 1995;102:426–430.
22. Jakobiec FA, Kirzhner M, Tollett MM, et al. Solitary epithelioid histiocytoma (reticulohistiocytoma) of the eyelid. *Arch Ophthalmol* 2011;129(11):1502–1504.

Angiomyxoma
23. Ali N, Child CS, Michaelides M, et al. Recurrence of a rare skin tumour: superficial angiomyxoma in the eyelid. *Can J Ophthalmol* 2011;46(2):205–206.
24. Yuen HK, Cheuk W, Luk FO, et al. Solitary superficial angiomyxoma in the eyelid. *Am J Ophthalmol* 2005;139(6):1141–1142.

EYELID JUVENILE FIBROMATOSIS, FIBROUS HISTIOCYTOMA, AND FIBROSARCOMA

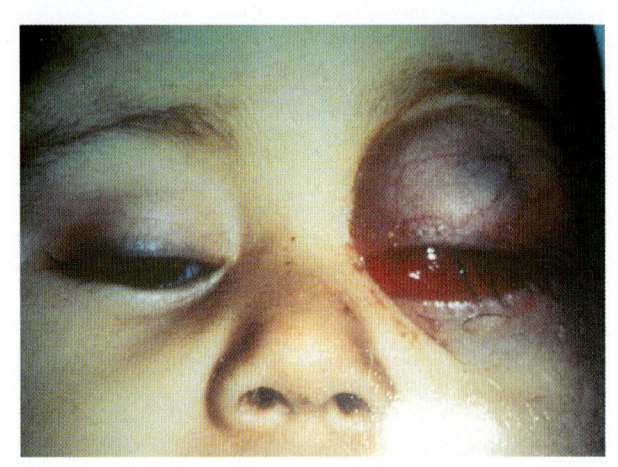

Figure 10.43. Juvenile fibromatosis in a 5-month-old child with massive involvement of upper eyelid and involvement of the orbit. The lesion was noted at birth and enlarged slowly.

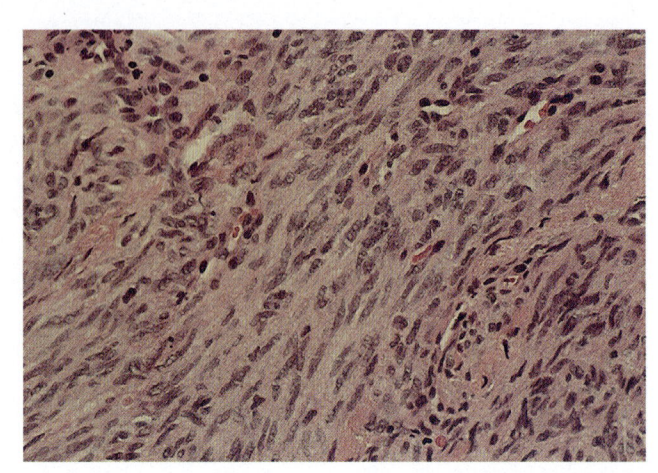

Figure 10.44. Histopathology of juvenile fibromatosis, showing closely compact spindle cells. (Hematoxylin–eosin ×150.) (Courtesy of Charles Lee, MD.)

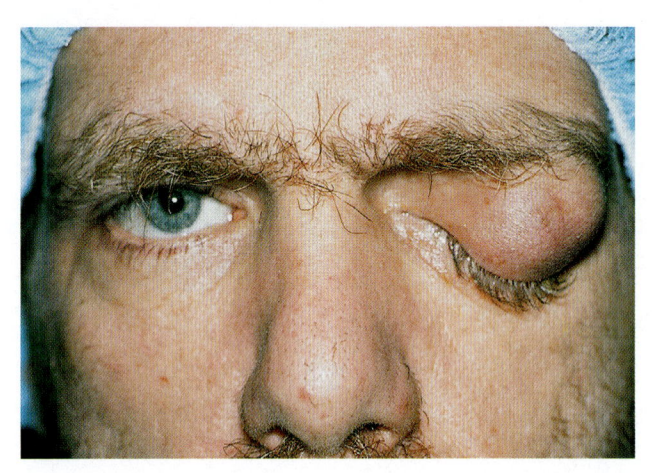

Figure 10.45. Fibrous histiocytoma of upper eyelid in a 37-year-old man. The lesion showed slow enlargement over 2 years. (Courtesy of Norman Charles, MD.)

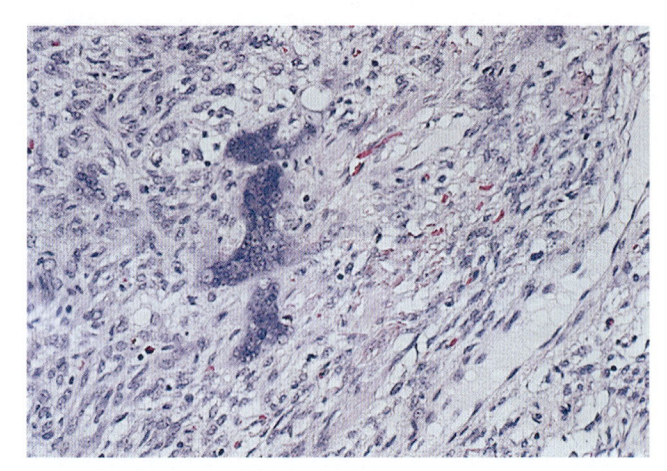

Figure 10.46. Histopathology of lesion shown in Figure 10.45. The mass is composed of fibroblasts, histiocytes, and large atypical hyperchromatic giant cells. (Hematoxylin–eosin ×175.) (Courtesy of Norman Charles, MD.)

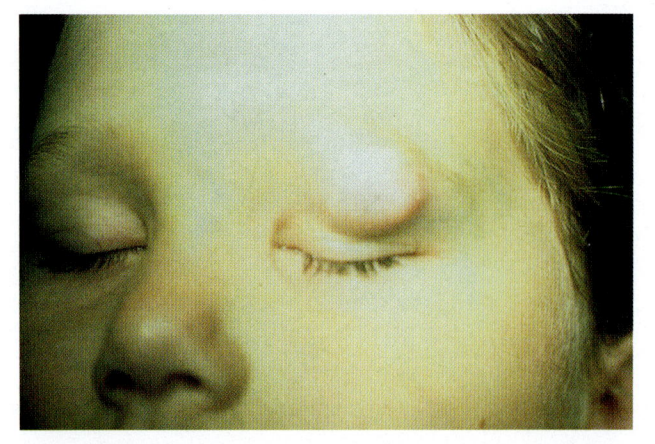

Figure 10.47. Fibrosarcoma of upper eyelid in an 8-year-old girl. It was successfully excised and there has been no recurrence after 15 years.

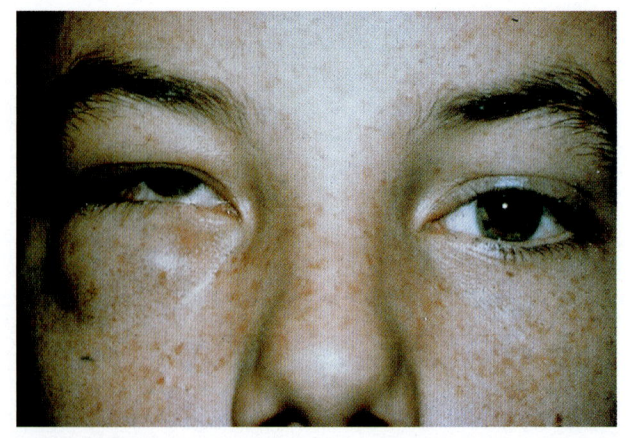

Figure 10.48. Recurrent fibrosarcoma of lower eyelid in a 15-year-old boy. The lesion was resected 8 years earlier and gradually returned. Orbital exenteration was subsequently performed. (Courtesy of Ahmed Hidayat, MD.)

Chapter 10 Eyelid Histiocytic, Myxoid, and Fibrous Lesions

EYELID MYXOMA AND MULTICENTRIC RETICULOHISTIOCYTOSIS

1. Grossniklaus HE, McLean IW, Gillespie JJ. Bilateral eyelid myxomas in Carney's complex. Br J Ophthalmol 2991;75:251–252.
2. Eagle RC Jr, Penne RA, Hneleski IS Jr. Eyelid involvement in multicentric reticulohistiocytosis. Ophthalmology 1995;102:426–430.

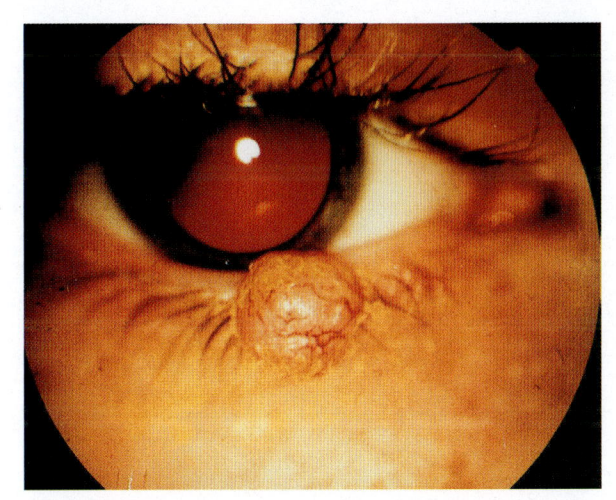

Figure 10.49. Myxoma of right lower eyelid in a 21-year-old man with Carney's complex. The patient also had spotty skin pigmentation and similar cutaneous lesions on ear and in groin. (Courtesy of Hans Grossniklaus, MD.)

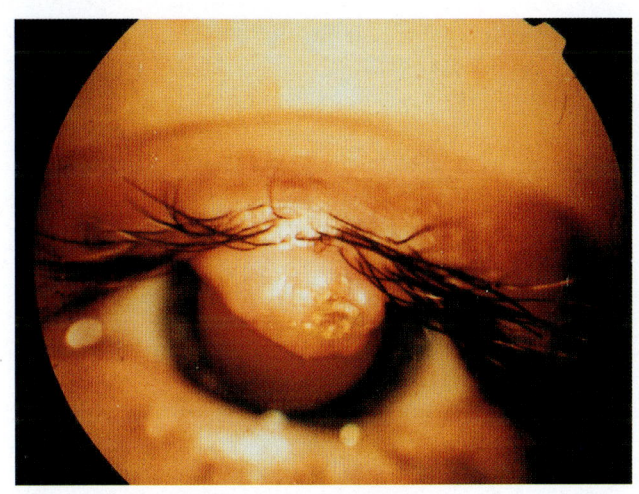

Figure 10.50. Myxoma of left upper eyelid in same patient shown in Figure 10.49. (Courtesy of Hans Grossniklaus, MD.)

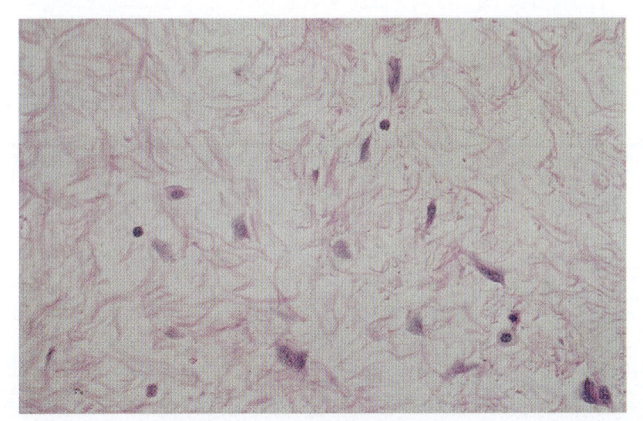

Figure 10.51. Histopathology of lesion shown in Figure 10.49, showing scattered spindle cells in a loose, myxoid stroma. (Hematoxylin–eosin ×200.) (Courtesy of Hans Grossniklaus, MD.)

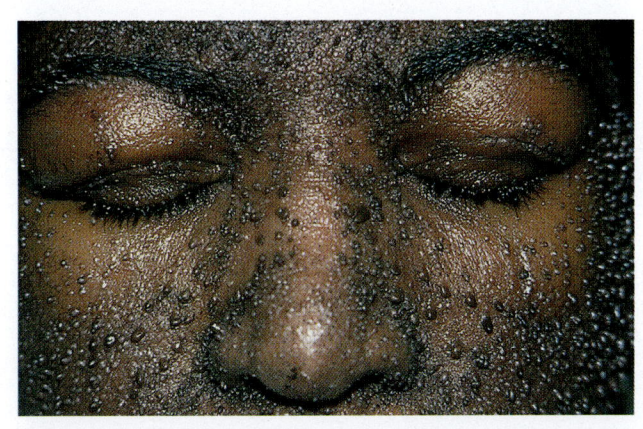

Figure 10.52. Facial and eyelid lesions in a 25-year-old woman with multicentric reticulohistiocytosis. (Courtesy of Robert Penne, MD.)

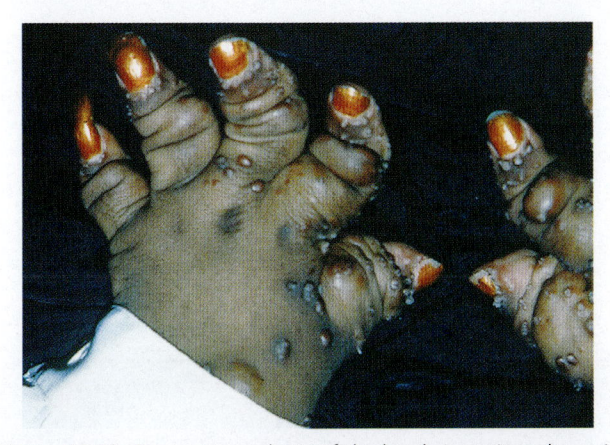

Figure 10.53. Destructive arthritis of the hands in patient shown in Figure 10.52. (Courtesy of Robert Penne, MD.)

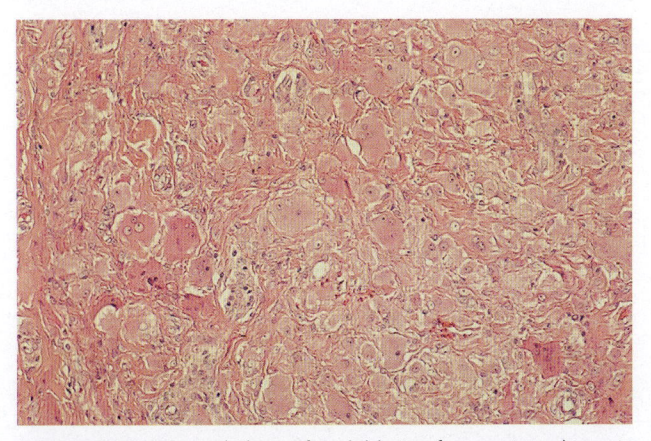

Figure 10.54. Histopathology of eyelid lesion from patient shown in Figure 10.52, showing histiocytic proliferation and giant cells. (Hematoxylin–eosin ×100.) (Courtesy of Ralph C. Eagle Jr, MD.)

CHAPTER 11

EYELID CYSTIC LESIONS SIMULATING NEOPLASMS

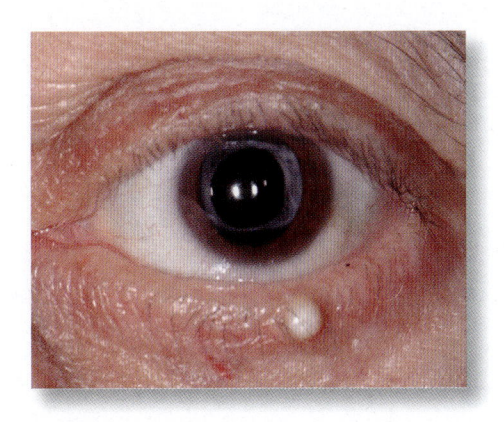

General Considerations

There are a number of cutaneous cystic lesions that can simulate neoplasms. In this section we discuss some of the more important ones that can affect the eyelids, beginning with eccrine hidrocystoma (1–11).

Eccrine hidrocystoma is a ductal retention cyst of an eccrine sweat gland. It appears to be more common in the eyelid region than elsewhere in the body. This tumor usually occurs on the cheeks and eyelids of adult women and may be similar clinically to other cutaneous cysts. In contrast to apocrine hidrocystoma, which is almost always solitary, eccrine hidrocystoma is more likely to be multiple. Eccrine hidrocystomas develop from retention of sweat. Heat, humidity, and perspiration can cause them to become larger, more numerous, and more symptomatic. Hence, they tend to increase in number and size in summer and decrease in winter.

Clinical Features

Clinically, eccrine hidrocystoma characteristically appears as a clear cystic translucent lesion, usually near the eyelid margin. The overlying skin is usually smooth and shiny (2,3). It may be indistinguishable clinically from apocrine hydrocystoma. This lesion can occasionally have a bluish color, a finding that is more common with apocrine hidrocystoma (to be discussed). Ultrasound biomicroscopy has been used to detect the cystic nature of the lesion and to differentiate it from melanoma and other solid tumors (5).

Pathology

Histopathologically, eccrine hidrocystoma is a clear cystic lesion lined by two layers of cuboidal epithelial cells. There is no evidence of apocrine decapitation secretion as seen with apocrine hidrocystoma. No myoepithelial cells are observed (1–11).

Management

Management includes observation or local excision. The cystic structure collapses if traumatized or surgically incised.

EYELID ECCRINE HIDROCYSTOMA

Selected References

Reviews
1. Elder D, Elenitsas R, Ragsdale BD. Tumors of the epidermal appendages. In: Elder D, Elenitsas R, Jaworsky C, et al., eds. *Lever's Histopathology of the Skin.* Philadelphia, PA: Lippincott-Raven; 1997:777–778.
2. Smith JD, Chernosky ME. Hidrocystomas. *Arch Dermatol* 1973;108:676–679.
3. Cordero AA, Montes LF. Eccrine hidrocystoma. *J Cutan Pathol* 1976;3:292–293.
4. Jakobiec FA, Zakka FR. A reappraisal of eyelid eccrine and apocrine hidrocystomas: microanatomic and immunohistochemical studies of 40 lesions. *Am J Ophthalmol* 2011;151(2):358–374.

Imaging
5. Furuta M, Shields CL, Danzig CJ, et al. Ultrasound biomicroscopy of eyelid eccrine hydrocystoma. *Can J Ophthalmol* 2007;42(5):750–751.

Case Reports
6. Yasaka N, Iozumi K, Nashiro K, et al. Bilateral periorbital eccrine hydrocystoma. *J Dermatol* 1994;21:490–493.
7. Al-Rohil RN, Meyer D, Slodkowska EA, et al. Pigmented Eyelid Cysts Revisited: Apocrine Retention Cyst Chromhidrosis. *Am J Dermatopathol* 2013;36(4):318–326.
8. Novitskaya E, Rene C, Dean A. Spontaneous haemorrhage in an eyelid hidrocystoma in a patient treated with clopidogrel. *Eye (Lond)* 2013;27(6):782–783.
9. Smith RJ, Kuo IC, Reviglio VE. Multiple apocrine hidrocystomas of the eyelids. *Orbit* 2012;31(2):140–142.
10. Hampton PJ, Angus B, Carmichael AJ. A case of Schöpf-Schulz-Passarge syndrome. *Clin Exp Dermatol* 2005;30(5):528–530.
11. Singh AD, McCloskey L, Parsons MA, et al. Eccrine hydrocystoma of the eyelid. *Eye (Lond)* 2005;19(1):77–79.

EYELID ECCRINE HIDROCYSTOMA

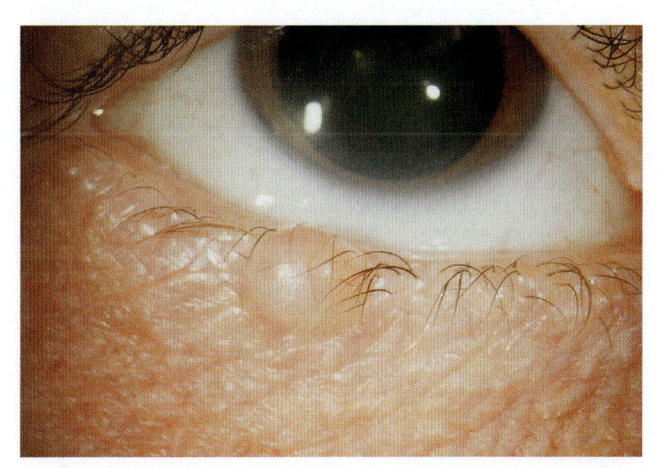

Figure 11.1. Solitary eccrine hidrocystoma of lower eyelid in a 62-year-old man.

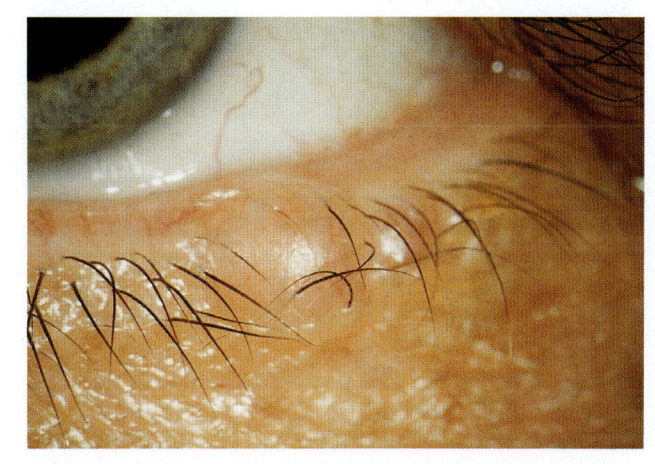

Figure 11.2. Solitary eccrine hidrocystoma of lower eyelid in a 67-year-old woman.

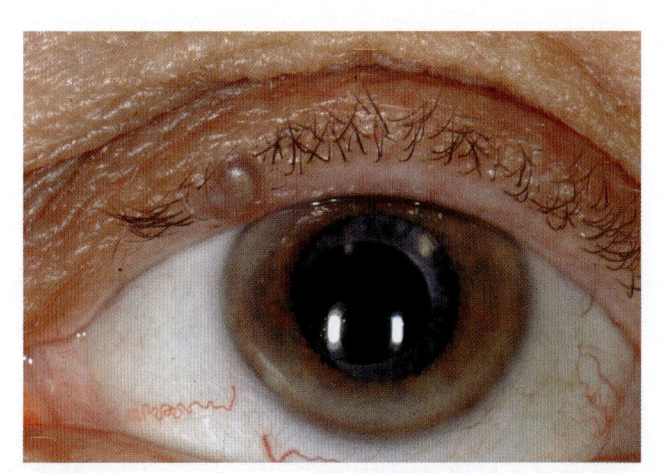

Figure 11.3. Slightly blue eccrine hidrocystoma of the left upper eyelid.

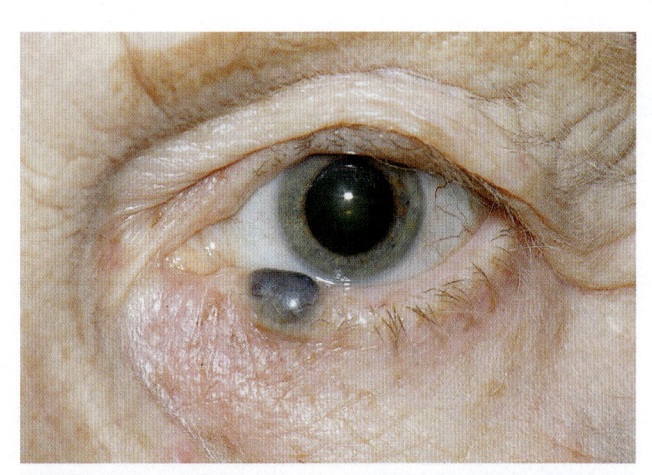

Figure 11.4. Blue-black eccrine hidrocystoma in a 75-year-old woman. This lesion appears pigmented, simulating a melanoma, a finding also common in apocrine hidrocystoma. Histopathologic studies confirmed eccrine hidrocystoma.

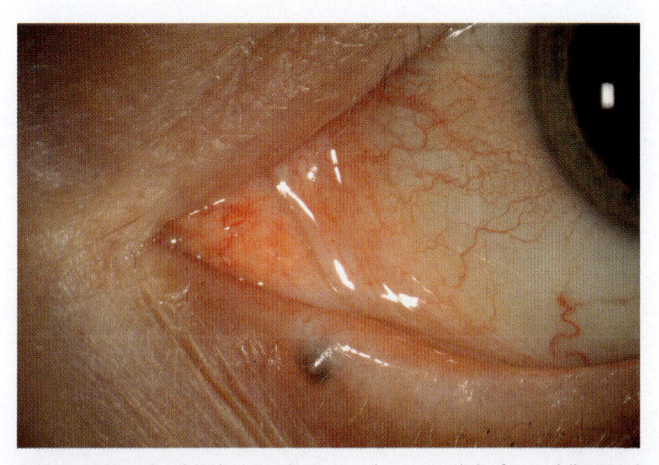

Figure 11.5. Blue-black cystic lesion on lower eyelid of a middle-aged woman. The lesion was excised.

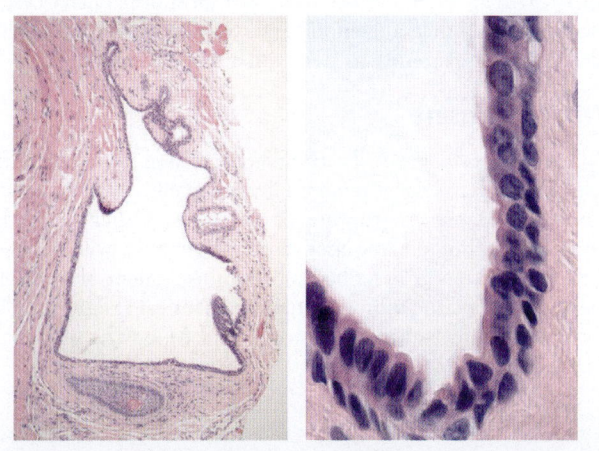

Figure 11.6. Photomicrograph of lesion shown in Figure 11.5, showing features of eccrine hidrocystoma. **Left picture** shows entire cyst removed intact. (Hematoxylin–eosin ×10.) **Right picture** shows double layer of epithelium lining the cyst. (Hematoxylin–eosin ×75.)

EYELID APOCRINE HIDROCYSTOMA

General Considerations

Apocrine hidrocystoma (apocrine cystadenoma; sudoriferous cyst) is a retention cyst of an apocrine gland (1–17). This cyst can develop from the apocrine glands of the eyelids (glands of Moll), in which case it usually occurs near the eyelid margin, corresponding to the orifices of Moll's glands. It is more common near the medial canthus. There is no gender predisposition. It generally occurs in adults, with a mean age of 55 years, but is occasionally seen in children.

Clinical Features

Apocrine hidrocystoma is a smooth or multiloculated cystic lesion that can develop on the eyelid, eyebrow, or near the medial or lateral canthus. It frequently has a bluish color and may resemble a blue nevus or melanoma. It can range from 1 mm to more than 1 cm in diameter.

Schöpf–Schulz–Passarge Syndrome

There is a variant of hereditary ectodermal dysplasia in which some cases have multiple apocrine hidrocystomas affecting both the upper and lower eyelids bilaterally. These patients can also demonstrate hypodontia, palmar–plantar hyperkeratosis, and onychodystrophy (10,11,14,15). This constellation of findings is called the Schöpf–Schulz–Passarge syndrome. Some cases appear isolated, while others have an autosomal-dominant or recessive pattern. This entity is described in more detail by Font et al. (11).

Pathology

Microscopically, apocrine hidrocystoma is a cystic lesion with a clear lumen lined by a double layer of cells. The innermost layer has apical snouts that project into the lumen, a characteristic feature of apocrine cells. The outermost layer consists of flattened myoepithelial cells. The cells also contain PAS-positive, diastase-resistant granules on their apical surfaces. Some authorities regard apocrine hidrocystoma as a form of papillary cystadenoma rather than a retention cyst, because the secretory cells do not appear flattened, as seen with a true retention cyst.

Management

Management is generally complete excision (4–6). Multiple lesions have been removed by an eyelid blepharoplasty approach to prevent rupture of the cysts. Other methods, including carbon dioxide laser vaporization, have been successful. A recent report described successful treatment of multiple periocular apocrine hidrocystomas by chemical ablation of the cyst epithelium with trichloroacetic acid (6,7). The prognosis is excellent.

Selected References

Reviews

1. Elder D, Elenitsas R, Ragsdale BD. Tumors of the epidermal appendages. In: Elder D, Elenitsas R, Jaworsky C, et al., eds. *Lever's Histopathology of the Skin*. Philadelphia, PA: Lippincott-Raven; 1997:769–770.
2. Smith JD, Chernosky ME. Apocrine hydrocystoma (cystadenoma). *Arch Dermatol* 1974;109:700.
3. Jakobiec FA, Zakka FR. A reappraisal of eyelid eccrine and apocrine hidrocystomas: microanatomic and immunohistochemical studies of 40 lesions. *Am J Ophthalmol* 2011;151(2):358–374.e2.

Management

4. Henderer JD, Tanenbaum M. Excision of multiple eyelid apocrine hidrocystomas via an en-bloc lower eyelid blepharoplasty incision. *Ophthalmic Surg Lasers* 2000;31:157–161.
5. del Pozo J, Garcia-Silva J, Pena-Penabad C, et al. Multiple apocrine hidrocystomas: treatment with carbon dioxide laser vaporization. *J Dermatol Treat* 2001;12:97–100.
6. Dailey RA, Saulny SM, Tower RN. Treatment of multiple apocrine hidrocystomas with trichloroacetic acid. *Ophthal Plast Reconstr Surg* 2005;21:148–150.
7. Shimizu A, Tamura A, Ishikawa O. Multiple apocrine hidrocystomas of the eyelids treated with trichloroacetic acid. *Eur J Dermatol* 2009;19(4):398–399.

Case Reports

8. Shields JA, Eagle RC Jr, Shields CL, et al. Apocrine hidrocystoma of the eyelid. *Arch Ophthalmol* 1993;111:866–867.
9. Combemale P, Kanitakis J, Dupin N, et al. Multiple Moll's gland cysts (apocrine hidrocystomas) of the eyelids. *Dermatology* 1997;194:195–196.
10. Schopf E, Schulz HJ, Passarge E. Syndrome of cystic eyelids, palmo-plantar keratosis, hypodontia, and hypotrichosis as a possible autosomal recessive trait. *Birth Defects* 1971;7:219–221.
11. Font RL, Stone MS, Schanzer C, et al. Apocrine hidrocystomas of the lids, hypodontia, palmar-plantar hyperkeratosis and onychodystrophy. *Arch Ophthalmol* 1986;104:1811–1813.
12. Alessi E, Gianotti R, Coggi A. Multiple apocrine hidrocystomas of the eyelids. *Br J Dermatol* 1997;137:642–645.
13. Mallaiah U, Dickinson J. Photo essay: bilateral multiple eyelid apocrine hidrocystomas and ectodermal dysplasia. *Arch Ophthalmol* 2001;119:186–187.
14. Gira AK, Robertson D, Swerlick RA. Multiple eyelid cysts with palmoplantar hyperkeratosis. Schopf-Schulz-Passarge syndrome. *Arch Dermatol* 2004;140:231–236.
15. Gira AK, Robertson D, Swerlick RA. Multiple eyelid cysts with palmoplantar hyperkeratosis. *Arch Dermatol* 2004;140:231–236.
16. Smith RJ, Kuo IC, Reviglio VE. Multiple apocrine hidrocystomas of the eyelids. *Orbit* 2012;31(2):140–142.
17. Milman T, Iacob C, McCormick SA. Hybrid cysts of the eyelid with follicular and apocrine differentiation: an under-recognized entity? *Ophthal Plast Reconstr Surg* 2008;24(2):122–125.

Chapter 11 Eyelid Cystic Lesions Simulating Neoplasms

● EYELID APOCRINE HIDROCYSTOMA

Depicted is a clinicopathologic correlation in an 18-year-old woman with a slightly larger bluish subcutaneous lesion in the nasal aspect of the right upper eyelid.

Shields JA, Eagle RC Jr, Shields CL, et al. Apocrine hidrocystoma of the eyelid. *Arch Ophthalmol* 1993;111:866–867.

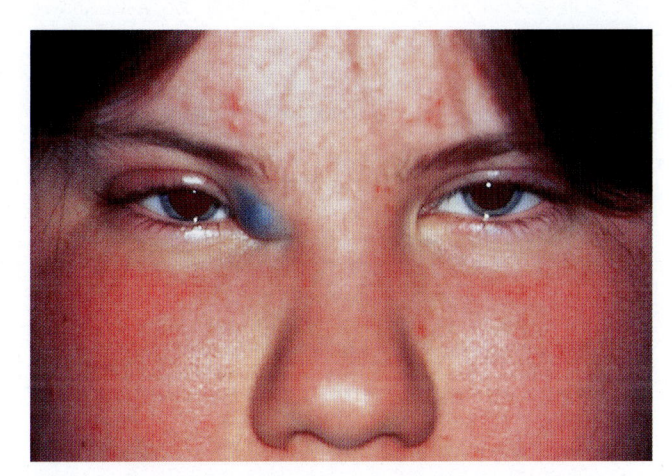

Figure 11.7. Facial appearance, showing the blue discoloration superonasal to the right eye in a teenage girl.

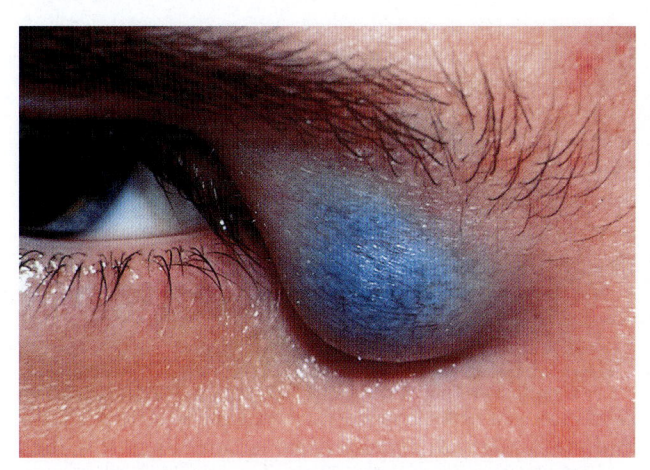

Figure 11.8. Closer view, showing lesion stretching the overlying skin.

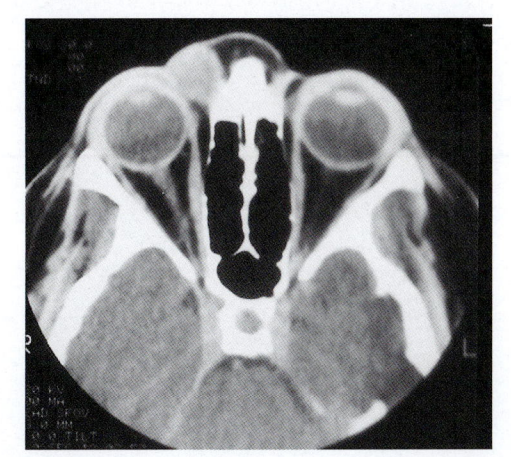

Figure 11.9. Axial computed tomogram of the lesion shown in Figure 11.8. Note the round cystic lesion anterior and medial to the globe.

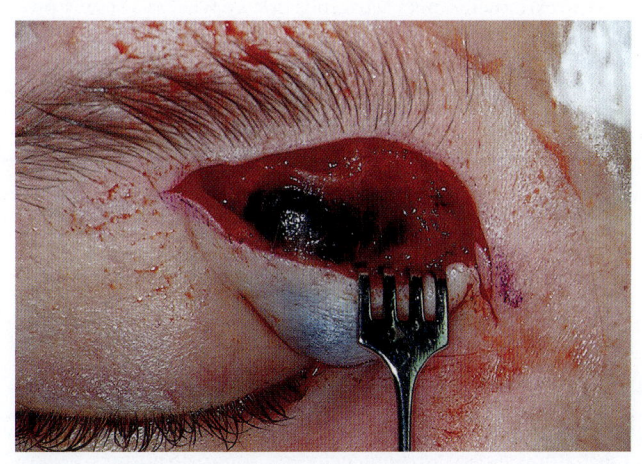

Figure 11.10. Exposure of lesion shown in Figure 11.7 at time of surgical removal. Note the blue color to the lesion.

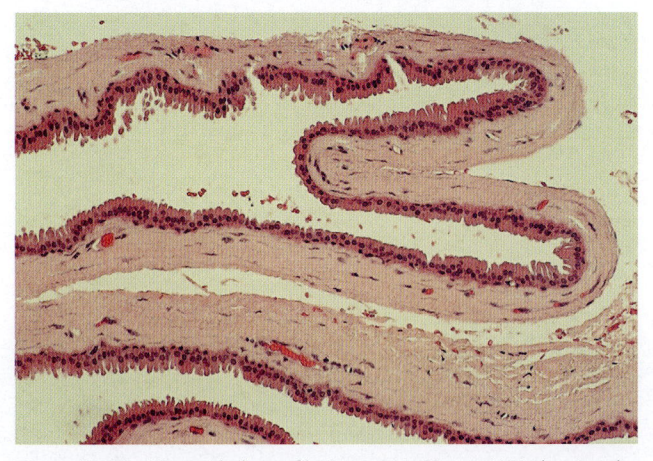

Figure 11.11. Histopathology of lesion seen in Figure 11.7, showing the collapsed cystic lesion with epithelial lining. (Hematoxylin–eosin ×10.)

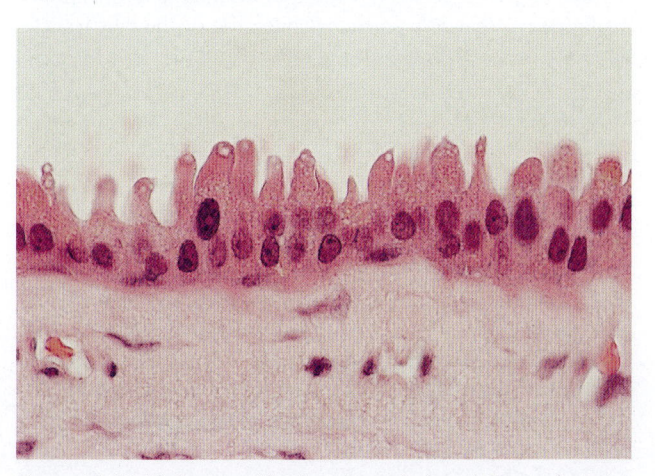

Figure 11.12. Higher-magnification photomicrograph better depicting double layer of epithelial cells lining the cyst. Note the apical snouts protruding from the inner layer into the lumen. (Hematoxylin–eosin ×200.)

EYELID SEBACEOUS CYST (PILAR CYST)

Sebaceous Cyst

The terminology regarding sebaceous cyst and epidermal inclusion cyst has been the subject of some disagreement (1–8). We have chosen to describe them as two different lesions. A sebaceous cyst is usually secondary to occlusion of the duct of a sebaceous gland and can occur on the eyelid and adjacent tissue. Perhaps the most common sebaceous cyst of the eyelid develops in the meibomian glands of the upper tarsus, from retention of meibomian gland material. Less often, it arises from the Zeis glands near the eyelid margin. Larger sebaceous cysts (pilar cysts) tend to arise in areas where there are numerous large hair follicles. Hence, it commonly develops on the scalp (90%), occasionally in the eyebrow area, and less often in the medial canthus and eyelid (1).

Clinical Features

Sebaceous cyst of meibomian gland appears as a focal, subcutaneous nodule with minimal or no inflammation. It is often small and of no serious clinical significance. However, it can develop secondary to inflammation, chalazion, or tumor (3,4).

The extrameibomian sebaceous cyst appears as a slowly progressive, smooth, yellow, opaque, freely movable, subcutaneous lesion, most often in the region of the eyebrow. It often contains a waxy comedo plug in the center. It is usually solitary, but can be multiple. It can occasionally rupture spontaneously, inciting an inflammatory response.

Pathology

Histopathologically, sebaceous cysts are characterized by an epithelial lining that does not possess intercellular bridges. The epithelial cells lose their nuclei and slough off into the lumen of the cyst (1). The lumen of the cyst usually contains predominantly homogeneous, eosinophilic material and less keratin. Calcification occurs in about 25% of cases (1). The cyst can rupture and incite a foreign body giant cell reaction. Concerning pathogenesis and nomenclature, some authorities believe that "sebaceous cyst" (pilar cyst) should be changed to trichilemmal cyst because it is now recognized their keratinization is analogous to that seen in the trichilemma of the hair follicles and they probably represent the same entity (2).

Management

A small, asymptomatic sebaceous cyst can be managed by observation or warm compresses. It eventually resolves in most cases. A larger or symptomatic lesion can be managed by surgical excision. An eyelid crease incision can be done adjacent to the cyst, which should be removed intact if possible. The wound should be allowed to heal or closed with fine absorbable sutures. If the cyst ruptures during surgery, an attempt should be made to remove all remaining epithelium of the cyst using curettage and irrigation. Recurrence is uncommon and the prognosis is generally excellent. In rare cases, extraocular sebaceous cyst has given rise to carcinoma (2,3).

Selected References

Reviews

1. Kirkham N. Tumors and cysts of the epidermis. In: Elder D, Elenitsas R, Jaworsky C, et al., eds. *Lever's Histopathology of the Skin*. Philadelphia, PA: Lippincott-Raven; 1997:695–696.

Case Reports

2. Pinkus H. Sebaceous cysts are trichilemmal cysts. *Arch Dermatol* 1969;99:544.
3. Bauer BS, Lewis VL Jr. Carcinoma arising in sebaceous and epidermoid cysts. *Ann Plast Surg* 1980;5:222–226.
4. Bauer B. Carcinoma arising in a sebaceous cyst. *IMJ Ill Med J* 1979;156:174–176.
5. Yonekawa Y, Jakobiec FA, Zakka FR, et al. Keratinizing cyst of the lacrimal punctum. *Cornea* 2013;32(6):883–885.
6. Kim HJ, Wojno TH, Grossniklaus HE. Multiple intratarsal keratinous cysts of the eyelid. *Ophthal Plast Reconstr Surg* 2012;28(5):e116.
7. Jakobiec FA, Zakka FR, Hatton MP. Eyelid basal cell carcinoma developing in an epidermoid cyst: a previously unreported event. *Ophthal Plast Reconstr Surg* 2010;26(6):491–494.
8. Jakobiec FA, Mehta M, Greenstein SH, et al. The white caruncle: sign of a keratinous cyst arising from a sebaceous gland duct. *Cornea* 2010;29(4):453–455.

Chapter 11 Eyelid Cystic Lesions Simulating Neoplasms

EYELID SEBACEOUS CYST

Clinically, sebaceous cyst can appear identical to epidermoid cyst and other cystic lesions. The diagnosis in some of these cases is presumptive; many have not come to histopathologic confirmation.

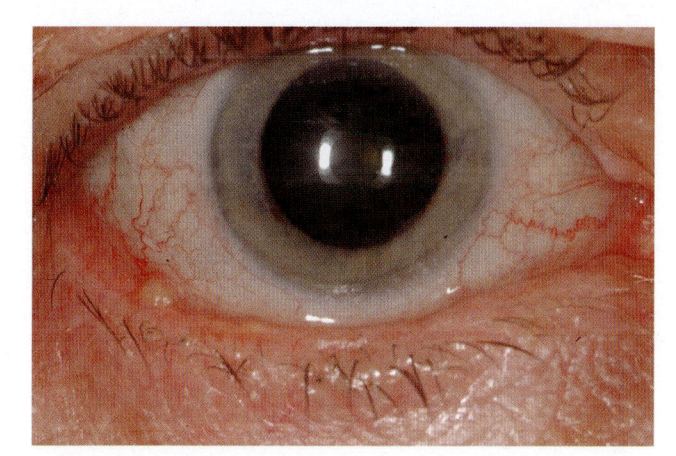

Figure 11.13. Subtle sebaceous cyst in temporal aspect of eyelid margin of right eye.

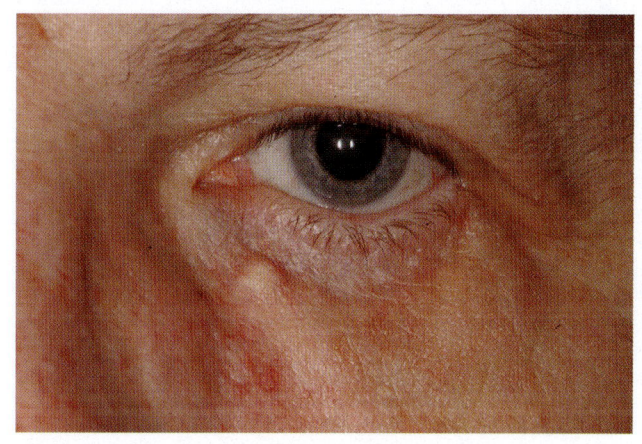

Figure 11.14. Sebaceous cyst below medial aspect of left lower eyelid.

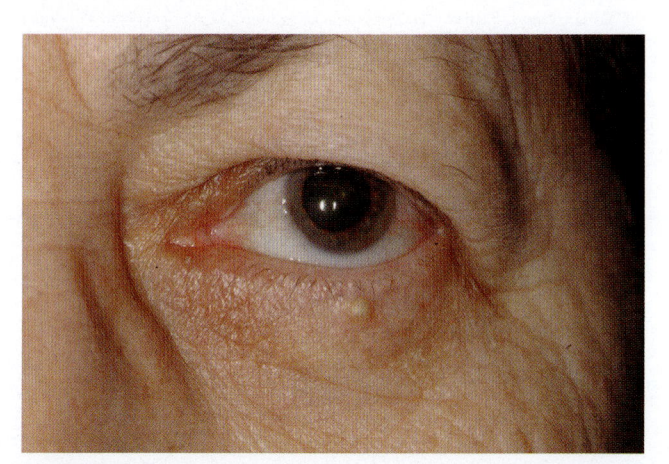

Figure 11.15. Sebaceous cyst near midportion of left lower eyelid.

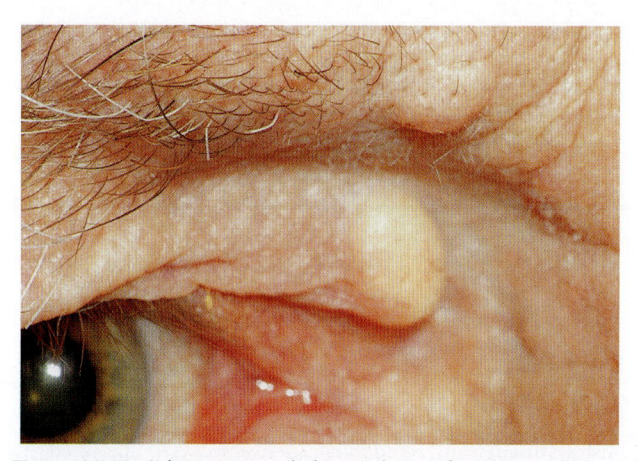

Figure 11.16. Sebaceous cyst below eyebrow of a 69-year-old man. Dispersed floating yellow material is present in the cyst.

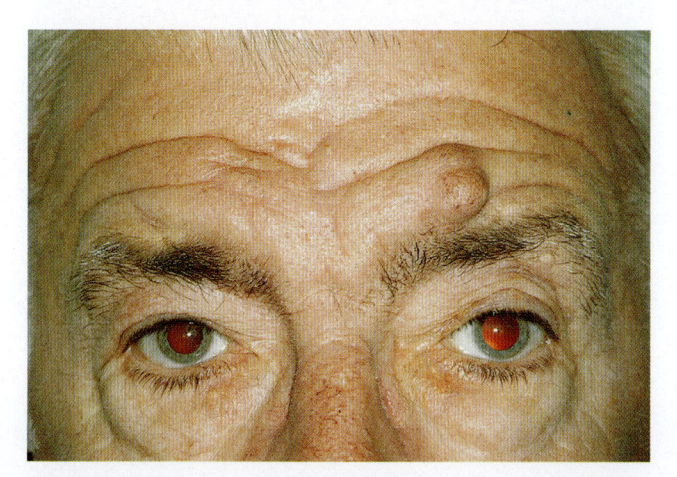

Figure 11.17. Sebaceous cyst above left eyebrow of a 71-year-old man.

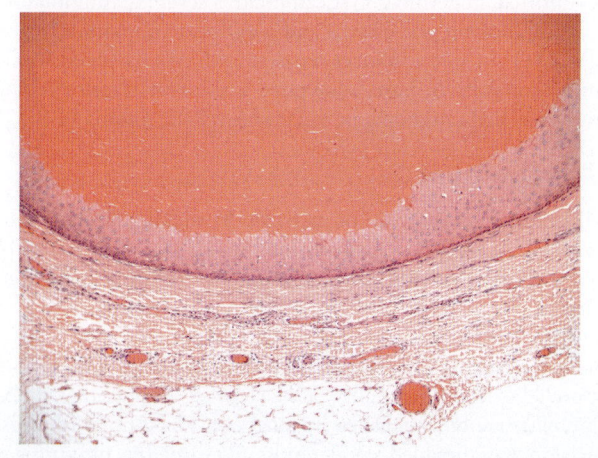

Figure 11.18. Histopathology of sebaceous cyst (pilar cyst), showing epithelial lining below and a lumen above with necrotic epithelial cells and keratin. (Hematoxylin–eosin ×20.)

EYELID EPIDERMAL INCLUSION CYST (EPIDERMOID CYST)

General Considerations

The overlap between sebaceous cyst and epidermal inclusion cyst was mentioned. Epidermal inclusion cyst is lined by epidermis and contains mostly desquamated keratin in its lumen (1–13). It can occur as a very small lesion (milium) or as a large lesion. Milium is a small retention cyst caused by obstruction of the orifices of the pilosebaceous units and rarely has clinical significance. The larger lesions are more clinically evident and can occur in the ocular region. Some authors prefer "infundibular cyst" because of some evidence that it originates from the infundibulum of a hair follicle (1).

Clinical Features

A milium appears as one or more small, gray-white, sometimes umbilicated lesions ranging from 1 to 3 mm in diameter (1,5,6). It often has a small keratin plug (blackhead) near the center. Due to their features and small size, milia are rarely considered in the differential diagnosis of solid eyelid tumors. A larger counterpart is the epidermal inclusion cyst.

Epidermal inclusion cyst is a smooth, soft, yellow, freely movable, subcutaneous lesion. It can be congenital or secondary to trauma or surgery (7). The cyst can spontaneously rupture and incite an inflammatory reaction. Occasionally, a periocular epidermoid cyst can become infected with bacteria, particularly *Staphylococcus aureus* and *Streptococcus pyogenes*. Carcinoma arising from epidermoid cyst is extremely rare on the eyelid (8).

Multiple epidermal inclusion cysts can be seen in patients with Muir–Torre syndrome or Gardner syndrome. In both syndromes, the epidermal inclusions are associated with bowel cancer and other internal and cutaneous lesions (1).

Pathology

Histopathologically, epidermal inclusion cysts are lined by keratinizing epithelium and contain liberated keratin. Unlike a dermoid cyst, the lining does not contain dermal appendages. A ruptured epidermoid cyst can incite a severe granulomatous reaction (keratin granuloma) and pseudocarcinomatous hyperplasia (1). In rare instances, epidermoid cyst has been found microscopically to have undergone malignant transformation into basal cell carcinoma or squamous cell carcinoma (1,9).

Management

Milium can be observed or managed by nicking the overlying skin with a scalpel or hypodermic needle and expressing the cyst contents with the same instrument or with a comedone extractor.

Concerning larger epidermal inclusion cyst, complete removal is desirable for a permanent cure and various approaches have been advocated (1,3,4,9). Epidermal inclusion cysts are best managed by local excision. An eyelid crease incision has provided good results (3), and the prognosis is excellent.

Selected References

Reviews

1. Kirkham N. Tumors and cysts of the epidermis. In: Elder D, Elenitsas R, Jaworsky C, et al., eds. *Lever's Histopathology of the Skin*. Philadelphia, PA: Lippincott-Raven; 1997:695–696.

Histopathology

2. Jakobiec FA, Mehta M, Iwamoto M, et al. Intratarsal keratinous cysts of the Meibomian gland: distinctive clinicopathologic and immunohistochemical features in 6 cases. *Am J Ophthalmol* 2010;149(1):82–94.

Management

3. Kronish JW, Dortzbach RK. Upper eyelid crease surgical approach to dermoid and epidermoid cysts in children. *Arch Ophthalmol* 1988;106:1625–1627.
4. Jordan DR. Multiple epidermal inclusion cysts of the eyelid: a simple technique for removal. *Can J Ophthalmol* 2002;37:39–40.

Case Reports

5. Ratnavel RC, Handfield-Jones SE, Norris PG. Milia restricted to the eyelids. *Clin Exp Dermatol* 1995;20:153–154.
6. Alapati U, Lynfield Y. Multiple papules on the eyelids. Primary milia. *Arch Dermatol* 1999;135:1545–1548.
7. Kronish JW, Sneed SR, Tse DT. Epidermal cysts of the eyelid. *Arch Ophthalmol* 1988;106:270.
8. Bauer BS, Lewis VL Jr. Carcinoma arising in sebaceous and epidermoid cysts. *Ann Plast Surg* 1980;5:222–226.
9. Ikeda I, Ono T. Basal cell carcinoma originating from an epidermoid cyst. *J Dermatol* 1990;17:643–646.
10. Lucarelli MJ, Ahn HB, Kulkarni AD, et al. Intratarsal epidermal inclusion cyst. *Ophthal Plast Reconstr Surg* 2008;24(5):357–359.
11. Jakobiec FA, Mehta M, Sutula F. Keratinous cyst of the palpebral conjunctiva. *Ophthal Plast Reconstr Surg* 2009;25(4):337–339.
12. Procianoy F, Golbert MB, Golbspan L, et al. Steatocystoma simplex of the eyelid. *Ophthal Plast Reconstr Surg* 2009;25(2):147–148.
13. Yuen HK, Wong AC, Wong AL, et al. Cholesteatoma palpebrae: an unusual cholesterol-filled cyst in the eyelid. *Ophthal Plast Reconstr Surg* 2006;22(2):148–150.

Chapter 11 Eyelid Cystic Lesions Simulating Neoplasms

● EYELID EPIDERMAL INCLUSION CYST

Clinically, epidermoid cyst can appear identical to sebaceous cyst and other cystic lesions. The diagnosis in some of these cases is presumptive; many have not come to histopathologic confirmation.

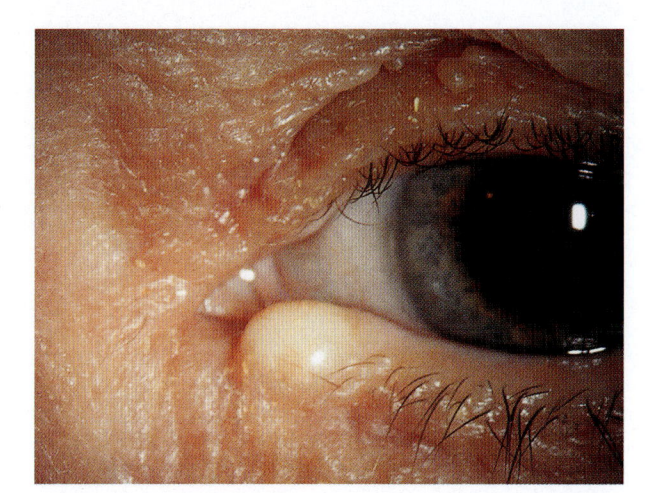

Figure 11.19. Epidermal inclusion cyst on lower eyelid of a 60-year-old woman.

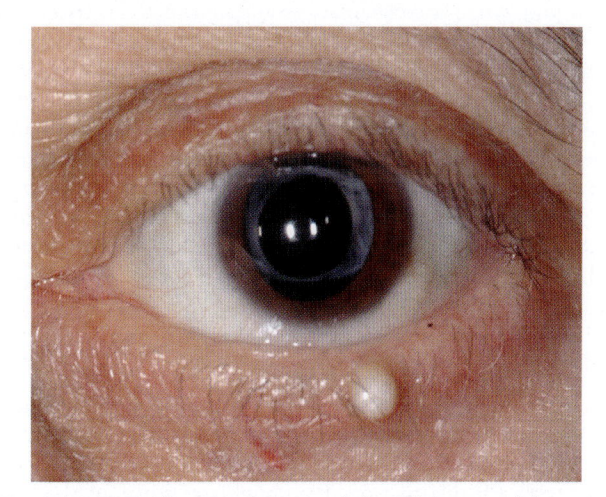

Figure 11.20. Epidermal inclusion cyst below left lower eyelid margin.

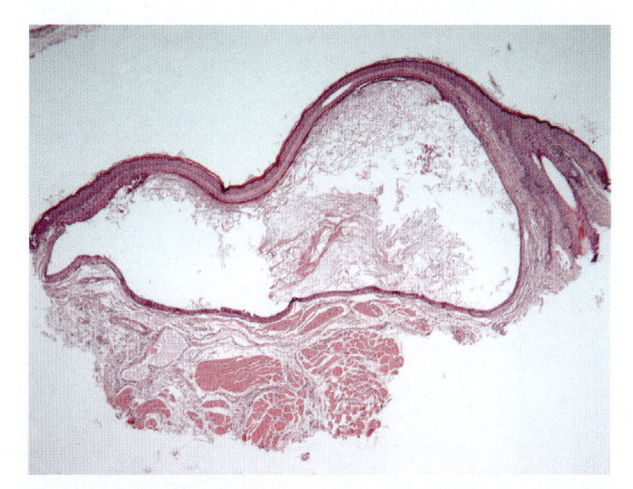

Figure 11.21. Low-magnification photomicrograph of lesion in Figure 11.20, showing epithelial-lined cyst with keratin in lumen. (Hematoxylin–eosin ×5.)

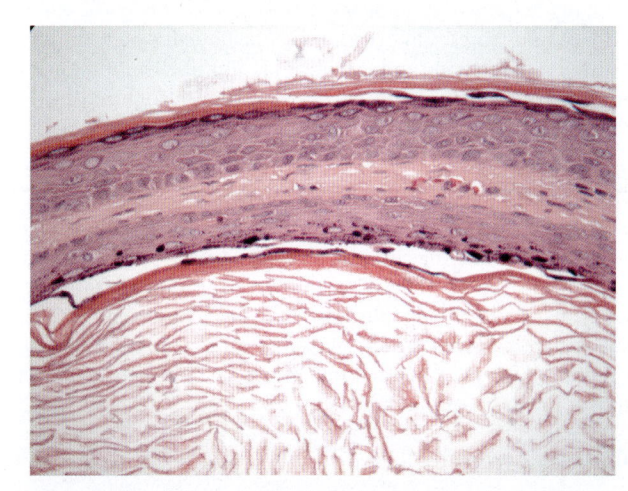

Figure 11.22. Higher-magnification photomicrograph showing cyst wall with epidermis (above) and keratin in lumen (below). (Hematoxylin–eosin ×25.)

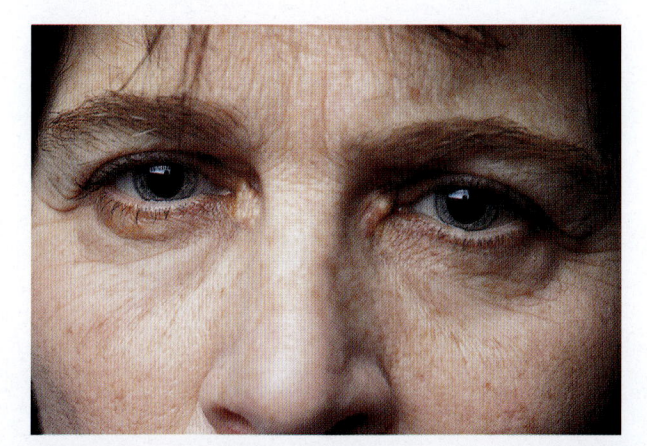

Figure 11.23. Multiple, bilateral epidermal inclusion cysts near medial canthus in a 52-year-old woman. Histopathology of excisional biopsy of all lesions confirmed the diagnosis.

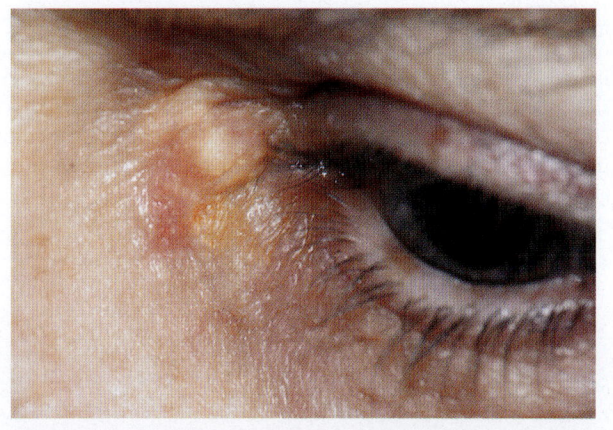

Figure 11.24. Close-up view of lesion near left medial canthus in patient shown in Figure 11.23. The lesions were excised with a good result.

EYELID DERMOID CYST

General Considerations

Dermoid cyst is a congenital cystic lesion that can affect the eyelid, orbit, or both (1–4). It generally occurs from entrapped ectoderm at a site of embryologic bony fusion. Most dermoid cysts in the ocular region occur at the bony orbital rim superotemporally at the site of the zygomaticofrontal suture and present as a rather firm subcutaneous mass beneath the lateral aspect of the upper eyelid and eyebrow. Hence, this condition is discussed in more detail in the section on orbital tumors. Because it often presents as a subcutaneous lesion near the eyelid, it is included here for completeness.

Clinical Features

Clinically, a dermoid cyst usually appears as a smooth, subcutaneous mass that is not movable because of its attachment to the underlying periosteum. It usually is located deep to the eyelid skin superotemporally and can occasionally be associated with a fistula that opens through the skin into the eyelid. Orbital computed tomography and magnetic resonance imaging demonstrate a nonenhancing mass that may cause secondary bony fossa. On occasion, a subcutaneous dermoid cyst transgresses the bone and extends in a dumbbell configuration into the orbit (1,4). Dermoid cyst has been recognized in the tarsus (3).

Pathology

Histopathologically, dermoid cyst is lined by stratified squamous epithelium that usually produces keratin that accumulates in the lumen. The wall of the cyst contains adnexal structures, particularly hair follicles, sebaceous glands, and eccrine sweat glands. Some dermoid cysts that come to histopathologic examination have a marked inflammatory response secondary to prior rupture of the cyst (1).

Management

A dermoid cyst can be managed by periodic observation or surgical excision. Most are eventually excised because of slow enlargement or for cosmetic considerations. Surgical excision should be done through an eyelid crease skin incision or infrabrow incision, with an attempt to remove the lesion intact. If a dermoid cyst ruptures at the time of surgical excision, then copious irrigation should be done and postoperative corticosteroids should be considered. Recurrence is uncommon after meticulous complete removal, but is known to occur after incomplete excision.

Selected References

Reviews

1. Shields JA, Kaden IH, Eagle RC Jr, et al. Orbital dermoid cysts. Clinicopathologic correlations, classification, and management. The 1997 Josephine E. Schueler Lecture. *Ophthal Plast Reconstr Surg* 1997;13:265–276.
2. Brownstein MH, Helwig EB. Subcutaneous dermoid cysts. *Arch Dermatol* 1973;107:237–239.

Case Reports

3. Koreen IV, Kahana A, Gausas RE, et al. Tarsal dermoid cyst: clinical presentation and treatment. *Ophthal Plast Reconstr Surg* 2009;25(2):146–147.
4. Emerick GT, Shields CL, Shields JA, et al. Chewing-induced visual impairment from a dumbbell dermoid cyst. *Ophthal Plast Reconstr Surg* 1997;13:57–61.

Chapter 11 Eyelid Cystic Lesions Simulating Neoplasms 205

● EYELID/ORBITAL DERMOID CYST: CLINICOPATHOLOGIC CORRELATION

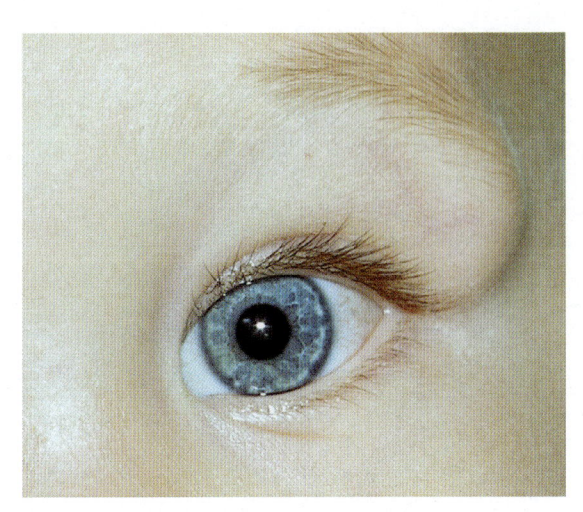

Figure 11.25. Typical dermoid cyst near lateral aspect to eyebrow in a 2-month-old child.

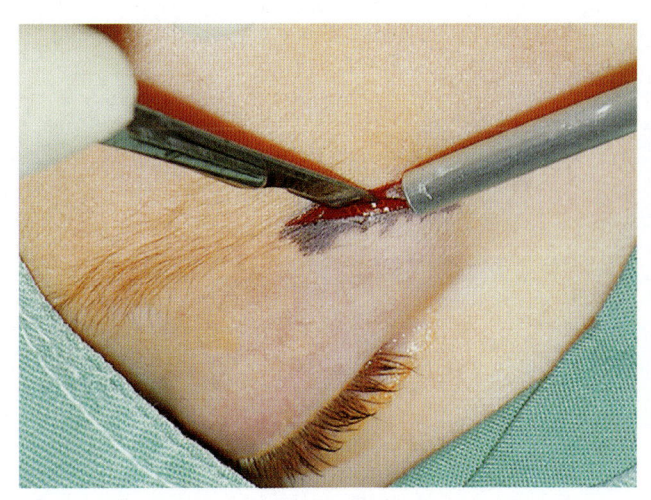

Figure 11.26. Infrabrow incision being performed to remove the lesion. Although the infrabrow incision has an excellent cosmetic result, we more often use an eyelid crease incision presently.

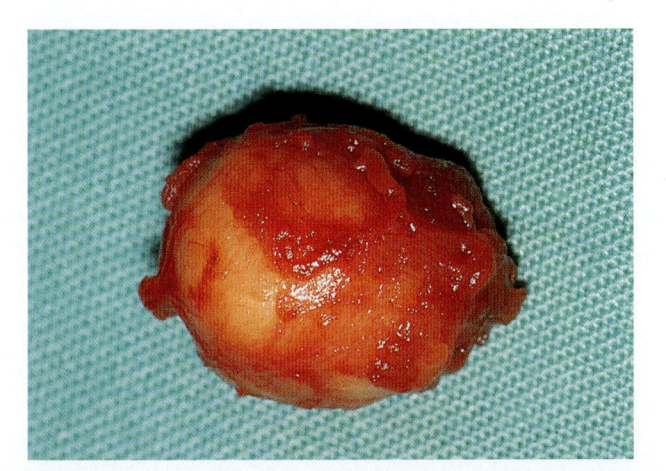

Figure 11.27. Gross appearance of resected specimen. The cyst was removed intact by careful dissection of the lesion from the underlying periosteum.

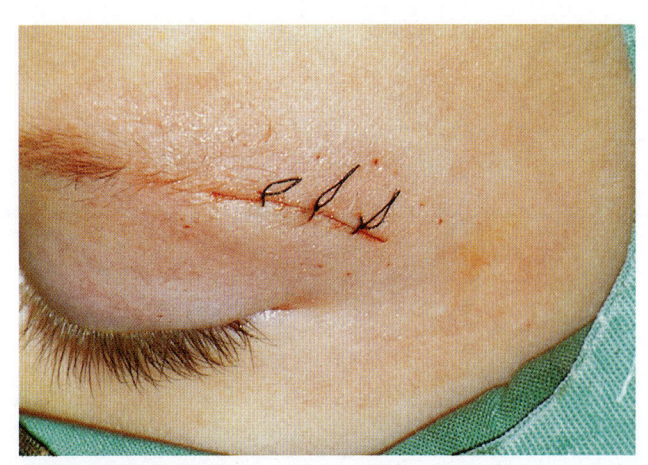

Figure 11.28. Appearance after skin closure.

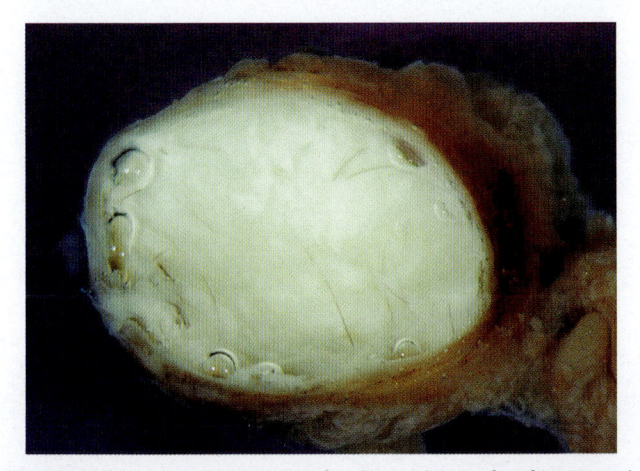

Figure 11.29. Gross appearance of a dermoid cyst after fixation and sectioning. Note the white, cheesy appearance of the material within the cyst.

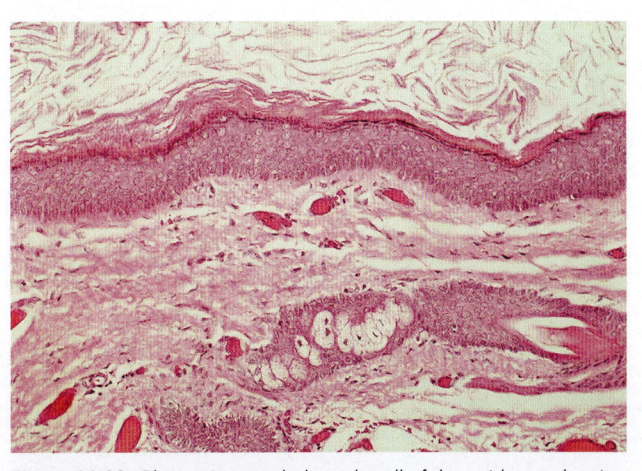

Figure 11.30. Photomicrograph through wall of dermoid cyst, showing the keratinizing epithelium, keratin within the lumen of the cyst (above), and sebaceous glands and hair shafts in the wall of the cyst (below). (Hematoxylin–eosin ×30.)

CHAPTER 12

EYELID INFLAMMATORY LESIONS SIMULATING NEOPLASMS

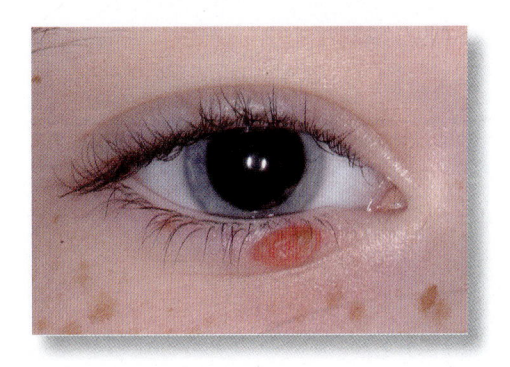

General Considerations

Molluscum contagiosum is an important cause of viral infection that can affect the eyelid and can sometimes simulate a neoplasm (1–11). Historically seen almost exclusively in young children, it was later recognized with greater frequency in adults with acquired immunodeficiency syndrome (AIDS) (3,6–11). In children, transmission results from direct contact (1). In adults, it is generally a sexually transmitted disease. It is a cutaneous pox virus infection that can produce lesions on face, trunk, and proximal extremities (1).

Clinical Features

Molluscum contagiosum infection typically occurs as one or more discrete, flesh-colored lesions that range from 1 to 5 mm in diameter. Each lesion typically has an umbilicated center, sometimes simulating basal cell carcinoma. A cheesy detritus can usually be expressed from this central pore. A chronic follicular conjunctivitis can also occur as a result of shedding of virus particles into the conjunctival fornix. If untreated, this can lead to a corneal pannus and can simulate trachoma. Eyelid molluscum contagiosum can also cause an eczematous-appearing periorbital dermatitis (1,6–9). In patients with human immunodeficiency virus infection, the lesions tend to be larger and more aggressive (6–11). Severe bilateral eyelid involvement can occur in immunosuppressed children (10). Eyelid molluscum contagiosum infection can occasionally be the first signs of AIDS (9).

Pathology

Histopathologically, the typical lesion shows invasive acanthosis and degeneration of epithelial cells that fill the central cavity. Numerous intracytoplasmic inclusion bodies (Henderson–Patterson bodies) are present within the cavity.

Management

The most commonly employed treatment is incision and expression or curettage of the central core (4). When the lesion is located on the eyelid margin, it can be excised by shaving. Cryotherapy and laser treatment have been employed mostly for extraocular lesions. Hyperfocal cryotherapy with local anesthesia is reported to be a safer method for multiple eyelid lesions in AIDS patients (5). Topical trichloroacetic acid tretinoin (Retin-A), salicylic acid, and cantharidin have been used. Once the lesion is completely eliminated, recurrence is rare.

EYELID MOLLUSCUM CONTAGIOSUM INFECTION

Selected References

Reviews

1. Plotik RD, Brown M. Molluscum contagiosum and papillomas. In: Mannis MJ, Macsai MS, Huntley AC, eds. *Eye and Skin Disease*. Philadelphia, PA: Lippincott Raven; 1996:489–494.
2. Vannas S, Lapinleimn K. Molluscum contagiosum in the skin caruncle, and conjunctiva. *Acta Ophthalmol* 1967;45:314–319.
3. Perez-Blazquez E, Villafruela I, Madero S. Eyelid molluscum contagiosum in patients with human immunodeficiency virus infection. *Orbit* 1999;18:75–81.

Management

4. Gonnering RS, Kronish JW. Treatment of periorbital molluscum contagiosum by incision and curettage. *Ophthalmic Surg* 1988;19:325–327.
5. Bardenstein DS, Elmets C. Hyperfocal cryotherapy of multiple molluscum contagiosum lesions in patients with the acquired immune deficiency syndrome. *Ophthalmology* 1995;102:1031–1034.

Case Reports

6. Pelaez CA, Gurbindo MD, Cortes C, et al. Molluscum contagiosum, involving the upper eyelids, in a child infected with HIV-1. *Pediatr AIDS HIV Infect* 1996;7:43–46.
7. Biswas J, Therese L, Kumarasamy N, et al. Lid abscess with extensive molluscum contagiosum in a patient with acquired immunodeficiency syndrome. *Indian J Ophthalmol* 1997;45:234–236.
8. Chattopadhyay DN, Basak SK, Ghose S. HIV-positive patient presented with giant molluscum contagiosum of the eyelid. *J Indian Med Assoc* 1997;95:202.
9. Leahey AB, Shane JJ, Listhaus A, et al. Molluscum contagiosum eyelid lesions as the initial manifestation of acquired immunodeficiency syndrome. *Am J Ophthalmol* 1997;124:240–241.
10. Katzman M, Emmets CA, Lederman MM. Molluscum contagiosum and the acquired immunodeficiency syndrome. *Ann Intern Med* 1985;102:413–414.
11. Charles NC, Friedberg DN. Epibulbar molluscum contagiosum in acquired immunodeficiency syndrome. *Ophthalmology* 1992;99:1123–1126.

EYELID MOLLUSCUM CONTAGIOSUM INFECTION

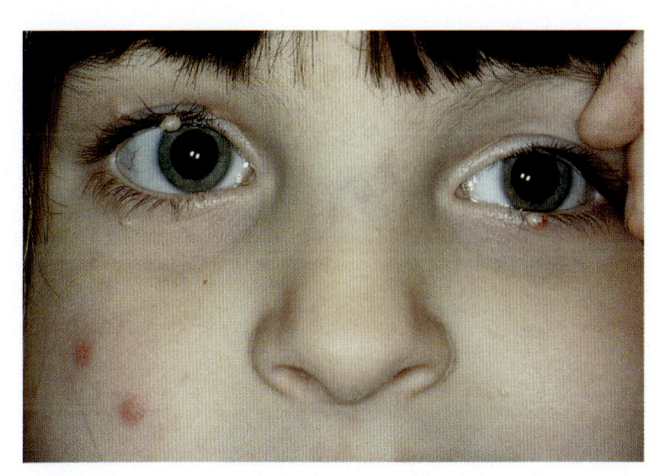

Figure 12.1. Molluscum contagiosum infection with lesions involving upper and lower eyelids and the cheek. (Courtesy of Sprague Eustis, MD.)

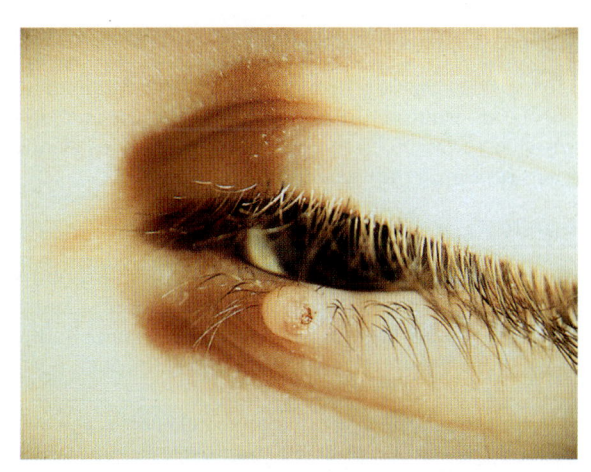

Figure 12.2. Closer view of left lower eyelid of the patient shown in Figure 12.1, revealing circumscribed papule with umbilicated center. (Courtesy of Sprague Eustis, MD.)

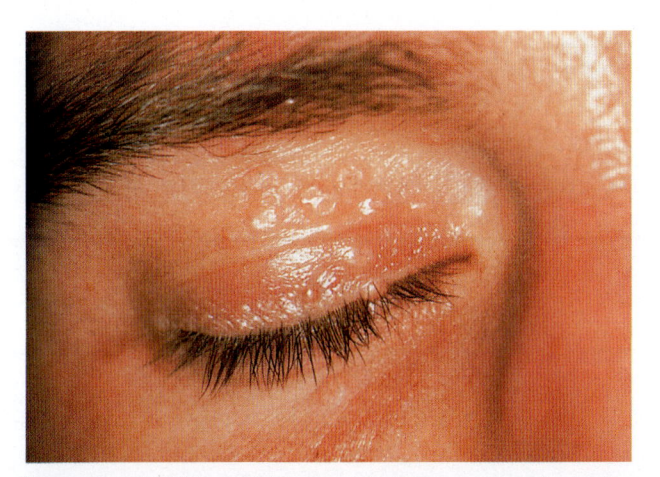

Figure 12.3. Multiple eyelid lesions of molluscum contagiosum in a 30-year-old man with AIDS. (Courtesy of Narsing Rao, MD.)

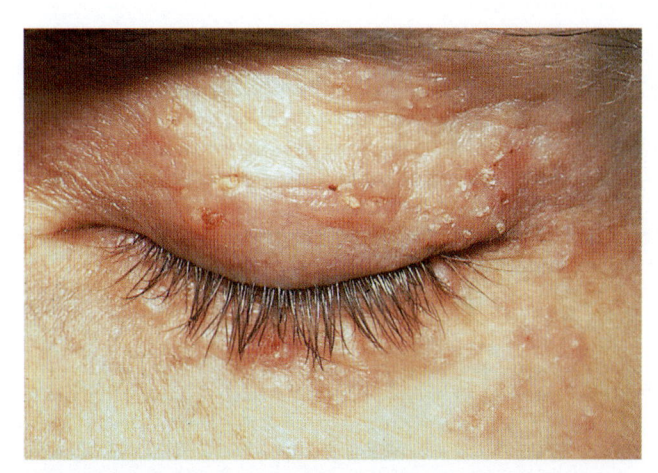

Figure 12.4. Eyelid involvement with molluscum contagiosum in a 34-year-old man with AIDS showing multifocal lesions. (Courtesy of Norman Charles, MD.)

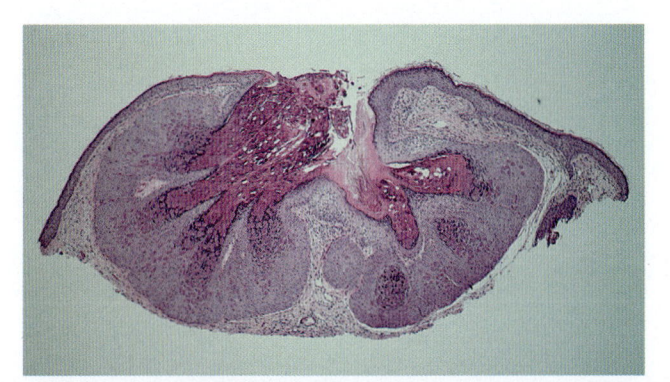

Figure 12.5. Histopathology of molluscum contagiosum lesion showing acanthosis and central core containing necrotic epithelial cells and inclusion bodies. (Hematoxylin–eosin ×5.)

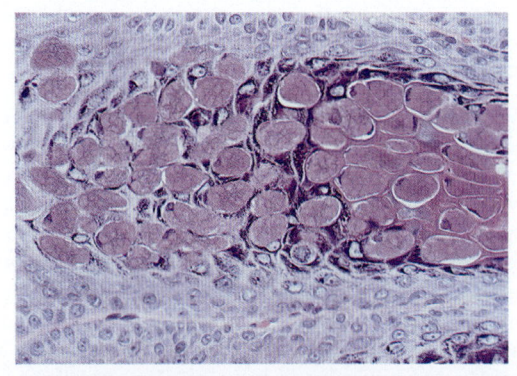

Figure 12.6. Higher-magnification photomicrograph of the central core of the lesion shown in Figure 12.5, demonstrating typical intranuclear inclusion bodies (Henderson–Patterson bodies). (Hematoxylin–eosin ×100.)

EYELID CHALAZION

General Considerations

Chalazion is a common lipogranulomatous inflammation of the sebaceous glands of the eyelids, most often the meibomian glands (1–28). It can also occur from the sebaceous glands of Zeis and appear on the eyelid margin.

Clinical Features

Chalazion usually occurs secondary to noninfectious obstruction of the ducts of the aforementioned sebaceous glands. It usually first appears as a firm, tender, erythematous lump in the tarsal plate. As it progresses, it may break through posteriorly and appear on the palpebral conjunctiva or it may drain anteriorly through the skin. A ruptured chalazion can sometimes incite production of granulation tissue in the form of a pyogenic granuloma. In some instances, pressure on the globe by a chalazion can induce significant refractive errors (17,18). More aggressive chalazions have been observed in patients with hyperimmunoglobulinemia E (Job's syndrome) (24,25), and tend to be more difficult to manage.

Chalazion generally has typical clinical features and the diagnosis can be made easily. It is reported that in 94% of cases the diagnosis is correctly made by the clinician. However, about 6% prove histopathologically to be other benign or malignant lesions (1); the most important is sebaceous carcinoma that can simulate a chalazion and is often misdiagnosed clinically and histopathologically (4,5). Several other malignant and benign eyelid conditions can closely mimic chalazion (1,19–22).

Pathology

Histopathologically, chalazion is characterized by a lipogranulomatous reaction to liberated lipid material. A connective tissue pseudocapsule is often present around the lesion. Round clear spaces in the lesion represent fat deposition. The granulomatous reaction with giant cells may be intermixed with acute and chronic inflammatory cells. Causative organisms are not usually identified, but secondary infection can occur, particularly in patients with Job's syndrome. The granulomas may resemble those seen with sarcoidosis, cat scratch disease, or tuberculosis.

Management

Management is generally hot compresses and good eyelid hygiene (6–16). Symptomatic lesions that do not resolve can be managed by incision and curettage, with special effort to remove the pseudocapsule. A conjunctival approach using a chalazion clamp with the lid everted is generally preferred. An eyelid incision can be used for anterior lesions that are eroding through the skin (6,14). Several techniques for local anesthesia for chalazion treatment have been reported (8–10). If the lesion is typical of chalazion, intralesional injection of corticosteroids can be effective in bringing about resolution (11–13,16). However, such injections should be done with great care, because inadvertent corneal penetration and traumatic cataract have been rarely recognized as complications of corticosteroid injection (11).

As mentioned, some malignant neoplasms, particularly sebaceous carcinoma, can simulate a chalazion (4,5). Hence, any tissue should be sent for histopathologic studies to exclude the possibility of malignancy. The prognosis for chalazion is excellent.

EYELID CHALAZION

Selected References

Reviews

1. Ozdal PC, Codere F, Callejo S, et al. Accuracy of the clinical diagnosis of chalazion. *Eye* 2004;18:135–138.
2. de Keizer RJ, Scheffer E. Masquerade of eyelid tumours. *Doc Ophthalmol* 1989; 72:309–321.
3. Hsu HC, Lin HF. Eyelid tumors in children: a clinicopathologic study of a 10-year review in southern Taiwan. *Ophthalmologica* 2004;218:274–277.
4. Shields JA, Demirci H, Marr BP, et al. Sebaceous carcinoma of the eyelids: personal experience with 60 cases (The 2003 J. Howard Stokes Lecture, part 2). *Ophthalmology* 2004;111:2151–2157.
5. Shields JA, Saktanasate J, Lally SE, et al. Sebaceous carcinoma of the ocular region. The 2014 Professor Winifred Mao Lecture. *Asia Pacific J Ophthalmol* 2015; in press.

Management

6. Shorr N, Kopelman JE. Modified chalazion surgery technique. In: Wesley RE, ed. *Techniques in Ophthalmic Plastic Surgery.* New York: John Wiley and Sons; 1986:7–9.
7. Smythe D, Hurwitz JJ, Tayfour F. The management of chalazion: a survey of Ontario ophthalmologists. *Can J Ophthalmol* 1990;25:252–255.
8. Li RT, Lai JS, Ng JS, et al. Efficacy of lignocaine 2% gel in chalazion surgery. *Br J Ophthalmol* 2003;87:157–159.
9. Wessels IF, Wessels GF. Lidocaine-prilocaine cream for local-anesthesia chalazion incision in children. *Ophthalmic Surg Lasers* 1996;27:431–433.
10. Bell RW, Butt ZA, Gardner RF. Warming lignocaine reduces the pain of injection during local anaesthetic eyelid surgery. *Eye* 1996;10:558–560.
11. Hosal BM, Zilelioglu G. Ocular complication of intralesional corticosteroid injection of a chalazion. *Eur J Ophthalmol* 2003;13:798–799.
12. Norris JH. Intralesional triamcinolone acetonide injection versus incision and curettage for primary chalazia: a prospective, randomized study. *Am J Ophthalmol* 2012;153(5):1005–1006.
13. Ben Simon GJ, Rosen N, Rosner M, et al. Intralesional triamcinolone acetonide injection versus incision and curettage for primary chalazia: a prospective, randomized study. *Am J Ophthalmol* 2011;151(4):714–718.e1.
14. Reifler DM, Leder DR. Eyelid crease approach for chalazion excision. *Ophthal Plast Reconstr Surg* 1989;5:63–67.
15. Korn EL. Laser chalazion removal. *Ophthalmic Surg* 1988;19:428–431.
16. Jain PK, Misuria V. Recent non-surgical approach in the treatment of chalazion. *Indian J Ophthalmol* 1988;36:34.

Case Reports

17. Cosar CB, Rapuano CJ, Cohen EJ, et al. Chalazion as a cause of decreased vision after LASIK. *Cornea* 2001;20:890–892.
18. Santa Cruz CS, Culotta T, Cohen EJ, et al. Chalazion-induced hyperopia as a cause of decreased vision. *Ophthalmic Surg Lasers* 1997;28:683–684.
19. Katowitz WR, Shields CL, Shields JA, et al. Pilomatrixoma of the eyelid simulating a chalazion. *J Pediatr Ophthalmol Strabismus* 2003;40:247–248.
20. Cunniffe G, Chang BY, Kennedy S, et al. Beware the empty curette! *Orbit* 2002;21:177–180.
21. Brookes JL, Bentley C, Verma S, et al. Microcystic adnexal carcinoma masquerading as a chalazion. *Br J Ophthalmol* 1998;82:196–197.
22. Shields JA, Guibor P. Neurilemoma of the eyelid resembling a recurrent chalazion. *Arch Ophthalmol* 1984;102:1650.
23. Donaldson MJ, Gole GA. Amblyopia due to inflamed chalazion in a 13-month-old infant. *Clin Exp Ophthalmol* 2005;33:332–333.
24. Destafeno JJ, Kodsi SR, Primack JD. Recurrent Staphylococcus aureus chalazion in hyperimmunoglobulinemia E (Job's) syndrome. *Am J Ophthalmol* 2004;138:1057–1058.
25. Crama N, Toolens AM, van der Meer JW, et al. Giant chalazion in the hyperimmunoglobulinemia E (hyper-IgE) syndrome. *Eur J Ophthalmol* 2004;14:258–260.
26. Mittal R, Tripathy D, Sharma S, et al. Tuberculosis of eyelid presenting as a chalazion. *Ophthalmology* 2013;120(5):1103.e1–e4.
27. Mukhopadhyay S, Shome S, Bar PK, et al. Ocular rhinosporidiosis presenting as recurrent chalazion. *Int Ophthalmol* 2012;DOI 10.1007/s10792-012-9625-2.
28. Al-Faky YH, Al Malki S, Raddaoui E. Hemangioendothelioma of the eyelid can mimic chalazion. *Oman J Ophthalmol* 2011;4(3):142–143.

Part 1 Tumors of the Eyelids

EYELID CHALAZION

In most instances, chalazion has a typical clinical presentation and the diagnosis is made with great certainty.

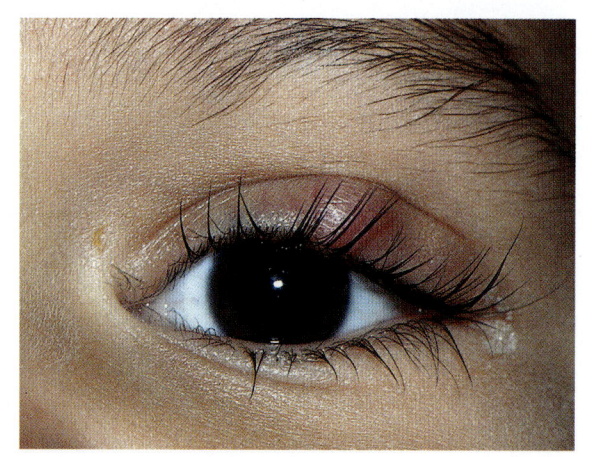

Figure 12.7. Small chalazion in center of upper eyelid in a 2-year-old boy.

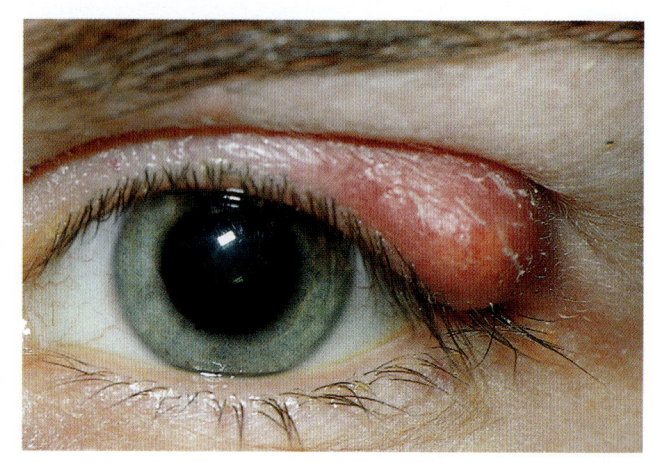

Figure 12.8. Chalazion near lateral aspect of upper eyelid in a 34-year-old woman.

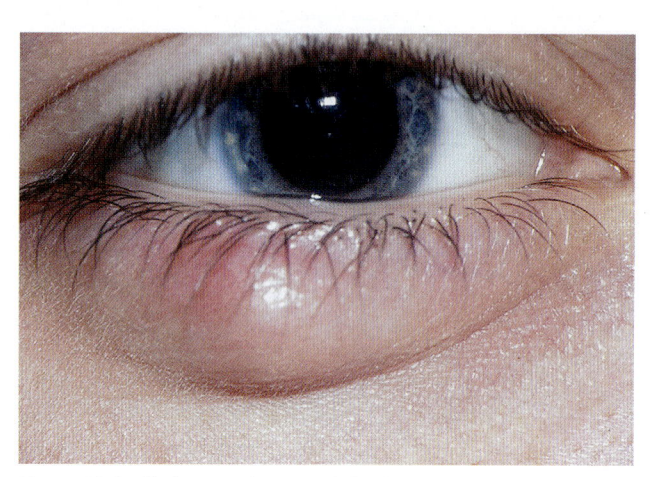

Figure 12.9. Chalazion in lower eyelid with secondary eyelid edema in a 21-year-old woman.

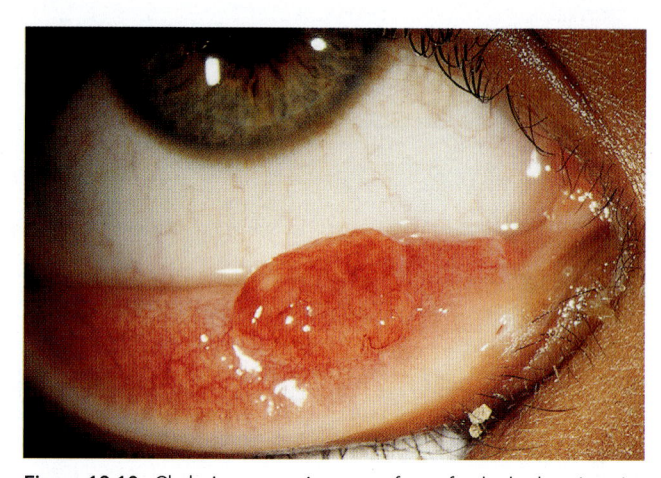

Figure 12.10. Chalazion appearing on surface of palpebral conjunctiva in a 15-year-old boy.

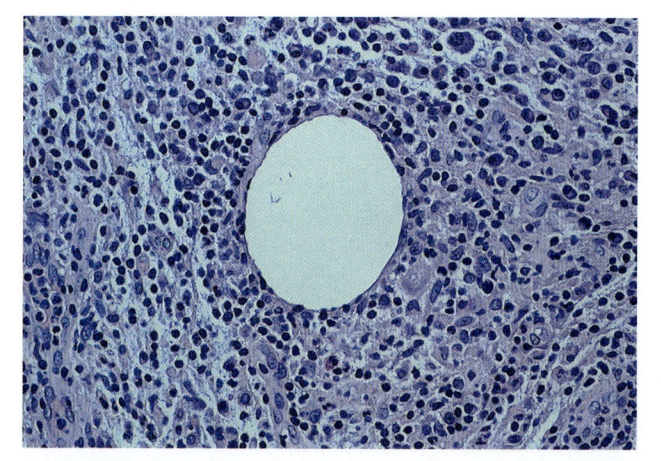

Figure 12.11. Photomicrograph of chalazion showing lipid globule surrounded by acute and chronic inflammatory cells. (Hematoxylin–eosin ×75.)

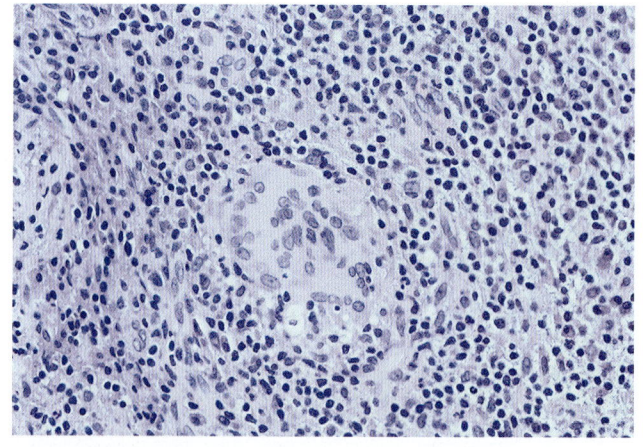

Figure 12.12. Photomicrograph of chalazion showing giant cell in area of granulomatous inflammation. (Hematoxylin–eosin ×75.)

EYELID CHALAZION: CLINICAL VARIATIONS

Chalazion can have a variety of clinical presentations in addition to a simple inflammatory nodule. It can erode through the skin or tarsal plate, producing an erosive or ulcerated appearance. A ruptured chalazion can assume a diffuse configuration without a distinct nodule. In some instances, it can cause diffuse thickening of the eyelid, simulating a blepharoconjunctivitis or sebaceous carcinoma.

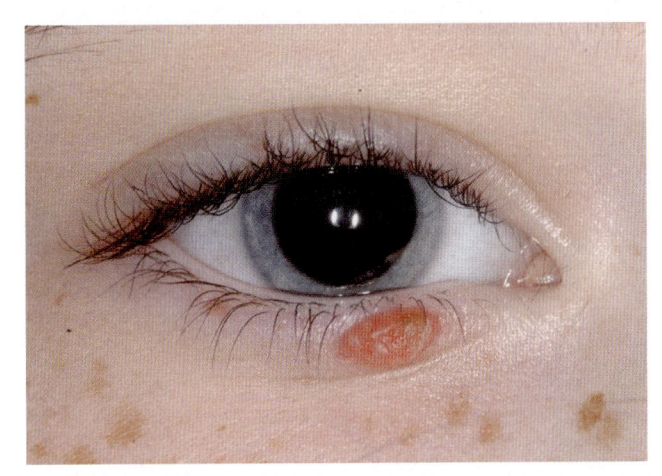

Figure 12.13. Chalazion of right lower eyelid in a child showing typical erosion of overlying skin.

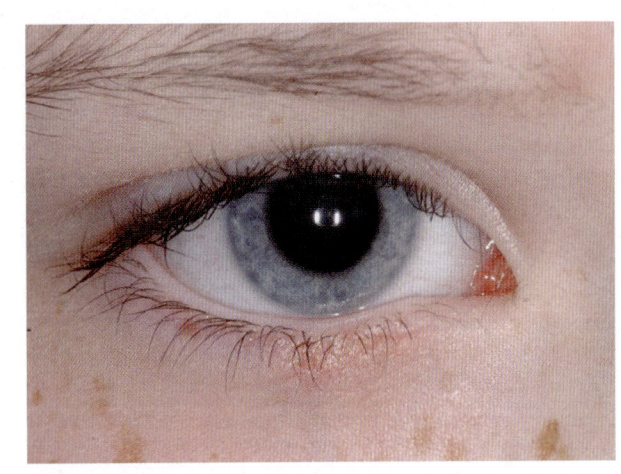

Figure 12.14. Same child 1 month later after treatment with antibiotic ointment and compresses, showing resolution of the lesion.

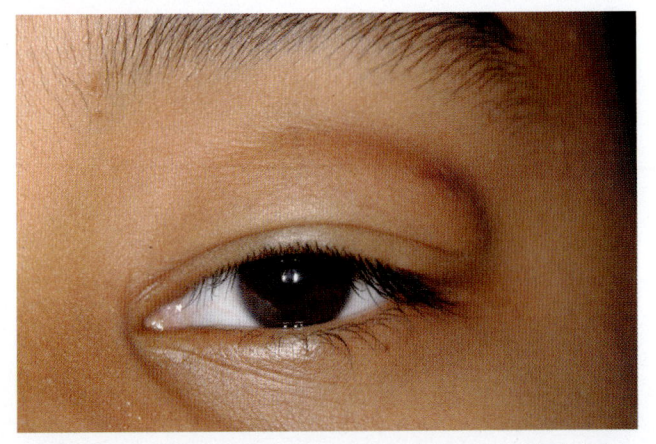

Figure 12.15. Diffuse edema of left upper eyelid in child with chalazion. The underlying chalazion was not readily evident because of the edema.

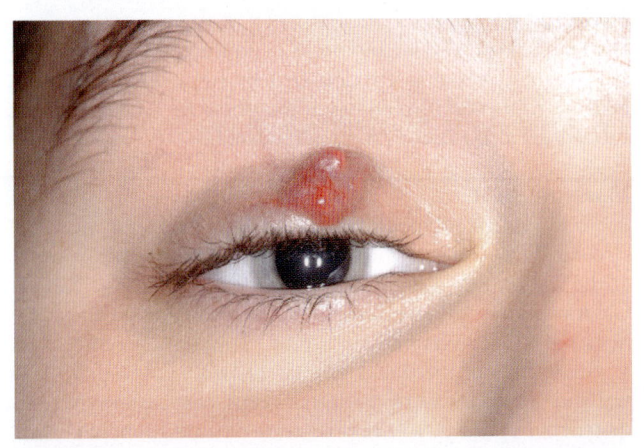

Figure 12.16. Erosive chalazion of right upper lid simulating a vascular tumor.

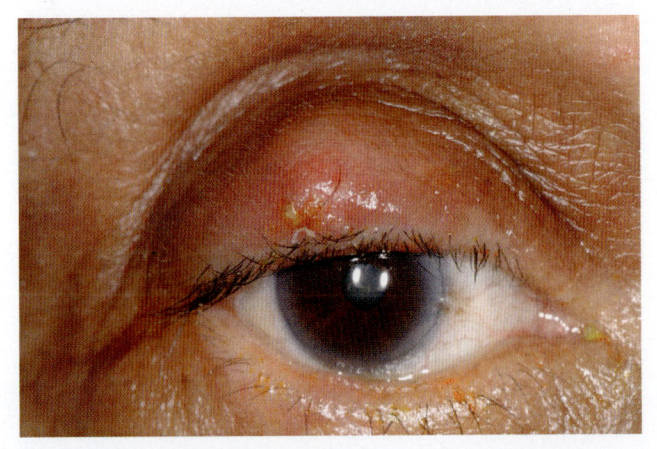

Figure 12.17. Upper lid chalazion with drainage through the skin.

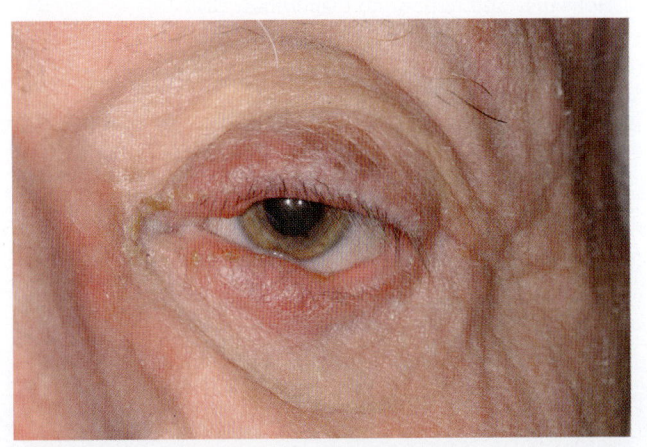

Figure 12.18. Elderly patient with chronic chalazion of upper and lower eyelids and some loss of cilia. In such patients, a diagnosis of sebaceous carcinoma should also be considered. In this case, sebaceous carcinoma was entertained, but the diagnosis of chalazion was confirmed histopathologically.

MISCELLANEOUS GRANULOMATOUS DISEASES

Eyelid Sarcoidosis

General Considerations
There are several idiopathic granulomatous inflammations that can also affect the eyelid and simulate a neoplasm. The two to be discussed briefly here are sarcoidosis and pseudorheumatoid nodule.

Sarcoidosis is an idiopathic disease characterized by noncaseating granulomatous inflammation. It can occur in many organs and all parts of the eye and adnexa (1–10). It can appear in the eyelid as an initial manifestation or in a patient with known systemic or ocular sarcoidosis (1–5).

Clinical Features
In the eyelid, sarcoidosis generally appears as one or more irregular, firm subcutaneous nodules. The adjacent conjunctiva can show numerous nodules or diffuse thickening, simulating a lymphoid infiltrate or viral conjunctivitis. On occasion, sarcoidosis has been reported to produce a more aggressive "destructive" lesion in the eyelid (7,8).

Pathology
Histopathologically, sarcoidosis is a noncaseating epithelioid cell granuloma that is characterized by histiocytes and giant cells (1). If no specific etiology is found for the inflammation, a diagnosis of sarcoidosis if often rendered.

Management
A biopsy is generally required to make the diagnosis of eyelid sarcoidosis. It is also known that a biopsy of suspicious areas of the adjacent conjunctiva can establish the diagnosis (9,10). Gallium scan may show lacrimal gland that may assist the diagnosis of the eyelid lesions.

Sarcoidosis of the eyelid, like sarcoidosis elsewhere, is generally responsive to oral or intralesional corticosteroids. The destructive eyelid variant may be more difficult to manage, but can show some response to corticosteroids and other immunosuppressive agents. There has been a suggestion that such lesions may also respond to thalidomide (8).

Selected References

Reviews
1. Zimmerman LE, Maumenee AE. Ocular aspects of sarcoidosis. *Am Rev Respir Dis* 1961;84:38–50.
2. Obernauf CD, Shaw HE, Sydnor CF, et al. Sarcoidosis and its ophthalmic manifestations. *Am J Ophthalmol* 1978;86:648–655.
3. Hall JG, Cohen KL. Sarcoidosis of the eyelid skin. *Am J Ophthalmol* 1995;119:100–101.
4. Gutman J, Shinder R. Orbital and adnexal involvement in sarcoidosis: analysis of clinical features and systemic disease in 30 cases. *Am J Ophthalmol* 2011;152(5):883.
5. Demirci H, Christianson MD. Orbital and adnexal involvement in sarcoidosis: analysis of clinical features and systemic disease in 30 cases. *Am J Ophthalmol* 2011;151(6):1074–1080.

Case Reports
6. Cacciatori M, McLaren KM, Kearns PP. Sarcoidosis presenting as a cutaneous eyelid mass. *Br J Ophthalmol* 1997;81:329–330.
7. Moin M, Kersten RC, Bernardini F, et al. Destructive eyelid lesions in sarcoidosis. *Ophthal Plast Reconstr Surg* 2001;17:123–125.
8. Karcioglu ZA. Re: "Destructive eyelid lesions in sarcoidosis". *Ophthal Plast Reconstr Surg* 2002;18:313.
9. Nichols CW, Eagle RC Jr, Yanoff M, et al. Conjunctival biopsy as an aid in the evaluation of the patient with suspected sarcoidosis. *Ophthalmology* 1980;87:287–291.
10. Dios E, Saornil MA, Herreras JM. Conjunctival biopsy in the diagnosis of ocular sarcoidosis. *Ocul Immunol Inflamm* 2001;9:59–64.

MISCELLANEOUS GRANULOMATOUS DISEASES

Eyelid Pseudorheumatoid Nodule (Granuloma Annulare)

General Considerations
Pseudorheumatoid nodule (granuloma annular) is an idiopathic, benign, self-limited, granulomatous disease that affects the head region of children and young adults (1–6). It is so named because of its histopathologic similarity to the subcutaneous nodule of rheumatoid arthritis or rheumatic fever. However, laboratory studies and follow-up on affected patients has failed to disclose a relationship with those conditions. The eyelid and adjacent ocular structures can be involved, with a predilection for the upper eyelid and lateral canthus.

Clinical Features
Pseudorheumatoid nodule can appear as one or more firm, movable, subcutaneous, tan-colored papules that may grow in a ring pattern. On occasion, it may be soft and fluctuant and appear cystic. It has a predilection for the lateral aspect of the upper eyelid and lateral canthus. The lesion pursues a benign course and may slowly regress without treatment in some cases.

Pathology
As mentioned, the lesions resemble the subcutaneous nodules seen with rheumatoid arthritis. There is generally a central area of necrobiotic collagen surrounded by a palisade of histiocytes and epithelioid cells.

Management
The diagnosis of eyelid pseudorheumatoid nodule is not often made clinically but is revealed on histopathologic examination of the excised lesion. In most instances, management has been simple excision or only observation. As mentioned, the lesions may gradually regress without treatment.

Selected References

Reviews
1. Rao NA, Font RL. Pseudorheumatoid nodules of the ocular adnexa. *Am J Ophthalmol* 1975;79:471–478.
2. Thornsberry LA, English JC 3rd. Etiology, diagnosis, and therapeutic management of granuloma annulare: an update. *Am J Clin Dermatol* 2013;14(4):279–290.
3. Lawton AW, Karesh JW. Periocular granuloma annulare. *Surv Ophthalmol* 1987;31:285–290.
4. Ross MJ, Cohen KL, Peiffer RL, et al. Episcleral and orbital pseudorheumatoid nodules. *Arch Ophthalmol* 1983;101:418–421.

Case Reports
5. Ferry AP. Subcutaneous granuloma annular ("pseudorheumatoid nodule") of the eyebrow. *J Pediatr Ophthalmol* 1977;14:154–157.
6. Mauriello JA Jr, Lambert WC, Mostafavi R. Granuloma annulare of the eyelid. *Ophthal Plast Reconstr Surg* 1996;12:141–145.

Eyelid Granulomatosis with Polyangiitis (Wegener's Granulomatosis)

General Considerations
Eyelid granulomatosis with polyangiitis, previously termed Wegener's granulomatosis (1–13) is a multisystem disease consisting of necrotizing granulomas and vasculitis of the upper respiratory tract, kidneys, and other organs. It can affect the nasal cavity and orbit and secondarily involve the eyelids.

Clinical Features
Eyelid involvement with granulomatosis with polyangiitis is usually secondary to severe orbital disease and this condition is discussed in other chapters of this volume. Orbital involvement is usually coexistent with sinus and nasal involvement. Eyelid involvement occurs secondary to vasculitis and can manifest as erythema, edema, irregular thickening, or ulceration of the eyelid (5). There is often severe inflammation of the tarsal conjunctiva that leads to secondary scarring of the eyelids (6,9). The limited form of granulomatosis with polyangiitis has presented with an ulcerated lesion of the eyelid (12). Occasionally, there is severe destruction of the eyelids (13). Bilateral yellow xanthelasma on the eyelids has also been described (10). Although several diagnostic laboratory tests have been used, the antineutrophil cytoplasmic antibody (ANCA) is both sensitive and specific in 60% to 90% of patients with this disease.

Pathology
Histopathologically, granulomatosis with polyangiitis is typified by vasculitis, necrosis, and granulomatous inflammation, usually with Langhan's type giant cells. Lymphocytes, plasma cells, neutrophils, and occasional eosinophils are also present.

Management
Eyelid granulomatosis with polyangiitis is generally treated by systemic corticosteroids, cyclophosphamide, and local palliative methods. The prognosis has improved with these methods (4,5). Many patients succumb to renal involvement or other complications. Orbital exenteration has sometimes been necessary for severe destructive lesions (7).

Selected References

Reviews
1. Hu CH, O'Laughlin S, Winklemann RK. Cutaneous manifestations of Wegener's granulomatosis. *Arch Dermatol* 1977;113:175–185.
2. Haynes BF, Fishman ML, Fauci AS, et al. The ocular manifestations of Wegener's granulomatosis. *Am J Med* 1977;63:131–136.
3. Bullen CL, Liesegang TJ, McDonald TH, et al. Ocular complications of Wegener's granulomatosis. *Ophthalmology* 1983;90:279–290.
4. Duffy M. Advances in diagnosis, treatment, and management of orbital and periocular Wegener's granulomatosis. *Curr Opin Ophthalmol* 1999;10:352–357.
5. Woo TL, Francis IC, Wilcsek GA, et al. Australasian Orbital and Adnexal Wegener's Study Group. Australasian orbital and adnexal Wegener's granulomatosis. *Ophthalmology* 2001;108:1535–1543.

Management
6. Robinson MR, Lee SS, Sneller MC, et al. Tarsal-conjunctival disease associated with Wegener's granulomatosis. *Ophthalmology* 2003;110:1770–1780.
7. Shields JA, Shields CL, Demirci H, et al. Experience with eyelid-sparing orbital exenteration: the 2000 Tullos O. Coston Lecture. *Ophthal Plast Reconstr Surg* 2001;17:355–361.

Case Reports
8. Koyama T, Matsuo N, Watanabe Y, et al. Wegener's granulomatosis with destructive ocular manifestations. *Am J Ophthalmol* 1984;98:736–740.
9. Jordan DR, Addison DJ. Wegener's granulomatosis. Eyelid and conjunctival manifestations as the presenting feature in two individuals. *Ophthalmology* 1994;101:602–607.
10. Tullo AB, Durrington P, Graham E, et al. Florid xanthelasmata (yellow lids) in orbital Wegener's granulomatosis. *Br J Ophthalmol* 1995;79:453–456.
11. Valmaggia C, Neuweiler J. Orbital involvement as the first manifestation in classic Wegener's granulomatosis. *Orbit* 2001;20:231–237.
12. Kubota T, Hirose H. Ocular changes in a limited form of Wegener's granulomatosis: patient with cutaneous ulcer of upper eyelid. *Jpn J Ophthalmol* 2003;47:398–400.
13. Cassells-Brown A, Morrell AJ, Davies BR, et al. Wegener's granulomatosis causing lid destruction: a further sight-threatening complication. *Eye* 2003;17:652–654.

EYELID GRANULOMAS: SARCOIDOSIS, PSEUDORHEUMATOID NODULE, AND GRANULOMATOSIS WITH POLYANGIITIS (WEGENER GRANULOMATOSIS)

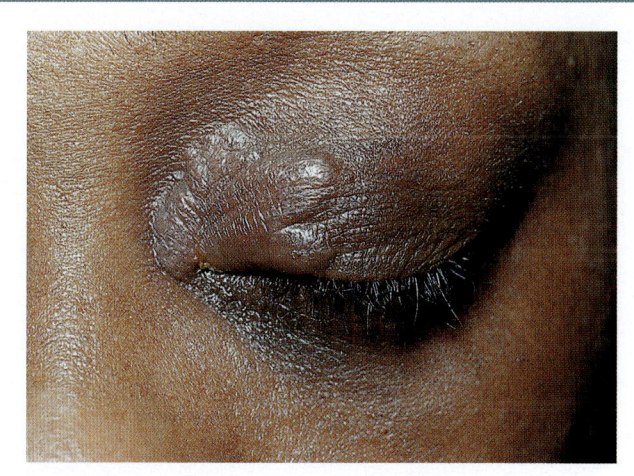

Figure 12.19. Sarcoidosis involving upper eyelid.

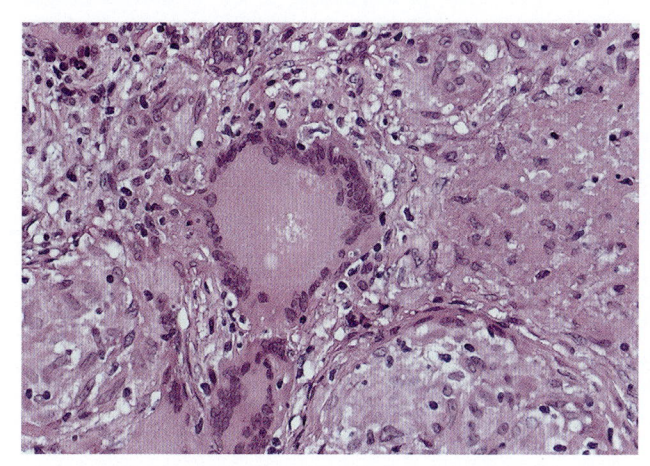

Figure 12.20. Histopathology of sarcoidosis, showing granulomatous inflammation with a giant cell. (Hematoxylin–eosin ×150.)

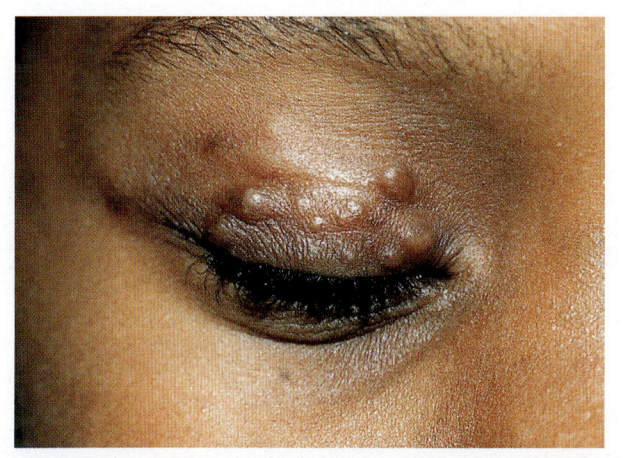

Figure 12.21. Pseudorheumatoid nodules (granuloma annulare) of upper eyelid in a 5-year-old girl. (Courtesy of Henry Ring, MD.)

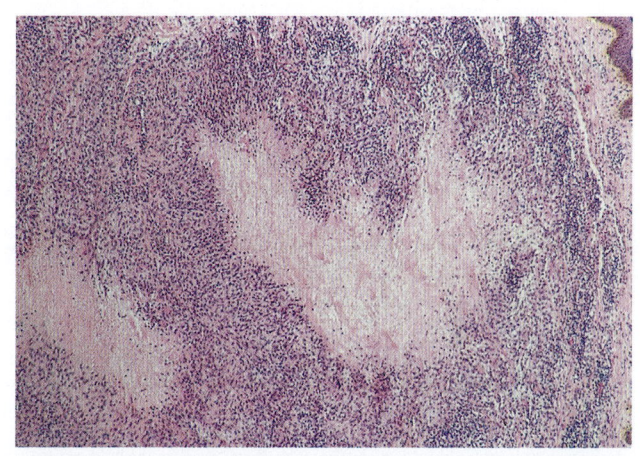

Figure 12.22. Histopathology of lesion shown in Figure 12.21, revealing chronic inflammation and necrobiosis of collagen. (Hematoxylin–eosin ×50.) (Courtesy of Henry Ring, MD.)

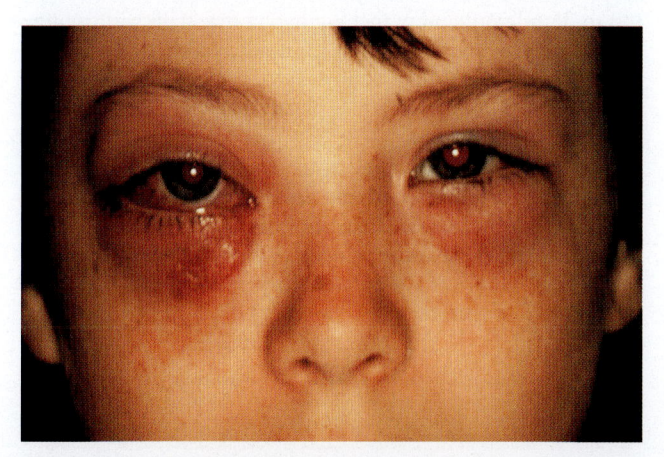

Figure 12.23. Granulomatosis with polyangiitis involving eyelids in a 10-year-old girl who also had renal involvement. (Courtesy of Tibor Farkas, MD.)

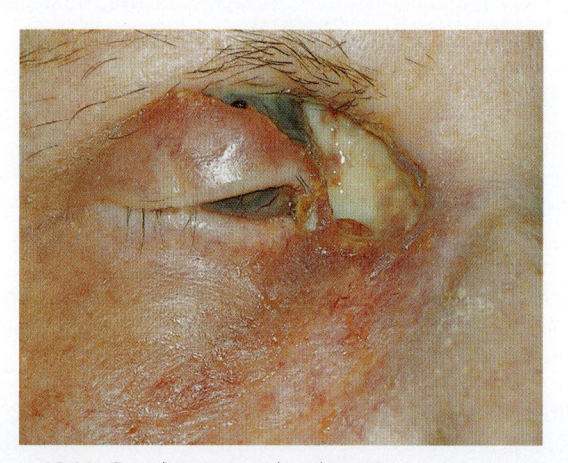

Figure 12.24. Granulomatosis with polyangiitis causing necrosis and erosion of medial aspect of eyelid in a 68-year-old woman.

EYELID MYCOTIC INFECTIONS

Eyelid Blastomycosis

General Considerations
Several mycotic infections, including blastomycosis, coccidioidomycosis, and mucormycosis can affect the eyelids. They generally originate in the lung and can secondarily involve the skin and eyelids by hematogenous dissemination. Examples of mycotic infections causing pseudoepitheliomatous hyperplasia are also depicted in Chapter 1.

Blastomycosis is an infectious disease caused by *Blastomyces dermatitidis* (1–6). The North American form is endemic in parts of the Eastern and Southern United States, especially Kentucky (2). It can affect any area of the skin including the face, eyelids, and conjunctiva (1–6).

Clinical Features
Eyelid involvement is characterized by a hyperkeratotic plaque that may be crusted and ulcerated. It can resemble squamous cell carcinoma or papilloma.

Pathology
Histopathologically, blastomycosis is characterized by marked pseudocarcinomatous hyperplasia with granulomatous inflammation containing Langhan's type giant cells. The organisms can be easily recognized microscopically.

Management
Treatment is with antifungal drugs like amphotericin B in standard doses. The prognosis varies with the extent of systemic disease.

Selected References
Reviews
1. Rucci J, Eisinger G, Miranda-Gomez G, et al. Blastomycosis of the head and neck. *Am J Otolaryngol* 2014;35:390–395.

Case Reports
2. Barr CC, Gamel JW. Blastomycosis of the eyelid. *Arch Ophthalmol* 1986;104;96–99.
3. Slack JW, Hyndiuk RA, Harris GJ, et al. Blastomycosis of the eyelid and conjunctiva. *Ophthal Plast Reconstr Surg* 1992;8:143–149.
4. Bartley GB. Blastomycosis of the eyelid. *Ophthalmology* 1995;102:2020–2023.
5. Mohney BG. Blastomycosis of the eyelid. *Ophthalmology* 1996;103:544–545.
6. Merin MR, Fung MA, Eisen DB, et al. Histoplasmosis presenting as a cutaneous malignancy of the eyelid. *Ophthal Plast Reconstr Surg* 2011;27(2):e41–e42.

Eyelid Coccidioidomycosis

General Considerations
Coccidioidomycosis is an infectious disease caused by *Coccidioides immitis*, which is endemic in areas of the Southwestern United States, particularly the San Joaquin Valley.

Clinical Features
Primary cutaneous coccidioidomycosis is rare and eyelid involvement has had little mention in the literature (1–3). It affects the eyelids in a similar manner to blastomycosis, as described. It can also be a cause of a uveitis.

Pathology
Histopathology shows a mixed granulomatous and suppurative reaction. Multinucleated giant cells contain spherules of *C. immitis*.

Management
Treatment is with antifungal drugs like amphotericin B in standard doses. The prognosis varies with the extent of systemic disease.

Selected References
Reviews
1. Borchers AT, Gershwin ME. The immune response in Coccidioidomycosis. *Autoimmun Rev* 2010;10:94–102.
2. Rodenbiker HT, Ganley JP. Review: ocular coccidioidomycosis. *Surv Ophthalmol* 1980;24:263–272.

Case Report
3. Irvine AR. Coccidioides granuloma of the lid. *Trans Am Acad Ophthalmol Otolaryngol* 1968;72:751–752.

Eyelid Mucormycosis

General Considerations
Mucormycosis (phycomycosis) generally occurs in patients with underlying systemic disease such as diabetic ketoacidosis, advanced malignancy, and other immunosuppressed states. It is discussed in greater detail in the section on orbital tumors. It often involves the respiratory tract and can secondarily affect the orbit with extension to the eyelids (1–3).

Clinical Features
Mucormycosis can produce necrosis of the orbital tissues and eyelids, leading to a black eschar. It may have a foul odor, which is suggestive of the diagnosis.

Pathology
Histopathologically, mucormycosis is characterized by acute inflammation, vascular thrombosis, necrosis, and numerous fungi. The organism is readily identified because of its large size (30 to 35 micron) and branching hypha that stain with routine hematoxylin and eosin. It tends to invade blood vessels and soft tissue (1–3).

Management
Management of eyelid/orbital mucormycosis is controversial. It is important to treat underlying disease, such as diabetic ketoacidosis, and to use debridement of necrotic tissue, amphotericin B, and other measures as necessary (1–3).

Selected References
Reviews
1. Camara-Lemarray CR, Gonzalez-Moreno E, Rodriguez-Gutierrez F, et al. Clinical features and outcome of mucormycosis. *Interdiscip Perspect Infect Dis* 2014;2014:562610.
2. Arndt S, Aschendorff A, Echternach M, et al. Rhino-orbital-cerebral mucormycosis and aspergillosis: differential diagnosis and treatment. *Eur Arch Otorhinolaryngol* 2009;266:71–76.
3. Gamaletsou MN, Sipsas NV, Roilides E, et al. Rhino-orbital-cerebral murcomycosis. *Curr Infect Dis Rep* 2012;14:423–434.

Chapter 12 Eyelid Inflammatory Lesions Simulating Neoplasms

● EYELID MYCOTIC INFECTIONS: COCCIDIOIDOMYCOSIS AND MUCORMYCOSIS

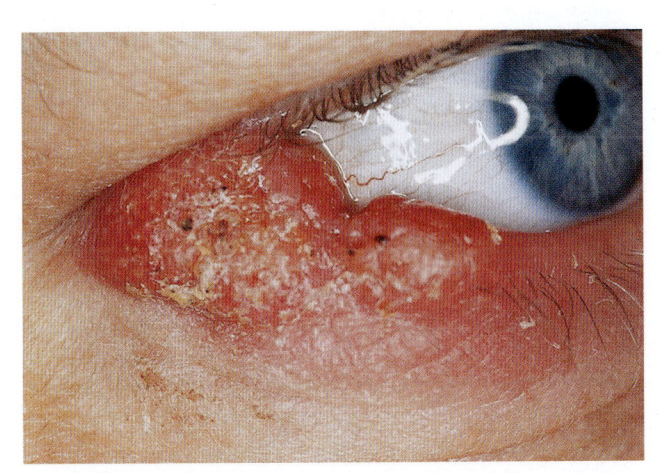

Figure 12.25. Blastomycosis of the eyelid in a 43-year-old man. He had a similar lesion on the forehead and pulmonary involvement. The eyelid lesion was originally suspected to be a chalazion. (Courtesy of R. Jean Campbell, MD.)

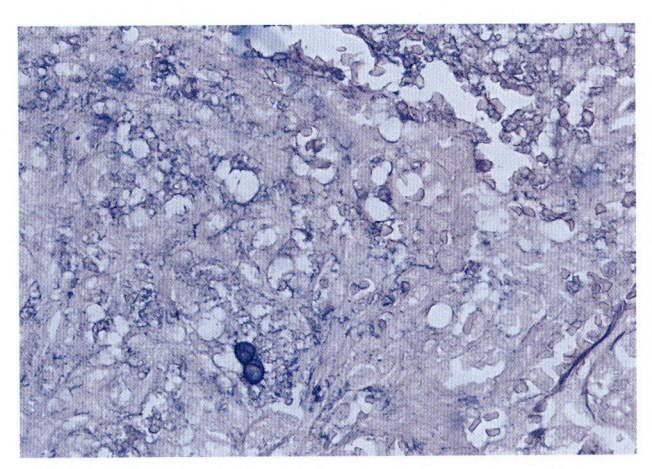

Figure 12.26. Histopathology of lesion shown in Figure 12.25, showing granulomatous inflammation and a yeast form inferiorly. (Gomori's methenamine silver ×200.)

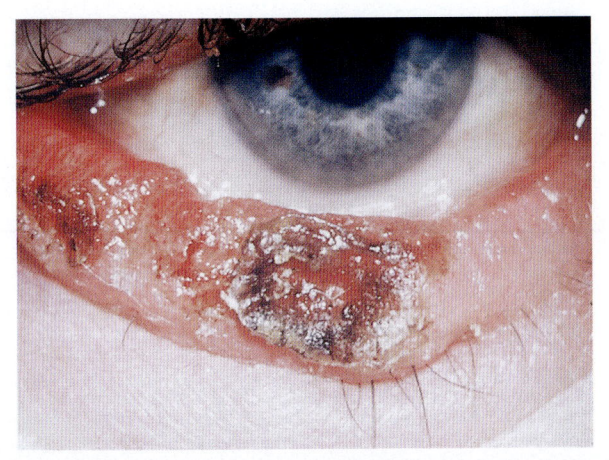

Figure 12.27. Coccidioidomycosis involving lower eyelid. (Courtesy of Armed Forces Institute of Pathology, Washington, DC.)

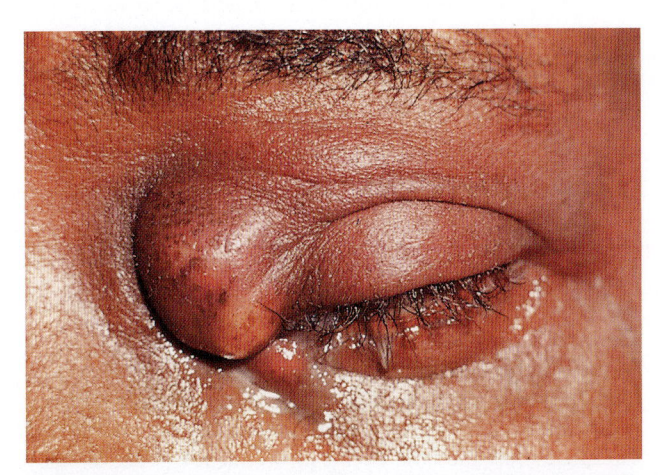

Figure 12.28. Mucormycosis involving medial canthus, upper eyelid, and orbit in a 53-year-old man with diabetic ketoacidosis. (Courtesy of Louis Karp, MD.)

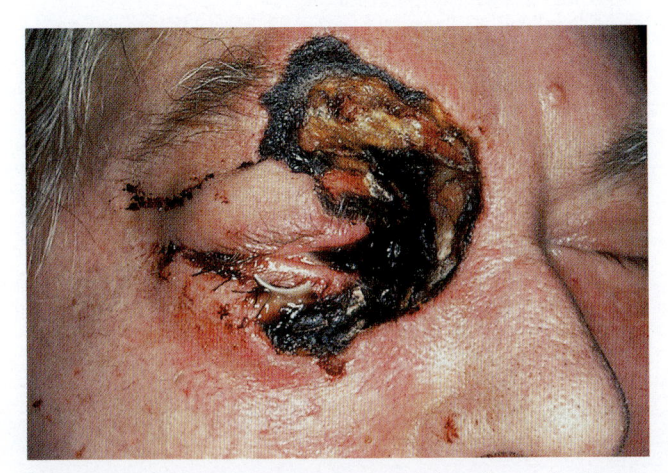

Figure 12.29. Mucormycosis involving medial canthus and orbit in a 60-year-old woman with diabetes who had multiple injuries from an automobile accident. (Courtesy of George Howard, MD.)

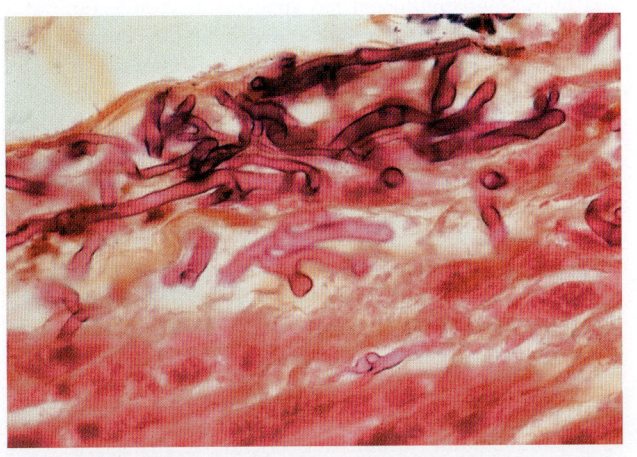

Figure 12.30. Histopathology of the lesion shown in Figure 12.29 demonstrating fungal organisms with large, branching, nonseptate hyphae. (Periodic acid-Schiff ×150.)

EYELID BACTERIAL INFECTIONS

Eyelid Abscess

General Considerations
In most cases, an abscess is easy to recognize and the diagnosis is made without difficulty. However, in some instances, a chronic abscess can simulate a neoplasm and some neoplasms may produce secondary inflammation or infection, masking the diagnosis of underlying eyelid tumor.

Clinical Features
A purulent abscess on the eyelid generally shows typical signs of infection, with acute onset, pain, redness, edema, and sometimes purulent drainage. It can occur after local trauma, systemic infection or, rarely, as secondary infection of a chalazion or tumor.

Pathology
Eyelid abscess is characterized by acute purulent infection with a massive infiltration by neutrophils. It can be secondary to a number of purulent organisms, but *Staphylococcus aureus* is a common cause.

Management
Treatment is with systemic antibiotics, sometimes combined with incision and drainage of large, symptomatic lesions. Culture and sensitivity studies can be taken to better direct treatment.

Necrotizing Fasciitis Involving Eyelid

General Considerations
Necrotizing fasciitis is characterized by a rapidly spreading infection resulting in necrosis of fascia, muscle, and subcutaneous fat. It can occur anywhere in subcutaneous tissue and can often affect the face. Eyelid involvement can occasionally develop (1–18).

Many cases of necrotizing fasciitis are idiopathic with no apparent predisposing cause (8). It can develop after surgical and nonsurgical trauma. It has appeared as an infection after blepharoplasty (12–14). It has occurred from direct spread from dacryocystitis. Predisposing debilitating disease like diabetes can play a role. In many cases, β-hemolytic streptococcus alone or in combination with other organisms has been identified.

Clinical Features
Necrotizing fasciitis can begin as a localized infection and rapidly progress to diffusely involve adjacent subcutaneous tissue. It appears as a diffuse thickening of the eyelid and surrounding facial skin with erythema and a blue discoloration owing to subcutaneous hemorrhage. The patient has pain and apprehension. Early detection is key and an algorithm has been developed (2).

Pathology
Histopathologically, necrotizing fasciitis is characterized by extensive inflammation and necrosis of subcutaneous tissue. There is a marked infiltration by acute inflammatory cells. With special stains or cultures, gram-positive bacteria are often identified as β-hemolytic streptococci.

Management
The treatment of necrotizing fasciitis is administration of appropriate antibiotics, often with surgical debridement and cultures. Some cases develop widespread systemic involvement and death has been reported in about 13% of cases despite vigorous treatment (7).

Selected References

Reviews
1. Hakkarainen TW, Kopari NM, Pham TN, et al. Necrotizing soft tissue infections: review and current concepts in treatment, systems of care, and outcomes. *Curr Probl Surg* 2014;51:344–362.
2. Malik V, Gadepalli C, Agrawal S, et al. An algorithm for early diagnosis of cervicofacial necrotising fasciitis. *Eur Arch Otorhinolaryngol* 2010;267:1169–1177.
3. Marshall DH, Jordan DR, Gilberg SM, et al. Periocular necrotizing fasciitis: a review of five cases. *Ophthalmology* 1997;104:1857–1862.

Management
4. Nallathambi MN, Ivatury RR, Rohman M, et al. Cranio-cervical necrotizing fasciitis: critical factors in management. *Can J Surg* 1987;30:61–63.
5. Luksich JA, Holds JB, Hartstein ME. Conservative management of necrotizing fasciitis of the eyelids. *Ophthalmology* 2002;109:2118–2122.

Case Reports
6. Walters R. A fatal case of necrotizing fasciitis of the eyelid. *Br J Ophthalmol* 1988;72:428–431.
7. Kronish JW, McLeish WM. Eyelid necrosis and periorbital necrotizing fasciitis. Report of a case and review of the literature. *Ophthalmology* 1991;98:92–98.
8. Williams SR, Carruth JA, Brightwell AP. Necrotizing fasciitis of the face without significant trauma. *Clin Otolaryngol* 1992;17:344–350.
9. Shayegani A, MacFarlane D, Kazim M, et al. Streptococcal gangrene of the eyelids and orbit. *Am J Ophthalmol* 1995;120:784–792.
10. Kent D, Atkinson PL, Patel B, et al. Fatal bilateral necrotising fasciitis of the eyelids. *Br J Ophthalmol* 1995;79:95–96.
11. Hunt L. Streptococcal necrotizing fasciitis of the eyelids and orbit. *Insight* 1996;21:96–97.
12. Ray AM, Bressler K, Davis RE, et al. Cervicofacial necrotizing fasciitis. A devastating complication of blepharoplasty. *Arch Otolaryngol Head Neck Surg* 1997;123:633–636.
13. Jordan DR, Mawn L, Marshall DH. Necrotizing fasciitis caused by group A streptococcus infection after laser blepharoplasty. *Am J Ophthalmol* 1998;125:265–266.
14. Suner IJ, Meldrum ML, Johnson TE, et al. Necrotizing fasciitis after cosmetic blepharoplasty. *Am J Ophthalmol* 1999;128:367–368.
15. Beerens AJ, Bauwens LJ, Leemans CR. A fatal case of craniofacial necrotizing fasciitis. *Eur Arch Otorhinolaryngol* 1999;256:506–509.
16. Goldberg RA, Li TG. Postoperative infection with group A beta-hemolytic streptococcus after blepharoplasty. *Am J Ophthalmol* 2002;134:908–910.
17. Lin PW, Lin HC. Facial necrotizing fasciitis following acute dacryocystitis. *Am J Ophthalmol* 2003;136:203–204.
18. Saonanon P, Tirakunwichcha S, Chierakul W. Case report of orbital cellulitis and necrotizing fasciitis from melioidosis. *Ophthal Plast Reconstr Surg* 2013;29(3):e81–e84.

Chapter 12 Eyelid Inflammatory Lesions Simulating Neoplasms

EYELID BACTERIAL INFECTIONS: ABSCESS AND NECROTIZING FASCIITIS

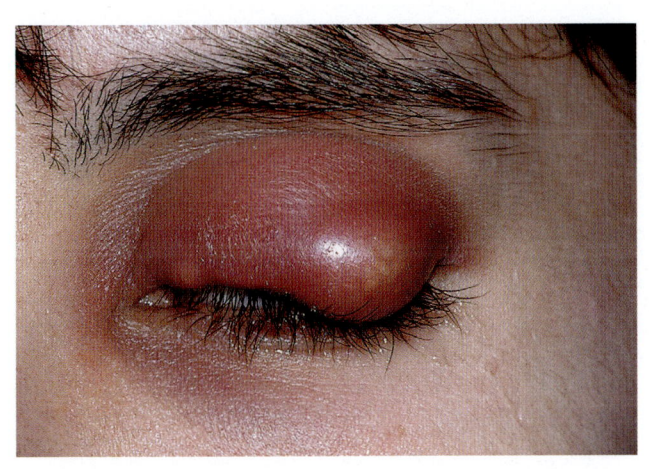

Figure 12.31. Purulent abscess of upper eyelid in a 20-year-old woman.

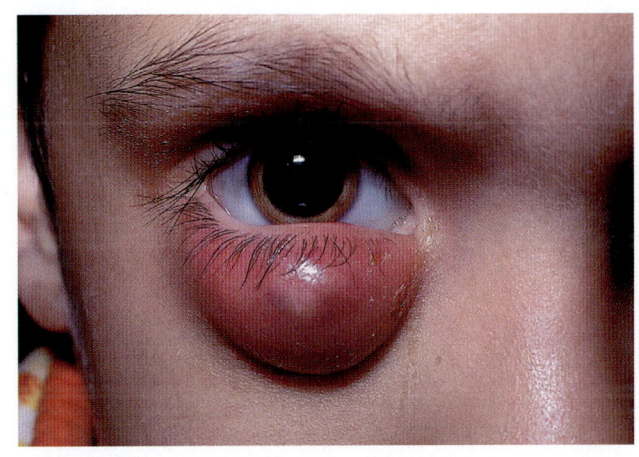

Figure 12.32. Purulent abscess of lower eyelid in a 14-year-old boy.

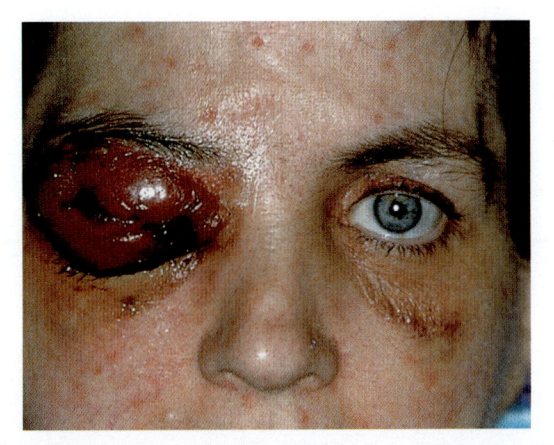

Figure 12.33. Necrotizing fasciitis involving upper eyelid and surrounding tissues. (Courtesy of David Addison, MD.)

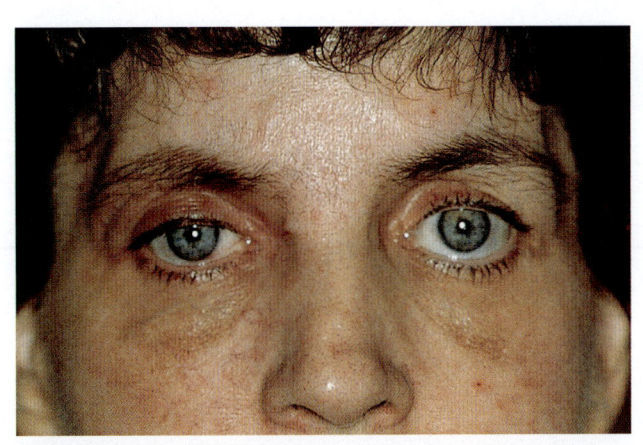

Figure 12.34. Appearance of patient shown in Figure 12.33 after debridement and appropriate antibiotics. (Courtesy of David Addison, MD.)

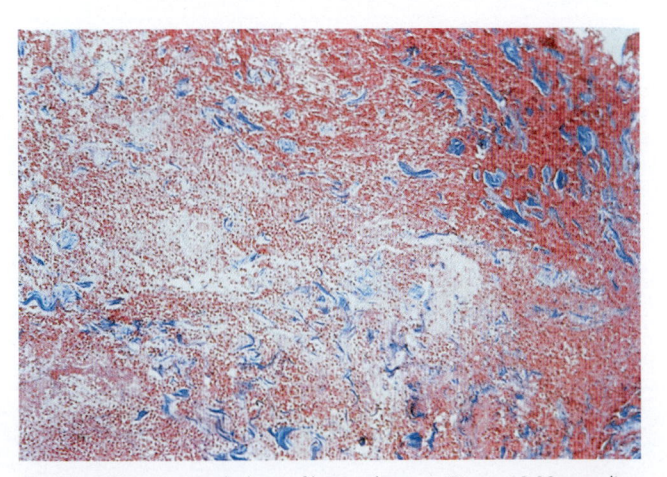

Figure 12.35. Histopathology of lesion shown in Figure 12.33 revealing inflammation and necrosis. (×100.) (Courtesy of David Addison, MD.)

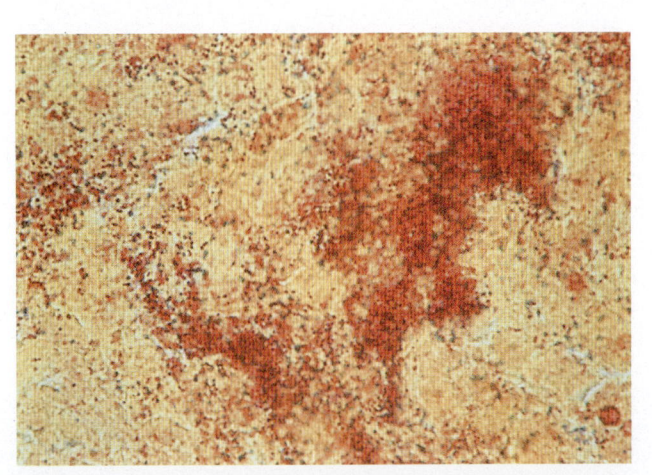

Figure 12.36. Histopathology of lesion shown in Figure 12.33 demonstrating gram-positive bacteria. (Gram stain ×100.) (Courtesy of David Addison, MD.)

CHAPTER 13

EYELID MISCELLANEOUS CONDITIONS SIMULATING NEOPLASMS

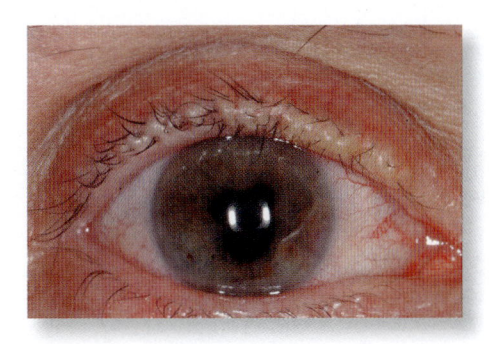

General Considerations

There are several tumors and pseudotumors that are difficult to classify. Examples discussed in this chapter include amyloidosis, lipoid proteinosis, granular cell tumor, malakoplakia, calcinosis cutis, and phakomatous choristoma.

Amyloidosis is characterized by deposition of a variety of abnormal proteins in many parts of the body (1). The eyelid is a preferred site in patients with primary systemic amyloidosis as well as those with systemic multiple myeloma, Waldenström's macroglobulinemia, and other monoclonal gammopathies (1–20).

Clinical Features

Eyelid involvement typically appears as multiple bilateral confluent papules that have a waxy pink or yellow color. The lesions tend to bleed spontaneously or following slight trauma. In many cases, there is blepharoptosis and thickening of the eyelid owing to diffuse involvement of the palpebral conjunctiva (11,13). In most instances, bilateral eyelid amyloidosis is associated with systemic amyloidosis, but amyloid deposition can also occur as an isolated phenomenon on the eyelids (10,14).

Pathology

Amyloid is an acellular, homogeneous, lightly eosinophilic material that is located in the dermis when the eyelid is involved. It is birefringent and shows a positive reaction with Congo red stain. Immunohistochemical studies have suggested an immunoglobulin light chain origin (12).

Management

Treatment of eyelid amyloidosis is controversial and difficult and should be directed toward the symptoms. Some lesions apparently remain stable for months and require no active treatment (15). Surgical excision of larger, cosmetically unacceptable eyelid lesions is appropriate (18). Some surgeons have reported successful removal of eyelid amyloid by meticulous dissection, leaving the anatomic planes of the eyelid intact (9). Although controversial, irradiation has been reported to cause regression of the lesions (8).

EYELID AMYLOIDOSIS

Selected References

Reviews

1. Real deAsua D, Galvan JM, Filigheddu MT, et al. Systemic AA amyloidosis: epidemiology, diagnosis, and management. *Clin Epidemiol* 2014;6:369–377.
2. Demirci H, Shields CL, Eagle RC Jr, et al. Conjunctival amyloidosis: report of six cases and review of the literature. *Surv Ophthalmol* 2006;51:419–433.
3. Al-Nuaimi D, Bhatt PR, Steeples L, et al. Amyloidosis of the orbita and adnexa. *Orbit* 2012;31:287–298.
4. Smith ME, Zimmerman LE. Amyloidosis of the eyelid and conjunctiva. *Arch Ophthalmol* 1966;75:42–50.
5. Natelson EA, Duncan WC, Macossay C, et al. Amyloidosis palbebrum. *Arch Intern Med* 1979;125:304–305.
6. Halasa AH. Amyloid disease of the eyelid and conjunctiva. *Arch Ophthalmol* 1965;74:298–301.
7. Brownstein MH, Elliott R, Helwig EB. Ophthalmologic aspects of amyloidosis. *Am J Ophthalmol* 1970;69:423–430.

Management

8. Pecora JL, Sambursky JS, Vargha Z. Radiation therapy in amyloidosis of the eyelid and conjunctiva: a case report. *Ann Ophthalmol* 1982;14:194–196.
9. Patrinely JR, Koch DD. Surgical management of advanced ocular adnexal amyloidosis. *Arch Ophthalmol* 1992;110:882–885.

Case Reports

10. Fett DR, Putterman AM. Primary localized amyloidosis presenting as an eyelid margin tumor. *Arch Ophthalmol* 1986;104:584–585.
11. Iijima S. Primary systemic amyloidosis: a unique case complaining of diffuse eyelid swelling and conjunctival involvement. *J Dermatol* 1992;19:113–118.
12. Olsen KE, Sandgren O, Sletten K, et al. Primary localized amyloidosis of the eyelid: two cases of immunoglobulin light chain-derived proteins, subtype lambda V respectively lambda VI. *Clin Exp Immunol* 1996;106:362–366.
13. Hill VE, Brownstein S, Jordan DR. Ptosis secondary to amyloidosis of the tarsal conjunctiva and tarsus. *Am J Ophthalmol* 1997;123:852–854.
14. Pelton RW, Desmond BP, Mamalis N, et al. Nodular cutaneous amyloid tumors of the eyelids in the absence of systemic amyloidosis. *Ophthalmic Surg Lasers* 2001;32:422–424.
15. Rodrigues G, Sanghvi V, Lala M. A rare cause of unilateral upper and lower eyelid swelling: isolated conjunctival amyloidosis. *Korean J Ophthalmol* 2001;15:38–40.
16. Goldstein DA, Schteingart MT, Birnbaum AD, et al. Bilateral eyelid ecchymosis and corneal crystals: an unusual presentation of multiple myeloma. *Cornea* 2005;24:757–758.
17. Landa G, Aloni E, Milshtein A, et al. Lid bleeding and atypical amyloidosis. *Am J Ophthalmol* 2004;138:495–496.
18. Stack RR, Vote BJ, Evans JL, et al. Bilateral ptosis caused by localized superficial eyelid amyloidosis. *Ophthalmol Plast Reconstr Surg* 2003;19:239–240.
19. Jacoby S, Toft PB, Prause JU, et al. Nodular amyloidosis of all four eyelids: first presenting symptom of Waldenström macroglobulinaemia. *Acta Ophthalmol* 2013;92(4):392–393.
20. Chee E, Kim YD, Lee JH, et al. Chronic eyelid swelling as an initial manifestation of myeloma-associated amyloidosis. *Ophthal Plast Reconstr Surg* 2013;29(1):e12–e14.

Chapter 13 Eyelid Miscellaneous Conditions Simulating Neoplasms 225

● EYELID AMYLOIDOSIS

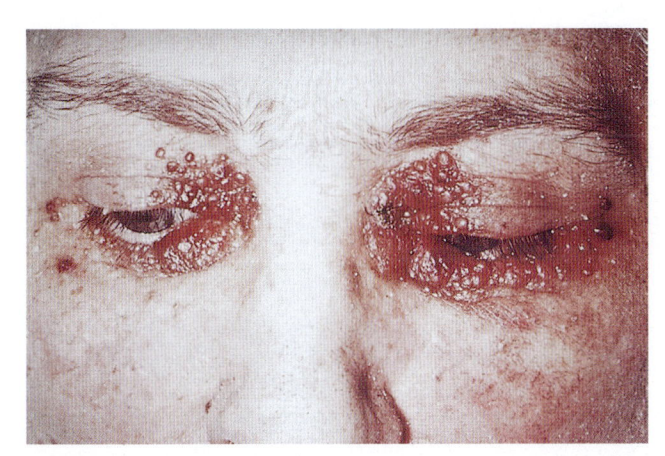

Figure 13.1. Bilateral eyelid involvement with amyloidosis. (Courtesy of Martin Brownstein, MD.)

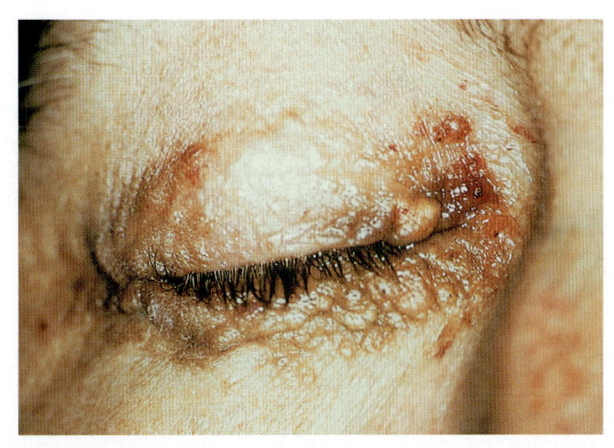

Figure 13.2. Eyelid amyloidosis in a 59-year-old man with multiple myeloma. (Courtesy of Myron Yanoff, MD.)

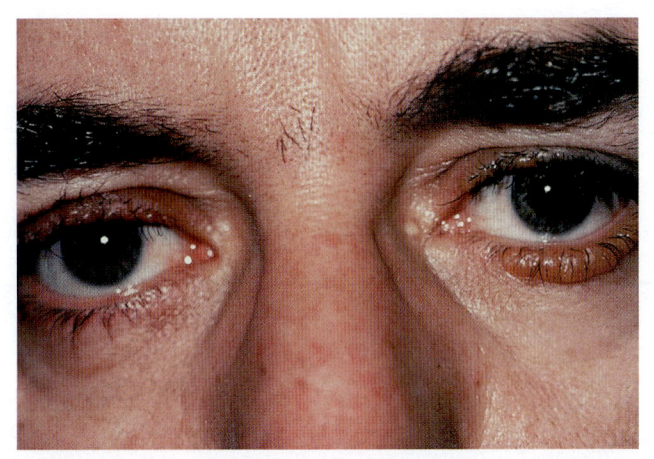

Figure 13.3. Eyelid margin amyloidosis in a 51-year-old man with no known systemic disease. There is involvement of all four eyelids, but it is most pronounced on the right upper eyelid and left lower eyelid. (Courtesy of David Barsky, MD and Thomas Spoor, MD.)

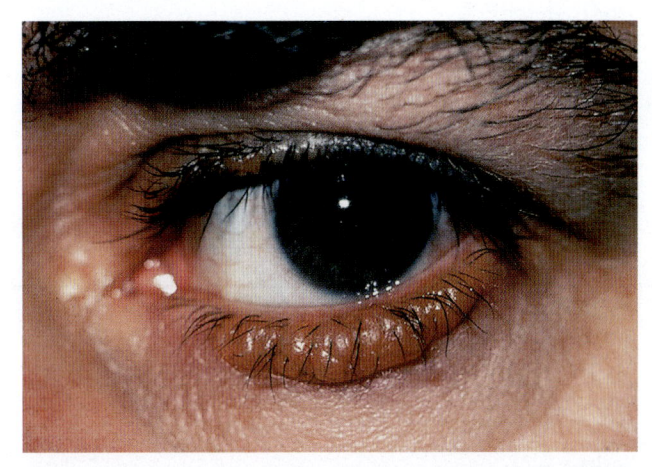

Figure 13.4. Closer view of lesion on left lower eyelid in patient shown in Figure 13.3. (Courtesy of David Barsky, MD and Thomas Spoor, MD.)

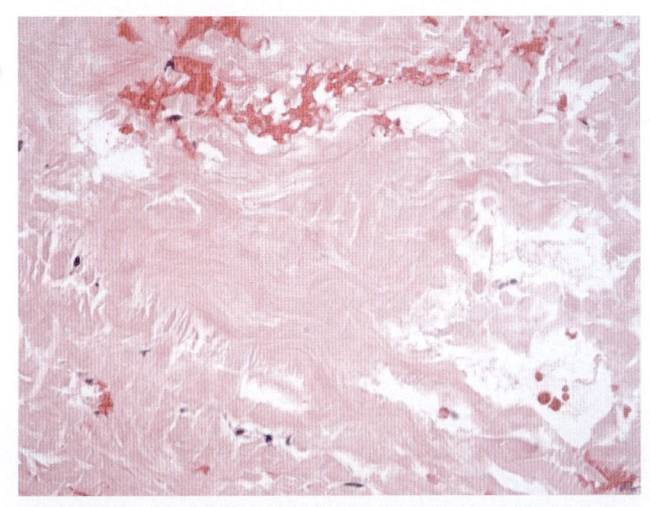

Figure 13.5. High-power photomicrograph of amyloid showing relatively acellular lightly eosinophilic material in the dermis. (Hematoxylin–eosin ×25.)

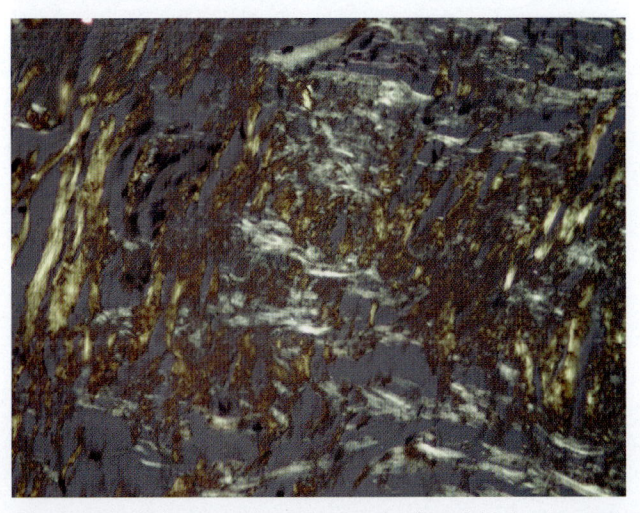

Figure 13.6. High-power photomicrograph of amyloid showing positive birefringence in polarized light. (Congo red ×25.)

EYELID LIPOID PROTEINOSIS (URBACH–WIETHE DISEASE)

General Considerations

Lipoid proteinosis (Urbach–Wiethe disease) is an uncommon autosomal-recessive condition characterized by numerous beaded papules and nodules that develop in the skin and mucous membranes and bilateral sickle-shaped skull calcifications on imaging studies (1–12). The eyelid lesions can occur in siblings and are believed to be pathognomonic (9).

Clinical Features

Eyelid involvement is characterized by multiple bilateral yellow-brown, waxy, hyperkeratotic papules. It can be clinically similar to amyloidosis. The lesions are often located along the eyelid margin and sometimes cause disruption of the cilia. It is wise to check the tongue, soft palate, and axilla for similar lesions and also check family members for the disease.

Pathology

Histopathologically, the lesions consist of a deposition of a hyaline material (glycoprotein, not lipid) in the dermis. The capillary walls are thickened. Electron microscopic studies have been performed, but the exact nature of the material remains unclear (4,5). Fibroblasts seem to play an active role in the synthesis of the substance.

Management

No treatment is effective, except for surgical removal of lesions that are cosmetically unacceptable. Carbon dioxide laser has been employed to eradicate the lesions (6).

Selected References

Reviews

1. Griffith DG, Salasche SJ, Clemons DE. Lipoid proteinosis. In: Griffith DG, Salasche SJ, Clemons DE, eds. *Cutaneous Abnormalities of the Eyelid and Face.* New York: McGraw-Hill; 1987:68.
2. Abtahi SM, Kianersi F, Abtahi MA, et al. Urbach-wiethe syndrome and the ophthalmologist: review of the literature and introduction of the first instance of bilateral uveitis. *Case Rep Med* 2012;2012:281516. doi: 10.1155/2012/281516. Epub 2012 Jul 31.
3. Hofer PA, Larsson PA, Goller H, et al. A clinical and histopathological study of twenty-seven cases of Urbach-Wiethe disease: dermatologic, gastroenterologic, neurophysiologic, ophthalmologic and roentgen diagnostic aspects, as well as the result of some clinico-chemical and histochemical examinations. *Acta Pathol Microbiol Scand* 1974;245:1–87.

Histopathology

4. Fabrizi G, Porfiri B, Borgioli M, et al. Urbach-Wiethe disease. Light and electron microscopic study. *J Cutan Pathol* 1980;7:8–20.
5. Dinakaran S, Desai SP, Palmer IR, et al. Lipoid proteinosis: clinical features and electron microscopic study. *Eye* 2001;15:666–668.

Management

6. Rosenthal G, Lifshitz T, Monos T, et al. Carbon dioxide laser treatment for lipoid proteinosis (Urbach-Wiethe syndrome) involving the eyelids. *Br J Ophthalmol* 1997;81:253.

Case Reports

7. Jensen AD, Khodadoust AA, Emery JM. Lipoid proteinosis. *Arch Ophthalmol* 1972;88:273–277.
8. Feiler-Ofry V, Levy A, Rogenbogen L, et al. Lipoid proteinosis (Urbach-Wiethe Syndrome). *Br J Ophthalmol* 1979;63:694–698.
9. Sharma V, Kashyap S, Betharia SM, et al. Lipoid proteinosis: a rare disorder with pathognomonic lid lesions. *Clin Exp Ophthalmol* 2004;32:110–112.
10. Al-Bitar Y, Samdani AJ. Lipoid proteinosis in two brothers with multiple organ involvement from Saudi Arabia. *Int J Dermatol* 2004;43:360–361.
11. Callizo M, Ibáñez-Flores N, Laue J, et al. Eyelid lesions in lipoid proteinosis or Urbach-Wiethe disease: case report and review of the literature. *Orbit* 2011;30(5):242–244.
12. Izadi F, Mahjoubi F, Farhadi M, et al. A novel missense mutation in exon 7 of the ECM1 gene in an Iranian lipoid proteinosis patient. *Genet Mol Res* 2012;11(4):3955–3960.

Chapter 13 Eyelid Miscellaneous Conditions Simulating Neoplasms

● EYELID LIPOID PROTEINOSIS (URBACH–WIETHE DISEASE)

Dinakaran S, Desai SP, Palmer IR, et al. Lipoid proteinosis: clinical features and electron microscopic study. *Eye* 2001;15:666–668.

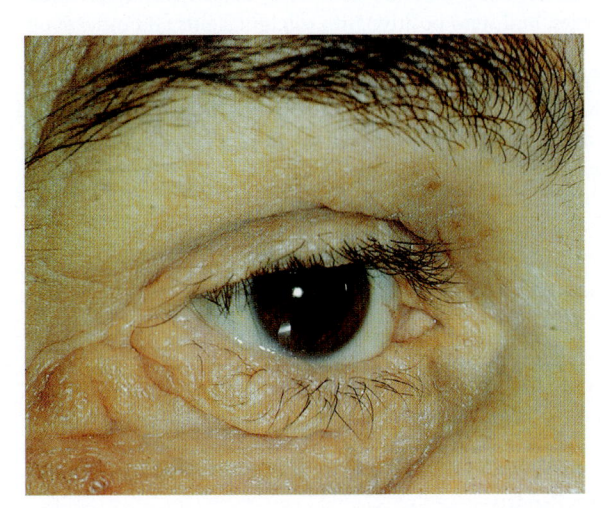

Figure 13.7. Lipoid proteinosis of lower eyelid in a 59-year-old woman who also had similar lesions on contralateral eyelids, elbows, and knees. There was a positive family history for this disease. (Courtesy of Richard Smith, MD.)

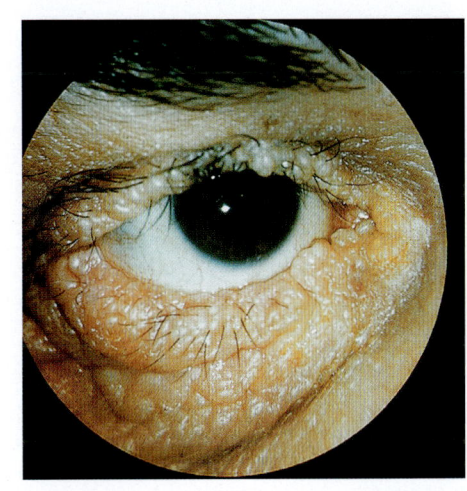

Figure 13.8. Closer view of the lesion shown in Figure 13.7. (Courtesy of Richard Smith, MD.)

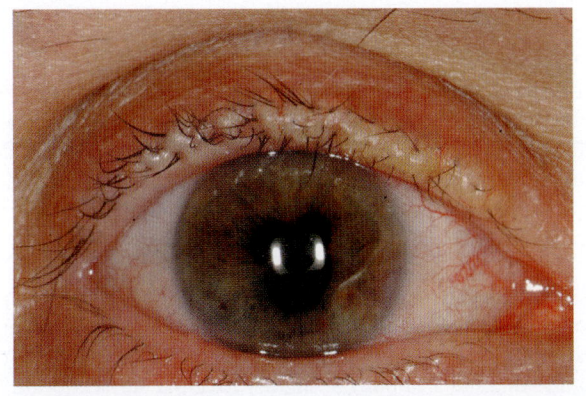

Figure 13.9. Lipoid proteinosis of upper and lower eyelid in an asymptomatic 45-year-old man.

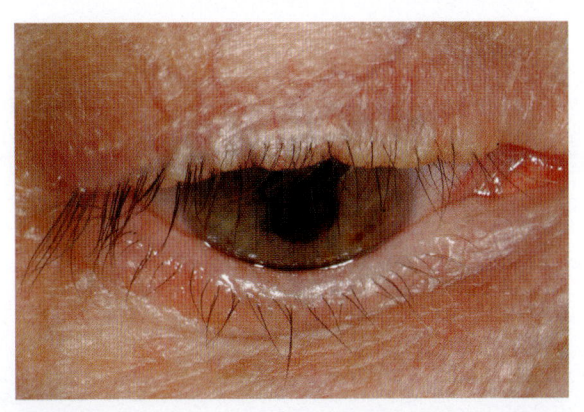

Figure 13.10. Closer view of patient in Figure 13.9 showing the irregular eyelid margin.

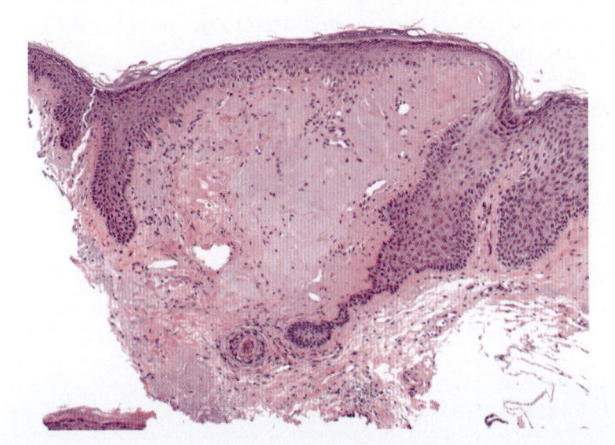

Figure 13.11. Low-power histopathology of lipoid proteinosis showing a thin zone of normal tissue in the superficial dermis and the reticular dermis is replaced by slightly basophilic amorphous hyaline material, with occasional cells resembling fibroblasts. (Hematoxylin–eosin ×20.) (Courtesy of Martha Farber, MD.)

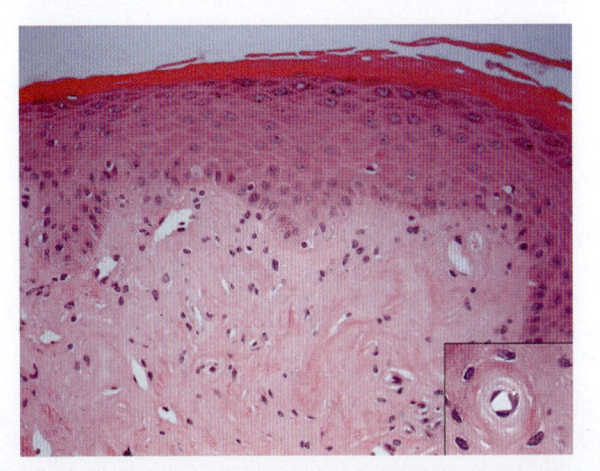

Figure 13.12. High-power histopathology of lipoid proteinosis showing amorphous material dermis with vascular cuffing of the material (*inset*). (Hematoxylin–eosin ×200.) (Courtesy of Seymour Brownstein, MD.)

MISCELLANEOUS OTHER PSEUDONEOPLASTIC EYELID LESIONS

Eyelid Granular Cell Tumor

General Considerations
Granular cell tumor (granular cell "myoblastoma") is an uncommon benign neoplasm that generally occurs on the tongue or skin. It was once considered to be of myoblastic origin; more recently, a Schwann cell origin has been postulated. It can occasionally originate in the eyelids, conjunctiva, caruncle, lacrimal sac, and orbit (1–6).

Clinical Features
The eyelid lesion generally appears as a solitary lump deep to the epidermis, often near the eyelid margin.

Pathology
Microscopically, it is composed of round to ovoid cells that have granular eosinophilic cytoplasm and eccentric nuclei. The cells are often embedded in dense collagenous tissue. Pseudoepitheliomatous hyperplasia is a common association (6). Immunohistochemical studies have detected S-100 protein in both the cytoplasm and nuclei, supporting the concept of a neurogenic origin for the neoplasm (3,4).

Management
Because there are no specific clinical features, the diagnosis of granular cell tumor is rarely made before histopathologic studies after biopsy or excision. However, like other solitary masses, the preferred treatment is complete local excision when possible.

Selected References

Case Reports
1. Friedman Z, Eden E, Neumann E. Granular cell myoblastoma of the eyelid margin. *Br J Ophthalmol* 1973;57:757–760.
2. Rubenzik R, Tenzel RR. Granular cell myoblastoma of the lid: case report. *Ann Ophthalmol* 1976;8:421–422.
3. Ishibashi T, Yoshitomi T, Ohnishi Y, et al. Granular cell tumor of the lower lid: histological and immunohistochemical studies. *Graefes Arch Clin Exp Ophthalmol* 1984;222:75–78.
4. Jaeger MJ, Green WR, Miller NR, et al. Granular cell tumor of the orbit and ocular adnexae. *Surv Ophthalmol* 1987;31:417–423.
5. Bregman DK, Hodges T, La Piana FG. Granular cell tumor of the eyelid. *Ann Ophthalmol* 1991;23:106–107.
6. Ferry AP. Granular cell tumor (myoblastoma) of the palpebral conjunctiva causing pseudoepitheliomatous hyperplasia of the conjunctival epithelium. *Am J Ophthalmol* 1981;91:234–238.

Eyelid Malakoplakia

General Considerations
Malakoplakia is an unusual condition in which plaquelike lesions appear in many parts of the body, presumably secondary to the presence of bacterial products occurring in patients who have debilitating disease. It rarely involves the eyelids (1–5).

Clinical Features
Clinically, the eyelid lesion is variable and can appear as a slightly tender or painful white-yellow nodule or as an ulcerated or draining mass.

Pathology
Histopathologically, there are peculiar laminated structures within foamy histiocytes (von Hansemann histiocytes) that contain typical basophilic inclusions, called Michaelis–Gutmann bodies, and stain positive with calcium stains and other stains.

Management
The diagnosis of this uncommon tumor is rarely made clinically. Like other circumscribed suspicious eyelid masses, the treatment is local excision. Medical management of the underlying infectious process is also suggested (3).

Selected References

Reviews
1. Kohl SK, Hans CP. Cutaneous malakoplakia. *Arch Pathol Lab Med* 2008;132:113–117.
2. Yousef GM, Naghibi B, Hamodat MM. Malakoplakia outside the urinary tract. *Arch Pathol Lab Med* 2007;131:297–300.

Management
3. Simpson C, Strong NP, Dickinson J, et al. Medical management of ocular malakoplakia. *Ophthalmology* 1992;99:192–196.

Case Reports
4. Addison DJ. Malakoplakia of the eyelid. *Ophthalmology* 1986;93:1064–1067.
5. Font RL, Bersani TA, Eagle RC. Malakoplakia of the eyelid. *Ophthalmology* 1988;95:61–68.

Eyelid Subepidermal Calcified Nodule

General Considerations
Subepidermal calcified nodule is a form of calcinosis cutis that most commonly occurs in children. It usually appears as a solitary verrucous nodule on the face, but multiple lesions are sometimes present. Eyelid involvement is rare, with only a few reported cases (1–6).

Clinical Features
Eyelid subepidermal calcified nodule usually appears as in early childhood or early adulthood as a solitary yellow-white, hard, nodule that has a smooth or slightly irregular surface (5–6).

Pathology
Microscopically, subepidermal calcified nodule consists of deposits of free calcium located deep to the dermis. The etiology and pathogenesis are poorly understood.

Management
Management is surgical excision. The prognosis is excellent.

Selected References

Reviews
1. Nico MM, Bergonse FN. Subepidermal calcified nodule: report of two cases and review of the literature. *Pediatr Dermatol* 2001;18:227–229.
2. Welborn MC, Gottschalk H, Bindra R. Juvenile dermatomyositis: A case of calcinosis cutis of the elbow and review of the literature. *J Pediatr Orthop* 2014 Nov 19. [Epub ahead of print.]

Case Reports
3. Tezuka T. Cutaneous calculus—its pathogenesis. *Dermatologica* 1980;161:191–199.
4. Cursiefen C, Junemann A. Subepidermal calcified nodule. *Arch Ophthalmol* 1998;116:1254–1255.
5. Nguyen J, Jakobiec FA, Hanna E, et al. Subepidermal calcified nodule of the eyelid. *Ophthalm Plasti Reconstr Surg* 2008;24:494–495.
6. Koylu MT, Uysal Y, Kucukevcilioglu M, et al. Bilateral symmetrical subepidermal calcified nodules of the eyelids. *Orbit* 2014;33:295–297.

MISCELLANEOUS EYELID LESIONS: GRANULAR CELL TUMOR, MALAKOPLAKIA, AND SUBEPIDERMAL CALCIFIED NODULE

1. Addison DJ. Malakoplakia of the eyelid. *Ophthalmology* 1986;93:1064–1067.
2. Font RL, Bersani TA, Eagle RC. Malakoplakia of the eyelid. *Ophthalmology* 1988;95:61–68.

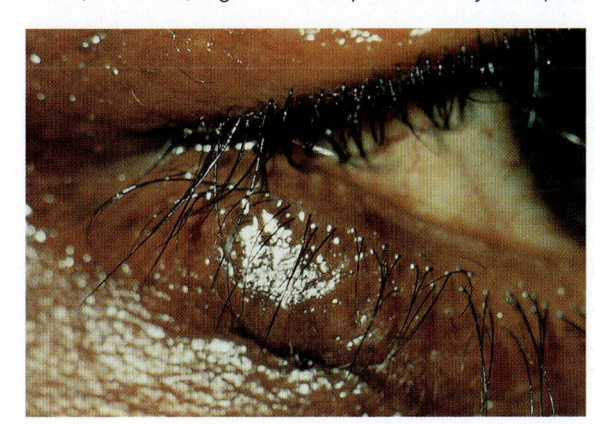

Figure 13.13. Granular cell tumor of eyelid. (Courtesy of Ralph C. Eagle, Jr, MD.)

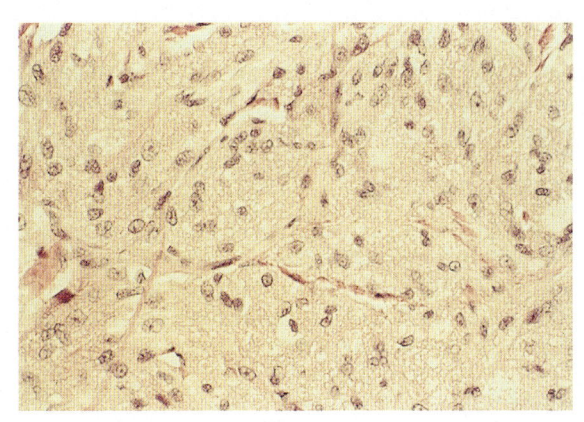

Figure 13.14. Photomicrograph of lesion shown in Figure 13.13 showing closely compact round cells with small round nuclei and granular cytoplasm. (Hematoxylin–eosin ×100.) (Courtesy of Ralph C. Eagle, Jr, MD.)

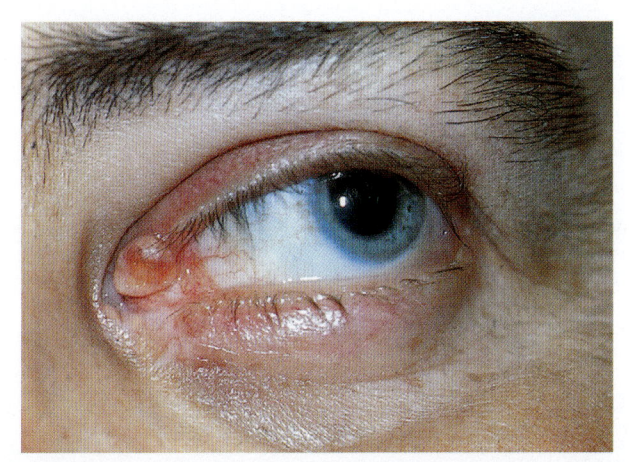

Figure 13.15. Malakoplakia near medial canthus. (Courtesy of David Addison, MD.)

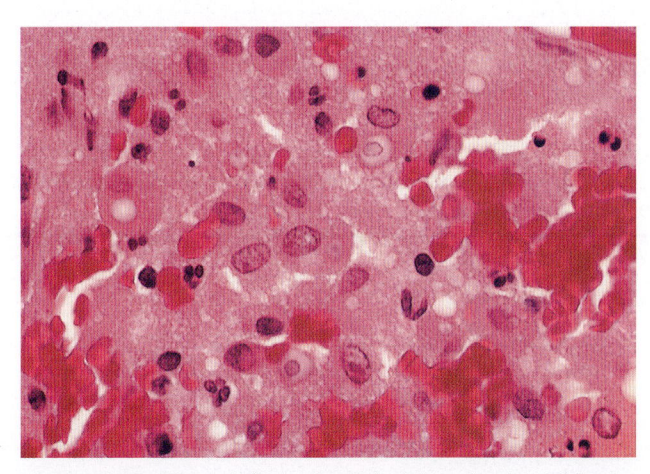

Figure 13.16. Histopathology of malakoplakia, showing Michaelis–Gutmann bodies within the histiocytes. (Periodic acid-Schiff ×350.) (Courtesy of Ralph C. Eagle, Jr, MD and Ramon L. Font, MD.)

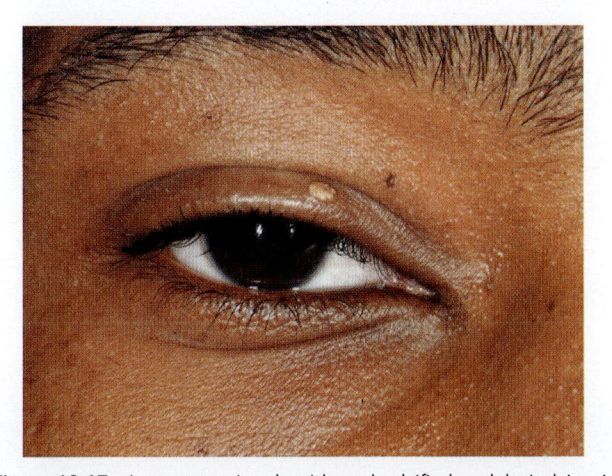

Figure 13.17. Asymptomatic subepidermal calcified nodule (calcinosis cutis) located on the upper eyelid in a 10-year-old boy.

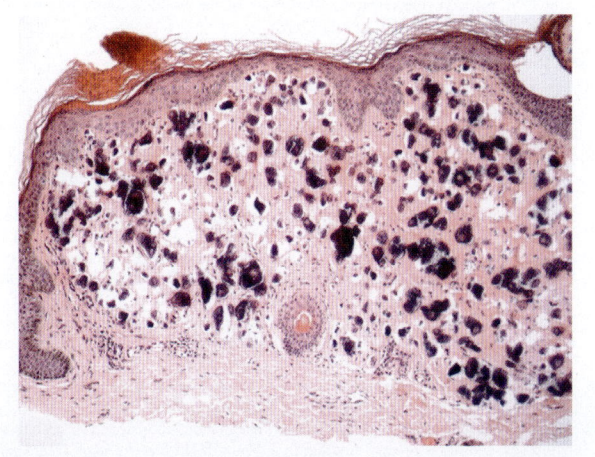

Figure 13.18. Histopathology of subepidermal calcified nodule shown in Figure 13.17, showing calcific deposits in dermis surrounded by amorphous material. (Hematoxylin–eosin ×50.)

EYELID PHAKOMATOUS CHORISTOMA

General Considerations

Phakomatous choristoma (Zimmerman's tumor) is a rare congenital lesion of lenticular (ocular lens) anlage that is invariably located in the deep eyelid or anterior orbit. Zimmerman (1) reported three cases in 1971 and a number of other cases have now been recorded (2–19).

Clinical Features

Clinically, phakomatous choristoma typically becomes apparent in the first few months of life as a smooth, firm, subcutaneous mass usually beneath the lower eyelid inferonasally. It is often diagnosed clinically as a dermoid cyst. Affected children have a normal lens in the eye.

Pathology

Histopathologically, the lesion is remarkably similar to the findings observed in congenital cataracts. It is believed to be a choristoma of lenticular anlage that probably results from displacement of the lens placode into the deeper mesodermal tissues of the lower eyelid. Special stains and immunohistochemical studies show positive reactivity for vimentin, S-100 protein, and periodic acid-Schiff. Immunohistochemical stains for cytokeratin and epithelial membrane antigen appear to be negative (3–9). One study showed intense immunoreactivity for all lens proteins (7). These findings, as well as ultrastructural observations, support the lenticular origin of the lesion.

Management

Management of phakomatous choristoma is local excision; recurrence has not been recognized; and the prognosis is excellent.

Selected References

Reviews

1. Zimmerman LE. Phakomatous choristoma of the eyelid. A tumor of lenticular anlage. *Am J Ophthalmol* 1971;71:169–177.
2. Filipic M, Silva M. Phakomatous choristoma of the eyelid: a tumor of lenticular anlage. *Arch Ophthalmol* 1972;88:173–175.

Histopathology

3. McMahon RT, Font RL, McLean IW. Phakomatous choristoma of the eyelid: electron microscopical confirmation of lenticular derivation. *Arch Ophthalmol* 1976;94:1778–1781.
4. Tripathi RC, Tripathi BJ, Ringus J. Phakomatous choristoma of the lower eyelid with psammoma body formation; a light and electron microscopic study. *Ophthalmology* 1981;88:1198–1206.
5. Sinclair-Smith CC, Emms M, Morris HB. Phakomatous choristoma of the lower eyelid. A light and ultrastructural study. *Arch Pathol Lab Med* 1989;113:1175–1177.
6. Rosenbaum PS, Kress Y, Slamovits TL, et al. Phakomatous choristoma of the eyelid. Immunohistochemical and electron microscopic observations. *Ophthalmology* 1992;99:1779–1784.
7. Ellis FJ, Eagle RC Jr, Shields JA, et al. Phakomatous choristoma (Zimmerman's tumor): Immunohistochemical confirmation of intrinsic lens proteins. *Ophthalmology* 1993;100:955–960.
8. Kamada Y, Sakata A, Nakadomari S, et al. Phakomatous choristoma of the eyelid: immunohistochemical observation. *Jpn J Ophthalmol* 1998;42:41–45.
9. Eustis HS, Karcioglu ZA, Dharma S, et al. Phakomatous choristoma: clinical, histopathologic and ultrastructural findings in a 4-month-old boy. *J Pediatr Ophthalmol Strabismus* 1990;17:208–211.

Case Reports

10. Greer CH. Phakomatous choristoma in the eyelid. *Aust J Ophthalmol* 1975;3:106–107.
11. Baggesen LH, Jensen OA. Phakomatous choristoma of the lower eyelid. A lenticular anlage tumor. *Ophthalmologica* 1977;175:231–235.
12. Peres LC, da Silva AR, Belluci AD, et al. Phakomatous choristoma of the orbit. *Orbit* 1998;17:47–53.
13. Seregard S. Phakomatous choristoma may be located in the eyelid or orbit or both. *Acta Ophthalmol Scand* 1999;77:343–346.
14. Shin HM, Song HG, Choi MY. Phakomatous choristoma of the eyelid. *Korean J Ophthalmol* 1999;13:133–137.
15. Blenc AM, Gomez JA, Lee MW, et al. Phakomatous choristoma: a case report and review of the literature. *Am J Dermatopathol* 2000;22:55–59.
16. Mencia-Gutierrez E, Gutierrez-Diaz E, Ricoy JR, et al. Eyelid phakomatous choristoma. *Eur J Ophthalmol* 2003;13:482–485.
17. Dithmar S, Schmack I, Volcker HE, et al. Phakomatous choristoma of the eyelid. *Graefes Arch Clin Exp Ophthalmol* 2004;242:40–43.
18. Verb SP, Roarty JD, Black EH, et al. Phakomatous choristoma: a rare orbital tumor presenting as an eyelid mass with obstruction of the nasolacrimal duct. *J AAPOS* 2009;13(1):85–87
19. Thaung C, Bonshek RE, Leatherbarrow B. Phakomatous choristoma of the eyelid: a case with associated eye abnormalities. *Br J Ophthalmol* 2006;90(2):245–246.

Chapter 13 Eyelid Miscellaneous Conditions Simulating Neoplasms

EYELID PHAKOMATOUS CHORISTOMA

A clinicopathologic correlation of a phakomatous choristoma is shown.

Ellis FJ, Eagle RC Jr, Shields JA, et al. Phakomatous choristoma (Zimmerman's tumor): immunohistochemical confirmation of intrinsic lens proteins. *Ophthalmology* 1993;100:955–960.

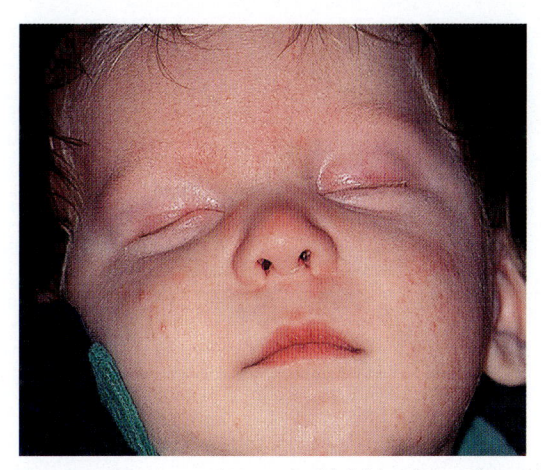

Figure 13.19. Appearance of 10-week-old child with mass beneath the right lower eyelid. The lesion was not visible, but was palpable as a hard subcutaneous lump.

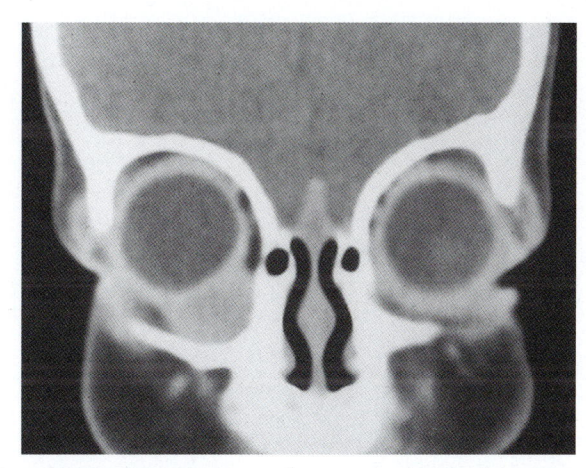

Figure 13.20. Coronal computed tomogram showing homogeneous mass in the eyelid and anterior orbit inferonasally.

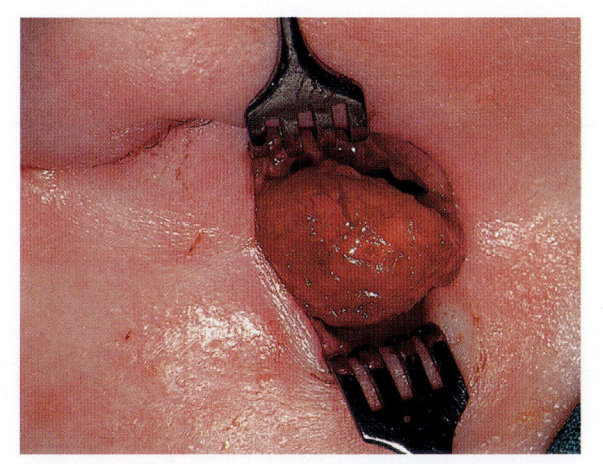

Figure 13.21. Exposure of the mass at time of surgical excision.

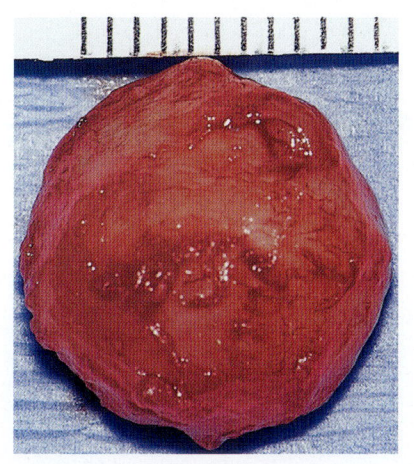

Figure 13.22. Appearance of mass removed intact.

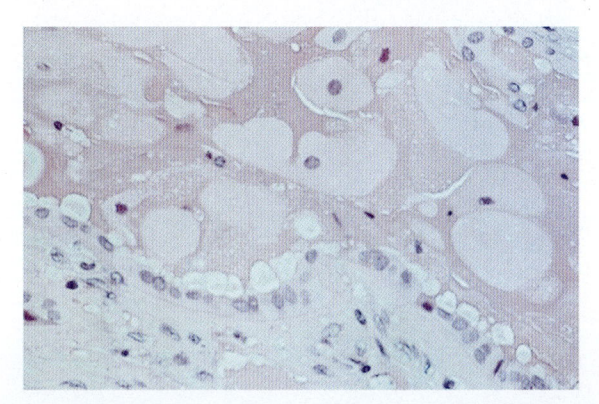

Figure 13.23. Photomicrograph showing lens epithelial-like cells surrounded by a thick basement membrane material and Wedl cells (bladder cells), similar to those seen in posterior subcapsular cataract. (Hematoxylin–eosin ×50.)

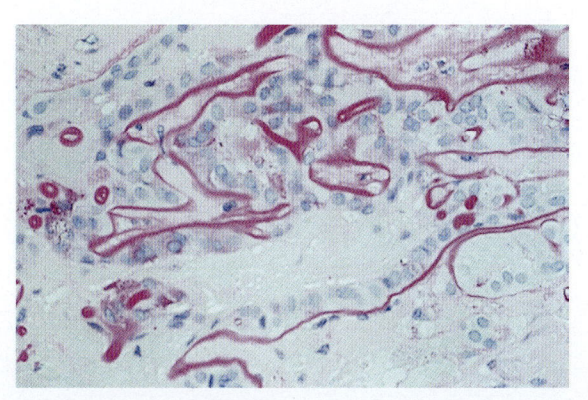

Figure 13.24. Periodic acid-Schiff stain showing the thick basement membrane enclosing the lens epithelial cells. (Periodic acid-Schiff ×100.)

TUMORS OF THE LACRIMAL DRAINAGE SYSTEM

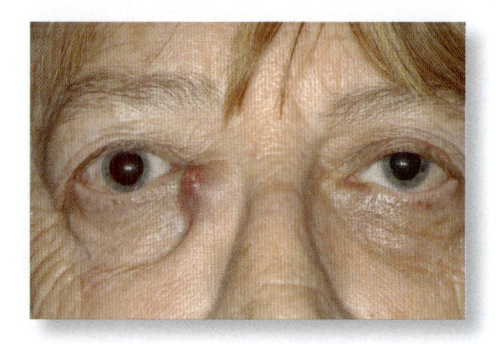

General Considerations

A variety of tumors can arise in the canaliculus, lacrimal sac, and the nasolacrimal duct, with the majority originating in the lacrimal sac. The section introduces the subject of tumors and pseudotumors of the lacrimal drainage system and provides some selected general references (1–13). Following that, a few of the specific lesions will be discussed, illustrated, and referenced in more detail.

Various surveys of lacrimal sac tumors and pseudotumors have shown considerable differences in the incidence of these lesions. In one series of 115 solid tumors of the lacrimal sac, 55% were malignant (1). The most common primary neoplasms of the lacrimal sac appear to be epithelial tumors, particularly squamous papilloma and squamous cell carcinoma. However, one study reported that non-Hodgkin's B-cell lymphoma was the most common lacrimal sac neoplasm (9). Other tumors and pseudotumors that have been reported less often in the lacrimal drainage system include melanoma, oncocytoma, hemangiopericytoma, solitary fibrous tumor, peripheral nerve tumors, angiofibroma, granular cell tumor, cavernous hemangioma, pleomorphic adenoma, adenocarcinoma, and adenoid cystic carcinoma. A series of 35 cases of nonepithelial tumors of the lacrimal sac revealed that fibrous histiocytoma was most common, followed by lymphoma and melanoma (2). Nonneoplastic conditions that can simulate lacrimal sac tumors include cyst, hematoma, pyogenic granuloma, juvenile xanthogranuloma, and sarcoidosis (10). In one analysis, routine biopsy of the lacrima sac at dacryocystorhinostomy for obstruction in 193 cases revealed 44 (23%) with normal histology, 146 (76%) with nonspecific chronic inflammation, and 3 (1.2%) with specific pathology of unsuspected sarcoidosis or papilloma (10). Most lacrimal sac tumors are uncommon and the pathology varies with the diagnosis. We will discuss them in general terms.

Clinical Features

Most neoplasms of the lacrimal sac are indistinguishable clinically and must be differentiated from the more common dacryocystitis. The latter occurs more often in infants or young children and is associated with inflammatory signs, is soft and fluctuant, and often has a purulent discharge that can be expressed with pressure. It generally is evident inferior to the medial canthus. In contrast, a solid neoplasm generally appears in adults as a progressive, firm, subcutaneous mass, usually, but not always superior to the medial canthus. Secondary epiphora, sometimes tinged with blood, is a common presenting feature (4). Melanoma can occur in the lacrimal sac as a de novo lesion or from epithelial extension from conjunctival melanoma, usually in association with primary acquired melanosis (PAM).

LACRIMAL DRAINAGE SYSTEM TUMORS

Diagnostic Approaches

Most tumors of the eyelid and conjunctiva can be appreciated clinically by direct visualization. However, those in the lacrimal sac are not so readily visible and imaging studies, including computed tomography (CT), magnetic resonance imaging (MRI), and dacryocystograms may provide more important information about the extent and nature of the lesion. Most tumors are initially circumscribed, defined by the walls of the lacrimal sac. Later, the more aggressive neoplasms lose their definition and become more diffuse or ill-defined on imaging studies.

Pathology

The histopathology of tumors and pseudotumors of the lacrimal sac is discussed under the same tumor categories in the eyelid and conjunctival sections of this atlas. The only exception is that squamous cell carcinoma of the lacrimal sac generally arises from an inverted papilloma and often has an invasive spindle cell component. There is controversy as to pathogenesis of hemangiopericytoma, fibrous histiocytoma, and solitary fibrous tumor, all of which have been reported to arise in the lacrimal sac. All are similar histopathologically and are discussed further in the section on orbital tumors. Human papillomavirus (HPV) appears to be involved in the pathogenesis of epithelial neoplasms of the lacrimal sac, with HPV type 11 reportedly associated with benign lesions and HPV type 18 reportedly associated with malignant lesions (12,13).

Management

The management of a lacrimal sac neoplasm varies with the clinical findings and suspected diagnosis. When possible, primary neoplasms are managed initially by complete surgical removal by dacryocystectomy. The specific surgical approach depends on the surgeon's preference. A nasal cutaneous approach (Lynch incision) or an endoscopic approach can provide adequate surgical exposure, depending on the suspected tumor.

Additional treatment may be required, depending on the final histopathologic diagnosis. More malignant epithelial tumors, lymphoma, and metastasis may require local irradiation or chemotherapy, depending on the specific diagnosis. Wide excision is important for papilloma, because lacrimal sac papilloma is invasive and has a high incidence of recurrence. In advanced cases, orbital or sinus exenteration may be necessary. Inflammatory conditions like juvenile xanthogranuloma and pyogenic granuloma can be treated with supplemental local or oral corticosteroids. Regardless of the diagnosis, subsequent reconstruction of the lacrimal drainage system can be undertaken, provided there is no tumor recurrence within a few months (8,9). The prognosis varies with the specific diagnosis.

LACRIMAL DRAINAGE SYSTEM TUMORS

Selected References

Reviews

1. Stefanyszyn MA, Hidayat AA, Pe'er JJ, et al. Lacrimal sac tumors. *Ophthal Plast Reconstr Surg* 1994;10:169–184.
2. Pe'er JJ, Stefanyszyn M, Hidayat AA. Nonepithelial tumors of the lacrimal sac. *Am J Ophthalmol* 1994;118:650–658.
3. Ryan SJ, Font RL. Primary epithelial neoplasms of the lacrimal sac. *Am J Ophthalmol* 1973;76:73–88.
4. Hornblass A, Jakobiec FA, Bosniak S, et al. The diagnosis and management of epithelial tumors of the lacrimal sac. *Ophthalmology* 1980;87:476–490.
5. Ni C, D'Amico DJ, Fan CQ, et al. Tumors of the lacrimal sac: a clinicopathological analysis of 82 cases. *Int Ophthalmol Clin* 1982;22:121–140.
6. Flanagan JC, Stokes DP. Lacrimal sac tumors. *Ophthalmology* 1978;85:1282–1287.
7. Anderson NG, Wojno TH, Grossniklaus HE. Clinicopathologic findings from lacrimal sac biopsy specimens obtained during dacryocystorhinostomy. *Ophthalmol Plast Reconstr Surg* 2003;19:173–176.

Management

8. Stokes DP, Flanagan JC. Dacryocystectomy for tumors of the lacrimal sac. *Ophthalmic Surg* 1977;8:85–90.
9. Parmar DN, Rose GE. Management of lacrimal sac tumours. *Eye* 2003;17:599–606.

Histopathology/Infectious Disease

10. Merkonidis C, Brewis C, Yuing M, et al. Is routine biopsy of the lacrimal sac wall indicated at dacryocystorhinostomy? A prospective study and literature review. *Br J Ophthalmol* 2005;89:1589–1591.
11. Pe'er J, Hidayat AA, Ilsar M, et al. Glandular tumors of the lacrimal sac. Their histopathologic patterns and possible origins. *Ophthalmology* 1996;103:1601–1605.
12. Madreperla SA, Green WR, Daniel R, et al. Human papillomavirus in primary epithelial tumors of the lacrimal sac. *Ophthalmology* 1993;100:569–573.
13. Nakamura Y, Mashima Y, Kameyama K, et al. Detection of human papillomavirus infection in squamous tumours of the conjunctiva and lacrimal sac by immunohistochemistry, in situ hybridisation, and polymerase chain reaction. *Br J Ophthalmol* 1997;81:308–313.

LACRIMAL SAC SQUAMOUS PAPILLOMA AND CARCINOMA

General Considerations

The most important primary epithelial neoplasms of lacrimal sac are squamous papilloma and squamous cell carcinoma with squamous papilloma often evolving into carcinoma (1–21). Unlike the benign, noninvasive papilloma of the eyelid skin described previously, papilloma of the lacrimal sac is usually of the inverted type, also called transitional cell carcinoma or Schneiderian papilloma, and is more invasive. It can arise primarily from the lacrimal sac or can extend into the sac from the nose or maxillary sinus.

Clinical Features

Both inverted papilloma and squamous cell carcinoma are slowly invasive and frequently recur after excision. Local intracranial extension can develop in more aggressive tumors, such as mucoepidermoid carcinoma (18). Transformation of inverted papilloma into squamous cell carcinoma occurs in 10% to 15% of cases, at which time the tumor becomes more locally invasive and can occasionally exhibit orbital recurrence, brain invasion, and distant metastasis (9).

Pathology

The histopathology of squamous papilloma and squamous cell carcinoma were discussed in the section on squamous neoplasms of the conjunctiva. Squamous cell carcinoma can also arise in the lacrimal sac de novo, without a prior papilloma. The mucoepidermoid variant of squamous cell carcinoma has also been found to arise primarily in the lacrimal sac (3,9,13,18).

Management

Management of lacrimal sac neoplasms was discussed in the previous section and involves methods of dacryocystectomy with full dissection of the nasolacrimal duct plus additional chemotherapy or radiotherapy as needed (6).

Selected References

Reviews

1. Stefanyszyn MA, Hidayat AA, Pe'er JJ, et al. Lacrimal sac tumors. *Ophthalmol Plast Reconstr Surg* 1994;10:169–184.
2. Ryan SJ, Font RL. Primary epithelial neoplasms of the lacrimal sac. *Am J Ophthalmol* 1973;76:73–88.
3. Hornblass A, Jakobiec FA, Bosniak S, et al. The diagnosis and management of epithelial tumors of the lacrimal sac. *Ophthalmology* 1980;87:476–490.
4. Ni C, D'Amico DJ, Fan CQ, et al. Tumors of the lacrimal sac: a clinicopathological analysis of 82 cases. *Int Ophthalmol Clin* 1982;22:121–140.
5. Coloma-Gonzalez I, Flores-Preciado J, Ceriotta A, et al. Lacrimal sac tumors presenting as lacrimal obstruction. Retrospective study in Mexican patients 2007–2012. *Arch Soc Esp Oftalmol* 2014;89:222–225.

Management

6. El-Sawy T, Frank SJ, Hanna E, et al. Multidisciplinary management of lacrimal sac/nasolacrimal duct carcinomas. *Ophthal Plast Reconstr Surg* 2013;29:454–457.

Histopathology/Infectious Disease

7. Nakamura Y, Mashima Y, Kameyama K. Human papilloma virus DNA detected in case of inverted squamous papilloma of the lacrimal sac. *Br J Ophthalmol* 1995;79:392–393.

Case Reports

8. Streeten BW, Carrillo R, Jamison R, et al. Inverted papilloma of the conjunctiva. *Am J Ophthalmol* 1979;88:1062–1066.
9. Elner VM, Burnstine MA, Goodman ML, et al. Inverted papillomas that invade the orbit. *Arch Ophthalmol* 1995;113:1178–1183.
10. Williams R, Ilsar M, Welham RA. Lacrimal canalicular papillomatosis. *Br J Ophthalmol* 1985;69:464–467.
11. Fechner RE, Sessions RB. Inverted papilloma of the lacrimal sac, the paranasal sinuses and the cervical region. *Cancer* 1977;40:2303–2308.
12. Katircioglu YA, Altiparmak UE, Akmansu H, et al. Squamous cell carcinoma of the lacrimal sac. *Orbit* 2003;22:151–153.
13. Kohn R, Nofsinger K, Freedman SI. Rapid recurrence of papillary squamous cell carcinoma of the canaliculus. *Am J Ophthalmol* 1981;92:363–367.
14. Bonder D, Fischer MJ, Levine MR. Squamous cell carcinoma of the lacrimal sac. *Ophthalmology* 1983;90:1133–1135.
15. Ni C, Wagoner MD, Wang W, et al. Mucoepidermoid carcinomas of the lacrimal sac. *Arch Ophthalmol* 1983;101:1572–1574.
16. Blake J, Mullaney J, Gillan J. Lacrimal sac mucoepidermoid carcinoma. *Br J Ophthalmol* 1986;70:681–685.
17. Anderson KK, Lessner AM, Hood I, et al. Invasive transitional cell carcinoma of the lacrimal sac arising in an inverted papilloma. *Arch Ophthalmol* 1994;112:306–307.
18. Khan JA, Sutula FC, Pilch BZ, et al. Mucoepidermoid carcinoma involving the lacrimal sac. *Ophthalmol Plast Reconstr Surg* 1988;4:153–157.
19. Bambirra EA, Miranda D, Rayes A. Mucoepidermoid tumor of the lacrimal sac. *Arch Ophthalmol* 1981;99:2149–2150.
20. Stephenson JA, Mayland DM, Ingall G, et al. Squamous cell carcinoma of the lacrimal sac. *Otolaryngol Head Neck Surg* 1988;99:524–527.
21. Fishman JR, Gladstone GJ, Jackson IT. Squamous cell carcinoma of the lacrimal sac. *Plast Reconstr Surg* 1993;92:1375–1379.

LACRIMAL SAC SQUAMOUS CELL PAPILLOMA AND CARCINOMA

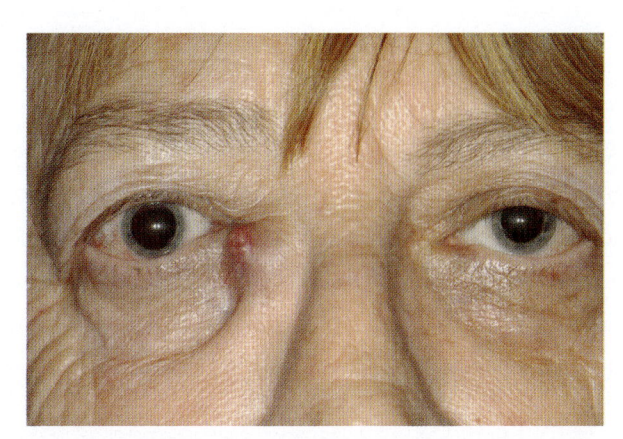

Figure 14.1. Squamous cell carcinoma of the right lacrimal sac appearing as a subcutaneous mass inferior to the medial canthus in an elderly woman. (Courtesy of Mary Stefanyszyn, MD.)

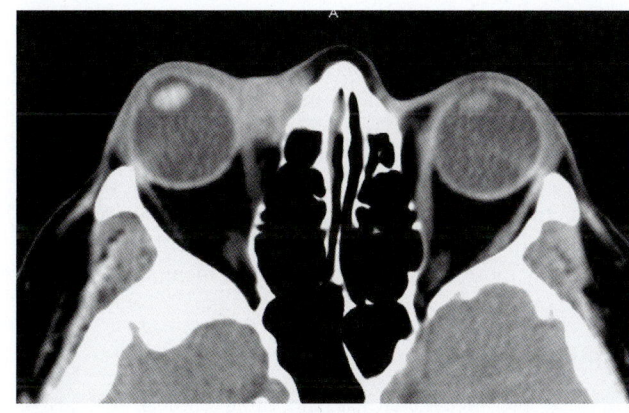

Figure 14.2. Axial computed tomography of the lesion shown in Figure 14.1, disclosing a 1-cm, soft tissue density in the region of the right lacrimal sac. (Courtesy of Mary Stefanyszyn, MD.)

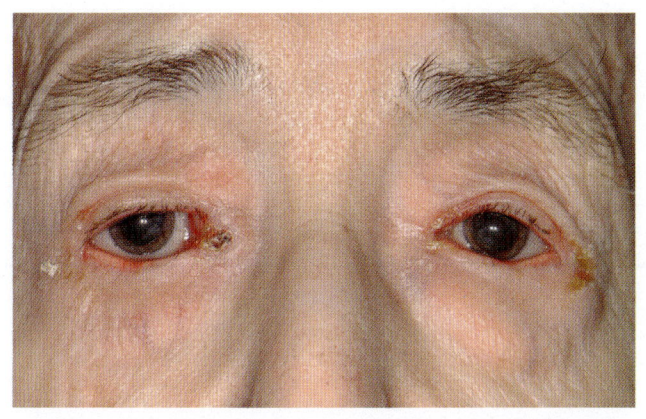

Figure 14.3. Squamous cell carcinoma of right lacrimal sac presenting as an erosive mass in right medial canthal region of an elderly man who had extensive exposure to sunlight. (Courtesy of David Bonder, MD and Mark R. Levine, MD.)

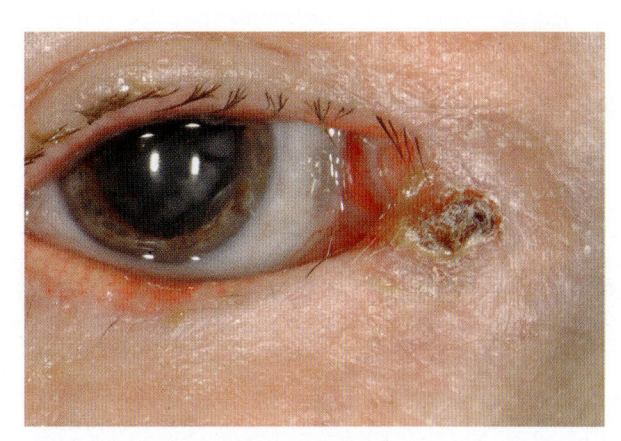

Figure 14.4. Closer view of lesion in Figure 14.3, showing fleshy mass in the medial canthal area and excoriation of the overlying skin. (Courtesy of David Bonder, MD and Mark R. Levine, MD.)

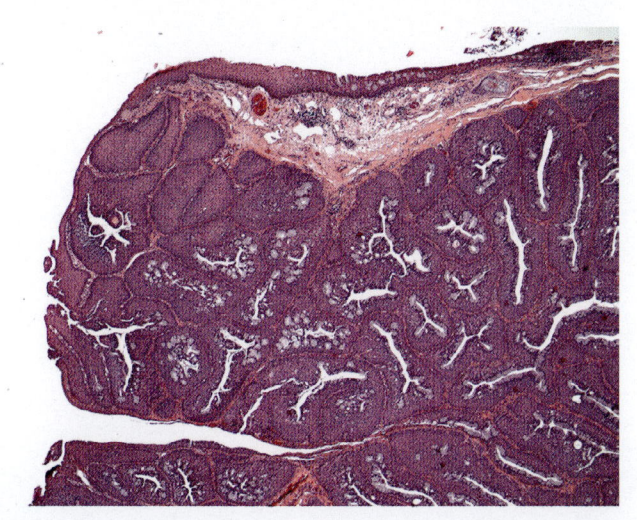

Figure 14.5. Histopathology of inverted squamous papilloma or early invasive squamous cell carcinoma of lacrimal sac, showing papillomatous lobules of tumor cells with intracellular mucin. (Hematoxylin–eosin ×20.)

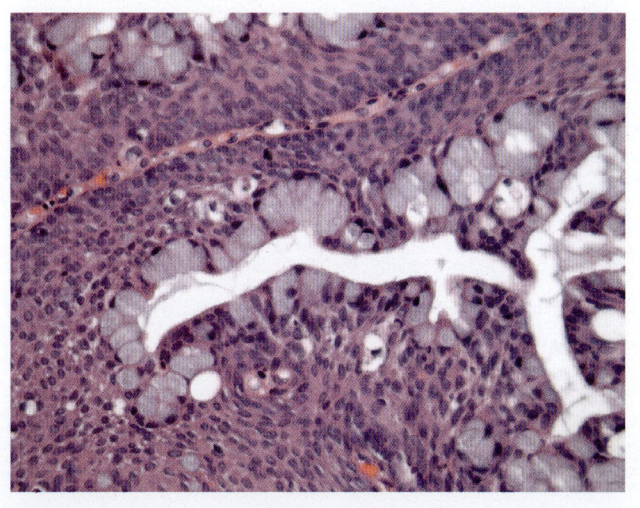

Figure 14.6. Higher magnification of lesion shown in Figure 14.5 demonstrating closely packed epithelial cells with mucin-containing cells near the ducts. (Hematoxylin–eosin ×175.)

LACRIMAL SAC MELANOMA

General Considerations

Primary malignant melanoma can occasionally develop in the lacrimal sac (1–17). Although its origin is disputed, it possibly arises from melanocytes located in the epithelium of the lacrimal drainage system or the underlying stroma. In some instances, lacrimal sac melanoma is secondary to seeding of conjunctiva melanoma into the canaliculus, particularly in patients with aggressive PAM of the conjunctiva (1,2). This is probably more likely following surgical manipulation of the conjunctival lesion.

Clinical Features

Lacrimal sac melanoma has the same clinical features as described in the section on clinical aspects of lacrimal sac tumors. In a patient with a lacrimal sac mass, the presence of conjunctival melanoma or PAM should arouse suspicion that the lacrimal sac lesion is a melanoma. Bleeding within the tumor can give it a darker blue appearance and bloody discharge from the punctum. MRI and CT can be helpful in detecting the extent of the neoplasm and presence of bone destruction secondary to the lesion (3,4).

Pathology

Histopathologically, the tumor is composed of malignant melanocytes, identical to conjunctival melanoma, previously discussed. Melanoma that extends to the lacrimal sac from the conjunctiva often shows no evidence of PAM, even though the original conjunctival melanoma notably arose from PAM (5).

Management

Management is generally wide surgical excision with dacryocystectomy. Orbital exenteration may be necessary in advanced cases. Prognosis is usually guarded because of potential for metastasis (1–17).

Selected References

Reviews

1. Robertson DM, Hungerford JL, McCartney A. Malignant melanomas of the conjunctiva, nasal cavity, and paranasal sinuses. *Am J Ophthalmol* 1989;108:440–442.
2. Shields CL, Markowitz JS, Belinsky I, et al. Conjunctival melanoma: outcomes based on tumor origin in 382 consecutive cases. *Ophthalmology* 2011;118:389–395.

Imaging

3. Gleizal A, Kodjikian L, Lebreton F, et al. Early CT-scan for chronic lacrimal duct symptoms—case report of a malignant melanoma of the lacrimal sac and review of the literature. *J Craniomaxillofac Surg* 2005;33:201–204.
4. Billing K, Malhotra R, Selva D, et al. Magnetic resonance imaging findings in malignant melanoma of the lacrimal sac. *Br J Ophthalmol* 2003;87:1187–1188.

Histopathology

5. Pujari A, Ali MJ, Mulay K, et al. The black lacrimal sac: a clinicopathological correlation of a malignant melanoma with anterior lacrimal crest infiltration. *Int Ophthalmol* 2014;34(1):111–115.

Case Reports

6. Yamade S, Kitagawa A. Malignant melanoma of the lacrimal sac. *Ophthalmologica* 1978;177:30–33.
7. Glaros D, Karesh JW, Rodrigues MM, et al. Primary malignant melanoma of the lacrimal sac. *Arch Ophthalmol* 1989;107:1244–1245.
8. Duguid IM. Malignant melanoma of the lacrimal sac. *Br J Ophthalmol* 1964;78:394–398.
9. Farkas TG, Lamberson RE. Malignant melanoma of the lacrimal sac. *Am J Ophthalmol* 1968;66:45–48.
10. Kuwabara H, Takeda J. Malignant melanoma of the lacrimal sac with surrounding melanosis. *Arch Pathol Lab Med* 1997;121:517–519.
11. Levine MR, Dinar Y, Davies R. Malignant melanoma of the lacrimal sac. *Ophthalmic Surg Lasers* 1996;27:318–330.
12. Lloyd WC, Leone CR Jr. Malignant melanoma of the lacrimal sac. *Acta Ophthalmol* 1993;71:273–276.
13. McNab AA, McKelvie P. Malignant melanoma of the lacrimal sac complicating primary acquired melanosis of the conjunctiva. *Ophthalmic Surg Lasers* 1997;28:501–504.
14. Lee HM, Kang HJ, Choi G, et al. Two cases of primary malignant melanoma of the lacrimal sac. *Head Neck* 2001;23:809–813.
15. Malik TY, Sanders R, Young JD, et al. Malignant melanoma of the lacrimal sac. *Eye* 1997;11:935–937.
16. Sendra-Tello J, Galindo-Campillo N, Rodriguez-Peralto JL, et al. Malignant melanoma of the lacrimal sac. *Otolaryngol Head Neck* 2004;131:334–336.
17. Sitole S, Zender CA, Ahmad AZ, et al. Lacrimal sac melanoma. *Ophthal Plast Reconstr Surg* 2007;23(5):417–419.

Chapter 14 Tumors of the Lacrimal Drainage System

LACRIMAL SAC MELANOMA

Melanoma of the lacrimal sac is similar histopathologically to melanoma of the conjunctiva.

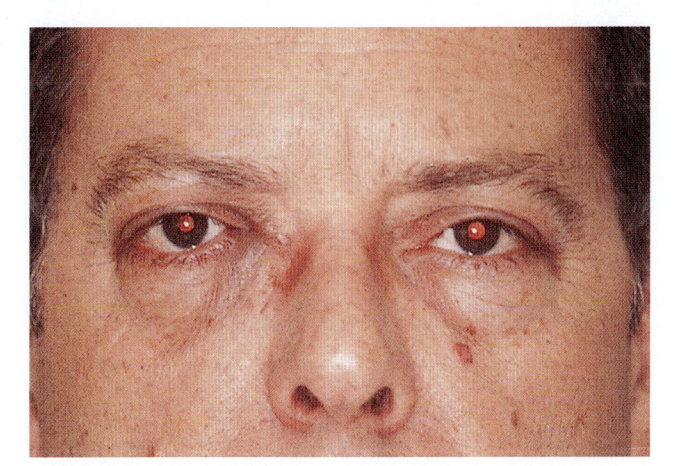

Figure 14.7. Malignant melanoma of right lacrimal sac in a 52-year-old man. (Courtesy of Francis LaPiana, MD and Ahmed Hidayat, MD.)

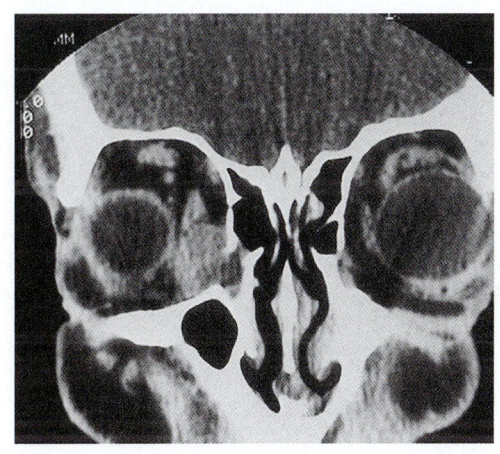

Figure 14.8. Coronal computed tomography of patient shown in Figure 14.7 demonstrating the solid mass nasal to the right eye. (Courtesy of Francis LaPiana, MD and Ahmed Hidayat, MD.)

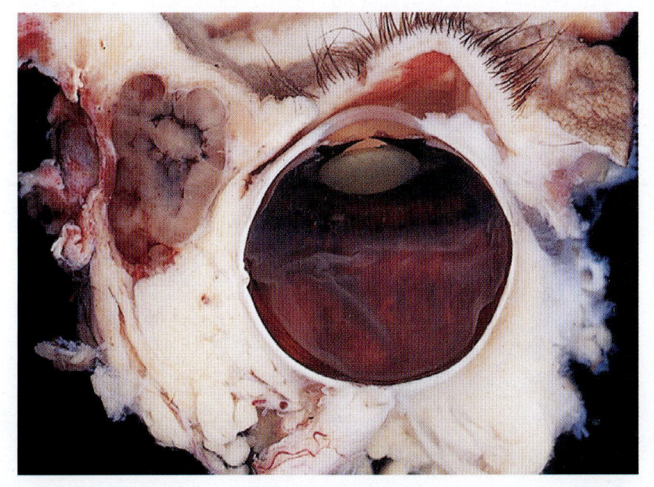

Figure 14.9. Exenteration specimen of patient shown in Figure 14.7 showing globe and brown mass adjacent to the globe inferiorly, arising from the lacrimal sac. (Courtesy of Francis LaPiana, MD and Ahmed Hidayat, MD.)

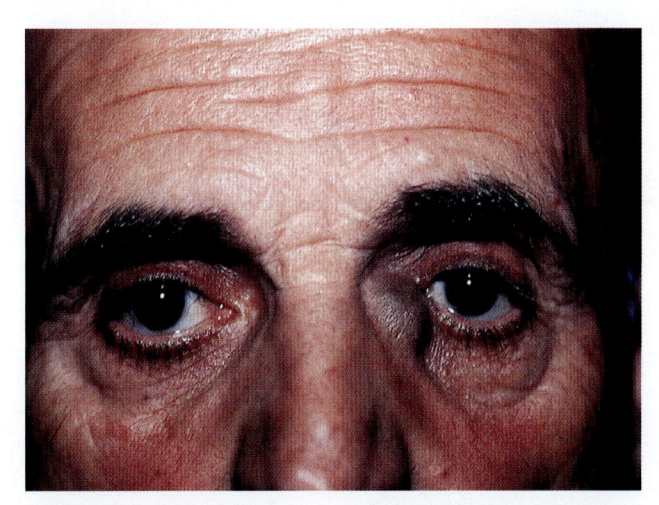

Figure 14.10. Malignant melanoma of left lacrimal sac in a middle-aged man. Note the dark color to the skin overlying the lesion. (Courtesy of Zeev Sinnreich, MD.)

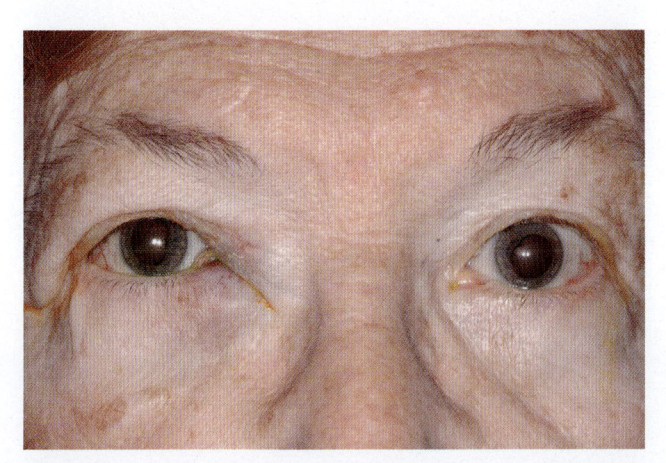

Figure 14.11. Malignant melanoma of right lacrimal sac in a 78-year-old woman.

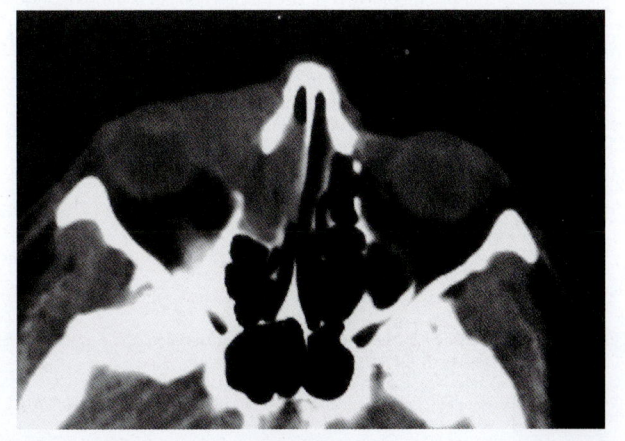

Figure 14.12. Computed tomography of patient shown in Figure 14.11 showing melanoma in region of lacrimal sac with extension into ethmoid and maxillary sinuses.

LACRIMAL SAC: MISCELLANEOUS TUMORS AND PSEUDOTUMORS

A number of other tumors and inflammations can also arise primarily in the lacrimal sac (1–39). Only selected examples are discussed and illustrated. As mentioned, benign papilloma can develop in the lacrimal sac and it can evolve, in some cases, into squamous cell carcinoma. Other reported lesions include leukemia and lymphoid hyperplasia lymphoid (3,36,38), oncocytoma (7–10), hemangiopericytoma, solitary fibrous tumor, and fibrous histiocytoma (11–19), peripheral nerve tumors (20,21), cysts (4,5,22,23), and others.

The clinical and histopathologic features of all lacrimal sac tumors and pseudotumors are similar and were discussed elsewhere. The management varies with the type of lesion, but is generally surgical removal by dacryocystectomy and subsequent reconstruction of the lacrimal drainage system.

Selected References

Reviews

1. Montalban A, Lietin B, Louvrier C, et al. Malignant lacrima sac tumors. *Eur Ann Otorhinolaryngol Head Neck Dis* 2010;127:165–172.
2. Tucker N, Chow D, Stockl F, et al. Clinically suspected primary acquired nasolacrimal duct obstruction: clinicopathologic review of 150 patients. *Ophthalmology* 1997;104:1882–1889.
3. Yip CC, Bartley GB, Habermann TM, et al. Involvement of the lacrimal drainage system by leukemia or lymphoma. *Ophthalmol Plast Reconstr Surg* 2002;18:242–246.
4. Hornblass A, Gabry JB. Diagnosis and treatment of lacrimal sac cysts. *Ophthalmology* 1979;86:1655–1661.
5. Hornblass A, Herschorn BJ. Lacrimal gland duct cysts. *Ophthalmic Surg* 1985;16:301–306.

Management

6. Parmar DN, Rose GE. Management of lacrimal sac tumours. *Eye* 2003;17:599–606.

Case Reports

7. Peretz WL, Ettinghausen SE, Gray GF. Oncocytic adenocarcinoma of the lacrimal sac. *Arch Ophthalmol* 1978;96:303–304.
8. Chen LJ, Liao SL, Kao SC, et al. Oncocytic adenomatous hyperplasia of the lacrimal sac: a case report and review of the literature. *Ophthalmol Plast Reconstr Surg* 1998;14:436–440.
9. Perlman JI, Specht CS, McLean IW, et al. Oncocytic adenocarcinoma of the lacrimal sac: report of a case with paranasal sinus and orbital extension. *Ophthalmic Surg* 1995;26:377–379.
10. Chow DR, Brownstein S, Codere F. Oncocytoma of the lacrimal sac associated with chronic dacryocystitis. *Can J Ophthalmol* 1996;31:249–251.
11. Charles NC, Palu RN, Jagirdar JS. Hemangiopericytoma of the lacrimal sac. *Arch Ophthalmol* 1998;116:1677–1680.
12. Rubin PA, Shore JW, Jakobiec FA, et al. Hemangiopericytoma of the lacrimal sac. *Ophthalmic Surg* 1992;23:562–563.
13. Roth SI, August CZ, Lissner GS, et al. Hemangiopericytoma of the lacrimal sac. *Ophthalmology* 1991;98:925–927.
14. Carnevali L, Trimarchi F, Rosso R, et al. Haemangiopericytoma of the lacrimal sac: a case report. *Br J Ophthalmol* 1988;72:782–785.
15. Gurney N, Chalkley T, O'Grady R. Lacrimal sac hemangiopericytoma. *Am J Ophthalmol* 1971;71:757–759.
16. Woo KI, Suh YL, Kim YD. Solitary fibrous tumor of the lacrimal sac. *Ophthalmol Plast Reconstr Surg* 1999;15:450–453.
17. Rumelt S, Kassif Y, Cohen I, et al. A rare solitary fibrous tumour of the lacrimal sac presenting as acquired nasolacrimal duct obstruction. *Eye* 2003;17:429–431.
18. Marback RL, Kincaid MC, Green WR, et al. Fibrous histiocytoma of the lacrimal sac. *Am J Ophthalmol* 1982;93:511–517.
19. Sen DK, Mohan H. Fibroma of the lacrimal sac. *J Pediatr Ophthalmol Strabismus* 1980;17:410–411.
20. Sen DK, Mohan H, Chatterjee PK. Neurilemmoma of the lacrimal sac. *Eye Ear Nose Throat Mon* 1971;50:179–180.
21. Bajaj MS, Nainiwal SK, Pushker N, et al. Neurofibroma of the lacrimal sac. *Orbit* 2002;21:205–208.
22. Mansour AM, Cheng KP, Mumma JV, et al. Congenital dacryocele. A collaborative review. *Ophthalmology* 1991;98:1744–1751.
23. Hornblass A, Gross ND. Lacrimal sac cyst. *Ophthalmology* 1987;94:706–708.
24. Asiyo MN, Stefani FH. Pyogenic granulomas of the lacrimal sac. *Eye* 1992;6:97–101.
25. Yen MT, Hipps WM. Nasolacrimal sac hematoma masquerading as an orbital mass. *Ophthalmol Plast Reconstr Surg* 2004;20:170–172.
26. Baredes S, Ludwin DB, Troublefield YL, et al. Adenocarcinoma ex-pleomorphic adenoma of the lacrimal sac and nasolacrimal duct: a case report. *Laryngoscope* 2003;113:940–942.
27. Yazici B, Setzen G, Meyer DR, et al. Giant cell angiofibroma of the nasolacrimal duct. *Ophthalmol Plast Reconstr Surg* 2001;17:202–206.
28. Sabet SJ, Tarbet KJ, Lemke BN, et al. Granular cell tumor of the lacrimal sac and nasolacrimal duct: no invasive behavior with incomplete resection. *Ophthalmology* 2000;107:1992–1994.
29. Mruthyunjaya P, Meyer DR. Juvenile xanthogranuloma of the lacrimal sac fossa. *Am J Ophthalmol* 1997;123:400–402.
30. Kincaid MC, Meis JM, Lee MW. Adenoid cystic carcinoma of the lacrimal sac. *Ophthalmology* 1989;96:1655–1658.
31. Parnell JR, Mamalis N, Davis RK, et al. Primary adenoid cystic carcinoma of the lacrimal sac: report of a case. *Ophthalmol Plast Reconstr Surg* 1994;10:124–129.
32. Howcroft MJ, Hurwitz JJ. Lacrimal sac fibroma. *Can J Ophthalmol* 1980;15:196–197.
33. Hurwitz JJ, Rodgers J, Doucet TW. Dermoid tumor involving the lacrimal drainage pathway: a case report. *Ophthalmic Surg* 1982;13:377–379.
34. Kaden IH, Shields JA, Shields CL, et al. Occult prostatic carcinoma metastatic to the medial canthal area. Diagnosis by immunohistochemistry. *Ophthalmol Plast Reconstr Surg* 1987;3:21–24.
35. Ferry AP, Kaltreider SA. Cavernous hemangioma of the lacrimal sac. *Am J Ophthalmol* 1990;110:316–318.
36. Schefler AC, Shields CL, Shields JA, et al. Lacrimal sac lymphoma in a child. *Arch Ophthalmol* 2003;121:1330–1333.
37. Anderson NG, Wojno TH, Grossniklaus HE. Clinicopathologic findings from lacrimal sac biopsy specimens obtained during dacryocystorhinostomy. *Ophthalmol Plast Reconstr Surg* 2003;19:173–176.
38. de Palma P, Ravalli L, Modestino R, et al. Primary lacrimal sac B-cell immunoblastic lymphoma simulating an acute dacryocystitis. *Orbit* 2003;22:171–175.
39. Arat YO, Font RL, Chaudhry IA, et al. Leiomyoma of the orbit and periocular region: a clinicopathologic study of four cases. *Ophthalmol Plast Reconstr Surg* 2005;21:16–22.

MISCELLANEOUS LACRIMAL SAC TUMORS: LEIOMYOMA, FIBROUS HISTIOCYTOMA, AND LYMPHOMA

Almost any soft tissue tumor can develop in the lacrimal sac, although such lesions are exceptionally uncommon. Examples are shown of leiomyoma, fibrous histiocytoma, and lymphoma.

1. Arat YO, Font RL, Chaudhry IA, Boniuk M. Leiomyoma of the orbit and periocular region: a clinicopathologic study of four cases. *Ophthalmol Plast Reconstr Surg* 2005;21:16–22.
2. Marback RL, Kincaid MC, Green WR, Iliff WJ. Fibrous histiocytoma of the lacrimal sac. *Am J Ophthalmol* 1982;93:511–517.
3. Schefler AC, Shields CL, Shields JA, et al. Lacrimal sac lymphoma in a child. *Arch Ophthalmol* 2003;121:1330–1333.

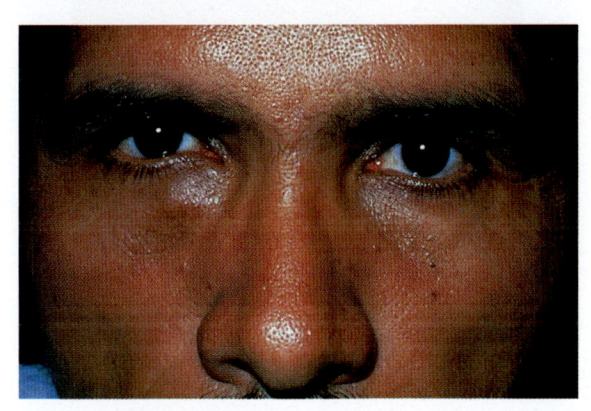

Figure 14.13. Leiomyoma of the lacrimal sac in a 43-year-old man. (Courtesy of Milton Boniuk, MD.)

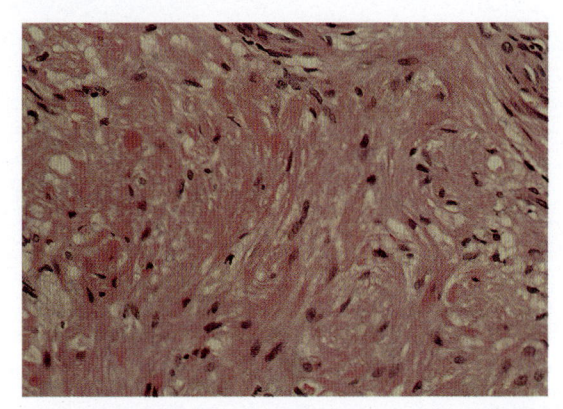

Figure 14.14. Histopathology of lesion shown in Figure 14.13 demonstrating spindle cell neoplasm with extracellular collagen, characteristic of leiomyoma. (Hematoxylin–eosin ×100.) (Courtesy of Milton Boniuk, MD.)

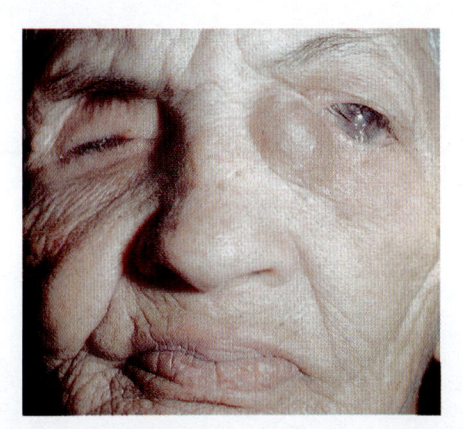

Figure 14.15. Lacrimal sac fibrous histiocytoma in a 62-year-old woman. (Courtesy of W. Richard Green, MD.)

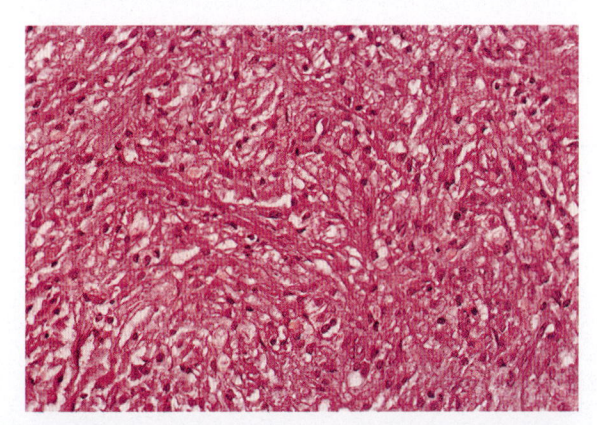

Figure 14.16. Histopathology of tumor shown in Figure 14.15 demonstrating spindle cells. Special studies confirmed fibrous histiocytoma. (Hematoxylin–eosin ×200.) (Courtesy of W. Richard Green, MD.)

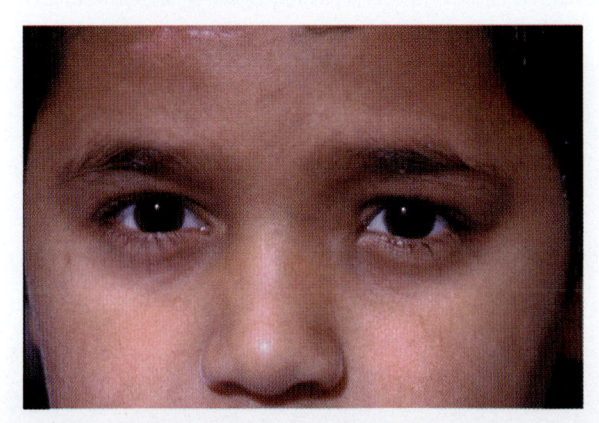

Figure 14.17. Mucosa-associated lymphoid tissue lymphoma in lacrimal sac of 10-year-old boy with mass in left medial canthal area. CT showed a circumscribed mass in the lacrimal sac.

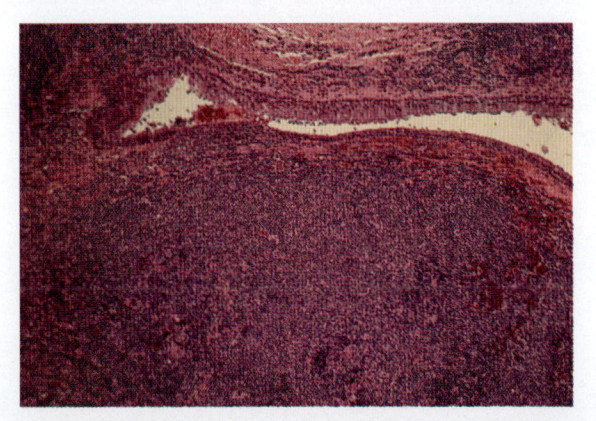

Figure 14.18. Histopathology of the mass from Figure 14.17 showing sheet of low-grade lymphocytes. The epithelium of the lacrimal sac is seen in superior portion of the field. The lesion was classified as a mucosa-associated lymphoid tissue lymphoma. (Hematoxylin–eosin ×50.)

LACRIMAL SAC INFLAMMATIONS AND INFECTIONS

Inflammations and infections are much more common than neoplasms in the lacrimal sac. However, they can often simulate true neoplasms.

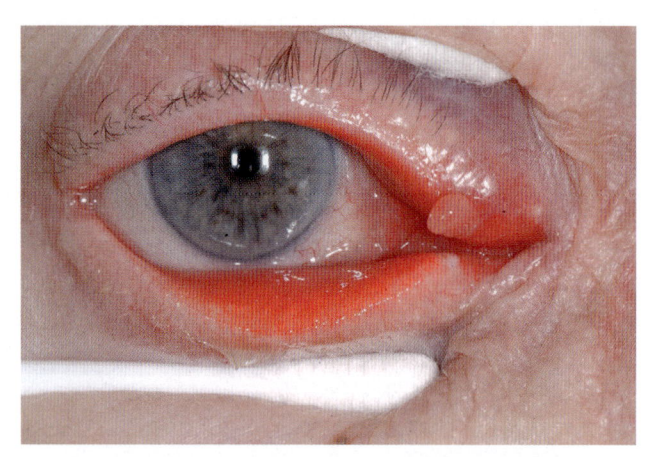

Figure 14.19. Pyogenic granuloma of lacrimal sac presenting as an outgrowth through the superior canaliculus. Note the associated severe conjunctivitis.

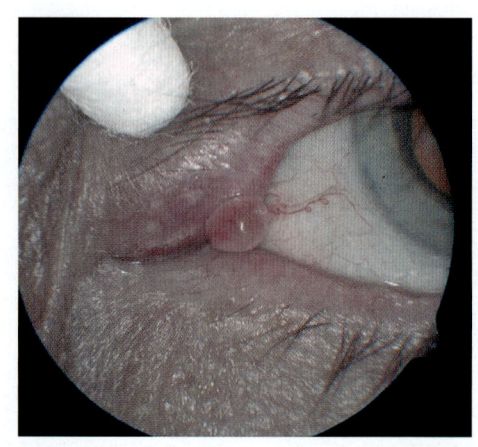

Figure 14.20. Pyogenic granuloma presenting through the superior canaliculus.

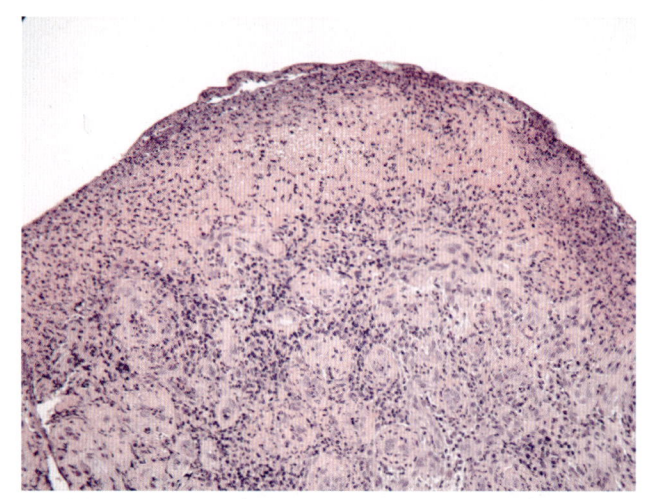

Figure 14.21. Low-magnification photomicrograph of lesion seen in Figure 14.20 showing infiltration of inflammatory cells. The occasional giant cells are atypical of pyogenic granuloma. (Hematoxylin–eosin ×10.)

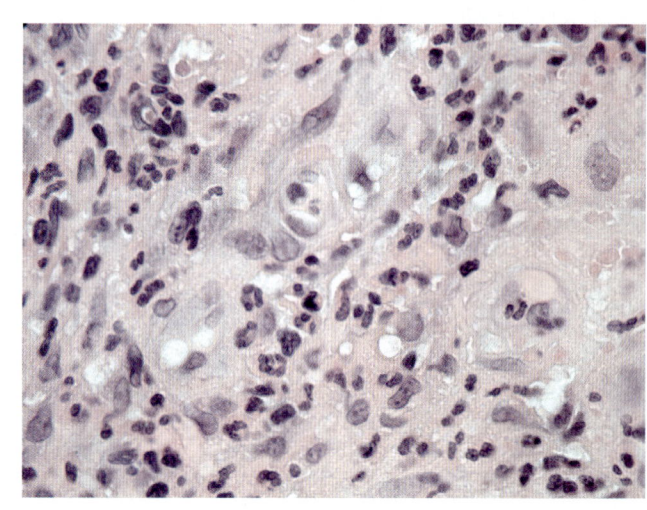

Figure 14.22. Higher magnification of lesion shown in Figure 14.21 showing acute and chronic inflammatory cells. (Hematoxylin–eosin ×100).

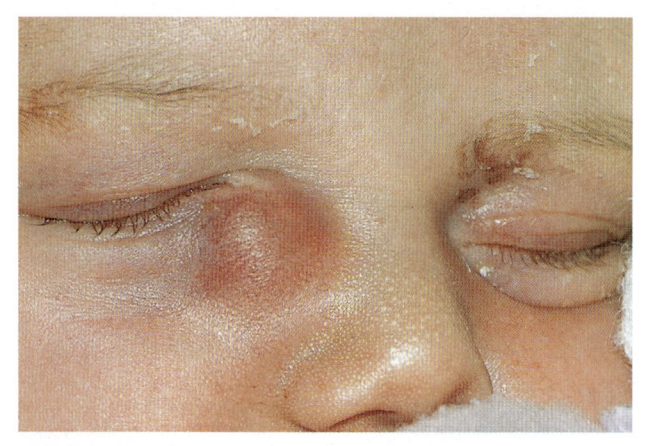

Figure 14.23. Acute dacryocystitis in an infant showing redness to skin over the lacrimal sac.

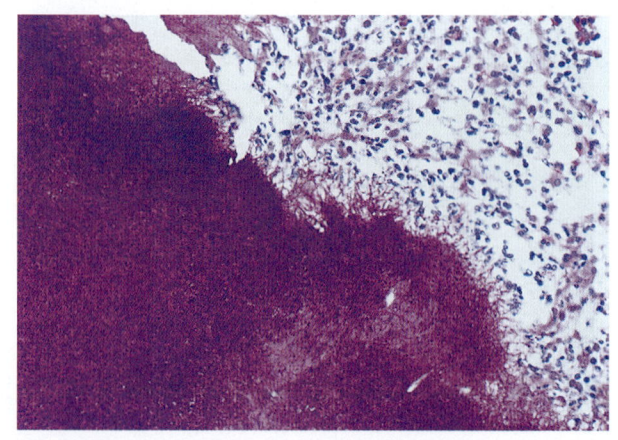

Figure 14.24. Histopathology of a dacryolith in an elderly patient with dacryocystitis secondary to actinomyces. The purple area down and to the left is a dense mass composed of fungi. (Hematoxylin–eosin ×10.)

CHAPTER 15

SURGICAL MANAGEMENT OF EYELID TUMORS

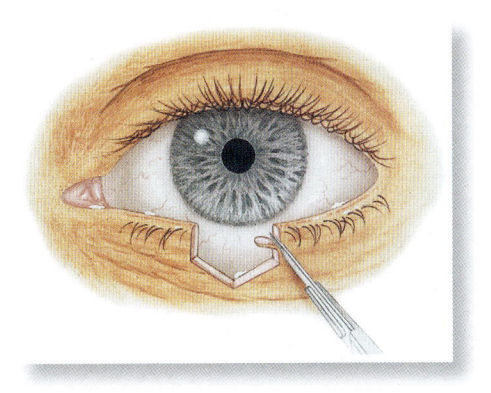

Surgical management of eyelid tumors can be complex. It involves knowledge of eyelid anatomy and experience with handling tumor tissue and cosmetic reconstruction. It is beyond the scope of this textbook and atlas to describe the fine details of surgical management of eyelid tumors. There are several excellent published articles (1–5) and textbooks (6) that cover surgery for eyelid tumors. In this chapter, we outline some of the basic surgical approaches to eyelid tumors.

In each patient with a suspicious eyelid lesion, the clinician must determine whether a biopsy is indicated and, if so, what kind of biopsy would be most appropriate. In the case of a large lesion (generally more than half of the eyelid) that is possibly malignant, an incisional biopsy is often warranted and a histopathologic diagnosis is obtained before extensive definitive surgery and reconstruction are undertaken. A small trephine punch is ideal for such a biopsy, although an incisional biopsy with a scalpel is also acceptable particularly for suspected basal cell carcinoma.

A probable benign tumor that is cosmetically unacceptable may be managed by a shaving biopsy. A highly probable malignant tumor that is small can be managed by primary excision with eyelid reconstruction, without risking a biopsy. This is particularly true for eyelid melanoma. An incisional diagnostic biopsy is generally acceptable for malignant tumors with low metastatic potential, such as basal cell carcinoma and squamous cell carcinoma. Frozen sections or chemosurgery are generally advisable to insure that margins are free of tumor before closure of the wound.

A skin graft or flap may be necessary in some cases to close the defect and minimize functional eyelid problems, such as cicatricial ectropion. Donor skin can be obtained from the upper eyelid of the ipsilateral or contralateral eye, retroauricular skin, or other sites, depending on the preference of the surgeon and the clinical circumstances. Larger malignant tumors may require wide surgical removal and extensive eyelid reconstruction. Some malignant eyelid tumors that invade the orbital soft tissues may require a subtotal or total orbital exenteration.

SURGICAL MANAGEMENT OF EYELID TUMORS

Selected References

Reviews

1. Mannor GE, Chern PL, Barnette D. Eyelid and periorbital skin basal cell carcinoma: oculoplastic management and surgery. *Int Ophthalmol Clin* 2009;49:1–16.
2. Rene C. Oculoplastics aspects of ocular oncology. *Eye* 2013;27:199–207.
3. Alghoul M, Pacella SJ, McClellan WT, et al. Eyelid reconstruction. *Plast Reconstr Surg* 2013;132:288e–302e.
4. Sullivan TJ. Topical therapies for periorbital cutaneous malignancies: indications and treatment regimens. *Curr Opin Ophthalmol* 2012;23:439–442.
5. Murchison AP, Walrath JD, Washington CV. Non-surgical treatments of primary, non-melanoma eyelid malignancies: a review. *Clin Experiment Ophthalmol* 2011;39:65–83.

Books

6. Basic and Clinical Science Course. *Section 7: Orbit, Eyelids, and Lacrimal System.* San Francisco, CA: American Academy of Ophthalmology; 2014–2015.

Chapter 15 Surgical Management of Eyelid Tumors

PUNCH BIOPSY, EXCISIONAL SHAVE BIOPSY, AND ELLIPTICAL EXCISION WITH SKIN GRAFT

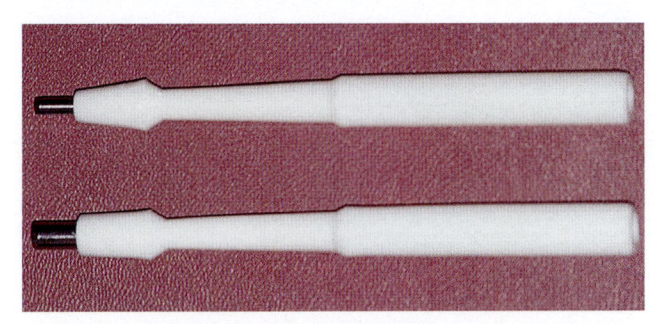

Figure 15.1. Examples of trephines to perform punch biopsy. Most biopsies are done with a 2-mm, 3-mm, or 4-mm diameter punch.

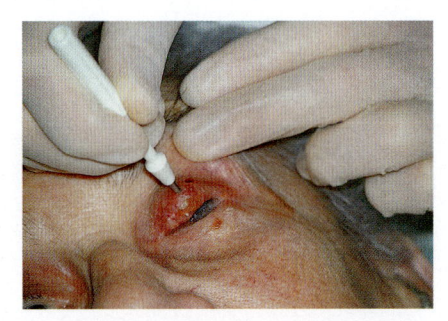

Figure 15.2. Technique of punch biopsy for diffuse lesion in upper eyelid suspected to be a large sebaceous gland carcinoma. That diagnosis was confirmed on histopathologic study of the punch biopsy.

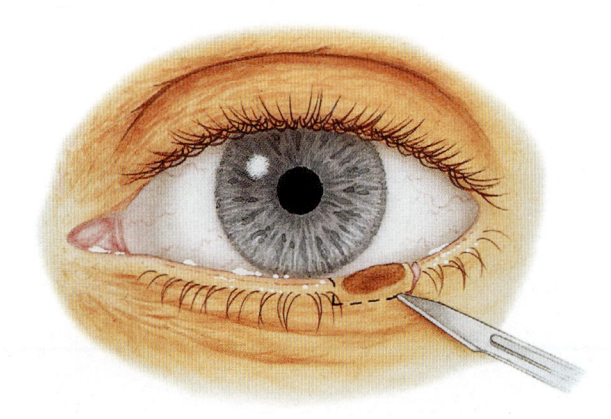

Figure 15.3. Technique of shaving excisional biopsy of lesion on eyelid margin.

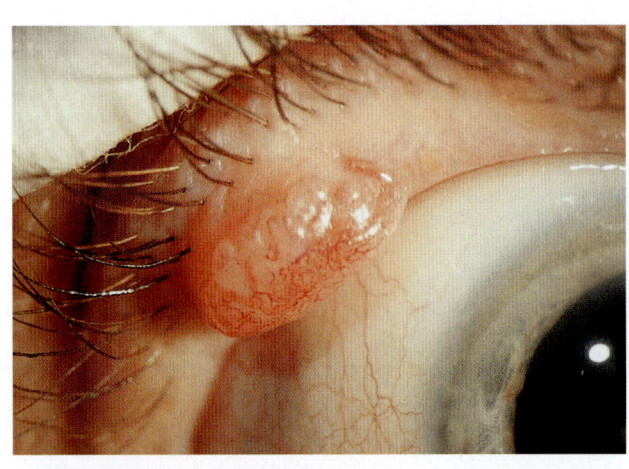

Figure 15.4. Lesion for which a shaving biopsy is appropriate. The differential diagnosis includes squamous papilloma and amelanotic nevus.

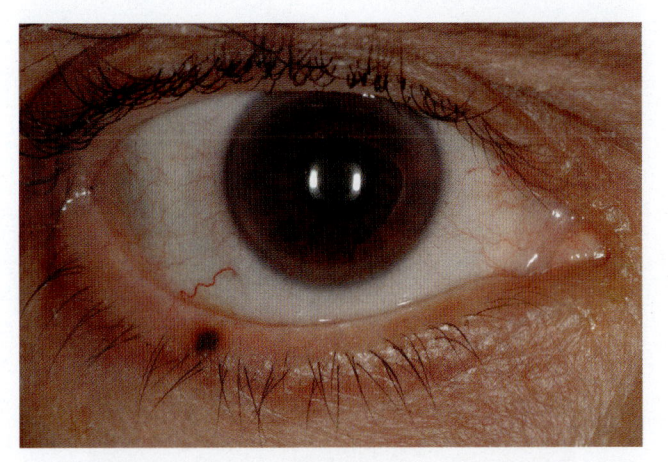

Figure 15.5. Newly found pigmented eyelid margin nevus for shave biopsy.

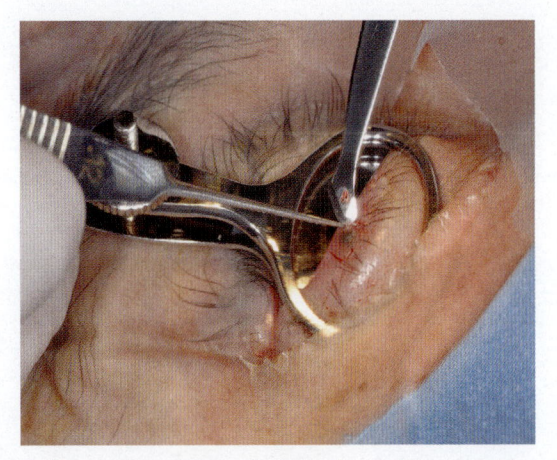

Figure 15.6. At shave biopsy the lesion is carefully shaved from the eyelid margin with intent to avoid removing tarsus. Chalazion clamp is used for hemostasis.

246 Part 1 Tumors of the Eyelids

● ELLIPTICAL EXCISION OF EYELID TUMOR

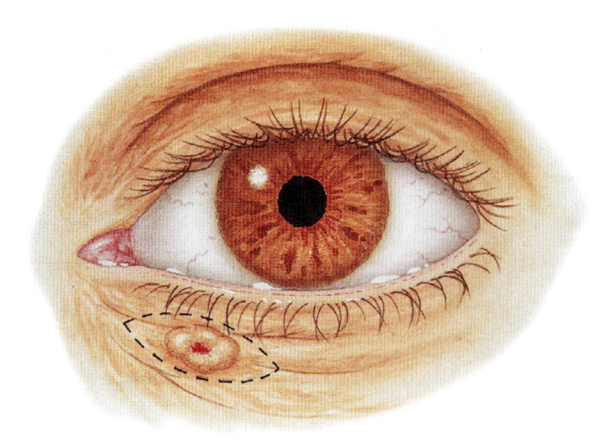

Figure 15.7. Lesion of lower eyelid where elliptical excision and primary closure is generally adequate. If it appears at the time of surgery that primary closure would cause ectropion of eyelid, then a rotational flap or skin graft, usually from the upper eyelid or retroauricular area, can be done.

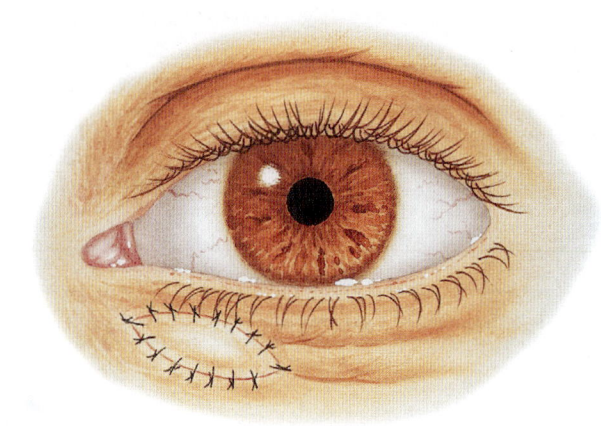

Figure 15.8. Skin graft sutured into position. This is shown for illustrative purposes only. Ordinarily, a skin graft would not be done for a defect as small as the one shown.

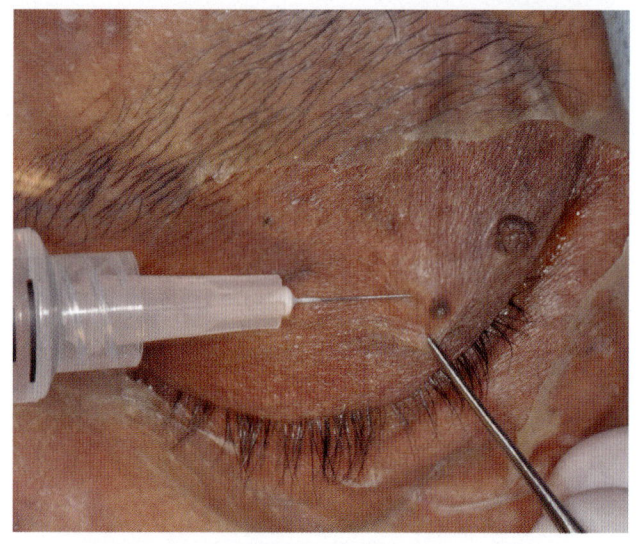

Figure 15.9. Two small upper eyelid seborrheic keratosis are removed using local anesthesia and elliptical excision.

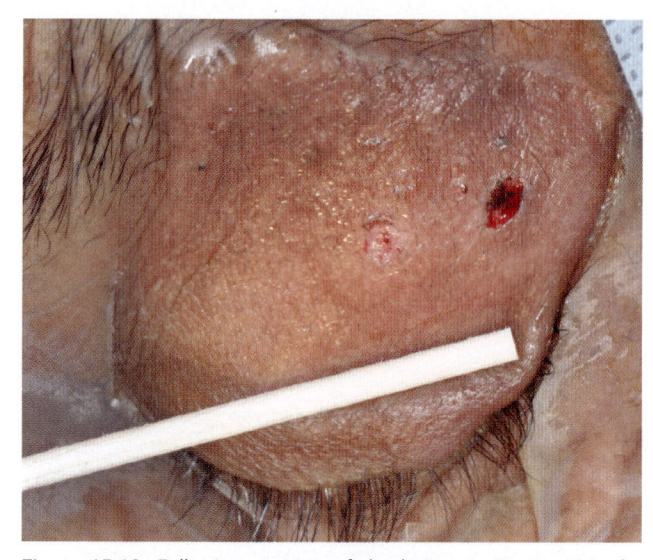

Figure 15.10. Following excision of the lesions in Figure 15.9, the wounds appear clean and require no suturing.

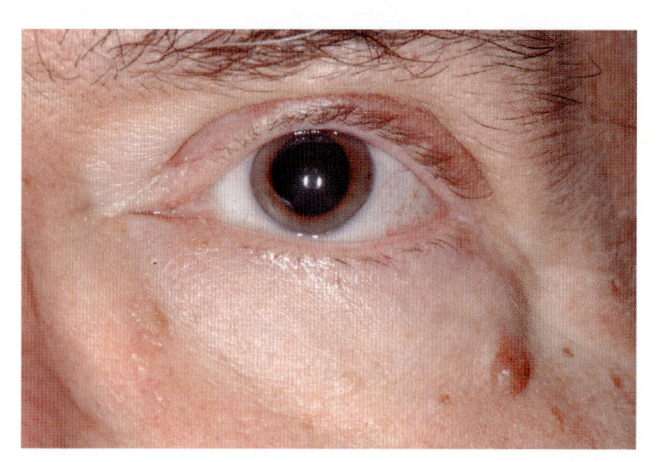

Figure 15.11. Larger seborrheic keratosis in inferior eyelid/cheek region.

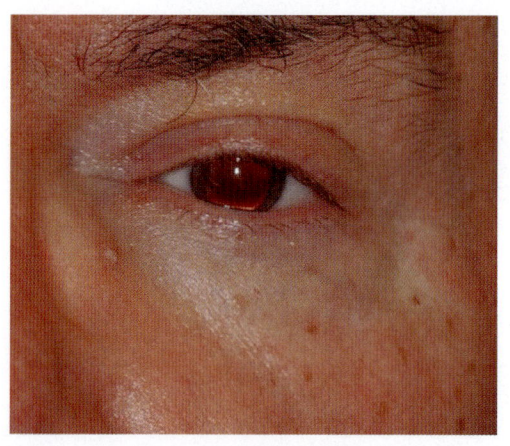

Figure 15.12. Following elliptical excision and primary suture closure of patient in Figure 15.11, the wound has healed well.

Chapter 15 Surgical Management of Eyelid Tumors   247

PENTAGONAL FULL-THICKNESS EXCISION OF EYELID TUMOR WITH SEMICIRCULAR FLAP RECONSTRUCTION

The same technique depicted here for the lower eyelid also applies to the upper eyelid, except that the direction of the semicircular flap is reversed.

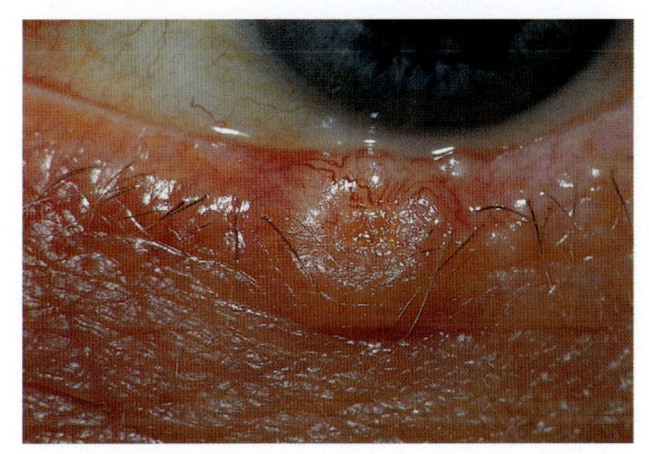

Figure 15.13. Basal cell carcinoma of lower eyelid where pentagonal excision is indicated.

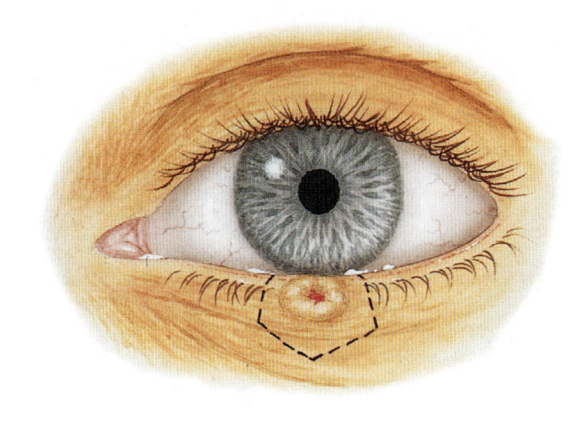

Figure 15.14. Outline of the planned pentagonal excision.

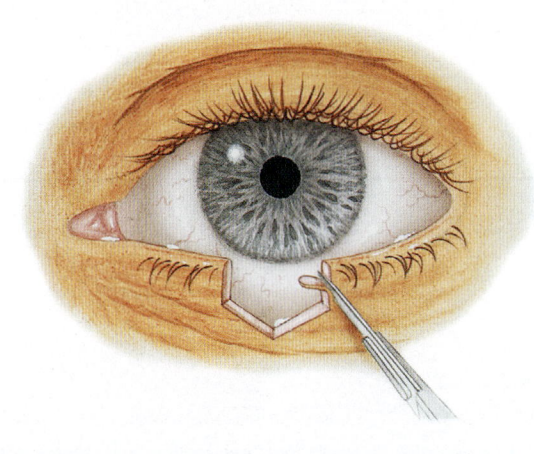

Figure 15.15. Lesion has been removed and marginal biopsy is being taken for frozen section readings. Frozen sections should be taken on temporal margin, nasal margin, and base.

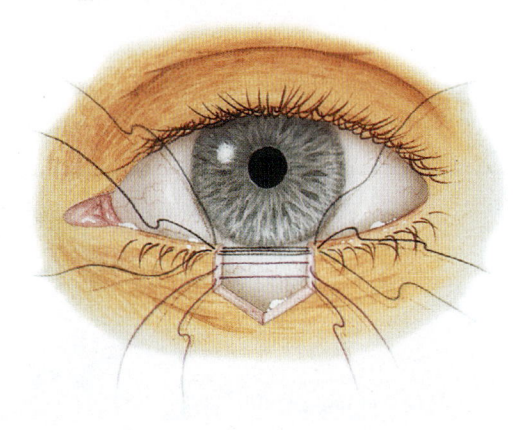

Figure 15.16. Eyelid margin and tarsal sutures have been placed. In this case, primary closure can be performed without a semicircular flap.

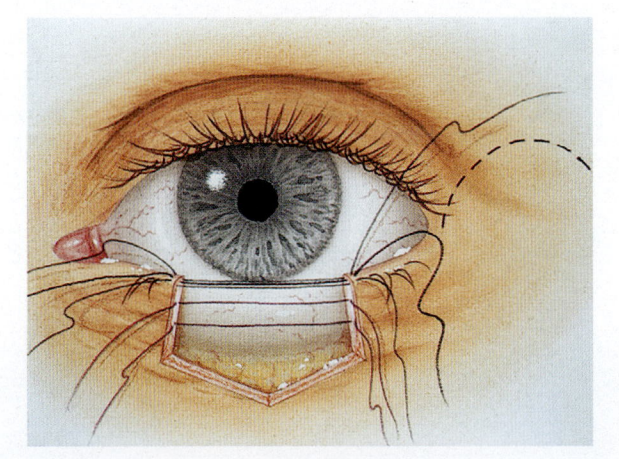

Figure 15.17. Slightly larger defect after tumor excision. The wound will not close easily, so a semicircular flap is designed temporally (dotted line).

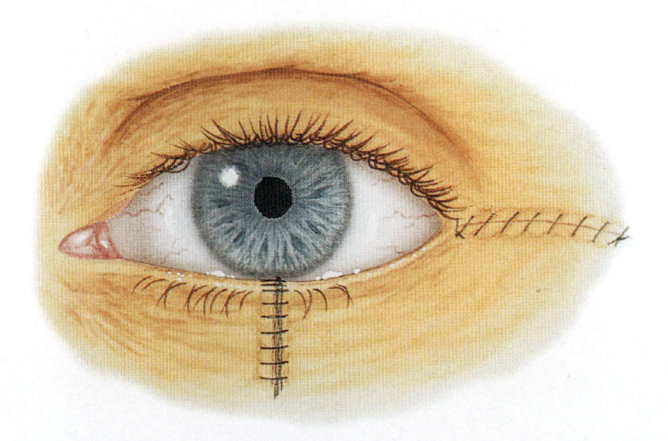

Figure 15.18. Final closure of eyelid defect and the semicircular flap. Nylon, silk, or absorbable sutures can be used, depending on the surgeons' preference.

Part 1 Tumors of the Eyelids

PENTAGONAL FULL-THICKNESS EXCISION OF EYELID TUMOR WITH PRIMARY CLOSURE

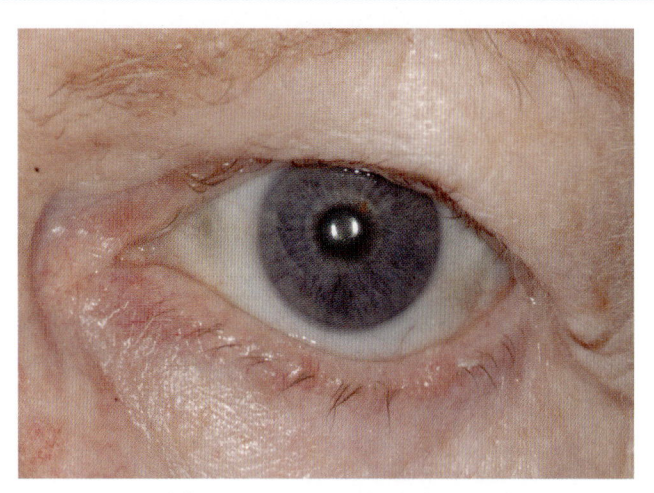

Figure 15.19. Subtle tumor on temporal right lower eyelid margin with irregular surface and loss of eyelashes, suspicious for basal cell carcinoma.

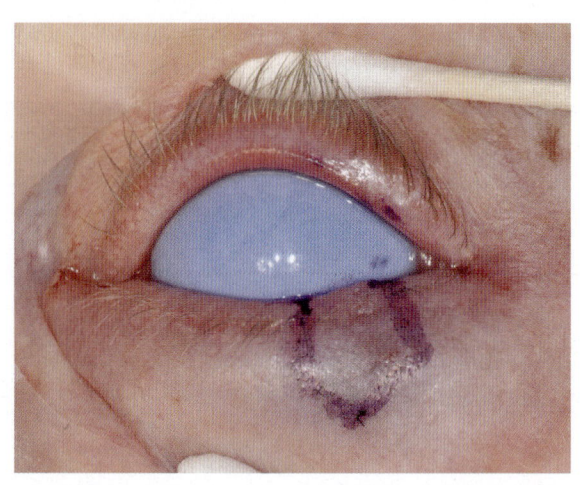

Figure 15.20. Surgical approach using scleral shell and pentagonal excision.

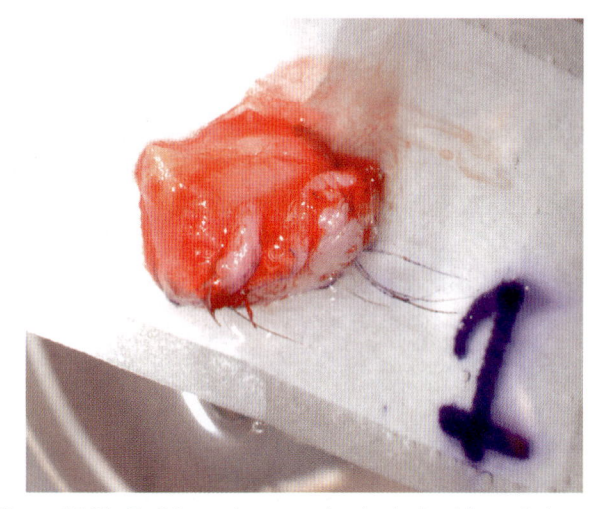

Figure 15.21. Eyelid mass is removed and submitted for pathology on cardboard in formalin. Histopathology confirms basal cell carcinoma.

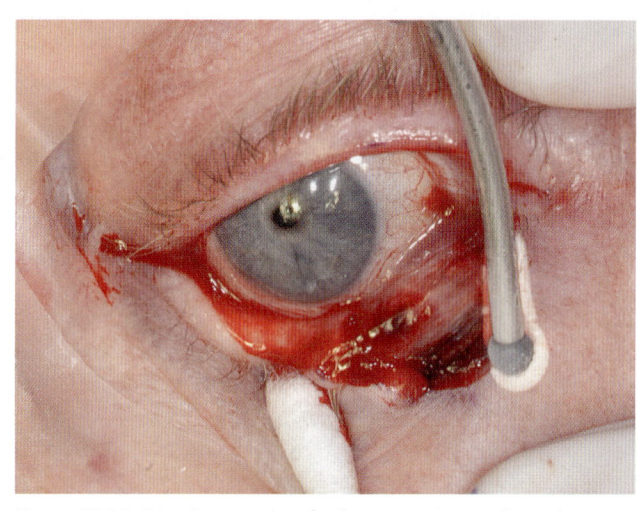

Figure 15.22. Margins are taken for frozen sections and cryotherapy is applied to the skin to minimize risk for recurrence.

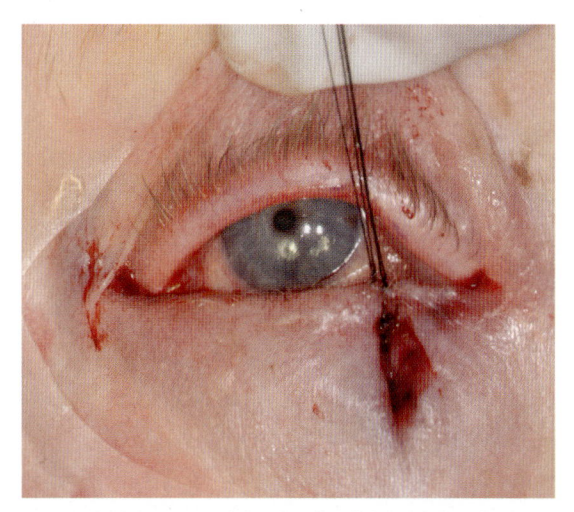

Figure 15.23. Closure is performed with vicryl sutures in the tarsus, silk sutures in eyelid margin (shown), and chromic sutures in anterior lamellar skin.

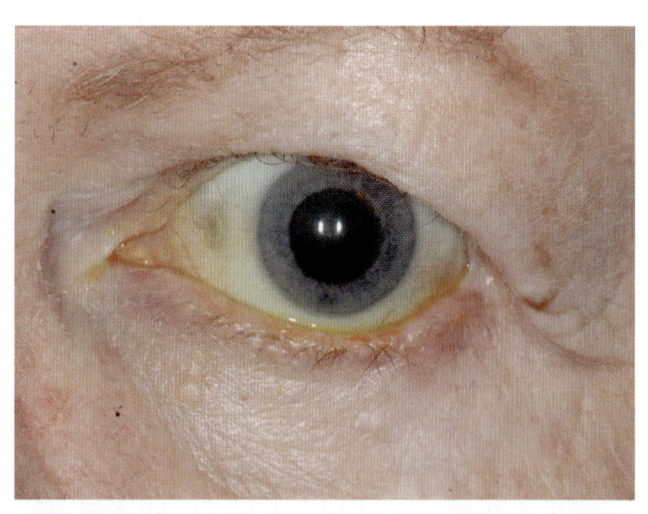

Figure 15.24. Four months later, the eyelid is completely healed without defect or tumor.

PART 2

TUMORS OF THE CONJUNCTIVA

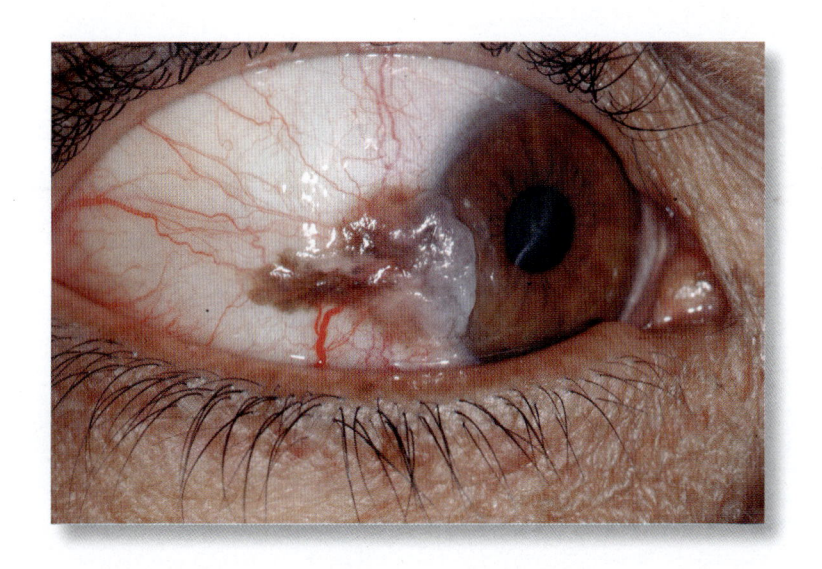

CONJUNCTIVAL AND EPIBULBAR CHORISTOMAS

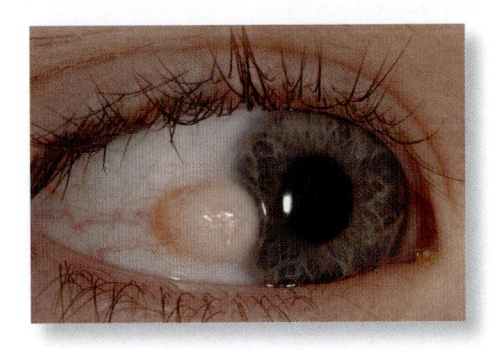

General Considerations

Most congenital tumors of the conjunctiva are choristomas, which are tumorous malformations composed of tissues not normally present at the involved site. A simple choristoma contains one type of tissue; a complex choristoma has more than one type. The main choristomatous tissues that occur in the conjunctiva include skin, bone, lacrimal gland, and cartilage (1–17). Most conjunctival choristomas are sporadic and nonhereditary. In a review of 262 children with conjunctival tumors, 10% were choristomas (3).

Both dermoid and dermolipoma are choristomas and often part of Goldenhar syndrome, which also includes auricular and vertebral anomalies. Dermoid is the second most common epibulbar choristoma, following dermolipoma (1,3). In the authors' clinical series of 1,643 conjunctival tumors in children and adults, there were 10 dermoids, accounting for 25% of all epibulbar choristomas and for <1% of all 1,643 lesions (1).

Clinical Features

Small dermoids are often asymptomatic, but larger lesions can cause irritation, astigmatism, and inadequate eyelid closure (8). It appears as a variably sized, yellow-white limbal mass inferotemporally but it can appear in other meridians. It can range from 2 to 15 mm in diameter and 0 to 10 mm in thickness. Fine white hairs often protrude from the lesion. There is often a yellow-white lipid line in the adjacent corneal stroma. A conjunctival dermoid can show extensive corneal involvement with little involvement of the adjacent conjunctiva (13). It can rarely arise from the caruncle (15). An unusual variant (ring dermoid syndrome) is bilateral, straddles the corneoscleral limbus for 360 degrees, and has an autosomal-dominant mode of inheritance (16).

Pathology

Histopathologically, dermoid is lined by stratified squamous epithelium. Deep to the epithelium is dense collagenous tissue in which pilosebaceous units, sweat glands, and fat are often identifiable (13). In rare instances, bone can be present within the dermoid (complex choristoma). It is possible that dermoid develops secondary to faulty eyelid fold closure embryologically with secondary entrapment of skin and mesenchyme.

Management

Smaller asymptomatic dermoids can be observed and larger lesions may require excision (9–12). Reasons for surgical removal include amblyopia, secondary astigmatism, encroachment on the visual axis, dellen formation, inadequate eyelid closure, and cosmetic considerations. Early removal is advocated for symptomatic lesions to achieve a better cosmetic outcome. However, it is believed that early removal does little to change the astigmatism that was present preoperatively (8). Removal can be achieved by superficial shaving or by deeper excision with lamellar keratoplasty for deeper lesions.

CONJUNCTIVAL DERMOID

Management can depend on extensiveness of dermoid. For grade I dermoid (superficial corneal involvement), observation is recommended, for grade II (full-thickness cornea with/without endothelial involvement) and grade III (with additional anterior chamber involvement), a combination of excision, lamellar keratoplasty, amniotic membrane and stem cell replacement are employed (9–11).

Selected References

Reviews

1. Shields CL, Demirci H, Karatza E, et al. Clinical survey of 1643 melanocytic and nonmelanocytic tumors of the conjunctiva. *Ophthalmology* 2004;111:1747–1754.
2. Shields CL, Shields JA. Tumors of the conjunctiva and cornea. *Surv Ophthalmol* 2004;49:3–24.
3. Shields CL, Shields JA. Conjunctival tumors in children. *Curr Opin Ophthalmol* 2007;18:351–360.
4. Cunha RP, Cunha MC, Shields JA. Epibulbar tumors in childhood. A survey of 282 biopsies. *J Pediatr Ophthalmol* 1987;24:249–254.
5. Elsas FJ, Green WR. Epibulbar tumors in childhood. *Am J Ophthalmol* 1975;79:1001–1007.
6. Dailey EG, Lubowitz RM. Dermoids of the limbus and cornea. *Am J Ophthalmol* 1962;53:661–665.
7. Burillon C, Durand L. Solid dermoids of the limbus and cornea. *Ophthalmologica* 1997;211:367–372.
8. Robb RM. Astigmatic refractive errors associated with limbal dermoids. *J Pediatr Ophthalmol Strabismus* 1996;33:241–243.

Management

9. Lang SJ, Bohringer D, Reinhard T. Surgical management of corneal limbal dermoids: Retrospective study of different techniques and use of Mitomycin C. *Eye* 2014;28:857–862.
10. Pirouzian A. Management of pediatric corneal limbal dermoids. *Clin Ophthalmol* 2013;7:607–614.
11. Pirouzian A, Holz H, Merrill K, et al. Surgical management of pediatric limbal dermoids with sutureless amniotic membrane transplantation and augmentation. *J Pediatr Ophthalmol Strabismus* 2012;49:114–119.
12. Mader TH, Stulting D. Technique for the removal of limbal dermoids. *Cornea* 1998;17:66–67.

Histopathology

13. Shields JA, Laibson PR, Augsburger JJ, et al. Central corneal dermoid. A clinicopathologic correlation and review of the literature. *Can J Ophthalmol* 1986;21:23–26.

Case Reports

14. Oakman JH, Lambert SR, Grossniklaus HE. Corneal dermoid: Case report and review of classification. *J Pediatr Ophthalmol Strabismus* 1993;30:388–391.
15. Ghafouri A, Rodgers IR, Perry HD. A caruncular dermoid with contiguous eyelid involvement: embryologic implications. *Ophthal Plast Reconstr Surg* 1998;14:375–377.
16. Mattos J, Contreras F, O'Donnell FE Jr. Ring dermoid syndrome. A new syndrome of autosomal dominantly inherited, bilateral, annular limbal dermoids with corneal and conjunctival extension. *Arch Ophthalmol* 1980;98:1059–1061.
17. Ferry AP, Hein HF. Epibulbar osseous choristoma within an epibulbar dermoid. *Am J Ophthalmol* 1970;70:764–766.

Chapter 16 Conjunctival and Epibulbar Choristomas

• CONJUNCTIVAL DERMOID

Conjunctival dermoid can occur as an isolated lesion or it can be a component of Goldenhar syndrome.

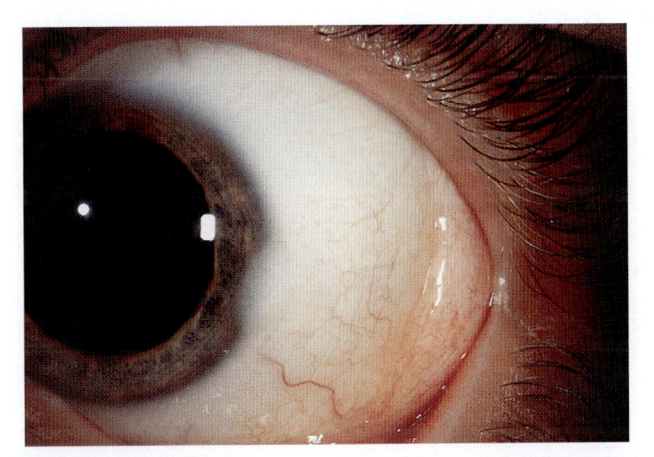

Figure 16.1. Typical round conjunctiva at the corneoscleral limbus inferotemporally.

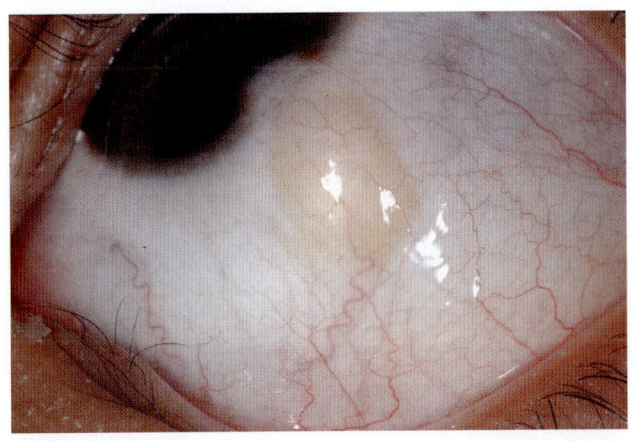

Figure 16.2. Ovoid conjunctival dermoid at limbus inferotemporally in a 12-year-old girl.

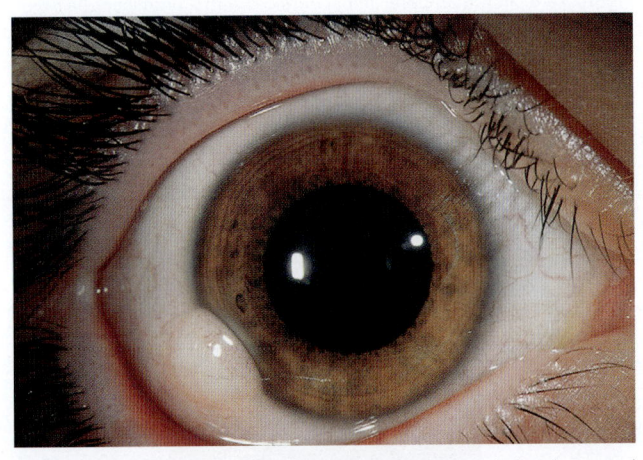

Figure 16.3. Inferotemporal conjunctival dermoid with fine hairs and telangiectasia.

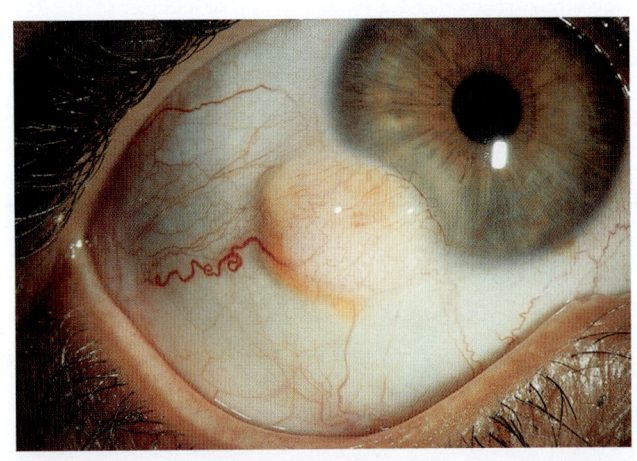

Figure 16.4. Larger limbal dermoid with a dilated blood vessel in a 47-year-old woman with Goldenhar syndrome.

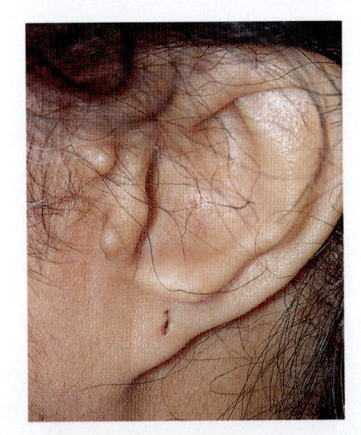

Figure 16.5. Preauricular skin appendages in the patient showing in Figure 16.4. The patient also had hearing loss, consistent with Goldenhar syndrome.

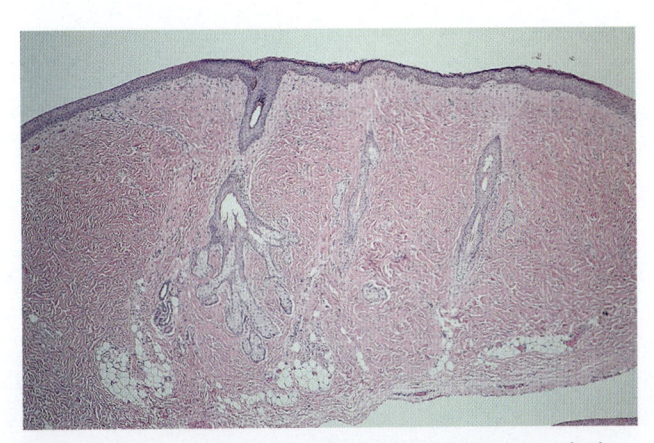

Figure 16.6. Histopathology of limbal dermoid showing several pilosebaceous units in dense collagenous tissue and foci of lipid. (Hematoxylin–eosin ×10.)

Part 2 Tumors of the Conjunctiva

CONJUNCTIVAL AND CORNEAL DERMOIDS

Dermoids and related choristomas can assume a variety of configurations and management varies with the type and extent of the lesion.

Shields JA, Laibson PR, Augsburger JJ, et al. Central corneal dermoid. A clinicopathologic correlation and review of the literature. Can J Ophthalmol 1986;21:23–26.

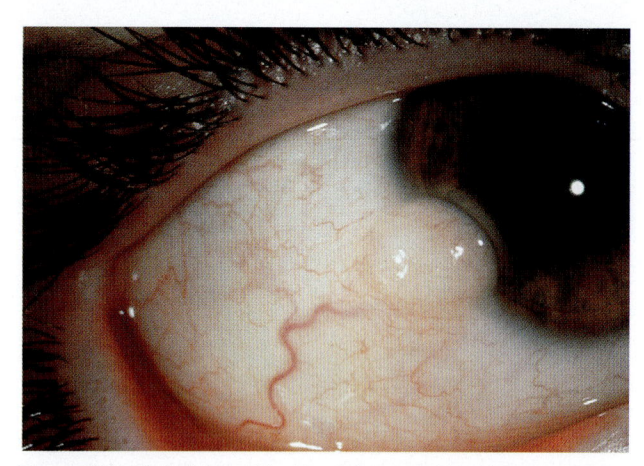

Figure 16.7. Limbal dermoid with subtle corneal lipid line.

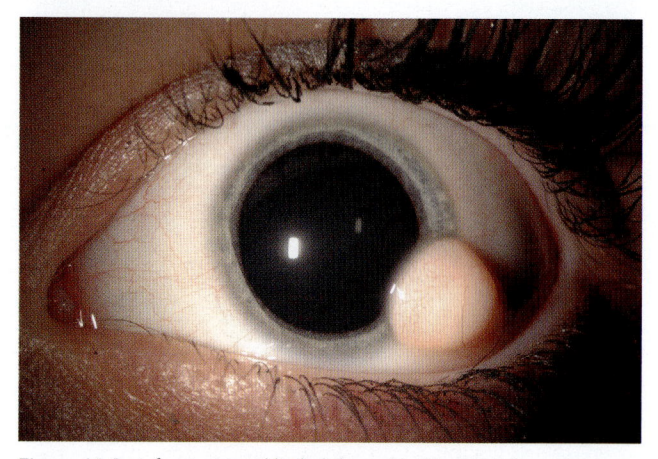

Figure 16.8. Inferotemporal limbal dermoid with a prominent hair.

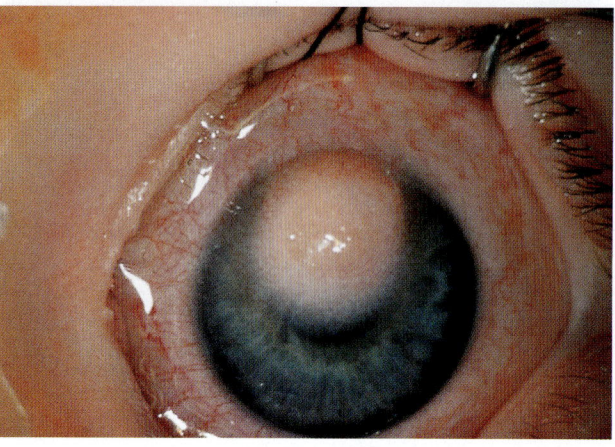

Figure 16.9. Corneal dermoid with minimal limbal involvement superiorly.

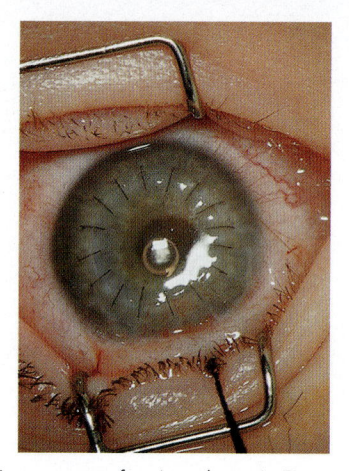

Figure 16.10. Appearance of patient shown in Figure 16.9 after penetrating keratoplasty. A lamellar keratoplasty was originally planned but it was found at the time of surgery that the lesion extended for full thickness of the corneal stroma.

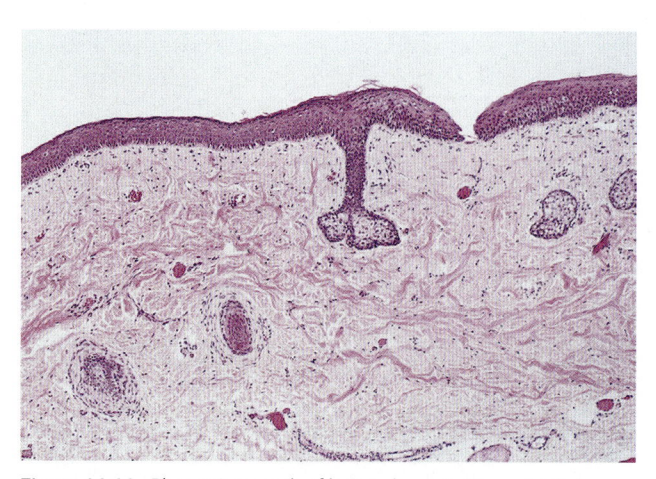

Figure 16.11. Photomicrograph of lesion shown in Figure 16.9 demonstrating pilosebaceous units. (Hematoxylin–eosin ×20.)

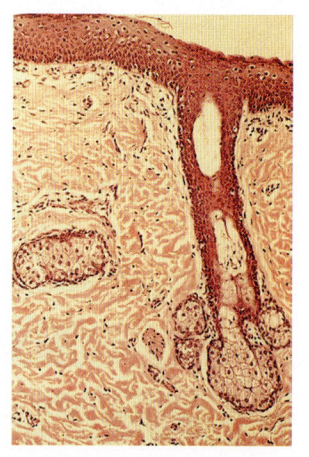

Figure 16.12. Photomicrograph of lesion shown in Figure 16.9 demonstrating pilosebaceous unit in a collagenous stroma within the disorganized corneal stroma. (Hematoxylin–eosin ×50.)

Chapter 16 Conjunctival and Epibulbar Choristomas 255

● CONJUNCTIVAL AND CORNEAL DERMOIDS: ATYPICAL VARIATIONS

Sometimes an epibulbar dermoid is more atypical and can have other tissues in addition to dermal elements, meeting criteria for a complex choristoma. Epibulbar dermoid is also known to extend through the limbus into the anterior chamber.

Oakman JH, Lambert SR, Grossniklaus HE. Corneal dermoid: case report and review of classification. *J Pediatr Ophthalmol Strabismus* 1993;30:388–391.

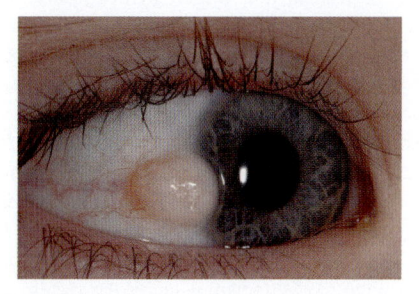

Figure 16.13. Limbal dermoid in a 7-year-old boy.

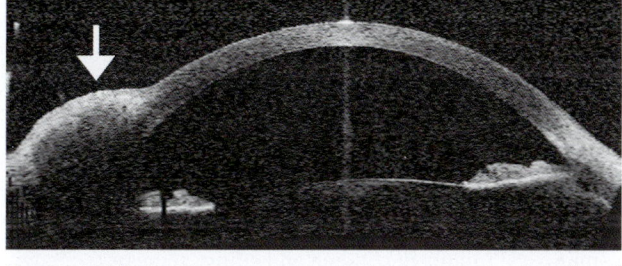

Figure 16.14. Anterior segment optical coherence tomography of lesion in Figure 16.13 demonstrating the solid dermoid at the limbus (*arrow*) with intact intraocular structures.

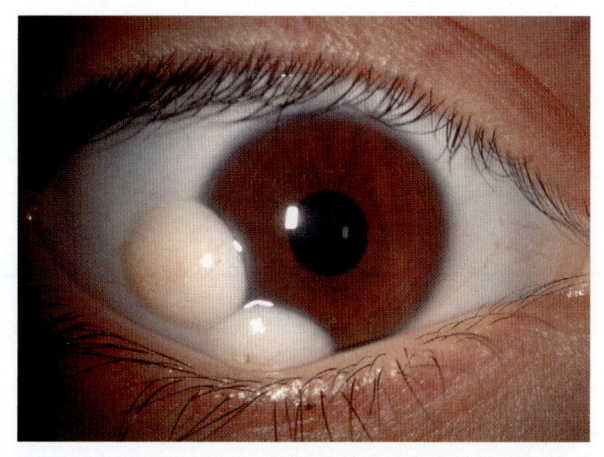

Figure 16.15. Bilobed corneal dermoid that was present at birth.

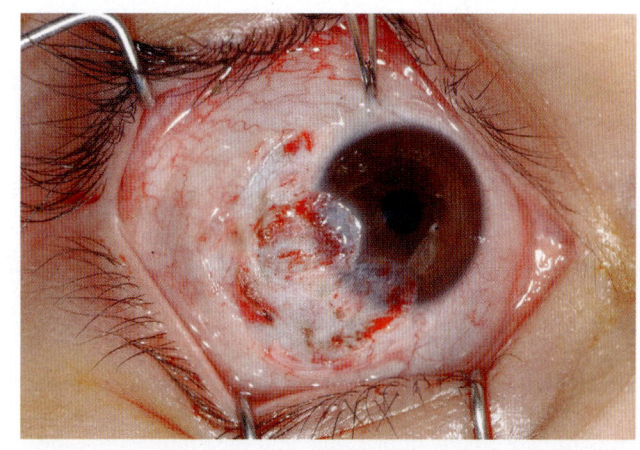

Figure 16.16. The patient in Figure 16.15 underwent surgical removal of the bilobed corneal dermoid at 15 years of age. Photograph taken at the time of surgery immediately after removal and before closure with sutures. The eye subsequently healed with minor white opacity in the peripheral cornea.

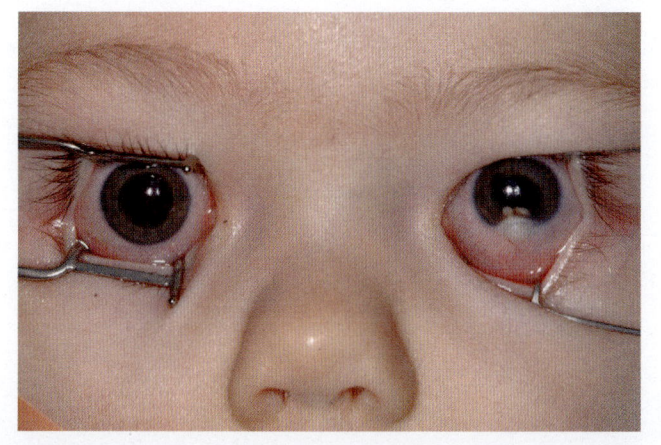

Figure 16.17. Both eyes of a baby at time of examination under anesthesia, showing atypical dermoid at the corneoscleral limbus inferiorly.

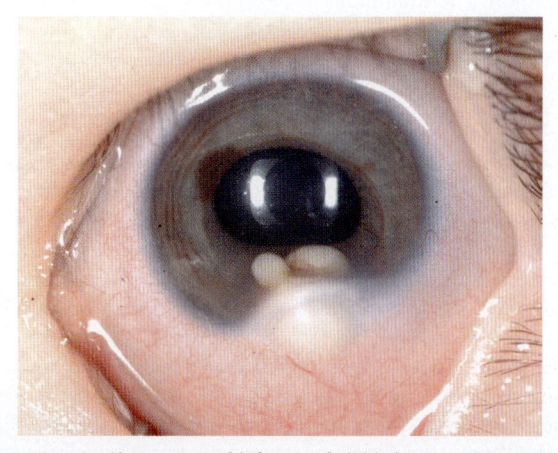

Figure 16.18. Closer view of left eye of child shown in Figure 16.17. The nodules in the anterior chamber were aspirated and they partially collapsed, a finding compatible with a cyst associated with the presumed solid dermoid. Cytopathology showed epithelial cells.

CONJUNCTIVAL/ORBITAL DERMOLIPOMA

General Considerations

In contrast to a dermoid, dermolipoma (lipodermoid) is less well defined and most often located in the superotemporal conjunctiva, often with extension posteriorly into the orbit (1–20). It can occasionally be atypical and even pedunculated. Like dermoid, it is frequently associated with Goldenhar syndrome. An analysis of 34 patients with dermolipoma found 12 (35%) with Goldenhar syndrome (6). It can also be a component of the organoid nevus syndrome (20). In the organoid nevus syndrome, the lesion usually has other heterotopic elements, most often cartilage and ectopic lacrimal gland tissue. Dermoid is the second most common epibulbar choristoma, following dermolipoma. In the authors' clinical series of 1,643 conjunctival tumors in children and adults, there were 23 dermolipomas, accounting for 58% of all epibulbar choristomas and for 1% of the 1,643 lesions (2). In a separate analysis of 262 conjunctival tumors in children, dermolipoma represented 5% (3).

Clinical Features

Dermolipoma is a congenital lesion that may not become clinically apparent until later in the first or second decade of life. It most often occurs in the superotemporal or inferotemporal conjunctival fornix. It is a sessile lesion that has a dull, yellow-pink color, with fine hairs protruding from the surface. On occasion, we have observed recurrent long black hairs protruding from a dermolipoma, presumably from a pilosebaceous unit within the lesion. Dermolipoma is not readily displaceable and can have regions of visible yellow lipid in its substance. It is often confused with herniated orbital fat. However, herniated orbital fat is more often bilateral, is a more butter-yellow color, lacks hairs, is readily displaceable into the orbit, and has brilliant lipid material deep to the conjunctival epithelium. The epithelial surface of a dermolipoma is usually smooth, but can occasionally be irregularly thickened. Dermolipoma can also simulate a neoplasm of the lacrimal gland.

Although dermolipoma is generally small and asymptomatic, it can occasionally be large and even pedunculated (11). In such cases, it may require excision for cosmetic reasons.

Pathology

Microscopically, dermolipoma is lined by stratified squamous epithelium that may be partially keratinized. The stroma consists of densely packed collagen fibers, similar to a dermoid, with deep lipid in some cases. Pilosebaceous units are not detected in many cases, despite the presence of small hairs. As mentioned, the stroma may occasionally contain other choristomatous elements such as bone, cartilage, and ectopic lacrimal gland (17,19). This is particularly true in the organoid nevus syndrome, to be discussed shortly (20). This is often unsuspected until the lesion is removed with the clinical diagnosis of "typical" dermolipoma.

Management

Dermolipoma is generally a nonprogressive, benign lesion that usually requires no treatment (8–10). Although it can usually be observed periodically, a larger, symptomatic lesion with ocular irritation may require excision and reconstruction. The surgical approach should be careful (8) to avoid damage to the lateral and superior rectus muscles, the levator muscle of the upper eyelid (9,13), and the lacrimal gland, as well as inherent fibrosis with scarring and retraction. It may be prudent to do a subtotal excision, removing only the ellipse of tissue that contains hair and avoiding removal of tissue posterior to the bony orbital rim. Doctor Crowell Beard has stated that, "The surgery of dermolipoma is fraught with dangers. It too often is followed by damage to the lacrimal secretory system, intractable diplopia, blepharoptosis, and perhaps other undesirable complications. Since these tumors are benign, the smallest amount of surgical debulking should be done to provide a cosmetically acceptable result. By being aware of this principle factors, the surgeon can avoid most complications" (8). Keratoconjunctivitis sicca has also been recognized as a potential complication of surgical excision of dermolipoma (18).

CONJUNCTIVAL/ORBITAL DERMOLIPOMA

Selected References

Reviews

1. Shields CL, Demirci H, Karatza E, et al. Clinical survey of 1643 melanocytic and nonmelanocytic tumors of the conjunctiva. *Ophthalmology* 2004;111:1747–1754.
2. Shields CL, Shields JA. Tumors of the conjunctiva and cornea. *Surv Ophthalmol* 2004;49:3–24.
3. Shields CL, Shields JA. Conjunctival tumors in children. *Curr Opin Ophthalmol* 2007;18:351–360.
4. Cunha RP, Cunha MC, Shields JA. Epibulbar tumors in childhood. A survey of 282 biopsies. *J Pediatr Ophthalmol* 1987;24:249–254.
5. Elsas FJ, Green WR. Epibulbar tumors in childhood. *Am J Ophthalmol* 1975;79:1001–1007.
6. Khong JJ, Hardy TG, McNab AA. Prevalence of oculo-auriculo-vertebral spectrum in dermolipoma. *Ophthalmology* 2013;120:1529–1532.

Imaging

7. Eijpe AA, Koornneef L, Bras J, et al. Dermolipoma: Characteristic CT appearance. *Doc Ophthalmol* 1990;74:321–328.

Management

8. Beard C. Dermolipoma surgery, or, "an ounce of prevention is worth a pound of cure." *Ophthal Plast Reconstr Surg* 1990;6:153–157.
9. Fry CL, Leone CR Jr. Safe management of dermolipomas. *Arch Ophthalmol* 1994;112:1114–1116.
10. Sa HS, Kim HK, Shin JH, et al. Dermolipoma surgery with rotational conjunctival flaps. *Acta Ophthalmol* 2012;90(1):86–90.

Case Reports

11. Ziavras E, Farber MG, Diamond GR. A pedunculated lipodermoid in oculoauriculovertebral dysplasia. *Arch Ophthalmol* 1990;108:1032–1033.
12. McNab AA. Subconjunctival fat prolapse. *Aust N Z J Ophthalmol* 1999;27:33–36.
13. Paris GL, Beard C. Blepharoptosis following dermolipoma surgery. *Ann Ophthalmol* 1973;5:697–699.
14. Mishriki YY. Bilateral eye tumors of long duration. Dermolipoma. *Postgrad Med* 2004;116:53–54.
15. Kiratli H, Tatlipinar S, Sanac AS, et al. Pseudo-Brown's syndrome secondary to a growing conjunctival dermolipoma. *J Pediatr Ophthalmol Strabismus* 2001;38:112–113.
16. Ganesh A, Rangaswamy M. Pedunculated dermolipoma with overlying upper lid coloboma and absent lateral canthus: cause and effect. *Eye* 1999;13:687–689.
17. Hered RW, Hiles DA. Epibulbar osseous choristoma and ectopic lacrimal gland underlying a dermolipoma. *J Pediatr Ophthalmol Strabismus* 1987;24:255–258.
18. Economidis I, Tragakis M, Mangouritsas N, et al. Keratoconjunctivitis sicca following excision of a dermolipoma of the lacrimal gland. *Ann Ophthalmol* 1978;1:1273–1278.
19. Daicker BC, Perren B. Epibulbar osteoma combined with dermolipoma. *Ophthalmologica* 1977;174:58–60.
20. Shields JA, Shields CL, Eagle RC Jr, et al. Ocular manifestations of the organoid nevus syndrome. *Ophthalmology* 1997;104:549–557.

Part 2 Tumors of the Conjunctiva

CONJUNCTIVAL DERMOLIPOMA

These lesions are presumed to be congenital and often have fine white hairs that are not seen in photographs but can be appreciated with slit-lamp biomicroscopy.

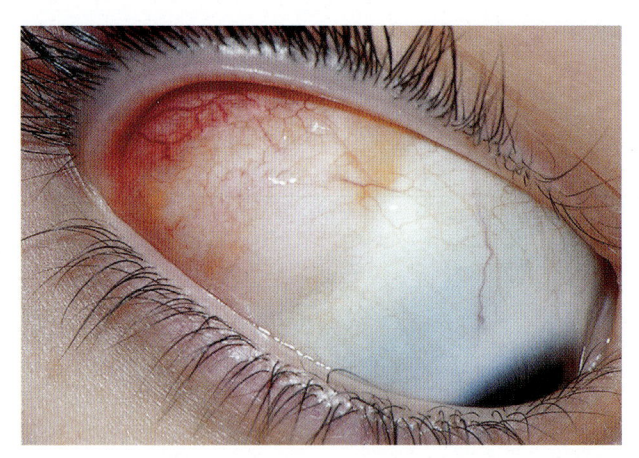

Figure 16.19. Sessile dermolipoma superotemporally in right eye of a 5-year-old girl.

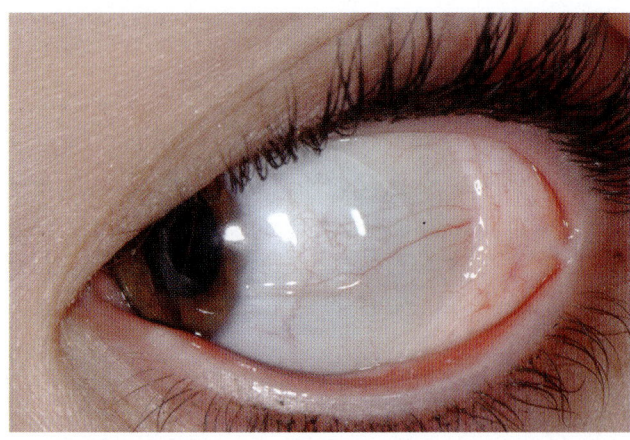

Figure 16.20. Sessile dermolipoma superotemporally in left eye of a young woman. Note that the curvature of the anterior margin is concave (curvature parallel to limbus), a feature often seen with dermolipoma. This helps to differentiate it from herniated orbital fat.

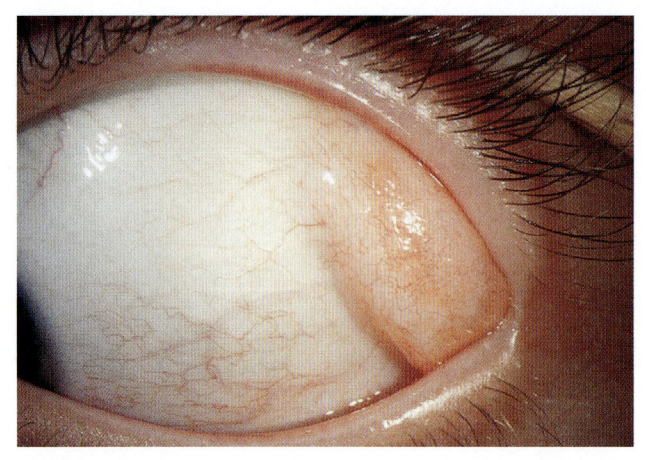

Figure 16.21. Rounded dermolipoma superotemporally in left eye of an 11-year-old boy.

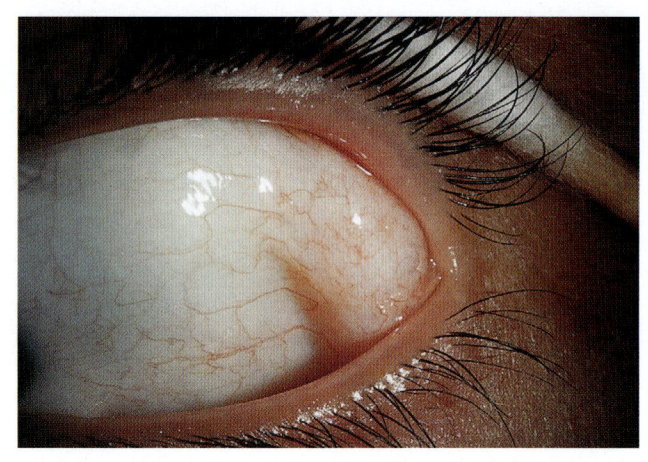

Figure 16.22. Rounded dermolipoma superotemporally in left eye of an 11-year-old girl.

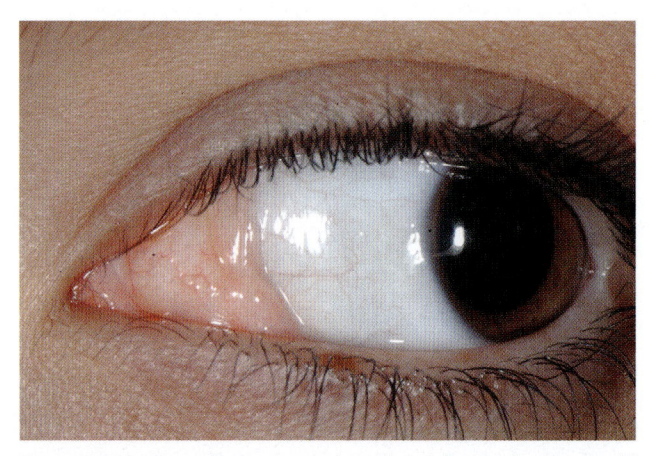

Figure 16.23. Dermolipoma located nasally in left eye of a 20-year-old woman. Note that the anterior edge of the lesion is concave, as seen in case shown in Figure 16.20.

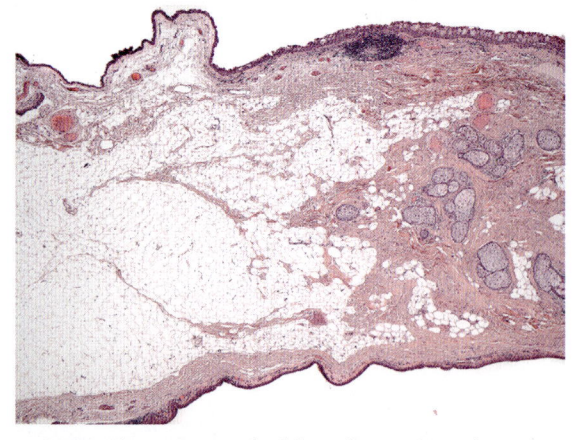

Figure 16.24. Photomicrograph of dermolipoma. Note the conjunctival epithelium with subepithelial collagenous tissue above and the fat cells below. There is more lipid in this case than in most dermolipomas. Some sebaceous glands are present to the right. (Hematoxylin–eosin ×25.)

CONJUNCTIVAL DERMOIDS AND DERMOLIPOMAS: BILOBED AND PEDUNCULATED VARIANTS

In some cases, dermoid and dermolipoma can overlap one another and have atypical bilobed or pedunculated configurations.

Ziavras E, Farber MG, Diamond GR. A pedunculated lipodermoid in oculoauriculovertebral dysplasia. *Arch Ophthalmol* 1990;108:1032–1033.

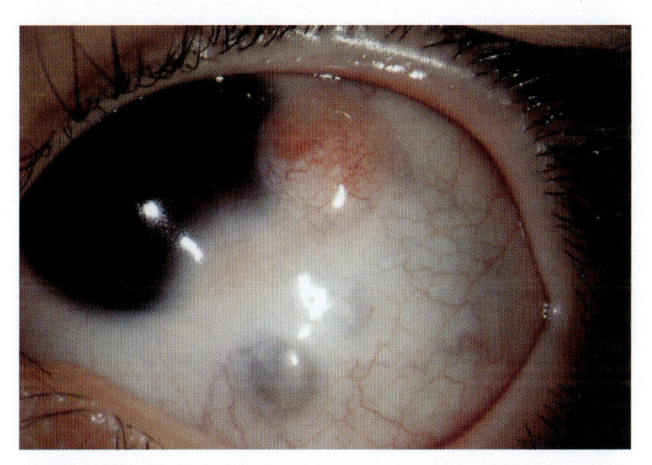

Figure 16.25. Bilobed limbal dermoid. The gray area inferiorly was not confirmed histopathologically and could be intrascleral cartilage. If so, it would meet the criteria for a complex choristoma.

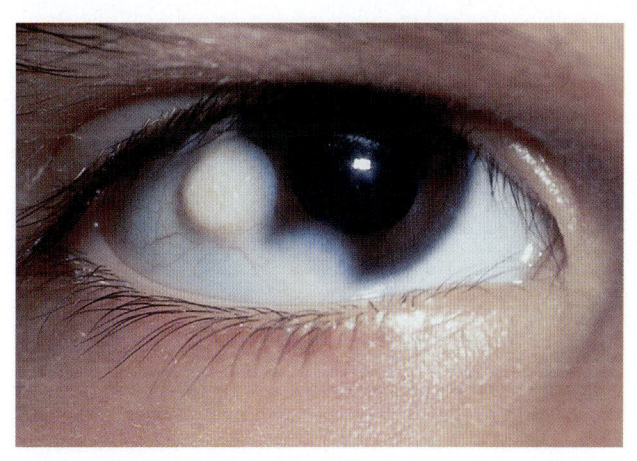

Figure 16.26. Bilobed corneal dermoid. The lesion more superiorly at limbus is fleshy and the lesion more inferiorly at limbus is white.

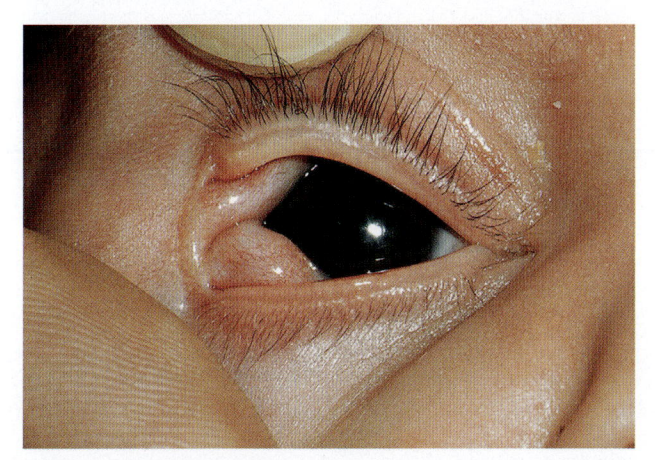

Figure 16.27. Bilobed dermoid replacing the lateral canthus, causing a lateral canthal defect (coloboma variant).

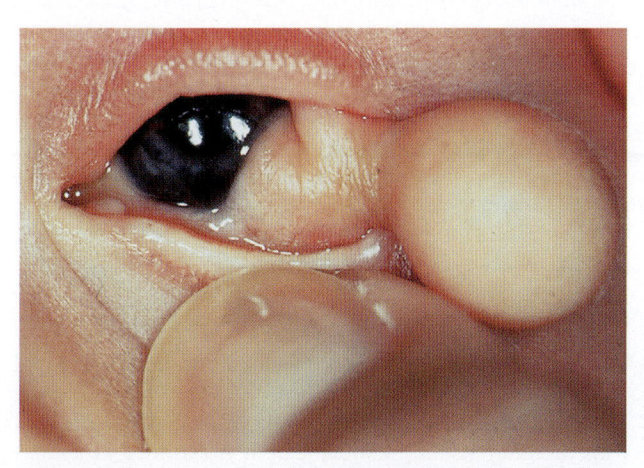

Figure 16.28. Large pedunculated dermolipoma arising from temporal conjunctiva and replacing skin of lateral canthus. The child had oculoauriculovertebral dysplasia, compatible with Goldenhar syndrome. (Courtesy of Elaine Ziavras, MD.)

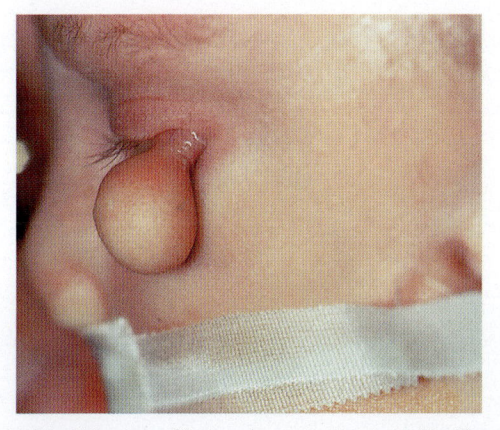

Figure 16.29. Side view of lesion shown in Figure 16.28. (Courtesy of Elaine Ziavras, MD.)

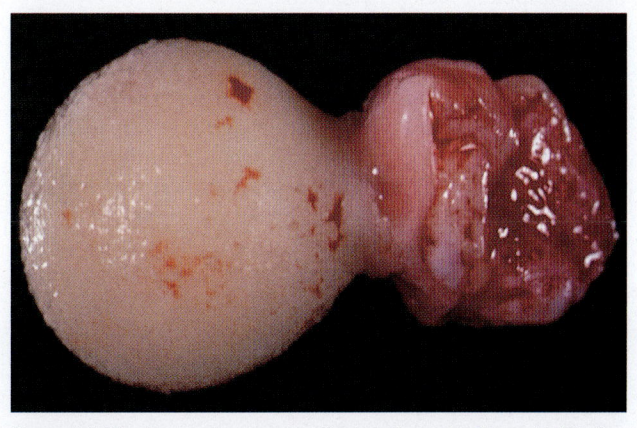

Figure 16.30. Gross appearance of lesion shown in Figure 16.28 after successful surgical removal. Histopathologically, the lesion had features consistent with a dermolipoma. (Courtesy of Elaine Ziavras, MD.)

EPIBULBAR OSSEOUS CHORISTOMA

General Considerations

Epibulbar osseous choristoma is a congenital simple choristoma consisting of pure bone on the surface of the globe. It is usually recognized in childhood and characteristically occurs in the superotemporal quadrant on or near the scleral surface, although there are several clinical variations (1–21). According to recent reviews, over 50 cases have been reported in the ophthalmic literature (3,4). In the authors' clinical series of 1,643 conjunctival tumors, there were two epibulbar osseous choristomas, accounting for 5% of all choristomas and for <1% of the 1,643 lesions (1). A more recent analysis of the authors' experience revealed 8 cases, with characteristic features, imaging, and outcomes (3).

Clinical Features

Epibulbar osseous choristoma is a rock-hard lesion usually located on the bulbar surface superotemporally. It is often firmly attached to the underlying sclera and can involve a rectus muscle. It may be palpable through the upper eyelid. It can be asymptomatic or it may produce conjunctival hyperemia or a mild foreign body sensation. It is generally a stable lesion that does not show appreciable growth. Although it is congenital, it may not become clinically apparent until later years. Most patients are <15 years old at the time of clinical diagnosis (3). More than 70% occur in females. The affected patient is generally asymptomatic but in rare instances, redness, foreign body sensation, or tearing can occur. The lesion is generally not associated with Goldenhar syndrome. Computed tomography (CT) or ultrasound biomicroscopy can demonstrate the lesion as being consistent with bone.

Pathology

Histopathologically, epibulbar osseous choristoma is composed of mature bone (3,5). Some cartilage (14), ectopic lacrimal gland (12), and dermolipoma tissue can be closely associated with the bony lesion, in which case it is classified as a complex choristoma. Although the embryogenesis is uncertain, it is speculated that it may correlate with the scleral ossicles seen in avian species and may represent abnormal activation of embryonic pluripotent mesenchymal cells (13).

Management

For asymptomatic lesions, periodic observation may be justified. If it is symptomatic or if it is of concern to the patient and family, then surgical excision is warranted. Complete removal of the mass via a conjunctival excision with dissection from the sclera is advisable. Because it is difficult to determine clinically how far the lesion extends into the sclera, the surgeon should be prepared to perform a scleral graft, although that is rarely necessary.

Selected References

Reviews
1. Shields CL, Demirci H, Karatza E, et al. Clinical survey of 1643 melanocytic and nonmelanocytic tumors of the conjunctiva. *Ophthalmology* 2004;111:1747–1754.
2. Shields CL, Shields JA. Tumors of the conjunctiva and cornea. *Surv Ophthalmol* 2004;49:3–24.
3. Shields CL, Qureshi A, Eagle RC Jr, et al. Epibulbar osseous choristoma in 8 patients. *Cornea* 2012;31(7):756–760.
4. Gayre GS, Proia AD, Dutton JJ. Epibulbar osseous choristoma: case report and review of the literature. *Ophthalmic Surg Lasers* 2002;33:410–415.

Histopathology
5. Shields JA, Eagle RC, Shields CL, et al. Epibulbar osseous choristoma. Computed tomography and clinicopathologic correlation. *Ophthalm Pract* 1997;15:110–112.

Case Reports
6. Boniuk M, Zimmerman LE. Episcleral osseous choristoma. *Am J Ophthalmol* 1961;53:290–296.
7. Beckman G, Sugar H. Episcleral osseous choristoma. *Arch Ophthalmol* 1964;71:377–378.
8. Roch LB, Milauskas AT. Epibulbar osteomas. *Arch Ophthalmol* 1968;79:578–579.
9. Ferry AP, Hein HF. Epibulbar osseous choristoma within an epibulbar dermoid. *Am J Ophthalmol* 1970;70:764–766.
10. Ortiz JM, Yanoff M. Epipalpebral conjunctival osseous choristoma. *Br J Ophthalmol* 1979;63:173–176.
11. Dreizen NG, Schachat AP, Shields JA, et al. Epibulbar osseous choristoma. *J Pediatr Ophthalmol Strabismus* 1983;20:247–249.
12. Hered RW, Hiles DA. Epibulbar osseous choristoma and ectopic lacrimal gland underlying a dermolipoma. *J Pediatr Ophthalmol Strabismus* 1987;24:255–258.
13. Gonnering RS, Fuerste FH, Lemke BN, et al. Epibulbar osseous choristomas with scleral involvement. *Ophthalmic Plast Reconstr Surg* 1988;4:63–66.
14. Melki TS, Zimmerman LE, Chavis RM, et al. A unique epibulbar osseous choristoma. *J Pediatr Ophthalmol Strabismus* 1990;27:252–254.
15. Santora DC, Biglan AW, Johnson BL. Episcleral osteocartilaginous choristoma. *Am J Ophthalmol* 1995;119:654–655.
16. Marback EF, Stout TJ, Rao NA. Osseous choristoma of the conjunctiva simulating extraocular extension of retinoblastoma. *Am J Ophthalmol* 2002;133:825–827.
17. Casady DR, Carlson JA, Meyer DR. Unusual complex choristoma of the lateral canthus. *Ophthal Plast Reconstr Surg* 2005;21:161–163.
18. Kim BJ, Kazim M. Bilateral asymmetrical epibulbar osseous choristoma. *Ophthalmology* 2006;113(3):456–458.
19. Tsai AS, Lee KY, Al Jajeh I, et al. Epibulbar osseous choristoma: a report of two cases. *Orbit* 2008;27(3):231–233.
20. Khan AO, Al-Hussein H, Al-Katan H. Osseous choristoma of the lateral canthus. *J AAPOS* 2007;11(5):502–503.
21. Verity DH, Rose GE, Uddin JM, et al. Epibulbar osseous choristoma: benign pathology simulating an intraorbital foreign body. *Orbit* 2007;26(1):29–32.

EPIBULBAR OSSEOUS CHORISTOMA

Shields CL, Qureshi A, Eagle RC Jr, et al. Epibulbar osseous choristoma in 8 patients. *Cornea* 2012;31(7):756–760.

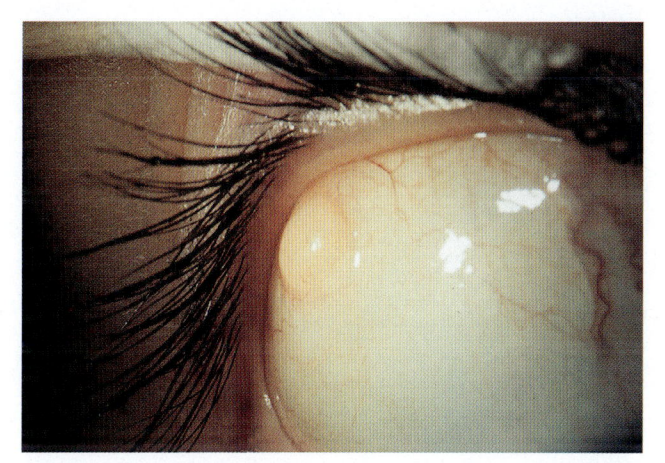

Figure 16.31. Typical epibulbar osseous choristoma in a 25-year-old woman.

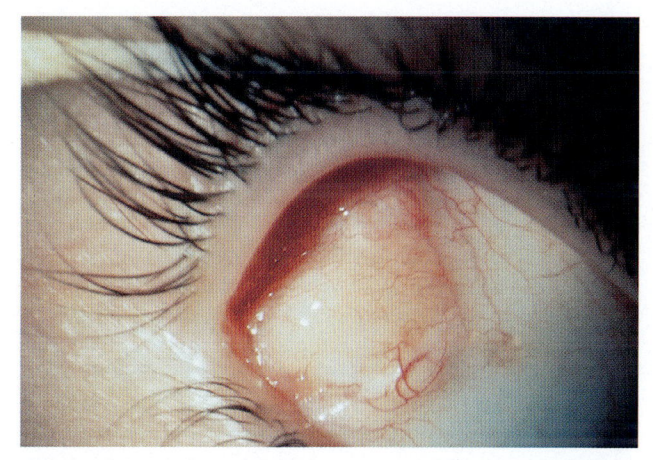

Figure 16.32. Typical epibulbar osseous choristoma in an 8-year-old boy.

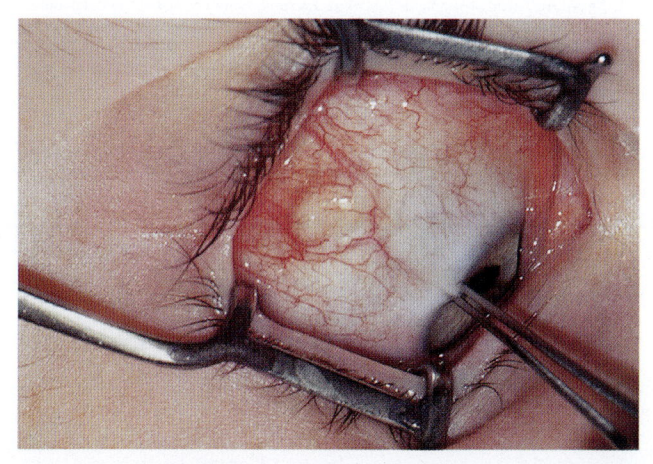

Figure 16.33. Typical epibulbar osseous choristoma in a 9-year-old girl.

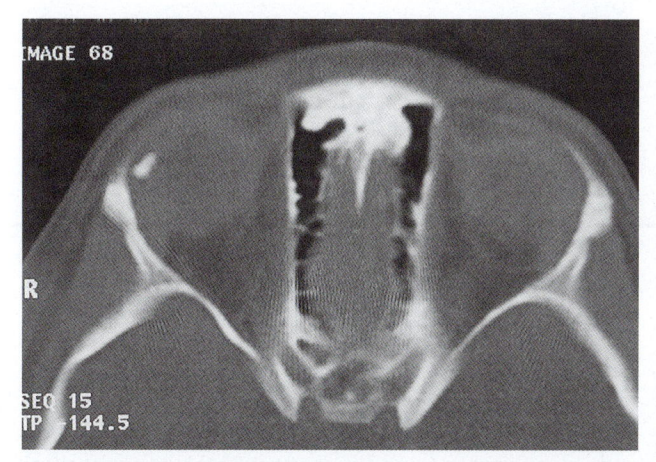

Figure 16.34. Axial computed tomography showing epibulbar lesion with features compatible with bone.

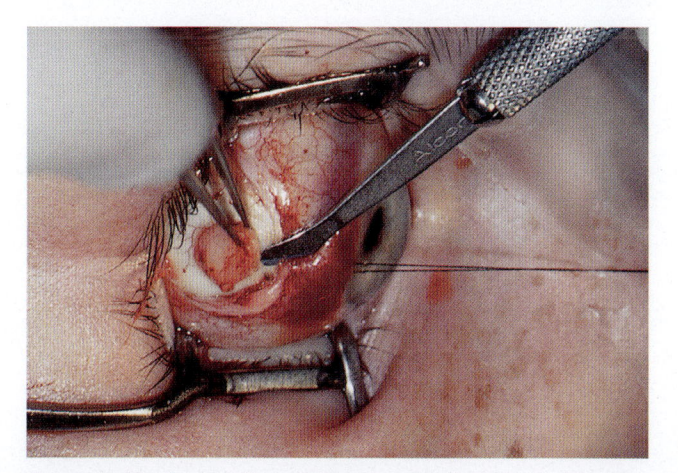

Figure 16.35. Surgical dissection of the mass from its attachment to the sclera.

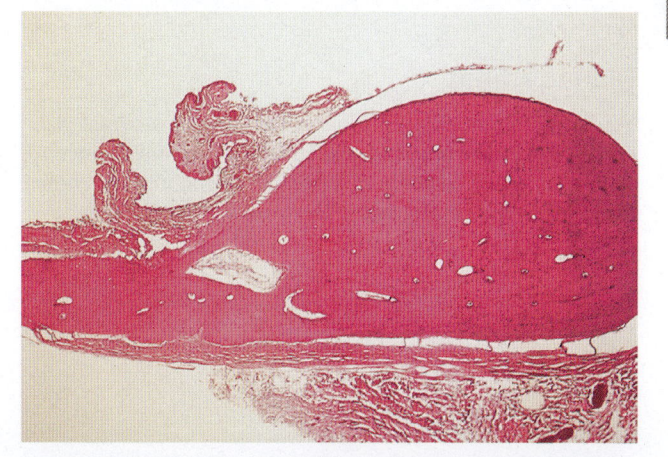

Figure 16.36. Photomicrograph of the specimen showing mature bone. Note some conjunctival tissue above and a thin layer of superficial sclera below. The lesion was adherent to both the conjunctiva and the sclera. (Hematoxylin–eosin ×10.)

LACRIMAL GLAND AND RESPIRATORY CHORISTOMAS OF CONJUNCTIVA

General Considerations

Other simple choristomas that have been observed in the conjunctiva are lacrimal gland choristoma and respiratory cyst choristoma. These choristomatous malformations are described here as simple choristomas. Strictly speaking, however, many of these lesions are composed mainly of one type of tissue but have small proportions of other tissues. Hence, they could rightfully be called complex, rather than simple, choristomas (1–13).

It is well known that small rests of ectopic lacrimal gland tissue can occasionally be present in the conjunctiva, separate from the accessory lacrimal glands of Krause and Wolfring. In some instances, such rests of ectopic lacrimal gland tissue may assume choristomatous proportions. It is of ophthalmic interest that lacrimal gland choristomas can occur in the anterior uveal tract (5,8) and orbit, as well as the conjunctiva (3). In the authors' clinical series of 1,643 conjunctival tumors, there was one lacrimal gland choristoma and no respiratory choristomas (1,2).

Clinical Features

Although there is little information about the clinical variations of this uncommonly diagnosed condition, it is likely that subtle cases may be subclinical and are never diagnosed. The clinically evident conjunctival lacrimal gland choristoma generally appears as a fairly distinct fleshy, pink lesion that resembles normal lacrimal gland. Likewise, respiratory choristoma can present as a pink, fleshy lesion near the limbus that can simulate a lymphoid infiltrate (12).

Pathology

Histopathologically, the lacrimal gland tissue is the same as that seen in the normal lacrimal gland. It may be associated with a papillomatous proliferation of squamous epithelium and hyperkeratosis (9). As the name implies, respiratory choristoma contains ducts and acini that are lined by respiratory epithelium.

Management

Small, asymptomatic lesions suspected of being lacrimal gland choristoma can be observed, and large or symptomatic ones can be excised locally. In advanced cases that extend into the cornea, keratoplasty may be necessary. The prognosis is excellent.

Selected References

Reviews
1. Shields CL, Demirci H, Karatza E, et al. Clinical survey of 1643 melanocytic and nonmelanocytic tumors of the conjunctiva. *Ophthalmology* 2004;111:1747–1754.
2. Shields CL, Shields JA. Tumors of the conjunctiva and cornea. *Surv Ophthalmol* 2004;49:3–24.

Histopathology/Cytopathology
3. Pokorny KS, Hyman BM, Jakobiec FA, et al. Epibulbar choristomas containing lacrimal tissue. Clinical distinction from dermoids and histologic evidence of an origin from the palpebral lobe. *Ophthalmology* 1987;94:1249–1257.
4. Alyahya GA, Bangsgaard R, Prause JU, et al. Occurrence of lacrimal gland tissue outside the lacrimal fossa: comparison of clinical and histopathological findings. *Acta Ophthalmol Scand* 2005;83:100–103.
5. Kobrin EG, Shields CL, Danzig C, et al. Intraocular lacrimal gland choristoma diagnosed by fine needle aspiration biopsy. *Cornea*. 2007;26:753–755.

Case Reports
6. Green WR, Zimmerman LE. Ectopic lacrimal gland tissue. *Arch Ophthalmol* 1967;78:318–327.
7. Pfaffenbach DD, Green WR. Ectopic lacrimal gland. *Int Ophthalmol Clin* 1971;3:149–159.
8. Shields JA, Eagle RC Jr, Shields CL, et al. Natural course and histopathologic findings of lacrimal gland choristoma of the iris and ciliary body. *Am J Ophthalmol* 1995;119:219–224.
9. Roth DB, Shields JA, Shields CL, et al. Lacrimal gland choristoma of the conjunctiva simulating a squamous cell carcinoma. *J Pediatr Ophthalmol Strabismus* 1994;31:62–64.
10. Kessing SV. Ectopic lacrimal gland tissue at the corneal limbus (glands of Manz?) *Acta Ophthalmol Scand* 1966;46:398–403.
11. Rao VA, Kwatra V, Puri A. Cyst of ectopic (choristomatous) lacrimal gland. *Indian J Ophthalmol* 1989;37:189–190.
12. Young TL, Buchi ER, Kaufman LM, et al. Respiratory epithelium in a cystic choristoma of the limbus. *Arch Ophthalmol* 1990;108:1736–1739.
13. Tuncer S, Araz B, Peksayar G, et al. Solitary lacrimal gland choristoma of the limbal conjunctiva. *Ophthalmic Surg Lasers Imaging* 2010;41:e1–e2.

LACRIMAL GLAND AND RESPIRATORY CHORISTOMAS OF CONJUNCTIVA

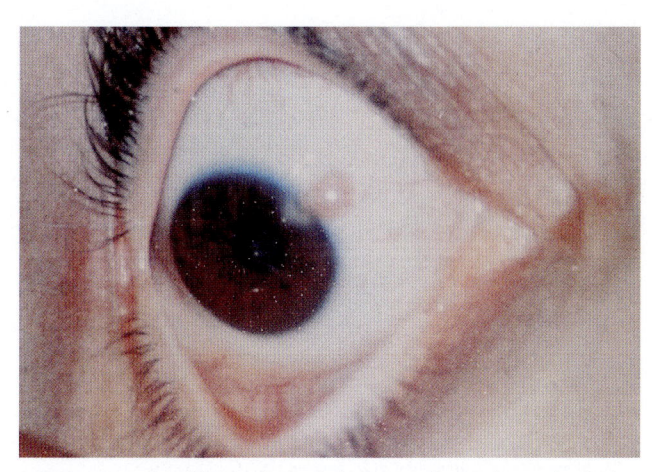

Figure 16.37. Small lacrimal gland choristoma located near the limbus in a 40-year-old woman. The lesion had apparently been present since birth. It was excised because of a foreign body sensation. The diagnosis was not suspected clinically. (Courtesy of Oscar Croxatto, MD.)

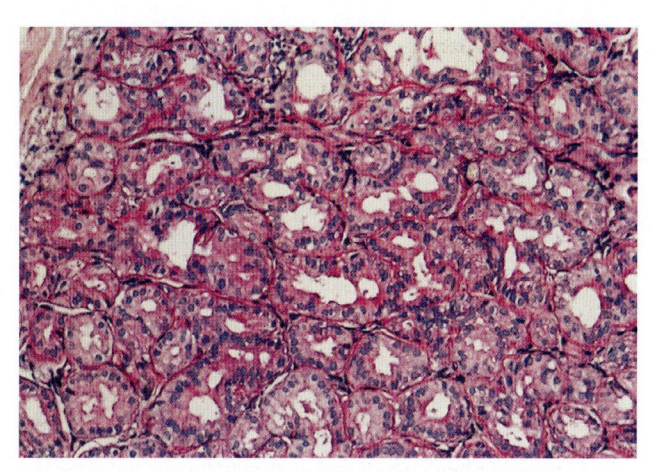

Figure 16.38. Histopathology of lesion shown in Figure 16.37, revealing normal lacrimal gland tissue. (Periodic acid-Schiff ×100.)

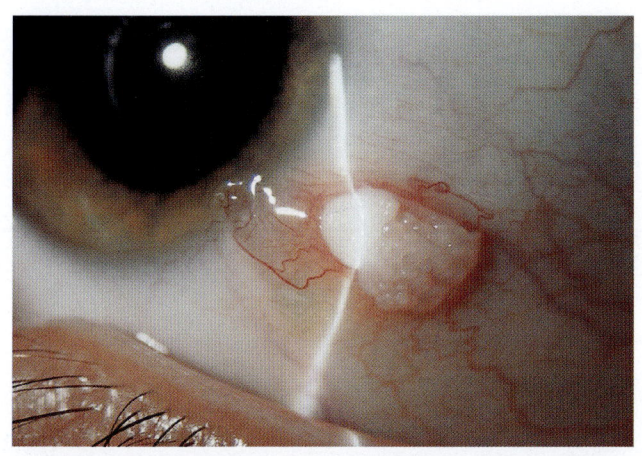

Figure 16.39. Hyperkeratotic lacrimal gland choristoma posterior to the limbus in a 13-year-old boy. The lesion was first noticed at age 18 months and had increased in size.

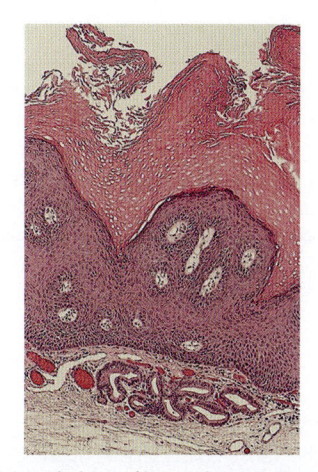

Figure 16.40. Histopathology of lesion shown in Figure 16.39 revealing normal lacrimal gland below, with overlying papillomatous proliferation of the epithelium and hyperkeratosis. (Hematoxylin–eosin ×15.)

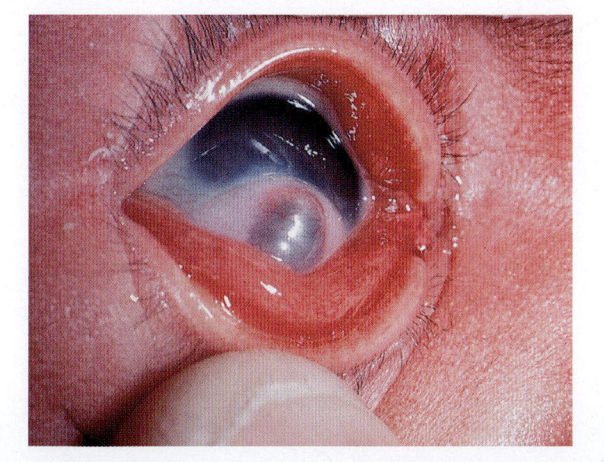

Figure 16.41. Choristomatous respiratory cyst involving inferior portion of cornea and conjunctiva in a 3-month-old infant who was noted to have sclerocorneal ectasia at birth. The lesion was excised with a penetrating keratoplasty procedure. (Courtesy of Mark Tso, MD.)

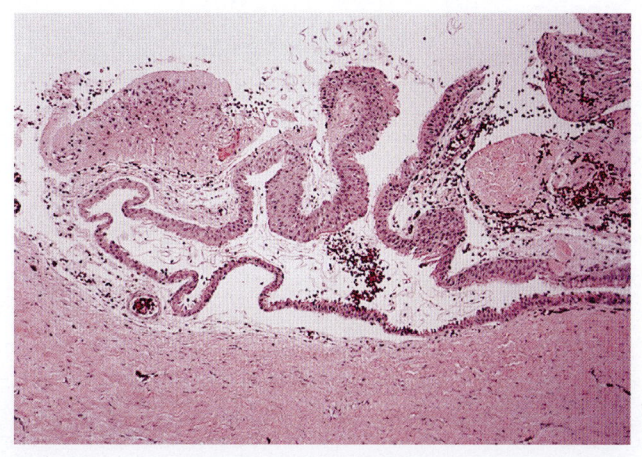

Figure 16.42. Histopathology of lesion shown in Figure 16.41 showing epithelial-lined cyst. The epithelium was of respiratory type. (Hematoxylin–eosin ×20.) (Courtesy of Mark Tso, MD.)

CONJUNCTIVAL COMPLEX CHORISTOMA

General Considerations

Complex choristoma of the conjunctiva is a congenital nonhereditary lesion that contains more than one tissue element. As mentioned, it may overlap with a simple choristoma, which can occasionally contain a small amount of a second tissue element. In the conjunctiva, the most frequent heterotopic tissues include skin, lipid, lacrimal gland, and cartilage. Complex choristoma has an association with an oculoneurocutaneous condition, most recently called the "organoid nevus syndrome" (1–3). The most common cutaneous feature of the organoid nevus syndrome is the sebaceous nevus of Jadassohn, which frequently affects the skin of the face, retroauricular area, and scalp. This was discussed in the eyelid section. This congenital cutaneous lesion can give rise later in life to basal cell carcinoma and other benign and malignant cutaneous tumors. The neurologic aspects of the organoid nevus syndrome include seizures and mental retardation, which occur secondary to arachnoid cysts and cerebral atrophy.

Clinical Features

The most common ocular features of the organoid nevus syndrome include the epibulbar complex choristoma and posterior sclerochoroidal cartilage that, based on ophthalmoscopy, ultrasonography, and CT, has been mistaken for choroidal osteoma (4,5). The epibulbar lesions can show considerable variation, ranging from a small, minimally symptomatic lesion to a large mass that involves the conjunctiva and covers a portion of the cornea (1–14). It can be obvious in the interpalpebral area or it can be hidden beneath the upper eyelid.

Pathology

Histopathologically, complex choristoma has highly variable elements, but the most characteristic features are a dermolipoma, often associated with ectopic lacrimal gland and mature hyaline cartilage.

Management

Smaller lesions can be observed. Large lesions that cover the cornea may require extensive surgery and reconstruction. Enucleation has been performed in some advanced cases (4,5).

Selected References

Reviews

1. Alfonso I, Howard C, Lopez PF, et al. Linear nevus sebaceous syndrome: A review. *J Clin Neuro-ophthalmol* 1987;7:170–177.
2. Solomon LM, Fretzin DF, Dewald RL. The epidermal nevus syndrome. *Arch Dermatol* 1968;97:273–285.
3. Roth AM, Keltner JL. Linear nevus sebaceous syndrome. *J Clin Neuro-ophthalmol* 1993;13:44–49.
4. Shields JA, Shields CL, Eagle RC Jr, et al. Ophthalmic features of the organoid nevus syndrome. *Trans Am Ophthalmol Soc* 1996;94:65–86.
5. Shields JA, Shields CL, Eagle RC Jr, et al. Ocular manifestations of the organoid nevus syndrome. *Ophthalmology* 1997;104:549–557.
6. Shields CL, Demirci H, Karatza E, et al. Clinical survey of 1643 melanocytic and nonmelanocytic tumors of the conjunctiva. *Ophthalmology* 2004;111:1747–1754.
7. Shields CL, Shields JA. Tumors of the conjunctiva and cornea. *Surv Ophthalmol* 2004;49:3–24.

Case Reports

8. Diven DG, Solomon AR, McNeely MC, et al. Nevus sebaceus associated with major ophthalmologic abnormalities. *Arch Dermatol* 1987;123:383–386.
9. Lambert HM, Sipperley JO, Shore JW, et al. Linear nevus sebaceous syndrome. *Ophthalmology* 1987;94:278–282.
10. Wilkes SR, Campbell RJ, Waller RR. Ocular malformation in association with ipsilateral facial nevus of Jadassohn. *Am J Ophthalmol* 1981;92:344–352.
11. Pe'er J, Ilsar M. Epibulbar complex choristoma associated with nevus sebaceous. *Arch Ophthalmol* 1995;113:1301–1304.
12. Mullaney PB, Weatherhead RG. Epidermal nevus syndrome associated with a complex choristoma and a bilateral choroidal osteoma. *Arch Ophthalmol* 1996;114:1292–1293.
13. Hayasaka S, Sekimoto M, Setogawa T. Epibulbar complex choristoma involving the bulbar conjunctiva and cornea. *J Pediatr Ophthalmol Strabismus* 1989;26:251–253.
14. Shields CN, Shields CL, Lin CJ, et al. Calcified scleral choristoma in organoid nevus syndrome simulating retinoblastoma. *J Pediatr Ophthalmol Strabismus* 2014;51:e1–e3.

EPIBULBAR COMPLEX CHORISTOMA: ASSOCIATION WITH ORGANOID NEVUS SYNDROME

Shields JA, Shields CL, Eagle RC Jr, et al. Ocular manifestations of the organoid nevus syndrome. *Ophthalmology* 1997;104: 549–557.

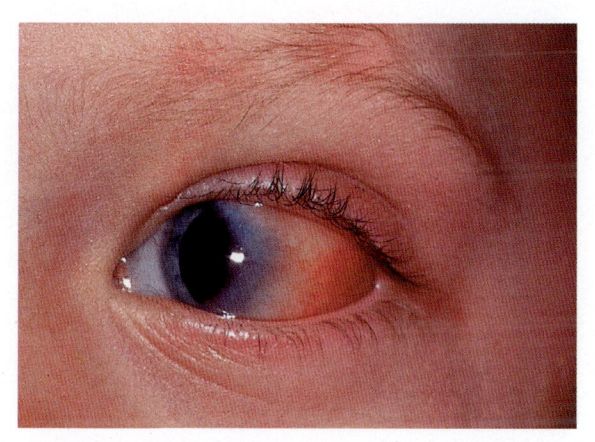

Figure 16.43. Epibulbar complex choristoma in a child with the organoid nevus syndrome. The diffuse lesion covers the lateral third of the cornea.

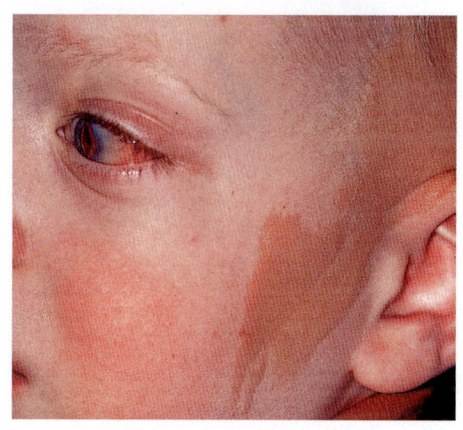

Figure 16.44. View of preauricular area of patient seen in Figure 16.43, showing tan sebaceous nevus.

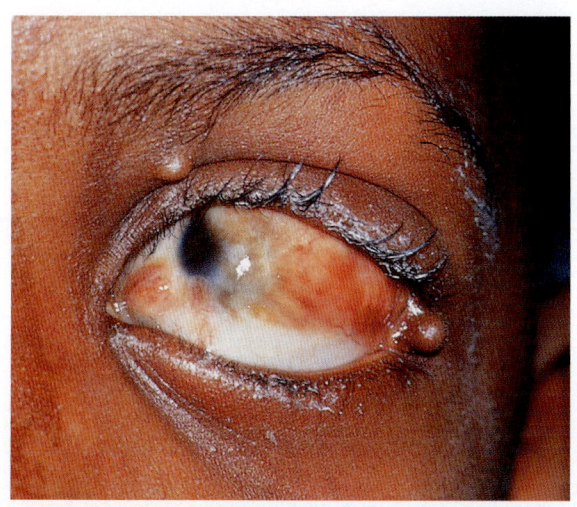

Figure 16.45. Epibulbar complex choristoma covering temporal conjunctiva and most of the cornea in a young African-American boy.

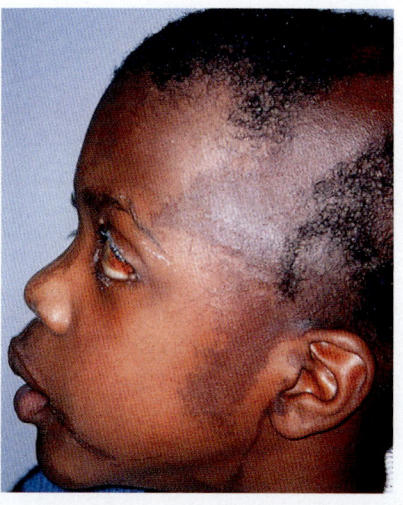

Figure 16.46. View of preauricular and scalp area of patient shown in Figure 16.45 demonstrating dark brown sebaceous nevus. Note the characteristic alopecia in the scalp, corresponding to the sebaceous nevus.

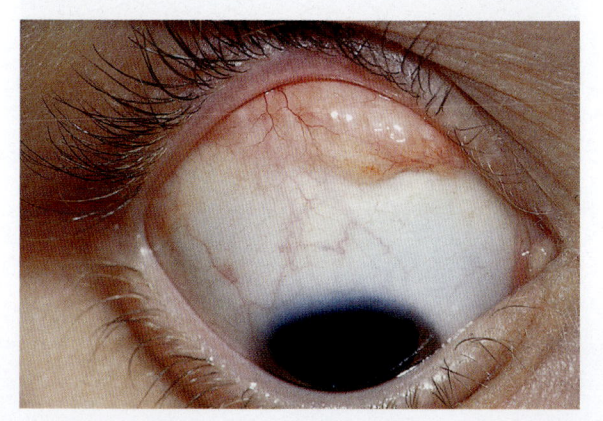

Figure 16.47. Complex choristoma in superior fornix of a child with sebaceous nevus. The child was believed to have idiopathic congenital blepharoptosis for several years before the forniceal lesion was discovered.

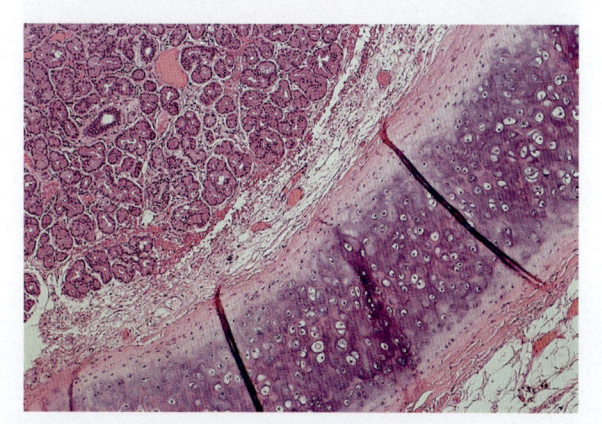

Figure 16.48. Histopathology of the lesion shown in Figure 16.45 disclosing lacrimal gland tissue above and cartilage below. (Hematoxylin–eosin ×25.)

EPIBULBAR COMPLEX CHORISTOMA: ASSOCIATION WITH ORGANOID NEVUS SYNDROME

Shields JA, Shields CL, Eagle RC Jr, et al. Ocular manifestations of the organoid nevus syndrome. *Ophthalmology* 1997;104:549–557.

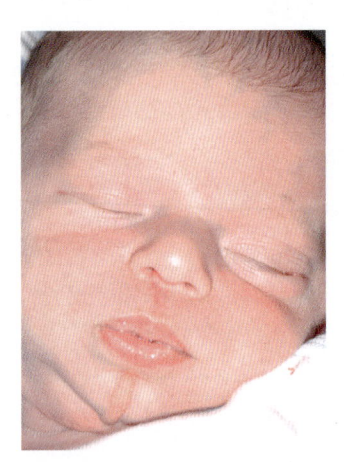

Figure 16.49. Linear nevus sebaceous in an infant involving the chin and extending into the neck.

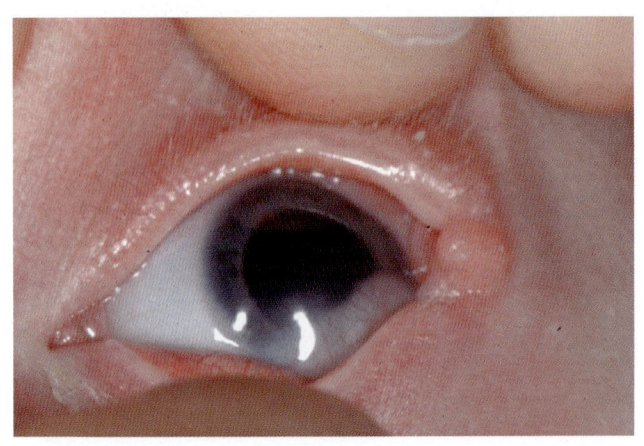

Figure 16.50. Close-up view of lateral canthus of left eye, showing congenital cutaneous nodule and maldevelopment of the lateral canthus. Note also the presumed complex choristoma at the corneoscleral limbus. The lesions were suspected to be choristomas, but no biopsy was done.

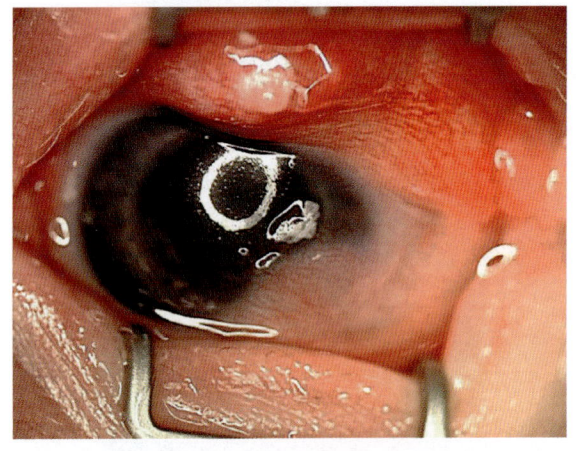

Figure 16.51. Appearance with eyelids open, showing better extensive complex choristoma seen in Figure 16.50. There is involvement of the forniceal conjunctiva superiorly and bulbar conjunctiva and cornea temporally.

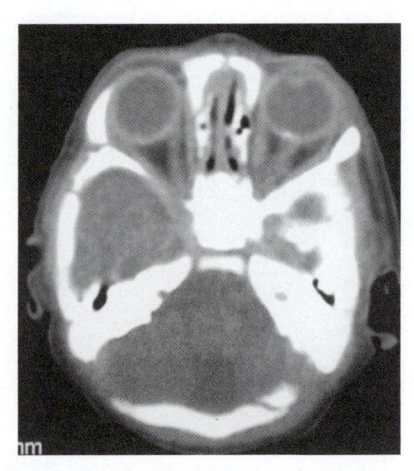

Figure 16.52. Axial CT scan showing bone density lesion in region of optic nerve head. Based on histopathology of a similar case, we believe that the lesion is most likely intrascleral cartilage.

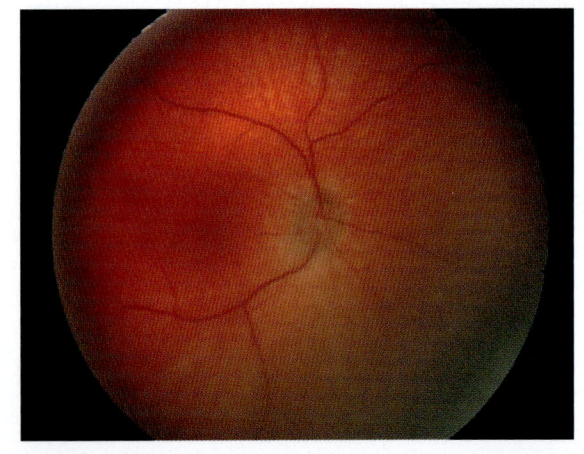

Figure 16.53. Fundus of right eye with relatively normal findings. Note the normal choroidal vascular pattern. The optic disc appears small and slightly atypical.

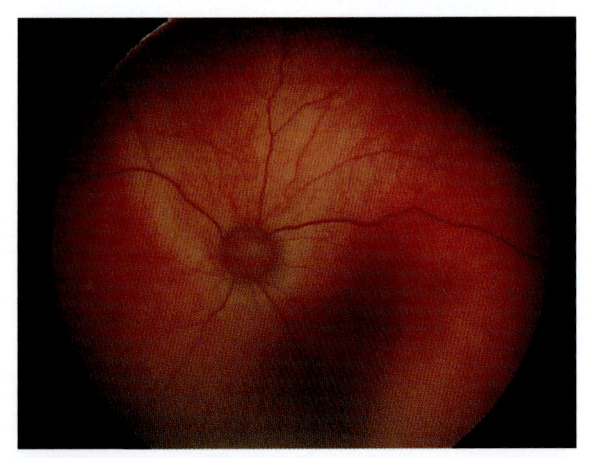

Figure 16.54. Fundus of left eye showing discoloration deep to retina. This is believed to correspond to scleral cartilage. The optic disc shows a coloboma.

CHAPTER 17

CONJUNCTIVAL BENIGN EPITHELIAL TUMORS

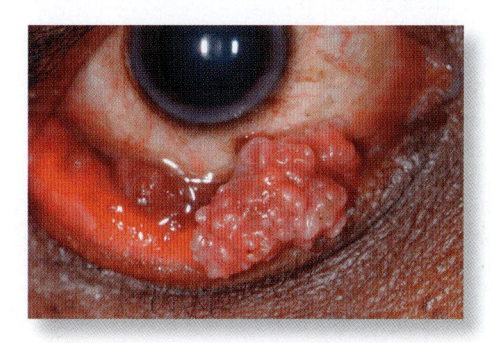

General Considerations

Conjunctival papilloma is a virus-induced lesion that generally affects children and young adults (1–27). We prefer to use the term "childhood papilloma" to distinguish it from the adult form that usually occurs in the elderly and generally has somewhat different clinical characteristics (3). In the authors' clinical series of 1,643 conjunctival tumors in children and adults, there were 5 childhood papillomas, accounting for 13% of benign epithelial lesions, and <1% of the 1,643 lesions (1). In a later separate analysis from our department on conjunctival papilloma based on age at examination in 10 children and 63 adults, we found the median age at presentation was 43 years (range 4 to 85 years) (3).

Clinical Features

Childhood conjunctival papilloma can be solitary or multiple and may assume a sessile or pedunculated configuration. In extreme cases, several lesions may become confluent, producing massive papillomatosis. Childhood conjunctival papilloma has a fleshy red appearance owing to the numerous fine vascular channels that ramify through the stroma beneath the epithelial surface of the lesion. It most often occurs in the inferior fornix or on the bulbar conjunctiva and rarely encroaches on the cornea. Occasionally, conjunctival papilloma can be pigmented and simulate a melanoma (21). This is more likely to occur in the adult form, which will be discussed in the next section. Conjunctival papilloma of childhood appears to have no malignant potential.

In an analysis of 10 pediatric patients with conjunctival papillomatosis, the tumor was unilateral in all cases but with multiple tumors in 30% (3). In that series the tumor(s) were most often located in the fornix (27%), caruncle (20%), plica (20%), or tarsal region (20%), and measured mean 8 mm in diameter (3). A comparison of conjunctival papilloma in those 10 children versus 63 adults revealed children with a higher incidence of multifocality, larger tumors, and recurrence following therapy (3). The authors warned that childhood papillomatosis can require multiple treatments and use of topical or injection interferon (3).

Pathology and Pathogenesis

Histopathologically, childhood conjunctival papilloma shows numerous vascularized papillary fronds lined by acanthotic epithelium, with minimal or no keratinization. The features of the conjunctival papilloma of adulthood are considered in the next section.

There has been a great deal of interest in the relationship between childhood conjunctival papilloma and infection with human papillomavirus (HPV). It often results from infection of the conjunctival epithelium with HPV, usually types 6 or 11.

CONJUNCTIVAL PAPILLOMA OF CHILDHOOD

Management

The management of childhood conjunctival papilloma has been the subject of considerable interest (3–12). Incompletely excised lesions can recur with aggressive behavior owing to surgically induced liberation of virus particles into the surrounding tissues. Double freeze-thaw cryotherapy can be an effective adjunct in eradicating childhood papilloma. For fairly circumscribed pedunculated lesions, we have employed cryotherapy to the lesion, lifting and freezing the entire lesion, and immediately cutting the normal conjunctival tissue at its base, followed by closure with absorbable sutures. Larger lesions may require surgical excision with complete removal of the mass and primary closure. A meticulous "no-touch" technique should be attempted, handling only the adjacent, clinically normal tissues. In the rare case where the conjunctival defect cannot be closed primarily, a mucous membrane or amniotic membrane graft may be necessary. Other reported methods of treatment (3–12) include laser treatment, dinitrochlorobenzene immunotherapy, α-interferon, and topical mitomycin chemotherapy 0.02%. We have observed dramatic response to recurrent papilloma to oral cimetidine (Tagamet) (11,12). Other nonsurgical treatments are topical or injection interferon alpha-2b, Mitomycin C, topical Cidofovir antiviral medication, and photodynamic therapy (3).

CONJUNCTIVAL PAPILLOMA OF CHILDHOOD

Selected References

Reviews

1. Shields CL, Demirci H, Karatza E, et al. Clinical survey of 1643 melanocytic and nonmelanocytic tumors of the conjunctiva. *Ophthalmology* 2004;111:1747–1754.
2. Shields CL, Shields JA. Tumors of the conjunctiva and cornea. *Surv Ophthalmol* 2004;49:3–24.
3. Kaliki S, Arepalli S, Shields CL, et al. Conjunctival papilloma. Features and outcomes based on age at initial examination. *JAMA Ophthalmol* 2013;131:585–593.

Management

4. Bosniak SL, Novick NL, Sachs ME. Treatment of recurrent squamous papillomata of the conjunctiva by carbon dioxide laser vaporization. *Ophthalmology* 1986;93:1078–1082.
5. Jackson WB, Beraja R, Codere F. Laser therapy of conjunctival papillomas. *Can J Ophthalmol* 1987;22:45–47.
6. Petrelli R, Cotlier E, Robins S, et al. Dinitrochlorobenzene immunotherapy of recurrent squamous papilloma of the conjunctiva. *Ophthalmology* 1981;88:1221–1225.
7. Harkey ME, Metz HS. Cryotherapy of conjunctival papillomata. *Am J Ophthalmol* 1968;66:872–874.
8. Lass JH, Foster CS, Grove AS, et al. Interferon-alpha therapy of recurrent conjunctival papillomas. *Am J Ophthalmol* 1987;103:294–301.
9. Yuen HK, Yeung EF, Chan NR, et al. The use of postoperative topical mitomycin C in the treatment of recurrent conjunctival papilloma. *Cornea* 2002;21:838–839.
10. Hawkins AS, Yu J, Hamming NA, et al. Treatment of recurrent conjunctival papillomatosis with mitomycin C. *Am J Ophthalmol* 1999;128:638–640.
11. Shields CL, Lally MR, Singh AD, et al. Oral cimetidine (Tagamet) for recalcitrant, diffuse conjunctival papillomatosis. *Am J Ophthalmol* 1999;128:362–364.
12. Chang SW, Huang ZL. Oral cimetidine adjuvant therapy for recalcitrant, diffuse conjunctival papillomatosis. *Cornea* 2006;25(6):687–690.

Histopathology

13. Lass HJ, Henson AB, Papale JJ, et al. Papillomavirus in human conjunctival papillomas. *Am J Ophthalmol* 1983;95:364–368.
14. Lass JH, Grove AS, Papale JJ, et al. Detection of human papillomavirus DNS sequences in conjunctival papillomas. *Am J Ophthalmol* 1983;96:670–674.
15. Naghashfar Z, McDonnell PJ, McDonnell JM, et al. Genital tract papillomavirus type 6 in recurrent conjunctival papilloma. *Arch Ophthalmol* 1986;104:1814–1815.
16. McDonnell PJ, McDonnell JM, Mounts P, et al. Demonstration of papillomavirus capsid antigen in human conjunctival neoplasia. *Arch Ophthalmol* 1986;104:1801–1805.
17. Karcioglu ZA, Issa TM. Human papilloma virus in neoplastic and non neoplastic conditions of the external eye. *Br J Ophthalmol* 1997;81:595–598.
18. Nakamura Y, Mashima Y, Kameyama K, et al. Detection of human papillomavirus infection in squamous tumours of the conjunctiva and lacrimal sac by immunohistochemistry, in situ hybridisation, and polymerase chain reaction. *Br J Ophthalmol* 1997;81:308–313
19. Sjo NC, Heegaard S, Prause JU, et al. Human papillomavirus in conjunctival papilloma. *Br J Ophthalmol* 2001;85:785–787.

Case Reports

20. Williams R, Ilsar M, Welham RA. Lacrimal canalicular papillomatosis. *Br J Ophthalmol* 1985;69:464–467.
21. Kremer I, Sandbank J, Weinberger D, et al. Pigmented epithelial tumours of the conjunctiva. *Br J Ophthalmol* 1992;76:294–296.
22. Streeten BW, Carrillo R, Jamison R, et al. Inverted papilloma of the conjunctiva. *Am J Ophthalmol* 1979;888:1062–1066.
23. Jakobiec FA, Harrison W, Aronian D. Inverted mucoepidermoid papillomas of the epibulbar conjunctiva. *Ophthalmology* 1987;94:283–287.
24. Miller DM, Brodell RT, Levine MR. The conjunctival wart: Report of a case and review of treatment options. *Ophthalmic Surg* 1994;25:545–548.
25. Jakobiec FA, Mendoza PR, Colby KA. Clinicopathologic and immunohistochemical studies of conjunctival large cell acanthoma, epidermoid dysplasia, and squamous papilloma. *Am J Ophthalmol* 2013;156(4):830–846.
26. Kalantzis G, Papaconstantinou D, Georgalas I, et al. Different types of conjunctival papilloma presenting in the same eye. *Orbit* 2010;29(5):266–268.
27. Sjö NC, von Buchwald C, Cassonnet P, et al. Human papillomavirus in normal conjunctival tissue and in conjunctival papilloma: Types and frequencies in a large series. *Br J Ophthalmol* 2007;91(8):1014–1015.

Part 2 Tumors of the Conjunctiva

CHILDHOOD CONJUNCTIVAL PAPILLOMA

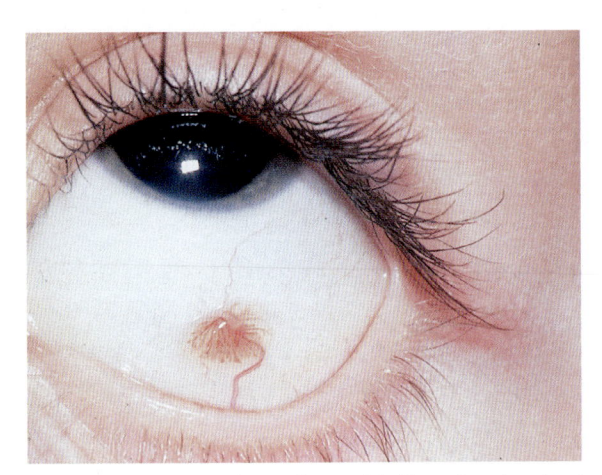

Figure 17.1. Solitary sessile papilloma of bulbar of conjunctiva in a 4-year-old boy.

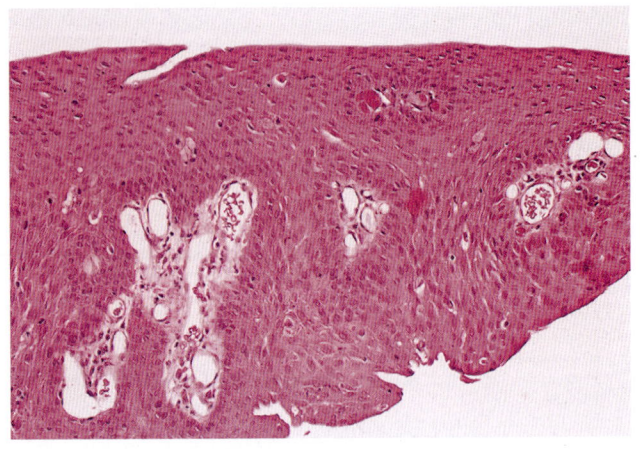

Figure 17.2. Histopathology of sessile papilloma seen in Figure 17.1 showing acanthotic epithelium with fibrovascular cores. (Hematoxylin–eosin ×10.)

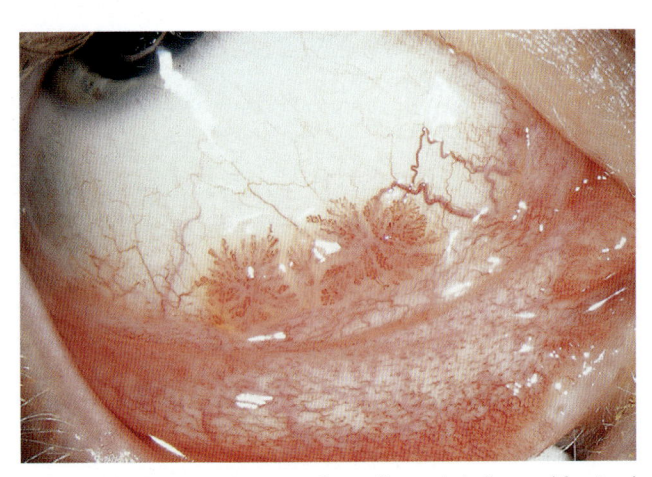

Figure 17.3. Two contiguous sessile papillomas in bulbar and forniceal conjunctiva in a 5-year-old child.

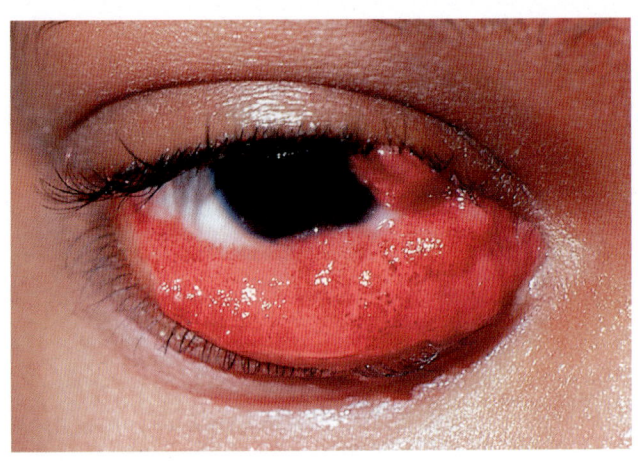

Figure 17.4. Extensive conjunctival papillomatosis in a young child. (Courtesy of Hobart Lerner, MD.)

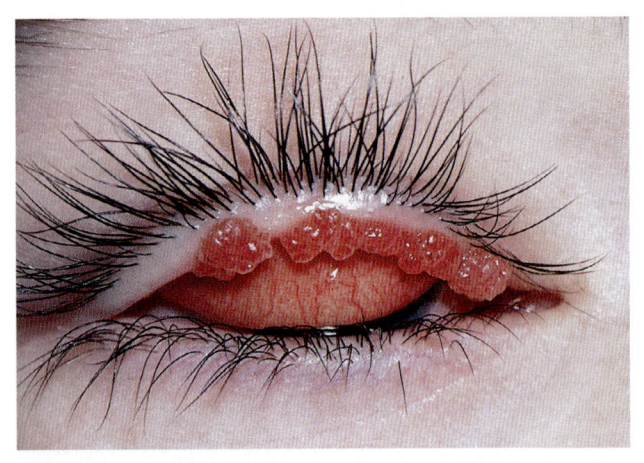

Figure 17.5. Multiple conjunctival papillomas arising from the palpebral conjunctiva and eyelid margin in a 4-year-old child.

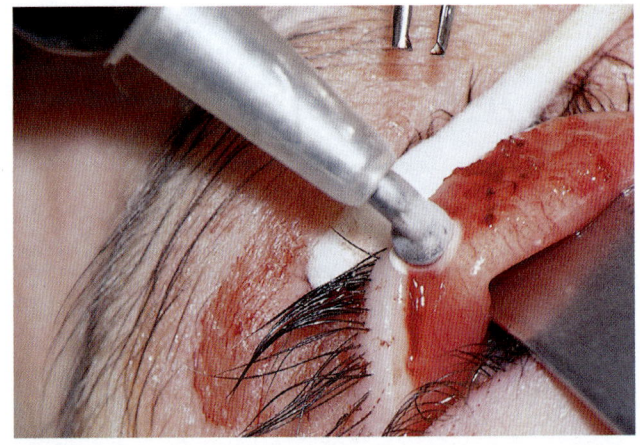

Figure 17.6. Cryotherapy being applied to the tumors shown in Figure 17.5.

CONJUNCTIVAL PAPILLOMA OF CHILDHOOD: MANAGEMENT WITH ORAL CIMETIDINE

Cimetidine is a histamine-2 receptor antagonist used to treat peptic ulcers. It also enhances the immune system by inhibiting suppressor T-cell function and augments delayed hypersensitivity. Although controversial, it has been used to treat selected cutaneous warts. We have found it to be useful for selected recalcitrant or recurrent conjunctival papillomatosis.

Shields CL, Lally MR, Singh AD, et al. Oral cimetidine (Tagamet) for recalcitrant, diffuse conjunctival papillomatosis. *Am J Ophthalmol* 1999;128:362–364.

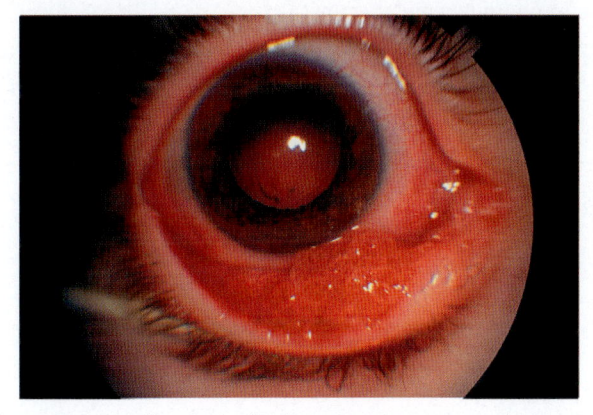

Figure 17.7. Papillomatosis of right conjunctiva in a young boy.

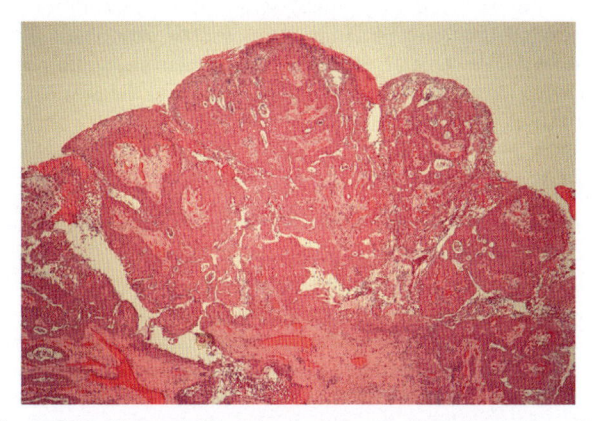

Figure 17.8. Histopathology after excision elsewhere, showing papillomatous lesion with acanthosis. (Hematoxylin–eosin ×10.)

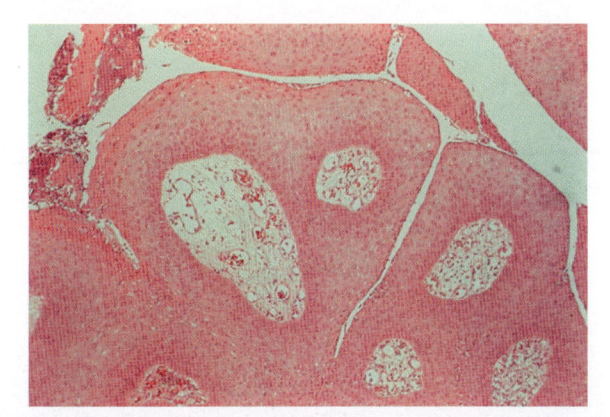

Figure 17.9. Higher-magnification photomicrograph showing fibrovascular cores within acanthotic epithelium. (Hematoxylin–eosin ×25.)

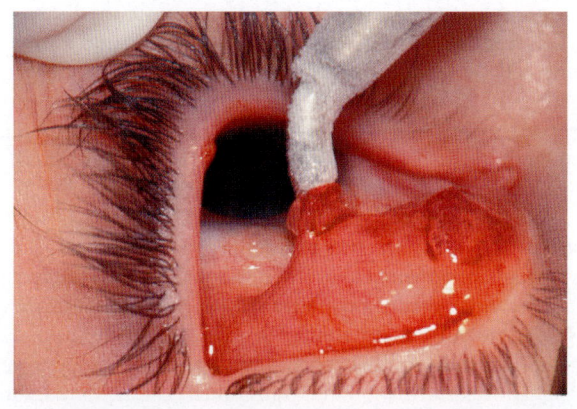

Figure 17.10. Cryotherapy being applied to a subsequent recurrence. This technique is often effective in controlling selected small conjunctival papillomas.

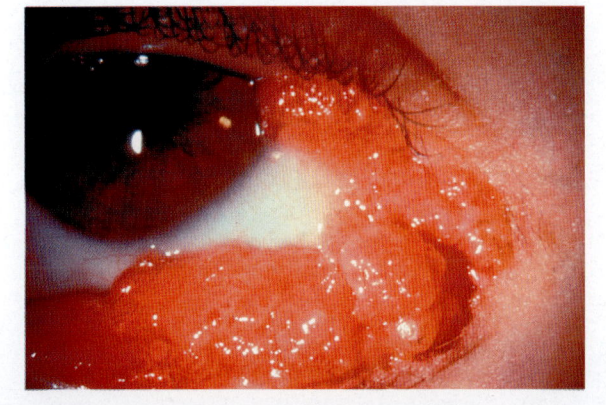

Figure 17.11. Massive recurrence about 6 months later. At this time, the patient was treated with oral cimetidine alone for 4 months.

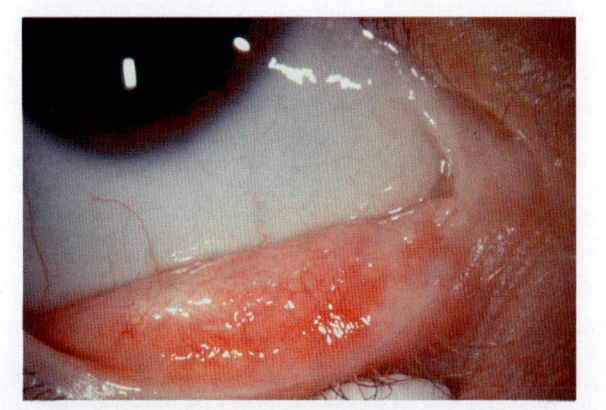

Figure 17.12. Appearance 10 months later showing marked resolution of the papilloma after treatment with cimetidine. The patient had no further recurrence after 5 years of follow-up.

CONJUNCTIVAL PAPILLOMA OF ADULTHOOD

General Considerations

Most textbooks do not differentiate the childhood from the adulthood types of conjunctival papilloma. Although the two types are similar, they also have some different characteristics (1–7). In the authors' clinical series of 1,643 conjunctival tumors in children and adults, there were 21 adult papillomas (1). In a later separate analysis on conjunctival papillomas in 73 cases, 10 were in children, 63 in adults, and the mean age at presentation was 43 years (range 4 to 85 years) (3).

Clinical Features

In contrast with the childhood type, adult papilloma usually occurs in young to elderly adults and may resemble squamous cell carcinoma or amelanotic melanoma clinically. Unlike the infectious papilloma of young children, it is more likely to be unilateral and solitary and is rarely multifocal (3). In an analysis of 63 adult patients with conjunctival papillomatosis, the tumor was unilateral in 97% of cases and with multifocality in 15%, was most often located in the caruncle (24%), fornix (18%), or plica (16%), and measured mean 6 mm in diameter (3).

Conjunctival papilloma can develop in adults who are immunosuppressed. It most often begins near the limbus or bulbar conjunctiva and can encroach on the cornea and even completely cover the cornea in some cases. It generally has a lighter pink color than the childhood type. In some individuals, particularly those with dark skin, a conjunctival papilloma may appear clinically pigmented owing to excessive melanocytes in the acanthotic epithelium.

In adults, conjunctival papilloma is probably also associated with HPV (3). Conjunctival papilloma of adulthood may have a low malignant potential to evolve into squamous cell carcinoma. However, occasionally a conjunctival papilloma can assume an inverted growth pattern similar to that seen in the nasal cavity and lacrimal sac. This variant has a greater tendency toward malignant transformation into transitional cell carcinoma, squamous cell carcinoma, or mucoepidermoid carcinoma.

Pathology

Histopathologically, the adult conjunctival papilloma is similar to the childhood variant and shows numerous vascularized papillary fronds lined by acanthotic epithelium. Mild hyperkeratosis is sometimes present. As mentioned, some papillomas have numerous melanocytes that impart a darker color to the lesion clinically. Using an immunoperoxidase technique, papillomavirus capsid antigen was found in nuclei of 23 conjunctival papillomas and 5 dysplasias and carcinomas (4). These results suggest that papillomavirus may play a role in the etiology of conjunctival papilloma, as well as dysplasia, and carcinoma.

Management

Surgical excision and supplemental cryotherapy seems to be the best treatment for adult conjunctival papilloma (3). The surgeon should not overestimate the extent of the lesion because it appears to cover the cornea. In most such cases, the lesion usually arises from a small base near the limbus and overlies the cornea, but does not invade the cornea. Hence, it can be lifted off the cornea and removed by severing the stalk near the limbus. Other methods of treatment include topical or injection of interferon alpha-2b, topical Mitomycin C, topical Cidofovir, or photodynamic therapy (3).

CONJUNCTIVAL PAPILLOMA OF ADULTHOOD

Selected References

Reviews
1. Shields CL, Demirci H, Karatza E, et al. Clinical survey of 1643 melanocytic and nonmelanocytic tumors of the conjunctiva. *Ophthalmology* 2004;111:1747–1754.
2. Shields CL, Shields JA. Tumors of the conjunctiva and cornea. *Surv Ophthalmol* 2004;49:3–24.
3. Kaliki S, Arepalli S, Shields CL, et al. Conjunctival papilloma. Features and outcomes based on age at initial examination. *JAMA Ophthalmol* 2013;131:585–593.

Histopathology
4. McDonnell PJ, McDonnell JM, Mounts P, et al. Demonstration of papillomavirus capsid antigen in human conjunctival neoplasia. *Arch Ophthalmol* 1986;104:1801–1805.

Case Reports
5. Kremer I, Sandbank J, Weinberger D, et al. Pigmented epithelial tumours of the conjunctiva. *Br J Ophthalmol* 1992;76:294–296.
6. Streeten BW, Carillo R, Jamison R, et al. Inverted papilloma of the conjunctiva. *Am J Ophthalmol* 1979;88:1062–1066.
7. Jakobiec FA, Harrison W, Aronian D. Inverted mucoepidermoid papillomas of the epibulbar conjunctiva. *Ophthalmology* 1987;94:283–287.

ADULT CONJUNCTIVAL PAPILLOMA

Illustrated are some adult onset papillomas that arose in extralimbal areas of the conjunctiva.

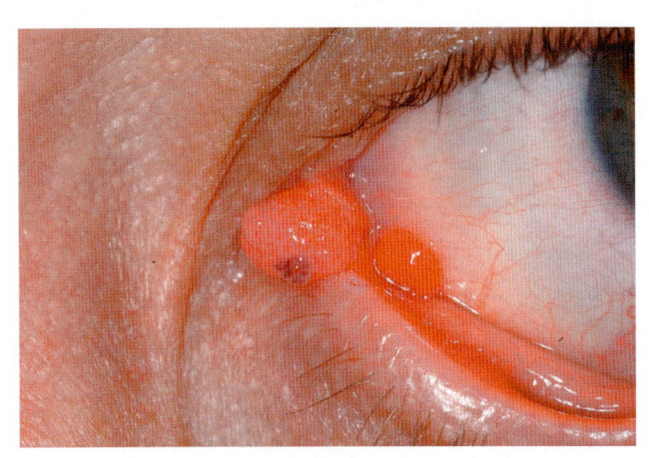

Figure 17.13. Eversion of lower eyelid of patient with conjunctival papillomas. Note the three separate papillomas, pedunculated ones on the caruncle and forniceal conjunctiva and a small sessile lesion one on the tarsal conjunctiva near the eyelid margin.

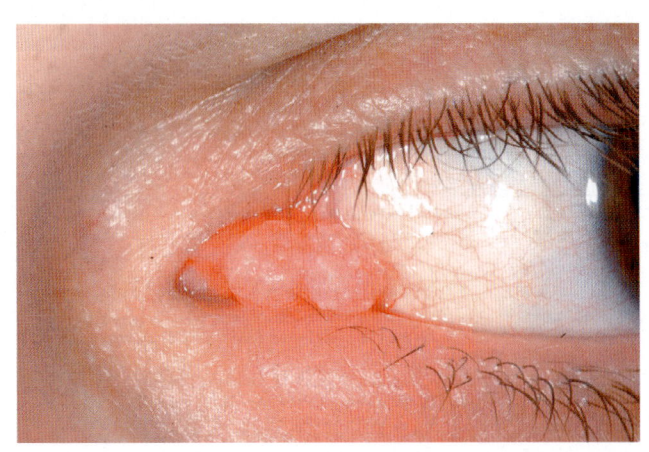

Figure 17.14. Bilobed squamous papilloma with a multinodular papillary configuration, located in the medial canthal region. The superficial white color is due to hyperkeratosis.

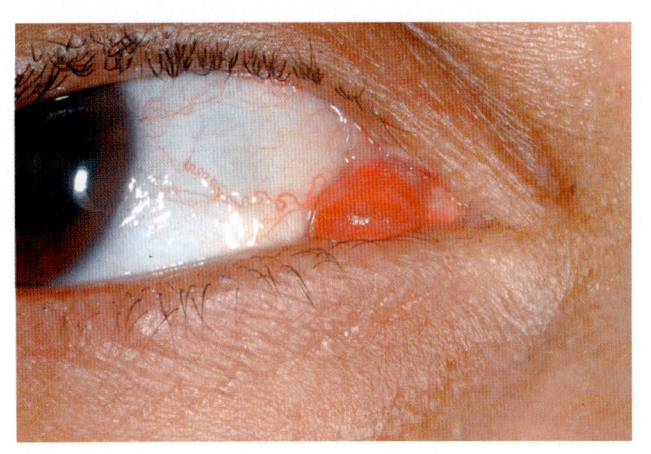

Figure 17.15. Squamous papilloma with a smooth surface and highly vascular appearance located in region of nasal conjunctiva and semilunar fold, simulating a pyogenic granuloma.

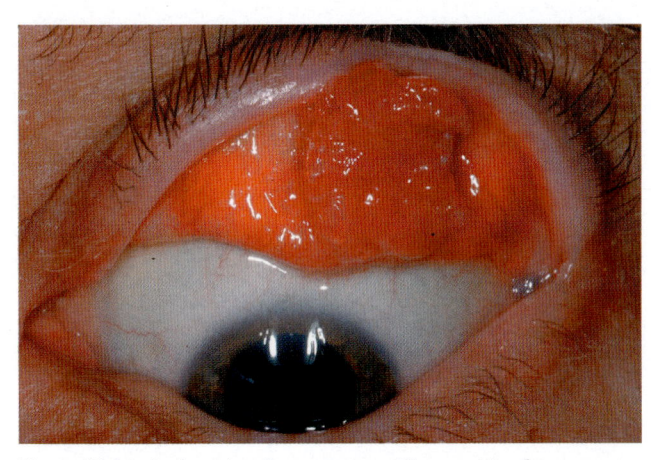

Figure 17.16. Pedunculated squamous papilloma arising from superior tarsal conjunctiva.

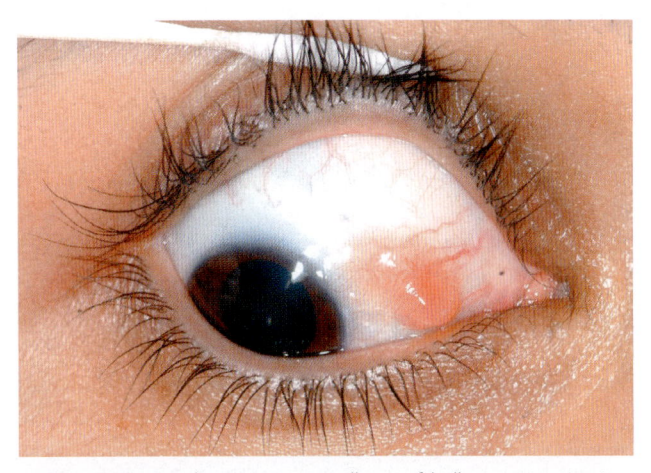

Figure 17.17. Sessile squamous papilloma of bulbar conjunctiva in a middle-aged woman. Note the straight radiating pattern of the blood vessels that characterize some papillomas.

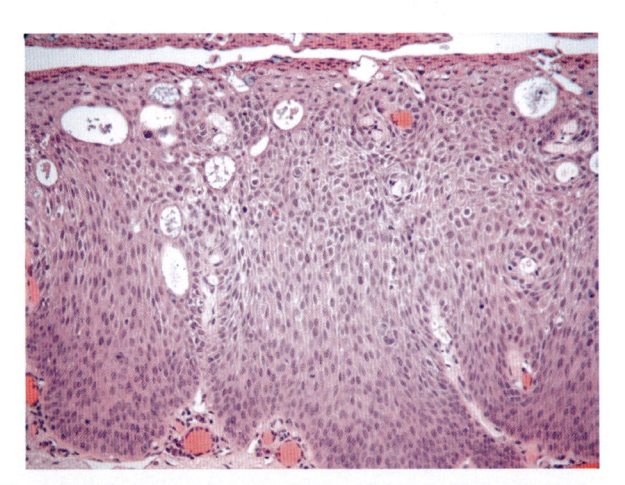

Figure 17.18. Histopathology of lesion shown in Figure 17.17 showing acanthosis owing to proliferation of spindle-shaped epithelial cells with mild pleomorphism and dysplasia. Note the pseudocysts within the tumor. (Hematoxylin–eosin ×25.)

ADULT CONJUNCTIVAL PAPILLOMA: ATYPICAL VARIATIONS

Kaliki S, Arepalli S, Shields CL, et al. Conjunctival papilloma. Features and outcomes based on age at initial examination. *JAMA Ophthalmol* 2013;131:585–593.

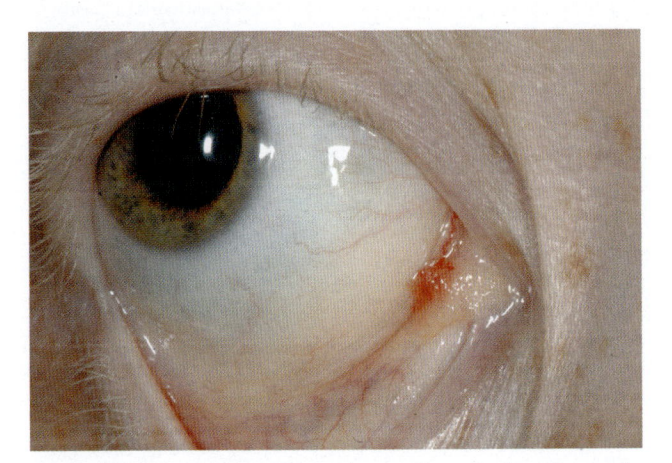

Figure 17.19. Nonpigmented vascular papilloma in the plica semilunaris of a Caucasian patient.

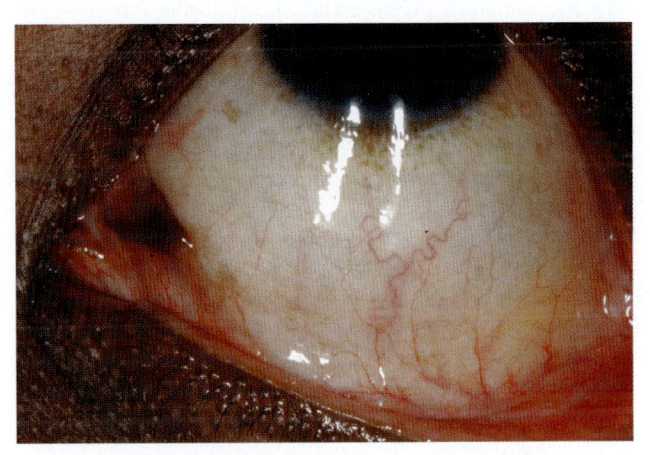

Figure 17.20. Pigmented papilloma in the plica semilunaris, simulating a nevus in an African-American patient.

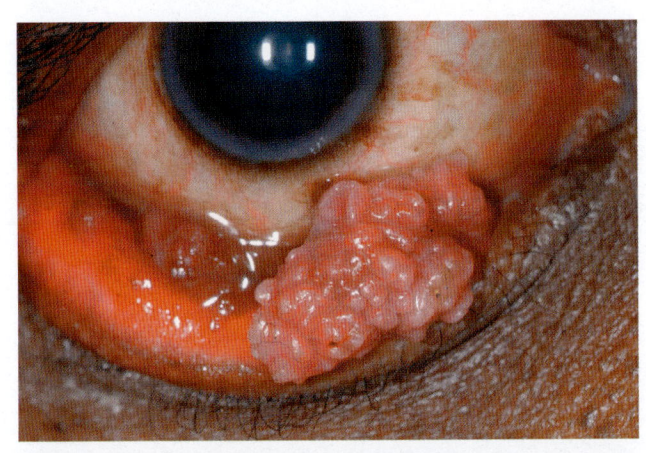

Figure 17.21. Large multinodular squamous papilloma in forniceal conjunctiva in an African American causing ectropion of lower eyelid. Note the complexion-related racial melanosis of the conjunctiva.

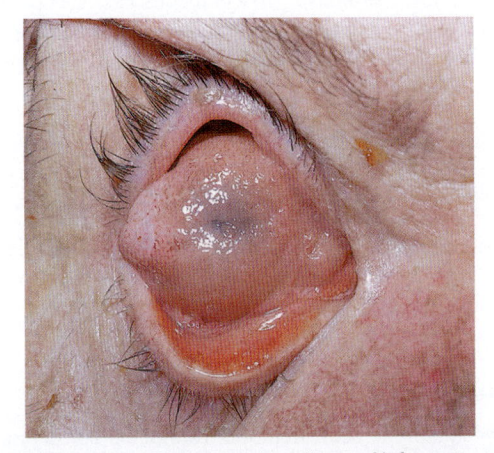

Figure 17.22. Extensive conjunctival papilloma of left eye in an elderly patient. This patient underwent orbital exenteration elsewhere because of histopathologic misdiagnosis of squamous cell carcinoma. Later review of the histopathology indicated the benign nature of the lesion.

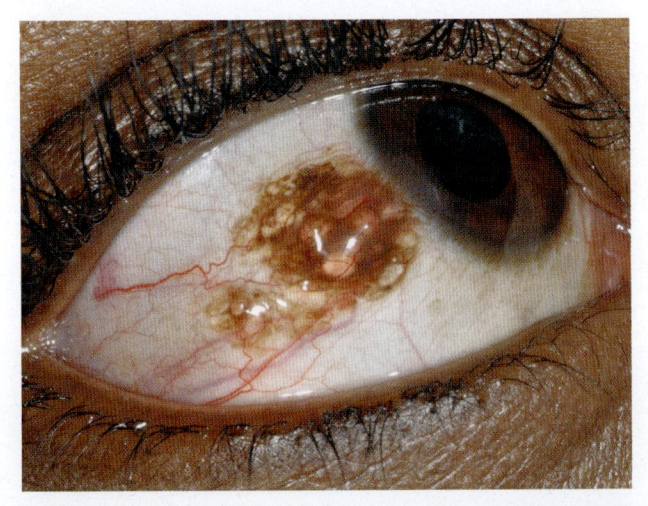

Figure 17.23. Pigmented mass in the conjunctiva simulating a cystic nevus in a Carribean American, but proven on histopathology to be an inverted papilloma.

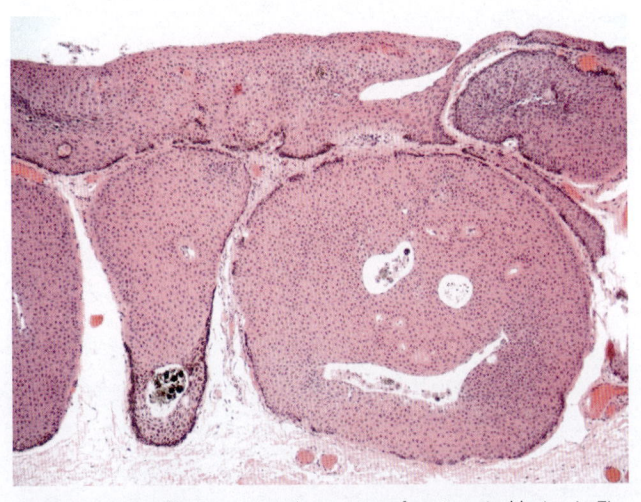

Figure 17.24. Following surgical resection of conjunctival lesion in Figure 17.23, the diagnosis of inverted papilloma twas established with features of surface acanthotic epithelial cells growing downward into the conjunctival stroma rather than the typical growth upward.

CONJUNCTIVAL PSEUDOEPITHELIOMATOUS HYPERPLASIA AND KERATOACANTHOMA

General Considerations

Like the epidermis of the eyelid, the epithelium of the conjunctiva can give rise to a benign, reactive, inflammatory proliferation of epithelial cells that can simulate carcinoma both clinically and histopathologically (pseudocarcinomatous hyperplasia, pseudoepitheliomatous hyperplasia [PEH]). PEH can arise from chronic inflammation, particularly over a pingueculum or pterygium or at the site of prior foreign body. Keratoacanthoma (KA) is a specific form of PEH that assumes a characteristic appearance (1–13). Although generally considered to be a benign condition, there is a belief that it may represent a variant of squamous cell carcinoma (see Chapter 1).

Clinical Features

In the conjunctiva, PEH (and its KA variant) is a rapidly progressive lesion that appears as an elevated mass with hyperkeratosis, similar to the better-known KA of the skin. In some cases, the conjunctival KA may have an umbilicated center with elevated margins similar to the cutaneous KA. It is important that this benign lesion be differentiated from squamous cell malignancy of the conjunctiva. In general, KA has a more rapid onset and more rapid progression.

Pathology

Histopathologically, PEH of the conjunctiva (and its variant KA) is characterized by massive acanthosis, hyperkeratosis, and parakeratosis of the conjunctival epithelium. Mitotic figures may be present, but cytologic atypia is generally lacking. It generally has more of an inflammatory reaction than a low-grade squamous cell carcinoma.

Management

Because squamous cell carcinoma cannot be ruled out clinically in most cases, treatment is generally complete excision and cryotherapy, similar to the technique used for squamous cell malignancies. The prognosis is excellent.

Selected References

Case Reports

1. Freeman RG, Cloud TM, Knox JM. Keratoacanthoma of the conjunctiva. A case report. *Arch Ophthalmol* 1961;65:817.
2. Bellamy ED, Allen JH, Hart NL. Keratoacanthoma of the conjunctiva. *Arch Ophthalmol* 1963;70:512.
3. Roth AM. Solitary keratoacanthoma of the conjunctiva. *Am J Ophthalmol* 1978;85:647–650.
4. Hamed LM, Wilson FM, Grayson M. Keratoacanthoma of the limbus. *Ophthalmic Surg* 1988;19:267.
5. Grossniklaus HE, Martin DF, Solomon AR. Invasive conjunctival tumor with keratoacanthoma features. *Am J Ophthalmol* 1990;109:736–737.
6. Munro S, Brownstein S, Liddy B. Conjunctival keratoacanthoma. *Am J Ophthalmol* 1993;116:654–655.
7. Schellini SA, Marques ME, Milanezi MF, et al. Conjunctival keratoacanthoma. *Acta Ophthalmol Scand* 1997;75:335–337.
8. Coupland SE, Heimann H, Kellner U, et al. Keratoacanthoma of the bulbar conjunctiva. *Br J Ophthalmol* 1998;82:586.
9. Tulvatana W, Pisarnkorskul P, Wannakrairot P. Solitary keratoacanthoma of the conjunctiva: Report of a case. *J Med Assoc Thai* 2001;84:1059–1064.
10. Hughes EH, Intzedy L, Dick AD, et al. Keratoacanthoma of the conjunctiva. *Eye* 2003;17:781–782.
11. Friedman RP, Morales A, Burnham TK. Multiple cutaneous and conjunctival keratoacanthomata. *Arch Dermatol* 1965;92:162–165.
12. Perdigao FB, Pierre-Filho Pde T, Natalino RJ, et al. Conjunctival keratoacanthoma. *Rev Hosp Clin Fac Med Sao Paulo* 2004;59:135–137.
13. Oellers P, Karp CL, Shah RR, et al. Conjunctival keratoacanthoma. *Br J Ophthalmol* 2014;98:275–276.

CONJUNCTIVAL PSEUDOEPITHELIOMATOUS HYPERPLASIA AND KERATOACANTHOMA

1. Hamid LM, Wilson FM II, Grayson M. Keratoacanthoma of the limbus. *Ophthalmic Surg* 1988;19:267–270.
2. Munro S, Brownstein S, Liddy B. Conjunctival keratoacanthoma. *Am J Ophthalmol* 1993;116:654–655.

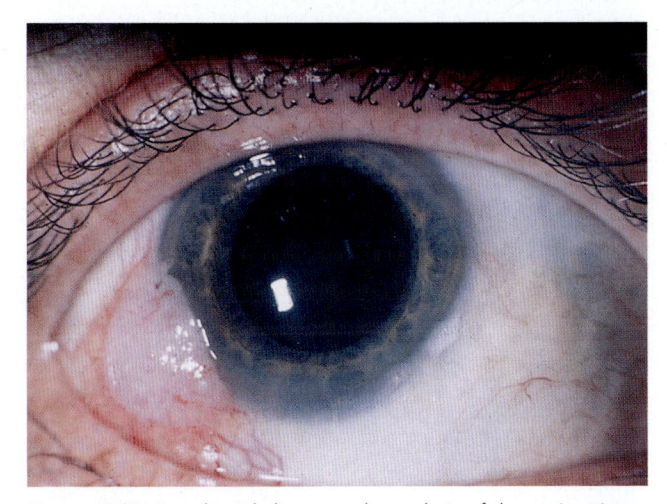

Figure 17.25. Pseudoepitheliomatous hyperplasia of the conjunctiva at the limbus inferotemporally. Note the leukoplakia secondary to hyperkeratosis. (Courtesy of Armed Forces Institute of Pathology, Washington, DC.)

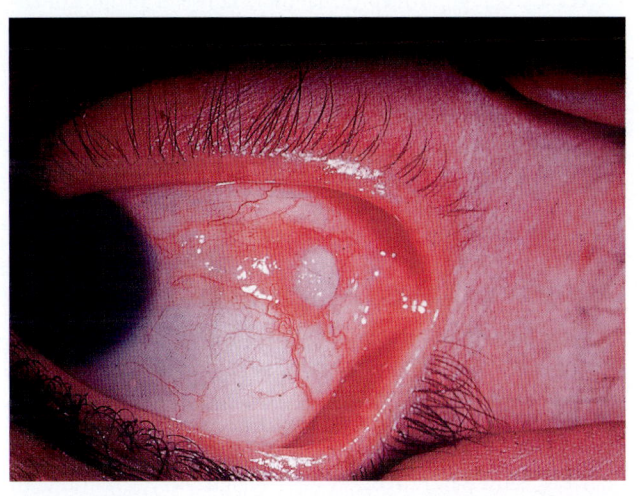

Figure 17.26. Keratoacanthoma of bulbar conjunctiva temporally showing leukoplakia. (Courtesy of Armed Forces Institute of Pathology, Washington, DC.)

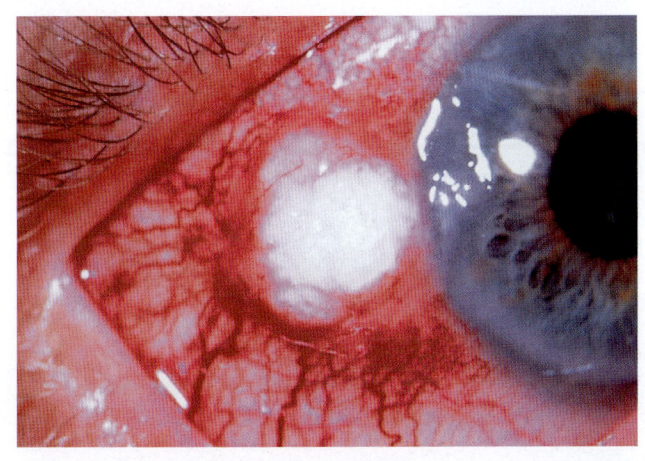

Figure 17.27. Keratoacanthoma of bulbar conjunctiva at the limbus. (Courtesy of Fred M. Wilson II, MD.)

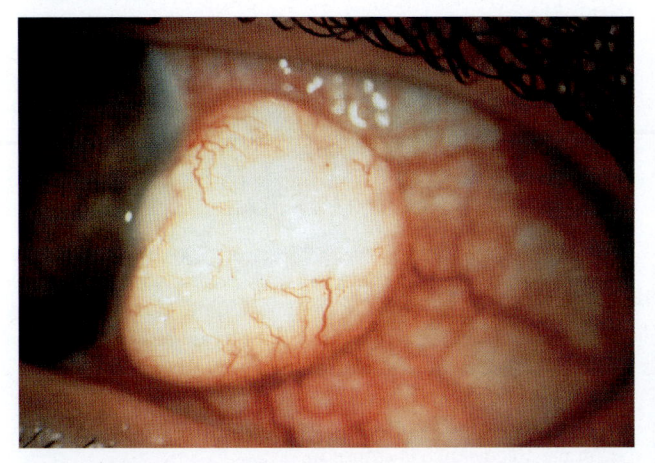

Figure 17.28. Keratoacanthoma of bulbar conjunctiva at the limbus in a 42-year-old man. Unlike squamous cell carcinoma, which evolves more slowly, this lesion grew rapidly. The intense white color is indicative of extensive keratinization on the surface of the lesion. (Courtesy of Seymour Brownstein, MD.)

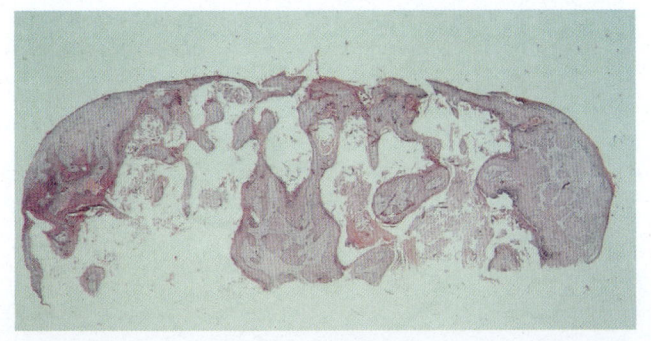

Figure 17.29. Histopathology of lesion in Figure 17.28, showing proliferation of squamous epithelium with invasive acanthosis and hyperkeratosis. (Hematoxylin–eosin ×10.) (Courtesy of Seymour Brownstein, MD.)

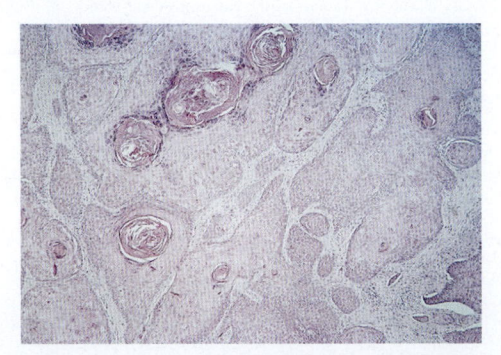

Figure 17.30. Higher-magnification view of lesion shown in Figure 17.28, showing invasive acanthosis with foci of keratin. (Hematoxylin–eosin ×100.) (Courtesy of Seymour Brownstein, MD.)

CONJUNCTIVAL HEREDITARY BENIGN INTRAEPITHELIAL DYSKERATOSIS

General Considerations

Hereditary benign intraepithelial dyskeratosis is an autosomal-dominant disorder that originally developed in an inbred isolate of Caucasians, African Americans, and Native Americans (1–11). This kindred, known as the Haliwa Indians, derive their name from their location in the counties of Halifax and Washington in North Carolina where the group originally resided. Hereditary benign intraepithelial dyskeratosis has subsequently been detected in several other parts of the United States and in patients who are not of Haliwa ancestry.

Clinical Features

Hereditary benign intraepithelial dyskeratosis develops in the first decade of life and is characterized by bilateral elevated fleshy plaques on the nasal or temporal perilimbal conjunctiva, often in a V-shape (3–11). Similar plaques can occur on the buccal mucosa. It can remain relatively asymptomatic or it can cause severe redness and foreign body sensation. In some instances, it can extend onto the cornea. It has no known malignant potential.

Pathology

Histopathologically, hereditary benign intraepithelial dyskeratosis is characterized by foci of markedly acanthotic and hyperkeratotic conjunctival epithelium with prominent dyskeratosis. The basement membrane is intact and the engorged stroma is chronically inflamed.

Management

Hereditary benign intraepithelial dyskeratosis has no known malignant potential. It does not usually require aggressive treatment. Smaller, less symptomatic lesions can be treated with ocular lubricants and judicious use of topical corticosteroids. Larger, symptomatic lesions can be managed by local resection with mucous membrane or amniotic membrane grafting if necessary. Recurrence is common.

Selected References

Reviews

1. Shields CL, Shields JA. Tumors of the conjunctiva and cornea. *Surv Ophthalmol* 2004;49:3–24.
2. Shields CL, Demirci H, Karatza E, et al. Clinical survey of 1643 melanocytic and nonmelanocytic tumors of the conjunctiva. *Ophthalmology* 2004;111:1747–1754.

Case Reports

3. Von Stallman L, Paton D. Hereditary benign intraepithelial dyskeratosis. I. Ocular manifestations. *Arch Ophthalmol* 1960;63:421–429.
4. Witco CJ, Shankle DH, Graham JB, et al. Hereditary benign intraepithelial dyskeratosis. II. Oral manifestations and hereditary transmission. *Arch Pathol* 1960;70:696–711.
5. Yanoff M. Hereditary benign intraepithelial dyskeratosis. *Arch Ophthalmol* 1968;79:291–293.
6. McLean IW, Riddle PJ, Scruggs JH, et al. Hereditary benign intraepithelial dyskeratosis. *Ophthalmology* 1981;88:164–168.
7. Reed JW, Cashwell LF, Klintworth GK. Corneal manifestations of hereditary benign intraepithelial dyskeratosis. *Arch Ophthalmol* 1979;97:297–300.
8. Shields CL, Shields JA, Eagle RC. Hereditary benign intraepithelial dyskeratosis. *Arch Ophthalmol* 1987;105:422–423.
9. Haisley-Royster CA, Allingham RR, Klintworth GK, et al. Hereditary benign intraepithelial dyskeratosis: Report of two cases with prominent oral lesions. *J Am Acad Dermatol* 2001;45:634–636.
10. Cai R, Zhang C, Chen R, et al. Clinicopathological features of a suspected case of hereditary benign intraepithelial dyskeratosis with bilateral corneas involved: A case report and mini review. *Cornea* 2011;30(12):1481–1484.
11. Cummings TJ, Dodd LG, Eedes CR, et al. Hereditary benign intraepithelial dyskeratosis: An evaluation of diagnostic cytology. *Arch Pathol Lab Med* 2008;132(8):1325–1328.

CONJUNCTIVAL HEREDITARY BENIGN INTRAEPITHELIAL DYSKERATOSIS

Hereditary benign intraepithelial dyskeratosis is an epithelial lesion of conjunctiva and other mucous membranes. A case example is shown.

Shields CL, Shields JA, Eagle RC. Hereditary benign intraepithelial dyskeratosis. *Arch Ophthalmol* 1987;105:422–423.

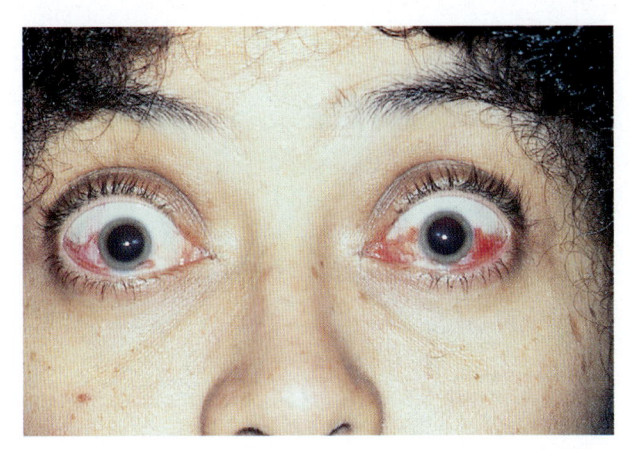

Figure 17.31. Hereditary benign intraepithelial dyskeratosis in a 37-year-old woman who had bilateral interpalpebral lesions present since age 3 years. She was a descendent of a Haliwa Indian tribe and traced her ancestry to North Carolina.

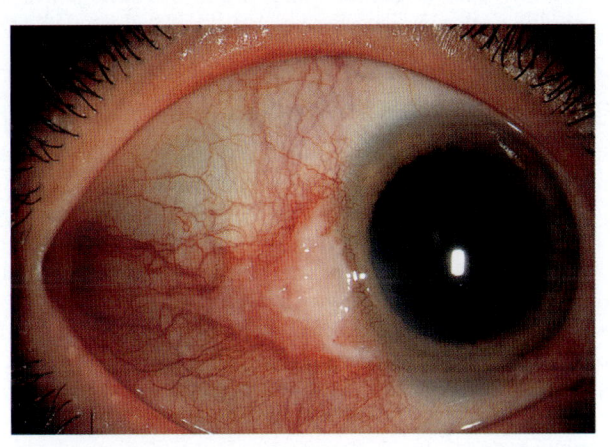

Figure 17.32. Close view of temporal lesion on the right eye, showing a white, frothy lesion near the limbus with marked hyperemia of the surrounding tissues.

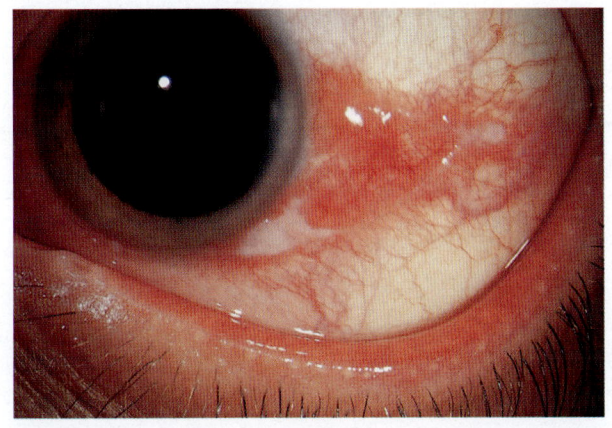

Figure 17.33. Close view of temporal lesion on the left eye showing similar features.

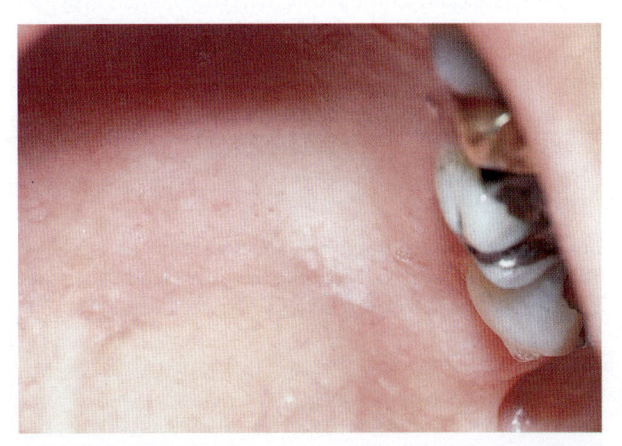

Figure 17.34. Similar lesion on the lateral aspect of the mucous membrane of the mouth.

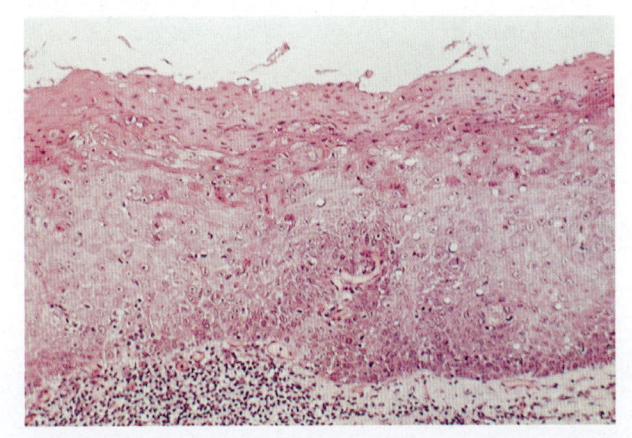

Figure 17.35. Histopathology of lesion in the right eye showing acanthosis and hyperkeratosis with inflammatory cells beneath the intact basement membrane. (Hematoxylin–eosin ×25.)

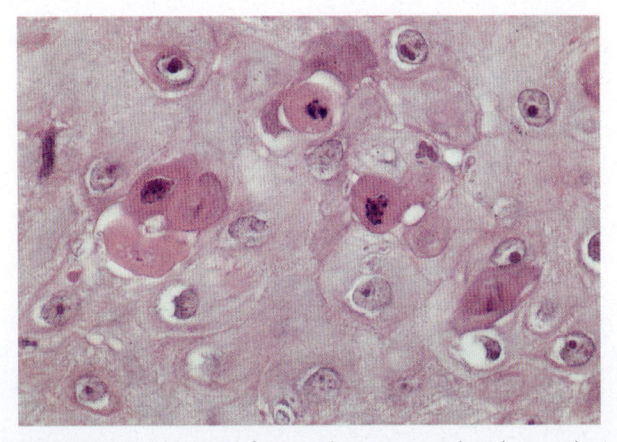

Figure 17.36. Higher-magnification photomicrograph in the acanthotic epithelium showing the large eosinophilic cells representing foci of dyskeratosis. (Hematoxylin–eosin ×250.)

CONJUNCTIVAL DACRYOADENOMA

General Considerations
Dacryoadenoma is a rare conjunctival tumor that presumably has its origin in children or young adults. Its clinical and histopathologic features have been reported by Jakobiec et al. (1).

Clinical Features
Dacryoadenoma appears as a fleshy pink lesion in the bulbar or palpebral conjunctiva. In one case, the lesion was first recognized in a 33-year-old patient as a salmon-colored mass in the inferior fornix (1). It was removed when the patient was 48 years old. It is uncertain whether the lesion had been present since birth in that patient. In another case, the lesion occurred in the bulbar conjunctiva as a darker red mass in a 14-year-old girl. In that case, the lesion had been present since birth and had slowly enlarged, according to the history. The clinical differential diagnosis includes lymphoma, conjunctival choristoma, and other pink- or salmon-colored masses in the conjunctiva.

Pathology
Histopathologically, conjunctival dacryoadenoma is a gland forming benign tumor that is believed to be of surface epithelial origin. The tumor appears to originate from the surface epithelium, proliferate inward into the stroma, and develop glandular lobules similar to those seen in normal lacrimal glands, except that they have abundant goblet cells.

Management
The diagnosis of conjunctival dacryoadenoma is rarely suspected clinically and can resemble lacrimal gland choristoma. Most such lesions have been excised. The prognosis is excellent.

Selected Reference
1. Jakobiec FA, Perry HD, Harrison W, et al. Dacryoadenoma. A unique tumor of the conjunctival epithelium. *Ophthalmology* 1989;96:1014–1020.

CONJUNCTIVAL DACRYOADENOMA

Jakobiec FA, Perry HD, Harrison W, et al. Dacryoadenoma. A unique tumor of the conjunctival epithelium. *Ophthalmology* 1989;96:1014–1020.

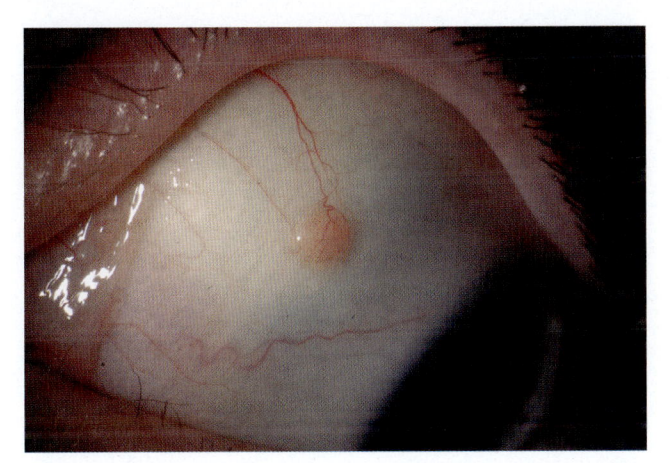

Figure 17.37. Dacryoadenoma of the superior bulbar conjunctiva.

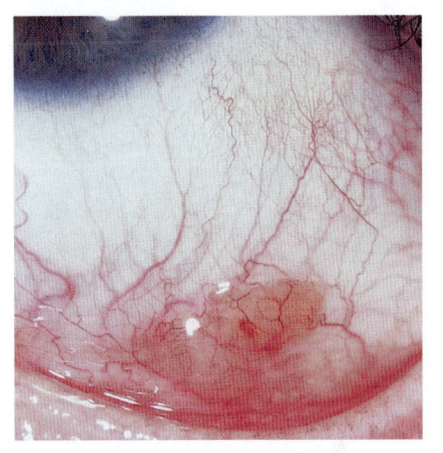

Figure 17.38. Dacryoadenoma of the forniceal conjunctiva. (Courtesy of Frederick Jakobiec, MD.)

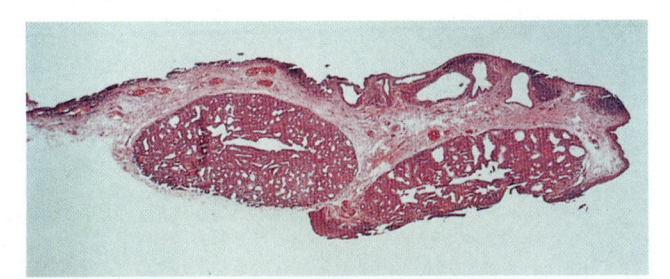

Figure 17.39. Histopathology of lesion in Figure 17.38, showing inward proliferation of the epithelial cells and a small opening to the surface. (Hematoxylin–eosin ×30.) (Courtesy of Frederick Jakobiec, MD.)

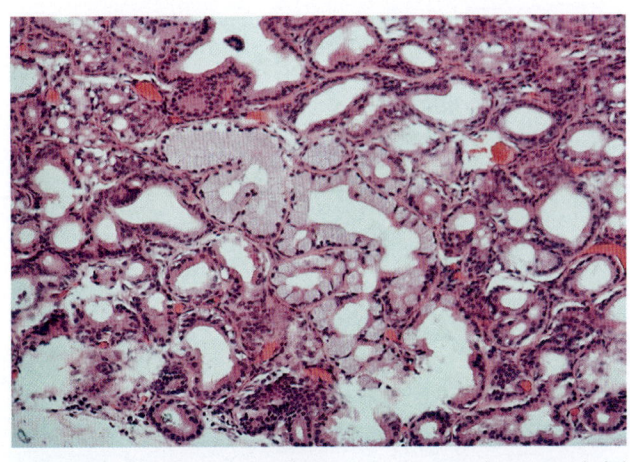

Figure 17.40. Histopathology of lesion in Figure 17.38, showing epithelial cell proliferation forming glandular units and basement membrane material. (Periodic acid-Schiff ×220.) (Courtesy of Frederick Jakobiec, MD.)

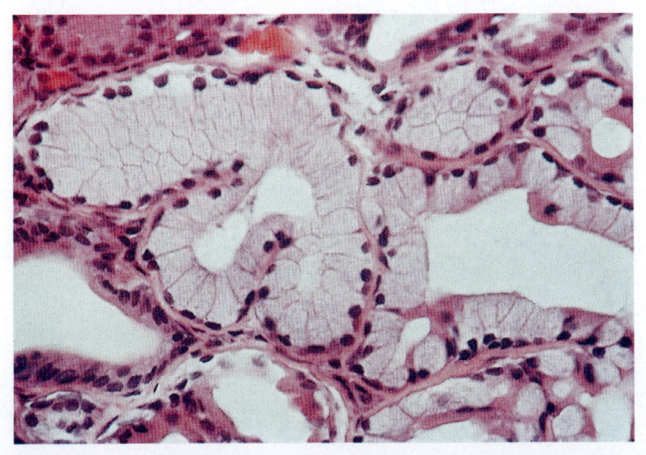

Figure 17.41. Histopathology of lesion in Figure 17.38, showing goblet cells with clear cytoplasm, suggestive of mucin secretion. (Hematoxylin–eosin ×300.) (Courtesy of Frederick Jakobiec, MD.)

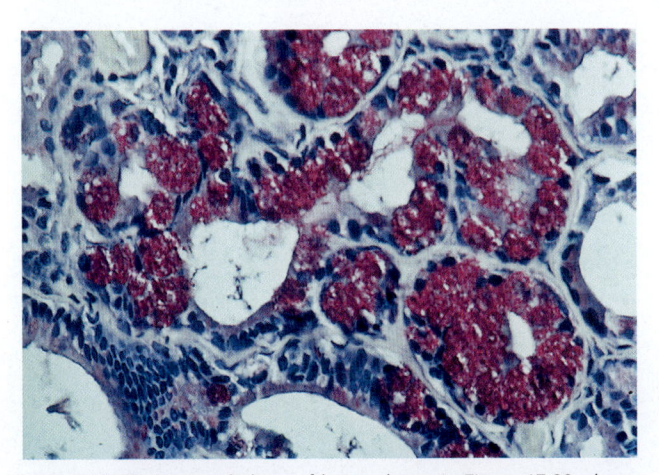

Figure 17.42. Histopathology of lesion shown in Figure 17.38, showing that the cells with the clear cytoplasm contain mucin. (Mucicarmine ×250.) (Courtesy of Frederick Jakobiec, MD.)

CHAPTER 18

PREMALIGNANT AND MALIGNANT LESIONS OF THE CONJUNCTIVAL EPITHELIUM

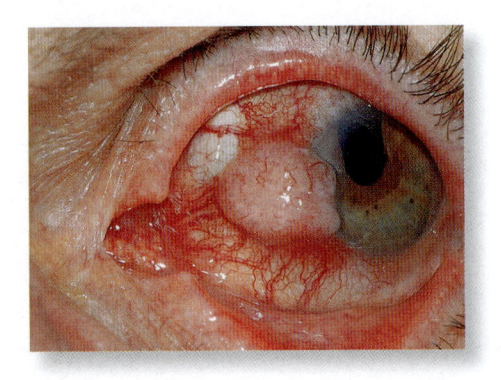

General Considerations

Several types of benign and malignant lesions can arise from the squamous epithelium of the conjunctiva. These lesions tend to form a spectrum ranging from those that are entirely benign, to those with low malignant potential, to more aggressive, malignant neoplasms. It is often difficult to differentiate clinically between the benign and malignant lesions. The majority of epithelial lesions seen in a clinical practice are low-grade proliferations with only a small chance of evolving into frank squamous cell carcinoma. Two of these are keratotic plaque and actinic keratosis (1–5). Because they may be impossible to differentiate clinically, they are considered together for this discussion. In the authors' clinical series of 1,643 conjunctival tumors, there were four keratotic plaques and four cases of actinic keratosis each representing less than 1% of the 1,643 cases (1).

Clinical Features

Both keratotic plaque and actinic keratosis can develop on the limbal or bulbar conjunctiva usually in the interpalpebral region. Clinically, the lesion appears as a flat, white plaque that appears gradually and shows no tendency toward aggressive growth. They can both resemble conjunctival intraepithelial neoplasia (CIN), squamous cell carcinoma, actinic granuloma, and other conditions (5).

Pathology

Pathologically, keratotic plaque consists of acanthosis of the epithelium with keratinization of the conjunctival epithelium and parakeratosis. Actinic keratosis (senile keratosis) is a similar proliferation of epithelium with prominent keratosis, often over a chronically inflamed pinguecula or pterygium. It can have a frothy or leukoplakic appearance and may be clinically similar to a keratotic plaque.

Management

Keratotic plaque and actinic keratosis of the conjunctiva are usually indistinguishable clinically from CIN, which has slightly greater potential to evolve into invasive squamous cell carcinoma. Therefore, the finding of leukoplakia in the conjunctiva is a relative indication for surgical excision and supplemental cryotherapy. However, it is also acceptable to follow some such lesions until progression is documented, particularly in elderly patients, because the prognosis is generally excellent, even for CIN.

CONJUNCTIVAL KERATOTIC PLAQUE AND ACTINIC KERATOSIS

Selected References

Reviews

1. Shields CL, Demirci H, Karatza E, et al. Clinical survey of 1643 melanocytic and nonmelanocytic tumors of the conjunctiva. *Ophthalmology* 2004;111:1747–1754.
2. Shields CL, Shields JA. Tumors of the conjunctiva and cornea. *Surv Ophthalmol* 2004;49:3–24.
3. Mauriello JA Jr, Napolitano J, McLean I. Actinic keratosis and dysplasia of the conjunctiva: a clinicopathological study of 45 cases. *Can J Ophthalmol* 1995;30:312–316.

Case Reports

4. Mortemousque B, Leger F, Brindeau C, et al. Actinic keratosis of the conjunctiva. Apropos of a clinical case. *J Fr Ophtalmol* 1998;215:458–461.
5. Mittal R, Meena M, Saha D. Actinic granuloma of the conjunctiva in young women. *Ophthalmology* 2013;120:1786–1789.

Chapter 18 Premalignant and Malignant Lesions of the Conjunctival Epithelium

CONJUNCTIVAL KERATOTIC PLAQUE AND ACTINIC KERATOSIS

These benign lesions can simulate neoplasia because of the leukoplakia produced by the keratosis.

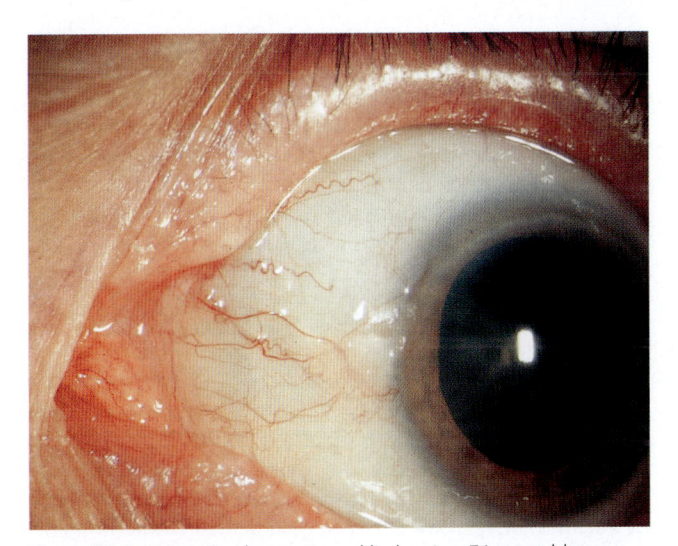

Figure 18.1. Keratotic plaque at nasal limbus in a 76-year-old man.

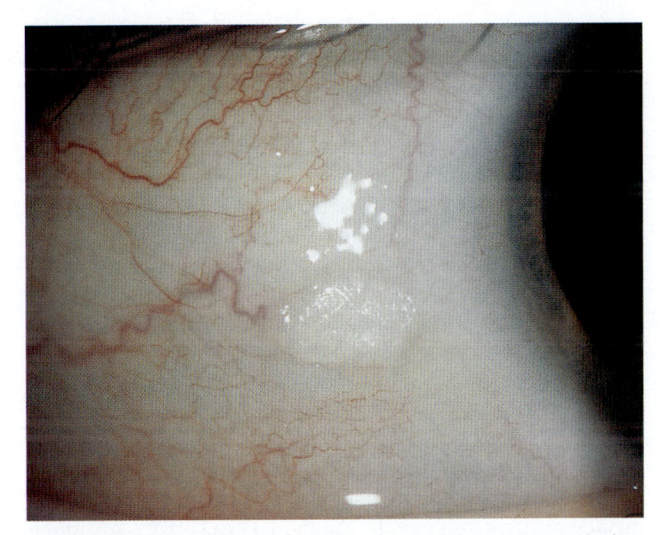

Figure 18.2. Keratotic plaque in bulbar conjunctiva posterior to the limbus in a 19-year-old man.

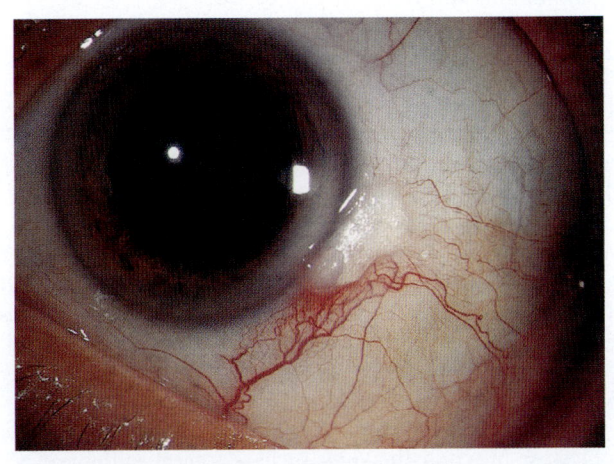

Figure 18.3. Keratosis associated with a pinguecula.

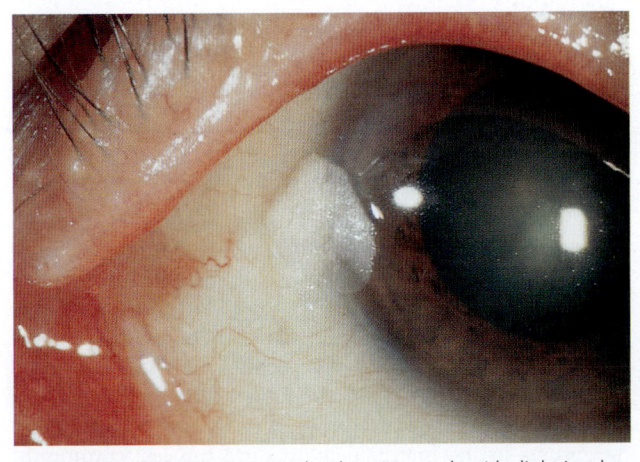

Figure 18.4. Keratosis associated with a pinguecula with slight involvement of the adjacent cornea.

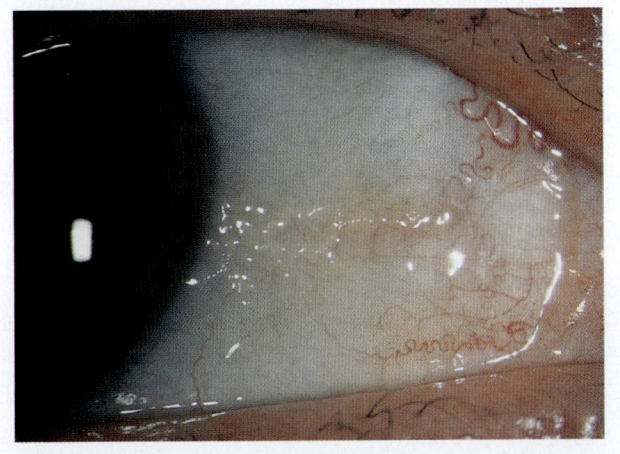

Figure 18.5. Diffuse keratosis associated with atypical pinguecula. The lesion showed peripheral corneal invasion after 15-year follow-up and proved to be keratosis and early dysplasia overlying a pinguecula.

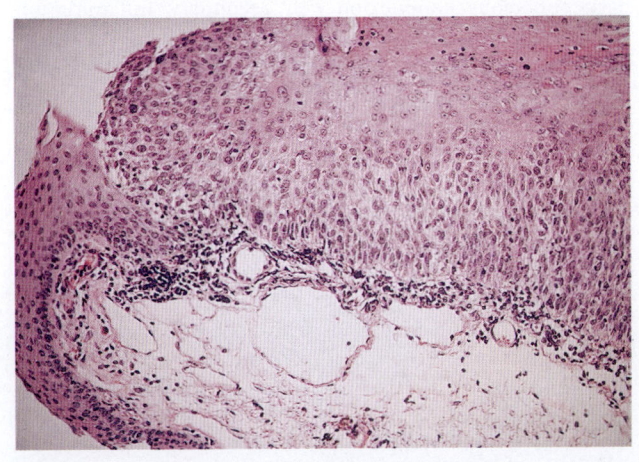

Figure 18.6. Histopathology of conjunctival keratotic plaque showing acanthosis and hyperkeratosis. (Hematoxylin–eosin ×80.)

CONJUNCTIVAL INTRAEPITHELIAL NEOPLASIA

General Considerations

Squamous cell neoplasia can be a localized, minimally aggressive lesion confined to the surface epithelium or a more aggressive tumor that transgresses the basement membrane and invades the adjacent tissues. The former has no potential to metastasize and is called CIN (1–37). The latter is called invasive squamous cell carcinoma and generally has a low potential for metastasis. In recent years, some authors have used the umbrella term "ocular surface squamous neoplasia" (OSSN) to include dysplasia, CIN, and invasive squamous cell carcinoma (6). We have preferred to use the term CIN and invasive squamous cell carcinoma, as they refer to degree of invasiveness of each type based on histopathology. However, if biopsy is not performed, then OSSN seems applicable. These lesions are initially confined to the epithelium (CIN) but can progress to invasive squamous cell carcinoma; therefore, CIN is generally considered to be a "precancerous" condition, rather than a true malignancy. The main predisposing factors include sunlight and human papillomavirus (HPV). Although results are conflicting, a recent study using polymerase chain reaction established the presence of HPV 16 or 18 in cases of CIN (34).

In the authors' clinical series of 1,643 conjunctival tumors, there were 71 cases of CIN, accounting for 39% of all premalignant and malignant epithelial lesions and for 4% of all conjunctival lesions (1).

Clinical Features

CIN is usually unilateral in fair-skinned, middle-aged or older patients who have had considerable exposure to sunlight (1–9). Rarely, it is found in children (36). Both CIN and invasive squamous cell carcinoma occur more frequently in immunosuppressed patients, particularly those with acquired immunodeficiency syndrome (AIDS) (8,34). Clinically, CIN has several variations, but usually appears as a fleshy, sessile, or minimally elevated lesion usually at the limbus in the interpalpebral fissure and less commonly in the forniceal or palpebral conjunctiva. Occasionally, this tumor can acquire pigmentation, especially in patients of dark cutaneous complexion (7). Secondary inflammation can lead to the misdiagnosis of atypical conjunctivitis before the neoplasm is suspected (37). Leukoplakia is usually absent or minimal; extensive leukoplakia should raise suspicion for invasive squamous cell carcinoma. Although greater thickness is believed to be a sign of malignant transformation we have seen thick tumors that remain within the epithelium. Hence, there are no consistent clinical criteria for distinguishing CIN from invasive squamous cell carcinoma. CIN can extend for a variable distance into the adjacent corneal epithelium, where it appears as a subtle advancing, gray, superficial opacity that may be relatively avascular or may have fine blood vessels. When the involvement is limited to the corneal epithelium with only minimal limbal involvement, it is called primary corneal dysplasia.

Diagnosis

Although the diagnosis of CIN is made histopathologically, it has sufficiently characteristic features that a diagnosis can be made clinically in most cases. Usually, conjunctival/corneal CIN is small and localized enough that primarily complete excision (discussed later) is the best method of establishing the diagnosis, and incisional biopsy is rarely indicated. However, some have advocated aspiration cytology (31) or impression/exfoliative cytology to establish the diagnosis (32,33).

Pathology

Histopathologically, mild CIN (dysplasia) is characterized by a partial thickness replacement of the epithelium by mildly anaplastic cells that lack normal maturation. Severe CIN (carcinoma in situ) is characterized by full-thickness replacement of the epithelium by similar cells. The basement membrane is intact. Both variants show a characteristic abrupt demarcation between the affected epithelium and the adjacent normal epithelium. In contrast with invasive carcinoma, hyperkeratosis and dyskeratosis are relatively uncommon findings.

Management

There are many reports that discuss management of CIN (10–30). Complete excision with adequate margins is the preferred initial treatment. For most localized lesions, we remove the growth with alcohol corneal epitheliectomy, partial lamellar sclerokeratoconjunctivectomy, and double freeze–thaw cryotherapy (10). This is the same technique used for localized squamous cell carcinoma and melanoma and it is discussed and illustrated in Chapter 25. Cryotherapy is almost always used as supplemental treatment and seems to provide better control. Low-dose irradiation with strontium-90 has been used in the past but is currently avoided.

The most recently employed nonsurgical methods include topical or injection therapies such as topical mitomycin C, interferon alpha-2b, 5-fluorouracil, or cidofovir for primary or recurrent/persistent cases (15–29). Topical or injection interferon alpha-2b has been immensely successful with few complications (21–28). Interferon is used for immunotherapy (complete primary treatment), immunoreduction (reduction of giant OSSN to allow smaller surgical resection), or immunoprevention (following surgery where margins were equivocal to prevent recurrence) (23–25,27). Similarly, mitomycin C and 5-fluorouracil can be used and are effective, but due to the nature of these chemotherapies, stem cell deficiency and other complications might occur.

However, our preference is primary surgical removal especially for a circumscribed tumor in an elderly person to save them the cost and difficulties of using the topical therapies for several weeks or months, particularly if hand–eye coordination is limited. The indications for surgical removal versus topical interferon is currently debated (14).

CONJUNCTIVAL INTRAEPITHELIAL NEOPLASIA

Selected References

Reviews
1. Shields CL, Demirci H, Karatza E, et al. Clinical survey of 1643 melanocytic and nonmelanocytic tumors of the conjunctiva. *Ophthalmology* 2004;111:1747–1754.
2. Shields CL, Shields JA. Tumors of the conjunctiva and cornea. *Surv Ophthalmol* 2004;49:3–24.
3. Grossniklaus HE, Green WR, Luckenbach M, et al. Conjunctival lesions in adults. A clinical and histopathologic review. *Cornea* 1987;6:78–116.
4. Erie JC, Campbell RF, Liesegang TJ. Conjunctival and corneal intraepithelial and invasive neoplasia. *Ophthalmology* 1986;93:176–183.
5. Lee GA, Hirst LW. Ocular surface squamous neoplasia. *Surv Ophthalmol* 1995;39:429–450.
6. Tunc M, Char DH, Crawford B, et al. Intraepithelial and invasive squamous cell carcinoma of the conjunctiva: analysis of 60 cases. *Br J Ophthalmol* 1999;83:98–103.
7. Shields CL, Manchandia A, Subbiah R, et al. Pigmented squamous cell carcinoma in situ of the conjunctiva in 5 cases. *Ophthalmology* 2008;115(10):1673–1678.
8. Shields CL, Ramasubramanian A, Mellen P, et al. Conjunctival squamous cell carcinoma arising in immunosuppressed patients (organ transplant, human immunodeficiency virus infection). *Ophthalmology* 2011;118:2133–2137.
9. Yousef YA, Finger PT. Squamous carcinoma and dysplasia of the conjunctiva and cornea: an analysis of 101 cases. *Ophthalmology* 2012;119(2):233–240.

Management
10. Shields JA, Shields CL, De Potter P. Surgical approach to conjunctival tumors. The 1994 Lynn B. McMahan Lecture. *Arch Ophthalmol* 1997;115:808–815.
11. Fraunfelder FT, Wingfield D. Management of intraepithelial conjunctival tumors and squamous cell carcinomas. *Am J Ophthalmol* 1983;95:359–363.
12. Tabin G, Levin S, Snibson G, et al. Later recurrences and necessity for long-term follow-up in corneal and conjunctival intraepithelial neoplasia. *Ophthalmology* 1997;104:485–492.
13. Zaki AA, Farid SF. Management of intraepithelial and invasive neoplasia of the cornea and conjunctiva: a long-term follow up. *Cornea* 2009;28(9):986–988.
14. Nanji AA, Moon CS, Galor A, et al. Surgical versus medical treatment of ocular surface squamous neoplasia: a comparison of recurrences and complications. *Ophthalmology* 2014;121:994–1000.

Mitomycin C
15. Frucht-Pery J, Rozenman Y. Mitomycin C therapy for corneal intraepithelial neoplasia. *Am J Ophthalmol* 1994;117:164–168.
16. Shields CL, Naseripour M, Shields JA. Topical mitomycin C for extensive, recurrent conjunctival squamous cell carcinoma. *Am J Ophthalmol* 2002;133:601–606.
17. Shields CL, Demirci H, Marr BP, et al. Chemoreduction with topical mitomycin C prior to resection of extensive squamous cell carcinoma of the conjunctiva. *Arch Ophthalmol* 2005;123:109–113.

5-Fluorouracil
18. Yeatts RP, Ford JG, Stanton CA, et al. Topical 5-fluorouracil in treating epithelial neoplasia of the conjunctiva and cornea. *Ophthalmology* 1995;102:1338–1344.
19. Yeatts RP, Engelbrecht NE, Curry CD, et al. 5-Fluorouracil for the treatment of intraepithelial neoplasia of the conjunctiva and cornea. *Ophthalmology* 2000;107:2190–2195.
20. Midena E, Angeli CD, Valenti M, et al. Treatment of conjunctival squamous cell carcinoma with topical 5-fluorouracil. *Br J Ophthalmol* 2000;84:268–272.

Interferon
21. Giaconi JA, Karp CL. Current treatment options for conjunctival and corneal intraepithelial neoplasia. *Ocul Surf* 2003;1:667–673.
22. Karp CL, Galor A, Chhabra S, et al. Subconjunctival/perilesional recombinant interferon α2b for ocular surface squamous neoplasia: a 10-year review. *Ophthalmology* 2010;117(12):2241–2246.
23. Shields CL, Kancherla S, Bianciotto CG, et al. Ocular surface squamous neoplasia (squamous cell carcinoma) of the socket: management of extensive tumors with interferon. *Ophthal Plast Reconstr Surg* 2011;27:247–250.
24. Shah S, Kaliki S, Kim HJ, et al. Topical interferon alpha 2b for management of ocular surface squamous neoplasia in 23 cases: outcomes based on American Joint Committee on Cancer (AJCC) classification. *Arch Ophthalmol* 2012;130:159–164.
25. Kim HJ, Shields CL, Shah SU, et al. Giant ocular surface squamous neoplasia managed with interferon alpha-2b as immunotherapy or immunoreduction. *Ophthalmology* 2012;119:938–944.
26. Nanji AA, Sayyad FE, Karp CL. Topical chemotherapy for ocular surface squamous neoplasia. *Curr Opin Ophthalmol* 2013;24(4):336–342.
27. Shields CL, Kaliki S, Kim HJ, et al. Interferon for ocular surface squamous neoplasia in 81 cases: outcomes based on the American Joint Committee on Cancer classification. *Cornea* 2013;32(3):248–256.
28. Besley J, Pappalardo J, Lee GA, et al. Risk factors for ocular surface squamous neoplasia recurrence after treatment with topical mitomycin C and interferon alpha-2b. *Am J Ophthalmol* 2014;157:287–293.

Others
29. Sherman MD, Feldman KA, Farahmand SM, et al. Treatment of conjunctival squamous cell carcinoma with topical cidofovir. *Am J Ophthalmol* 2002;134:432–433.
30. Damani MR, Shah AR, Karp CL, et al. Treatment of ocular surface squamous neoplasia with topical aloe vera drops. *Cornea* 2015;34(1):87–89.

Histopathology/Cytopathology/Infectious Disease
31. Grossniklaus HE, Stulting RD, Gansler T, et al. Aspiration cytology of the conjunctival surface. *Acta Cytol* 2003;47:239–246.
32. Semenova EA, Milman T, Finger PT, et al. The diagnostic value of exfoliative cytology vs histopathology for ocular surface squamous neoplasia. *Am J Ophthalmol* 2009;148(5):772–778.e1.
33. Spinak M, Friedman AH. Squamous cell carcinoma of the conjunctiva. Value of exfoliative cytology in diagnosis. *Surv Ophthalmol* 1977;21:351–355.
34. Scott IU, Karp CL, Nuovo GJ. Human papillomavirus 16 and 18 expression in conjunctival intraepithelial neoplasia. *Ophthalmology* 2002;109:542–547.
35. Aoki S, Kubo E, Nakamura S, et al. Possible prognostic markers in conjunctival dysplasia and squamous cell carcinoma. *Jpn J Ophthalmol* 1998;42:256–261.

Case Reports
36. Linwong M, Herman SJ, Rabb MF. Carcinoma in situ of the corneal limbus in an adolescent girl. *Arch Ophthalmol* 1972;87:48–51.
37. Akpek EK, Polcharoen W, Chan R, et al. Ocular surface neoplasia masquerading as chronic blepharoconjunctivitis. *Cornea* 1999;18:282–288.

CONJUNCTIVAL INTRAEPITHELIAL NEOPLASIA: FLESHY AND PAPILLOMATOUS CONFIGURATIONS

Some cases of CIN lack leukoplakia and can simulate inflammation or sessile papilloma. Clinical and histopathologic examples of CIN are shown.

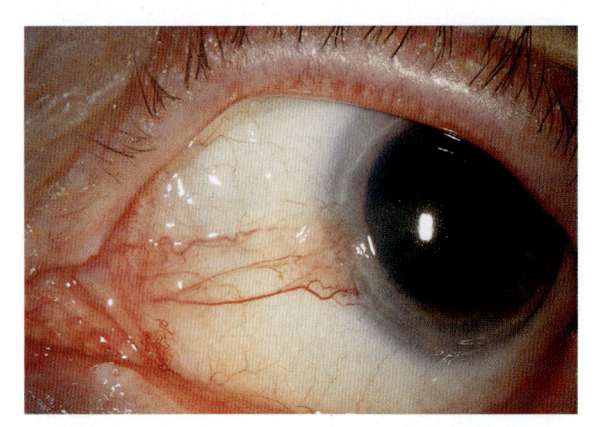

Figure 18.7. Small conjunctival intraepithelial neoplasia near limbus, simulating inflammation, in a 77-year-old man.

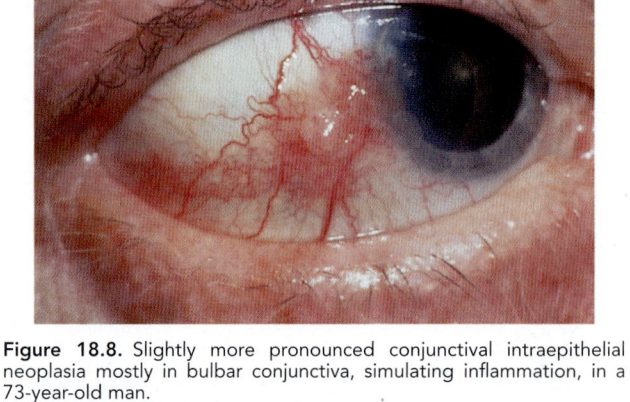

Figure 18.8. Slightly more pronounced conjunctival intraepithelial neoplasia mostly in bulbar conjunctiva, simulating inflammation, in a 73-year-old man.

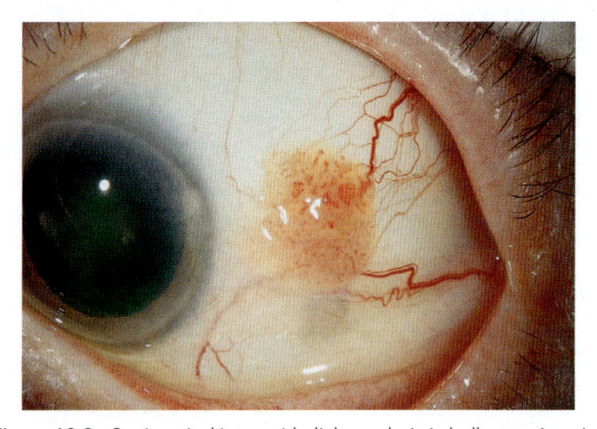

Figure 18.9. Conjunctival intraepithelial neoplasia in bulbar conjunctiva simulating a sessile papilloma in a 73-year-old woman.

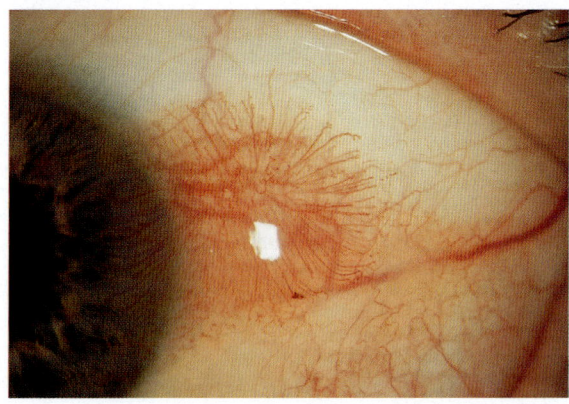

Figure 18.10. Conjunctival intraepithelial neoplasia simulating a sessile papilloma in a 52-year-old man who had extensive exposure to sunlight for many years. The lesion was removed successfully but recurred twice over the next 10 years, requiring additional surgical procedures and cryotherapy. Eventually, superficial corneal invasion developed and the patient was treated successfully with topical mitomycin C.

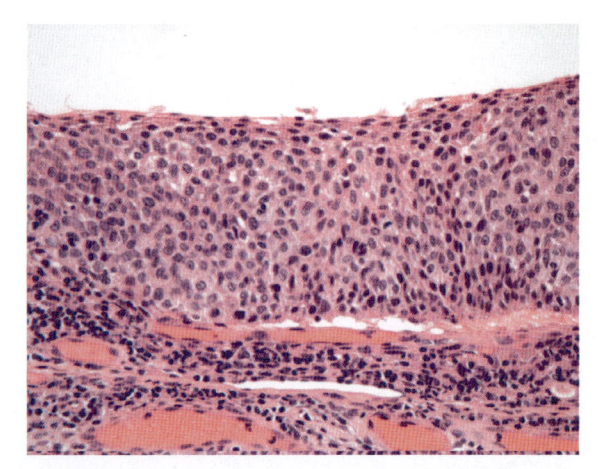

Figure 18.11. Histopathology of conjunctival intraepithelial neoplasia showing almost full-thickness replacement of the epithelium by neoplastic squamous cells. Chronic inflammatory cells are present in the underlying stroma. (Hematoxylin–eosin ×50.)

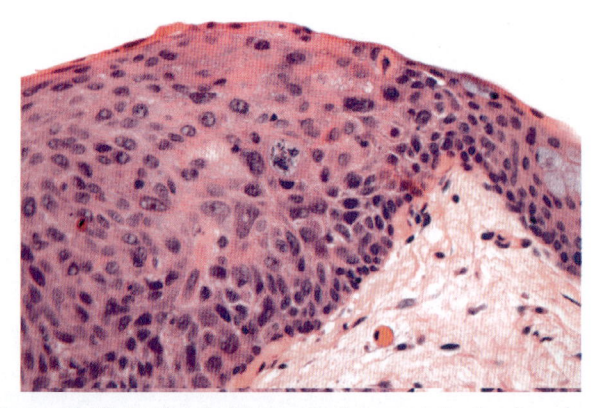

Figure 18.12. Conjunctival intraepithelial neoplasia showing abrupt transition from the normal conjunctival epithelium (to the right) to the tumor (to the left). (Hematoxylin–eosin ×40.)

Chapter 18 Premalignant and Malignant Lesions of the Conjunctival Epithelium

CONJUNCTIVAL INTRAEPITHELIAL NEOPLASIA (CIN): LEUKOPLAKIA

Leukoplakia (white plaque) over a conjunctival lesion generally suggests the process of keratosis of the involved epithelium.

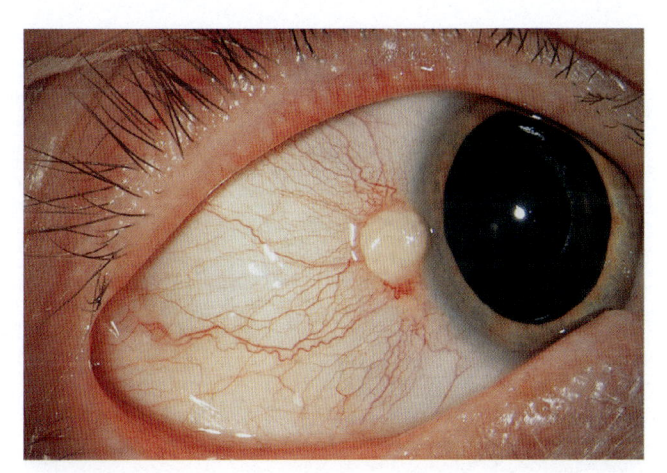

Figure 18.13. Round lesion near limbus in a 56-year-old woman.

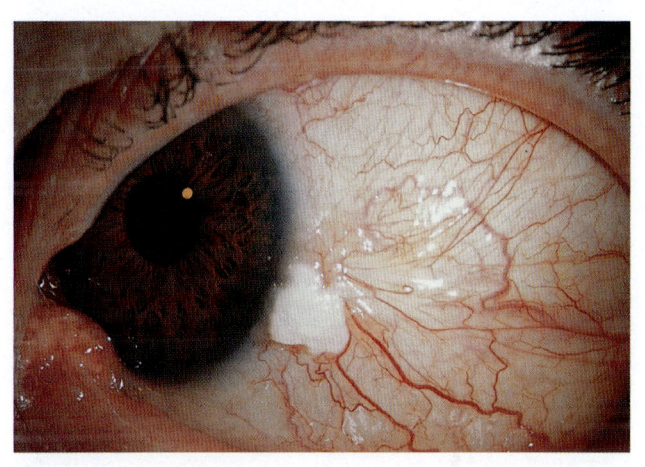

Figure 18.14. Slightly irregular lesion near limbus in a 57-year-old man.

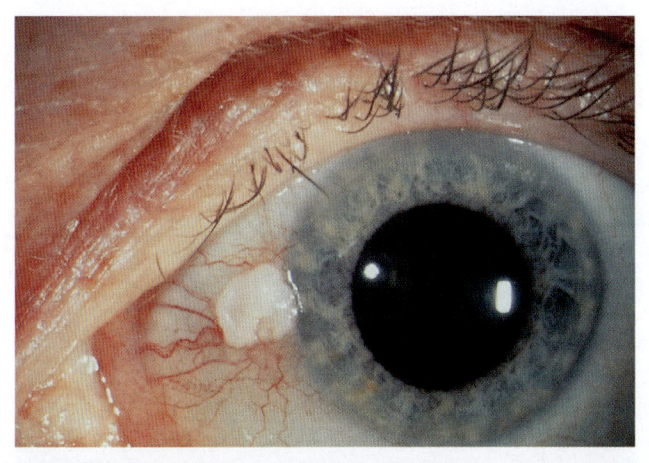

Figure 18.15. Slightly irregular lesion near limbus in a 55-year-old woman.

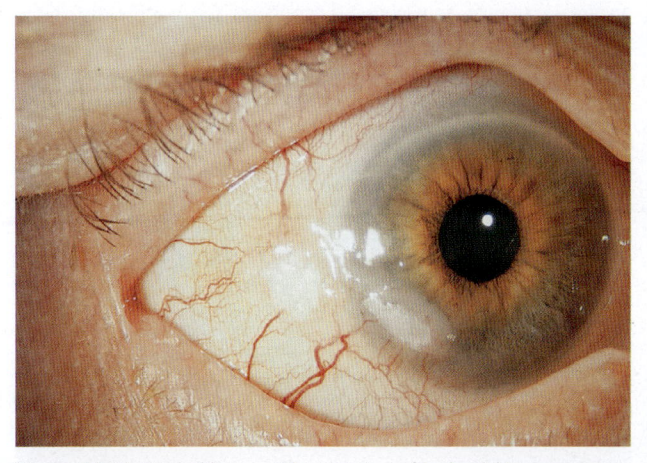

Figure 18.16. Limbal lesion with extension of leukoplakia onto cornea in a 65-year-old man.

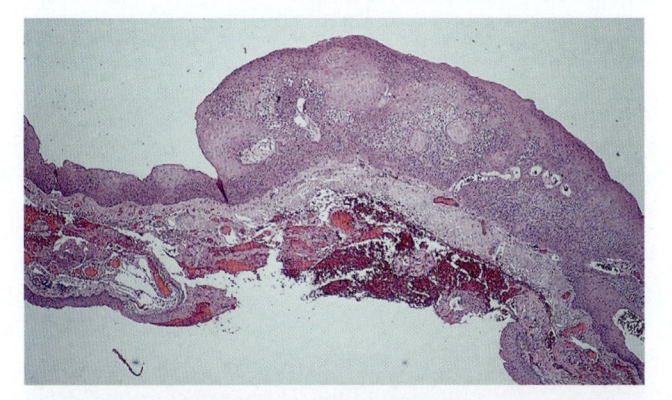

Figure 18.17. Histopathology of conjunctival intraepithelial neoplasia showing abrupt transition between the normal epithelium and the thickened abnormal epithelium. (Hematoxylin–eosin ×10.)

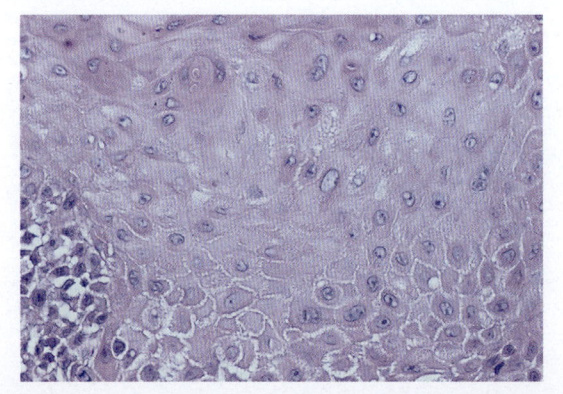

Figure 18.18. Histopathology of conjunctival intraepithelial neoplasia showing abnormal epithelial cells with mitotic activity. (Hematoxylin–eosin ×200.)

TUMORS OF THE CONJUNCTIVA

CONJUNCTIVAL INTRAEPITHELIAL NEOPLASIA: VARIOUS CLINICAL LOCATIONS AT LIMBUS

In some cases, the tumor is confined to the epithelium microscopically, despite a very thick clinical appearance. CIN was documented histopathologically in each of these cases.

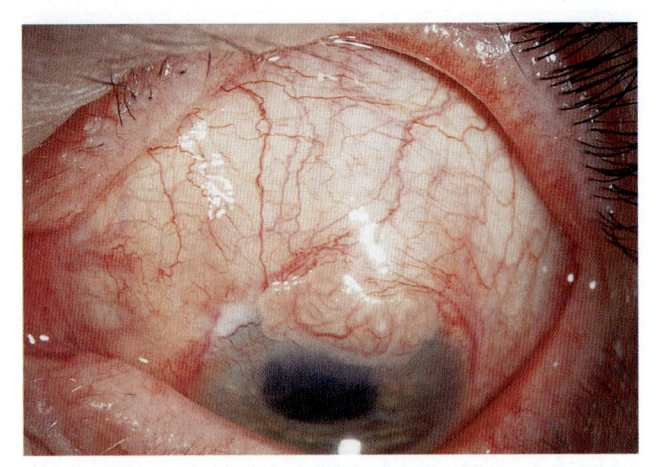

Figure 18.19. Nodular vascular lesion arising from the superior limbus and secondarily invading the cornea in a 64-year-old man. This is an atypical location for squamous cell neoplasms; the majority arise in the interpalpebral area.

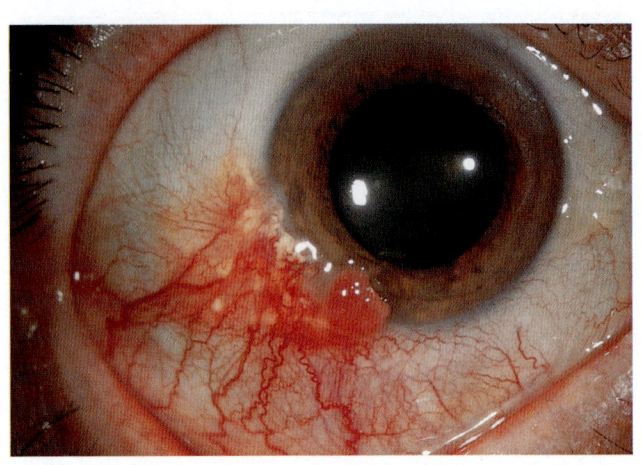

Figure 18.20. Lesion with irregular, fleshy nodules in the peripheral cornea in a 61-year-old woman.

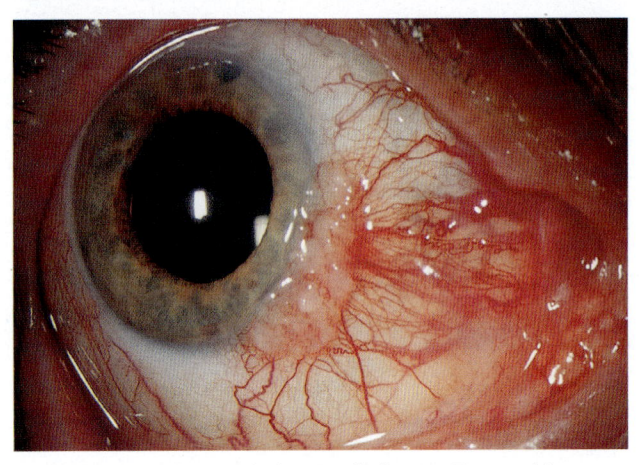

Figure 18.21. Frothy vascular lesion at limbus in a 71-year-old man.

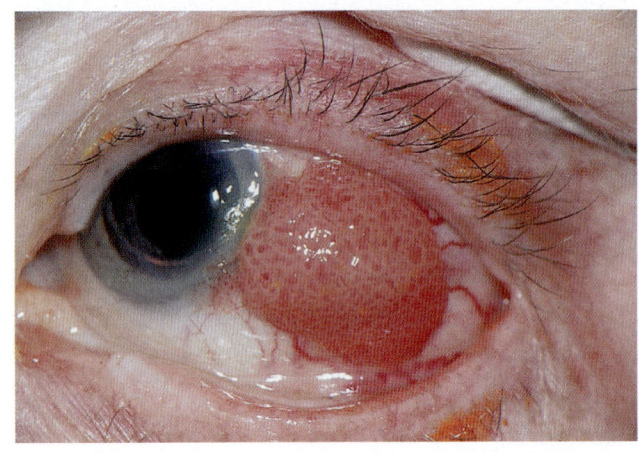

Figure 18.22. Large, pedunculated lesion arising from limbal area and overhanging the cornea in an 85-year-old woman. Histopathologically, the lesion was confined to the epithelium and had not invaded the stroma despite marked elevation.

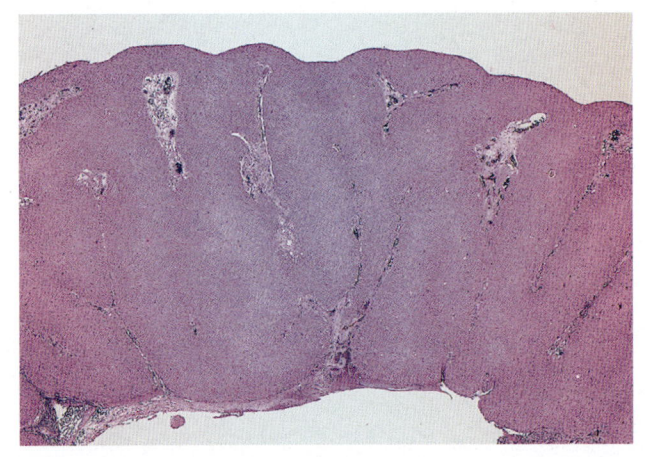

Figure 18.23. Photomicrograph of lesion shown in Figure 18.22. Note the thickened epithelium with the intact basement membrane below. (Hematoxylin–eosin ×15.)

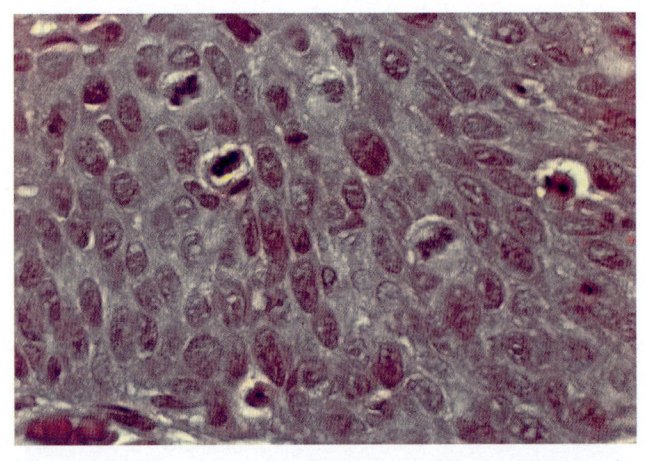

Figure 18.24. Photomicrograph of lesion shown in Figure 18.22. Note the malignant epithelial cells with mitotic activity. (Hematoxylin–eosin ×200.)

Chapter 18 Premalignant and Malignant Lesions of the Conjunctival Epithelium

CONJUNCTIVAL INTRAEPITHELIAL NEOPLASIA: SUPERFICIAL CORNEAL INVASION

Corneal invasion can sometimes be very subtle and is best detected with slit-lamp biomicroscopy. It appears as a translucent gray area at the level of the corneal epithelium. Vascularity may be minimal or absent. It should be carefully mapped, depicted on a large drawing prior to surgical excision or other management. These cases were documented histopathologically to be CIN.

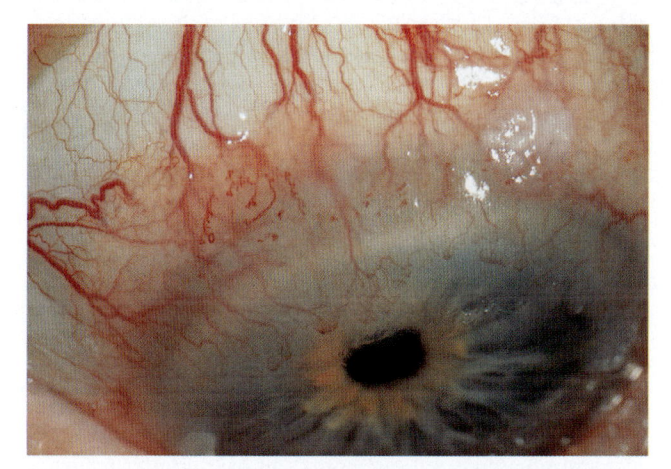

Figure 18.25. Diffuse conjunctival intraepithelial neoplasia with corneal invasion, simulating an inflammatory pannus in a 78-year-old man.

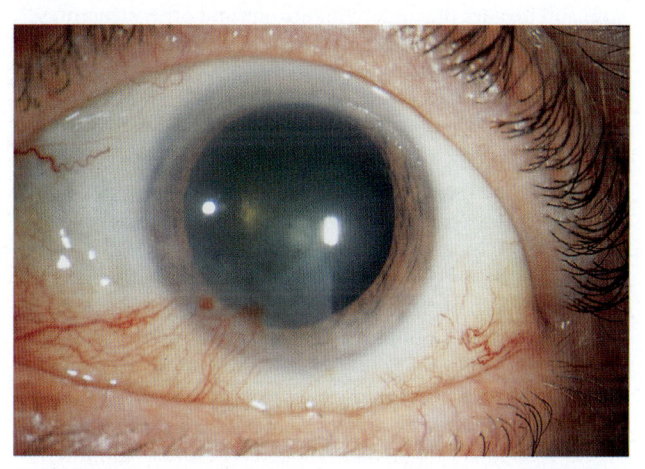

Figure 18.26. Subtle involvement of the inferonasal quadrant of the cornea in a 69-year-old man.

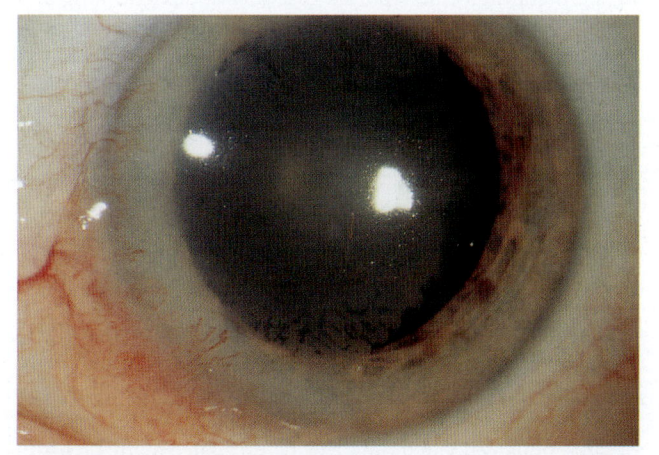

Figure 18.27. Involvement of nasal 70% of cornea with subtle conjunctival intraepithelial neoplasia in a 73-year-old man. Note the fine vertical line to the right separating the abnormal from the normal corneal epithelium.

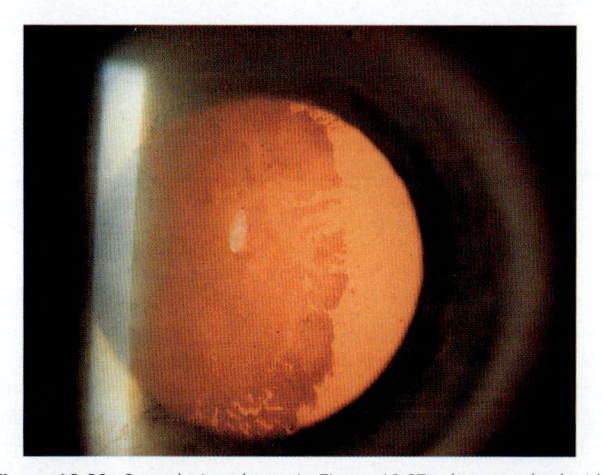

Figure 18.28. Same lesion shown in Figure 18.27, photographed with retroillumination of the anterior segment. Note the irregular border of the progressive corneal involvement.

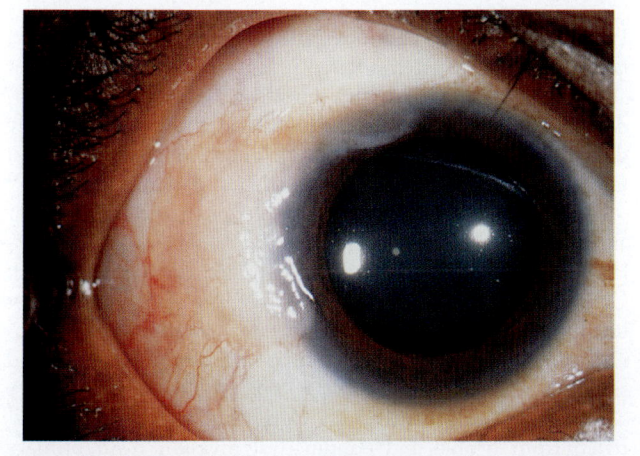

Figure 18.29. Corneal invasion of squamous cell carcinoma in a 60-year-old African-American woman. This condition is considerably less common in dark-skinned individuals.

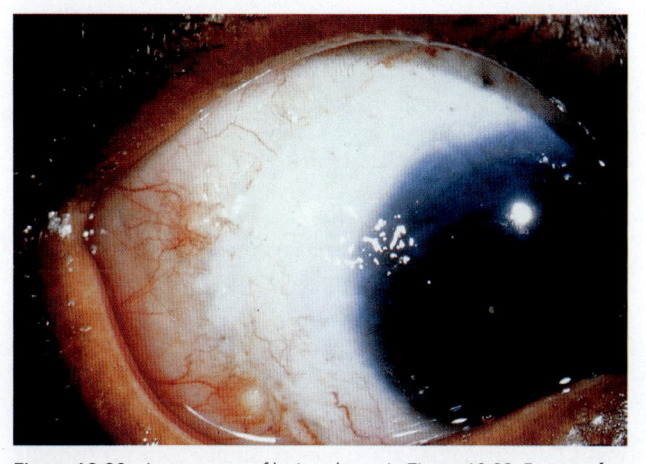

Figure 18.30. Appearance of lesion shown in Figure 18.29, 5 years after surgical resection, showing good result without recurrence.

CONJUNCTIVAL INVASIVE SQUAMOUS CELL CARCINOMA

General Considerations

When CIN breaches the basement membrane of the epithelium and invades the underlying stroma and other structures, it is classified as invasive squamous cell carcinoma, another well-known neoplasm that has received extensive attention in the literature (1–68). The discussion of CIN also applies to invasive squamous cell carcinoma, which is a continuation of the spectrum of the same disease.

Invasive squamous cell carcinoma of the conjunctiva occurs with much less frequency than CIN, with an incidence that varies from 0.02 to 3.5 per 100,000. A rough summary of reported cases suggests that about 75% occur in men, 75% are diagnosed in older patients (>60 years old), and more than 75% occur at the limbus (1,2). It occurs with greater frequency in patients with xeroderma pigmentosum, atopic eczema, and other conditions that predispose to epithelial malignancies. The dysfunction of T lymphocytes seen in these disorders may play a role in the malignant transformation of conjunctival epithelium. Various HPV subtypes have been associated with some tumors (45).

In the authors' clinical series of 1,643 conjunctival tumors, there were 108 cases of invasive squamous cell carcinoma, accounting for 60% of all malignant epithelial tumors and for 7% of the 1,643 lesions (1). The frequency of this condition varies depending on patient age, sun exposure, race, and system immune system.

Clinical Features

The clinical presentation of invasive squamous cell carcinoma is similar to that of CIN and, in many instances, they cannot be differentiated clinically. Like CIN, invasive squamous cell carcinoma is most common in the interpalpebral region of elderly Caucasian men, but can occur in younger individuals, both genders, and all races. It is more aggressive in immunosuppressed patients, particularly those with AIDS. The tumor displays a wide array of clinical appearances and can be a circumscribed, gelatinous, sessile, papillomatous mass with varying amounts of leukoplakia. Large, dilated conjunctival blood vessels frequently feed and drain the mass. Squamous cell carcinoma can be locally invasive into the globe and orbit, but metastasis occurs in less than 1% of patients. However, it can extend locally to cover the cornea and invade the orbit and globe. Intraocular invasion can cause uncontrollable glaucoma that may necessitate enucleation.

Occasionally, squamous cell carcinoma can present as a diffuse, flat, poorly delineated neoplasm without distinct tumefaction. In such cases, it may be confused clinically with conjunctivitis, keratoconjunctivitis, scleritis, or pagetoid invasion of sebaceous carcinoma.

Two less common, but aggressive variations of conjunctival squamous cell carcinoma, the mucoepidermoid (54–63) and spindle cell (64–68) forms, deserve special consideration. These account for fewer than 5% of cases of conjunctival squamous cell carcinoma. These tumors display a greater capacity for aggressive local behavior. They must be differentiated from conventional conjunctival squamous cell carcinoma, which carries a more favorable prognosis.

Mucoepidermoid carcinoma characteristically occurs in elderly individuals, usually over 70 years of age. However, it has been reported to originate in the caruncle and secondarily invade the orbit and paranasal sinuses (58). It is more aggressive than conventional squamous cell carcinoma, with a tendency toward intraocular and orbital invasion. The intraocular component has been known to produce a large intraocular mucinous cyst in the supraubveal space (63). It may have a more yellow, globular, cystic appearance than typical squamous cell carcinoma. It is important to be cognizant of this variant. In some cases, the mucinous component is not apparent in the original specimen, but can be more pronounced in the recurrence. Sometimes, the mucinous cysts are not apparent in the epibulbar tumor, and only the intraocular component shows appreciable mucin production (61,62).

Spindle cell carcinoma tends to be more locally invasive than standard squamous cell carcinoma and has a greater tendency to metastasize (66). Fewer than 20 cases have been reported in the literature. One reported case metastasized to lung and bone; the patient expired 14 months after the original diagnosis (66). The treatment is similar to that of standard squamous cell carcinoma, but wider excision is advisable.

Diagnosis

As with CIN, invasive squamous cell carcinoma is often small and localized enough that primarily complete excision is the most appropriate treatment. An incisional biopsy to establish the diagnosis is not usually indicated unless the tumor is large and diffuse. In such instances, map biopsies, similar to that used for conjunctival involvement of sebaceous carcinoma, may be advisable.

As mentioned in the section on CIN, some authors have advocated impression/exfoliative cytology to establish the diagnosis (46,47). In addition, the depth of limbal invasion of squamous cell carcinoma can be estimated with high-frequency ultrasonography (ultrasound biomicroscopy).

Pathology

Histopathologically, conjunctival squamous cell carcinoma is typically a fairly well-differentiated neoplasm composed of abnormal epithelial cells with mitotic activity and keratin production. Occasionally, a squamous cell carcinoma is very poorly differentiated and shows bizarre, pleomorphic cells, giant cells, numerous mitotic figures, acanthosis, and dyskeratosis.

Mucoepidermoid carcinoma has an epidermoid component and variable quantities of mucin. The cells have clear, vacuolated cytoplasm and eccentric nuclei (signet ring cells) (54–63). Caution should be employed in making the diagnosis; another uncommon condition – benign pseudoadenomatous hyperplasia – may contain abundant mucin-secreting goblet cells and simulate mucoepidermoid carcinoma. In addition, primary conjunctival mucoepidermoid carcinoma must be differentiated from orbital and conjunctival invasion from primary mucoepidermoid carcinoma in the paranasal sinuses.

CONJUNCTIVAL INVASIVE SQUAMOUS CELL CARCINOMA

Spindle cell carcinoma is composed of pleomorphic spindle cells that may be indistinguishable from fibroblasts with light microscopy and may be misdiagnosed as fibrosarcoma. Immunohistochemistry and electron microscopy can be used to confirm the epithelial origin of the cells (64–68).

Classification

The American Joint Committee on Cancer (AJCC) classification for OSSN provides a method to group stages of disease for outcome measurements (Table 18.1).

Management

The initial treatment of invasive squamous cell carcinoma should be similar to that described in the prior section for the less invasive in situ variations. Many cases can be cured by surgical resection, topical chemotherapy, or topical/injection immunotherapy (16–43). However, more advanced cases may require in-depth surgical removal into the orbit or eyelids and with reconstruction.

We prefer complete surgical removal with alcohol corneal epitheliectomy, partial lamellar sclerokeratoconjunctivectomy, and double freeze–thaw cryotherapy to the surrounding conjunctival margins (16). Occasionally, an amniotic membrane graft is necessary for reconstruction of large defects following surgical removal of tumor.

Some of the same supplemental methods used for CIN may also be used for mild forms of invasive squamous cell carcinoma and for minor superficial recurrence after surgical resection. Hence topical mitomycin C, 5-fluorouracil, interferon *alpha*-2b (particularly for recurrent or persistent cases), and cidofovir, can be attempted in selected cases (21–35). Our favored nonsurgical approach is with topical interferon for immunotherapy (complete primary treatment), immunoreduction (reduction of giant squamous cell carcinoma to allow smaller surgical resection), or immunoprevention (following surgery where margins were equivocal to prevent recurrence) (29–32,34). Similarly, mitomycin C and 5-fluorouracil can be effective, but these chemotherapy agents can lead to complications, particularly limbal stem cell deficiency.

Multiple local recurrences can be a problem with management of conjunctival squamous cell carcinoma, because of conjunctival scarring from surgical procedures. In cases with local recurrence, we have often employed techniques of custom-designed plaque radiotherapy for invasive tumors with success in globe salvage (15,38).

Table 18.1 American Joint Committee on Cancer (AJCC) classification of ocular surface squamous neoplasia

Clinical stage	Definition
Primary tumor (T)	
TX	Tumor cannot be assessed
T0	Tumor absent
Tis	Tumor present as carcinoma in situ/conjunctival intraepithelial neoplasia
T1	Tumor present with largest basal diameter ≤5 mm
T2	Tumor present with largest basal diameter >5 mm, no invasion of adjacent structures[a]
T3	Tumor invades adjacent structures excluding the orbit
T4	Tumor invades the orbit with or without further extension
T4a	Tumor invades orbital soft tissues, without bone invasion
T4b	Tumor invades bone
T4c	Tumor invades adjacent paranasal sinuses
T4d	Tumor invades brain
Regional lymph nodes (N)	
NX	Regional lymph nodes cannot be assessed
N0	Regional lymph node metastasis absent
N1	Regional lymph node metastasis present
Distant metastasis (M)	
Mx	Distant metastasis cannot be assessed
M0	Distant metastasis present
M1	Distant metastasis present

[a]Adjacent structures include cornea, forniceal conjunctiva, palpebral conjunctiva, tarsal conjunctiva, intraocular compartments, caruncle, lacrimal punctum and canaliculi, plica, anterior or posterior eyelid lamellae, and/or eyelid margin.
mm, millimeters.
From Edge SB, Byrd DR, Compton CC, et al., eds. Carcinoma of the conjunctiva. In: *AJCC Cancer Staging Manual*. 7th ed. New York: Springer; 2010:531–537.

The management of more advanced disease may require more aggressive treatment, because extensive invasion can lead to blindness or death. For small degrees of orbital invasion into the anterior orbital tissues, local resection and/or irradiation may be warranted. Plaque brachytherapy is an option to control small gross or microscopic residual tumor. More extensive orbital invasion usually requires orbital exenteration. An eyelid-sparing exenteration can be performed in most cases of orbital extension of conjunctival squamous cell carcinoma (43).

Intraocular invasion of conjunctival squamous cell carcinoma is notorious for simulating anterior uveitis, often resulting in a delay in diagnosis (15,52). Any patient who has a history of excision of conjunctival squamous cell carcinoma who develops "uveitis" and elevated intraocular pressure should be considered to have intraocular invasion of the tumor until proven otherwise. If the intraocular invasion is diffuse, modified enucleation should be done, removing the involved conjunctiva along with the globe. On rare occasions, when the intraocular component is circumscribed without seeding, local eye wall resection can be employed (68).

Prognosis

Overall, the prognosis for conjunctival squamous cell carcinoma is quite good. With the modern techniques described, the local recurrence rate is about 5% and regional lymph node metastasis is only about 1% to 2% (4,34). As mentioned, the prognosis seems to be worse in patients with mucoepidermoid or spindle cell variants and in patients who are immunosuppressed, particularly those with AIDS.

Selected References

Reviews

1. Shields CL, Demirci H, Karatza E, et al. Clinical survey of 1643 melanocytic and nonmelanocytic tumors of the conjunctiva. *Ophthalmology* 2004;111:1747–1754.
2. Shields CL, Shields JA. Tumors of the conjunctiva and cornea. *Surv Ophthalmol* 2004;49:3–24.
3. Grossniklaus HE, Green WR, Luckenbach M, et al. Conjunctival lesions in adults. A clinical and histopathologic review. *Cornea* 1987;6:78–116.
4. Erie JC, Campbell RF, Liesegang TJ. Conjunctival and corneal intraepithelial and invasive neoplasia. *Ophthalmology* 1986;93:176–183.
5. Lee GA, Hirst LW. Ocular surface squamous neoplasia. *Surv Ophthalmol* 1995;39:429–450.
6. Tunc M, Char DH, Crawford B, et al. Intraepithelial and invasive squamous cell carcinoma of the conjunctiva: analysis of 60 cases. *Br J Ophthalmol* 1999;83:98–103.
7. Shields CL, Manchandia A, Subbiah R, et al. Pigmented squamous cell carcinoma in situ of the conjunctiva in 5 cases. *Ophthalmology* 2008;115(10):1673–1678.
8. Shields CL, Ramasubramanian A, Mellen P, et al. Conjunctival squamous cell carcinoma arising in immunosuppressed patients (organ transplant, human immunodeficiency virus infection). *Ophthalmology* 2011;118:2133–2137.
9. Yousef YA, Finger PT. Squamous carcinoma and dysplasia of the conjunctiva and cornea: an analysis of 101 cases. *Ophthalmology* 2012;119(2):233–240.
10. Cervantes G, Rodriguez AA Jr, Leal AG. Squamous cell carcinoma of the conjunctiva: clinicopathological features in 287 cases. *Can J Ophthalmol* 2002;37:14–19.
11. McKelvie PA, Daniell M, McNab A, et al. Squamous cell carcinoma of the conjunctiva: a series of 26 cases. *Br J Ophthalmol* 2002;86:168–173.
12. Tulvatana W, Bhattarakosol P, Sansopha L, et al. Risk factors for conjunctival squamous cell neoplasia: a matched case-control study. *Br J Ophthalmol* 2003;87:396–398.
13. Lee SB, Au Eong KG, Saw SM, et al. Eye cancer incidence in Singapore. *Br J Ophthalmol* 2000;84:767–770.
14. Heinz C, Fanihagh F, Steuhl KP. Squamous cell carcinoma of the conjunctiva in patients with atopic eczema. *Cornea* 2003;22:135–137.
15. Shields JA, Shields CL, Gunduz K, et al. Intraocular invasion of squamous cell carcinoma of the conjunctiva in five patients. The 1998 Pan American Lecture. *Ophthalmic Plast Reconstr Surg* 1999;15:153–160.

Management/Surgery

16. Shields JA, Shields CL, De Potter P. Surgical approach to conjunctival tumors. The 1994 Lynn B. McMahan Lecture. *Arch Ophthalmol* 1997;115:808–815.
17. Tabin G, Levin S, Snibson G, et al. Later recurrences and necessity for long-term follow-up in corneal and conjunctival intraepithelial neoplasia. *Ophthalmology* 1997;104:485–492.
18. Zaki AA, Farid SF. Management of intraepithelial and invasive neoplasia of the cornea and conjunctiva: a long-term follow up. *Cornea* 2009;28(9):986–988.
19. Nanji AA, Moon CS, Galor A, et al. Surgical versus medical treatment of ocular surface squamous neoplasia: a comparison of recurrences and complications. *Ophthalmology* 2014;121:994–1000.
20. Peksayar G, Altan-Yaycioglu R, Onal S. Excision and cryosurgery in the treatment of conjunctival malignant epithelial tumours. *Eye* 2003;17:228–232.

Mitomycin C

21. Frucht-Pery J, Rozenman Y. Mitomycin C therapy for corneal intraepithelial neoplasia. *Am J Ophthalmol* 1994;117:164–168.
22. Frucht-Pery J, Rozenman Y, Pe'er J. Topical mitomycin-C for partially excised conjunctival squamous cell carcinoma. *Ophthalmology* 2002;109:548–552.
23. Shields CL, Naseripour M, Shields JA. Topical mitomycin C for extensive, recurrent conjunctival squamous cell carcinoma. *Am J Ophthalmol* 2002;133:601–606.
24. Shields CL, Demirci H, Marr BP, et al. Chemoreduction with topical mitomycin C prior to resection of extensive squamous cell carcinoma of the conjunctiva. *Arch Ophthalmol* 2005;123:109–113.

5-Fluorouracil

25. Yeatts RP, Ford JG, Stanton CA, et al. Topical 5-fluorouracil in treating epithelial neoplasia of the conjunctiva and cornea. *Ophthalmology* 1995;102:1338–1344.
26. Yeatts RP, Engelbrecht NE, Curry CD, et al. 5-Fluorouracil for the treatment of intraepithelial neoplasia of the conjunctiva and cornea. *Ophthalmology* 2000;107:2190–2195.
27. Midena E, Angeli CD, Valenti M, et al. Treatment of conjunctival squamous cell carcinoma with topical 5-fluorouracil. *Br J Ophthalmol* 2000;84:268–272.

Interferon

28. Giaconi JA, Karp CL. Current treatment options for conjunctival and corneal intraepithelial neoplasia. *Ocul Surf* 2003;1:667–673.
29. Karp CL, Galor A, Chhabra S, et al. Subconjunctival/perilesional recombinant interferon α2b for ocular surface squamous neoplasia: a 10-year review. *Ophthalmology* 2010;117(12):2241–2246.
30. Shields CL, Kancherla S, Bianciotto CG, et al. Ocular surface squamous neoplasia (squamous cell carcinoma) of the socket: management of extensive tumors with interferon. *Ophthal Plast Reconstr Surg* 2011;27:247–250.
31. Shah S, Kaliki S, Kim HJ, et al. Topical interferon alpha 2b for management of ocular surface squamous neoplasia in 23 cases: outcomes based on American Joint Committee on Cancer (AJCC) classification. *Arch Ophthalmol* 2012;130:159–164.
32. Kim HJ, Shields CL, Shah SU, et al. Giant ocular surface squamous neoplasia managed with interferon alpha-2b as immunotherapy or immunoreduction. *Ophthalmology* 2012;119:938–944.
33. Nanji AA, Sayyad FE, Karp CL. Topical chemotherapy for ocular surface squamous neoplasia. *Curr Opin Ophthalmol* 2013;24(4):336–342.
34. Shields CL, Kaliki S, Kim HJ, et al. Interferon for ocular surface squamous neoplasia in 81 cases: outcomes based on the American Joint Committee on Cancer classification. *Cornea* 2013;32(3):248–256.
35. Besley J, Pappalardo J, Lee GA, et al. Risk factors for ocular surface squamous neoplasia recurrence after treatment with topical mitomycin C and interferon alpha-2b. *Am J Ophthalmol* 2014;157:287–293.

Radiotherapy

36. Lommatzsch P. Beta-ray treatment of malignant epithelial tumors of the conjunctiva. *Am J Ophthalmol* 1976;81:198–206.
37. Walsh-Conway N, Conway RM. Plaque brachytherapy for the management of ocular surface malignancies with corneoscleral invasion. *Clin Experiment Ophthalmol* 2009;37(6):577–583.
38. Arepalli S, Kaliki S, Shields CL, et al. Plaque radiotherapy for scleral-invasive conjunctival squamous cell carcinoma: analysis of 15 eyes. *JAMA Ophthalmol* 2014;132:691–696.

Others

39. Sherman MD, Feldman KA, Farahmand SM, et al. Treatment of conjunctival squamous cell carcinoma with topical cidofovir. *Am J Ophthalmol* 2002;134:432–433.
40. Finger PT, Chin KJ. Refractory squamous cell carcinoma of the conjunctiva treated with subconjunctival ranibizumab (Lucentis): a two-year study. *Ophthal Plast Reconstr Surg* 2012;28(2):85–89.
41. Damani MR, Shah AR, Karp CL, et al. Treatment of ocular surface squamous neoplasia with topical aloe vera drops. *Cornea* 2014;15(1):87–89.
42. Maalouf TJ, Dolivet G, Angioi KS, et al. Sentinel lymph node biopsy in patients with conjunctival and eyelid cancers: experience in 17 patients. *Ophthal Plast Reconstr Surg* 2012;28(1):30–34.
43. Shields JA, Shields CL, Demirci H, et al. Experience with eyelid-sparing orbital exenteration. The 2000 Tullos O. Coston Lecture. *Ophthal Plast Reconstr Surg* 2001;17:355–361.

Histopathology/Cytopathology/Infectious Disease

44. Grossniklaus HE, Stulting RD, Gansler T, et al. Aspiration cytology of the conjunctival surface. *Acta Cytol* 2003;47:239–246.
45. McDonnell JM, Mayr AJ, Martin WG. DNA of human papillomavirus type 26 in dysplastic and malignant lesions of the conjunctiva and cornea. *N Engl J Med* 1989;320:1442–1446.
46. Semenova EA, Milman T, Finger PT, et al. The diagnostic value of exfoliative cytology vs histopathology for ocular surface squamous neoplasia. *Am J Ophthalmol* 2009;148(5):772–778.
47. Spinak M, Friedman AH. Squamous cell carcinoma of the conjunctiva. Value of exfoliative cytology in diagnosis. *Surv Ophthalmol* 1977;21:351–355.
48. Aoki S, Kubo E, Nakamura S, et al. Possible prognostic markers in conjunctival dysplasia and squamous cell carcinoma. *Jpn J Ophthalmol* 1998;42:256–261.

Case Reports

49. Mahmood MA, Al-Rajhi A, Riley F, et al. Sclerokeratitis: an unusual presentation of squamous cell carcinoma of the conjunctiva. *Ophthalmology* 2001;108:553–558.
50. Cha SB, Shields CL, Shields JA, et al. Massive precorneal extension of squamous cell carcinoma of the conjunctiva. *Cornea* 1993;12:537–540.
51. Panda A, Sharma N, Sen S. Massive corneal and conjunctival squamous cell carcinoma. *Ophthalmic Surg Lasers* 2000;31:71–72.
52. Nicholson DH, Herschler J. Intraocular extension of squamous cell carcinoma of the conjunctiva. *Arch Ophthalmol* 1977;95:843–846.
53. Johnson TE, Tabbara KF, Weatherhead RG, et al. Secondary squamous cell carcinoma of the orbit. *Arch Ophthalmol* 1997;115:75–78.
54. Rao NA, Font RL. Mucoepidermoid carcinoma of the conjunctiva: a clinicopathologic study of five cases. *Cancer* 1976;38:1699–1709.
55. Hwang IP, Jordan DR, Brownstein S, et al. Mucoepidermoid carcinoma of the conjunctiva: a series of three cases. *Ophthalmology* 2000;107:801–805.
56. Biswas J, Datta M, Subramaniam N. Mucoepidermoid carcinoma of the conjunctiva of the lower lid—report of a case. *Indian J Ophthalmol* 1996;44:231–233.
57. Carrau RL, Stillman E, Canaan RE. Mucoepidermoid carcinoma of the conjunctiva. *Ophthal Plast Reconstr Surg* 1994;10:163–168.
58. Margo CE, Weitzenkorn DE. Mucoepidermoid carcinoma of the conjunctiva: report of a case in a 36-year-old with paranasal sinus invasion. *Ophthalmic Surg* 1986;17:151–154.
59. Gamel JW, Eiferman RA, Guibor P. Mucoepidermoid carcinoma of the conjunctiva. *Arch Ophthalmol* 1984;102:730–731.
60. Hwang IP, Jordan DR, Brownstein S, et al. Mucoepidermoid carcinoma of the conjunctiva: a series of three cases. *Ophthalmology* 2000;107:801–805.
61. Searl SS, Krigstein HJ, Albert DM, et al. Invasive squamous cell carcinoma with intraocular mucoepidermoid features. Conjunctival carcinoma with intraocular invasion and diphasic morphology. *Arch Ophthalmol* 1982;100:109–111.
62. Brownstein S. Mucoepidermoid carcinoma of the conjunctiva with intraocular invasion. *Ophthalmology* 1981;88:1126–1130.
63. Gunduz K, Shields CL, Shields JA, et al. Intraocular neoplastic cyst from mucoepidermoid carcinoma of the conjunctiva. *Arch Ophthalmol* 1998;116:1521–1523.
64. Cohen BH, Green R, Iliff NT, et al. Spindle cell carcinoma of the conjunctiva. *Arch Ophthalmol* 1980;98:1809–1813.
65. Ni C, Guo BK. Histological types of spindle cell carcinoma of the cornea and the conjunctiva. *Chin Med J* 1990;103:915.
66. Seregard S, Kock E. Squamous spindle cell carcinoma of the conjunctiva; fatal outcome of a pterygium-like lesion. *Acta Ophthalmol Scand* 1995;73:464–466.
67. Schubert HD, Farris RL, Green WR. Spindle cell carcinoma of the conjunctiva. *Graefes Arch Clin Exp Ophthalmol* 1995;233:52–53.
68. Shields JA, Eagle RC, Grossniklaus H, et al. Invasive spindle cell carcinoma of the conjunctiva managed by full thickness eye wall resection. *Cornea* 2007;26:1014–1016.

CONJUNCTIVAL SQUAMOUS CELL CARCINOMA: SUNLIGHT EXPOSURE

Examples are illustrated.

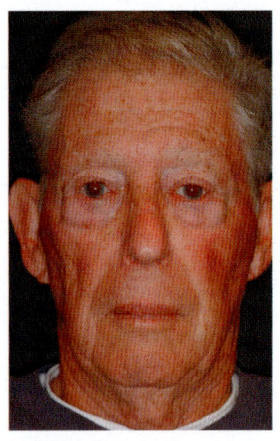

Figure 18.31. Facial appearance of elderly man showing slight rosacea of skin and actinic changes.

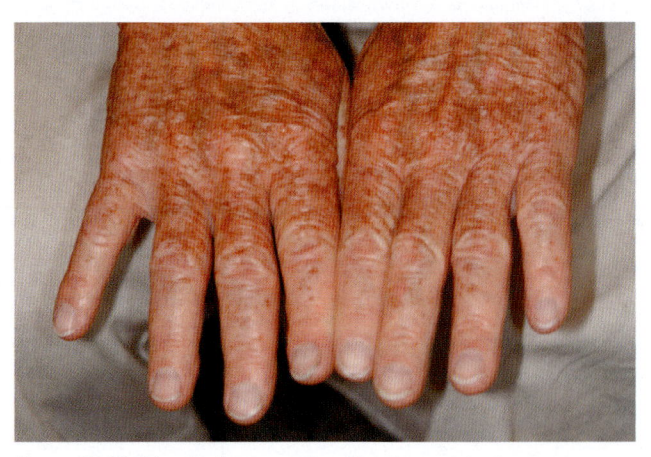

Figure 18.32. Hands of same patient showing actinic changes.

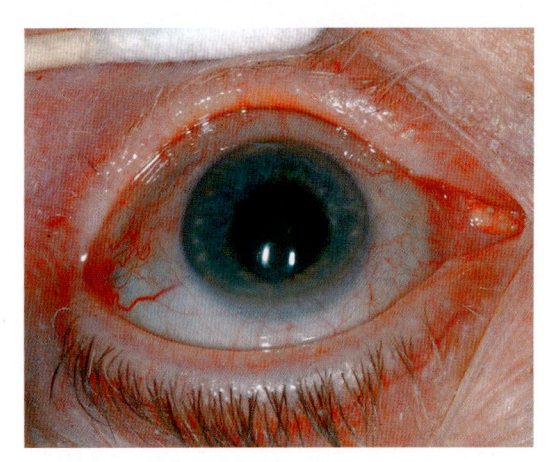

Figure 18.33. Close-up of right eye of same patient, showing small temporal pinguecula, also a result of sun exposure.

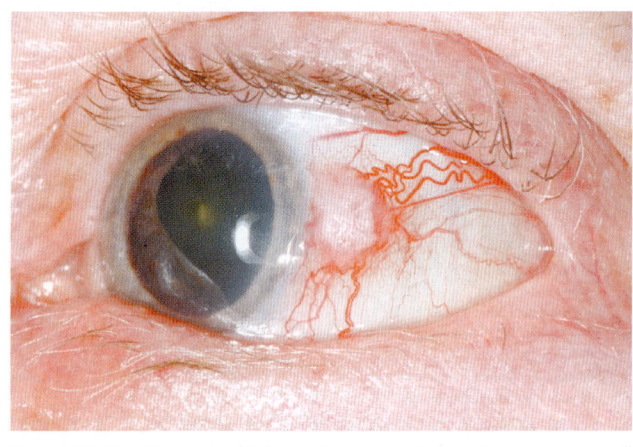

Figure 18.34. Close-up of left eye showing early invasive squamous cell carcinoma. The diagnosis was confirmed histopathologically.

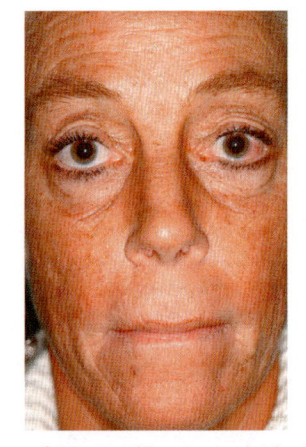

Figure 18.35. Face of 40-year-old woman who had a long history of sun exposure.

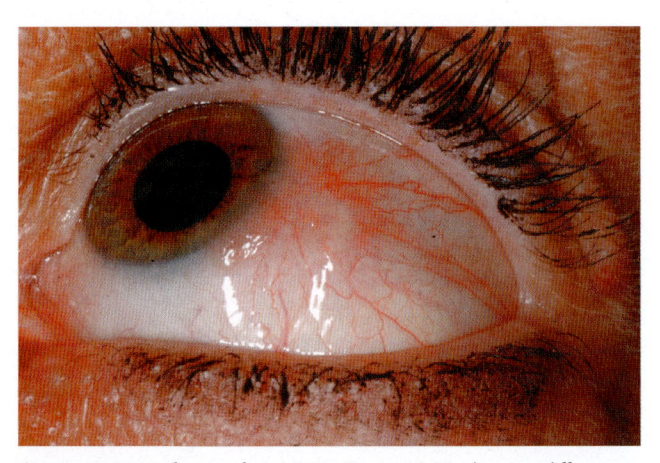

Figure 18.36. Left eye of patient in Figure 18.35, showing diffuse sessile squamous cell carcinoma of conjunctiva.

Chapter 18 Premalignant and Malignant Lesions of the Conjunctival Epithelium

CONJUNCTIVAL SQUAMOUS CELL CARCINOMA: EARLY INVASIVE TYPE

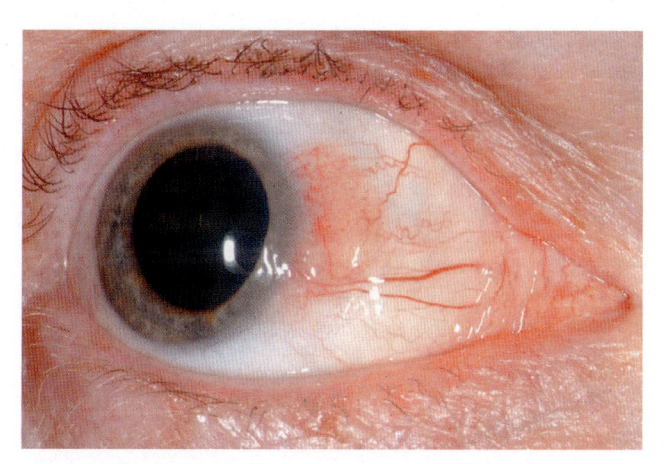

Figure 18.37. Sessile papillomatous squamous cell carcinoma at nasal limbus in elderly patient. Note the slight corneal invasion and the feeder vessels.

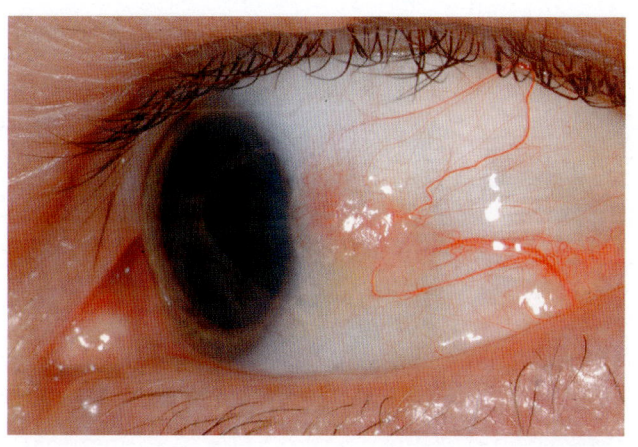

Figure 18.38. Sessile gelatinous squamous cell carcinoma at nasal limbus in elderly patient. There is slight corneal involvement and feeder vessels similar to those shown in Figure 18.37.

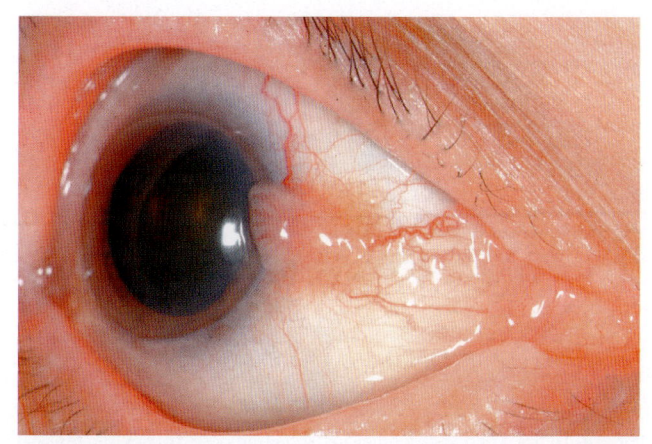

Figure 18.39. Slightly more elevated squamous cell carcinoma with early corneal invasion.

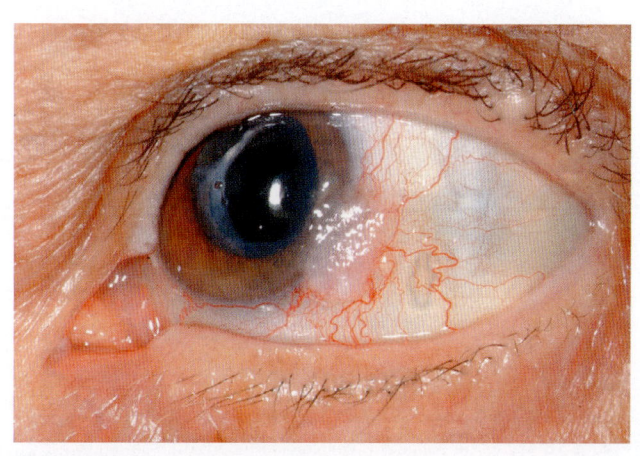

Figure 18.40. Squamous cell carcinoma with leukoplakia in elderly patient who had prior cataract surgery. Note the markedly dilated blood vessels that supply and drain the lesion.

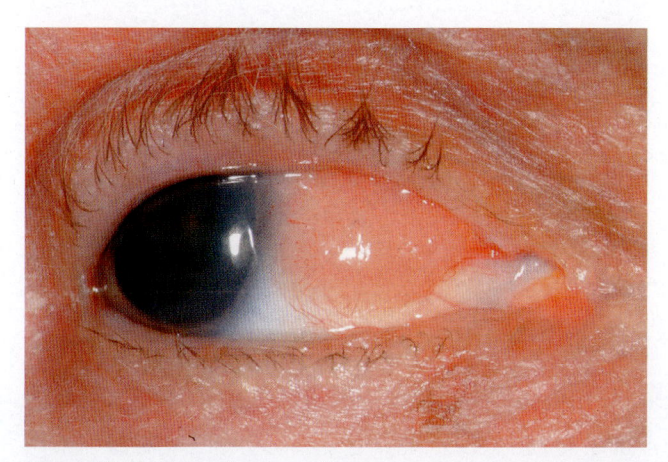

Figure 18.41. Larger fleshy, papillomatous squamous cell carcinoma touching limbus in nasal conjunctiva.

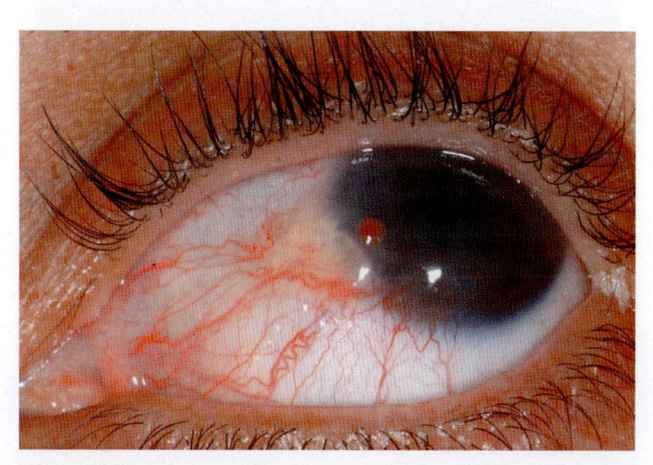

Figure 18.42. Invasive squamous cell carcinoma in a patient with AIDS.

CONJUNCTIVAL SQUAMOUS CELL CARCINOMA: ADVANCED INVASIVE TYPE

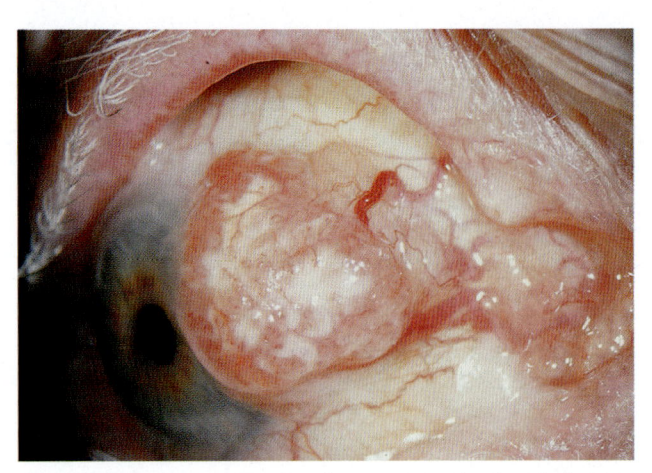

Figure 18.43. Large squamous cell carcinoma arising from limbus in a 75-year-old man.

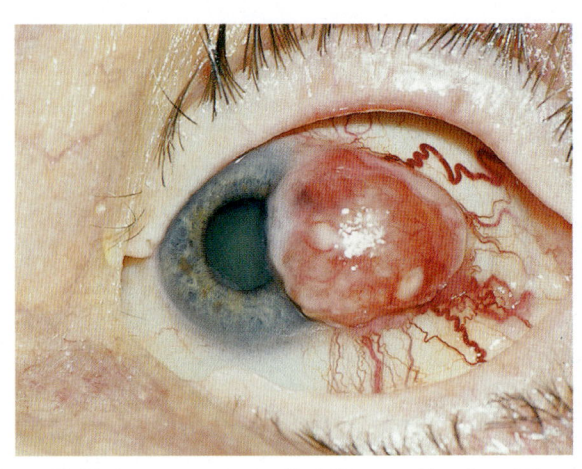

Figure 18.44. Large squamous cell carcinoma arising from limbus in a 74-year-old woman.

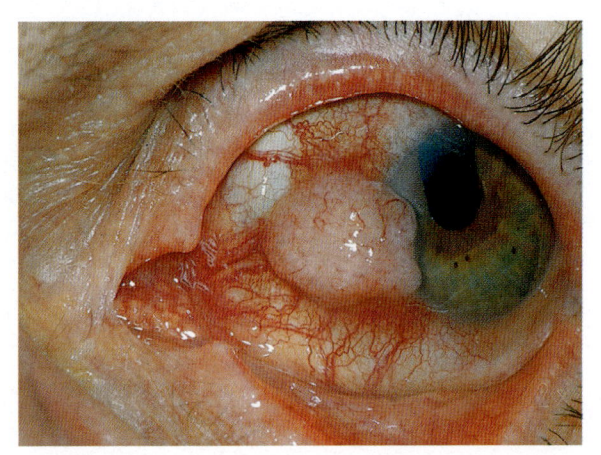

Figure 18.45. Large squamous cell carcinoma arising from limbus in an 83-year-old man who had prior cataract surgery. The tumor can sometimes grow through a surgical wound and lead to intraocular involvement.

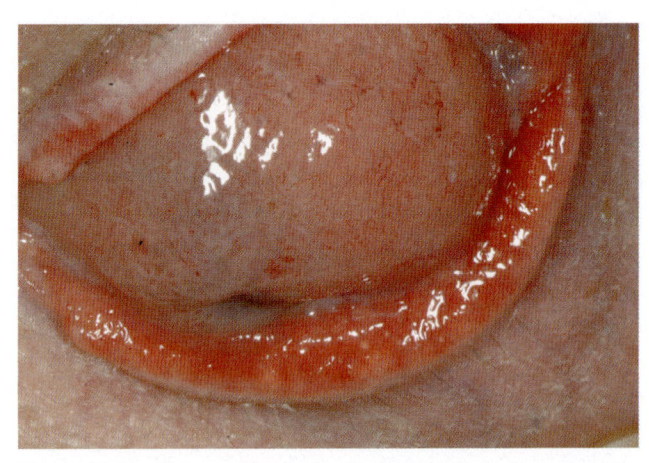

Figure 18.46. Giant papillomatous squamous cell carcinoma causing chronic mucous discharge in an 88-year-old man.

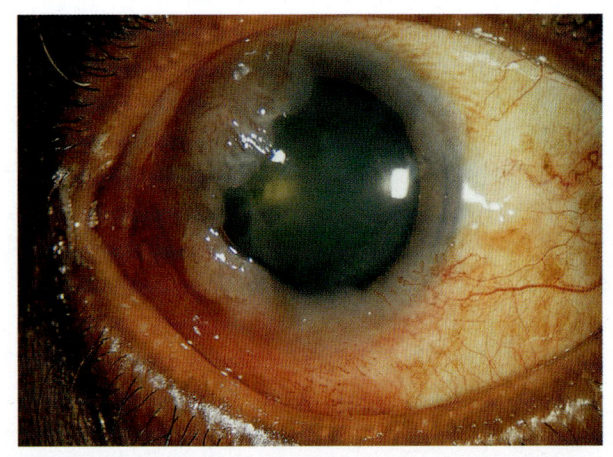

Figure 18.47. Squamous cell carcinoma assuming a ring growth pattern at the limbus in a 61-year-old African-American woman. Histopathologically, the lesion was mostly in the epithelium with minimal stromal invasion.

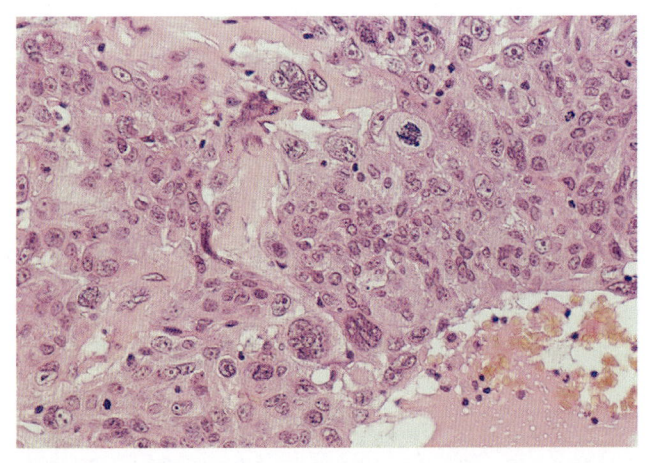

Figure 18.48. Histopathology of squamous cell carcinoma showing anaplastic squamous cells. (Hematoxylin–eosin ×250.)

CONJUNCTIVAL SQUAMOUS CELL CARCINOMA: INVOLVEMENT OF TARSAL CONJUNCTIVA

It is important to evert the eyelid in patients with conjunctival squamous cell carcinoma to detect involvement of palpebral conjunctiva.

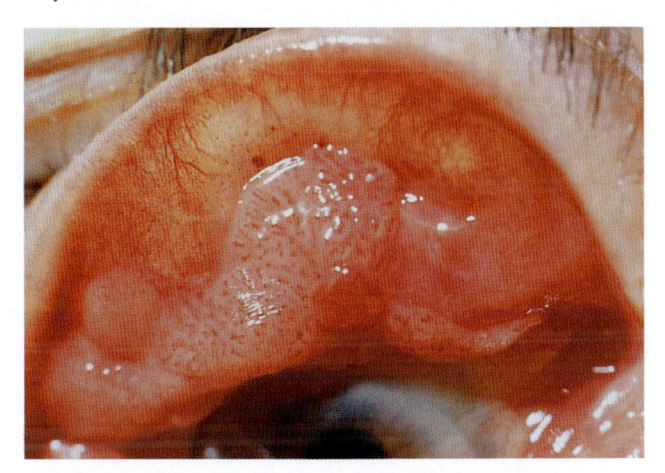

Figure 18.49. Multinodular squamous cell carcinoma arising from superior palpebral conjunctiva in a 71-year-old man.

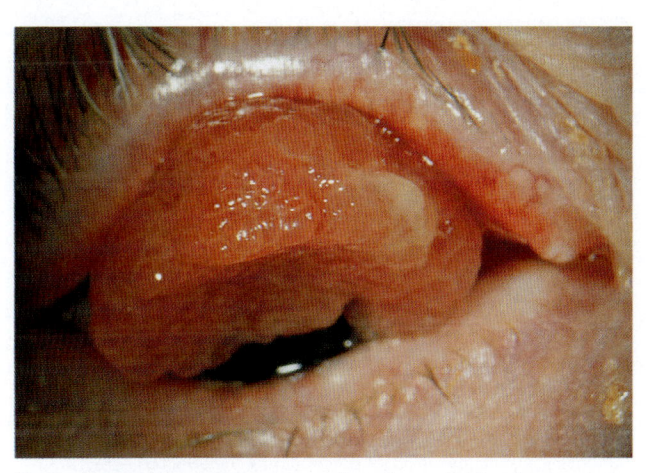

Figure 18.50. Massive squamous cell carcinoma arising from superior palpebral conjunctiva and conforming to the opposing corneal surface in an 87-year-old man.

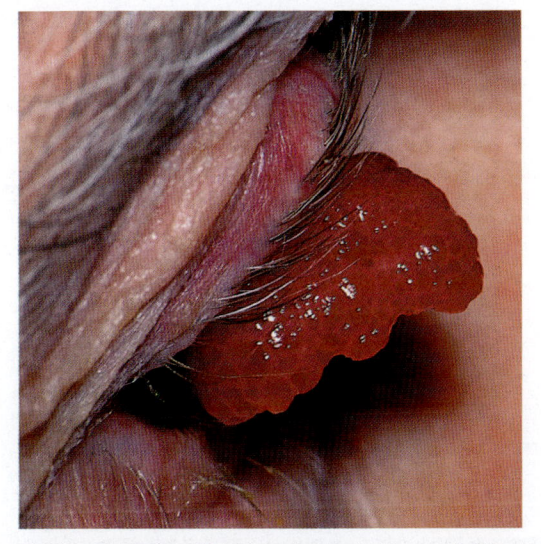

Figure 18.51. Side view of lesion shown in Figure 18.50 showing pedunculated configuration of lesion.

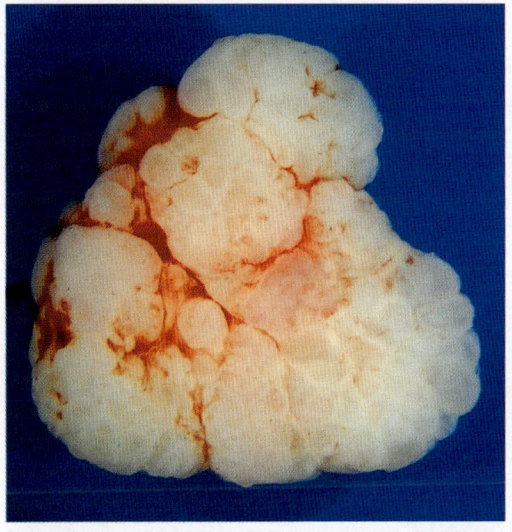

Figure 18.52. Gross appearance of lesion shown in Figure 18.50 after excision and mucous membrane graft.

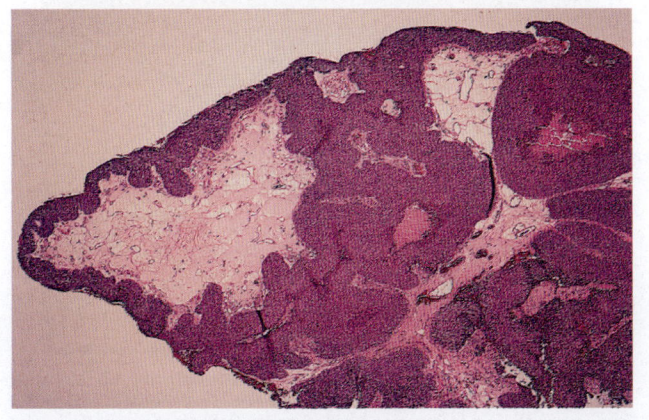

Figure 18.53. Histopathology of lesion shown in Figure 18.50 showing invasive cords of malignant epithelial cells. Despite the large size of the lesion, most of the tumor remained intraepithelial, with only moderate stromal invasion. (Hematoxylin–eosin ×5.)

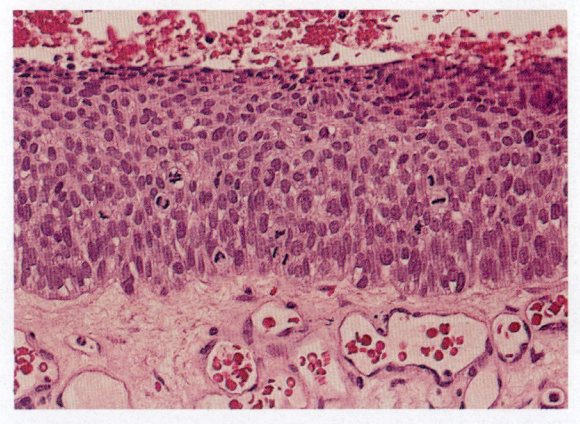

Figure 18.54. Photomicrograph of lesion shown in Figure 18.50 showing area of intraepithelial involvement with intact basement membrane. (Hematoxylin–eosin ×75.)

CONJUNCTIVAL SQUAMOUS CELL CARCINOMA: EXTENSIVE PAPILLOMATOUS CORNEAL INVOLVEMENT

In some cases, a conjunctival squamous cell carcinoma can extend to cover the entire corneal surface. An example in a 73-year-old man is shown.

Cha SB, Shields CL, Shields JA, et al. Massive precorneal extension of squamous cell carcinoma of the conjunctiva. *Cornea* 1993;12:537–540.

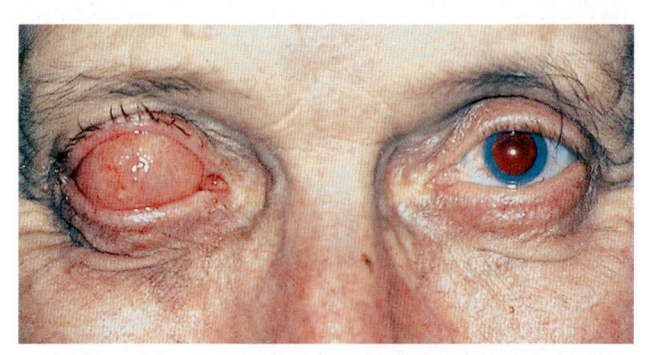

Figure 18.55. Appearance of lesion filling the palpebral aperture. The patient's visual acuity was light perception in the affected eye.

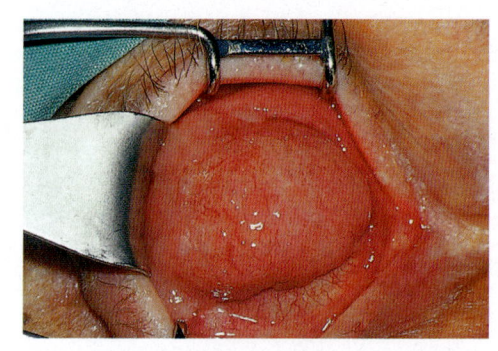

Figure 18.56. Close view of lesion showing papilloma-like mass.

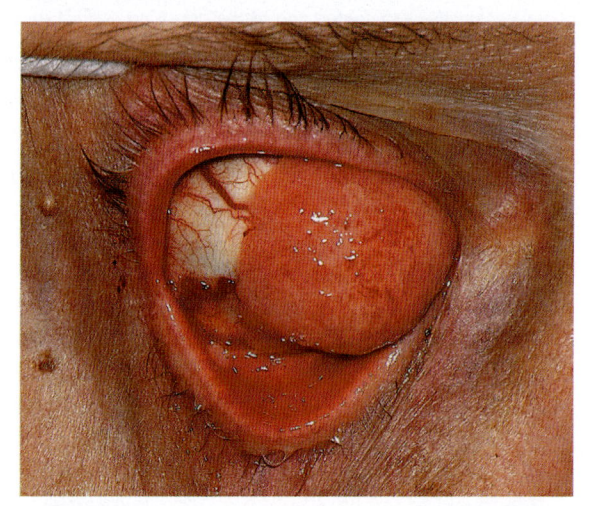

Figure 18.57. The peripheral portion of the bulbar conjunctiva is not involved with tumor, suggesting that the lesion arose from the limbus. Note the dilated feeder blood vessels.

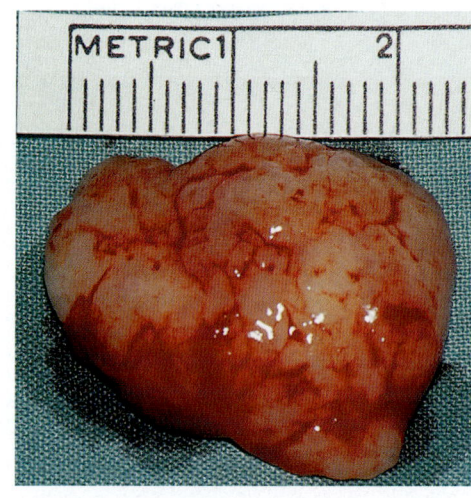

Figure 18.58. Gross appearance of lesion after resection.

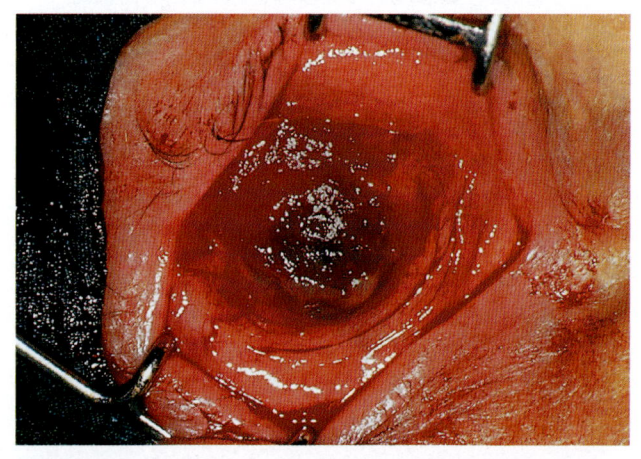

Figure 18.59. Appearance immediately after tumor removal, showing hemorrhagic pseudomembrane on corneal surface. This was easily dissected from the cornea.

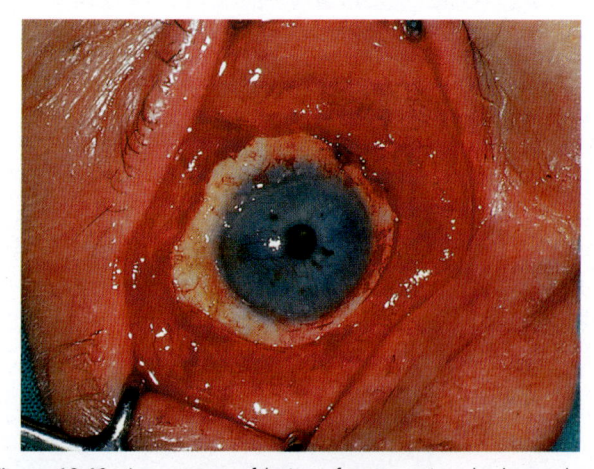

Figure 18.60. Appearance of lesion after removing the hemorrhagic pseudomembrane showing clear cornea. His vision was 20/30 1 day after surgery. This lesion also proved to be largely intraepithelial, with only moderate stromal invasion by the tumor.

Chapter 18 Premalignant and Malignant Lesions of the Conjunctival Epithelium

CONJUNCTIVAL SQUAMOUS CELL CARCINOMA: ATYPICAL VARIATIONS

Shields CL, Manchandia A, Subbiah R, et al. Pigmented squamous cell carcinoma in situ of the conjunctiva in 5 cases. *Ophthalmology* 2008;115(10):1673–1678.

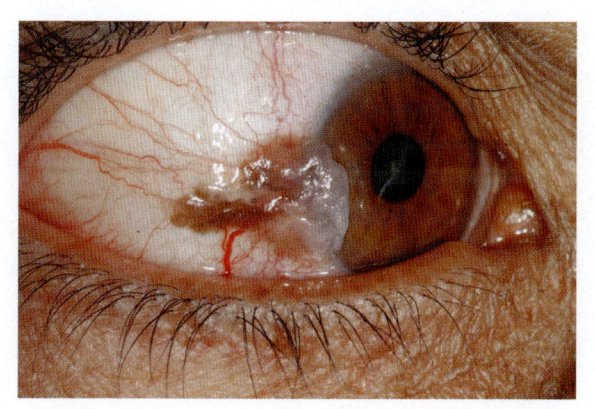

Figure 18.61. Pigmented and leukoplakic papillomatous squamous cell carcinoma in a Hispanic man.

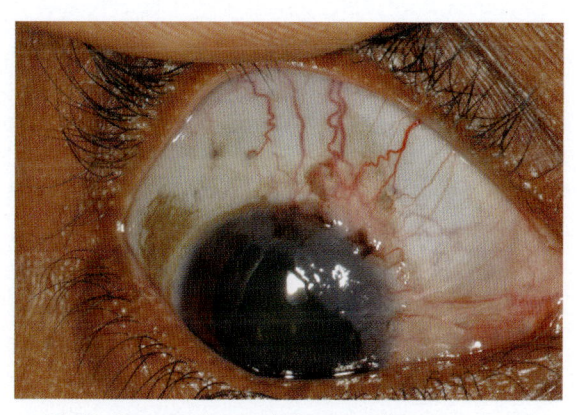

Figure 18.62. Pigmented and gelatinous papillomatous squamous cell carcinoma in a 43-year-old African-American woman. Note the adjacent conjunctival complexion-related melanosis.

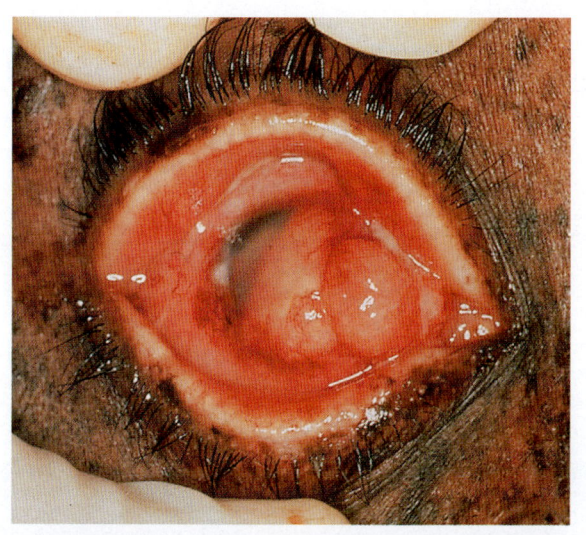

Figure 18.63. Large squamous cell carcinoma of conjunctiva in a 16-year-old South African male with xeroderma pigmentosum. (Courtesy of David Sevel.)

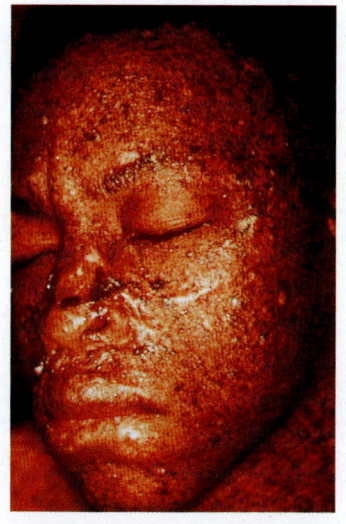

Figure 18.64. Face of patient shown in Figure 18.63. Note the numerous cutaneous tumors consistent with xeroderma pigmentosum. (Courtesy of David Sevel.)

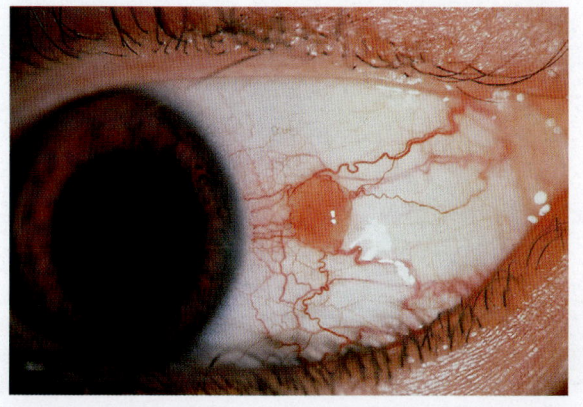

Figure 18.65. Spindle cell carcinoma of conjunctiva appearing as a reddish mass in the bulbar conjunctiva of a 30-year-old woman. (Courtesy of Hermann Schubert, MD.)

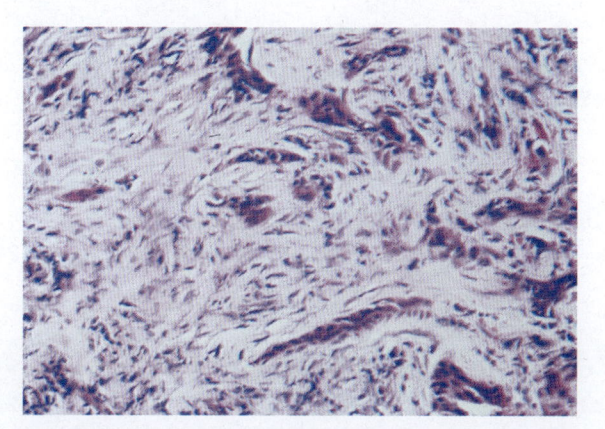

Figure 18.66. Histopathology of lesion shown in Figure 18.65 showing spindle cells invading the stroma. The lesion showed connection to the epithelium in other sections and immunohistochemical studies confirmed the epithelial derivation of the neoplasm. (Hematoxylin–eosin ×150.) (Courtesy of Hermann Schubert, MD.)

CONJUNCTIVAL SPINDLE CELL CARCINOMA: EN BLOC EYE WALL RESECTION

Shields JA, Eagle RC, Grossniklaus H, et al. Invasive spindle cell carcinoma of the conjunctiva managed by full-thickness eye wall resection. *Cornea* 2007;26:1014–6.

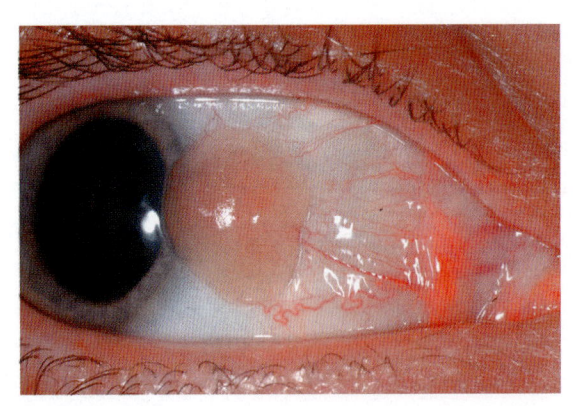

Figure 18.67. Clinical appearance of mass in nasal conjunctiva of right eye. The lesion shown here is a recurrence after prior excision elsewhere and diagnosis of spindle cell carcinoma of the conjunctiva was made.

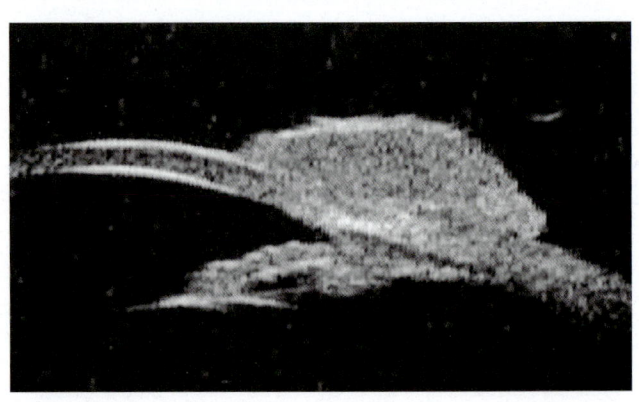

Figure 18.68. Ultrasound biomicroscopy revealing epibulbar limbal mass with extension through peripheral cornea to Descemet's membrane.

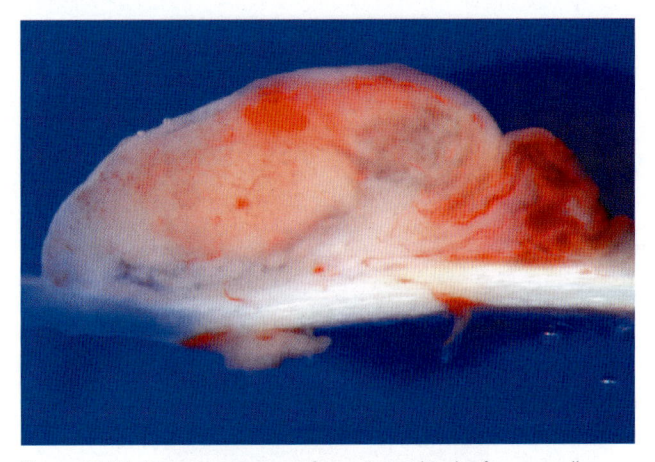

Figure 18.69. Gross appearance of mass immediately after eye wall resection showing well-defined mass with deep invasion through the limbus.

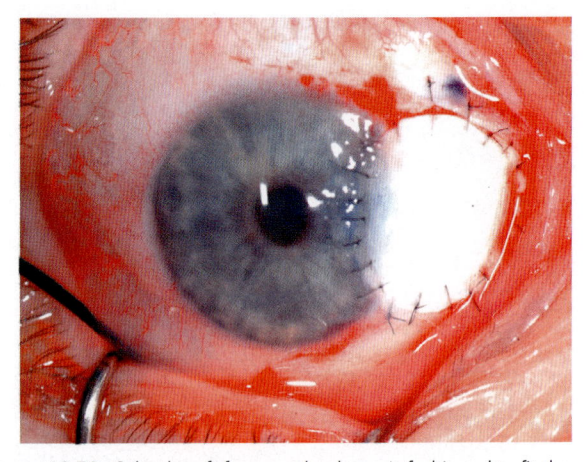

Figure 18.70. Scleral graft from eye bank eye is fashioned to fit the eye defect and is sutured in place.

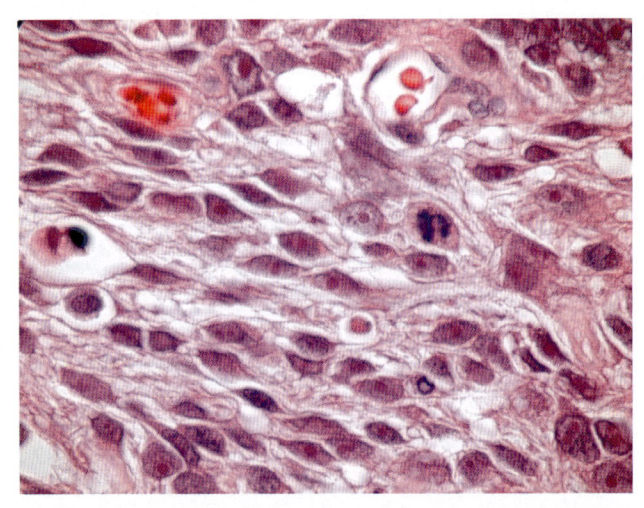

Figure 18.71. Photomicrograph showing spindle cells. In some sections, there was continuity with the surface epithelium. (Hematoxylin–eosin ×150.)

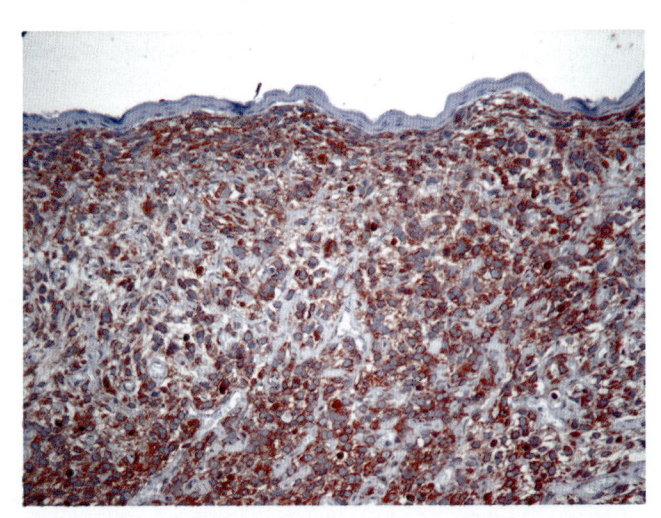

Figure 18.72. Immunohistochemical stain for vimentin, showing positive reaction. The lesion was weakly positive with epithelial markers. These findings are consistent with reported cases of conjunctival spindle cell carcinoma. (Vimentin ×75.)

Chapter 18 Premalignant and Malignant Lesions of the Conjunctival Epithelium

CONJUNCTIVAL SQUAMOUS CELL CARCINOMA: ORBITAL INVASION

In some instances squamous cell carcinoma of the conjunctiva can grow posteriorly into the orbit, causing displacement of the globe. Such an occurrence in a 70-year-old African-American man is illustrated.

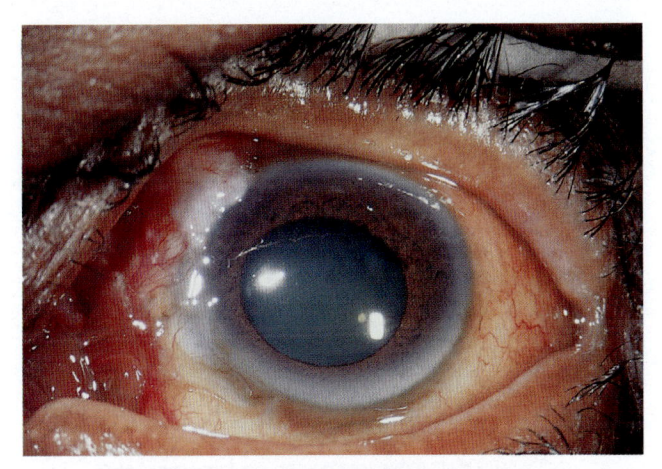

Figure 18.73. Diffuse conjunctival squamous cell carcinoma nasally in the left eye at the time of initial presentation.

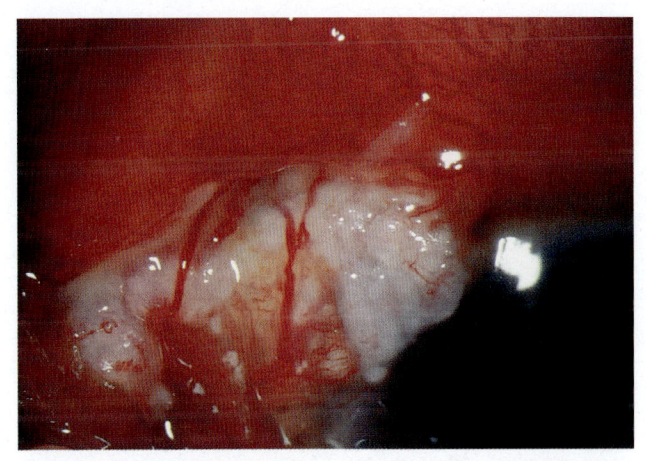

Figure 18.74. Closer view of lesion, demonstrating marked leukoplakia.

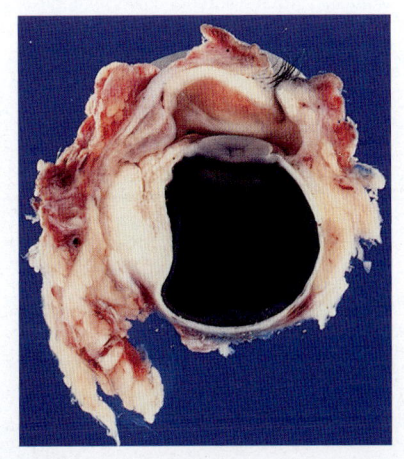

Figure 18.75. Section of exenteration specimen, revealing the ovoid white orbital mass compressing the globe.

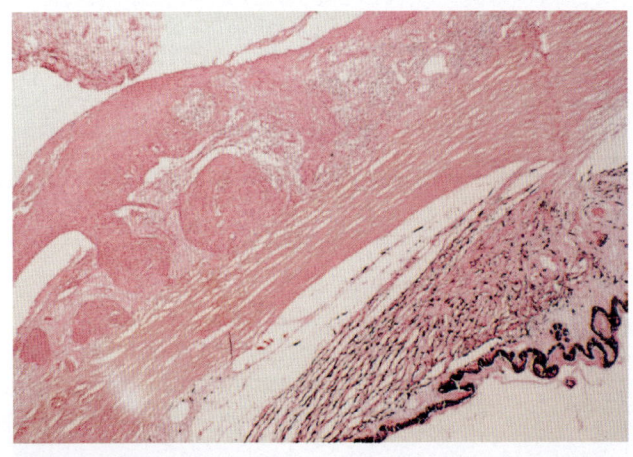

Figure 18.76. Histopathology of epibulbar mass, demonstrating invasive squamous cell carcinoma invading the sclera at the limbus. (Hematoxylin–eosin ×25.)

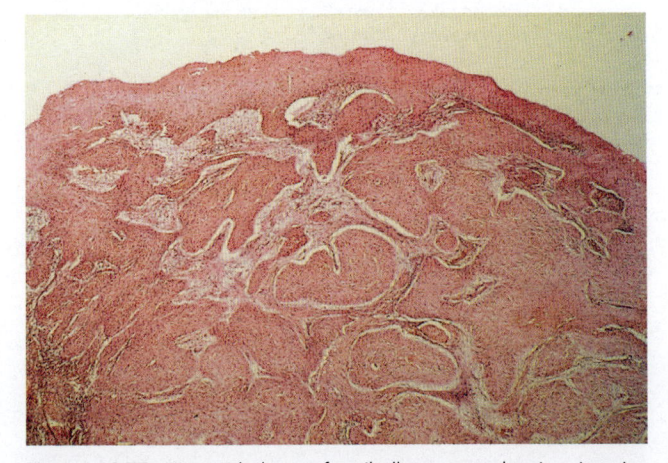

Figure 18.77. Histopathology of epibulbar mass showing invasive squamous cell carcinoma. (Hematoxylin–eosin ×50.)

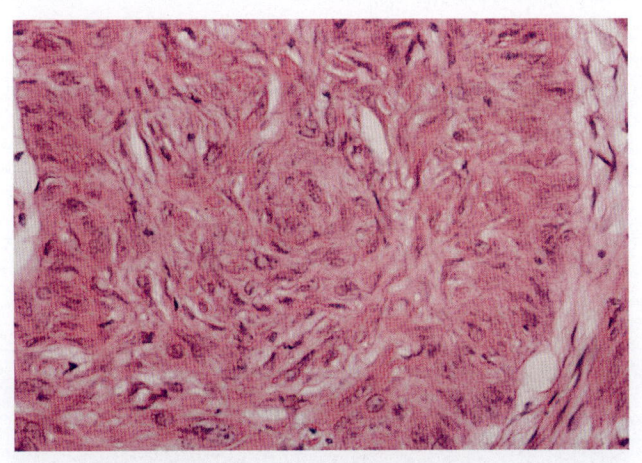

Figure 18.78. Histopathology of orbital mass showing invasive squamous cell carcinoma. (Hematoxylin–eosin ×150.)

CONJUNCTIVAL SQUAMOUS CELL CARCINOMA: INTRAOCULAR INVASION

In some instances, squamous cell carcinoma of the conjunctiva can grow through the cornea and sclera in the limbal region to enter the anterior chamber where the tumor shows continued proliferation, often producing signs of iritis and uncontrollable secondary glaucoma. Two such examples are illustrated.

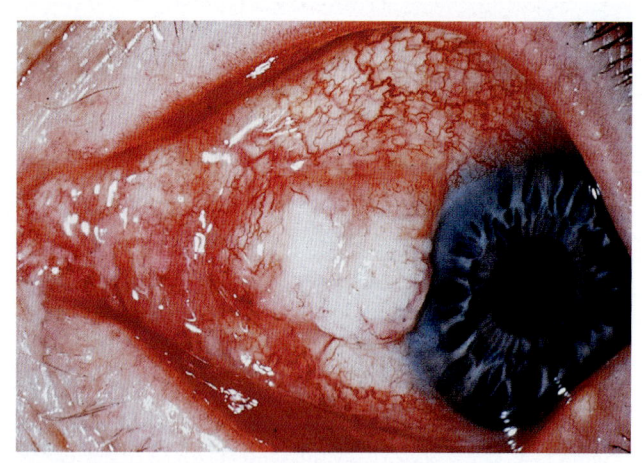

Figure 18.79. White lesion at limbus in a 70-year-old man. The lesion had been excised previously and the diagnosis of dysplasia was made. The patient had painful glaucoma secondary to intraocular invasion.

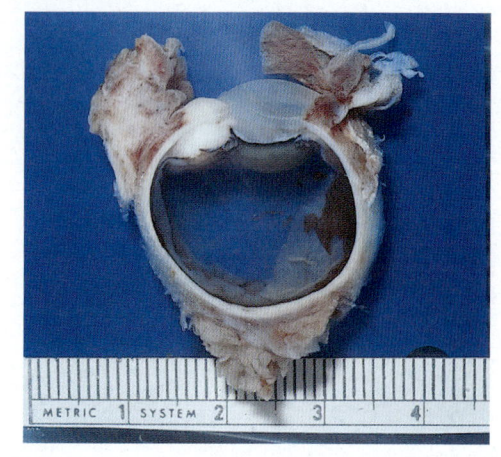

Figure 18.80. Section of eye shown in Figure 18.79 after modified enucleation with removal of much of the conjunctiva. Note the white epibulbar mass with extension into the anterior chamber angle and ciliary body.

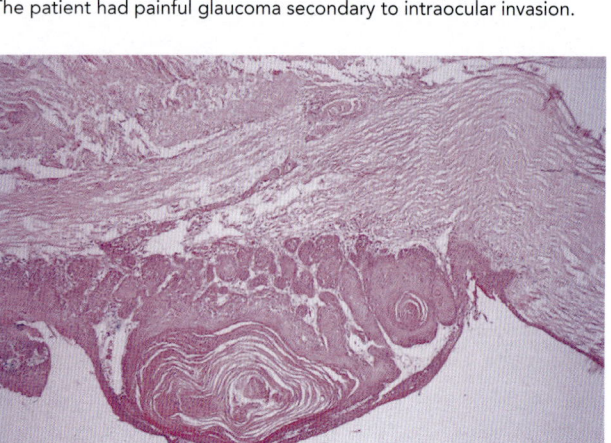

Figure 18.81. Photomicrograph of anterior chamber region, showing intraocular squamous cell carcinoma with intraocular production of keratin. (Hematoxylin–eosin ×10.)

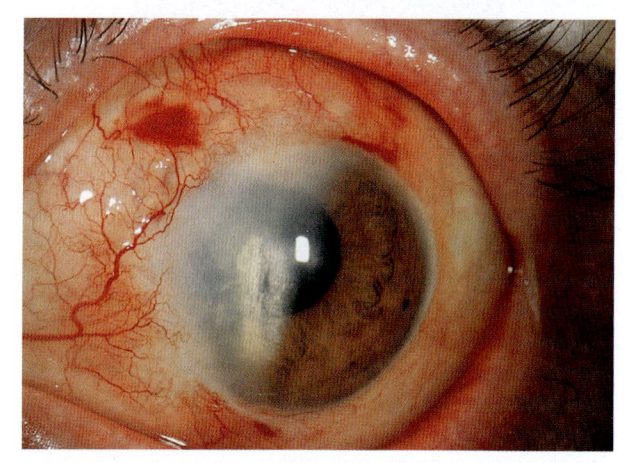

Figure 18.82. Diffuse white conjunctival and corneal lesion in a 55-year-old woman who had undergone prior excisions elsewhere of squamous cell carcinoma of conjunctiva. The patient had severe secondary glaucoma and gonioscopy showed extensive angle involvement with dense white tumor. The eye was enucleated.

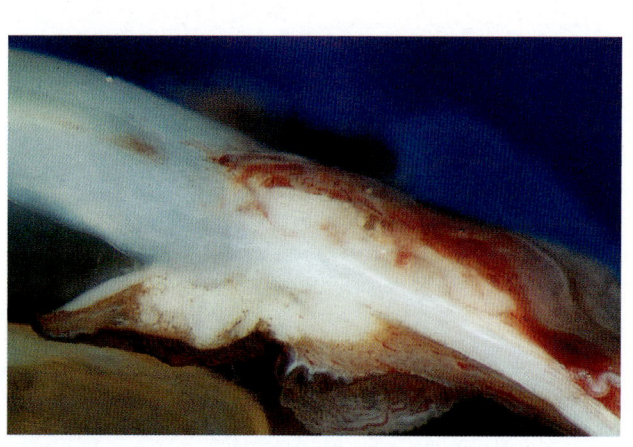

Figure 18.83. Gross photograph of ciliary body region showing intraocular invasion by solid white tumor tissue.

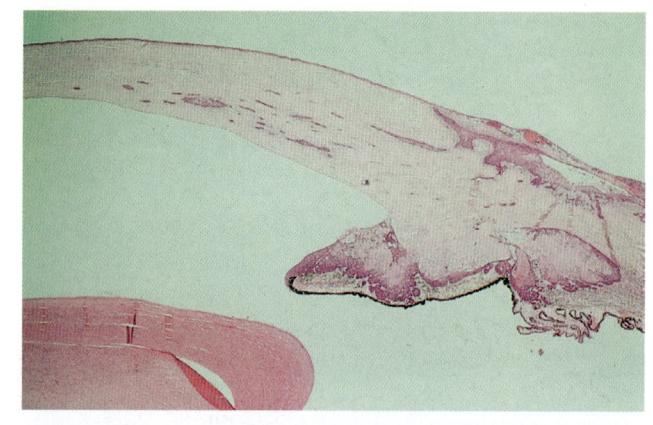

Figure 18.84. Low-magnification photomicrograph showing tumor cells at limbus and within the cornea, sclera, ciliary body, and iris. (Hematoxylin–eosin ×8.)

CONJUNCTIVAL MUCOEPIDERMOID SQUAMOUS CELL CARCINOMA: INTRAOCULAR INVASION

Mucoepidermoid carcinoma is an aggressive variant of squamous cell carcinoma that has a tendency toward aggressive invasion of adjacent structures, including the orbit and the globe.

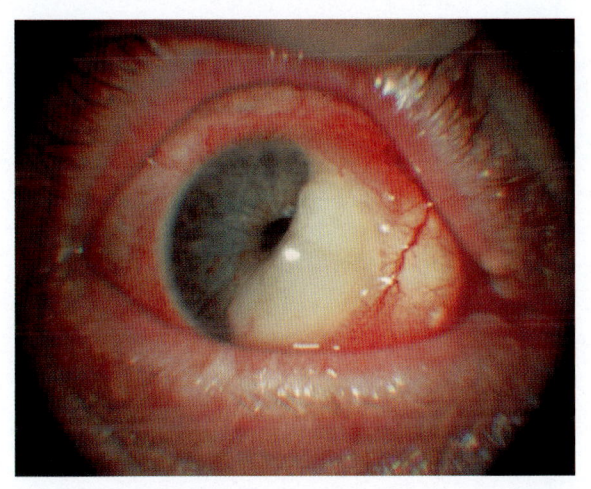

Figure 18.85. Mucoepidermoid carcinoma of conjunctiva in a 70-year-old man. A conjunctival squamous cell neoplasm was previously removed from the same site. (Courtesy of Seymour Brownstein, MD.)

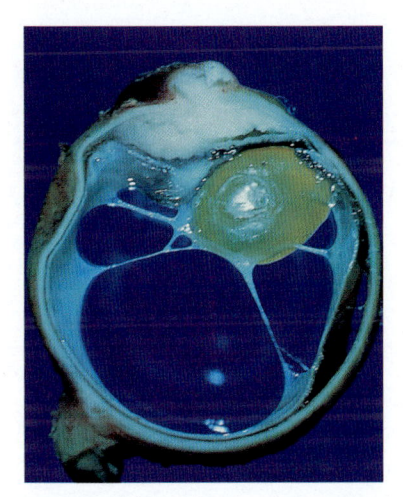

Figure 18.86. Sectioned globe after enucleation showing intraocular invasion of the mass and subluxation of the lens. (Courtesy of Seymour Brownstein, MD.)

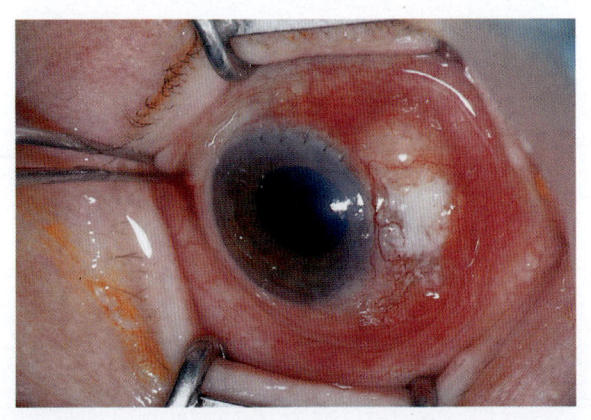

Figure 18.87. Mucoepidermoid carcinoma of the conjunctiva temporally in the right eye of a 91-year-old woman. The lesion was excised and cryotherapy performed.

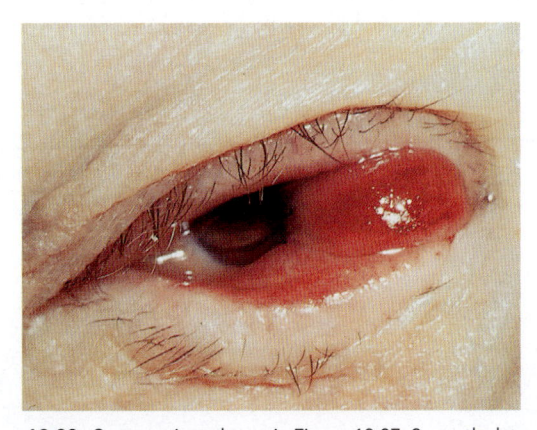

Figure 18.88. Same patient shown in Figure 18.87, 3 months later, with a fleshy recurrence.

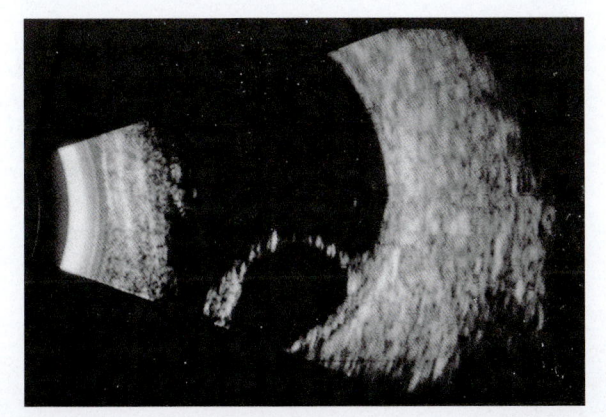

Figure 18.89. B-scan ultrasonogram of the globe showing a cystic intraocular lesion due to an epithelial-lined cyst secondary to intraocular invasion of the limbal tumor. A modified enucleation was performed.

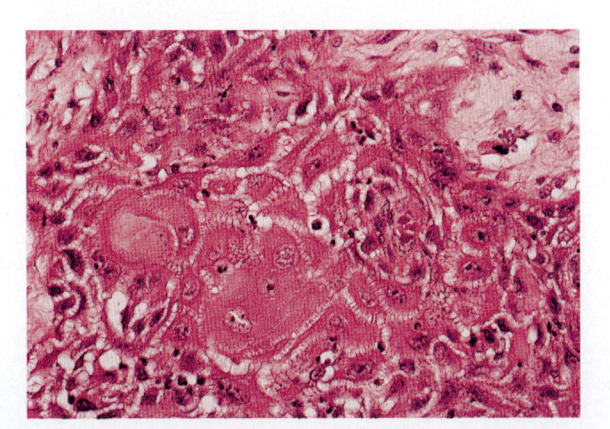

Figure 18.90. Photomicrograph of epibulbar mass showing invasive squamous cell carcinoma. Similar cells lined the intraocular cyst. Other areas showed marked mucin deposition. (Hematoxylin–eosin ×200.)

CONJUNCTIVAL MELANOCYTIC LESIONS

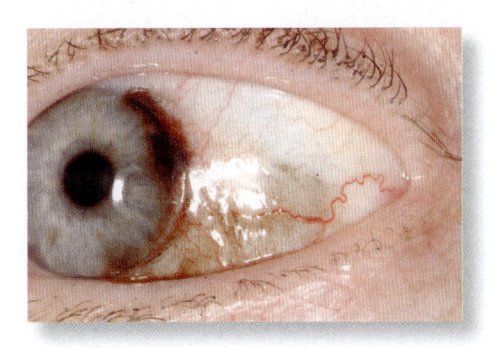

General Considerations

Nevus is the most common melanocytic conjunctival tumor (1–35). In the authors' clinical series of 1,643 conjunctival tumors, there were 454 nevi, accounting for 52% of conjunctival melanocytic lesions and for 28% of the 1,643 lesions (1). In our clinical series of conjunctival tumors in 262 children, there were 175 (67%) melanocytic tumors and 148 (56%) nevi (5).

There is controversy as to whether conjunctival nevi are congenital or acquired. It generally becomes clinically apparent in the first or second decade of life (3,4). The nevus begins as a small nest of melanocytes in the basal layer of the epithelium, at which stage it is called a "junctional" nevus. In the second to third decade of life, the cells gradually migrate into the underlying stroma to form a "compound" nevus. At this stage, characteristic pseudocysts form in the lesion. By the third to fourth decade, the lesion has migrated to reside entirely in the stroma, forming a "subepithelial" nevus. It is helpful to consider these three types as stages in the evolution of a nevus, rather than distinct types.

Melanocytic nevus of the conjunctiva is generally sporadic with no systemic associations. However, lentigines and nevi are rarely associated with Carney complex and the dysplastic nevus syndrome (DNS) (26,27). Carney complex is also mentioned in the sections on eyelid and conjunctival myxomas in this atlas. The DNS is an autosomal-dominant entity characterized by numerous dysplastic cutaneous nevi and a high incidence of cutaneous melanoma. There may be an increased incidence of conjunctival nevi (and melanoma) in association with DNS (26).

Clinical Features

A study of 410 consecutive cases of conjunctival nevi seen by the authors revealed that 89% occurred in Caucasians, 6% in African Americans, and 5% in Asian, Hispanic, or Indian patients (4). The nevus contained clinically evident pigment in 84% and was clinically amelanotic in 16%. The tumor was located in the bulbar conjunctiva in 72%, caruncle in 15%, semilunar fold in 11%, and fornix, tarsus, and cornea in 1% each. About 90% were located in the interpalpebral area with relative equal distribution nasally and temporally. Malignant transformation was estimated to be less than 1%, a finding that is similar to other series (3).

Conjunctival nevus is usually a discrete lesion within the bulbar conjunctiva, generally in the sun-exposed region of the interpalpebral area. Nevus can range from deeply pigmented to completely amelanotic. Cysts are commonly found within nevus and are especially visible in pigmented nevi. The cysts can displace the pigment to the side. Over time, a nevus can become more pigmented, leading to misinterpretation of growth or malignant transformation into melanoma. However, true increase in size can occur in young children, but it is usually minimal. Such enlargement does not necessarily mean malignant transformation into melanoma. When nevus is not pigmented, the presence of multiple, clear cystic spaces within the lesion, using slit-lamp biomicroscopy, help to differentiate nevus from papilloma, lymphoma, and amelanotic melanoma, which generally do not have cysts. Lymphangioma, on the

CONJUNCTIVAL MELANOCYTIC NEVUS

other hand, can have cyst-like spaces and resemble a diffuse amelanotic nevus.

Another common clinical variant is what the authors call a speckled nevus. It is less well defined and appears as a patchy area of pigmentation in the conjunctiva. It may closely resemble primary acquired melanosis (PAM), to be discussed shortly, except that it generally occurs in younger individuals and sometimes contains subtle clear cysts, a finding not seen with PAM.

In rare cases, a blue nevus can occur in the conjunctiva. This is believed to be congenital and appears clinically as a blue to black, circumscribed or slightly ill-defined lesion deep to the conjunctival epithelium that differs from the more diffuse scleral or episcleral melanocytosis (4,28–31). Conjunctival blue nevus can have a diffuse growth pattern and resemble PAM. Such a diffuse blue nevus can rarely undergo malignant transformation into melanoma (28).

Although most nevi develop in the interpalpebral region near the limbus, they can also be located in the extralimbal bulbar conjunctiva, semilunar fold, or caruncle. In rare instances, nevus can apparently be confined to the palpebral conjunctiva (21) or cornea (22). Such locations should raise suspicion that the lesion is an early melanoma (4,20).

In some instances, a conjunctival nevus can assume an irregular, diffuse configuration extending for over 10 to 20 mm of the conjunctival surface and with numerous cysts. Such a giant cystic nevus can occupy an entire quadrant of the conjunctiva and simulate melanoma (10). The multicystic appearance can mislead the clinical toward the diagnosis of lymphangioma (10). A relatively common occurrence with conjunctival nevus is secondary inflammation, which may simulate primary conjunctivitis or episcleritis (35). However, slit-lamp biomicroscopy often discloses the typical cysts that characterize the nevus.

Pathology

The histopathologic classification of nevi is discussed in the literature (4,14–19). Although most pathologists accustomed to evaluating ocular tissues can make the diagnosis without difficulty, there are some cases where the lesion has borderline malignant features and even experienced ocular pathologists may have difficulty classifying the lesion as benign or malignant (33). Histopathologically, a conjunctival nevus is composed of a diffuse infiltration or distinct nests of benign melanocytes near the basal layer of the epithelium. Depending on their relationship to the layers of the conjunctiva, they are most often classified as junctional, compound, or deep (4). Depending on their cytology and other features, they may be classified as dysplastic nevus, spindle cell nevus, epithelioid cell nevus, balloon cell nevus, blue nevus, or a combination of these variants (24,28–34).

A blue nevus is uncommon in the conjunctiva. It may be identical to the typical congenital or acquired nevus, except that it is more likely to be deep to the conjunctival epithelium, sometimes partially attached to the sclera. It may be dark brown or black and it is less likely to contain cysts (28–31).

On occasion, a conjunctival nevus shows features of both a conventional nevus and deeper dendritic cells that characterize a blue nevus. Such a lesion has been called a "combined" nevus. It has recently been stressed that such a nevus may be more common than previously suspected and must be differentiated from a melanoma (17).

Currently used immunohistochemical techniques can be used to differentiate melanocytic lesions from nonmelanocytic conditions. However, the popular melanoma-specific antigen (HMB-45) generally shows a positive reaction with both nevus and melanoma and cannot be reliably used to differentiate benign from malignant melanocytic lesions (18).

CONJUNCTIVAL MELANOCYTIC NEVUS

Management

The best initial management for a small, typical conjunctival nevus is usually periodic observation with photographic documentation. If growth is documented, local excision of the lesion should be considered. However, relative indications for earlier excision include atypical location in the forniceal or palpebral conjunctiva or cornea, nutrient blood vessels, larger lesion that contains no cysts, positive family history of conjunctival or cutaneous melanoma, distinct onset of the lesion in middle age or later in life, insistence of the patient or parents, and cancerophobia. In addition, any recurrence of a previously excised conjunctival nevus should be removed. Such a recurrence should raise the possibility of malignant transformation. We have sometimes removed a small lesion believed clinically to be a nevus and were surprised to find that it was a melanoma histopathologically.

If a lesion shows suspicious change or growth, it is important that an excisional biopsy be done, using a reported technique, described later in this chapter and illustrated in Chapter 25 (12). As a general rule, incisional biopsy is contraindicated in lesions that can be resected entirely in one procedure. The resection technique that we employ is the same as that used for malignant neoplasms, like squamous cell carcinoma, and other lesions near the limbus. It involves a "no touch" technique using a partial alcohol epitheliectomy, removal of the main tumor by partial lamellar sclerokeratoconjunctivectomy, double freeze-thaw cryotherapy, and conjunctivoplastic reconstruction (12).

Selected References

Reviews

1. Shields CL, Demirci H, Karatza E, et al. Clinical survey of 1643 melanocytic and nonmelanocytic tumors of the conjunctiva. *Ophthalmology* 2004;111:1747–1754.
2. Shields CL, Shields JA. Tumors of the conjunctiva and cornea. *Surv Ophthalmol* 2004;49:3–24.
3. Gerner N, Norregaard JC, Jensen OA, et al. Conjunctival naevi in Denmark 1960–1980. A 21-year follow-up study. *Acta Ophthalmol Scand* 1996;74:334–337.
4. Shields CL, Fasiudden A, Mashayekhi A, et al. Conjunctival nevi: clinical features and natural course in 410 consecutive patients. *Arch Ophthalmol* 2004;122:167–175.
5. Shields CL, Shields JA. Conjunctival tumors in children. *Curr Opin Ophthalmol* 2007;18:351–360.
6. Rodriguez-Sains RS. Pigmented conjunctival neoplasms. *Orbit* 2002;21:231–238.
7. McDonnell JM, Carpenter JD, Jacobs P, et al. Conjunctival melanocytic lesions in children. *Ophthalmology* 1989;96:986–993.
8. Kabukcuoglu S, McNutt NS. Conjunctival melanocytic nevi of childhood. *J Cutan Pathol* 1999;26:248–252.
9. Farber M, Schutzer P, Mihm MC Jr. Pigmented lesions of the conjunctiva. *J Am Acad Dermatol* 1998;38:971–978.
10. Shields CL, Regillo AC, Mellen PL, et al. Giant conjunctival nevus: clinical features and natural course in 32 cases. *JAMA Ophthalmol* 2013;131(7):857–863.

Imaging

11. Bianciotto C, Shields CL, Guzman JM, et al. Assessment of anterior segment tumors with ultrasound biomicroscopy versus anterior segment optical coherence tomography in 200 cases. *Ophthalmology* 2011;118(7):1297–1302.

Management

12. Shields JA, Shields CL, De Potter P. Surgical management of circumscribed conjunctival melanomas. *Ophthal Plast Reconstr Surg* 1998;14:208–215.
13. Shin KH, Hwang JH, Kwon JW. Argon laser photoablation of superficial conjunctival nevus: results of a 3-year study. *Am J Ophthalmol* 2013;155(5):823–828.

Histopathology

14. Grossniklaus HE, Green WR, Luckenbach M, et al. Conjunctival lesions in adults. A clinical and histopathologic review. *Cornea* 1987;6:78–116.
15. Folberg R, Jakobiec FA, Bernardino VB, et al. Benign conjunctival melanocytic lesions. Clinicopathologic features. *Ophthalmology* 1989;96:436–461.
16. Jakobiec FA, Folberg R, Iwamoto T. Clinicopathologic characteristics of premalignant and malignant melanocytic lesions of the conjunctiva. *Ophthalmology* 1989;96:147–166.
17. Crawford JB, Howes EL Jr, Char DH. Combined nevi of the conjunctiva. *Arch Ophthalmol* 1999;117:1121–1127.
18. Glasgow BJ, McCall LC, Foos RY. HMB-45 antibody reactivity in pigmented lesions of the conjunctiva. *Am J Ophthalmol* 1990;109:696–700.
19. Mudhar HS, Smith K, Talley P, et al. Fluorescence in situ hybridisation (FISH) in histologically challenging conjunctival melanocytic lesions. *Br J Ophthalmol* 2013;97(1):40–46.

Case Reports

20. Buckman G, Jakobiec FA, Folberg R, et al. Melanocytic nevi of the palpebral conjunctiva. An extremely rare location usually signifying melanoma. *Ophthalmology* 1988;95:1053–1057.
21. Kim HJ, McCormick SA, Nath S, et al. Melanocytic nevi of the tarsal conjunctiva: clinicopathologic case series with review of literature. *Ophthal Plast Reconstr Surg* 2010;26(6):438–442.
22. Shields JA, Shields CL, Eagle RC Jr, et al. Compound nevus of the cornea simulating a foreign body. *Am J Ophthalmol* 2000;130:235–236.
23. Rosenfeld SI, Smith ME. Benign cystic nevus of the conjunctiva. *Ophthalmology* 1983;90:1459–1461.
24. Pfaffenbach DD, Green WR, Maumenee AE. Balloon cell nevus of the conjunctiva. *Ophthalmology* 1972;87:192–195.
25. Jakobiec FA, Zuckerman BD, Berlin AJ, et al. Unusual melanocytic nevi of the conjunctiva. *Am J Ophthalmol* 1985;100:100–103.
26. Friedman RJ, Rodriguez-Sains R, Jakobiec F. Ophthalmologic oncology: conjunctival malignant melanoma in association with sporadic dysplastic nevus syndrome. *J Dermatol Surg Oncol* 1987;13:31–34.
27. Carney JA. Carney complex: the complex of myxomas, spotty pigmentation, endocrine overactivity, and schwannomas. *Semin Dermatol* 1995;14:90–98.
28. Demirci H, Shields CL, Shields JA, et al. Malignant melanoma arising from unusual conjunctival blue nevus. *Arch Ophthalmol* 2000;118:1581–1584.
29. Blicker JA, Rootman J, White VA. Cellular blue nevus of the conjunctiva. *Ophthalmology* 1992;99:1714–1717.
30. Eller AW, Bernardino VB. Blue nevi of the conjunctiva. *Ophthalmology* 1983;90:1469–1471.
31. Berman EL, Shields CL, Sagoo MS, et al. Multifocal blue nevus of the conjunctiva. *Surv Ophthalmol* 2008;53(1):41–49.
32. Seregard S. Pigmented spindle cell naevus of reed presenting in the conjunctiva. *Acta Ophthalmol Scand* 2000;78:104–106.
33. Margo CE, Roper DL, Hidayat AA. Borderline melanocytic tumor of the conjunctiva: diagnostic and therapeutic considerations. *J Pediatr Ophthalmol Strabismus* 1991;28:268–270.
34. Kantelip B, Boccard R, Nores JM, et al. A case of conjunctival Spitz nevus: review of literature and comparison with cutaneous locations. *Ann Ophthalmol* 1989;21:176–179.
35. Zamir E, Mechoulam H, Micera A, et al. Inflamed juvenile conjunctival naevus: clinicopathological characterisation. *Br J Ophthalmol* 2002;86:28–30.

Chapter 19 Conjunctival Melanocytic Lesions

CONJUNCTIVAL MELANOCYTIC NEVUS: PIGMENTED TYPE

Most conjunctival nevi are pigmented and located near the limbus in the interpalpebral region. Characteristic clear cysts in the lesion strongly support the diagnosis of compound nevus. Conjunctival nevus can be completely pigmented, partly pigmented, or nonpigmented.

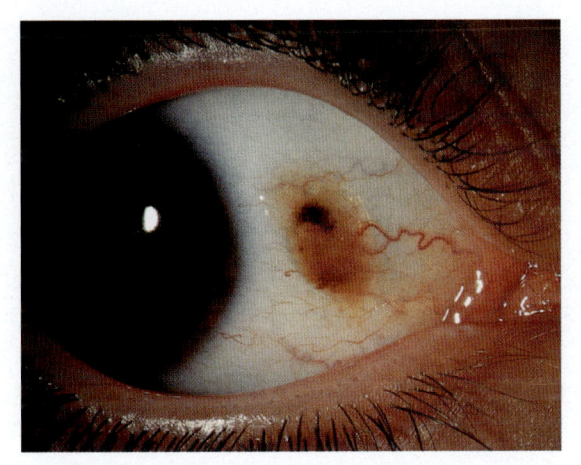

Figure 19.1. Typical conjunctival nevus in a 43-year-old man.

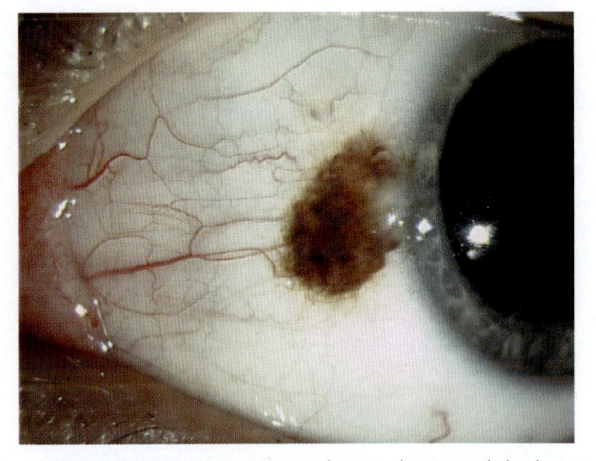

Figure 19.2. Characteristic conjunctival nevus showing subtle clear cystic spaces.

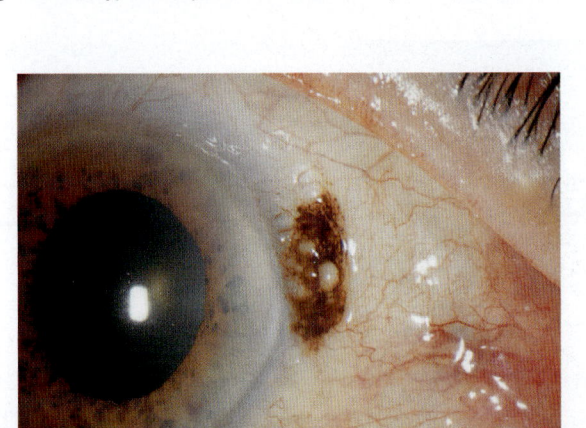

Figure 19.3. Characteristic conjunctival nevus with more distinct clear cystic spaces.

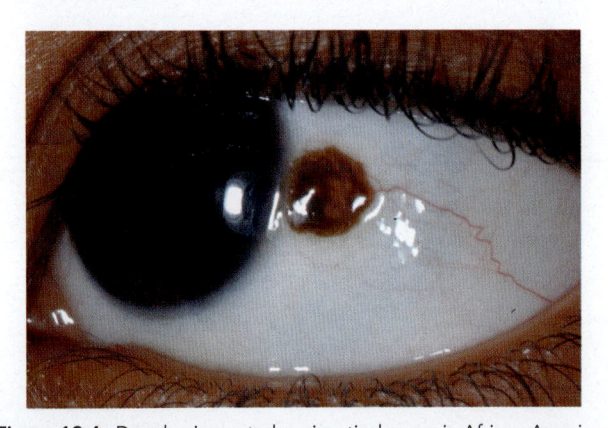

Figure 19.4. Deeply pigmented conjunctival nevus in African-American child. Note the associated dilated conjunctival blood vessel.

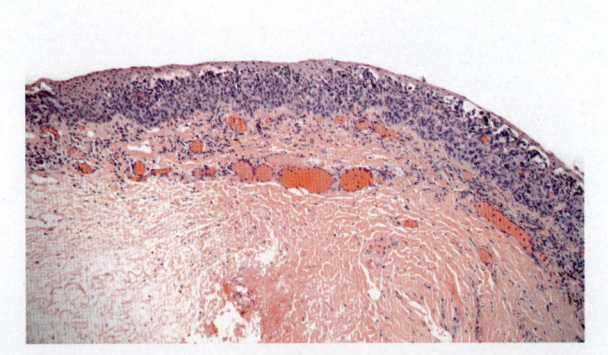

Figure 19.5. Histopathology of functional conjunctival nevus showing diffuse atypical melanocytes in the deeper layers of the conjunctival epithelium. In this case, there are no large cysts. (Hematoxylin–eosin ×10.)

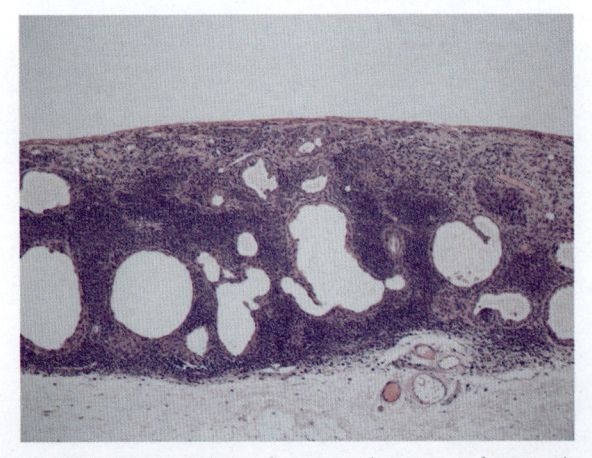

Figure 19.6. Histopathology of compound conjunctival nevus showing numerous cysts within the lesion, lined by conjunctival epithelium. (Hematoxylin–eosin ×20.)

TUMORS OF THE CONJUNCTIVA

CONJUNCTIVAL MELANOCYTIC NEVUS: NONPIGMENTED TYPE

Some conjunctival melanocytic nevi have no apparent pigment on clinical examination. Typical cysts within the lesion on slit-lamp examination, however, should suggest the diagnosis of nevus. All of the lesions shown here had typical cysts, but cysts are not appreciated in every case. Such an amelanotic nevus can become inflamed periodically and be confused with conjunctivitis or episcleritis.

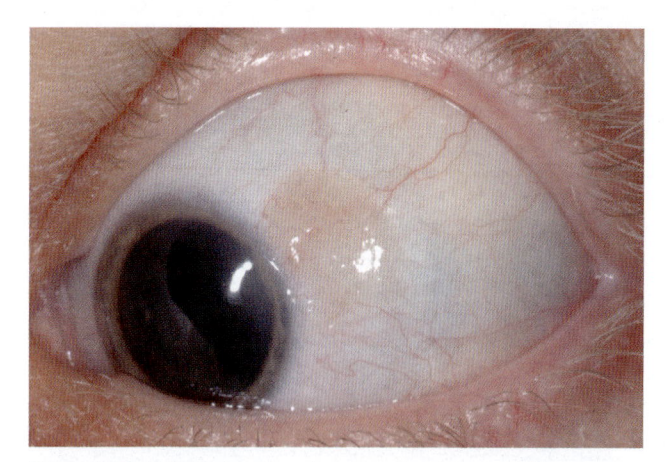

Figure 19.7. Light pink conjunctival nevus in a 13-year-old boy.

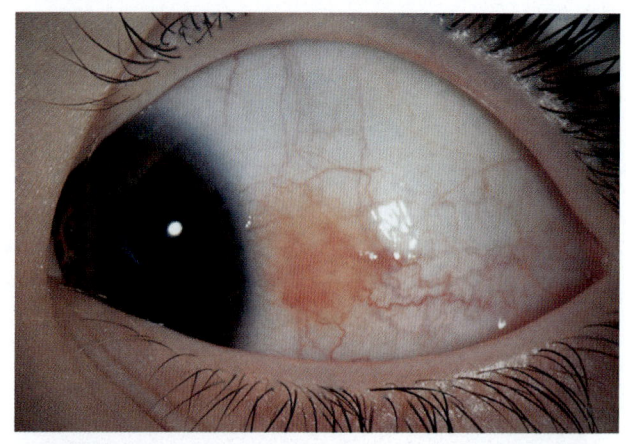

Figure 19.8. Nonpigmented conjunctival nevus near limbus in a 50-year-old man.

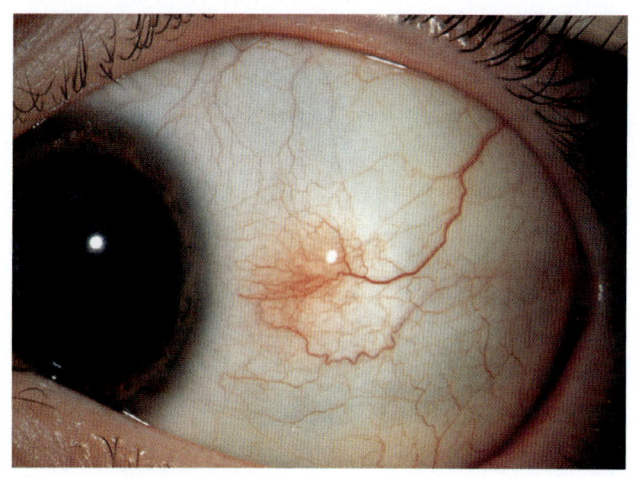

Figure 19.9. Subtle conjunctival nevus with slightly prominent feeder vessel in a 20-year-old man.

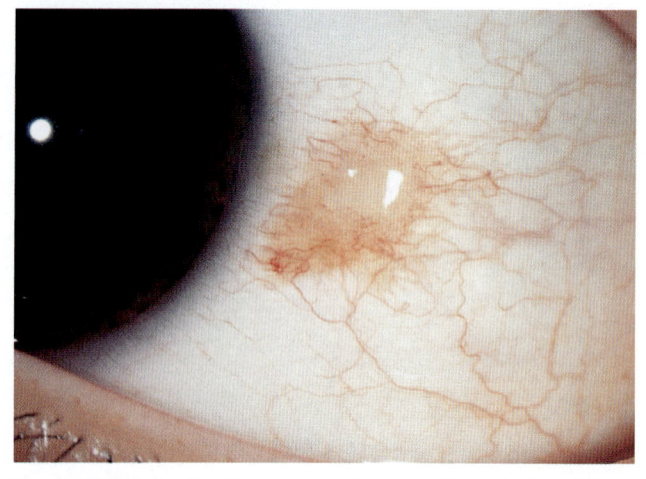

Figure 19.10. Amelanotic conjunctival nevus with minimal peripheral pigmentation in a 13-year-old girl.

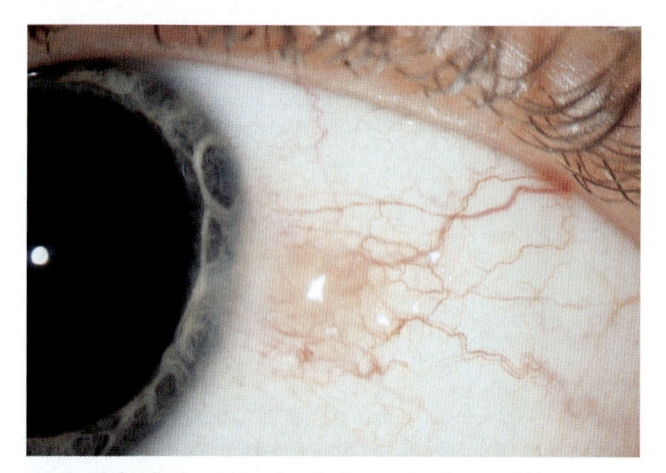

Figure 19.11. Light pink conjunctival nevus in a 9-year-old boy.

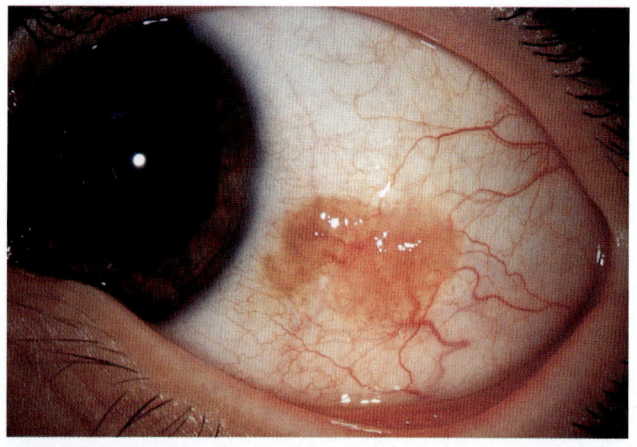

Figure 19.12. Larger, more irregular, salmon-colored conjunctival nevus in a 14-year-old boy.

CONJUNCTIVAL MELANOCYTIC NEVUS: PARTIALLY PIGMENTED TYPE

In some instances, a conjunctival nevus is only partly pigmented. The presence of even minimal pigmentation should strongly suggest that the lesion is a melanocytic nevus.

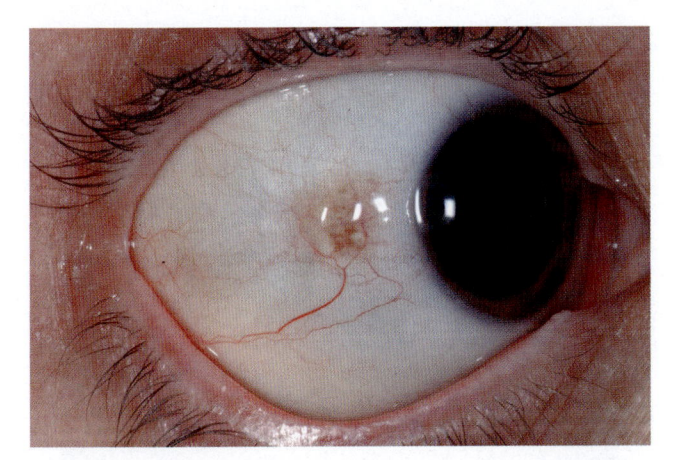

Figure 19.13. Slightly pigmented conjunctival nevus on temporal bulbar conjunctiva. Note the dilated blood vessel.

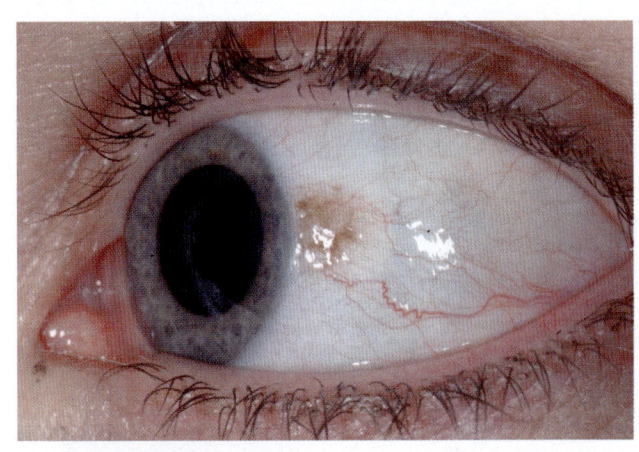

Figure 19.14. Slightly pigmented conjunctival nevus at limbus with mildly dilated vessels.

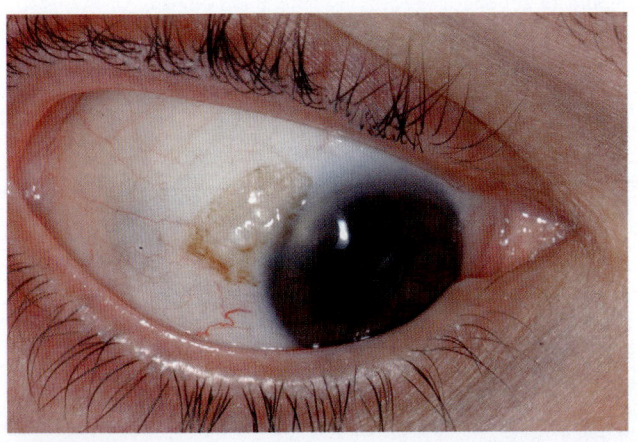

Figure 19.15. Partially pigmented cystic conjunctival nevus with corneal stroma opacity.

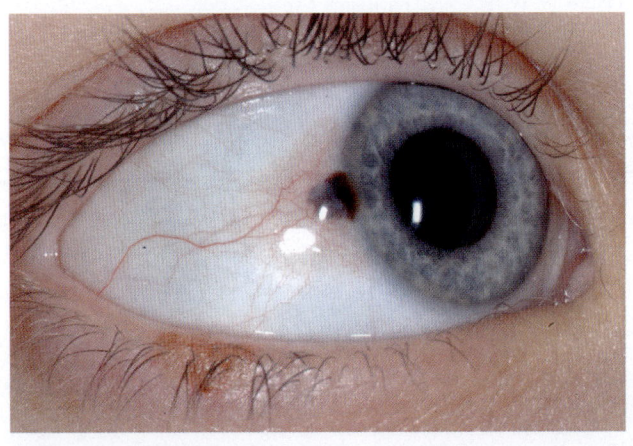

Figure 19.16. Mostly nonpigmented conjunctival nevus with well-defined central focus of pigmentation.

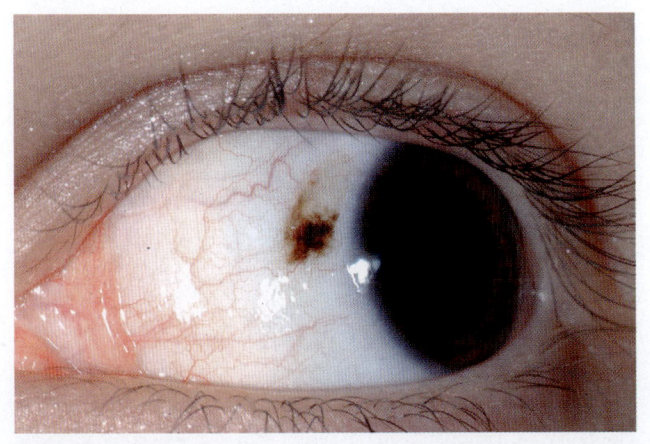

Figure 19.17. Conjunctival nevus with pigmented inferior portion and nonpigmented superior portion.

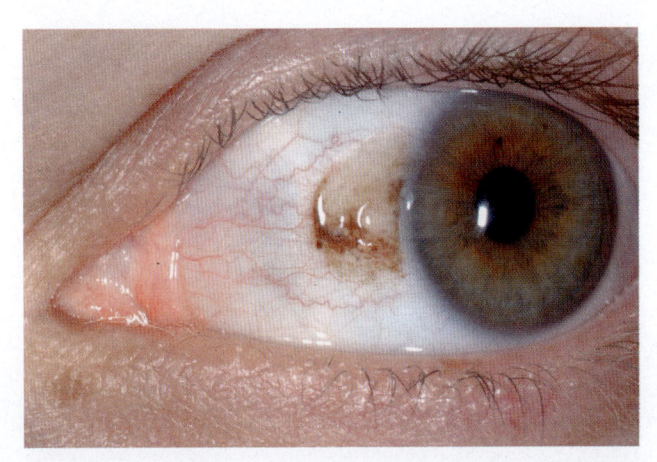

Figure 19.18. Gelatinous nonpigmented conjunctival nevus with irregular rim of pigmentation.

CONJUNCTIVAL MELANOCYTIC NEVUS: CLINICAL VARIATIONS

Conjunctival nevi can vary in size, color, and location. Occasionally, a conjunctival nevus may be apparently confined to the cornea. There are some atypical clinical and histopathologic variations of conjunctival nevus. Selected examples include the speckled nevus that might resemble PAM, epithelioid cell nevus, corneal nevus.

Shields JA, Shields CL, Eagle RC Jr, et al. Compound nevus of the cornea simulating a foreign body. *Am J Ophthalmol* 2000;130:235–236.

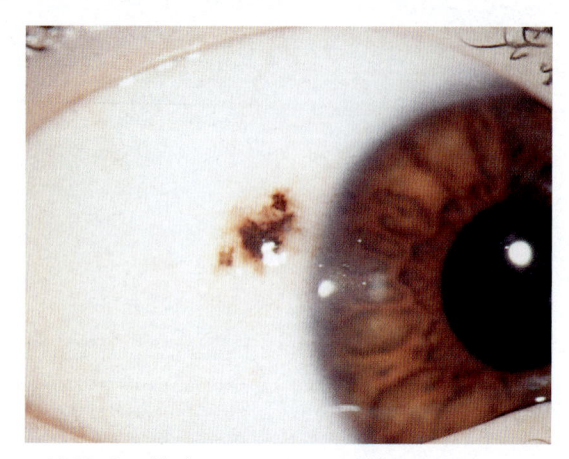

Figure 19.19. Speckled nevus in a 7-year-old boy.

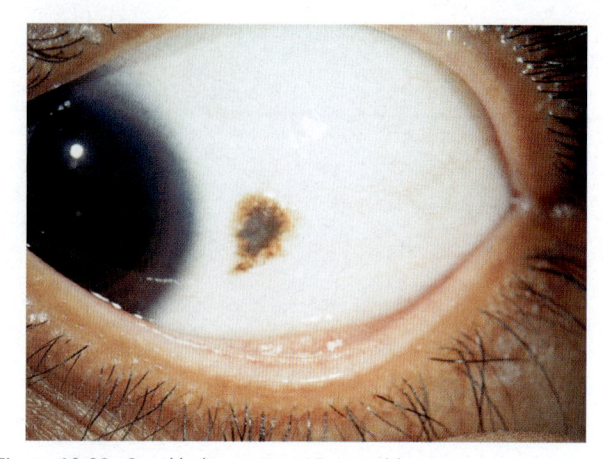

Figure 19.20. Speckled nevus in a 33-year-old woman.

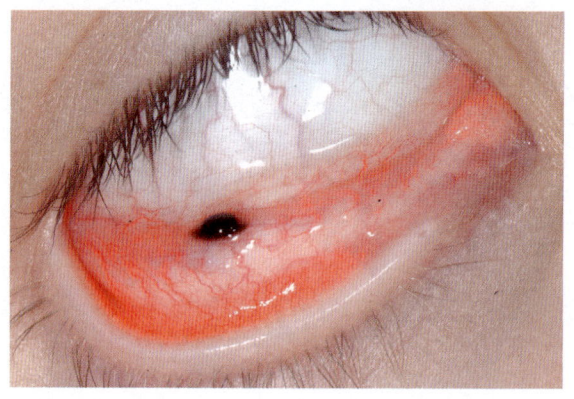

Figure 19.21. Example of epithelioid cell nevus. Deeply pigmented nevus in inferior fornix of a 12-year-old girl.

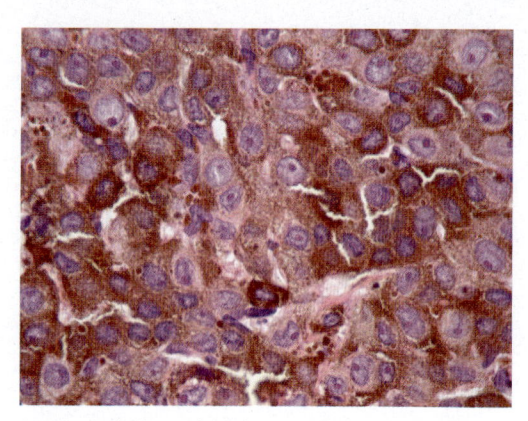

Figure 19.22. Pathology of the lesion shown in Figure 19.21 showing large, round, pigmented cells with abundant cytoplasm uniform nuclei, prominent uniform nucleoli, and lack of mitotic activity. (Hematoxylin–eosin ×250.)

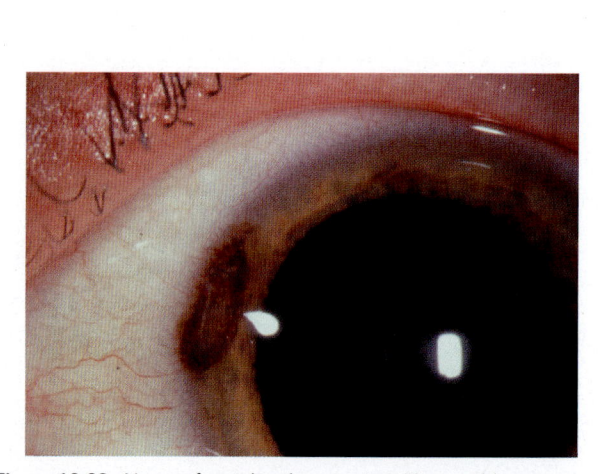

Figure 19.23. Nevus of peripheral cornea in a 22-year-old man, resembling a rusty corneal foreign body.

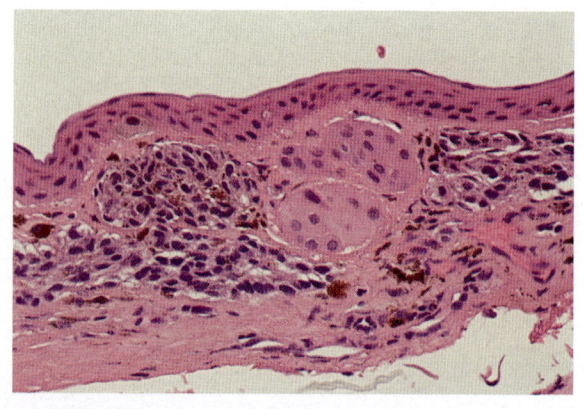

Figure 19.24. Histopathology of lesion shown in Figure 19.23 showing clusters of deep nevus cells within the peripheral corneal stroma. (Hematoxylin–eosin ×50.)

Chapter 19 Conjunctival Melanocytic Lesions

● CONJUNCTIVAL MELANOCYTIC NEVUS: EXTRALIMBAL LOCATION

Nevi can often be located in the extralimbal bulbar conjunctiva, semilunar fold (plica semilunaris), and the caruncle. Caruncular lesions are discussed and illustrated later.

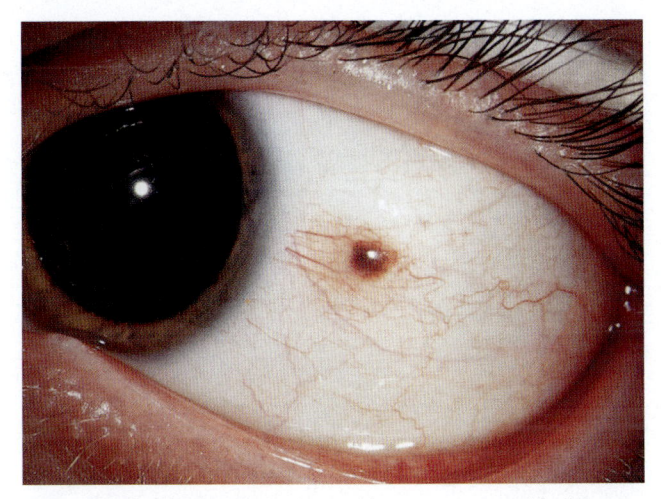

Figure 19.25. Small, slightly elevated lesion in temporal bulbar conjunctiva in a 20-year-old man.

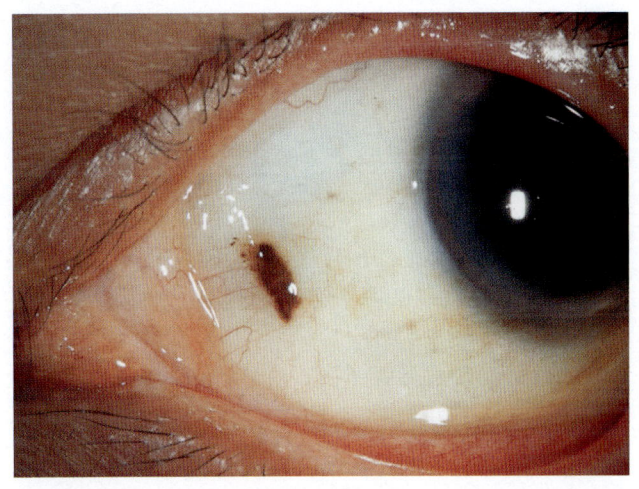

Figure 19.26. Nevus in nasal bulbar conjunctiva just central to the semilunar fold in a 43-year-old man. Note the dusting of pigment around the main lesion.

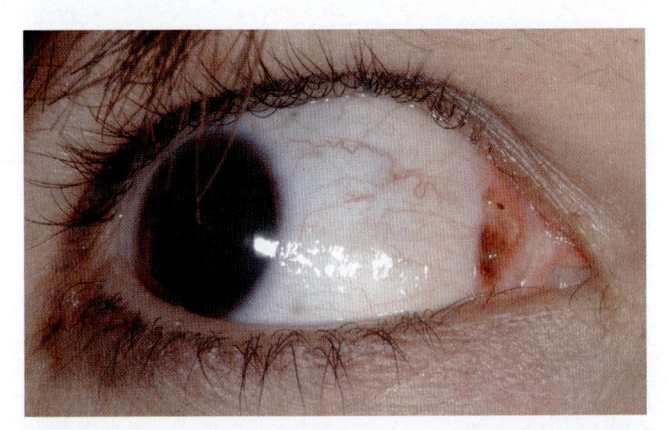

Figure 19.27. Lightly pigmented nevus of semilunar fold in young woman.

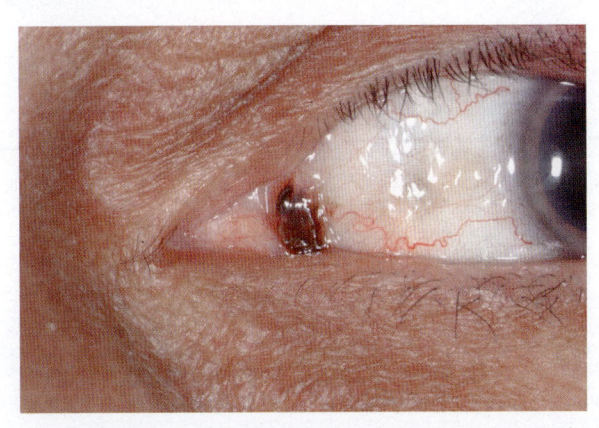

Figure 19.28. More heavily pigmented conjunctival nevus in semilunar fold of left eye.

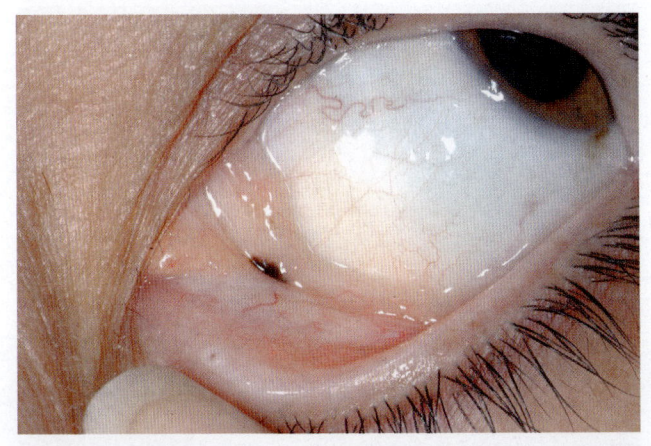

Figure 19.29. Nevus in inferonasal conjunctival fornix in a middle-aged woman.

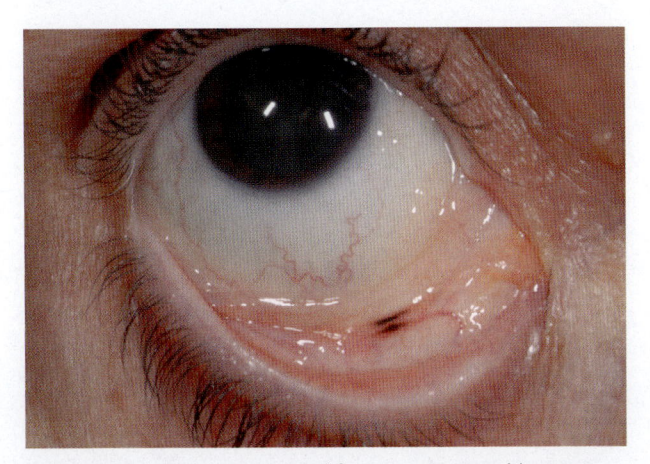

Figure 19.30. Nevus in conjunctival fornix in a 30-year-old woman.

CONJUNCTIVAL MELANOCYTIC NEVUS: ATYPICAL CASES WITH PROMINENT CYSTS AND LARGE SIZE (GIANT NEVUS)

In some instances, the cysts within a conjunctival nevus can be quite prominent and the nevus can be large and cystic suggesting the diagnosis of a lymphangioma.

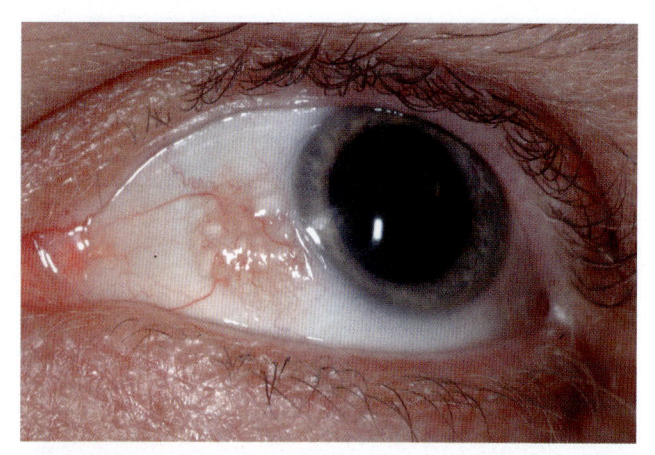

Figure 19.31. Amelanotic cystic conjunctival nevus near limbus.

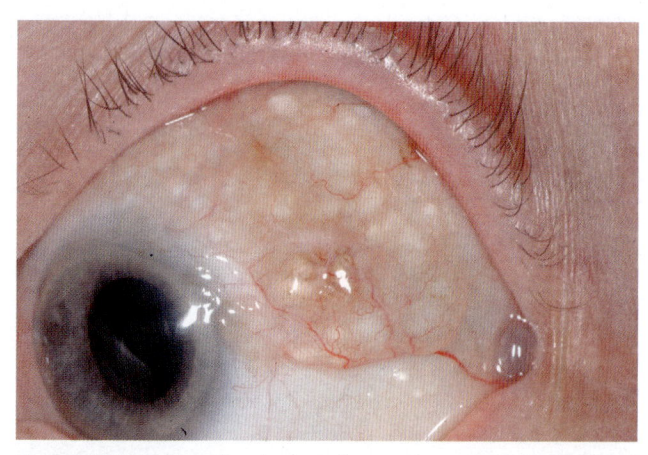

Figure 19.32. Minimally pigmented extensive superior conjunctival nevus with cysts.

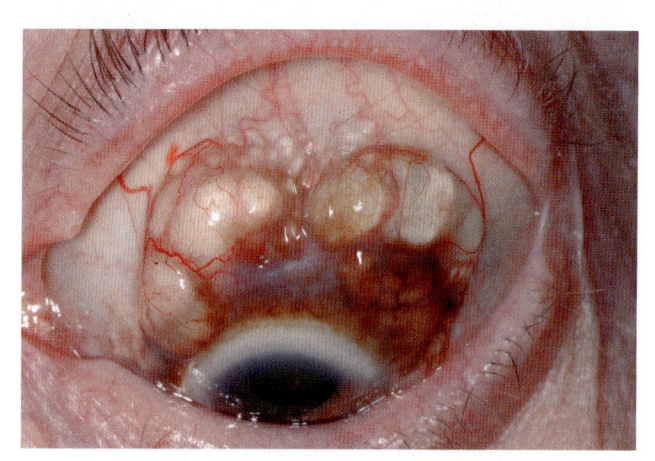

Figure 19.33. Pigmented conjunctiva with giant cysts in an elderly man. The lesion had been present and unchanged since childhood.

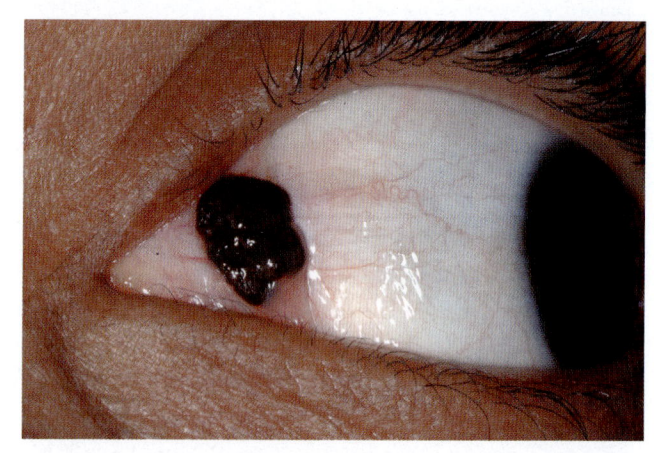

Figure 19.34. Dark black, heavily pigmented cystic nevus of conjunctival semilunar fold in an African-American patient. The cysts were obscured by the dense pigment but were evident on slit-lamp biomicroscopy.

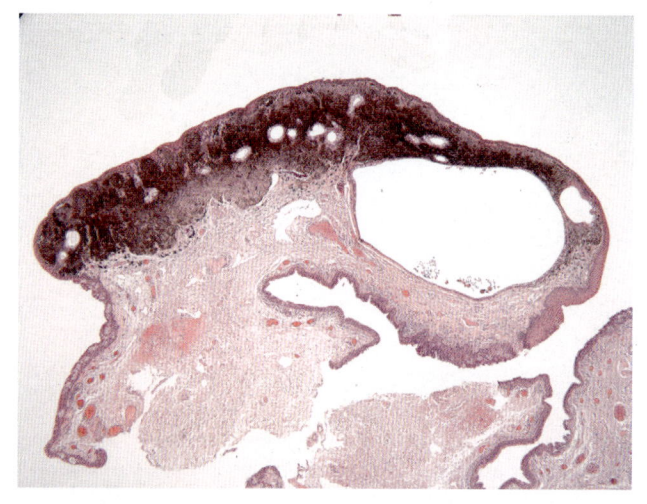

Figure 19.35. Low-magnification photomicrograph of lesion shown in Figure 19.34 depicting superficial pigment and deep cyst. Goblet cells lining the cyst are barely visible. (Hematoxylin–eosin ×25.)

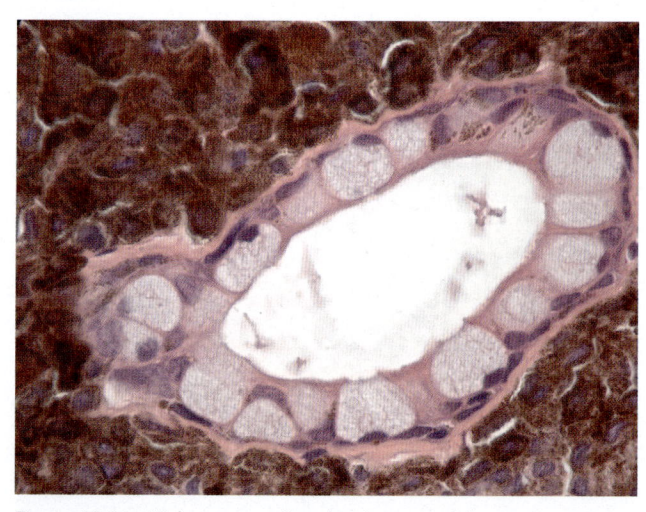

Figure 19.36. Higher-power view showing one of the cystic structures with very evident goblet cells. (Hematoxylin–eosin ×150.)

CONJUNCTIVAL MELANOCYTIC NEVUS: BLUE NEVUS VARIANT

A blue nevus may be similar to a typical acquired nevus except that it is located deeper in the stroma and episcleral tissues and it generally lacks cysts. Examples are illustrated.

Berman EL, Shields CL, Sagoo MS, et al. Multifocal blue nevus of the conjunctiva. *Surv Ophthalmol* 2008;53(1):41–49.

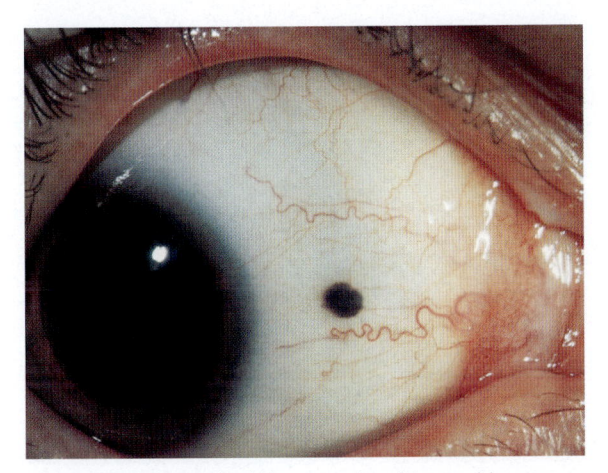

Figure 19.37. Dark episcleral blue nevus in a 45-year-old woman.

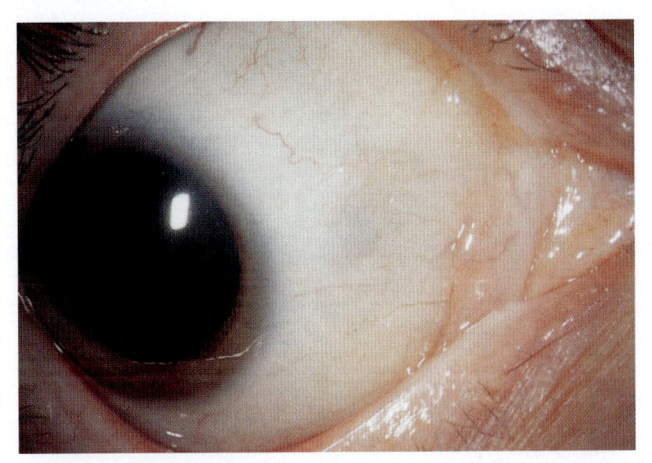

Figure 19.38. Appearance of area shown in Figure 19.37, 1 year after excision of lesion with no tumor recurrence.

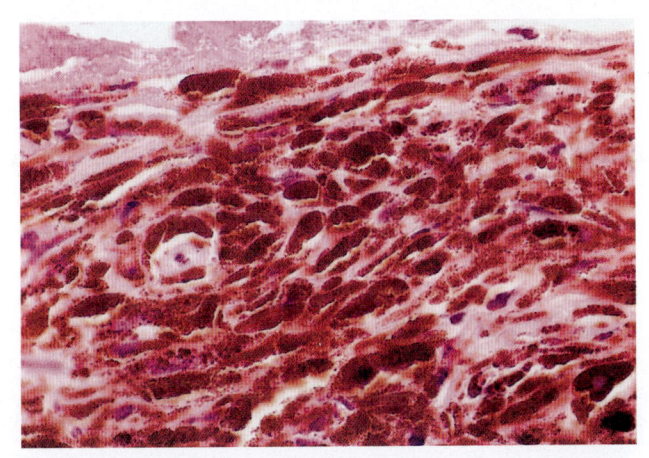

Figure 19.39. Histopathology of same lesion, showing the closely compact deeply pigmented melanocytes. (Hematoxylin–eosin ×100.)

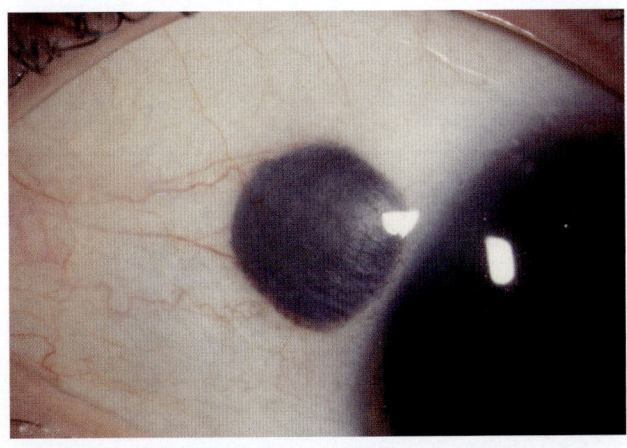

Figure 19.40. Large, ovoid blue nevus superotemporal to limbus.

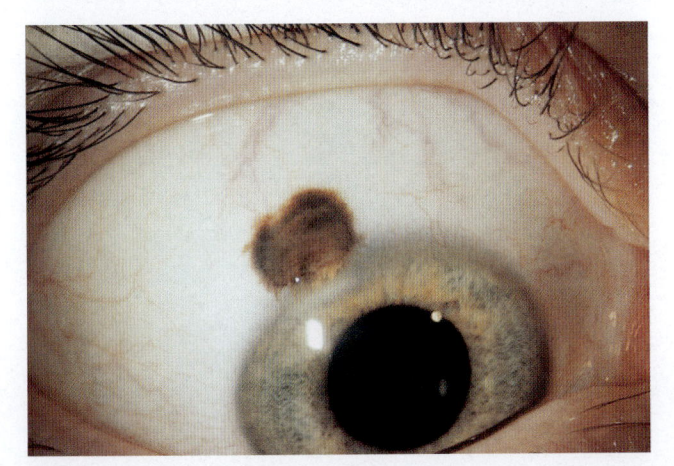

Figure 19.41. Cellular blue nevus located near limbus superiorly in a 38-year-old man. This lesion was more brown than gray, but had histopathologic features of a deep blue nevus.

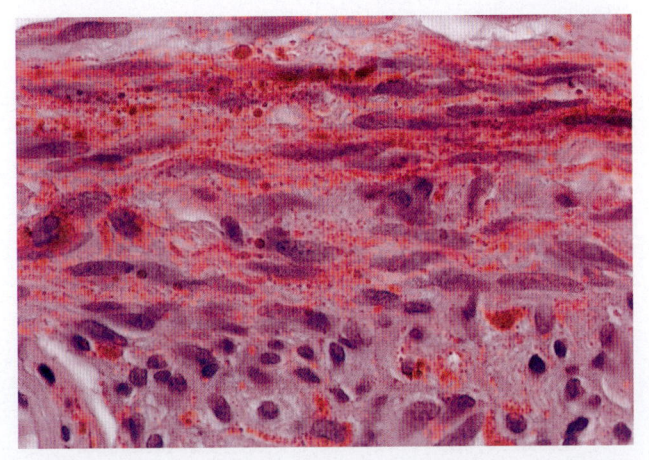

Figure 19.42. Histopathology of lesion shown in Figure 19.41, showing densely packed tumor cells in the stroma. (Hematoxylin–eosin ×200.)

CONJUNCTIVAL MELANOCYTIC NEVUS: GIANT TYPE

Conjunctival nevus range from a small lesion of only 1 mm or less to a large mass that encompasses a quadrant, hemisphere, or the entire conjunctival surface. Such large lesions, over 10 mm, are arbitrarily termed giant nevus. Below are some examples.

Shields CL, Regillo AC, Mellen PL, et al. Giant conjunctival nevus: clinical features and natural course in 32 cases. *JAMA Ophthalmol* 2013;131(7):857–863.

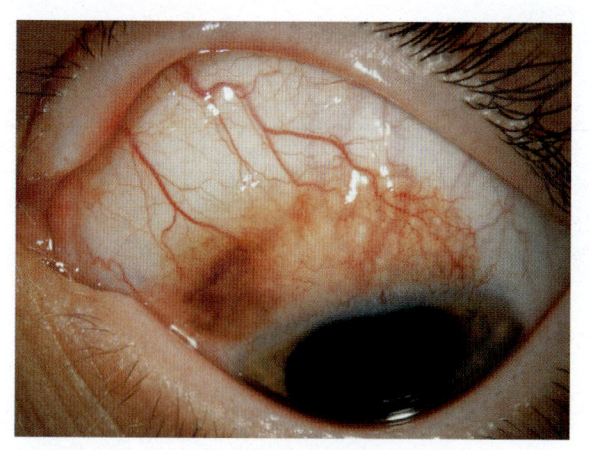

Figure 19.43. Lightly pigmented large diffuse nevus of 14-mm basal dimension, at superior limbus in a 13-year-old boy.

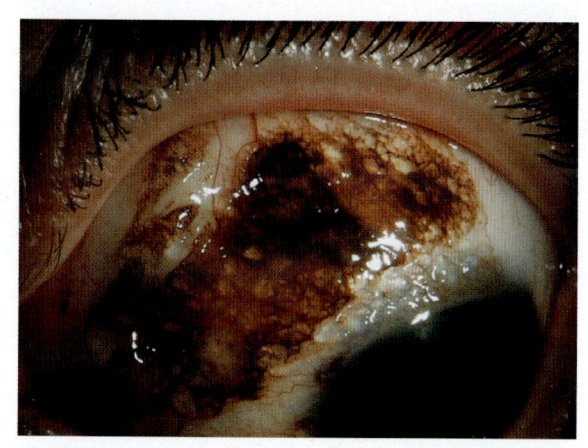

Figure 19.44. Deeply pigmented giant diffuse nevus of 20-mm basal dimension, located superonasally in a 43-year-old man. Note the numerous large cysts that are evident in the lesion.

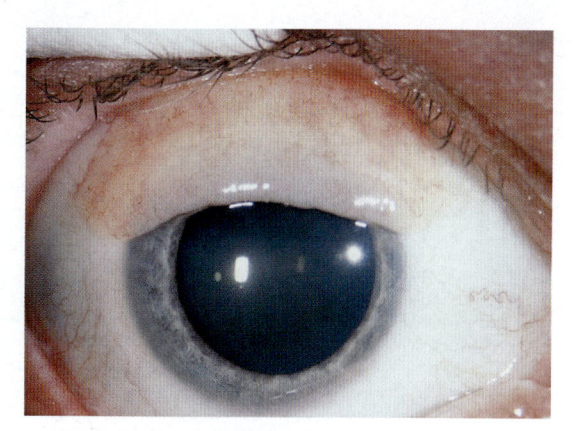

Figure 19.45. Amelanotic diffuse nevus measuring 14 mm in basal dimension, located in the superior conjunctiva of a 42-year-old man. The thickened lesion actually overhangs the cornea for about 2 mm, an exceptional finding for a conjunctival nevus.

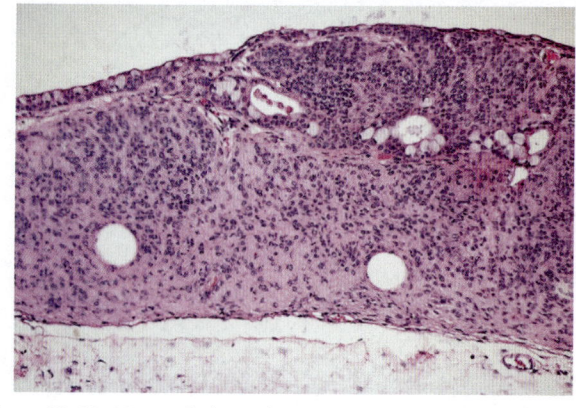

Figure 19.46. Histopathology of lesion shown in Figure 19.45 showing densely packed amelanotic nevus cells, mostly in the stroma, with cystic spaces. (Hematoxylin–eosin ×15.)

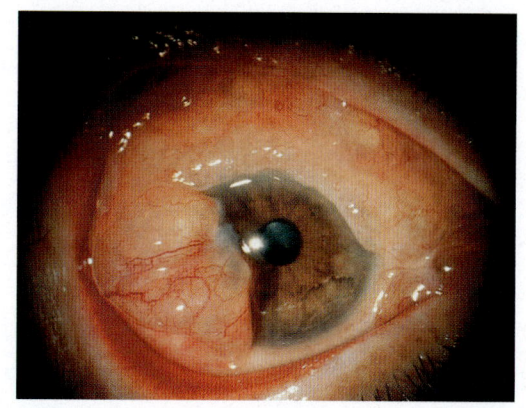

Figure 19.47. Massive amelanotic, cystic nevus in a 51-year-old man. The lesion was similar clinically to a lymphangioma or lymphoma. (Courtesy of Morton Smith, MD.)

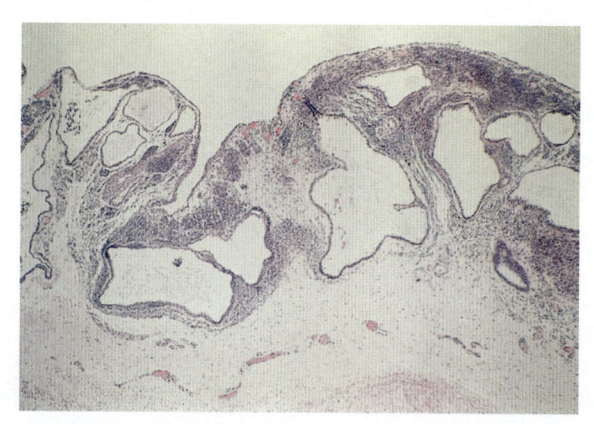

Figure 19.48. Histopathology of lesion in Figure 19.47, showing nevus cells and large, epithelial-lined cystic spaces. (Hematoxylin–eosin ×50.) (Courtesy of Morton Smith, MD.)

Chapter 19 Conjunctival Melanocytic Lesions

CONJUNCTIVAL MELANOCYTIC NEVUS IN NON-CAUCASIANS

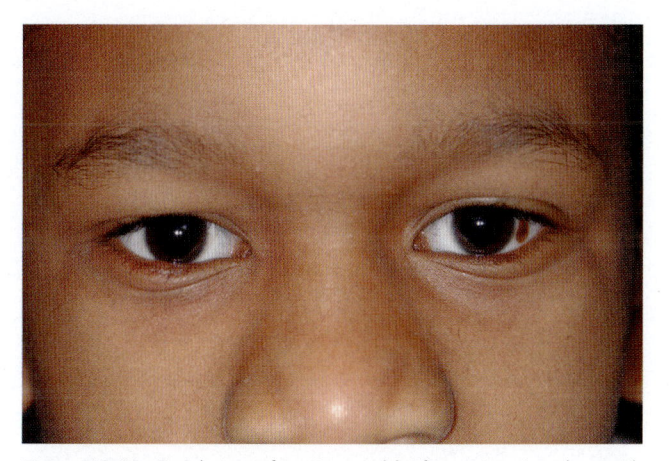

Figure 19.49. Facial view of an 8-year-old African-American boy with obvious conjunctival nevus temporally in left eye.

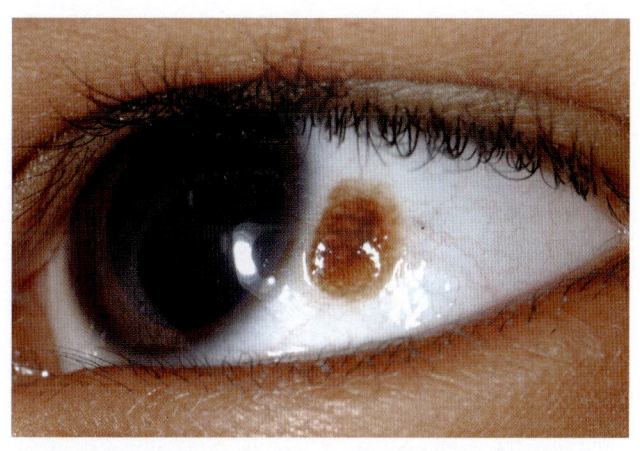

Figure 19.50. Close-up view of lesion shown in Figure 19.49 depicting the conjunctival nevus and a trace of racial melanosis at limbus.

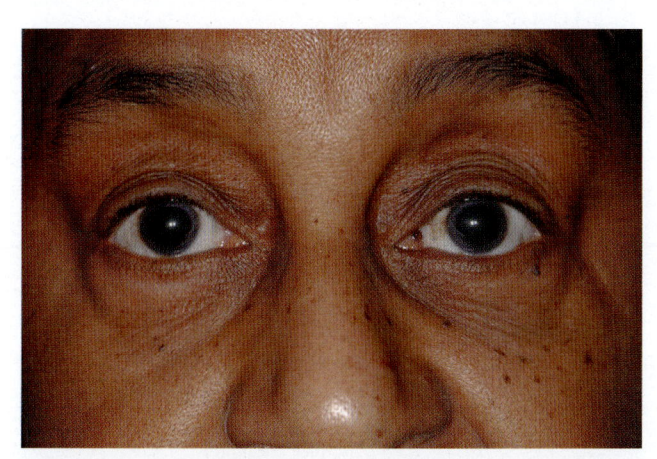

Figure 19.51. Facial view of 83-year-old African-American woman with conjunctival nevus located near semilunar fold in the left eye, as well as bilateral racial melanosis.

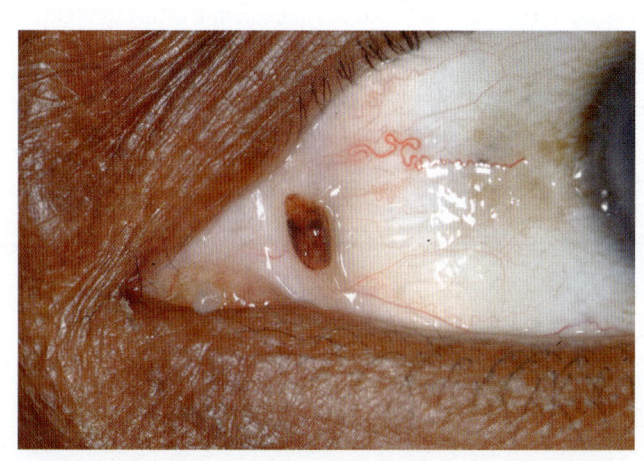

Figure 19.52. Close-up view of lesion shown in Figure 19.51. Note the circumscribed nevus at semilunar fold and unrelated racial melanosis near the limbus.

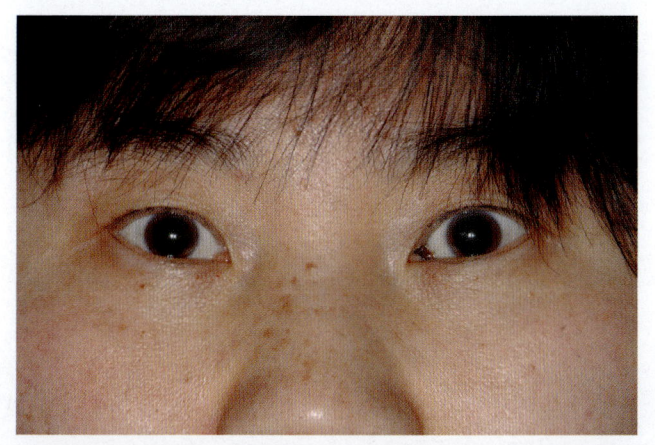

Figure 19.53. Facial view of middle-aged Asian woman with pigmentation in left semilunar fold.

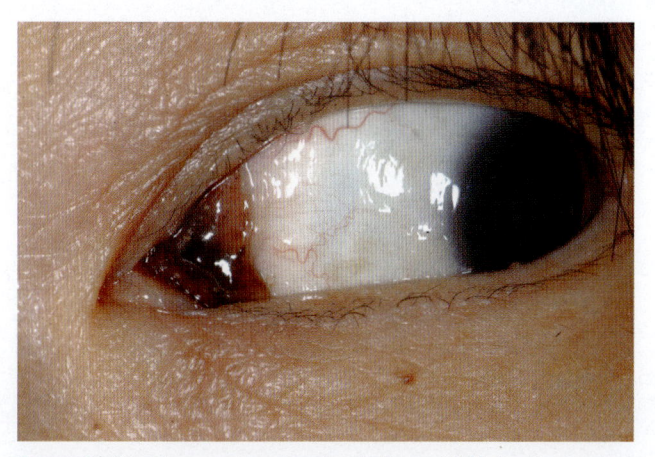

Figure 19.54. Close-up view of patient in Figure 19.53 showing involvement of entire semilunar fold. The lesion was suspicious for melanoma but proved histopathologically to be a nevus.

TUMORS OF THE CONJUNCTIVA

OCULAR MELANOCYTOSIS: SCLERAL AND EPISCLERAL PIGMENT

General Considerations

Congenital episcleral melanocytosis can occur as a solitary lesion but, in a clinical setting, it is more often seen as a component of ocular melanocytosis or oculodermal melanocytosis (nevus of Ota) (1–18). Oculodermal melanocytosis is discussed under the subject of pigmented lesions of the eyelids. Because of the association of the condition with uveal melanoma, it is also discussed in the *Atlas of Intraocular Tumors*. It is mentioned here because, although not strictly in the conjunctiva, it is included in the differential diagnosis of conjunctival nevus and PAM of the conjunctiva.

Clinical Features

Clinically, the lesions appear as irregular geographic patches of scleral and episcleral pigmentation that can range from distinct brown to gray in color (Table). The pigment can be randomly distributed or it can follow a sector distribution, sometimes corresponding to similar sector pigmentation of the uveal tract (6). Although we have not observed it in our tumor clinic, reports from other facilities have shown that this condition has a 10% incidence of elevated intraocular pressure or true glaucoma, which can occasionally be congenital or late congenital (5). Hyperpigmentation of the palatal mucosa and tympanic membrane can be associated with oculodermal melanocytosis.

Diagnostic Approaches

The diagnosis can usually be made readily with external ocular examination and slit-lamp biomicroscopy. To help differentiate it from a conjunctival lesion, one can move the conjunctiva with a cotton-tipped applicator. The overlying conjunctiva can be moved over the lesion without distorting it, confirming that it is located deep to the conjunctiva. Fundus examination should be done to exclude uveal melanoma. Uveal melanoma that arises from ocular melanocytosis carries a more serious prognosis that melanoma from nevus or de novo (8,9).

Pathology

The scleral and episcleral lesion consists of deeply pigmented dendritic melanocytes with benign cytologic features. In most cases of ocular melanocytosis, the pigmentation involves the sclera and the underlying uveal tract. There is evidence that ocular melanocytosis manifests mutations in G proteins (GNAQ, GNA11) that could lead to melanoma (13).

Management

No management is necessary for the scleral and episcleral pigmentation of ocular melanocytosis. As mentioned, the patient should be followed for the development of uveal melanoma or secondary glaucoma. There have been a few reports on laser therapy to reduce the ocular pigmentation for cosmetic reasons (11).

Selected References

Reviews

1. Shields CL, Demirci H, Karatza E, et al. Clinical survey of 1643 melanocytic and nonmelanocytic tumors of the conjunctiva. *Ophthalmology* 2004;111:1747–1754.
2. Shields CL, Shields JA. Tumors of the conjunctiva and cornea. *Surv Ophthalmol* 2004;49:3–24.
3. Singh AD, De Potter P, Fijal BA, et al. Lifetime prevalence of uveal melanoma in Caucasian patients with ocular (dermal) melanocytosis. *Ophthalmology* 1998;105:195–198.
4. Teekhasaenee C, Ritch R, Rutnin U, et al. Ocular findings in oculodermal melanocytosis. *Arch Ophthalmol* 1990;108:1114–1120.
5. Teekhasaenee C, Ritch R, Rutnin U, et al. Glaucoma in oculodermal melanocytosis. *Ophthalmology* 1990;97:562–570.
6. Shields CL, Qureshi A, Mashayekhi A, et al. Sector (partial) oculo(dermal) melanocytosis in 89 eyes. *Ophthalmology* 2011;118(12):2474–2479.
7. Shields CL, Kligman BE, Suriano M, et al. Phacomatosis pigmentovascularis of cesioflammea type in 7 patients: combination of ocular pigmentation (melanocytosis or melanosis) and nevus flammeus with risk for melanoma. *Arch Ophthalmol* 2011;129(6):746–750.
8. Shields CL, Kaliki S, Livesey M, et al. Association of ocular and oculodermal melanocytosis with rate of uveal melanoma metastasis. Analysis of 7872 consecutive eyes. *JAMA Ophthalmology* 2013;131(8):993–1003.
9. Mashayekhi A, Kaliki S, Walker B, et al. Metastasis from uveal melanoma associated with congenital ocular melanocytosis: A matched study. *Ophthalmology* 2013;120:1465–1468.

Imaging

10. Pellegrini M, Shields CL, Arepalli S, et al. Choroidal melanocytosis evaluation with enhanced depth imaging optical coherence tomography. *Ophthalmology* 2014;121(1):257–261.

Management

11. Kim JY, Hong JT, Lee SH, et al. Surgical reduction of ocular pigmentation in patients with oculodermal melanocytosis. *Cornea* 2012;31:520–524.

Histopathology/Genetics

12. Zimmerman LE. Melanocytes, melanocytic nevi and melanocytomas. The Jonas S. Friedenwald Memorial Lecture. *Invest Ophthalmol* 1965;4:11–41.
13. Van Raamsdonk CD, Griewank KG, Crosby MB, et al. Mutations in GNA11 in uveal melanoma. *N Engl J Med* 2010;363:2191–2199.

Case Reports

14. Kiratli H, Bilgig S, Satilmis M. Ocular melanocytosis associated with intracranial melanoma. *Br J Ophthalmol* 1996;80:1025.
15. Kiratli H, Irkec M. Melanocytic glaucoma in a child associated with ocular melanocytosis. *J Pediatr Ophthalmol Strabismus* 1997;34:380–381.
16. Donoso LA, Shields JA, Nagy RM. Epibulbar lesions simulating extraocular extension of uveal melanomas. *Ann Ophthalmol* 1982;14:1120–1123.
17. Louwagie CR, Baratz KH, Pulido JS, et al. Episcleral melanoma as a complication of ocular melanocytosis. *Graefes Arch Clin Exp Ophthalmol* 2008;246(9):1351–1353.
18. Shields CL, Eagle RC, Ip MS, et al. Two discrete uveal melanomas in a child with ocular melanocytosis. *Retina* 2006;26(6):684–687.

Chapter 19 Conjunctival Melanocytic Lesions

SCLERAL INVOLVEMENT WITH CONGENITAL OCULAR MELANOCYTOSIS

The scleral pigmentation of congenital ocular melanocytosis has typical features and location. It must be differentiated from other diffuse epibulbar pigmentary conditions like PAM and complexion-related pigmentation. Unlike these other conditions, it is attached to the sclera and does not move with manipulation of the conjunctiva.

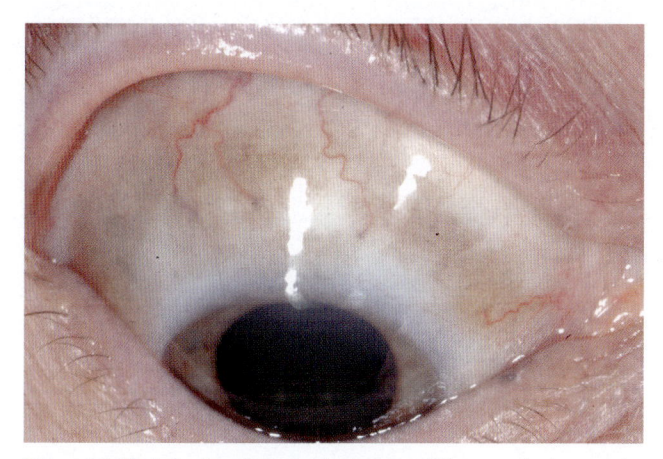

Figure 19.55. Scleral melanocytosis showing diffuse patchy brown pigment in superior aspect of the right eye.

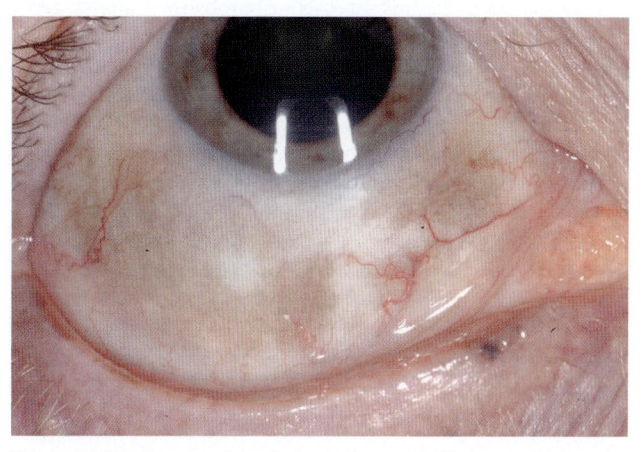

Figure 19.56. Same patient shown in Figure 19.55 demonstrating pigment in the inferior aspect of the right eye.

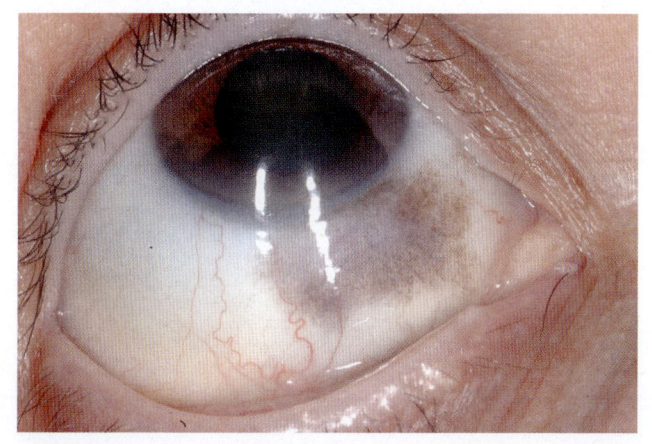

Figure 19.57. Sector scleral melanocytosis inferonasally in the right eye. Note the corresponding sector iris melanocytosis.

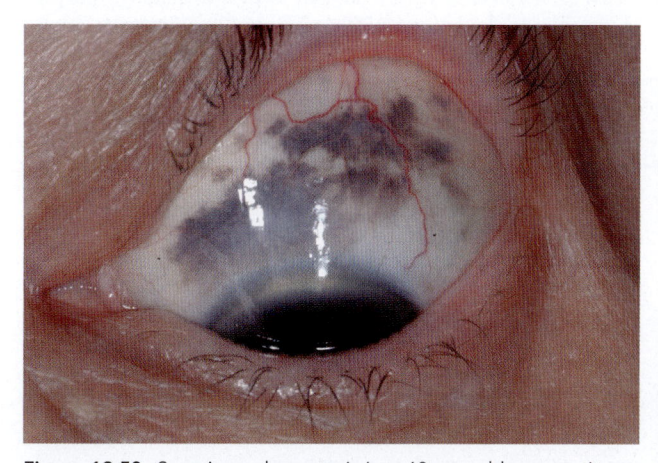

Figure 19.58. Superior melanocytosis in a 60-year-old woman. It was followed for more than 20 years without change.

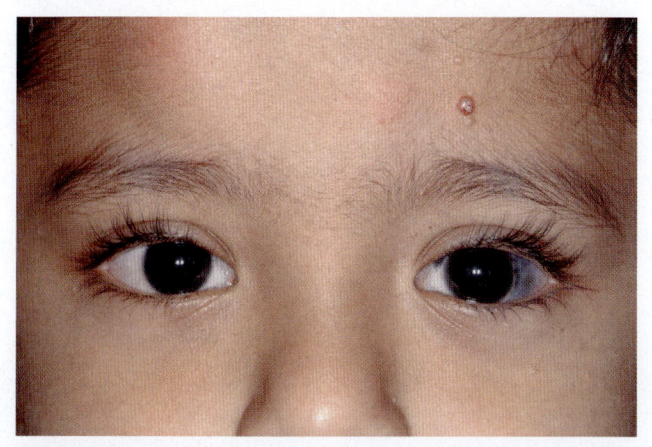

Figure 19.59. Face view of young child with blue-gray discoloration of sclera.

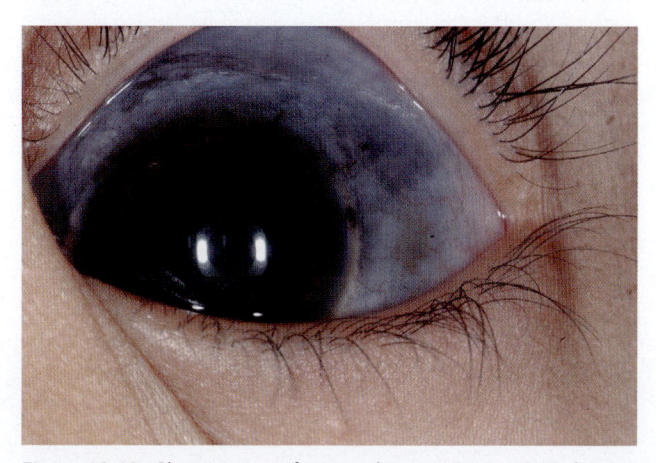

Figure 19.60. Close-up view of person shown in Figure 19.59 showing extensive blue-gray melanocytosis.

COMPLEXION-RELATED CONJUNCTIVAL PIGMENTATION (COMPLEXION-ASSOCIATED MELANOSIS, RACIAL MELANOSIS)

General Considerations

Complexion-related conjunctival pigmentation (complexion-associated melanosis [CAM]) is probably a better term than the commonly used "racial melanosis." This rather typical but variable pigmentation is not confined to a single race, but is said to be present in approximately 95% of African Americans, 35% of Asians, 30% of Hispanics, and 5% of Caucasians (1–5). In one study of conjunctival melanosis, tiny regions of pigmentation were found on the ocular surface in patients of European descent (Caucasians) in 36% of cases (4). They found CAM in Caucasians, most often those of southern European ancestry, with dark brown hair, facial nevi, pingueculae or pterygia, hypertension, and cigarette smoking (4). Although CAM is not a true tumor, it is included because it must be differentiated from other diffuse epibulbar pigmented conditions like conjunctival PAM, ocular melanocytosis, and diffuse conjunctival melanoma.

Clinical Features

CAM is characterized by bilateral, diffuse or patchy, flat pigmentation of the conjunctiva that is more common and pronounced in dark-skinned individuals. The pigmentation is most concentrated near the corneoscleral limbus where it may appear as spoke-like linear opacities oriented obliquely to the limbus. CAM is usually fairly symmetric, but can be more pronounced in one eye. In such cases, it must be differentiated from PAM, which can occasionally occur in dark-skinned individuals and can rarely give rise to conjunctival melanoma in such cases.

Pathology

CAM is characterized histopathologically by hyperpigmentation of the basal cells of the conjunctival epithelium. There is no evidence of melanocytic hyperplasia or atypia.

Management

If the diagnosis of CAM is suspected clinically, no treatment is necessary. The concerned patient should be assured that it is most likely a benign condition that has no proven tendency to undergo malignant change. However, if CAM is more advanced and asymmetric, biopsy should be considered by the technique described under the section on management of PAM. We have seen several cases of conjunctival melanoma develop adjacent to CAM in dark-skinned individuals, as biopsy and treatment should be done in suspicious atypical cases.

Selected References

Reviews

1. Shields CL, Demirci H, Karatza E, et al. Clinical survey of 1643 melanocytic and nonmelanocytic tumors of the conjunctiva. *Ophthalmology* 2004;111:1747–1754.
2. Shields CL, Shields JA. Tumors of the conjunctiva and cornea. *Surv Ophthalmol* 2004;49:3–24.
3. Henkind P, Friedman AH. External ocular pigmentation. *Int Ophthalmol Clin* 1971;11:87–111.
4. Gloor P, Alexandrakis G. Clinical characterization of primary acquired melanosis. *Invest Ophthalmol Vios Sci* 1995;36:1721–1729.

Imaging

5. Messmer EM, Machert MJ, Zapp DM, et al. In vivo confocal microscopy of pigmented conjunctival tumors. *Graefes Arch Clin Exp Ophthalmol* 2006;244:1437–1445.

COMPLEXION-RELATED CONJUNCTIVAL PIGMENTATION ("RACIAL MELANOSIS")

Complexion-related conjunctival pigmentation ("racial melanosis") can be difficult to differentiate clinically and histopathologically from PAM of the conjunctiva, a subject to be discussed in the next section.

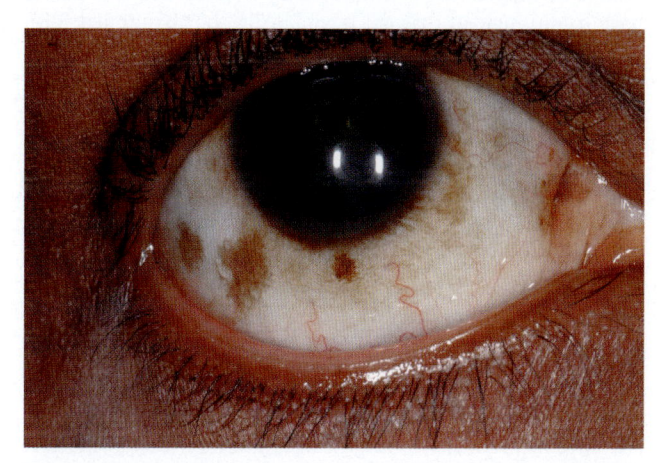

Figure 19.61. Patchy complexion-related conjunctival pigmentation in right eye. Note the characteristic linear spoke-like deposits of pigment oriented perpendicular to limbus.

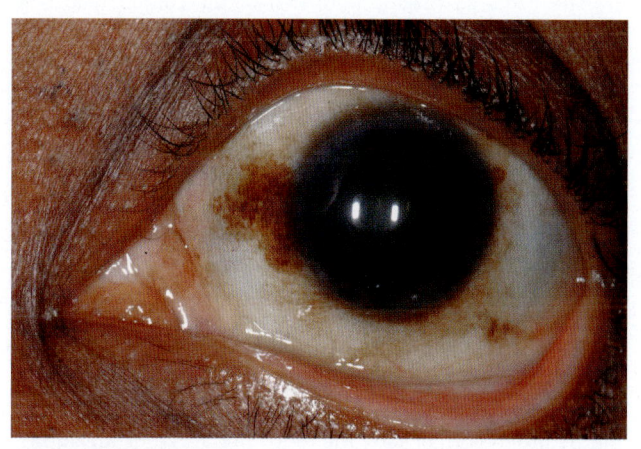

Figure 19.62. Patchy complexion-related conjunctival pigmentation in left eye of patient in Figure 19.61 showing similar findings as in the right eye.

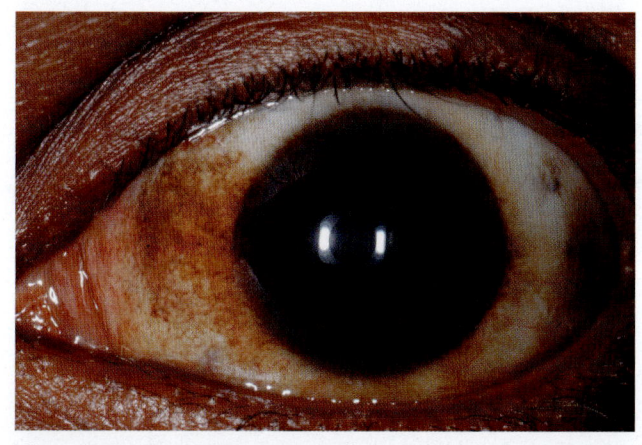

Figure 19.63. More extensive complexion-related conjunctival pigmentation in an African-American subject.

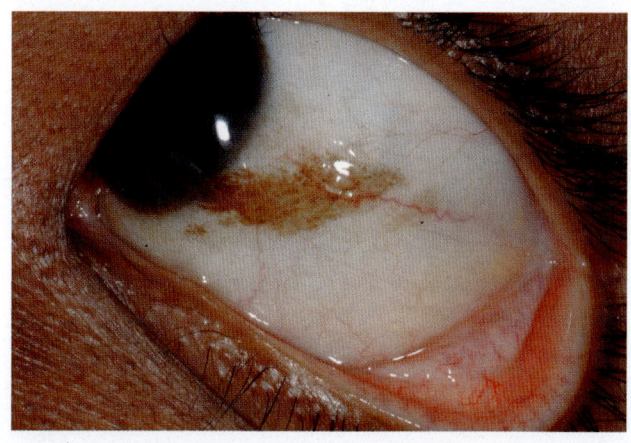

Figure 19.64. Atypical linear presumed complexion-related conjunctival pigmentation in an African-American patient. This may be difficult to differentiate from primary acquired melanosis.

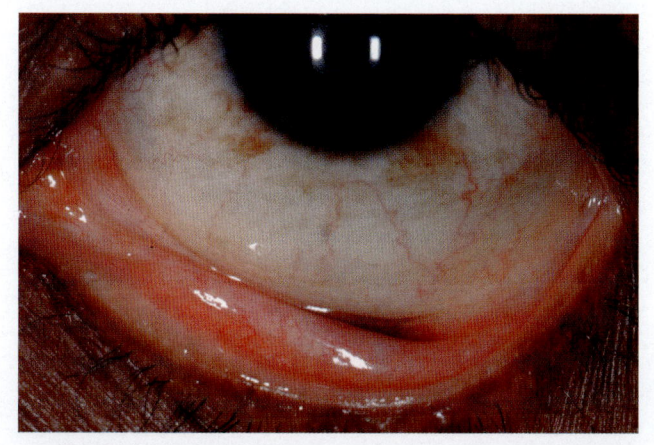

Figure 19.65. Complexion-related conjunctival pigmentation simulating primary acquired melanosis in an African-American patient.

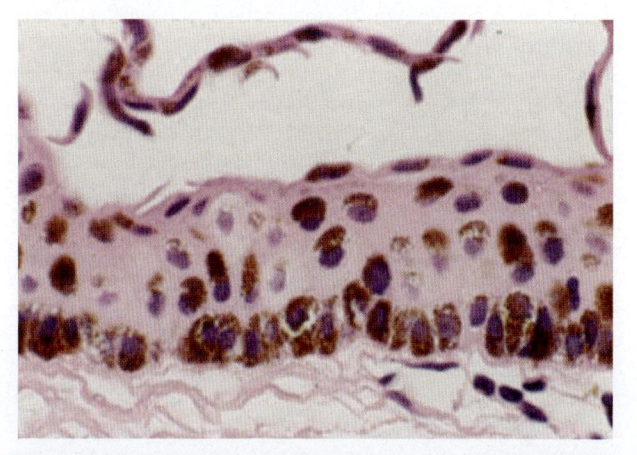

Figure 19.66. Histopathology of complexion-related conjunctival pigmentation demonstrating the dense pigmentation of the basal layer of conjunctival epithelium and some pigmented cells more superficially in the epithelium. (Hematoxylin–eosin ×100.)

CONJUNCTIVAL PRIMARY ACQUIRED MELANOSIS

General Considerations

Primary acquired melanosis (PAM) of the conjunctiva is an important condition that has been the subject of great interest to ophthalmologists and ophthalmic pathologists (1–38). In the authors' clinical series of 1,643 conjunctival tumors, there were 180 cases of PAM, accounting for 25% of conjunctival melanocytic lesions and for 11% of the 1,643 lesions (1).

Historically, the terminology for this condition has been a source of controversy (23). Based on early observations, Reese (6) noted that this condition had a tendency to evolve into melanoma and he called this entity "precancerous melanosis." Later, he estimated that 17% of his patients with "precancerous melanosis" developed conjunctival melanoma. This prompted many ophthalmologists to treat small areas of PAM very aggressively with wide conjunctival excisions and even radical neck dissections (23). Zimmerman (7) was alarmed by this trend and he proposed replacing the term "precancerous melanosis" with "benign-acquired melanosis" in hopes of discouraging radical treatment for many lesions that would remain benign. He proposed dividing this condition into two stages, with stage I representing intraepithelial disease and stage II representing malignant melanoma. He had subclassifications of these two stages based on cellular atypia and invasiveness.

Subsequently, attempts were made to equate PAM with cutaneous melanoma, using the Clark classification of melanoma. This was based on a comparison of PAM with lentigo maligna. This proved to be problematic and the World Health Organization, under the guidance of Zimmerman, later accepted the term "PAM," which is in current use.

A study by Folberg et al. (21) provided additional information as to prediction of evolution of PAM into melanoma. In a series of 41 cases with long-term follow-up, 23 (32%) progressed to melanoma. None of the lesions without cytologic atypia evolved into melanoma, whereas 46% of those with atypia progressed to melanoma. The authors acknowledged that their study of biopsy specimens submitted to the Armed Forces Institute of Pathology might not reflect the true clinical situation. The true prevalence of PAM in the general population is not known. In one analysis, Seregard et al. estimated that prevalence of PAM in the general population at 8%, but it is difficult to know if this is overestimation of true PAM (4).

We reported on 311 eyes with PAM in 276 patients and confirmed the relationship of PAM to the development of melanoma. As in prior reports, no patient developed melanoma if they had PAM without atypia or with mild atypia. Of those with severe atypia, 21% developed melanoma (3).

Most clinical ophthalmologists have employed the term "PAM" loosely and the differentiation from the more benign complexion-associated melanosis (CAM, racial melanosis) can be challenging. There are no set criteria, but, in general, CAM is bilateral, symmetric, and in patients with dark complexion, whereas PAM is unilateral, asymmetric, and in fair-skinned persons (Table). PAM carries a risk for melanoma whereas CAM generally does not.

There is also debate in the histopathology of PAM. Ackerman et al. believe that PAM is actually "melanoma in situ" and have recommended that the term "PAM" be abandoned (28). However, ophthalmic pathologists still use the term PAM, and we have chosen to use that term herein.

The etiology of PAM is uncertain, but exposure to sunlight may play a role (38). Although a relationship to DNS has been suggested, a large matched study from Denmark revealed no statistical relationship between PAM and DNS (4). PAM and conjunctival melanoma have been seen in patients with neurofibromatosis, raising speculation that it may have a developmental relationship to the neural crest (37).

Clinical Features

In contrast to conjunctival nevus, which generally becomes clinically apparent in childhood, PAM is acquired and usually appears gradually in middle age, although we have seen it occasionally in teenagers and young adults. It usually appears as unilateral, noncystic patches of brown pigmentation in the superficial aspect of any portion of the conjunctiva and peripheral cornea. It can be solitary, patchy, diffuse, or multifocal. When located in the bulbar or forniceal conjunctiva, it is freely movable with conjunctival manipulation, but when it involves the palpebral conjunctiva or corneal epithelium, it is not movable. PAM frequently extends for variable distances into the corneal epithelium, where it appears as speckled, superficial pigmentation that is usually avascular. Corneal involvement, although it may be avascular, should nevertheless raise the possibility of malignant transformation in the nearby conjunctiva (31) (Table 19.1).

Melanoma arising from PAM can rarely extend through the lacrimal canaliculus into the lacrimal sac (33,36) or through the limbal emissaries into the eye (32), necessitating removal of the lacrimal drainage system or modified enucleation, respectively. PAM can simultaneously affect the eyelid margin and even the eyelid skin. In such instances, it is almost identical clinically and histopathologically to lentigo maligna, a benign precursor of cutaneous melanoma, which was discussed in the eyelid section.

PAM can occasionally be nonpigmented, in which case the affected conjunctiva can appear almost normal or minimally thickened. Amelanotic PAM can be difficult to recognize clinically and histopathologically (3,34,35). The areas of amelanotic PAM can be multifocal, making diagnosis and management even more difficult.

Pathology

Histopathologically, PAM is composed of abnormal melanocytes in the basal layers of the epithelium. The histopathologic fine points of PAM are discussed in more detail in the literature (3,20–29). Briefly, PAM without atypia is defined as melanin pigmentation of the basal epithelium with or without hyperplasia of cytologically benign melanocytes. In contrast, PAM with atypia has similar pigmentary changes, but with cytologically atypical melanocytes. It is recommended that pathologists

CONJUNCTIVAL PRIMARY ACQUIRED MELANOSIS

attempt to classify the melanocytes as having atypia or no atypia based on these features. PAM with atypia can appear almost identical microscopically to a junctional nevus (23). Hence, the clinician should provide the pathologist with a history, including the patient's age and a clinical description or photographs of the lesion. PAM with atypia has a significant chance of evolving into conjunctival melanoma, whereas PAM without atypia has an extremely small chance of turning malignant. However, PAM without atypia can theoretically progress to PAM with atypia, which in turn can progress to malignant melanoma.

As mentioned, immunohistochemical techniques can be used to differentiate melanocytic lesions from nonmelanocytic conditions. HMB-45 generally shows a positive reaction with both nevus and melanoma and a less intense reaction with PAM (26,27). The cells of PAM have been shown to be estrogen-receptor negative (26).

Patients treated with topical mitomycin C (MMC) chemotherapy (discussed subsequently) have been shown microscopically to develop nuclear enlargement and hyperchromasia that may simulate recurrent or residual tumor (19). However, these changes are located in the superficial, rather than the basal, layer of the epithelium as seen with PAM with atypia (19).

Management

PAM without atypia presumably has little chance of evolving into melanoma, whereas PAM with atypia has a significantly greater chance of doing so. Unfortunately, there are no highly reliable clinical criteria for differentiating PAM without atypia from PAM with atypia. Because small patches of melanosis are common in the population, it would be unreasonable to biopsy all lesions. However, there are criteria that we believe are helpful in determining which lesions might require surgical intervention. Although each case must be individualized, our relative indications for biopsy and active treatment include one or more of the following:

1. Lesion diameter ≥5 mm;
2. Documented progression of the lesion;
3. Thickness of the lesion;
4. Distinct nodule arising within the lesion (pigmented or nonpigmented);
5. Nutrient vessels to the lesion;
6. Involvement of the cornea;
7. Involvement of palpebral conjunctiva;
8. Dysplastic nevus syndrome in the affected patient or close relatives;
9. Personal history of cutaneous or uveal melanoma; and
10. Patient cancerophobia.

The presence of a nodule arising in PAM deserves further comment. We strongly recommend that any nodule, whether clinically pigmented or amelanotic, that arises in the setting of PAM be removed completely intact using a "no-touch" approach. Incisional biopsy to establish a diagnosis is generally contraindicated.

Mild PAM (less than 1 clock hour of conjunctival involvement), can usually be initially managed by observation and active management withheld until the described criteria are met. A report from our department revealed that the most important clinical factor in predicting transformation of PAM into melanoma was extent of PAM (3). Each clock hour imparted 1.7 times relative risk for transformation (3). Hence, large areas of PAM that are 3 or more clock hours are generally excised or treated with other methods.

Moderately suspicious PAM, particularly if there has been progression of the disease, should be managed by biopsy (excisional biopsy if possible). At the time of surgery, additional small map biopsies should be taken in uninvolved quadrants of the conjunctiva to determine if there are atypical melanocytes that could potentially give rise to melanoma. During the same surgical procedure, double freeze-thaw cryotherapy should then be applied to the residual involved conjunctiva to devitalize melanocytes that could spawn melanoma (9–12,13).

It is stressed that these are relative criteria and there may be an argument for treating some lesions even earlier. On a few occasions, we have removed a small lesion, because of patient insistence, that we would have followed in the past and were surprised to find histopathologically that the lesion was a malignant melanoma. Based on such experiences, we sometimes suggest that a lesion that does not meet these criteria be treated by complete surgical removal combined with surrounding alcohol treatment and heavy double freeze-thaw cryotherapy. The argument is fortified by the fact that most small lesions are surgically accessible and can be managed with local anesthesia, complications are rare, and the cosmetic results are satisfactory.

Extensive and suspicious PAM should be managed by alcohol corneal epitheliectomy to remove the corneal pigment, surgical removal of suspicious areas, followed by quadratic map biopsies, and cryotherapy. The map biopsies are important, because clinically normal conjunctiva can occasionally harbor amelanotic PAM (11,12). The presence of PAM with atypia in map biopsies should prompt additional treatment, usually with topical chemotherapy. When removing the corneal pigmented component careful scrolling of epithelium off of the corneal surface without cutting Bowman's membrane is advised (see Chapter 25). Bowman's membrane serves as a barrier to prevent intraocular invasion of tumor.

In recent years, there has been increasing interest in topical chemotherapy, especially MMC, for PAM (13–18). Although doses of MMC can vary from 0.01% to 0.04% from center to center, we have used 0.04% drops three times daily for 1 week and then no medication for 1 week, repeating the on–off cycle two to three times. For selected cases of PAM giving rise to superficial melanoma, our group and others have used wide surgical removal of the lesion in one piece combined with amniotic membrane allograft and followed by topical chemotherapy (26,27). It should be noted that topical MMC is toxic and should not be started until the ocular surface is completely healed.

Table 19.1 Differential diagnosis of pigmented conjunctival and epibulbar lesions

Diagnosis	Anatomic location	Color	Depth	Margins	Laterality	Other features	Progression
Nevus	Interpalpebral limbus	Brown or yellow	Stroma	Well defined	Uni	Cysts	<1% progress to conjunctival melanoma
Ocular melanocytosis	Bulbar conjunctiva	Gray	Episclera	Ill defined	Uni > Bi	Congenital, often with periocular skin pigmentation	<1% progress to uveal melanoma
Complexion-associated melanosis (CAM) (racial melanosis)	Limbus > bulbar > palpebral conjunctiva	Brown	Epithelium	Ill defined	Bi	Flat, no cysts	Rarely progression to melanoma
Primary acquired melanosis (PAM)	Bulbar > forniceal > palpebral conjunctiva	Brown	Epithelium	Ill defined	Uni	Flat, no cysts	Progression to melanoma in nearly 50% cases that show cellular atypia
Melanoma	Anywhere	Brown or pink	Stroma	Well defined	Uni	Vascular nodule, dilated feeder vessels, can be nonpigmented	32% develop metastasis by 15 yrs

Uni, unilateral; Bi, bilateral.

Selected References

Reviews
1. Shields CL, Demirci H, Karatza E, et al. Clinical survey of 1643 melanocytic and nonmelanocytic tumors of the conjunctiva. *Ophthalmology* 2004;111:1747–1754.
2. Shields CL, Shields JA. Tumors of the conjunctiva and cornea. *Surv Ophthalmol* 2004;49:3–24.
3. Shields JA, Shields CL, Eagle RC Jr, et al. Primary acquired melanosis of the conjunctiva. Experience with 311 eyes. The 2006 Zimmerman Lecture. *Ophthalmology* 2008;115(3):511–519.
4. Seregard S, Trampe E, Mansson-Brahme E, et al. Prevalence of primary acquired melanosis and nevi of the conjunctiva and uvea in the dysplastic nevus syndrome. A case-control study. *Ophthalmology* 1995;102:1524–1529.
5. Damato B, Coupland SE. Conjunctival melanoma and melanosis: a reappraisal of terminology, classification and staging. *Clin Experiment Ophthalmol* 2008;36(8):786–795.
6. Reese AB. Precancerous and cancerous melanosis. *Am J Ophthalmol* 1966;61:1272–1277.
7. Zimmerman LE. Criteria for management of melanosis. *Arch Ophthalmol* 1966;76:307–308.

Imaging
8. Messmer EM, Mackert MJ, Zapp DM, et al. In vivo confocal microscopy of pigmented conjunctival tumors. *Graefes Arch Clin Exp Ophthalmol* 2006;244(11):1437–1445.

Management
9. Brownstein S, Jakobiec FA, Wilkinson RD, et al. Cryotherapy for precancerous melanosis (atypical melanocytic hyperplasia of the conjunctiva). *Arch Ophthalmol* 1981;99:1224–1231.
10. Jakobiec FA, Rini FJ, Fraunfelder FT, et al. Cryotherapy for conjunctival primary acquired melanosis and malignant melanoma. Experience with 62 cases. *Ophthalmology* 1988;95:1058–1070.
11. Shields JA, Shields CL, De Potter P. Surgical approach to conjunctival tumors. The 1994 Lynn B. McMahan Lecture. *Arch Ophthalmol* 1997;115:808–815.
12. Shields JA, Shields CL, De Potter P. Surgical management of circumscribed conjunctival melanomas. *Ophthalmic Plast Reconstr Surg* 1998;14:208–215.
13. Shields CL, Shields JA, Armstrong T. Management of conjunctival and corneal melanoma with surgical excision, amniotic membrane allograft, and topical chemotherapy. *Am J Ophthalmol* 2001;132:576–578.
14. Paridaens D, Beekhuis H, van Den Bosch W, et al. Amniotic membrane transplantation in the management of conjunctival malignant melanoma and primary acquired melanosis with atypia. *Br J Ophthalmol* 2001;85:658–661.
15. Frucht-Pery J, Pe'er J. Use of mitomycin C in the treatment of conjunctival primary acquired melanosis with atypia. *Arch Ophthalmol* 1996;114:1261–1264.
16. Demirci H, McCormick SA, Finger PT. Topical mitomycin chemotherapy for conjunctival malignant melanoma and primary acquired melanosis with atypia: clinical experience with histopathologic observations. *Arch Ophthalmol* 2000;118:885–891.
17. Shields CL, Demirci H, Shields JA, et al. Dramatic regression of conjunctival and corneal acquired melanosis with topical mitomycin C. *Br J Ophthalmol* 2002;86:244–245.
18. Yuen VH, Jordan DR, Brownstein S, et al. Topical mitomycin treatment for primary acquired melanosis of the conjunctiva. *Ophthal Plast Reconstr Surg* 2003;19:149–151.
19. Salomao DR, Mathers WD, Sutphin JE, et al. Cytologic changes in mimicking malignancy after topical mitomycin C chemotherapy. *Ophthalmology* 1999;106:1756–1760.

Histopathology
20. Folberg R, McLean IW, Zimmerman LE. Conjunctival melanosis and melanoma. *Ophthalmology* 1984;91:673–678.
21. Folberg R, McLean IW, Zimmerman LE. Primary acquired melanosis of the conjunctiva. *Hum Pathol* 1985;16:129–135.
22. Folberg R, McLean IW. Primary acquired melanosis and melanoma of the conjunctiva; terminology, classification, and biologic behavior. *Hum Pathol* 1986;17:652–654.
23. Folberg R, Jakobiec FA, Bernardino VB, et al. Benign conjunctival melanocytic lesions. Clinicopathologic features. *Ophthalmology* 1989;96:436–461.
24. Jakobiec FA, Folberg R, Iwamoto T. Clinicopathologic characteristics of premalignant and malignant melanocytic lesions of the conjunctiva. *Ophthalmology* 1989;96:147–166.
25. Sharara NA, Alexander RA, Luthert PJ, et al. Differential immunoreactivity of melanocytic lesions of the conjunctiva. *Histopathology* 2001;39:426–431.
26. Chowers I, Livni N, Frucht-Pery J, et al. Immunostaining of the estrogen receptor in conjunctival primary acquired melanosis. *Ophthalmic Res* 1999;31:210–212.
27. Glasgow BJ, McCall LC, Foos RY. HMB-45 antibody reactivity in pigmented lesions of the conjunctiva. *Am J Ophthalmol* 1990;109:696–700.
28. Ackerman AB, Sood R, Koenig M. Primary acquired melanosis of the conjunctiva is melanoma in situ. *Mod Pathol* 1991;4:253–263.
29. Dratviman-Storobinsky O, Cohen Y, Frenkel S, et al. Lack of oncogenic GNAQ mutations in melanocytic lesions of the conjunctiva as compared to uveal melanoma. *Invest Ophthalmol Vis Sci* 2010;51(12):6180–6182.
30. Vereecken G, Gobert A, De Laey JJ, et al. Primary acquired melanosis and melanoma of the conjunctiva. *Bull Soc Belge Ophthalmol* 1996;263:97–100.

Case Reports
31. Tuomaala S, Aine E, Saari KM, et al. Corneally displaced malignant conjunctival melanomas. *Ophthalmology* 2002;109:914–919.
32. Wenkel H, Rummelt V, Naumann GO. Malignant melanoma of the conjunctiva with intraocular extension. *Arch Ophthalmol* 2000;118:557–560.
33. McNab AA, McKelvie P. Malignant melanoma of the lacrimal sac complicating primary acquired melanosis of the conjunctiva. *Ophthalmic Surg Lasers* 1997;28:501–504.
34. Paridaens AD, McCartney AC, Hungerford JL. Multifocal amelanotic conjunctival melanoma and acquired melanosis sine pigmento. *Br J Ophthalmol* 1992;76:163–165.
35. Jay V, Font RL. Conjunctival amelanotic malignant melanoma arising in primary acquired melanosis sine pigmento. *Ophthalmology* 1998;105:191–194.
36. Robertson DM, Hungerford JL, McCartney A. Malignant melanomas of the conjunctiva, nasal cavity, and paranasal sinuses. *Am J Ophthalmol* 1989;108:440–442.
37. To KW, Rabinowitz SM, Friedman AH, et al. Neurofibromatosis and neural crest neoplasms: primary acquired melanosis and malignant melanoma of the conjunctiva. *Surv Ophthalmol* 1989;33:373–379.
38. Yu GP, Hu DN, McCormick S, et al. Conjunctival melanoma: Is it increasing in the United States? *Am J Ophthalmol* 2003;135:800–806.

CONJUNCTIVAL PRIMARY ACQUIRED MELANOSIS: MILD INVOLVEMENT

Such small patches of pigmentation are common in the general population, and can usually be safely observed unless progression is documented. PAM without atypia, PAM with atypia, and melanoma arising from PAM represents a spectrum and may not be easy to differentiate clinically.

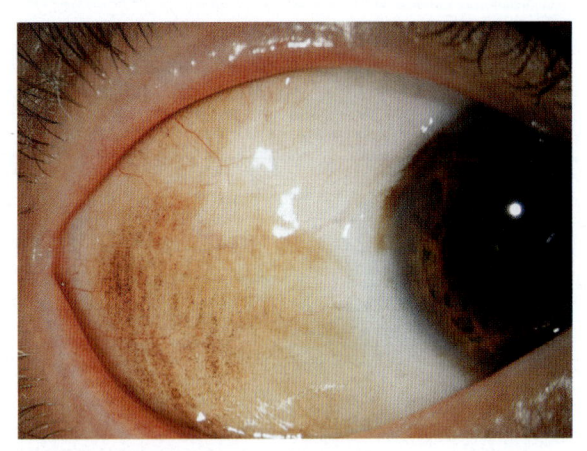

Figure 19.67. Primary acquired melanosis in temporal conjunctiva in a 46-year-old woman.

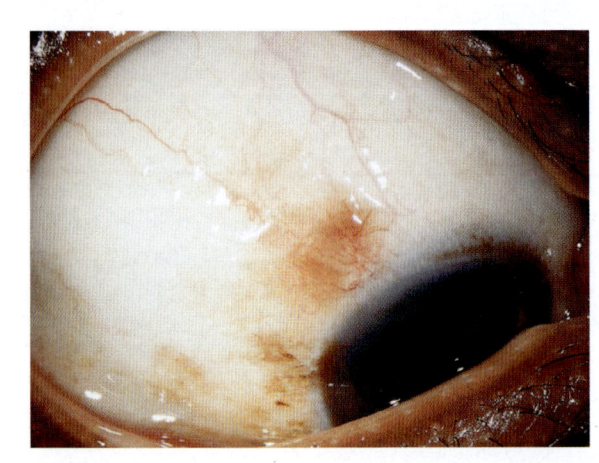

Figure 19.68. Primary acquired melanosis in superotemporal conjunctiva of a 52-year-old woman.

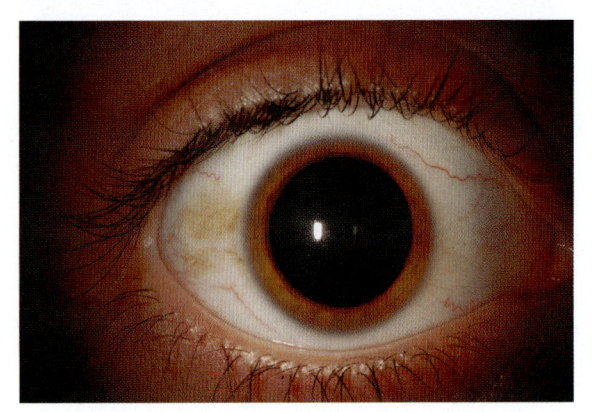

Figure 19.69. Subtle primary acquired melanosis at temporal limbal involvement in a young Caucasian woman.

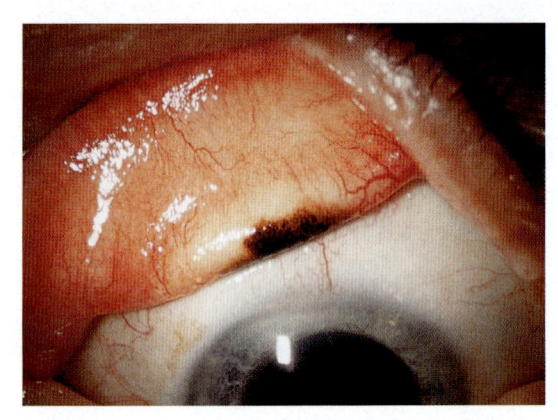

Figure 19.70. Primary acquired melanosis (PAM) involving the tarsal conjunctiva shown with eyelid everted in a 62-year-old man. PAM or melanoma in such a location often remains undetected unless the eyelid is everted and carefully inspected.

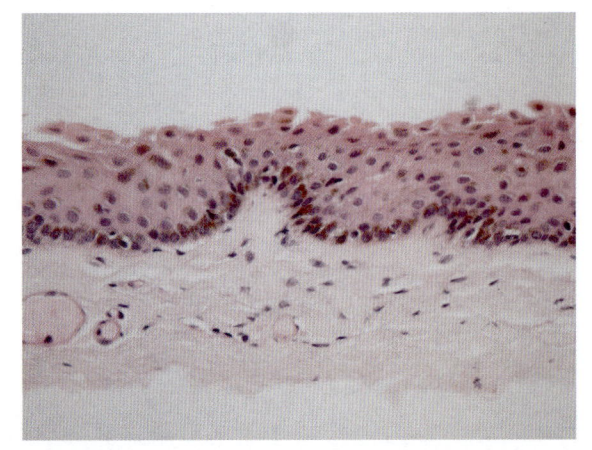

Figure 19.71. Histopathology of primary acquired melanosis without atypia. There is an increased number of melanocytes in the basal layer of the epithelium, but the cells and their nuclei are of uniform size. (Hematoxylin–eosin ×150.)

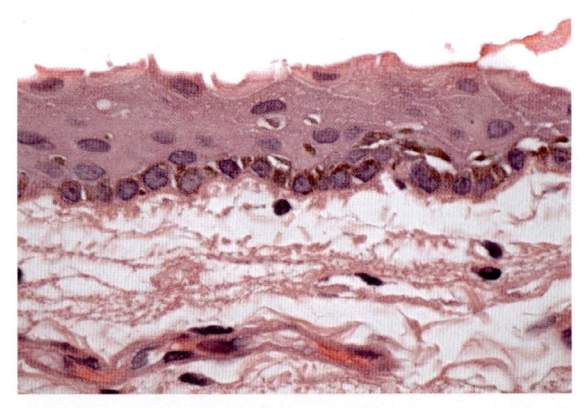

Figure 19.72. Histopathology of conjunctival primary acquired melanosis with mild atypia. The nuclei have some variation in size and shape. (Hematoxylin–eosin ×250.)

Chapter 19 Conjunctival Melanocytic Lesions

CONJUNCTIVAL PRIMARY ACQUIRED MELANOSIS: SEVERE ATYPIA

Some PAM lesions are more suspicious and the patient should be advised that staging biopsies and cryotherapy are warranted, depending on other clinical circumstances, such as patient age, general health, degree of apprehension, and status of the opposite eye. The diagnosis was made histopathologically in all of the cases shown, but some clinicians and pathologists would likely call these lesions "melanoma in situ."

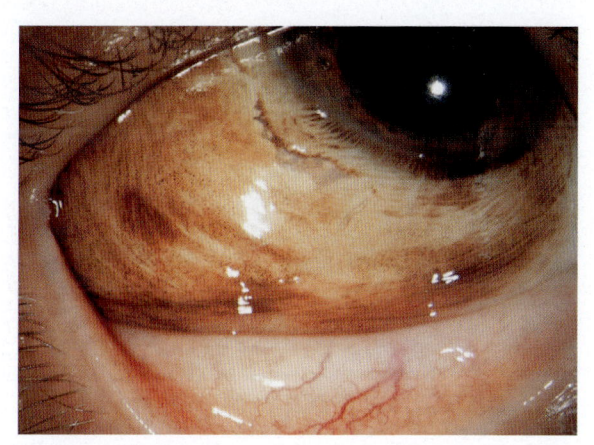

Figure 19.73. Diffuse primary acquired melanosis inferiorly in a 48-year-old woman.

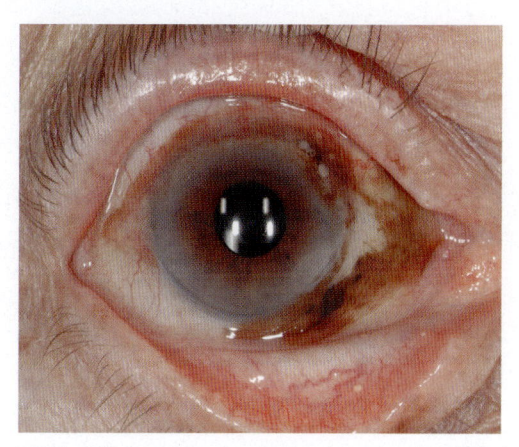

Figure 19.74. Diffuse primary acquired melanosis with mild limbal corneal involvement in an older man.

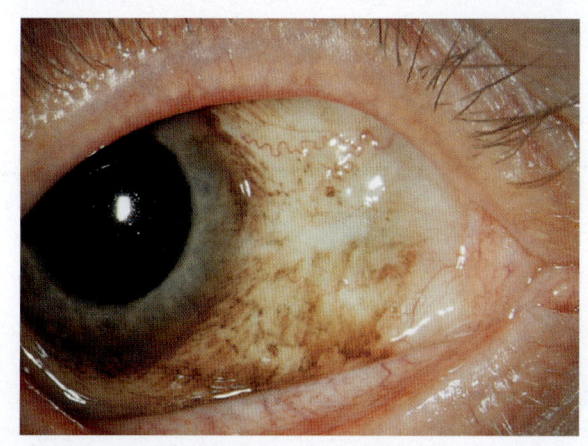

Figure 19.75. Nasal primary acquired melanosis with minimal corneal involvement in a 63-year-old man.

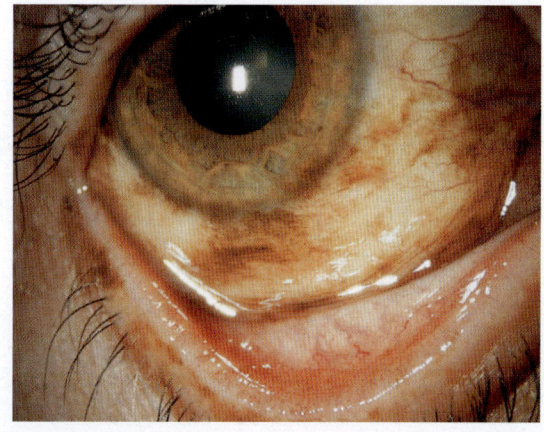

Figure 19.76. Primary acquired melanosis with early corneal involvement in a 66-year-old woman.

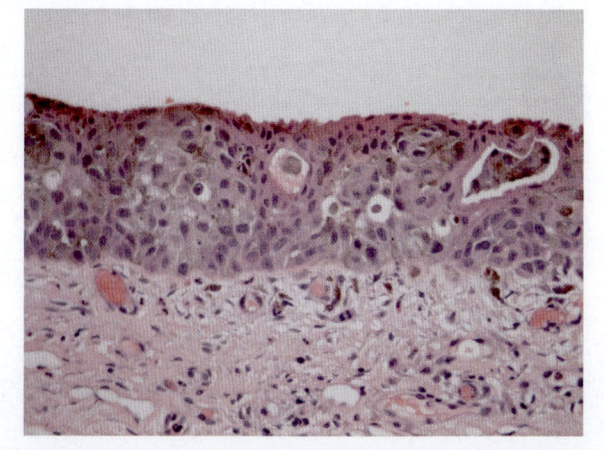

Figure 19.77. Histopathology of conjunctival primary acquired melanosis with severe atypia. The epithelioid cells replace most of the thickness of the epithelium, cell walls are fairly distinct, and the nuclei show considerable variation in size and shape. (Hematoxylin–eosin ×250.)

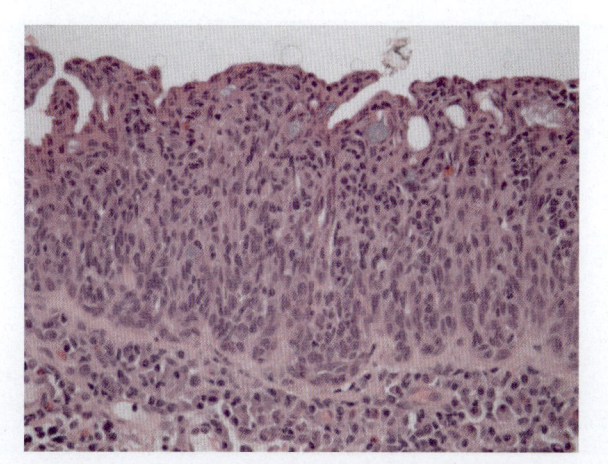

Figure 19.78. Histopathology of severe primary acquired melanosis sine pigmento. The abnormal cells that replace the epithelium are void of pigment. Clinically, such a lesion is characterized by amelanotic thickening of the conjunctiva without visible pigment. (Hematoxylin–eosin ×250.)

CONJUNCTIVAL PRIMARY ACQUIRED MELANOSIS: DEVELOPMENT OF EARLY MELANOMA

The diagnosis was confirmed as melanoma histopathologically in all of the cases shown.

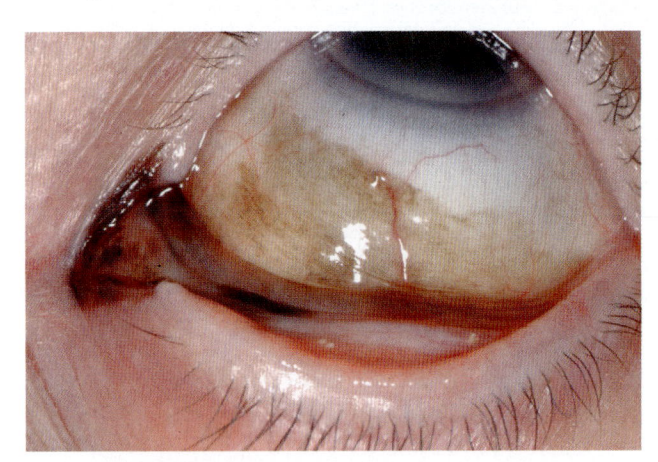

Figure 19.79. Diffuse primary acquired melanosis in inferior fornix with forniceal and medial canthal melanoma.

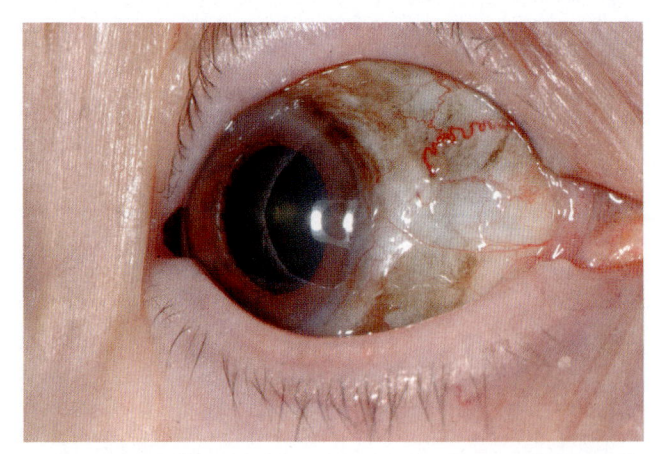

Figure 19.80. Diffuse primary acquired melanosis giving rise to early invasive melanoma at limbus.

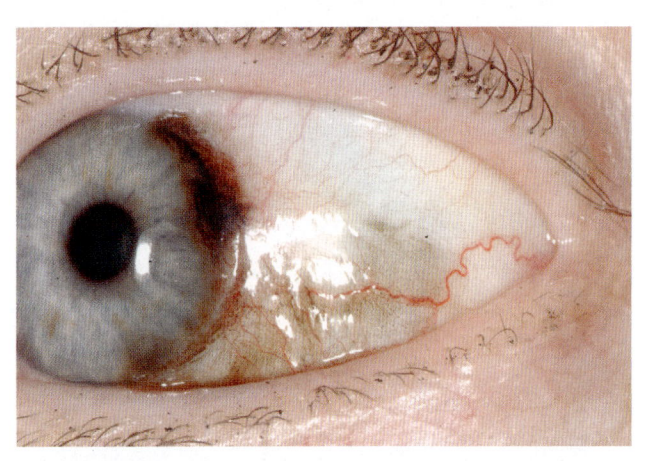

Figure 19.81. Diffuse primary acquired melanosis giving rise to more darkly pigmented flat melanoma at the limbus.

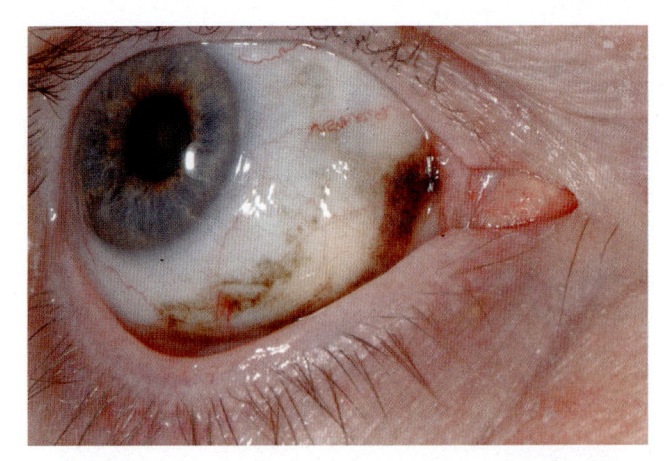

Figure 19.82. Diffuse bulbar and forniceal primary acquired melanosis with early melanoma in medial bulbar conjunctiva.

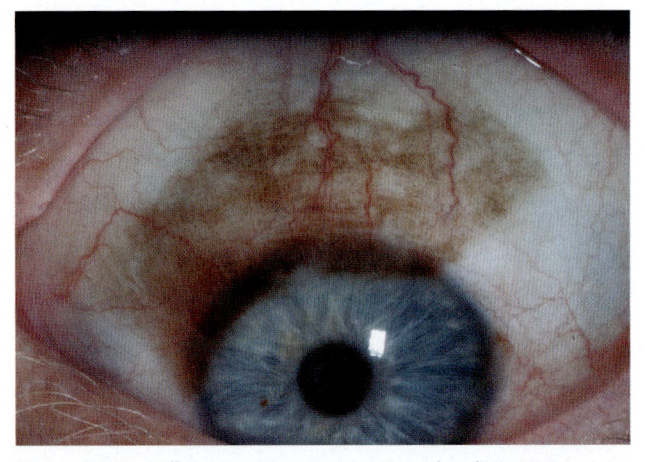

Figure 19.83. Diffuse superior primary acquired melanosis giving rise to more densely pigmented flat melanoma at the limbus region.

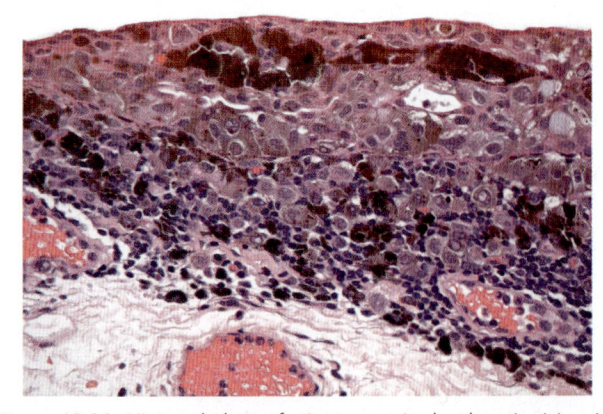

Figure 19.84. Histopathology of primary acquired melanosis giving rise to melanoma. (Hematoxylin–eosin ×250.)

CONJUNCTIVAL PRIMARY ACQUIRED MELANOSIS: DEVELOPMENT OF OBVIOUS MELANOMA

PAM that appears thicker, slightly nodular, and invades the cornea should be considered highly suspicious for early melanoma; appropriate surgical excision, biopsies, and cryotherapy are warranted. Most patients with such findings are found to have early malignant melanoma based on histopathologic examination. The diagnosis of invasive melanoma was confirmed histopathologically in all of these cases.

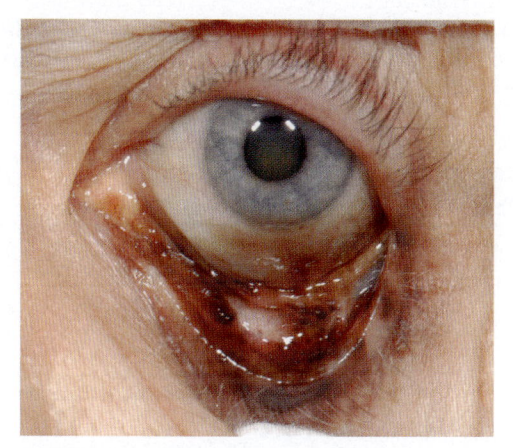

Figure 19.85. Melanoma arising on tarsal conjunctiva from severe primary acquired melanosis in an elderly woman. Note the cutaneous lentigo maligna at the eyelid margin.

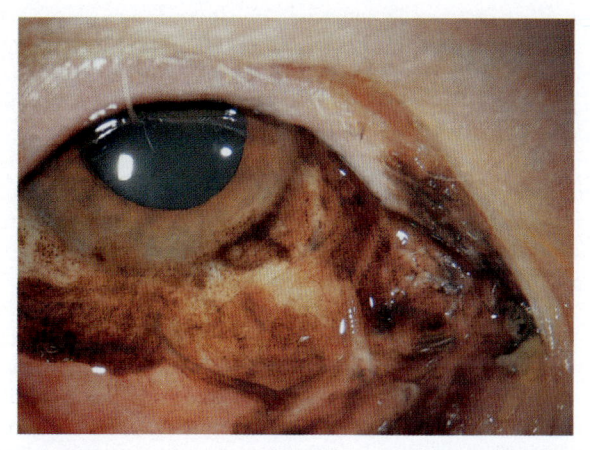

Figure 19.86. Melanoma arising from severe primary acquired melanosis in an 80-year-old woman. Note the involvement of the adjacent skin of the eyelid (lentigo maligna).

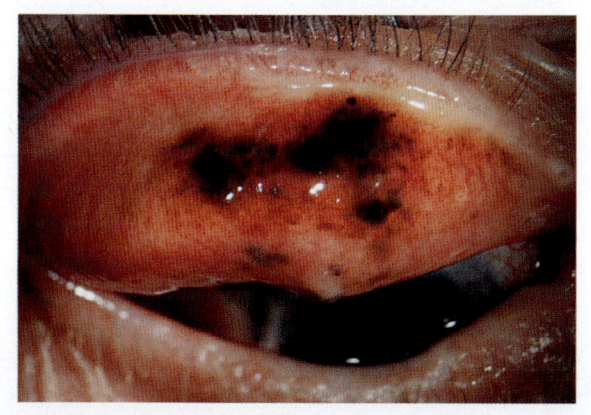

Figure 19.87. Severe primary acquired melanosis (PAM) in superior tarsus giving rise to melanoma in a 73-year-old man. All patients with PAM should have eversion (and double eversion if possible) of the eyelid on every office visit, to detect such occult disease.

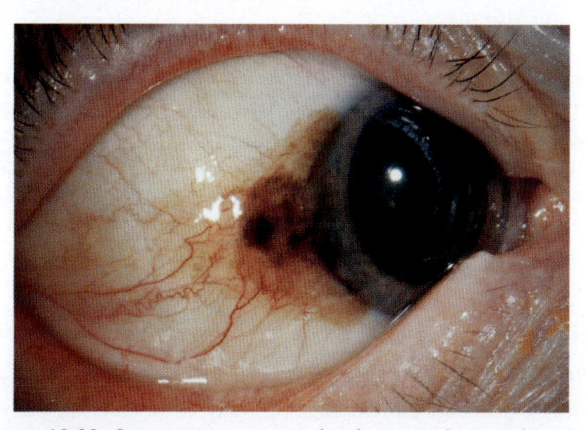

Figure 19.88. Severe primary acquired melanosis with corneal involvement, giving rise to early melanoma in a 73-year-old woman.

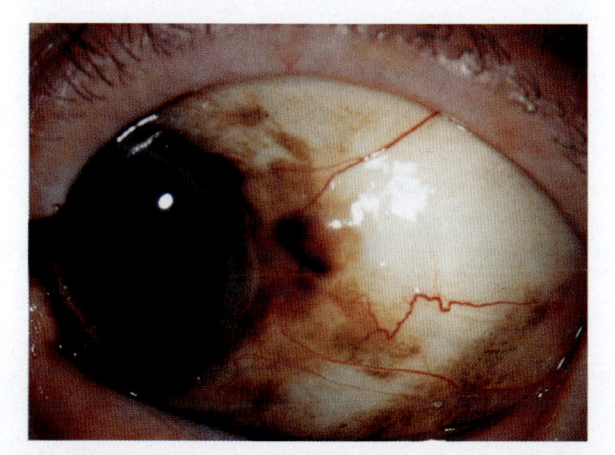

Figure 19.89. Severe primary acquired melanosis posterior to the limbus giving rise to early melanoma in an 80-year-old woman.

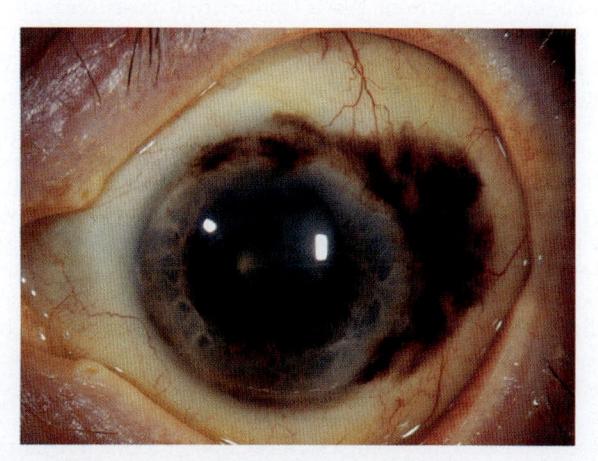

Figure 19.90. Severe primary acquired melanosis with corneal involvement giving rise to early melanoma in an 81-year-old man.

CONJUNCTIVAL MALIGNANT MELANOMA

General Considerations

Conjunctival melanoma has been the subject of many publications, a few of which are cited here (1–44). There has been a marked increase in incidence of cutaneous melanoma in recent years, and there has also been trend for increased incidence of conjunctival melanoma. A report on data collected through the Surveillance, Epidemiology, and End Results (SEER) program suggested a twofold increase in conjunctival melanoma from 0.27/million population in 1973 to 0.54/million population in 1999 in the USA (10). Data collected from Finland over the same 26 years showed exactly the same twofold increase in the incidence of conjunctival melanoma, predominantly in males (10,11).

In a large series on 382 consecutive cases of conjunctival melanoma, the malignancy arose from PAM in 74%, pre-existing nevus in 7%, and de novo in 19% (4). Conjunctival melanoma has been occasionally associated with conditions like blue nevus (42), xeroderma pigmentosum (40), and neurofibromatosis (44). There has been some concern that sunlight can be an etiologic factor (10,11), but that does not explain the occasional occurrence of melanoma in the fornices or palpebral conjunctiva (4).

Conjunctival melanoma is more common in lighter-skinned individuals. However, we have seen a number of African-American patients with conjunctival melanoma (4). There appears to be no predilection for gender and this neoplasm is more common in middle-aged or elderly individuals. However, we have seen several patients in the second decade of life with conjunctival melanoma. It occurs at a younger age in patients with xeroderma pigmentosum and the other syndromes discussed.

Clinical Features

Clinically, conjunctival melanoma varies from case to case, but it is generally a pigmented or fleshy, elevated conjunctival lesion that is usually located in the bulbar conjunctiva near the nasal or temporal limbus. In some cases it may be more diffuse or multiple, with ill-defined margins, particularly when the melanoma arises from PAM. Conjunctival melanoma occasionally originates in the fornical or palpebral conjunctiva. It is also possible for a conjunctival melanoma to develop secondary to continuous touch from an eyelid margin melanoma (41).

Conjunctival melanoma can be amelanotic, making it more difficult to differentiate from squamous cell carcinoma, lymphoma, and other nonpigmented conditions. Curiously, amelanotic melanoma can sometimes arise within an area of deeply pigmented PAM. It has been our observation that when a conjunctival melanoma recurs after prior excision, it is usually amelanotic clinically. Hence, recurrent melanoma can be also sometimes confused clinically with several nonpigmented lesions, particularly pyogenic granuloma.

Conjunctival melanoma can recur locally, particularly if resection has been incomplete. It can exhibit regional metastasis, most often to the preauricular and submandibular lymph nodes. We have rarely observed regional lymph node metastasis before the diagnosis of the primary conjunctival tumor. Distant metastasis by hematogenous spread can occur in brain, liver, skin, and bone.

There is a unifying classification for conjunctival melanoma based on the American Joint Committee for Cancer (AJCC) (Table 19.2).

Table 19.2 American Joint Committee on Cancer (AJCC) classification of conjunctival melanoma

Clinical stage	Definition
Primary tumor (T)	
Tx	Tumor extent cannot be assessed
T0	Tumor absent
T(is)	Tumor confined to conjunctival epithelium
T1	Tumor of bulbar conjunctiva
T1a	≤1 quadrant
T1b	>1 but ≤2 quadrants
T1c	>2 but ≤3 quadrants
T1d	>3 quadrants
T2	Tumor of palpebral conjunctiva, forniceal conjunctiva and/or caruncle
T2a	≤1 quadrant but not involving caruncle
T2b	≥1 quadrant but not involving caruncle
T2c	≤1 quadrant and involving caruncle
T2d	≥1 quadrant and involving caruncle
T3	Tumor with local invasion
T3a	Invasion into globe
T3b	Invasion into eyelid
T3c	Invasion into orbit
T3d	Invasion into paranasal sinus
T4	Invasion into brain
Regional lymph node (N)	
Nx	Regional lymph nodes cannot be assessed
N0a	Regional lymph node involvement absent, biopsy done
N0b	Regional lymph node involvement absent, no biopsy done
N1	Regional lymph node metastasis present
Distant metastasis (M)	
Mx	Distant metastasis cannot be assessed
M0	Distant metastasis absent
M1	Distant metastasis present

From Edge SB, Byrd DR, Compton CC, et al., eds. Malignant melanoma of the conjunctiva. In: *AJCC Cancer Staging Manual.* 7th ed. New York: Springer; 2010:539–546.

CONJUNCTIVAL MALIGNANT MELANOMA

Differential Diagnosis

Lesions known to simulate conjunctival melanoma include conjunctival nevus, PAM, ocular melanocytosis, racial pigmentation, squamous cell carcinoma, extraocular extension of ciliary body melanoma, and most other discrete or diffuse conjunctival tumors. Because these lesions are discussed in detail elsewhere in these textbooks, their differentiating features are not repeated here. In addition, other nonneoplastic simulating lesions include conjunctival foreign body, hematoma, epithelial inclusion cyst, argyrosis, and other conditions listed in Chapter 24. The clinician should be cognizant of these simulating lesions whenever the diagnosis of melanoma is entertained.

Pathology

Conjunctival melanoma is composed of variably pigmented malignant melanocytes. The cells may range from relatively low-grade spindle cells to more anaplastic epithelioid cells (31–36). This tumor initially affects the basal area of the epithelium but readily invades the stroma where it has access to conjunctival lymphatic channels. There may be microscopic evidence of PAM or a pre-existing nevus.

Immunophenotype studies have shown that conjunctival melanoma expresses S-100 protein, tyrosinase, melan-A, HMB-45 and HMB 50 combination, and microphthalmia conscription factor at high levels, suggesting that these are good diagnostic markers for this tumor (34,35). In most instances, however, the diagnosis can be made based on routine histopathologic examination, and such studies are not usually necessary.

More recent evaluation on the genetics of conjunctival melanoma have revealed that this malignancy commonly harbors BRAF mutation, a mutation found with cutaneous melanoma but not uveal melanoma (37,38). In addition, Koopmans et al. observed that mutations in telomerase reverse transcriptase (TERT) were found in 41% of conjunctival melanomas, 8% of conjunctiva PAM with atypia, and 0% of PAM without atypia or conjunctival nevi (39). This suggests that TERT promoter mutations could play a role in the progression of conjunctival melanoma.

Management

The management of conjunctival melanoma varies with the clinical findings. Classic limbal lesions are best removed primarily by alcohol corneal epitheliectomy, wide partial lamellar scleroconjunctivectomy, double freeze-thaw cryotherapy, and primary conjunctival closure (23–26) (see Chapter 25). Larger lesions that extend into the forniceal region may require wider excision with primary closure or a graft from the opposite conjunctiva, buccal mucosa, or amniotic membrane (26,27). Lesions that extend into the globe may require a modified enucleation and those that extend into the orbit may require orbital exenteration (30). The role of orbital exenteration for conjunctival melanoma with orbital invasion is controversial. However, when the lesion has invaded the deeper orbital soft tissues, we currently believe that exenteration is justified. The eyelid-sparing orbital exenteration is usually possible in such cases, because invasive conjunctival melanoma does not usually extend to involve the anterior lamellae of the eyelid (30).

Radiotherapy using teletherapy or brachytherapy can be employed for management of conjunctival melanoma (28). We have found that unshielded plaque radiotherapy, using conformer plaque, can treat the entire bulbar, forniceal, and palpebral surfaces to prevent melanoma recurrence.

Conjunctival melanoma can recur locally and metastasize to regional lymph nodes, brain, and other organs. Complete early excision, combined with the aforementioned ancillary techniques, offers the best chance of cure. Recurrent lesions are associated with a worse prognosis (4,6). On initial and follow-up office visits, it is important to check the conjunctival fornices and lacrimal puncta, and to palpate the bony orbital rim, because anterior orbital recurrence can appear in that location. The patient should undergo palpation for enlarged lymph nodes at each office visit and should have periodic systemic evaluations to detect distant metastasis to liver, brain, and other organs.

The role of prophylactic lymph node dissection for patients with conjunctival melanoma is controversial (18–21,29). To avoid extensive lymph node dissection, there has been interest in preoperative lymphoscintigraphy for identification of sentinel lymph nodes and selectively removing those nodes for histopathologic evaluation. There is still insufficient data to determine the value of such selected sentinel node biopsy.

Prognosis

The overall mortality rate for patients with conjunctival melanoma is about 25% (4). There have been a number of reports on clinical and histopathologic factors predictive of recurrence, metastasis, and mortality (3–8,36). At 10-year follow-up, conjunctival melanoma that arise de novo carry double the risk for metastasis (49%) compared to those arising from nevus (26%) or PAM (25%) (4). According to the AJCC classification, 10-year risk for metastasis was 3% for stage I, 0% for stage II, 54% for stage III, and 100% for stage IV (5).

Selected References

Reviews

1. Shields CL, Demirci H, Karatza E, et al. Clinical survey of 1643 melanocytic and nonmelanocytic tumors of the conjunctiva. *Ophthalmology* 2004;111:1747–1754.
2. Shields CL, Shields JA. Tumors of the conjunctiva and cornea. *Surv Ophthalmol* 2004;49:3–24.
3. Seregard S. Conjunctival melanoma. *Surv Ophthalmol* 1998;42:321–350.
4. Shields CL, Markowitz JS, Belinsky I, et al. Conjunctival melanoma. Outcomes based on tumor origin in 382 consecutive cases. *Ophthalmology* 2011;118:389–395.
5. Shields CL, Kaliki S, Al-Daamash S, et al. American Joint Committee on Cancer (AJCC) Clinical Classification Predicts Conjunctival Melanoma Outcomes. *Ophthalm Plast Reconstr Surg* 2012;5:313–323.
6. Shields CL, Shields JA, Gunduz K, et al. Conjunctival melanoma: risk factors for recurrence, exenteration, metastasis and death in 150 consecutive patients. *Arch Ophthalmol* 2000;118:1497–1507.
7. De Potter P, Shields CL, Shields JA, et al. Clinical predictive factors for development of recurrence and metastasis in conjunctival melanoma: a review of 68 cases. *Br J Ophthalmol* 1993;77:624–630.
8. Liesegang TJ, Campbell RJ. Mayo Clinic experience with conjunctival melanomas. *Arch Ophthalmol* 1980;98:1385–1389.
9. Inskip PD, Devesa SS, Fraumeni JF Jr. Trends in the incidence of ocular melanoma in the United States, 1974–1998. *Cancer Causes Control* 2003;14:251–257.
10. Yu GP, Hu DN, McCormick S, et al. Conjunctival melanoma: Is it increasing in the United States? *Am J Ophthalmol* 2003;135:800–806.
11. Tuomaala S, Kivela T. Conjunctivla melanoma: Is it increasing in the United States? *Am J Ophthalmol* 2003;136:1189–1190.
12. Damato B, Coupland SE. Conjunctival melanoma and melanosis: a reappraisal of terminology, classification and staging. *Clin Experiment Ophthalmol* 2008;36(8):786–795.
13. Shields JA, Shields CL, Eagle RC Jr, et al. Primary acquired melanosis of the conjunctiva. Experience with 311 eyes. The 2006 Zimmerman Lecture. *Ophthalmology* 2008;115(3):511–519.
14. Shields CL, Fasiudden A, Mashayekhi A, et al. Conjunctival nevi: clinical features and natural course in 410 consecutive patients. *Arch Ophthalmol* 2004;122:167–175.
15. Shields CL, Regillo AC, Mellen PL, et al. Giant conjunctival nevus: clinical features and natural course in 32 cases. *JAMA Ophthalmol* 2013;131(7):857–863.
16. Rodriguez-Sains RS. Pigmented conjunctival neoplasms. *Orbit* 2002;21:231–238.

Imaging

17. Bianciotto C, Shields CL, Guzman JM, et al. Assessment of anterior segment tumors with ultrasound biomicroscopy versus anterior segment optical coherence tomography in 200 cases. *Ophthalmology* 2011;118(7):1297–1302.
18. Amato M, Esmaeli B, Ahmadi MA, et al. Feasibility of preoperative lymphoscintigraphy for identification of sentinel lymph nodes in patients with conjunctival and periocular skin malignancies. *Ophthal Plast Reconstr Surg* 2003;19:102–106.
19. Esmaeli B, Eicher S, Popp J, et al. Sentinel lymph node biopsy for conjunctival melanoma. *Ophthal Plast Reconstr Surg* 2001;17:436–442.
20. Esmaeli B. Sentinel node biopsy as a tool for accurate staging of eyelid and conjunctival malignancies. *Curr Opin Ophthalmol* 2002;13:317–323.
21. Wilson MW, Fleming JC, Fleming RM, et al. Sentinel node biopsy for orbital and ocular adnexal tumors. *Ophthal Plast Reconstr Surg* 2001;17:338–344.

Management

22. Jakobiec FA, Rini FJ, Fraunfelder FT, et al. Cryotherapy for conjunctival primary acquired melanosis and malignant melanoma. Experience with 62 cases. *Ophthalmology* 1988;95:1058–1070.
23. Shields JA, Shields CL, Augsberger JJ. Current options in the management of conjunctival melanomas. *Orbit* 1986;6:25–30.
24. Shields JA, Shields CL, De Potter P. Surgical approach to conjunctival tumors. The 1994 Lynn B. McMahan Lecture. *Arch Ophthalmol* 1997;115:808–815.
25. Shields JA, Shields CL, De Potter P. Surgical management of circumscribed conjunctival melanomas. *Ophthalmic Plast Reconstr Surg* 1998;14:208–215.
26. Shields CL, Shields JA, Armstrong T. Management of conjunctival and corneal melanoma with surgical excision, amniotic membrane allograft, and topical chemotherapy. *Am J Ophthalmol* 2001;132:576–578.
27. Paridaens D, Beekhuis H, van Den Bosch W, et al. Amniotic membrane transplantation in the management of conjunctival malignant melanoma and primary acquired melanosis with atypia. *Br J Ophthalmol* 2001;85:658–661.
28. Cohen VM, Papastefanou VP, Liu S, et al. The use of strontium-90 Beta radiotherapy as adjuvant treatment for conjunctival melanoma. *J Oncol* 2013;2013:349162.
29. Cohen VM, Tsimpida M, Hungerford JL, et al. Prospective study of sentinel lymph node biopsy for conjunctival melanoma. *Br J Ophthalmol* 2013;97(12):1525–1529.
30. Shields JA, Shields CL, Demirci H, et al. Experience with eyelid-sparing orbital exenteration: the 2000 Tullos O. Coston Lecture. *Ophthal Plast Reconstr Surg* 2001;17:355–361.

Histopathology/Genetics

31. Folberg R, McLean IW, Zimmerman LE. Malignant melanoma of the conjunctiva. *Hum Pathol* 1985;16:136–143.
32. Folberg R, McLean IW. Primary acquired melanosis and melanoma of the conjunctiva; terminology, classification, and biologic behavior. *Hum Pathol* 1986;17:652–654.
33. Jakobiec FA, Folberg R, Iwamoto T. Clinicopathologic characteristics of premalignant and malignant melanocytic lesions of the conjunctiva. *Ophthalmology* 1989;96:147–166.
34. Sharara NA, Alexander RA, Luthert PJ, et al. Differential immunoreactivity of melanocytic lesions of the conjunctiva. *Histopathology* 2001;39:426–431.
35. Iwamoto S, Burrows RC, Grossniklaus HE, et al. Immunophenotype of conjunctival melanomas: comparisons with uveal and cutaneous melanomas. *Arch Ophthalmol* 2002;120:1625–1629.
36. Anastassiou G, Heiligenhaus A, Bechrakis N, et al. Prognostic value of clinical and histopathological parameters in conjunctival melanomas: a retrospective study. *Br J Ophthalmol* 2002;86:163–167.
37. Gear H, Williams H, Kemp EG, et al. BRAF mutations in conjunctival melanoma. *Invest Ophthalmol Vis Sci* 2004;45:2484–2488.
38. Spendlove HE, Damato BE, Humphreys J, et al. BRAF mutations are detectable in conjunctival but not uveal melanomas. *Melanoma Res* 2004;14:449–452.
39. Koopmans AE, Ober K, Dubbink HJ, et al. Prevalence and implications of TERT promoter mutation in uveal and conjunctival melanoma and in benign and premalignant conjunctival melanocytic lesions. *Invest Ophthalmol Vis Sci* 2014;55:6024–6030.

Case Reports

40. Mehta C, Gupta CN, Krishnaswamy M. Malignant melanoma of conjunctiva with xeroderma pigmentosa. *Indian J Ophthalmol* 1996;44:165–166.
41. Giblin ME, Shields CL, Shields JA, et al. Primary eyelid malignant melanoma associated with primary conjunctival malignant melanoma. *Aust N Z J Ophthalmol* 1988;16:127–131.
42. Demirci H, Shields CL, Shields JA, et al. Malignant melanoma arising from unusual conjunctival blue nevus. *Arch Ophthalmol* 2000;118:1581–1584.
43. Shields JA, Shields CL, Luminais S, et al. Differentiation of pigmented conjunctival squamous cell carcinoma from melanoma. *Ophthalmic Surg Lasers Imaging* 2003;34:406–408.
44. To KW, Rabinowitz SM, Friedman AH, et al. Neurofibromatosis and neural crest neoplasms: primary acquired melanosis and malignant melanoma of the conjunctiva. *Surv Ophthalmol* 1989;33:373–379.

CONJUNCTIVAL MELANOMA: EVOLUTION FROM PRIMARY ACQUIRED MELANOSIS

Melanoma that arises from PAM can assume any of a number of presentations. It can be anywhere in the bulbar or palpebral conjunctiva and can be pigmented or nonpigmented. In some cases, the melanoma may be hidden beneath the upper eyelid, underscoring the necessity of everting the upper eyelid in all patients with PAM.

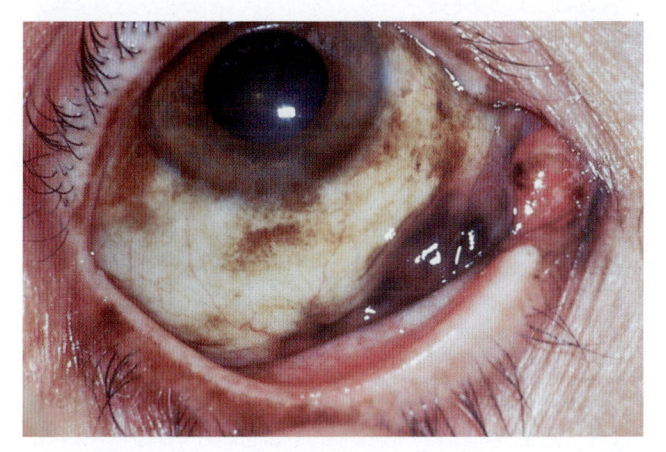

Figure 19.91. Melanoma arising from diffuse primary acquired melanosis in inferior fornix in a 69-year-old woman.

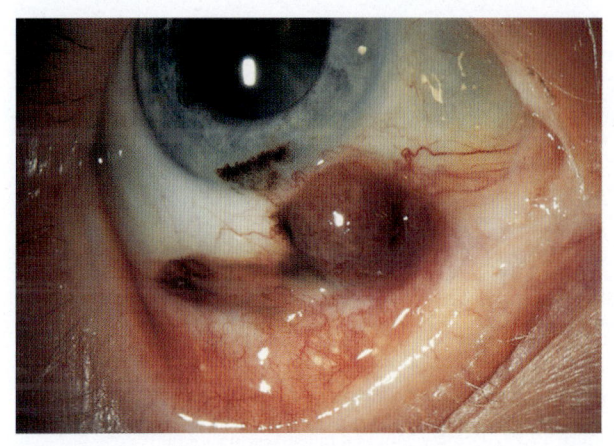

Figure 19.92. Nodular melanoma arising from localized primary acquired melanosis in inferior fornix in an 81-year-old man.

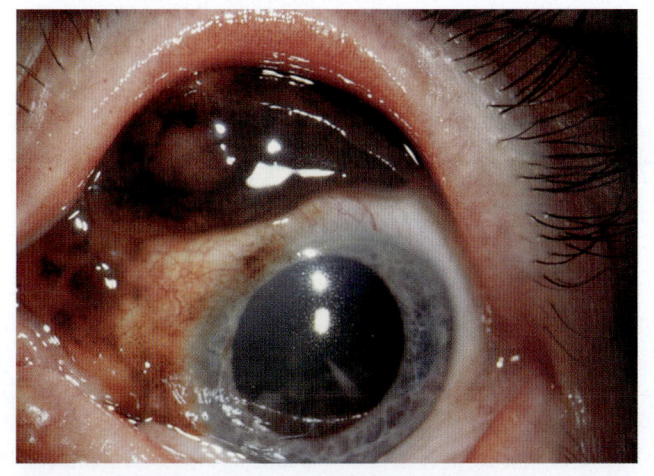

Figure 19.93. Diffuse, pigmented melanoma arising in superior fornix in a 74-year-old woman with primary acquired melanosis.

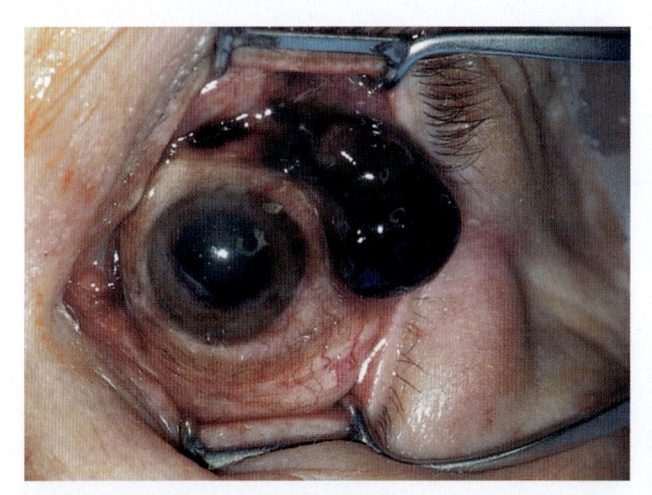

Figure 19.94. Pedunculated, pigmented melanoma arising in superior fornix in an 80-year-old woman with primary acquired melanosis.

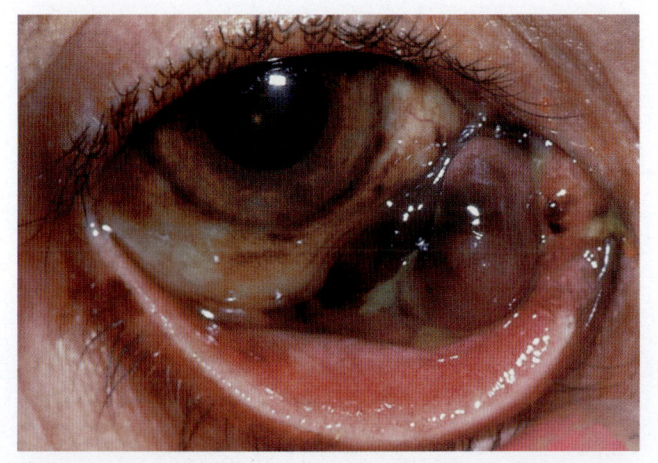

Figure 19.95. Variably pigmented melanoma arising in inferior fornix in a 70-year-old woman with primary acquired melanosis.

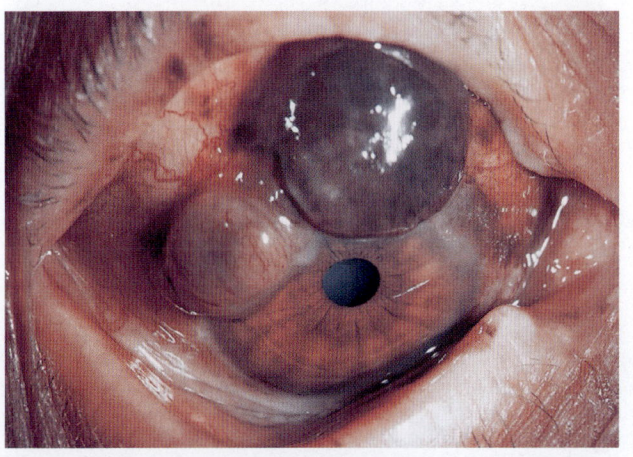

Figure 19.96. Bilobed pedunculated melanoma arising near limbus in an 82-year-old woman with primary acquired melanosis. Note that one lobe is minimally pigmented and the other is markedly pigmented.

CONJUNCTIVAL MELANOMA: EVOLUTION FROM PRIMARY ACQUIRED MELANOSIS

Melanoma that arises from PAM can be subtle, amelanotic, and sometimes extend to cover the cornea, suggesting a primary corneal tumor.

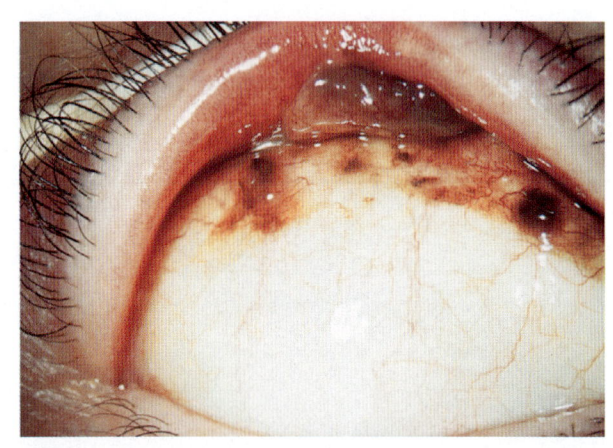

Figure 19.97. Primary acquired melanosis in superior fornix, giving rise to a nodular melanoma in a 55-year-old woman. A hidden lesion like this can be easily overlooked clinically, stressing the need to carefully examine the superior fornix in such patients.

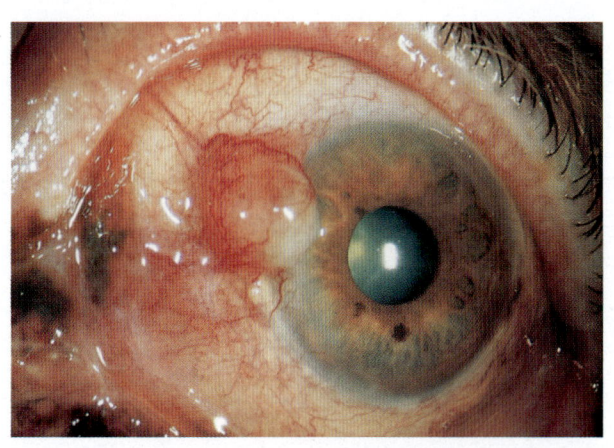

Figure 19.98. Amelanotic melanoma arising from amelanotic primary acquired melanosis in an 86-year-old man. Note that there is pigmentation near the medial canthus, but most of the conjunctival PAM is without evident pigment.

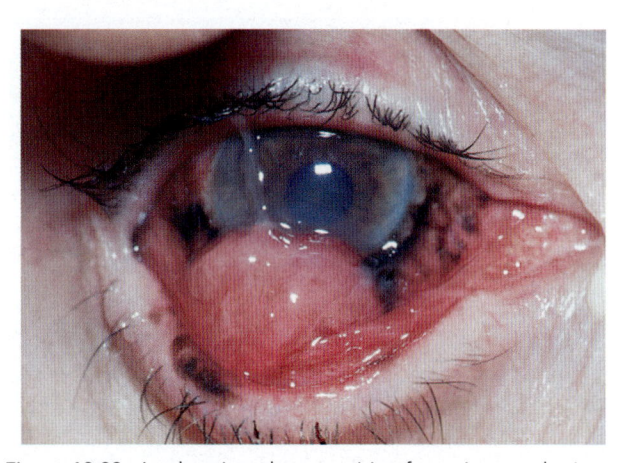

Figure 19.99. Amelanotic melanoma arising from pigmented primary acquired melanosis in a 61-year-old woman.

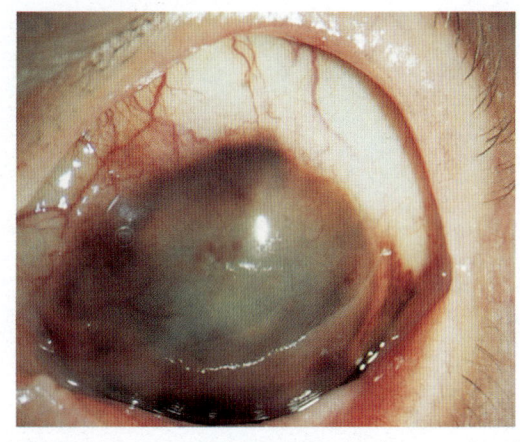

Figure 19.100. Aggressive melanoma covering the cornea in a 79-year-old woman. The patient had extensive primary acquired melanosis in the bulbar conjunctiva. She declined treatment.

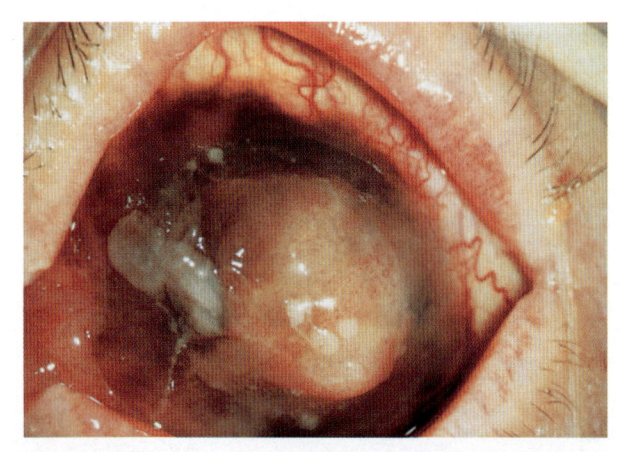

Figure 19.101. Appearance of lesion shown in Figure 19.100 after 2 years. The corneal pigmentation has grown extensively into a melanoma completely covering the cornea. The patient still refused treatment because of severe cardiovascular disease.

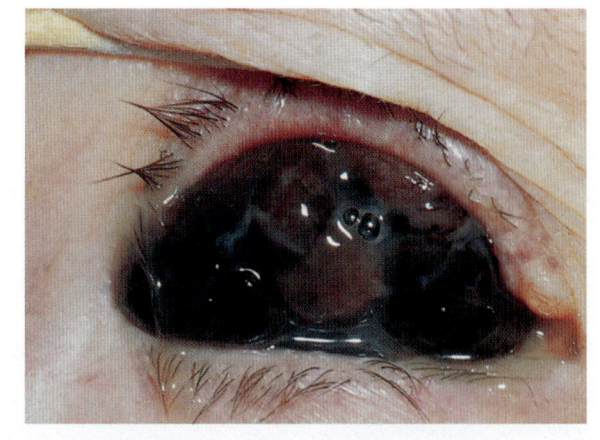

Figure 19.102. Massive, diffuse melanoma arising from primary acquired melanosis and filling the entire palpebral fissure in an 87-year-old woman, who did not seek medical care until lesion was far advanced.

Chapter 19 Conjunctival Melanocytic Lesions

CONJUNCTIVAL MELANOMA IN NON-CAUCASIANS

Primary acquired melanosis and conjunctival melanoma occur predominantly in light-skinned individuals and are rare in African-American patients.

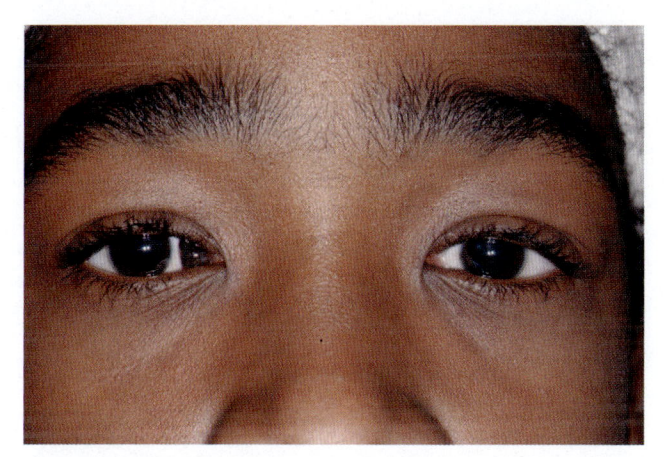

Figure 19.103. Conjunctival melanoma in the nasal conjunctiva in an African-American teenager.

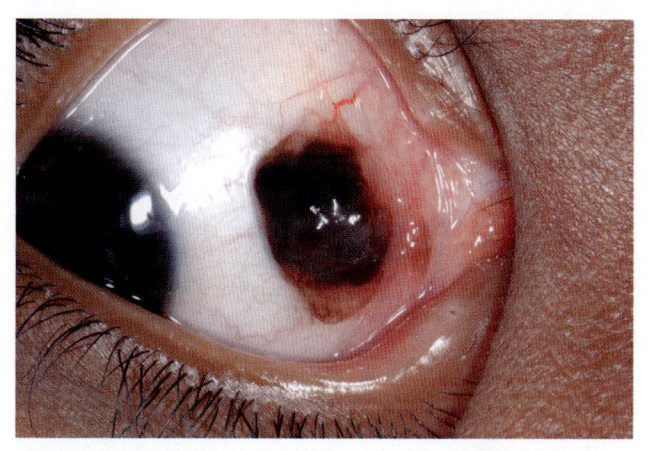

Figure 19.104. Closer view of lesion shown in Figure 19.103. It appeared clinically and pathologically that the lesion arose de novo with no convincing evidence of pre-existing complexion-related conjunctival pigmentation, primary acquired melanosis, or nevus.

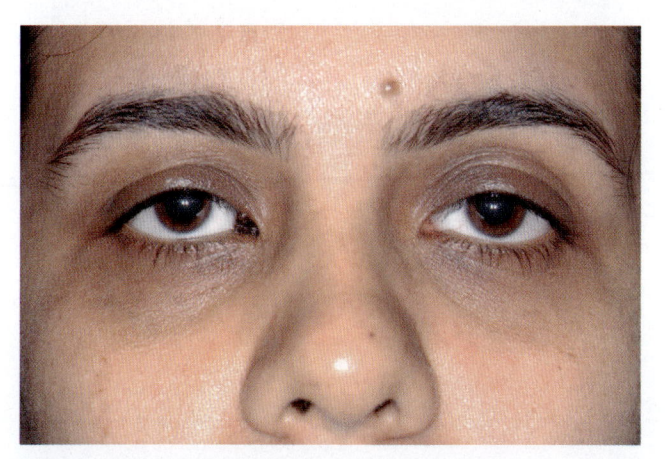

Figure 19.105. Conjunctival melanoma in medial conjunctiva and caruncle of right eye in a middle-aged Asian-Indian woman.

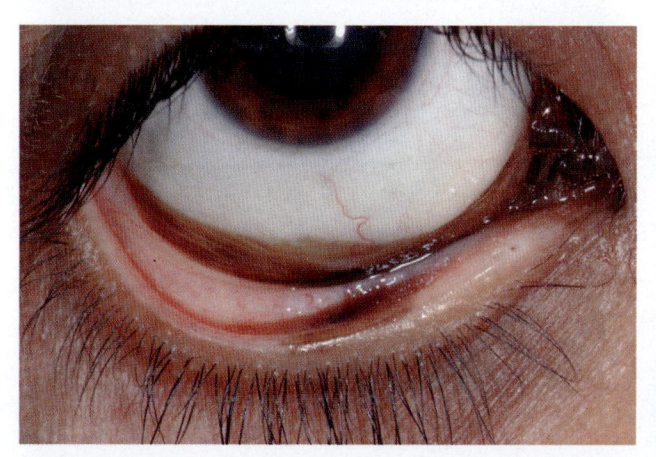

Figure 19.106. Closer view of lesion shown in Figure 19.105 with eversion of lower eyelid, disclosing diffuse melanoma presumably arising from primary acquired melanosis.

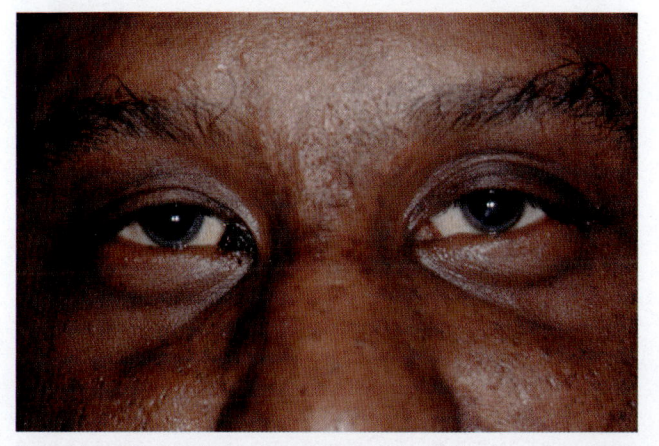

Figure 19.107. Facial appearance of 48-year-old African-American man showing pigmented mass in medial canthus of right eye.

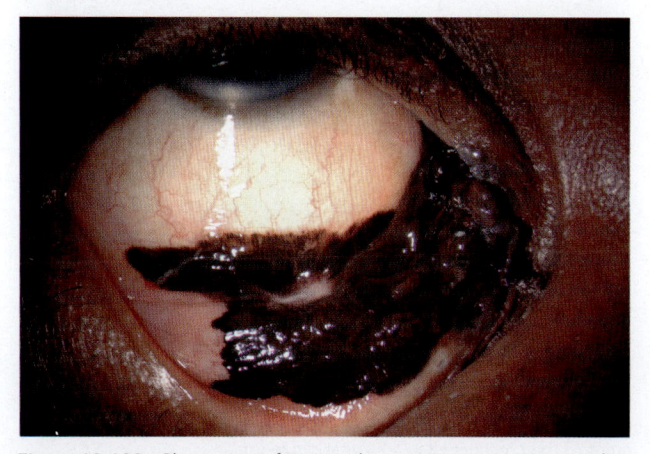

Figure 19.108. Closer view of patient shown in Figure 19.107 revealing full extent of deeply pigmented melanoma diffusely involving caruncle, palpebral, and forniceal conjunctiva. Pathology showed poorly differentiated invasive melanoma.

TUMORS OF THE CONJUNCTIVA

CONJUNCTIVAL MELANOMA: TUMORS POSSIBLY ARISING DE NOVO

In some instances, it may be difficult to determine clinically and histopathologically whether a melanoma arose from primary acquired melanosis pre-existing nevus, or de novo. Such melanomas can assume a wide variety of clinical configurations.

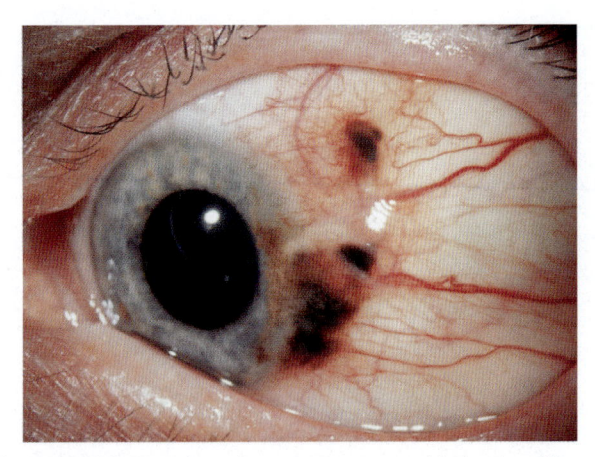

Figure 19.109. Irregular melanoma near temporal limbus in a 45-year-old man.

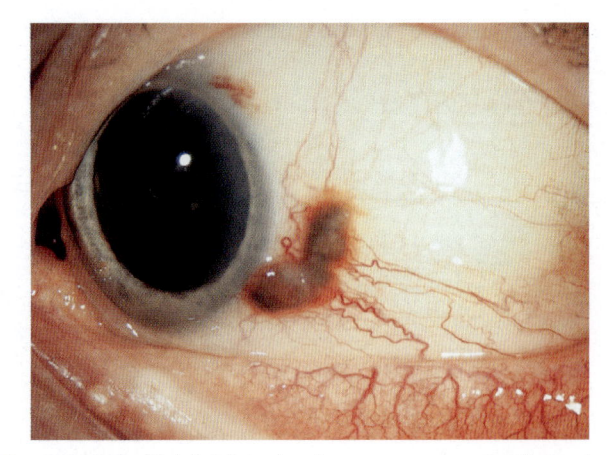

Figure 19.110. Slightly bilobed melanoma near temporal limbus in a 50-year-old man.

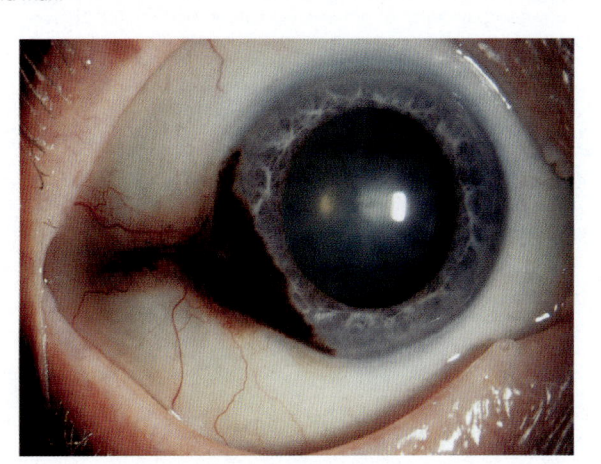

Figure 19.111. Peculiar-shaped melanoma extending from near the lateral canthus to the cornea in a 78-year-old man.

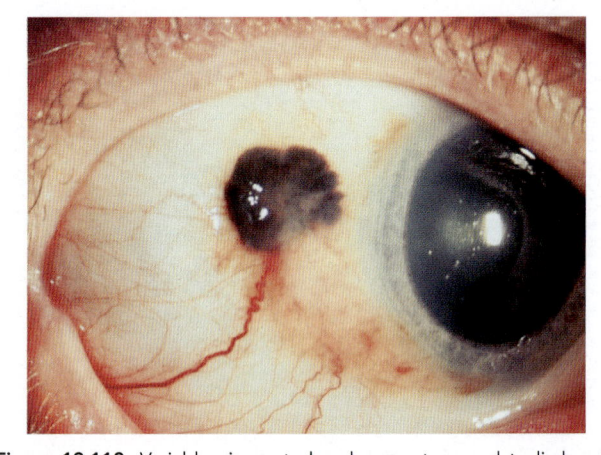

Figure 19.112. Variably pigmented melanoma temporal to limbus in a 71-year-old man. Note that the pigmented superior portion of the tumor has a large feeder vessel and the amelanotic inferior portion has less evident feeder vessels.

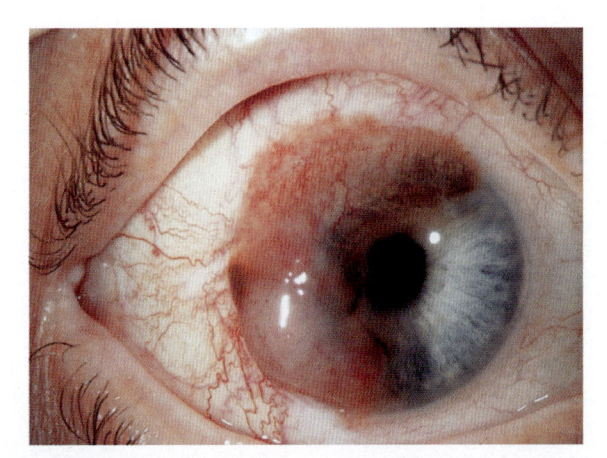

Figure 19.113. Melanoma affecting cornea with only minimal involvement of the conjunctiva in a 74-year-old woman.

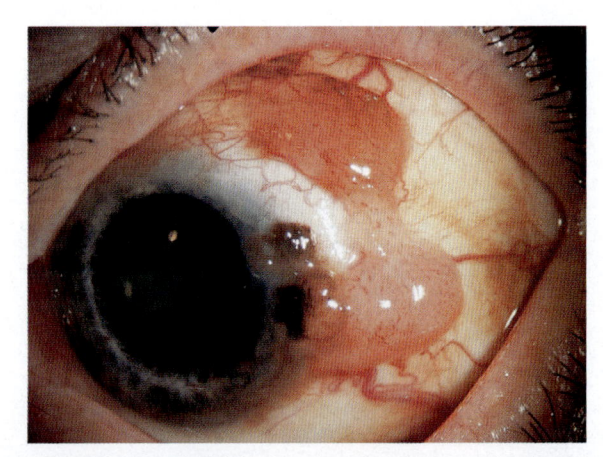

Figure 19.114. Irregular bilobed amelanotic melanoma with only minimal pigment near the limbus in a 60-year-old man. This was a recurrence since the patient had a prior excision of a pigmented lesion at another institution.

Chapter 19 Conjunctival Melanocytic Lesions

● CONJUNCTIVAL MELANOMA: PRESUMABLY ARISING FROM NEVUS AND DE NOVO

Although most conjunctival melanomas in a clinical practice arise from primary acquired melanosis, many present as a circumscribed lesion unassociated with PAM. If the patient has no history of a prior nevus, then it may be difficult to determine whether the lesion arose from an unrecognized nevus or if it arose de novo.

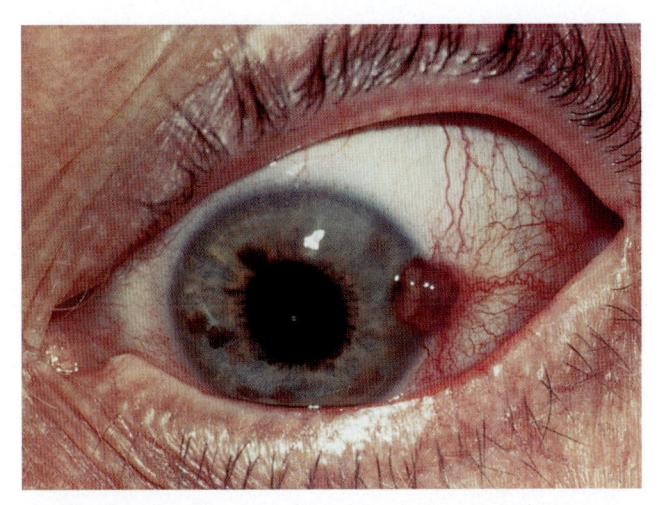

Figure 19.115. Circumscribed melanoma at limbus, arising from a pre-existing nevus in a 51-year-old woman. She gave a history of a prior nevus at that site for many years, confirmed with inspection of prior photographs.

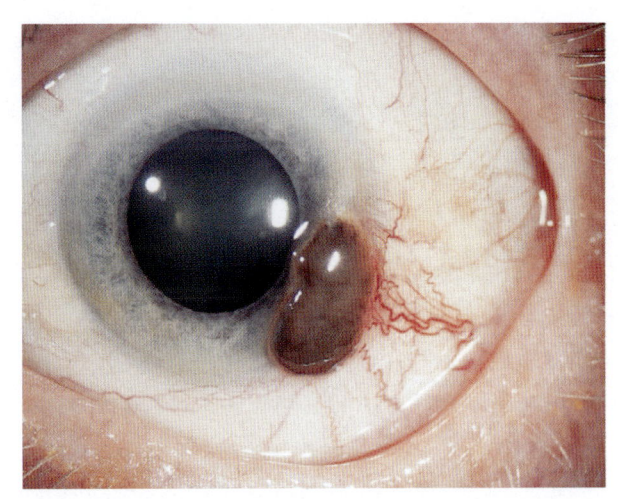

Figure 19.116. Oval-shaped melanoma at the limbus in a 67-year-old man who had no known history of a prior nevus.

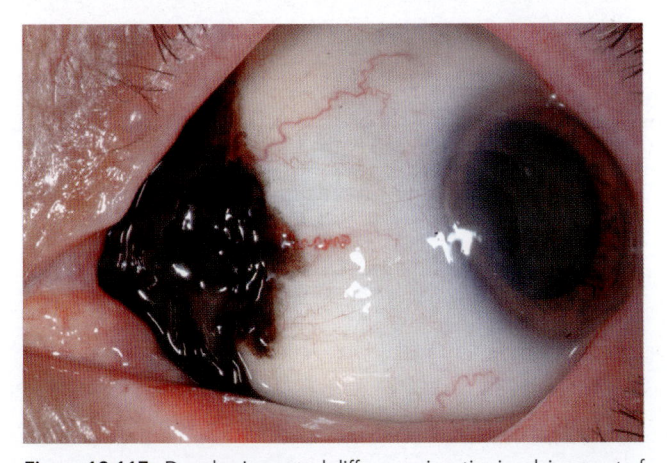

Figure 19.117. Deeply pigmented diffuse conjunctiva involving most of the medial conjunctiva, mostly in the semilunar fold.

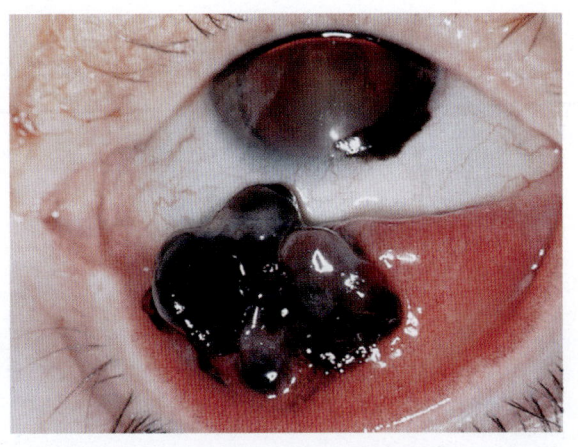

Figure 19.118. Irregular nodular melanoma arising from inferior forniceal conjunctiva. (Courtesy of Don Nicholson, MD.)

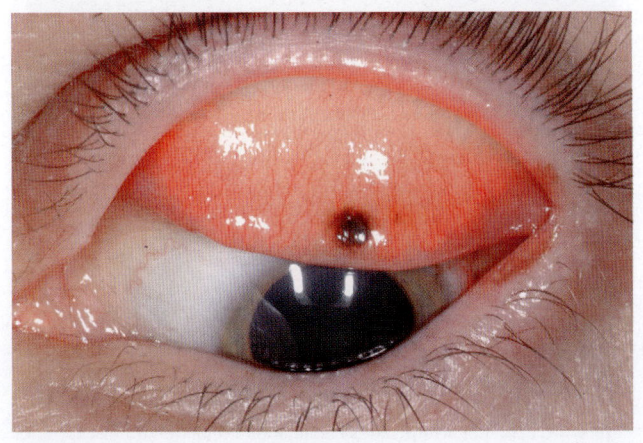

Figure 19.119. Small circumscribed melanoma arising from superior tarsal conjunctiva of left eye. Melanoma was confirmed histopathologically.

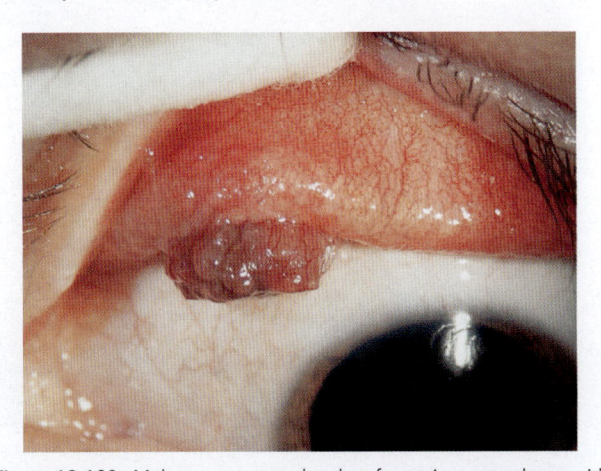

Figure 19.120. Melanoma at upper border of superior tarsus shown with eyelid everted in a 31-year-old man. He presented with what appeared to be a subcutaneous nodule in upper eyelid. All such patients should have double eversion of the eyelid and examination of the superior fornix.

TUMORS OF THE CONJUNCTIVA

CONJUNCTIVAL MELANOMA: AMELANOTIC VARIATIONS

In some instances, a conjunctival melanoma can occur as a solitary, clinically amelanotic tumor without convincing clinical evidence of primary acquired melanosis. In some such cases, the tumor may have arisen from amelanotic PAM. When a pigmented melanoma recurs after local resection, the recurrence is often amelanotic and may be confused with pyogenic granuloma.

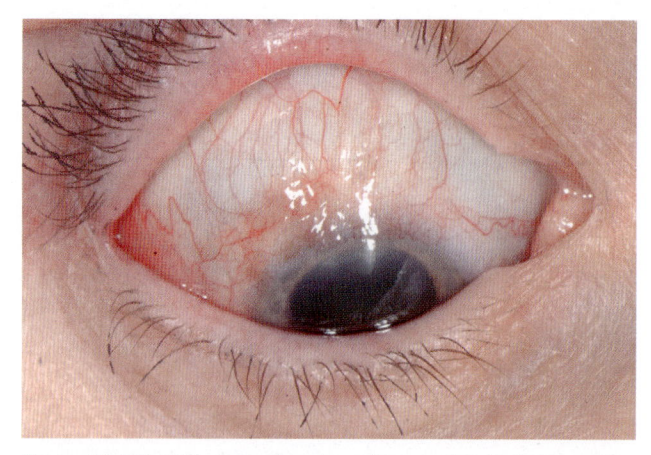

Figure 19.121. Diffuse amelanotic melanoma that had shown slow growth near superior limbus in a 65-year-old woman. The clinical diagnosis was nevus, but histopathology revealed unequivocal melanoma.

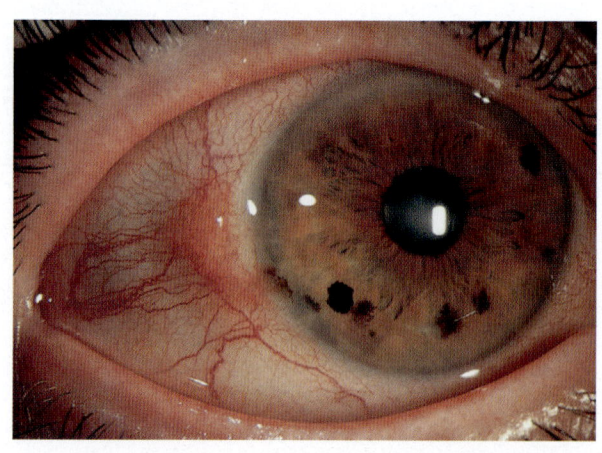

Figure 19.122. Circumscribed amelanotic conjunctival melanoma near the temporal limbus.

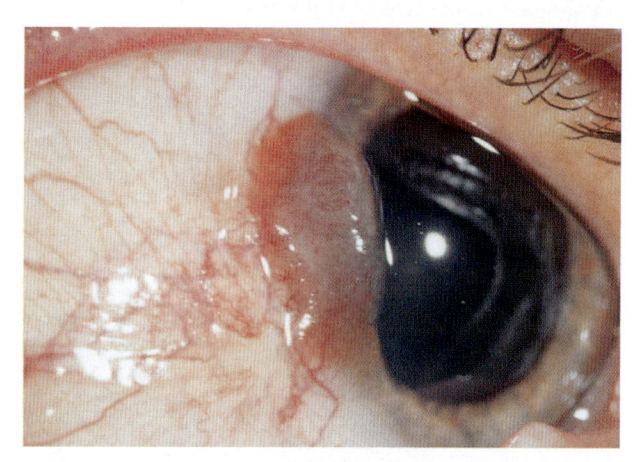

Figure 19.123. Oval-shaped amelanotic melanoma at nasal limbus in a 51-year-old man.

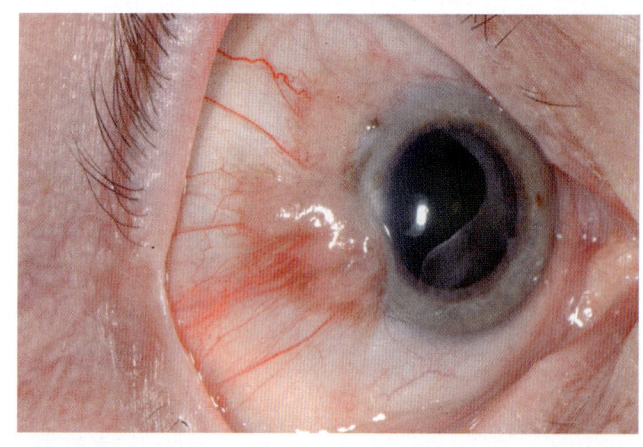

Figure 19.124. Diffuse, irregular conjunctival melanoma located temporally in the right eye.

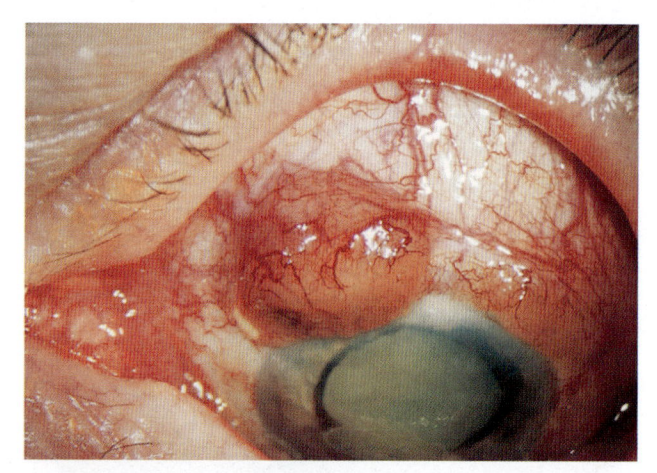

Figure 19.125. Recurrent amelanotic melanoma near superior limbus in a 70-year-old woman. A pigmented melanoma had been previously excised from the same location.

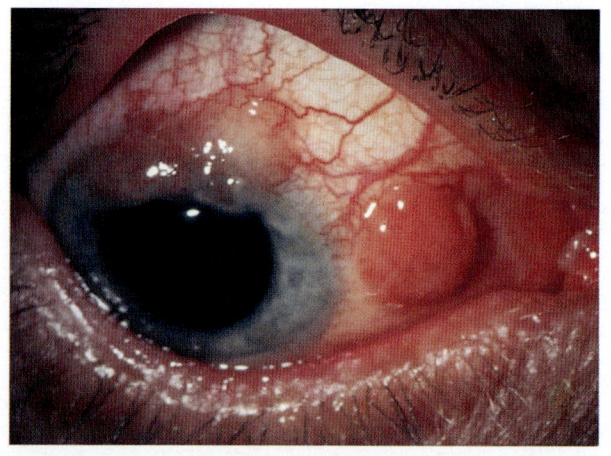

Figure 19.126. Recurrent diffuse amelanotic melanoma near superior limbus in a 70-year-old woman. A pigmented melanoma had been previously excised from the same location.

Chapter 19 Conjunctival Melanocytic Lesions

● CONJUNCTIVAL MELANOMA: ALCOHOL EPITHELIECTOMY, SURGICAL RESECTION, AND CRYOTHERAPY. RESULTS OF TREATMENT

These tumors were removed by partial lamellar sclerokeratoconjunctivectomy and cryotherapy. With carefully planned surgery, most circumscribed melanomas can be cured, in contrast with melanoma arising from primary acquired melanosis where the recurrence rate is generally greater.

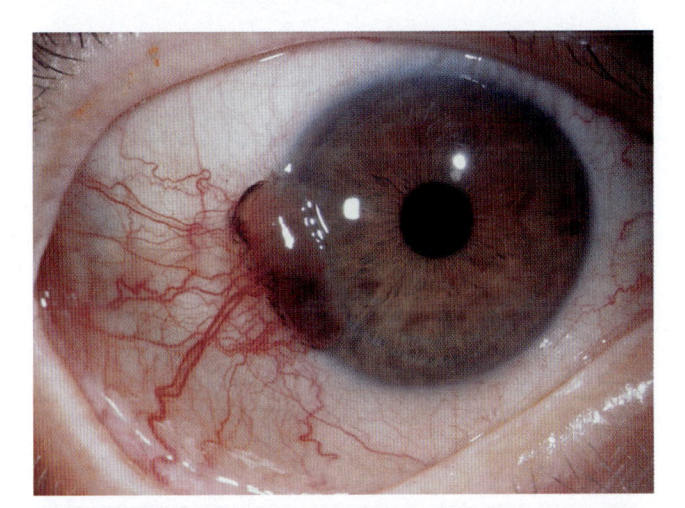

Figure 19.127. Limbal melanoma in a 60-year-old man.

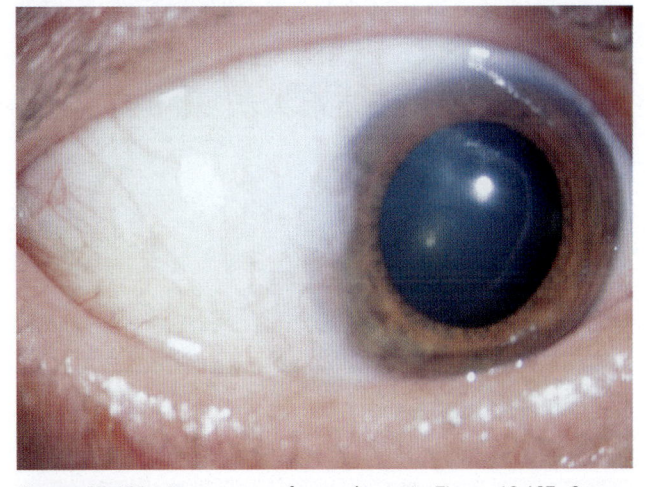

Figure 19.128. Appearance of area shown in Figure 19.127, 2 years after surgery, showing no evidence of recurrence.

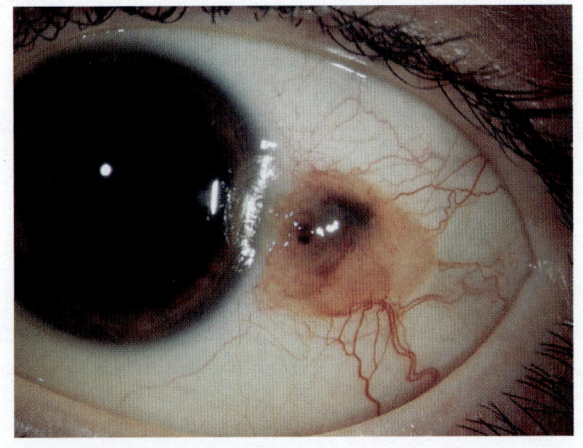

Figure 19.129. Limbal melanoma in a 45-year-old woman.

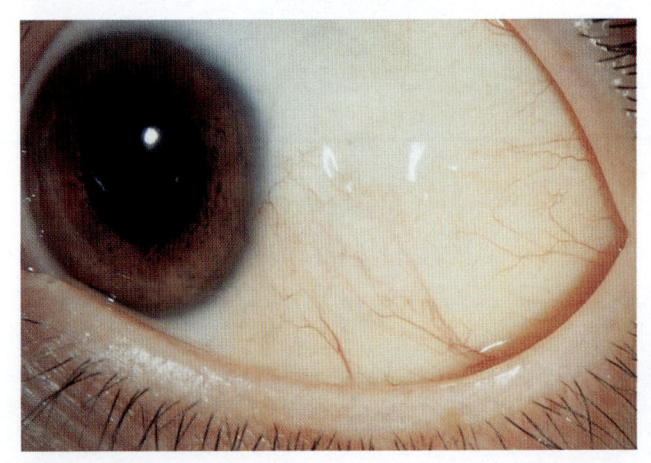

Figure 19.130. Appearance of area shown in Figure 19.129, 13 years later, showing no recurrence.

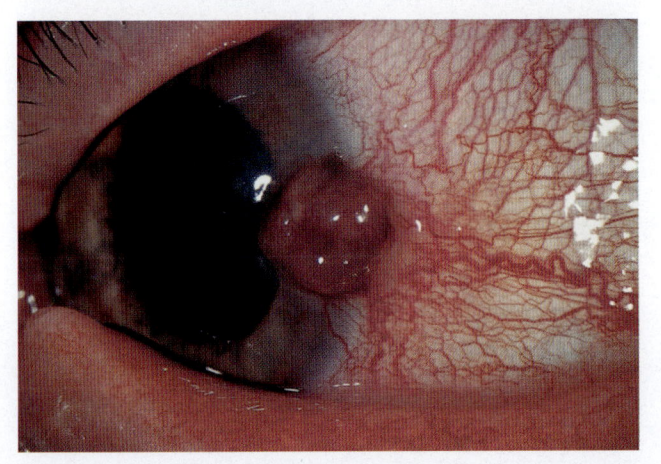

Figure 19.131. Limbal melanoma in a 57-year-old woman.

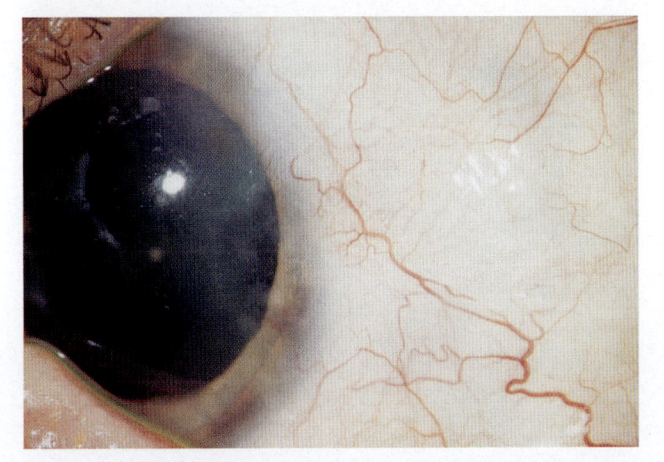

Figure 19.132. Appearance of area shown in Figure 19.131, 2 years after surgery, showing no recurrence.

Part 2 Tumors of the Conjunctiva

● CONJUNCTIVAL MELANOMA: DIFFUSE TUMORS BEFORE AND AFTER TREATMENT

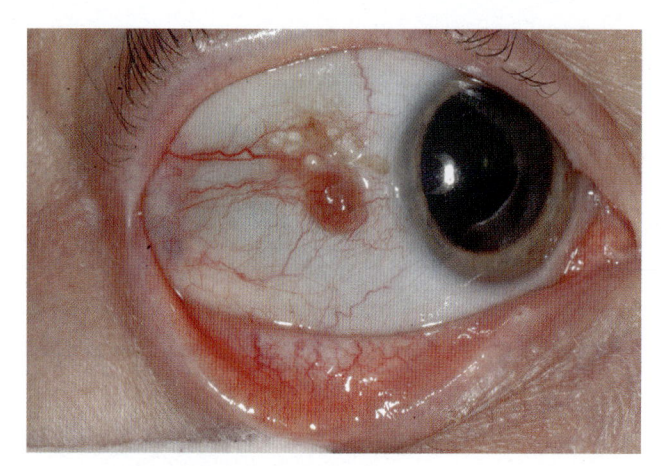

Figure 19.133. Temporal conjunctival melanoma with solid component inferiorly and cystic nevoid component superiorly.

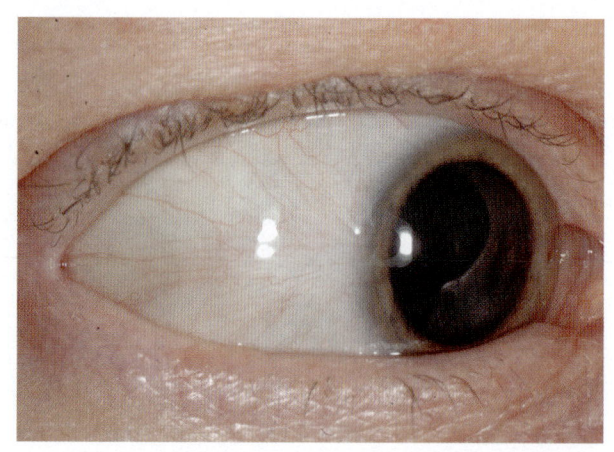

Figure 19.134. Appearance of same area seen in Figure 19.133, 1 month after surgery. The scar is well healed and vascularized with no residual tumor.

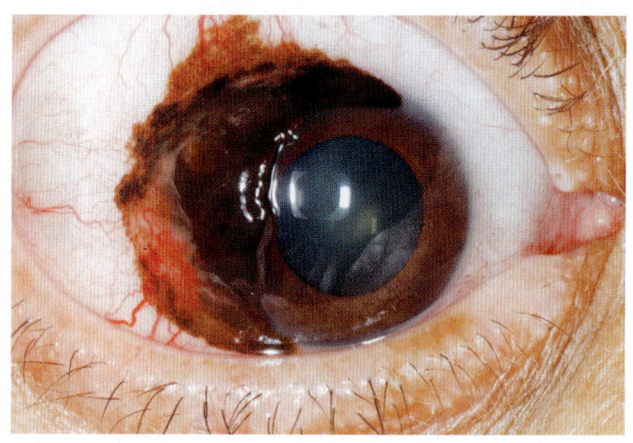

Figure 19.135. Aggressive diffuse conjunctival melanoma replacing the temporal limbal conjunctiva and invading the cornea.

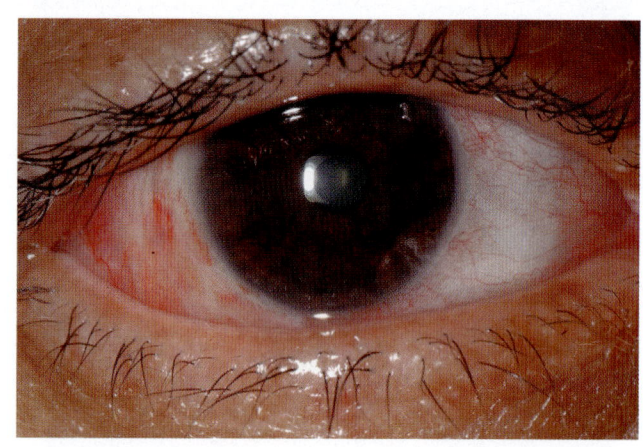

Figure 19.136. Appearance about 1 month after surgery showing no residual tumor and a clear cornea.

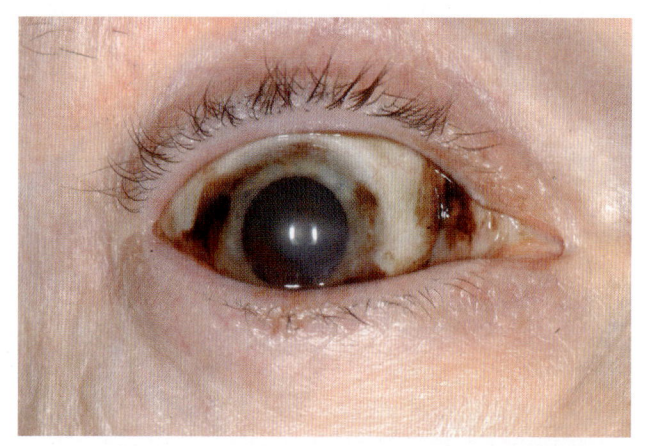

Figure 19.137. Multiple areas of diffuse conjunctival melanoma arising from primary acquired melanosis.

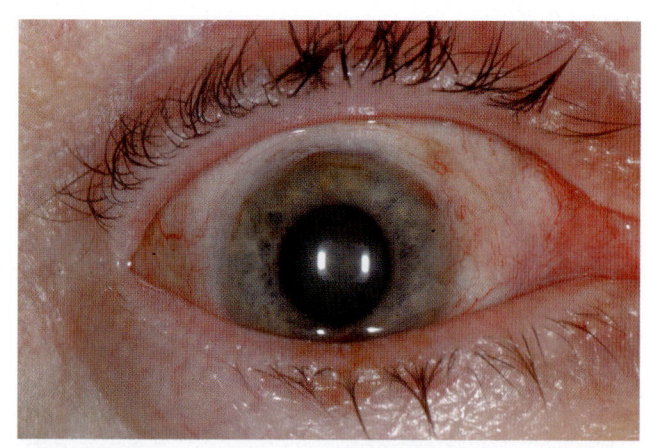

Figure 19.138. Posttreatment appearance of eye shown in Figure 19.137. Note that there is no residual or recurrent tumor. The very subtle residual pigmentation was treated and controlled with double freeze-thaw cryotherapy.

CONJUNCTIVAL MELANOMA: CLINICOPATHOLOGIC CORRELATION OF TUMOR WITH SCLERAL INVASION

Lesions that are suspicious and adherent to the underlying tissues at the limbus should be removed along with a superficial scleral base. If not done, the patient has chance of developing intraocular recurrence of the tumor. This case demonstrates the importance of the scleral dissection.

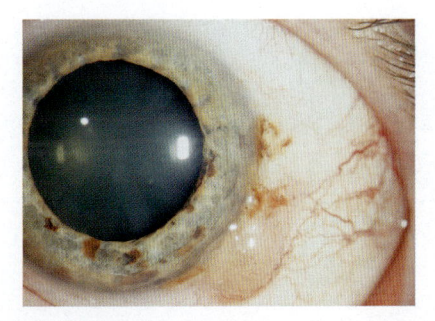

Figure 19.139. Preoperative appearance of amelanotic melanoma near the limbus, associated with mild primary acquired melanosis in a 66-year-old woman.

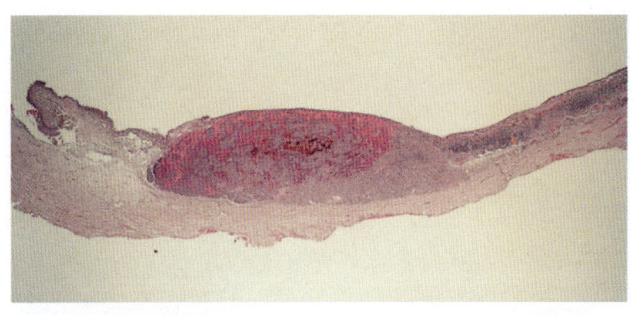

Figure 19.140. Photomicrograph of resected tumor and scleral base. (Hematoxylin–eosin ×5.)

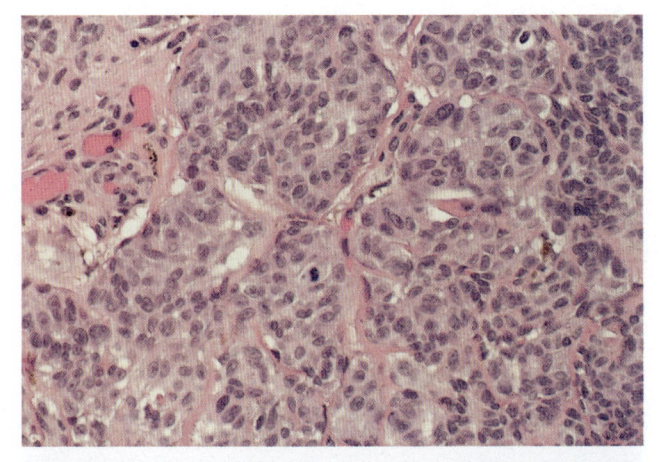

Figure 19.141. Histopathology showing melanoma cells. (Hematoxylin–eosin ×100.)

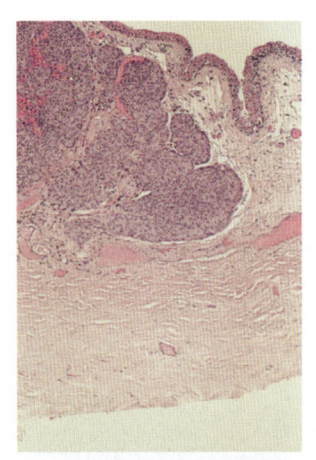

Figure 19.142. Photomicrograph showing margin of tumor to the left and the normal conjunctival tissue to the right. (Hematoxylin–eosin ×25.)

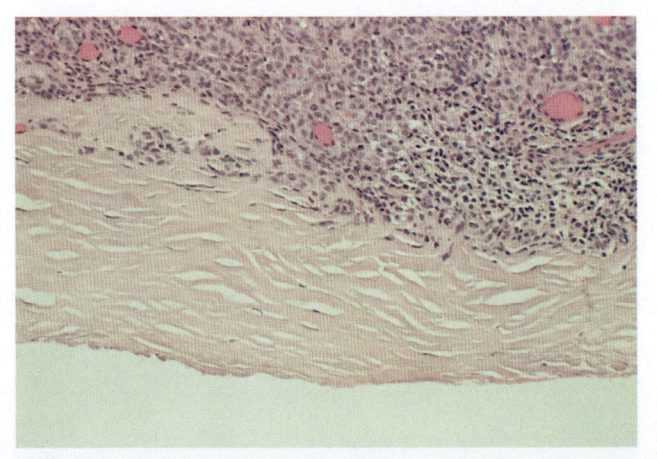

Figure 19.143. Histopathology of sclera immediately beneath the tumor showing tumor cells infiltrating the scleral lamellae. (Hematoxylin–eosin ×75.)

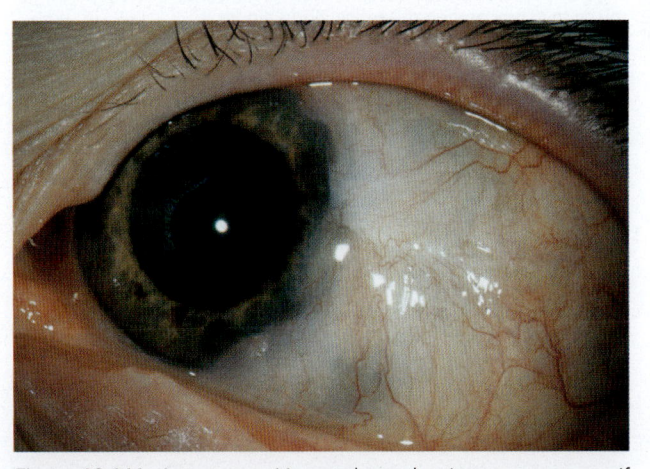

Figure 19.144. Appearance 11 years later, showing no recurrence. If the superficial scleral tissues had not been removed, the patient would probably have intraocular recurrence and secondary glaucoma. The elderly patient is free of tumor after 20 years.

CONJUNCTIVAL MELANOMA: LOCALIZATION FOR SENTINEL LYMPH NODE BIOPSY

To avoid extensive lymph node dissection in the head and neck region, there has been interest in preoperative lymphoscintigraphy for identification of sentinel lymph nodes and selectively removing those nodes for histopathologic evaluation. There are still insufficient data as to whether identification and biopsy of such lymph nodes is of benefit.

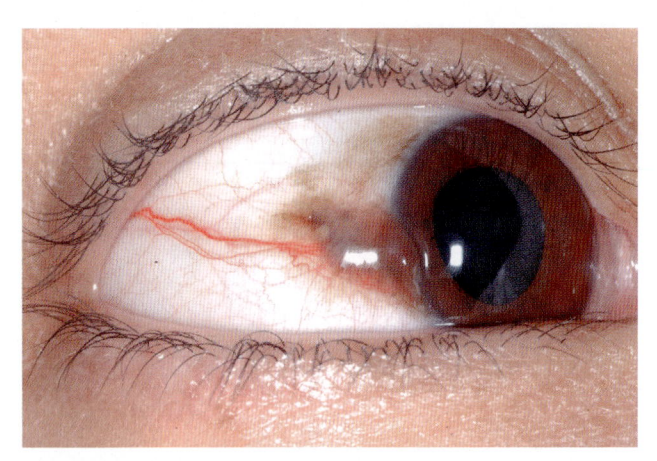

Figure 19.145. Conjunctival melanoma arising from primary acquired melanosis in temporal conjunctiva.

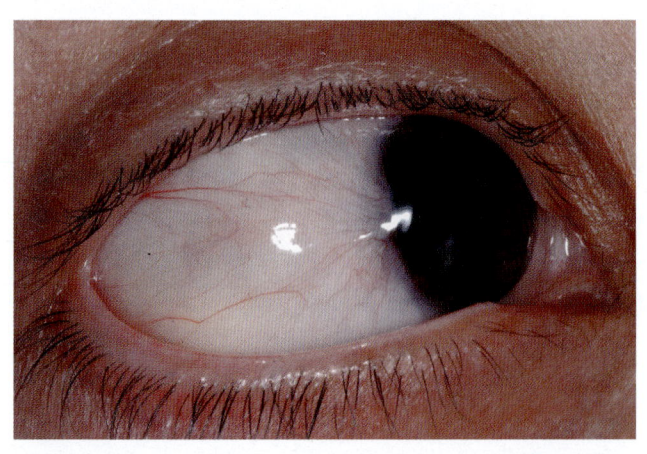

Figure 19.146. Area shown in Figure 19.145, 1 year after removal showing no recurrent tumor. The patient elected to have sentinel lymph node biopsy.

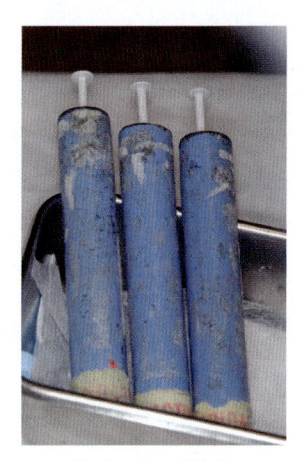

Figure 19.147. Isotope (Technetium-99) in containers prepared for injection in preparation of sentinel node biopsy.

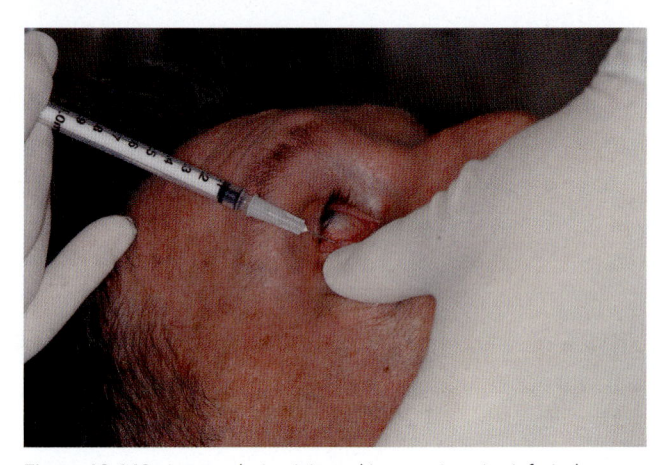

Figure 19.148. Isotope being injected into conjunctiva inferiorly.

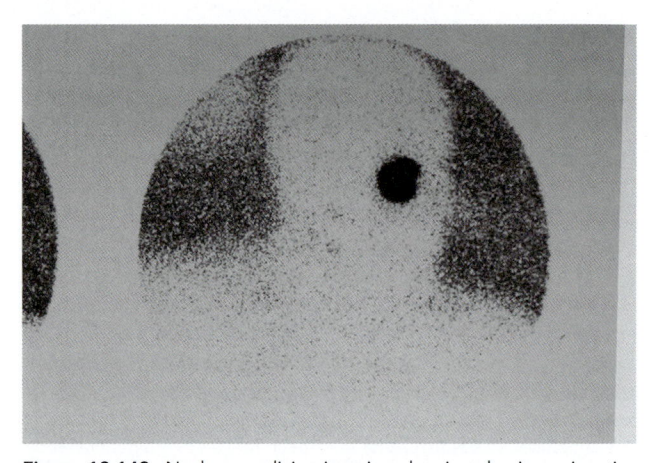

Figure 19.149. Nuclear medicine imaging showing dye in conjunctiva immediately after injection in same patient.

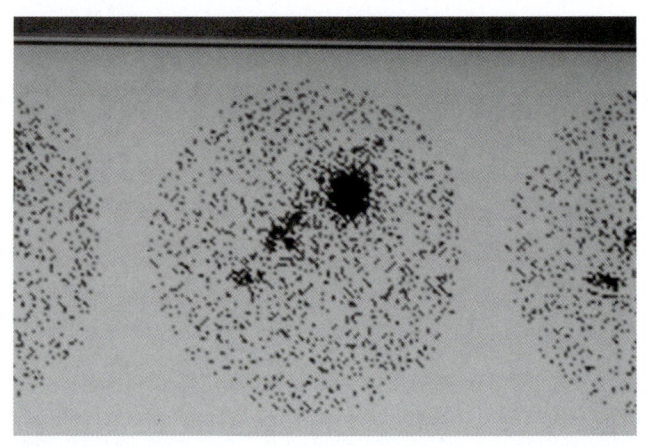

Figure 19.150. A later view demonstrating location of chain of lymph nodes.

CONJUNCTIVAL MELANOMA: PLAQUE RADIOTHERAPY FOR ADVANCED, RECURRENT TUMOR

Plaque radiotherapy is often used as an alternative to orbital exenteration for advanced recurrent melanoma and conjunctival squamous cell carcinoma. It is usually appropriate for older patients who have minimal residual tumor that is not easily resectable and who have useful vision in the affected eye. Plaque design depends on the clinical findings and is individualized for each case. The plaque can be shielded or unshielded depending on the clinical distribution of the tumor.

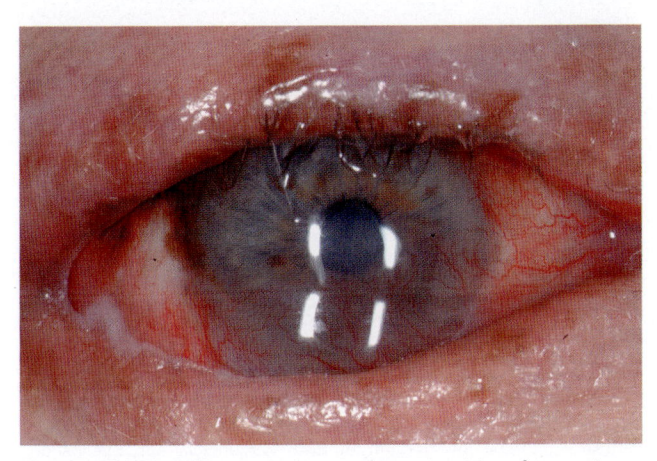

Figure 19.151. Diffuse recurrent melanoma arising from primary acquired melanosis. Six prior excisions had been done and topical chemotherapy had been employed. Nevertheless, there was diffuse multifocal recurrence. There is justification for plaque radiotherapy, rather than orbital exenteration, in some such cases.

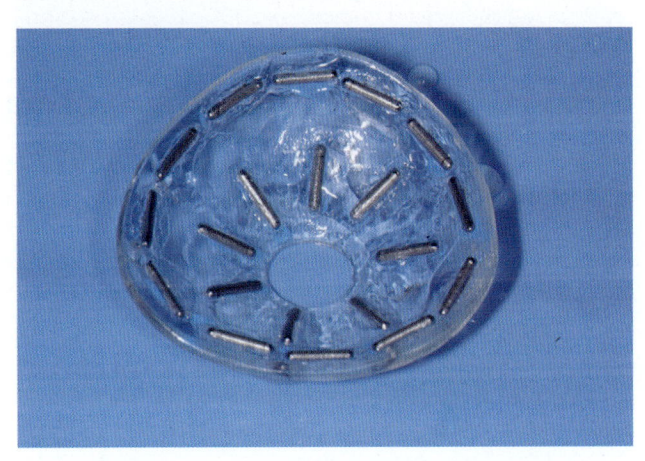

Figure 19.152. Design of donut-shaped plaque with central hole to spare the cornea and placement of the I-125 seeds in the plaque.

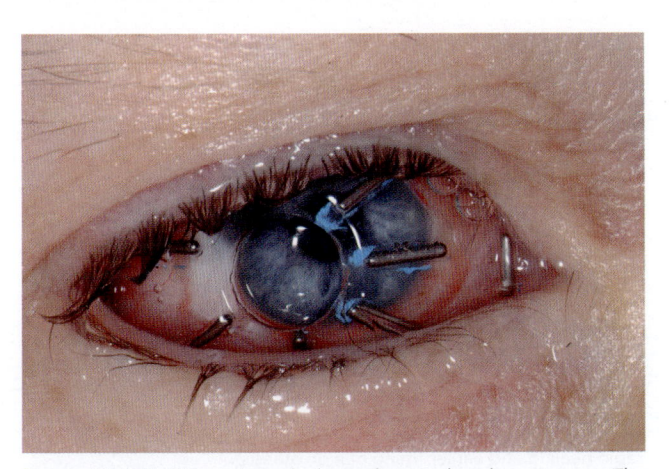

Figure 19.153. Donut-shaped plaque being placed on cornea. The plaque is fixed into one position and a patch and protective metal shield is placed while the plaque is on the eye.

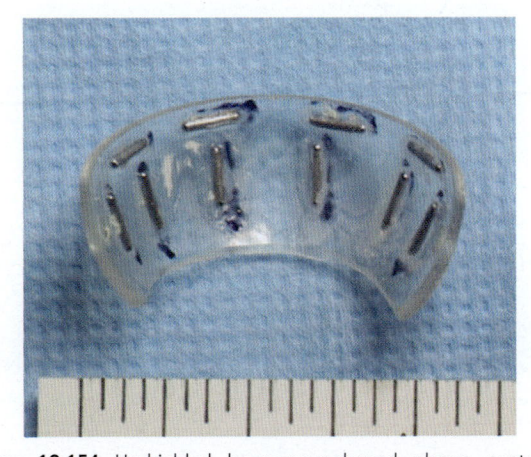

Figure 19.154. Unshielded boomerang-shaped plaque containing I-125 seeds. A plaque with this design is used for tumors that involve less than one-half of the circumference of the conjunctiva.

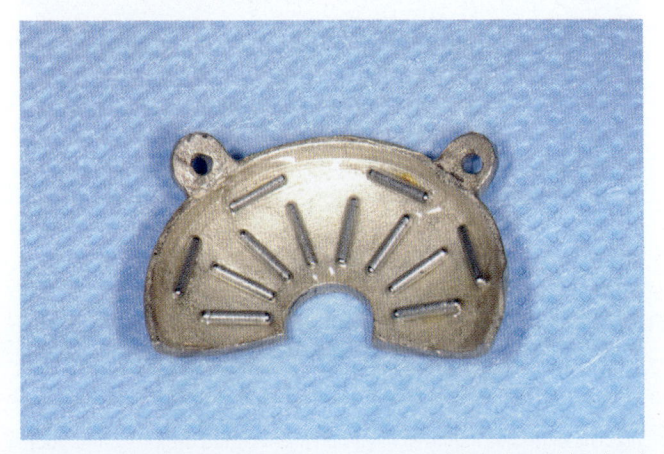

Figure 19.155. Shielded half-donut plaque used for selected localized tumors that involve less than one-half of the circumference of the conjunctiva. The two holes are used for suture placement to the underlying sclera.

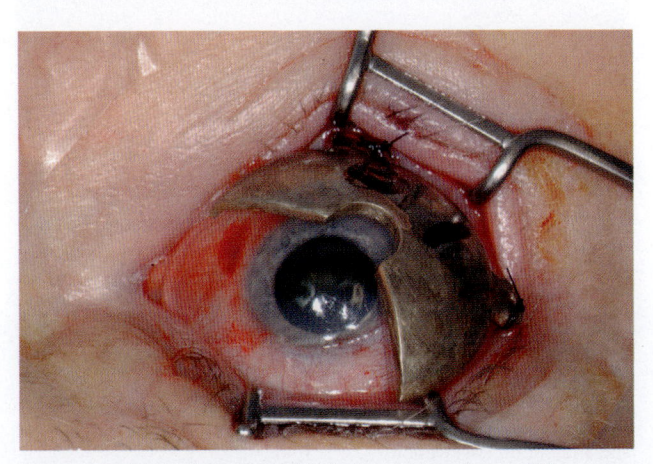

Figure 19.156. Half-donut shielded plaque placed over diffuse recurrence of conjunctival melanoma.

346   Part 2 Tumors of the Conjunctiva

CONJUNCTIVAL MELANOMA: ORBITAL EXENTERATION

Two patients are shown in whom there was recurrence for multiple surgical procedures that had been done elsewhere for conjunctival melanoma before referral for orbital exenteration.

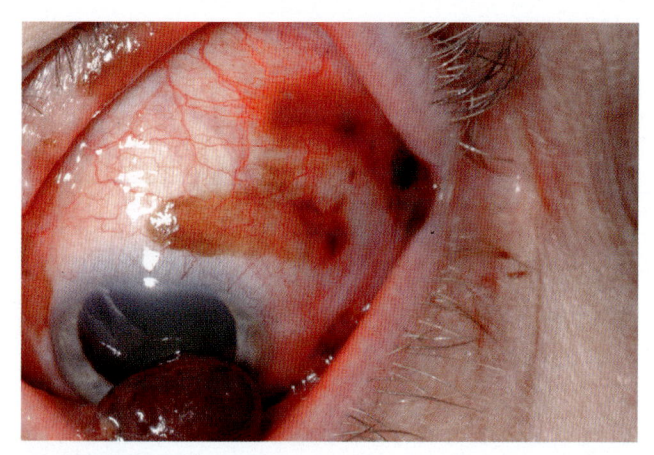

Figure 19.157. Diffuse conjunctiva that has recurred after attempted resections elsewhere.

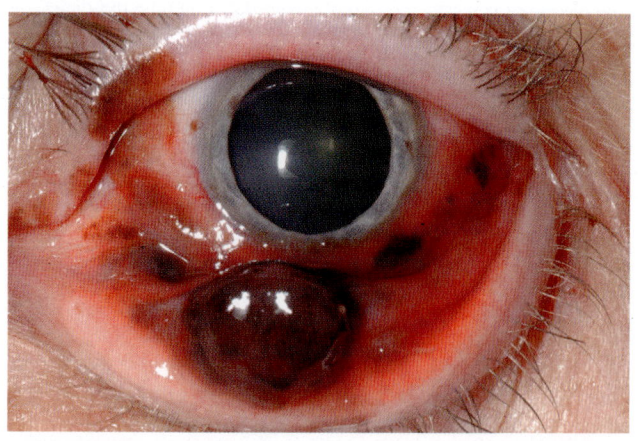

Figure 19.158. Another view of patient shown in Figure 19.157. Note diffuse multifocal involvement of both conjunctiva and eyelids and the pigmented nodular melanoma arising from the inferior fornix. The patient chose to have orbital exenteration after extensive counseling.

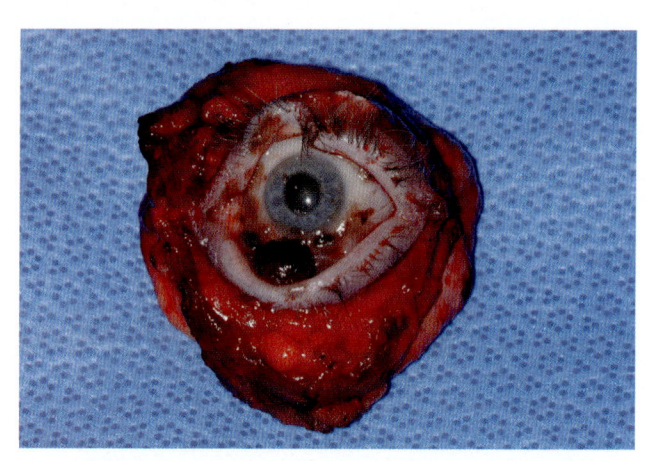

Figure 19.159. Anterior view of specimen following orbital exenteration showing same tumors depicted in Figure 19.158.

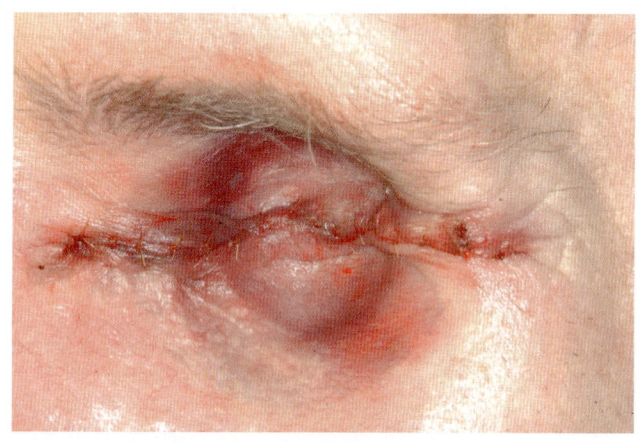

Figure 19.160. Eyelids sutured together immediately after the orbital contents were removed. The eyelid-sparing exenteration offers more rapid healing and earlier fitting of a prosthesis.

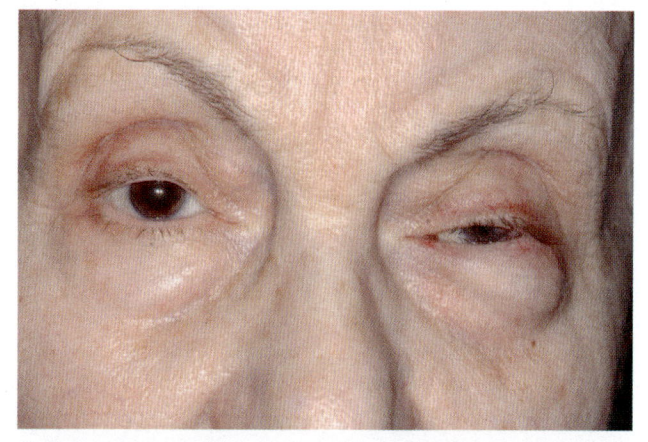

Figure 19.161. Another patient with recurrent conjunctival melanoma involving inferotemporal orbit and presenting as a mass beneath eyelid and anterior orbital invasion.

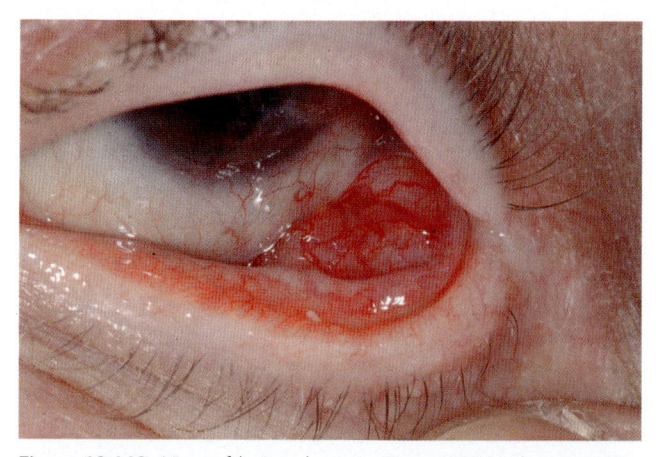

Figure 19.162. View of lesion shown in Figure 19.161 demonstrating nonpigmented melanoma presenting in inferotemporal conjunctival fornix. The extensive nature of the lesion necessitated orbital exenteration.

Chapter 19 Conjunctival Melanocytic Lesions

CONJUNCTIVAL MELANOMA: METASTASIS TO PREAURICULAR LYMPH NODES AND BRAIN

Conjunctival melanoma has a tendency to metastasize to regional lymph nodes, brain, and other organs. The metastasis usually appears months or years after the primary treatment of the conjunctival melanoma. Occasionally, however, the metastasis is evident prior to the diagnosis of the primary conjunctival tumor. There is nearly 25% 5-year mortality rate from conjunctival melanoma.

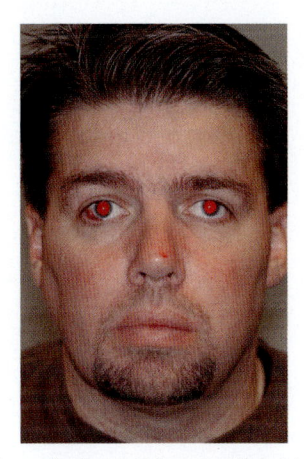

Figure 19.163. Face of 40-year-old man with conjunctival melanoma that was present for 2 years and for which he did not seek treatment. Note the enlarged preauricular lymph node, representing regional metastasis, that was first detected on our examination.

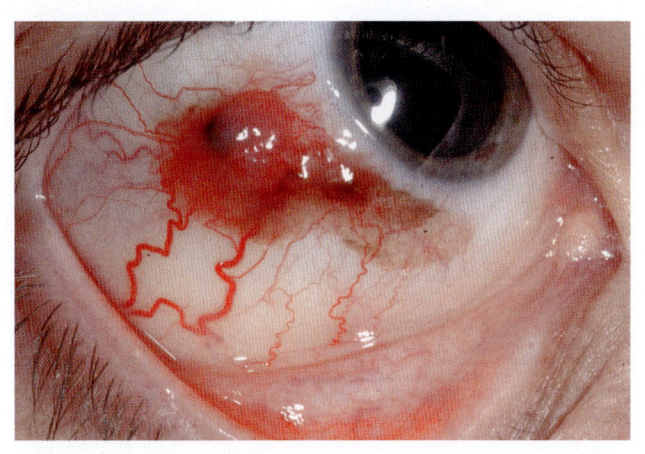

Figure 19.164. Closer view of conjunctival melanoma in patient shown in Figure 19.163. This is a rare example where the conjunctival melanoma had metastasized to regional lymph nodes before it was treated.

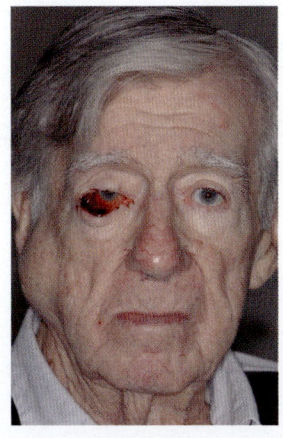

Figure 19.165. Conjunctival melanoma in right eye of an 85-year-old man with a large preauricular lymph node secondary to metastasis from conjunctiva. Note the very large preauricular subcutaneous mass.

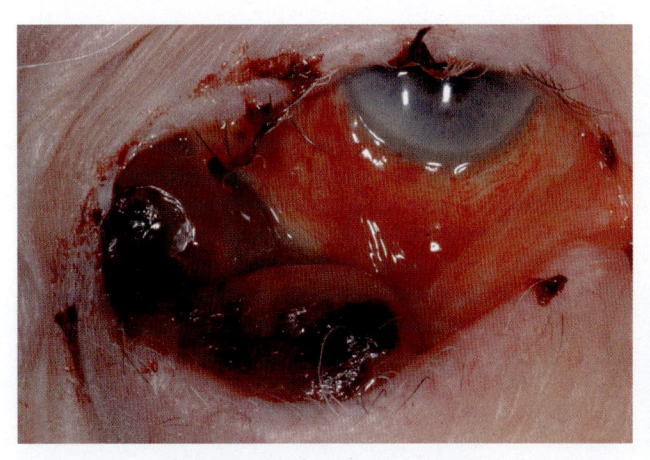

Figure 19.166. Close-up view of patient shown in Figure 19.165 showing extensive conjunctival melanoma. The patient had undergone several resections for recurrent conjunctival melanoma.

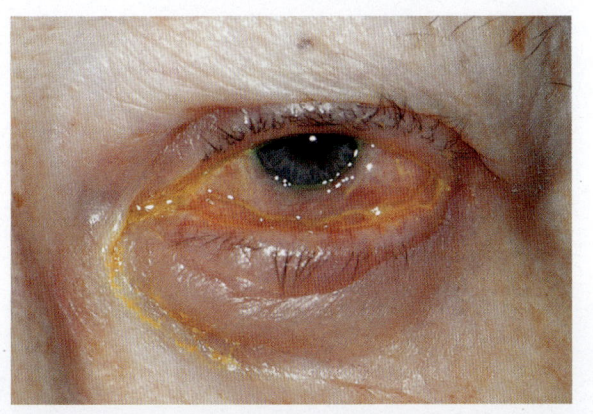

Figure 19.167. Appearance of diffuse amelanotic recurrence of conjunctival melanoma of an 80-year-old woman who had excision elsewhere 3 years earlier of a small pigmented melanoma near limbus. Computed tomography showed diffuse melanoma in anterior orbit, encasing the globe. Orbital exenteration was performed.

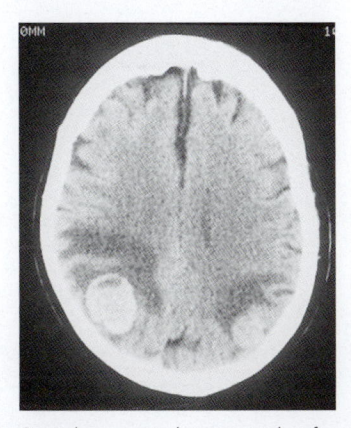

Figure 19.168. Cranial computed tomograph of patient shown in Figure 19.167, 1 year after orbital exenteration, showing intracranial metastasis.

CHAPTER 20

VASCULAR TUMORS AND RELATED LESIONS OF THE CONJUNCTIVA

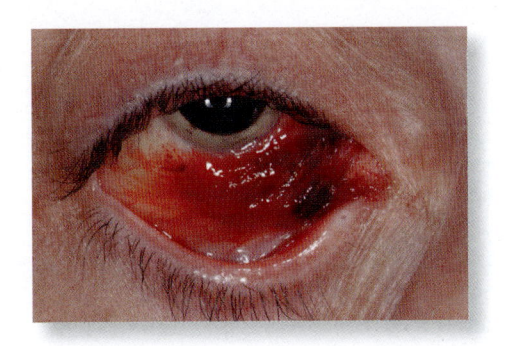

General Considerations

There are a few important vascular tumor and related lesions that can occur in the conjunctiva, including pyogenic granuloma, lymphangioma, varix, capillary hemangioma, cavernous hemangioma, and Kaposi sarcoma (KS). In the authors' clinical series of 1,643 conjunctival tumors, there were 63 vascular lesions, accounting for 4% of the 1,643 lesions (1).

Pyogenic granuloma is a common and well-known condition (1–18). In the authors' series of 1,643 conjunctival tumors, the 11 pyogenic granulomas accounted for 18% of 63 conjunctival vascular lesions and for less than 1% of the 1,643 lesions (1).

The classification and terminology of pyogenic granuloma has been the source of considerable confusion. Some pathologists prefer to classify it as exuberant granulation tissue of "pyogenic granuloma type," which is the term employed by our pathologist (Ralph C. Eagle, Jr., MD, personal communication). Others prefer the term "acquired capillary hemangioma, pyogenic granuloma type." Some dermatologists term this lesion an "acquired lobular capillary hemangioma" (5,6), which does not easily apply to the lesions seen in the conjunctiva. Until a more accurate name is agreed upon, we have chosen to continue to use the conventional term "pyogenic granuloma," even though it is a misnomer. In actuality, it is a proliferative fibrovascular response (granulation tissue) to prior tissue insult by inflammation or trauma (surgical or nonsurgical). It is most commonly seen at a traumatic wound site or near a suture line after surgery for chalazion, pterygium, strabismus, or enucleation. It has been recognized at the site of a dermis fat graft used after enucleation (11). It can also occur as a primary response to a chalazion, even if there is no history of prior surgery. It has been recognized in patients who wear contact lenses, presumably from chronic inflammation or from retention of a "lost" contact lens (10). Rarely, it appears to be entirely primary, without any underlying cause or event.

Pyogenic granuloma is usually confined to the conjunctiva, but it has also occurred on the cornea (7,12). A report of 14 corneal pyogenic granulomas showed that there was usually an underlying cause and a precipitating event. Predisposing conditions included indolent corneal ulceration, dry eye syndrome, trachoma, trichiasis, alkali burn, multiple topical drug use, previous orbital irradiation, and ocular cicatricial pemphigoid. The precipitating event was usually a persistent epithelial defect secondary to those predisposing conditions (7). It has also occurred at the surgical site after blepharoplasty (13), after corneal transplantation (12), and after injection of antivascular endothelial growth factor therapy (18).

CONJUNCTIVAL PYOGENIC GRANULOMA

Clinical Features

Clinically, pyogenic granuloma generally has a rapid onset and progression usually follows an apparent insult. It can assume any of several clinical variations. It is usually an elevated fleshy red-pink mass that often has a florid blood supply from the adjacent conjunctiva. The shape of the lesion can vary considerably from case to case, ranging from round to ovoid, broad based, and even mushroom shaped. Elevation of the margin of a pyogenic granuloma with a cotton-tipped applicator often reveals that the lesion is pedunculated, with an underlying stalk of blood vessels and connective tissue.

Pathology

Microscopically, pyogenic granuloma is composed of granulation tissue with lymphocytes, plasma cells, scattered neutrophils, and numerous small-caliber blood vessels. As mentioned, it is often pointed out that the term "pyogenic granuloma" is a misnomer; the lesion is neither pyogenic nor granulomatous.

Management

Pyogenic granuloma sometimes responds to topical corticosteroids, but many cases ultimately require surgical excision. We have found that shaving excision at the small base, followed by cautery and cryotherapy is usually effective, but recurrence is not uncommon. In the rare case of recurrence and continued growth, low-dose brachytherapy with a radioactive plaque has been effective (8).

CONJUNCTIVAL PYOGENIC GRANULOMA

Selected References

Reviews
1. Shields CL, Demirci H, Karatza E, et al. Clinical survey of 1643 melanocytic and nonmelanocytic tumors of the conjunctiva. *Ophthalmology* 2004;111:1747–1754.
2. Shields CL, Shields JA. Tumors of the conjunctiva and cornea. *Surv Ophthalmol* 2004;49:3–24.
3. Shields JA, Mashayekhi A, Kligmen B, et al. Vascular tumors of the conjunctiva in 140 cases. The 2010 Melvin Rubin Lecture. *Ophthalmology* 2011;118:1747–1753.
4. Ferry AP. Pyogenic granulomas of the eye and ocular adnexa: a study of 100 cases. *Trans Am Ophthalmol Soc* 1989;87:327–347.
5. Mills SE, Cooper PH, Fechner RE. Lobular capillary hemangioma, the underlying lesion of pyogenic granuloma: a study of 73 cases from the oral and nasal mucous membranes. *Am J Surg Pathol* 1980;4:471–479.
6. Patrice SJ, Wiss K, Mulliken JB. Pyogenic granuloma (lobular capillary hemangioma): a clinicopathologic study of 178 cases. *Pediatr Dermatol* 1991;8:267–276.
7. Cameron JA, Mahmood MA. Pyogenic granulomas of the cornea. *Ophthalmology* 1995;102:1681–1687.

Management
8. Gunduz K, Shields CL, Shields JA, et al. Plaque radiotherapy for recurrent conjunctival pyogenic granuloma. *Arch Ophthalmol* 1998;116:538–539.

Case Reports
9. Fryer RH, Reinke KR. Pyogenic granuloma: a complication of transconjunctival incisions. *Plast Reconstr Surg* 2000;105:1565–1566.
10. Horton JC, Mathers WD, Zimmerman LE. Pyogenic granuloma of the palpebral conjunctiva associated with contact lens wear. *Cornea* 1990;9:359–361.
11. Liszauer AD, Brownstein S, Codere F. Pyogenic granuloma on a dermis fat graft in acquired anophthalmic orbits. *Am J Ophthalmol* 1987;104:641–644.
12. DePotter P, Tardio DJ, Shields CL, et al. Pyogenic granuloma of the cornea after penetrating keratoplasty. *Cornea* 1992;11:589–591.
13. Soll SM, Lisman RD, Charles NC, et al. Pyogenic granuloma after transconjunctival blepharoplasty: a case report. *Ophthal Plast Reconstr Surg* 1993;9:298–301.
14. Espinoza GM, Lueder GT. Conjunctival pyogenic granuloma after strabismus surgery. *Ophthalmology* 2005;112:1283–1286.
15. Akova YA, Demirhan B, Cakmakci S, et al. Pyogenic granuloma: a rare complication of silicone punctal plugs. *Ophthalmic Surg Lasers* 1999;30:584–585.
16. Murphy BA, Dawood GS, Margo CE. Acquired capillary hemangioma of the eyelid in an adult. *Am J Ophthalmol* 1997;124:403–404.
17. D'Hermies F, Meyer A, Morel X, et al. Conjunctival pyogenic granuloma in a patient with chalazions. *J Fr Ophthalmol* 2003;26:1085–1088.
18. Jung JJ, Della Torre KE, Fell MR. Presumed pyogenic granuloma associated with intravitreal antivascular endothelial growth factor therapy. *Open Ophthalmol J* 2011;5:59–62.

CONJUNCTIVAL PYOGENIC GRANULOMA: PRIMARY (IDIOPATHIC) TYPE

In some cases, pyogenic granuloma can appear in the conjunctiva as a spontaneous lesion, without an evident cause. Some may be related to ruptured chalazion of which the patient was unaware; others may develop secondary to subclinical trauma or other insults.

Ferry AP. Pyogenic granulomas of the eye and ocular adnexa: a study of 100 cases. *Trans Am Ophthalmol Soc* 1989;87:327–347.

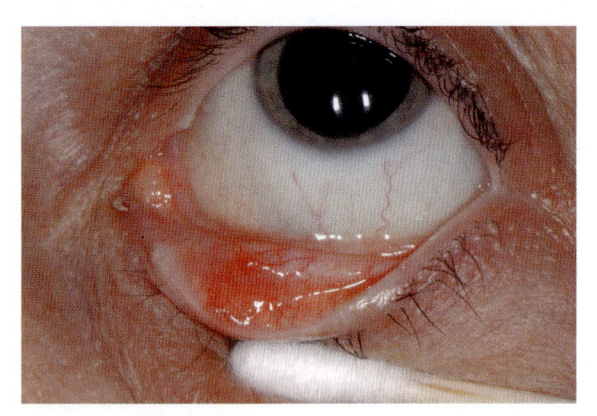

Figure 20.1. Small pyogenic granuloma in inferior fornix.

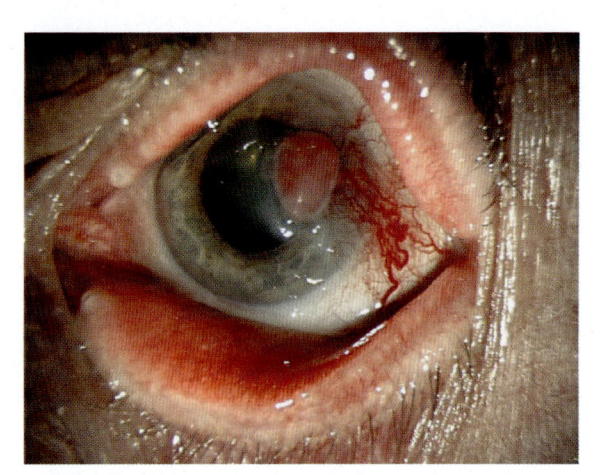

Figure 20.2. Spontaneous pyogenic granuloma arising from conjunctiva inferiorly in a 66-year-old woman. The lesion was very pedunculated and was connected by a stalk to the underlying conjunctiva.

Figure 20.3. Pyogenic granuloma of the cornea. The etiology was uncertain. Note the dilated feeder vessels.

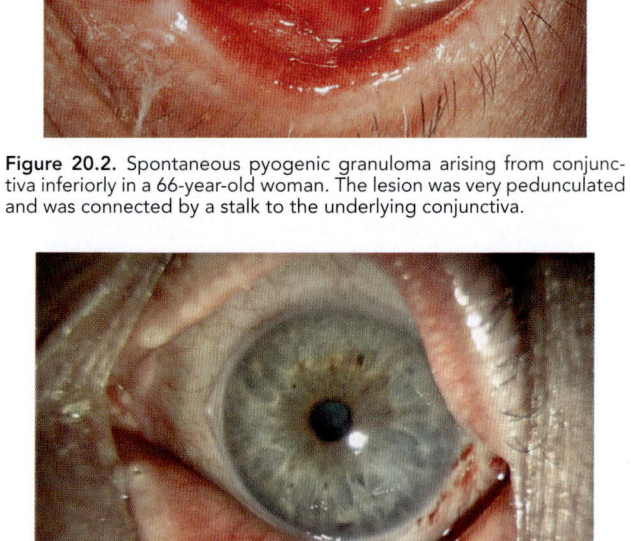

Figure 20.4. Appearance of eye shown in Figure 20.3, 1 year after superficial surgery to remove the lesion. The cornea is clear and the feeder vessels have mostly resolved.

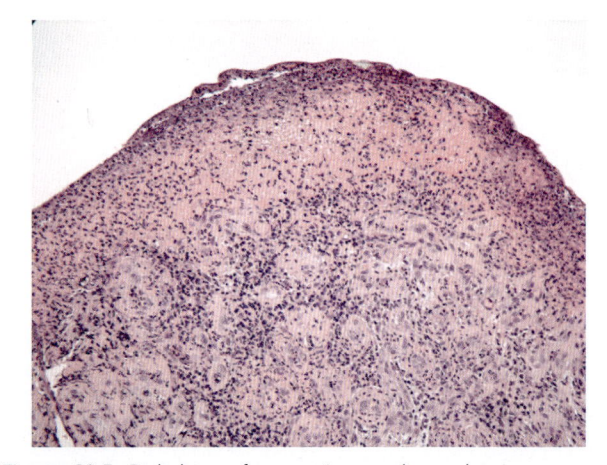

Figure 20.5. Pathology of pyogenic granuloma showing compact inflammatory cells and granulation. (Hematoxylin–eosin ×20.)

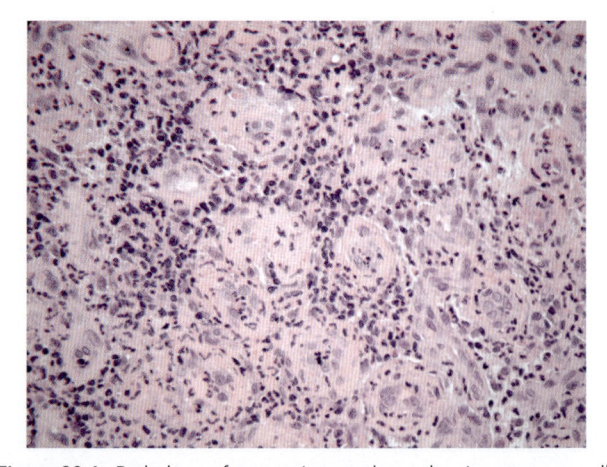

Figure 20.6. Pathology of pyogenic granuloma showing compact cells with mixture of acute and chronic inflammatory cells. There is a suggestion of granulomatous inflammation, which is unusual for a typical pyogenic granuloma. (Hematoxylin–eosin ×100.)

SECONDARY CONJUNCTIVAL PYOGENIC GRANULOMA: TREATMENT WITH PLAQUE RADIOTHERAPY

In many instances, pyogenic granuloma is due to an apparent underlying cause, such as prior ocular surgery, trauma, or ruptured chalazion. Surgical procedures that can be associated with the development of pyogenic granuloma include procedures for strabismus, pterygium, retinal detachment, and procedures like corneal transplant, and enucleation. In some instances, pyogenic granuloma can involve the cornea.

1. DePotter P, Tardio DJ, Shields CL, et al. Pyogenic granuloma of the cornea after penetrating keratoplasty. *Cornea* 1992;11:589–591.
2. Gunduz K, Shields CL, Shields JA, et al. Plaque radiotherapy for recurrent conjunctival pyogenic granuloma. *Arch Ophthalmol* 1998;116:538–539.

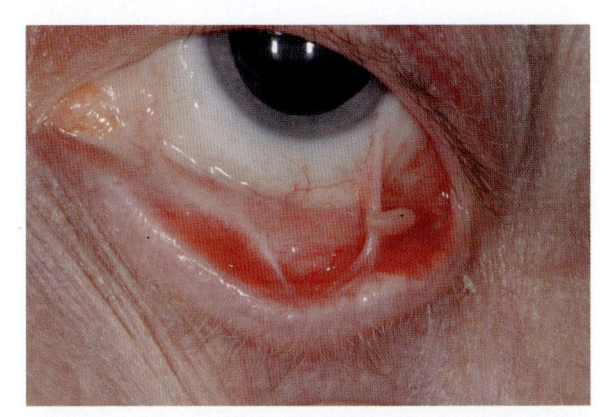

Figure 20.7. Pedunculated pyogenic granuloma that developed after uncomplicated surgical removal and cryotherapy of primary acquired melanosis of the inferior fornix.

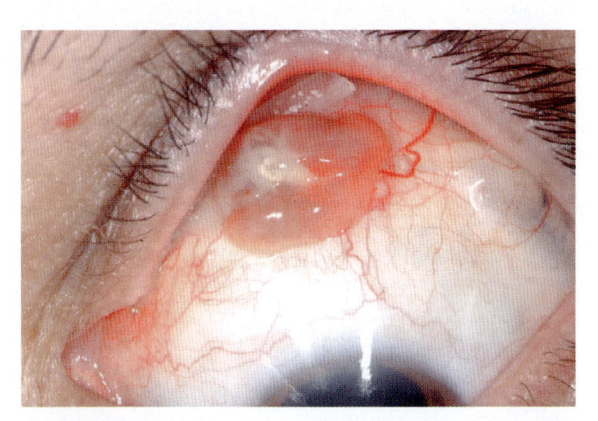

Figure 20.8. Pyogenic granuloma that developed as a reaction to scleral buckling procedure for rhegmatogenous retinal detachment. Note the exposed silicone band just posterior to the lesion.

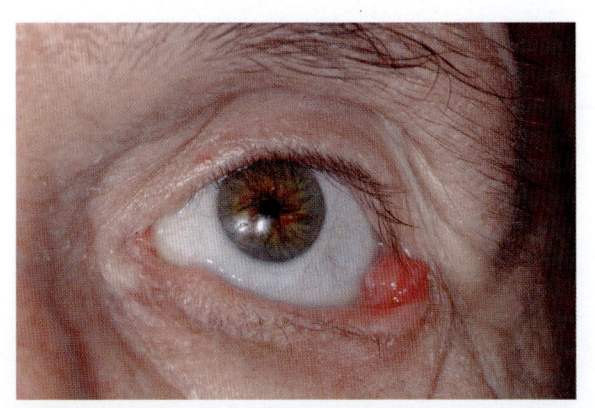

Figure 20.9. Pyogenic granuloma in lateral canthal region that possibly developed from irritation by a slightly poor-fitting prosthesis after enucleation for uveal melanoma.

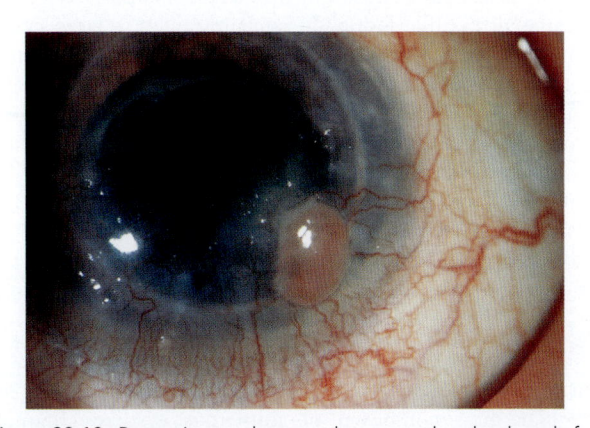

Figure 20.10. Pyogenic granuloma on the cornea that developed after penetrating keratoplasty.

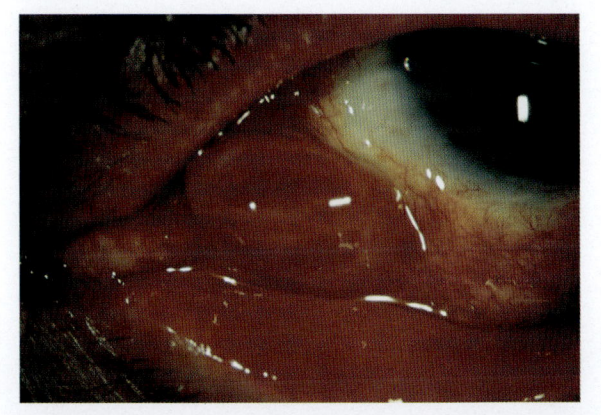

Figure 20.11. Pyogenic granuloma at the resection margin of prior pterygium surgery in a 65-year-old man. This lesion recurred twice and was excised each time after failure of corticosteroid treatment. It was then treated with application of a radioactive plaque giving 1,000 cGy.

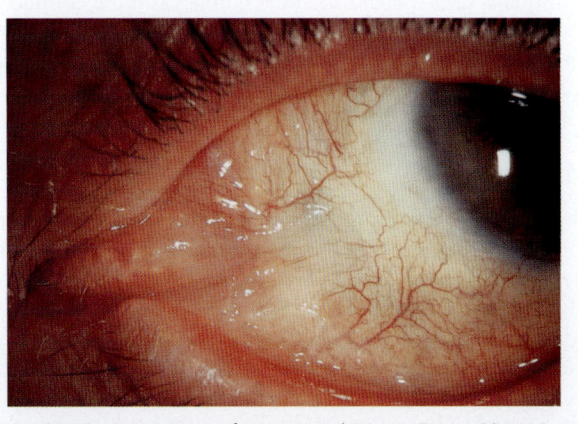

Figure 20.12. Appearance of same eye shown in Figure 20.11, 1 year after plaque radiotherapy. There has been no further recurrence after plaque brachytherapy.

CONJUNCTIVAL LYMPHANGIECTASIA AND LYMPHANGIOMA

General Considerations

In some instances, the lymphatic channels in the conjunctiva are dilated and prominent, a condition called "lymphangiectasia." When the vascular lesion forms a distinct mass, it is called a "lymphangioma" (1–17). Although it is usually a unilateral, sporadic occurrence, it has been recognized as part of Turner's syndrome and Nonne–Milroy–Meige disease (13). In the authors' clinical series of 1,643 conjunctival tumors, there were 15 lymphangiomas, accounting for 24% of conjunctival vascular lesions and for less than 1% of the 1,643 lesions (1).

Clinical Features

When there is bleeding into the lymph channels, it is called "hemorrhagic lymphangiectasia" (14). When lymphangiectasia assumes tumorous proportions, it is called "lymphangioma." Conjunctival lymphangioma can occur as either a solitary conjunctival lesion or as multifocal conjunctival lesions. In most instances, the conjunctival lymphangioma represents a superficial component of a deeper diffuse orbital lymphangioma. The lymph channels in a lymphangioma may contain clear fluid (lymph), in which case it appears as a multiloculated, cystlike lesion. In such instances, a large cystic compound nevus of the conjunctiva may be clinically similar to lymphangioma (7). Usually, when it becomes clinically apparent in the first decade of life it has undergone bleeding into the cystoid spaces and appears as a multiloculated blue-red mass containing variable-sized, clear, dilated vascular channels (13–17). When this blood is present in many of the cystic spaces, the lesion has been called a "chocolate cyst" as the blood gradually turns to a brown color. At that stage, the lesion may resemble a cavernous hemangioma.

Pathology

Histopathologically, lymphangioma is a nonencapsulated, irregular mass composed of numerous cystlike channels that contain clear fluid, blood, or a combination of the two (4). The ectatic channels are lined by somewhat attenuated endothelial cells. Separating the channels is loose connective tissue that contains aggregates of small lymphocytes, sometimes forming a lymph follicle. In contrast with cavernous hemangioma, smooth muscle is generally lacking or sparse in lymphangioma.

Management

The treatment of conjunctival lymphangioma may be difficult because surgical resection or radiotherapy cannot completely eradicate the mass. The carbon dioxide laser has been advocated as a helpful adjunct to prevent excessive bleeding in surgical debulking of the tumor (10). However, it probably provides little benefit over standard surgical debulking and cautery. Fractionated β irradiation using a strontium-90 applicator has been used to treat an unresectable conjunctival lymphangioma, but this technique is rarely used today (12). Currently, large unresectable, hemorrhagic lymphangiomas are managed with aspiration and tissue glue injection, which offers a temporary or permanent cure. More extensive lesions can be treated with percutaneous drainage and internal sclerotherapy with resultant collapse of the vascular mass and sclerosis (9).

CONJUNCTIVAL LYMPHANGIECTASIA AND LYMPHANGIOMA

Selected References

Reviews

1. Shields CL, Demirci H, Karatza E, et al. Clinical survey of 1643 melanocytic and nonmelanocytic tumors of the conjunctiva. *Ophthalmology* 2004;111:1747–1754.
2. Shields CL, Shields JA. Tumors of the conjunctiva and cornea. *Surv Ophthalmol* 2004;49:3–24.
3. Shields JA, Mashayekhi A, Kligman B, et al. Vascular tumors of the conjunctiva in 140 cases. The 2010 Melvin Rubin Lecture. *Ophthalmology* 2011;118:1747–1753.
4. Jones IS. Lymphangiomas of the ocular adnexa. An analysis of sixty-two cases. *Am J Ophthalmol* 1961;51:481–509.
5. Rootman J, Hay E, Graeb D, et al. Orbital-adnexal lymphangiomas. A spectrum of hemodynamically isolated vascular hamartomas. *Ophthalmology* 1986;93:1558–1570.
6. Welch J, Srinivasan S, Lyall D, et al. Conjunctival lymphangiectasai: a report of 11 cases and review of the literature. *Surv Ophthalmol* 2012;57:136–148.
7. Shields CL, Regillo A, Mellen PL, et al. Giant conjunctival nevus: Clinical features and natural course in 32 cases. *JAMA Ophthalmol* 2013;131:857–863.

Imaging

8. Daya SM, Papdopoulos R. Ocular coherence tomography in lymphangiectasia. *Cornea* 2011;30:1170–1172.

Management

9. Hill RH, Shiels WE, Foster JA, et al. Percutaneous drainage and ablation as first line therapy for macrocystic and microcystic orbital lymphatic malformations. *Ophthal Plast Reconstr Surg* 2012;28:119–125.
10. Jordan DR, Anderson RL. Carbon dioxide (CO_2) laser therapy for conjunctival lymphangioma. *Ophthalmic Surg* 1987;18:728–730.
11. Han KE, Choi CY, Seo KY. Removal of lymphangiectasis using high-frequency radio wave electrosurgery. *Cornea* 2013;32:547–549.
12. Behrendt S, Bernsmeier H, Randzio G. Fractionated beta-irradiation of a conjunctival lymphangioma. *Ophthalmologica* 1991;203:161–163.

Case Reports

13. Perry HD, Cossari AJ. Chronic lymphangiectasis in Turner's syndrome. *Br J Ophthalmol* 1986;70:396–399.
14. Jampol LM, Nagpal KC. Hemorrhagic lymphangiectasia of the conjunctiva. *Am J Ophthalmol* 1978;85:4–29.
15. Goble RR, Frangoulis MA. Lymphangioma circumscriptum of the eyelids and conjunctiva. *Br J Ophthalmol* 1990;74:574–575.
16. Quezada AA, Shields CL, Wagner RS, et al. Lymphangioma of the conjunctiva and nasal cavity in a child presenting with diffuse subconjunctival hemorrhage and nosebleeds. *J Ped Ophthalmol Strabism* 2007;44:180–182.
17. Seca M, Borges P, Reimão P, et al. Conjunctival lymphangioma: a case report and brief review of the literature. *Case Rep Ophthalmol Med* 2012;2012:836573.

CONJUNCTIVAL LYMPHANGIECTASIA AND LYMPHANGIOMA

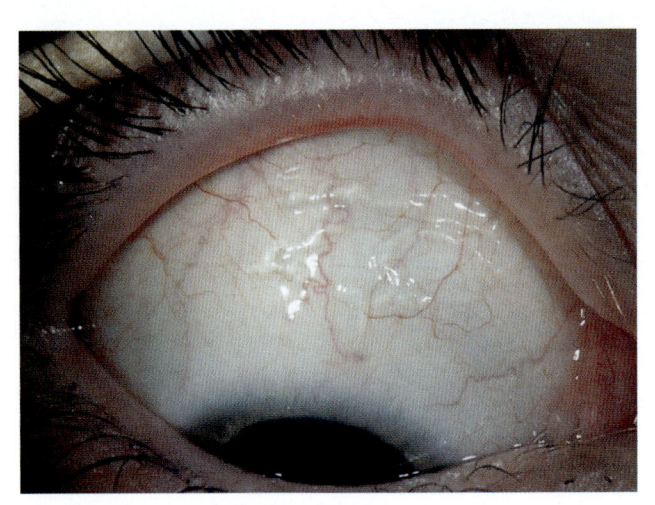

Figure 20.13. Conjunctival lymphangiectasia in a 24-year-old woman.

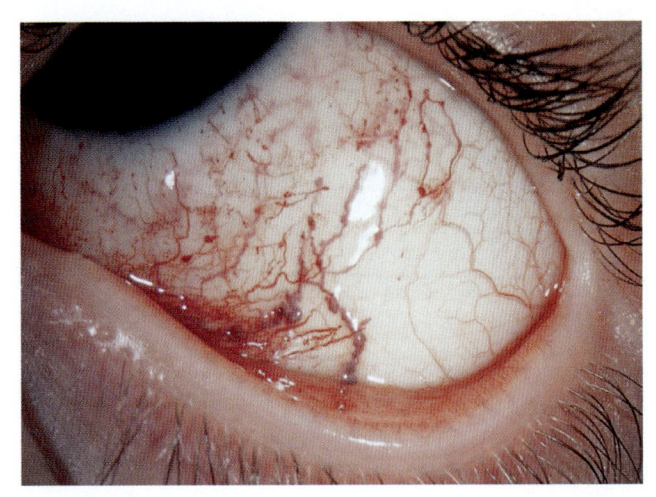

Figure 20.14. Conjunctival hemorrhagic lymphangiectasia in a 10-year-old boy.

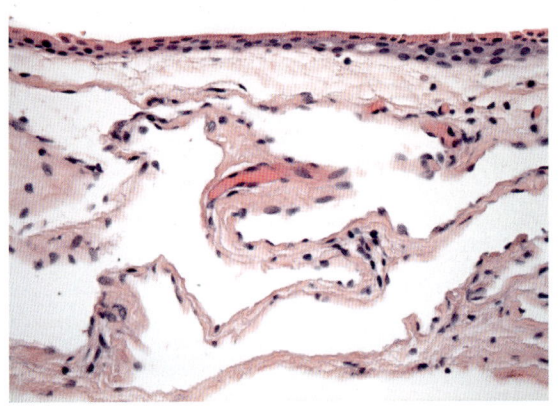

Figure 20.15. Histopathology of conjunctival lymphangiectasia, showing bloodless ectatic vascular channels lined by thin endothelial cells. In cases like this, it may be difficult to differentiate lymphangiectasia from small lymphangioma, but such differentiation is not clinically important. (Hematoxylin–eosin ×50.)

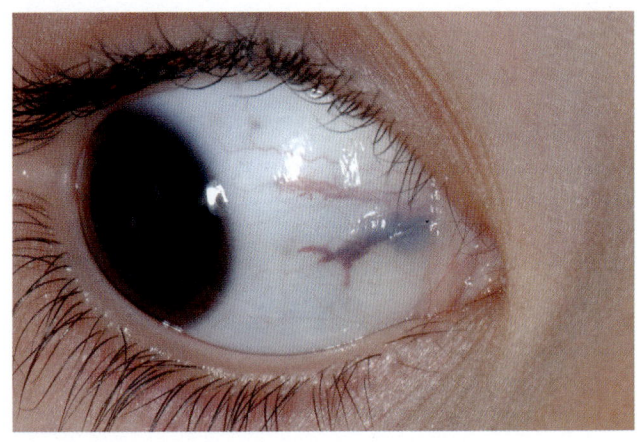

Figure 20.16. Conjunctival lymphangiectasia near medial canthus. This likely represents conjunctival extension from a more extensive anterior orbital lesion.

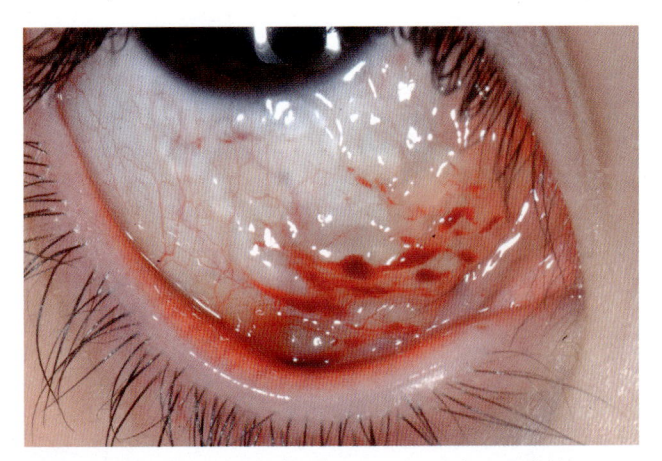

Figure 20.17. Hemorrhagic lymphangioma in inferonasal fornix in a 5-year-old girl.

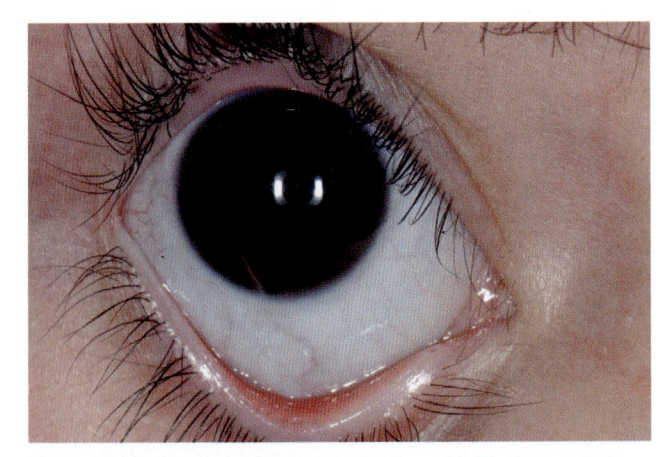

Figure 20.18. Same patient depicted in Figure 20.17 a few weeks later, showing complete spontaneous resolution of the hemorrhage. Some clear lymphatic channels persist.

Chapter 20 Vascular Tumors and Related Lesions of the Conjunctiva 357

CONJUNCTIVAL LYMPHANGIOMA

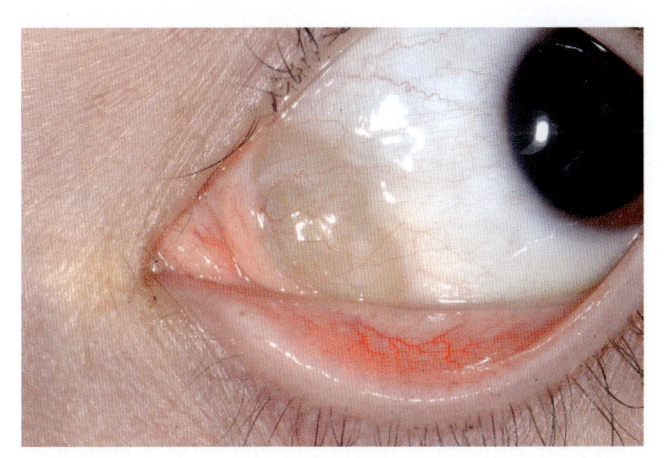

Figure 20.19. Cystic, nonhemorrhagic lymphangioma in a young adult woman. It has remained asymptomatic for years.

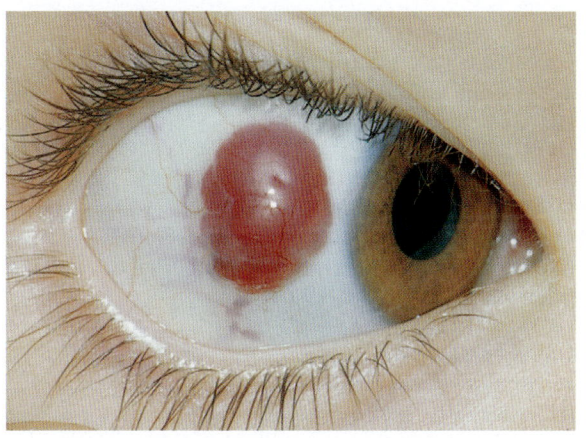

Figure 20.20. Localized lymphangioma that was present at birth. This was originally diagnosed as a cavernous hemangioma, but the diagnosis was disputed; some pathologists favor the diagnosis of lymphangioma. Detection of a separate ipsilateral orbital lymphangioma 8 years later led to a more definitive diagnosis of lymphangioma.

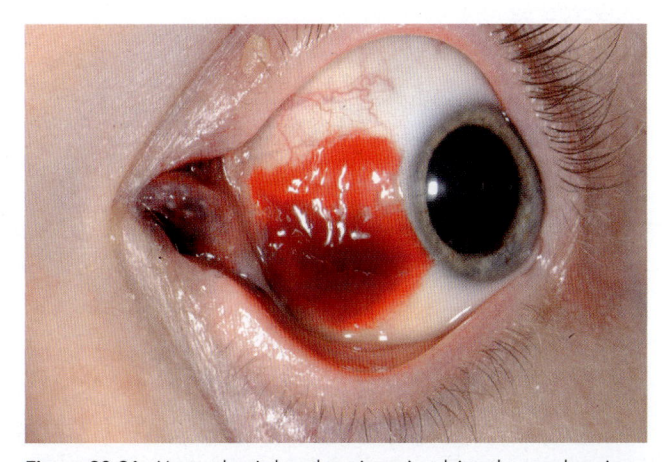

Figure 20.21. Hemorrhagic lymphangioma involving the nasal conjunctiva in the caruncle of a 40-year-old man.

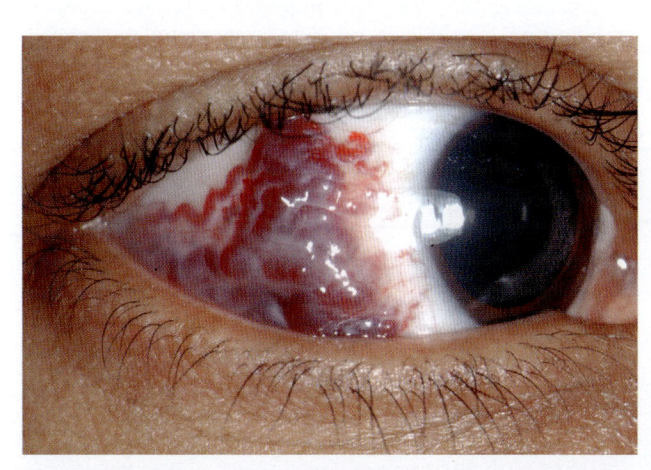

Figure 20.22. Diffuse conjunctival lymphangioma with extensive bleeding in a 30-year-old woman. Note the blue color of the lower eyelid, indicating subcutaneous anterior orbital involvement by the tumor.

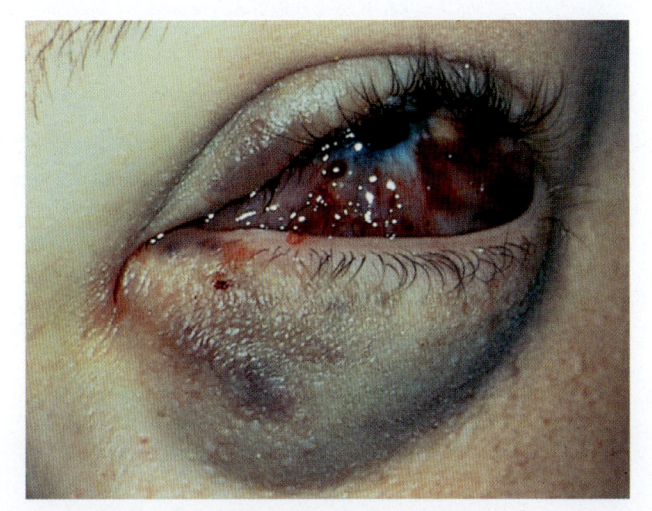

Figure 20.23. Large, diffuse conjunctival lymphangioma with orbital involvement and proptosis in a 30-year-old woman.

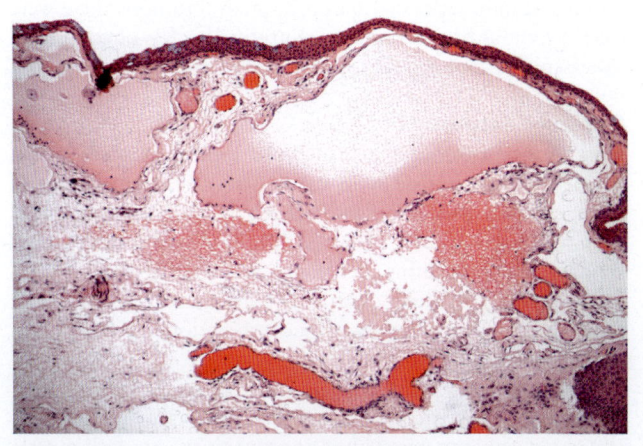

Figure 20.24. Histopathology of lymphangioma showing large dilated vascular channels filled with lymph and blood. (Hematoxylin–eosin ×100.)

MISCELLANEOUS VASCULAR LESIONS OF THE CONJUNCTIVA: VARIX, CAVERNOUS HEMANGIOMA, MACROVESSELS, SENTINEL VESSELS, AND ACQUIRED SESSILE HEMANGIOMA

Several additional vascular tumors and related conditions can develop in the conjunctiva (1–16).

Conjunctival Varix

General Considerations
Varix is a venous malformation that can occur in the orbit and conjunctiva (1–6,10,11,17). It is covered in more detail in the section on orbital tumors.

Clinical Features
Conjunctival varix usually is an anterior extension of an orbital varix. It may be directly visible as large, distinct blood vessels or it may be deeper and have a diffuse faint blue-black color. It is generally movable and not fixed to the sclera.

Pathology
Histopathologically, varix is composed of venous channels, ranging from one dilated vessel to more complex channels. Thrombosis and hyalinization are frequent (17). Pathologists often have difficulty differentiating varix, lymphangioma, and cavernous hemangioma because their features can overlap. Some authorities believe that varix and lymphangioma represent separate entities (5), whereas others believe that they are a spectrum of one condition (6).

Management
Varix that affects the conjunctiva is often asymptomatic and requires no treatment. When it is symptomatic or a cosmetic consideration, surgical excision is warranted. The surgeon must be prepared for considerable bleeding and extension of the conjunctival component posteriorly into the orbit.

Cavernous Hemangioma

General Considerations
Cavernous hemangioma is a fairly common orbital tumor. It is relatively uncommon in the conjunctiva (1–3,12–14). In the authors' clinical series of 1,643 conjunctival tumors, there were four cavernous hemangiomas, accounting for 8% of conjunctival vascular lesions and for less than 1% of the 1,643 lesions (1).

Clinical Features
Conjunctival cavernous hemangioma appears at any age as a red or blue lesion, usually in the stroma. It can be solitary or it can occur in association with other cavernous hemangiomas, such as Sturge–Weber syndrome (8), blue rubber bleb nevus syndrome (15), or diffuse neonatal hemangiomatosis (16). The literature is not entirely clear as to whether such lesions are a pure cavernous hemangioma or a combination of types.

Pathology
Conjunctival cavernous hemangioma is composed of dilated, congested veins separated by connective tissue. Smooth muscle may be present in the walls of the blood vessels.

Management
Conjunctival cavernous hemangioma can be managed by periodic observation or local resection. It is important to be sure that it does not represent conjunctival extension of an orbital hemangioma.

Conjunctival Macrovessels and Episcleral Sentinel Vessels

The epibulbar surface can sometimes develop large, dilated and sometimes tortuous blood vessels. They can represent a normal variation without clinical significance or they can be a hallmark of an underlying ciliary body neoplasm, usually a malignant melanoma. A patient with a prominent episcleral blood vessel should be appropriately evaluated for a ciliary body neoplasm. A similar sentinal vessel can be in association with iris arteriovenous communication (7).

Selected References

Reviews
1. Shields CL, Demirci H, Karatza E, et al. Clinical survey of 1643 melanocytic and nonmelanocytic tumors of the conjunctiva. *Ophthalmology* 2004;111:1747–1754.
2. Shields CL, Shields JA. Tumors of the conjunctiva and cornea. *Surv Ophthalmol* 2004;49:3–24.
3. Shields JA, Mashayekhi A, Kligman B, et al. Vascular tumors of the conjunctiva in 140 cases. The 2010 Melvin Rubin Lecture. *Ophthalmology* 2011;118:1747–1753.
4. Welch J, Srinivasan S, Lyall D, et al. Conjunctival lymphangiectasai: a report of 11 cases and review of the literature. *Surv Ophthalmol* 2012;57:136–148.
5. Rootman J, Hay E, Graeb D, et al. Orbital-adnexal lymphangiomas. A spectrum of hemodynamically isolated vascular hamartomas. *Ophthalmology* 1986;93:1558–1570.
6. Wright JF, Sullivan TJ, Garner A, et al. Orbital venous anomalies. *Ophthalmology* 1997;104:905–913.
7. Shields JA, Streicher TF, Spirkova JH, et al. Arteriovenous malformation of the iris in 14 cases. The 2004 Alvaro Rodriguez Gold Medal Award Lecture. *Arch Ophthalmol* 2006;124:370–375.
8. Sullivan TJ, Clarke MP, Morin JD. The ocular manifestations of the Sturge-Weber syndrome. *J Pediatr Ophthalmol Strabismus* 1992;29:349–356.
9. Shields JA, Kligman BE, Mashayekhi A, et al. Acquired sessile hemangioma of the conjunctiva: a report of 10 cases. *Am J Ophthalmol* 2011;152(1):55–59.

Case Reports
10. Shields JA, Eagle RC Jr, Shields CL, et al. Orbital varix presenting as a subconjunctival mass. *Ophthal Plast Reconstr Surg* 1995;11:37–38.
11. Margo CE, Rowda J, Barletta J. Bilateral conjunctival varix thrombosis associated with habitual headstanding. *Am J Ophthalmol* 1992;113:726–727.
12. Ullman SS, Nelson LB, Shields JA, et al. Cavernous hemangioma of the conjunctiva. *Orbit* 1988;6:261–265.
13. Rao MR, Patankar VL, Reddy V. Cavernous haemangioma of conjunctiva (a case report). *Indian J Ophthalmol* 1989;3:37–38.
14. Bajaj MS, Nainiwal SK, Pushker N, et al. Multifocal cavernous hemangioma: a rare presentation. *Orbit* 2003;22:155–159.
15. Crompton JL, Taylor D. Ocular lesions in the blue rubber bleb naevus syndrome. *Br J Ophthalmol* 1981;65:133–137.
16. Chang CW, Rao NA, Stout JT. Histopathology of the eye in diffuse neonatal hemangiomatosis. *Am J Ophthalmol* 1998;125:868–870.
17. Jakobiec FA, Werdich XQ, Chodosh J, et al. An analysis of conjunctival and periocular venous malformations: clinicopathologic and immunohistochemical features with a comparison of racemose and cirsoid lesions. *Surv Ophthalmol* 2014;9:236–244.

CONJUNCTIVAL VARIX, CAVERNOUS HEMANGIOMA, MACROVESSELS, AND SENTINEL VESSELS

1. Shields JA, Eagle RC Jr, Shields CL, et al. Orbital varix presenting as a subconjunctival mass. *Ophthal Plast Reconstr Surg* 1995;11:37–38.
2. Shields JA, Streicher TFE, Spirkova JHJ, et al. Arteriovenous malformation of the iris in 14 cases. The 2004 Alvaro Rodriguez Gold Medal Award Lecture. *Arch Ophthalmol* 2006;124:370–375.

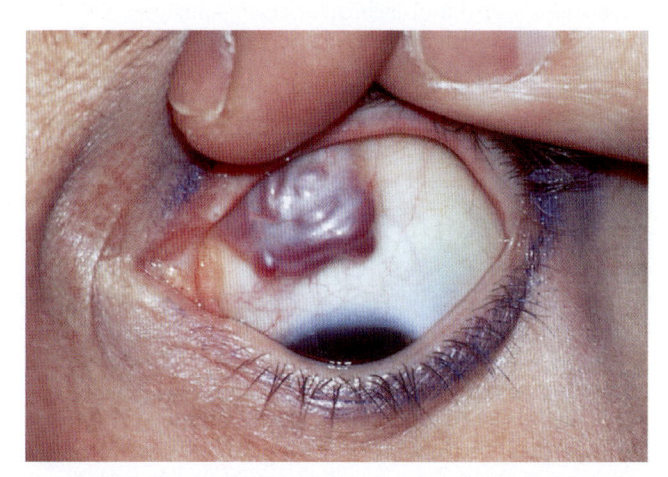

Figure 20.25. Varix in superior bulbar conjunctiva in a 44-year-old woman. The lesion extended posteriorly into the anterior portion of the orbit.

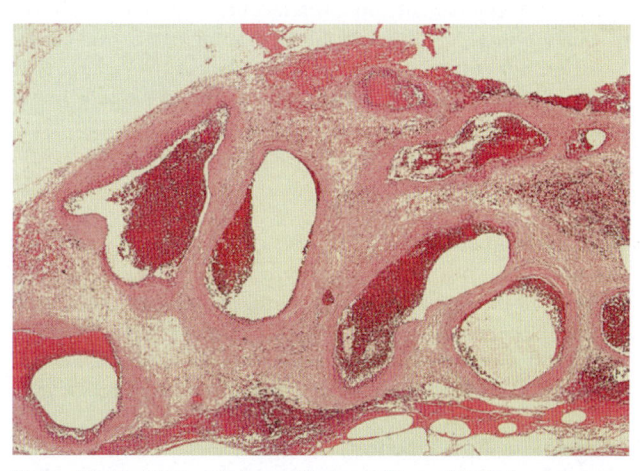

Figure 20.26. Histopathology of lesion in Figure 20.25 showing large, dilated, congested veins. (Hematoxylin–eosin ×40.)

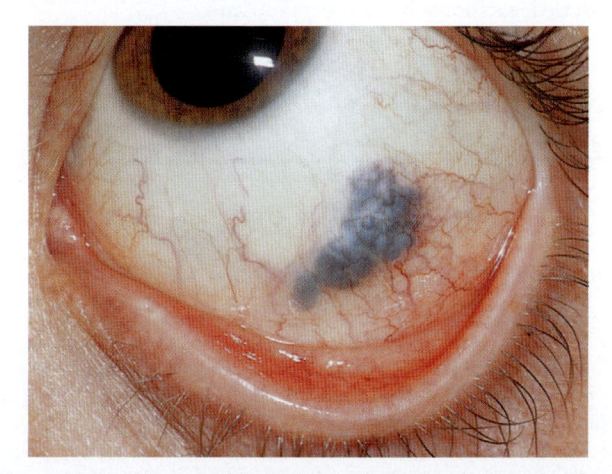

Figure 20.27. Cavernous hemangioma attached to the scleral surface. This teenage girl first noticed the lesion while inserting a contact lens.

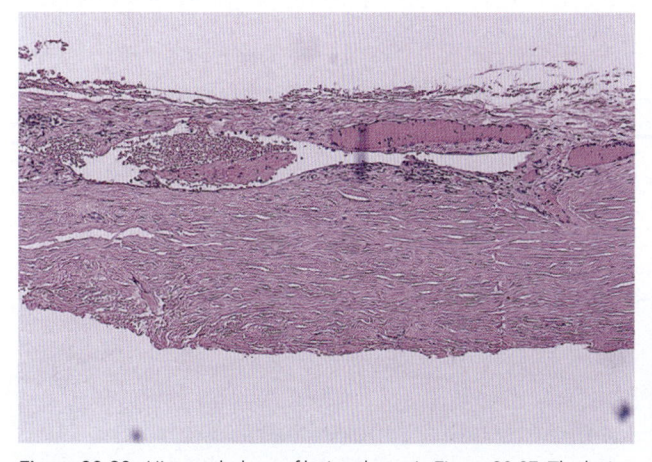

Figure 20.28. Histopathology of lesion shown in Figure 20.27. The lesion partially collapsed during surgical removal. (Hematoxylin–eosin ×10.)

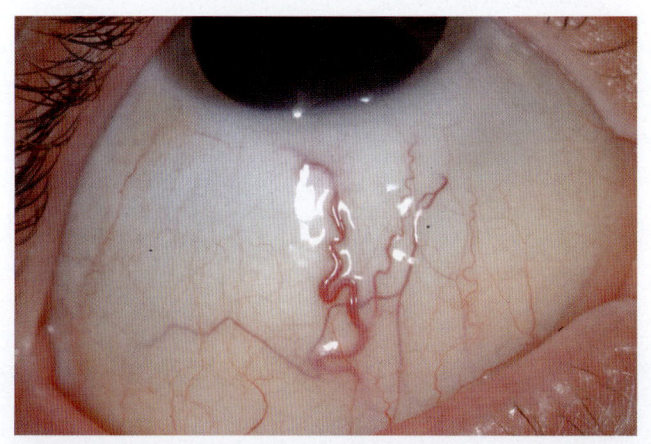

Figure 20.29. Episcleral macrovessel located inferiorly in an otherwise normal eye. This vascular lesion is presumed to be a congenital malformation and is not associated with ciliary body melanoma. However, detailed examination to exclude a ciliary body melanoma is mandatory in such cases. Such a vessel can also be seen with an iris arteriovenous communication.

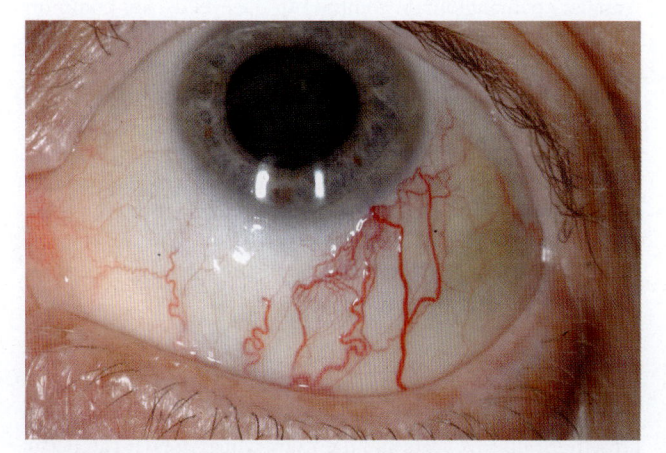

Figure 20.30. Shown for comparison is an episcleral sentinel blood vessel overlying a ciliary body malignant melanoma.

CONJUNCTIVAL ACQUIRED SESSILE HEMANGIOMA AND CAPILLARY HEMANGIOMA

Acquired Sessile Hemangioma

General Considerations
Acquired sessile hemangioma is a recently reported condition that has typical clinical and histopathologic features (1–4). Based on our clinical experience with 10 cases, we believe that it is more common than previously recognized because many such lesions are relatively small and asymptomatic, and likely to be overlooked (3,4). In an earlier study from our department, there were no recorded cases of sessile hemangioma (1).

Clinical Features
Acquired sessile hemangioma generally appears in adulthood as a flat array of intertwining or coiling, mildly dilated blood vessels on the bulbar conjunctiva surface. This lesion has a small feeding artery and draining vein. This lesion generally remains asymptomatic and stable, but can rarely show minimal enlargement.

Diagnostic Approaches
The diagnosis is clinically made based on the recognition of typical clinical features. Fluorescein angiography shows rapid filling with leakage of dye from the deeper feeding artery and diffuse staining of the lesion.

Pathology
In one case that we studied histopathologically following surgical resection at the time of removal of ipsilateral unrelated conjunctival papilloma we found closely packed, slightly dilated cavernous blood vessels multilayered atop each other and immediately beneath the conjunctiva (4).

Management
Acquired sessile hemangioma usually remains asymptomatic and stable. This lesion is usually managed with observation.

Conjunctival Capillary Hemangioma

General Considerations
Capillary hemangioma is common in the eyelids, less common in the orbit, and uncommon in the conjunctiva (1–9). In the authors' clinical series of 1,643 conjunctival tumors, the 10 capillary hemangiomas accounted for 16% of conjunctival vascular lesions and less than 1% of the 1,643 lesions (1,3). It typically has an onset in infancy, but a rare form of capillary hemangioma may develop as an acquired lesion in older adults, similar to the cherry hemangioma seen on the eyelids. There is sometimes overlap clinically histopathologically among capillary hemangioma, cavernous hemangioma, and lymphangioma, making precise categorization difficult.

Clinical Features
Like its eyelid counterpart, conjunctival capillary hemangioma generally appears at or shortly after birth and shows progressive growth for up to 2 years and then slowly regresses. It can occur anywhere in the conjunctiva and appears as a distinct or diffuse red conjunctival mass. It can occur as an isolated lesion or it can be seen in association with a periocular cutaneous capillary hemangioma. Conjunctival involvement can also be seen in association with diffuse neonatal hemangiomatosis, which is sometimes a fatal condition (9).

Pathology
Histopathologically, conjunctival capillary hemangioma is composed of lobules of proliferating endothelial cells separated by thin fibrous septa. Lesions that have shown spontaneous regression are less vascular and contain more fibrous tissue.

Management
The management of infantile conjunctival capillary hemangioma is generally observation, with the assumption that the lesion will regress. In our experience, most have been small and asymptomatic. In the rare case where the lesion is larger and potentially amblyogenic, treatment with oral or intralesional corticosteroids has been used in the past, but currently, most clinicians prefer the use of oral propranolol to hasten resolution (7,8). If other tumors, like rhabdomyosarcoma, cannot be excluded, excisional biopsy is appropriate.

Selected References

Reviews
1. Shields CL, Demirci H, Karatza E, et al. Clinical survey of 1643 melanocytic and nonmelanocytic tumors of the conjunctiva. *Ophthalmology* 2004;111:1747–1754.
2. Shields CL, Shields JA. Tumors of the conjunctiva and cornea. *Surv Ophthalmol* 2004;49:3–24.
3. Shields JA, Mashayekhi A, Kligman B, et al. Vascular tumors of the conjunctiva in 140 cases. The 2010 Melvin Rubin Lecture. *Ophthalmology* 2011;118:1747–1753.
4. Shields JA, Kligman BE, Mashayekhi A, et al. Acquired sessile hemangioma of the conjunctiva: A report of 10 cases. *Am J Ophthalmol* 2011;152:55–59.
5. Wright JF, Sullivan TJ, Garner A, et al. Orbital venous anomalies. *Ophthalmology* 1997;104:905–913.
6. Rootman J, Hay E, Graeb D, et al. Orbital-adnexal lymphangiomas. A spectrum of hemodynamically isolated vascular hamartomas. *Ophthalmology* 1986;93:1558–1570.

Management
7. Cheng JF, Gole GA, Sullivan TJ. Propranolol in the management of periorbital infantile haemangioma. *Clin Experiment Ophthalmol* 2010;38:547–553.
8. Thoumazet F, Leaute-Labreze C, Colin J, et al. Efficacy of systemic propranolol for severe infantile haemangioma of the orbit and eyelid: a case study of eight patients. *Br J Ophthalmol* 2011;96:370–374.

Histopathology
9. Chang CW, Rao NA, Stout JT. Histopathology of the eye in diffuse neonatal hemangiomatosis. *Am J Ophthalmol* 1998;125:868–870.

CONJUNCTIVAL CONGENITAL CAPILLARY HEMANGIOMA, ACQUIRED SESSILE HEMANGIOMA, AND VARIX

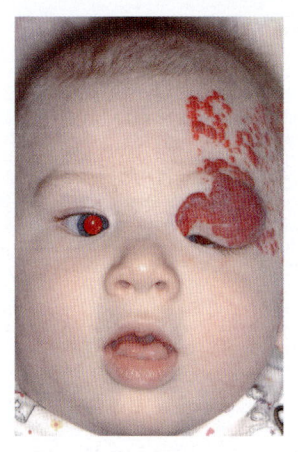

Figure 20.31. Congenital capillary hemangioma of upper eyelid and forehead.

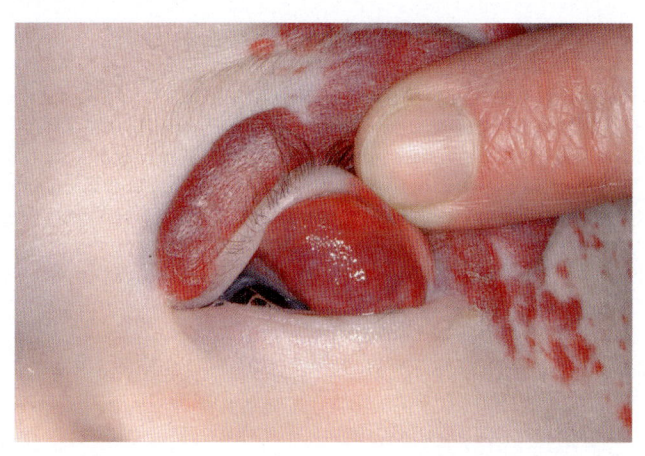

Figure 20.32. Same child shown in Figure 20.31 with eversion of the left upper eyelid revealing a large tarsal capillary hemangioma.

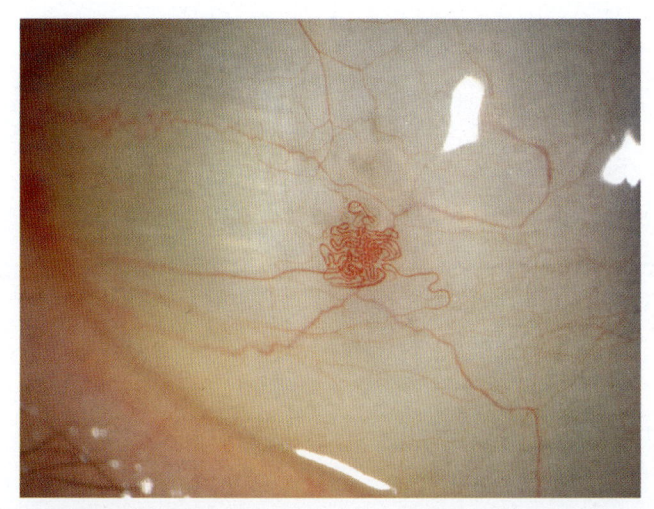

Figure 20.33. Clinical appearance of acquired sessile hemangioma of conjunctiva in an adult.

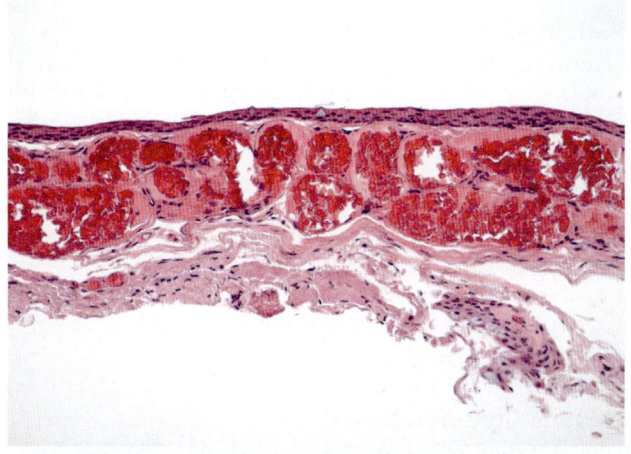

Figure 20.34. Histopathology of lesion shown in Figure 20.33 demonstrating ectatic stromal vessels filled with red blood cells and surrounded by endothelium, consistent with sessile hemangioma.

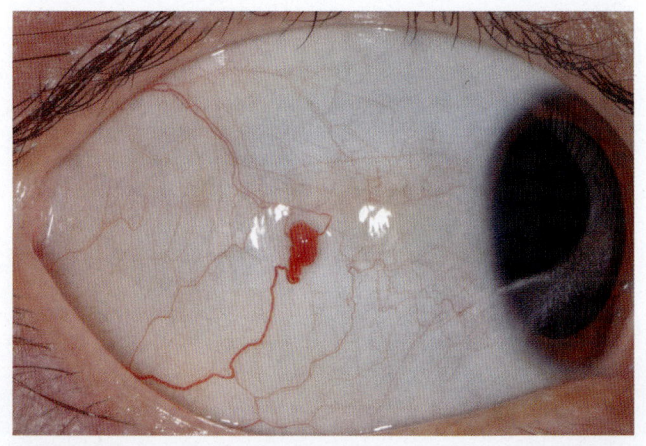

Figure 20.35. Red conjunctival mass in a young man, classified as a varix.

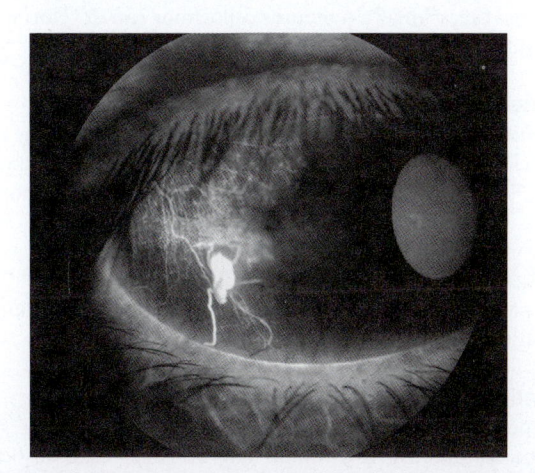

Figure 20.36. Fluorescein angiography of lesion shown in Figure 20.35 demonstrating large vascular lake, consistent with diagnosis of varix.

CONJUNCTIVAL HEMANGIOPERICYTOMA AND GLOMANGIOMA (GLOMUS TUMOR)

Conjunctival Hemangiopericytoma

General Considerations
Historically, hemangiopericytoma has been known as a neoplasm derived from vascular pericytes. In recent years, the true existence of a tumor derived from pericytes has been challenged and some authorities believe that previously reported cases of hemangiopericytoma may be variants of solitary fibrous tumor. Until that issue is resolved, we continue to include conjunctival hemangiopericytoma. In the orbit, it is reported to show a benign or malignant clinical course and to metastasize in 12% to 45% of cases. Hemangiopericytoma confined to the conjunctiva is rare (1–7).

Clinical Features
Conjunctival hemangiopericytoma appears as an elevated or pedunculated reddish-pink mass that has no distinct clinical features. It shows slow, progressive growth and often is continuous with a more posterior orbital component.

Pathology
Hemangiopericytoma is a tumor composed of an abnormal proliferation of pericytes that surround blood vessels. With routine light microscopy, a characteristic feature is the "staghorn" branching of the blood vessels in the tumor.

Management
The diagnosis is rarely made clinically and the recommended treatment is wide excision and close clinical follow-up.

Conjunctival Glomangioma (Glomus Tumor)

General Considerations
Glomus tumor (glomangioma) is a relatively common vascular lesion that arises from the glomus body, a specialized structure that is usually found in the hand and that has a thermoregulatory function. It was discussed in the section on eyelid tumors. Occasionally, a glomus cell tumor can develop in the conjunctiva.

Clinical Features
Conjunctival glomus tumor can appear as a reddish-blue mass that closely resembles a lymphangioma (1,2,8,9). It is uncommon, but may have a predisposition to affect the insertions of rectus muscles (9).

Pathology
The pathology of glomus tumor is discussed in the section on eyelid tumors.

Management
Glomus tumor can be surgically excised or simply observed. In the conjunctiva this tumor may be larger than suspected clinically and may extend into the orbit (9).

Selected References

Reviews
1. Shields CL, Demirci H, Karatza E, et al. Clinical survey of 1643 melanocytic and nonmelanocytic tumors of the conjunctiva. *Ophthalmology* 2004;111:1747–1754.
2. Shields CL, Shields JA. Tumors of the conjunctiva and cornea. *Surv Ophthalmol* 2004;49:3–24.
3. Shields JA, Mashayekhi A, Kligman B, et al. Vascular tumors of the conjunctiva in 140 cases. The 2010 Melvin Rubin Lecture. *Ophthalmology* 2011;118:1747–1753.
4. Folpe AL, Fanburg-Smith JC, Miettinen M, et al. Atypical and malignant glomus tumors: analysis of 52 cases, with a proposal for the reclassification of glomus tumors. *Am J Surg Pathol* 2001;25:1–12.

Histopathology
5. Stout AP, Murray MR. Hemangiopericytoma; a vascular tumor featuring Zimmerman's pericytes. *Ann Surg* 1942;116:16–33.

Case Reports
6. Sujatha S, Sampath R, Bonshek RE, et al. Conjunctival haemangiopericytoma. *Br J Ophthalmol* 1994;78:497–499.
7. Grossniklaus HE, Green WR, Wolff SM, et al. Hemangiopericytoma of the conjunctiva. Two cases. *Ophthalmology* 1986;93:265–267.
8. Charles NC. Multiple glomus tumors of the face and eyelid. *Arch Ophthalmol* 1976;94:1283–1285.
9. Shields JA, Eagle RC Jr, Marr BP, et al. Orbital glomangioma involving two ocular rectus muscles. *Am J Ophthalmol* 2006;142:511–513.

CONJUNCTIVAL HEMANGIOPERICYTOMA AND GLOMANGIOMA

1. Grossniklaus HE, Green WR, Wolff SM, et al. Hemangiopericytoma of the conjunctiva. Two cases. *Ophthalmology* 1986;93:265–267.
2. Shields JA, Eagle RC Jr, Shields CL, et al. Orbital-conjunctival glomangiomas involving two ocular rectus muscles. *Am J Ophthalmol* 2006;142:511–513.

Figure 20.37. Hemangiopericytoma arising from the inferior fornix in a 40-year-old woman. (Courtesy of Hans Grossniklaus, MD.)

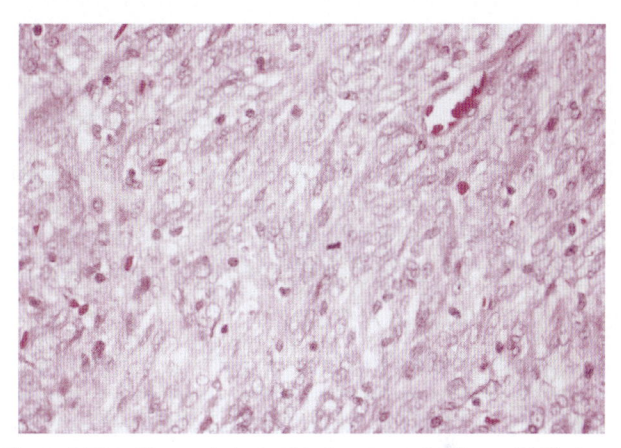

Figure 20.38. Histopathology of lesion shown in Figure 20.37 showing solid tumor composed of spindle-shaped cells and blood vessels. (Hematoxylin–eosin ×63.)

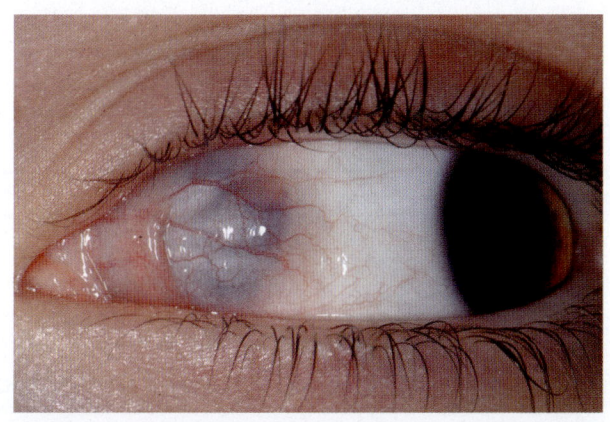

Figure 20.39. Conjunctival glomangiomas in a 17-year-old boy. Clinical appearance of one lesion, located in the conjunctival and subconjunctival tissues at insertion of medial rectus muscle.

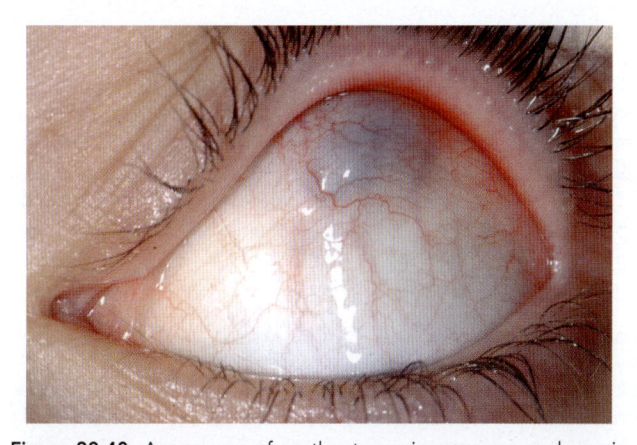

Figure 20.40. Appearance of another tumor in same eye as shown in Figure 20.39 in downgaze, showing similar lesion in region of superior rectus muscle.

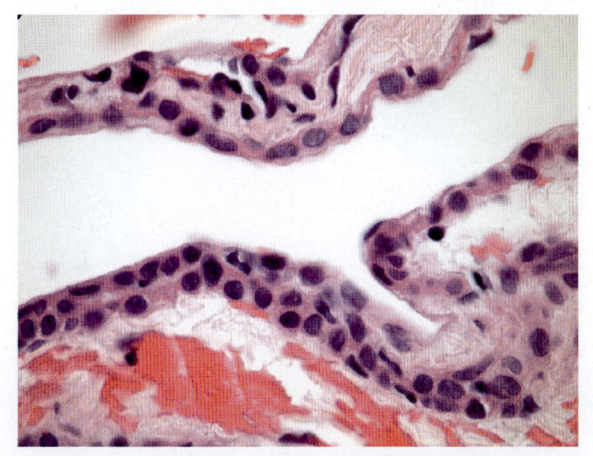

Figure 20.41. Photomicrograph of lesion seen in Figure 20.39 showing vascular lumen ringed by characteristic cuboidal glomus cells. (Hematoxylin–eosin ×200.)

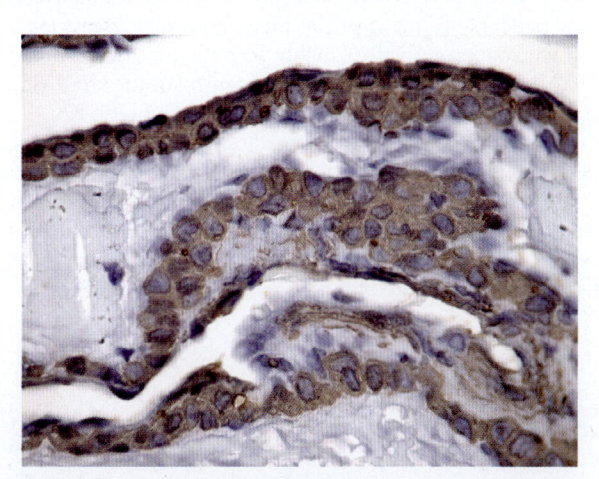

Figure 20.42. Immunohistochemistry, showing positive reaction to muscle-specific actin. Vimentin stain was also positive and epithelial and endothelial cell markers were nonreactive. (Hematoxylin–eosin ×200.)

CONJUNCTIVAL KAPOSI SARCOMA

General Considerations

Some general aspects of KS were discussed in the section on eyelid tumors. KS can also develop in the conjunctiva (1–20). In the authors' clinical series of 1,643 conjunctival tumors, the nine KS accounted for 14% of conjunctival vascular lesions and for less than 1% of the 1,643 lesions (1). Until a few years ago, 20% of patients with acquired immunodeficiency syndrome (AIDS) had ocular involvement and, of those, 20% had conjunctival involvement (4,5). Today, ocular KS is diagnosed less often, perhaps owing to more effective treatment of AIDS in more medically advanced countries.

Clinical Features

In the conjunctiva, KS has the same systemic associations as in the eyelids, but has a different clinical appearance. Conjunctival involvement can be the first sign of AIDS (17,18) or it can be completely unrelated to AIDS (19). It appears as one or more painless, reddish vascular masses that may become confluent and resemble hemorrhagic conjunctivitis (1–20).

Pathology

KS is a malignant vascular tumor composed of spindle-shaped cells with elongated oval nuclei, well-formed capillary channels, and vascular slits containing blood but without an endothelial lining (13). Staining for factor VIII–related antigen is positive and electron microscopy can sometimes detect Weibel–Palade bodies, supporting the concept of an endothelial cell derivation of the tumor (13,17). This malignancy is believed related to infection with Herpes virus type 8 (7).

Management

Conjunctival KS is responsive to chemotherapy and low-dose radiotherapy. Doses ranging from 800 to 2,000 cGy (8–11) have been advocated for conjunctival KS. Interferon-α-2a has also been used (12). Such treatment should be coordinated with infectious disease specialists and general oncologists. Currently, most patients are managed by their infectious disease physician with increase in their highly active antiretroviral therapy (HAART), which leads to improved control of the viral-stimulated malignancy and hence causes involution of the KS.

Sometimes, if the lesion is small and circumscribed, local excision is feasible. When the diagnosis is uncertain, biopsy can be done to exclude simple conjunctival hemorrhage or other hemorrhagic neoplasms. Incomplete excision has been associated with regression of residual tumor (5,7). The affected patient should also be evaluated for life-threatening visceral disease.

Selected References

Reviews
1. Shields CL, Demirci H, Karatza E, et al. Clinical survey of 1643 melanocytic and nonmelanocytic tumors of the conjunctiva. *Ophthalmology* 2004;111:1747–1754.
2. Shields CL, Shields JA. Tumors of the conjunctiva and cornea. *Surv Ophthalmol* 2004;49:3–24.
3. Shields JA, Mashayekhi A, Kligman B, et al. Vascular tumors of the conjunctiva in 140 cases. The 2010 Melvin Rubin Lecture. *Ophthalmology* 2011;118:1747–1753.
4. Holland GN, Pepose JS, Pettit TH, et al. Acquired immune deficiency syndrome. Ocular manifestations. *Ophthalmology* 1983;90;859–873.
5. Jeng BH, Holland GN, Lowder CY, et al. Anterior segment and external ocular disorders associated with human immunodeficiency virus disease. *Surv Ophthalmol* 2007;52(4):329–368.
6. Palestine AG, Rodrigues MM, Macher AM, et al. Ophthalmic involvement in acquired immunodeficiency syndrome. *Ophthalmology* 1984;91:1092–1099.
7. Verma V, Shen D, Sieving PC, et al. The role of infectious agents in the etiology of ocular adnexal neoplasia. *Surv Ophthalmol* 2008;53(4):312–331.

Management
8. Dugel PU, Gill PS, Frangieh GT, et al. Treatment of ocular adnexal Kaposi's sarcoma in acquired immune deficiency syndrome. *Ophthalmology* 1992;99:1127–1132.
9. Kirova YM, Belembaogo E, Frikha H, et al. Radiotherapy in the management of epidemic Kaposi's sarcoma: a retrospective study of 643 cases. *Radiother Oncol* 1998;46:19–22.
10. Ghabrial R, Quivey JM, Dunn JP Jr, et al. Radiation therapy of acquired immunodeficiency syndrome-related Kaposi's sarcoma of the eyelids and conjunctiva. *Arch Ophthalmol* 1992;110:1423–1426.
11. Brunt AM, Phillips RH. Strontium-90 for conjunctival AIDS-related Kaposi's sarcoma: the first case report. *Clin Oncol* 1990;2:118–119.
12. Hummer J, Gass JD, Huang AJ. Conjunctival Kaposi's sarcoma treated with interferon alpha-2a. *Am J Ophthalmol* 1993;116:502–503.

Histopathology
13. Weiter JJ, Jakobiec FA, Iwamoto T. The clinical and morphologic characteristics of Kaposi's sarcoma of the conjunctiva. *Am J Ophthalmol* 1980;89:546–552.

Case Reports
14. Lieberman PH, Llovera IN. Kaposi's sarcoma of the bulbar conjunctiva. *Arch Ophthalmol* 1972;88:44–45.
15. Nicholson DH, Lane L. Epibulbar Kaposi sarcoma. *Arch Ophthalmol* 1978;96:95–96.
16. Murray N, McCluskey P, Wakefield D, et al. Isolated bulbar conjunctival Kaposi's sarcoma. *Aust N Z J Ophthalmol* 1994;22:81–82.
17. Macher AM, Palestine A, Masur H, et al. Multicentric Kaposi's sarcoma of the conjunctiva in a male homosexual with acquired immunodeficiency syndrome. *Ophthalmology* 1983;90:879–884.
18. Shuler JD, Holland GN, Miles SA, et al. Kaposi sarcoma of the conjunctiva and eyelids associated with the acquired immunodeficiency syndrome. *Arch Ophthalmol* 1989;107:858–862.
19. Fogt F, Sulewski M, Meralli F, et al. Conjunctival Kaposi's sarcoma in a nonimmunocompromised patient. *Can J Ophthalmol* 2007;42:310–311.
20. Reiser BJ, Mok A, Kukes G, et al. Non-AIDS-related Kaposi sarcoma involving the tarsal conjunctiva and eyelid margin. *Arch Ophthalmol* 2007;125(6):838–840.

CONJUNCTIVAL KAPOSI SARCOMA IN PATIENTS WITH AIDS AND IMMUNOCOMPETENT PATIENTS

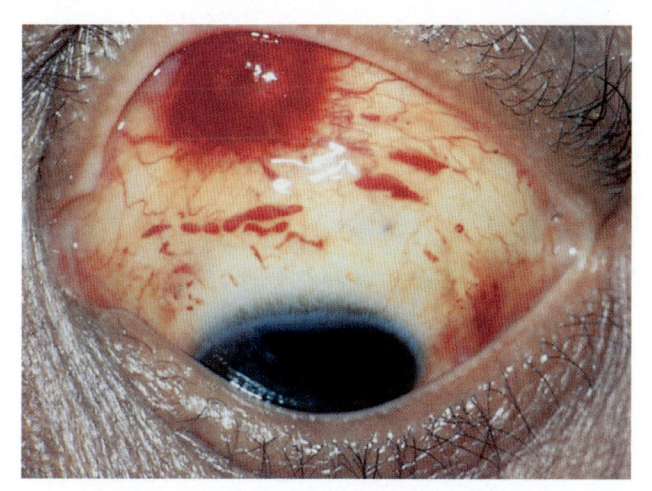

Figure 20.43. Solitary KS of the conjunctiva in a 51-year-old man with AIDS. The referral diagnosis was hemorrhagic conjunctivitis.

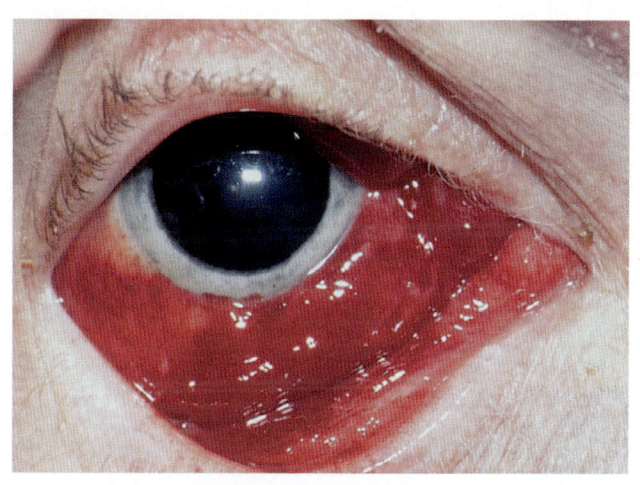

Figure 20.44. Diffuse multinodular KS in the lower conjunctiva of a 43-year-old man with AIDS.

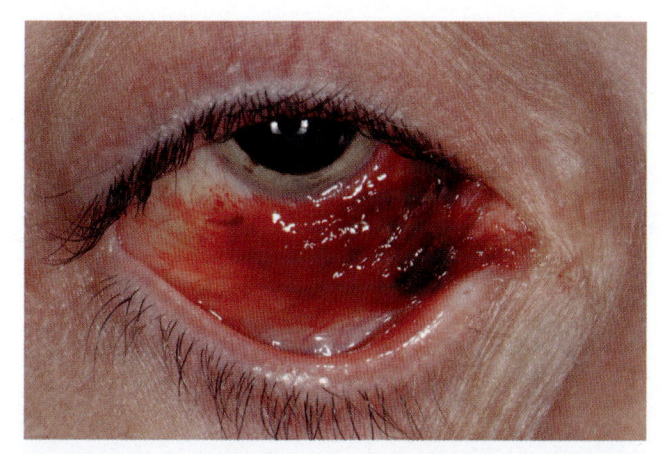

Figure 20.45. Multifocal KS of the conjunctiva in a middle-aged man with AIDS. The patient was treated with injection interferon and improvement in highly active antiretroviral therapy (HAART).

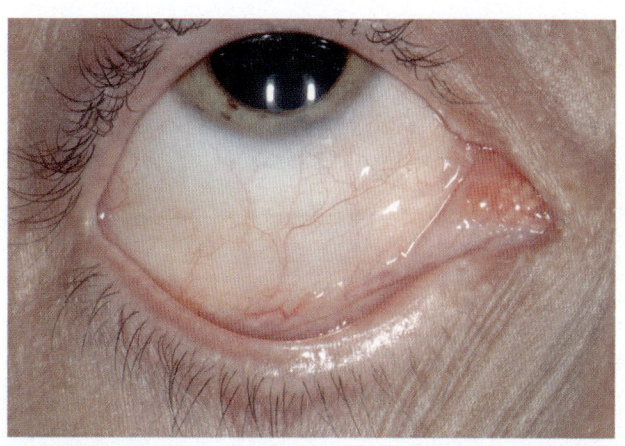

Figure 20.46. Following nonsurgical therapy, the KS in Figure 20.45 completely resolved.

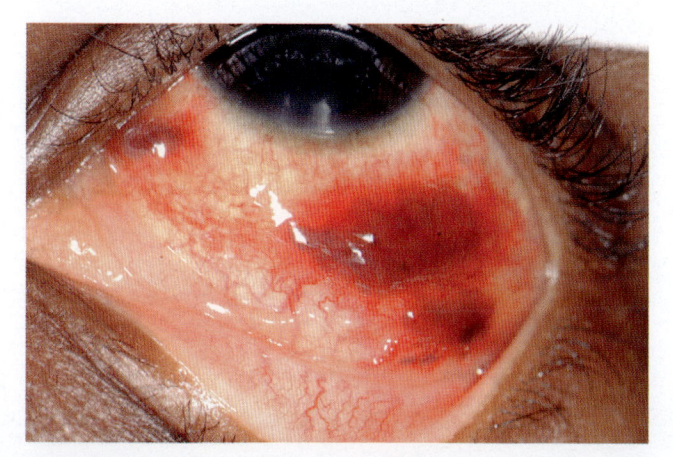

Figure 20.47. Diffuse, multifocal KS in conjunctiva of a presumably immunocompetent patient.

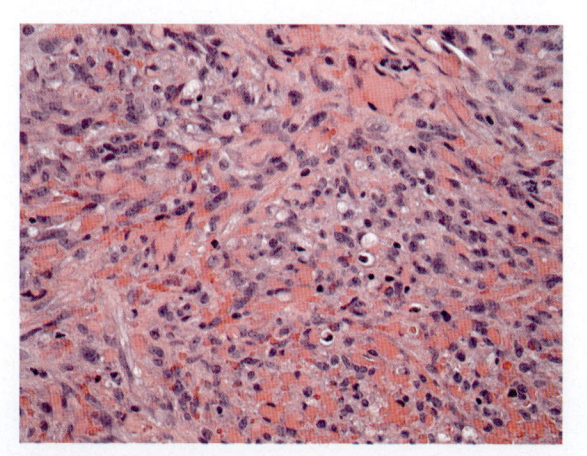

Figure 20.48. Histopathology of lesion shown in Figure 20.47 showing malignant spindle-shaped cells and slitlike vascular spaces. (Hematoxylin–eosin ×200.)

CONJUNCTIVAL NEURAL, XANTHOMATOUS, FIBROUS, MYXOMATOUS, AND LIPOMATOUS TUMORS

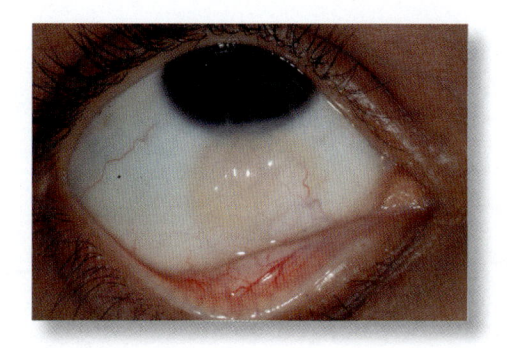

Several related soft tissue tumors appear to derive from neural, histiocytic, fibrous myxomatous, or lipomatous elements of the conjunctiva. These can have distinct features or overlap considerably in their cellular constituents. They are discussed briefly, beginning with neuroma and neurofibroma.

General Considerations

Neural tumors like simple neuroma and neurofibroma can occur in the conjunctiva (1–12). The best known simple neuromas are the soft mucosal neural tumors that appear in the conjunctiva and other mucous membranes in patients with multiple endocrine neoplasia type 2b (6,10–12). Such patients have prominent corneal nerves in 100% of cases. Because of the high association with life-threatening medullary thyroid carcinoma, ophthalmologists should be familiar with these conjunctival lesions. These benign neural tumors are generally asymptomatic and usually require no treatment. We have seen a patient with this uncommon disorder but have not been able to obtain acceptable photographs.

Neurofibroma is a peripheral nerve sheath tumor that can occur in the conjunctiva as a solitary mass or as a diffuse or plexiform variety associated with von Recklinghausen's neurofibromatosis (NF-1) (3–5,7–9). Conjunctival and orbital neurofibromas can be divided into solitary, diffuse, and plexiform types. The solitary type is not usually associated with NF-1, the diffuse type is sometimes associated with NF-1, and the plexiform type is generally considered to be almost pathognomonic of NF-1. There was only one neurofibroma in our clinical series of 1,643 conjunctival tumors.

Clinical Features

Solitary conjunctival neurofibroma appears as a yellow-gray sessile or dome-shaped mass located in the conjunctival stroma. The sessile variant can have poorly defined margins. The plexiform variant is an ill-defined, firm, irregular mass that has been likened to a bag of worms. The conjunctival plexiform neurofibroma is often in continuity with the same lesion of the eyelid and orbit.

CONJUNCTIVAL NEUROMA AND NEUROFIBROMA

Pathology

Histopathologically, diffuse and plexiform neurofibromas are composed of bundles of enlarged nerves with proliferation of Schwann cells and endoneural fibroblasts in a mucoid matrix. A distinct perineural sheath defines the individual tumor cores. The localized neurofibroma lacks a perineural sheath and is encapsulated. It can sometimes be difficult to differentiate from other spindle cell tumors and special stains for axons may help make the diagnosis in such cases (6).

Management

Solitary tumors appear as slowly enlarging elevated stromal masses that can be managed by complete surgical resection. The plexiform type can be extremely difficult to remove intact and debulking procedures are often necessary. This can result in extensive scarring. The systemic prognosis is good; malignant transformation is extremely rare.

Selected References

Reviews

1. Shields CL, Demirci H, Karatza E, et al. Clinical survey of 1643 melanocytic and nonmelanocytic tumors of the conjunctiva. *Ophthalmology* 2004;111:1747–1754.
2. Shields CL, Shields JA. Tumors of the conjunctiva and cornea. *Surv Ophthalmol* 2004;49:3–24.
3. Brownstein S, Little JM. Ocular neurofibromatosis. *Ophthalmology* 1983;91:1595–1599.
4. Krohel GB, Rosenberg PN, Wright J, et al. Localized orbital neurofibromas. *Am J Ophthalmol* 1985;100:458–464.
5. Kobrin JL, Blodi FC, Weingiest TA, et al. Ocular and orbital manifestations of neurofibromatosis. *Surv Ophthalmol* 1979;24:45–51.

Histopathology

6. Riley FC Jr, Robertson DM. Ocular histopathology in multiple endocrine neoplasia type 2b. *Am J Ophthalmol* 1981;91:57–64.

Case Reports

7. Perry HD. Isolated episcleral neurofibroma. *Ophthalmology* 1982;89:1095–1098.
8. Dabezies OH Jr, Penner RJ. Neurofibroma or neurilemoma of the bulbar conjunctiva. *Arch Ophthalmol* 1961;66:73–75.
9. Kalina PH, Bartley GB, Campbell RJ, et al. Isolated neurofibromas of the conjunctiva. *Am J Ophthalmol* 1991;111:694–698.
10. Jacobs JM, Hawes MJ. From eyelid bumps to thyroid lumps: report of a MEN type IIb family and review of the literature. *Ophthal Plast Reconstr Surg* 2001;17:195–201.
11. Robertson DM, Sizemore GW, Gordon H. Thickened corneal nerves as a manifestation of multiple endocrine neoplasia. *Trans Sect Ophthalmol Am Acad Ophthalmol Otolaryngol* 1975;79:772–787.
12. Shields JA, Shields CL, Perez N. Choroidal metastasis from medullary thyroid carcinoma in multiple endocrine neoplasia. *Am J Ophthalmol* 2002;134:607–609.

CONJUNCTIVAL NEUROFIBROMA

Perry HD. Isolated episcleral neurofibroma. *Ophthalmology* 1982;89:1095–1098.

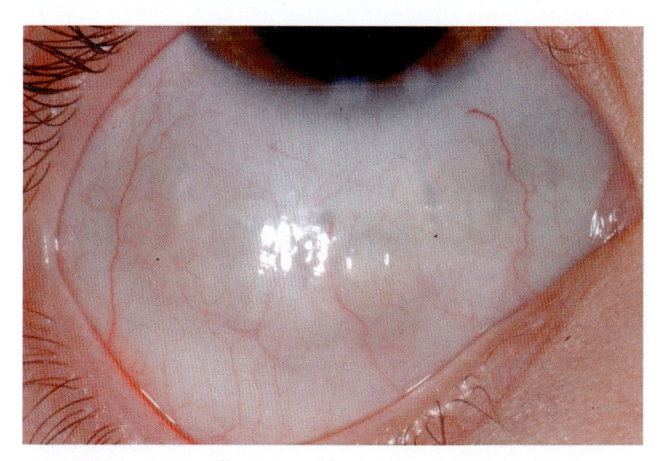

Figure 21.1. Subtle diffuse neurofibroma of the inferior bulbar conjunctiva in a young girl with NF-1.

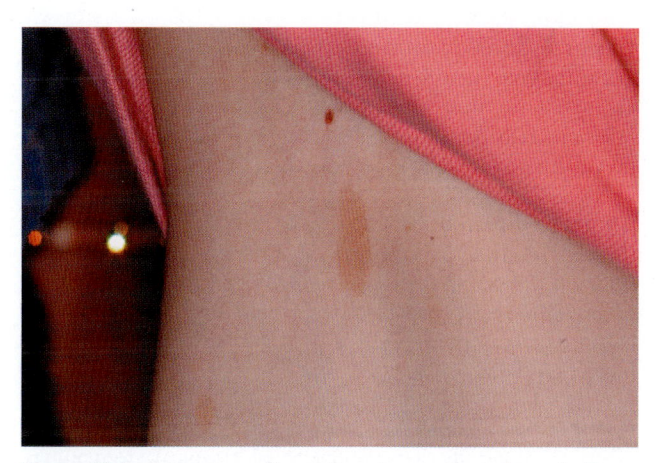

Figure 21.2. Cutaneous café-au-lait spot on patient shown in Figure 21.1.

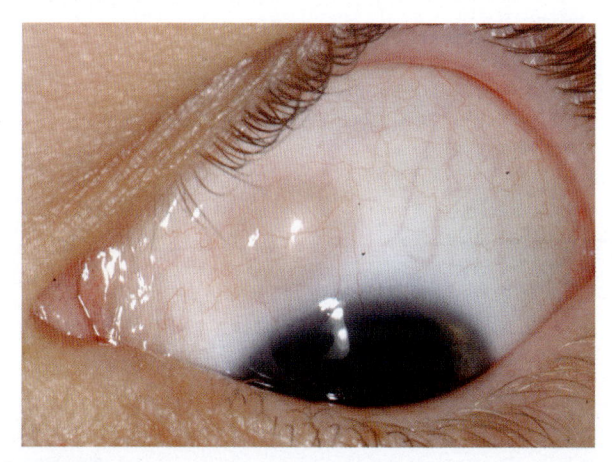

Figure 21.3. Involvement of superior aspect of conjunctiva with episcleral neurofibroma in a boy with NF-1.

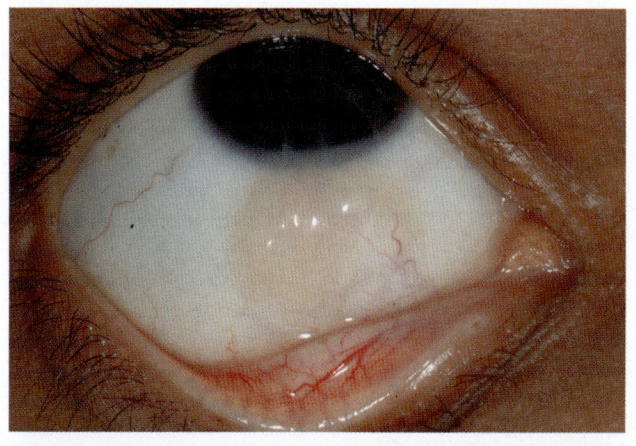

Figure 21.4. Involvement of inferior conjunctiva with episcleral neurofibroma in a teenage boy with documented NF-1.

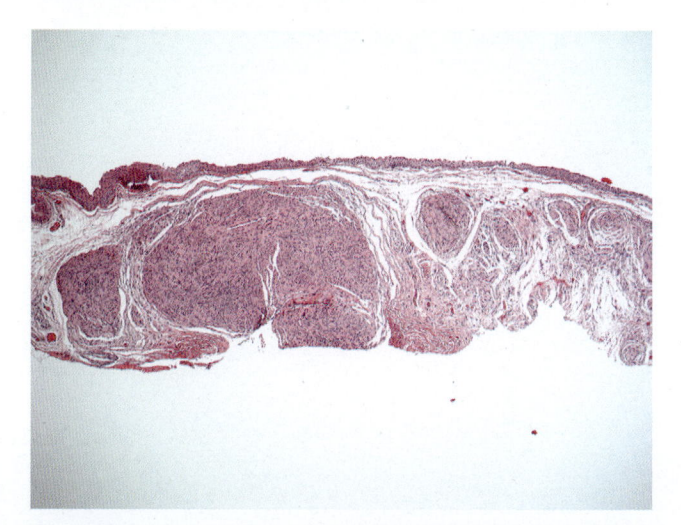

Figure 21.5. Histopathology of neurofibroma in Figure 21.4 showing closely compact spindle cells. (Hematoxylin–eosin ×10.)

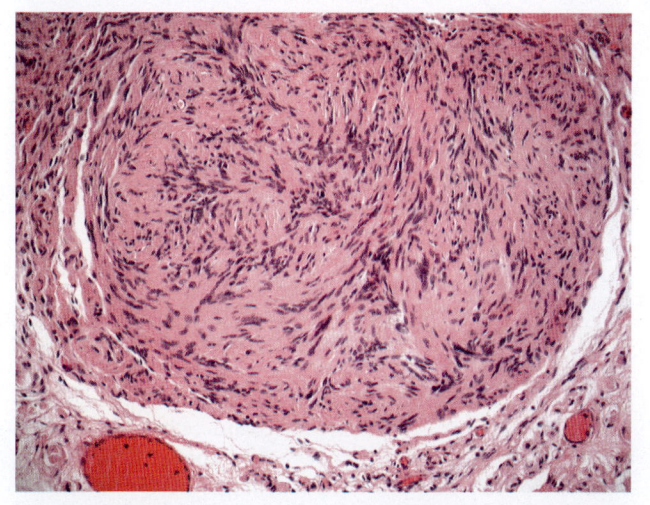

Figure 21.6. Higher-magnification photomicrograph of lesion shown in Figure 21.5 documenting enlarged nerve bundle with numerous spindle-shaped cells. (Hematoxylin–eosin ×100.)

CONJUNCTIVAL SCHWANNOMA AND GRANULAR CELL TUMOR

Conjunctival Schwannoma

General Considerations
Schwannoma (neurilemoma) is a benign peripheral nerve sheath tumor that is composed of a pure proliferation of Schwann cells. It is a relatively common soft tissue tumor of the orbit and can occasionally occur in the conjunctiva (1–6).

Clinical Features
In the conjunctiva, schwannoma presents as a light pink-yellow, elevated mass that generally lies in the stroma of the bulbar conjunctiva or episcleral tissues. It is a slow-growing lesion that may have mildly dilated conjunctival or episcleral nutrient vessels.

Pathology
Histopathologically, it is composed of a typical arrangement of spindle cells, usually forming an Antoni A or B pattern and Verocay bodies (1). Ultrastructurally, the cytoplasm of the cells contains areas of wide-spacing collagen, a typical feature of Schwann cells.

Management
The best management of conjunctival schwannoma is complete surgical resection. It is important to completely excise the lesion within its capsule, because of the possibility of recurrence after incomplete excision. Malignant peripheral nerve sheath tumor (malignant schwannoma) has been known to arise in the orbit, but, to our knowledge, has not been reported in the conjunctiva.

Conjunctival Granular Cell Tumor

General Considerations
Granular cell tumor is an uncommon neoplasm for which the pathogenesis is uncertain and disputed. Although it was previously believed to be a tumor of muscle origin, a Schwann cell origin for this tumor has been most recently popularized (7,8).

Clinical Features
In the conjunctiva, like in the orbit, granular cell tumor is clinically indistinguishable from most other well-circumscribed, nonpigmented conjunctival neoplasms.

Pathology
Microscopically, granular cell tumor consists of cords and lobules of round, benign cells with a pronounced granular cytoplasm. Pseudoepitheliomatous hyperplasia of the overlying conjunctival epithelium is a recognized feature of this tumor. Based on electron microscopic studies, it has been suggested that the cells may be modified Schwann cells, although the precise histogenesis of the tumor is still disputed. A malignant variation of this tumor may be indistinguishable from alveolar soft part sarcoma. Granular cell tumor is rarely diagnosed clinically.

Management
Like other slowly progressive, circumscribed, benign tumors, the best management is complete surgical excision. The prognosis is good.

Selected References
Reviews/Series
1. Demirci H, Shields CL, Eagle RC Jr, et al. Epibulbar schwannoma in a 17-year-old boy and review of the literature. *Ophthal Plast Reconstr Surg* 2010;26:48–50.
2. Charles NC, Fox DM, Avendano JA, et al. Conjunctival neurilemoma. Report of 3 cases. *Arch Ophthalmol* 1997;115:547–549.

Case Reports
3. Dabezies OH Jr, Penner RJ. Neurofibroma or neurilemoma of the bulbar conjunctiva. *Arch Ophthalmol* 1961;66:73–75.
4. Vincent NJ, Cleasby GW. Schwannoma of the bulbar conjunctiva. *Arch Ophthalmol* 1968;80:641–642.
5. Le Marc'hadour F, Romanet JP, Fdili A, et al. Schwannoma of the bulbar conjunctiva. *Arch Ophthalmol* 1996;114:1258–1260.
6. Oshima K, Kitada M, Yamadori I. Neurilemoma of the bulbar conjunctiva. *Jpn J Ophthalmol* 2007;51:68–69.
7. Ferry AP. Granular cell tumor (myoblastoma) of the palpebral conjunctiva causing pseudoepitheliomatous hyperplasia of the conjunctival epithelium. *Am J Ophthalmol* 1981;91:234–237.
8. Charles NC, Fox DM, Glasberg SS, et al. Epibulbar granular cell tumor. Report of a case and review of the literature. *Ophthalmology* 1977;104:1454–1456.

Chapter 21 Conjunctival Neural, Xanthomatous, Fibrous, Myxomatous, and Lipomatous Tumors

CONJUNCTIVAL SCHWANNOMA AND GRANULAR CELL TUMOR

Conjunctival tumors of Schwann cell origin and presumed Schwann cell origin include schwannoma (neurilemoma) and granular cell tumor, respectively.

1. Le Marc'hadour F, Romanet JP, Fdili A, et al. Schwannoma of the bulbar conjunctiva. *Arch Ophthalmol* 1996;114:1258–1260.
2. Charles NC, Fox DM, Glasberg SS, et al. Epibulbar granular cell tumor. Report of a case and review of the literature. *Ophthalmology* 1977;104:1454–1456.

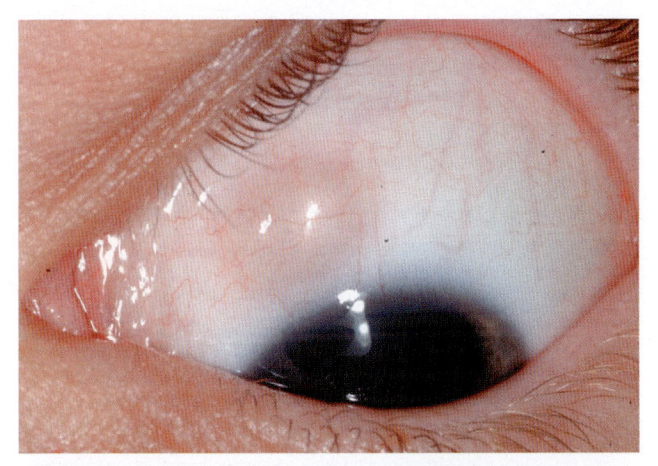

Figure 21.7. Epibulbar schwannoma in a 15-year-old boy. The lesion appeared and enlarged slowly over several weeks.

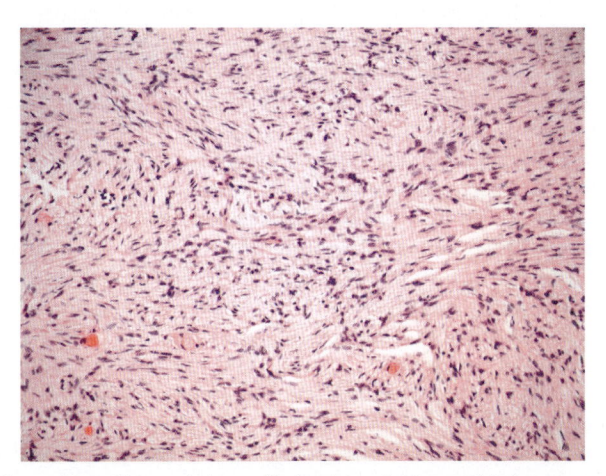

Figure 21.8. Histopathology of lesion shown in Figure 21.7 demonstrating mostly Antoni A pattern of schwannoma. (Hematoxylin–eosin ×80.)

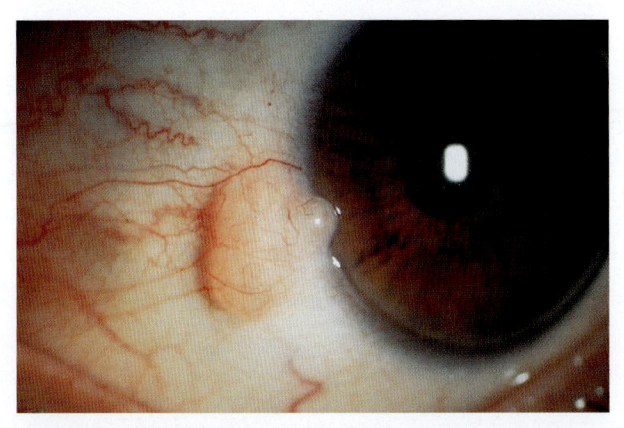

Figure 21.9. Epibulbar schwannoma in a 37-year-old man. (Courtesy of Francois Le Marc'hadour, MD.)

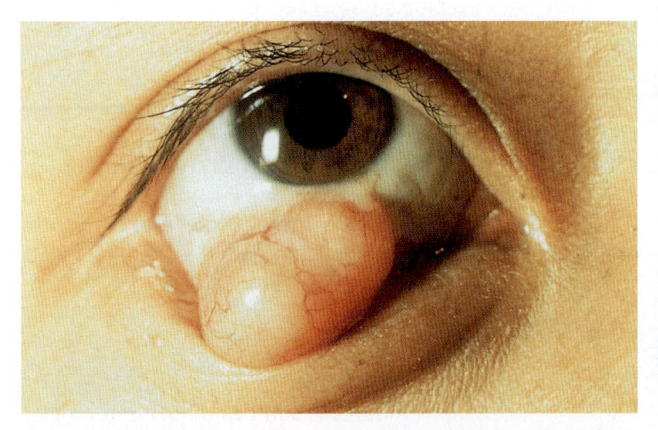

Figure 21.10. Bilobed epibulbar schwannoma arising from inferior forniceal conjunctiva in a 19-year-old woman. (Courtesy of José Avendano, MD.)

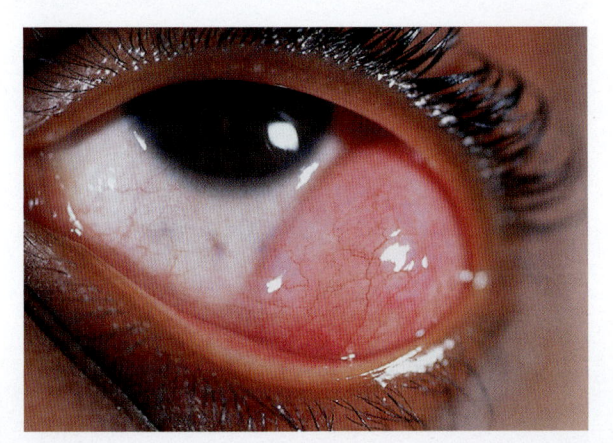

Figure 21.11. Granular cell tumor arising inferotemporally in the left eye of a 5-year-old girl. (Courtesy of Drs Norman Charles and David Fox.)

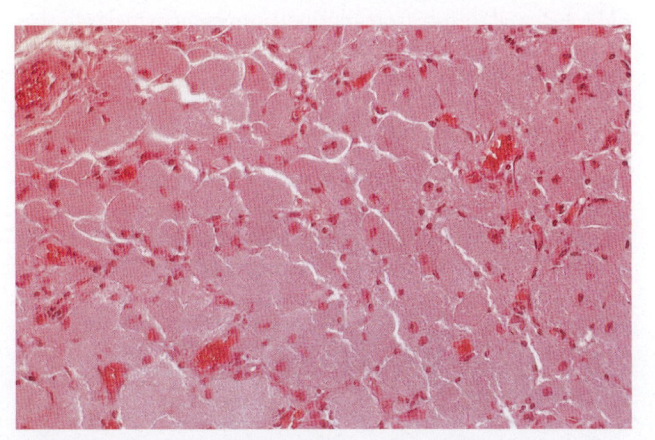

Figure 21.12. Histopathology of lesion shown in Figure 21.11 demonstrating large round cells with pink granular cytoplasm. (Hematoxylin–eosin ×200.) (Courtesy of Drs Norman Charles and David Fox.)

CONJUNCTIVAL FIBROUS HISTIOCYTOMA

General Considerations

Fibrous histiocytoma (FH), a tumor containing a variable combination of fibroblasts and histiocytes, can occur as a primary neoplasm of the conjunctiva (1–20). In the authors' clinical series of 1,643 conjunctival tumors, the four FHs accounted for 57% of fibrous tumors and for less than 1% of the 1,643 lesions (3). We subsequently reported a personal series of six patients (1). The mean patient age at diagnosis was 37 years (median, 38; range, 12 to 72 years). Surgical resection was performed in all cases and histopathology demonstrated benign FH in four and malignant FH in two cases (1).

Several years ago, FH emerged as one of the more important soft tissue tumors of the orbit. The reason for its apparent increased frequency was explained by the fact that the tumor was previously misdiagnosed as hemangiopericytoma, meningioma, schwannoma, neurofibroma, fibrosarcoma, and other spindle cell neoplasms. Confusion still exists as to the classification of this tumor and, more recently, a number of FH have been reclassified as solitary fibrous tumors (18). Hence, the validity of some of the case reports is debatable. Like the same tumor in the orbit, FH of the conjunctiva can be benign, locally aggressive, or malignant. Malignant lesions are locally aggressive but rarely metastasize (12–16).

Clinical Features

Clinically, conjunctival FH can be well-circumscribed or have rather ill-defined margins. It is most often located at the corneoscleral limbus and frequently extends to involve the cornea. It can be present deep in the conjunctiva and be attached to the sclera. The lesion has a yellow color owing to the presence of histiocytes. Conjunctival FH has occurred in young patients with xeroderma pigmentosum (13,17).

Pathology

Microscopically, FH characteristically shows a variable mixture of spindle-shaped fibroblasts and ovoid histiocytes, often arranged in a storiform pattern. The histiocytes stain positive for lipid. Variable amounts of collagen are often present. The FH is believed to arise from pluripotent mesenchymal cells that have the capacity to differentiate toward both fibroblasts and histiocytes.

Management

The best management of conjunctival FH is complete surgical excision (4). This is true for all circumscribed tumors that are accessible to total removal. Lesions that extend deeply into the peripheral cornea may require keratoplasty. The diagnosis is not usually made clinically, but microscopically after surgical excision.

Selected References

Reviews

1. Kim HJ, Shields CL, Eagle RC Jr, et al. Fibrous histiocytoma of the conjunctiva: report of 6 cases. *Am J Ophthalmol* 2006;142:1036–1043.
2. Font RL, Hidayat AA. Fibrous histiocytoma of the orbit. A clinicopathologic study of 150 cases. *Hum Pathol* 1982;13:199–209.
3. Shields CL, Demirci H, Karatza E, et al. Clinical survey of 1643 melanocytic and nonmelanocytic tumors of the conjunctiva. *Ophthalmology* 2004;111:1747–1754.

Management

4. Mietz H, Severin M, Arnold G, et al. Management of fibrous histiocytoma of the corneoscleral limbus: report of a case and review of the literature. *Graefes Arch Clin Exp Ophthalmol* 1997;235:87–91.

Case Reports

5. Jakobiec FA. Fibrous histiocytoma of the corneoscleral limbus. *Am J Ophthalmol* 1974;78:700–706.
6. Faludi JE, Kenyon K, Green WR. Fibrous histiocytoma of the corneoscleral limbus. *Am J Ophthalmol* 1975;80:619–624.
7. Litricin O. Fibrous histiocytoma of the corneosclera. *Arch Ophthalmol* 1983;101:426–428.
8. Lahoud S, Brownstein S, Laflamme MY. Fibrous histiocytoma of the corneoscleral limbus and conjunctiva. *Am J Ophthalmol* 1988;106:579–583.
9. Nores JM, Kantelip B, Souedan M, et al. Fibrous histiocytoma of the conjunctiva. *Ophthalmologica* 1989;199:47–49.
10. Kiratli H, Ruacan S. Fibrous histiocytoma of the conjunctiva. *Can J Ophthalmol* 2003;38:504–506.
11. Margo C, Horton M. Malignant fibrous histiocytoma of the conjunctiva with metastasis. *Am J Ophthalmol* 1989;107:433–434.
12. Pe'er J, Levinger S, Ilsar M, et al. Malignant fibrous histiocytoma of the conjunctiva. *Br J Ophthalmol* 1990;74:624–628.
13. Pe'er J, Levinger S, Chirambo M, et al. Malignant fibrous histiocytoma of the skin and the conjunctiva in xeroderma pigmentosum. *Arch Pathol Lab Med* 1991;115:910–914.
14. Balestrazzi E, Ventura T, Delle Noci N, et al. Malignant conjunctival epibulbar fibrous histiocytoma with orbital invasion. *Eur J Ophthalmol* 1991;1:23–27.
15. Roth AM. Malignant fibrous histiocytoma of the ocular adnexa. *Metab Pediatr Syst Ophthalmol* 1993;16:5–8.
16. Allaire GS, Corriveau C, Teboul N. Malignant fibrous histiocytoma of the conjunctiva. *Arch Ophthalmol* 1999;117:685–687.
17. Brodovsky SC, Dexter DF, Willis WE. Epibulbar fibrous histiocytoma in a child. *Can J Ophthalmol* 1996;31:130–132.
18. Pe'er J, Maly A, Deckel Y, et al. Solitary fibrous tumor of the conjunctiva. *Arch Ophthalmol* 2007;125(3):423–426.
19. Hsu JK, Cavanagh HD, Green WR. An unusual case of elastofibroma oculi. *Cornea* 1997;16(1):112–119.
20. Wood JW, Elliott JH, Lawrence GA. Conjunctival fibrous xanthoma. *Arch Ophthalmol* 1970;84(3):306–311.

Chapter 21 Conjunctival Neural, Xanthomatous, Fibrous, Myxomatous, and Lipomatous Tumors

CONJUNCTIVAL FIBROUS HISTIOCYTOMA

Fibrous histiocytoma of the conjunctiva can assume a variety of clinical appearances.

Kim HJ, Shields CL, Eagle RC Jr, et al. Fibrous histiocytoma of the conjunctiva: report of 6 cases. *Am J Ophthalmol* 2006;142:1036–1043.

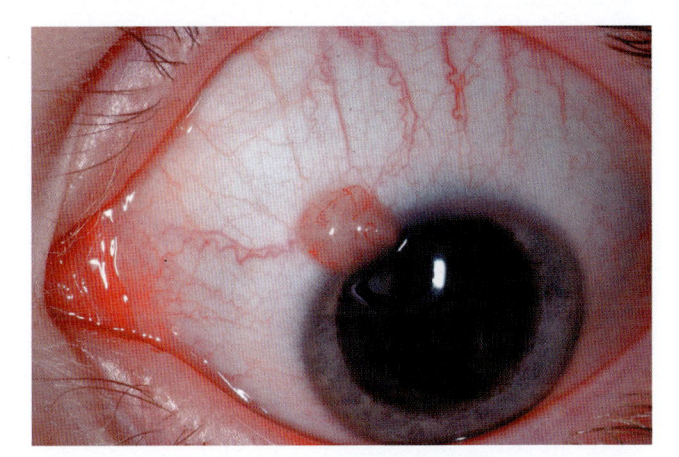

Figure 21.13. Localized fibrous histiocytoma at limbus superonasally in an 8-year-old boy.

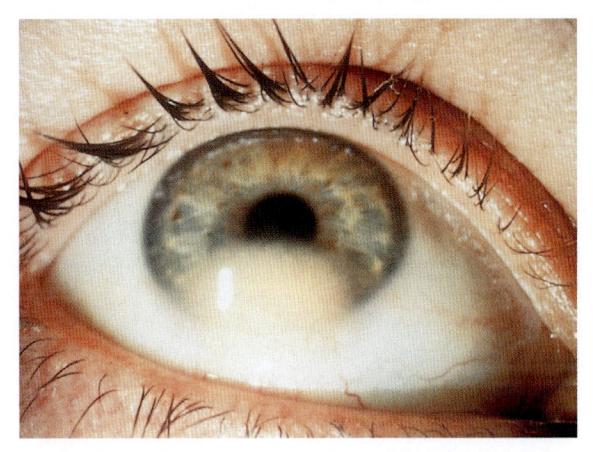

Figure 21.14. Well-circumscribed, yellow-white fibrous histiocytoma located at the limbus inferiorly in a 27-year-old woman.

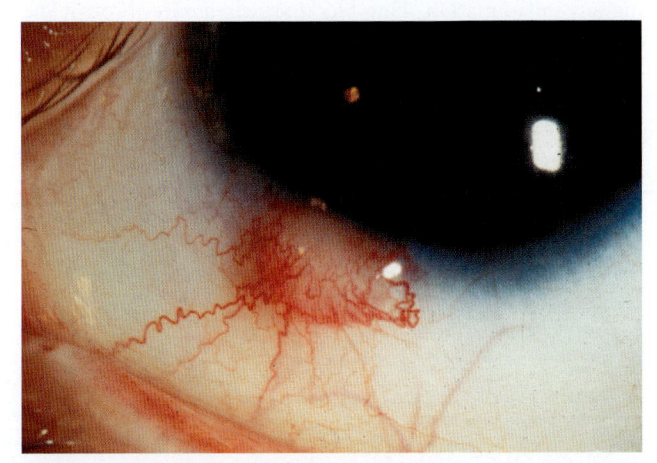

Figure 21.15. Fibrous histiocytoma at limbus inferonasally. Note the dilated tortuous conjunctival feeder blood vessels.

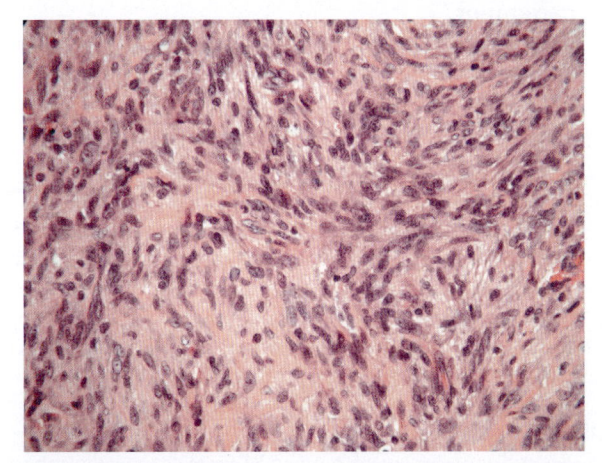

Figure 21.16. Histopathology of conjunctival fibrous histiocytoma. Note the characteristic bland spindle cells. (Hematoxylin–eosin ×150.)

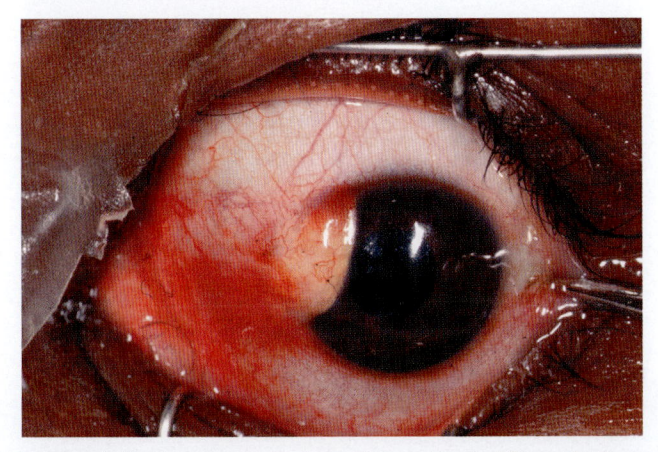

Figure 21.17. More aggressive appearing conjunctival fibrous histiocytoma located and limbus with secondary corneal invasion. The yellow portion of the tumor in the cornea suggested mucoepidermoid carcinoma.

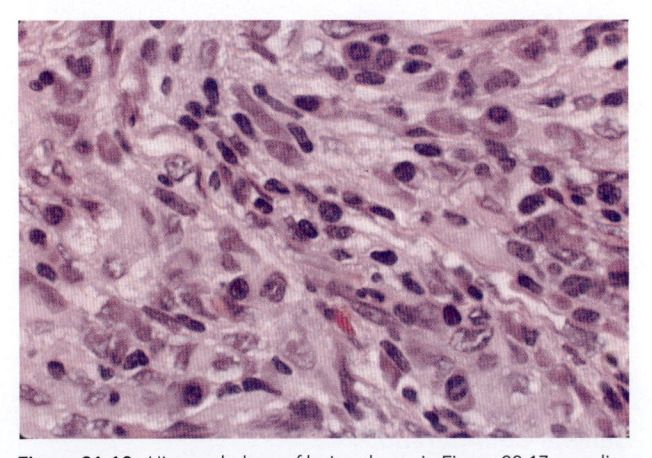

Figure 21.18. Histopathology of lesion shown in Figure 22.17 revealing more atypical spindle cells, suggesting low-grade malignant transformation. (Hematoxylin–eosin ×175.)

CONJUNCTIVAL MISCELLANEOUS LESIONS: FIBROMA, NODULAR FASCIITIS, AND JUVENILE XANTHOGRANULOMA

Conjunctival Fibroma

General Considerations
Miscellaneous conjunctival lesions discussed here include fibroma, nodular fasciitis, and juvenile xanthogranuloma (JXG) (1–14). Fibroma often occurs in subcutaneous tissue but it is very rare in the conjunctiva (1,2,5–8). In the authors' clinical series of 1,643 conjunctival tumors, two fibromas were identified (1).

Clinical Features
Conjunctival fibroma generally develops in adulthood and can be nodular or diffuse. It can be bilateral and appear as a progressive fluffy white lesion (8).

Pathology
Fibroma is composed of closely compact fibroblasts and collagen. It is speculated to arise from Tenon's fascia (5). A rare variant, elastofibroma oculi, contains lobules of fat, tissue not normally found in the conjunctival stroma (7,8).

Management
The best management is surgical resection. Larger, more diffuse lesions may be impossible to remove entirely.

Conjunctival Nodular Fasciitis

General Considerations
Nodular fasciitis (pseudosarcomatous fasciitis) is an idiopathic, benign nodular proliferation of connective tissue that involves the superficial fascia. It is important that this inflammatory condition be differentiated clinically and histopathologically from malignant spindle cell neoplasms. In the ocular region it usually affects the eyelids, but can develop in the orbit or conjunctiva (3,9).

Clinical Features
The age at diagnosis ranges from 3 to 81 years. It generally appears as a solitary episcleral nodule that may show signs of inflammation.

Pathology
Microscopically it is a proliferation of primitive fibroblasts. Most cases of nodular fasciitis in the ocular area are not diagnosed until tissue is obtained for microscopic assessment.

Management
The circumscribed lesion is usually completely excised because the possibility of a malignant neoplasm cannot be excluded on clinical grounds. The role of corticosteroids or radiotherapy in the management is unclear. Although recurrence is known, the prognosis is good.

Conjunctival Juvenile Xanthogranuloma

General Considerations
JXG is an idiopathic cutaneous eruption of childhood characterized by solitary or multiple, yellow-red, transient papules (4,10–14). In the ocular region, it is best known for causing an iris mass that can produce a spontaneous hyphema. It can also affect the eyelid, conjunctiva, and orbital tissues. In the authors' clinical series of 1,643 conjunctival tumors, only one JXG was identified (1).

Clinical Features
Conjunctival involvement usually occurs as a solitary lesion unassociated with the skin eruption. It appears as a yellow, elevated lesion, usually near the corneoscleral limbus in any quadrant. Although cutaneous and iris JXG classically appear in infancy or childhood, JXG on the conjunctiva often appear as a solitary mass and can have its onset in adulthood (11,14). This adult-onset xanthogranuloma seems to be identical clinically and histopathologically to the infantile or juvenile form.

Pathology
Histopathologically, JXG is a mass composed of lipid histiocytes, chronic inflammatory cells, and Touton giant cells, which typically have a ring of lipid around a focus of granulomatous inflammation. Fine blood vessels ramify through the lesion.

Management
Most conjunctival JXG lesions have been excised because the diagnosis was uncertain clinically. However, if the diagnosis is suspected clinically, a period of observation is justified as this lesion, when cutaneous, can resolve without treatment. Topical, injection, or oral corticosteroids can be employed for cases that do not resolve. Recurrence after complete excision is rare.

Selected References
Reviews
1. Shields CL, Demirci H, Karatza E, et al. Clinical survey of 1643 melanocytic and nonmelanocytic tumors of the conjunctiva. *Ophthalmology* 2004;111:1747–1754.
2. Shields CL, Shields JA. Tumors of the conjunctiva and cornea. *Surv Ophthalmol* 2004;49:3–24.
3. Font RL, Zimmerman LE. Nodular fasciitis of the eye and adnexa. A report of ten cases. *Arch Ophthalmol* 1966;75:475–481.
4. Zimmerman LE. Ocular lesions of juvenile xanthogranuloma (nevoxanthoendothelioma). *Trans Am Acad Ophthalmol Otolaryngol* 1965;69:412–442.

Case Reports
5. Herschorn BJ, Jakobiec FA, Hornblass A, et al. Epibulbar subconjunctival fibroma: a tumor possibly arising from Tenon's capsule. *Ophthalmology* 1983;90:1490–1494.
6. Jakobiec FA, Sacks E, Lisman RL, et al. Epibulbar fibroma of the conjunctival substantia propria. *Arch Ophthalmol* 1988;106:661–664.
7. Austin P, Jakobiec FA, Iwamoto T, et al. Elastofibroma oculi. *Arch Ophthalmol* 1983;101:1575–1579.
8. Hsu JK, Cavanagh HD, Green WR. An unusual case of elastofibroma oculi. *Cornea* 1997;16:112–119.
9. Ferry AP, Sherman SE. Nodular fasciitis of the conjunctiva apparently originating in the fascia bulbi (Tenon's capsule). *Am J Ophthalmol* 1974;78:514–517.
10. Yanoff M, Perry HD. Juvenile xanthogranuloma of the corneoscleral limbus. *Arch Ophthalmol* 1995;113:915–917.
11. Kobayashi A, Shirao Y, Takata Y, et al. Adult-onset limbal juvenile xanthogranuloma. *Arch Ophthalmol* 2002;120:96–97.
12. Nordentoft B, Andersen SR. Juvenile xanthogranuloma of the cornea and conjunctiva. *Acta Ophthalmol (Copenh)* 1967;45:720–726.
13. Olmo N, Barrio-Barrio J, Moreno-Montanes J, et al. Conjunctival juvenile xanthogranuloma in a preschool child. *Ocul Immunol Inflamm* 2013;21:403–404.
14. Kim MS, Kim SA, Sa HS. Old-age-onset subconjunctival juvenile xanthogranuloma without limbal involvement. *BMC Ophthalmol* 2014;14:24. doi: 10.1186/1471-2415-14-24. PMID: 24602225

Chapter 21 Conjunctival Neural, Xanthomatous, Fibrous, Myxomatous, and Lipomatous Tumors

● CONJUNCTIVAL NODULAR FASCIITIS AND JUVENILE XANTHOGRANULOMA

All of the cases below were confirmed histopathologically after biopsy or surgical excision.

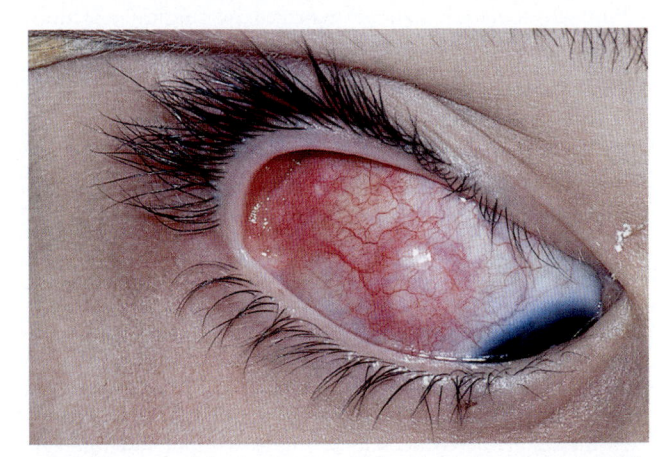

Figure 21.19. Nodular fasciitis in epibulbar tissues superotemporally in an 11-year-old boy.

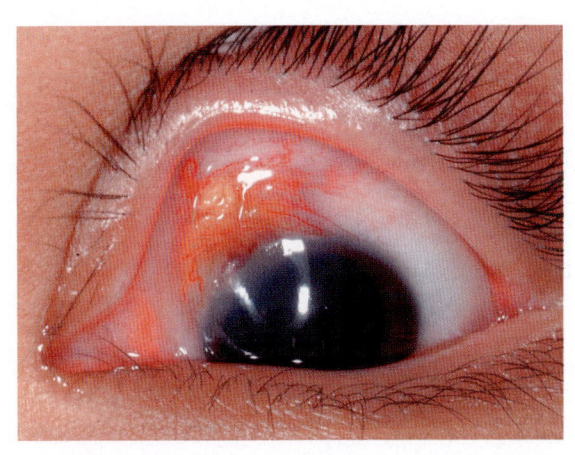

Figure 21.20. Conjunctival nodular fasciitis in superonasal quadrant of a 23-year-old woman.

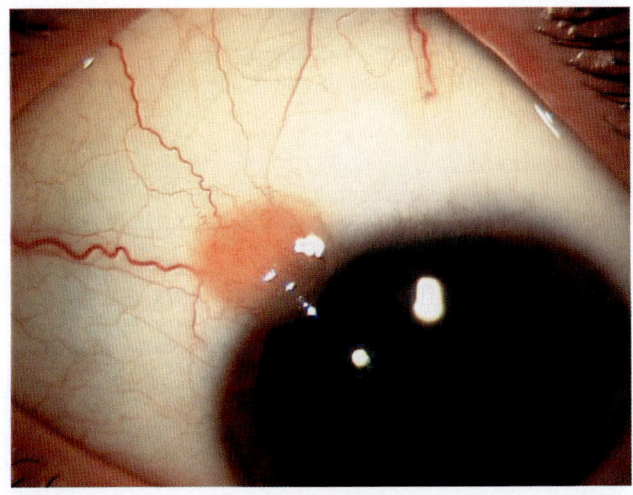

Figure 21.21. Small limbal juvenile xanthogranuloma of the conjunctiva in a child.

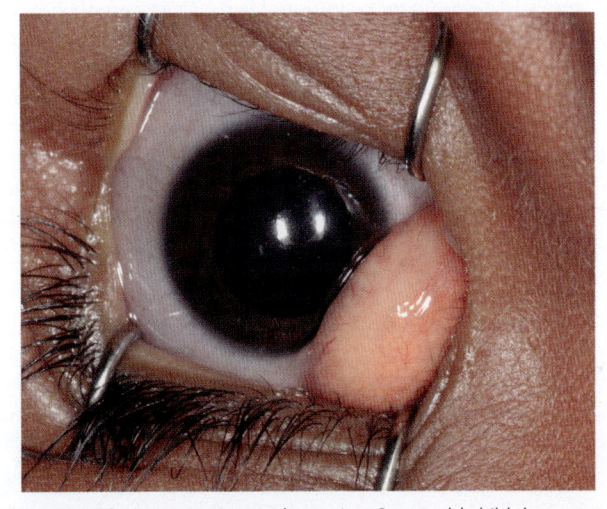

Figure 21.22. Large conjunctival mass in a 2-year-old child that proved to be juvenile xanthogranuloma.

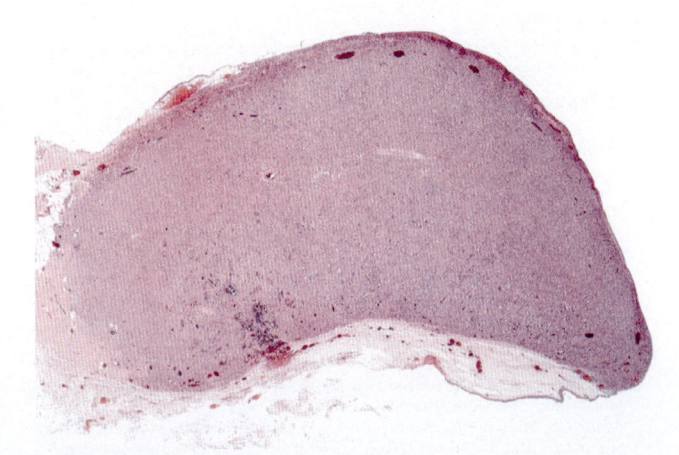

Figure 21.23. Low-power histopathology of conjunctival juvenile xanthogranuloma of patient in Figure 21.22 showing cellular mass. (Hematoxylin–eosin ×10.)

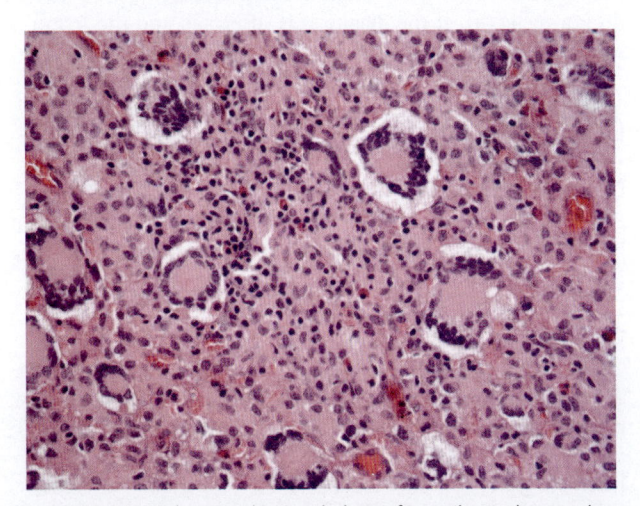

Figure 21.24. High-power histopathology of juvenile xanthogranuloma in Figure 21.22 documenting numerous Touton giant cells, eosinophils, chronic lymphocytes, and macrophages. (Hematoxylin–eosin ×100.)

CONJUNCTIVAL MISCELLANEOUS LESIONS: MYXOMA, LIPOMA, AND RETICULOHISTIOCYTOMA

Conjunctival Myxoma

General Considerations
Myxoma is a benign neoplasm presumably derived from primitive mesenchyme. It usually occurs in the heart, but can arise in the orbit, eyelid, and conjunctiva (1–9). Conjunctiva myxoma is a condition of adulthood with no predisposition for gender. In the authors' clinical series of 1,643 conjunctival tumors, one myxoma was identified (1).

Clinical Features
Conjunctival myxoma appears as a soft, freely movable, pink-white lesion usually found in the temporal bulbar conjunctiva. Unlike nevus and lymphangioma, which may appear similar, myxoma characteristically does not have cysts. However, the clear lesion can sometimes resemble a conjunctival cyst (4).

Carney Complex
Conjunctival and eyelid myxoma can occur in association with an autosomal-dominant condition called Carney complex, characterized by myxomas, spotty pigmentation of skin and mucous membranes, endocrine overactivity, and schwannomas (10,11). Typical sites for the myxomas are heart, skin, and breast. Most conjunctival myxomas have been solitary, without systemic evidence of Carney complex. However, any myxoma of the eyelid or conjunctiva should prompt evaluation for cardiac myxoma, a life-threatening condition. Eyelid and conjunctival myxomas can become apparent long before cardiac myxoma is recognized.

Pathology
Myxoma is a hypocellular lesion consisting of sparse stellate and spindle-shaped cells interspersed in a myxoid stroma. Cytoplasmic vacuoles are often present. Scattered mast cells may be present. Special stains and electron microscopy may help to differentiate myxoma from similar lesions like myxoid liposarcoma, spindle cell lipoma, myxoid neurofibroma, and rhabdomyosarcoma (5).

Management
Management is generally surgical resection; most excised lesions do not recur (4). If the diagnosis is suspected and the lesion is small and asymptomatic, observation only may be appropriate.

Conjunctival Lipoma

General Considerations
Although lipoma is occasionally seen in the orbit, conjunctival lipoma is rare and has usually been of the pleomorphic type (12,13). The etiology is unknown.

Clinical Features
Clinically, pleomorphic lipoma occurs in adults and has a similar appearance to the myxoma described. It may have a yellow color owing to the presence of lipid.

Pathology
Lipoma shows loose myxoid connective with pleomorphic lipocytes, often with a spindle cell configuration.

Management
Conjunctival lipoma can be managed by surgical resection. Recurrence after complete surgical resection is unlikely.

Conjunctival Reticulohistiocytoma

General Considerations
Reticulohistiocytoma is a rare benign histiocytic lesion that is often a part of a systemic disorder known as multicentric reticulohistiocytosis.

Clinical Features
Although multiple lesions can occur on the eyelid in association with multicentric reticulohistiocytosis (14), cases reported in the conjunctiva have been in adults and appeared as localized masses at the corneoscleral limbus without systemic evidence of multicentric reticulohistiocytosis (15).

Pathology
Reticulohistiocytoma is composed of large mononuclear or multinucleated cells with fine granular cytoplasm. It differs from JXG in that it occurs in adults and lacks Touton giant cells histopathologically (14).

Management
Management is complete surgical resection. The role of corticosteroids is unknown.

Selected References

Reviews

1. Shields CL, Demirci H, Karatza E, et al. Clinical survey of 1643 melanocytic and nonmelanocytic tumors of the conjunctiva. *Ophthalmology* 2004;111:1747–1754.
2. Shields CL, Shields JA. Tumors of the conjunctiva and cornea. *Surv Ophthalmol* 2004;49:3–24.
3. Patrinely JR, Green WR. Conjunctival myxoma. A clinicopathologic study of four cases and a review of the literature. *Arch Ophthalmol* 1983;101:1426–1430.
4. Pe'er J, Hidayat AA. Myxomas of the conjunctiva. *Am J Ophthalmol* 1986;102:80–86.
5. Demirci H, Shields CL, Eagle RC Jr, et al. Report of conjunctival myxoma case and review of the literature. *Arch Ophthalmol* 2006;124:735–738.
6. Horie Y, Ikawa S, Okamoto I, et al. Myxoma of the conjunctiva: a case report and a review of the literature. *Jpn J Ophthalmol* 1995;39:77–82.

Histopathology

7. Mottow-Lippa L, Tso MO, Sugar J. Conjunctival myxoma. A clinicopathologic study. *Ophthalmology* 1983;90:1452–1458.

Case Reports

8. Pe'er J, Ilsar M, Hidayat A. Conjunctival myxoma: a case report. *Br J Ophthalmol* 1984;68:618–622.
9. Soong T, Soong V, Salvi SM, et al. Primary corneal myxoma. *Cornea* 2008;27:1186–1188.
10. Kennedy RH, Flanagan JC, Eagle RC Jr, et al. The Carney complex with ocular signs suggestive of cardiac myxoma. *Am J Ophthalmol* 1991;111:699–702.
11. Carney JA. Carney complex: the complex of myxomas, spotty pigmentation, endocrine overactivity, and schwannomas. *Semin Dermatol* 1995;14:90–98.
12. Bryant J. Pleomorphic lipoma of the bulbar conjunctiva. *Ann Ophthalmol* 1987;19:148–149.
13. Streeten BW. Pleomorphic lipoma of the conjunctiva. Presented at the Eastern Ophthalmic Pathology Society, 1991.
14. Eagle RC Jr, Penne RA, Hneleski IS Jr. Eyelid involvement in multicentric reticulohistiocytosis. *Ophthalmology* 1995;102:426–430.
15. Allaire GS, Hidayat AA, Zimmerman LE, et al. Reticulohistiocytoma of the limbus and cornea. A clinicopathologic study of two cases. *Ophthalmology* 1990;97:1018–1022.

Chapter 21 Conjunctival Neural, Xanthomatous, Fibrous, Myxomatous, and Lipomatous Tumors

CONJUNCTIVAL MYXOMA, LIPOMA, AND RETICULOHISTIOCYTOMA

1. Demirci H, Shields CL, Eagle RC Jr, et al. Report of conjunctival myxoma case and review of the literature. *Arch Ophthalmol* 2006;124:735–738.
2. Eagle RC Jr, Penne RA, Hneleski IS Jr. Eyelid involvement in multicentric reticulohistiocytosis. *Ophthalmology* 1995;102:426–430.

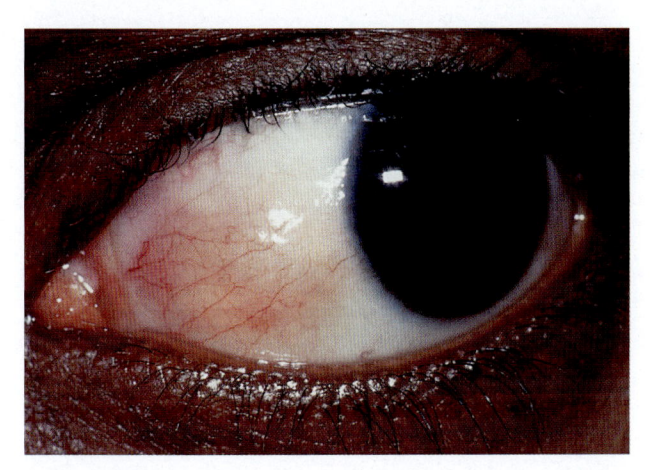

Figure 21.25. Conjunctival myxoma of nasal conjunctiva in a 31-year-old man.

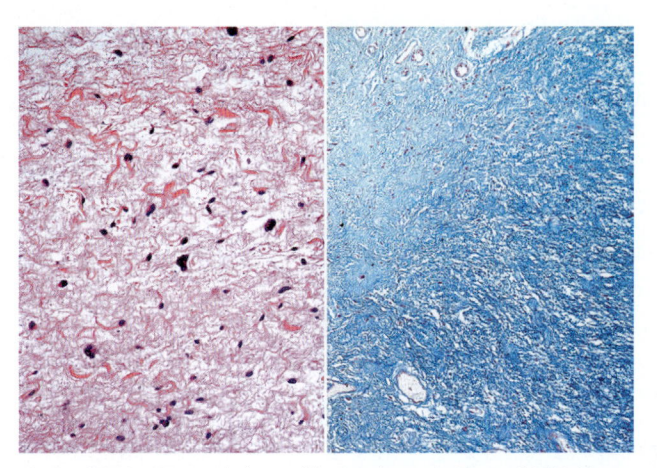

Figure 21.26. Histopathology of lesion shown in Figure 21.25. Hematoxylin and eosin stain on the left shows spindle-shaped cells in loose myxoid stroma. Alcian blue stain on the right shows positive reaction to mucin. (×150.)

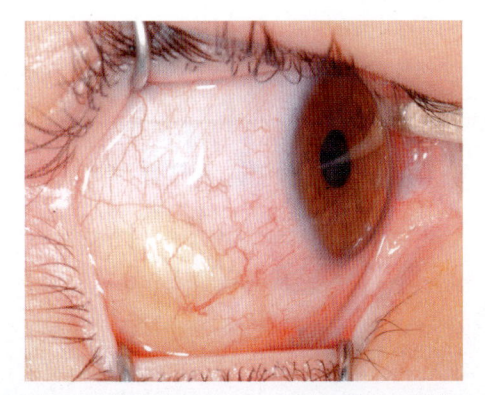

Figure 21.27. Conjunctival lipoma in a child with familial hypercholesterolemia.

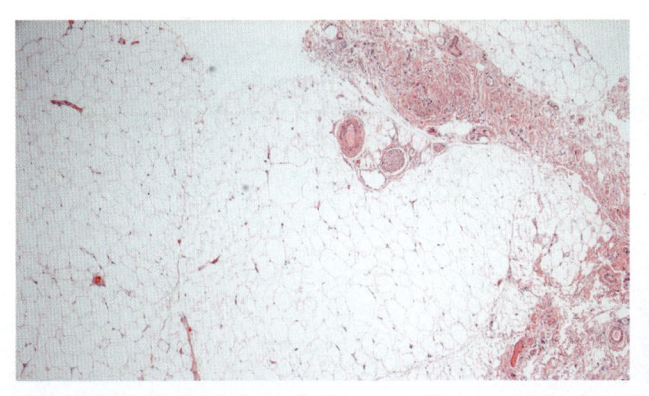

Figure 21.28. Histopathology of a conjunctival lipoma showing round benign lipocytes. (Hematoxylin–eosin ×100.)

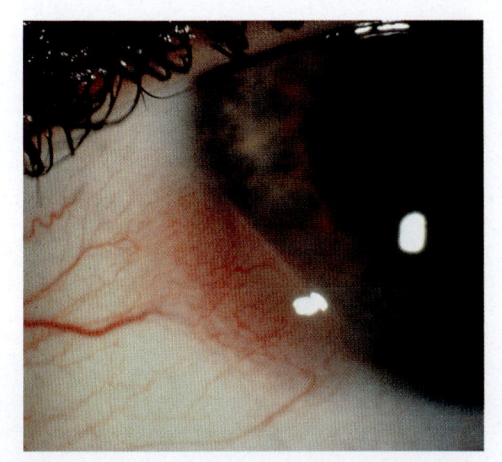

Figure 21.29. Localized reticulohistiocytosis at the limbus in a 21-year-old woman.

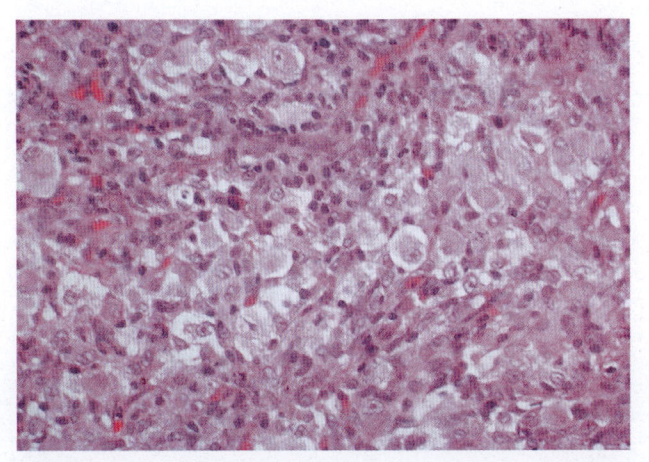

Figure 21.30. Histopathology of lesion shown in Figure 21.19 showing large histiocytes with a granular cytoplasm. (Hematoxylin–eosin ×150.)

CONJUNCTIVAL LYMPHOID, LEUKEMIC, AND METASTATIC TUMORS

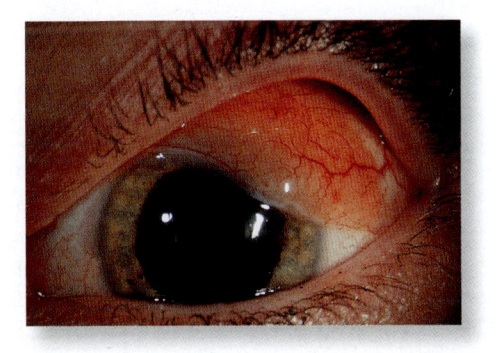

General Considerations

A lymphoid tumor can occur in the conjunctiva as an isolated condition or it can be a manifestation of systemic lymphoma (1–30). In the authors' clinical series of 1,643 conjunctival tumors, there were 128 lymphoid lesions, accounting for 8% of conjunctival tumors (1). The details of classification, clinical features, histopathologic characteristics, and prognosis are discussed elsewhere (3–6,11,12) and are beyond the scope of this chapter. It is traditional to divide lymphoid infiltrates into benign reactive lymphoid hyperplasia (BRLH) and malignant lymphoma. It is not usually possible to differentiate the BRLH and lymphoma clinically; the histopathologic differential is also sometimes difficult. Hence, they are discussed collectively here. There is a tumor, node, metastasis (TNM) classification of ocular adnexal lymphoma based on the American Joint Commission on Cancer classification (Table 22-1).

In recent years, there has been increasing emphasis on the fact that many conjunctival "lymphomas" are low-grade B-cell lymphomas of the mucosa-associated lymphoid tumor (MALT) type (12). There is also some controversy as to the role of inflammation (conjunctivitis) in the pathogenesis of MALT lymphoma, also known as extranodal marginal zone lymphoma (ENMZL). MALT lymphoma is best known to occur in the stomach. The gastric lesion appears to have an association with *Helicobacter pylori* infection. There is currently an increasing interest in the relationship between conjunctival MALT lymphoma and *H. pylori*. If such a relationship is established, antibiotics may prove to be an effective initial management.

Plasmacytoma and closely related lymphoplasmacytoid tumors can rarely arise in the conjunctiva (8,9,25–30). In a sense, plasmacytoma is a neoplasm that is related to a lymphoma in that the plasma cell is a highly differentiated form type of B lymphocyte. Tumors composed of malignant plasma cells are often associated with multiple myeloma, in which cases the disease is manifested mainly in bone. However, soft tissue plasmacytoma can also occur as part of multiple myeloma or as a solitary lesion. Extraskeletal plasmacytoma can occasionally be the first sign of myeloma. Because lymphoma and plasmacytoma are so similar clinically, they are discussed together in this chapter.

Clinical Features

Clinically, a lymphoid tumor is usually a diffuse, slightly elevated fleshy pink mass that has been likened to smoked salmon. It is generally located in the forniceal or bulbar conjunctiva, but occasionally occurs at the limbus. It does not seem to have a predilection for the interpalpebral conjunctiva like squamous

CONJUNCTIVAL LYMPHOID AND PLASMACYTIC TUMORS

Table 22.1 American Joint Committee on Cancer (AJCC) classification of ocular adnexal lymphoma

Clinical stage	Definition
Primary tumor (T)	
Tx	Tumor extent cannot be assessed
T0	Tumor absent
T1	Tumor in conjunctiva
T1a	Tumor in bulbar conjunctiva
T1b	Tumor in palpebral, forniceal, caruncular conjunctiva
T1c	Tumor extensive in conjunctiva
T2	Tumor in orbit
T2a	Tumor in orbit anteriorly
T2b	Tumor in orbit and lacrimal gland
T2c	Tumor in orbit posteriorly
T2d	Tumor in orbit and nasolacrimal system
T3	Tumor in preseptal eyelid
T4	Tumor in orbit plus additional bone or brain
T4a	Tumor in additional nasopharynx
T4b	Tumor in additional bone
T4c	Tumor in additional sinuses
T4d	Tumor in additional brain
Regional lymph node (N)	
Nx	Regional lymph nodes cannot be assessed
N0	Regional lymph node involvement absent
N1	Regional lymph node ipsilateral involvement present
N2	Regional lymph node contralateral/bilateral involvement present
N3	Regional lymph node remote from ocular region present
N4	Central lymph node involvement present
Distant metastasis (M)	
M0	Distant metastasis cannot be assessed
M1a	Distant involvement in noncontiguous tissue (parotid, lung, liver, spleen, kidney, breast)
M1b	Distant involvement in bone marrow
M1c	Both M1a and M1b present

From Edge SB, Byrd DR, Compton CC, et al., eds. Carcinoma of the conjunctiva. In: *AJCC Cancer Staging Manual*. 7th ed. New York, NY: Springer; 2010:583–589.

the patient with a conjunctival lymphoid infiltrate as to the chances of developing systemic lymphoma. A review of 117 patients who presented with such a conjunctival lesion revealed that 31% eventually developed systemic lymphoma overall (3). If the lymphoid infiltrate was unilateral, the chance of systemic lymphoma was 17% and if the lymphoid infiltrate was bilateral, the chances for systemic lymphoma were 47% (3). The authors use these figures in counseling the patient with a conjunctival lymphoid infiltrate. With longer follow-up, it is most likely that a higher percent of affected patients would develop systemic lymphoma.

The clinical features of conjunctival plasmacytoma are probably identical to those previously described for lymphoma. The lesion can present as a localized or diffuse salmon-colored infiltration (8,25–30).

Pathology

Histopathologically, a lymphoid tumor is composed of solid sheets of lymphocytes and the lesion is classified as BRLH, atypical lymphoid hyperplasia, or malignant lymphoma, depending on the degree of cellular anaplasia. The benign and atypical lymphoid hyperplasia are less likely to be associated with systemic lymphoma and the malignant lymphoid tumor is more likely to be associated with systemic lymphoma. Although there is much overlap, BRLH is generally polymorphic, with well-differentiated lymphocytes and plasma cells. In general, lymphoma tends to be more monomorphic. Immunohistochemistry may be helpful in determining whether the lesions are monoclonal or polyclonal. However, it seems that immunohistochemistry has limitations in determining prognosis; many monoclonal lesions may follow a benign clinical course. Most conjunctival lymphomas are non-Hodgkin's B-cell lymphomas; Hodgkin's lymphoma and T-cell lymphoma affect the conjunctiva less frequently (20).

Plasmacytoma is composed of rather uniform large round to ovoid cells with abundant cytoplasm, displaced nucleus, clumping of nuclear chromatin, prominent nucleoli, and variable mitotic activity.

cell carcinoma. It usually has a mild vascular supply, but large dilated conjunctival nutrient vessels can be apparent in larger tumors. Although conjunctival lymphoma usually has a smooth surface, it can have a multinodular appearance and resemble follicular conjunctivitis.

It is not usually possible to differentiate clinically between a benign and malignant lymphoid tumor. Therefore, biopsy is necessary to help establish the diagnosis and a systemic evaluation should be done in all affected patients to exclude the presence of systemic lymphoma. It is also important to counsel

CONJUNCTIVAL LYMPHOID AND PLASMACYTIC TUMORS

Management

If the conjunctival lesion is small and circumscribed, an excisional biopsy and supplemental cryotherapy can be performed and no further treatment may be necessary. If a conjunctival lymphoid lesion is large and cannot be excised completely, we recommend a generous biopsy, histopathologic staging, and then treatment with chemotherapy or radiotherapy. However, we biopsy enough tissue for diagnosis, but not so much as to require grafting. This seems logical since conjunctival lymphoma is sensitive to radiotherapy, chemotherapy, and biologic therapy and wide excision seems unnecessary. Others have suggested that larger lesions should be excised, even if amniotic membrane transplant is necessary to close the defect (14).

Follow tumor biopsy and confirmation histopathologically, further treatment should be given. If the patient has systemic lymphoma, then treatment should include systemic chemotherapy or rituximab. Rituximab has been quite successful in selected cases (17). If the lesion is solitary, with no systemic lymphoma, external beam irradiation is generally the treatment of choice, but rituximab or chemotherapy are considered. All types of lymphoma are particularly sensitive to radiotherapy. The dose of external beam irradiation ranges from 2,000 cGy for benign lesions to 4,000 cGy for more malignant lesions.

We have seen several patients with low-grade MALT lymphoma of the conjunctiva who had little or no residual tumor after biopsy and who were reluctant to undergo irradiation because they were asymptomatic. We have simply observed the lesion in a number of such patients and have been impressed that the majority of them show no progression and the patient remains asymptomatic. A recent report described some patients who actually had regression of the lesion after biopsy only (15). Although it remains controversial, we currently believe that periodic observation may be the preferred treatment in some cases. In patients with extensive residual tumor or with progression after biopsy, however, radiotherapy is generally advisable.

There is increasing interest in the role of antibiotics in the management of conjunctival lymphoma. In rare cases, the tumor responds completely to a course of antibiotics (18). In most cases, the antibiotics are given to help protect the patient from systemic lymphoma.

Management of conjunctival plasmacytoma is similar to that for lymphoma. The patient should be evaluated initially and periodically for multiple myeloma and monoclonal gammopathy. The conjunctival lesion can be completely excised if small and localized. Larger, more aggressive lesions respond to irradiation or chemotherapy that is given for the systemic disease (25–30).

Selected References

Reviews

1. Shields CL, Demirci H, Karatza E, et al. Clinical survey of 1643 melanocytic and nonmelanocytic tumors of the conjunctiva. *Ophthalmology* 2004;111:1747–1754.
2. Shields CL, Shields JA. Tumors of the conjunctiva and cornea. *Surv Ophthalmol* 2004;49:3–24.
3. Shields CL, Shields JA, Carvalho C, et al. Conjunctival lymphoid tumors: clinical analysis of 117 cases and relationship to systemic lymphoma. *Ophthalmology* 2001;108:979–984.
4. Coupland SE, Krause L, Delecluse HJ, et al. Lymphoproliferative lesions of the ocular adnexa. Analysis of 112 cases. *Ophthalmology* 1998;105:1430–1441.
5. Malek SN, Hatfield AJ, Flinn IW. MALT Lymphomas. *Curr Treat Options Oncol* 2003;4:269–279.
6. Lauer SA. Ocular adnexal lymphoid tumors. *Curr Opin Ophthalmol* 2000;11: 361–366.
7. Bardenstein DS. Ocular adnexal lymphoma: classification, clinical disease, and molecular biology. *Ophthalmol Clin North Am* 2005;18:187–197.
8. Adkins JW, Shields JA, Shields CL, et al. Plasmacytoma of the eye and orbit. *Int Ophthalmol* 1996–1997;20:339–343.
9. Knapp AJ, Gartner S, Henkind P. Multiple myeloma and its ocular manifestations. *Surv Ophthalmol* 1987;31:343–351.
10. Stacy RC, Jakobiec FA, Schoenfield L, et al. Unifocal and multifocal reactive lymphoid hyperplasia vs follicular lymphoma of the ocular adnexa. *Am J Ophthalmol* 2010;150(3):412–426.
11. Coupland SE, White VA, Rootman J, et al. A TNM-based clinical staging system of ocular adnexal lymphomas. *Arch Pathol Lab Med* 2009;133(8):1262–1267.
12. Coupland S, Heegaard S. Can conjunctival lymphoma be a clinical diagnosis? *Br J Ophthalmol* 2014;98:574–575.
13. Beykin G, Pe'er J, Amir G, et al. Paediatric and adolescent elevated conjunctival lesions in the plical area: lymphoma or reactive lymphoid hyperplasia? *Br J Ophthalmol* 2014;98:645–650.

Management

14. Kobayashi A, Takahira M, Yamada A, et al. Fornix and conjunctiva reconstruction by amniotic membrane in a patient with conjunctival mucosa-associated lymphoid tissue lymphoma. *Jpn J Ophthalmol* 2002;46:346–348.
15. Matsuo T, Yoshino T. Long-term follow-up results of observation of radiation for conjunctival malignant lymphoma. *Ophthalmology* 2004;111:1233–1237.
16. Bianciotto C, Shields CL, Lally SE, et al. CyberKnife radiosurgery for the treatment of intraocular and periocular lymphoma. *Arch Ophthalmol* 2010;128(12): 1561–1567.
17. Zinzani PL, Alinari L, Stefoni V, et al. Rituximab in primary conjunctiva lymphoma. *Leuk Res* 2005;29:107–108.
18. Abramson DH, Rollins I, Coleman M. Periocular mucosa-associated lymphoid/low grade lymphomas: treatment with antibiotics. *Am J Ophthalmol* 2005;140:729–730.

Case Reports

19. Yeung L, Tsao YP, Chen PY, et al. Combination of adult inclusion conjunctivitis and mucosa-associated lymphoid tissue (MALT) lymphoma in a young adult. *Cornea* 2004;23:71–75.
20. Shields CL, Shields JA, Eagle RC. Rapidly progressive T-cell lymphoma of the conjunctiva. *Arch Ophthalmol* 2002;120:508–509.
21. Lee DH, Sohn HW, Park SH, et al. Bilateral conjunctival mucosa-associated lymphoid tissue lymphoma misdiagnosed as allergic conjunctivitis. *Cornea* 2001;20: 427–429.
22. Scullica L, Manganelli C, Turco S, et al. Bilateral non-Hodgkin lymphoma of the conjunctiva. *Eye* 1999;13:379–380.
23. Obata H, Mori K, Tsuru T. Subconjunctival mucosa-associated lymphoid tissue (MALT) lymphoma arising in Tenon's capsule. *Graefes Arch Clin Exp Ophthalmol* 2006;244:118–121.
24. Chang YC, Chang CH, Liu YT, et al. Spontaneous regression of a large-cell lymphoma in the conjunctiva and orbit. *Ophthal Plast Reconstr Surg* 2004;20:461–463.
25. Tetsumoto K, Iwaki H, Inoue M. IgG-kappa extramedullary plasmacytoma of the conjunctiva and orbit. *Br J Ophthalmol* 1993;77:255–257.
26. Lugassy G, Rozenbaum D, Lifshitz L, et al. Primary lymphoplasmacytoma of the conjunctiva. *Eye* 1992;6:326–327.
27. Kremer I, Flex D, Manor R. Solitary conjunctival extramedullary plasmacytoma. *Ann Ophthalmol* 1990;22:126–130.
28. Seddon JM, Corwin JM, Weiter JJ, et al. Solitary extramedullary plasmacytoma of the palpebral conjunctiva. *Br J Ophthalmol* 1982;66:450–454.
29. Benjamin I, Taylor H, Spindler J. Orbital and conjunctival involvement in multiple myeloma. Report of a case. *Am J Clin Pathol* 1975;63:811–817.
30. Jampol LM, Marsh JC, Albert DM, et al. IgA associated lymphoplasmacytic tumor involving the conjunctiva, eyelid, and orbit. *Am J Ophthalmol* 1975;79:279–284.

CONJUNCTIVAL BENIGN REACTIVE LYMPHOID HYPERPLASIA

Both benign and malignant lymphoid tumors have an identical clinical appearance in the conjunctiva. Biopsy and staging are necessary to determine the malignancy of these lesions. The lesions illustrated here were found histopathologically to be low-grade lymphoid lesions, and were categorized as BRLH. They all have the typical salmon pink color.

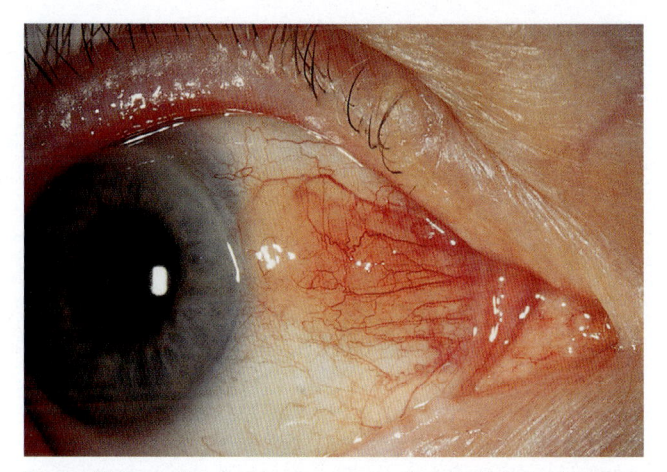

Figure 22.1. Conjunctival benign reactive lymphoid hyperplasia presenting as a sessile lesion in the vicinity of the medial rectus muscle in an 83-year-old woman.

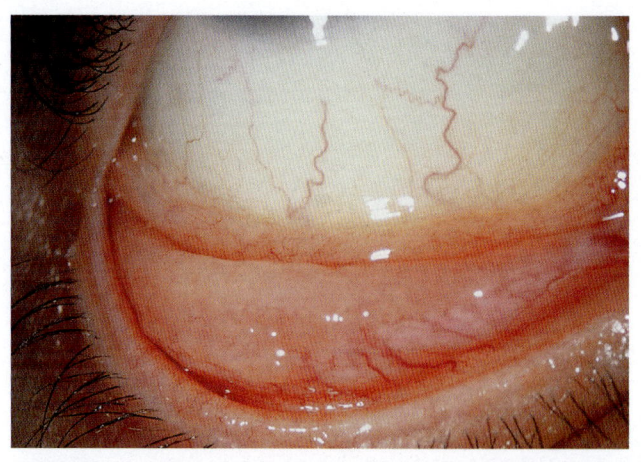

Figure 22.2. Conjunctival benign reactive lymphoid hyperplasia presenting as a horizontal fusiform lesion in inferior fornix in a 50-year-old man.

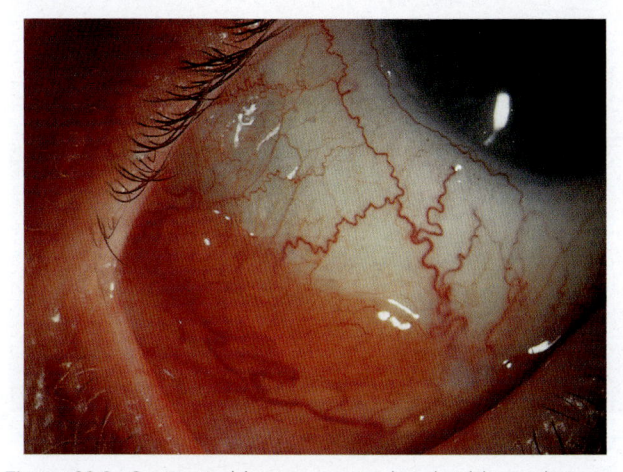

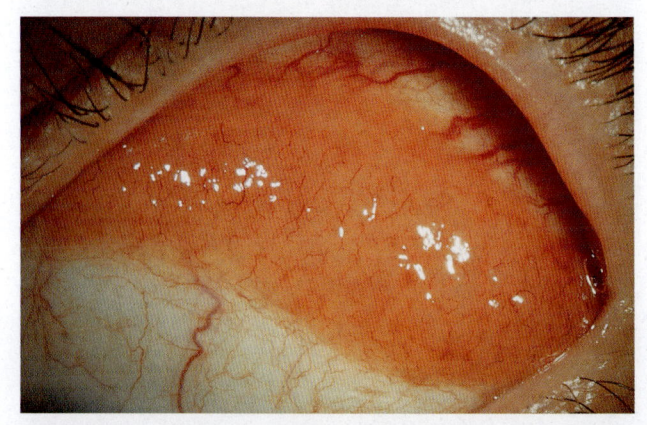

Figure 22.3. Conjunctival benign reactive lymphoid hyperplasia presenting as a placoid, slightly elevated mass in forniceal and bulbar conjunctiva in a 70-year-old woman.

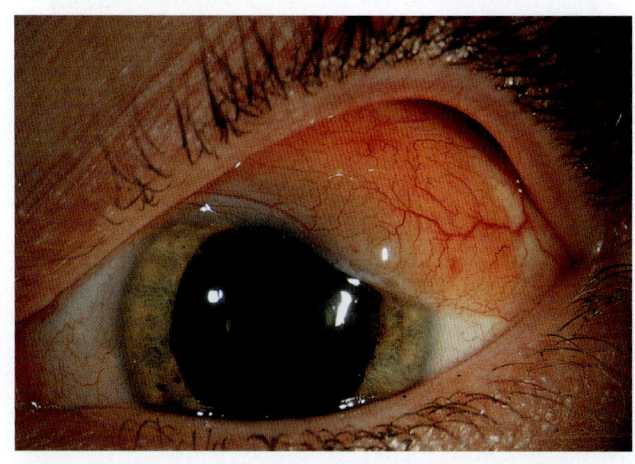

Figure 22.4. Conjunctival benign reactive lymphoid hyperplasia presenting as a diffuse lesion superotemporally in a 55-year-old woman.

Figure 22.5. Conjunctival benign reactive lymphoid hyperplasia presenting as a diffuse elevated mass in the superior bulbar conjunctiva in a 38-year-old man.

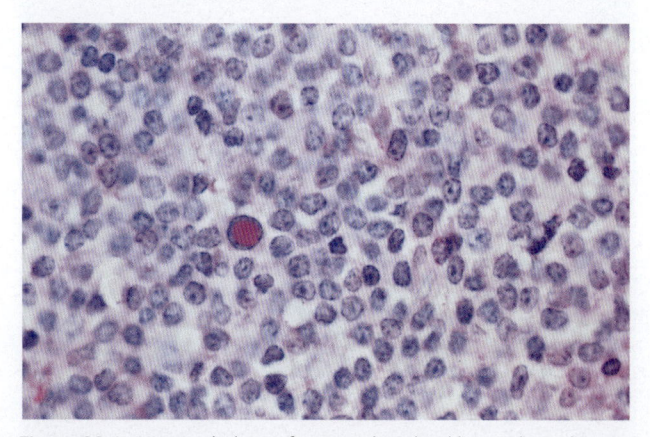

Figure 22.6. Histopathology of reactive lymphoid hyperplasia showing well-differentiated uniform lymphocytes. Near the center of the field, note the cell with the large intranuclear inclusion body, referred to as a Dutcher body. (Hematoxylin–eosin ×200.)

CONJUNCTIVAL NON-HODGKIN'S LYMPHOMA

Most lymphomas of the conjunctiva are of the B-cell non-Hodgkin's type with a characteristic salmon pink color. Most patients do not have systemic lymphoma initially, but some will be found on subsequent evaluation or follow-up to have systemic lymphoma. The lesions shown here were found histopathologically to be malignant lymphoma.

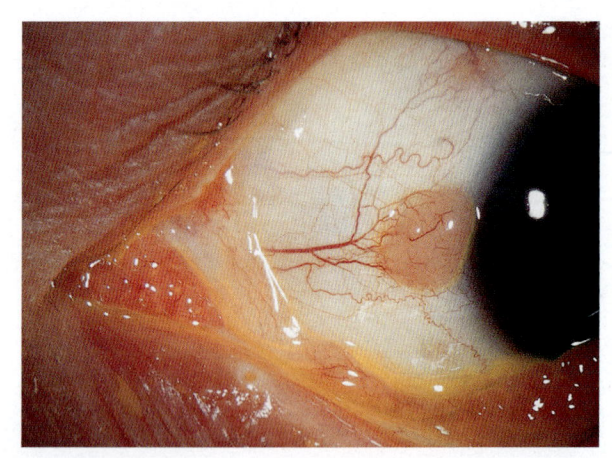

Figure 22.7. Conjunctival lymphoma presenting as a circumscribed mass near the limbus in a 43-year-old woman.

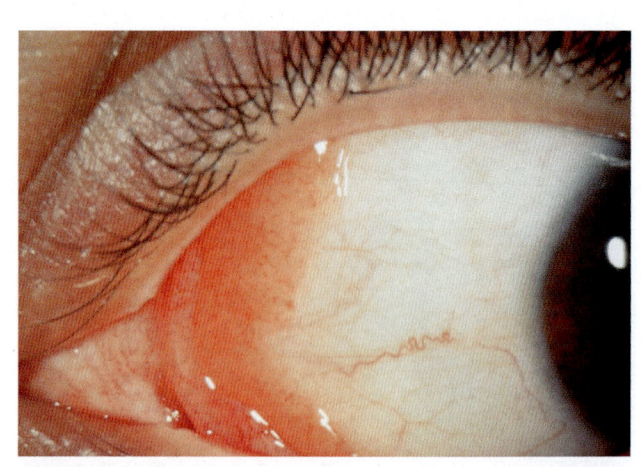

Figure 22.8. Diffuse lymphoma affecting medial aspect of conjunctiva in a 39-year-old woman.

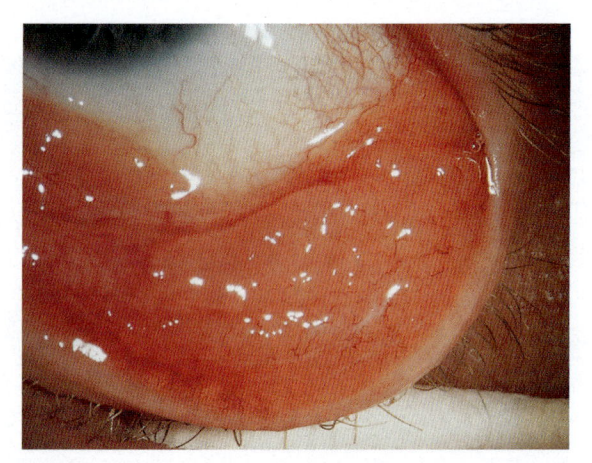

Figure 22.9. Irregular, multinodular lymphoma in inferior conjunctiva in a 40-year-old man.

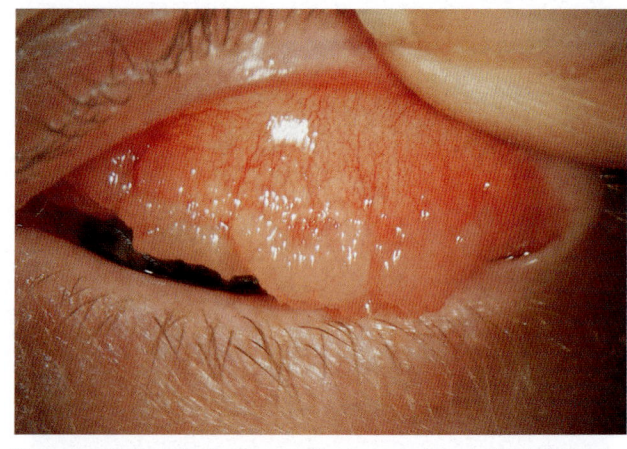

Figure 22.10. Irregular lymphoma affecting superior palpebral conjunctiva.

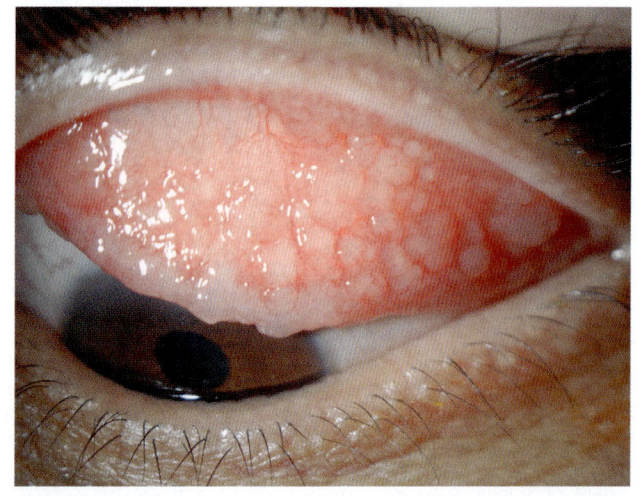

Figure 22.11. Diffuse lymphoma affecting tarsal conjunctiva in an older man.

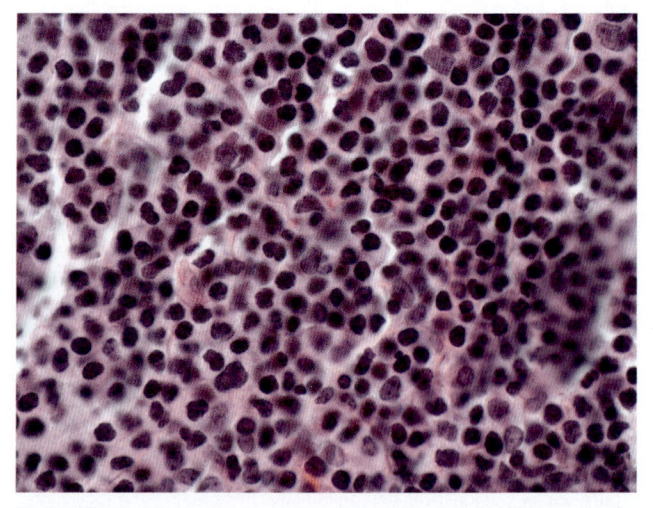

Figure 22.12. Histopathology of malignant lymphoma showing monotonous lymphoid cells and some with prominent nucleoli. (Hematoxylin–eosin ×200.)

Chapter 22 Conjunctival Lymphoid, Leukemic, and Metastatic Tumors

CONJUNCTIVAL LYMPHOMA: ATYPICAL FORMS AND RESPONSE TO RADIOTHERAPY

Although most conjunctival lymphomas are classified as B-cell type, T-cell lymphoma, and Hodgkin's lymphoma can occasionally affect the conjunctiva. Most lymphomas show a good response to radiotherapy.

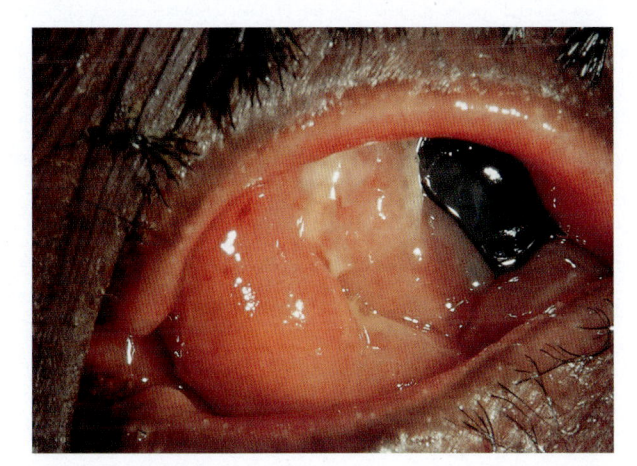

Figure 22.13. Conjunctival involvement in a 72-year-old woman with systemic T-cell lymphoma.

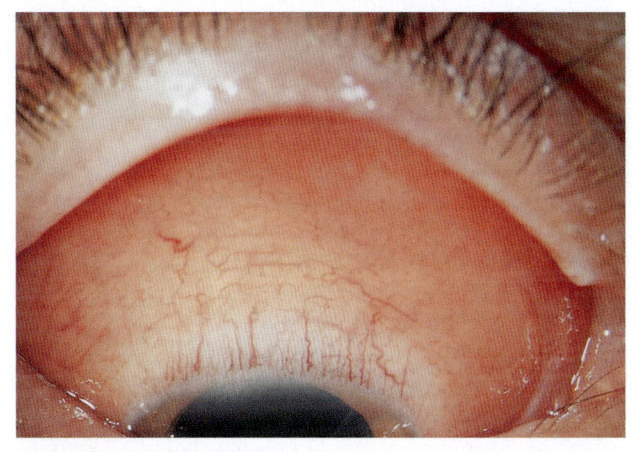

Figure 22.14. Diffuse infiltration of conjunctiva in a 61-year-old patient with Hodgkin's lymphoma.

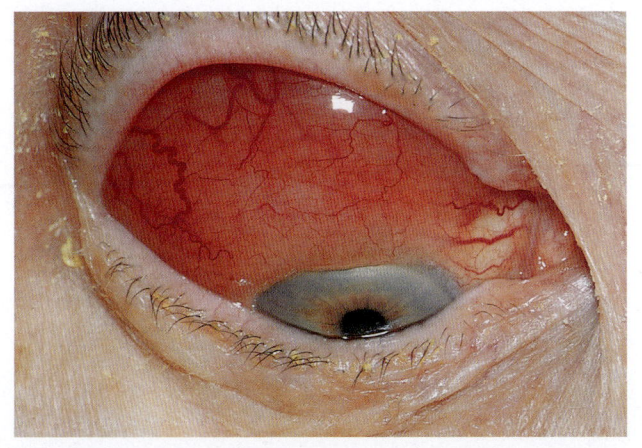

Figure 22.15. Large, diffuse B-cell lymphoma in an 82-year-old woman.

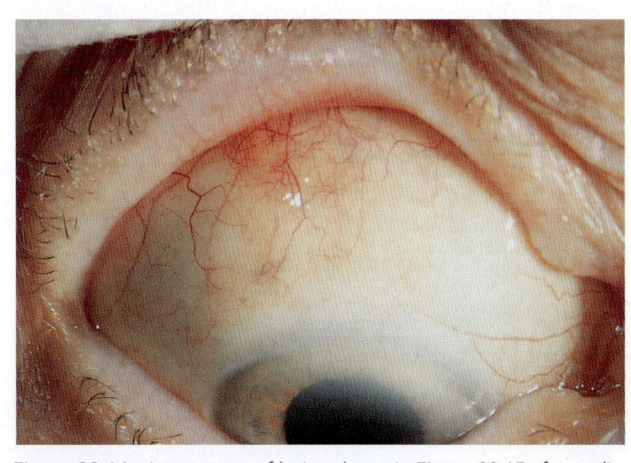

Figure 22.16. Appearance of lesion shown in Figure 22.15 after radiotherapy.

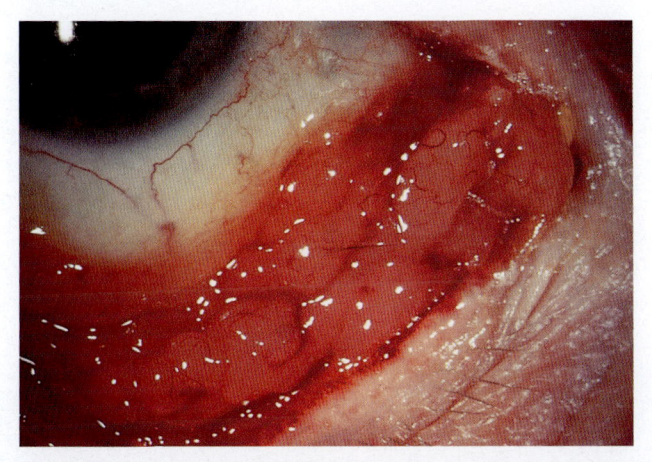

Figure 22.17. Extensive multinodular lymphoma involving inferior conjunctiva in a 76-year-old man.

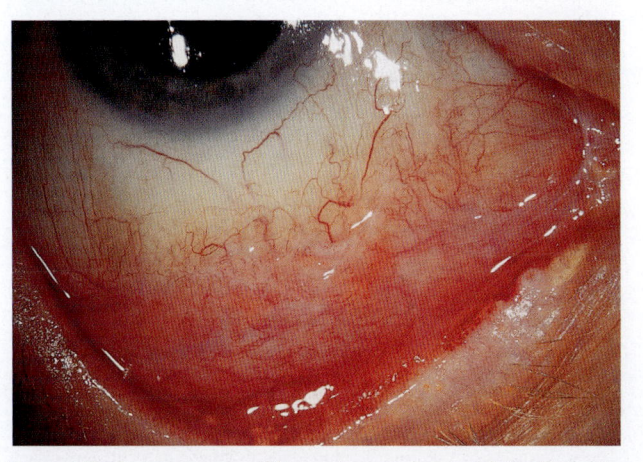

Figure 22.18. Appearance of lesion shown in Figure 22.17 after radiotherapy demonstrating improvement.

CONJUNCTIVAL POSTTRANSPLANT LYMPHOPROLIFERATIVE DISORDER

General Considerations

Posttransplant lymphoproliferative disorder (PTLD) is an important entity that consists of a polyclonal or monoclonal lymphocytic proliferation, or both that occurs in about 3% of organ transplant recipients who undergo intensive immunosuppression treatment (1–10). Some affected patients have had prior infection with Epstein–Barr virus (EBV) and EBV has been implicated using Southern blot, polymerase chain reaction, and in situ hybridization techniques on affected tissue (3–10). It can affect several tissues including central nervous system, gastrointestinal tract, cervical lymph nodes, and tonsils. More cases are being recognized in the ocular region, including the conjunctiva and orbit (5–10).

Clinical Features

PTLD can occur in the orbit, eyelid, conjunctiva, uveal tract, and retina. Conjunctival PTLD presents clinically like other lymphoid neoplasms discussed previously and is not elaborated upon further here. It should be suspected in any immunosuppressed transplant patient who presents with a salmon-colored lesion in the conjunctiva.

Pathology

Although histopathologic and immunohistochemical characteristics vary, the cells are of lymphocytes of B-cell lineage and vary from well-differentiated to poorly differentiated lesions. A pathology classification of PTLD has been proposed and can be used in predicting prognosis (4).

Management

Treatment of conjunctival involvement by PTLD should depend on the extent of involvement and histopathologic features. An attempt should be made to decrease the immunosuppression and allow the host immune system to recover. As with other orbital lymphoid tumors, small localized lesions can be excised and large lesions can be confirmed by biopsy and treated with irradiation. Newer treatment strategies involve the use of rituximab (3). The prognosis varies with the extent of disease with some patients experiencing complete recovery and others having a fatal outcome.

Selected References

Reviews
1. Shields CL, Demirci H, Karatza E, et al. Clinical survey of 1643 melanocytic and nonmelanocytic tumors of the conjunctiva. *Ophthalmology* 2004;111:1747–1754.
2. Shields CL, Shields JA. Tumors of the conjunctiva and cornea. *Surv Ophthalmol* 2004;49:3–24.

Management
3. Iu LP, Yeung JC, Loong F, et al. Successful treatment of intraocular post-transplant lymphoproliferative disorder with intravenous rituximab. *Pediatr Blood Cancer* 2015;62:169–172.

Histopathology
4. Knowles DM, Cesarman E, Chadburn A, et al. Correlative morphologic and molecular genetic analysis demonstrates three distinct categories of posttransplantation lymphoproliferative disorders. *Blood* 1995;85:552–565.

Case Reports
5. Strazzabosco M, Corneo B, Iemmolo RM, et al. Epstein-Barr virus-associated post-transplant lympho-proliferative disease of donor origin in liver transplant recipient. *J Hepatol* 1997;269:26–34.
6. Douglas RS, Goldstein SM, Katowitz JA, et al. Orbital presentation of posttransplantation lymphoproliferative disorder: a small case series. *Ophthalmology* 2002;109:2351–2355.
7. Pomeranz HD, McEvoy LT, Lueder GT. Orbital tumor in a child with posttransplantation lymphoproliferative disorder. *Arch Ophthalmol* 1996;114:1422–1423.
8. Clark WL, Scott IU, Murray TG, et al. Primary intraocular posttransplantation lymphoproliferative disorder. *Arch Ophthalmol* 1998;116:1667–1669.
9. Chan SM, Hutnik CM, Heathcote JG, et al. Iris lymphoma in a pediatric cardiac transplant recipient: clinicopathologic findings. *Ophthalmology* 2000;107:1479–1482.
10. Walton RC, Onciu MM, Irshad FA, et al. Conjunctival pos-transplantation lymphoproliferative disorder. *Am J Ophthalmol* 2007;143:1050–1051.

Chapter 22 Conjunctival Lymphoid, Leukemic, and Metastatic Tumors 387

● CONJUNCTIVAL POSTTRANSPLANT LYMPHOPROLIFERATIVE DISORDER

A case is illustrated of conjunctival PTLD related to EBV.

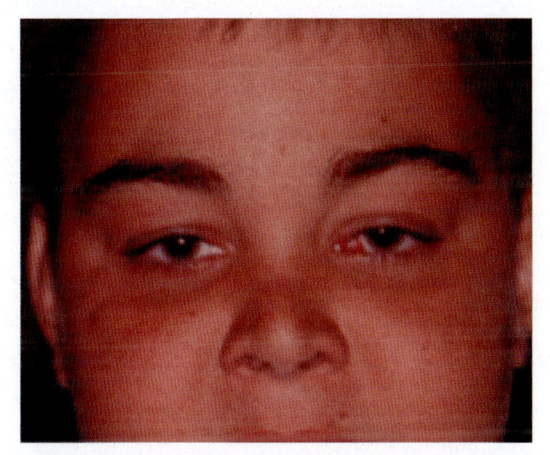

Figure 22.19. Facial appearance of a young boy with a mass in medial canthal region. He had a history of reflux nephropathy hypodysplasia and had undergone renal transplantation 6 months earlier.

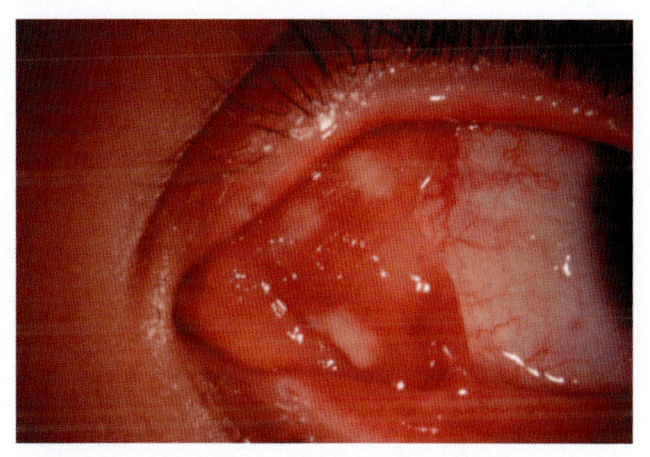

Figure 22.20. Closer view of red-pink mass in the medial canthus.

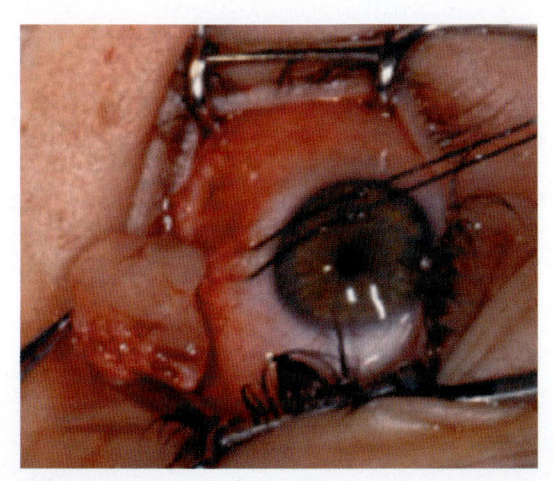

Figure 22.21. Gross appearance of mass at the time of surgical removal.

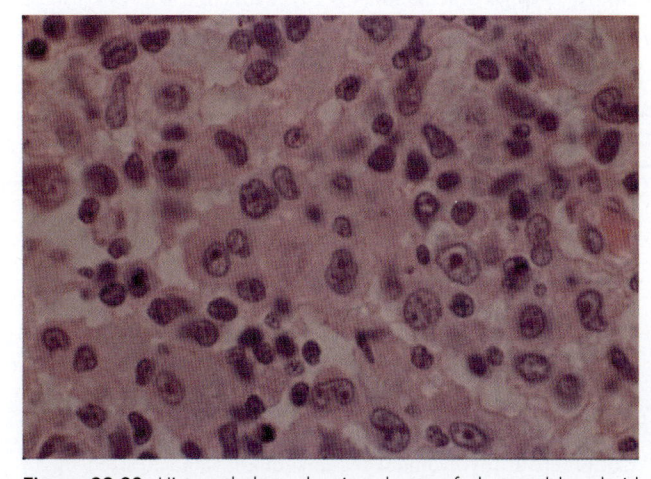

Figure 22.22. Histopathology showing sheets of abnormal lymphoid cells and plasma cells. (Hematoxylin–eosin ×200.)

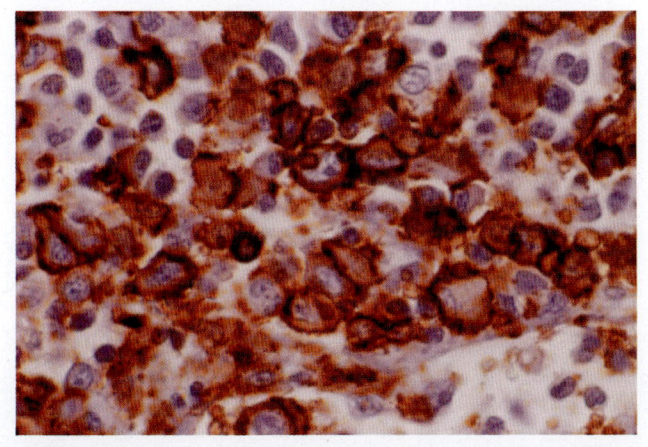

Figure 22.23. Immunohistochemistry showing positive reaction to CD 20. (×250.)

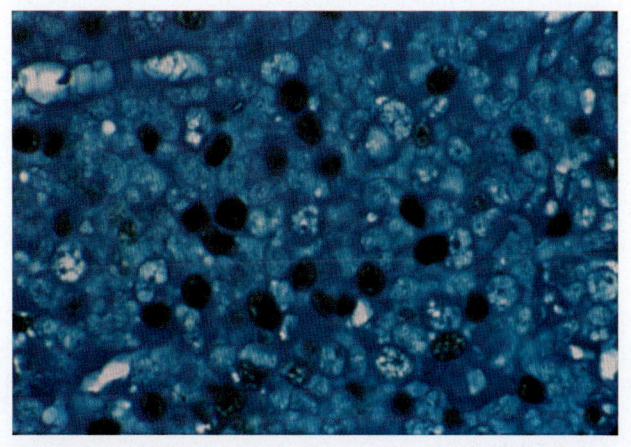

Figure 22.24. Positive in situ hybridization reaction for EBV showing black nuclear staining. (×250.)

CONJUNCTIVAL LEUKEMIA

General Considerations

Leukemia is a complex disease with continually changing classification. Virtually all types of leukemia can affect the ocular structures. Improved methods of diagnosis and treatment of the leukemias has led to prolonged survival of affected patients. Hence, there has been an increase in the variability of ocular presentations. Leukemic involvement of the ocular adnexal tissues usually involves the orbit and less often extends to involve the conjunctiva and eyelid. Orbital and adnexal involvement can occur as granulocytic sarcoma ("chloroma"), which is an infiltration of the soft tissues with myeloid leukemia in children. Conjunctival involvement in patients with leukemia usually takes the form of subconjunctival hemorrhage rather than direct infiltration of the tissues with leukemic cells. However, direct infiltration of the conjunctival tissues by leukemic cells is well known (1–19). Most early reviews of ocular manifestations of leukemia discuss the intraocular and orbital manifestations, but hardly mention conjunctival involvement (3). However, there are documented reports of conjunctival involvement by almost all types of leukemia (3–19). Leukemic cells can also be observed in the conjunctiva at autopsy in patients who apparently had no clinical evidence of a conjunctival mass. Conjunctival involvement can occur at any age, depending on the type of leukemia. It is often an early sign of relapse of previously treated disease.

Clinical Features

In most instances, leukemic infiltration of the conjunctiva has a similar appearance to lymphoma. However, it often has a more red color, probably due to hemorrhage within a leukemic infiltration, which rarely occurs with lymphoma. It may have a tendency to appear in the perilimbal tissues near the cornea.

Pathology

Conjunctival involvement by leukemia is characterized by an infiltration of the conjunctival stroma by leukemic cells. The characteristics of the cells vary with the type of leukemia. Special stains and immunohistochemistry may assist in characterizing the nature of the leukemia.

Management

The management of conjunctival leukemia involves treatment of the systemic disease with appropriate chemotherapy as part of the systemic treatment. For cases that do not respond to such treatment, low-dose radiotherapy can be very effective.

Selected References

Reviews

1. Shields CL, Demirci H, Karatza E, et al. Clinical survey of 1643 melanocytic and nonmelanocytic tumors of the conjunctiva. *Ophthalmology* 2004;111:1747–1754.
2. Shields CL, Shields JA. Tumors of the conjunctiva and cornea. *Surv Ophthalmol* 2004;49:3–24.
3. Kincaid MC, Green WR. Ocular and orbital involvement in leukemia. *Surv Ophthalmol* 1983;27:211–232.
4. Sharma T, Grewal J, Gupta S, et al. Ophthalmic manifestations of acute leukaemias: the ophthalmologist's role. *Eye* 2004;7:663–672.

Case Reports

5. Font RL, Mackay B, Tang R. Acute monocytic leukemia recurring as bilateral perilimbal infiltrates. *Ophthalmology* 1985;92:1681–1685.
6. Mansour AM, Traboulsi EI, Frangieh GT, et al. Caruncular involvement in myelomonocytic leukemia: a case report. *Med Pediatr Oncol* 1985;13:46–47.
7. Rodgers R, Weiner M, Friedman AH. Ocular involvement in congenital leukemia. *Am J Ophthalmol* 1986;101:730–732.
8. Tsumura T, Sakaguchi M, Shiotani N, et al. A case of acute myelomonocytic leukemia with subconjunctival tumor. *Jpn J Ophthalmol* 1991;35:226–231.
9. Fujikawa LS, Salahuddin SZ, Ablashi D, et al. Human T-cell leukemia/lymphotropic virus type III in the conjunctival epithelium of a patient with AIDS. *Am J Ophthalmol* 1985;100:507–509.
10. Lee DA, Su WP. Acute myelomonocytic leukemia cutis presenting as a conjunctival lesion. *Int J Dermatol* 1985;24:369–370.
11. Takahashi K, Sakuma T, Onoe S, et al. Adult T-cell leukemia with leukemic cell infiltration in the conjunctiva. *Doc Ophthalmol* 1993;83:255–260.
12. Cook BE Jr, Bartley GB. Acute lymphoblastic leukemia manifesting in an adult as a conjunctival mass. *Am J Ophthalmol* 1997;124:104–105.
13. Douglas RS, Goldstein SM, Nichols C. Acute myelogenous leukaemia presenting as a conjunctival lesion and red eye. *Acta Ophthalmol Scand* 2002;80:671–672.
14. Mori A, Deguchi HE, Mishima K, et al. A case of uveal, palpebral, and orbital invasions in adult T-Cell leukemia. *Jpn J Ophthalmol* 2003;47:599–602.
15. Campagnoli MF, Parodi E, Linari A, et al. Conjunctival mass: an unusual presentation of acute lymphoblastic leukemia relapse in childhood. *J Pediatr* 2003;142:211.
16. Nau J, Shields CL, Shields JA, et al. Acute myeloid leukemia manifesting initially as a conjunctival mass in a patient with acquired immunodeficiency syndrome. *Arch Ophthalmol* 2002;120:1741–1742.
17. Shah SB, Reichstein DA, Lally SE, et al. Persistent bloody tears as the initial manifestation of conjunctival chloroma associated with chronic myelogenous leukemia. *Graefes Arch Clin Exp Ophthalmol* 2013;251(3):991–992.
18. Shinder R. Ocular myeloid sarcoma in a 10-year-old child. *J AAPOS* 2012;16(2):213.
19. Lee SS, Robinson MR, Morris JC, et al. Conjunctival involvement with T-cell prolymphocytic leukemia: report of a case and review of the literature. *Surv Ophthalmol* 2004;49(5):525–536.

Chapter 22 Conjunctival Lymphoid, Leukemic, and Metastatic Tumors

• CONJUNCTIVAL LEUKEMIC INFILTRATE

The conjunctiva can be involved by any form of leukemia. The conjunctival infiltrate is very similar to that seen with lymphomas.

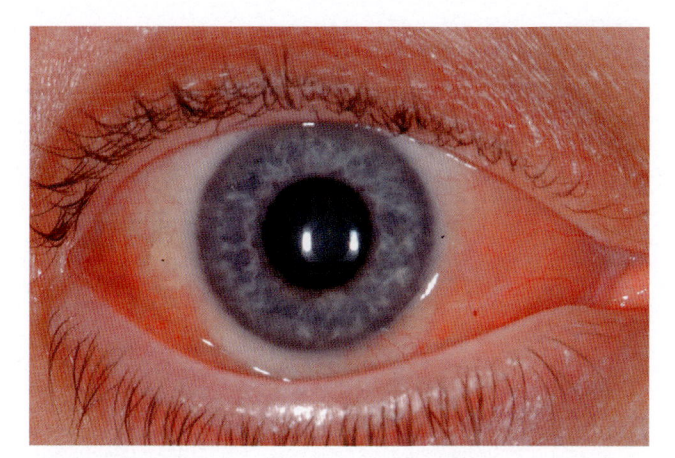

Figure 22.25. Diffuse conjunctival leukemic infiltrate in right eye of a 60-year-old man with chronic lymphocytic leukemia.

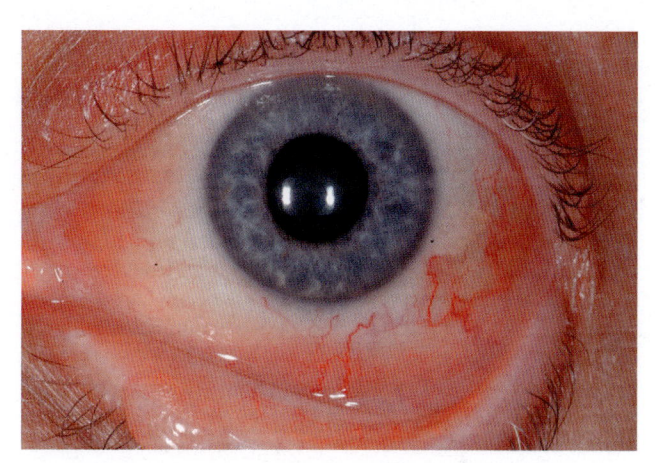

Figure 22.26. Left eye of patient shown in Figure 22.25 showing similar leukemic infiltrate as seen in the right eye.

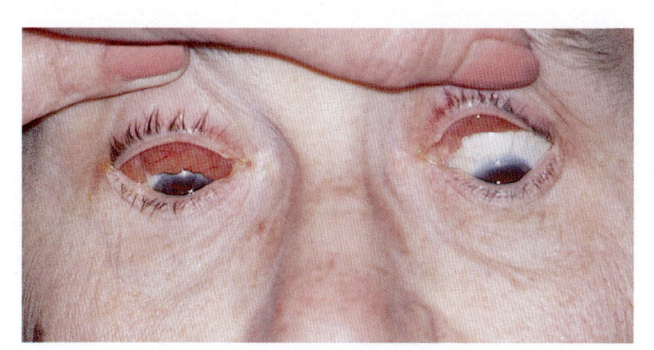

Figure 22.27. Bilateral superior conjunctival involvement with chronic lymphocytic leukemia in a 72-year-old woman.

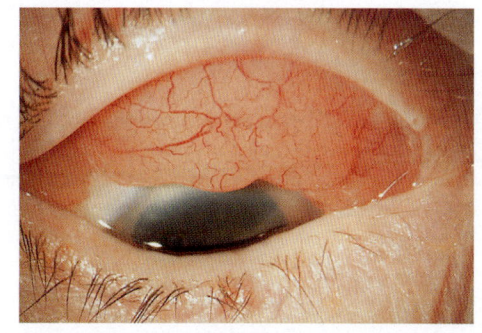

Figure 22.28. Closer view of infiltration in patient shown in Figure 22.27.

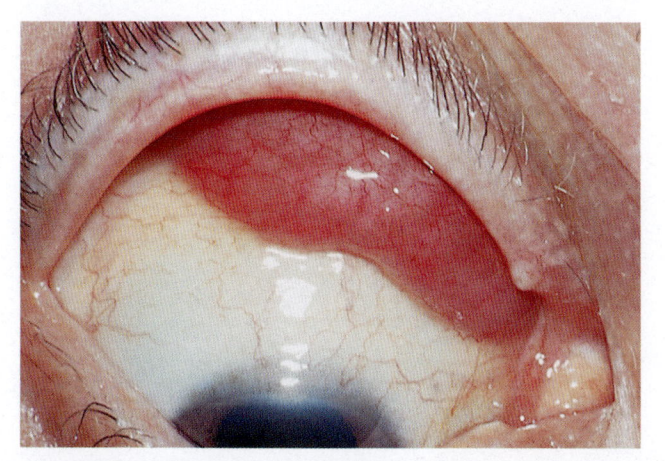

Figure 22.29. Infiltration of the superior conjunctival tissues with chronic lymphocytic leukemia in an 87-year-old man.

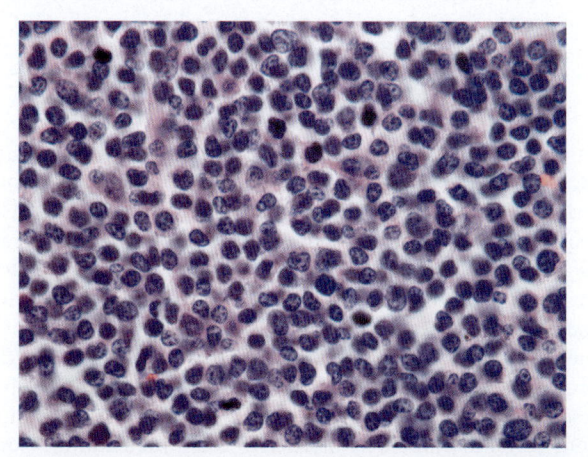

Figure 22.30. Histopathology of lesion shown in Figure 22.25, showing sheets of mononuclear cells with round to oval uniform nuclei. (Hematoxylin–eosin ×200.)

CONJUNCTIVAL METASTATIC TUMORS

General Considerations

Most metastatic cancer to the ocular region involves the uveal tract and orbit. Eyelid and conjunctival metastasis are less common and individual cases are often reported (1–11). Among 2,455 conjunctival lesions that came to biopsy in one series, there was only one case of metastasis (3). In a recent report of 1,643 conjunctival lesions, there were 13 cases of conjunctival metastasis (1). In an earlier report of 10 cases of conjunctival metastasis, the primary tumor was in breast in 4, lung in 2, cutaneous melanoma in 2, larynx in 1, and undetermined in 1 (4). Most patients have a history of a primary malignancy, but sometimes the conjunctival metastasis is the initial manifestation of a systemic cancer (6,7,9).

Some neoplasms can reach the conjunctiva and episcleral tissue by direct spread from an adjacent structure, such as the eyelid, orbital, or sinuses. We prefer to call such contiguous spread a "secondary conjunctival tumor" rather than a true metastasis. Sebaceous carcinoma of the eyelid and uveal melanoma, and orbital rhabdomyosarcoma are examples. These specific tumors are discussed in other sections of this atlas and in the other atlases.

Clinical Features

Clinically, conjunctival metastasis appears as a rapidly growing, sessile or nodular mass that has a yellow or fleshy color. The lesion can be diffuse or multifocal. Melanoma metastatic to the conjunctiva is usually pigmented, but can be nonpigmented (1,4,9).

Pathology

Histopathologically, conjunctival metastasis varies with the primary tumor and the degree of differentiation of the metastasis focus. Some lesions, like melanoma, breast cancer, or renal cell carcinoma, have characteristic features (4–11). Poorly differentiated tumors may require immunohistochemistry to assist in confirming the primary site of involvement.

Management

In addition to management of the primary neoplasm, the conjunctival metastasis may require specific management. A small lesion may be removed by local excision. Larger lesions may require an incisional biopsy to confirm the diagnosis. Needle biopsy can be performed, but it generally yields less tissue, thus making the diagnosis more difficult. If the patient is receiving specific chemotherapy for the primary lesion, a conjunctival metastasis can be observed for a period of time to assess the response to chemotherapy. If conjunctival metastasis does not respond to chemotherapy, it can be treated with irradiation with 3,000 to 4,000 cGy of external beam irradiation. Plaque brachytherapy is another option in selected cases.

Selected References

Reviews
1. Shields CL, Demirci H, Karatza E, et al. Clinical survey of 1643 melanocytic and nonmelanocytic tumors of the conjunctiva. *Ophthalmology* 2004;111:1747–1754.
2. Shields CL, Shields JA. Tumors of the conjunctiva and cornea. *Surv Ophthalmol* 2004;49:3–24.
3. Grossniklaus HE, Green WR, Luckenbach M, et al. Conjunctival lesions in adults. A clinical and histopathologic review. *Cornea* 1987;6:78–116.
4. Kiratli H, Shields CL, Shields JA, et al. Metastatic tumors to the conjunctiva. Report of ten cases. *Brit J Ophthalmol* 1996;80:5–8.

Case Reports
5. Ortiz JM, Esterman B, Paulson J. Uterine cervical carcinoma metastasis to subconjunctival tissue. *Arch Ophthalmol* 1995;113:1362–1363.
6. Shields JA, Gunduz K, Shields CL, et al. Conjunctival metastasis as the initial manifestation of lung cancer. *Am J Ophthalmol* 1997;124:399–400.
7. Shields JA, Shields CL, Eagle RC Jr, et al. Diffuse ocular metastases as an initial sign of metastatic lung cancer. *Ophthalmic Surg Lasers* 1998;29:598–601.
8. Tokuyama J, Kubota T, Otani Y, et al. Rare case of early mucosal gastric cancer presenting with metastasis to the bulbar conjunctiva. *Gastric Cancer* 2002;5:102–106.
9. Shields JA, Shields CL, Eagle RC Jr, et al. Conjunctival metastasis as initial sign of disseminated cutaneous melanoma. *Ophthalmology* 2004;111:1933–1934.
10. Bianciotto C, Shields CL, Guzman JM, et al. Assessment of anterior segment tumors with ultrasound biomicroscopy versus anterior segment optical coherence tomography in 200 cases. *Ophthalmology* 2011;118(7):1297–1302.
11. Shields JA, Eagle RC, Gausas RE, et al. Retrograde metastasis of cutaneous melanoma to conjunctival lymphatics. *Arch Ophthalmol* 2009;127:1122–1123.

Chapter 22 Conjunctival Lymphoid, Leukemic, and Metastatic Tumors

● CONJUNCTIVAL METASTASIS

1. Kiratli H, Shields CL, Shields JA, et al. Metastatic tumors to the conjunctiva. Report of ten cases. *Brit J Ophthalmol* 1996;80:5–8.
2. Shields JA, Gunduz K, Shields CL, et al. Conjunctival metastasis as the initial manifestation of lung cancer. *Am J Ophthalmol* 1997;124:399–400.

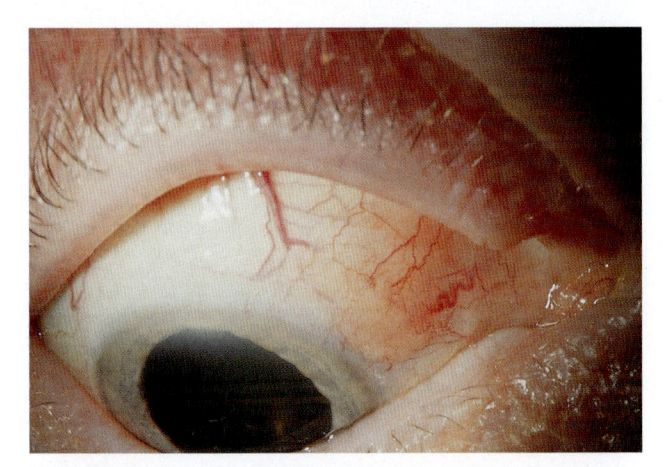

Figure 22.31. Breast cancer metastatic to the conjunctiva in a 60-year-old woman.

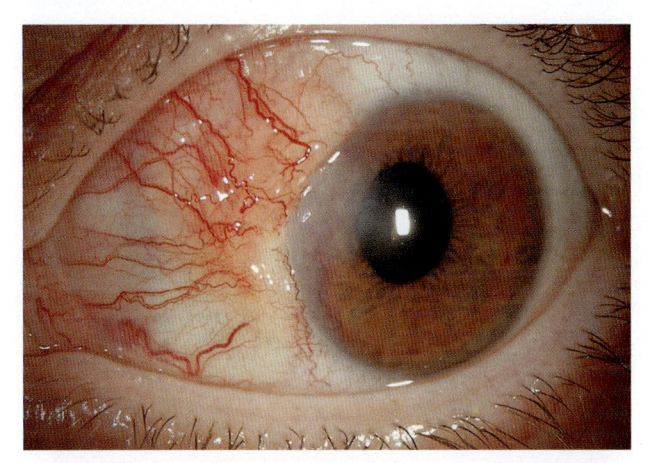

Figure 22.32. Breast cancer metastatic to the conjunctiva in a 55-year-old woman.

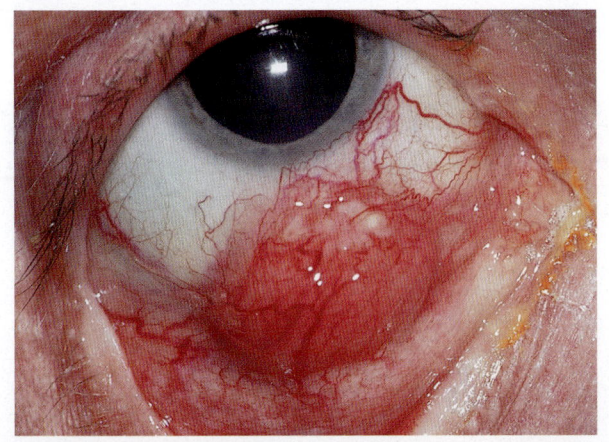

Figure 22.33. Lung cancer metastatic to the conjunctiva in a 55-year-old man. Subsequent systemic evaluation revealed the primary lung cancer.

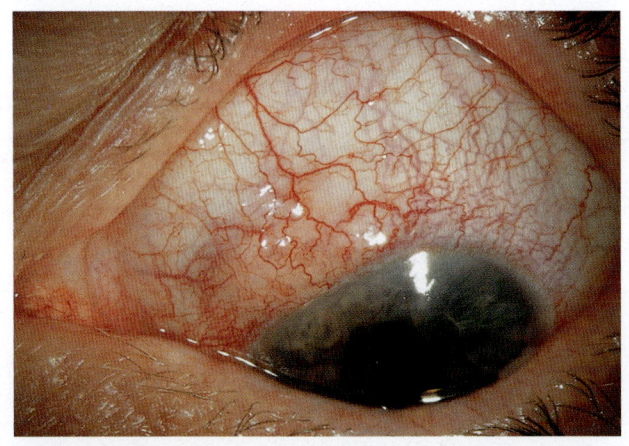

Figure 22.34. Metastatic carcinoid tumor to the conjunctiva in a 56-year-old woman.

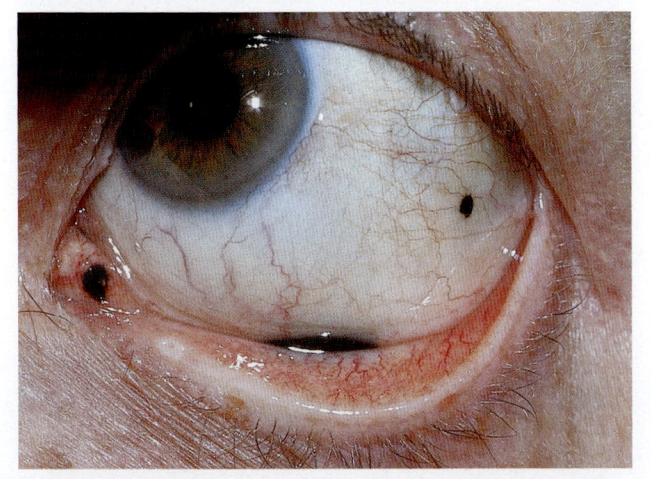

Figure 22.35. Metastatic cutaneous melanoma to the conjunctiva presenting as multiple pigmented lesions in a 60-year-old man.

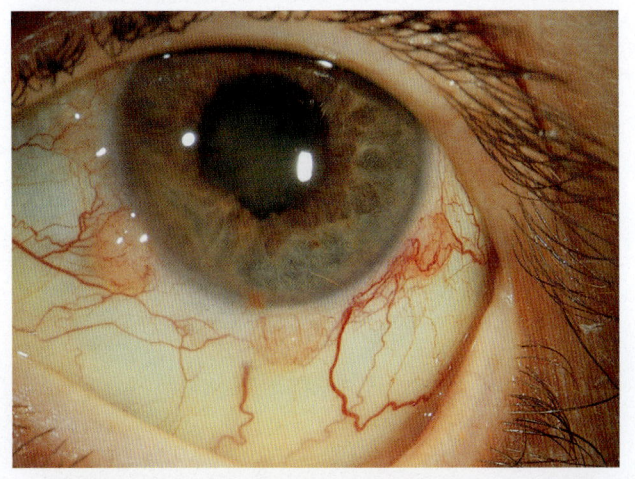

Figure 22.36. Metastatic cutaneous melanoma to the conjunctiva presenting as nonpigmented masses near the limbus in a 54-year-old woman.

CONJUNCTIVAL METASTASIS FROM CUTANEOUS MELANOMA

Conjunctival metastasis from cutaneous melanoma can be the initial manifestation of metastatic disease. It can sometimes show unusual patterns of metastasis, including involvement of the palpebral conjunctiva.

Shields JA, Shields CL, Eagle RC Jr, et al. Conjunctival metastasis as initial sign of disseminated cutaneous melanoma. *Ophthalmology* 2004;111:1933–1934.

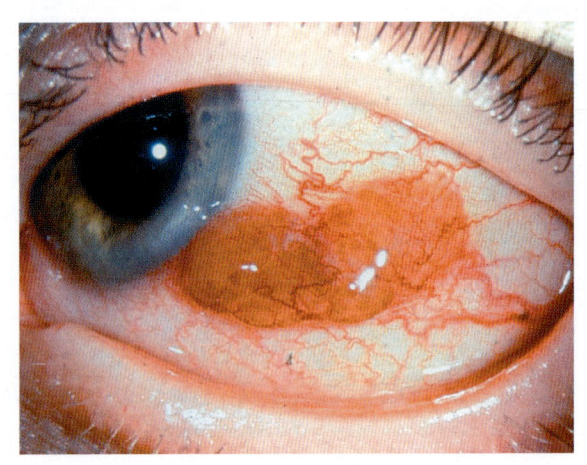

Figure 22.37. Tan-colored mass in bulbar conjunctiva of a 48-year-old woman with a history of cutaneous melanoma. She had no known metastasis at time of ocular presentation, but was subsequently found to have widespread metastases.

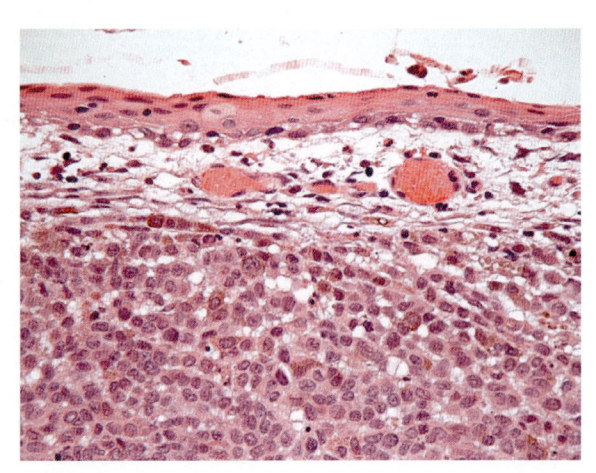

Figure 22.38. Low-magnification photomicrograph of lesion in Figure 22.37. Note that the tumor cells are deep to the epithelium in the stroma. (Hematoxylin–eosin ×150.)

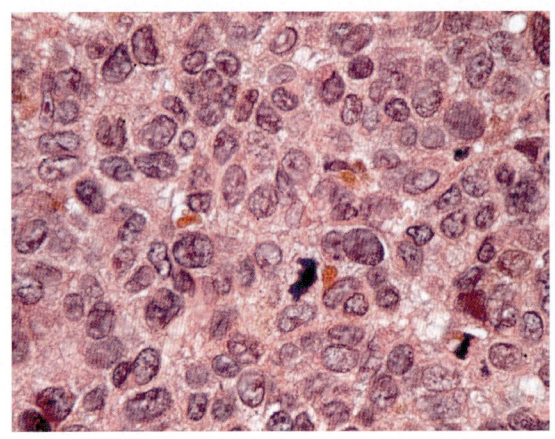

Figure 22.39. Higher magnification of lesion in Figure 22.38 showing the epithelioid melanoma cells. Note the mitotic figures. (Hematoxylin–eosin ×250.)

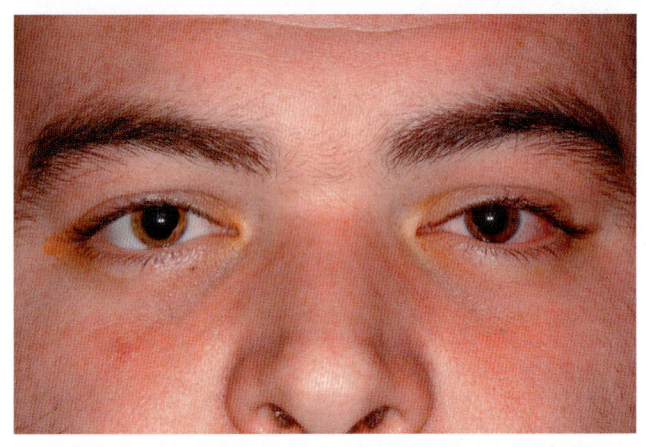

Figure 22.40. Face of 34-year-old man with widespread metastases from cutaneous melanoma.

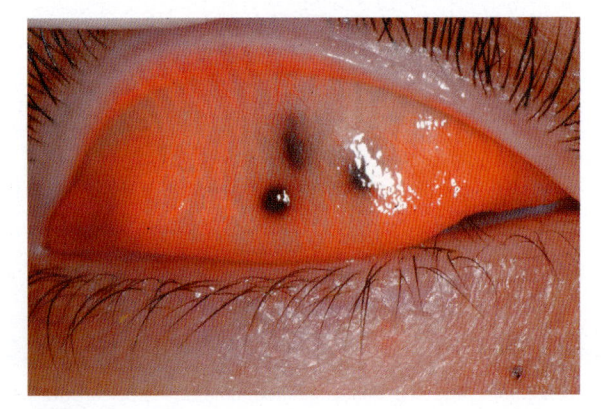

Figure 22.41. Everted right upper eyelid showing multiple foci of metastatic melanoma on the tarsal conjunctiva.

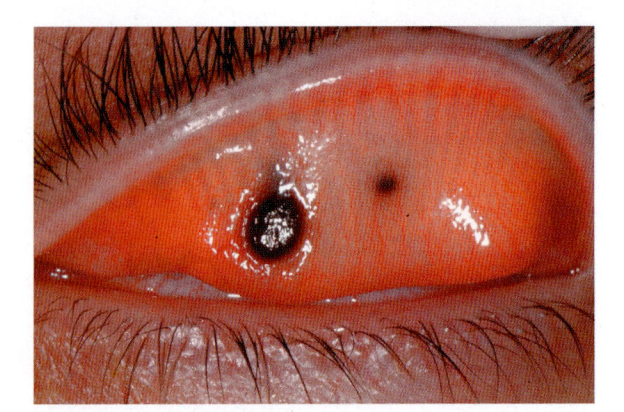

Figure 22.42. Everted left upper eyelid showing multiple foci of metastatic melanoma on the tarsal conjunctiva.

CARUNCULAR TUMORS

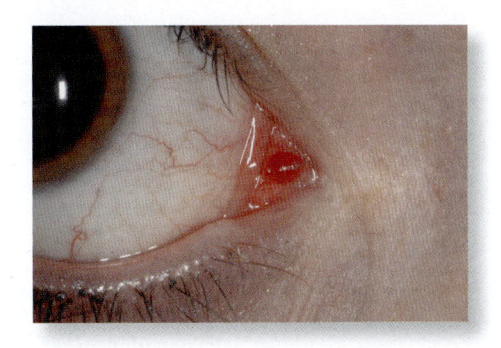

General Considerations

The caruncle lies at the inner canthus nasal to the plica semilunaris. It has a nonkeratinizing epithelial lining similar to conjunctival epithelium. However, the caruncle harbors cutaneous elements such as hair follicles, sebaceous glands, sweat glands, and accessory lacrimal gland. Consequently, the caruncle can spawn a tumor or cyst that may be similar to one found in the skin, conjunctiva, or lacrimal gland (1–27).

Approximately 95% of caruncular lesions that are suspicious enough to warrant surgical excision prove to be benign, with the majority being either papilloma or melanocytic nevus. Only 5% of biopsied tumors of the caruncle are malignant (1,3). In our early series of 57 excised caruncular tumors, a breakdown of lesions is as follows: papilloma 32%, melanocytic nevus 24%, pyogenic granuloma 9%, inclusions cyst 7%, chronic inflammation 7%, and oncocytoma 4% (3). In a later series on 93 cases, the tumor category is listed in Table 23-1.

Clinical Features

Clinically, a caruncular tumor presents as an enlargement of the caruncle as a distinct mass arising from or displacing the caruncle. The clinical appearance varies with the type of tumor. Papilloma generally appears as a frondlike mass with fine vascular tufts visible clinically in the central core of each frond (1–3). Caruncular nevus usually appears at about puberty, is variably pigmented, and may show slight change in size or color with time. It generally contains clear cysts best seen with slit-lamp biomicroscopy (1–3). Caruncular melanoma appears as a variably pigmented, usually noncystic, solid mass (27).

Oncocytoma is a benign tumor that is believed to originate from transformed glandular epithelial cells, particularly in the lacrimal gland, salivary glands, and other organs. When it occurs in the caruncle, it appears as an asymptomatic, slowly growing, reddish-blue solid or cystic mass (15–21). It most often occurs in older individuals.

Several sebaceous gland tumors and cysts can arise from the caruncle. Sebaceous gland hyperplasia and sebaceous adenoma may resemble each other clinically, appearing as a smooth or multinodular yellow mass. Sebaceous gland carcinoma in the ocular area usually arises from the sebaceous gland of the tarsus (meibomian glands) or cilia (Zeis glands), but they can arise from the sebaceous gland of the caruncle (8,26). Sebaceous gland carcinoma can be aggressive and can metastasize.

Other lesions that can occasionally develop in the caruncle include metastatic carcinoid neoplasms, cavernous hemangioma, Kaposi sarcoma, lymphoma, adenosquamous carcinoma and dacryops, and dermoid tumor (1–3,22–25).

Pathology

The pathology of caruncular tumors is similar to the same tumors of the conjunctiva and is discussed in those sections. Oncocytoma is composed of benign epithelial cells with abundant eosinophilic granular cytoplasm. Electron microscopy shows large numbers of abnormal mitochondria.

CARUNCULAR TUMORS

Table 23.1 Types of tumors in the caruncle in a series of 93 cases

Tumor category	Number (%), n = 93 cases
Choristomatous	0 (0%)
Epithelial benign	7 (18%)
Epithelial premalignant/malignant	2 (1%)
Melanocytic	66 (8%)
Vascular	1 (2%)
Fibrous	1 (14%)
Neural	0 (0%)
Xanthomatous	0 (0%)
Myxomatous	0 (0%)
Lipomatous	0 (0%)
Lacrimal gland	4 (33%)
Lymphoma	1 (2%)
Leukemic	0 (0%)
Metastatic	0 (0%)
Secondary	1 (2%)
Nonneoplastic simulating lesions	10 (5%)

From Shields CL, Demirci H, Karatza E, et al. Clinical survey of 1643 melanocytic and nonmelanocytic tumors of the conjunctiva. Ophthalmology 2004;111:1747–1754.

Management

Management of a caruncular tumor is complete surgical excision when possible. We generally deliver subcaruncular local anesthesia and perform an incision through the normal surrounding conjunctiva approximately 1 to 2 mm outside the tumor margin using microscopic technique. In some cases, the medial rectus muscle is hooked to prevent severing, especially if the tumor extends deep into the orbit. The tumor is removed intact using a minimal manipulation or "no touch" method. Supplemental cryotherapy is applied to the remaining conjunctival margins. Squamous papilloma requires special precautions because, like that in the caruncle, disruption of the lesion can theoretically lead to shedding of viral particles into the surrounding tissue. Pedunculated papilloma is sometimes managed by clamping the base of the mass with a hemostat and cutting beneath the hemostat, removing the tumor intact. Another alternative is to freeze the lesion using a cryoprobe and cutting its base. Suspected malignant tumors like melanoma and sebaceous carcinoma require wider excision and heavy cryotherapy, because they have a greater capacity to invade into the deeper tissue. We often use punctal plugs in cases of primary acquired melanosis and melanoma to prevent seeding of tumor cells into the nasolacrimal drainage system.

Selected References

1. Shields CL, Demirci H, Karatza E, et al. Clinical survey of 1643 melanocytic and nonmelanocytic tumors of the conjunctiva. *Ophthalmology* 2004;111:1747–1754.
2. Shields CL, Shields JA. Tumors of the conjunctiva and cornea. *Surv Ophthalmol* 2004;49:3–24.
3. Shields CL, Shields JA, White D, et al. Types and frequency of lesions of the caruncle. *Am J Ophthalmol* 1986;102:771–778.
4. Luthra CL, Doxanas MT, Green WR. Lesions of the caruncle. A clinicopathologic study. *Surv Ophthalmol* 1978;23:183–195.
5. Shields CL, Shields JA. Tumors of the caruncle. In: Shields JA, ed. Update on malignant ocular tumors. *Int Ophthalmol Clin* 1993;33:31–36.
6. Kaeser PF, Uffer S, Zografos L, et al. Tumors of the caruncle: a clinicopathologic correlation. *Am J Ophthalmol* 2006;142:448–455.
7. Shields CL, Fasiudden A, Mashayekhi A, et al. Conjunctival nevi: clinical features and natural course in 410 consecutive patients. *Arch Ophthalmol* 2004;122:167–175.
8. Shields JA, Demirci H, Marr BP, et al. Sebaceous carcinoma of the eyelids. Personal experience with 60 cases. The 2003 J. Howard Stokes Lecture. *Ophthalmology* 2004;111:2151–2157.
9. Kiratli H, Shields CL, Shields JA, et al. Metastatic tumors to the conjunctiva. Report of ten cases. *Br J Ophthalmol* 1996;80:5–8.
10. Say EA, Shields CL, Bianciotto C, et al. Oncocytic lesions (oncocytoma) of the ocular adnexa: report of 15 cases and review of literature. *Ophthal Plast Reconstr Surg* 2012;28(1):14–21.

Imaging

11. Uysal Y, Shields CL, Mashayekhi A, et al. Ultrasound biomicroscopy of cystic and solid caruncular oncocytoma. *Arch Ophthalmol* 2006;124:1650–1652.

Histopathology

12. Morgan MB, Truitt CA, Romer C, et al. Ocular adnexal oncocytoma: a case series and clinicopathologic review of the literature. *Am J Dermatopathol* 1998;20:487–490.

Case Reports

13. Streeten BW, Carrillo R, Jamison R, et al. Inverted papilloma of the conjunctiva. *Am J Ophthalmol* 1979;88:1062–1066.
14. Kalski RS, Lomeo MD, Kirchgraber PR, et al. Caruncular malignant melanoma in a Black patients. *Ophthal Surg* 1995;26:139–141.
15. Deutsch AR, Duckworth JK. Onkocytoma (oxyphilic adenoma) of the caruncle. *Am J Ophthalmol* 1967;64:458–461.
16. Biggs SL, Font RL. Oncocytic lesions of the caruncle and other ocular adnexa. *Arch Ophthalmol* 1977;95:474–478.
17. Rennie IG. Oncocytomas (oxyphil adenomas) of the lacrimal caruncle. *Br J Ophthalmol* 1980;64:935–938.
18. Lamping KA, Albert DM, Ni C, et al. Oxyphil cell adenomas. *Arch Ophthalmol* 1984;102:263–264.
19. Shields CL, Shields JA, Arbizo V, et al. Oncocytoma of the caruncle. *Am J Ophthalmol* 1986;102:315–319.
20. Orcutt JC, Matsko TH, Milam AH. Oncocytoma of the caruncle. *Ophthal Plast Reconstr Surg* 1992;8:300–302.
21. Chang WJ, Nowinski TS, Eagle RC Jr. A large oncocytoma of the caruncle. *Arch Ophthalmol* 1995;113:382.
22. Gritz DC, Rao NA. Metastatic carcinoid tumor diagnosis from a caruncular mass. *Am J Ophthalmol* 1991;112:470–471.
23. Nylander AG, Atta HR. Adenosquamous carcinoma of the lacrimal caruncle: a case report. *Br J Ophthalmol* 1986;70:864–866.
24. Ghafouri A, Rodgers IR, Perry HD. A caruncular dermoid with contiguous eyelid involvement: embryologic implications. *Ophthal Plast Reconstr Surg* 1998;14:375–377.
25. Rossman D, Arthurs B, Odashiro A, et al. Basal cell carcinoma of the caruncle. *Ophthal Plast Reconstr Surg* 2006;22:313–314.
26. Shields JA, Shields CL, Marr BP, et al. Sebaceous carcinoma of the caruncle. *Cornea* 2006;25(7):858–859.
27. Shields JA, Lim R, Lally SL, et al. Malignant melanoma presenting as pedunculated lesion of the caruncle. *JAMA Ophthalmol* 2015; in press.

CARUNCULAR PAPILLOMA

Papilloma of the caruncle has many features similar to conjunctival papilloma, as discussed. It can occur at any age. The adult form seems to be more common in the caruncle.

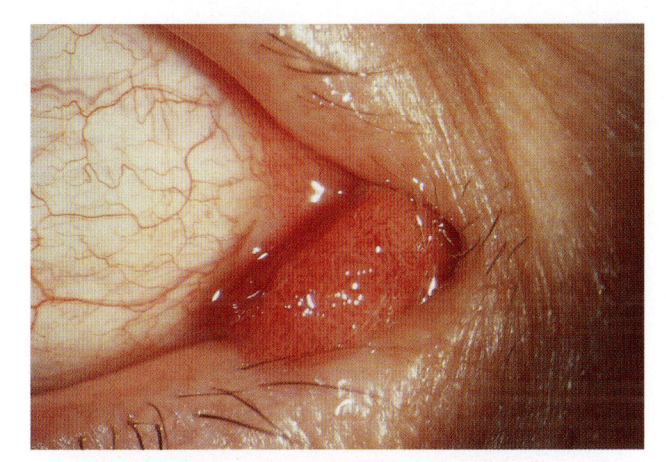

Figure 23.1. Papilloma of caruncle in a 31-year-old woman.

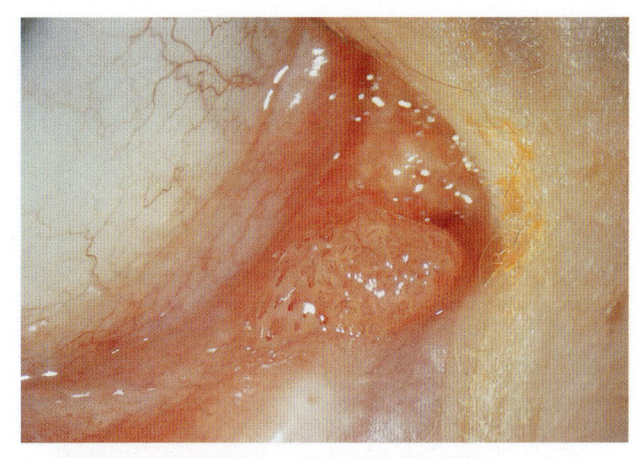

Figure 23.2. Papilloma of caruncle in a 15-year-old girl.

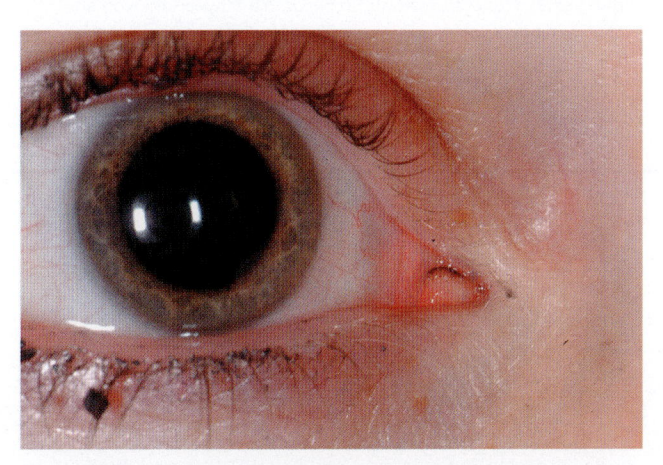

Figure 23.3. Papilloma of caruncle in a 49-year-old woman.

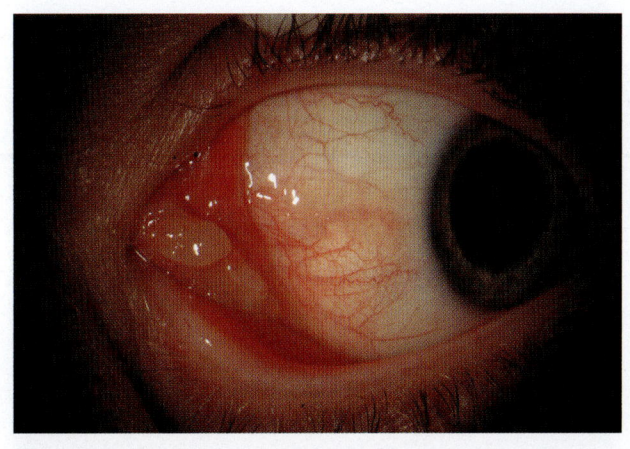

Figure 23.4. Multinodular caruncular papilloma in a young man.

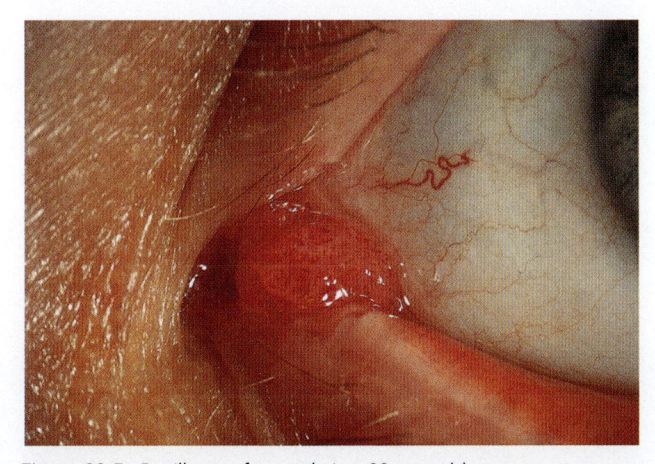

Figure 23.5. Papilloma of caruncle in a 33-year-old woman.

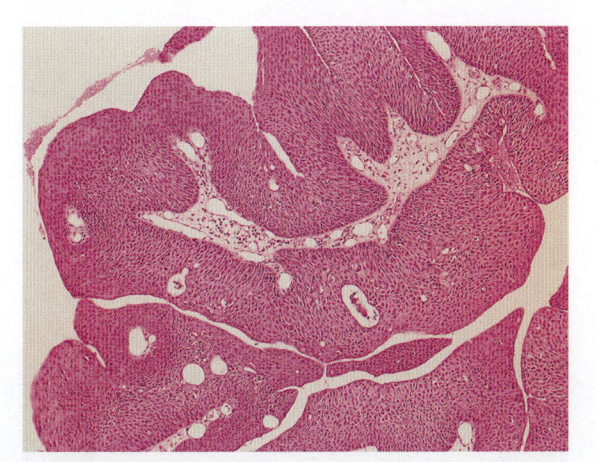

Figure 23.6. Histopathology of papilloma shown in Figure 23.5. (Hematoxylin–eosin ×10.)

396   Part 2 Tumors of the Conjunctiva

CARUNCULAR NEVUS

Caruncular nevus has many features similar to conjunctival nevus discussed previously. Most have some degree of pigmentation and contain clear cysts when viewed with slit-lamp biomicroscopy.

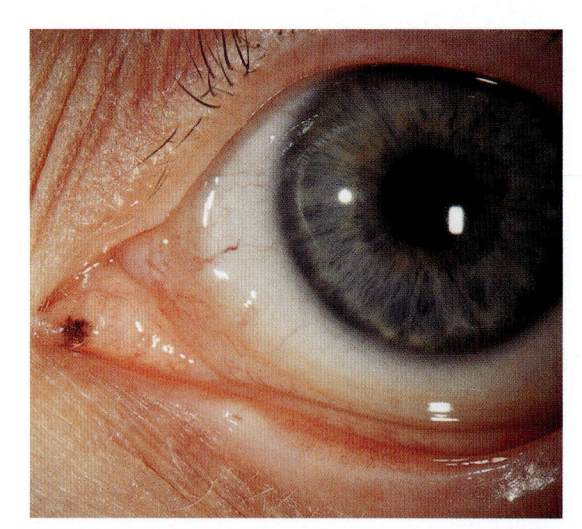

Figure 23.7. Small noncystic caruncular nevus in a 40-year-old woman.

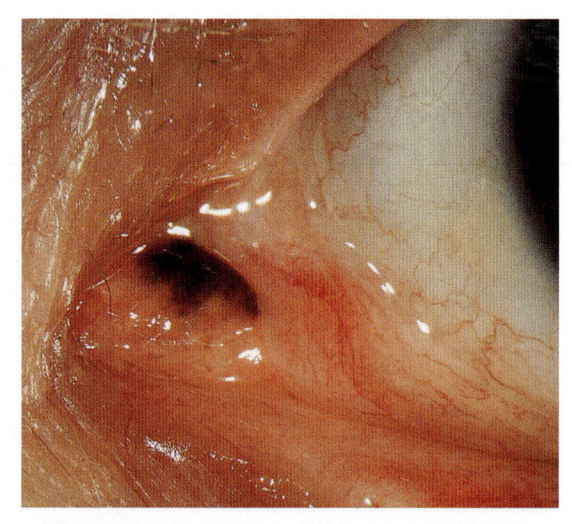

Figure 23.8. Noncystic caruncular nevus in a 50-year-old woman.

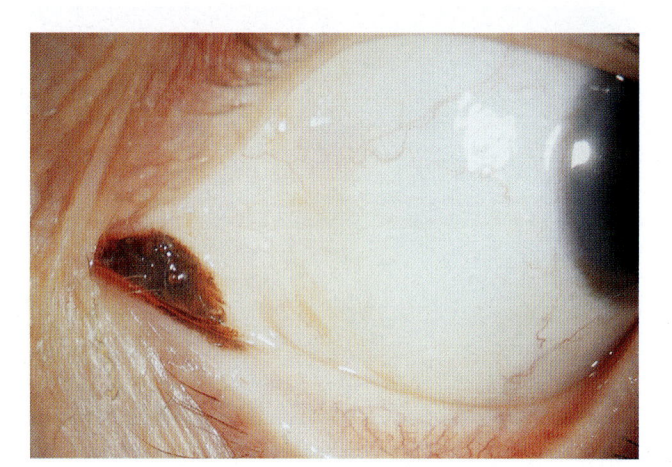

Figure 23.9. Cystic caruncular nevus in a 47-year-old woman.

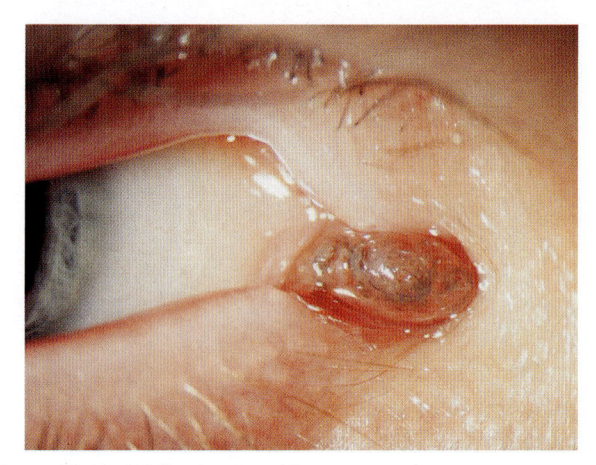

Figure 23.10. Mildly pigmented large caruncular nevus in a 17-year-old man.

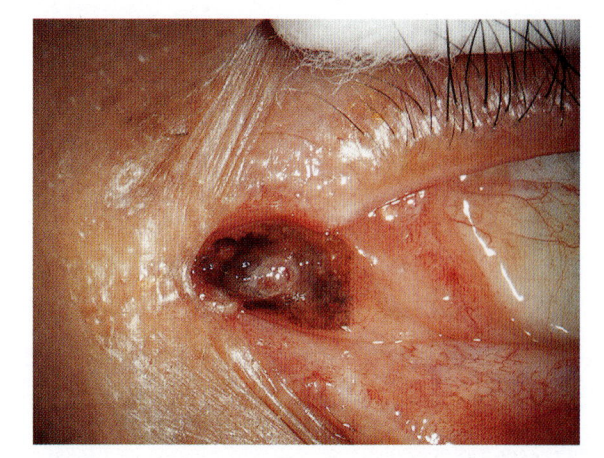

Figure 23.11. Caruncular nevus in a 68-year-old patient.

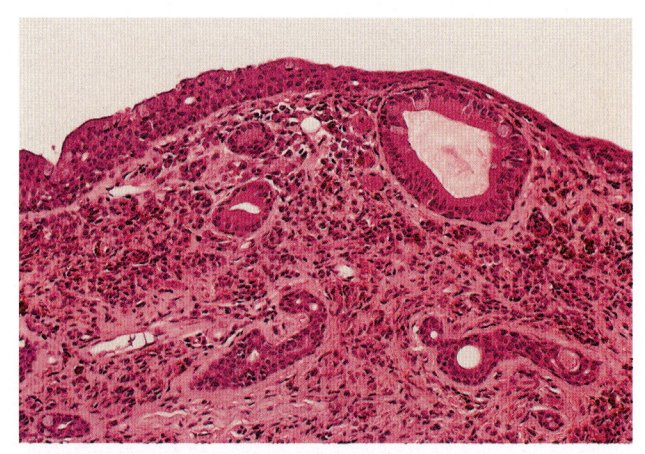

Figure 23.12. Histopathology of lesion shown in Figure 23.11, depicting cystic structures and nevus cells in stroma of the caruncle. (Hematoxylin–eosin ×100.)

Chapter 23 Caruncular Tumors 397

CARUNCULAR MELANOMA

Caruncular melanoma has many features similar to conjunctival melanoma. It can arise from primary acquired melanosis, pre-existing nevus, or de novo. Unlike nevus, it is generally larger, noncystic, and demonstrates slowly progressive growth. It can exhibit local invasion, regional lymph node metastasis, or distant hematogenous metastasis.

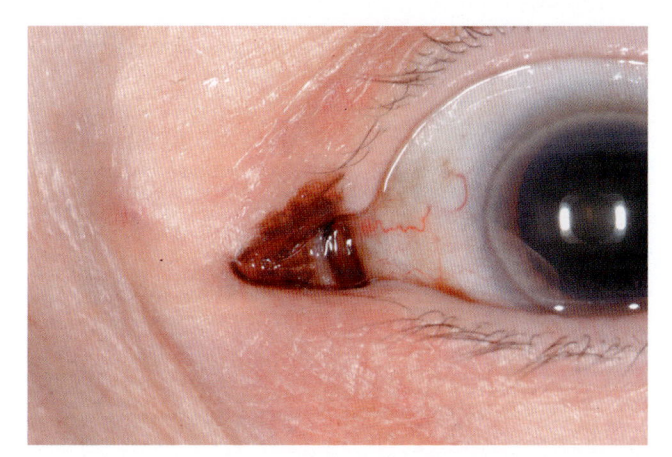

Figure 23.13. Caruncular melanoma with involvement of the adjacent eyelid skin.

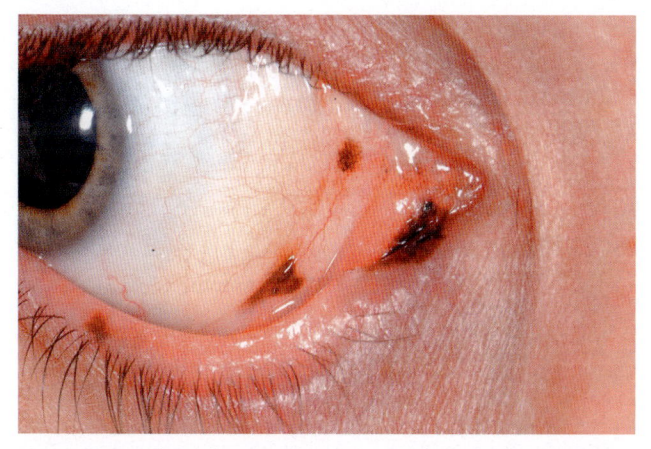

Figure 23.14. Flat melanoma affecting part of the caruncle with involvement of the adjacent eyelid margin. Note also the associated primary acquired melanosis of the conjunctiva.

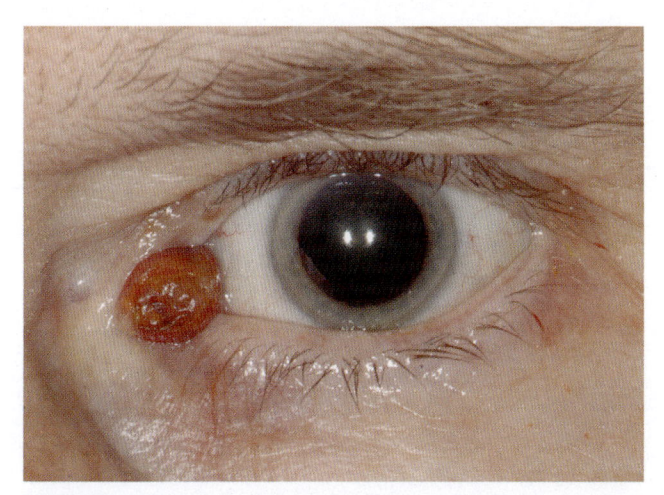

Figure 23.15. Ulcerated caruncular amelanotic melanoma in an elderly man.

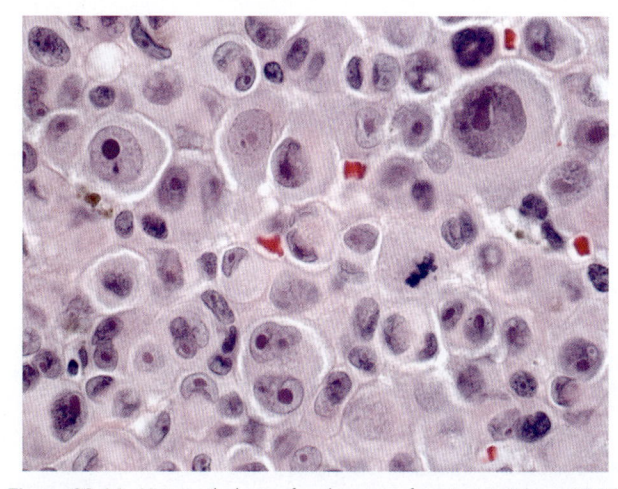

Figure 23.16. Histopathology of melanoma of patient in Figure 23.15, demonstrating highly anaplastic melanoma cells with pleomorphism, prominent nucleoli, and mitotic activity. (Hematoxylin–eosin ×250.)

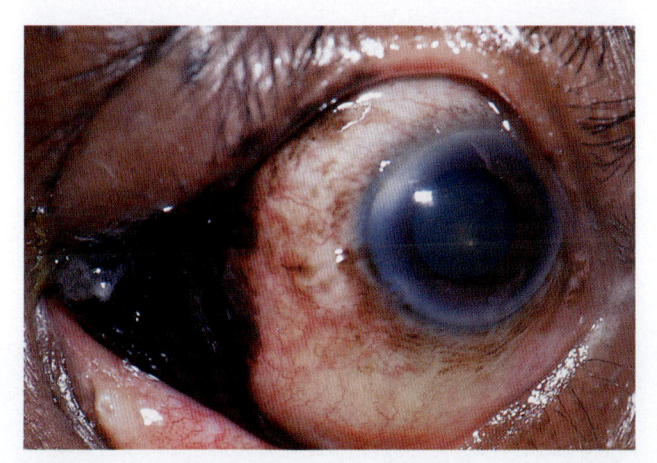

Figure 23.17. Caruncular melanoma arising from primary acquired melanosis in a 71-year-old African-American patient.

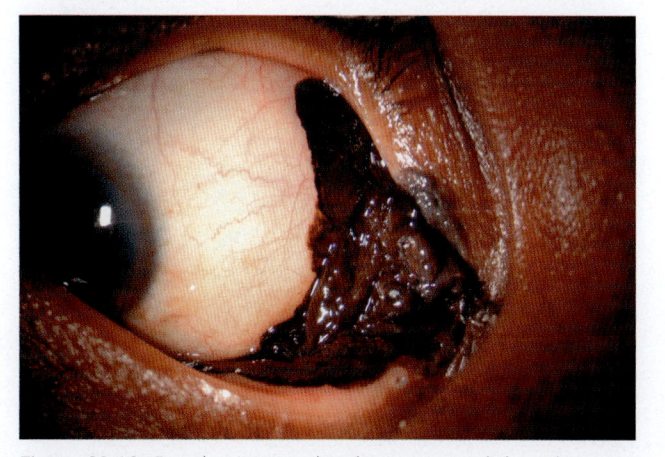

Figure 23.18. Deeply pigmented melanoma in medial canthus, presumably arising from conjunctival primary acquired melanosis in an African-American man.

CARUNCULAR ONCOCYTOMA

Oncocytoma is a rather common lesion of the lacrimal gland, where it generally remains asymptomatic. In the caruncle, it is more likely to become clinically apparent as a solid or cystic mass.

Shields CL, Shields JA, Arbizo V, et al. Oncocytoma of the caruncle. *Am J Ophthalmol* 1986;102:315.

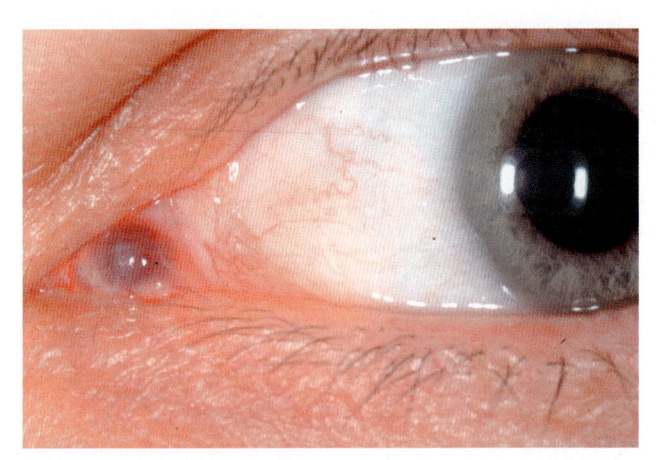

Figure 23.19. Caruncular oncocytoma. Note the blue color and cystic appearance.

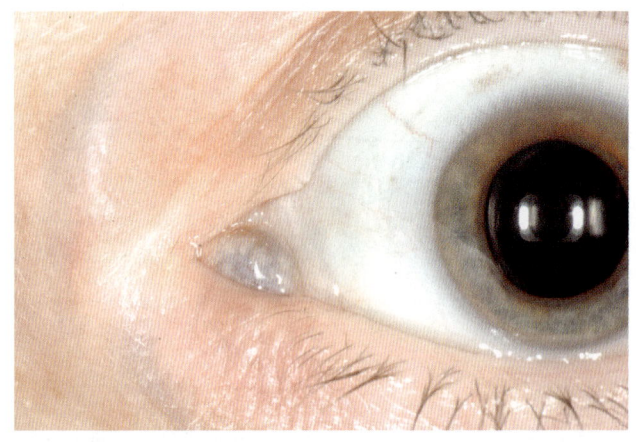

Figure 23.20. Caruncular oncocytoma with a blue cystic appearance color in an elderly woman.

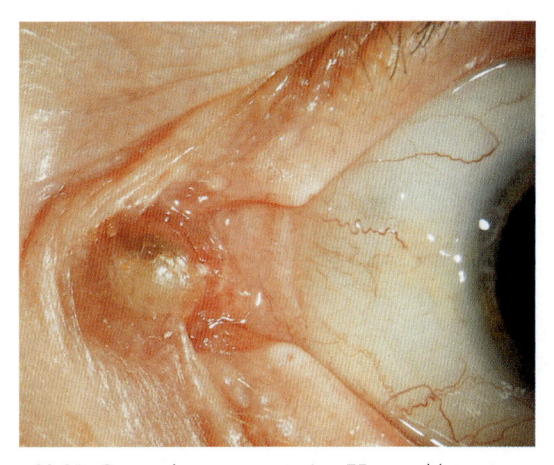

Figure 23.21. Caruncular oncocytoma in a 75-year-old man.

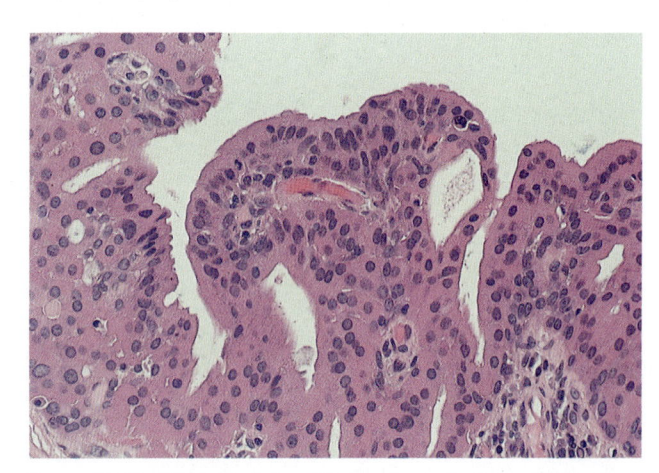

Figure 23.22. Histopathology of lesion shown in Figure 23.21, showing lining of cystic area with epithelial cells with granular cytoplasm. (Hematoxylin–eosin ×75.)

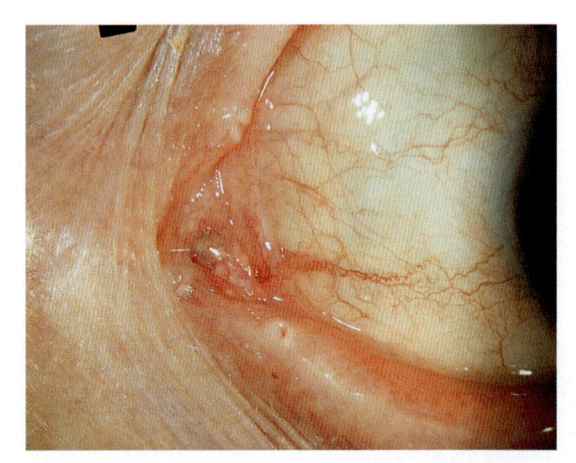

Figure 23.23. Caruncular oncocytoma in a 78-year-old woman.

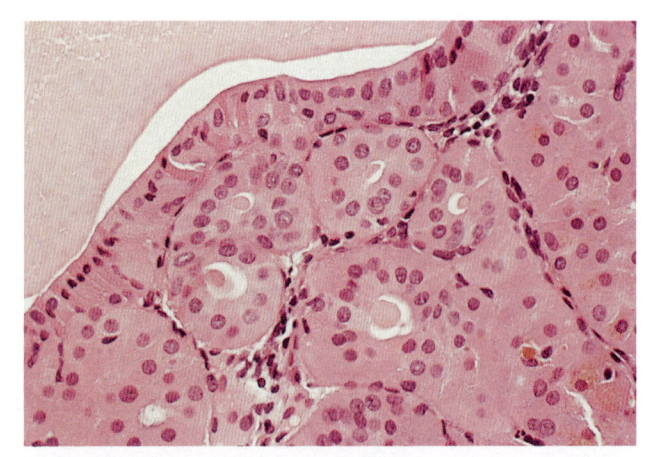

Figure 23.24. Histopathology of lesion shown in Figure 23.23, showing the lining of cystic area with uniform epithelial cells with granular cytoplasm with acini formation. (Hematoxylin–eosin ×90.)

CARUNCULAR SEBACEOUS TUMORS

Because the caruncle has numerous sebaceous glands, it is not surprising that the sebaceous gland cyst, hyperplasia, adenoma, and carcinoma can arise in that tissue.

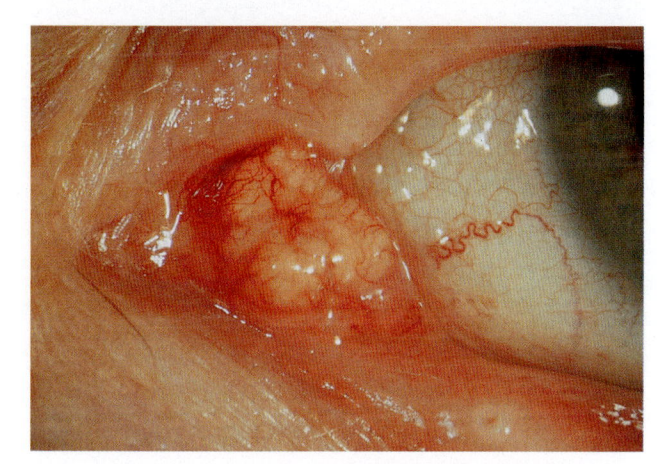

Figure 23.25. Sebaceous gland hyperplasia of the caruncle in a 60-year-old woman.

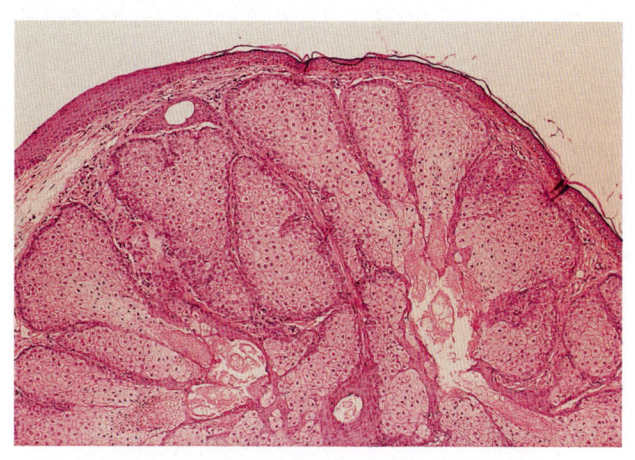

Figure 23.26. Histopathology of lesion depicted in Figure 23.25, showing lobules of well-differentiated sebaceous glands. (Hematoxylin–eosin ×50.)

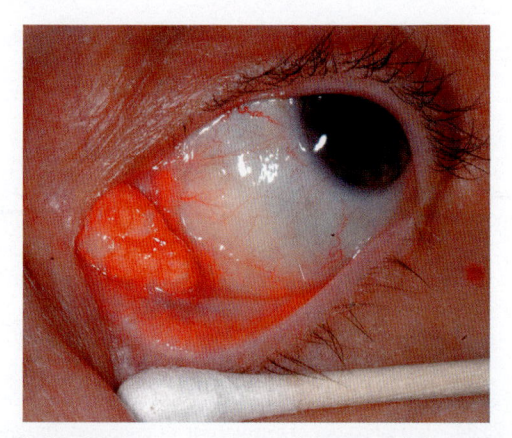

Figure 23.27. Sebaceous carcinoma of the caruncle in a 68-year-old woman. Note the clinical similarity to the sebaceous gland hyperplasia shown in Figure 23.25.

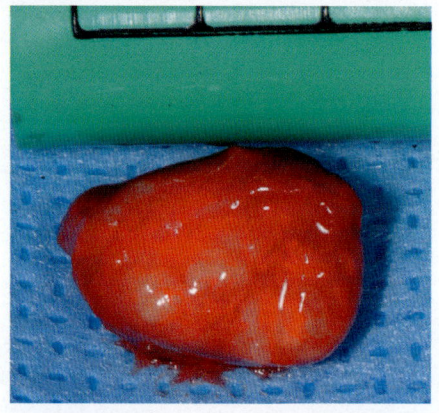

Figure 23.28. Gross appearance of excised lesion in Figure 23.27. The mass was excised intact.

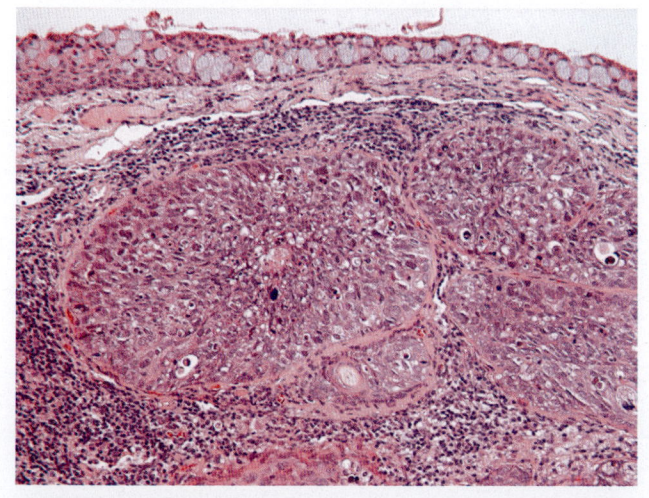

Figure 23.29. Photomicrograph of lesion shown in Figure 23.27, demonstrating lobule of malignant sebaceous cells. Note the rather intense infiltration of lymphocytes. The overlying conjunctival epithelium shows goblet cells but no epithelial invasion by the neoplasm. (Hematoxylin–eosin ×75.)

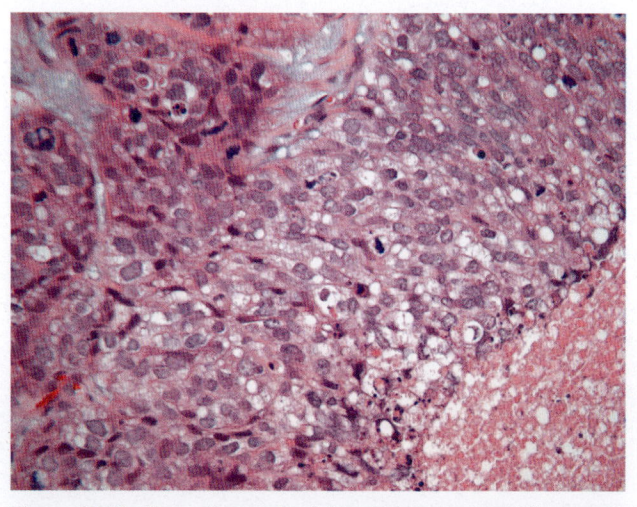

Figure 23.30. Photomicrograph of same lesion showing higher-magnification view of malignant cells. Note the vacuolated cytoplasm of the tumor cells and several mitotic figures. (Hematoxylin–eosin ×150.)

CARUNCULAR CYSTS

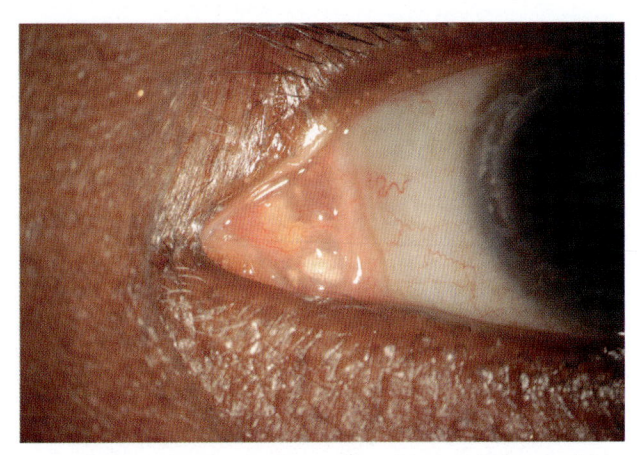

Figure 23.31. Inclusion cyst of caruncle. In this case the lesion is blue.

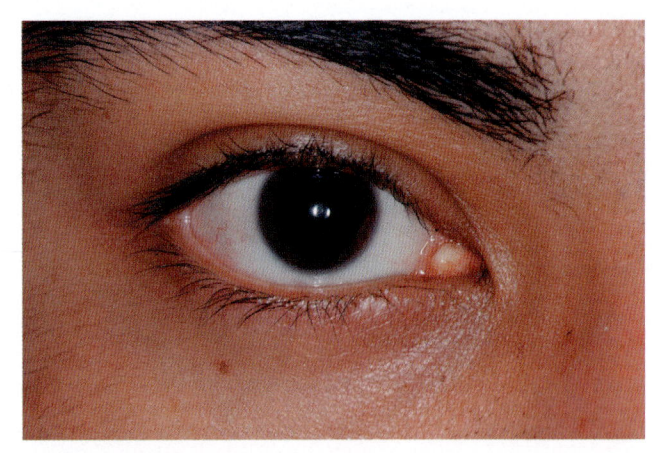

Figure 23.32. Sebaceous cyst. The diagnosis was uncertain but the yellow color suggested a sebaceous cyst.

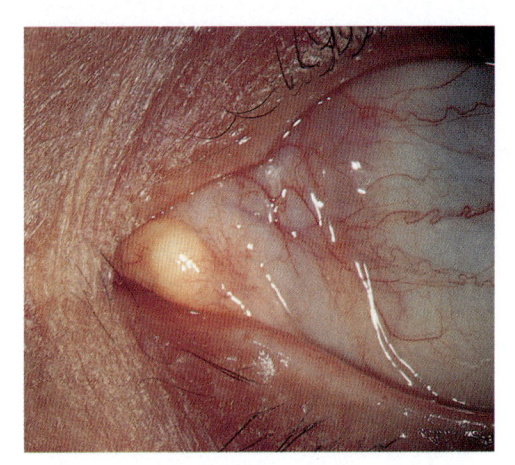

Figure 23.33. Sebaceous cyst of the caruncle in a 49-year-old woman.

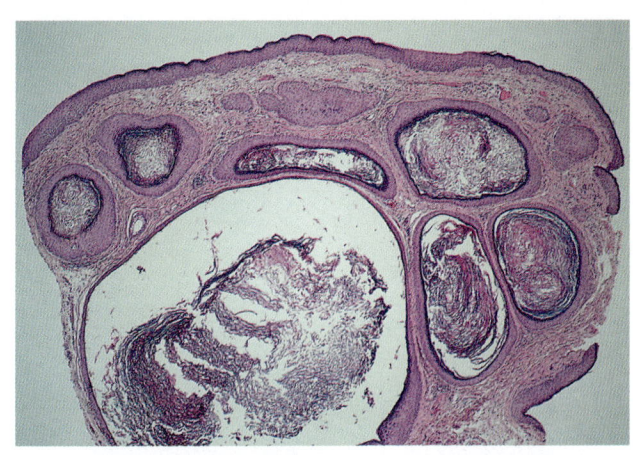

Figure 23.34. Histopathology of a caruncular inclusion cyst. The lesion has keratin in the lumen. It was uncertain as to whether the lesion should be classified as a sebaceous cyst or epidermoid cyst. (Hematoxylin–eosin ×15.)

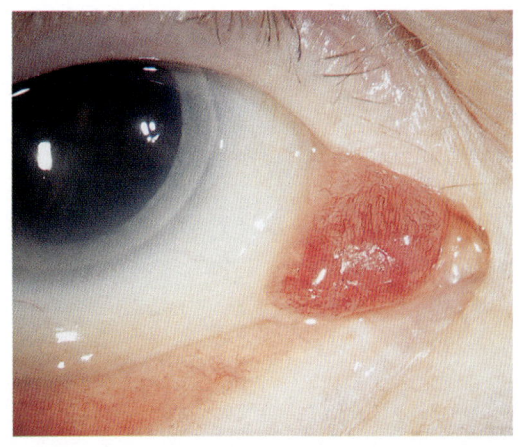

Figure 23.35. Epithelial inclusion cyst of caruncle in an 82-year-old woman.

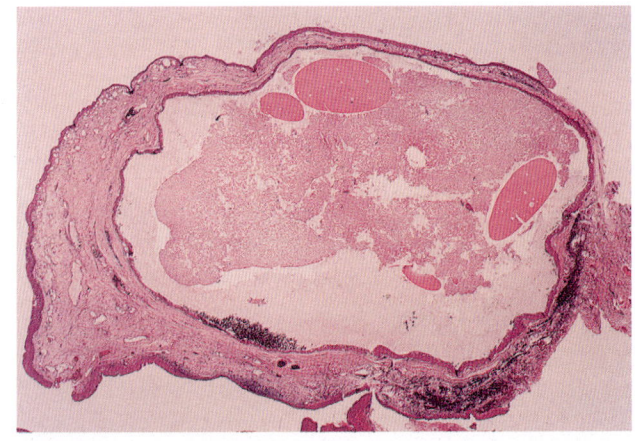

Figure 23.36. Histopathology of lesion shown in Figure 23.35, showing epithelial-lined cyst with epithelial debris in the lumen. (Hematoxylin–eosin ×15.)

MISCELLANEOUS CARUNCULAR TUMORS

Several eyelid and conjunctival lesions that were previously described can also occur in the caruncle. These include pyogenic granuloma, Kaposi sarcoma, cavernous hemangioma, lymphoma, and fibroma.

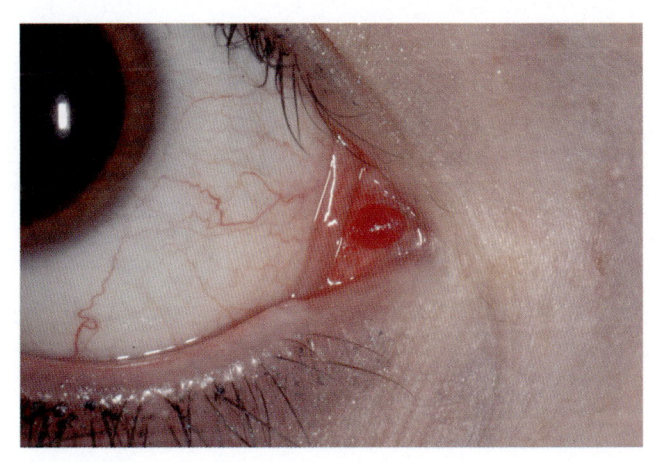

Figure 23.37. Pyogenic granuloma of the caruncle in a young woman.

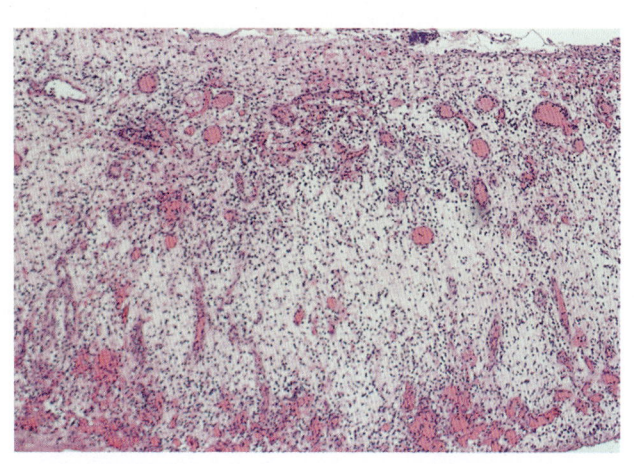

Figure 23.38. Histopathology of pyogenic granuloma showing fine vascular channels and acute and chronic inflammatory cells. (Hematoxylin–eosin ×75.)

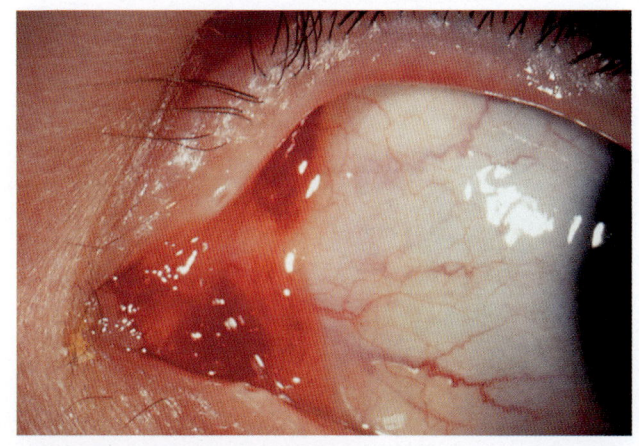

Figure 23.39. Kaposi sarcoma of the caruncle in a 34-year-old man with acquired immunodeficiency syndrome.

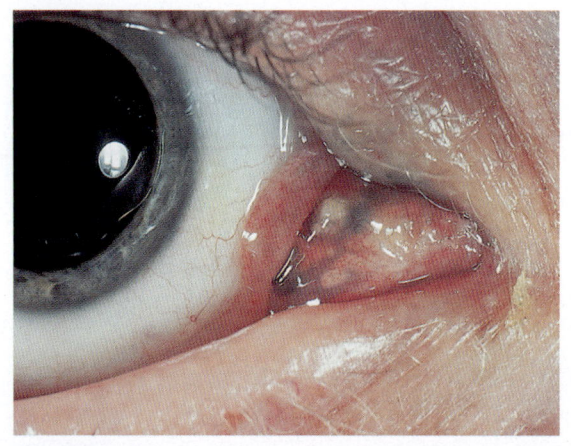

Figure 23.40. Cavernous hemangioma of the caruncle. (Courtesy of Andrew Ferry, MD.)

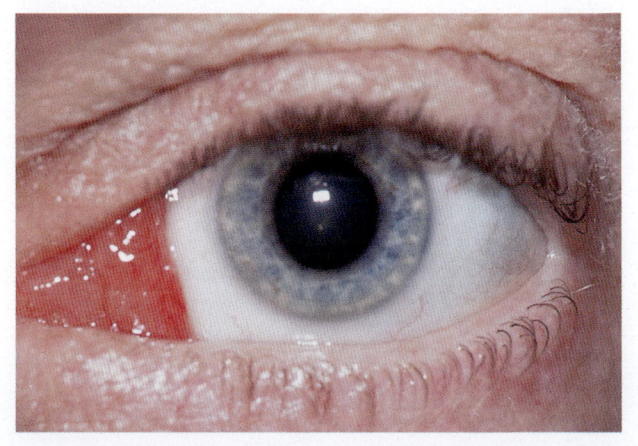

Figure 23.41. Lymphoma affected mainly the caruncle with some involvement of the adjacent conjunctiva in a 54-year-old man.

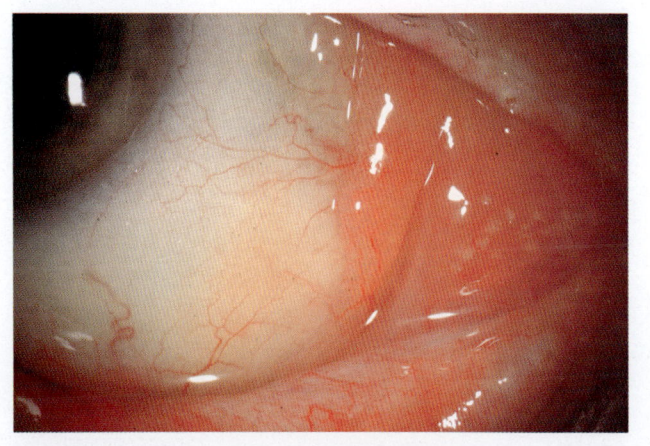

Figure 23.42. Diffuse mass in caruncle and plica region that proved on biopsy to be benign reactive lymphoid hyperplasia.

CHAPTER 24

MISCELLANEOUS LESIONS THAT SIMULATE CONJUNCTIVAL NEOPLASMS

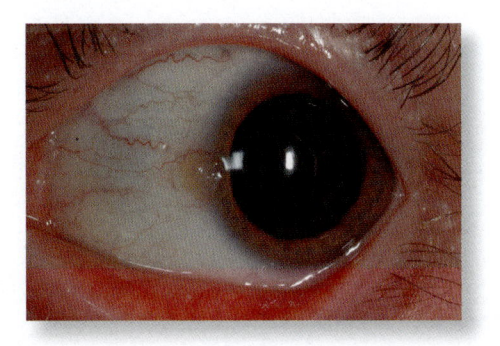

General Considerations

Several primary cystic lesions can occur in the conjunctiva (1–14). Although conjunctival epithelial inclusion cyst is a common lesion, surprisingly little has been written on this subject and it is only mentioned briefly in the literature. It is usually stationary and recognized readily on slit-lamp examination as a clear, round cyst, deep to the epithelium. Observation, marsupialization, or surgical excision is recommended. Occasionally a conjunctival inclusion cyst becomes large and symptomatic and extends into the orbit. In such cases, surgical excision is necessary (9,10). In other instances, a conjunctival inclusion cyst can be larger or atypical and the possibility of a neoplasm prompts surgical excision.

Clinical Features

Clinically, a conjunctival inclusion cyst is a smooth, thin-walled lesion. It may contain clear or slightly turbid fluid. In some instances, epithelial debris secreted into the lumen of the cyst can deposit inferiorly and assume a "pseudohypopyon" appearance. Particularly in dark-skinned patients, a cyst can be lined with pigment, leading to clinical suspicion of malignant melanoma (3). Conjunctival-orbital cyst has been observed in patients with mucous membrane disorders, like Steven–Johnson syndrome (4).

Although most conjunctival cysts are simple inclusion cysts, there are many causes of a cystic lesion of the conjunctiva, including epithelial implantation cysts from surgical or nonsurgical trauma and parasitic cysts. Some tumors, like lymphangioma and diffuse conjunctival nevus, can be highly cystic (15,16).

Pathology

Histopathologically, an epithelial inclusion cyst is usually lined by conjunctival epithelium. The lumen can be clear or it can contain mucinous material, epithelial debris, and occasionally keratin. In some instances, the keratin or sebaceous debris can gravitate inferiorly to form an intracystic "pseudohypopyon."

Management

In most instances, a conjunctival inclusion cyst can be followed and the lesion may eventually disappear. Larger lesions that produce symptoms or raise suspicion of a neoplasm can be excised locally. Some authors have recommended using indocyanine green solution to facilitate visualization of the cyst during surgery. The prognosis is generally excellent. Sometimes, a cyst may show progressive enlargement and become so extensive that excision may be necessary.

CONJUNCTIVAL EPITHELIAL INCLUSION CYST

Selected References

Reviews

1. Shields CL, Demirci H, Karatza E, et al. Clinical survey of 1643 melanocytic and nonmelanocytic tumors of the conjunctiva. *Ophthalmology* 2004;111:1747–1754.
2. Shields CL, Shields JA. Tumors of the conjunctiva and cornea. *Surv Ophthalmol* 2004;49:3–24.

Case Reports

3. Jahnle R, Shields JA, Bernardino V, et al. Pigmented conjunctival inclusion cyst simulating a malignant melanoma. *Am J Ophthalmol* 1985;100:483–484.
4. Desai V, Shields CL, Shields JA. Orbital cyst in a patient with Stevens Johnson syndrome. *Cornea* 1992;11:592–594.
5. Bouncier T, Monin C, Baudrimont M, et al. Conjunctival inclusion cyst following pars plana vitrectomy. *Arch Ophthalmol* 2003;121:1067.
6. Raina UK, Jain S, Arora R, et al. Photographic documentation of spontaneous extrusion of a subconjunctival cysticercus cyst. *Clin Exp Ophthalmol* 2002;30:361–362.
7. Kobayashi A, Saeki A, Nishimura A, et al. Visualization of conjunctival cyst by indocyanine green. *Am J Ophthalmol* 2002;133:827–828.
8. Agarwal M, Amitava AK. Spontaneous expulsion of a subconjunctival cysticercus cyst. *J Pediatr Ophthalmol Strabismus* 2000;37:371–372.
9. Basar E, Pazarli H, Ozdemir H, et al. Subconjunctival cyst extending into the orbit. *Int Ophthalmol* 1998;22:341–343.
10. Shields JA, Shields CL. Orbital cysts of childhood—classification, clinical features and management. The 2002 Angeline Parks lecture. *Surv Ophthalmol* 2004;49:281–299.
11. Song JJ, Finger PT, Kurli M, et al. Giant secondary conjunctival inclusion cysts: a late complication of strabismus surgery. *Ophthalmology* 2006;113(6):1049.
12. Jakobiec FA, Mehta M, Sutula F. Keratinous cyst of the palpebral conjunctiva. *Ophthal Plast Reconstr Surg* 2009;25(4):337–339.
13. Pereira LS, Hwang TN, McCulley TJ. Marsupialization of orbital conjunctival inclusion cysts related to strabismus surgery. *J Pediatr Ophthalmol Strabismus* 2009;46(3):180–181.
14. Mendoza PR, Jakobiec FA, Yoon MK. Keratinous cyst of the palpebral conjunctiva: new observations. *Cornea* 2013;32(4):513–516.

Differential Diagnosis

15. Shields CL, Fasiudden A, Mashayekhi A, et al. Conjunctival nevi: Clinical features and natural course in 410 consecutive patients. *Arch Ophthalmol* 2004;122:167–175.
16. Shields CL, Regillo A, Mellen PL, et al. Giant conjunctival nevus: clinical features and natural course in 32 cases. *JAMA Ophthalmol* 2013;131:857–863.

Chapter 24 Miscellaneous Lesions That Simulate Conjunctival Neoplasms

CONJUNCTIVAL EPITHELIAL INCLUSION CYST

1. Shields CL, Demirci H, Karatza E, et al. Clinical survey of 1643 melanocytic and nonmelanocytic tumors of the conjunctiva. *Ophthalmology* 2004;111:1747–1754.
2. Jahnle R, Shields JA, Bernardino V, et al. Pigmented conjunctival inclusion cyst simulating a malignant melanoma. *Am J Ophthalmol* 1985;100:483–484.

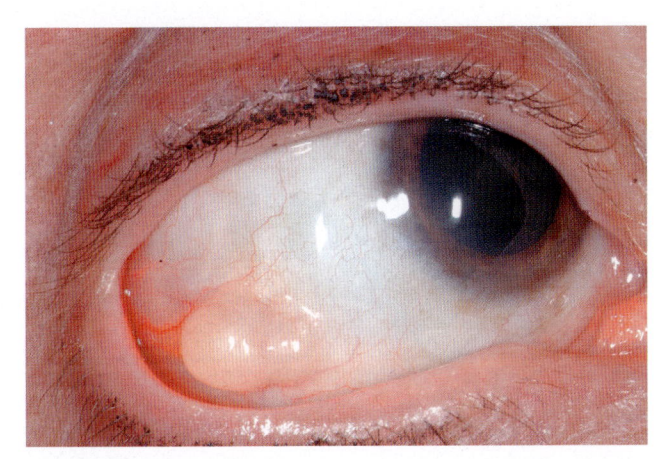

Figure 24.1. Inferotemporal epithelial inclusion cyst in bulbar conjunctiva in a middle-aged woman.

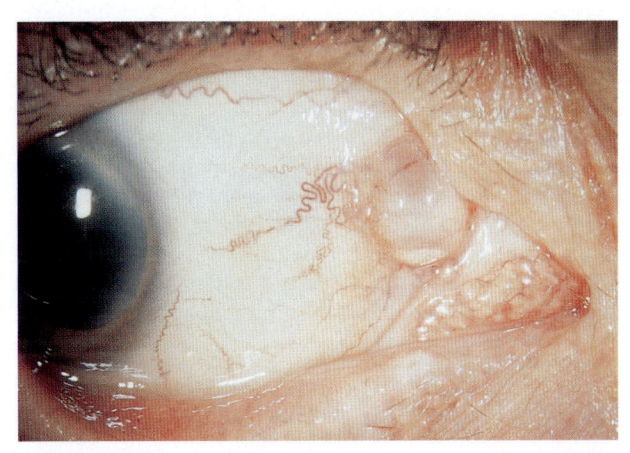

Figure 24.2. Nasal conjunctival inclusion cyst with layered epithelial debris in the lumen, forming a "pseudohypopyon" in a 61-year-old man.

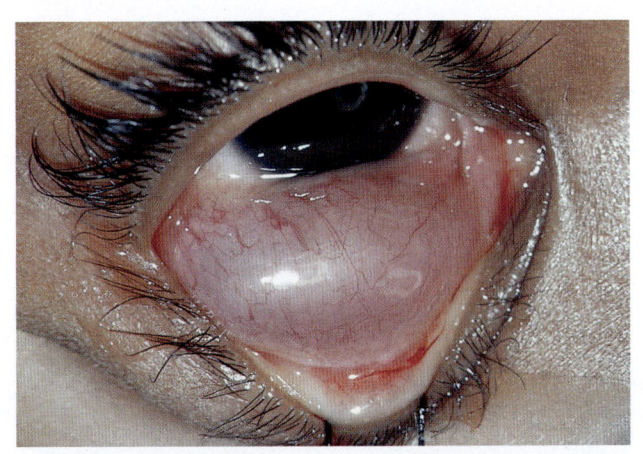

Figure 24.3. Giant epithelial inclusion involving the inferior conjunctiva in a 5-year-old girl. With meticulous dissection, the cyst was removed, leaving intact the overlying surface epithelium.

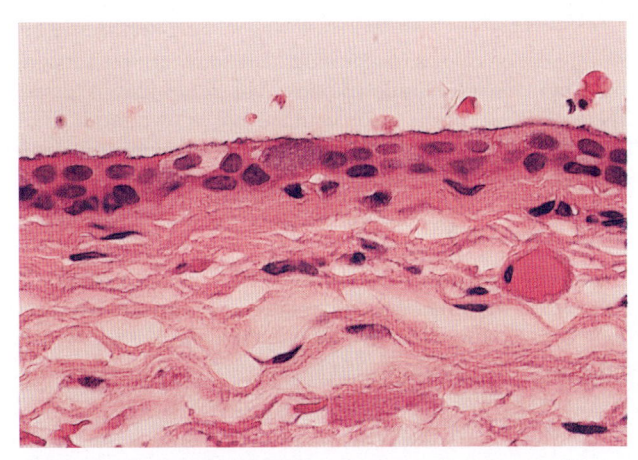

Figure 24.4. Histopathology of lesion in Figure 24.3, showing the nonkeratinizing epithelium lining the cyst. (Hematoxylin–eosin ×10.)

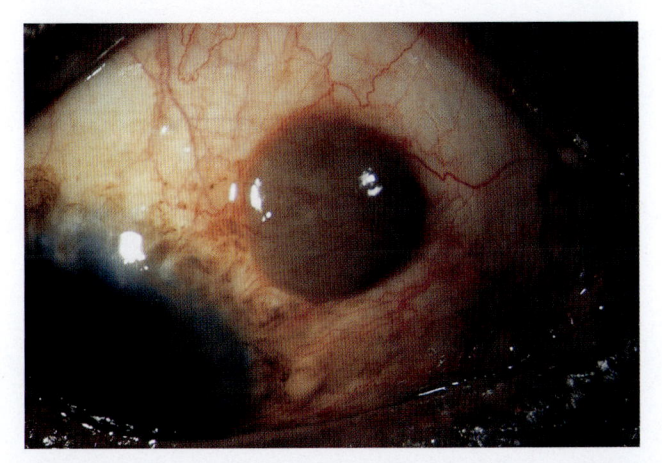

Figure 24.5. Pigmented epithelial inclusion cyst simulating a conjunctival melanoma in a 62-year-old African-American patient.

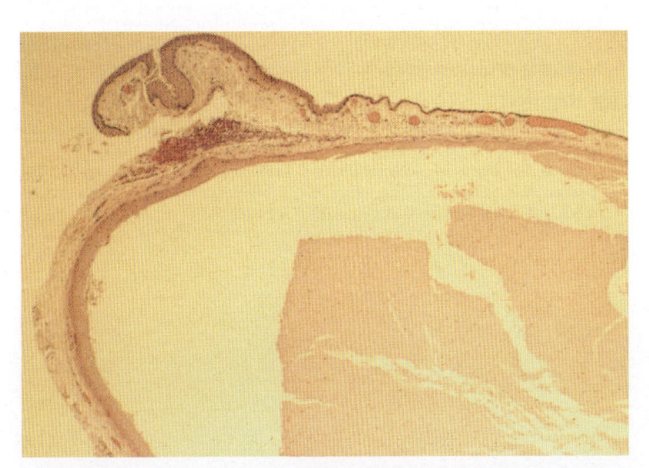

Figure 24.6. Histopathology of lesion shown in Figure 24.5. Much of the melanotic appearance was due to pigment in the surface epithelium over the cyst, rather than pigment in the wall of the cyst. (Hematoxylin–eosin ×10.)

CONJUNCTIVAL ORGANIZING HEMATOMA ("HEMATIC CYST"; "HEMATOCELE")

General Considerations

Organizing hematoma is a circumscribed blood clot that can simulate a pigmented tumor. In the ocular area, the lesion is best known to occur under the periosteum of the orbit, often after overt or occult trauma (1–5). Although the terms "hematic cyst" or "hematocele" were previously used by most authors, it has recently been stressed that, because it lacks a true epithelial lining, the term "cyst" is inappropriate and "organizing hematoma" is the preferred terminology. In the conjunctiva, an organizing hematoma can occur spontaneously, after surgical or nonsurgical trauma. Bleeding around an implant for retinal detachment repair can occasionally be confused with conjunctival melanoma (4). Orbital and conjunctival cysts occur occasionally in the anophthalmic orbit following enucleation.

Clinical Features

Organizing hematoma is often dark in color, suggesting a malignant melanoma (1,2,4). However, it generally lacks feeder vessels or episcleral sentinel vessels.

Pathology

Histopathologically, an organizing hematoma is a pseudocyst, lined by a pseudocapsule composed of dense fibrous tissue. The central part of the lesion contains breakdown products of blood including cholesterol and a golden-yellow bile pigment called hematoidin (4).

Management

Organizing hematoma can be observed if blood is expected. However, if the lesion does not resolve and produces a foreign body sensation or other symptoms, then surgical excision is justified.

Selected References

Reviews

1. Shields JA, Mashayekhi A, Kligman BE, et al. Vascular tumors of the conjunctiva in 140 cases. *Ophthalmology* 2011;118:1747–1753.
2. Welch J, Srinivasan S, Lyall D, et al. Conjunctival lymphangiectasia: a report of 11 cases and review of the literature. *Surv Ophthalmol* 2012;57:136–148.
3. Shapiro A, Tso MO, Putterman AM, et al. A clinicopathologic study of hematic cysts of the orbit. *Am J Ophthalmol* 1986;102:237–241.

Case Reports

4. Lieb WE, Shields JA, Shields CL, et al. Postsurgical hematic cyst simulating a conjunctival malignant melanoma. *Retina* 1990;10:63–67.
5. Quezada AA, Shields CL, Wagner RS, et al. Lymphangioma of the conjunctiva and nasal cavity in a child presenting with diffuse subconjunctival hemorrhage and nosebleeds. *J Pediatr Ophthalmol Strabismus* 2007;44:180–182.

CONJUNCTIVAL ORGANIZING HEMATOMA SECONDARY TO SILICONE SPONGE FOR RETINAL DETACHMENT REPAIR

Chronic bleeding around a sponge used for retinal detachment repair can simulate a conjunctival melanoma, as occurred in this 75-year-old man 15 years after retinal detachment surgery.

Lieb WE, Shields JA, Shields CL, et al. Postsurgical hematic cyst simulating a conjunctival malignant melanoma. *Retina* 1990;10:63–67.

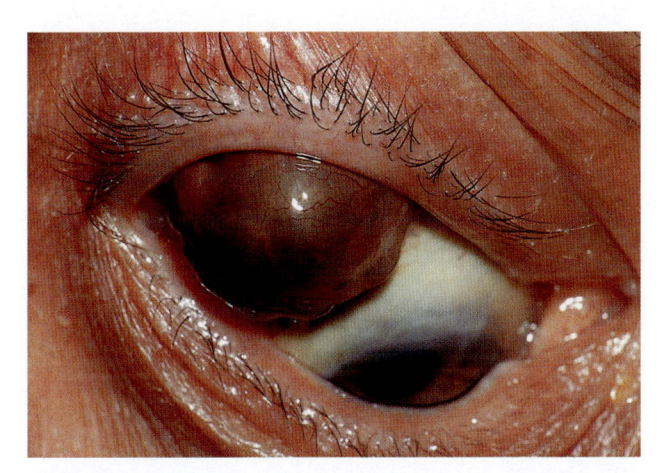

Figure 24.7. Dome-shaped pigmented mass in conjunctiva superotemporally. Note the lack of large feeding and draining blood vessels that would generally be evident in a true melanoma.

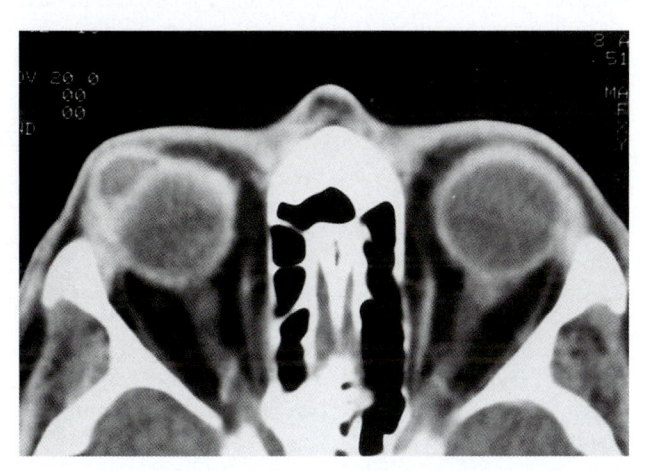

Figure 24.8. Axial computed tomograph showing that the lesion in Figure 24.7 has a cystic, rather than a solid, appearance.

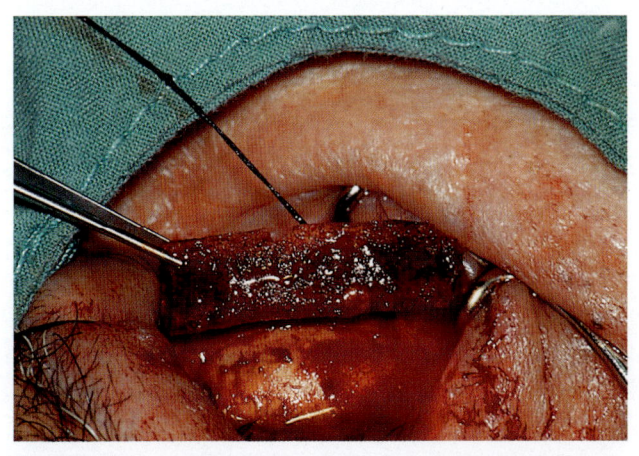

Figure 24.9. View of the sponge used in prior retinal detachment surgery several years earlier, surrounded by blood at the time of surgical removal.

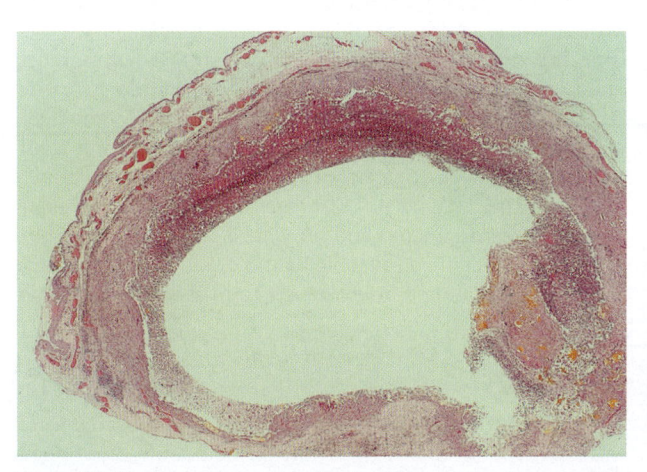

Figure 24.10. Photomicrograph showing clear space that was filled with blood products before their liberation at surgery and during histopathologic processing. (Hematoxylin–eosin ×5.)

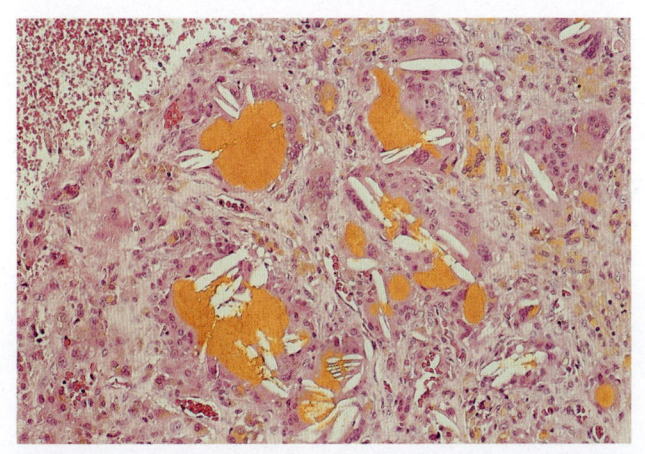

Figure 24.11. Histopathology from wall of cystoid lesion showing foreign body giant cells surrounded by cholesterol clefts and golden-yellow hematoidin pigment. (Hematoxylin–eosin ×100.)

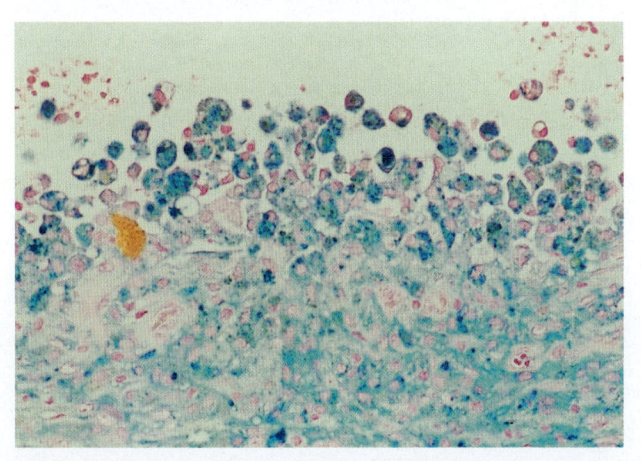

Figure 24.12. Histopathology of cells lining the inner wall of the cysts, showing histiocytes with positive cytoplasmic staining for iron. (Prussian blue stain ×125.)

CONJUNCTIVAL FOREIGN BODY

General Considerations
Several types of foreign body can lodge in the conjunctiva and simulate a neoplasm (1–12). It can result from overt trauma or it can be present without an antecedent history of injury. It is most frequent in carpenters, construction workers, and others with occupations that might subject them to foreign objects. It is important to take a careful history when a foreign body is suspected because the lesion may be noticed many years after the trauma, which may have been forgotten by the patient. Metallic foreign bodies are often dark in color and can be clinically confused with primary acquired melanosis or circumscribed melanoma.

A peculiar form of foreign body is the synthetic fiber granuloma (5–8). It results from the implantation of filamentous synthetic fibers in the conjunctival fornix. It is most often seen in infants and young children who sleep in close contact with toys, such as teddy bears, that have synthetic fibers containing titanium, barium, or zinc.

Clinical Features
The clinical appearance of a conjunctival foreign body varies with the type of foreign object. It is an irregular mass that appears to contain hairs, sometimes suggesting a dermoid, dermolipoma, or caterpillar hairs. However, the hairlike structures are actually synthetic fibers from the toy. Clinically, a metallic foreign body can be black, brown, or gray, suggesting a primary melanoma or extraocular extension of a uveal melanoma. Mascara pigment used to accentuate the eyelashes can rarely imbed in the conjunctiva and simulate a melanoma (9). Some workers have acquired silver pigmentation of their conjunctiva resembling melanoma or melanosis from work-related exposures (12).

Pathology
The pathology of a conjunctival foreign body necessarily varies with the type of object. Most foreign bodies are birefringent with polarized light. With regard to the synthetic fiber granuloma, the hairlike fibers induce an intense granulomatous inflammatory reaction with foreign body giant cells surrounding the foreign material.

Management
Treatment is generally surgical removal. A small, asymptomatic foreign body can be observed without surgical excision.

CONJUNCTIVAL FOREIGN BODY

Selected References

Reviews

1. Shields CL, Demirci H, Karatza E, et al. Clinical survey of 1643 melanocytic and nonmelanocytic tumors of the conjunctiva. *Ophthalmology* 2004;111:1747–1754.
2. Shields CL, Shields JA. Tumors of the conjunctiva and cornea. *Surv Ophthalmol* 2004;49:3–24.
3. Shields CL, Demirci H, Marr BP, et al. Expanding MIRAgel™ scleral buckle simulating an orbital tumor in 4 cases. *Ophthal Plast Reconstr Surg* 2005;21:32–38.

Case Reports

4. Guy JR, Rao NA. Graphite foreign body of the conjunctiva simulating melanoma. *Cornea* 1986;4:263–265.
5. Weinberg JC, Eagle RC, Font RL, et al. Conjunctival synthetic fiber granuloma. A lesion that resembles conjunctivitis nodosa. *Ophthalmology* 1984;91:867.
6. Shields JA, Augsburger JJ, Stechschulte J, et al. Synthetic fiber granuloma of the conjunctiva. *Am J Ophthalmol* 1985;99:598–600.
7. Lueder GT. Synthetic fiber granuloma. *Arch Ophthalmol* 1995;113(7):848–849.
8. Ferry AP. Synthetic fiber granuloma. 'Teddy bear' granuloma of the conjunctiva. *Arch Ophthalmol* 1994;112(10):1339–1341.
9. Shields JA, Marr BP, Shields CL, et al. Conjunctival mascaroma masquerading as melanoma. *Cornea* 2005;24:496–497.
10. Portero A, Carreño E, Galarreta D, et al. Corneal inflammation from pine processionary caterpillar hairs. *Cornea* 2013;32(2):161–164.
11. Lin PH, Wang NK, Hwang YS, et al. Bee sting of the cornea and conjunctiva: management and outcomes. *Cornea* 2011;30(4):392–394.
12. Zografos L, Uffer S, Chamot L. Unilateral conjunctival-corneal argyrosis simulating conjunctival melanoma. *Arch Ophthalmol* 2003;121:1483–1487.

CONJUNCTIVAL FOREIGN BODY

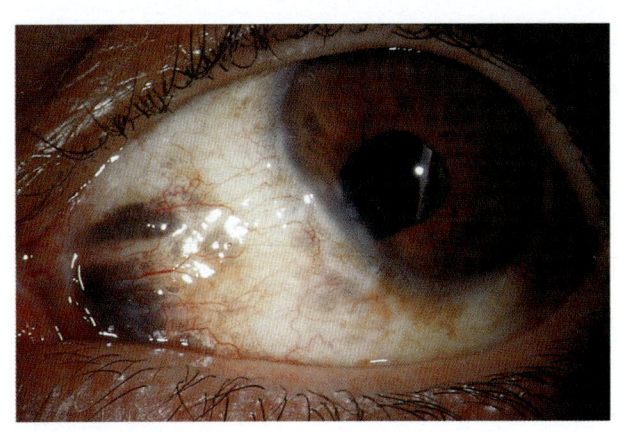

Figure 24.13. Diffuse, dark gray conjunctival lesion in a 51-year-old man who was referred with the diagnosis of conjunctival melanoma arising from primary acquired melanosis. Further history revealed that the patient had been hit in the eye with shrapnel during military activities many years earlier.

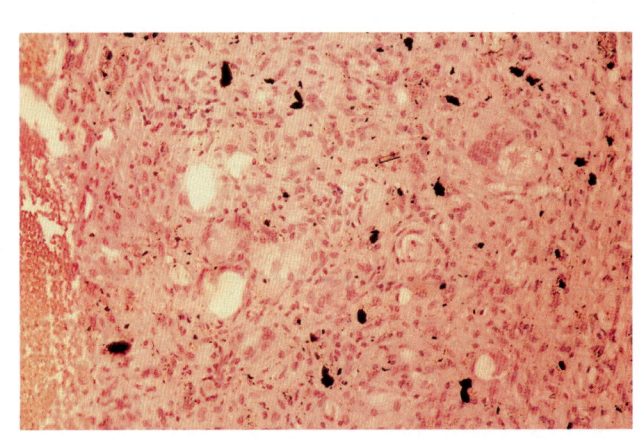

Figure 24.14. Histopathology of the lesion in Figure 24.14, showing tissue containing metallic fragments that stained positive for iron. (Hematoxylin–eosin ×100.)

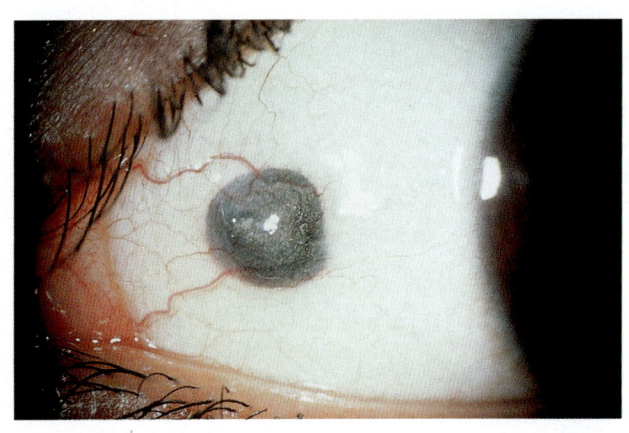

Figure 24.15. Large, gray-black conjunctival lesion in a 24-year-old man referred with the diagnosis of conjunctival melanoma. History revealed that he had been hit in the eye with a pencil at age 7 years. The lesion had gradually enlarged over the last 5 years. (Courtesy of Narsing Rao, MD.)

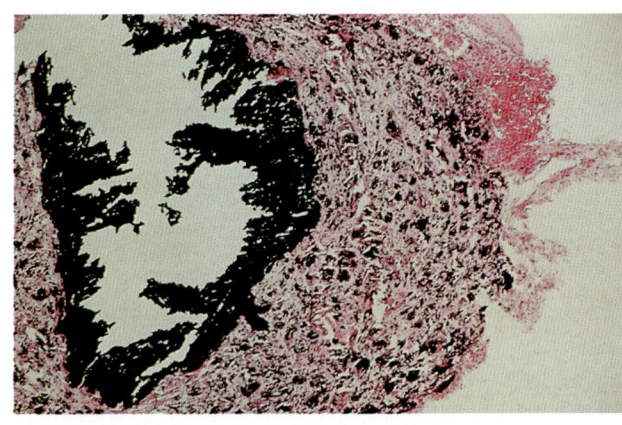

Figure 24.16. Histopathology of the lesion seen in Figure 24.15, showing inflammatory reaction around lead foreign body. (Hematoxylin–eosin ×15.)

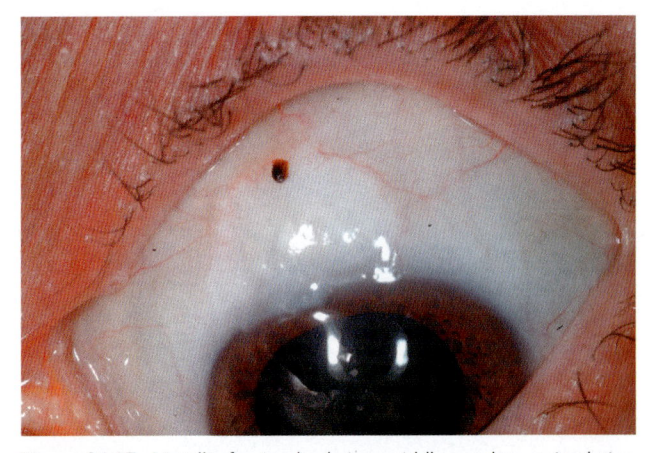

Figure 24.17. Metallic foreign body in a middle-aged man simulating nevus or melanoma. Note the rust deposit on superior margin, suggestive of metallic foreign body. The filtering bleb, performed for glaucoma, is unrelated to the foreign body in this case.

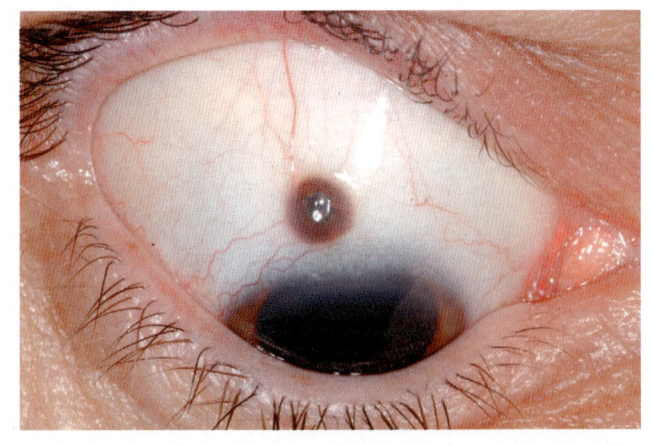

Figure 24.18. Bulbar conjunctiva of right eye of another patient. The lesion was removed and documented to be a metallic foreign body.

Chapter 24 Miscellaneous Lesions That Simulate Conjunctival Neoplasms

● CONJUNCTIVAL FOREIGN BODY

Miscellaneous foreign materials can occur in the conjunctiva and simulate a neoplasm. Unusual examples are shown of synthetic fiber granuloma, MIRAgel retinal detachment implant, and mascara simulating melanoma.

1. Shields CL, Demirci H, Karatza E, et al. Clinical survey of 1643 melanocytic and nonmelanocytic tumors of the conjunctiva. *Ophthalmology* 2004;111:1747–1754.
2. Shields CL, Demirci H, Marr BP, et al. Expanding MIRAgel™ scleral buckle simulating an orbital tumor in 4 cases. *Ophthal Plast Reconstr Surg* 2005;21:32–38.
3. Shields JA, Marr BP, Shields CL, et al. Conjunctival mascaroma masquerading as melanoma. *Cornea* 2005;24:496–497.

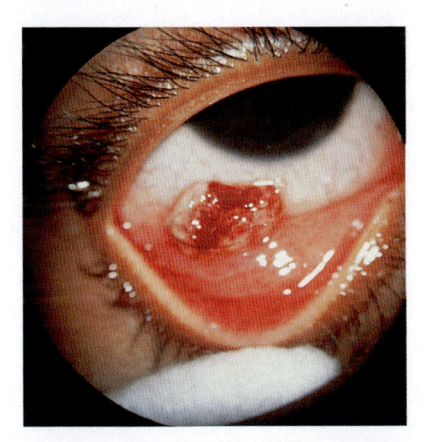

Figure 24.19. Synthetic fiber granuloma in the inferior conjunctiva in a 26-month-old child. The child had slept with a toy teddy bear.

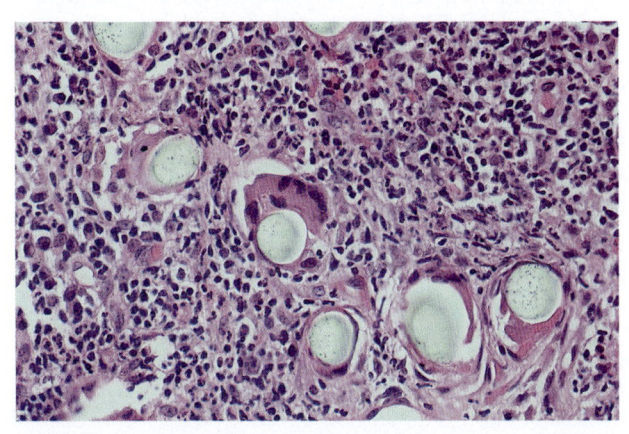

Figure 24.20. Histopathology of lesion shown in Figure 24.19. Note the hairlike structures that are inducing a foreign body inflammatory response with giant cells. (Hematoxylin–eosin ×40.)

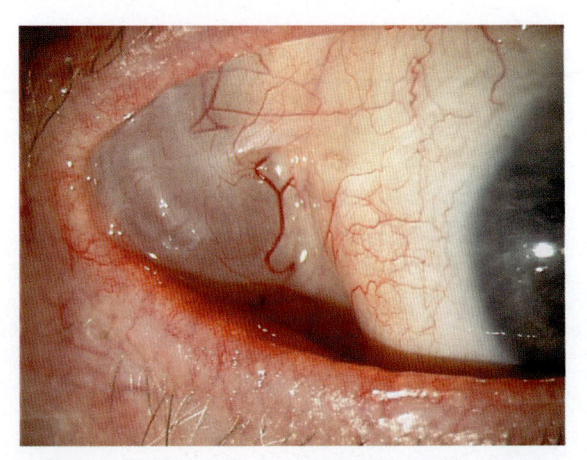

Figure 24.21. MIRAgel retinal detachment implant simulating a neoplasm.

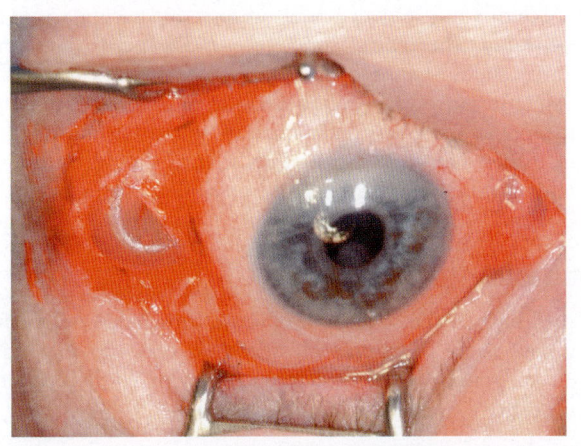

Figure 24.22. MIRAgel implant shown in Figure 24.21 exposed at time of surgical removal.

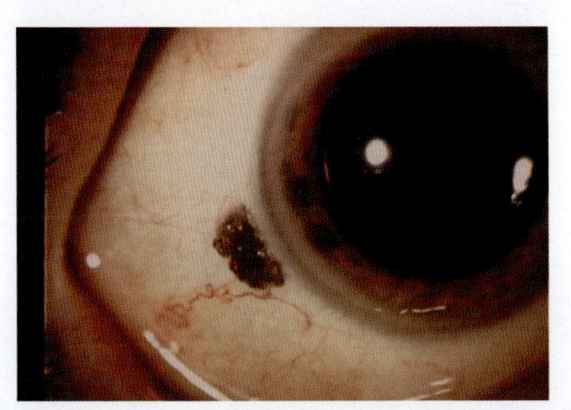

Figure 24.23. Mascara deposit ("mascaroma") near limbus simulating conjunctiva melanoma in a patient who used excessive mascara.

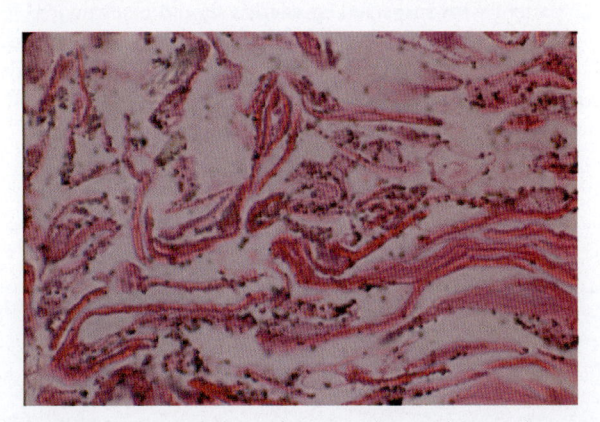

Figure 24.24. Histopathology of mascara deposit showing deposition of mascara in superficial layer of keratin corresponding to the black lesion seen clinically in Figure 24.23. (Hematoxylin–eosin ×50.)

EPISCLERITIS AND SCLERITIS SIMULATING NEOPLASMS

General Considerations

Episcleritis and scleritis can be elevated and vascular, and simulate an amelanotic conjunctival neoplasm, particularly conjunctival squamous cell carcinoma. Nodular episcleritis is a benign, often painful inflammatory condition. It is idiopathic in most instances, but can be related to several inflammatory conditions, including rheumatoid arthritis. It lasts about 2 to 3 weeks, after which it spontaneously resolves (1–4). It has a tendency to recur.

Clinical Features

The acute onset and progression and the associated pain are usually sufficient to differentiate episcleritis from a primary neoplasm, which is usually nonpainful and more slowly progressive. One tumor that can have a similarly rapid onset and pain is metastatic carcinoma to the conjunctiva, which is a rare condition. Episcleritis can be localized (nodular) or diffuse (3).

Scleritis is often a deeper inflammation that may be granulomatous or nongranulomatous in nature (1,2). Almost half of affected patients will be found to have other systemic disease, particularly connective tissue disease such as rheumatoid arthritis. Other cases remain idiopathic despite systemic evaluation (4). Scleritis can lead to scleral necrosis and secondary uveal staphyloma. The typical appearance and associated systemic findings should help to differentiate scleritis from neoplasm. In some instances, however, a necrotic intraocular melanoma can produce secondary inflammation of the sclera and adjacent tissues. Hence, a patient with scleritis should undergo a fundus examination to exclude the possibility of an intraocular neoplasm.

Pathology

Depending on the state of the disease, episcleritis or scleritis can have acute or chronic inflammatory cells and may have signs of granulomatous inflammation with epithelioid and giant cells.

Management

The patient with suspected episcleritis should be evaluated for the known causes of inflammation, such as rheumatoid arthritis and other known granulomatous inflammations. If the lesion does not resolve on systemic or topical corticosteroids, then excisional biopsy may be warranted.

Selected References

1. Homanyounfar G, Nardone N, Borkar DS, et al. Incidence of scleritis and episcleritis: results for the Pacific Ocular Inflammation Study. *Am J Ophthalmol* 2013;156: 752–758.
2. Rothschild PR, Pagnous C, Seror R, et al. Ophthalmologic manifestations of systemic necrotizing vasculitides at diagnosis: a retrospective study of 1286 patients and review of the literature. *Semin Arthritis Rheum* 2013;42:507–514.
3. Watson PG. The diagnosis and management of scleritis. *Ophthalmology* 1980;87: 716–720.
4. Rao NA, Marak GE, Hidayat AA. Necrotizing scleritis. A clinicopathologic study of 41 cases. *Ophthalmology* 1985;92;1542–1549.

Chapter 24 Miscellaneous Lesions That Simulate Conjunctival Neoplasms

EPISCLERITIS AND SCLERITIS

Shields CL, Demirci H, Karatza E, et al. Clinical survey of 1643 melanocytic and nonmelanocytic tumors of the conjunctiva. *Ophthalmology* 2004;111:1747–1754.

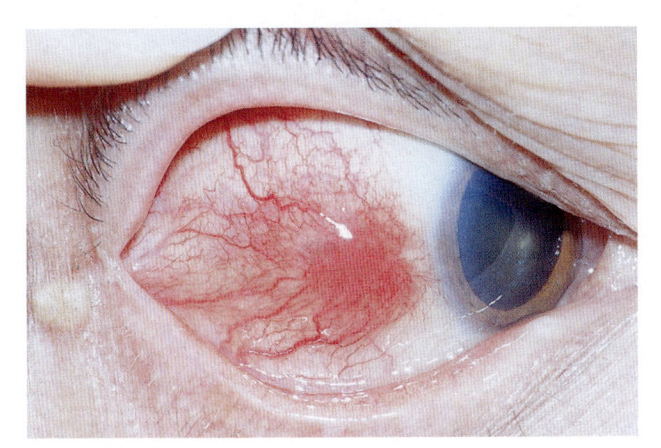

Figure 24.25. Diffuse episcleritis in a 67-year-old man.

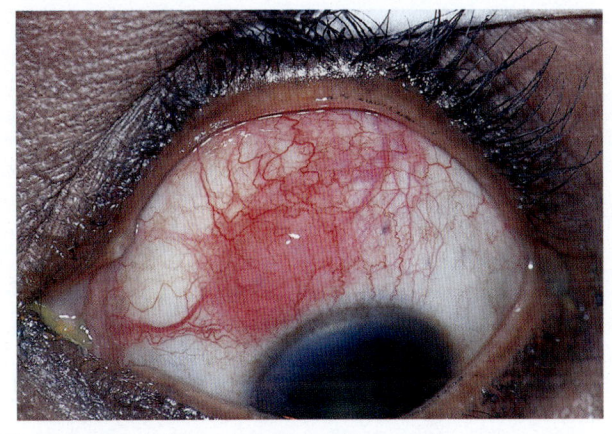

Figure 24.26. Nodular episcleritis in a 61-year-old woman.

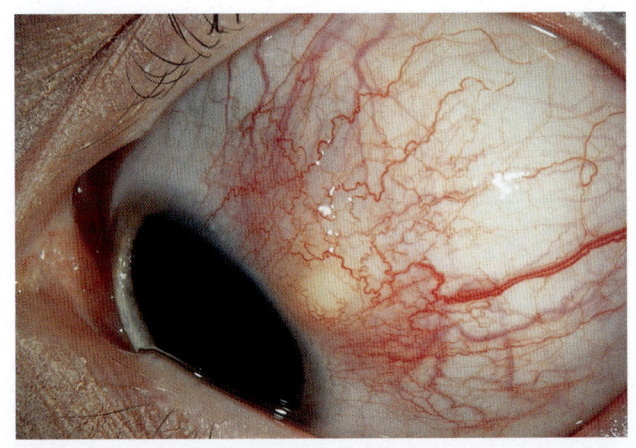

Figure 24.27. Nodular scleritis near the limbus in a 25-year-old woman.

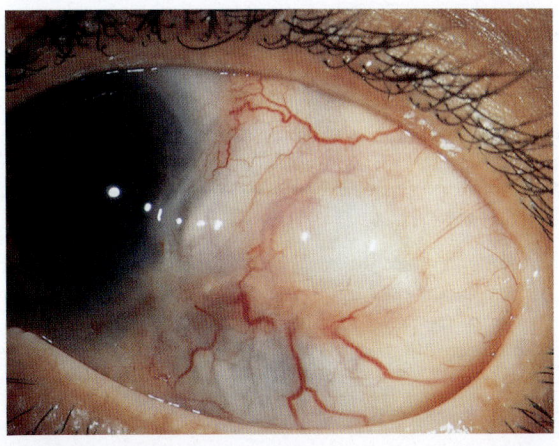

Figure 24.28. Nodular scleritis simulating a nonpigmented neoplasm in a 63-year-old woman.

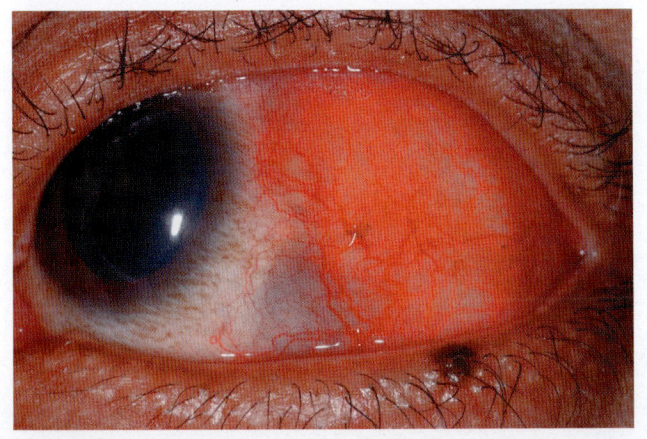

Figure 24.29. Diffuse inflammation of conjunctiva and sclera of uncertain etiology in an elderly African-American patient. Systemic evaluation for sarcoidosis was negative. Biopsy was eventually done.

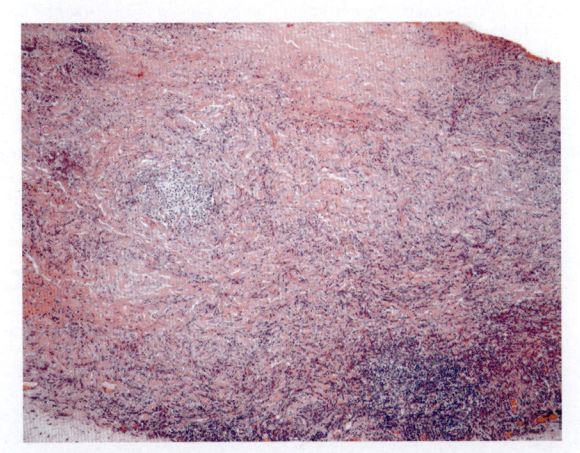

Figure 24.30. Histopathology of lesion shown in Figure 24.29, revealing diffuse infiltration of chronic inflammatory cells in the sclera. The patient had no systemic diseases that could be related to the ocular process. (Hematoxylin–eosin ×50).

CONJUNCTIVAL CHURG–STRAUSS ALLERGIC GRANULOMATOSIS SIMULATING CONJUNCTIVAL NEOPLASM

General Considerations

Churg–Strauss syndrome is an uncommon systemic disease characterized by asthma, eosinophilia, and vasculitis (1–6). Systemic involvement can lead to renal and cardiac failure as well as peripheral neuropathy, and often has a fatal outcome. The differentiation of Churg–Strauss syndrome from vasculitides like Wegener's granulomatosis and periarteritis nodosa have been described (2). Conjunctival involvement is now known to be a feature of Churg–Strauss syndrome, in which case it can simulate a neoplasm (2–7).

Clinical Features

It tends to be unilateral and appears as a pink, nodular, inflammatory thickening that has a predilection for the upper tarsal conjunctiva, but can involve any part of the bulbar or palpebral conjunctiva. It can simulate squamous cell carcinoma of the conjunctiva or conjunctival involvement with invasive sebaceous gland carcinoma of the eyelid.

Pathology

Histopathologically, the affected tissues show granulomatous inflammation with eosinophils and necrotizing vasculitis. There is noncaseating, granulomatous inflammation with lymphocytes, plasma cells, giant cells, and numerous eosinophils.

Management

The lesion must be differentiated from conjunctival involvement by sebaceous carcinoma or other diffuse neoplasms. If neoplasm is excluded, the conjunctival involvement can often be controlled with local or systemic corticosteroids, but chemotherapy may be required for more severe systemic involvement.

Selected References

Reviews

1. Churg J, Strauss L. Allergic granulomatosis, allergic angiitis, and periarteritis nodosa. *Am J Pathol* 1951;27:277–301.
2. Robin JB, Schanzlin DJ, Meisler DM, et al. Ocular involvement in the respiratory vasculitides. *Surv Ophthalmol* 1985;30:127–140.
3. Cury D, Breakey AS, Payne BF. Allergic granulomatous angiitis associated with uveoscleritis and papilledema. *Arch Ophthalmol* 1955;55:261–266.

Case Reports

4. Meisler DM, Stock EL, Wertz RD, et al. Conjunctival inflammation and amyloidosis in allergic granulomatosis and angiitis (Churg-Strauss syndrome). *Am J Ophthalmol* 1981;91:216–219.
5. Shields CL, Shields JA, Rozanski T. Conjunctival involvement in the Churg-Strauss syndrome. *Am J Ophthalmol* 1986;102:601–605.
6. Margolis R, Kosmorsky GS, Lowder CY, et al. Conjunctival involvement in Churg-Strauss syndrome. *Ocul Immunol Inflamm* 2007;15:113–115.
7. Yaman A, Ozbek Z, Saatci AO, et al. Topical steroids in the management of Churg-Strauss syndrome involving the conjunctiva. *Cornea* 2007;26(4):498–500.

CONJUNCTIVAL CHURG–STRAUSS ALLERGIC GRANULOMATOSIS

1. Meisler DM, Stock EL, Wertz RD, et al. Conjunctival inflammation and amyloidosis in allergic granulomatosis and angiitis (Churg-Strauss syndrome). *Am J Ophthalmol* 1981;91:216–219.
2. Shields CL, Shields JA, Rozanski T. Conjunctival involvement in the Churg-Strauss syndrome. *Am J Ophthalmol* 1986;102:601–605.

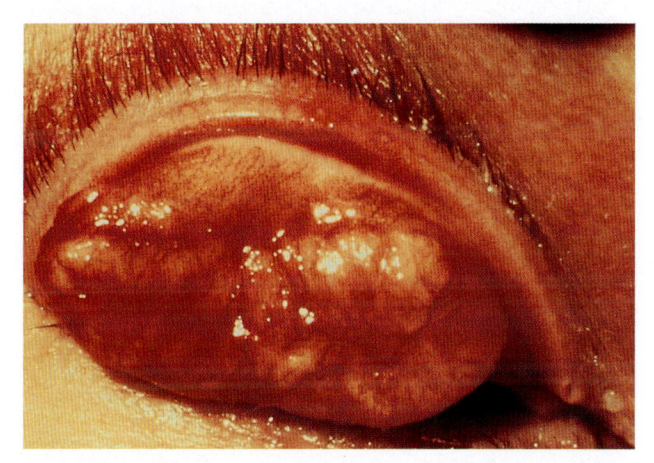

Figure 24.31. Diffuse nodular thickening of the upper palpebral conjunctiva in a 32-year-old woman. (Courtesy of David Meisler, MD and Richard O'Grady, MD.)

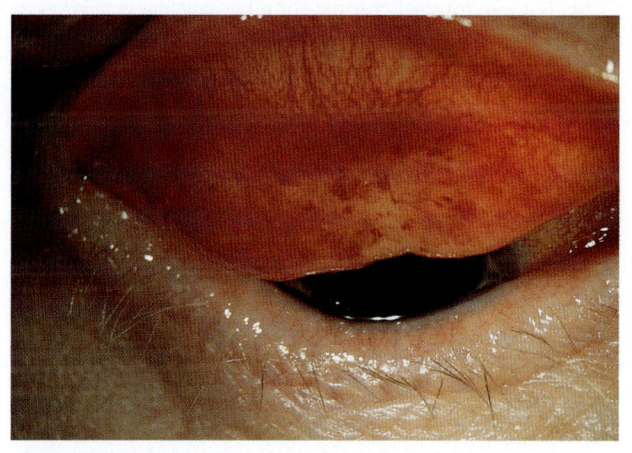

Figure 24.32. Thickening and hyperemia of the upper tarsus in a 64-year-old man with Churg–Strauss syndrome.

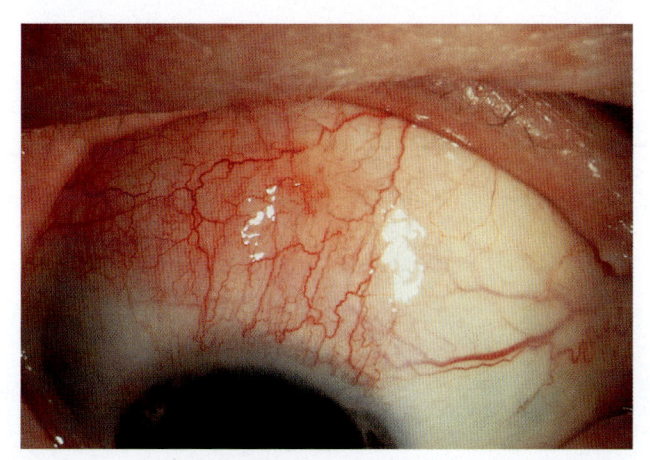

Figure 24.33. Involvement of the upper bulbar conjunctiva in the patient shown in Figure 24.32.

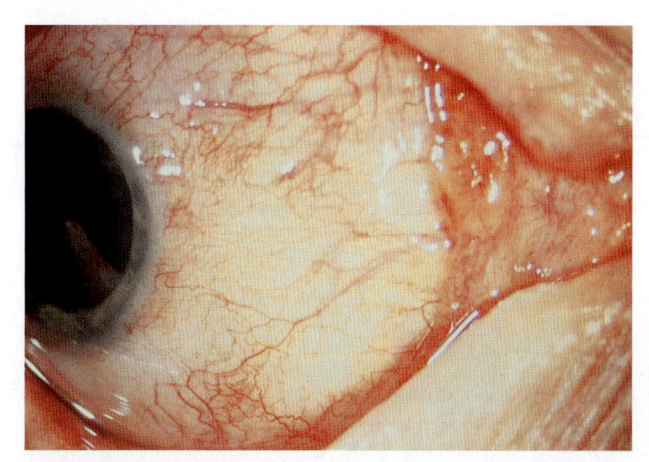

Figure 24.34. Subtle thickening of the semilunar fold in the patient shown in Figure 24.32.

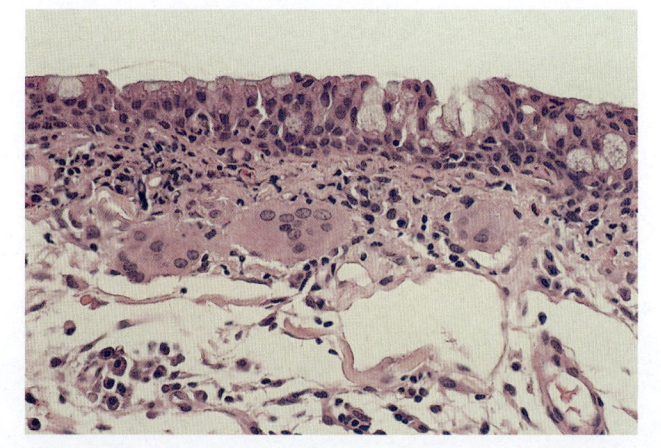

Figure 24.35. Histopathology of lesion shown in Figure 24.32. Note the granulomatous reaction with giant cells immediately beneath the conjunctival epithelium and scattered plasma cells and eosinophils. (Hematoxylin–eosin ×100.)

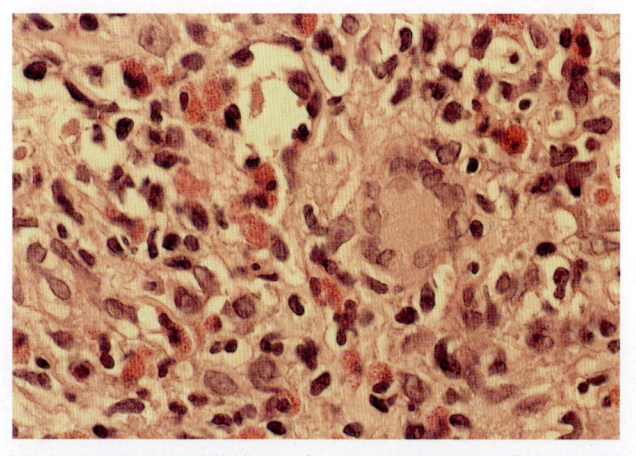

Figure 24.36. Histopathology of conjunctival stroma from patient shown in Figure 24.32. Note the granulomatous inflammation with abundant eosinophils. (Hematoxylin–eosin ×200.)

CONJUNCTIVAL LIGNEOUS CONJUNCTIVITIS

General Considerations

Ligneous conjunctivitis (chronic pseudomembranous conjunctivitis) is a rare form of chronic conjunctivitis characterized by fibrin-rich, woodylike pseudomembranous lesions that usually occur on the tarsal conjunctiva. The lesions may be either unilateral or bilateral (1–10). It usually occurs in childhood with a median age at onset of 5 years, but it can develop in adulthood. It can have its onset after trauma or surgery, particularly for pterygium or pinguecula (3). Affected patients can have similar lesions in the mouth and upper respiratory system, indicating that it is a systemic disease. It has traditionally been presumed to be an autoimmune disease and an autosomal-recessive hereditary pattern has been postulated (10). Systemic plasminogen deficiency has recently been linked to ligneous conjunctivitis in humans and mice (5).

Clinical Features

It appears as a unilateral or bilateral, woody induration of the palpebral conjunctiva, but it can also affect the bulbar and limbal conjunctiva. The lesions are often yellow, white, or red and they can assume a variety of configurations ranging from sessile to pedunculated (1–3).

Pathology

Histopathologically, the conjunctival epithelium is thinned and focally replaced by necrotic fibrinous tissue that may be entrapped in the stroma (7). There are numerous chronic inflammatory cells and new blood vessels in the tissue. The material resembles amyloid, but stains for amyloid are routinely negative (8).

Management

Larger lesions are generally removed surgically and residual or small lesions are treated with topical cyclosporine, corticosteroids, plasmin, or plasminogen (3–6). Amniotic membrane grafting has been used successfully to replace the diseased conjunctiva (6).

Selected References

Reviews

1. Hidayat AA, Riddle PJ. Ligneous conjunctivitis: a clinicopathologic study of 17 cases. *Ophthalmology* 1987;94:949–959.
2. Spencer LM, Straatsma BR, Foos RY. Ligneous conjunctivitis. *Arch Ophthalmol* 1968;80:365–367.
3. Schuster V, Seregard S. Ligneous conjunctivitis. *Surv Ophthalmol* 2003;48:369–388.

Management

4. Rubin BI, Holland EJ, de Smet MD, et al. Response of reactivated ligneous conjunctivitis to topical cyclosporine (letter). *Am J Ophthalmol* 1991;112:95–96.
5. Heidemann DG, Williams GA, Hartzer M, et al. Treatment of ligneous conjunctivitis with topical plasmin and topical plasminogen. *Cornea* 2003;22:760–762.
6. Barabino S, Rolando M. Amniotic membrane transplantation in a case of ligneous conjunctivitis. *Am J Ophthalmol* 2004;137:752–753.

Histopathology

7. Eagle RC Jr, Brooks JS, Katowitz JA, et al. Fibrin as a major constituent of ligneous conjunctivitis. *Am J Ophthalmol* 1986;101:493–494.
8. Holland EJ, Chan CC, Kuwabara T, et al. Immunohistologic findings and results of treatment with cyclosporine in ligneous conjunctivitis. *Am J Ophthalmol* 1989;107:160–166.

Case Reports

9. Girard LJ, Veselinovic A, Font RL. Ligneous conjunctivitis after pinguecula removal in an adult. *Cornea* 1989;8:7–14.
10. Batemen JB, Pettit TH, Isenberg SJ, et al. Ligneous conjunctivitis: an autosomal recessive disorder. *J Pediatr Ophthalmol Strabismus* 1986;23:137–140.

Chapter 24 Miscellaneous Lesions That Simulate Conjunctival Neoplasms 417

CONJUNCTIVAL LIGNEOUS CONJUNCTIVITIS

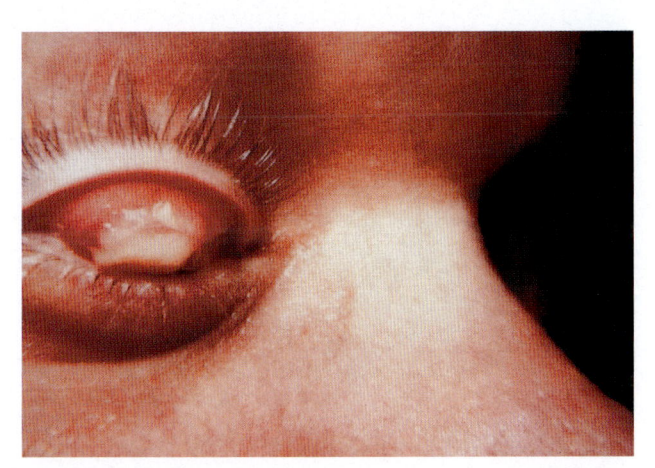

Figure 24.37. Ligneous conjunctivitis of upper palpebral conjunctiva in a 15-year-old boy. (Courtesy of Drs. Charles Steinmetz and Ralph C. Eagle, Jr.)

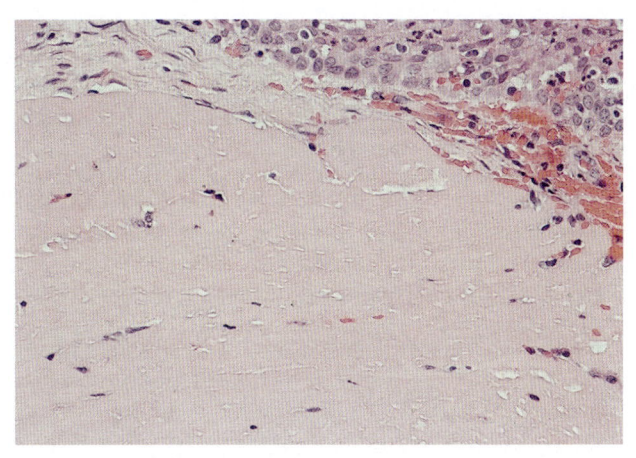

Figure 24.38. Histopathology of lesion in Figure 24.37, showing lightly eosinophilic, amorphous material. (Hematoxylin–eosin ×100.) (Courtesy of Drs. Charles Steinmetz and Ralph C. Eagle Jr.)

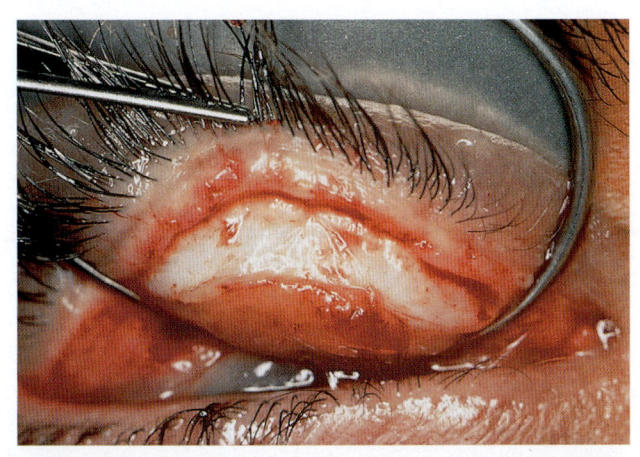

Figure 24.39. Ligneous conjunctivitis of upper palpebral conjunctiva in a 34-year-old woman. (Courtesy of Drs. Douglas Cameron and Edward Holland.)

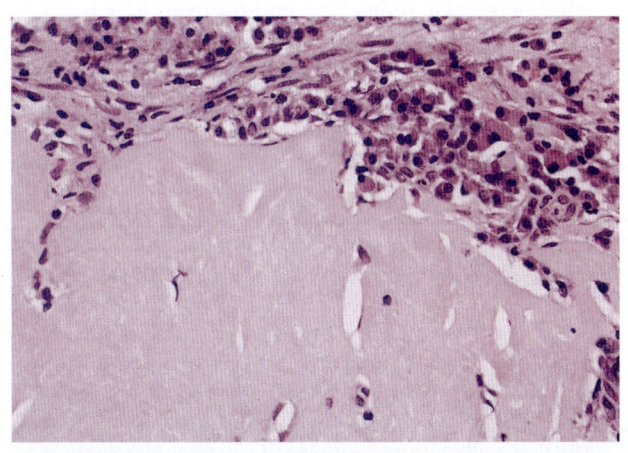

Figure 24.40. Histopathology of lesion in Figure 24.39, showing lightly eosinophilic, amorphous material and chronic inflammatory cells. (Hematoxylin–eosin ×100.) (Courtesy of Drs. Douglas Cameron and Edward Holland.)

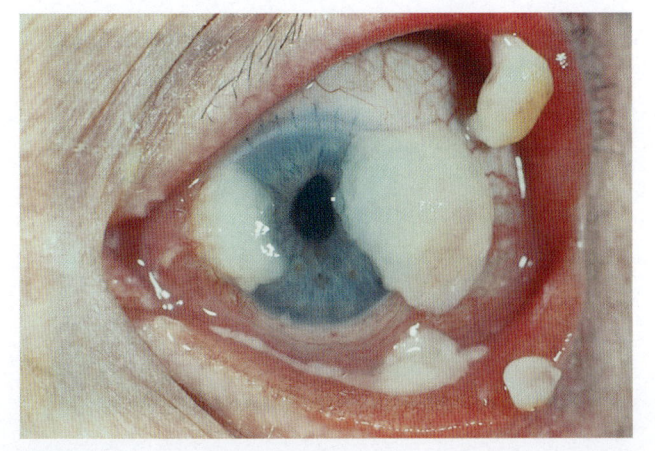

Figure 24.41. Ligneous conjunctivitis involving the palpebral and limbal conjunctiva in a 68-year-old woman. She had cataract surgery and pterygium about 5 months before the onset of these lesions. (Courtesy of Henry Perry, MD.)

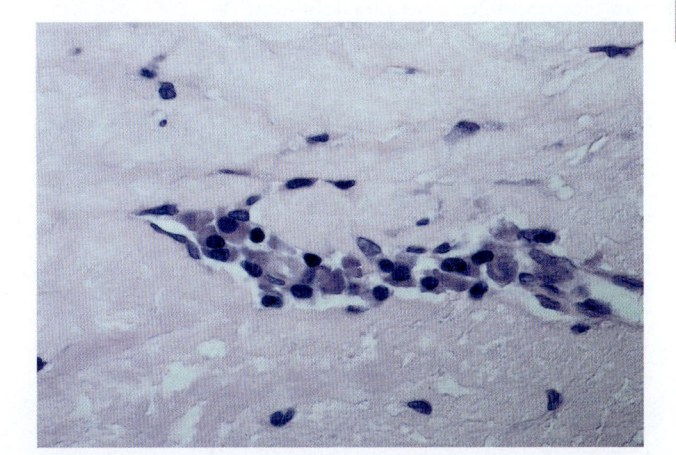

Figure 24.42. Histopathology of lesion in Figure 24.41, showing chronic inflammatory cells within the fibrinous material. (Hematoxylin–eosin ×100.) (Courtesy of Henry Perry, MD.)

CONJUNCTIVAL MISCELLANEOUS INFECTIOUS LESIONS THAT SIMULATE NEOPLASMS

There are numerous conjunctival or episcleral infectious lesions that can occasionally simulate a conjunctival neoplasm (1–9). Selected examples to be illustrated include staphylococcal scleral abscess, molluscum conjunctivitis, tuberculosis, atypical mycobacterium infection, and rhinosporidiosis.

A purulent abscess can sometimes affect the anterior or posterior sclera. It can be red owing to severe inflammation. In many cases, the reason for localization of the infection in the sclera is unknown. Management involves prompt and aggressive antibiotic therapy and draining of the abscess may be necessary (3,9).

Molluscum contagiosum is a viral infection that is well known to involve the eyelids. It often produces an associated follicular conjunctivitis. Occasionally, molluscum contagiosum causes a localized conjunctival lesion that resembles an epithelial tumor of the conjunctiva. Conjunctival molluscum contagiosum infection is seen more frequently in immunosuppressed patients (4).

Tuberculosis can affect the conjunctiva and sclera and can resemble a tumor. It is a granulomatous inflammation that can sometimes assume tumorous proportions. Ocular involvement can be the first and only sign of systemic tuberculosis (5). Atypical mycobacterium infection of the conjunctiva is rarely seen. We are aware of an unusual case of a patient with a white lesion near the limbus that proved to be *Mycobacterium chelonae* infection (4).

Rhinosporidiosis is a fungal infection that can rarely affect either the palpebral or limbal conjunctiva. It can appear clinically as a fleshy, pink nodule that may closely resemble an epithelial neoplasm. However, it contains small, white, cystoid spherules that would not be seen with primary epithelial neoplasms (7).

There has also been a report of a conjunctival mycotic infection that resembled a melanoma (9). *Serratia marcescens* is an opportunistic, gram-negative bacillus that was once considered to be nonpathogenic in humans, but we have managed a patient with a *S. marcescens* abscess of the conjunctiva that clinically resembled a lymphoid infiltrate (9).

CONJUNCTIVAL MISCELLANEOUS INFECTIOUS LESIONS THAT SIMULATE NEOPLASMS

Selected References

Reviews
1. Shields CL, Demirci H, Karatza E, et al. Clinical survey of 1643 melanocytic and nonmelanocytic tumors of the conjunctiva. *Ophthalmology* 2004;111:1747–1754.
2. Shields CL, Shields JA. Tumors of the conjunctiva and cornea. *Surv Ophthalmol* 2004;49:3–24.

Case Reports
3. Kiratli H, Shields JA, Shields CL, et al. Localized transcleral staphylococcal abscess simulating a neoplasm. *German J Ophthalmol* 1995;4:302–305.
4. Charles NC, Friedberg DN. Epibulbar molluscum contagiosum in acquired immunodeficiency syndrome. *Ophthalmology* 1992;99:1123–1126.
5. Regillo C, Shields CL, Shields JA, et al. Ocular tuberculosis. *JAMA* 1991;266:1490.
6. Margo CE. Atypical mycobacterium infection of the conjunctiva. Presented at the Eastern Ophthalmic Pathology Meeting. 1995.
7. Reidy JJ, Sudesh S, Klafter AB, et al. Infection of the conjunctiva by Rhinosporidium seeberi. *Surv Ophthalmol* 1997;41:409–413.
8. Laquis SJ, Wilson MW, Haik BG, et al. Conjunctival mycosis masquerading as melanoma. *Am J Ophthalmol* 2002;134:117–118.
9. Shields JA, Shields CL, Eagle RC Jr, et al. Localized infection by Serratia marcescens simulating a conjunctival neoplasm. *Am J Ophthalmol* 2000;129:247–248.

CONJUNCTIVAL MISCELLANEOUS INFECTIOUS LESIONS THAT SIMULATE NEOPLASMS

1. Kiratli H, Shields JA, Shields CL, et al. Localized transcleral staphylococcal abscess simulating a neoplasm. *German J Ophthalmol* 1995;4:302–305.
2. Charles NC, Friedberg DN. Epibulbar molluscum contagiosum in acquired immunodeficiency syndrome. *Ophthalmology* 1992;99:1123–1126.
3. Reidy JJ, Sudesh S, Klafter AB, et al. Infection of the conjunctiva by Rhinosporidium seeberi. *Surv Ophthalmol* 1997;41:409–413.
4. Regillo C, Shields CL, Shields JA, et al. Ocular tuberculosis. *JAMA* 1991;266:1490.

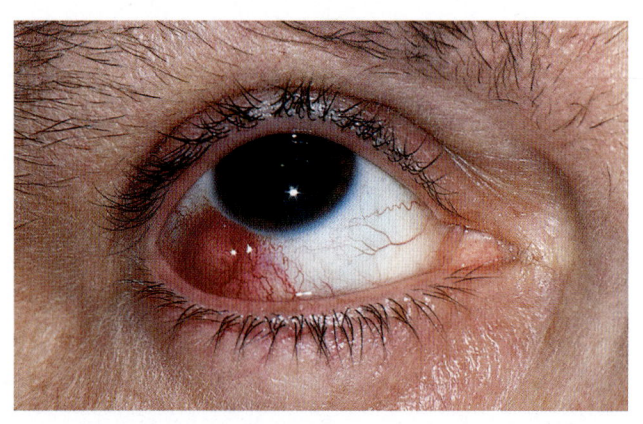

Figure 24.43. Spontaneous staphylococcal abscess in a 47-year-old woman. The lesion extended through the sclera necessitating a scleral graft. The patient had an excellent recovery after antibiotic treatment.

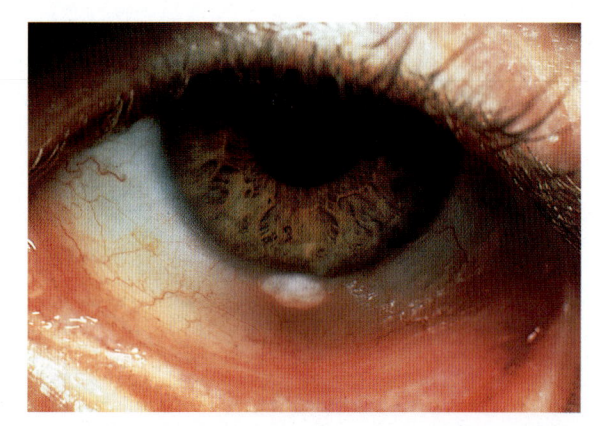

Figure 24.44. Solitary lesion of molluscum contagiosum at the inferior limbus in a patient with acquired immunodeficiency syndrome. (Courtesy of Norman Charles, MD.)

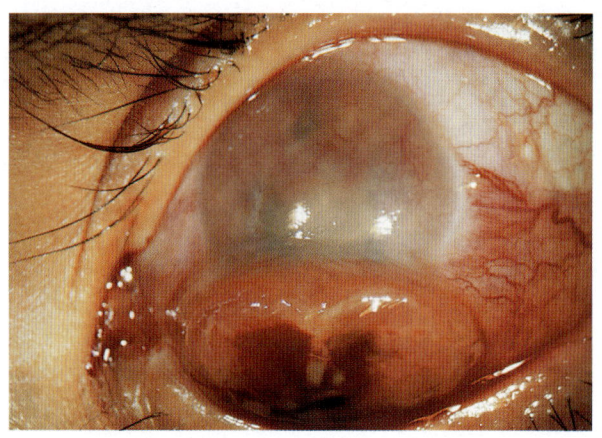

Figure 24.45. Large tuberculous granuloma involving the conjunctiva and sclera inferior to the limbus in a 29-year-old woman from Ecuador. The patient had no known history of findings of tuberculosis, but had been treated for uveitis that was believed to be secondary to sarcoidosis. The blind, painful eye was enucleated and the acid-fast organisms were demonstrated microscopically.

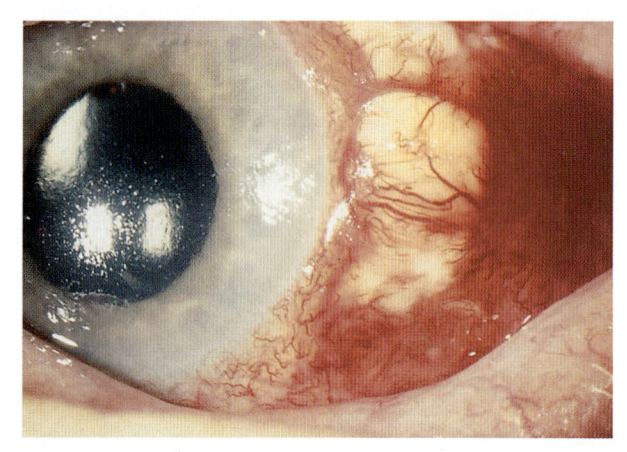

Figure 24.46. Conjunctival infection with *Mycobacterium chelonae* simulating a squamous cell neoplasm. The patient had previously undergone excision and irradiation for a squamous cell carcinoma of the ipsilateral upper eyelid. (Courtesy of Curtis Margo, MD.)

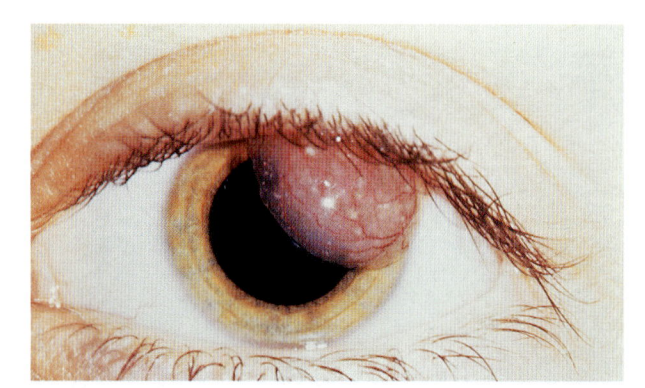

Figure 24.47. Conjunctival mass secondary to rhinosporidiosis in an 11-year-old boy. (Courtesy of James Reidy, MD.)

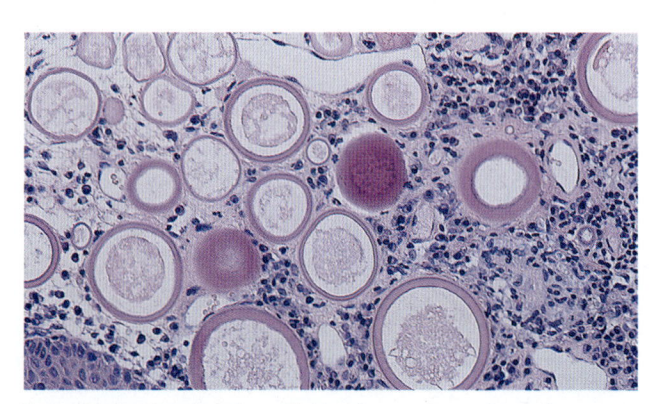

Figure 24.48. Histopathology of lesion shown in Figure 24.47, demonstrating multiple sporangia surrounded by chronic inflammatory cells in the subepithelial region. (Hematoxylin–eosin ×50.) (Courtesy of James Reidy, MD.)

Chapter 24 Miscellaneous Lesions That Simulate Conjunctival Neoplasms

CONJUNCTIVAL MISCELLANEOUS INFECTIOUS LESIONS THAT SIMULATE NEOPLASMS

Shields JA, Shields CL, Eagle RC Jr, et al. Localized infection by Serratia marcescens simulating a conjunctival neoplasm. *Am J Ophthalmol* 2000;129:247–248.

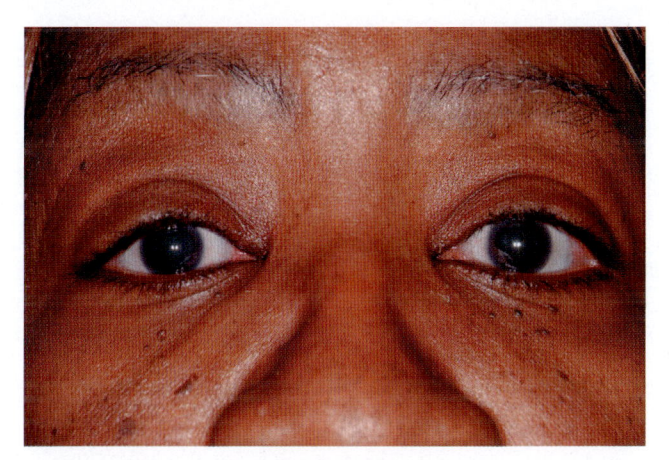

Figure 24.49. Facial appearance of African-American man showing slight conjunctival redness temporally in left eye.

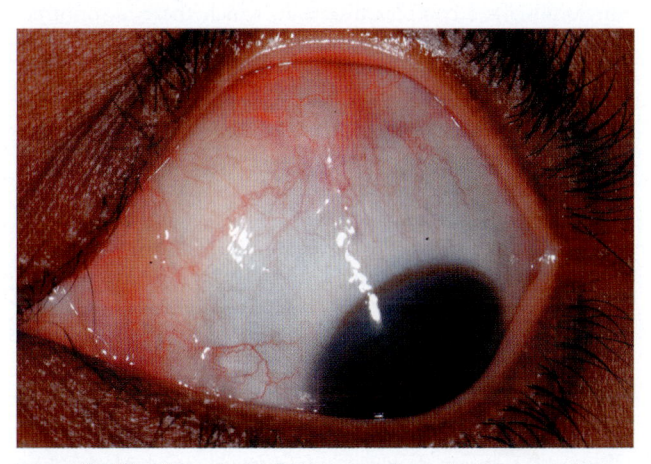

Figure 24.50. Closer view of conjunctiva in patient shown in Figure 24.49. Sarcoidosis was confirmed on conjunctival biopsy. The patient had systemic sarcoidosis but no other ocular involvement.

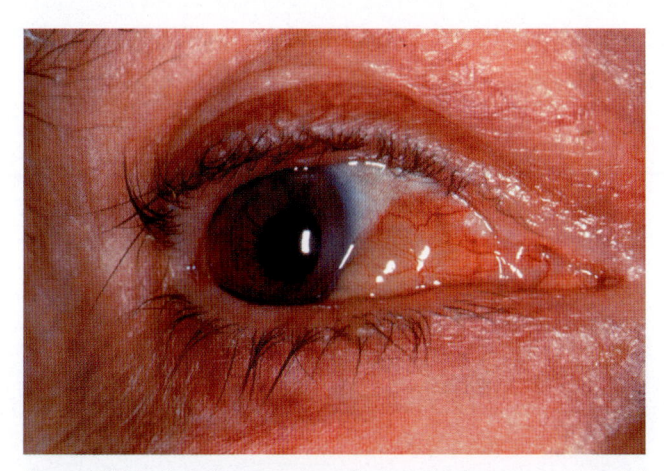

Figure 24.51. *Serratia marcescens* abscess simulating a conjunctival lymphoma. This yellow-pink lesion is in the bulbar conjunctiva of an elderly man who had prior cataract and glaucoma surgery.

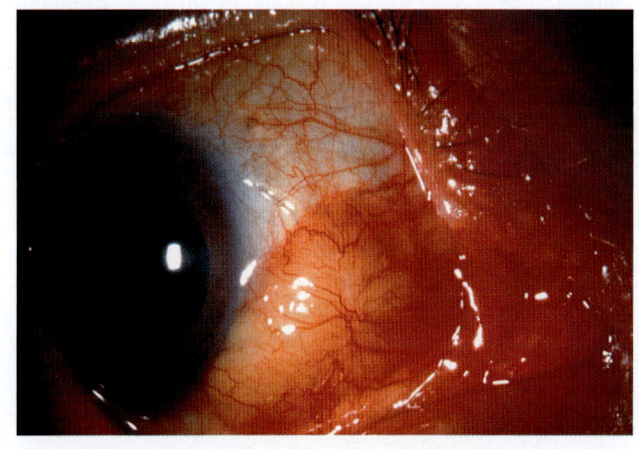

Figure 24.52. Closer view of lesion shown in Figure 24.51.

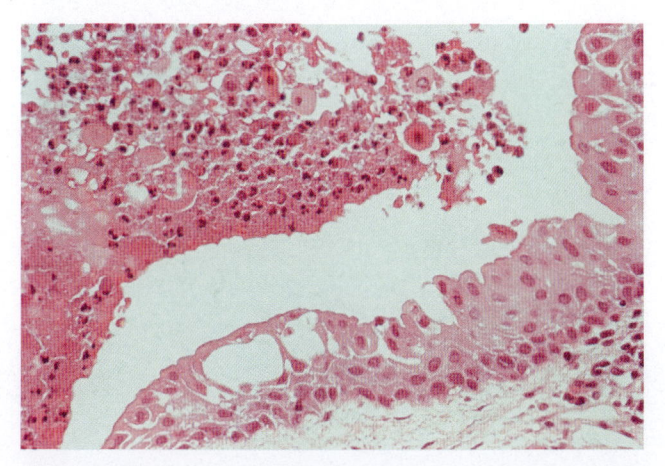

Figure 24.53. Photomicrograph of same lesion depicted in Figure 24.51, showing conjunctival epithelium (*below*) and contents of the cystic lesion (*above*). The cells in the cyst are mostly neutrophils, confirming an abscess. (Hematoxylin–eosin ×50.)

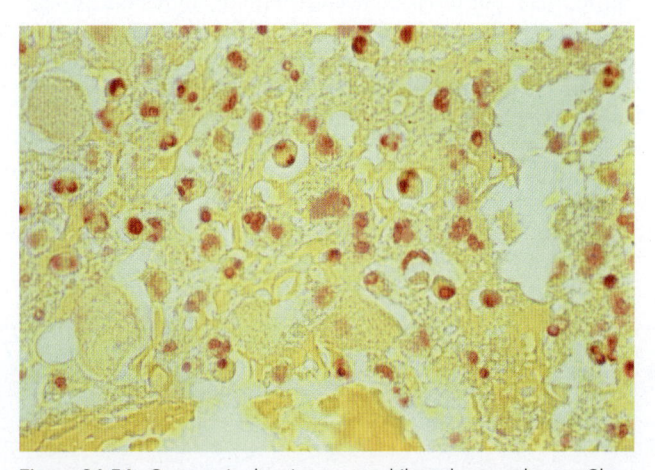

Figure 24.54. Gram stain showing neutrophils and macrophages. Close scrutiny disclosed numerous intracellular gram-negative rods compatible with *Serratia marcescens*. (Gram stain ×250.) *S. marcescens* was identified.

CONJUNCTIVAL AMYLOIDOSIS

General Considerations

Amyloidosis is a complex disease in which there is abnormal deposition of a variety of unrelated proteins in many parts of the body. The eyelid and conjunctiva are often involved in patients with amyloidosis (1–20). Conjunctival involvement almost always appears as primary localized deposition in the absence of antecedent or coexisting adnexal disease. However, conjunctival involvement has been recognized as the presenting sign of systemic amyloidosis (17). Secondary amyloidosis of the conjunctiva, which is less common, has been seen after long-standing inflammation of the ocular adnexa, particularly trachoma (7), after strabismus surgery (6), in association with systemic multiple myeloma (3), lymphoma (3,11,15), and Churg–Strauss syndrome (8).

Clinical Features

Clinically, primary localized conjunctival amyloidosis characteristically occurs in healthy, young or middle-aged adults without evidence of systemic amyloidosis. It can occur anywhere in the conjunctiva as unilateral or bilateral, confluent fusiform or polypoidal papules that have a waxy or yellow color. Blepharoptosis is a well-known presenting sign; the lesion is often located in the upper tarsus. Conjunctival amyloidosis frequently causes hemorrhage, either spontaneously or following slight trauma (1–20).

Pathology

Histopathologically, hematoxylin and eosin stains show an acellular, homogeneous, lightly eosinophilic material in the dermis. The material is birefringent and shows a positive reaction with Congo red stain and other stains for amyloid, findings that confirm the diagnosis.

Management

There is currently no highly effective treatment. Surgical excision of larger, cosmetically unacceptable lesions seems to be appropriate, but often uninvolved surface epithelium is sacrificed and major conjunctival reconstruction is necessary (4). We have devised a method to unroof the region of amyloidosis, remove the amyloid tissue, then close unaffected epithelial tissue to spare large reconstructions.

CONJUNCTIVAL AMYLOIDOSIS

Selected References

Reviews

1. Richlin JJ, Kuwabara T. Amyloid disease of the eyelid and conjunctiva. *Arch Ophthalmol* 1962;67:138–142.
2. Smith ME, Zimmerman LE. Amyloidosis of the eyelid and conjunctiva. *Arch Ophthalmol* 1966;75:42–50.
3. Demirci H, Shields CL, Eagle RC Jr, et al. Conjunctival amyloidosis: report of six cases and review of the literature. *Surv Ophthalmol.* 2006;51:419–433.

Management

4. Patrinely JR, Koch DD. Surgical management of advanced ocular adnexal amyloidosis. *Arch Ophthalmol* 1992;110:882–885.

Case Reports

5. Rodrigues MM, Cullen G, Shannon G. Primary localised conjunctival amyloidosis following strabismus surgery. *Can J Ophthalmol* 1976;11:177–179.
6. Blodi FC, Apple DJ. Localized conjunctival amyloidosis. *Am J Ophthalmol* 1979;88:346–350.
7. Chumbley LC, Peacock OS. Amyloidosis of the conjunctiva—an unusual complication of trachoma. A case report. *S Afr Med J* 1977;52:897.
8. Meisler DM, Stock EL, Wertz RD, et al. Conjunctival inflammation and amyloidosis in allergic granulomatosis and angiitis (Churg-Strauss syndrome). *Am J Ophthalmol* 1981;91:216–219.
9. Purcell JJ Jr, Birkenkamp R, Tsai CC, et al. Conjunctival involvement in primary systemic nonfamilial amyloidosis. *Am J Ophthalmol* 1983;95:845–847.
10. Borodic GE, Beyer-Mechule CK, Millin J, et al. Immunoglobulin deposition in localized conjunctival amyloidosis. *Am J Ophthalmol* 1984;98:617–622.
11. Marsh WM, Streeten BW, Hoepner JA, et al. Localized conjunctival amyloidosis associated with extranodal lymphoma. *Ophthalmology* 1987;94:61–64.
12. O'Donnell B, Wuebbolt G, Collin R. Amyloidosis of the conjunctiva. *Aust N Z J Ophthalmol* 1995;23:207–212.
13. Moorman CM, McDonald B. Primary (localised non-familial) conjunctival amyloidosis; three case reports. *Eye* 1997;11:603–606.
14. Hill VE, Brownstein S, Jordan DR. Ptosis secondary to amyloidosis of the tarsal conjunctiva and tarsus. *Am J Ophthalmol* 1997;123:852–854.
15. Setoguchi M, Hoshii Y, Takahashi M, et al. Conjunctival amyloidosis associated with a low-grade B-cell lymphoma. *Amyloid* 1999;6:210–214.
16. Lee HM, Naor J, DeAngelis D, et al. Primary localized conjunctival amyloidosis presenting with recurrence of subconjunctival hemorrhage. *Am J Ophthalmol* 2000;129:245–247.
17. Shields JA, Eagle RC, Shields CL, et al. Systemic amyloidosis presenting as a mass of the conjunctival semilunar fold. *Am J Ophthalmol* 2000;130:523–525.
18. Chaturvedi P, Lala M, Desai S, et al. A rare case of both eyelids swelling: isolated conjunctival amyloidosis. *Indian J Ophthalmol* 2000;48:56–57.
19. Kamal S, Goel R, Bodh SA, et al. Primary localized amyloidosis presenting as a tarsal mass: report of two cases. *Middle East Afr J Ophthalmol* 2012;19(4):426–428.
20. Spitellie PH, Jordan DR, Gooi P, et al. Primary localized conjunctival amyloidosis simulating a lymphoproliferative disorder. *Ophthal Plast Reconstr Surg* 2008;24(5):417–419.

CONJUNCTIVAL AMYLOIDOSIS

Conjunctival amyloidosis can have several clinical variations. In all of the following examples, the diagnosis was made histopathologically after excision or biopsy and the systemic evaluation for amyloidosis was negative.

Demirci H, Shields CL, Eagle RC Jr, et al. Conjunctival amyloidosis: report of 6 cases and review of the literature. *Surv Ophthalmol* 2006;51:419–433.

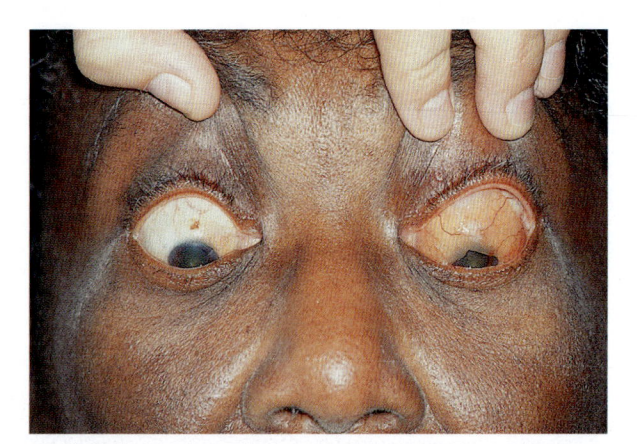

Figure 24.55. Primary unilateral diffuse amyloidosis in a 68-year-old woman with no known systemic disease.

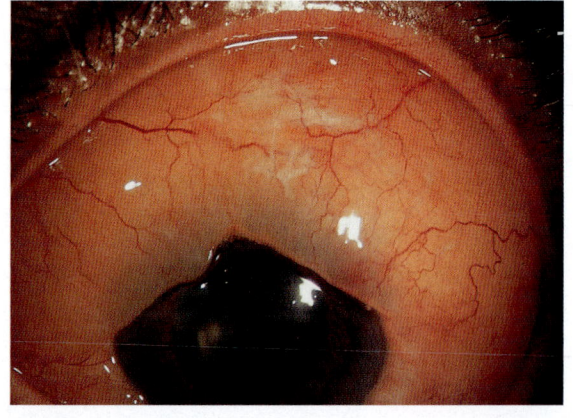

Figure 24.56. Closer view of affected left eye in patient shown in Figure 24.55. Note the waxy pink-yellow thickening of the conjunctiva.

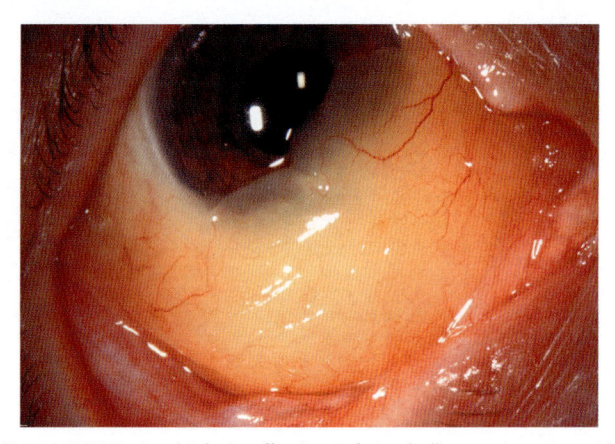

Figure 24.57. Amyloidosis affecting inferior bulbar conjunctiva with extension over cornea in a 69-year-old Caucasian woman.

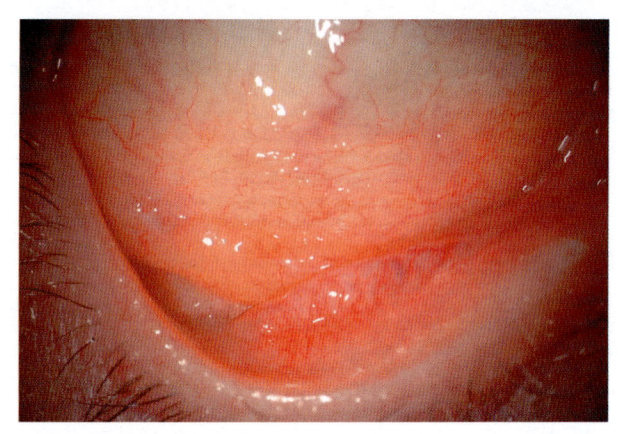

Figure 24.58. Conjunctival amyloidosis in inferior conjunctival fornix in a 50-year-old woman, appearing as a subtle pink thickening of the affected tissue. The first clinical diagnosis was lymphoma, but amyloidosis was a secondary consideration.

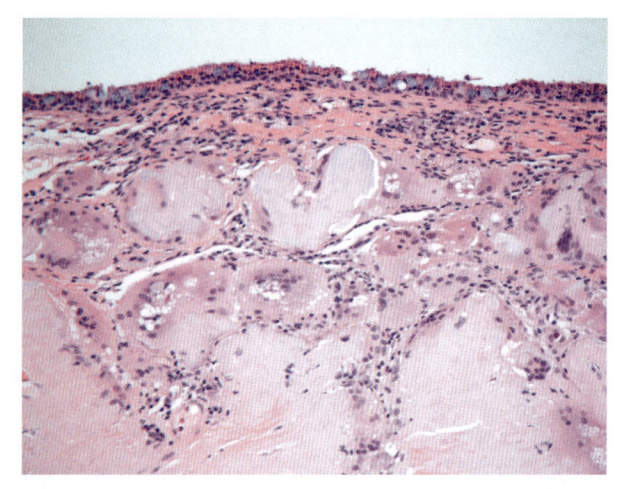

Figure 24.59. Photomicrograph of lesion shown in Figure 24.58 demonstrating lightly eosinophilic material compatible with amyloidosis deep to the conjunctival epithelium. (Hematoxylin–eosin ×50.)

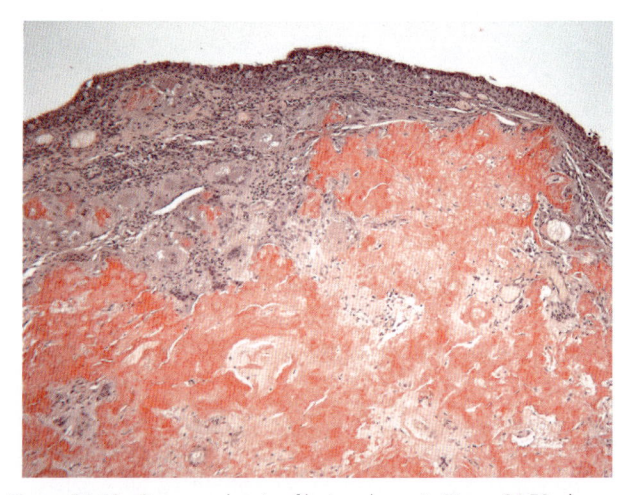

Figure 24.60. Congo red stain of lesion shown in Figure 24.58, demonstrating typical positive staining reaction of amyloid material. (×50.)

Chapter 24 Miscellaneous Lesions That Simulate Conjunctival Neoplasms

CONJUNCTIVAL AMYLOIDOSIS

In most instances, conjunctival amyloidosis is an isolated phenomenon with no demonstrable relationship to systemic amyloidosis. However, on occasion, it can be the initial manifestation of occult systemic amyloidosis. Sometimes, conjunctival amyloidosis can be bilateral and symmetrical.

Shields JA, Eagle RC, Shields CL, et al. Systemic amyloidosis presenting as a mass of the conjunctival semilunar fold. *Am J Ophthalmol* 2000;130:523–525.

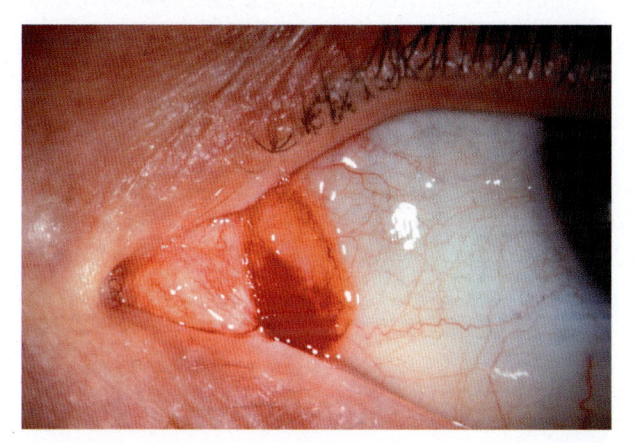

Figure 24.61. Pink mass occupying the semilunar fold nasally in the right eye of a middle-aged man.

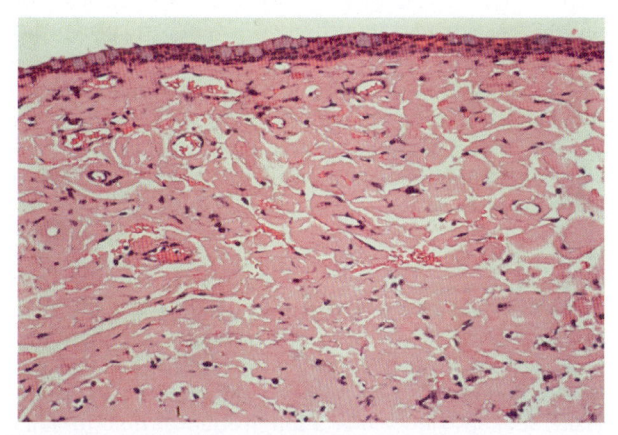

Figure 24.62. Histopathology of lesion shown in Figure 24.61, revealing the acellular material typical of amyloidosis. (Hematoxylin–eosin ×75.)

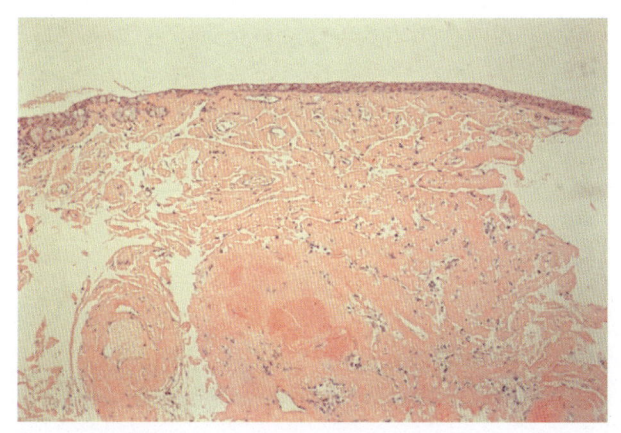

Figure 24.63. Positive Congo red stain of lesion shown in Figure 24.62. (×7.)

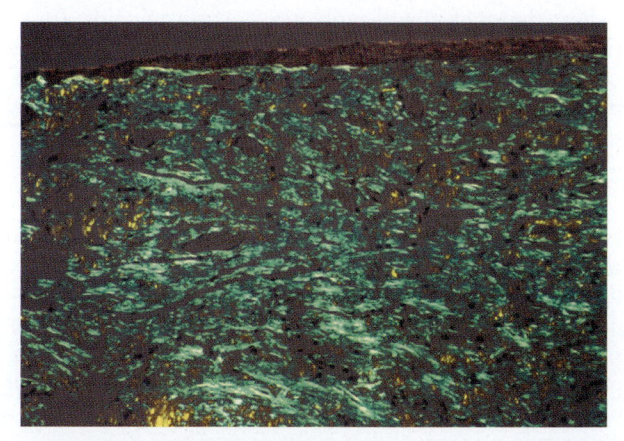

Figure 24.64. Typical apple-green birefringence of lesion shown in Figure 24.62. This patient initially had a negative systemic evaluation but later was found to have systemic amyloidosis. (×20.)

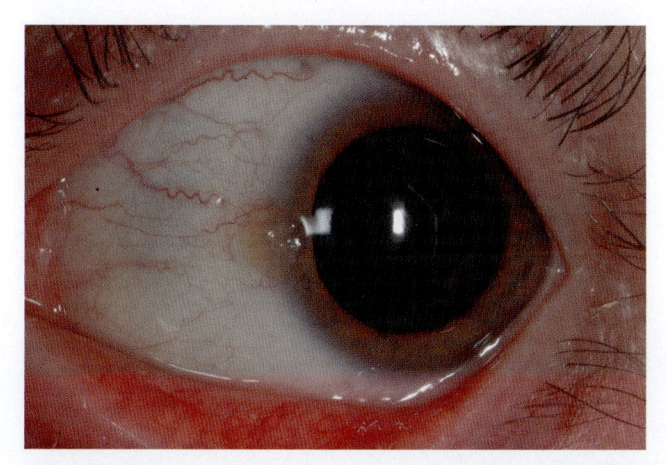

Figure 24.65. Focal amyloidosis at limbus in a middle-aged woman.

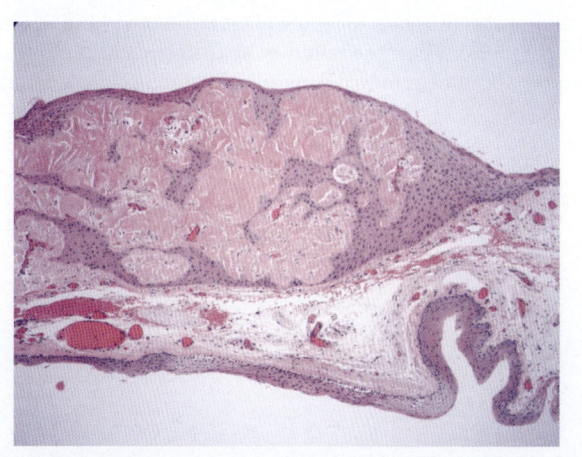

Figure 24.66. Histopathology of lesion shown in Figure 24.65, demonstrating lightly eosinophilic acellular mass in the conjunctival stroma. (Hematoxylin–eosin ×100.)

PINGUECULA

General Considerations

Selected degenerative actinic lesions that can simulate a conjunctival neoplasm include pinguecula and pterygium. Although these lesions are usually readily recognized by the experienced clinician, they can sometimes be atypical and simulate a malignant conjunctival neoplasm, particularly squamous cell carcinoma. Indeed, it is not uncommon for a lesion suspected to be squamous cell carcinoma to be found on histopathologic examination to be a benign lesion. Conversely, it is also common for the surgeon to remove a "typical" pinguecula or pterygium that, on subsequent histopathologic examination, is found to be a squamous cell carcinoma or melanoma.

Clinical Features

Clinically, pinguecula is a localized, yellow-gray, slightly elevated lesion that is usually located bilaterally near the limbus nasally, temporally or both (1–8). It can be unilateral or bilateral, symmetrical or asymmetrical. This typical subtle lesion usually develops slowly over a long period of time in adults who have had considerable exposure to sunlight or a dusty environment. It may become inflamed periodically and require a short course of topical antibiotics or corticosteroids. Larger symptomatic or cosmetically bothersome lesions can be surgically excised for cosmetic reasons. For lesions that are more suspicious, in which malignancy is a consideration, wider surgical removal is warranted.

Pathology

Histopathologically, pinguecula consists of a zone of thickened conjunctival stroma that is largely replaced by amorphous, lightly eosinophilic, granular-appearing material resembling degenerated collagen interspersed with abnormal elastic tissue (7,8). The overlying epithelium usually shows mild atrophy, but may rarely show hyperkeratosis or parakeratosis or both. Ultrastructural studies appear to support the fact that a pinguecula is a form of elastotic degeneration (7,8).

Management

In most cases, it is best to follow pingueculum without surgical intervention. When the lesion is of cosmetic concern to the patient, it can be removed surgically. Recurrence is common.

Selected References

Reviews

1. Shields CL, Shields JA. Tumors of the conjunctiva and cornea. *Surv Ophthalmol* 2004;49:3–24.
2. Shields CL, Demirci H, Karatza E, et al. Clinical survey of 1643 melanocytic and nonmelanocytic tumors of the conjunctiva. *Ophthalmology* 2004;111:1747–1754.
3. Norn MS. Prevalence of pinguecula in Greenland and in Copenhagen, and its relation to pterygium and spheroid degeneration. *Acta Ophthalmol (Copenh)* 1979;57:96–105.
4. Mimura T, Usui T, Obata H, et al. Severity and determinants of pinguecula in a hospital-based population. *Eye Contact Lens* 2011;37:31–35.
5. Ozer PA, Altiparmak UE, Yalniz Z, et al. Prevalence of pinguecula and pterygium in patients with thyroid orbitopathy. *Cornea* 2010;29:659–663.
6. Dong N, Li W, Lin H, et al. Abnormal epithelial differentiation and tear film alteration in pinguecula. *Invest Ophthalmol Vis Sci* 2009;50:2710–2715.

Histopathology

7. Ledoux-Corbusier M, Danis P. Pinguecula and actinic elastosis. An ultrastructural study. *J Cutan Pathol* 1979;6:404–413.
8. Austin P, Jakobiec FA, Iwamoto T. Elastodysplasia and elastodystrophy as the pathologic bases of ocular pterygia and pinguecula. *Ophthalmology* 1983;90:96–109.

Chapter 24 Miscellaneous Lesions That Simulate Conjunctival Neoplasms

CONJUNCTIVAL PINGUECULA

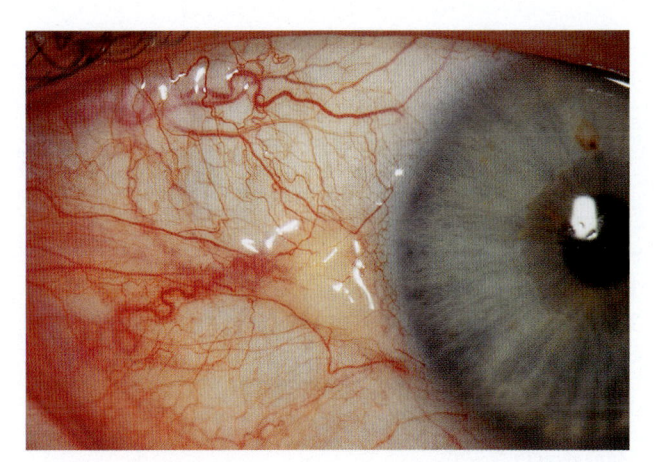

Figure 24.67. Slightly inflamed pinguecula nasally in a 51-year-old man.

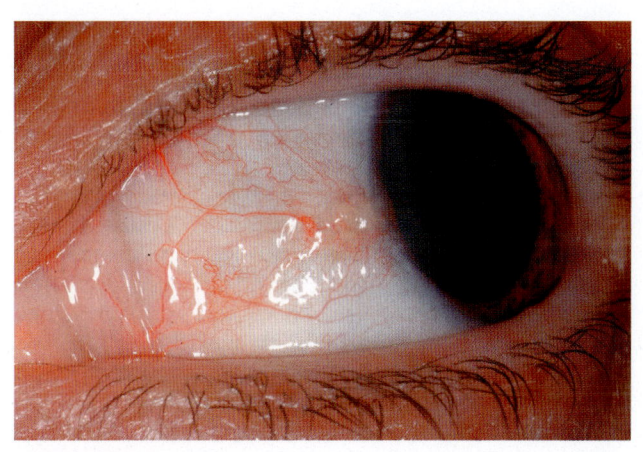

Figure 24.68. Nasally located, yellow-pink pinguecula with increased vascularity in adjacent conjunctiva.

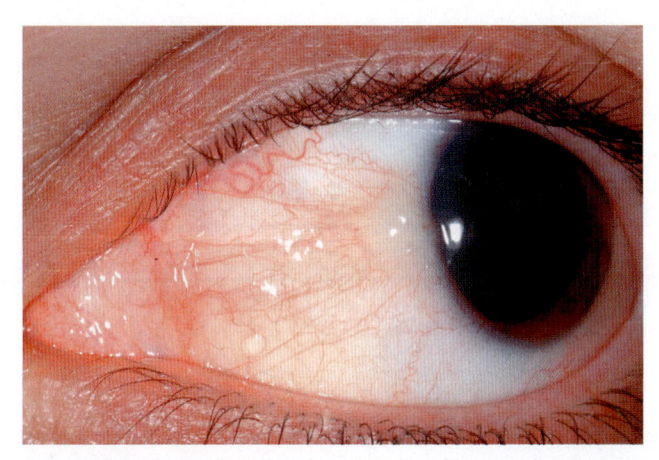

Figure 24.69. Nasally located pinguecula similar to the one shown in Figure 24.68.

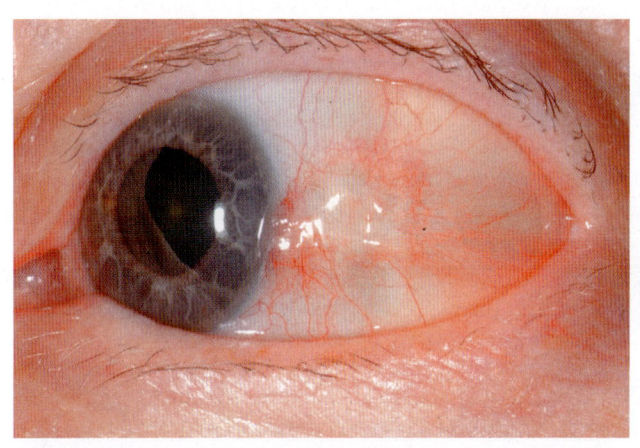

Figure 24.70. Pinguecula at temporal limbus.

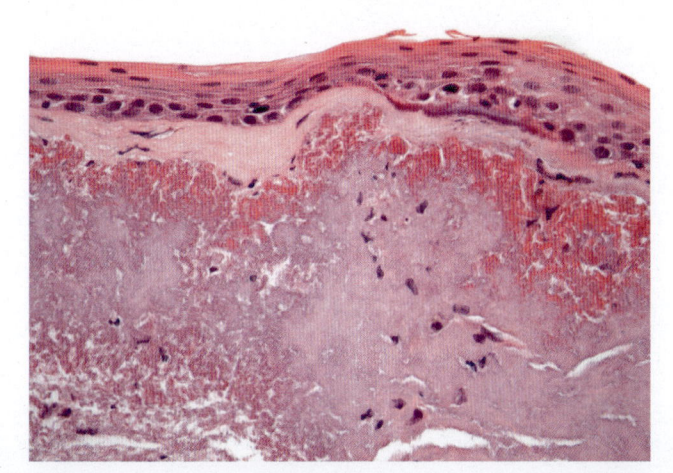

Figure 24.71. Histopathology of a pinguecula showing amorphous material replacing much of the superficial stroma. (Hematoxylin–eosin ×50.)

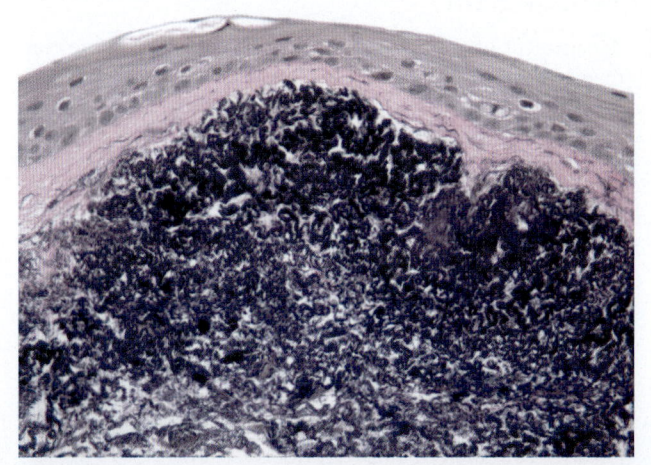

Figure 24.72. Verhoeff–Van Gieson stain of pinguecula, showing positive reaction for elastic tissue in same lesion shown in Figure 24.71. (×50.) Special studies have shown that it is not true elastic tissue, but rather degenerated collagen.

PTERYGIUM

General Considerations

Pterygium, like pinguecula, is a very common conjunctival/corneal lesion that is presumably related to chronic sunlight exposure. It is more common among those living in tropical areas, but is known to occur in any climate. It tends to invade the cornea, unlike pinguecula, which characteristically does not extend for any appreciable distance into the cornea (1–11).

This condition can induce corneal astigmatism and visual impairment. A meta-analysis of pooled prevalence worldwide revealed 10% of the population affected with pterygium, higher in men than women (4). The pooled odds ratio was 2.32 for male gender and 1.76 for outdoor activity.

Clinical Features

Pterygium generally begins near the nasal limbus but it starts temporally and can occur both nasally and temporally and be a unilateral or a bilateral lesion. However, it assumes a pattern of very slow growth into the superficial cornea. A typical feature is dragging of conjunctival tissue and blood vessels across the cornea, giving it a winglike appearance. The word pterygium means "bat wing," emphasizing this appearance. The growth is usually very slow but, given sufficient time, it can encroach on the visual axis and cause visual disturbance.

Pathology

Histopathologically, pterygium has features very similar to pinguecula. There is a zone of thickened conjunctival stroma that is largely replaced by amorphous, lightly eosinophilic, granular-appearing material resembling degenerated collagen interspersed with abnormal elastic tissue. Corneal epithelium is usually identified in specimen. Recent information on ischemic tissue injury and progenitor cell tropism were contributors to the development of pterygium (5). Others have found gene and protein abnormalities in pterygium (6).

Management

Management of pterygium has been the subject of some controversy (7–11). Many surgeons have had a great deal of experience with this condition, and there is no widespread agreement as to the best approach. Minor asymptomatic pterygium can often be followed without treatment. However, if it is bothersome or cosmetic problem, or if it shows progression across the cornea toward the visual axis with progressive astigmatism, then surgical excision is warranted. Options in management have been recently reviewed by Hirst (7). Most recent articles have suggested that the older technique of removing the lesion and leaving bare scleral is no longer widely accepted. More recent articles recommend removal and corneoconjunctival autograft transplantation (7–11). For recurrent pterygia, some authors have recommended amniotic membrane transplantation with conjunctival autograft (8).

Selected References

Reviews

1. Shields CL, Shields JA. Tumors of the conjunctiva and cornea. *Surv Ophthalmol* 2004;49:3–24.
2. Shields CL, Demirci H, Karatza E, et al. Clinical survey of 1643 melanocytic and nonmelanocytic tumors of the conjunctiva. *Ophthalmology* 2004;111:1747–1754.
3. Ozer PA, Altiparmak UE, Yalniz Z, et al. Prevalence of pinguecula and pterygium in patients with thyroid orbitopathy. *Cornea* 2010;29:659–663.
4. Liu L, Wu J, Geng J, et al. Geographical prevalence and risk factors for pterygium: a systemic review and meta-analysis. *BJM Open* 2013;3:e003787.

Histopathology/Genetics

5. Kim KW, Ha HS, Kim JC. Ischemic tissue injury and progenitor cell tropism: significant contributors to the pathogenesis of pterygium. *Histol Histopathol* 2015;30(3):311–320.
6. Hou A, Lan W, Law KP, et al. Evaluation of global differential gene and protein expression in primary pterygium: S100A8 and S100A9 as possible drivers of a signaling network. *PLoS One* 2014;9(5):e97402.

Management

7. Hirst LW. The treatment of pterygium. *Surv Ophthalmol* 2003;48:145–180.
8. Shimazaki J, Kosaka K, Shimmura S, et al. Amniotic membrane transplantation with conjunctival autograft for recurrent pterygium. *Ophthalmology* 2003;110:119–124.
9. Sangwan VS, Murthy SI, Bansal AK, et al. Surgical treatment of chronically recurring pterygium. *Cornea* 2003;22:63–65.
10. Frau E, Labetoulle M, Lautier-Frau M, et al. Corneo-conjunctival autograft transplantation for pterygium surgery. *Acta Ophthalmol Scand* 2004;82:59–63.
11. Kurian A, Reghunadhan I, Nair KG. Autologous blood versus fibrin glue for conjunctival autograft adherence in sutureless pterygium surgery: a randomized controlled trial. *Br J Ophthalmol* 2015;99(4):464–470.

Chapter 24 Miscellaneous Lesions That Simulate Conjunctival Neoplasms

● PTERYGIUM

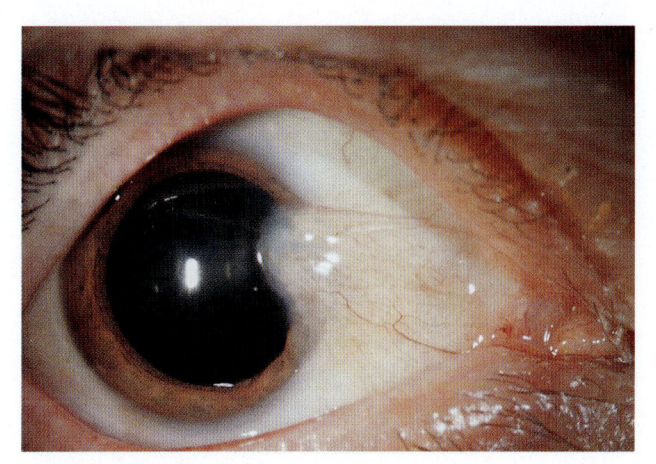

Figure 24.73. Typical pterygium in a 50-year-old man.

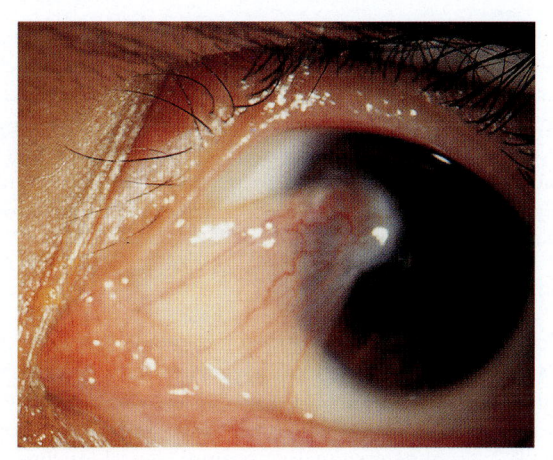

Figure 24.74. Recurrent pterygium in a 31-year-old man.

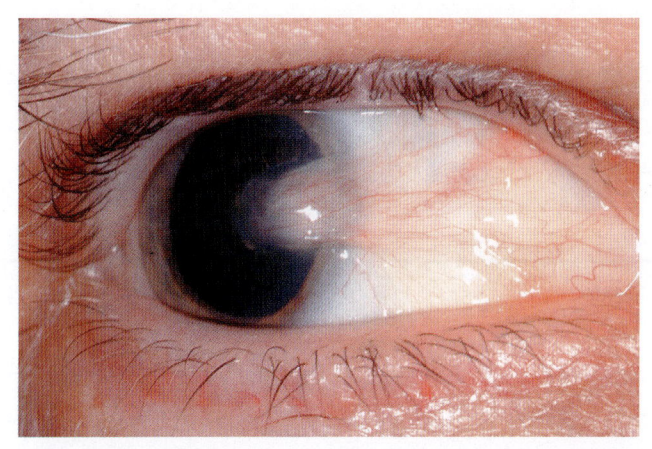

Figure 24.75. Nasal pterygium extending to central portion of cornea.

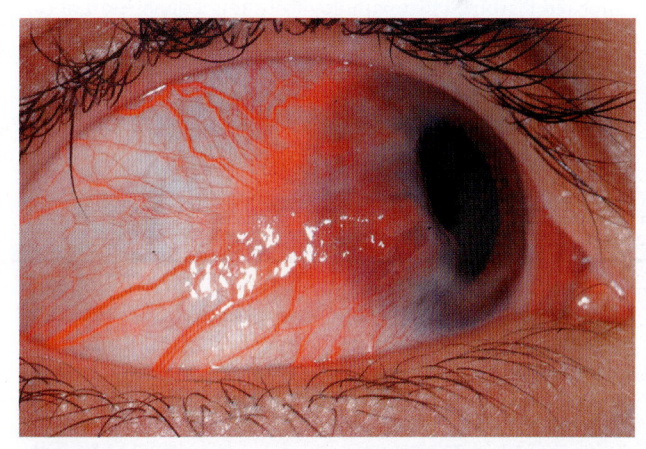

Figure 24.76. Pterygium with severe secondary inflammation.

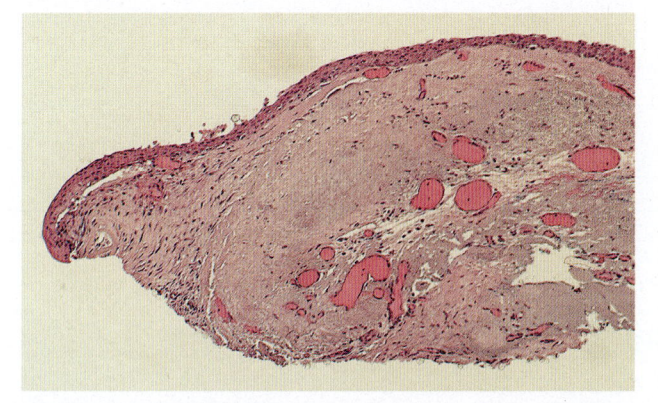

Figure 24.77. Histopathology of a pterygium, showing thickened amorphous tissue beneath the conjunctival and corneal epithelium. (Hematoxylin–eosin ×25.)

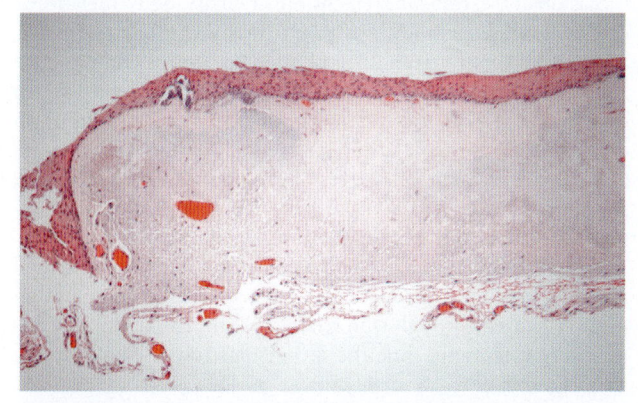

Figure 24.78. Histopathology of chronic pterygium showing slight basophilia of the actinic changes in the stroma. There is a small amount of dystrophic calcification near the basement membrane of the conjunctival epithelium. (Hematoxylin–eosin ×25.)

CONJUNCTIVAL AND SCLERAL MISCELLANEOUS LESIONS THAT SIMULATE PIGMENTED MELANOMA

There are several dark lesions that can occur in the epibulbar tissue and simulate melanoma (1–12). Some of these, such as metallic foreign body, have been mentioned. Others include pigmented Axenfeld nerve loop, ocular melanocytosis, argyrosis, and epinephrine deposition. Three other lesions that are sometimes initially diagnosed as possible conjunctival melanoma include the calcified scleral plaque, uveal staphyloma, and extraocular extension of ciliary body melanoma.

Calcified Scleral Plaque

Calcified scleral plaque, also called focal senile translucency of the sclera (7) or Cogan's plaque, is a gray, intrascleral lesion that occurs near the insertions of the medial and lateral rectus muscles in elderly patients. It is usually seen clinically and occasionally is prominent enough to prompt referral for suspected melanoma. In other cases, these calcified plaques are found with computed tomography of the orbit that is performed for unrelated reasons. Histopathologically, it is a deposition of calcium forming a plaque in the anterior or midportion of the sclera. No treatment is generally necessary.

Staphyloma

Staphyloma is bulging of uveal tissue through a congenital or acquired defect in the sclera. Congenital staphyloma is usually idiopathic, whereas acquired staphyloma is most often secondary to rheumatoid scleritis or other connective tissue disorders that induce scleral thinning (8,11). It can be differentiated from conjunctival melanoma and extraocular extension of uveal melanoma by transillumination. Uveal staphyloma transmits light readily, whereas pigmented melanoma blocks transmission of light.

Extraocular Extension of Ciliary Body Melanoma

Occasionally, extraocular extension of ciliary body melanoma can be confused clinically with a primary conjunctival melanoma. Conversely, epibulbar pigmented lesions can be confused with extraocular extension of uveal melanoma (4). In contrast with conjunctival melanoma, extrascleral extension of uveal melanoma lies deep to the conjunctiva and may be associated with large, dilated sentinel blood vessels. In addition, slit-lamp biomicroscopy, ophthalmoscopy, and ultrasonography should reveal the underlying intraocular tumor.

Other cases of ciliary body melanoma can show scleral necrosis following plaque radiotherapy, leading to a brown mass visualized through thin sclera (6). This can resemble conjunctival melanoma, but the intraocular tumor will confirm the diagnosis of uveal melanoma.

Selected References

Reviews
1. Shields CL, Shields JA. Tumors of the conjunctiva and cornea. *Surv Ophthalmol* 2004;49:3–24.
2. Shields CL, Demirci H, Karatza E, et al. Clinical survey of 1643 melanocytic and nonmelanocytic tumors of the conjunctiva. *Ophthalmology* 2004;111:1747–1754.
3. Shields CL, Markowitz JS, Belinsky I, et al. Conjunctival melanoma. Outcomes based on tumor origin in 382 consecutive cases. *Ophthalmology* 2011;118:389–395.
4. Shields CL, Kaliki S, Furuta M, et al. Clinical spectrum and prognosis of uveal melanoma based on age at presentation in 8033 cases. *Retina* 2012;32:1363–1372.
5. Shields CL, Regillo A, Mellen PL, et al. Giant conjunctival nevus: Clinical features and natural course in 32 cases. *JAMA Ophthalmol* 2013;131:857–863.
6. Kaliki S, Shields CL, Rojanaporn D, et al. Scleral necrosis following plaque radiotherapy of uveal melanoma: A case-control study. *Ophthalmology* 2013;120:1004–1011.

Case Reports
7. Cogan DB, Kuwabara T. Focal senile translucency of the sclera. *Arch Ophthalmol* 1959;62:604–610.
8. Watson PG. The diagnosis and management of scleritis. *Ophthalmology* 1980;87:716–720.
9. Donoso LA, Shields JA. Epibulbar lesions simulating extraocular extension of uveal melanomas. *Ann Ophthalmol* 1982;14:1120–1123.
10. Margo CE. Episcleral pseudomelanoma: late complication of scleral tunnel incision. *Am J Ophthalmol* 2003;135:387–389.
11. Shields JA, Shields CL, Lavrich J. Congenital anterior scleral staphyloma in an otherwise normal eye. *J Pediatr Ophthalmol Strabismus* 2003;40:108–109.
12. Marr BP, Shields JA, Shields CL, et al. Uveal prolapse following cataract extraction simulating melanoma. *Ophthalmic Surg Lasers Imaging* 2008;39:250–251.

Chapter 24 Miscellaneous Lesions That Simulate Conjunctival Neoplasms

SCLERAL STAPHYLOMA AND UVEAL PROLAPSE THAT SIMULATE MELANOMA

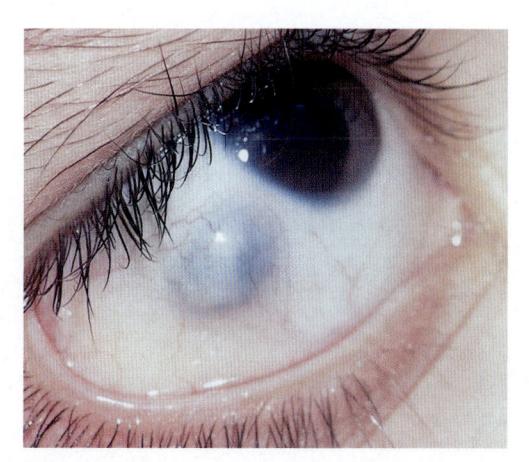

Figure 24.79. Congenital uveal staphyloma in an 11-year-old boy.

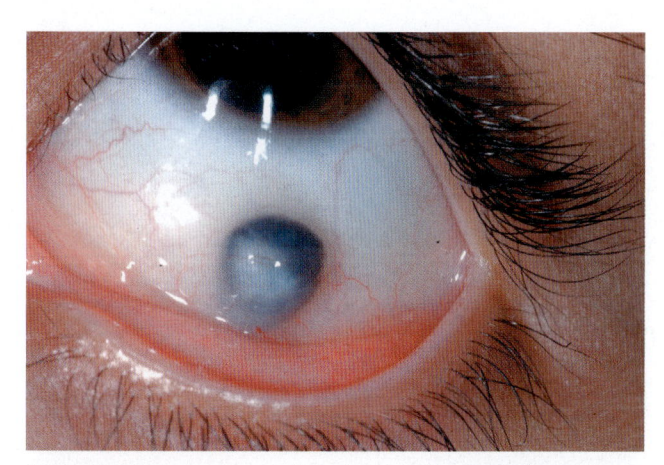

Figure 24.80. Congenital uveal staphyloma in a young girl.

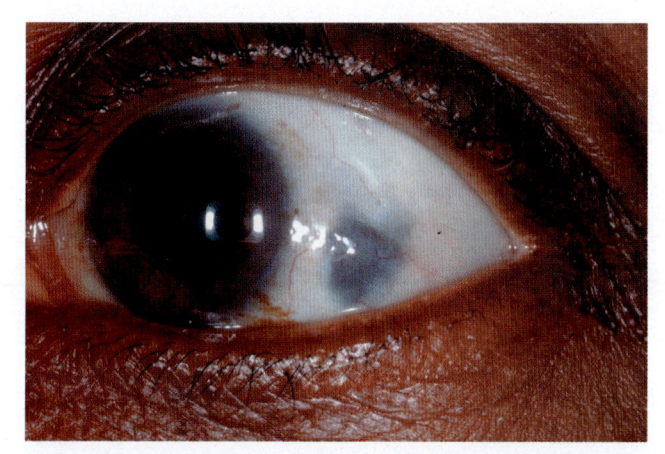

Figure 24.81. Temporal staphyloma of uncertain cause in an African-American woman.

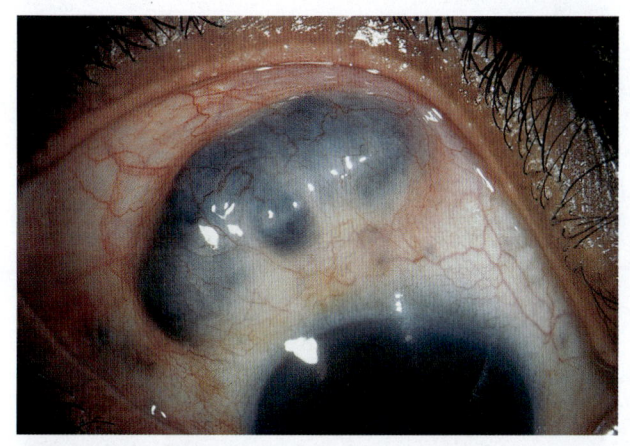

Figure 24.82. Acquired uveal staphyloma in a 60-year-old woman with a history of rheumatoid arthritis.

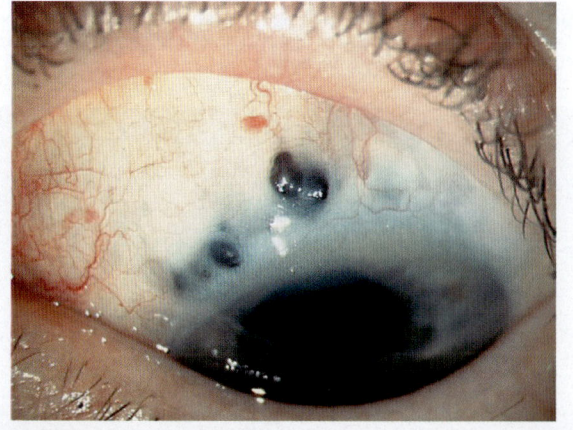

Figure 24.83. Multifocal staphyloma in an elderly patient with rheumatoid arthritis.

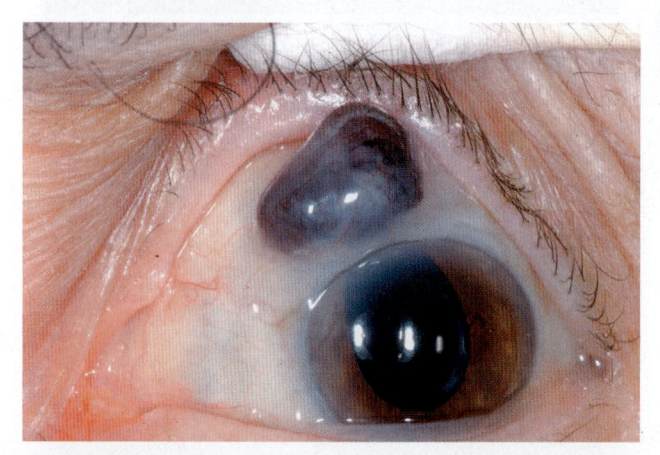

Figure 24.84. Superior uveal prolapse after cataract surgery simulating conjunctival melanoma and extraocular extension of ciliary body melanoma.

CONJUNCTIVAL MISCELLANEOUS LESIONS THAT SIMULATE MELANOMA

1. Shields JA, Marr BP, Shields CL, et al. Conjunctival mascaroma masquerading as melanoma. *Cornea* 2005;24:496–497.
2. Kaliki S, Shields CL, Rojanaporn D, et al. Scleral necrosis following plaque radiotherapy of uveal melanoma: a case-control study. *Ophthalmology* 2013;120:1004–1011.

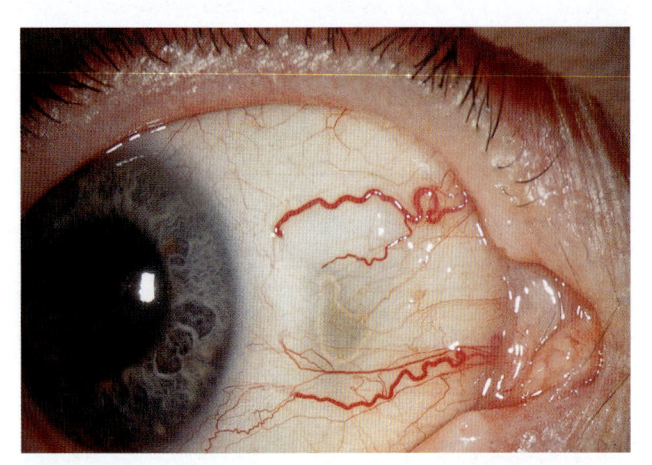

Figure 24.85. Calcified scleral plaque in a 75-year-old woman.

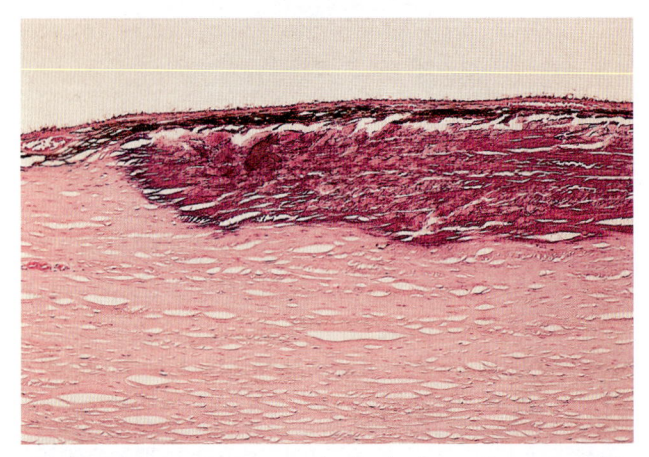

Figure 24.86. Histopathology of scleral plaque showing acellular basophilic plaque, typical of calcium, in anterior portion of sclera. (Hematoxylin–eosin ×20.)

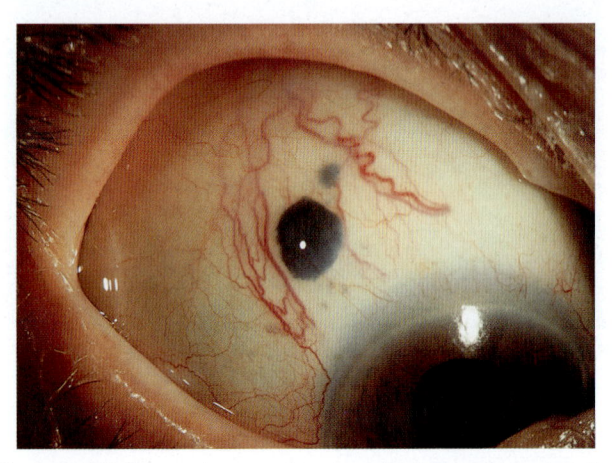

Figure 24.87. Extraocular extension of uveal melanoma. Note the adjacent sentinel vessels.

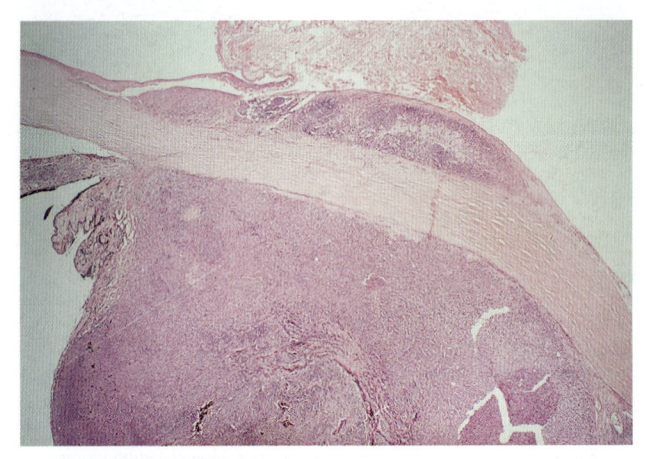

Figure 24.88. Histopathology of extraocular extension of ciliary body melanoma. Note the intraocular tumor (*below*) and the episcleral nodule of tumor (*above*). (Hematoxylin–eosin ×15.)

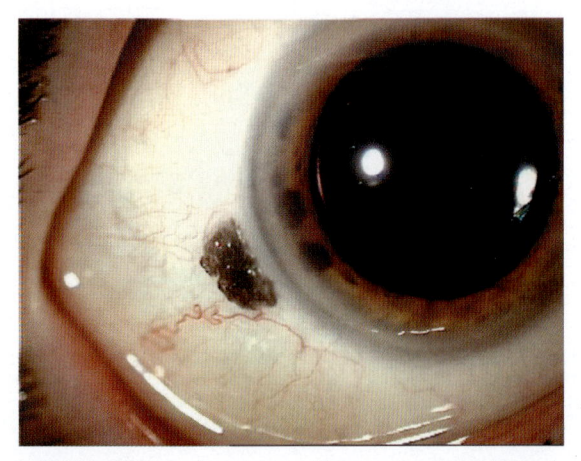

Figure 24.89. Mascara deposit in a middle-aged woman who had used mascara excessively for many years. The lesion was removed and mascara was identified.

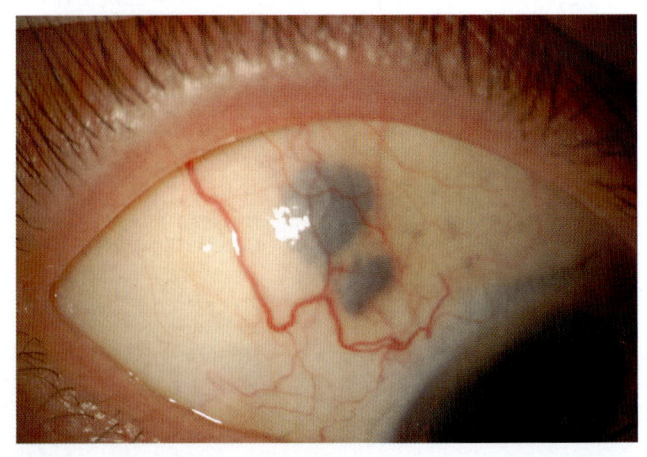

Figure 24.90. Sub-Tenon's fascia scleral necrosis following plaque radiotherapy for ciliary body melanoma simulating conjunctival melanoma or extrascleral extension of ciliary body melanoma.

CHAPTER 25

SURGICAL MANAGEMENT OF CONJUNCTIVAL TUMORS

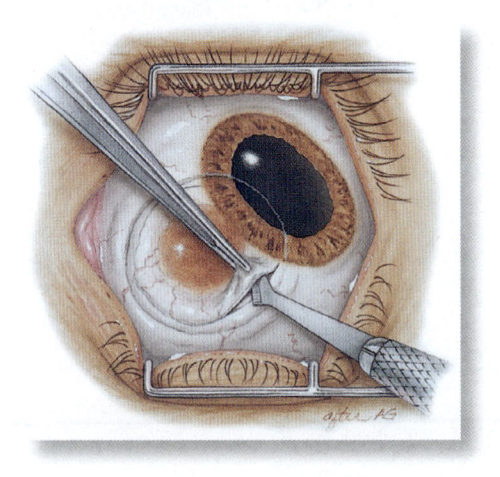

It is important that malignant or potentially malignant conjunctival tumors be completely removed with as little manipulation as possible. The most appropriate surgical method differs with limbal tumors, extralimbal tumors, and primary acquired melanosis (PAM) as well as the type of tumor (1–19). Some tumors are only managed with surgical resection whereas others can be treated with cryotherapy, topical Mitomycin C, topical 5-fluoruracil, or topical/injection interferon alpha-2b (8–18). Tumors locally invasive into the eye may require plaque radiotherapy (19).

The surgical techniques are reported in detail in the literature (2–6) and are briefly described herein. In all cases, the "no touch" technique is used whereby the tumor itself is not handled. Only surrounding healthy tissue is grasped. Limbal lesions are generally best managed by localized alcohol corneal epitheliectomy, removal of the main mass by a partial lamellar scleroconjunctivectomy, and supplemental double freeze thaw cryotherapy. Tumors located in the extralimbal conjunctiva are managed by alcohol application, wide circumferential surgical resection, and cryotherapy.

There are no rigid methods for the management of PAM of the conjunctiva. In general, it is best managed by alcohol epitheliectomy, removal of suspicious pigmented foci, quadratic staging biopsies, and cryotherapy from the underside of the conjunctiva. In all cases, a "no touch" method is used and direct manipulation of the tumor is avoided in an effort to prevent tumor cell seeding into a new area (2–7). During this surgery, it is often prudent to place punctual plugs in the upper and lower canaliculus to prevent seeding of tumor cells in the lacrimal drainage system.

Certain ancillary approaches are employed in conjunction with primary surgical resection of selected conjunctival lesions. These methods include mucous membrane or amniotic membrane grafting, topical chemotherapy or immunotherapy (9–18), and radiotherapy (19). Grafting is used following a large resection of more than 3 clock hours of conjunctival tissue with extensive conjunctival defect. Topical Mitomycin C, 5-fluoroacil, and interferon are used primarily as alternatives to surgical resection of superficial lesions of the bulbar conjunctiva and cornea, particularly conjunctival/corneal intraepithelial neoplasia and PAM. These agents can be used as a primary therapy or secondary therapy. In addition, they can be employed as neoadjuvant therapy to reduce a large tumor size in preparation for surgery. Radiotherapy is used primarily for cases of squamous cell carcinoma, melanoma, or other conjunctival neoplasms in which further surgical excision is not feasible to achieve good tumor control and in which orbital exenteration is becoming the only therapeutic option.

SURGICAL MANAGEMENT OF CONJUNCTIVAL TUMORS

Regarding topical chemotherapy, we have primarily employed Mitomycin C for PAM and interferon alpha-2b for OSSN. Mitomycin C is administered by applying one drop of 0.04% mitomycin four times daily for 7 days. We strategize with 1 week of medicine, then 1 week for healing without medicine, then we repeat both weeks and check the patient at 1 month. This is important as Mitomycin C can be toxic to the corneal surface. For interferon, we use 1 million units/cc eye drop four times daily for 3 to 6 months. Patients are examined on 3-month basis. Interferon alpha-2b rarely causes side effects. Topical chemotherapy has been highly successful in controlling selected superficial conjunctival malignancies. For conjunctival melanoma or deep tumors, we generally avoid topical medications and only use surgical approach.

Selected References

Reviews

1. Shields CL, Demirci H, Karatza E, et al. Clinical survey of 1643 melanocytic and nonmelanocytic tumors of the conjunctiva. *Ophthalmology* 2004;111:1747–1754.
2. Shields CL, Shields JA. Tumors of the conjunctiva and cornea. *Surv Ophthalmol* 2004;49:3–24.

Management/Surgery

3. Shields JA, Shields CL, DePotter P. Surgical approach to conjunctival tumors. The 1994 Lynn B. McMahan Lecture. *Arch Ophthalmol* 1997;115:808–815.
4. Shields JA, Shields CL, De Potter P. Surgical management of circumscribed conjunctival melanomas. *Ophthal Plast Reconstr Surg* 1998;14:208–215.
5. Shields CL, Shields JA. Overview of tumors of the conjunctiva and cornea. In: Foster CS, Azar DT, Dohlman CL, eds. *Smolin and Thoft's The Cornea*. 4th ed. Philadelphia, PA: Lippincott, Williams & Wilkins; 2005:735–755.
6. Shields JA, Shields CL. Tumors of the conjunctiva. In: Stephenson CM, ed. *Ophthalmic Plastic, Reconstructive and Orbital Surgery*. Stoneham, MA: Butterworth-Heinemann; 1997:260–261.
7. Shields CL, Markowitz JS, Belinsky I, et al. Conjunctival melanoma. Outcomes based on tumor origin in 382 consecutive cases. *Ophthalmology* 2011;118:389–395.
8. Nanji AA, Moon CS, Galor A, et al. Surgical versus medical treatment of ocular surface squamous neoplasia: a comparison of recurrences and complications. *Ophthalmology* 2014;121:994–1000.

Mitomycin C

9. Frucht-Pery J, Rozenman Y. Mitomycin C therapy for corneal intraepithelial neoplasia. *Am J Ophthalmol* 1994;117:164–168.
10. Shields CL, Naseripour M, Shields JA. Topical Mitomycin C for extensive, recurrent conjunctival squamous cell carcinoma. *Am J Ophthalmol* 2002;133:601–606.
11. Shields CL, Demirci H, Marr BP, et al. Chemoreduction with topical Mitomycin C prior to resection of extensive squamous cell carcinoma of the conjunctiva. *Arch Ophthalmol* 2005;123:109–113.

5-Fluorouracil

12. Yeatts RP, Engelbrecht NE, Curry CD, et al. 5-Fluorouracil for the treatment of intraepithelial neoplasia of the conjunctiva and cornea. *Ophthalmology* 2000;107:2190–2195.
13. Midena E, Angeli CD, Valenti M, et al. Treatment of conjunctival squamous cell carcinoma with topical 5-fluorouracil. *Br J Ophthalmol* 2000;84:268–272.

Interferon

14. Karp CL, Galor A, Chhabra S, et al. Subconjunctival/perilesional recombinant interferon α2b for ocular surface squamous neoplasia: a 10-year review. *Ophthalmology*. 2010;117(12):2241–2246.
15. Shields CL, Kancherla S, Bianciotto CG, et al. Ocular surface squamous neoplasia (squamous cell carcinoma) of the socket: Management of extensive tumors with interferon. *Ophthal Plast Reconstr Surg* 2011;27:247–250.
16. Shah S, Kaliki S, Kim HJ, et al. Topical interferon alpha 2b for management of ocular surface squamous neoplasia in 23 cases: Outcomes based on American Joint Committee on Cancer (AJCC) classification. *Arch Ophthalmol* 2012;130:159–164.
17. Kim HJ, Shields CL, Shah SU, et al. Giant ocular surface squamous neoplasia managed with interferon alpha-2b as immunotherapy or immunoreduction. *Ophthalmology* 2012;119:938–944.
18. Shields CL, Kaliki S, Kim HJ, et al. Interferon for ocular surface squamous neoplasia in 81 cases: Outcomes based on the American Joint Committee on Cancer classification. *Cornea* 2013;32(3):248–256.

Radiotherapy

19. Arepalli S, Kaliki S, Shields CL, et al. Plaque radiotherapy for scleral-invasive conjunctival squamous cell carcinoma: an analysis of 15 eyes. *JAMA Ophthalmol* 2014;132(6):691–696.

Chapter 25 Surgical Management of Conjunctival Tumors   435

● SURGICAL RESECTION OF CIRCUMSCRIBED CONJUNCTIVAL TUMORS NEAR LIMBUS

Surgical planning and technique are very important in management of conjunctival tumors. Depicted is the drawing that is done in the clinic and placed in the operating room at the time of surgery. The surgical steps are shown in the drawings.

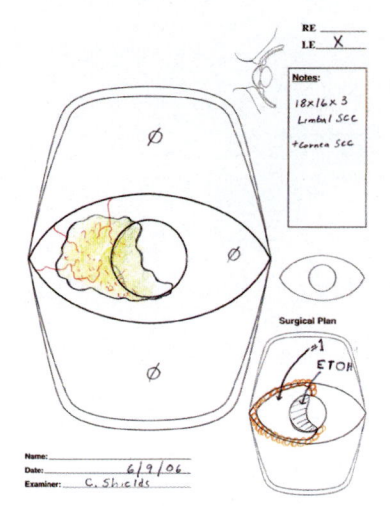

Figure 25.1. Large drawing of circumscribed limbal and corneal tumor. The large drawing is done in the office at slit-lamp examination and is used in all cases at the time of surgery. The drawing shows the extent of corneal involvement, as seen in the office using slit-lamp biomicroscopy. Number 1 is the extent of the lesion to be resected. The orange color is used to indicate the extent of cryotherapy, done immediately after tumor is removed. ETOH indicates the area where absolute alcohol is applied.

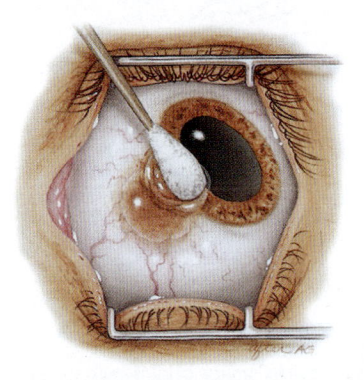

Figure 25.2. Alcohol being applied with a cotton-tipped applicator to a conjunctival melanoma with peripheral corneal invasion. A small cellulose sponge is more often used today.

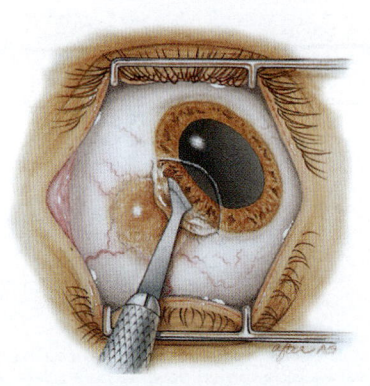

Figure 25.3. Localized corneal epitheliectomy being performed with a small scalpel using a gentle, controlled scrolling technique. The corneal epithelium is gently everted and laid on the surface of the main tumor at and behind the limbus.

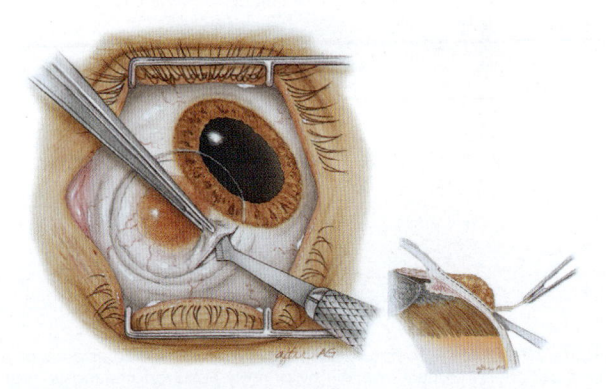

Figure 25.4. A superficial scleral groove has been made around the tumor base, which is being removed by dissecting a thin layer of superficial sclera immediately beneath the tumor and just posterior to the limbus. *Inset* shows side view of depth of superficial scleral dissection.

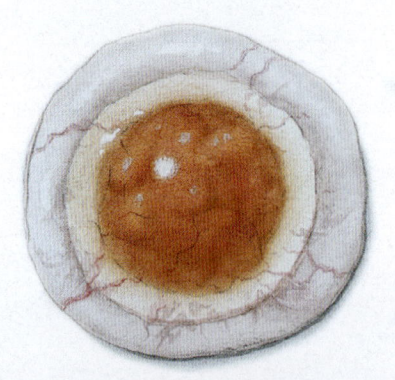

Figure 25.5. The tumor has been removed and placed flatly on a piece of sterile cardboard on the operating table. After a few seconds, it is placed in this flat position in fixative and allowed to float in that position. The same principle applies to other conjunctival and iris lesions that are removed surgically.

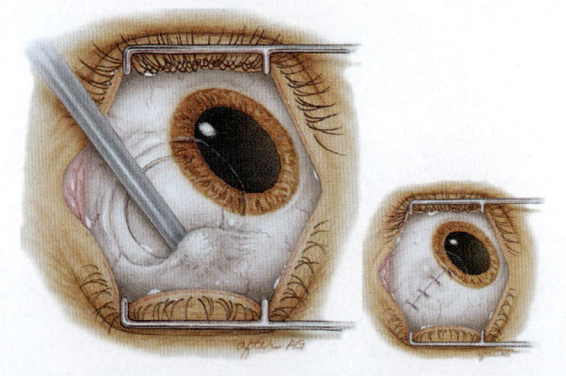

Figure 25.6. After the tumor has been removed and placed in fixative, double freeze thaw cryotherapy is applied from underneath the conjunctiva in an outward direction. *Inset* shows closure with absorbable sutures.

SURGICAL MANAGEMENT OF PRIMARY ACQUIRED MELANOSIS AND MELANOMA OF CONJUNCTIVA

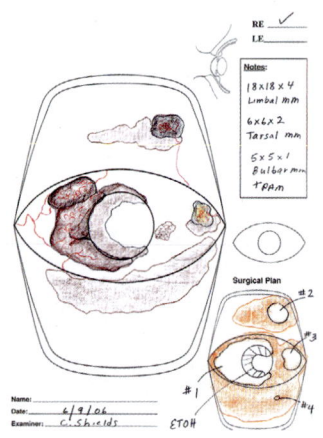

Figure 25.7. Large drawing of extensive primary acquired melanosis, possibly giving rise to melanoma. The large drawing is done in the office at slit-lamp examination and is used in all cases at the time of surgery. The drawing shows the extent of corneal involvement, as seen in the office using slit-lamp biomicroscopy. Number 1 shows the extent of the lesion to be resected. The orange color is used to indicate the extent of cryotherapy. In cases of PAM, heavy widespread cryotherapy is applied. ETOH indicates the area where absolute alcohol will be applied.

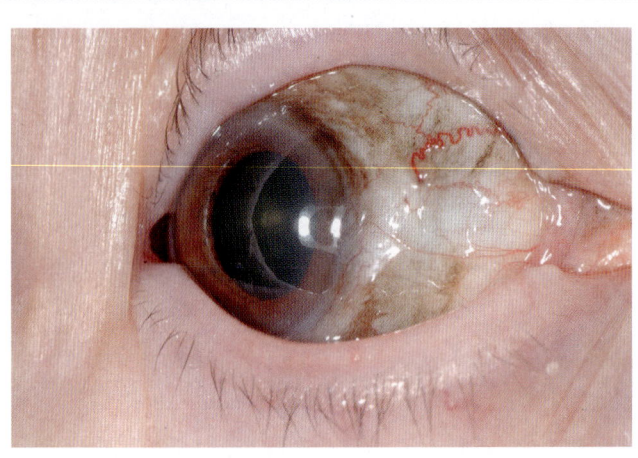

Figure 25.8. Diffuse conjunctival primary acquired melanosis in another case giving rise to melanoma that would be removed by the methods shown in steps below.

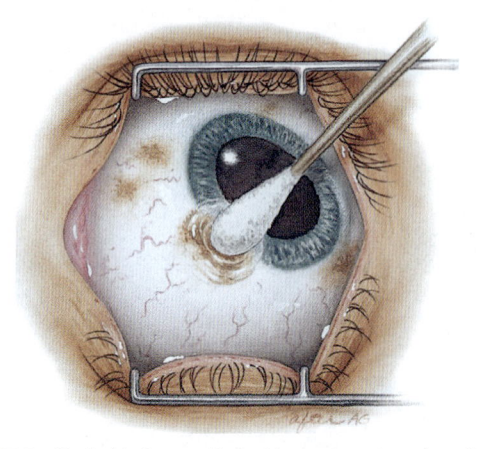

Figure 25.9. Alcohol being applied with a cotton-tipped applicator to treat peripheral corneal invasion by primary acquired melanosis. Note several additional small nodules of pigmentation in other areas of the conjunctiva.

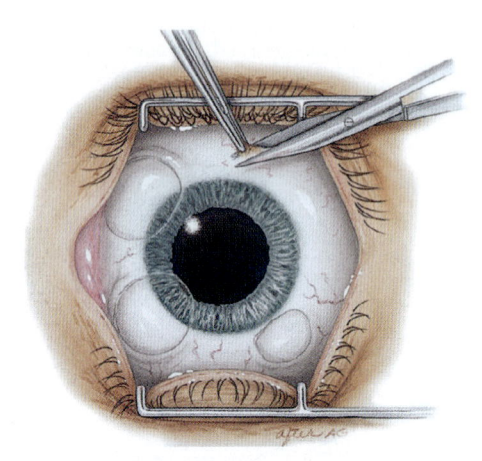

Figure 25.10. All nodular pigmented areas have been removed by a circular conjunctival excision carried down to bare sclera. A small staging map biopsy is being taken from the bulbar conjunctiva near the fornix. Such a biopsy is generally taken in all four quadrants even though the conjunctiva appears to be clinically normal in that area.

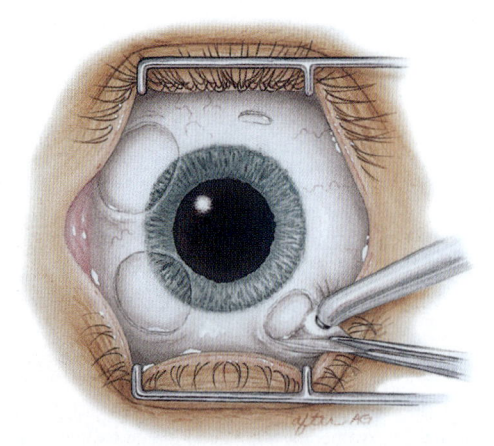

Figure 25.11. Cryotherapy being applied from beneath the conjunctiva in an outward direction. The conjunctiva is being everted with forceps.

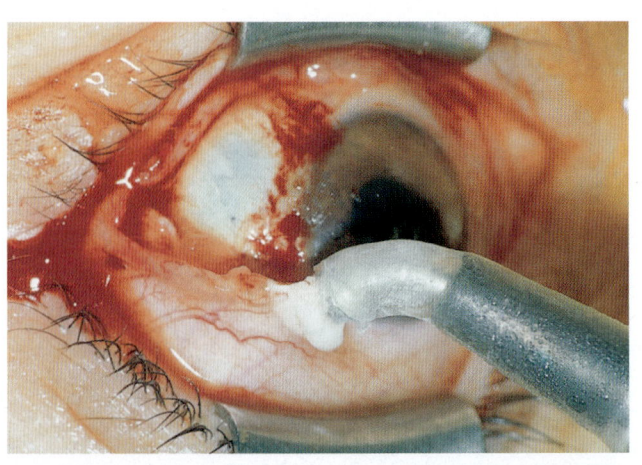

Figure 25.12. Photograph showing proper application of cryotherapy.

RESULTS OF SURGICAL MANAGEMENT OF CONJUNCTIVAL TUMORS

Although the surgical technique necessarily varies with the clinical circumstances, such lesions are generally removed by partial corneal epitheliectomy with absolute alcohol followed by tumor removal by partial lamellar sclerokeratoconjunctivectomy using a "no touch" technique and surrounding double freeze thaw cryotherapy.

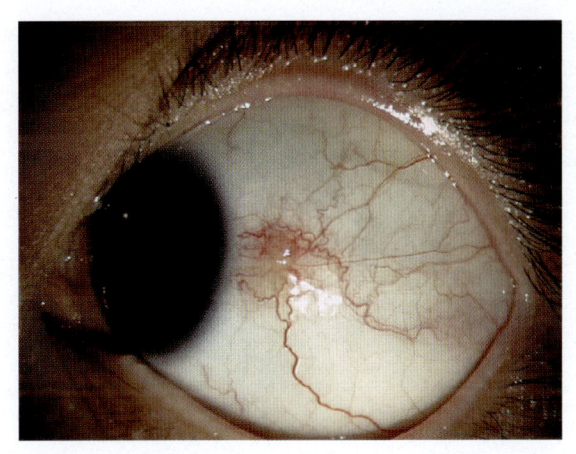

Figure 25.13. Conjunctival epithelial neoplasia near limbus before surgical excision. Clinically, the lesion resembles a pinguecula but proved histopathologically to be in situ squamous cell carcinoma.

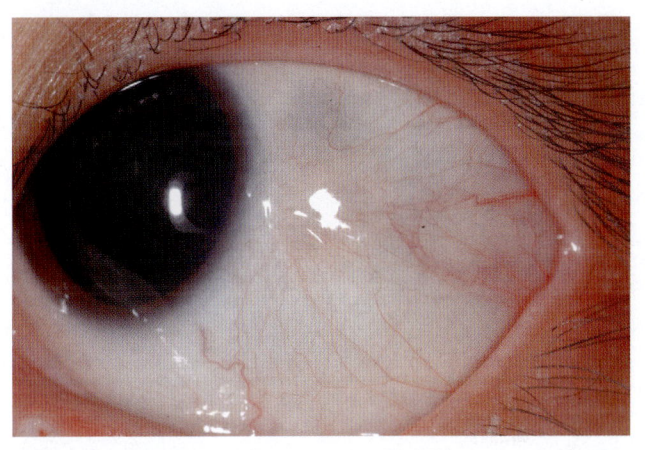

Figure 25.14. Same area shown in Figure 25.13 about 1 year after surgical removal of the lesion and cryotherapy. Note that the area of the lesion looks normal.

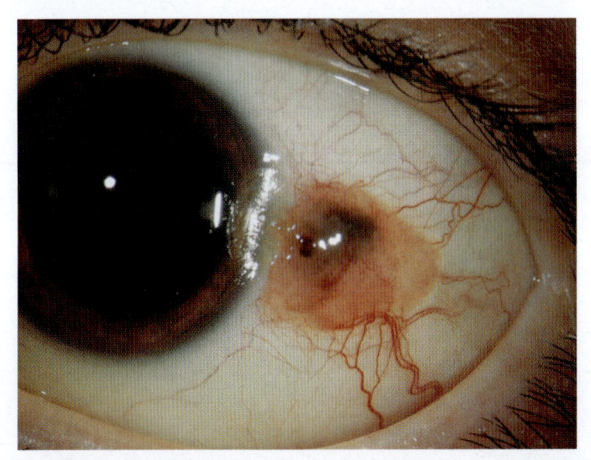

Figure 25.15. Melanoma of bulbar conjunctiva with peripheral corneal invasion in a 45-year-old woman.

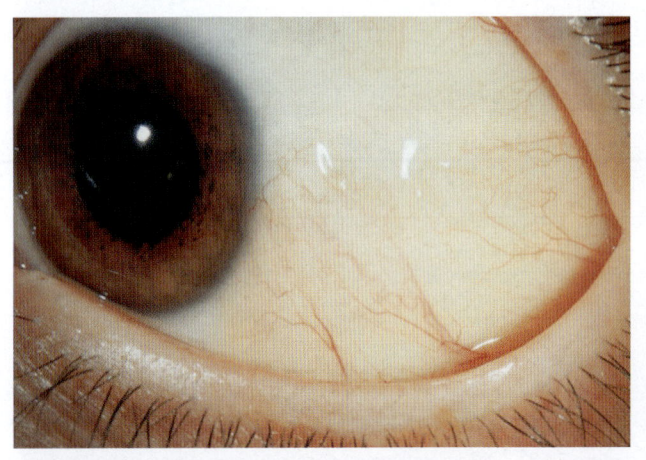

Figure 25.16. Appearance of area shown in Figure 25.15, 13 years later, after resection and cryotherapy, showing no recurrence.

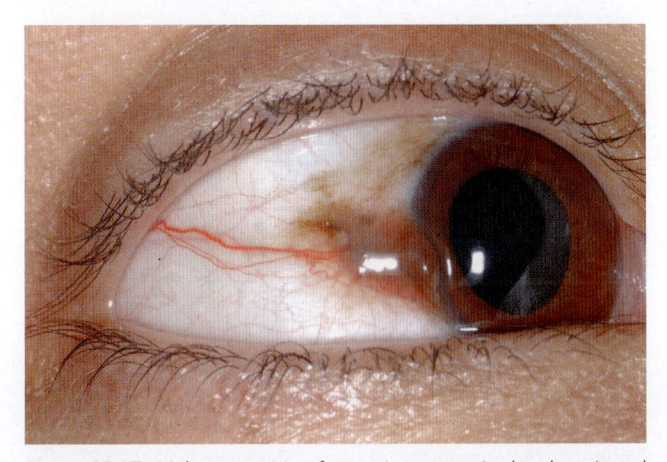

Figure 25.17. Melanoma arising from primary acquired melanosis and secondarily invading the cornea.

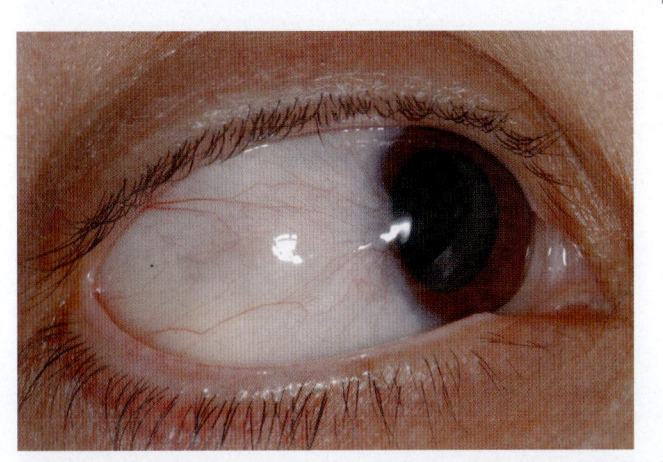

Figure 25.18. Appearance of same area 6 months after removal and cryotherapy, showing excellent result with no tumor recurrence.

TREATMENT OF CONJUNCTIVAL MALIGNANCIES WITH TOPICAL CHEMOTHERAPY AND INTERFERON

Topical chemotherapy can sometimes be used as ancillary treatment for conjunctival malignancies, particularly squamous cell carcinoma, PAM, and superficial melanoma. It is generally used after incomplete surgical resection or recurrence, but can be employed as a primary treatment, particularly in older individuals who are poor candidates for surgery.

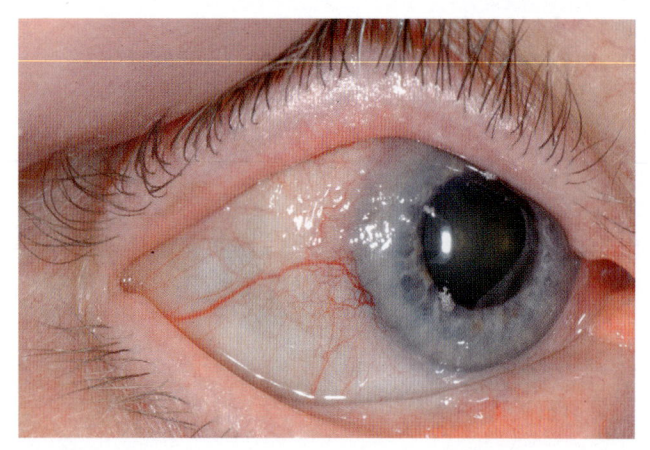

Figure 25.19. Appearance of recurrent conjunctival squamous cell carcinoma with corneal invasion before treatment with topical Mitomycin C.

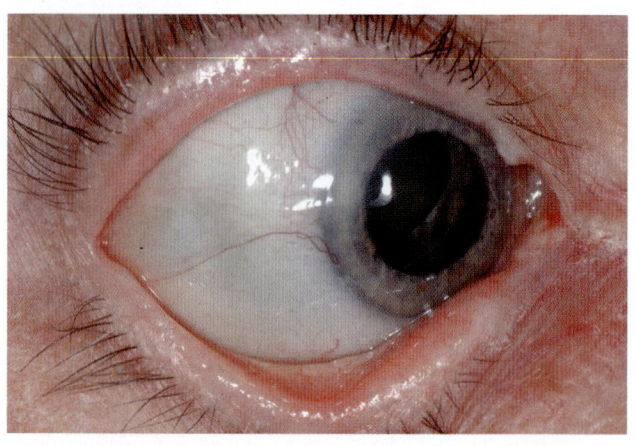

Figure 25.20. After 2 weeks of topical Mitomycin C treatment, the tumor showed a dramatic response. This photograph was taken 9 months after treatment, still showing no recurrence.

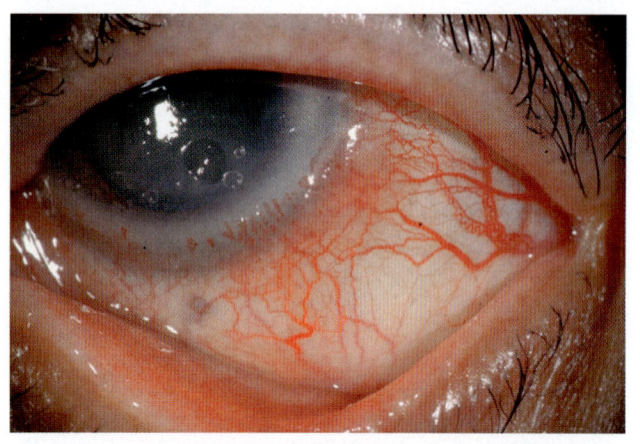

Figure 25.21. Diffuse squamous cell carcinoma involving limbal conjunctiva and cornea for 6 clock hours. A small biopsy confirmed the diagnosis.

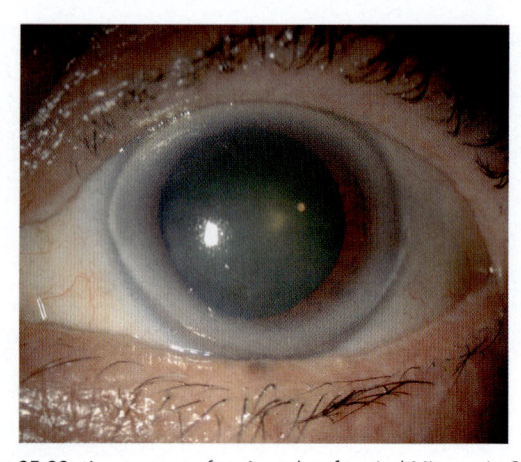

Figure 25.22. Appearance after 4 weeks of topical Mitomycin C treatment showing complete resolution of the tumor.

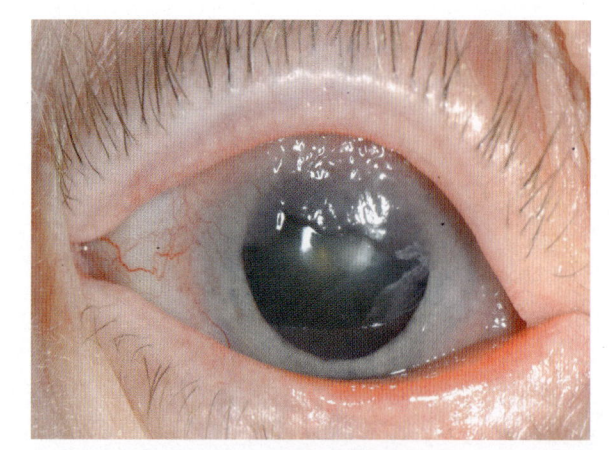

Figure 25.23. Appearance of squamous cell carcinoma involving superior bulbar conjunctiva for 8 clock hours of cornea in an elderly man from a nursing home.

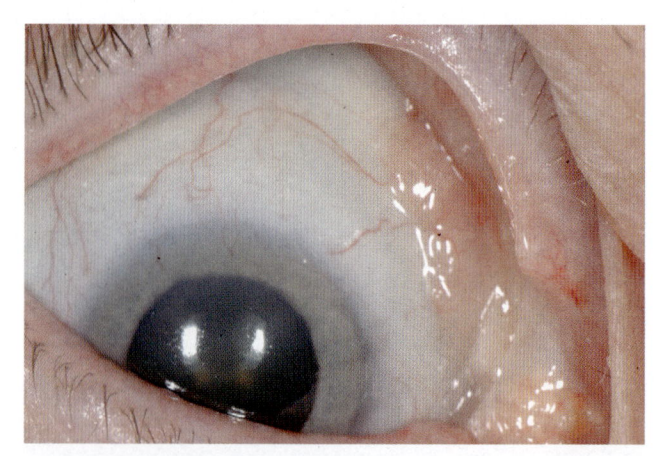

Figure 25.24. Appearance of lesion shown in Figure 25.23 after 4 months of daily topical interferon treatment. Note the complete response of the corneal portion of the lesion.

SUPPLEMENTAL TREATMENT OF CONJUNCTIVAL NEOPLASMS WITH PLAQUE RADIOTHERAPY

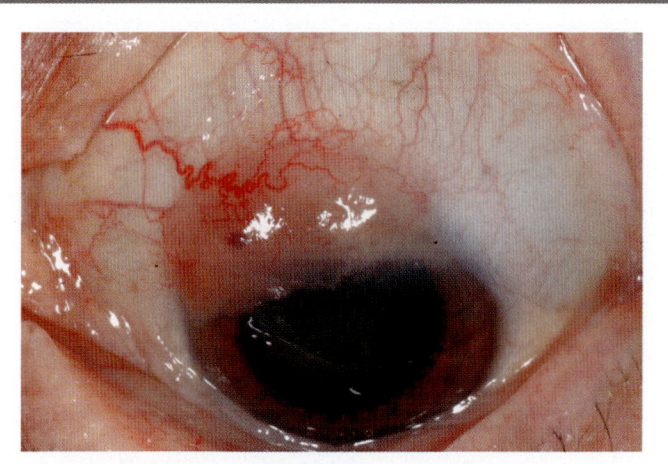

Figure 25.25. Amelanotic limbal conjunctival melanoma in 70-year-old man.

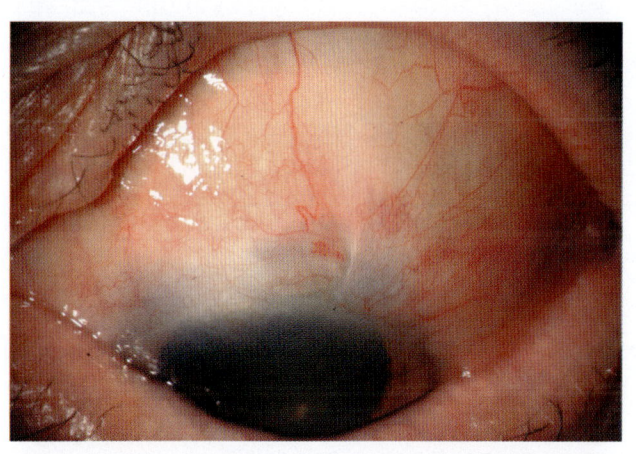

Figure 25.26. After surgical resection, the wound has healed well but histopathology showed extensive scleral invasion and possible positive superior margin.

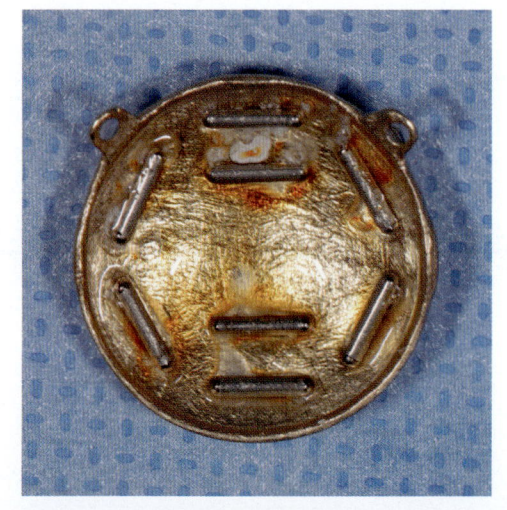

Figure 25.27. Design of plaque that will be used to treat residual scleral invasion of melanoma in patient shown in Figure 25.25.

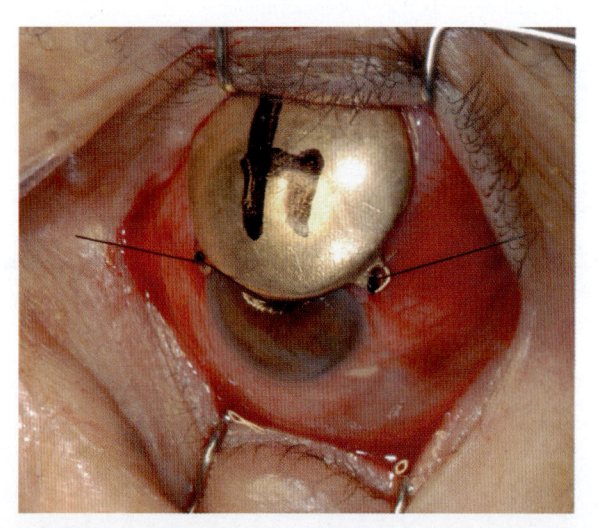

Figure 25.28. Plaque applied to eye designed to deliver dose of 60 gray to the tumor site.

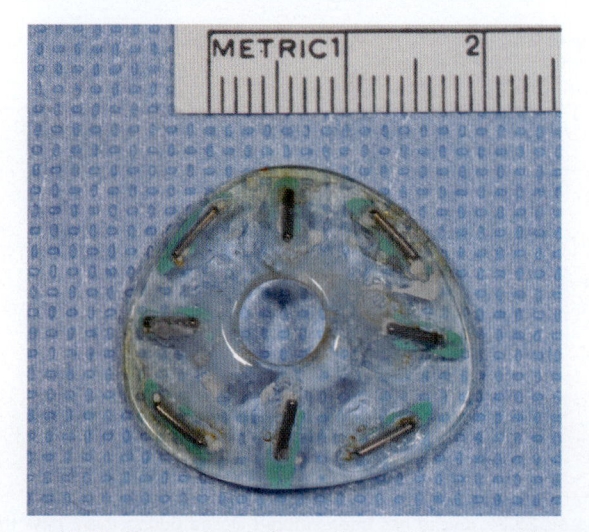

Figure 25.29. Plaque design for patients with more widespread involvement. The plaque is not shielded so that all tarsal and palpebral conjunctiva will receive adequate dose. The I-125 seeds are placed circumferentially in this case.

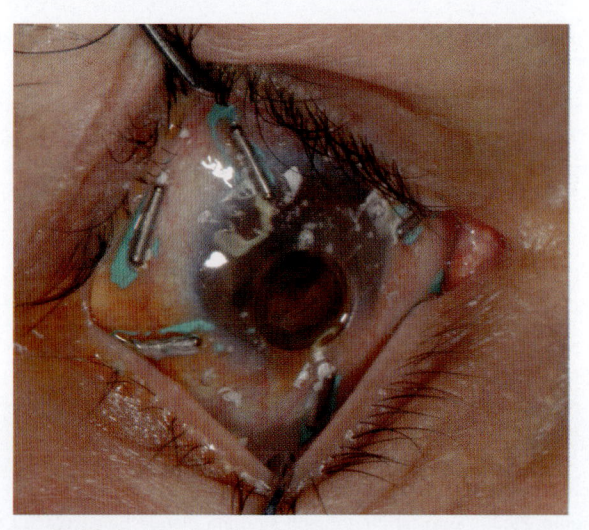

Figure 25.30. Unshielded plaque placed on eye to treat residual conjunctival melanoma.

SUPPLEMENTAL TREATMENT OF EXTENSIVE CONJUNCTIVAL NEOPLASM WITH PLAQUE BRACHYTHERAPY

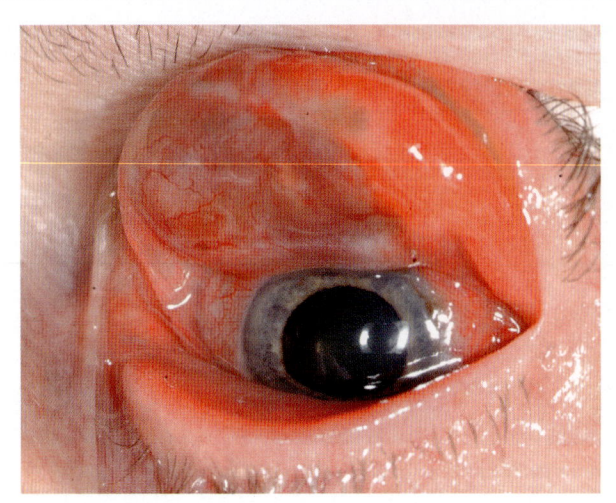

Figure 25.31. Recurrent amelanotic conjunctival melanoma occupying entire superior fornix in a 60-year-old woman.

Figure 25.32. At time of surgery, tumor was removed totally with postlamellar dissection of eyelid.

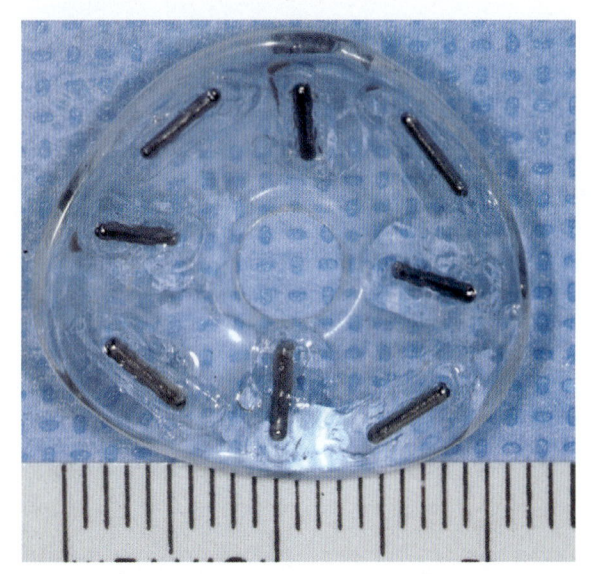

Figure 25.33. Design of plaque to treat entire surface of conjunctiva; the patient had multiple prior recurrences in all quadrants.

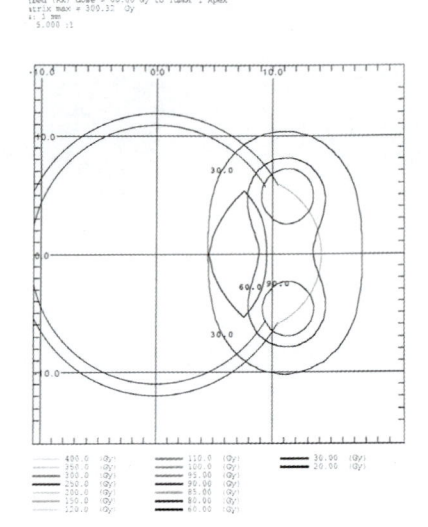

Figure 25.34. Radiation dose plot showing distribution of radiation to anterior segment of the eye.

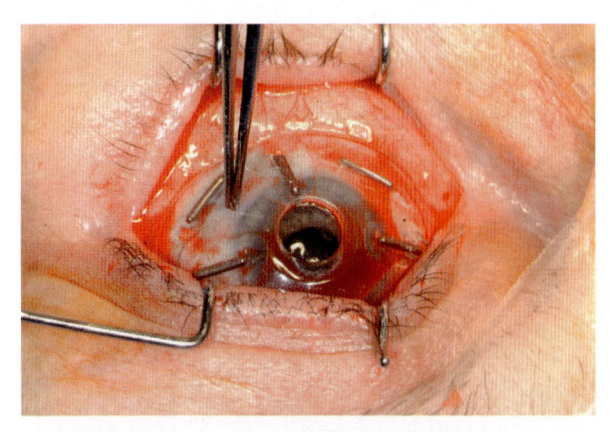

Figure 25.35. Surgical photograph showing plaque being placed on eye.

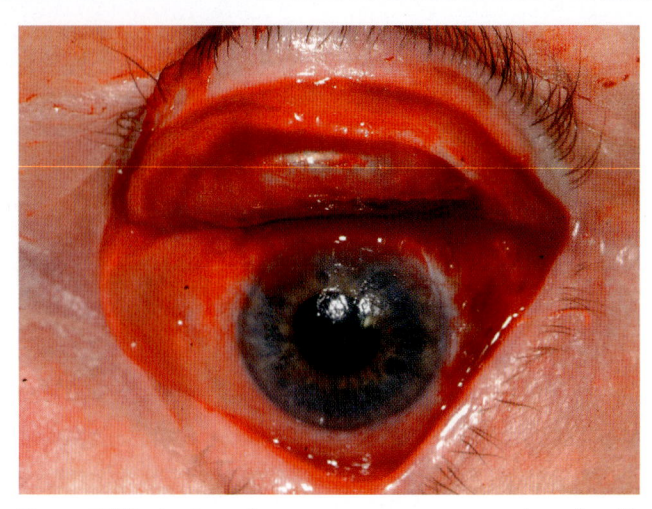

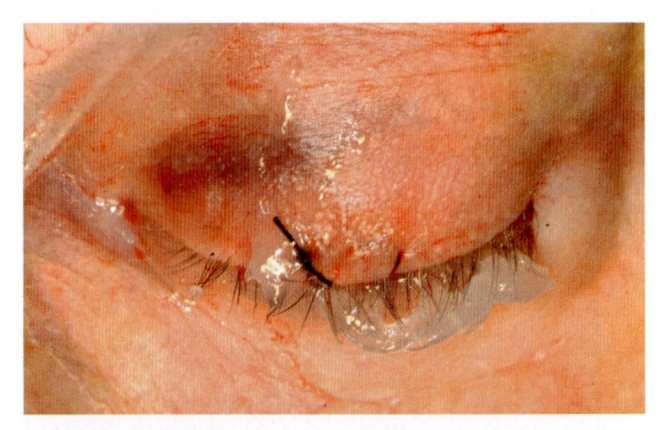

Figure 25.36. Eyelid has been sutured closed during the 7 days that plaque will remain on the eye.

PART 3

TUMORS OF THE ORBIT

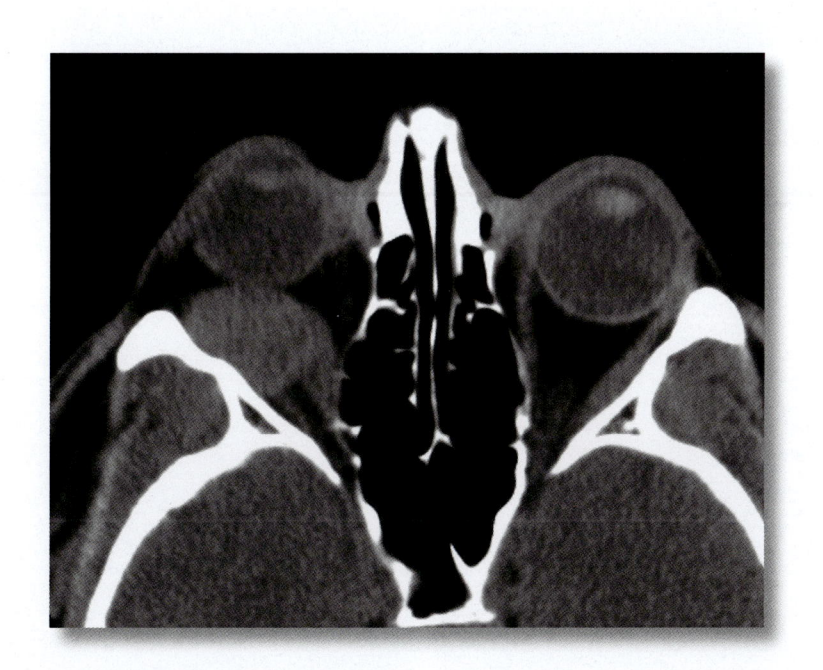

CHAPTER 26

INFLAMMATORY ORBITAL LESIONS THAT SIMULATE NEOPLASMS

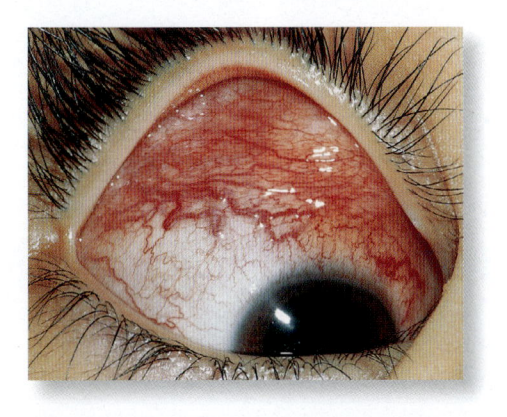

General Considerations

There are a number of orbital inflammatory processes that are important in the differential diagnosis of orbital tumors. The most important of these are thyroid-related ophthalmopathy (TRO) and idiopathic nongranulomatous orbital inflammation (INOI) (inflammatory pseudotumor, idiopathic orbital inflammatory syndrome [IOIS]). In addition, there are a number of bacterial, fungal, and idiopathic granulomatous disorders that can occur in the orbit.

TRO is a common autoimmune disorder usually associated with hyperthyroidism. The diverse nomenclature for this intriguing entity has been confusing and inconsistent and includes Graves disease, Graves orbitopathy, Graves ophthalmopathy, thyroid eye disease, thyroid orbitopathy, thyroid ophthalmopathy, dysthyroid orbitopathy, dysthyroid ophthalmopathy, thyroid-related orbitopathy, thyroid-associated orbitopathy, and thyroid-associated ophthalmopathy. We have chosen to use the term "thyroid-related ophthalmopathy" because the condition is generally related to thyroid dysfunction and affects other ocular structures (eyelids, conjunctiva) in addition to the orbit.

TRO typically affects the extraocular muscles and has rather characteristic features. In some cases, it can simulate a neoplasm clinically and radiographically. Numerous chapters and articles have addressed the clinical features, pathogenesis, pathology, and management of TRO and only some of the more important or recent ones are cited here (1–20).

Clinical Features

Clinically, the patient with TRO usually shows characteristic unilateral or bilateral proptosis, eyelid retraction, eyelid lag on downgaze, eyelid edema, and conjunctival hyperemia and edema. In more advanced cases, the patient can develop diplopia, exposure keratopathy, and optic disc edema owing to compression of the optic nerve in the orbit.

Diagnostic Approaches

Although there are many laboratory tests to assess thyroid gland function and diagnose TRO, the main ones used by most clinicians are tri-iodothyronine (T3), total and free thyroxine (T4), and thyroid-stimulating hormone (TSH). Orbital imaging studies have become highly reliable methods of diagnosing TRO. Computed tomography (CT) and magnetic resonance imaging (MRI) show characteristic enlargement of rectus muscles without appreciable involvement of the muscle tendons and orbital fat. Ultrasonography has been largely replaced by these superior imaging techniques (9,10).

THYROID-RELATED OPHTHALMOPATHY

Pathology

On surgical inspection or gross examination, the extraocular muscles are enlarged, firm, and rubbery. Histopathology reveals infiltration of the affected enlarged muscles by lymphocytes, plasma cells, and scattered mast cells (19).

Management

Depending on the severity of the disease and the complications, management of TRO can include observation, corticosteroids, radiotherapy, tarsorrhaphy, and orbital decompression. These treatment approaches are discussed in detail in the literature (11–18).

THYROID-RELATED OPHTHALMOPATHY

Selected References

Reviews
1. Bartalena L, Wiersinga WM, Pinchera A. Graves' ophthalmopathy: State of the art and perspectives. *J Endocrinol Invest* 2004;27:295–301.
2. Prabhakar BS, Bahn RS, Smith TJ. Current perspective on the pathogenesis of Graves' disease and ophthalmopathy. *Endocr Rev* 2003;24:802–835.
3. Chavis PS. Thyroid and the eye. *Curr Opin Ophthalmol* 2002;13:352–356.
4. Hatton MP, Rubin PA. The pathophysiology of thyroid-associated ophthalmopathy. *Ophthalmol Clin North Am* 2002;15:113–119.
5. Bradley EA. Graves ophthalmopathy. *Curr Opin Ophthalmol* 2001;12:347–351.
6. Bahn RS. Understanding the immunology of Graves' ophthalmopathy. Is it an autoimmune disease? *Endocrinol Metab Clin North Am* 2000;29:287–296.
7. Wang Y, Smith TJ. Current concepts in the molecular pathogenesis of thyroid-associated ophthalmopathy. *Invest Ophthalmol Vis Sci* 2014;55:1735–1748.
8. Edmunds MR, Huntback J, Durrani OM. Are ethnicity, social grade, and social deprivation associated with severity of thyroid-associated ophthalmopathy? *Ophthal Plast Reconstr Surg* 2014;30:241–245.

Imaging
9. Konuk O, Atasever T, Unal M, et al. Orbital gallium-67 scintigraphy in Graves' ophthalmopathy. *Thyroid* 2002;12:603–608.
10. Rabinowitz MP, Carrasco JR. Update on advanced imaging options for thyroid-associated orbitopathy. *Saudi J Ophthalmol* 2012;26(4):385–392.

Management
11. Bartalena L, Pinchera A, Marcocci C. Management of Graves' ophthalmopathy: reality and perspectives. *Endocr Rev* 2000;21:168–199.
12. Clauser L, Galie M, Sarti E, et al. Rationale of treatment in Graves ophthalmopathy. *Plast Reconstr Surg* 2001;108:1880–1894.
13. Gorman CA, Garrity JA, Fatourechi V, et al. The aftermath of orbital radiotherapy for Graves' ophthalmopathy. *Ophthalmology* 2002;109:2100–2107.
14. Gorman CA, Garrity JA, Fatourechi V, et al. A prospective, randomized, double-blind, placebo-controlled study of orbital radiotherapy for Graves' ophthalmopathy. *Ophthalmology* 2001;108:1523–1534.
15. Chu YK, Kim SJ, Lee SY. Surgical treatment modalities of thyroid ophthalmopathy. *Korean J Ophthalmol* 2001;15:128–132.
16. Inoue Y, Tsuboi T, Kouzaki A, et al. Ophthalmic surgery in dysthyroid ophthalmopathy. *Thyroid* 2002;12:257–263.
17. Larsen DA, Ehlers N, Bek T. Thyroid-associated orbitopathy (TAO) treated by lateral orbital decompression. *Acta Ophthalmol Scand* 2004;82:108–109.
18. Hahn E, Paperriere N, Millar BA, et al. Orbital radiation therapy for Graves ophthalmopathy: measuring clinical efficacy and impact. *Pract Radiat Oncol* 2014;4:233–239.

Histopathology
19. Hufnagel TJ, Hickey WF, Cobbs WH, et al. Immunohistochemical and ultrastructural studies on the exenterated orbital tissues of a patient with Grave's disease. *Ophthalmology* 1984;91:1411–1419.

Case Reports
20. Hornbeak DM, Tamhankar MA, Eckstein LA. No light perception vision from compressive thyroid orbitopathy. *Orbit* 2014;33:72–74.

THYROID-RELATED OPHTHALMOPATHY

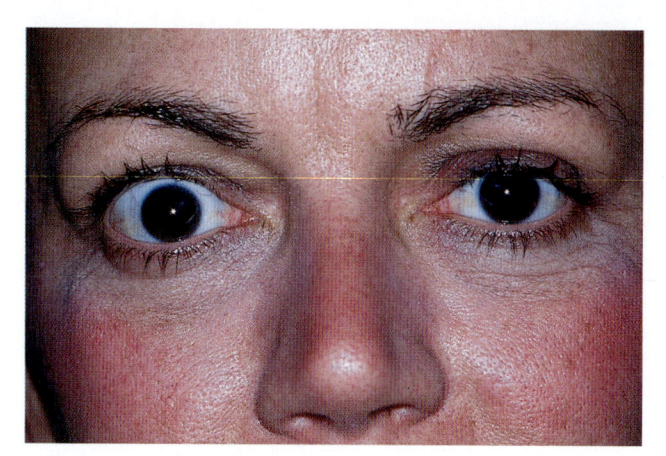

Figure 26.1. Thyroid-related ophthalmopathy with characteristic proptosis and eyelid retraction affecting mainly the right eye in a 35-year-old woman.

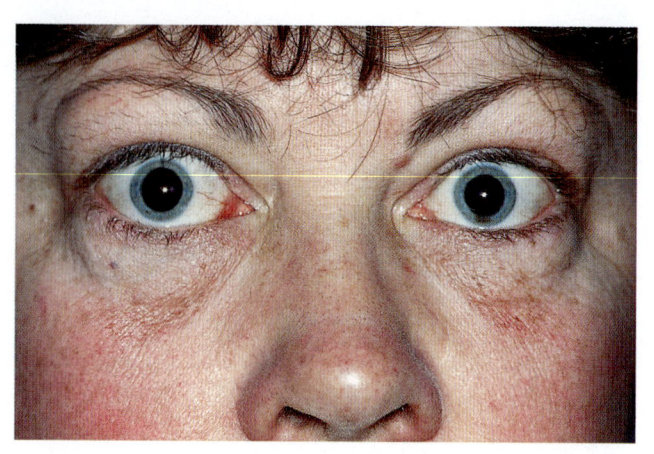

Figure 26.2. Thyroid-related ophthalmopathy with bilateral symmetric proptosis and eyelid retraction in a 43-year-old woman.

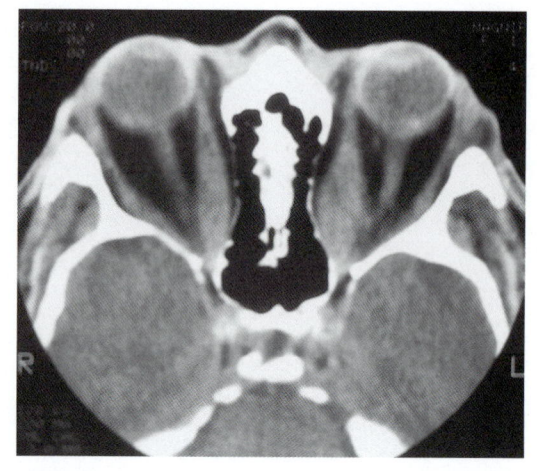

Figure 26.3. Axial computed tomography showing typical enlargement of extraocular muscles with sparing of the tendons. In this case, the medial rectus muscles are mainly involved.

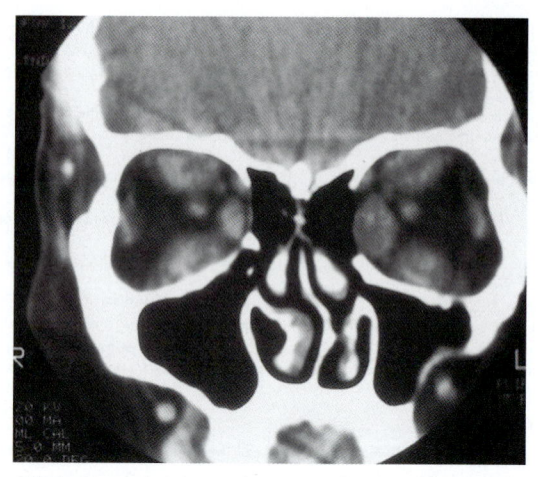

Figure 26.4. Coronal computed tomography through the midportion of the orbit, showing enlargement of several rectus muscles.

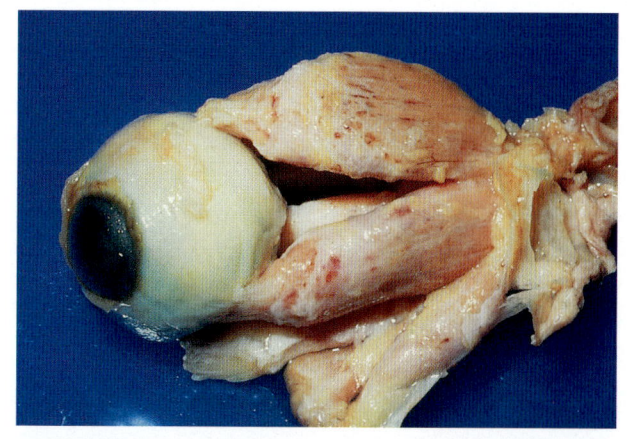

Figure 26.5. Gross specimen of globe and extraocular muscles removed postmortem from a patient with severe TRO. Note the marked enlargement of all rectus muscles. (Courtesy of Ralph C. Eagle, Jr, MD.)

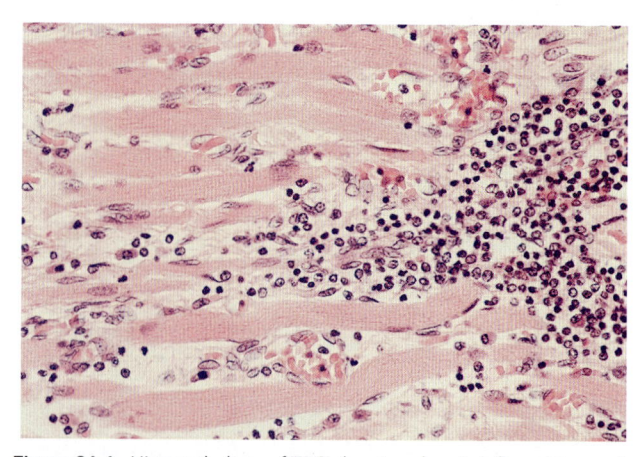

Figure 26.6. Histopathology of TRO showing chronic inflammatory cells infiltrating the extraocular muscle. (Hematoxylin–eosin ×100.) (Courtesy of Ralph C. Eagle, Jr, MD.)

Chapter 26 Inflammatory Orbital Lesions That Simulate Neoplasms 447

● THYROID-RELATED OPHTHALMOPATHY: CLINICAL AND RADIOLOGIC VARIATIONS

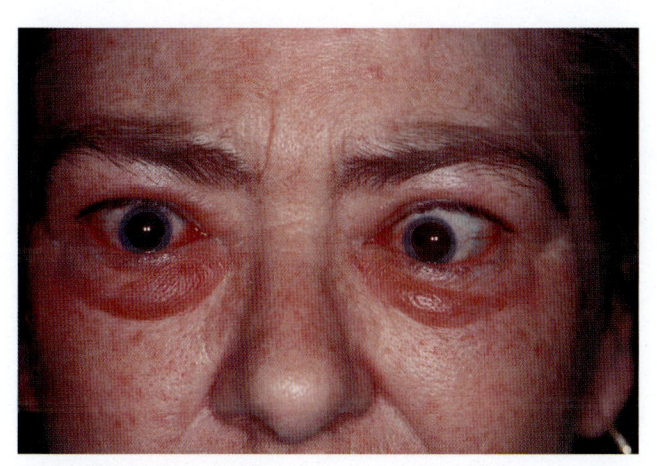

Figure 26.7. Middle-aged woman with typical eyelid edema, eyelid retraction, and left esotropia.

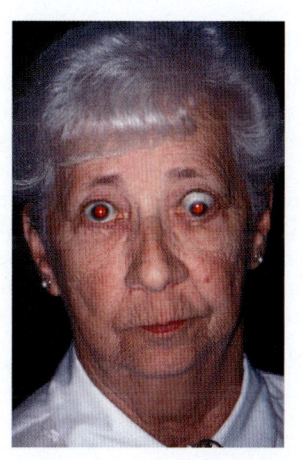

Figure 26.8. Woman with retraction of right upper eyelid and more severe involvement of the left eye with downward displacement of the globe.

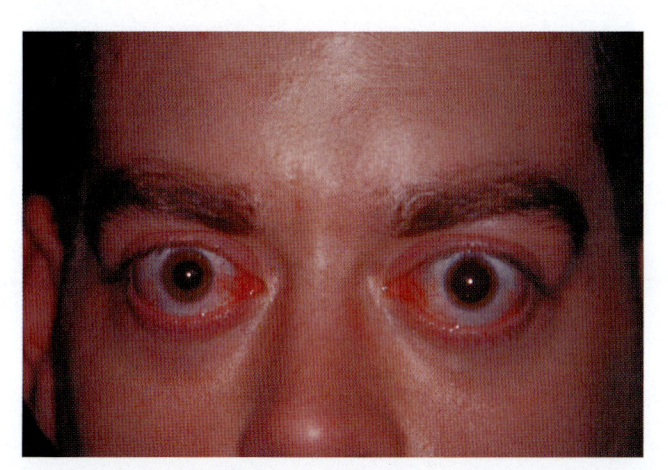

Figure 26.9. Bilateral eyelid retraction producing typical "thyroid stare" in a 27-year-old man.

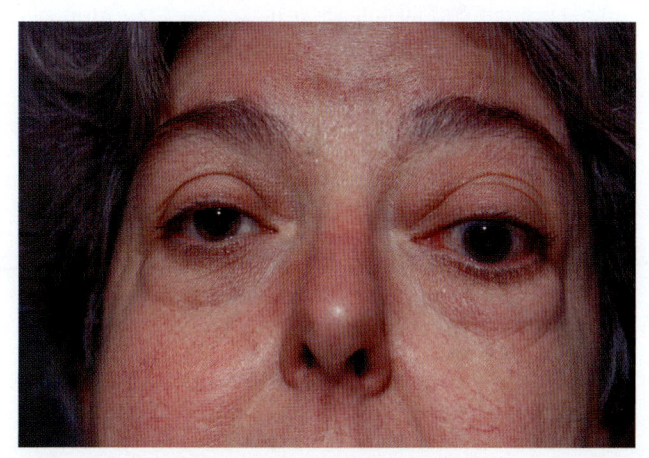

Figure 26.10. Unilateral TRO involving left orbit in a 57-year-old woman. In this instance, there is proptosis of left eye with less edema and eyelid retraction.

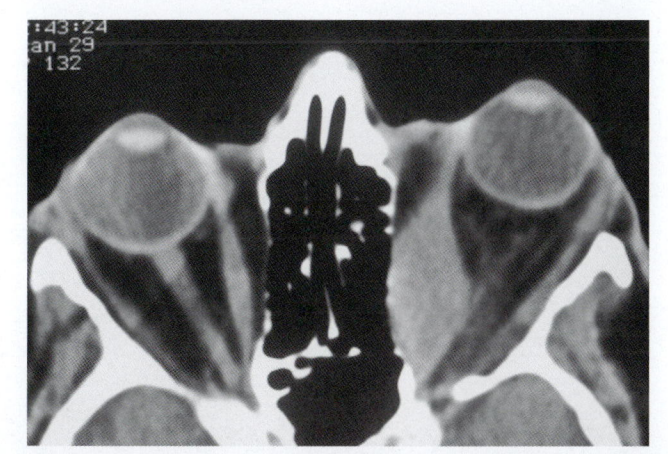

Figure 26.11. Axial computed tomography of patient shown in Figure 26.10, demonstrating marked enlargement of left medial rectus muscle but no evident enlargement of other extraocular muscles. Note the sparing of the tendon of the rectus muscle. Myositis from non-TRO causes would be more likely to affect the tendon.

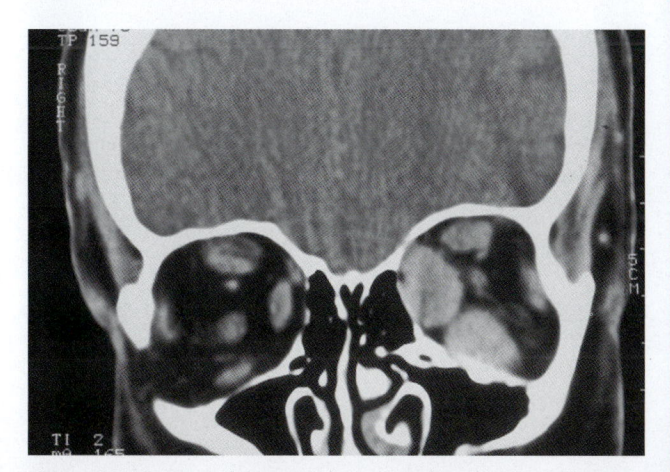

Figure 26.12. Coronal computed tomography of patient shown in Figure 26.10, demonstrating marked enlargement of left medial and inferior rectus muscles in left eye.

ORBITAL CELLULITIS

General Considerations

Acute orbital cellulitis is an infection of the soft tissues of the orbit and adjacent structures. It can affect children or adults. It most commonly occurs as a result of infectious extension from the ethmoid or frontal sinuses (1–9). However, it can also develop by contiguous spread from sites of trauma or infection, including dacryocystitis and conjunctivitis. Mucocele and mucopyocele, which can also extend into the orbit from the sinuses, are discussed in Chapter 27. Infectious orbital inflammation has been classified into five categories (2):

Group 1: Preseptal cellulitis
Group 2: Orbital cellulitis
Group 3: Subperiosteal abscess
Group 4: Orbital abscess
Group 5: Cavernous sinus thrombosis

Based on traditional terminology, we use the umbrella term "orbital cellulitis" to include all of these categories. Although the classification suggests an orderly progression, that is not necessarily the case and clinical onset can vary considerably.

Clinical Features

The clinical findings in orbital cellulitis vary with the inciting cause and the category and severity of the disease. The patient can present with any combination of pain, eyelid edema, conjunctival hyperemia, discharge, proptosis, displacement of the globe, and diplopia. Cavernous sinus thrombosis (group 5) can induce severe symptoms and was often fatal before the advent of antibiotics. In some instances, an orbital abscess can be localized and simulate a cyst or neoplasm. In a child, rhabdomyosarcoma and other malignant tumors can produce inflammatory signs and should be considered in the differential diagnosis (6). It should also be remembered that necrotic retinoblastoma can cause secondary inflammatory signs and simulate orbital cellulitis (7,8).

Diagnostic Approaches

History and physical examination should be directed toward detecting an inciting cause. Imaging studies like CT and MRI can detect primary infection of the sinuses, determine the extent of the orbital disease, and allow classification of the infectious process.

Pathology

The pathology of orbital cellulitis varies with the cause of the infection and the inciting organism. Histopathologically, the tissues are infiltrated or replaced by acute and chronic inflammatory cells and the inciting organisms can often be identified. Most common organisms include *Streptococcus* species, *Staphylococcus aureus*, and *Staphylococcus epidermidis*. *Haemophilus influenzae* was previously the most common cause, especially among children. However, it has become uncommon since the introduction of specific vaccines.

Management

Treatment generally involves microscopic study and cultures of the discharge and appropriate antibiotic therapy (9). Surgical drainage is often helpful. The prognosis is generally good unless severe cavernous sinus thrombosis develops.

Selected References

Reviews
1. Murphy C, Livingstone I, Foot B, et al. Orbital cellulitis in Scotland: Current incidence, aetiology, management and outcomes. *Br J Ophthalmol* 2014;98:1575–1578.
2. Chandler JR, Langenbrunner DJ, Stevens ER. The pathogenesis of orbital complications in acute sinusitis. *Laryngoscope* 1970;80:1414–1428.
3. Shovlin JP. Orbital infections and inflammations. *Curr Opin Ophthalmol* 1998;9:41–48.
4. Tovilla-Canales JL, Nava A, Tovilla y Pomar JL. Orbital and periorbital infections. *Curr Opin Ophthalmol* 2001;12:335–341.
5. Hornblass A, Herschorn BJ, Stern K, et al. Orbital abscess. *Surv Ophthalmol* 1984;29:169–178.
6. Cota N, Chandna A, Abernethy LJ. Orbital abscess masquerading as a rhabdomyosarcoma. *J AAPOS* 2000;4:318–320.
7. Shields JA, Shields CL, Suvarnamani C, et al. Retinoblastoma manifesting as orbital cellulitis. *Am J Ophthalmol* 1991;112:442–449.
8. Mullaney PB, Karcioglu ZA, Huaman AM, et al. Retinoblastoma associated orbital cellulitis. *Br J Ophthalmol* 1998;82:517–521.
9. Lee S, Yen MT. Management of preseptal and orbital cellulitis. *Saudi J Ophthalmol* 2011;25:21–29.

Chapter 26 Inflammatory Orbital Lesions That Simulate Neoplasms

ORBITAL CELLULITIS AND ABSCESS

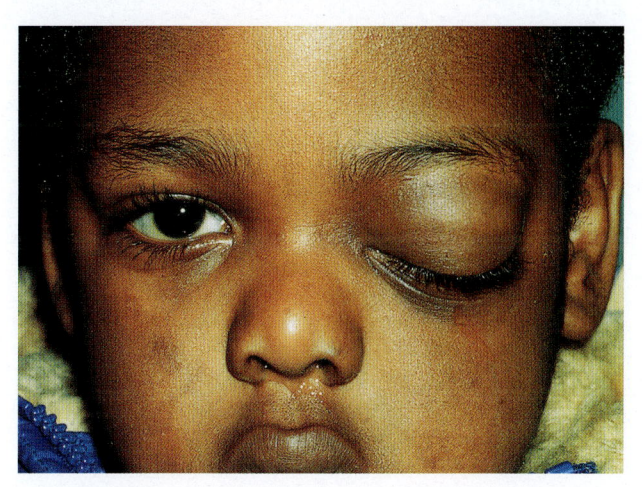

Figure 26.13. Acute orbital cellulitis secondary to ethmoid sinusitis and subperiosteal abscess in a 3-year-old child, showing eyelid swelling and blepharoptosis.

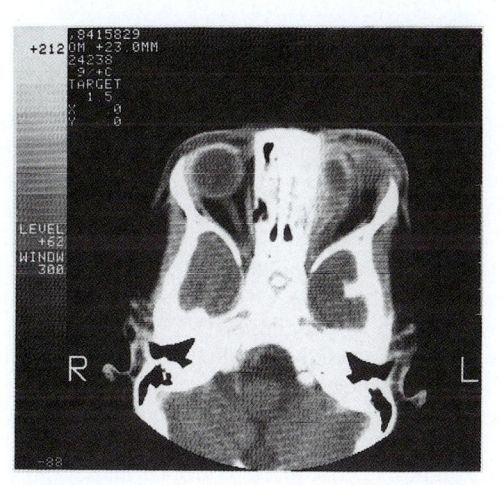

Figure 26.14. Axial computed tomography of patient shown in Figure 26.13, demonstrating ethmoiditis and left subperiosteal abscess.

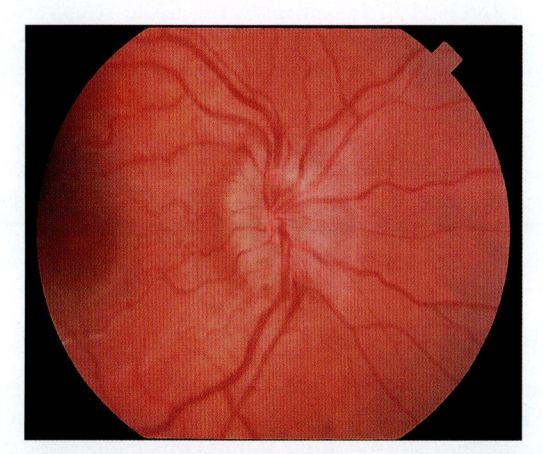

Figure 26.15. Fundus photograph showing edema and hyperemia of right optic disc in an 8-year-old girl with circumscribed orbital abscess compressing the optic nerve.

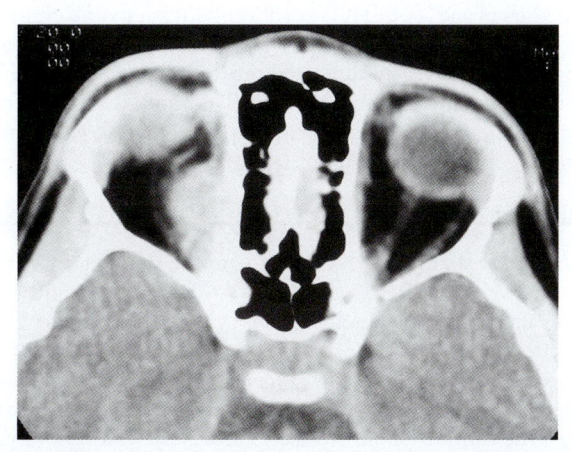

Figure 26.16. Axial computed tomography of patient shown in Figure 26.15, revealing circumscribed lesion in orbit. The peripheral aspects of the lesion demonstrated gadolinium enhancement with magnetic resonance imaging.

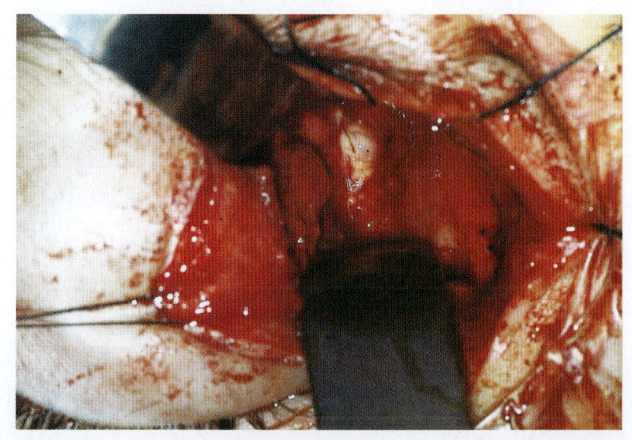

Figure 26.17. Surgical view showing yellow purulent material coming from abscess discovered at the time of surgical exploration. No organisms were found on stains and cultures.

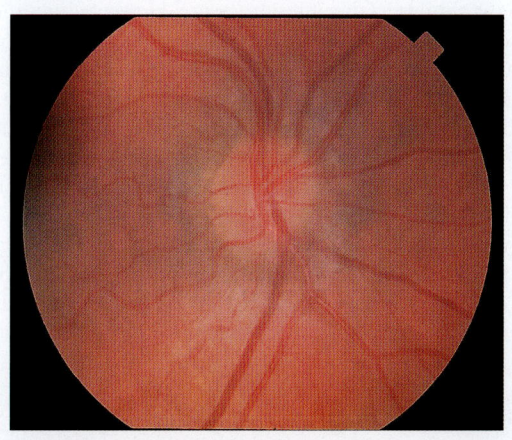

Figure 26.18. Appearance of optic disc 2 months later. The disc edema resolved rapidly after drainage of the abscess and treatment with broad-spectrum antibiotics.

ORBIT: IDIOPATHIC NONGRANULOMATOUS ORBITAL INFLAMMATION (INFLAMMATORY PSEUDOTUMOR, IDIOPATHIC ORBITAL INFLAMMATORY SYNDROME)

General Considerations

"Nonspecific orbital inflammation (NOI)" is traditionally used to describe a nongranulomatous inflammatory process within the orbit that has no demonstrable cause (1–20). The term "pseudotumor" is sometimes applied to this condition. However, that term can apply to any lesion that simulates a neoplasm, including granulomatous inflammation, abscess, and amyloidosis. Therefore, we prefer to avoid "pseudotumor," and prefer to call this condition INOI or IOIS (14). There is considerable confusion regarding this condition and the definition, terminology, and classification will most certainly change as it is better understood and more specific etiologies are identified.

In the authors' series of 1,264 orbital masses, 98 cases of INOI accounted for 74% of inflammatory-infectious diseases and for 8% of all orbital lesions (1). In a study of orbital tumors in older patients, it accounted for 8% of lesions among patients >60 years of age (12). INOI can affect both adults and children (3). The mean age at diagnosis is about 45 years with an age range of 2 to 92 years. About 25% are bilateral (8). Depending on the tissues involved and the orbital location, INOI has been divided into subcategories, including myositis, dacryoadenitis, anterior, diffuse, and posterior (apical) (2).

Clinical Features

The clinical features of INOI vary with the subcategory of the disease. Myositis affects one or more rectus muscles and produces acute onset of pain that is worse with eye movements, and injection of the muscle insertion. Central vision is usually preserved. Dacryoadenitis shows superotemporal eyelid and conjunctival swelling, pain, and a tender mass in the lacrimal gland area. The central vision is usually intact. The anterior variant is characterized by pain, eyelid edema, conjunctival chemosis, and limitation of ocular motility. Affected patients can have signs of diffuse uveitis and retinal detachment, findings similar to Harada disease. The diffuse variant demonstrates symptoms and signs similar to the anterior variety. However, the findings are more severe and proptosis is more pronounced. The apical variant of INOI causes more severe pain, visual loss, and motility disturbance, but less anterior segment inflammation. The pain is particularly severe with ocular movement. The painful ophthalmoplegia is similar to the Tolosa–Hunt syndrome (10).

In some instances, INOI can extend beyond the orbit into the paranasal sinuses and brain. Some such patients may have only minimal symptoms and signs to suggest neurologic extension, but it can be recognized on neuroimaging (19). Severe cases can rarely present with central retinal artery and vein obstruction secondary to compression of the globe or the vascular structures in the orbit (20).

Differential Diagnosis

The differential diagnosis of INOI includes a variety of inflammatory and neoplastic conditions. Myositis can closely resemble thyroid-associated orbitopathy or metastatic carcinoma. Any variant must be differentiated from lymphoma, metastatic carcinoma, and other circumscribed or diffuse orbital masses.

Diagnostic Approaches

Findings on CT and MRI vary with the location and extent of involvement. Myositis shows enlargement of one or more rectus muscles, often with involvement of the muscle tendons, a finding that helps to differentiate it from thyroid-related orbitopathy, in which the tendons are spared. Dacryoadenitis shows enlargement of the lacrimal gland and inflammatory signs and may cause findings similar to a ruptured dermoid cyst. Anterior and diffuse involvements show an ill-defined mass and choroidal thickening and retinal detachment. The apical variant shows a diffuse or ill-defined mass at the orbital apex with compression of nerves and muscles. As mentioned, neuroimaging studies can sometimes detect extraorbital extension of INOI (19). In patients with classic symptoms and signs, an orbital biopsy is generally not indicated unless the lesion fails to respond to medical therapy (see Management).

Pathology

Histopathologically, the affected tissues in INOI are infiltrated by chronic inflammatory cells, mainly lymphocytes and plasma cells without granulomatous inflammation. In children, there are generally more eosinophils. More chronic cases show marked fibrosis and sclerosis.

Management

If the diagnosis INOI is suspected clinically, the first course of management is oral corticosteroids (usually 80 to 100 mg of prednisone daily for adults and less for children) for about 5 days followed by gradual tapering of the medication. Most cases show a dramatic response unless the lesion has extensive fibrosis. If there is a poor response to steroids, then carefully planned incisional biopsy is warranted to exclude a malignant neoplasm. If the diagnosis is established histopathologically, then corticosteroid-resistant cases can be treated with cytotoxic agents or radiotherapy. Recurrence is common and a second course of treatment is often necessary (10). Orbital exenteration rarely becomes necessary because of severe fibrosis or unrelenting pain.

There has been recent interest in the use of infliximab, an anti-tumor monoclonal antibody directed against tumor necrosis factor-α (15,16). It was used primarily in recalcitrant cases of myositis after failure of standard treatments. It has also been administered for severe bilateral cases. More patients and longer follow-up are necessary to determine the efficacy of this method of treatment.

ORBIT: IDIOPATHIC NONGRANULOMATOUS ORBITAL INFLAMMATION (INFLAMMATORY PSEUDOTUMOR, IDIOPATHIC ORBITAL INFLAMMATORY SYNDROME)

Selected References

Reviews

1. Shields JA, Shields CL, Scartozzi R. Survey of 1264 patients with orbital tumors and simulating lesions: the 2002 Montgomery Lecture, part 1. *Ophthalmology* 2004;111:997–1008.
2. Rootman J, Nugent R. The classification and management of acute orbital pseudotumors. *Ophthalmology* 1982;89:1040–1048.
3. Mottow LS, Jakobiec FA. Idiopathic inflammatory orbital pseudotumor in childhood. I. Clinical characteristics. *Arch Ophthalmol* 1978;96:1410–1416.
4. Mombaerts I, Koornneef L. Current status in the treatment of orbital myositis. *Ophthalmology* 1997;104:402–408.
5. Mannor GE, Rose GE, Moseley IF, et al. Outcome of orbital myositis. Clinical features associated with recurrence. *Ophthalmology* 1997;104:409–414.
6. Foley MR, Moshfeghi DM, Wilson MW, et al. Orbital inflammatory syndromes with systemic involvement may mimic metastatic disease. *Ophthal Plast Reconstr Surg* 2003;19:324–327.
7. Gordon LK. Diagnostic dilemmas in orbital inflammatory disease. *Ocul Immunol Inflamm* 2003;11:3–15.
8. Yuen SJ, Rubin PA. Idiopathic orbital inflammation: distribution, clinical features, and treatment outcome. *Arch Ophthalmol* 2003;121:491–499.
9. Jacobs D, Galetta S. Diagnosis and management of orbital pseudotumor. *Curr Opin Ophthalmol* 2002;13:347–351.
10. Wasmeier C, Pfadenhauer K, Rosler A. Idiopathic inflammatory pseudotumor of the orbit and Tolosa-Hunt syndrome—are they the same disease? *J Neurol* 2002;249:1237–1241.
11. Yuen SJ, Rubin PA. Idiopathic orbital inflammation: ocular mechanisms and clinicopathology. *Ophthalmol Clin North Am* 2002;15:121–126.
12. Demirci H, Shields CL, Shields JA, et al. Orbital tumors in the older adult population. *Ophthalmology* 2002;109:243–248.
13. Espinoza GM. Orbital inflammatory pseudotumors: etiology, differential diagnosis, and management. *Curr Rheumatol Rep* 2010;12:443–447.
14. Shields JA, Shields CL. Orbital pseudotumor versus idiopathic nongranulomatous orbital inflammation. Commentary. *Ophthal Plast Reconstr Surg* 2013;29(5)349.

Management

15. Wilson MW, Shergy WJ, Haik BG. Infliximab in the treatment of recalcitrant idiopathic orbital inflammation. *Ophthal Plast Reconstr Surg* 2004;20:381–383.
16. Garrity JA, Coleman AW, Matteson EL, et al. Treatment of recalcitrant idiopathic orbital inflammation (chronic orbital myositis) with infliximab. *Am J Ophthalmol* 2004;138:925–930.

Case Reports

17. Oguz KK, Kiratli H, Oguz O, et al. Multifocal fibrosclerosis: a new case report and review of the literature. *Eur Radiol* 2002;12:1134–1138.
18. Reittner P, Riepl T, Goritschnig T, et al. Bilateral orbital pseudotumour due to Ormond's disease: MR imaging and CT findings. *Neuroradiology* 2002;44:272–274.
19. Mahr MA, Salomao DR, Garrity JA. Inflammatory orbital pseudotumor with extension beyond the orbit. *Am J Ophthalmol* 2004;138:396–400.
20. Foroozan R. Combined central retinal artery and vein occlusion from orbital inflammatory pseudotumour. *Clin Exp Ophthalmol* 2004;32:435–437.

IDIOPATHIC NONGRANULOMATOUS ORBITAL INFLAMMATION IN ADULTHOOD

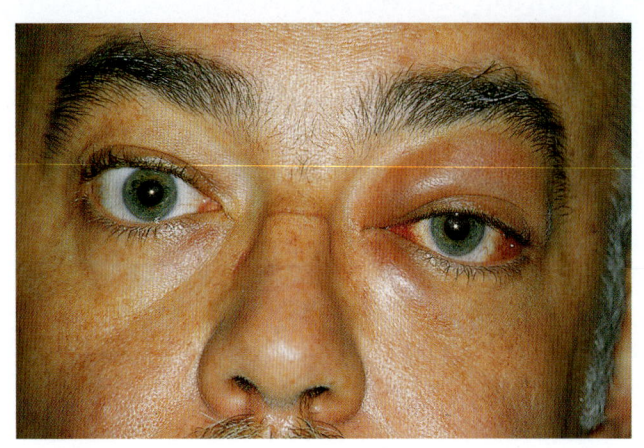

Figure 26.19. Acute orbital inflammation. Proptosis, eyelid edema, and conjunctival hyperemia in a 48-year-old man with acute ocular pain and visual loss.

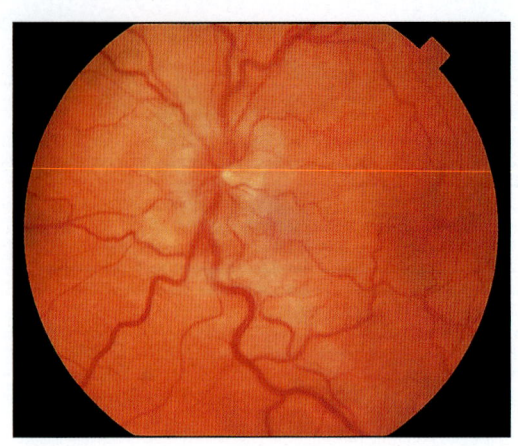

Figure 26.20. Fundus appearance of left eye of patient shown in Figure 26.19, demonstrating optic disc edema secondary to compression of the left optic nerve.

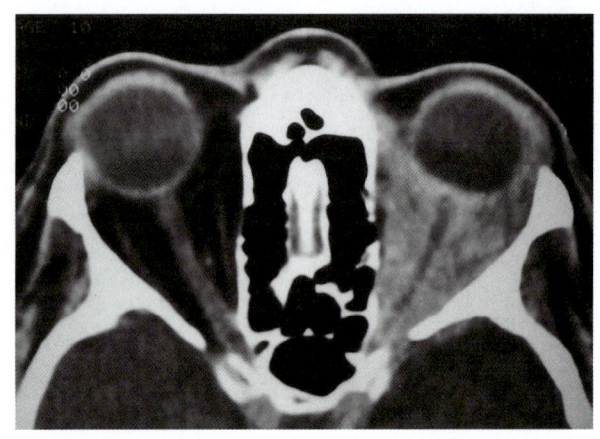

Figure 26.21. Axial computed tomography of patient shown in Figure 26.19, demonstrating diffuse involvement of all orbital tissues with compression of the optic nerve.

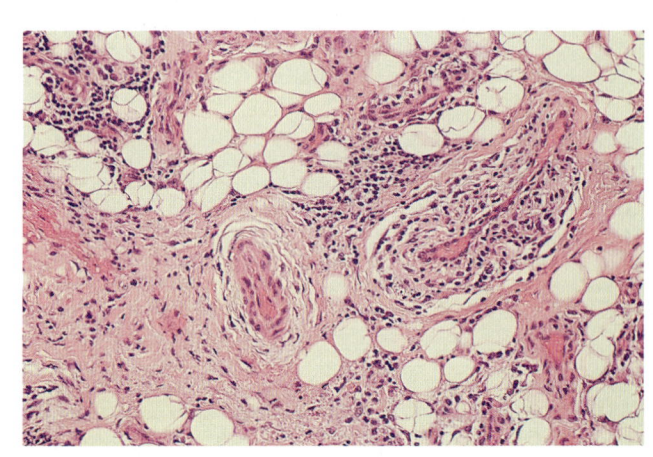

Figure 26.22. Histopathology of mass shown in Figure 26.19, demonstrating chronic nongranulomatous inflammation in the orbital fat. (Hematoxylin–eosin ×50.)

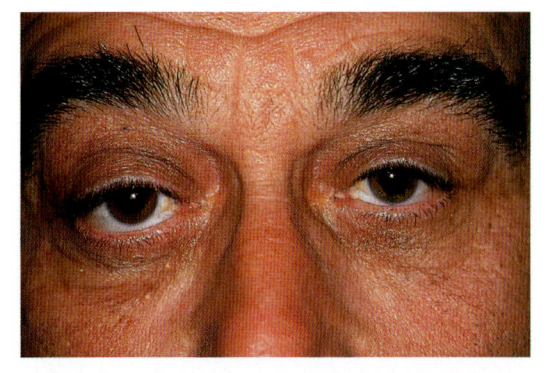

Figure 26.23. Chronic orbital inflammation. Bilateral proptosis, worse on right side, in a 57-year-old man with chronic, low-grade, bilateral ocular pain.

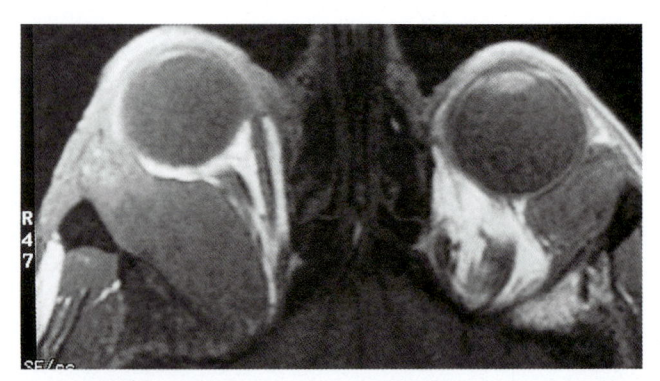

Figure 26.24. Axial magnetic resonance imaging in T1-weighted image of patient shown in Figure 26.23. Note the bilateral orbital masses involving the lacrimal glands, lateral rectus muscles, and adjacent soft tissues. Histopathologic examination of biopsy specimen confirmed the diagnosis of sclerosing idiopathic inflammation.

Chapter 26 Inflammatory Orbital Lesions That Simulate Neoplasms 453

IDIOPATHIC NONGRANULOMATOUS ORBITAL INFLAMMATION CLINICAL AND RADIOLOGIC SPECTRUM

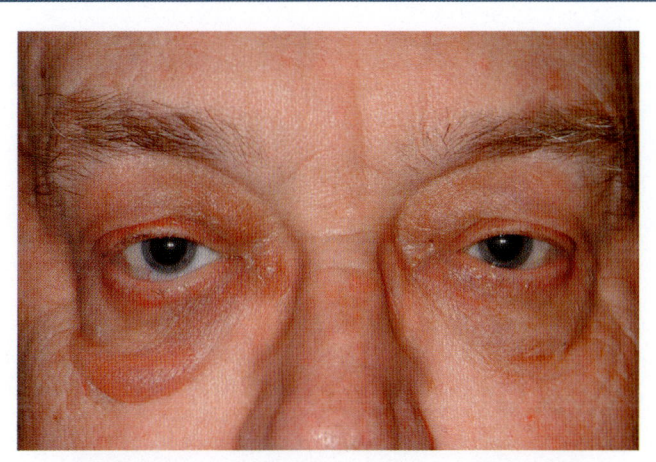

Figure 26.25. Myositic variant of INOI. Elderly man with right proptosis and edema of upper and lower eyelids, but no redness. He had only minimal right orbital pain.

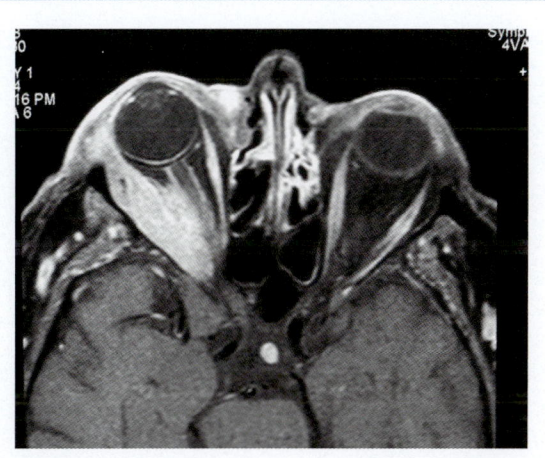

Figure 26.26. Axial magnetic resonance imaging, of patient seen in Figure 26.25, T1-weighted image with fat suppression and gadolinium enhancement, showing enlarged, enhancing lateral rectus muscle with involvement of adjacent soft tissue.

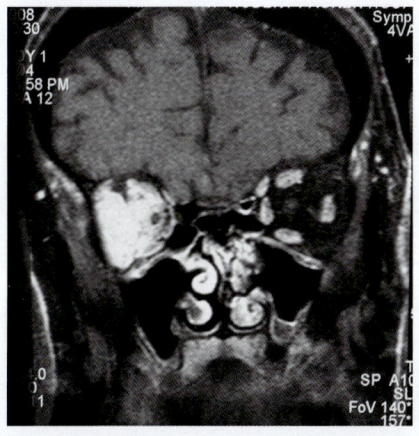

Figure 26.27. Coronal magnetic resonance imaging with similar settings of patient seen in Figure 26.25. Note marked enhancement of lateral rectus muscle and medial displacement of the optic nerve.

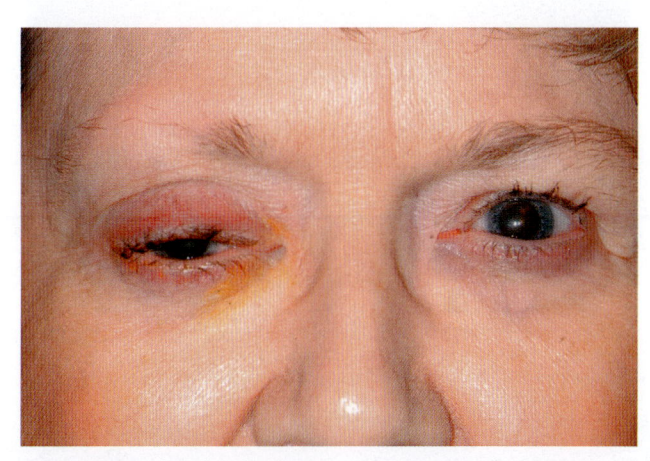

Figure 26.28. Middle-aged woman with blepharoptosis and redness of the right upper and lower eyelids.

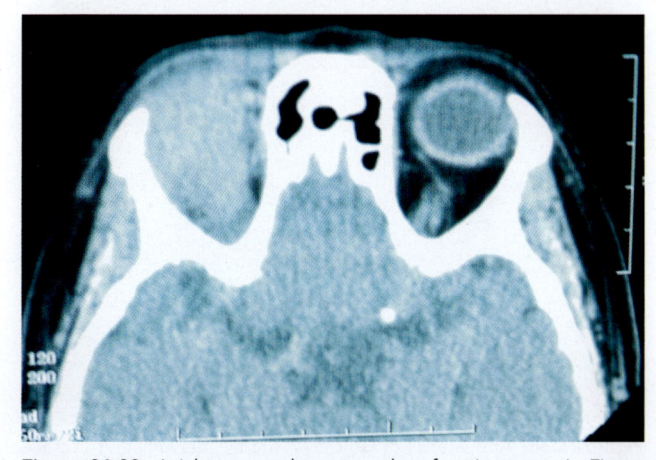

Figure 26.29. Axial computed tomography of patient seen in Figure 26.28, showing diffuse mass in superior orbit.

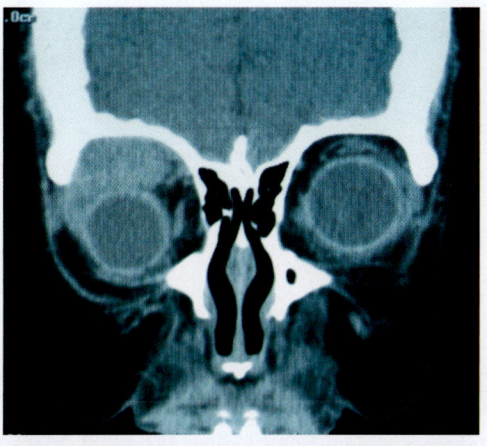

Figure 26.30. Coronal computed tomography of patient seen in Figure 26.28, showing diffuse superior orbital mass.

Part 3 Tumors of the Orbit

IDIOPATHIC NONGRANULOMATOUS ORBITAL INFLAMMATION IN CHILDHOOD

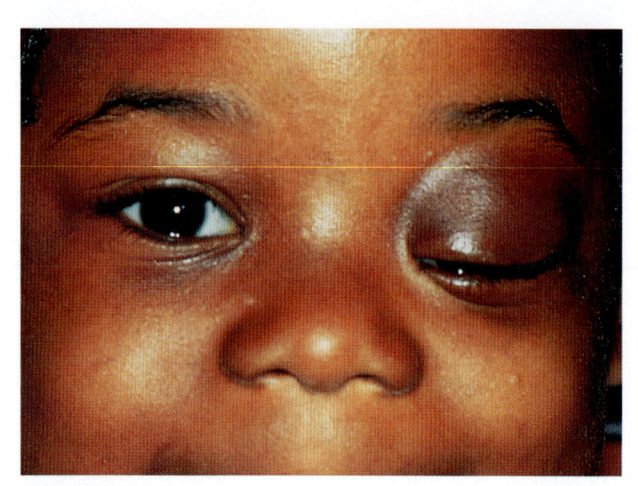

Figure 26.31. Acute swelling and ptosis of left upper eyelid in a 4-year-old child.

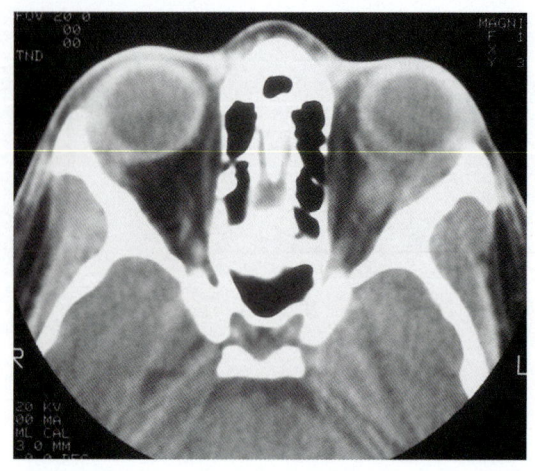

Figure 26.32. Axial computed tomography showing diffuse, ill-defined inflammation of the soft tissue of the left orbit.

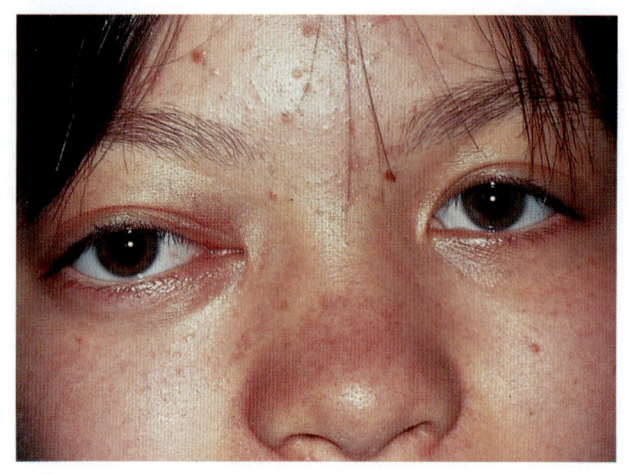

Figure 26.33. Proptosis and lateral displacement of the right eye in a 12-year-old girl with eyelid edema and mild pain.

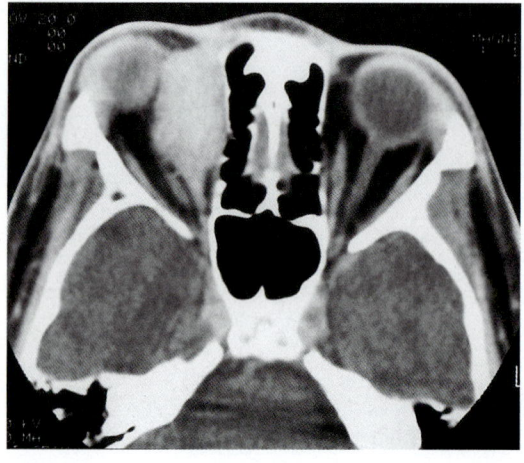

Figure 26.34. Axial computed tomography of patient shown in Figure 26.33, revealing marked enlargement of right medial rectus muscle. The lesion responded to oral corticosteroids.

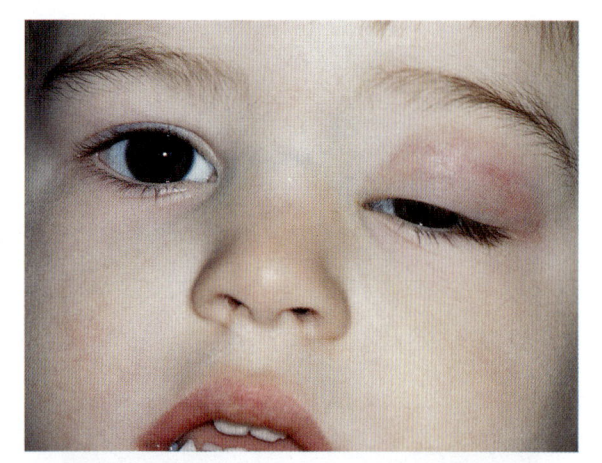

Figure 26.35. Proptosis, eyelid edema, and eyelid hyperemia in a 2-year-old child.

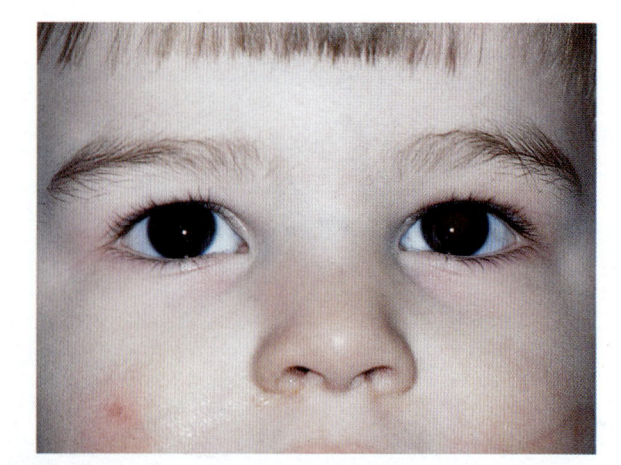

Figure 26.36. Appearance of same child shortly after initiating a course of oral corticosteroids, showing dramatic improvement in the inflammation. The pain subsided. A biopsy was not necessary.

Chapter 26 Inflammatory Orbital Lesions That Simulate Neoplasms

NONSPECIFIC ACUTE ORBITAL MYOSITIS

This is a variant of INOI that exclusively affects the extraocular muscles, often one specific muscle. The preferred treatment is systemic corticosteroids and recurrences are common. Radiotherapy may not be effective in preventing recurrence.

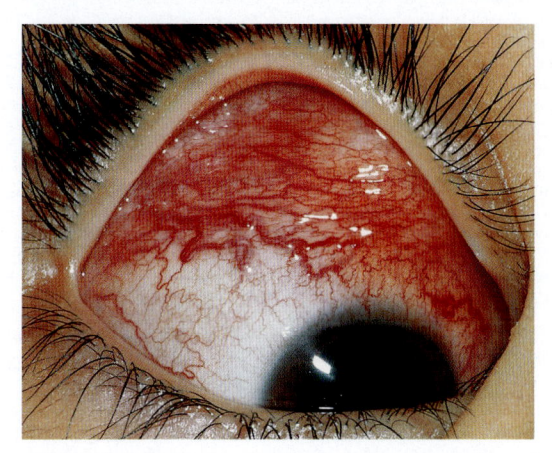

Figure 26.37. Acute redness secondary to a mass in superior epibulbar tissues in an 8-year-old boy. Rhabdomyosarcoma was a diagnostic consideration, biopsy was performed, and nongranulomatous inflammation was found.

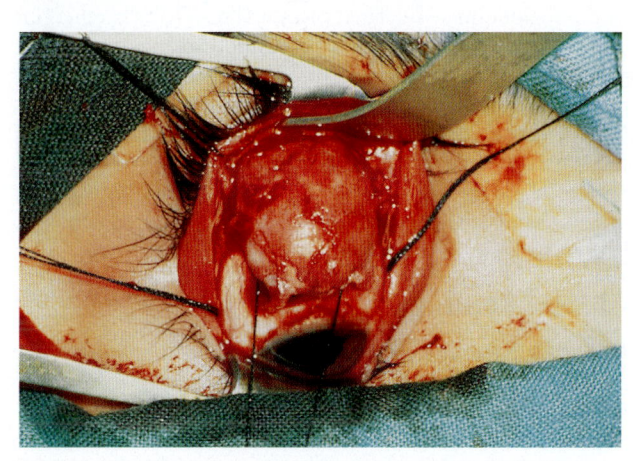

Figure 26.38. Surgical view of area shown in Figure 26.37. Note that a suture has been placed beneath the superior rectus and the exposed mass appears to involve the muscle itself. Histopathology revealed nongranulomatous inflammation.

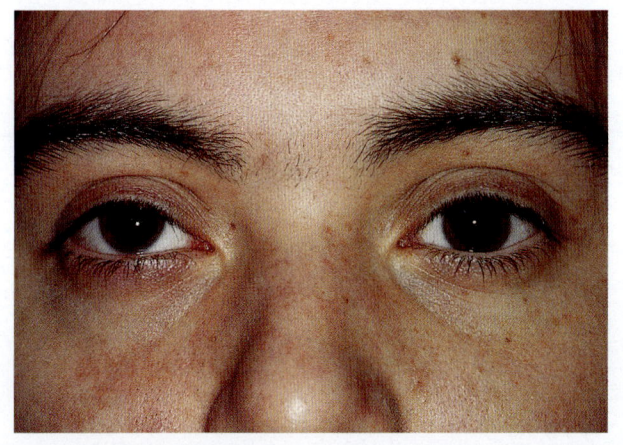

Figure 26.39. Proptosis of the right eye and blepharoptosis of right upper eyelid in a 34-year-old man.

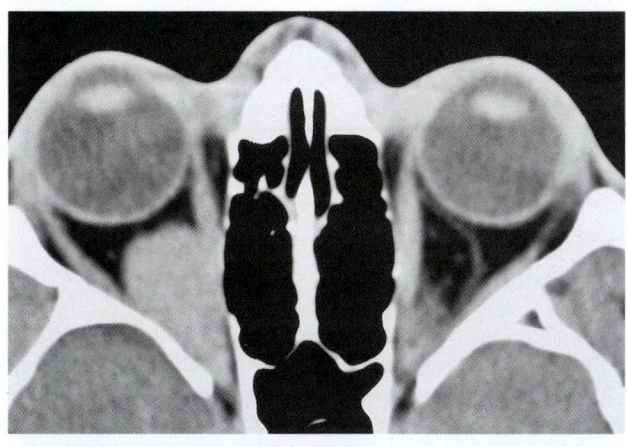

Figure 26.40. Axial computed tomography of patient shown in Figure 26.39. Note the smooth mass that appears to be in the muscle cone.

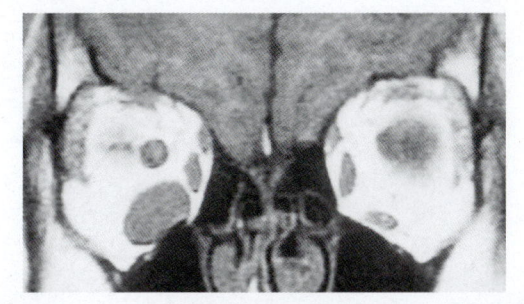

Figure 26.41. Coronal magnetic resonance imaging of patient shown in Figure 26.39, depicting the mass to correspond to an enlarged right inferior rectus muscle. Oral corticosteroids were given and tapered.

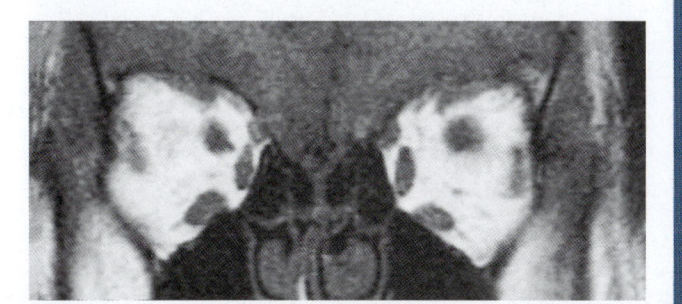

Figure 26.42. Coronal magnetic resonance imaging done 3 weeks later. There was a dramatic clinical response with the inferior rectus muscle returning to normal size.

TUMORS OF THE ORBIT

IMMUNOGLOBULIN G4–RELATED DISEASE (IgG4-RD)

General Considerations

Immunoglobulin G4–related disease (IgG4-RD) is emerging as an increasingly important idiopathic inflammatory disorder (1–6). This was first recognized as a form of autoimmune pancreatitis and later multisystem involvement was identified. Organs that can become involved include the pancreas, liver, biliary tract, lung, kidneys, retroperitoneum, lymph nodes, parotid gland, thyroid gland, and ocular adnexa. Some cases of INOI and orbital lymphoproliferative disorders are proven later to be IgG4-RD (2).

Clinical Features

IgG4-RD generally presents with indolent swelling in the periocular region. According to a study from Japan, patients tend to display frequent lacrimal gland involvement with commonly bilateral disease, evidence of inflammatory disease elsewhere in the body, and high recurrence rate following therapy (2). The mean age at presentation was 55 years and there were no patients under 20 years of age. The most frequent periocular site of involvement was lacrimal gland (84%), orbital soft tissues (19%), extraocular muscles (19%), and less often the eyelid and infraorbital and supraorbital nerves (2,5). Conjunctival involvement was rarely found. Most studies indicate bilateral involvement in 50% to 85%.

Diagnostic Approaches

The diagnosis is established on the basis of clinical multisystem involvement, histopathologic features, and the elevated IgG4 serum levels.

Pathology

Histopathology of this condition reveals diffuse lymphoplasmacytes and high IgG4 positive plasma cell infiltration (>30 IgG4 positive cells per high power field) and a positive IgG4:IgG cell ratio >40% with either fibrosis or sclerosis (2).

Management

The management of IgG4-RD generally involves oral or injection corticosteroids. Occasionally the serum IgG4 levels decrease following therapy. Recurrent disease may require repeat corticosteroids, radiotherapy, or rituximab therapy (6).

Selected References

1. Wallace ZS, Deshapande V, Stone JH. Ophthlamic manifestations of IgG4-related disease: single center experience and literature review. *Semin Arthritis Rheum* 2014;43:806–817.
2. Yu WK, Kao SC, Yang CF, et al. Ocular adnexal IgG4-related disease: clinical features, outcome, and factors associated with response to systemic steroids. *Jpn J Ophthalmol* 2014;59(1):8–13.
3. Andrew NH, Sladden N, Kearney DJ, et al. An analysis of IgG4-related disease (IgG4-RD) among idiopathic orbital inflammations and benign lymphoid hyperplasias using two consensus-based diagnostic criteria for IgG4-RD. *Br J Ophthalmol* 2014;99(3):376–381.
4. Hagaya C, Tsuboi H, Yokosawa M, et al. Clincipathological features of IgG4-related disease complicated with orbital involvement. *Mod Rheumatol* 2014;24:471–476.
5. Plaza JA, Garrity JA, Dogan A, et al. Orbital inflammation with IgG4-positive plasma cells: manifestation of IgG4 systemic disease. *Arch Ophthalmol* 2011;129:421–428.

Case Reports

6. Chen TS, Figueira E, Lau OC, et al. Successful "medical" orbital decompression with adjunctive rituximab for severe visual loss in IgG4-related orbital inflammatory disease with orbital myositis. *Ophthal PLast Reconstr Surg* 2014;30:e122–e125.

ORBITAL TUBERCULOSIS

General Considerations

Although tuberculosis (TB) has remained relatively uncommon in North America, it remains a major worldwide disease. Involvement of TB in the orbit and periocular region is particularly uncommon in the United States (1–18). It can occur as a periostitis that affects the bones in young adults, causing a chronic cold abscess or a fistula. It can also occur as an isolated orbital or lacrimal gland granuloma derived from the bloodstream, or it can extend into the orbit from the adjacent nasal cavity or sinuses. In such cases, it becomes important in the differential diagnosis of orbital tumors. TB can be confined to the orbital area or it can be associated with pulmonary or extrapulmonary TB. Occasionally, atypical mycobacteria, other than classic TB, can affect the orbit. These other mycobacteria can be difficult to differentiate from true TB.

In an analysis of periocular TB from an eye hospital in the United Kingdom, there were 9 cases over 10 years and manifestations included periocular dermatitis (n = 3), dacryocystitis (n = 2), and orbital cellulitis (n = 4) (1). All patients were immunocompetent and three had previous TB. A complete course of antituberculous medications resolved the findings (1).

Clinical Features

Clinically, orbital TB or other mycobacterial infections can present like other orbit inflammations or tumors and have no distinct features. It can appear as a distinct mass or as an ill-defined diffuse process.

Diagnostic Approaches

If orbital TB is a diagnostic consideration, the patient should have medical evaluation for active TB, particularly a chest x-ray and skin testing. Open or fine-needle biopsy can be used to confirm the diagnosis (6).

Pathology

Histopathologically, TB is generally a caseating granuloma with characteristic Langhans giant cells. The diagnosis can be made by appropriate systemic evaluation and orbital biopsy. Polymerase chain reaction can be used to for amplification of the *Mycobacterium tuberculosis* genome (5).

Management

Treatment includes appropriate antituberculous therapy to which orbital involvement responds favorably (1–4).

Selected References

Reviews

1. Salam T, Uddin JM, Collin JR, et al. Periocular tuberculous disease:Experience from a UK eye hospital. *Br J Ophthalmol* 2014;99(5):582–585.
2. Sen DK. Tuberculosis of the orbit and lacrimal gland: a clinical study of 14 cases. *J Pediatr Ophthalmol Strabismus* 1980;17:232–238.
3. Madge SN, Prabhakaran VC, Shome D, et al. Orbital tuberculosis: a review of the literature. *Orbit* 2008;27(4):267–277.
4. Khurana S, Pushker N, Naik SS, et al. Orbital tuberculosis in a paediatric population. *Trop Doct* 2014;44:148–151.

Histopathology/Microbiology

5. Biswas J, Roy Chowdhury B, Krishna Kumar S, et al. Detection of *Mycobacterium tuberculosis* by polymerase chain reaction in a case of orbital tuberculosis. *Orbit* 2001;20:69–74.
6. Dhaliwal U, Arora VK, Singh N, et al. Clinical and cytopathologic correlation in chronic inflammations of the orbit and ocular adnexa: a review of 55 cases. *Orbit* 2004;23(4):219–225.

Case Reports

7. Pillai S, Malone TJ, Abad JC. Orbital tuberculosis. *Ophthal Plast Reconstr Surg* 1995;11:27–31.
8. Khalil MK, Lindley S, Matouk E. Tuberculosis of the orbit. *Ophthalmology* 1985;92:1624–1627.
9. D'Souza P, Garg R, Dhaliwal RS, et al. Orbital-tuberculosis. *Int Ophthalmol* 1994;18:149–152.
10. Mehra KS, Pattanayak SP, Saroj G. Tuberculoma of orbit. *Indian J Ophthalmol* 1992;40:90–91.
11. Maurya OP, Patel R, Thakur V, et al. Tuberculoma of the orbit–a case report. *Indian J Ophthalmol* 1990;38:191–192.
12. Sheridan PH, Edman JB, Starr SE. Tuberculosis presenting as an orbital mass. *Pediatrics* 1981;67:874–875.
13. Spoor TC, Harding SA. Orbital tuberculosis. *Am J Ophthalmol* 1981;91:644–647.
14. Maria DL, Mundada SH. Sub-periosteal tuberculoma of the left lateral wall of orbit. *Indian J Ophthalmol* 1981;29:47–49
15. Aversa do Souto A, Fonseca AL, Gadelha M, et al. Optic pathways tuberculoma mimicking glioma: case report. *Surg Neurol* 2003;60:349–353.
16. van Assen S, Lutterman JA. Tuberculous dacryoadenitis: a rare manifestation of tuberculosis. *Neth J Med* 2002;60:327–329.
17. Aggarwal D, Suri A, Mahapatra AK. Orbital tuberculosis with abscess. *J Neuroophthalmol* 2002;22:208–210.
18. Shome D, Honavar SG, Vemuganti GK, et al. Orbital tuberculosis manifesting with enophthalmos and causing a diagnostic dilemma. *Ophthal Plast Reconstr Surg* 2006;22(3):219–221.

Chapter 26 Inflammatory Orbital Lesions That Simulate Neoplasms 459

ORBITAL TUBERCULOSIS

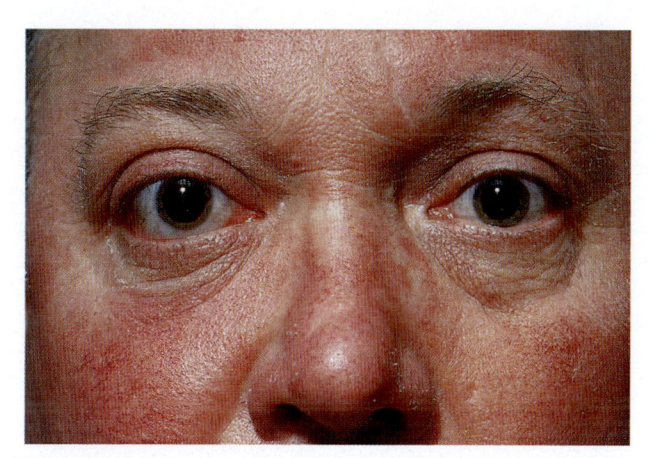

Figure 26.43. Proptosis of the right eye in an otherwise healthy 51-year-old man.

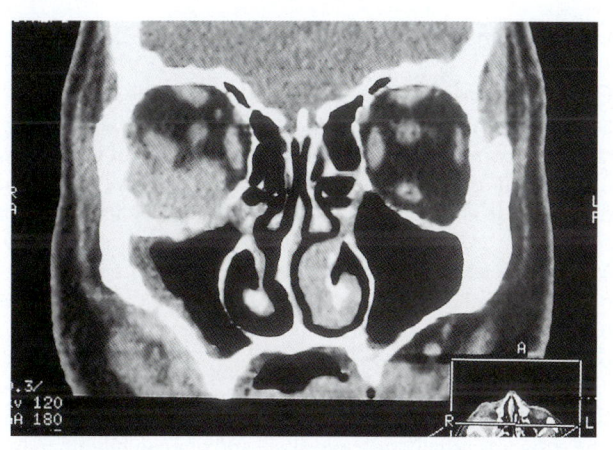

Figure 26.44. Coronal computed tomography of patient shown in Figure 26.43, depicting diffuse mass in the inferior and posterior aspects of the orbit. Biopsy showed granulomatous inflammation and acid-fast organisms compatible with tuberculosis or atypical mycobacteria.

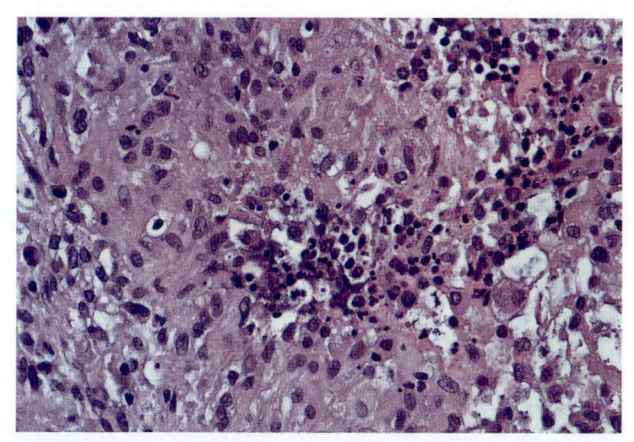

Figure 26.45. Histopathology of lesion shown in Figure 26.43, revealing histiocytes within a necrotizing granuloma. (Hematoxylin–eosin ×150.)

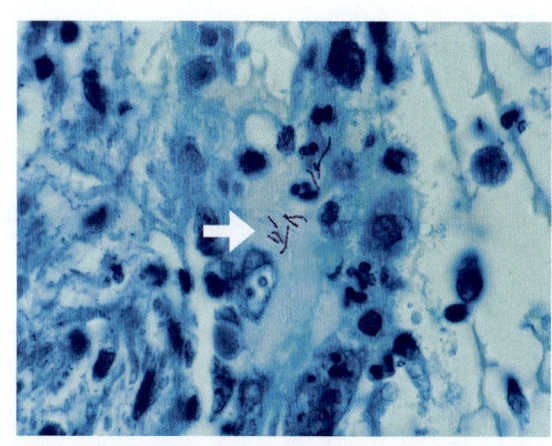

Figure 26.46. Histopathology of orbital TB showing acid-fast organisms (*arrow*). (Acid-fast stain ×200.)

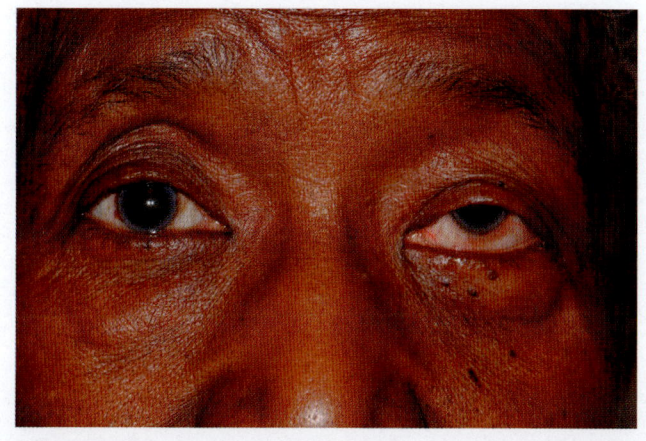

Figure 26.47. Facial view of an elderly African-American woman showing upward displacement of left eye and no appreciable inflammatory signs.

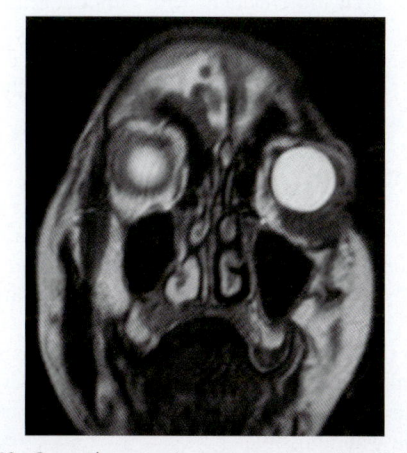

Figure 26.48. Coronal magnetic resonance imaging in T2-weighted image of patient shown in Figure 26.47. An inferotemporal mass is seen as a low signal area. Biopsy demonstrated acid-fast organisms and the patient responded to tuberculosis medications.

ORBITAL MYCOTIC INFECTIONS: ASPERGILLOSIS AND MUCORMYCOSIS

Orbital Mucormycosis

General Considerations
Several mycotic infections can occur in the orbit. Mucormycosis (phycomycosis) is perhaps the best known of the orbital mycoses. It mostly occurs in patients who have advanced disease such as diabetic ketoacidosis, malignancies, or other conditions associated with immunosuppression (1–6). Mucormycosis originates in the nose and sinuses and secondarily invades the orbit. In rare instances, certain species of mucormycosis have been reported to develop in immunocompetent individuals (1,6).

Clinical Features
The patient is usually systemically ill and often debilitated. The most common underlying illnesses include diabetes mellitus, hematological malignancies, hematopoietic stem cell transplantation, and solid-organ transplantation. Sporangiospores of mucormycosis are deposited in the nasal turbinates and paranasal sinuses and the relatively incompetent neutrophils, monocytes, and macrophages allow the spores to proliferate and invade tissue (2). This leads to angioinvasion, thrombosis, and tissue necrosis. Clinically, there is fairly rapid onset of orbital inflammation with proptosis, diplopia, and ophthalmoplegia. A characteristic black eschar develops in the involved areas, particularly the periorbital skin, owing to tissue necrosis. Early diagnosis of this life-threatening condition is critical to prevent brain invasion and death.

Diagnostic Approaches
The diagnosis can be made by clinical suspicion in these clinical settings and an orbital or sinus biopsy of the most accessible tissue.

Pathology
Histopathologically, the organism is a large (30 to 50 micron) nonseptate, branching hypha that stains with hematoxylin and eosin, but is even more evident with periodic acid-Schiff and specific fungal stains such as Gomori methenamine silver stain. The organisms have a tendency to invade the orbital blood vessels leading to necrosis. Many neutrophils are usually present in the area of involvement (2).

Management
The optimal therapy orbital mucormycosis involves multidisciplinary approach that relies on prompt institution of antifungal medication, reversal of underlying predisposing condition, and surgical debridement of necrotic tissue (1–6). Initiation of treatment is urgent because the disease is frequently fatal owing to invasion through the orbital tissue and into the intracranial cavity. Sino-orbital exenteration might be necessary to completely control the disease, but there is a trend toward avoiding exenteration when possible.

Selected References
Reviews
1. Jung H, Park SK. Indolent mucormycosis of the paranasal sinus in immunocompetent patients: are antifungal drugs needed? *J Laryngol Otol* 2013;127:872–875.
2. Gamaletsou MN, Sipsas NV, Roilides E, et al. Rino-orbital-cerebral mucormycosis. *Curr Infect Dis Rep* 2012;14:423–434.
3. Mbarek C, Zribi S, Khamassi K, et al. Rinocerebral mucormycosis: five cases and a literature review. *B-ENT* 2011;7:189–193.
4. Peterson KL, Wang M, Canalis RF, et al. Rhinocerebral mucormycosis: evolution of the disease and treatment options. *Laryngoscope* 1997;107:855–862.
5. Luna JD, Ponssa XS, Rodriguez SD, et al. Intraconal amphotericin B for the treatment of rhino-orbital mucormycosis. *Ophthalmic Surg Lasers* 1996;27:706–708.
6. Fairley C, Sullivan TJ, Bartley P, et al. Survival after rhino-orbital-cerebral mucormycosis in an immunocompetent patient. *Ophthalmology* 2000;107:555–558.

ORBITAL ASPERGILLOSIS—ALLERGIC FUNGAL SINUSITIS

General Considerations

Aspergillosis is an important mycotic infection that is best known in ophthalmology to cause endophthalmitis, but can also infect the orbit (1–21). It is caused by any of several species of the genus *Aspergillus,* which are opportunistic organisms that normally reside in the oropharynx and sinuses, particularly in the ethmoid and sphenoid sinuses. Unlike mucormycosis, which appears in debilitated patients, orbital aspergillosis often develops in otherwise healthy individuals (1). Orbital extension from aspergillosis can develop secondary to allergic fungal sinusitis (AFS) (3,16). AFS is a disease characterized by recurrent sinusitis, eosinophilia, and increased serum immunoglobulin E levels. Patients are typically young and have a history of asthma and nasal polyposis. Orbital involvement by AFS owing to aspergillosis has been recognized with increasing frequency in recent years.

Clinical Features

Unlike mucormycosis, aspergillosis can more often infect the orbit of ostensibly healthy individuals, but it also develops in patients who are immunocompromised. The clinical manifestations may be very similar to those of mucormycosis with the exception that aspergillosis usually has a more insidious onset and slow course. The infection may become organized into a rather defined mass called an "aspergilloma." Aspergillosis has been known to develop as a mass in the orbital apex, with minimal sinus involvement, a situation that is difficult to manage and can lead to death. The AFS variant can simulate a primary nasal or sinus neoplasm.

In an analysis of 35 cases by Mody et al., the mean age at presentation was 38 years and duration of symptoms was 1 year (1). The findings included proptosis (23%), mass (13%), dysmotility (71%), and poor visual acuity to no light perception (8%). Imaging showed infiltrative orbital mass with bone destruction (63%). Diagnosis was made by histopathology and microbiology evaluation, detecting *Aspergillus flavus* (86%) or fumigatus (14%). Treatment was medical management (51%) or surgical debulking (49%), leading to patient survival in 94% (1).

Diagnostic Approaches

CT or MRI generally shows a diffuse mass in the sinuses with secondary unilateral or bilateral orbital extension. The diagnosis can be suspected on the basis of the clinical findings but fine needle aspiration or incisional biopsy can be employed to establish a definitive diagnosis.

Pathology

Histopathologically, there is an intense inflammatory reaction with lymphocytes, plasma cells, epithelioid cells, and giant cells sometimes with areas of caseation necrosis and Charcot–Leyden crystals, which are peculiar eosinophilic needle–shaped crystalline structures that characterize this inflammation. The organism is a septate hypha form branching at a characteristic 45-degree angle. The walls of aspergillus stain positively with silver stains for fungi.

Management

The management of orbital aspergillosis is wide surgical debridement of the involved sinuses and orbital tissues, combined with amphotericin B or itraconazole in appropriate doses (1,6,7). Corticosteroids can be successful in cases of AFS (3,16). Extension of the infectious process into the brain can cause death. Hence, eyelid-sparing orbital exenteration is sometimes advocated for posterior orbital lesions, regardless of the functional status of the eye (8,19). For anterior orbital lesions, wide debridement without exenteration may be justified (1,6,7,19).

Selected References

Reviews

1. Mody KH, Ali MJ, Bemuganti GK, et al. Orbital aspergillosis in immunocompetent patients. *Br J Ophthalmol* 2014;98:1379–1384.
2. Panda NK, Balaji P, Chakrabarti A, et al. Paranasal sinus aspergillosis: its categorization to develop a treatment protocol. *Mycoses* 2004;47:277–283.
3. Chang WJ, Tse DT, Bressler KL, et al. Diagnosis and management of allergic fungal sinusitis with orbital involvement. *Ophthal Plast Reconstr Surg* 2000;16:72–74.
4. Liu JK, Schaefer SD, Moscatello AL, et al. Neurosurgical implications of allergic fungal sinusitis. *J Neurosurg* 2004;100:883–890.
5. Michaels L, Lloyd G, Phelps P. Origin and spread of allergic fungal disease of the nose and paranasal sinuses. *Clin Otolaryngol* 2000;25:518–525.

Management

6. Harris GJ, Will BR. Orbital aspergillosis. Conservative debridement and local amphotericin irrigation. *Ophthal Plast Reconstr Surg* 1989;5(3):207–211.
7. Dhiwakar M, Thakar A, Bahadur S. Invasive sino-orbital aspergillosis: surgical decisions and dilemmas. *J Laryngol Otol* 2003;117:280–285.
8. Shields JA, Shields CL, Demirci H, et al. Experience with eyelid-sparing orbital exenteration: the 2000 Tullos O. Coston Lecture. *Ophthal Plast Reconstr Surg* 2001;17:355–361.

Case Reports

9. Nakamaru Y, Fukuda S, Maguchi S, et al. A case of invasive aspergillosis of the paranasal sinuses with a feature of allergic Aspergillus sinusitis. *Otolaryngol Head Neck Surg* 2002;126:204–205.
10. Nenoff P, Kellermann S, Horn LC, et al. Case report. Mycotic arteritis due to *Aspergillus fumigatus* in a diabetic with retrobulbar aspergillosis and mycotic meningitis. *Mycoses* 2001;44:407–414.
11. Ugurlu S, Maden A, Sefi N, et al. *Aspergillus niger* infection of exenterated orbit. *Ophthal Plast Reconstr Surg* 2001;17:452–453.
12. Palacios E, Valvassori G, D'Antonio M. Aggressive invasive fungal sinusitis. *Ear Nose Throat J* 2000;79:842.
13. Oyarzabal MF, Chevretton EB, Hay RJ. Semi-invasive allergic aspergillosis of the paranasal sinuses. *J Laryngol Otol* 2000;114:290–292.
14. Johnson TE, Casiano RR, Kronish JW, et al. Sino-orbital aspergillosis in acquired immunodeficiency syndrome. *Arch Ophthalmol* 1999;117:57–64.
15. Facer ML, Ponikau JU, Sherris DA. Eosinophilic fungal rhinosinusitis of the lacrimal sac. *Laryngoscope* 2003;113:210–214.
16. Chang W, Shields CL, Shields JA, et al. Bilateral orbital involvement with massive allergic fungal sinusitis. *Arch Ophthalmol* 1996;114:767–768.
17. Hutnik CM, Nicolle DA, Munoz DG. Orbital aspergillosis. A fatal masquerader. *J Neuro-Ophthalmol* 1997;17:257–261.
18. Klapper SR, Lee AG, Patrinely JR, et al. Orbital involvement in allergic fungal sinusitis. *Ophthalmology* 1997;104:2094–2100.
19. Kusaka K, Shimamura I, Ohashi Y, et al. Long term survival of patient with invasive aspergillosis involving orbit, paranasal sinus, and central nervous system. *Br J Ophthalmol* 2003;87:791–792.
20. Yumoto E, Kitani S, Okamura H, et al. Sino-orbital aspergillosis associated with total ophthalmoplegia. *Laryngoscope* 1985;95(2):190–192.
21. Dortzbach RK, Segrest DR. Orbital aspergillosis. *Ophthalmic Surg* 1983;14(3):240–244.

ORBITAL MYCOTIC INFECTIONS: ASPERGILLOSIS AND MUCORMYCOSIS

Chang W, Shields CL, Shields JA, et al. Bilateral orbital involvement with massive allergic fungal sinusitis. *Arch Ophthalmol* 1996;114:767–768.

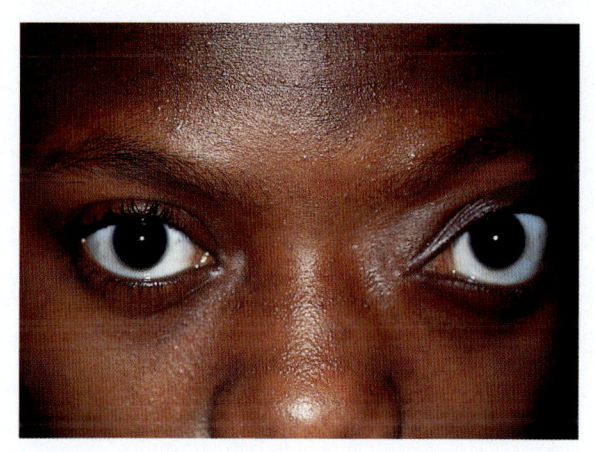

Figure 26.49. Allergic fungal sinusitis secondary to aspergillosis. Proptosis of left eye in an 11-year-old girl.

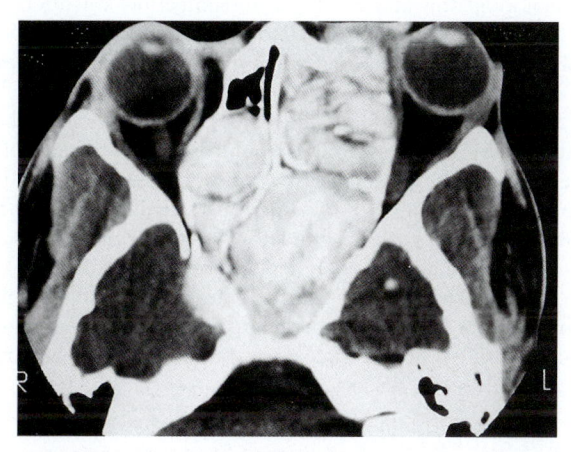

Figure 26.50. Axial computed tomography of patient in Figure 26.49, showing contrast-enhancing soft tissue lesion filling and expanding the ethmoid sinus, sphenoid sinus, and nasal cavity, and encroaching on both orbits.

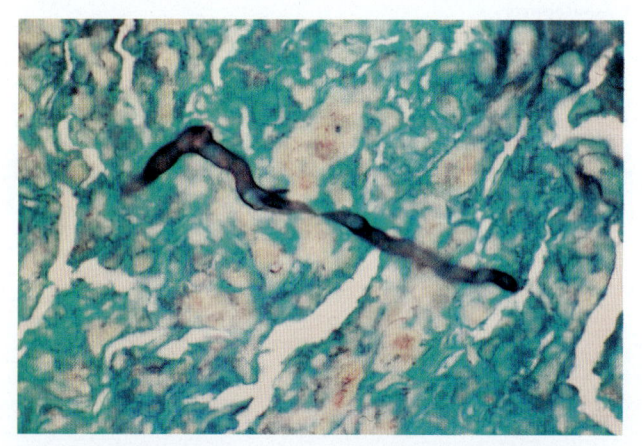

Figure 26.51. Fungus stain of same specimen, more clearly demonstrating the organisms. (Gomori methenamine silver ×250.)

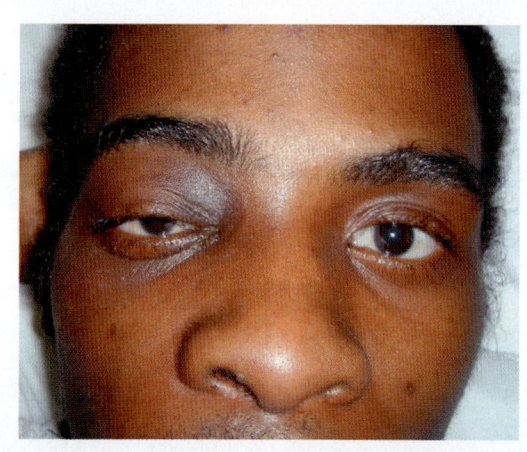

Figure 26.52. Sino-orbital mucormycosis. Facial appearance of 23-year-old man with poorly controlled diabetes mellitus, who developed pain, headache, rhinorrhea, chills, and lethargy. Note the right proptosis, eyelid edema and right nasal discharge. (Courtesy of Stephen Soll, MD.)

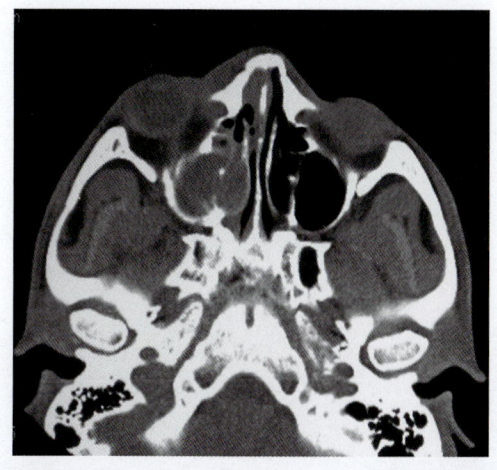

Figure 26.53. Axial computed tomography of patient seen in Figure 26.52, showing abscess in ethmoid region with bone destruction and orbital invasion. (Courtesy of Stephen Soll, MD.)

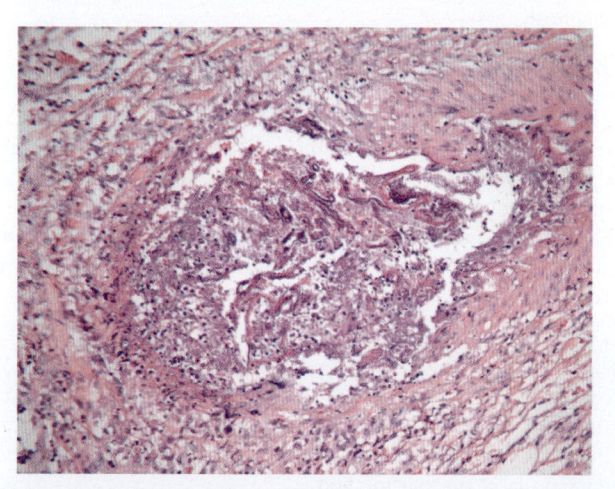

Figure 26.54. Histopathology of biopsy from lesion shown in Figure 26.53, demonstrating a thrombus in orbital blood vessels with numerous fungi. (Hematoxylin–eosin ×50.) (Courtesy of Ralph C. Eagle, Jr, MD.)

ORBITAL SARCOIDOSIS

General Considerations

Several idiopathic granulomatous inflammations can affect the orbit. Considered here are sarcoidosis, granulomatosis with polyangiitis (Wegener granulomatosis), and Kimura disease (1–15).

Sarcoidosis is a systemic disease of unknown etiology characterized by granulomatous inflammation involving lungs, liver, spleen, skin, bone marrow, and ocular structures. It is more common in African Americans. Ocular involvement occurs in 20% of patients with known systemic sarcoidosis and is sometimes the initial manifestation of systemic disease. Isolated ocular involvement, with no detectable systemic disease, can also occur (3). Granulomatous uveitis is the most common ocular manifestation of sarcoidosis, but orbital involvement is occasionally seen (1–15).

Clinical Features

The most common form of orbital involvement by sarcoidosis is subacute, chronic dacryoadenitis, although it can occur as an isolated mass apart from the lacrimal gland in patients with no evidence of systemic or intraocular sarcoidosis (3). Sarcoid granuloma can resemble a neoplasm. When it occurs bilaterally in the lacrimal and the salivary glands, it is sometimes referred to as Mikulicz syndrome, although this syndrome can have other etiologies. The association of fever, parotid gland enlargement, and uveitis is termed Heerfordt syndrome (uveoparotid fever), which can be a presenting manifestation of sarcoidosis.

Diagnostic Approaches

If orbital sarcoidosis is a diagnostic consideration, evaluation for systemic sarcoidosis should include physical examination, chest x-ray, serum angiotensin-converting enzyme (ACE), and a gallium scan (7). Elevated ACE is strongly suggestive of the sarcoidosis. Positive ACE and gallium scans are >95% accurate in diagnosing sarcoidosis (7). Orbital CT or MRI show a unilateral or bilateral mass of the lacrimal gland, simulating a lacrimal gland neoplasm. Biopsy of any suspicious conjunctival nodules or biopsy of the lacrimal gland can also support the diagnosis.

Pathology

Histopathologically, sarcoidosis is characterized by noncaseating granulomas with epithelioid cells and giant cells. To diagnose presumed sarcoidosis, one must do special stains and other appropriate studies to exclude tubercle bacilli, fungi, foreign bodies, and other causes of granulomatous inflammation. If these are not found and the histopathologic findings are compatible with sarcoidosis, then the diagnosis can be made.

Management

Systemic corticosteroids are considered to be the best treatment for suspected orbital sarcoidosis. It is possible that local injection of corticosteroids can be effective, but there are few data available on that method.

Selected References

Reviews
1. Demirci H, Christianson MD. Orbital and adnexal involvement in sarcoidosis: analysis of clinical features and systemic disease in 30 cases. Am J Ophthalmol 2011;151(6):1074–1080.
2. Mavrikakis I, Rootman J. Diverse clinical presentations of orbital sarcoid. Am J Ophthalmol 2007;144(5):769–775.
3. Rabinowitz MP, Halfpenny CP, Bedrossian EH Jr. The frequency of granulomatous lacrimal gland inflammation as a cause of lacrimal gland enlargement in patients without a diagnosis of systemic sarcoidosis. Orbit 2013;32(3):151–155.
4. Collison JM, Miller NR, Green WR. Involvement of orbital tissues by sarcoid. Am J Ophthalmol 1986;102:302–307.
5. Khan JA, Hoover DL, Giangiacomo J, et al. Orbital and childhood sarcoidosis. J Pediatr Ophthalmol Strabismus 1986;23:190–194.
6. Hoover DL, Khan JA, Giangiacomo J. Pediatric ocular sarcoidosis. Surv Ophthalmol 1986;30:215–228.

Imaging
7. Power WJ, Neves RA, Rodriguez A, et al. The value of combined serum angiotensin-converting enzyme and gallium scan in diagnosing ocular sarcoidosis. Ophthalmology 1995;102:2007–2011.
8. Mafee MF, Dorodi S, Pai E. Sarcoidosis of the eye, orbit, and central nervous system. Role of MR imaging. Radiol Clin North Am 1999;37:73–87.

Management
9. Rabinowitz MP, Murchison AP. Orbital sarcoidosis treated with hydroxychloroquine. Orbit 2011;30(1):13–15.

Case Reports
10. Salvage DR, Spencer JA, Batchelor AG, et al. Sarcoid involvement of the supraorbital nerve: MR and histologic findings. AJNR Am J Neuroradiol 1997;18:1785–1787.
11. Mombaerts I, Schlingemann RO, Goldschmeding R, et al. Idiopathic granulomatous orbital inflammation. Ophthalmology 1996;103:2135–2141.
12. Raskin EM, McCormick SA, Maher EA, et al. Granulomatous idiopathic orbital inflammation. Ophthal Plast Reconstr Surg 1995;11:131–135.
13. Imes RK, Reifschneider JS, O'Connor LE. Systemic sarcoidosis presenting initially with bilateral orbital and upper lid masses. Ann Ophthalmol 1988;20:466–467.
14. Segal EI, Tang RA, Lee AG, et al. Orbital apex lesion as the presenting manifestation of sarcoidosis. J Neuroophthalmol 2000;20:156–158.
15. Tawfik HA, Assem M, Elkafrawy MH, et al. Scar sarcoidosis developing 16 years after complete excision of an eyelid basal carcinoma. Orbit 2008;27(6):438–440.

Chapter 26 Inflammatory Orbital Lesions That Simulate Neoplasms

ORBITAL SARCOIDOSIS

Orbital sarcoidosis most often involves the lacrimal gland. Less commonly, it affects extraocular muscles or other orbital tissues. Depicted is a case involving lacrimal gland and another case involving extraocular muscle. Although more common in African Americans, both patients shown are Caucasians.

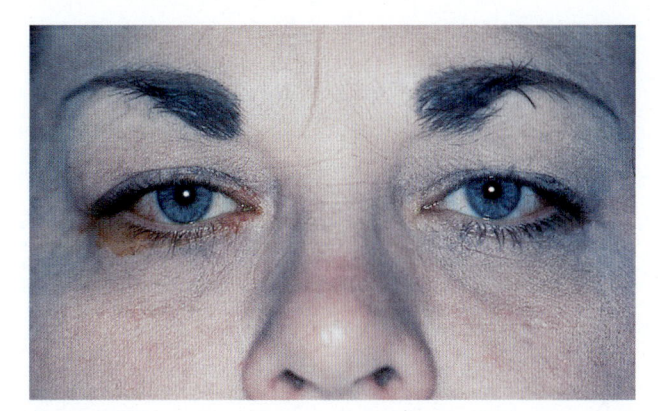

Figure 26.55. Swelling of temporal aspect of right upper eyelid in a 42-year-old woman. Systemic evaluation was unrevealing and angiotensin-converting enzyme level was normal. (Courtesy of Daniel Albert, MD, Morton Smith, MD, and Nasreen Syed, MD.)

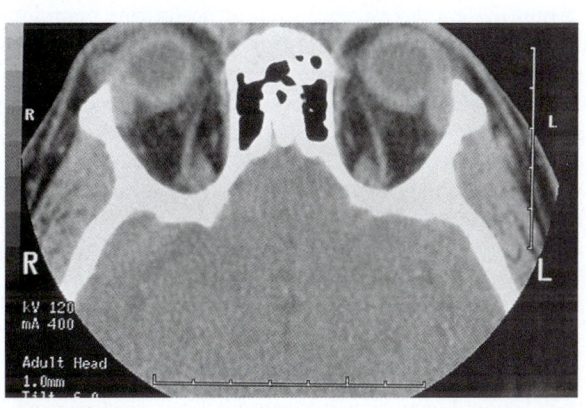

Figure 26.56. Axial computed tomography of patient shown in Figure 26.55, demonstrating an irregular mass in the right lacrimal gland. There may be slight enlargement of the left lacrimal gland as well.

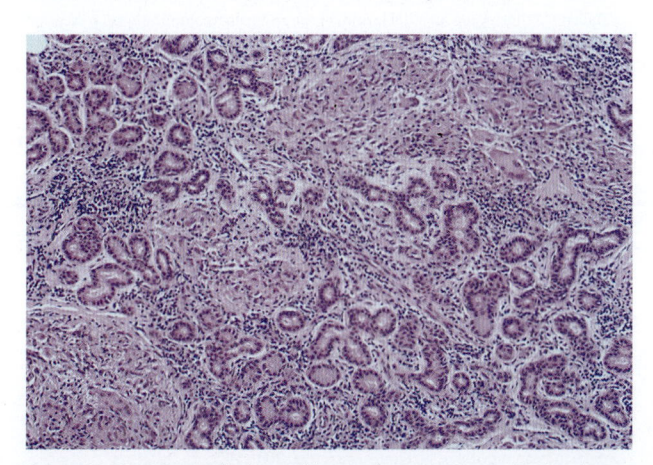

Figure 26.57. Histopathology of lesion shown in Figure 26.55, demonstrating noncaseating granuloma compatible with sarcoidosis involving the lacrimal gland. (Hematoxylin–eosin ×50.) Note the epithelioid cell granulomas with characteristic giant cells.

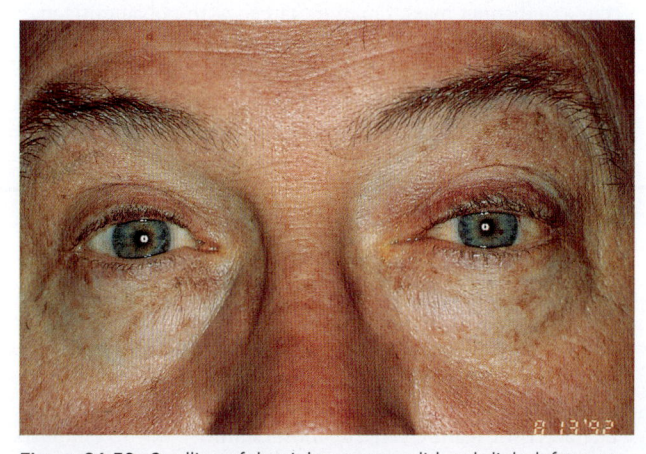

Figure 26.58. Swelling of the right upper eyelid and slight left proptosis in a 47-year-old man with a history of pulmonary sarcoidosis and a highly positive angiotensin-converting enzyme. (Courtesy of Ronan Conlon, MD, and Keith Carter, MD.)

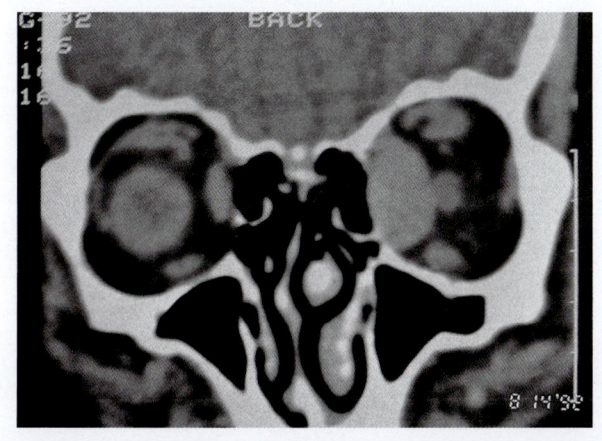

Figure 26.59. Coronal computed tomography of patient shown in Figure 26.58, revealing circumscribed enlargement of the medial rectus muscle.

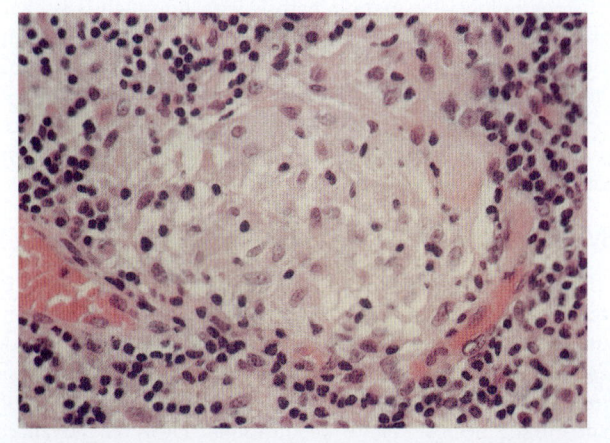

Figure 26.60. Photomicrograph of lesion shown in Figure 26.58, demonstrating a noncaseating epithelioid cell granuloma. (Hematoxylin–eosin ×150.)

ORBITAL GRANULOMATOSIS WITH POLYANGIITIS (WEGENER GRANULOMATOSIS)

General Considerations

Granulomatosis with polyangiitis (Wegener granulomatosis) is a multisystem disease consisting of necrotizing granulomas and vasculitis of the respiratory tract, generalized small vessel vasculitis, and focal necrotizing glomerulonephritis, can show ocular involvement in about 50% of cases (1–16). This condition can involve the orbit as a part of widespread disease or as limited form without the characteristic renal involvement. Orbital involvement can occur at any age and can be bilateral. The orbit was affected in 40 of 140 patients with granulomatosis with polyangiitis (Wegener granulomatosis) in one series (7). In a study of 15 cases with orbital involvement, 12 were limited to the orbit and 3 had associated systemic disease (11).

Clinical Features

Orbital granulomatosis with polyangiitis is characterized by pain, proptosis, motility disturbance, erythematous edema of the eyelids, and characteristic scleral necrosis. Although many cases demonstrate diffuse orbital inflammation, it can also occur as a distinct mass. Granulomatosis with polyangiitis may be similar clinically to NOI, metastatic carcinoma, and lymphoma. However, scleral necrosis with scleral melting, characteristic of granulomatosis with polyangiitis, does not usually occur with these other conditions. This scleral necrosis may be similar to that seen with rheumatoid scleritis.

Diagnostic Approaches

Positive titers for cytoplasmic anti-neutrophil cytoplasmic antibody (c-ANCA) are helpful in establishing the diagnosis. However, false-negative and false-positive results do occur. In some cases c-ANCA is initially negative but becomes positive as the disease progresses (4). Orbital imaging shows a diffuse orbital mass. With MRI, a marked decrease in the T2 signal is a characteristic feature (7). The most definitive way to establish the diagnosis is with a biopsy.

Pathology

Histopathologically, granulomatosis with polyangiitis is characterized by a granulomatous inflammation with multinucleated Langhans giant cells and necrotizing vasculitis. This inflammation typically affects the walls of the blood vessels and produces fibrinoid necrosis. There are numerous lymphocytes and plasma cells and some polymorphonuclear leukocytes, but eosinophils are uncommon.

Management

The orbital diagnosis should generally be made by a biopsy of the most accessible involved tissue. The management of granulomatosis with polyangiitis with systemic cyclophosphamide and corticosteroids has dramatically improved the prognosis for many patients. Newer alternatives include rituximab and anti-tumor necrosis factor medications. However, advanced cases may require orbital exenteration. Patients with the limited form of the disease generally have a better prognosis because they do not have renal involvement.

Selected References

Reviews

1. Santiago YM, Fay A. Wegener's granulomatosis of the orbit: a review of clinical features and updates in diagnosis and treatment. *Semin Ophthalmol* 2011;26(4–5):349–355.
2. Tan LT, Davagnanam I, Isa H, et al. Clinical and imaging features predictive of orbital granulomatosis with polyangiitis and the risk of systemic involvement. *Ophthalmology* 2014;121:1304–1309.
3. Rothschild PR, Pagnous C, Seror R, et al. Ophthalmologic manifestations of systemic necrotizing vasculitides at diagnosis a retrospective study of 1286 patients and review of the literature. *Semin Arthritis Rheum* 2013;42:507–514.
4. Perry SR, Rootman J, White VA. The clinical and pathologic constellation of Wegener's granulomatosis of the orbit. *Ophthalmology* 1997;104:683–694.
5. DeRemee RA. Sarcoidosis and Wegener's granulomatosis: a comparative analysis. *Sarcoidosis* 1994;11:7–18.
6. Lie JT. Wegener's granulomatosis: histological documentation of common and uncommon manifestations in 216 patients. *Vasa* 1997;26:261–270.
7. Haynes BF, Fishman ML, Fauci AS, et al. The ocular manifestations of Wegener's granulomatosis. Fifteen years experience and review of the literature. *Am J Med* 1977;63:131–141.
8. Fechner FP, Faquin WC, Pilch BZ. Wegener's granulomatosis of the orbit: a clinicopathological study of 15 patients. *Laryngoscope* 2002;112:1945–1950.
9. Bullen CL, Liesegang TJ, McDonald TJ, et al. Ocular complications of Wegener's granulomatosis. *Ophthalmology* 1983;90:279–290.

Imaging

10. McKinnon SG, Gentry LR. Systemic diseases involving the orbit. *Semin Ultrasound CT MR* 1998;19:292–308.
11. Courcoutsakis NA, Langford CA, Sneller MC, et al. Orbital involvement in Wegener's granulomatosis: MR findings in 12 patients. *J Comput Assist Tomogr* 1997;21:452–458.

Histopathology

12. Isa H, Lightman S, Luthert PJ, et al. Histopathological features predictive of a clinical diagnosis of ophthalmic granulomatosis with polyangiitis (GPA). *Int J Clin Exp Pathol* 2012;5(7):684–689.

Case Reports

13. Ziakas NG, Boboridis K, Gratsonidis A, et al. Wegener's granulomatosis of the orbit in a 5-year-old child. *Eye* 2004;18:658–660.
14. Chan AS, Yu DL, Rao NA. Eosinophilic variant of Wegener granulomatosis in the orbit. *Arch Ophthalmol* 2011;129(9):1238–1240.
15. Bhatia A, Yadava U, Goyal JL, et al. Limited Wegener's granulomatosis of the orbit: a case study and review of literature. *Eye (Lond)* 2005;19(1):102–104.
16. Knoch DW, Lucarelli MJ, Dortzbach RK, et al. Limited Wegener granulomatosis with 40 years of follow-up. *Arch Ophthalmol* 2003;121(11):1640–1642.

Chapter 26 Inflammatory Orbital Lesions That Simulate Neoplasms 467

● ORBITAL GRANULOMATOSIS WITH POLYANGIITIS (WEGENER GRANULOMATOSIS)

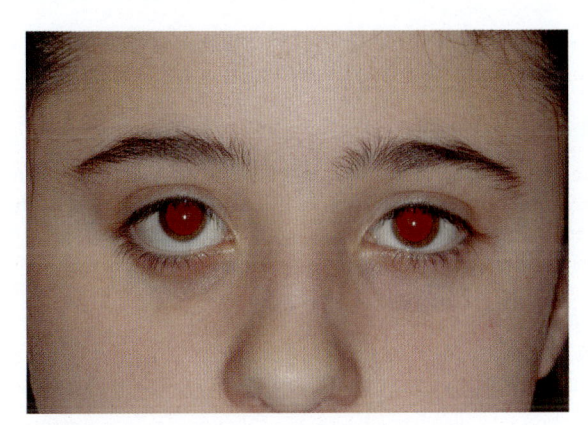

Figure 26.61. Slight right proptosis in a 9-year-old girl.

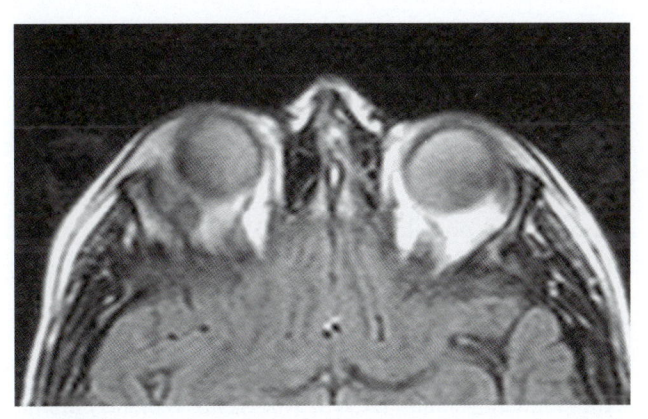

Figure 26.62. T1-weighted magnetic resonance imaging of patient in Figure 26.61, showing right lacrimal fossa mass.

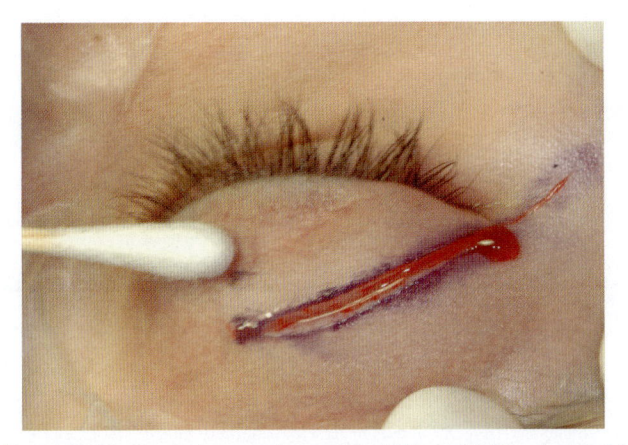

Figure 26.63. Surgical approach to patient in Figure 26.61, using eyelid crease incision.

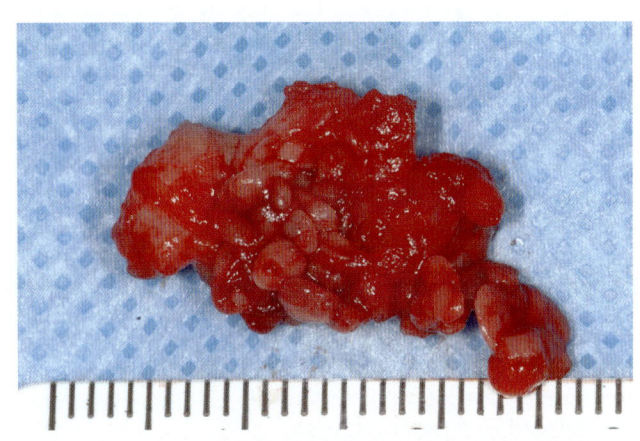

Figure 26.64. Ill-defined adherent mass was removed.

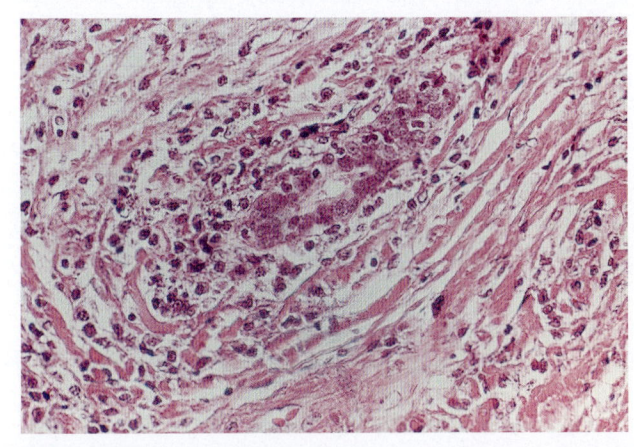

Figure 26.65. Histopathology of granulomatosis with polyangiitis showing necrotizing vasculitis. (Hematoxylin–eosin ×100.)

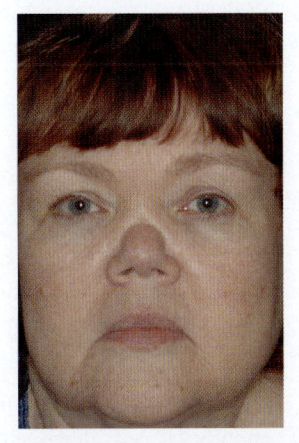

Figure 26.66. Chronic granulomatosis with polyangiitis in a woman demonstrating the "saddle nose deformity" from a perforated septum, characteristic of this disease.

KIMURA DISEASE AND ANGIOLYMPHOID HYPERPLASIA WITH EOSINOPHILIA

General Considerations

"Kimura disease" and "angiolymphoid hyperplasia with eosinophilia" (ALHE) have been used interchangeably in the Western literature to define an entity characterized clinically by skin lesions, blood and tissue eosinophilia, bronchial asthma, renal disease, and rather characteristic histopathologic features, and occasional orbital involvement (1–13). However, recent reports have strongly suggested that Kimura disease and ALHE should be considered as two separate entities, based on histopathologic differences (1,3). True Kimura disease is more common in the head and neck areas of young adult Asians who often have eosinophilia in the peripheral blood and increased serum immunoglobulin E levels. True ALHE is more common in Caucasians and more often limited to the head and neck region. Both diseases can cause proptosis, eyelid swelling, ocular dysmotility, or a palpable mass. These two conditions can show similar clinical features, but they are distinguished on histopathology (9).

Clinical Features

Kimura disease tends to occur in young adult, male Asians as a discrete nodules or localized swelling in the head and neck region, commonly with lymphadenopathy (3). It can be unilateral or bilateral. Blood eosinophilia is commonly present and elevated IgE is often found. ALHE tends to manifest in young to middle-aged persons of all races as nodules or erythematous papules of about 1 cm diameter in the head and neck region and without lymphadenopathy (3). Eosinophilia and IgE are uncommon in ALHE.

Diagnostic Approaches

On imaging, Kimura disease tends to show a noncircumscribed mass, whereas ALHE tends to be more circumscribed (3). Both can show a diffuse soft tissue mass that may be impossible to differentiate from NOI, lymphoma, or metastatic carcinoma. The diagnosis is generally made histopathologically after orbital biopsy.

Pathology

Histopathologically, Kimura disease is noncircumscribed, located in the subcutaneous tissue or muscle and with minor vascular proliferation demonstrating endothelium of flat to low appearance (1–3). There are abundant lymphocytes and plasma cells, with lymphoid follicles, and eosinophilic infiltration, occasionally with eosinophilic abscess. Sclerosis is prominent in all stages.

ALHE shows a more circumscribed mass in the dermis or subcutaneous tissue with florid vascular proliferation demonstrating "chubby" endothelial cells described as cuboidal or dome-shaped. Lymphocytes and plasma cells can be sparse to heavy infiltration and lymphoid follicles might be present. Eosinophils are sparse to abundant, but eosinophilic abscess is rare. Sclerosis is rarely found. The histopathologic differential diagnosis of these conditions includes angiosarcoma, granulomatosis with polyangiitis, Churg–Strauss syndrome, pyogenic granuloma, and other similar entities.

Management

The best management of orbital ALHE and Kimura disease of the orbit is complete surgical excision when possible. The therapeutic role of systemic corticosteroids and radiotherapy is not clearly established, but should be considered in difficult cases.

Selected References

Reviews

1. Buggage RR, Spraul CW, Wojno TH, et al. Kimura disease of the orbit and ocular adnexa. *Surv Ophthalmol* 1999;44:79–91.
2. Azari AA, Kanavi MR, Lucarelli M, et al. Angiolymphoid hyperplasia with eosinophilia of the orbit and ocular adnexa: report of 5 cases. *JAMA Ophthalmol* 2014;132:633–636.
3. Seregard S. Angiolymphoid hyperplasia with eosinophila should not be confused with Kimura's disease. *Acta Ophthalmologica Scan* 2001;79:91–93.

Management

4. Baker MS, Avery RB, Johnson CR, et al. Methotrexate as an alternative treatment for orbital angiolymphoid hyperplasia with eosinophilia. *Orbit* 2012;31(5):324–326.

Case Reports

5. Shetty AK, Beaty MW, McGuirt WF, et al. Kimura's disease a diagnostic challenge. *Pediatrics* 2002;110:e39.
6. Kodama T, Kawamoto K. Kimura's disease of the lacrimal gland. *Acta Ophthalmol Scand* 1998;76:374–377.
7. Shields CL, Shields JA, Glass RM. Bilateral orbital involvement in angiolymphoid hyperplasia with eosinophilia. Kimura's disease. *Orbit* 1990;9:89–95.
8. Sheren SB, Custer PL, Smith ME. Angiolymphoid hyperplasia with eosinophilia of the orbit associated with obstructive airway disease. *Am J Ophthalmol* 1989;108:167–169.
9. Smith DL, Kincaid MC, Nicolitz E. Angiolymphoid hyperplasia with eosinophilia (Kimura's disease) of the orbit. *Arch Ophthalmol* 1988;106:793–795.
10. Francis IC, Kappagoda MB, Smith J, et al. Kimura's disease of the orbit. *Ophthal Plast Reconstr Surg* 1988;4:235–239.
11. Hidayat AA, Cameron JD, Font RL, et al. Angiolymphoid hyperplasia with eosinophilia (Kimura's disease) of the orbit and ocular adnexa. *Am J Ophthalmol* 1983;96:176–189.
12. Cunniffe G, Alonso T, Dinarès C, et al. Angiolymphoid hyperplasia with eosinophilia of the eyelid and orbit: the Western cousin of Kimura's disease? *Int Ophthalmol* 2014;34:107–110.
13. Alder B, Proia A, Liss J. Distinct, bilateral epithelioid hemangioma of the orbit. *Orbit* 2013;32(1):51–53.

Chapter 26 Inflammatory Orbital Lesions That Simulate Neoplasms

ORBITAL ANGIOLYMPHOID HYPERPLASIA WITH EOSINOPHILIA AND KIMURA DISEASE

A clinicopathologic correlation of orbital involvement with angiolymphoid hyperplasia with eosinophilia in a Caucasian woman and a second case of Kimura disease in an Asian boy is depicted.

Shields CL, Shields JA, Glass RM. Bilateral orbital involvement in angiolymphoid hyperplasia with eosinophilia (Kimura's disease). *Orbit* 1990;9:89–95.

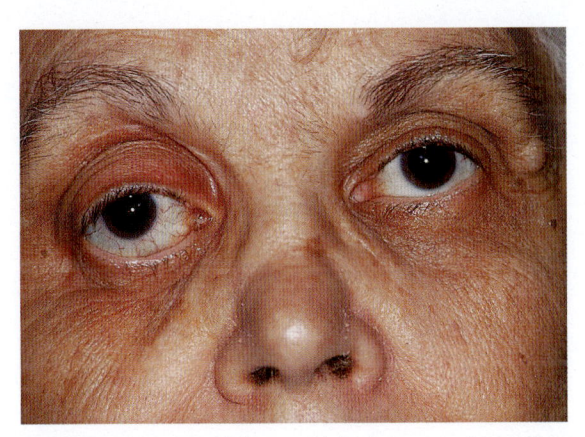

Figure 26.67. Proptosis and downward displacement of the right eye in a 55-year-old woman with ALHE.

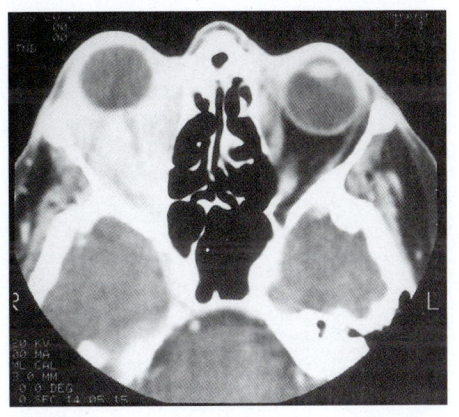

Figure 26.68. Axial computed tomography of patient in Figure 26.67, showing massive soft tissue involvement with ALHE of the right orbit and less severe involvement of the left orbit.

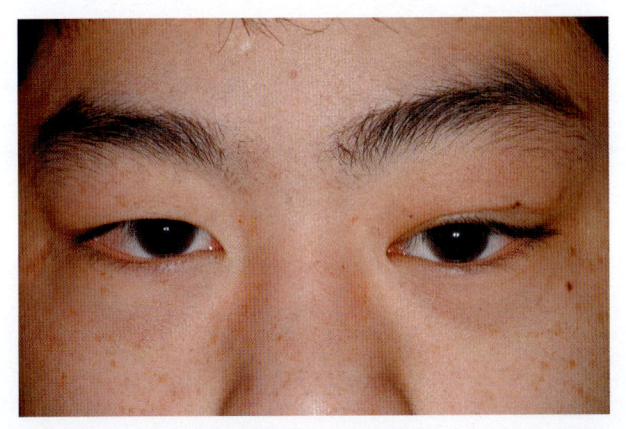

Figure 26.69. Facial appearance of 14-year-old Asian boy with fullness of both upper eyelids from Kimura disease.

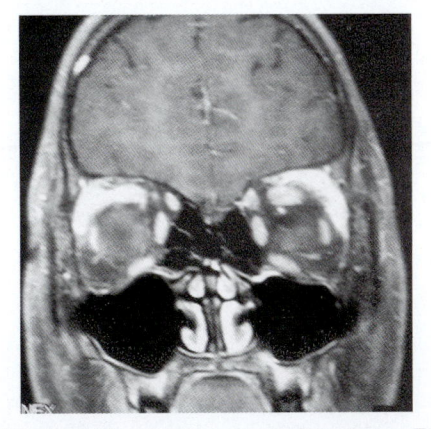

Figure 26.70. Coronal magnetic resonance imaging on T1-weighted image with fat suppression of patient shown in Figure 26.69. Note the diffuse enhancing lesions in lacrimal glands and surrounding tissue in both eyes. This patient with Kimura disease was treated with corticosteroids with poor response; the tumors were removed surgically from both orbits in separate operations.

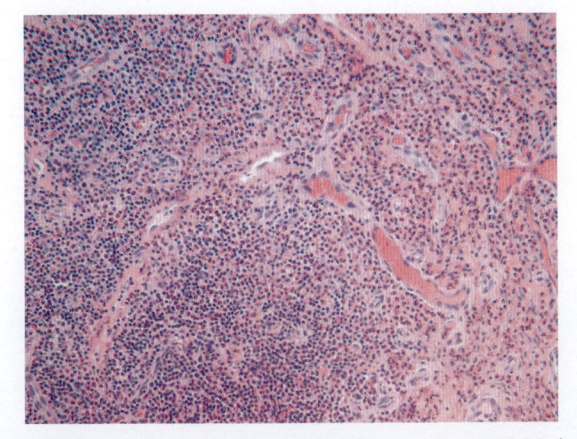

Figure 26.71. Photomicrograph of lesion shown in Figure 26.70 shows diffuse infiltration of lymphocytes and eosinophils with many small blood vessels. (Hematoxylin–eosin ×200.)

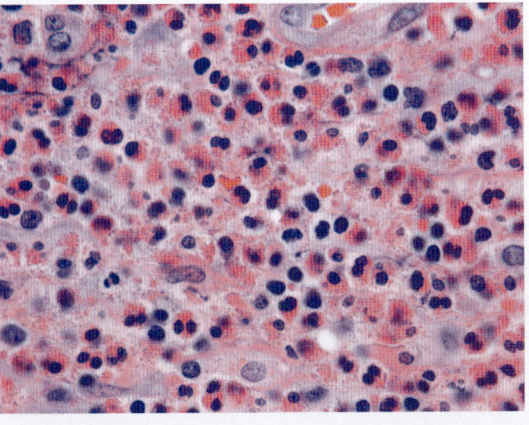

Figure 26.72. Higher power photomicrograph of same lesion, better depicting admixture of eosinophils and small lymphocytes, typical of Kimura disease. (Hematoxylin–eosin ×200.)

CHAPTER 27

ORBITAL CYSTIC LESIONS

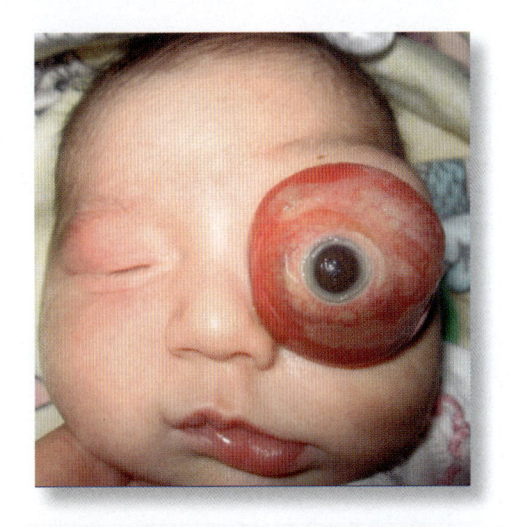

General Considerations

Cystic lesions in the orbit are fairly common (1–23). In the authors' series of 1,264 orbital masses seen on the Oncology Service at Wills Eye Hospital, the 70 orbital cysts seen accounted for 6% of all orbital lesions (1). Dermoid cyst was the most common, accounting for 26 cases, or 37% of all cystic lesions (1). Overall, about 61% of head and neck dermoid cysts occur in the periorbital region (1–9). This congenital lesion forms from epithelial cells that are entrapped during embryogenesis beneath the surface epithelium, often near bony sutures. Orbital dermoid cysts have been classified into juxtasutural, sutural, and soft tissue variants, with subcategories of each (1–3). In a clinicopathologic series of 197 cases from the Oncology Service and Pathology Department of Wills Eye Hospital, it was found that about 70% were located superotemporally at the zygomaticofrontal suture, 20% superonasally at the maxillofrontal suture, and 5% in the nasal soft tissue; other locations were less common (3).

Clinical Features

Orbital dermoid cyst classically occurs as a firm, fixed subcutaneous lesion near the orbital rim superotemporally in a young child. Less often, it develops at the orbital rim superonasally or in the deeper orbital soft tissues. Such a soft tissue nasal cyst is generally derived from conjunctival epithelium and is sometimes call a "conjunctivoid" (6). In most cases, there is a visible and palpable mass beneath the skin. The less common deep orbital cyst causes proptosis and/or displacement of the globe and is sometimes referred to as a "giant dermoid cyst" (13–17). The anterior dermoid can rupture spontaneously or after trauma and produce a subcutaneous inflammatory reaction that resembles cellulitis or dacryoadenitis. A draining cutaneous fistula can develop in such cases (22).

Diagnostic Approaches

The classic dermoid cyst can usually be diagnosed on the basis of the clinical appearance of a subcutaneous mass superotemporally at the orbital rim. However, the findings are not pathognomonic and other less common benign and malignant lesions can have a similar appearance. Imaging studies show a cystic lesion with enhancement of the wall but no significant enhancement of the lumen. Adjacent bone changes, usually a smooth fossa, are demonstrated in about 85% of cases (10). Fluid levels and calcification are frequently seen (10,21). In some instances, a dermoid cyst can have extraorbital and intraorbital components that are connected through a defect in bone (dumbbell dermoid) (11).

ORBITAL DERMOID CYST

Pathology

Histopathologically, orbital dermoid cyst is lined by surface epithelium (epidermis or conjunctiva). Cysts lined by conjunctival epithelium are more often found in the orbital soft tissue nasally. The cyst wall can contain dermal appendages, sebaceous glands, and sweat glands, features that are diagnostic of a dermoid cyst. The cyst lumen contains desquamated epithelial cells, sebaceous material, and hair.

Management

Management of orbital dermoid cyst ranges from observation to surgical excision, with most being removed surgically because the patient presents with a visible lesion or ocular symptoms owing to rupture of the cyst and secondary orbital inflammation. An anteriorly located orbital dermoid cyst can be excised by way of a cutaneous or conjunctival approach. An eyelid crease incision may provide a better cosmetic result. A deeper cyst may require a lateral orbitotomy. If such a deep cyst cannot be removed intact, it can be aspirated and more easily removed in a collapsed state. Care should be taken to avoid surgical rupture of the cyst if possible. If rupture occurs, vigorous irrigation and instillation of antibiotics or corticosteroids is advisable to prevent postoperative inflammation. The prognosis for vision and life are excellent.

ORBITAL DERMOID CYST

Selected References

Reviews

1. Shields JA, Shields CL, Scartozzi R. Survey of 1264 patients with orbital tumors and simulating lesions: the 2002 Montgomery Lecture, part 1. *Ophthalmology* 2004;111:997–1008.
2. Shields JA, Bakewell B, Augsburger DG, et al. Space-occupying orbital masses in children. A review of 250 consecutive biopsies. *Ophthalmology* 1986;93:379–384.
3. Shields JA, Kaden IH, Eagle RC Jr, et al. Orbital dermoid cysts. Clinicopathologic correlations, classification, and management. The 1997 Josephine E. Schueler Lecture. *Ophthal Plast Reconstr Surg* 1997;13:265–276.
4. Pryor SG, Lewis JE, Weaver AL, et al. Pediatric dermoid cysts of the head and neck. *Otolaryngol Head Neck Surg* 2005;132:938–942.
5. Shields JA, Shields CL. Orbital cysts of childhood—classification, clinical features, and management. The 2003 Angeline Parks Lecture. *Surv Ophthalmol* 2004;49: 281–299.
6. Jakobiec FA, Bonanno PA, Sigelman J. Conjunctival adnexal cysts and dermoids. *Arch Ophthalmol* 1978;96:1404–1409.
7. Sathananthan N, Moseley IF, Rose GE, et al. The frequency and clinical significance of bone involvement in outer canthus dermoid cysts. *Br J Ophthalmol* 1993;77: 789–794.
8. Sherman RP, Rootman J, Lapointe JJ. Orbital dermoids: Clinical presentation and management. *Br J Ophthalmol* 1984;68:642–652.
9. Mee JJ, McNab AA, McKelvie P. Respiratory epithelial orbital cysts. *Clin Exp Ophthalmol* 2002;30:356–360.

Imaging

10. Chawda SJ, Moseley IF. Computed tomography of orbital dermoids: a 20-year review. *Clin Radiol* 1999;54:821–825.

Case Reports

11. Emerick GT, Shields CL, Shields JA, et al. Chewing-induced visual impairment from a dumbbell dermoid cyst. *Ophthal Plast Reconstr Surg* 1997;13:57–61.
12. Shields JA, Augsburger JJ, Donoso LA. Orbital dermoid cyst of conjunctival origin. *Am J Ophthalmol* 1986;101:726–729.
13. Bickler-Bluth ME, Custer PL, Smith ME. Giant dermoid cyst of the orbit. *Arch Ophthalmol* 1987;105:1434–1435.
14. Grove AS Jr. Giant dermoid cysts of the orbit. *Ophthalmology* 1979;86: 1513–1520.
15. Pollard ZF, Calhoun J. Deep orbital dermoid with draining sinus. *Am J Ophthalmol* 1975;79:310–313.
16. Niederhagen B, Reich RH, Zentner J. Temporal dermoid with intracranial extension: report of a case. *J Oral Maxillofac Surg* 1998;56:1352–1354.
17. Leonardo D, Shields CL, Shields JA, et al. Recurrent giant orbital dermoid of infancy. *J Pediatr Ophthalmol Strabismus* 1994;31:50–52.
18. Sathananthan N, Moseley IF, Rose GE, et al. The frequency and clinical significance of bone involvement in outer canthus dermoid cysts. *Br J Ophthalmol* 1993;77: 789–794.
19. Kronish JW, Dortzbach RK. Upper eyelid crease surgical approach to dermoid and epidermoid cysts in children. *Arch Ophthalmol* 1988;106:1625–1627.
20. Samuelson TW, Margo CE, Levy MH, et al. Zygomaticofrontal suture defect associated with orbital dermoid cyst. *Surv Ophthalmol* 1988;33:127–130.
21. Karatza E, Shields CL, Shields JA, et al. Calcified orbital cyst in an adult simulating a malignant lacrimal gland tumor. *Ophthal Plast Reconstr Surg* 2004;20:397–399.
22. Wells TS, Harris GJ. Orbital dermoid cyst and sinus tract presenting with acute infection. *Ophthal Plast Reconstr Surg* 2004;20:465–467.
23. Dutton JJ, Fowler AM, Proia AD. Dermoid cyst of conjunctival origin. *Ophthal Plast Reconstr Surg* 2006;22(2):137–139.

ORBITAL DERMOID CYST: TYPICAL CASE OF EPIDERMAL ORIGIN

Most dermoid cysts in the orbital region are located superotemporally near the zygomaticofrontal suture. A typical case with imaging, surgical approach, and pathology is shown.

Shields JA, Kaden IH, Eagle RC Jr, et al. Orbital dermoid cysts. Clinicopathologic correlations, classification, and management. The 1997 Josephine E. Schueler Lecture. *Ophthal Plast Reconstr Surg* 1997;13:265–276.

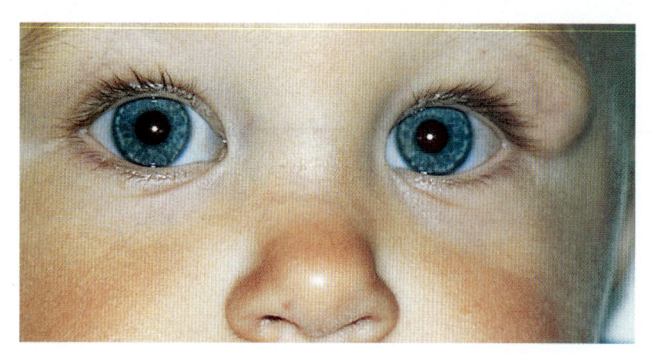

Figure 27.1. Characteristic left superotemporal subcutaneous mass in a 2-month-old boy.

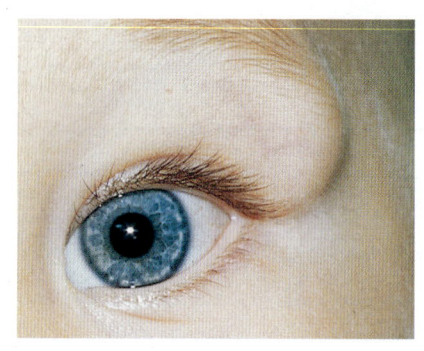

Figure 27.2. Closer view of the lesion.

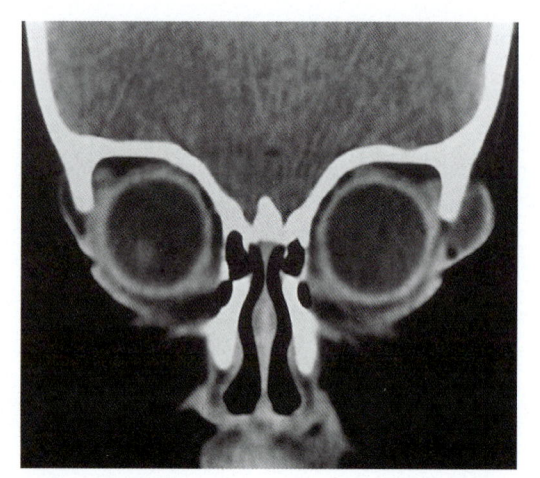

Figure 27.3. Coronal CT showing cystic lesion at the orbital rim. The lumen of the cyst is hypointense, similar to vitreous and orbital fat.

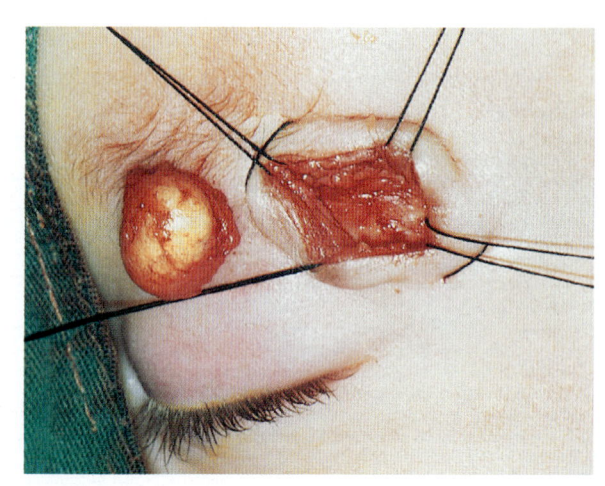

Figure 27.4. The cyst (to the *left*) has been removed by a cutaneous approach. One can use either an infrabrow or eyelid crease incision. The posterior aspect of the cyst is often adherent to the periosteum, requiring meticulous dissection to remove the cyst intact.

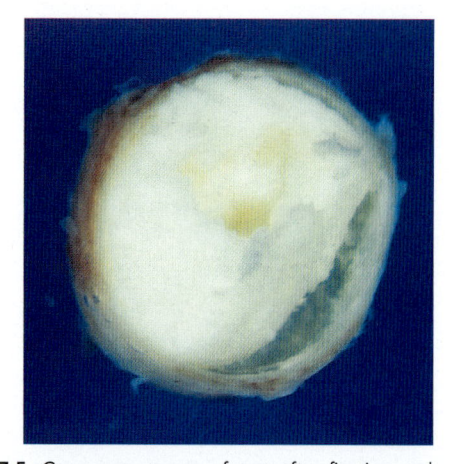

Figure 27.5. Gross appearance of cyst after fixation and sectioning. Note the capsule and the yellow material in the lumen.

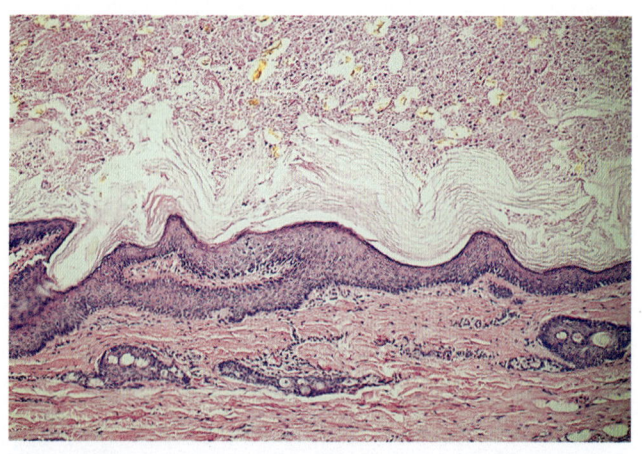

Figure 27.6. Histopathology through the cyst wall (*below*) and the lumen (*above*). The cyst is lined by keratinizing epithelium and has dermal elements (hair follicles and sebaceous glands) in the wall (*below*) and in the lumen (*above*). (Hematoxylin–eosin ×25.)

ORBITAL DERMOID CYST: LESION OF CONJUNCTIVAL ORIGIN IN A CHILD

Dermoid cysts lined by conjunctival epithelium usually occur in the orbital soft tissues nasally. It is possible that they originate from primitive epithelium destined to form the adult caruncle. In contrast with the typical dermoid cyst shown previously, this type is generally recognized in older children or adults.

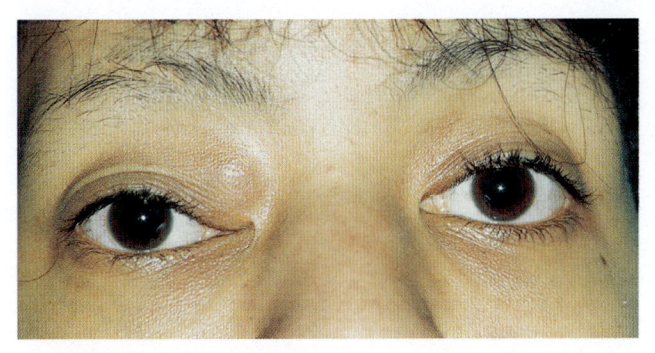

Figure 27.7. Soft tissue subcutaneous mass superonasally on right side in a 17-year-old woman.

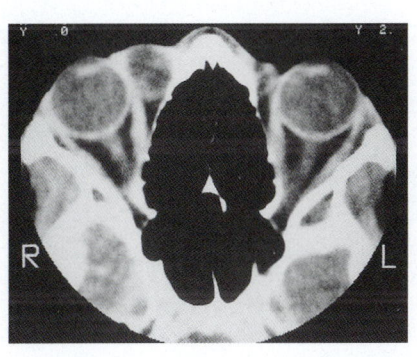

Figure 27.8. Axial computed tomography showing cystic nature of the lesion.

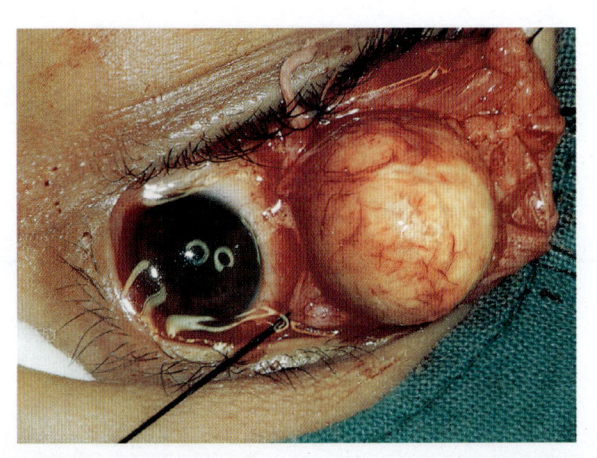

Figure 27.9. Cyst has been exposed and removed through a superonasal conjunctival approach.

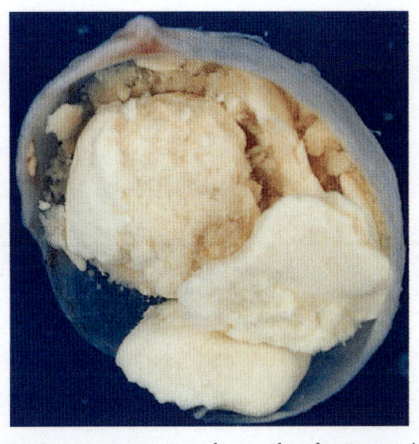

Figure 27.10. Gross appearance of cyst after fixation and sectioning. Note the very thin capsule and the yellow material in the lumen.

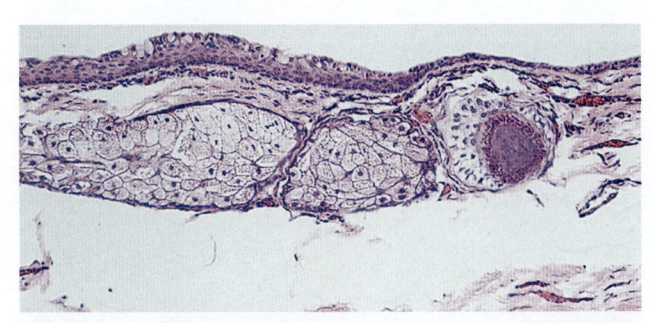

Figure 27.11. Photomicrograph showing wall of cyst with nonkeratinizing epithelium with goblet cells, hair shafts, and sebaceous glands. (Hematoxylin–eosin ×25.)

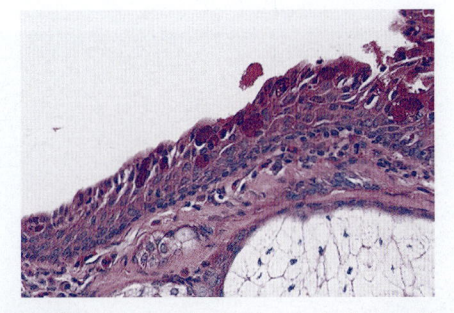

Figure 27.12. Photomicrograph showing wall of cyst with nonkeratinizing epithelium containing Periodic acid-Schiff–positive goblet cells. (Periodic acid-Schiff ×50.)

ORBITAL DERMOID CYST: LESION OF CONJUNCTIVAL ORIGIN IN AN ADULT

Although orbital dermoid cysts are congenital, the soft tissue dermoid cyst of conjunctival origin may lie dormant for many years before clinical detection. Such cysts have been recognized in patients >70 years old. A clinicopathologic correlation in a 50-year-old patient is shown.

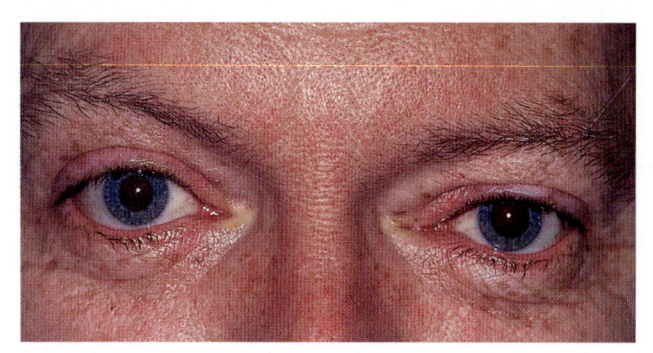

Figure 27.13. Slight blepharoptosis and inferotemporal displacement of left eye in a 50-year-old man.

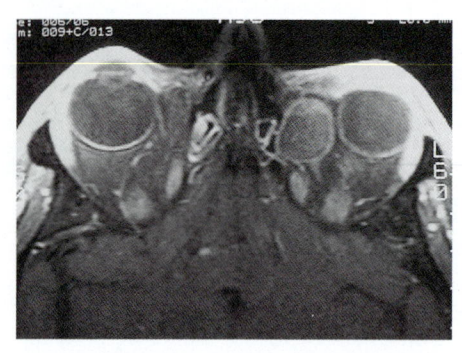

Figure 27.14. Axial magnetic resonance imaging in T1-weighted image, showing temporal displacement of left eye by cystic mass.

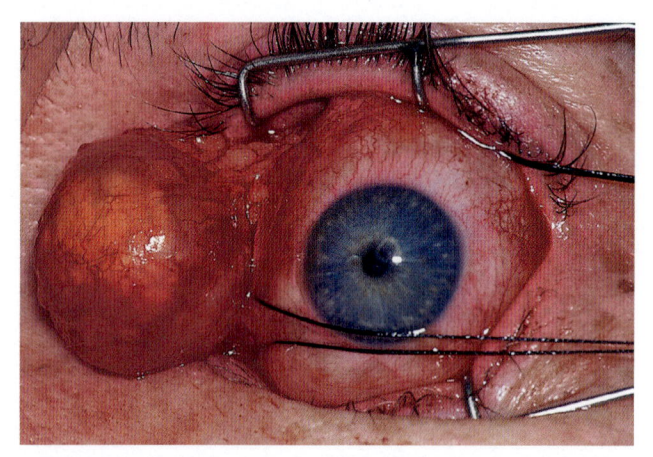

Figure 27.15. Lesion being removed intact by way of a forniceal incision in the conjunctiva. It was easily delivered by sharp and blunt orbital dissection.

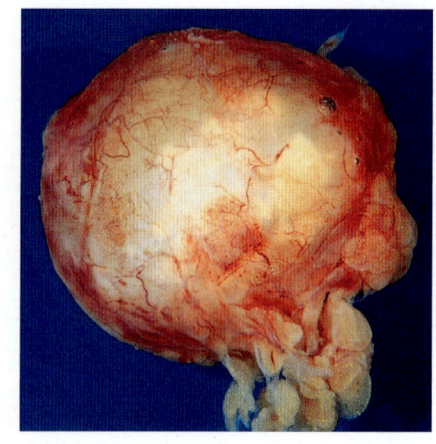

Figure 27.16. Gross appearance of the intact cyst after excision. Note the yellow material deep to the thin capsule.

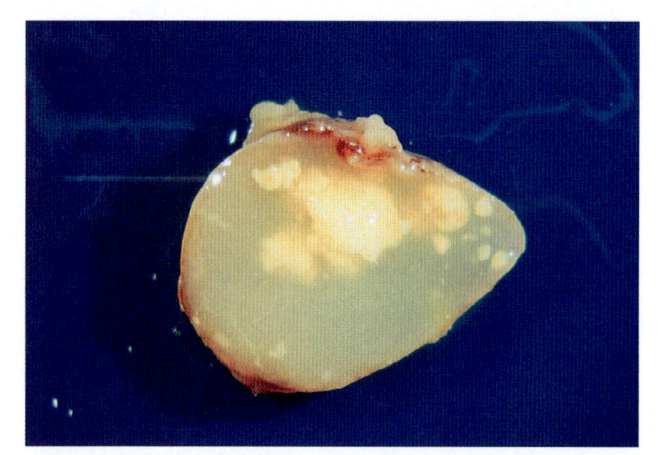

Figure 27.17. Gross appearance of cyst after fixation and sectioning. Note the very thin capsule and the yellow material in the lumen.

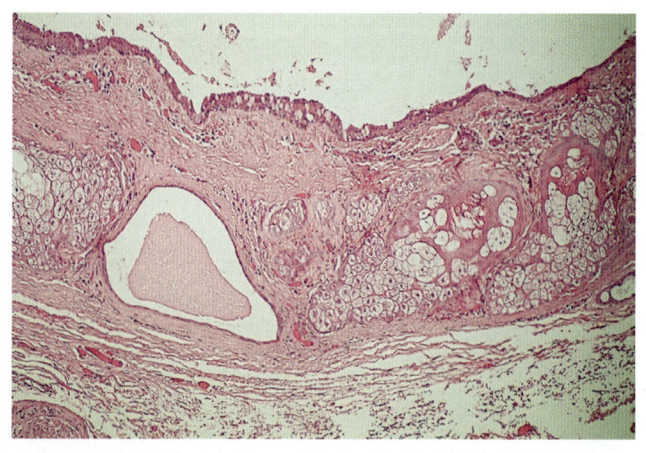

Figure 27.18. Histopathology through the cyst wall (*below*) and the lumen (*above*). The cyst is lined by nonkeratinizing epithelium with goblet cells and has dermal elements in the wall and in the lumen. (Hematoxylin–eosin ×40.)

ORBITAL DERMOID CYST: DUMBBELL TYPE

Dumbbell dermoid cysts are characterized by two cystic components connected by a channel through the adjacent bone, at the site of a bony suture. Like other subcutaneous dermoid cysts, they can break through the epidermis and produce a draining fistula.

Emerick GT, Shields CL, Shields JA, et al. Chewing-induced visual impairment from a dumbbell dermoid cyst. *Ophthal Plast Reconstr Surg* 1997;13:57–61.

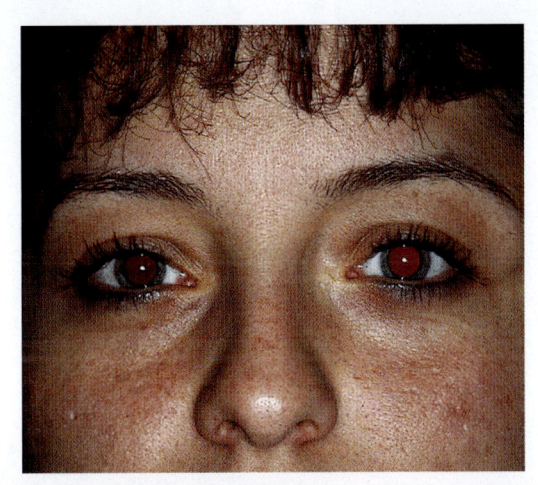

Figure 27.19. Subcutaneous mass temporal to left eye in a 29-year-old woman.

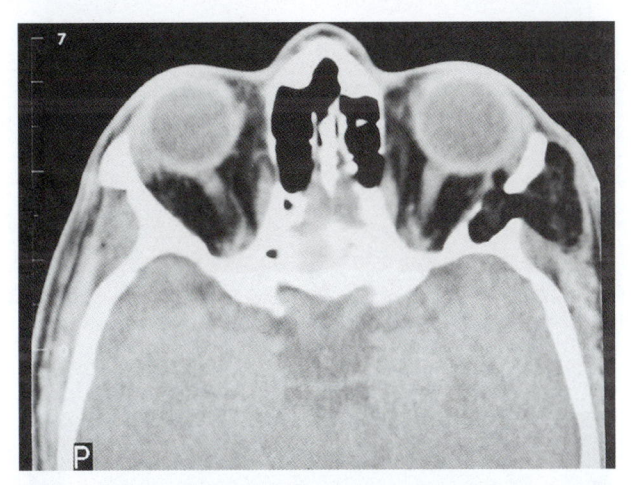

Figure 27.20. Axial computed tomography of patient shown in Figure 27.19, showing bilobed cystic lesion communicating through an enlarged zygomaticofrontal suture. Note that the lumen of the lesion is dark, similar to orbital fat. The lesion was excised piecemeal.

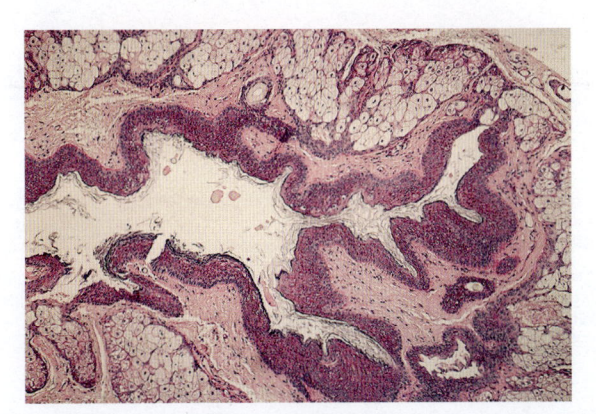

Figure 27.21. Histopathology of excised cyst shown in Figure 27.20, demonstrating the keratinizing epithelium with numerous sebaceous glands in the wall. (Hematoxylin–eosin ×40.)

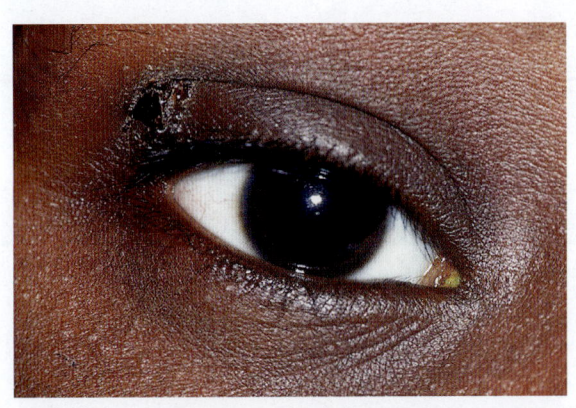

Figure 27.22. Draining cutaneous fistula superotemporal to right eye in an 8-year-old boy. Such a fistula in this location is highly suggestive of a ruptured dermoid cyst.

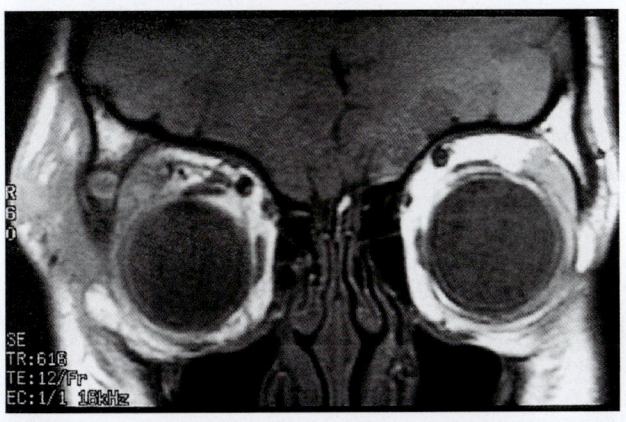

Figure 27.23. Coronal magnetic resonance imaging in T1-weighted image of patient shown in Figure 27.22, revealing the bony defect connecting the two irregular lobes of the cyst.

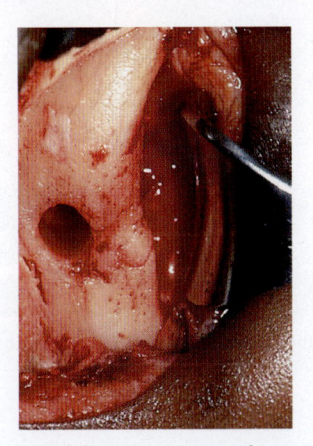

Figure 27.24. Osseous defect seen at time of surgery after piecemeal removal of the dermoid cyst in patient shown in Figure 27.22.

ORBITAL DERMOID CYST: DUMBBELL TYPE, SURGICAL RESECTION

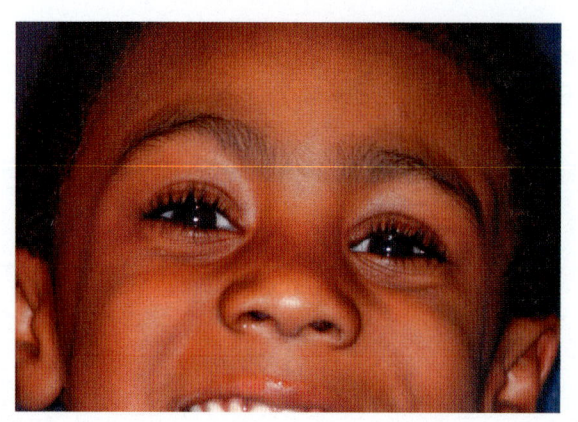

Figure 27.25. Facial appearance of 6-year-old boy. There was minimal soft tissue subcutaneous swelling temporal to left eye.

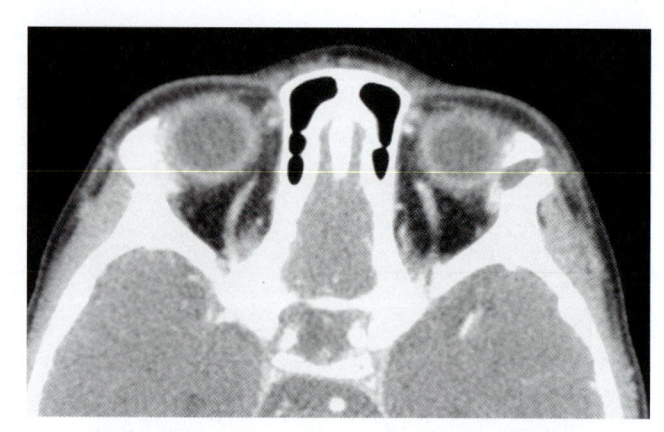

Figure 27.26. Axial computed tomography showing osseous defect in zygoma of left eye (to the *right* in the image). Note the normal bone on the contralateral side.

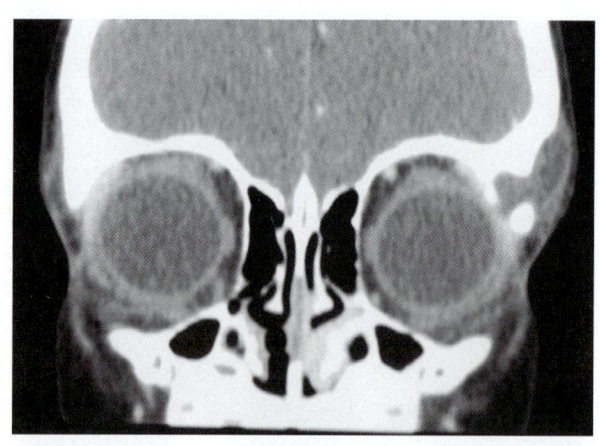

Figure 27.27. Coronal computed tomography more clearly showing the osseous defect.

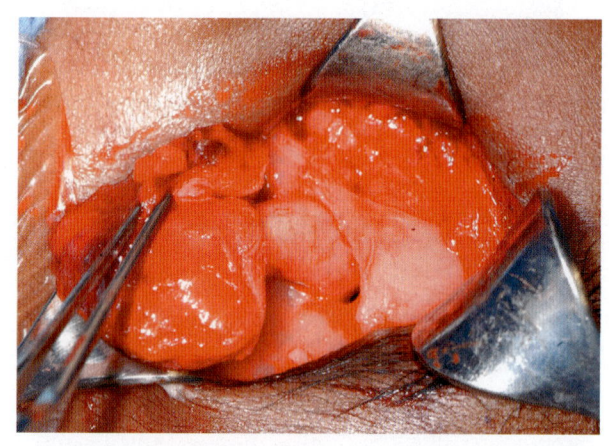

Figure 27.28. Surgical photograph showing subcutaneous component of the cyst (retracted with forceps to the left) and the tubular component of the cyst passing through the bony defect (in the center).

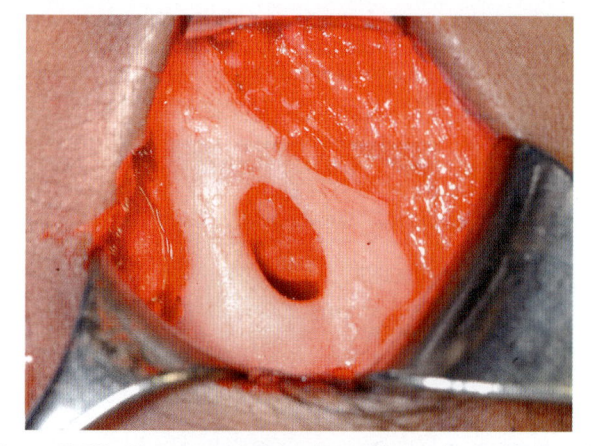

Figure 27.29. After removal of the dermoid cyst, the oval hole in the bone is clearly visualized.

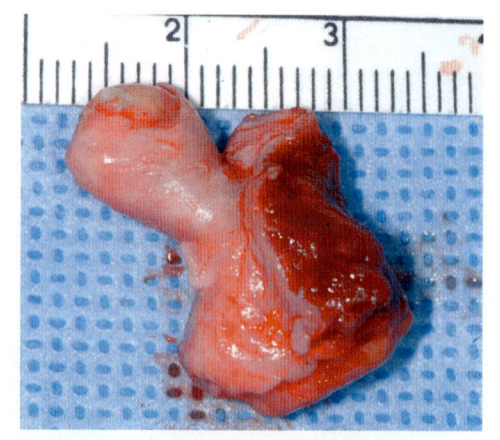

Figure 27.30. Gross appearance of the bilobed dermoid cyst immediately after surgical removal. The component up and to the left represents the tubular intraosseous component of the lesion.

ORBITAL DERMOID CYST: DEEP ORBITAL TYPE

Large dermoid cysts located in the posterior orbit pose more of a diagnostic and therapeutic challenge. Such cysts can slowly grow to a large size at a young age and can recur after excision. A clinicopathologic correlation is depicted.

Leonardo D, Shields CL, Shields JA, et al. Recurrent giant orbital dermoid of infancy. *J Pediatr Ophthalmol Strabismus* 1994;31:50–52.

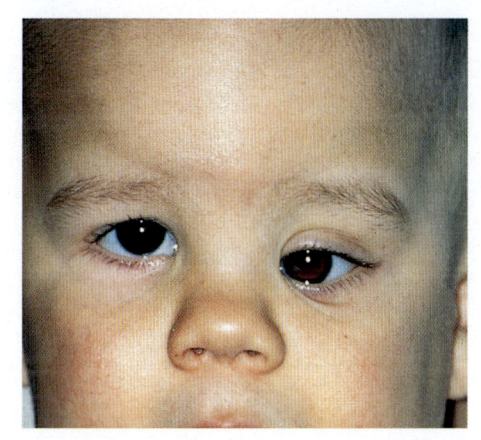

Figure 27.31. Proptosis and downward displacement of the left eye in a 2-year-old boy. The findings were noted shortly after birth and had become progressively worse.

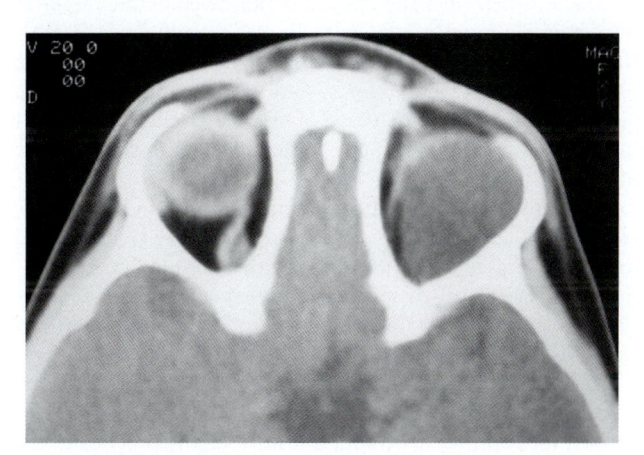

Figure 27.32. Axial computed tomography showing large superior orbital mass in the left orbit.

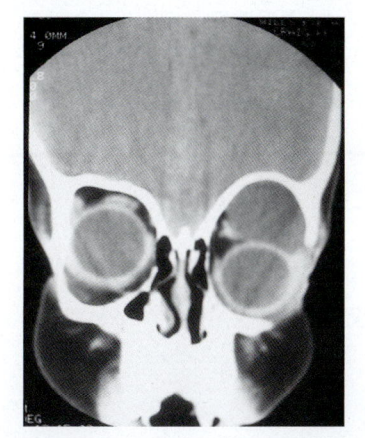

Figure 27.33. Coronal computed tomography showing mass above the globe. Note that the orbit is larger and there is superior displacement of the orbital roof.

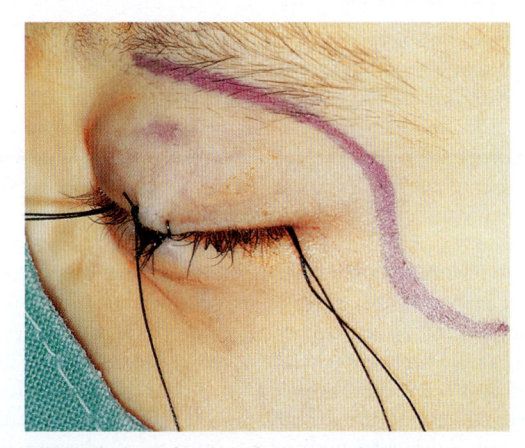

Figure 27.34. Outline of incision for lateral orbitotomy.

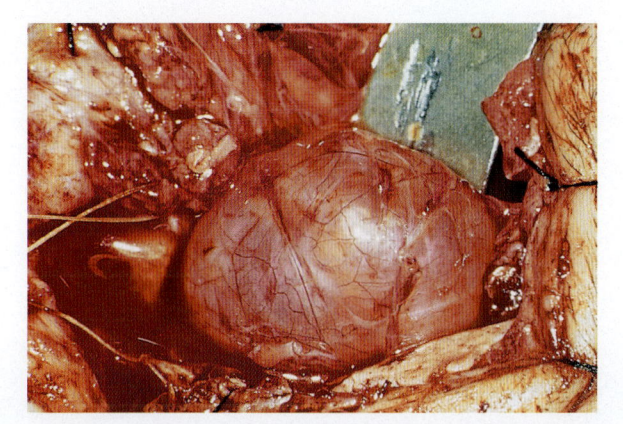

Figure 27.35. Cystic mass exposed after lateral orbitotomy. It was aspirated and removed.

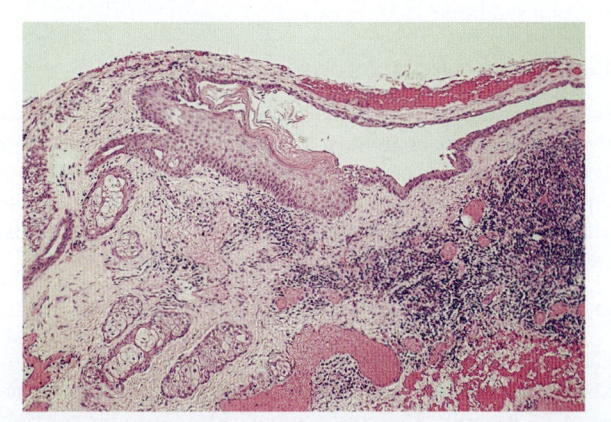

Figure 27.36. Histopathology of a portion of the collapsed cyst showing features of a dermoid cyst. Although most of the cyst was lined by nonkeratinizing epithelium similar to conjunctiva, a small portion of it showed keratinizing epithelium. The lesion recurred in the temporal orbit about 2 years later and was excised surgically with a good result. (Hematoxylin–eosin ×25.)

ORBITAL SIMPLE PRIMARY CYST OF CONJUNCTIVAL ORIGIN

General Considerations

Simple epithelial cysts can be classified according to the type of epithelium that lines the cyst. This can be epidermis, respiratory epithelium, glandular epithelium, or conjunctiva (1–15). In the authors' series of 1,264 orbital masses, the 12 simple epithelial cysts accounted for 17% of cystic lesions and for 1% of all orbital lesions. Each type of cyst has similar clinical and imaging features and only the conjunctival epithelial cysts are described here (1–8).

A simple orbital cyst of conjunctival origin can be primary, without an apparent cause, or it can be secondary to surgical or nonsurgical trauma. In contrast with a dermoid cyst of conjunctival origin (discussed previously), a simple cyst of conjunctival origin does not contain dermal appendages within its walls. In a review of 128 cases of conjunctival adnexal and dermoid cysts, there were 5 simple conjunctival cysts (5). In another series of 11 conjunctival cysts of the orbit, 6 were presumed to be primary, without a history of antecedent surgery or trauma (6).

Clinical Features

A primary conjunctival cyst can become apparent at any age, with patient ages in one series ranging from 4 to 45 years old at the time of diagnosis (5). The patient usually presents with a soft, fluctuant mass in the anterior superonasal aspect of the orbit, without visual loss, proptosis, or displacement of the globe. As the cyst enlarges, it can induce pain, tenderness, motility disturbance, displacement of the globe, and refractive error. The features of a secondary conjunctival cyst vary with the type of prior surgery or trauma. After strabismus surgery, the cyst may be visible near the insertion of the affected rectus muscle, but can extend deeper into the orbital soft tissues (9). After retinal detachment surgery, it can be located deeper in the orbit and affect a rectus muscle (11). After enucleation, it may appear as an asymptomatic mass in the anophthalmic orbit or it may cause difficulty with retention of the ocular prosthesis (7). This type of cyst can also occur in the anterior aspect of the orbit after conjunctival inflammations such as Stevens–Johnson syndrome (13).

Diagnostic Approaches

In many instances, the diagnosis of the orbital cyst of conjunctival origin can be established by direct visualization of a clear cyst that appears in the conjunctival region. Computed tomography and magnetic resonance imaging generally demonstrate a clear, nonenhancing cyst that is confined to orbital soft tissues without bone erosion.

Pathology and Pathogenesis

Conjunctival epithelial cyst is lined by attenuated nonkeratinizing stratified squamous epithelium without adnexal structures in its wall. The epithelium characteristically contains mucous-secreting goblet cells identical to those found in the conjunctiva. It is believed that such cysts occur as a result of misdirected cleavage of mesoderm during formation of the superior conjunctival fornix (8).

Management

The management of a suspected conjunctival orbital cyst necessarily varies from case to case. A small asymptomatic cyst can be followed without treatment. However, most larger cysts should be removed surgically, with an attempt to completely excise the lesion without disrupting its epithelial lining. This can usually be accomplished with meticulous dissection by an anterior orbital approach, depending on the size and location of the lesion.

ORBITAL SIMPLE PRIMARY CYST OF CONJUNCTIVAL ORIGIN

Selected References

Reviews

1. Shields JA, Shields CL, Scartozzi R. Survey of 1264 patients with orbital tumors and simulating lesions: the 2002 Montgomery Lecture, part 1. *Ophthalmology* 2004;111:997–1008.
2. Shields JA, Bakewell B, Augsburger DG, et al. Space-occupying orbital masses in children. A review of 250 consecutive biopsies. *Ophthalmology* 1986;93:379–384.
3. Shields JA, Kaden IH, Eagle RC Jr, et al. Orbital dermoid cysts. Clinicopathologic correlations, classification, and management. The 1997 Josephine E. Schueler Lecture. *Ophthal Plast Reconstr Surg* 1997;13:265–276.
4. Shields JA, Shields CL. Orbital cysts of childhood—classification, clinical features, and management. The 2003 Angeline Parks Lecture. *Surv Ophthalmol* 2004;49:281–299.
5. Jakobiec FA, Bonanno PA, Sigelman J. Conjunctival adnexal cysts and dermoids. *Arch Ophthalmol* 1978;96:1404–1409.
6. Goldstein MH, Soparkar CN, Kersten RC, et al. Conjunctival cysts of the orbit. *Ophthalmology* 1998;105:2056–2060.
7. Smit TJ, Koornneef L, Zonneveld FW. Conjunctival cysts in anophthalmic orbits. *Br J Ophthalmol* 1991;75:342–343.
8. Rose GE, O'Donnell BA. Congenital orbital cysts associated with the common sheath of superior rectus and levator palpebrae superioris muscles. *Ophthalmology* 1995;102:135–138.

Case Reports

9. Metz HS, Searl S, Rosenberg P, et al. Giant orbital cyst after strabismus surgery. *JAAPOS* 1999;3:185–187.
10. Basar E, Pazarli H, Ozdemir H, et al. Subconjunctival cyst extending into the orbit. *Int Ophthalmol* 1998;22:341–343.
11. De Potter P, Kunin AW, Shields CL, et al. Massive orbital cyst of the lateral rectus muscle after retinal detachment surgery. *Ophthal Plast Reconstr Surg* 1993;9:292–297.
12. Johnson DW, Bartley GB, Garrity JA, et al. Massive epithelium-lined cyst after scleral buckling. *Am J Ophthalmol* 1992;113:439–444.
13. Desai V, Shields CL, Shields JA. Orbital cyst in a patient with Stevens Johnson syndrome. *Cornea* 1992;11:592–594.
14. Boynton JR, Searl SS, Ferry AP, et al. Primary nonkeratinized epithelial ("conjunctival") orbital cysts. *Arch Ophthalmol* 1992;110:1238–1242.
15. McCarthy RW, Beyer CK, Dallow RL, et al. Conjunctival cysts of the orbit following enucleation. *Ophthalmology* 1981;88:30–35.

ORBITAL CYST OF CONJUNCTIVAL ORIGIN: PRIMARY IDIOPATHIC TYPE

Some orbital cysts are lined by conjunctival epithelium without dermal elements in the cyst wall. A cyst of this type is called a "simple conjunctival epithelial cyst of the orbit." Such a cyst can occur as an idiopathic lesion or it can be secondary to implantation of conjunctival epithelium after surgical or nonsurgical trauma. A clinicopathologic correlation of the idiopathic variant is shown.

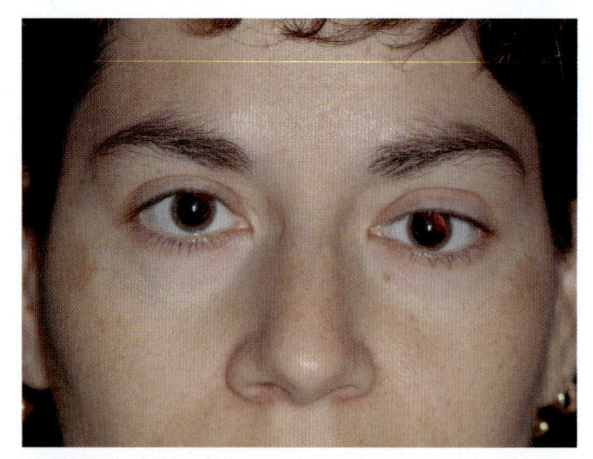

Figure 27.37. Facial appearance of a 36-year-old woman with proptosis and downward displacement of left eye.

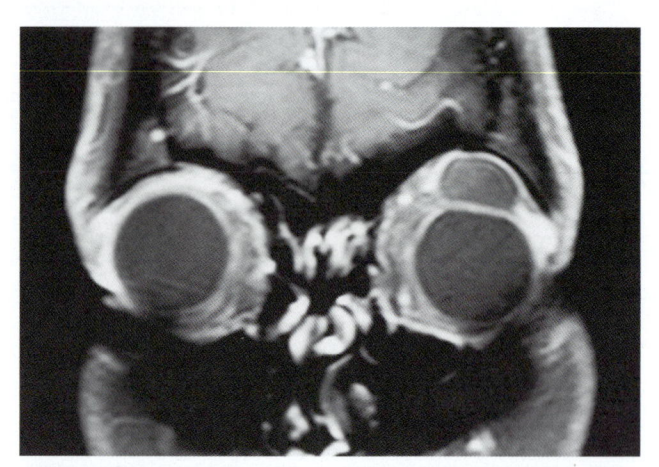

Figure 27.38. T1-weighted magnetic resonance imaging, coronal orientation, delineating the circumscribed cyst in the superior orbit.

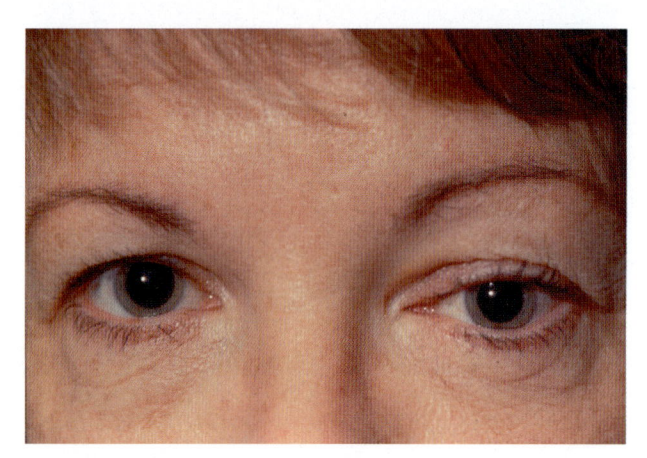

Figure 27.39. Facial appearance of a 52-year-old woman with proptosis and downward displacement of left eye.

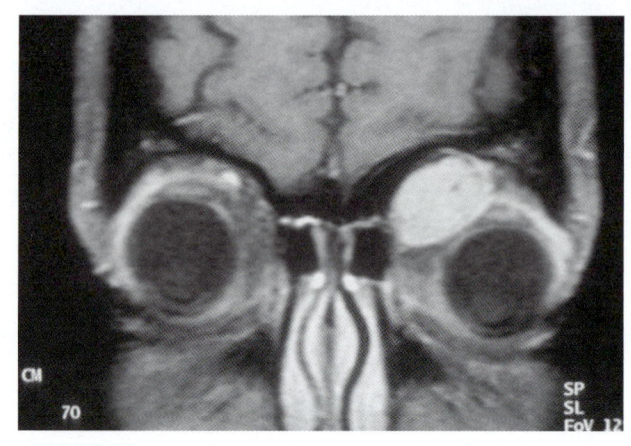

Figure 27.40. Coronal magnetic resonance imaging in T1-weighted image delineating the mass in the orbit superonasally.

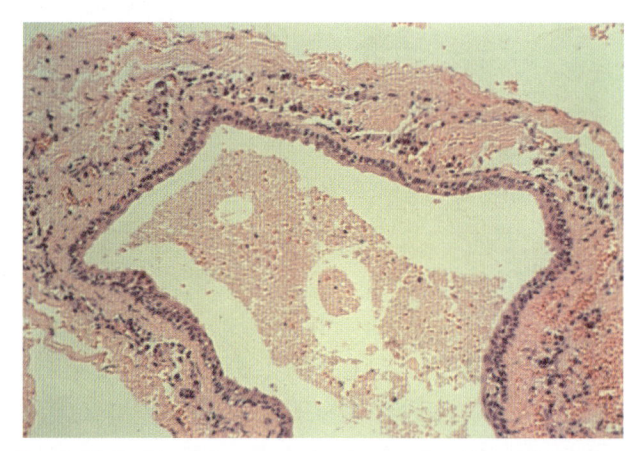

Figure 27.41. Photomicrograph showing cyst lined by nonkeratinizing stratified epithelium compatible with conjunctival epithelium. No goblet cells are appreciated in this field. The lumen contains necrotic cellular debris. (Hematoxylin–eosin ×25.)

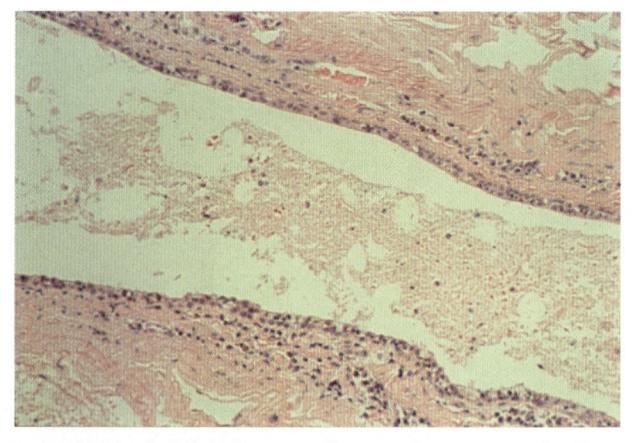

Figure 27.42. Slightly higher magnification photomicrograph of same lesion showing mild infiltration of chronic inflammatory cells in the cyst wall but no dermal structure. (Hematoxylin–eosin ×25.)

Chapter 27 Orbital Cystic Lesions 483

ORBITAL CYST OF CONJUNCTIVAL ORIGIN: SECONDARY TYPE, AFTER ENUCLEATION

An orbital cyst can develop in an anophthalmic orbit following enucleation for any cause. It presumably arises from rests of conjunctival epithelium. Depicted is a clinicopathologic correlation of an orbital conjunctival cyst that developed years after enucleation for retinoblastoma.

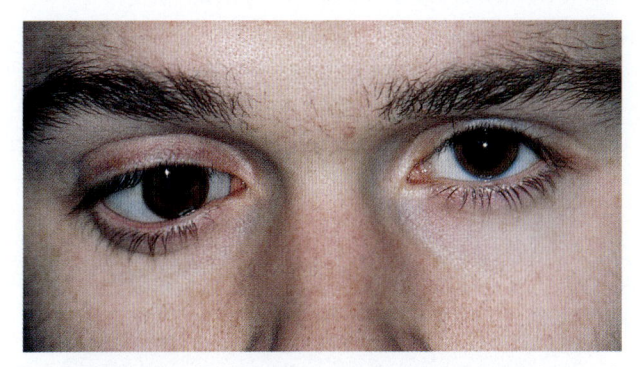

Figure 27.43. Downward displacement and proptosis of the enucleation prosthesis in an 18-year-old man who underwent enucleation elsewhere for retinoblastoma 16 years earlier.

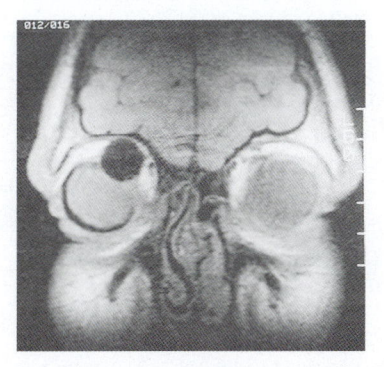

Figure 27.44. Coronal magnetic resonance imaging showing large cyst, the size of a normal globe, displacing the silastic ball implant superonasally.

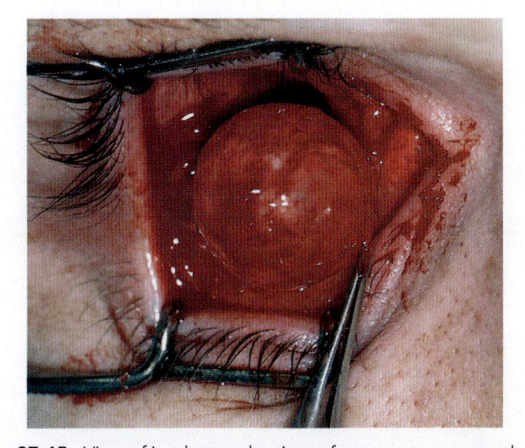

Figure 27.45. View of implant at the time of surgery to remove the cyst.

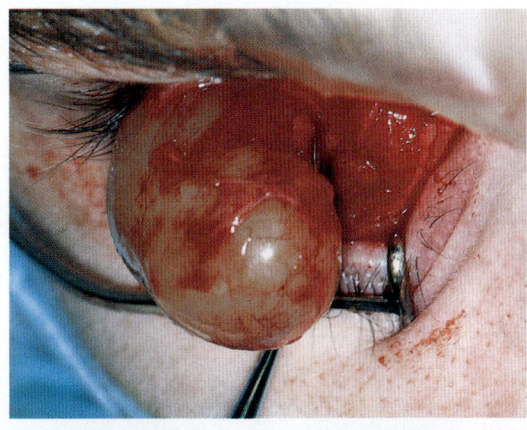

Figure 27.46. View of the large cyst that is being removed after the implant was taken out.

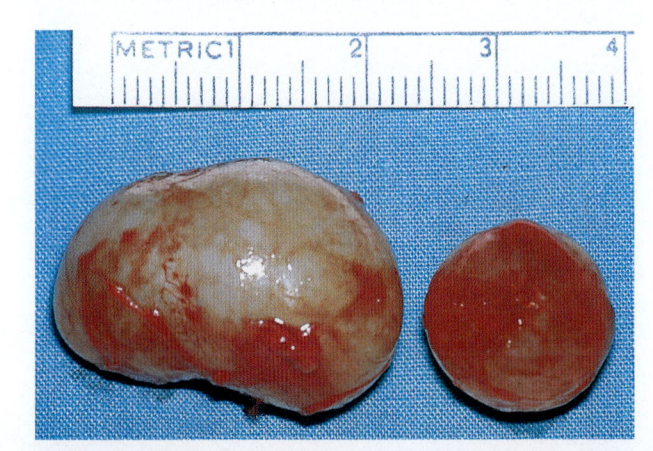

Figure 27.47. Appearance of cyst (to the *left*) and the removed implant (to the *right*) immediately after surgical removal.

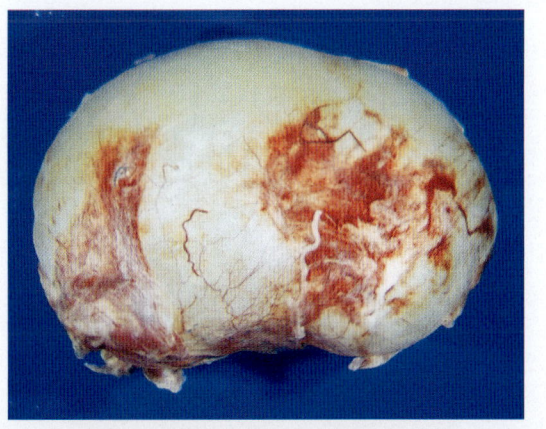

Figure 27.48. Gross view of the cyst after fixation. The clear cyst was lined by conjunctival epithelium.

ORBITAL CYST OF CONJUNCTIVAL ORIGIN: SECONDARY TYPE, AFTER RETINAL DETACHMENT SURGERY

An orbital cyst can develop after retinal detachment surgery, presumably from displacement of conjunctival epithelium into the deeper orbital tissues. A clinicopathologic correlation is shown.

De Potter P, Kunin AW, Shields CL, et al. Massive orbital cyst of the lateral rectus muscle after retinal detachment surgery. *Ophthal Plast Reconstr Surg* 1993;9:292–297.

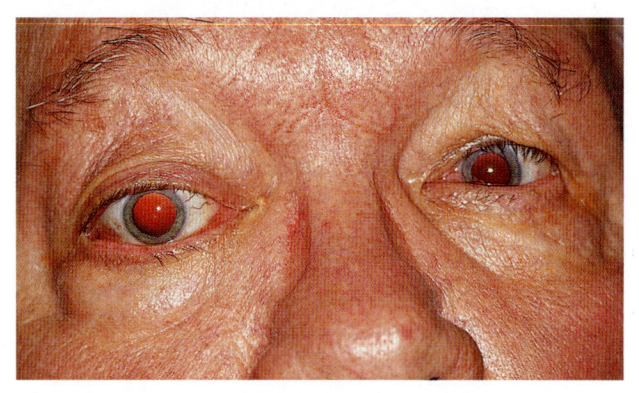

Figure 27.49. Proptosis of the right eye in a 76-year-old man who had undergone ipsilateral retinal detachment surgery several years earlier.

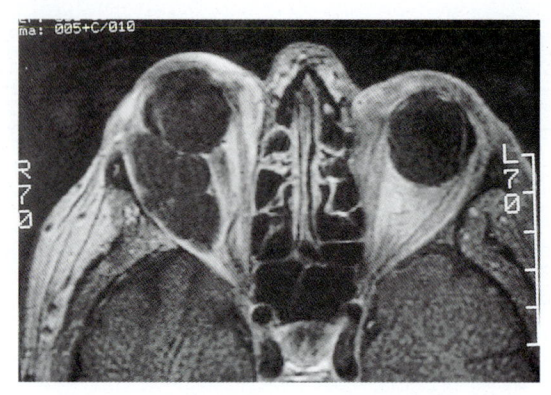

Figure 27.50. Axial magnetic resonance imaging in T1-weighted image, showing irregular cyst in lateral portion of orbit.

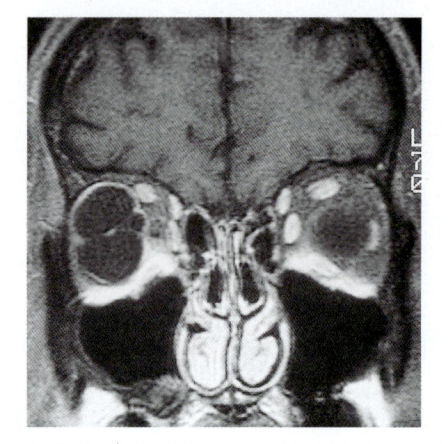

Figure 27.51. Coronal magnetic resonance imaging in T1-weighted image showing the cyst.

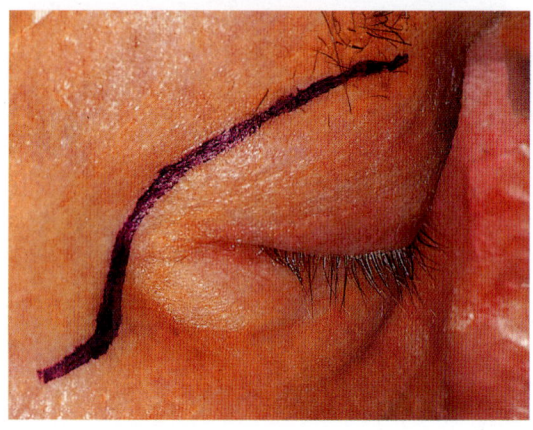

Figure 27.52. Outline of superotemporal orbitotomy incision to remove the cyst.

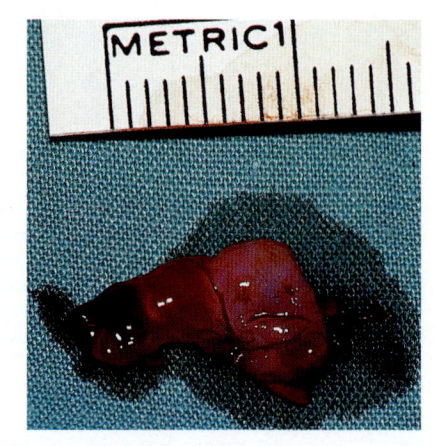

Figure 27.53. A portion of the collapsed cyst is shown after it was aspirated and removed piecemeal.

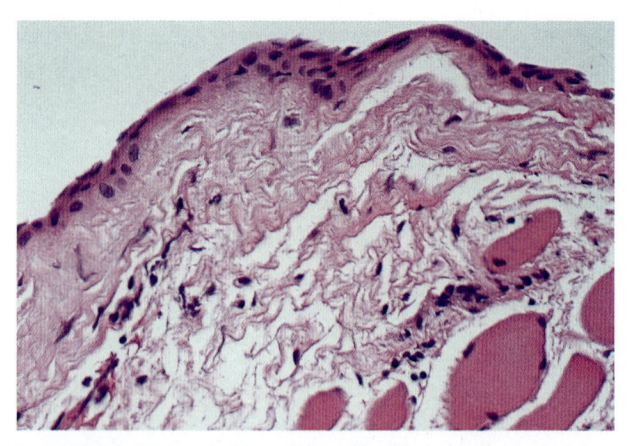

Figure 27.54. Histopathology of the wall of the cyst showing nonkeratinizing epithelium. (Hematoxylin–eosin ×25.)

ORBITAL CYST: SIMPLE CONJUNCTIVAL TYPE ASSOCIATED WITH STEVENS–JOHNSON SYNDROME

It is possible that adhesions between the tarsal and bulbar conjunctiva can entrap conjunctival epithelium and lead to a cyst. That may have been the mechanism in this case.

Desai V, Shields CL, Shields JA. Orbital cyst in a patient with Stevens-Johnson syndrome. *Cornea* 1992;11:592–594.

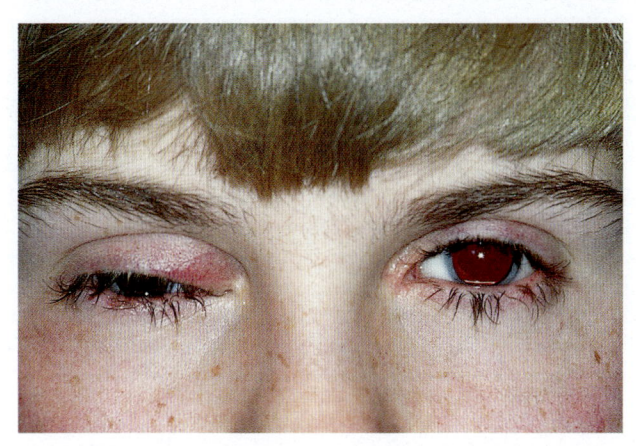

Figure 27.55. Blepharoptosis of an irritated, uncomfortable right eye in a 10-year-old girl who had Stevens–Johnson syndrome with severe ocular involvement. The cyst had recurred after simple aspiration.

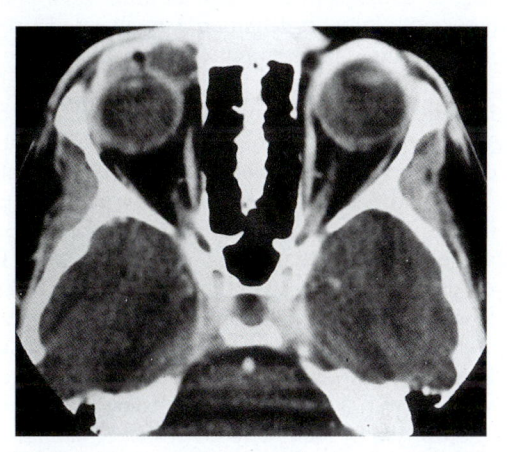

Figure 27.56. Axial computed tomography showing cystic lesion superior and nasal to the globe.

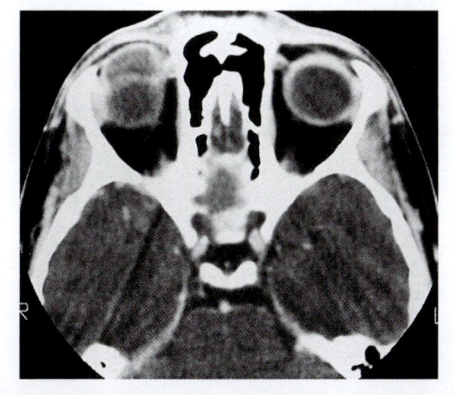

Figure 27.57. Axial computed tomography at a higher level, showing extent of the cyst.

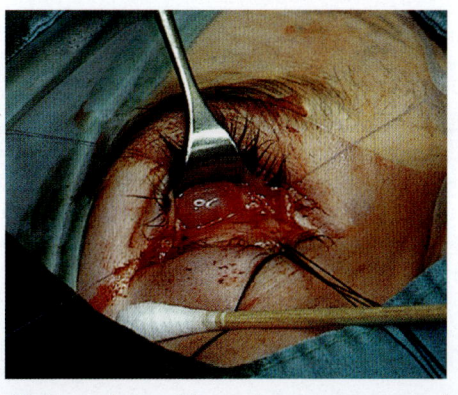

Figure 27.58. Surgical view of the cyst beneath the superior fornix. The cyst was removed and a buccal mucous membrane graft was done.

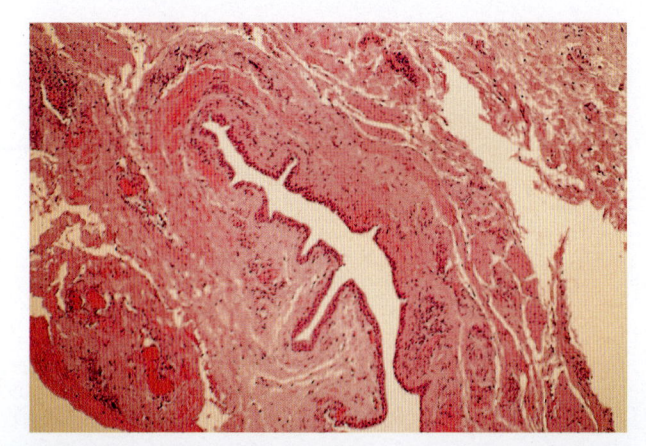

Figure 27.59. Histopathology showing nonkeratinizing epithelium surrounded by dense fibrosis secondary to chronic inflammation. (Hematoxylin–eosin ×10.)

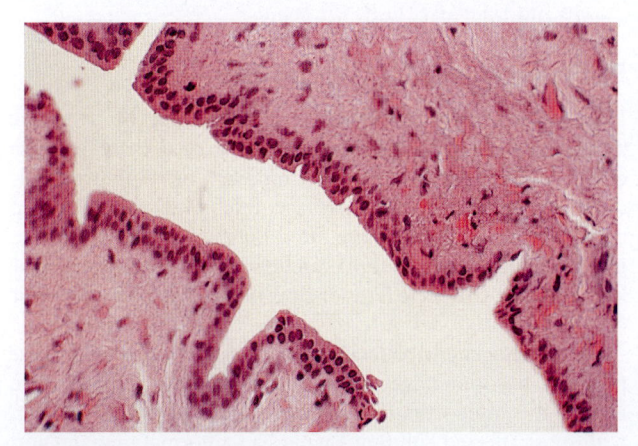

Figure 27.60. Histopathology on slightly higher power, showing nonkeratinizing epithelium. (Hematoxylin–eosin ×30.)

ORBITAL TERATOMA (TERATOMATOUS CYST)

General Considerations

Teratoma is a congenital, multicystic mass that most often occurs in the gonads but can occur in other sites, including the orbit (1–28). By strict definition, a true teratoma contains histologic structures representing all three embryonic germ layers: ectoderm, mesoderm, and endoderm. Orbital teratoma is sufficiently uncommon that individual case reports are usually cited in the literature. In a review of literature in 1980 the authors cited 51 reported cases of true orbital teratoma (20). Almost all of the reported cases were unilateral, but there are occasional reports of bilateral cases. There appears to be a 2:1 female preponderance and a slight preference for the left eye. Although teratomas in other parts of the body have been known to undergo malignant transformation, teratomas that are confined to the orbit are generally benign. Malignant transformation of pure orbital teratoma has been reported, but there is controversy as to the validity of some of those reports (18,22). Surprisingly, there were no orbital teratomas among the 1,264 consecutive orbital space–occupying lesions seen on the oncology service (1).

Clinical Features

The child with an orbital teratoma characteristically presents with severe unilateral proptosis at birth. The proptosis may increase over the first few days or weeks and compression of the globe can produce corneal exposure and visual loss. Larger lesions can produce severe disfigurement of the orbit and midface. The globe is usually pushed forward and upward by the mass and there may be marked conjunctival chemosis and eyelid swelling. The tumor can extend to involve the temporal fossa and other adjacent orbital tissues. When the lesion is smaller, the globe is often normal.

Diagnostic Approaches

The diagnosis of orbital teratoma should be considered in any child with a large mass present at birth. Computed tomography and magnetic resonance imaging reveal enlarged orbit with a cystic, multiloculated soft tissue mass.

Pathology and Pathogenesis

Histopathologically, teratoma is characterized by complex arrangement of various tissues, including clear cysts lined by either epidermis, gastrointestinal mucosal, or respiratory epithelium. Islands of hyaline cartilage, cerebral tissue, epidermal cysts, and choroid plexus are often present. In extremely rare instances, an orbital teratoma can be so well differentiated that it resembles a complete fetus or a portion of a fetus in the orbit (8).

The pathogenesis of teratoma is unclear, but it seems that primitive pluripotent germ cells in the orbital area differentiate toward the adult structures involved. The stimulus is unclear, with most affected children having had a normal prenatal and birth history.

Management

The unsightly appearance of many orbital teratomas at birth has often prompted orbital exenteration either for cosmetic reasons or because a malignant tumor was suspected. In some cases, however, a number of less advanced orbital teratomas have been removed surgically, with preservation of the eye (4,14). It may be helpful to first aspirate the fluid from a larger cyst to decrease the size of the mass and facilitate complete removal. Some cases managed in this manner have had excellent functional and cosmetic results (14). In advanced cases, modified exenteration of the orbital contents may still be necessary.

Although orbital teratoma is usually cytologically benign, local invasion of cranio-orbital teratoma can lead to death. Prompt diagnosis and careful surgical planning can also result in a favorable visual outcome. Neglected or advanced lesions can produce irreversible vision loss.

ORBITAL TERATOMA (TERATOMATOUS CYST)

Selected References

Reviews

1. Shields JA, Shields CL, Scartozzi R. Survey of 1264 patients with orbital tumors and simulating lesions: the 2002 Montgomery Lecture, part 1. *Ophthalmology* 2004;111:997–1008.
2. Shields JA, Bakewell B, Augsburger DG, et al. Space-occupying orbital masses in children. A review of 250 consecutive biopsies. *Ophthalmology* 1986;93:379–384.
3. Shields JA, Kaden IH, Eagle RC Jr, et al. Orbital dermoid cysts. Clinicopathologic correlations, classification, and management. The 1997 Josephine E. Schueler Lecture. *Ophthal Plast Reconstr Surg* 1997;13:265–276.
4. Shields JA, Shields CL. Orbital cysts of childhood—classification, clinical features, and management. The 2003 Angeline Parks Lecture. *Surv Ophthalmol* 2004;49:281–299.
5. Bonavolontà G, Strianese D, Grassi P, et al. An analysis of 2,480 space-occupying lesions of the orbit from 1976 to 2011. *Ophthal Plast Reconstr Surg* 2013;29(2):79–86.
6. Weiss AH, Greenwald MJ, Margo CE, et al. Primary and secondary orbital teratomas. *J Pediatr Ophthalmol Strabismus* 1989;26:44–49.
7. Gunalp I, Gunduz K. Cystic lesions of the orbit. *Int Ophthalmol* 1996–1997;20:273–277.

Histopathology

8. Kivela T, Tarkkanen A. Orbital germ cell tumors revisited: a clinicopathological approach to classification. *Surv Ophthalmol* 1994;38:541–554.
9. Assalian A, Allaire G, Codere F, et al. Congenital orbital teratoma: a clinicopathological case report including immunohistochemical staining. *Can J Ophthalmol* 1994;29:30–33.

Case Reports

10. Prause JU, Borgesen SE, Carstensen H, et al. Cranio-orbital teratoma. *Acta Ophthalmol Scand Suppl* 1996;219:53–56.
11. Levin ML, Leone CR Jr, Kincaid MC. Congenital orbital teratomas. *Am J Ophthalmol* 1986;102:476–481.
12. Mamalis N, Garland PE, Argyle JC, et al. Congenital orbital teratoma: a review and report of two cases. *Surv Ophthalmol* 1985;30:41–46.
13. Berlin AJ, Rich LS, Hahn JF. Congenital orbital teratoma. *Childs Brain* 1983;10:208–216.
14. Chang DF, Dallow RL, Walton DS. Congenital orbital teratoma: report of a case with visual preservation. *J Pediatr Ophthalmol Strabismus* 1980;17:88–95.
15. Ide CH, Davis WE, Black SP. Orbital teratoma. *Arch Ophthalmol* 1978;96:2093–2096.
16. Barishak YR, Mashiah M. Congenital teratoma of the orbit. *J Pediatr Ophthalmol* 1977;14:217–220.
17. Barber JC, Barber LF, Guerry D 3rd, et al. Congenital orbital teratoma. *Arch Ophthalmol* 1974;91:45–48.
18. Soares EJ, Lopes KD, Andrade JD, et al. Orbital malignant teratoma. A case report. *Orbit* 1983;2:235–242.
19. Ferry AP. Teratoma of the orbit: a report of two cases. *Surv Ophthalmol* 1965;10:434–443.
20. Chang DF, Dallow RL, Walton DS. Congenital orbital teratoma; report of a case with visual preservation. *J Pediatr Ophthalmol Strabismus* 1980;17:33–35.
21. Lee JC, Jung SM, Chao AS, et al. Congenital mixed malignant germ cell tumor involving cerebrum and orbit. *J Perinat Med* 2003;31:261–265.
22. Mahesh L, Krishnakumar S, Subramanian N, et al. Malignant teratoma of the orbit: a clinicopathological study of a case. *Orbit* 2003;22:305–309.
23. Sreenan C, Johnson R, Russell L, et al. Congenital orbital teratoma. *Am J Perinatol* 1999;16:251–255.
24. Gnanaraj L, Skibell BC, Coret-Simon J, et al. Massive congenital orbital teratoma. *Ophthal Plast Reconstr Surg* 2005;21:445–447.
25. Singh M, Singh U, Gupta A, et al. Primary orbital teratoma with tooth in an adult: a rare association with cataract and corectopia. *Orbit* 2013;32(5):327–329.
26. Chawla B, Chauhan K, Kashyap S. Mature orbital teratoma with an ectopic tooth and primary anophthalmos. *Orbit* 2013;32(1):67–69.
27. Hassan HM, Mc Andrew PT, Yagan A, et al. Mature orbital teratoma presenting as a recurrent orbital cellulitis with an ectopic tooth and sphenoid malformation-a case report. *Orbit* 2008;27(4):309–312.
28. Kivelä T, Merenmies L, Ilveskoski I, et al. Congenital intraocular teratoma. *Ophthalmology* 1993;100(5):782–791.

ORBITAL TERATOMA (TERATOMATOUS CYST) DISCOVERED IN UTERO

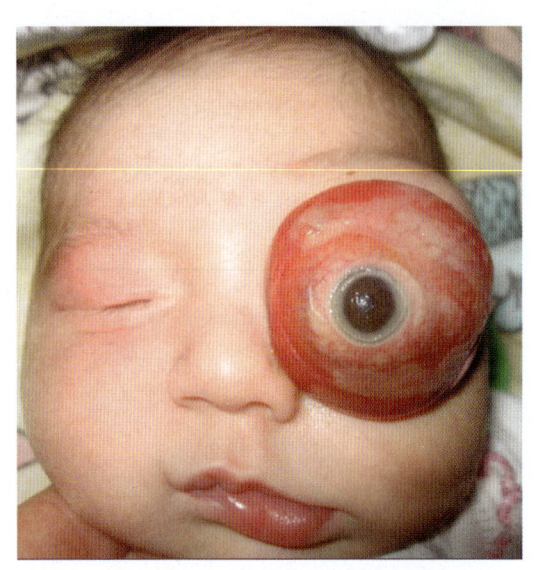

Figure 27.61. Orbital teratoma causing severe proptosis and chemosis in a newborn baby. (Courtesy of Samuray Tuncer, MD.)

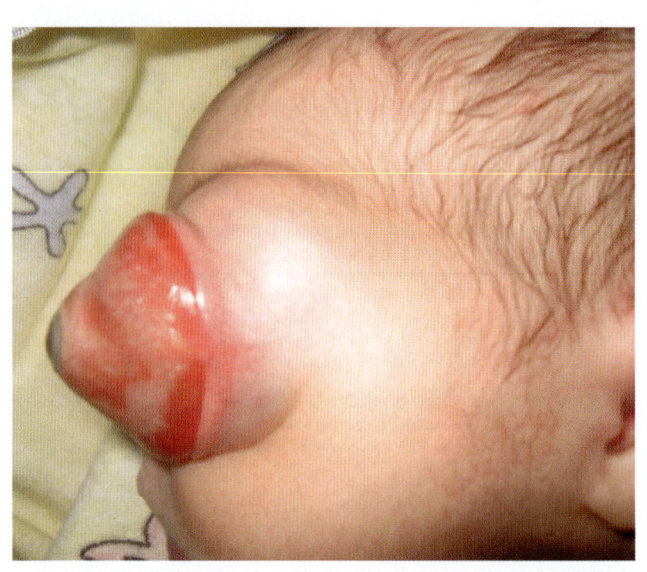

Figure 27.62. Profile view of newborn shown in Figure 27.61, demonstrating marked proptosis and orbital congestion.

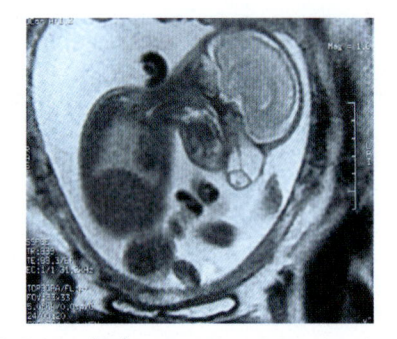

Figure 27.63. Prior to birth, magnetic resonance imaging depicted the massive proptosis while the child was in utero.

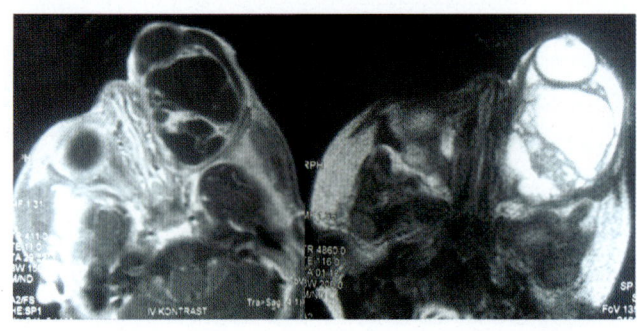

Figure 27.64. Magnetic resonance imaging following birth showing the multicystic massive tumor on T1- (*left*) and T2- (*right*) weighted images.

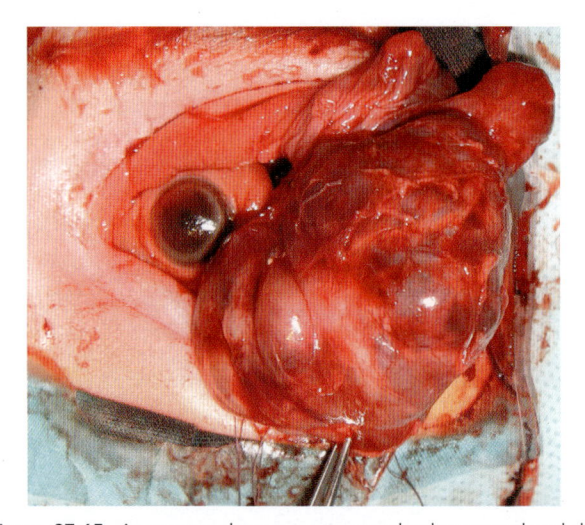

Figure 27.65. At surgery, the mass was completely resected and the globe salvaged.

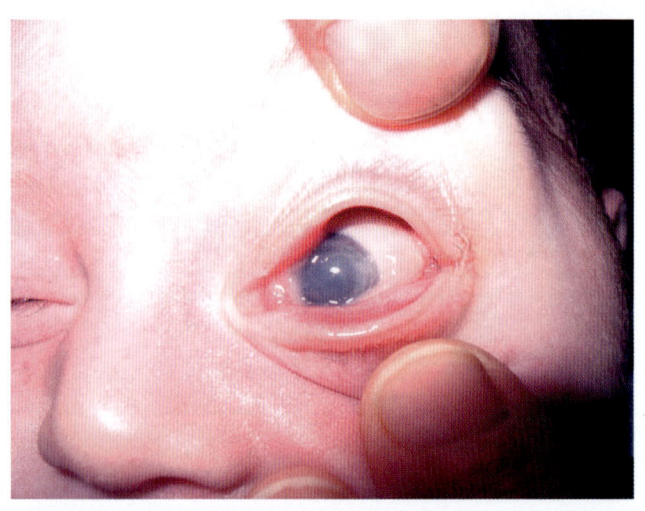

Figure 27.66. One month following surgery of patient in Figure 27.61, the globe appears intact and the eyelid swelling has reduced.

ORBITAL TERATOMA (TERATOMATOUS CYST)

Chang DF, Dallow RL, Walton DS. Congenital orbital teratoma; report of a case with visual preservation. *J Pediatr Ophthalmol Strabismus* 1980;17:33–35.

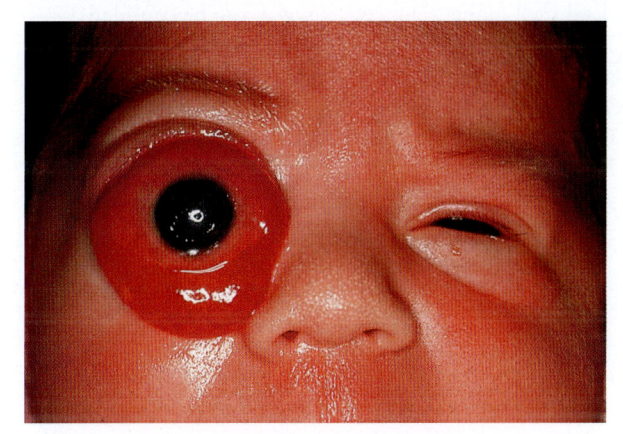

Figure 27.67. Newborn child with marked proptosis and chemosis secondary to orbital teratoma. (Courtesy of David Walton, MD.)

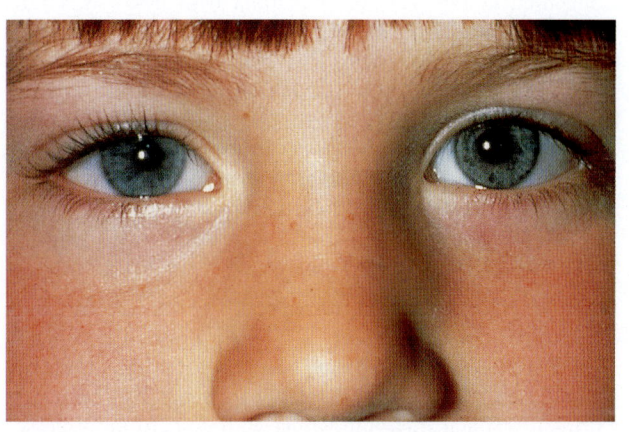

Figure 27.68. Appearance of child shown in Figure 27.67 several years later. The retrobulbar tumor was removed successfully and the eye was saved. (Courtesy of David Walton, MD.)

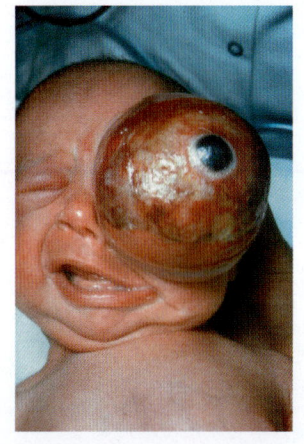

Figure 27.69. Massive orbital teratoma in a newborn. (Courtesy of A.M. Verbeck, MD.)

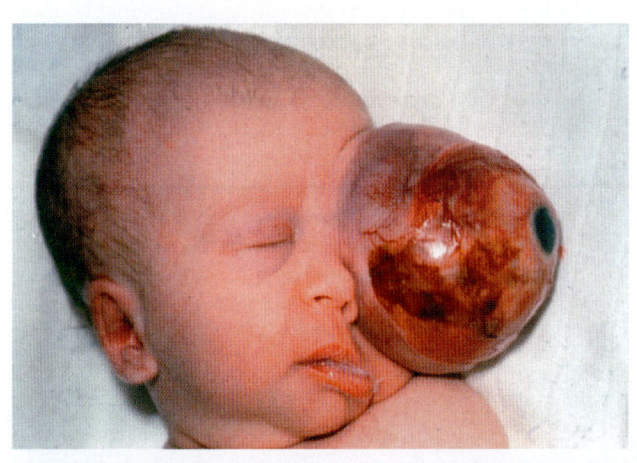

Figure 27.70. Side view of patient shown in Figure 27.69. (Courtesy of A.M. Verbeck, MD.)

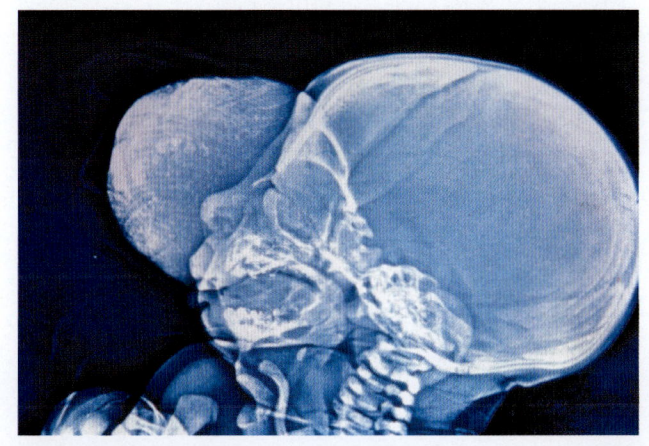

Figure 27.71. X-ray of same patient showing large mass. (Courtesy of A.M. Verbeck, MD.)

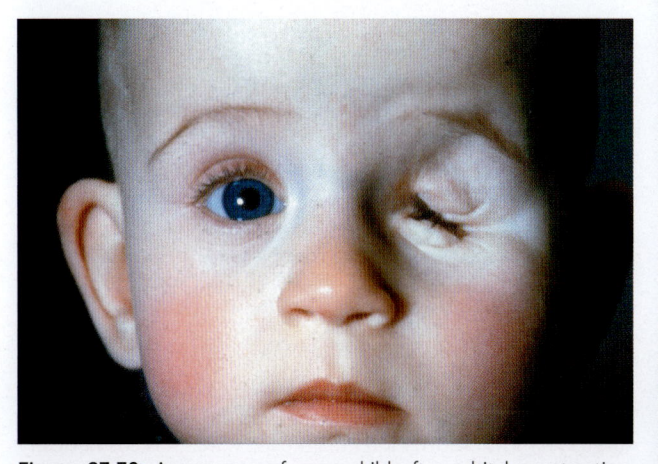

Figure 27.72. Appearance of same child after orbital exenteration. (Courtesy of A.M. Verbeck, MD.)

ORBITAL CONGENITAL CYSTIC EYE

General Considerations

Congenital cystic eye ("anophthalmia with cyst") is a rare, benign orbital lesion that results from failure of invagination of the primary optic vesicle. The cystic structure actually represents the primitive optic vesicle that failed to undergo differentiation into its adult components (1–22). There were no cases of this rare entity among the authors' series of 1,264 consecutive space-occupying lesions of the orbit (1). Using ultrasonography, the diagnosis can be established prenatally.

Clinical Features

The affected child can be systemically healthy or can have other associated defects such as cleft lip or basal encephalocele. When associated with such nonocular abnormalities, congenital cystic eye can be bilateral (15). It has also been seen with contralateral microphthalmia with cyst, to be discussed subsequently (7). Congenital cystic eye has been in association with Fraser syndrome (cryptophthalmos, abnormal genitalia, mental deficiency, renal agenesis, and abnormal ears) (20). Congenital cystic eye appears clinically as a soft, variably sized, bluish orbital mass that is evident at the time of birth. It can be located behind the upper or lower eyelid, or both.

The extraocular muscles may be attached to the cystic structure in a normal or anomalous pattern, although the lesion does not move like a normal eye. Congenital cystic eye can be differentiated from a colobomatous cyst (microphthalmos with cyst) because the latter is associated with a small but recognizable eye and it usually enlarges inferiorly, displacing the lower eyelid, rather than the upper eyelid.

Diagnostic Approaches

The diagnosis of congenital cystic eye is based mainly on the history and clinical features described. The presence of a congenital, soft, blue subcutaneous mass in an orbit without an otherwise recognizable eye should suggest the clinical diagnosis. Ultrasonography, computed tomography, and magnetic resonance imaging reveal a solitary cystic or semisolid orbital mass.

Pathology and Pathogenesis

The pathology of congenital cystic eye varies from case to case. It is usually lined by dense fibrous connective tissue resembling sclera, to which skeletal muscle and adipose tissue are attached. The inner aspect of the cyst is lined by immature retinal tissue. The lens is absent, owing to a developmental failure of the lens placode. An optic nerve–like structure, which extends posteriorly from the mass, consists of fibrous astrocytes without neurons. The pathogenesis is apparently a failure of invagination of the optic vesicle.

Management

In most instances, congenital cystic eye has been managed by surgical removal shortly after diagnosis. When it is cosmetically unsightly, surgical excision with placement of a ball implant and a prosthesis can improve the appearance. If the lesion is small and not bulging through the palpebral fissure, a cosmetic scleral shell, rather than cyst removal, can be considered.

Selected References

Reviews

1. Shields JA, Shields CL, Scartozzi R. Survey of 1264 patients with orbital tumors and simulating lesions: the 2002 Montgomery Lecture, part 1. *Ophthalmology* 2004;111: 997–1008.
2. Shields JA, Bakewell B, Augsburger DG, et al. Space-occupying orbital masses in children. A review of 250 consecutive biopsies. *Ophthalmology* 1986;93:379–384.
3. Shields JA, Kaden IH, Eagle RC Jr, et al. Orbital dermoid cysts. Clinicopathologic correlations, classification, and management. The 1997 Josephine E. Schueler Lecture. *Ophthal Plast Reconstr Surg* 1997;13:265–276.
4. Shields JA, Shields CL. Orbital cysts of childhood—classification, clinical features, and management. The 2003 Angeline Parks Lecture. *Surv Ophthalmol* 2004;49: 281–299.
5. Bonavolontà G, Strianese D, Grassi P, et al. An analysis of 2,480 space-occupying lesions of the orbit from 1976 to 2011. *Ophthal Plast Reconstr Surg* 2013;29(2): 79–86.

Management

6. Subramaniam N, Udhay P, Mahesh L. Prepucial skin graft for forniceal and socket reconstruction in complete cryptophthalmos with congenital cystic eye. *Ophthal Plast Reconstr Surg* 2008;24(3):227–229.

Histopathology

7. Waring GO III, Roth AM, Rodrigues MM. Clinicopathologic correlation of microphthalmos with cyst. *Am J Ophthalmol* 1976;82:714–721.
8. Mehta M, Pushker N, Sen S, et al. Congenital cystic eye: a clinicopathologic study. *J Pediatr Ophthalmol Strabismus* 2010;47 Online:e1–e4.
9. Chaudhry IA, Shamsi FA, Elzaridi E, et al. Congenital cystic eye with intracranial anomalies: a clinicopathologic study. *Int Ophthalmol* 2007;27(4):223–233.

Case Reports

10. Singer JR, Droste PJ, Hassan AS. Congenital cystic eye in utero: novel prenatal magnetic resonance imaging findings. *JAMA Ophthalmol* 2013;131;1092–1095.
11. Mansour AM, Li HK. Congenital cystic eye. *Ophthalmic Plast Reconstr Surg* 1996;12:104–105.
12. Gupta P, Malik KP, Goel R. Congenital cystic eye with multiple dermal appendages: a case report. *BMC Ophthalmol* 2003;3:7.
13. Robb RM, Anthony DC. Congenital cystic eye: recurrence after initial surgical removal. *Ophthalmic Genet* 2003;24:117–123.
14. Hayashi N, Repka MX, Ueno H, et al. Congenital cystic eye: report of two cases and review of the literature. *Surv Ophthalmol* 1999;44:173–179.
15. Goldberg SH, Farber MG, Bullock JD, et al. Bilateral congenital ocular cysts. *Ophthalmic Paediatr Genet* 1991;12:1231–1238.
16. Gupta VP, Chaturvedi KU, Sen DK, et al. Congenital cystic eyeball. *Indian J Ophthalmol* 1990;38:205–206.
17. Baghdassarian SA, Tabbara KF, Matta CS. Congenital cystic eye. *Am J Ophthalmol* 1973;76:269–275.
18. Helveston EM, Malone E Jr, Lashmet MH. Congenital cystic eye. *Arch Ophthalmol* 1970;84:622–624.
19. Dollfus MA, Marx P, Langlois J, et al. Congenital cystic eyeball. *Am J Ophthalmol* 1968;66:504–509.
20. Amrith S, Lee Y, Lee J, et al. Congenital orbito-palpebral cyst in a case of Fraser syndrome. *Orbit* 2003;22:279–283.
21. Guthoff R, Klein R, Lieb WE. Congenital cystic eye. *Graefes Arch Clin Exp Ophthalmol* 2004;242:268–271.
22. Raina UK, Tuli D, Arora R, et al. Congenital cystic eyeball. *Ophthalmic Surg Lasers* 2002;33:262–263.

ORBITAL CONGENITAL CYSTIC EYE DISCOVERED IN UTERO

Singer JR, Droste PJ, Hassan AS. Congenital cystic eye in utero: Novel prenatal magnetic resonance imaging findings. *JAMA Ophthalmol* 2013;131:1092–1095.

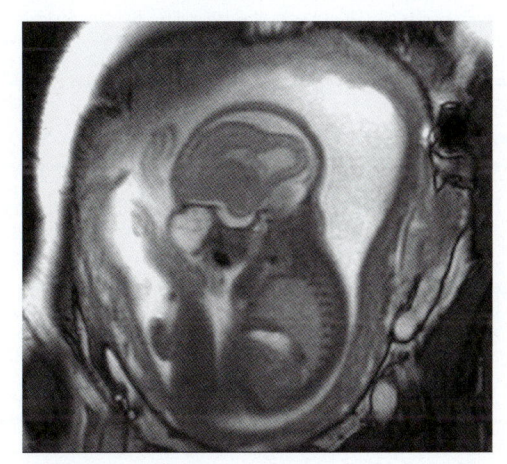

Figure 27.73. Fetus with large cystic orbital mass found on magnetic resonance imaging while in utero. (Courtesy of Singer JR, MD, Droste PJ, MD, and Hassan AS, MD.)

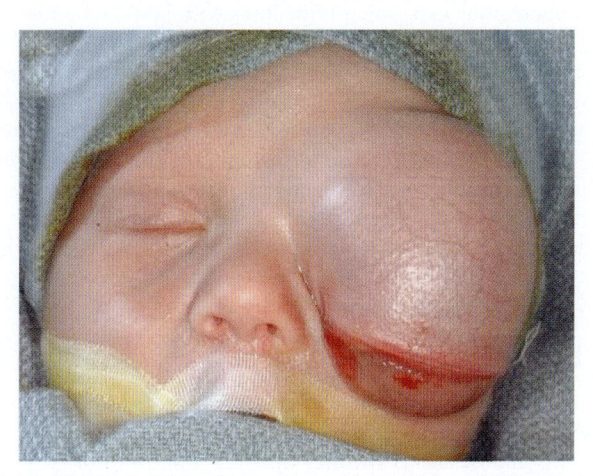

Figure 27.74. At birth, the massive orbital tumor caused extensive upper eyelid stretching and no view of the globe.

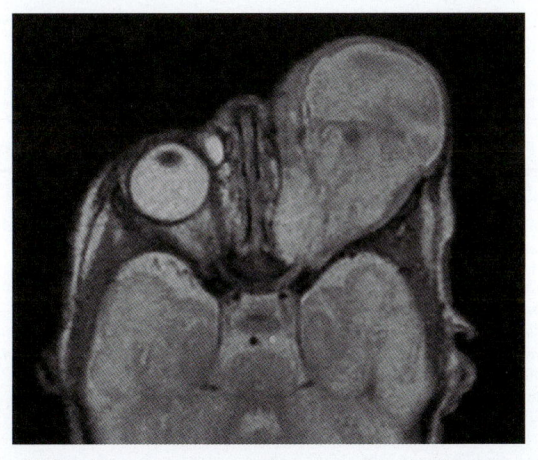

Figure 27.75. Magnetic resonance imaging of the newborn revealed a large mass and no normal eye structures.

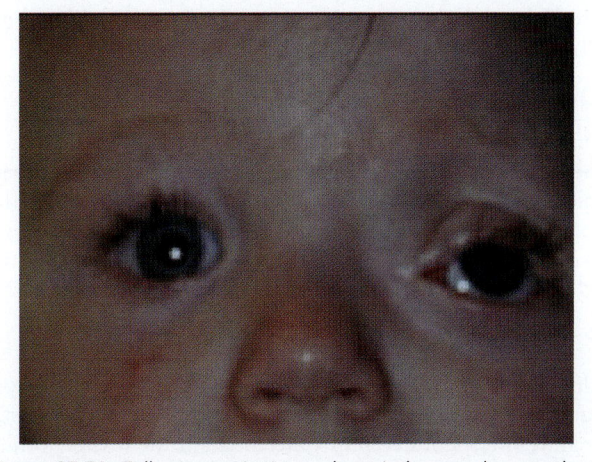

Figure 27.76. Following aspiration and surgical removal, a prosthesis was fitted with good cosmetic appearance at 1 year old.

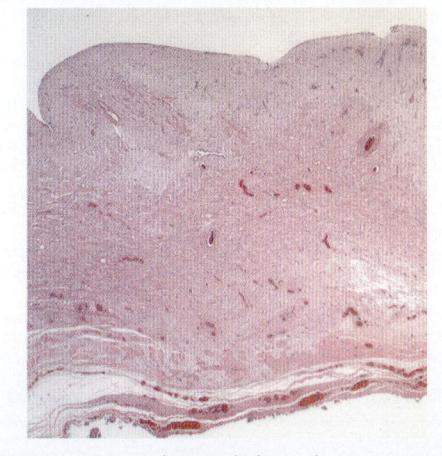

Figure 27.77. Low-power histopathology showing neuroglial tissue with connective tissue in the wall and the cystic space lined by ependymal epithelium. (Hematoxylin–eosin ×2.)

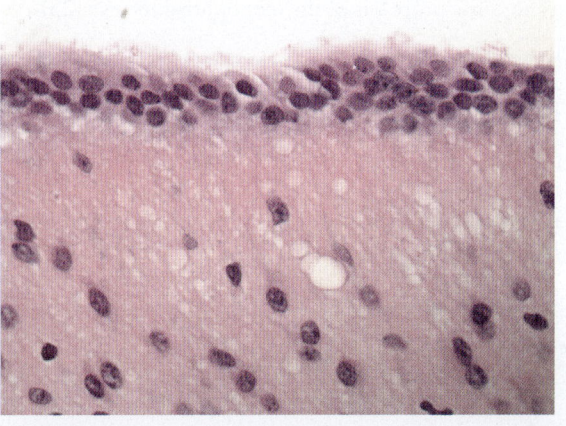

Figure 27.78. High-power histopathology of the wall demonstrating the microvilli on the surface of ependymal epithelium. (Hematoxylin–eosin ×60.)

ORBITAL COLOBOMATOUS CYST (MICROPHTHALMOS WITH CYST)

General Considerations

Colobomatous cyst (microphthalmos with cyst) is a congenital abnormality that consists of a small, malformed eye with a coloboma through which a cystic herniation of glial tissue protrudes into the orbit (1–32). It is present at birth and is usually nonheritable, although familial cases have been documented (24). There appears to be no predisposition for gender or laterality, but the condition is sometimes bilateral (18). It can occur in association with systemic anomalies, particularly when it is bilateral and familial. It has been observed in a patient with an optic nerve and chiasmal glioma, polycystic kidney, trisomy 13, and Edward syndrome (17,22).

Clinical Features

Clinical findings vary by case. The small eye and anterior segment abnormalities may prevent a view of the fundus. The coloboma almost always involves the optic disc, with or without uveal involvement. There may be a visible or palpable mass behind the lower eyelid, corresponding to the inferonasal location of the coloboma through which neuroglial tissue protrudes. The microphthalmic eye may be difficult to visualize. Occasionally, the cyst may protrude through the palpebral fissure.

Diagnostic Approaches

Diagnosis can be facilitated by ultrasonography and computed tomography. B-scan ultrasonography shows the microphthalmic eye, coloboma, and orbital cystic structure adjacent to the coloboma (6). Orbital CT and magnetic resonance imaging demonstrate a round or irregular cystic lesion adjacent to the microphthalmic eye (7).

Pathology and Pathogenesis

The orbital cyst is composed of two layers. The inner layer consists of primitive neuroretinal tissue that may show retinal architecture, photoreceptor differentiation, or rosette formation. The outer layer is continuous with the sclera and contains vascularized connective tissue, sometimes with foci of cartilage (12,13). In some instances, glial tissue may proliferate later in life and cause proptosis of the microphthalmic eye (23).

Management

If the cyst is cosmetically unacceptable, it can be managed by aspiration (9). If it recurs, repeated aspiration may sometimes bring about a permanent cure. In many cases, removal of the cyst and the microphthalmic eye with fitting of a prosthesis may be necessary. It is also possible in some cases to excise the cyst and leave the eye in place (8).

Selected References

Reviews
1. Shields JA, Shields CL, Scartozzi R. Survey of 1264 patients with orbital tumors and simulating lesions: the 2002 Montgomery Lecture, part 1. *Ophthalmology* 2004;111:997–1008.
2. Shields JA, Bakewell B, Augsburger DG, et al. Space-occupying orbital masses in children. A review of 250 consecutive biopsies. *Ophthalmology* 1986;93:379–384.
3. Shields JA, Kaden IH, Eagle RC Jr, et al. Orbital dermoid cysts. Clinicopathologic correlations, classification, and management. The 1997 Josephine E. Schueler Lecture. *Ophthal Plast Reconstr Surg* 1997;13:265–276.
4. Shields JA, Shields CL. Orbital cysts of childhood—classification, clinical features, and management. The 2003 Angeline Parks Lecture. *Surv Ophthalmol* 2004;49:281–299.
5. Awan KJ. Intraocular and extraocular colobomatous cysts in adults. *Ophthalmologica* 1986;192:76–81.

Imaging
6. Fisher YL. Microphthalmos with ocular communicating orbital cyst-ultrasonic diagnosis. *Ophthalmology* 1978;85:1208–1211.
7. Weiss A, Greenwald M, Martinez C. Microphthalmos with cyst: Clinical presentations and computed tomographic findings. *J Pediatr Ophthalmol Strabismus* 1985;22:6–12.

Management
8. Polito E, Leccisotti A. Colobomatous ocular cyst excision with globe preservation. *Ophthal Plast Reconstr Surg* 1995;11:288–292.
9. Raynor M, Hodgkins P. Microphthalmos with cyst. Preservation of the eye by repeated aspiration. *J Pediatr Ophthalmol Strabismus* 2001;38:245–246.
10. Subramaniam N, Udhay P, Mahesh L. Prepucial skin graft for forniceal and socket reconstruction in complete cryptophthalmos with congenital cystic eye. *Ophthal Plast Reconstr Surg* 2008;24(3):227–229.

Histopathology
11. Lieb W, Rochels R, Gronemeyer U. Microphthalmos with colobomatous orbital cyst: clinical, histological, immunohistological, and electronmicroscopic findings. *Br J Ophthalmol* 1990;74(1):59–62.
12. Waring GO II, Roth AM, Rodrigues MM. Clinicopathologic correlation of microphthalmos with cyst. *Am J Ophthalmol* 1976;82:714–721.
13. Meyer E, Zonis S, Gdal-On M. Microphthalmos with orbital cyst. A clinicopathological report. *J Pediatr Ophthalmol* 1977;14:38–41.
14. Mehta M, Pushker N, Sen S, et al. Congenital cystic eye: a clinicopathologic study. *J Pediatr Ophthalmol Strabismus* 2010;47 Online:e1–e4.
15. Chaudhry IA, Shamsi FA, Elzaridi E, et al. Congenital cystic eye with intracranial anomalies: a clinicopathologic study. *Int Ophthalmol* 2007;27(4):223–233.

Case Reports
16. Porges Y, Gershoni-Baruch R, Leibu R, et al. Hereditary microphthalmia with colobomatous cyst. *Am J Ophthalmol* 1992;114:30–34.
17. Magni R, Pierro L, Brancato R. Microphthalmos with colobomatous orbital cyst in trisomy 13. *Ophthalmic Paediatr Genet* 1991;12:39–42.
18. Demirci H, Singh AD, Shields JA, et al. Bilateral microphthalmos and orbital cyst. *Eye* 2003;17:273–276.
19. Arstikaitis M. A case report of bilateral microphthalmos with cysts. *Arch Ophthalmol* 1969;82:480–482.
20. Bonner J, Ide CH. Astrocytoma of the optic nerve and chiasm associated with microphthalmos and orbital cyst. *Br J Ophthalmol* 1974;58:828–831.
21. Foxman S, Cameron JD. The clinical implications of bilateral microphthalmos with cyst. *Am J Ophthalmol* 1984;97:632–638.
22. Guterman C, Abboud E, Mets MB. Microphthalmos with cyst and Edwards' syndrome. *Am J Ophthalmol* 1990;109:228–230.
23. Nowinski T, Shields JA, Augsburger JJ, et al. Exophthalmos secondary to massive intraocular gliosis in a patient with a colobomatous cyst. *Am J Ophthalmol* 1984;97:641–643.
24. Makley TA Jr, Battles M. Microphthalmos with cyst. Report of two cases in the same family. *Surv Ophthalmol* 1969;13:200–206.
25. Ehlers N. Cryptophthalmos with orbito-palpebral cyst and microphthalmos. *Acta Ophthalmol* 1966;44:84–94.
26. Pushker N, Tinwala S, Khurana S, et al. Bilateral microphthalmos with unilateral superior cyst in a child with autism and CHARGE syndrome. *Int Ophthalmol* 2013;33(2):195–198.
27. Hornby S, Gilbert C. Orbital cyst and bilateral colobomatous microphthalmos. *Br J Ophthalmol* 2008;92(11):1568–1569.
28. Decock CE, Breusegem CM, Van Aken EH, et al. High beta-trace protein concentration in the fluid of an orbital cyst associated with bilateral colobomatous microphthalmos. *Br J Ophthalmol* 2007;91(6):836.
29. Demirci H, Peksayar G, Demirci FY, et al. Bilateral microphthalmos with colobomatous orbital cyst. *J Pediatr Ophthalmol Strabismus* 2002;39(2):110–113.
30. Garcia LM, Castro E, Foster JA, et al. Colobomatous microphthalmia and orbital neuroglial cyst: case report. *Ophthalmic Genet* 2002;23(1):37–42.
31. Kurbasic M, Jones FV, Cook LN. Bilateral microphthalmos with colobomatous orbital cyst and de-novo balanced translocation t(3;5). *Ophthalmic Genet* 2000;21(4):239–242.
32. Porges Y, Gershoni-Baruch R, Leibu R, et al. Hereditary microphthalmia with colobomatous cyst. *Am J Ophthalmol* 1992;114(1):30–34.

ORBITAL COLOBOMATOUS CYST

Weiss A, Greenwald M, Martinez C. Microphthalmos with cyst: clinical presentations and computed tomographic findings. *J Pediatr Ophthalmol Strabismus* 1985;22:6–12.

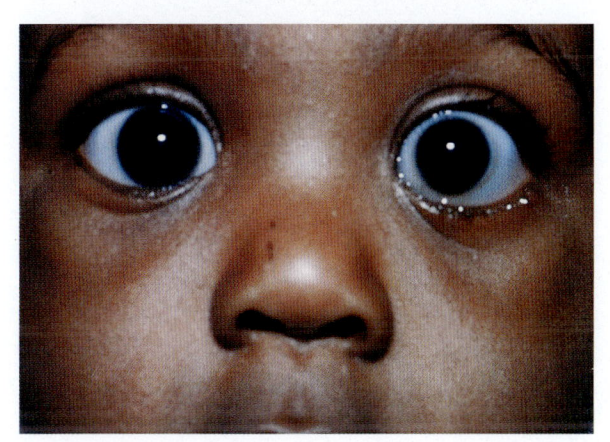

Figure 27.79. Microphthalmia of left eye in a young child. (Courtesy of William Dickerson, MD.)

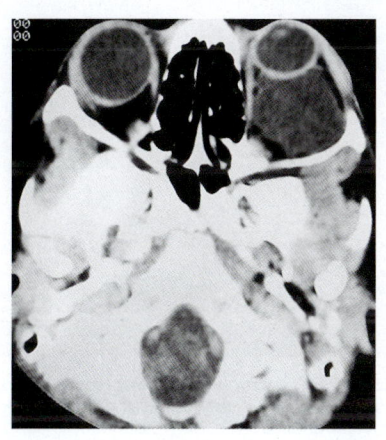

Figure 27.80. Axial computed tomography of patient shown in Figure 27.79, demonstrating a small eye with a large retrobulbar cyst. (Courtesy of William Dickerson, MD.)

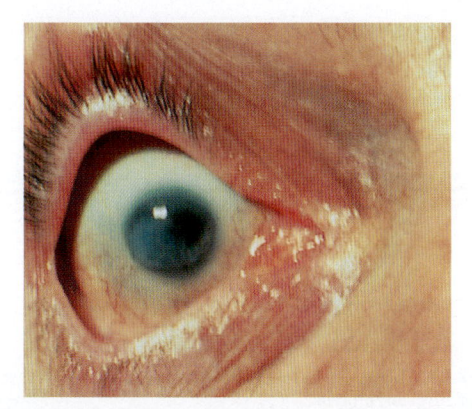

Figure 27.81. Microphthalmia of right eye in a 57-year-old man. It was present since birth. (Courtesy of Avery Weiss, MD.)

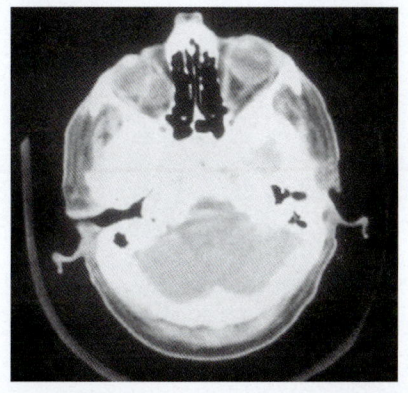

Figure 27.82. Axial computed tomography of patient shown in Figure 27.81, revealing a cystic lesion posterior to the microphthalmic eye. (Courtesy of Avery Weiss, MD.)

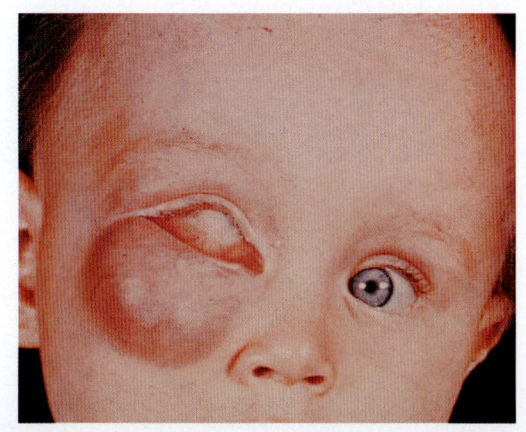

Figure 27.83. Typical appearance of colobomatous cyst with upward displacement of the microphthalmic eye and protrusion of the lower eyelid secondary to a large inferior orbital cyst. (Courtesy of Lorenz Zimmerman, MD, and Armed Forces Institute of Pathology.)

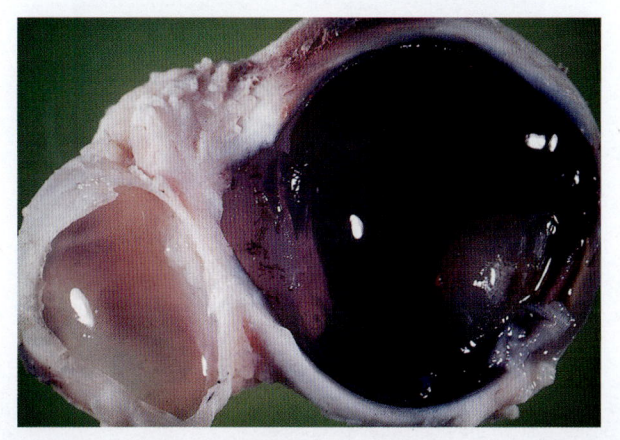

Figure 27.84. Gross appearance of microphthalmic eye (to the right) and colobomatous cyst (to the left). (Courtesy of Lorenz Zimmerman, MD, and Armed Forces Institute of Pathology.)

ORBITAL COLOBOMATOUS CYST: BILATERAL OCCURRENCE, CLINICOPATHOLOGIC CORRELATION

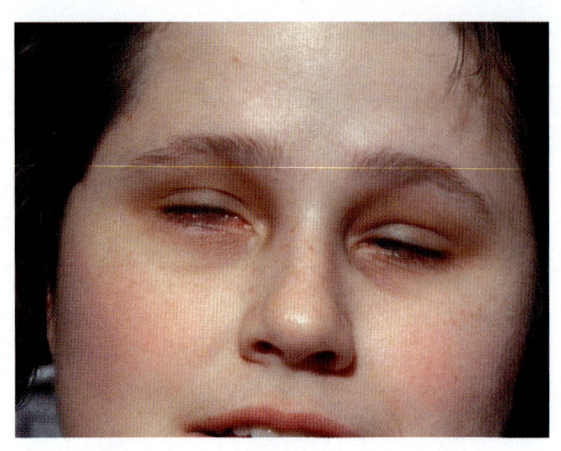

Figure 27.85. Bilateral microphthalmia in a young woman with bilateral colobomatous cysts. The condition was present since birth and the patient recently experienced recurrent bouts of pain and inflammation and requested bilateral enucleation to relieve pain and achieve a better cosmetic appearance.

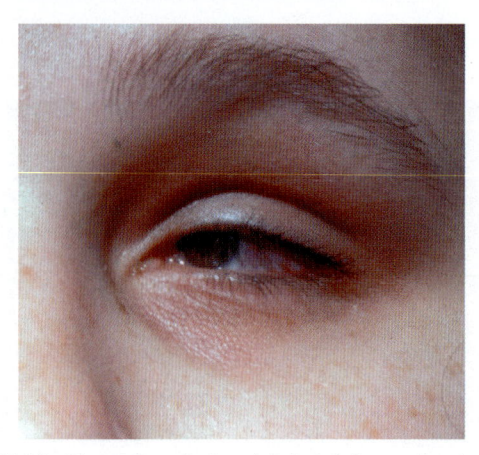

Figure 27.86. Closer view of microphthalmic left eye, showing enophthalmos and small cornea.

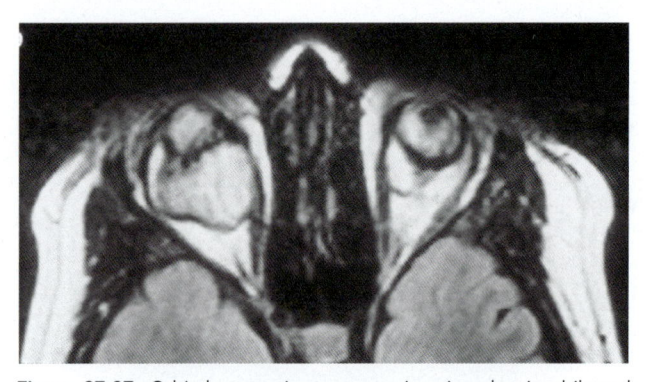

Figure 27.87. Orbital magnetic resonance imaging showing bilateral microphthalmia and orbital cysts.

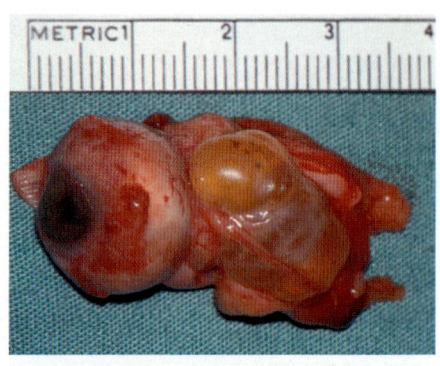

Figure 27.88. Gross appearance of right eye and orbital cyst immediately after surgical removal.

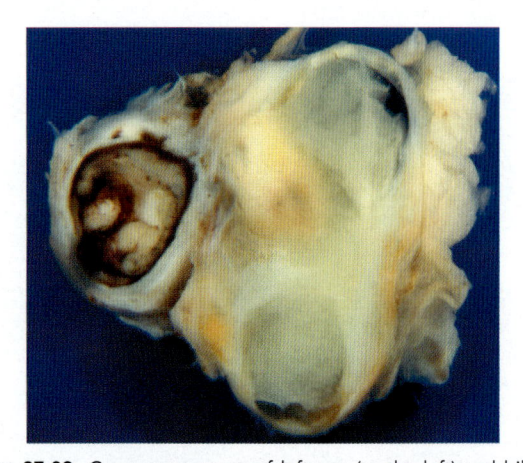

Figure 27.89. Gross appearance of left eye (to the left) and bilobed orbital cyst (to the right) after sectioning.

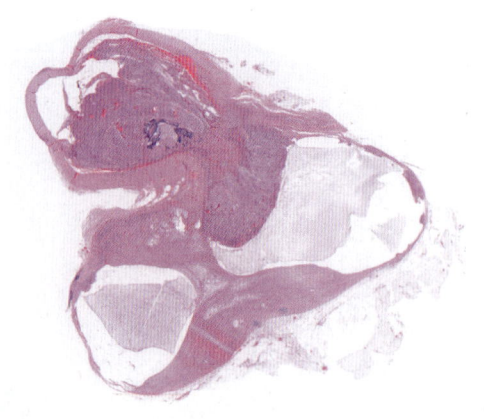

Figure 27.90. Low-magnification view of specimen shown in Figure 27.89, correlating with the gross appearance. The globe (to the left and up) is more than half filled with reactive glial tissue which contains dystrophic calcification. One component of the bilobed cyst (to the right and down) is partly filled with glial tissue that is continuous with the intraocular glial tissue via the coloboma.

ORBITAL COLOBOMATOUS CYST: CLINICAL VARIATIONS, ULTRASONOGRAPHY, AND PATHOLOGY

Colobomatous cyst can have a variety of clinical manifestations. In long-standing cases, the globe and the cystic structure can be replaced by massive gliosis.

Nowinski T, Shields JA, Augsburger JJ, et al. Exophthalmos secondary to massive intraocular gliosis in a patient with a colobomatous cyst. *Am J Ophthalmol* 1984;97:641–643.

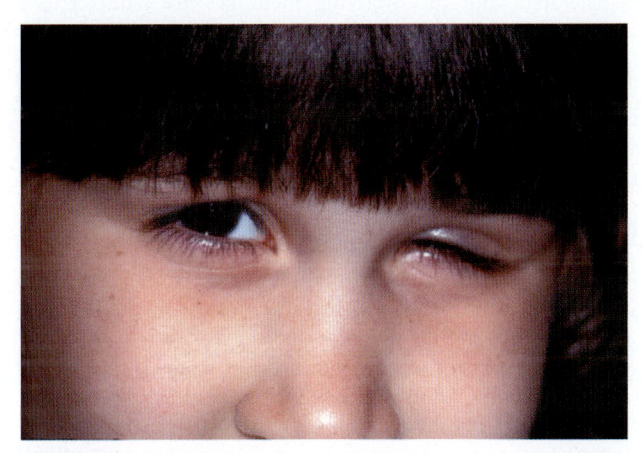

Figure 27.91. Microphthalmia associated with colobomatous cyst of left eye in a young girl.

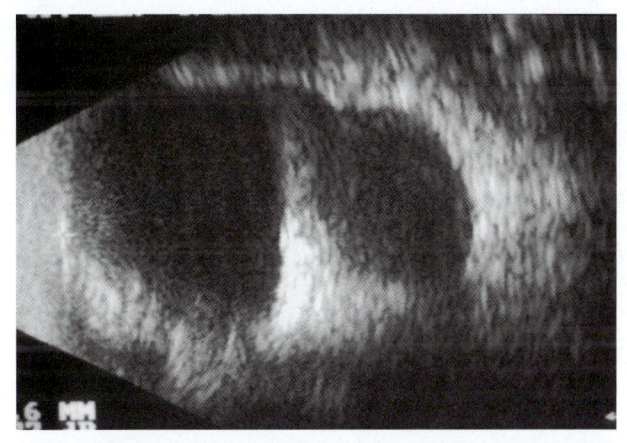

Figure 27.92. B-scan ultrasonogram in patient shown if Figure 27.91. The globe is to the left and the echographically clear cyst is to the right.

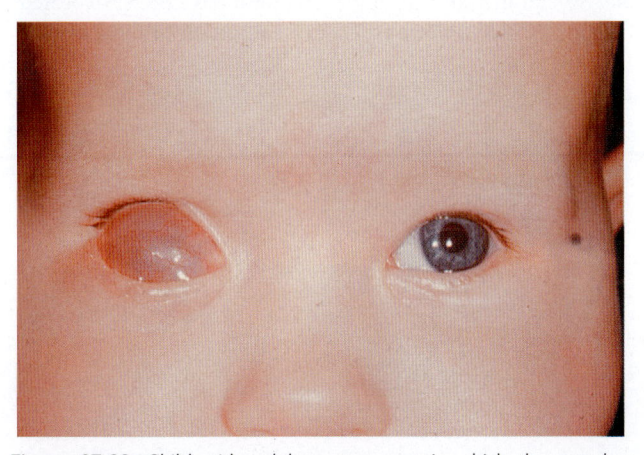

Figure 27.93. Child with colobomatous cyst in which the cyst has enlarged forward and upward to cover the small cornea. (Courtesy of Torrence Makley, MD.)

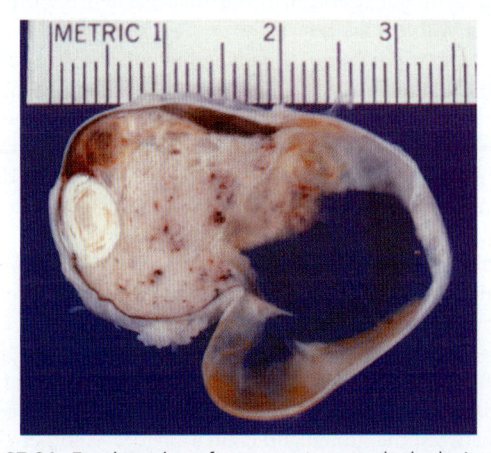

Figure 27.94. Enucleated eye from a young man who had microphthalmia with orbital cyst, who later developed proptosis of the microphthalmic eye. Note the glial tissue that has filled the globe (to the left) and part of the orbital cyst (to the right).

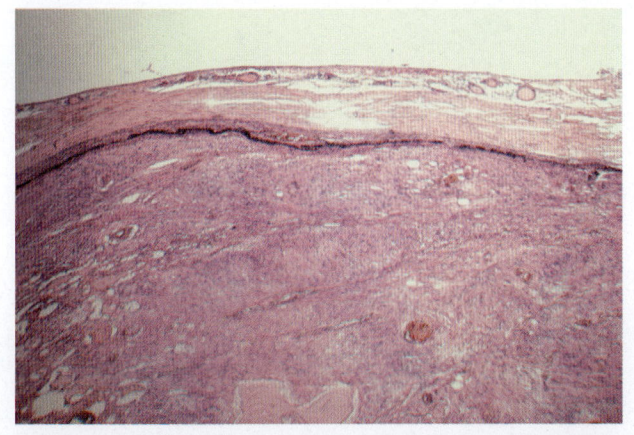

Figure 27.95. Histopathology of Figure 27.94, showing sclera (*above*) and glial tissue filling the globe (*below*). The massive gliosis developed from the retina and there is a thin remaining retinal pigment epithelium between the glial tissue and the sclera. (Hematoxylin–eosin ×20.)

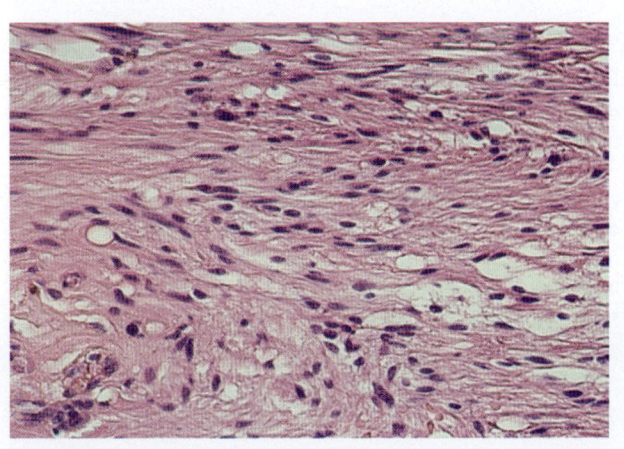

Figure 27.96. Higher magnification of massive proliferation of glial cells within the globe. (Hematoxylin–eosin ×100.)

ORBITAL CEPHALOCELE

General Considerations

Congenital or acquired defects in the orbital bones may be associated protrusion of meningeal (meningocele) or brain tissue (cephalocele) (1–20). We generally use the broad term "cephalocele" to define both types. It is possible that the incidence of orbital cephalocele is higher than implied in the ophthalmic literature, because small, minimally symptomatic lesion may not be subjected to biopsy and others may be managed by neurosurgeons or otolaryngologists and are not referred to an ophthalmology facility (4). Although there are a number of variations of cephalocele, two general types that involve the orbit are anterior (ethmoidal) cephalocele and posterior (sphenoidal) cephalocele.

Clinical Features

Anterior cephalocele most often protrudes through a defect between the frontal and lacrimal bones. It characteristically appears at or shortly after birth as a fluctuant, smooth swelling on the side of the nose near the medial canthus. In some cases, the lesion can be bilateral (11). If it is more posterior, it can produce temporal and downward displacement of the globe without a visible mass externally.

Posterior cephalocele usually protrudes into the orbit through the superior orbital fissure or the optic foramen. Consequently, it is slower in onset than the anterior type. The globe is usually displaced forward and downward; ocular motility may be limited. It can sometimes be seen in patients with neurofibromatosis, who can develop similar herniation secondary to dysplasia or absence of the sphenoid bone.

A characteristic feature of either type of cephalocele is rhythmical pulsations. In the case of anterior cephalocele, the pulsation is seen immediately beneath the skin. In the case of posterior orbital cephalocele, it occurs as pulsating proptosis. Such pulsations can also be seen with carotid-cavernous fistula, neurofibromatosis, and other lesions associated with an osseous defect between the orbital and cranial cavities. Another clinical feature is diplastic optic disc, often morning glory disc (13–15). Several ocular abnormalities can occur in association with either type of cephalocele. These are detailed elsewhere (4).

Diagnostic Approaches

It is important to make the clinical diagnosis of cephalocele rather than recognizing the diagnosis after biopsy. Careful inspection should be done to look for pulsating proptosis, which can be quite subtle. Using standard roentgenography, computed tomography, or magnetic resonance imaging, the orbital cystic or solid mass, consistent with brain, and the osseous defect can be demonstrated. In some instances, there may be no demonstrable osseous defect and such cases may be classified as ectopic brain tissue in the orbit (4,16,17).

Pathology and Pathogenesis

Histopathology reveals brain tissue with overlying thinned meninges. In long-standing lesions, the brain tissue may be degenerated, and the overlying meninges are reduced to a strand of condensed tissue containing tiny calcified spherules (psammoma bodies). Orbital cephaloceles are believed to be developmental abnormalities in which there is failure of fusion between certain orbital bones. This allows the developing brain and overlying meninges to protrude into the orbital cavity through the osseous defect.

Management

If a cephalocele is suspected clinically and the diagnosis substantiated with CT, then the decision must be made regarding whether to observe the lesion periodically or to remove it surgically. This decision should generally be made jointly by the ophthalmologist, neurosurgeon, and otolaryngologist. If the lesion is small and involves only a small portion of the posterior orbit, then it may be prudent to withhold treatment and follow the course of the lesion. Such a lesion often remains stable. Several methods of surgical removal have been advocated. Postoperative antibiotic coverage is important in these cases.

ORBITAL CEPHALOCELE

Selected References

Reviews

1. Shields JA, Shields CL, Scartozzi R. Survey of 1264 patients with orbital tumors and simulating lesions: the 2002 Montgomery Lecture, part 1. *Ophthalmology* 2004;111:997–1008.
2. Shields JA, Bakewell B, Augsburger DG, et al. Space-occupying orbital masses in children. A review of 250 consecutive biopsies. *Ophthalmology* 1986;93:379–384.
3. Shields JA, Kaden IH, Eagle RC Jr, et al. Orbital dermoid cysts. Clinicopathologic correlations, classification, and management. The 1997 Josephine E. Schueler Lecture. *Ophthal Plast Reconstr Surg* 1997;13:265–276.
4. Shields JA, Shields CL. Orbital cysts of childhood—classification, clinical features, and management. The 2003 Angeline Parks Lecture. *Surv Ophthalmol* 2004;49:281–299.
5. Islam N, Mireskandari K, Burton BJ, et al. Orbital varices, cranial defects, and encephaloceles: an unrecognized association. *Ophthalmology* 2004;111:1244–1247.
6. Rojvachiranonda N, David DJ, Moore MH, et al. Frontoethmoidal encephalomeningocele: new morphological findings and a new classification. *J Craniofac Surg* 2003;14:847–858.

Case Reports

7. Crenshaw A, Borsetti M, Nelson RJ, et al. Massive plexiform neurofibroma with associated meningo-encephalocoele and occipital bone defect presenting as a cervical mass. *Br J Plast Surg* 2003;56:514–517.
8. Kapadia SB, Janecka IP, Curtin HD, et al. Diffuse neurofibroma of the orbit associated with temporal meningocele and neurofibromatosis-1. *Otolaryngol Head Neck Surg* 1998;119:652–655.
9. Weizman Z, Tenembaum A, Perlman M, et al. Orbital meningocele presenting as periorbital cellulitis. *Childs Brain* 1981;8:207–210.
10. Rodrigues M, Shannon G. Orbital meningoencephalocele in a healthy adult. *Can J Ophthalmol* 1977;12:63–65.
11. Chohan BS, Chandra P, Parmar IP, et al. Orbital meningoencephalocele communicating with the lacrimal sac. A case report. *Clin Pediatr (Philadelphia)* 1974;13:330–332.
12. Acers TE. Encephalocele. *Arch Ophthalmol* 1965;73:84–85.
13. Itakura T, Miyamoto K, Uematsu Y, et al. Bilateral morning glory syndrome associated with sphenoid encephalocele. Case report. *J Neurosurg* 1992;77:949–951.
14. Koenig SB, Naidich TP, Lissner G. The morning glory syndrome associated with sphenoidal encephalocele. *Ophthalmology* 1981;89:1368–1373.
15. Tuft SJ, Clemett RS. Dysplastic optic discs in association with transsphenoidal encephalocele and hypopituitary dwarfism. A case report. *Aust J Ophthalmol* 1983;11:309–313.
16. Newman NJ, Miller NR, Green WR. Ectopic brain in the orbit. *Ophthalmology* 1986;93:268–272.
17. Call NB, Baylis HI. Cerebellar heterotopia in the orbit. *Arch Ophthalmol* 1980;98:717–719.
18. Caprioli J, Lesser RL. Basal encephalocele and morning glory syndrome. *Br J Ophthalmol* 1983;67:349–351.
19. Pushker N, Mehta M, Bajaj MS, et al. Nasoethmoidal cephalocele with bilateral orbital extension presenting as bilateral lower eyelid mass. *J Pediatr Ophthalmol Strabismus* 2010;47(1):64.
20. Kumar R, Verma A, Sharma K, et al. Post-traumatic pseudomeningocele of the orbit in a young child. *J Pediatr Ophthalmol Strabismus* 2003;40(2):110–112.

ORBITAL CEPHALOCELE: ANTERIOR (ETHMOIDAL) TYPE

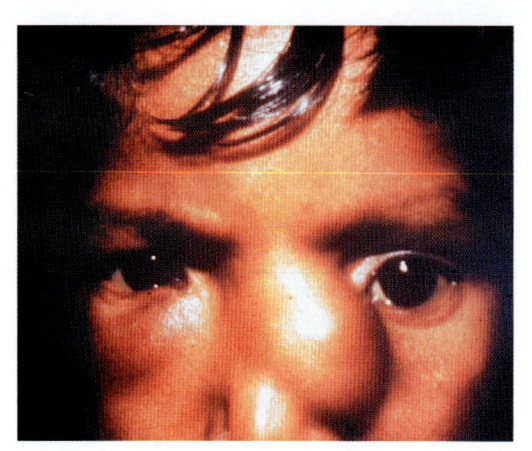

Figure 27.97. Anterior meningoencephalocele in a young child, showing the smooth subcutaneous mass in the region of the left medial canthus and nose. (Courtesy of Armed Forces Institute of Pathology, Washington, DC.)

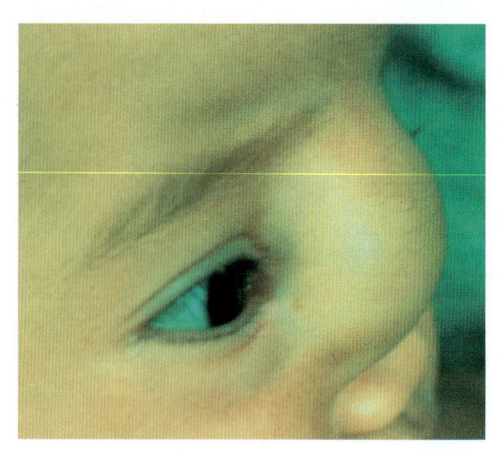

Figure 27.98. Side view of another anterior cephalocele.

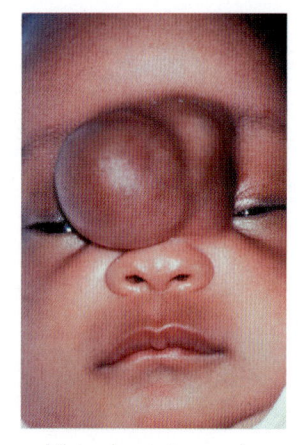

Figure 27.99. Larger bilateral anterior meningoencephalocele in an infant. (Courtesy of Darrell Wolfley, MD.)

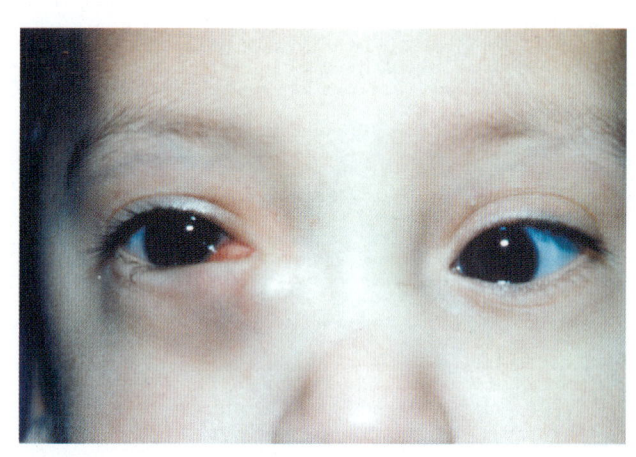

Figure 27.100. Anterior orbital (ethmoidal) cephalocele. Subcutaneous fluctuant mass below medial canthal region of right eye of a baby. (Courtesy of Polly McKinstry, MD.)

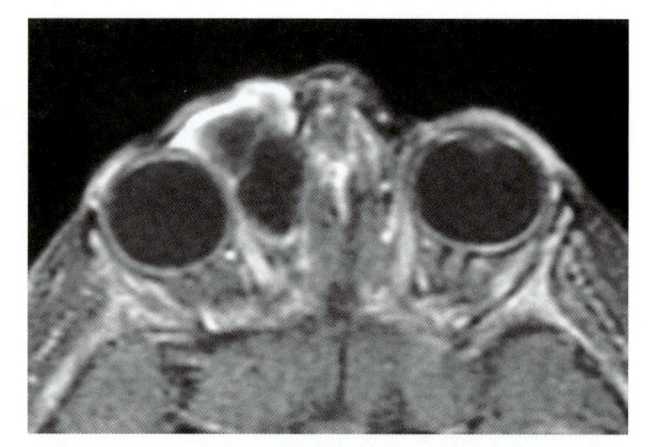

Figure 27.101. Axial magnetic resonance imaging in T1-weighted image showing mass in medial orbit and ethmoid region in patient shown in Figure 27.100. The mass is isodense, similar to vitreous and brain. (Courtesy of Polly McKinstry, MD.)

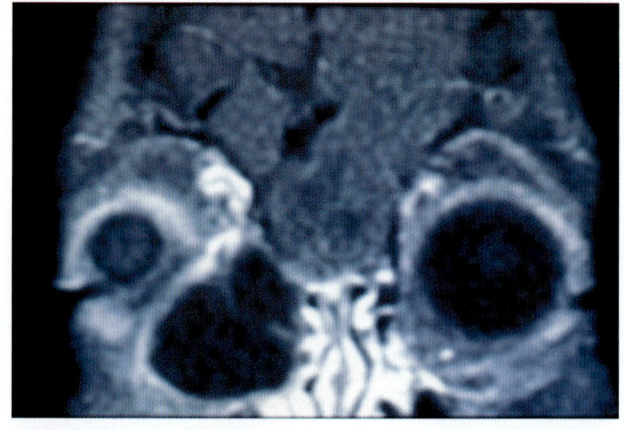

Figure 27.102. Coronal magnetic resonance imaging in T1-weighted image showing the same mass. (Courtesy of Polly McKinstry, MD.)

Chapter 27 Orbital Cystic Lesions

ORBITAL CEPHALOCELE: POSTERIOR (SPHENOIDAL) TYPE

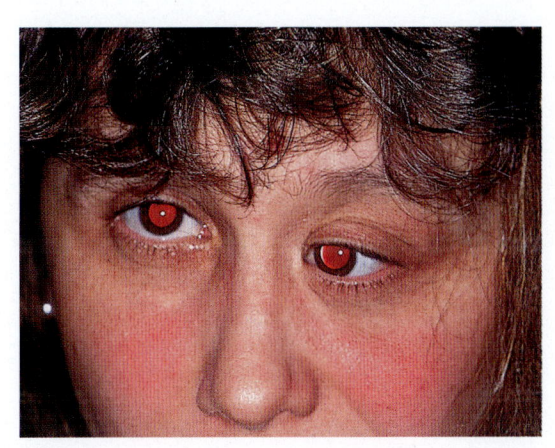

Figure 27.103. Marked proptosis and downward displacement of the left eye secondary to a posterior orbital meningoencephalocele in a 37-year-old woman who had neurofibromatosis and absence of the sphenoid wing.

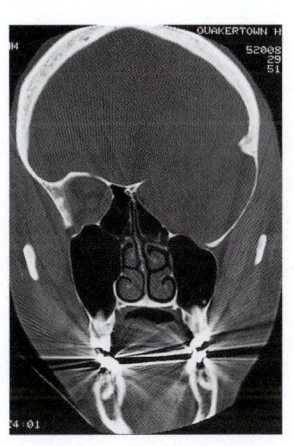

Figure 27.104. Coronal computed tomography of patient shown in Figure 27.103, demonstrating marked herniation of brain into the posterior orbit through the area of bony absence.

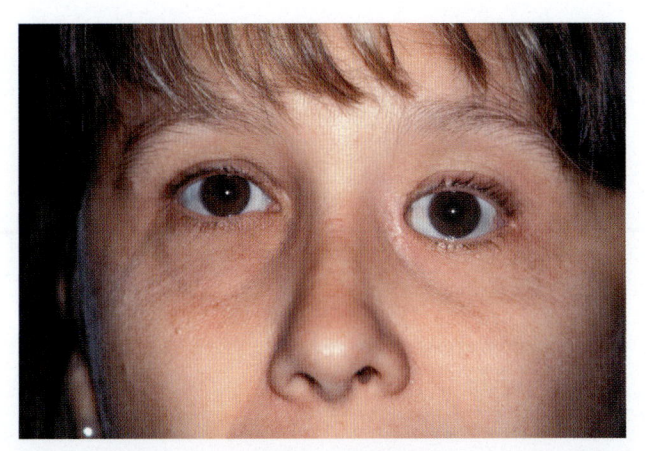

Figure 27.105. Postoperative face appearance of patient shown in Figure 27.103 after craniofacial reconstruction. There was considerable cosmetic improvement.

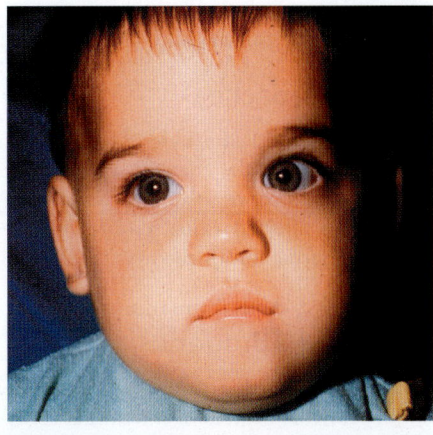

Figure 27.106. Sphenoid cephalocele. Proptosis of left eye in a young child.

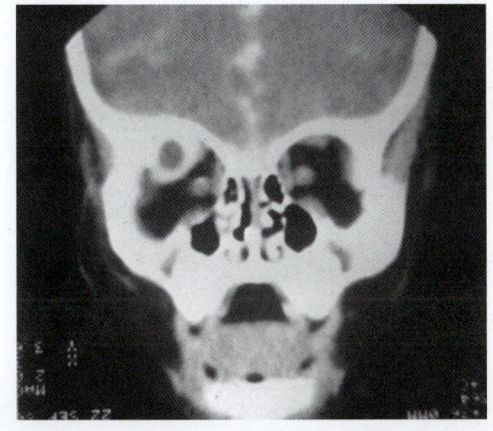

Figure 27.107. Coronal computed tomography of child shown in Figure 27.106, demonstrating superior orbital cephalocele. This was a surprise and unrelated finding in a child with unilateral retinoblastoma in the fellow eye.

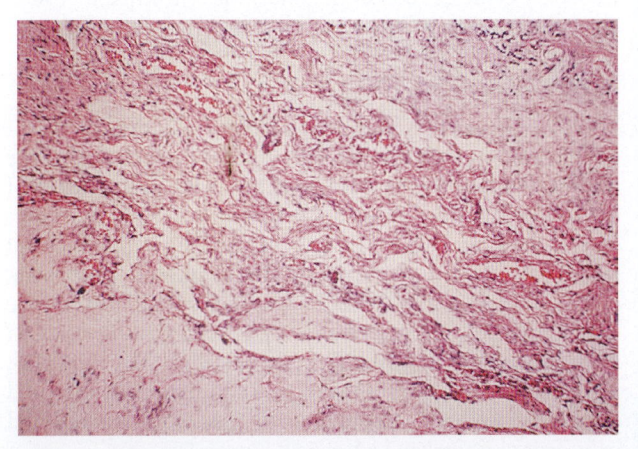

Figure 27.108. Histopathology of cephalocele showing mature brain tissue. (Hematoxylin–eosin ×50.)

ORBITAL MUCOCELE

General Considerations

Orbital mucocele is a cystic lesion containing mucus that usually arises from a chronically inflamed paranasal sinus that secondarily invades the orbit (1–18). If a mucocele becomes secondarily infected and contains pus, it is called a "mucopyocele." Mucocele typically occurs in adults with chronic sinusitis. When it develops in childhood, it is more commonly associated with cystic fibrosis and a child with mucocele should be evaluated for that disease (18). In the authors' series of 1,264 consecutive space occupying orbital lesions, the 11 mucoceles accounted for 17% of the 70 cystic lesions and for 1% of all lesions (1).

Clinical Features

Mucocele occurs most often in the frontal or ethmoid sinuses. A frontoethmoidal mucocele tends to produce slowly progressive proptosis with downward and temporal displacement of the globe. A nontender, slightly fluctuant mass may be visible and palpable beneath the orbital rim superonasally. Most patients experience some pain, usually due to chronic sinusitis.

Diagnostic Approaches

In addition to the clinical features described, the diagnosis of mucocele can be made by the changes on computed tomography or magnetic resonance imaging, which demonstrates opacification of the affected sinus, erosion of the adjacent orbital bones, and herniation of the cyst through the osseous defect into the orbit (7).

Pathology and Pathogenesis

Pathologically, mucocele is lined by pseudostratified columnar epithelium. Variable degrees of inflammation are present. Mucus or pus occupies the lumen of the lesion. Regarding pathogenesis, it is possible that chronic inflammation of the sinus leads to gradual obstruction of the outlet of the sinus and secondary cystic dilation of the sinus, with subsequent erosion through the orbital bones.

Management

The management of mucocele or mucopyocele is usually surgical and often requires marsupialization or exenteration of the involved sinuses (8–18). Management begins with imaging of the mucocele using computed tomography or magnetic resonance imaging. Surgical marsupialization through endonasal endoscopic sinus surgery is a conservative and minimally invasive method to restore sinus drainage without obliterating the sinus architecture (13). Past techniques such as obliteration of the sinus cavity with dermis fat graft is generally not employed. Appropriate antibiotics should be administered before and after surgery. The visual prognosis is good after removal and treatment of frontal and ethmoidal mucoceles.

ORBITAL MUCOCELE

Selected References

Reviews

1. Shields JA, Shields CL, Scartozzi R. Survey of 1264 patients with orbital tumors and simulating lesions: the 2002 Montgomery Lecture, part 1. *Ophthalmology* 2004;111: 997–1008.
2. Shields JA, Bakewell B, Augsburger DG, et al. Space-occupying orbital masses in children. A review of 250 consecutive biopsies. *Ophthalmology* 1986;93:379–384.
3. Moriyama H, Nakajima T, Honda Y. Studies on mucocoeles of the ethmoid and sphenoid sinuses: analysis of 47 cases. *J Laryngol Otol* 1992;106:23–27.
4. Ormerod LD, Weber AL, Rauch SD, et al. Ophthalmic manifestations of maxillary sinus mucoceles. *Ophthalmology* 1987;94:1013–1019.
5. Bier H, Ganzer U. Involvement of the orbit in diseases of the paranasal sinuses. *Neurosurg Rev* 1990;13:109–112.
6. Perugini S, Pasquini U, Menichelli F, et al. Mucoceles in the paranasal sinuses involving the orbit: CT signs in 43 cases. *Neuroradiology* 1982;23:133–139.

Imaging

7. Vashist S, Goulatia RK, Dayal Y, et al. Radiological evaluation of mucocoele of the paranasal sinuses. *Br J Radiol* 1985;58:959–963.

Management

8. Molteni G, Spinelli R, Panigatti S, et al. Voluminous frontoethmoidal mucocele with epidural involvement. Surgical treatment by coronal approach. *Acta Otorhinolaryngol Ital* 2003;23:185–190.
9. Lai PC, Liao SL, Jou JR, et al. Transcaruncular approach for the management of frontoethmoid mucoceles. *Br J Ophthalmol* 2003;87:699–703.
10. Conboy PJ, Jones NS. The place of endoscopic sinus surgery in the treatment of paranasal sinus mucocoeles. *Clin Otolaryngol* 2003;28:207–210.
11. Weitzel EK, Hollier LH, Calzada G, et al. Single stage management of complex fronto-orbital mucoceles. *J Craniofac Surg* 2002;13:739–745.
12. Shah A, Meyer DR, Parnes S. Management of frontoethmoidal mucoceles with orbital extension: is primary orbital reconstruction necessary? *Ophthal Plast Reconstr Surg* 2007;23(4):267–271.
13. Serrano E, Klossek JM, Percodani J, et al. Surgical management of paranasal sinus mucoceles: a long-term study of 60 cases. *Otolaryngol Head Neck Surg* 2004;131: 133–140.

Case Reports

14. Garber PF, Abramson AL, Stallman PT, et al. Globe ptosis secondary to maxillary sinus mucocele. *Ophthal Plast Reconstr Surg* 1995;11:254–260.
15. Sharma GD, Doershuk CF, Stern RC. Erosion of the wall of the frontal sinus caused by mucopyocele in cystic fibrosis. *J Pediatr* 1994;124:745–747.
16. Hasegawa M, Kuroishikawa Y. Protrusion of postoperative maxillary sinus mucocele into the orbit: case reports. *Ear Nose Throat J* 1993;72:752–754.
17. Curtin HD, Rabinov JD. Extension to the orbit from paraorbital disease. The sinuses. *Radiol Clin North Am* 1998;36:1201–1213.
18. Levine MR, Kim Y, Witt W. Frontal sinus mucopyocele in cystic fibrosis. *Ophthalmic Plast Reconstr Surg* 1988;4:221–225.

502   Part 3 Tumors of the Orbit

ORBITAL MUCOCELE

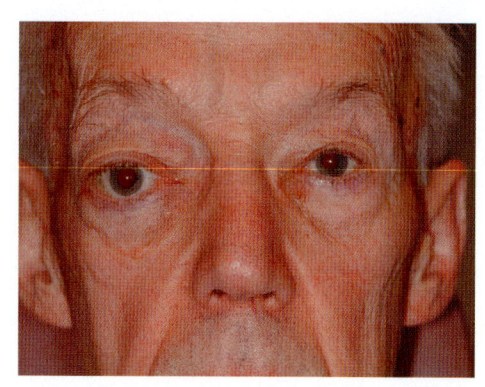

Figure 27.109. Fluctuant superonasal mass above the right eye in an elderly man. Note the typical downward and lateral displacement of the globe.

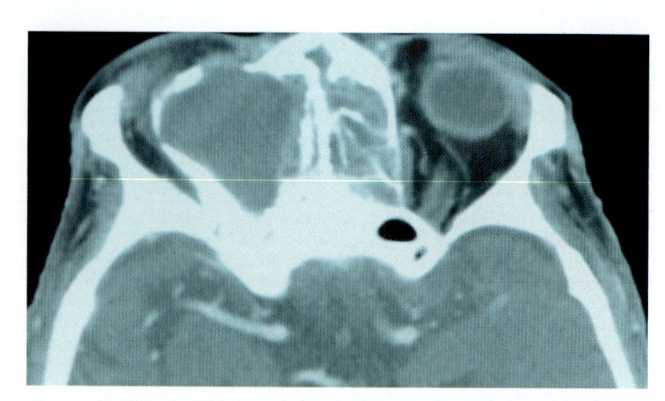

Figure 27.110. Axial computed tomography of patient shown in Figure 27.109. Note the cloudy ethmoid sinuses and displacement of ethmoid bone far into the orbit by a large opaque cystic mass.

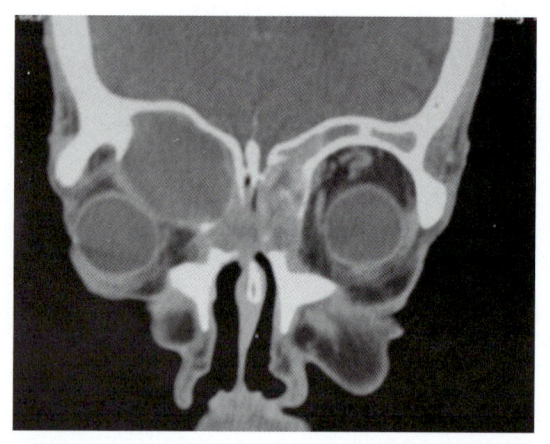

Figure 27.111. Coronal computed tomography of same patient shown in Figure 27.109, disclosing mucocele arising from frontal and ethmoid sinuses and replacing the tissue in the superonasal aspect of the orbit.

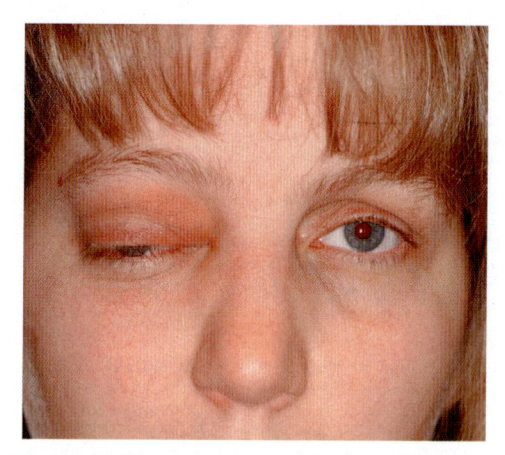

Figure 27.112. Middle-aged woman with blepharoptosis, proptosis, and downward displacement of right eye.

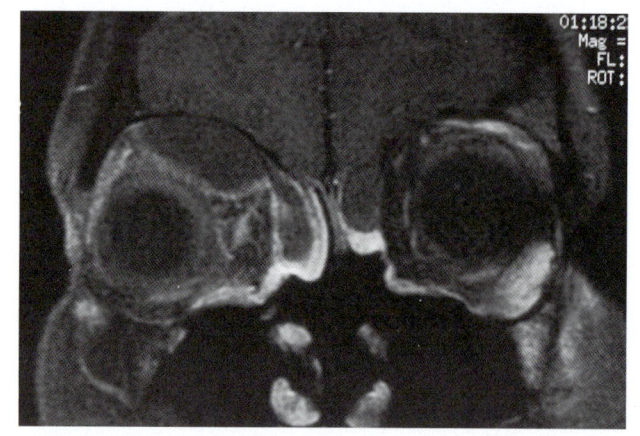

Figure 27.113. Magnetic resonance imaging in T1-weighted image with fat suppression of patient shown in Figure 27.112. Note the superior hypointense orbital mucocele arising from frontal and ethmoid sinuses.

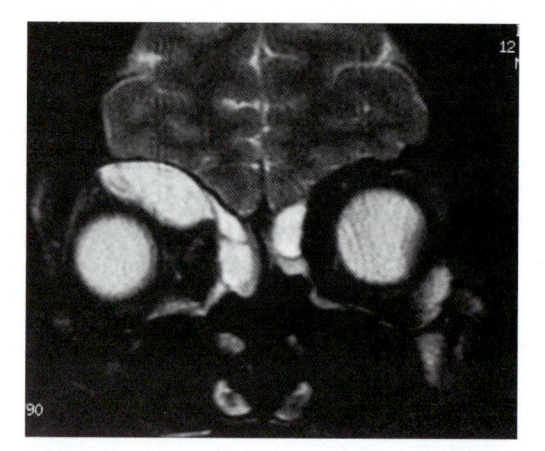

Figure 27.114. Magnetic resonance imaging in T2-weighted image of patient shown in Figure 27.112. Note that the contents of the cyst are isointense to vitreous.

Chapter 27 Orbital Cystic Lesions

ORBITAL MUCOCELE: CLINICAL, IMAGING, AND HISTOPATHOLOGIC CORRELATIONS

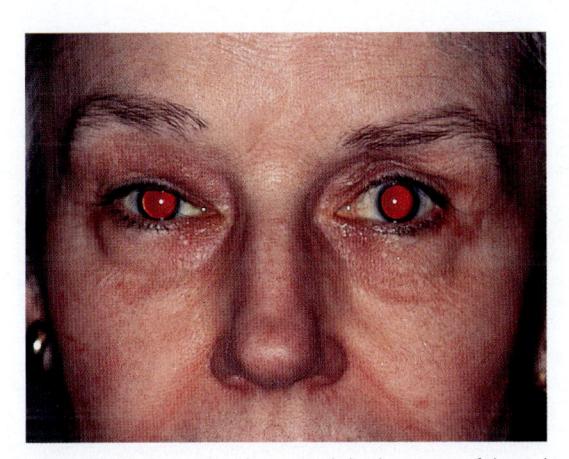

Figure 27.115. Downward and temporal displacement of the right eye in 66-year-old woman.

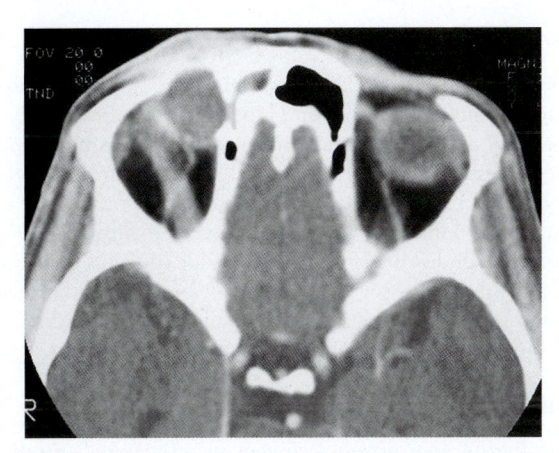

Figure 27.116. Axial computed tomography of patient shown in Figure 27.115. Note the cloudy sinus and the cystic structure in the superonasal portion of the orbit.

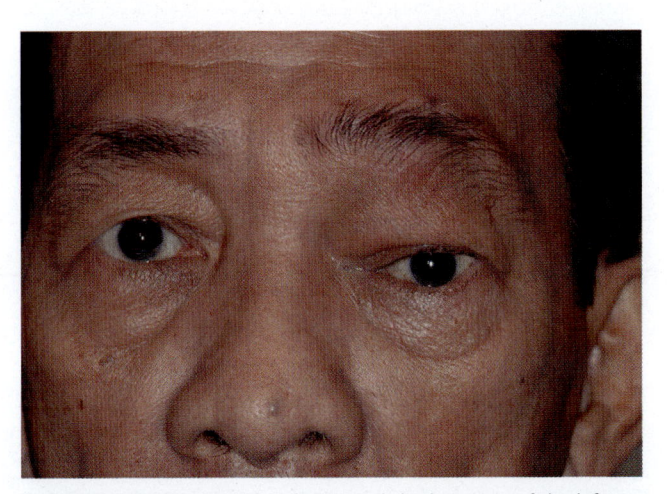

Figure 27.117. Downward and temporal displacement of the left eye in 66-year-old man.

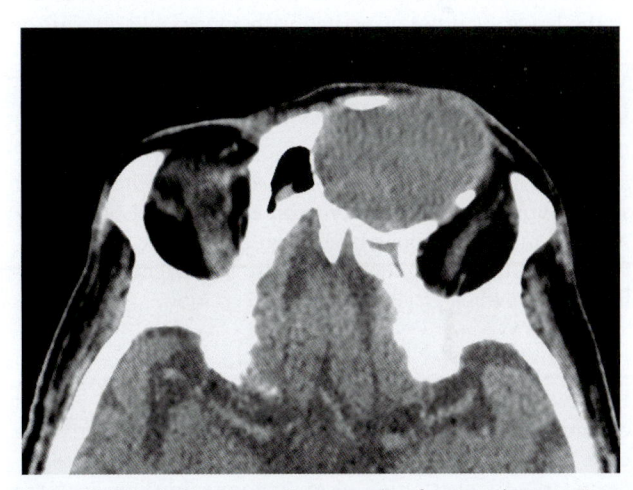

Figure 27.118. Axial computed tomography of patient shown in Figure 27.117, showing large ethmoid mucocele eroding the orbital wall and entering the superonasal portion of the orbit.

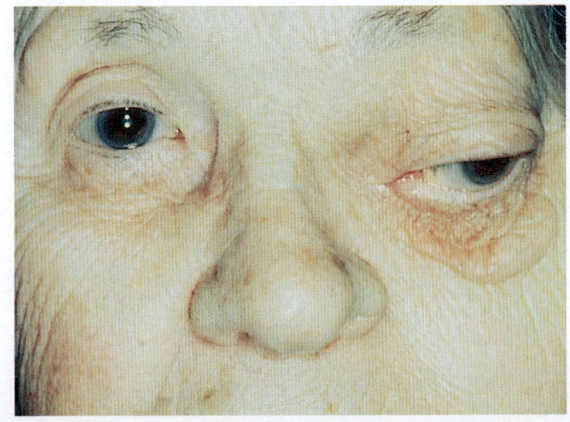

Figure 27.119. Downward and temporal displacement of the left eye in an 84-year-old woman with a long history of sinusitis and proptosis. (Courtesy of John Bullock, MD.)

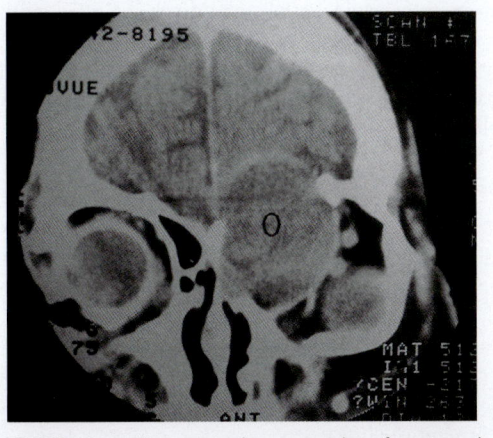

Figure 27.120. Coronal computed tomography of patient shown in Figure 27.119, showing a 4-cm cystic mass with bony destruction and marked inferotemporal displacement of the globe. (Courtesy of John Bullock, MD.)

ORBITAL RESPIRATORY EPITHELIAL CYST

General Considerations

Orbital mucoceles that develop secondary to sinusitis are lined by sinus respiratory epithelium. However, there are other types of orbital cysts that are unassociated with sinusitis but are also lined by respiratory epithelium (1–10). They can be congenital or acquired. The congenital choristomatous respiratory cyst occurs as a nonhereditary developmental malformation. An acquired respiratory cyst can be idiopathic (perhaps congenital and previously unrecognized) or it can occur after trauma. It differs from a mucocele in that the affected patient does not have sinusitis and may not display severe inflammatory signs.

Clinical Features

A respiratory cyst, whether congenital or acquired, produces symptoms similar to other cysts, with unilateral proptosis and occasional pain. The degree of proptosis and direction of globe displacement depends on the size and orbital location of the lesion. It is not associated with appreciable sinusitis or mucocele.

Diagnostic Approaches

With computed tomography or magnetic resonance imaging, an orbital respiratory cyst may be similar to other cysts. It shows a round or ovoid lesion with enhancement of the cyst wall and minimal or no enhancement of the lumen. A respiratory cyst is rarely diagnosed clinically. The diagnosis is established histopathologically after surgical excision.

Pathology and Pathogenesis

Respiratory cyst is lined by thin pseudostratified ciliated columnar epithelium with goblet cells and its lumen contains mucus. It is believed in most cases to be a choristoma, secondary to sequestration of respiratory epithelium into the orbit during intrauterine development of the paranasal sinuses (5). There is usually no history of trauma or sinusitis and the lesion is located in the temporal orbit, findings that suggest a choristomatous origin, rather than displaced nasal epithelium. In the case of secondary respiratory cysts, however, there is a history of trauma or sinus surgery. In such instances, the cyst may have developed from orbital implantation of nasal sinus epithelium.

Management

The best management of a symptomatic orbital respiratory cyst is complete excision. Aspiration of the cyst can be done, but that leaves epithelial cells that can lead to recurrence. As mentioned, the specific diagnosis is rarely made clinically but is made at the time of histopathologic evaluation following excisional or incisional biopsy. Because the diagnosis is not usually made clinically, most symptomatic lesions are excised, which is the treatment of choice.

Selected References

Reviews

1. Shields JA, Shields CL, Scartozzi R. Survey of 1264 patients with orbital tumors and simulating lesions: the 2002 Montgomery Lecture, part 1. *Ophthalmology* 2004;111:997–1008.
2. Shields JA, Bakewell B, Augsburger DG, et al. Space-occupying orbital masses in children. A review of 250 consecutive biopsies. *Ophthalmology* 1986;93:379–384.
3. Shields JA, Kaden IH, Eagle RC Jr, et al. Orbital dermoid cysts. Clinicopathologic correlations, classification, and management. The 1997 Josephine E. Schueler Lecture. *Ophthal Plast Reconstr Surg* 1997;13:265–276.
4. Shields JA, Shields CL. Orbital cysts of childhood—classification, clinical features, and management. The 2003 Angeline Parks Lecture. *Surv Ophthalmol* 2004;49:281–299.

Case Reports

5. Newton C, Dutton JJ, Klintworth GK. A respiratory epithelial choristomatous cyst of the orbit. *Ophthalmology* 1985;9:1754–1757.
6. James RC, Lines R, Wright JE. Respiratory epithelium lined cysts presenting in the orbit without associated mucocele formation. *Br J Ophthalmol* 1986;70:387–390.
7. Mee JJ, McNab AA, McKelvie P. Respiratory epithelial orbital cysts. *Clin Exp Ophthalmol* 2002;30:356–360.
8. Morris WR, Fleming JC. Respiratory choristomatous cysts in the temporal orbit. *Ophthal Plast Reconstr Surg* 2001;17:462–464.
9. Neves RB, Yeatts RP, Martin TJ. Pneumo-orbital cyst after orbital fracture repair. *Am J Ophthalmol* 1998;125:879–880.
10. Eggert JE, Harris GJ, Caya JG. Respiratory epithelial cyst of the orbit. *Ophthal Plast Reconstr Surg* 1988;4:101–104.

ORBITAL RESPIRATORY EPITHELIAL CYST

Newton C, Dutton JJ, Klintworth GK. A respiratory epithelial choristomatous cyst of the orbit. *Ophthalmology* 1985;9:1754–1757.

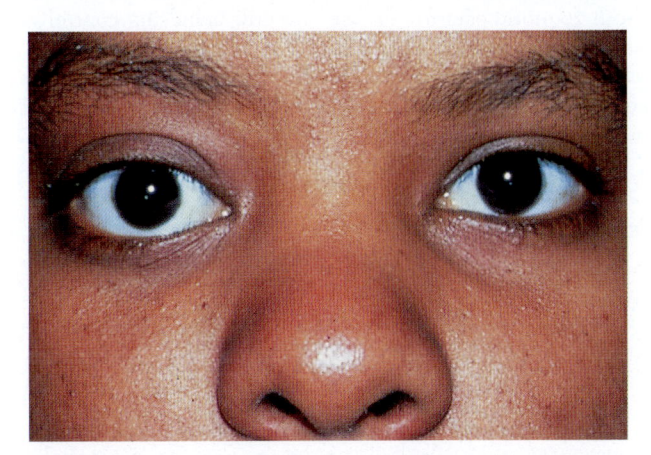

Figure 27.121. Proptosis of the right eye in a 23-year-old woman. It was noted at age 4 years, had been slowly progressive, and had produced intermittent episodes of pain. (Courtesy of Jonathan Dutton, MD.)

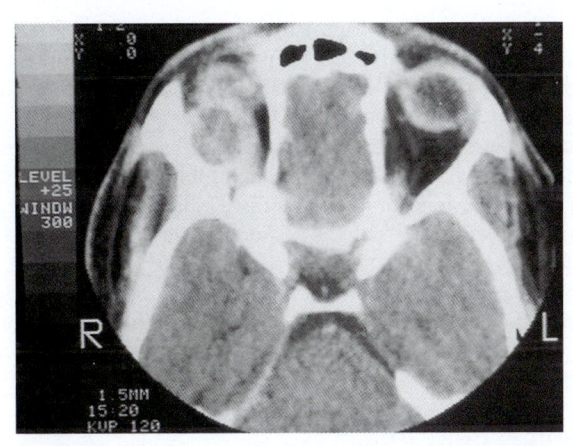

Figure 27.122. Axial computed tomography of patient shown in Figure 27.121, revealing a cystic lesion producing anterior and downward displacement of the right eye. (Courtesy of Jonathan Dutton, MD.)

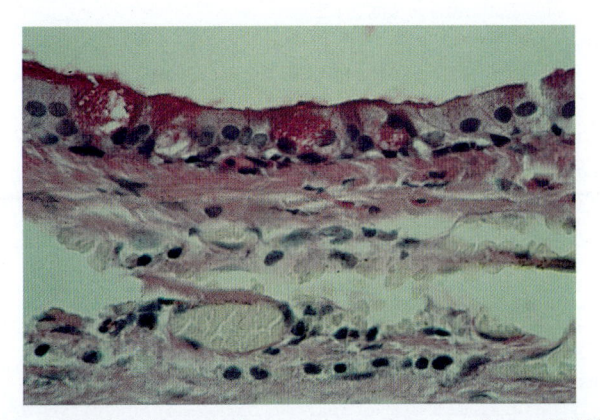

Figure 27.123. Histopathology of lesion shown in Figure 27.121, demonstrating the respiratory epithelium with goblet cells. (Periodic acid-schiff ×200.)

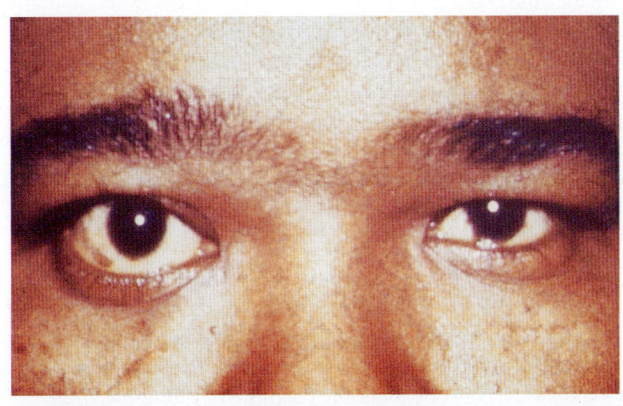

Figure 27.124. Proptosis of the right eye in a 37-year-old man. Proptosis had been present for most of his life, but it had recently become progressively worse. (Courtesy of William R. Morris, MD.)

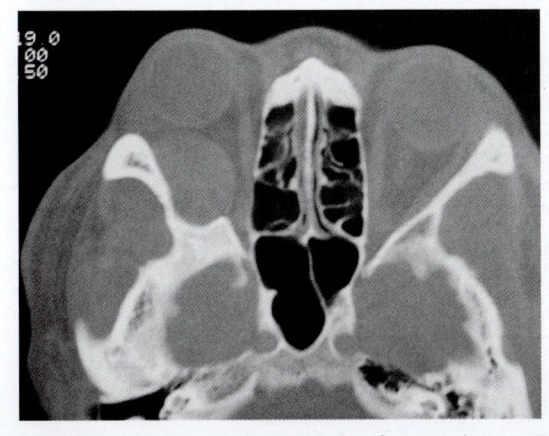

Figure 27.125. Axial computed tomography of patient shown in Figure 27.125, revealing a homogeneous mass causing proptosis of the right eye. The lesion was excised. (Courtesy of William R. Morris, MD.)

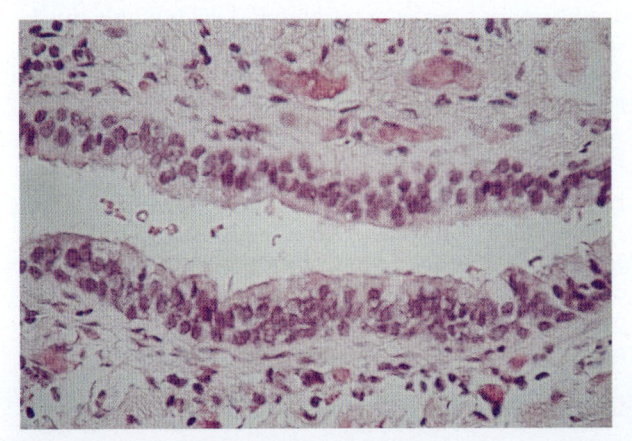

Figure 27.126. Histopathology of lesion shown in Figure 27.125, demonstrating the ciliated respiratory epithelium that lined the mass. (Hematoxylin–eosin ×200.) (Courtesy of William R. Morris, MD.)

ORBITAL PARASITIC CYSTS

General Considerations

Even though it is an inflammatory condition, orbital parasitic infestation is discussed in this chapter because of its importance in the differential diagnosis of orbital cystic lesions (1–27). Sporadic cases occur in North America and Europe but it occurs more often in endemic countries like Iran, Lebanon, Spain, Iraq, India, and in parts of Africa and Central and South America. No cases were encountered among the 1,264 orbital space–occupying lesions seen by the authors on the Oncology Service at Wills Eye Hospital (1).

Most parasitic cysts in the orbit are due to infestation of orbital tissue by the larvae of the tapeworms, *Taenia echinococcus* (hydatid cyst) and *Taenia solium* (cysticercosis). Because of their clinical similarities, they are discussed together.

Clinical Features

The patient with a parasitic orbital cyst can present with a variety of symptoms and signs, including any combination of painless proptosis, oculomotor palsies, eyelid edema, optic disc edema, and, sometimes, optic atrophy. With either hydatid cyst or cysticercosis, the rectus muscles are involved alone or in conjunction with brain and systemic involvement (16,11). Although the cysts are usually solitary, one patient had 15 separate cysts in one orbit (21). The orbital lesions can be bilateral. It is of ophthalmic interest that subretinal and vitreal involvement with cysticercosis can also occur.

Diagnostic Approaches

The clinical findings as described in a patient who lives in an endemic area for cysticercosis or echinococcosis should suggest the diagnosis. A history of eating poorly cooked pork supports the diagnosis of cysticercosis and a history of close contact with dogs should arouse concern about the diagnosis of echinococcosis.

Orbital ultrasonography can show a cystic lesion, usually in the anterior portion of the orbit, often with dense material in the lumen (9,11). Computed tomography and magnetic resonance imaging demonstrate a well-defined cystic mass with a density similar to water or cerebrospinal fluid. Within the cyst is a dense structure that represents the viable or dead larva. The predilection for extraocular muscles is often verified with neuroimaging studies (11,16).

Pathology

Pathology of the echinococcal or cysticercosis cyst reveals a thick fibrous wall with external layers of acellular material called the ectocyst and an inner structure containing the larvae called the endocyst (19). The material within the cyst may contain many scolices of the larvae. The pathogenesis of the orbital parasitic cyst is related to the life cycle of the larvae.

Management

Management is surgical removal, which may require a lateral orbitotomy for deeply located lesions. Supplemental medical therapy with oral albendazole appears to be beneficial (12,18). Both zoonotic parasitic diseases are now achieving control of the hosts to reduce human infection using new and highly effective vaccines capable of preventing infections. This vaccine approach will likely reduce global burden of human infections with cysticercus and echinococcus.

Selected References

Reviews

1. Shields JA, Shields CL, Scartozzi R. Survey of 1264 patients with orbital tumors and simulating lesions: the 2002 Montgomery Lecture, part 1. *Ophthalmology* 2004;111:997–1008.
2. Shields JA, Bakewell B, Augsburger DG, et al. Space-occupying orbital masses in children. A review of 250 consecutive biopsies. *Ophthalmology* 1986;93:379–384.
3. Shields JA, Kaden IH, Eagle RC Jr, et al. Orbital dermoid cysts. Clinicopathologic correlations, classification, and management. The 1997 Josephine E. Schueler Lecture. *Ophthal Plast Reconstr Surg* 1997;13:265–276.
4. Shields JA, Shields CL. Orbital cysts of childhood—classification, clinical features, and management. The 2003 Angeline Parks Lecture. *Surv Ophthalmol* 2004;49:281–299.
5. Templeton AC. Orbital tumors in African children. *Br J Ophthalmol* 1971;55:254–261.
6. Gomez Morales A, Croxatto JO, Crovetto L, et al. Hydatid cysts of the orbit. A review of 35 cases. *Ophthalmology* 1988;95:1027–1032.
7. Benazzou S, Arkha Y, Derraz S, et al. Orbital hydatid cyst: review of 10 cases. *J Craniomaxillofac Surg* 2010;38:274–278.

Imaging

8. Hamza R, Touibi S, Jamoussi M, et al. Intracranial and orbital hydatid cysts. *Neuroradiology* 1982;22:211–214.
9. Murthy H, Kumar A, Verma L. Orbital cysticercosis—an ultrasonic diagnosis. *Acta Ophthalmol (Copenh)* 1990;68:612–614.

Management

10. Akhan O, Bilgic S, Akata D, et al. Percutaneous treatment of an orbital hydatid cyst: a new therapeutic approach. *Am J Ophthalmol* 1998;125:877–879.
11. Sekhar GC, Honavar SG. Myocysticercosis: experience with imaging and therapy. *Ophthalmology* 1999;106:2336–2340.
12. Sihota R, Honavar SG. Oral albendazole in the management of extraocular cysticercosis. *Br J Ophthalmol* 1994;78:621–623.
13. Lightowlers MW. Cysticercosis and echinococcosis. *Curr Top Microbiol Immunol* 2013;365:315–335.

Case Reports

14. Sekhar GC, Lemke BN. Orbital cysticercosis. *Ophthalmology* 1978;104:2599–2604.
15. Bonavolonta G, Tranfa F. An unusual orbital cyst. *Orbit* 1984;3:179–182.
16. Kiratli H, Bilgic S, Ozturkmen C, et al. Intramuscular hydatid cyst of the medial rectus muscle. *Am J Ophthalmol* 2003;135:98–99.
17. Betharia SM, Pushker N, Sharma V, et al. Disseminated hydatid disease involving orbit, spleen, lung and liver. *Ophthalmologica* 2002;216:300–304.
18. Sihota R, Sharma T. Albendazole therapy for a recurrent orbital hydatid cyst. *Indian J Ophthalmol* 2000;48:142–143.
19. Apple DJ, Fajoni ML, Garland PE, et al. Orbital hydatid cyst. *J Pediatr Ophthalmol Strabismus* 1981;17:380–383.
20. Baghdassarian SA, Zakharia H. Report of three cases of hydatid cyst of the orbit. *Am J Ophthalmol* 1971;71:1081–1084.
21. Pirooz MS. Hydatid cysts of the orbit. *Orbit* 1983;2:65–68.
22. Pluschke M, Bennett G. Orbital cysticercosis. *Aust N Z J Ophthalmol* 1998;26:333–336.
23. Sundaram PM, Jayakumar N, Noronha V. Extraocular muscle cysticercosis—a clinical challenge to the ophthalmologists. *Orbit* 2004;23:255–262.
24. Gulliani BP, Dadeya S, Malik KP, et al. Bilateral cysticercosis of the optic nerve. *J Neuroophthalmol* 2001;21:217–218.
25. Hanioglu S, Saygi S, Yazar Z, et al. Orbital hydatid cyst. *Can J Ophthalmol* 1997;32:334–337.
26. Bagheri A, Fallahi MR, Yazdani S, et al. Two different presentations of orbital echinococcosis: a report of two cases and review of the literature. *Orbit* 2010;29:51–56.
27. Murthy R, Honavar SG, Vemuganti GK, et al. Polycystic echinococcosis of the orbit. *Am J Ophthalmol* 2005;140:561–563.

ORBITAL HYDATID CYST

Bonavolonta G, Tranfa F. An unusual orbital cyst. *Orbit* 1984;3:179–182.

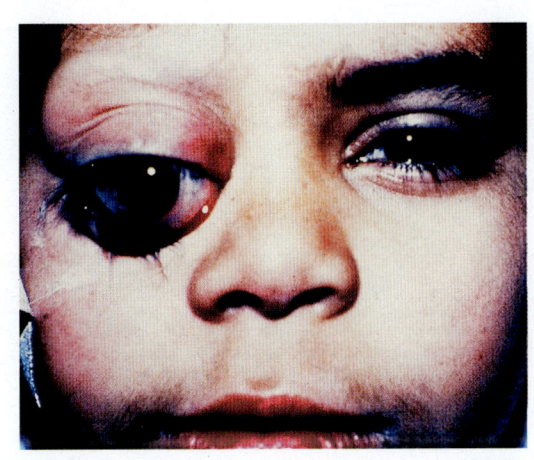

Figure 27.127. Proptosis and downward displacement of right eye secondary to orbital hydatid cyst in a 6-year-old girl. There was 17 mm of proptosis, total impairment of ocular motility and vision of finger counting in the affected right eye. (Courtesy of J. Oscar Croxatto, MD.)

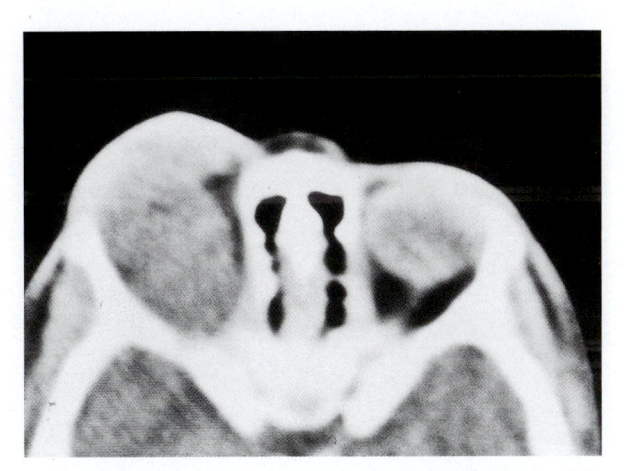

Figure 27.128. Axial computed tomography of patient shown in Figure 27.127, demonstrating large cystic mass in the orbit causing marked proptosis and displacement of the globe. (Courtesy of J. Oscar Croxatto, MD.)

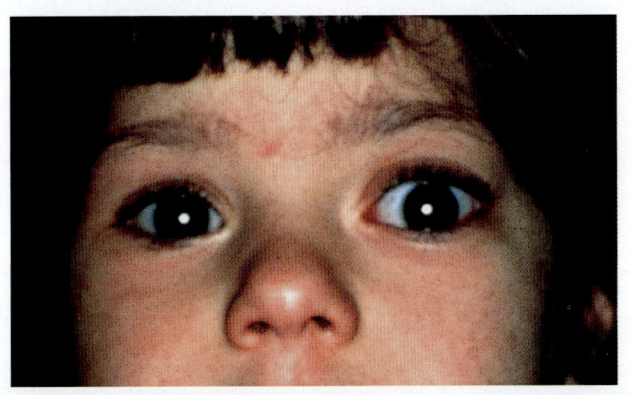

Figure 27.129. Proptosis of left eye in a 4-year-old girl. (Courtesy of Giulio Bonavolonta, MD.)

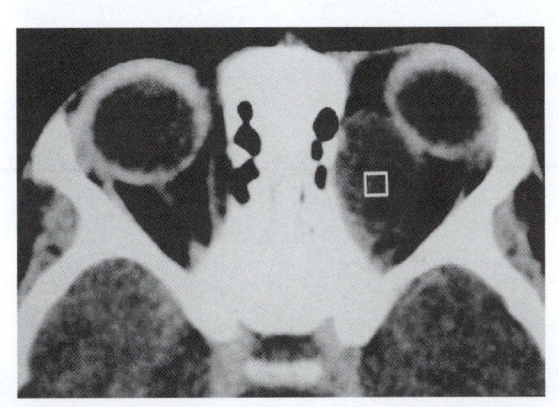

Figure 27.130. Orbital computed tomography demonstrating the cystic mass in the orbit (marked with a *square*). (Courtesy of Giulio Bonavolonta, MD.)

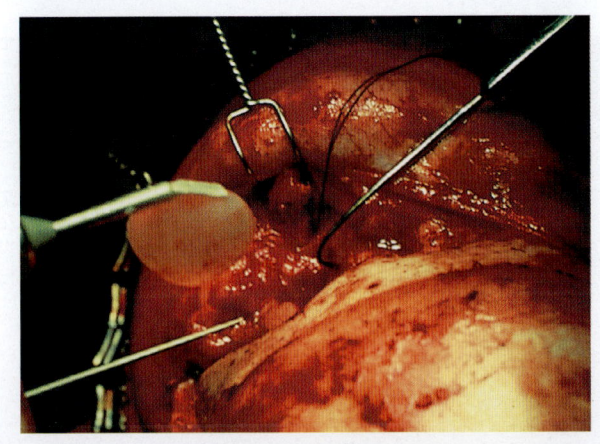

Figure 27.131. After surgical exposure, the cyst is being removed with an erisophake. (Courtesy of Giulio Bonavolonta, MD.)

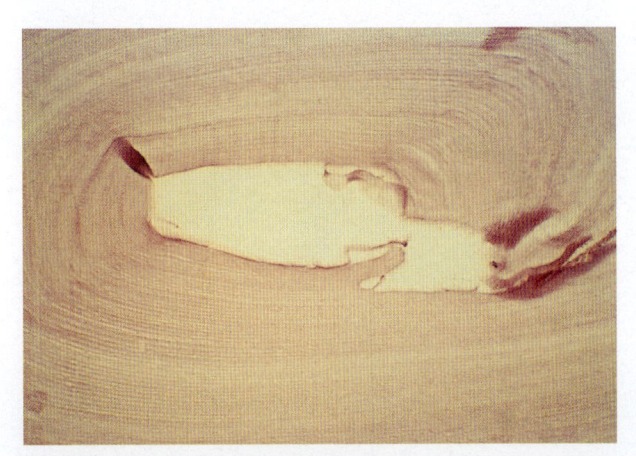

Figure 27.132. Histopathology of lesion shown in Figure 27.131, demonstrating the capsule of the cyst composed of acellular hyaline material. (Hematoxylin–eosin ×250.) (Courtesy of Giulio Bonavolonta, MD.)

ORBITAL HYDATID CYST

A case is shown in a young man from India.

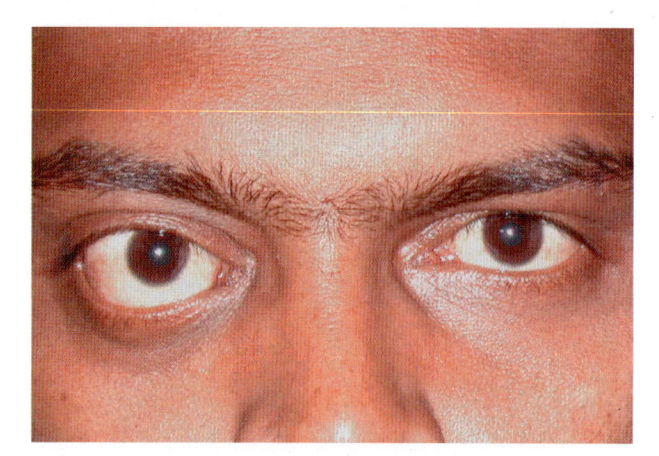

Figure 27.133. Proptosis of right eye in a 30-year-old male of 1 year duration. Visual acuity was 20/100 in the right eye. (Courtesy of Drs Santosh Honavar, Milind Naik, and Geeta Vemuganti, Hyderabad, India.)

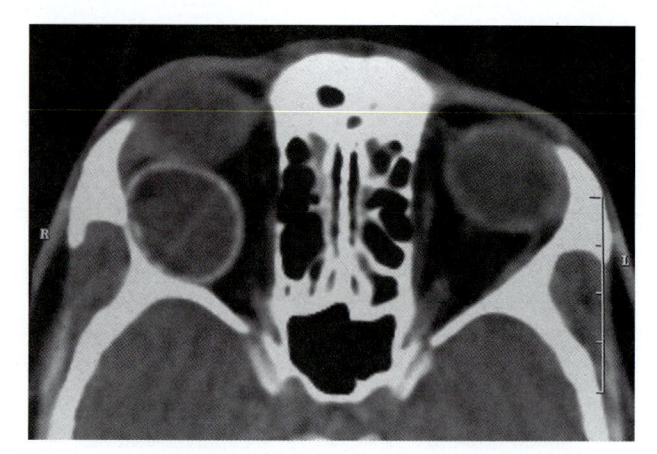

Figure 27.134. Axial computed tomography shows revealed a large cystic extraconal mass in the right orbit with bone scalloping. (Courtesy of Drs Santosh Honavar, Milind Naik, and Geeta Vemuganti, Hyderabad, India.)

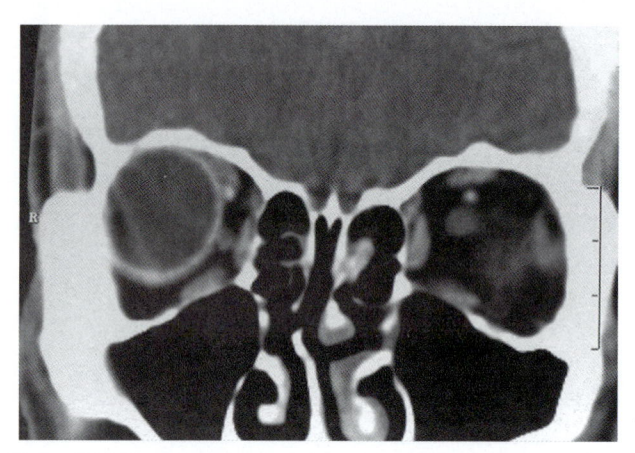

Figure 27.135. Coronal computed tomography shows sharply defined round cyst in the midportion of the orbit. (Courtesy of Drs Santosh Honavar, Milind Naik, and Geeta Vemuganti, Hyderabad, India.)

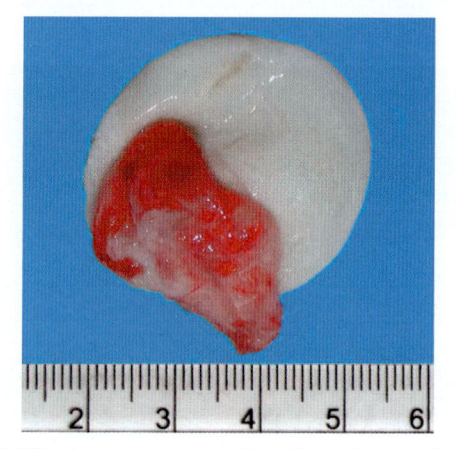

Figure 27.136. Appearance of partly collapsed cysts after surgical removal. The cyst ruptured during surgery and was aspirated. The collapsed cyst was removed with cryoextraction. The patient was treated with oral albendazole and prednisolone. (Courtesy of Drs Santosh Honavar, Milind Naik, and Geeta Vemuganti, Hyderabad, India.)

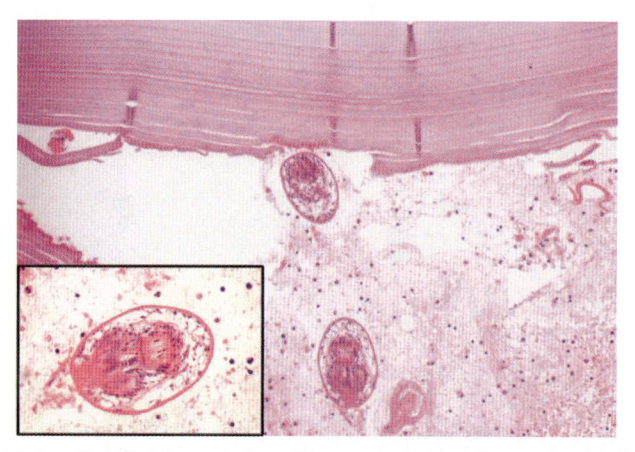

Figure 27.137. Histopathology shows laminated membrane of hydatid cyst. *Inset* shows a single scolex. (Hematoxylin–eosin ×200.) (Courtesy of Drs Santosh Honavar, Milind Naik, and Geeta Vemuganti, Hyderabad, India.)

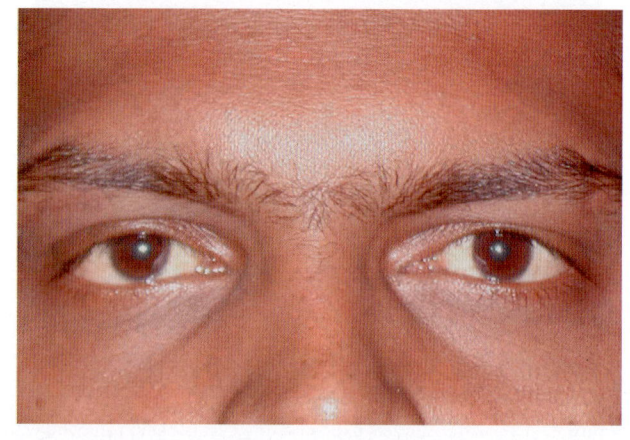

Figure 27.138. Postoperative appearance of patient. The proptosis is gone and visual acuity improved to 20/30. (Courtesy of Drs Santosh Honavar, Milind Naik, and Geeta Vemuganti, Hyderabad, India.)

ORBITAL VASCULAR AND HEMORRHAGIC LESIONS

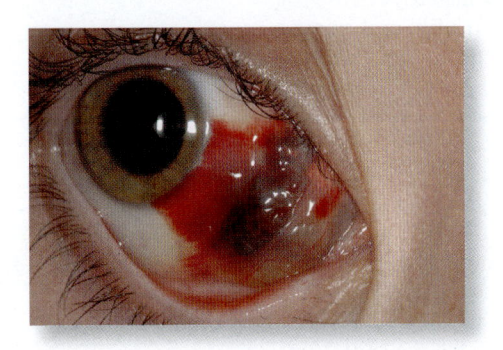

General Considerations

Capillary hemangioma (benign hemangioendothelioma; strawberry hemangioma) is an important cutaneous vascular tumor of childhood. In the ocular region, it usually begins on the eyelid but it can also occur in the orbit (1–23). About 7% of ocular adnexal capillary hemangiomas arise in the orbit posterior to the orbital septum (5). In the authors' series, orbital capillary hemangioma accounted for 1% of all biopsied orbital lesions in all age groups (2) and for 4% of all orbital biopsies in children (3). In a more recent series of 1,264 consecutive space-occupying orbital lesions, the 36 capillary hemangiomas accounted for 17% of the 213 vascular lesions and for 3% of all lesions (1).

Clinical Features

In the orbit, capillary hemangioma is usually apparent shortly after birth as a soft mass deep to the skin. It is more pronounced when the child strains or cries. Occasionally, it occurs in the deeper portions of the orbit without eyelid signs. Associated hemangioma on the periocular skin facilitates making the orbital diagnosis. The main complications are amblyopia and strabismus. Lesions >1 cm in diameter are more likely to cause these complications, whereas lesions <1 cm in diameter are considerably less likely to do so (22). The lesion usually shows enlargement for 1 to 2 years and then undergoes gradual regression, similar to eyelid capillary hemangioma. Orbital capillary hemangioma may be associated with large visceral hemangiomas, which can cause platelet entrapment and thrombocytopenia, a condition called the Kasabach–Merritt syndrome.

Orbital capillary hemangioma is rare in adults. However, an orbital tumor with similar histopathologic features has been reported to arise in the medial rectus muscle of a 73-year-old woman (21).

Diagnostic Approaches

With computed tomography (CT) and magnetic resonance imaging (MRI), orbital capillary hemangioma varies from case to case. It can be a round or ovoid circumscribed mass or an irregular or diffuse mass. It shows marked homogeneous enhancement with contrast agents. This tumor should be differentiated from malignant rhabdomyosarcoma that can have similar features and should be included in the differential diagnosis. However, rhabdomyosarcoma rarely is present in infancy but generally occurs in children aged between 5 and 15 years.

Pathology and Pathogenesis

Histopathologically, orbital capillary hemangioma is composed of lobules of proliferating small vascular channels separated by thin fibrous septa. The pathogenesis of capillary hemangioma has been largely unknown. However, it has been recognized that placenta and capillary hemangiomas have unique immunohistochemical similarities (19,20). This has led to speculation

ORBITAL CAPILLARY HEMANGIOMA

that infantile hemangiomas could be of placental origin. Two theories have been proposed to explain this hemangioma–placental connection. First, angioblasts could proliferate toward placental tissue in the site where the hemangioma develops. A second intriguing theory is that cells of placental origin could embolize to the target areas (19,20).

Management

Initial management of orbital capillary hemangioma should include refraction and occlusive patching treatment for associated amblyopia. If there is no threat to vision, the lesion can be cautiously observed. In our hands, approximately 90% to 95% of infants with hemangioma are monitored without therapy.

Oral or local injection of corticosteroids can hasten regression of the lesion (11–14). Ultrasound guidance has been used to accurately place the needle in the tumor (13). However, corticosteroids have a number of potential complications, including retinal artery obstruction, linear perilymphatic subcutaneous fat atrophy, eyelid depigmentation, eyelid necrosis, and adrenal gland suppression (12,14). Interferon-α2b has also been reported to be effective in hastening tumor regression (15,16). Surgical excision is an appropriate treatment for select well-circumscribed tumors (8–10).

The most recent advance in therapy is the use of the beta blocker, propranolol (17,18). This acts to stimulate involution of the tumor over a relatively shorter period of time. Propranolol can be given orally or topically, depending on the depth of the tumor.

ORBITAL CAPILLARY HEMANGIOMA

Selected References

Reviews
1. Shields JA, Shields CL, Scartozzi R. Survey of 1264 patients with orbital tumors and simulating lesions: The 2002 Montgomery Lecture, part 1. *Ophthalmology* 2004;111:997–1008.
2. Shields JA, Bakewell B, Augsburger JJ, et al. Classification and incidence of space-occupying lesions of the orbit. A survey of 645 biopsies. *Arch Ophthalmol* 1984;102:1606–1611.
3. Shields JA, Bakewell B, Augsburger JJ, et al. Space-occupying orbital masses in children: A review of 250 consecutive biopsies. *Ophthalmology* 1986;93:379–384.
4. Gunalp I, Gunduz K. Vascular tumors of the orbit. *Doc Ophthalmol* 1995;89:337–345.
5. Haik BG, Jakobiec FA, Ellsworth RM, et al. Capillary hemangioma of the lids and orbit: an analysis of the clinical features and therapeutic results in 101 cases. *Ophthalmology* 1979;86:760–792.
6. Schwartz SR, Blei F, Ceisler E, et al. Risk factors for amblyopia in children with capillary hemangiomas of the eyelids and orbit. *J AAPOS* 2006;10(3):262–268.

Imaging
7. Kavanagh EC, Heran MK, Peleg A, et al. Imaging of the natural history of an orbital capillary hemangioma. *Orbit* 2006;25(1):69–72.

Management
8. Aldave AJ, Shields CL, Shields JA. Surgical excision of selected amblyogenic periorbital capillary hemangiomas. *Ophthalmic Surg Lasers* 1999;30:754–757.
9. Deans RM, Harris GJ, Kivlin JD. Surgical dissection of capillary hemangiomas. An alternative to intralesional corticosteroids. *Arch Ophthalmol* 1992;110:1743–1747.
10. Levi M, Schwartz S, Blei F, et al. Surgical treatment of capillary hemangiomas causing amblyopia. *J AAPOS* 2007;11(3):230–234.
11. Egbert JE, Paul S, Engel WK, et al. High injection pressure during intralesional injection of corticosteroids into capillary hemangiomas. *Arch Ophthalmol* 2001;119:677–683.
12. O'Keefe M, Lanigan B, Byrne SA. Capillary haemangioma of the eyelids and orbit: a clinical review of the safety and efficacy of intralesional steroid. *Acta Ophthalmol Scand* 2003;81:294–298.
13. Neumann D, Isenberg SJ, Rosenbaum AL, et al. Ultrasonographically guided injection of corticosteroids for the treatment of retroseptal capillary hemangiomas in infants. *JAAPOS* 1997;1:34–40.
14. Goyal R, Watts P, Lane CM, et al. Adrenal suppression and failure to thrive after steroid injections for periocular hemangioma. *Ophthalmology* 2004;111:389–395.
15. Wilson MW, Hoehn ME, Haik BG, et al. Low-dose cyclophosphamide and interferon alfa 2a for the treatment of capillary hemangioma of the orbit. *Ophthalmology* 2007;114(5):1007–1011.
16. Hastings MM, Milot J, Barsoum-Homsy M, et al. Recombinant interferon alfa-2b in the treatment of vision-threatening capillary hemangiomas in childhood. *JAAPOS* 1997;1:226–230.
17. Thoumazet F, Léauté-Labrèze C, Colin J, et al. Efficacy of systemic propranolol for severe infantile haemangioma of the orbit and eyelid: a case study of eight patients. *Br J Ophthalmol* 2012;96(3):370–374.
18. Chambers CB, Katowitz WR, Katowitz JA, et al. A controlled study of topical 0.25% timolol maleate gel for the treatment of cutaneous infantile capillary hemangiomas. *Ophthal Plast Reconstr Surg* 2012;28:103–106.

Histopathology
19. North PE, Waner M, Mizeracki A, et al. A unique microvascular phenotype shared by juvenile hemangiomas and human placenta. *Arch Dermatol* 2001;137:559–570.
20. North PE, Waner M, Brodsky MC. Are infantile hemangiomas of placental origin? *Ophthalmology* 2002;109:633–634.
21. Cockerham KP, Sachs DM, Cockerham GC, et al. Orbital hemangioblastoma arising in a rectus muscle. *Ophthal Plast Reconstr Surg* 2003;19:248–250.
22. Ceisler E, Blei F. Ophthalmic issues in hemangiomas of infancy. *Lymphat Res Biol* 2003;1:321–330.
23. Aletaha M, Salour H, Bagheri A, et al. Successful treatment of orbital hemangioma with propranolol in a 5-year-old girl. *Orbit* 2012;31(1):18–20.

ORBITAL CAPILLARY HEMANGIOMA

Orbital capillary hemangioma can occur in the deep orbit and produce proptosis or displacement of the globe or it can occur in the anterior portion of the orbit and present as a reddish-blue, fluctuant, subcutaneous eyelid mass. The more common cutaneous eyelid capillary hemangioma is discussed in this text.

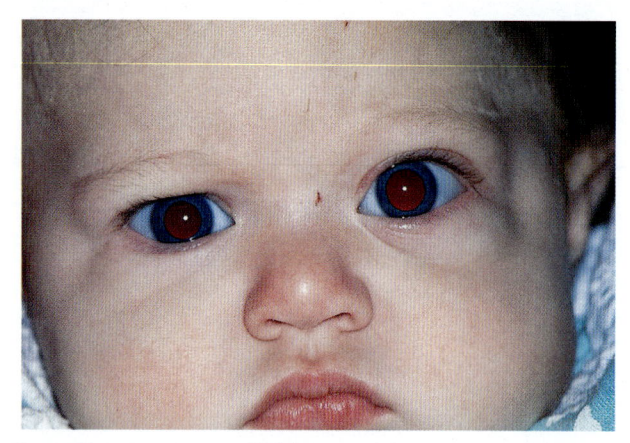

Figure 28.1. Prominence of left lower eyelid secondary to orbital capillary hemangioma in a 4-month-old girl.

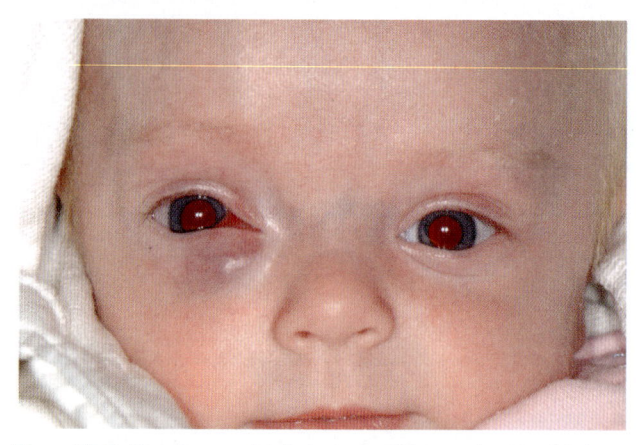

Figure 28.2. Prominence of right lower eyelid secondary to orbital capillary hemangioma in a 3-month-old girl.

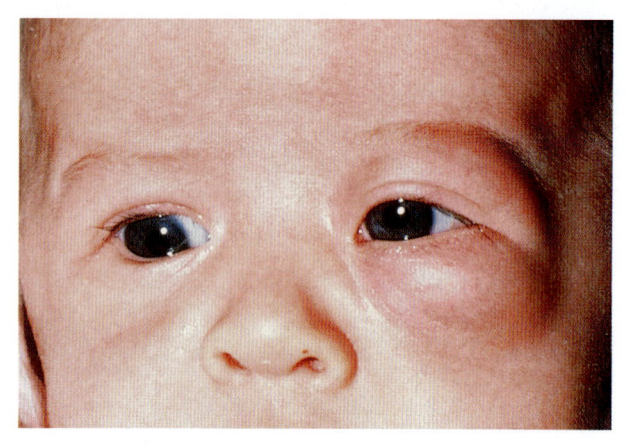

Figure 28.3. Prominence of left lower and upper eyelids secondary to orbital capillary hemangioma in a 1-year-old girl.

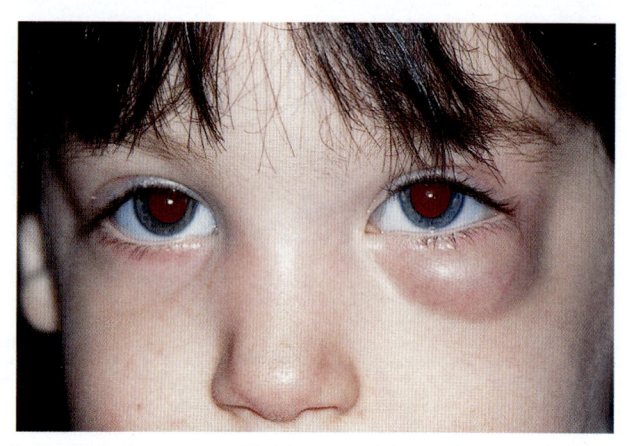

Figure 28.4. Prominence of left lower eyelid secondary to orbital capillary hemangioma in a 2-year-old girl.

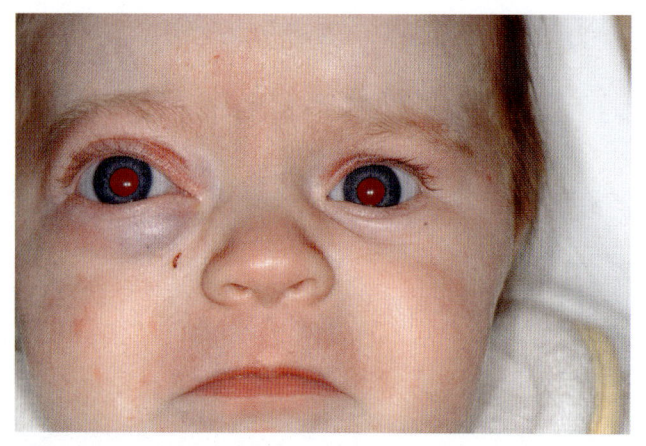

Figure 28.5. Prominence of right lower eyelid from orbital capillary hemangioma in a 2-month-old boy.

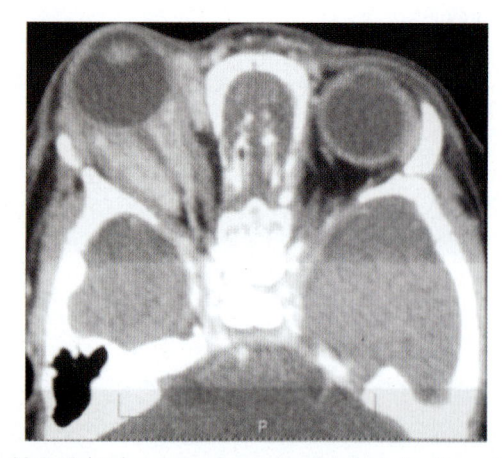

Figure 28.6. Orbital computed tomography displaying the entire right orbit of patient in Figure 28.5 filled with infantile capillary hemangioma.

Chapter 28 Orbital Vascular and Hemorrhagic Lesions 513

ORBITAL CAPILLARY HEMANGIOMA: CLINICAL VARIATIONS AND REGRESSION

Orbital capillary hemangioma can have a variety of clinical manifestations. A common feature of infantile capillary hemangiomas, however, is their tendency to grow rapidly in infancy and then to stabilize and gradually regress.

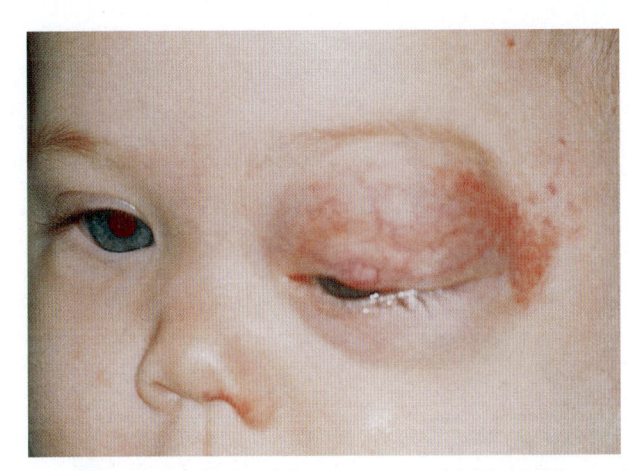

Figure 28.7. Proptosis of the left eye in a 4-month-old girl. The associated cutaneous hemangioma should suggest an orbital hemangioma as the cause of the proptosis.

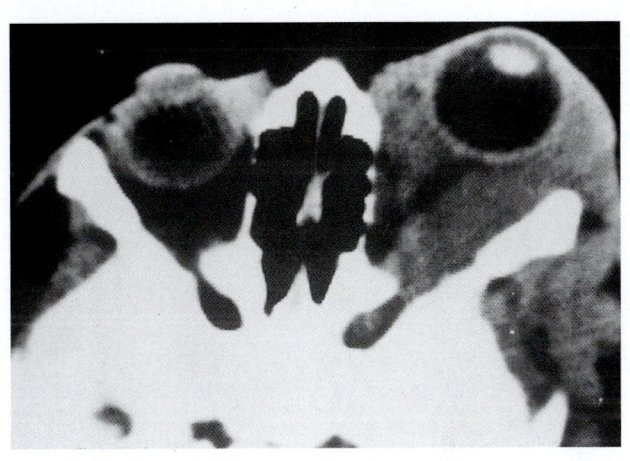

Figure 28.8. Axial computed tomography of patient shown in Figure 28.7. Note the diffuse involvement of the orbital soft tissues.

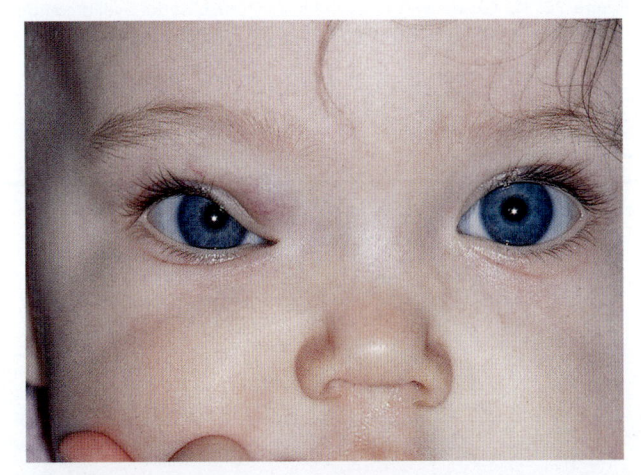

Figure 28.9. Characteristic subcutaneous mass superonasal to the right eye in a 5-month-old girl.

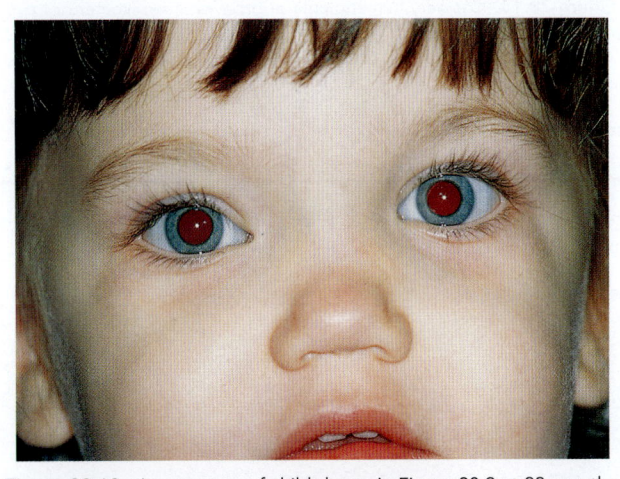

Figure 28.10. Appearance of child shown in Figure 28.9 at 23 months. The lesion has regressed without treatment.

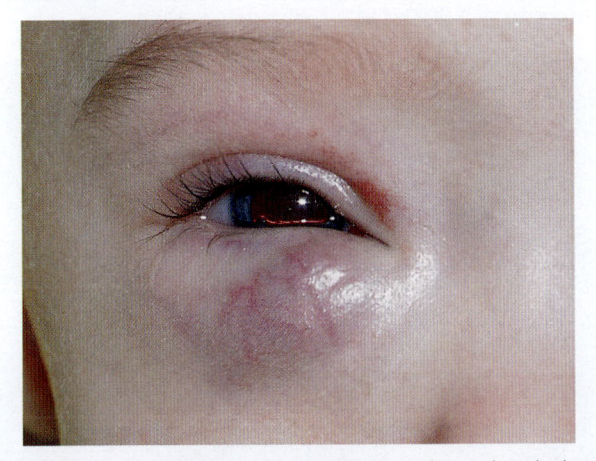

Figure 28.11. Reddish-blue subcutaneous mass beneath right lower eyelid in a 4-month-old boy.

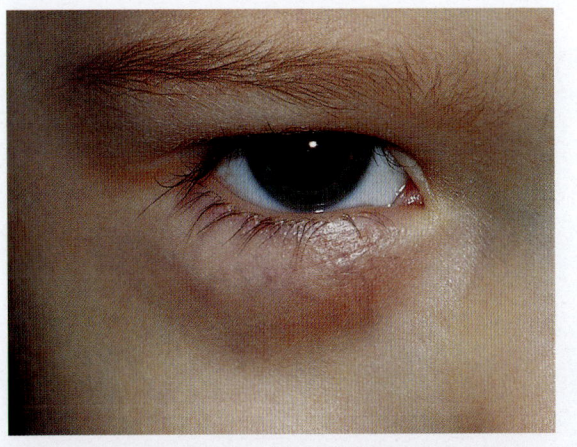

Figure 28.12. Appearance of child shown in Figure 28.11 at 24 months. The lesion has shown regression without treatment.

ORBITAL CAPILLARY HEMANGIOMA: SIMULTANEOUS EYELID AND ADNEXAL INVOLVEMENT

In some instances, a capillary hemangioma of the eyelid can be associated with orbital capillary hemangioma and extraocular cutaneous hemangiomas.

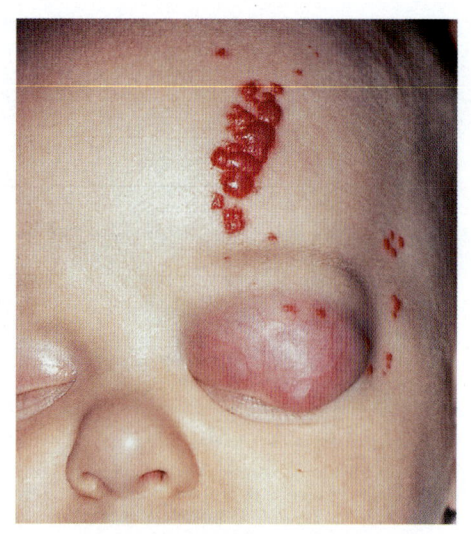

Figure 28.13. Capillary hemangioma of orbit with involvement of eyelid and forehead.

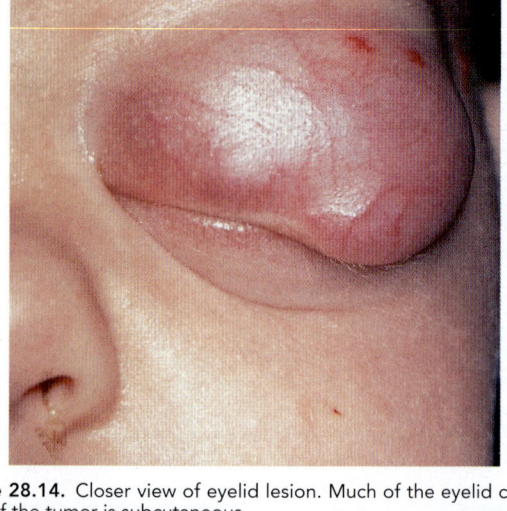

Figure 28.14. Closer view of eyelid lesion. Much of the eyelid component of the tumor is subcutaneous.

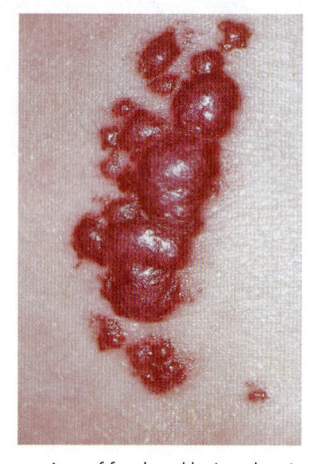

Figure 28.15. Closer view of forehead lesion showing red lobular mass.

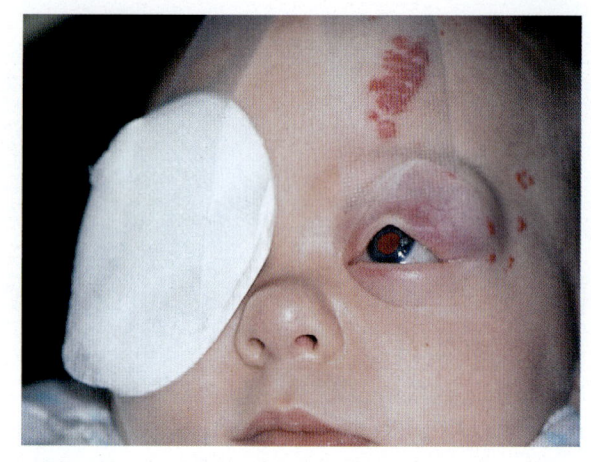

Figure 28.16. Management of patient with patching of opposite eye and opening the affected eyelid with tape to forehead.

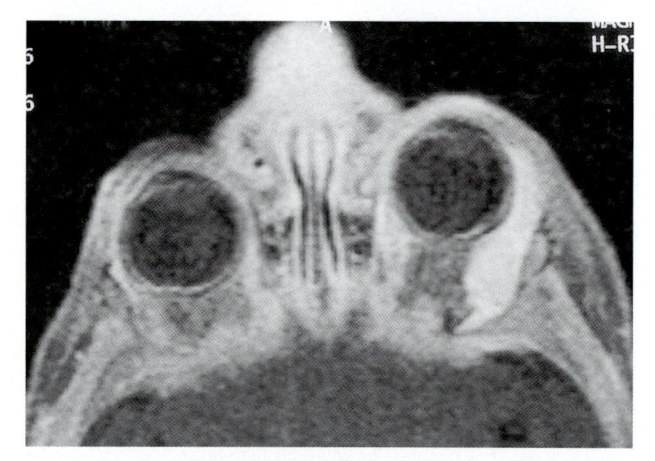

Figure 28.17. Magnetic resonance imaging in T1-weighted image showing enhancement of superotemporal orbital mass.

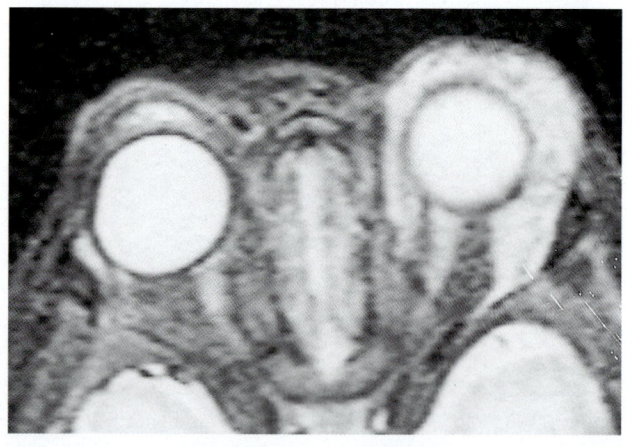

Figure 28.18. Magnetic resonance imaging in T2-weighted image showing extensive hyperintense orbital mass.

ORBITAL CAPILLARY HEMANGIOMA: SURGICAL RESECTION

In a very young infant, surgical excision may be the best treatment of a large, anterior, well-circumscribed orbital capillary hemangioma producing significant ocular signs and symptoms and that is destined to show further growth and visual loss. A clinicopathologic correlation is shown.

Aldave AJ, Shields CL, Shields JA. Surgical excision of selected amblyogenic periorbital capillary hemangiomas. *Ophthalmic Surg Lasers* 1999;30:754–757.

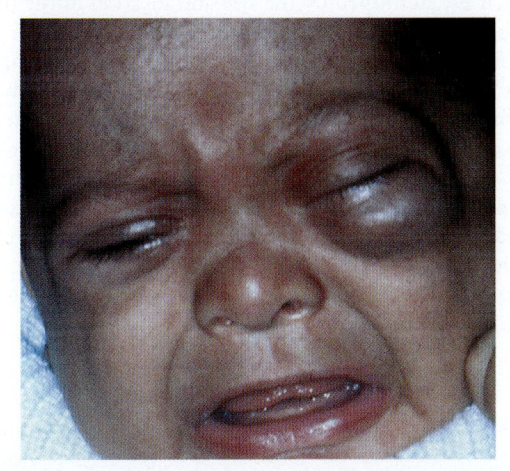

Figure 28.19. Extensive inferior orbital mass producing a prominent blue appearance to the left lower eyelid in an infant girl. The lesion was growing rapidly.

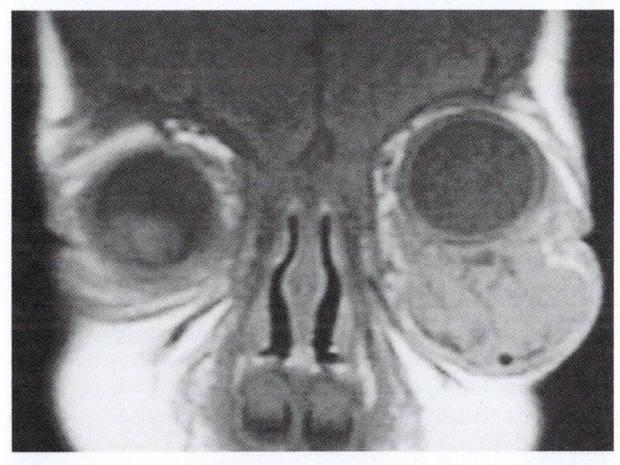

Figure 28.20. Coronal magnetic resonance imaging in T1-weighted image showing large but fairly well-circumscribed inferior orbital mass with upward displacement of the left eye. The mass was removed by way of an eyelid crease incision.

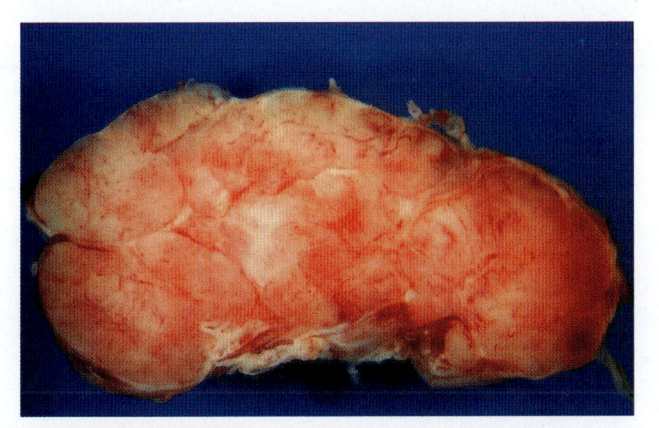

Figure 28.21. Appearance of the lesion after surgical excision and bisection, showing that the lesion was removed intact.

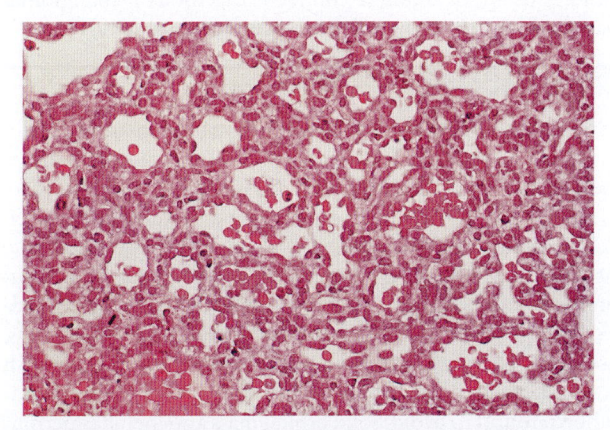

Figure 28.22. Low-magnification photomicrograph showing lobules of proliferating endothelial cells with fine blood vessels. (Hematoxylin–eosin ×75.)

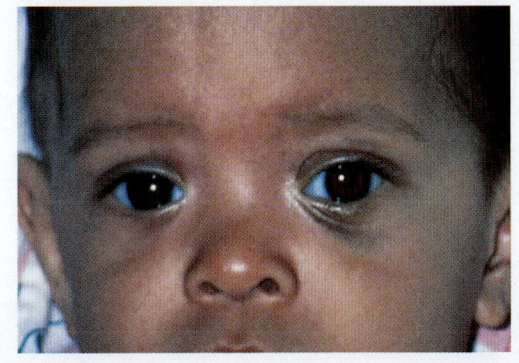

Figure 28.23. Appearance of same child 7 weeks after surgery showing good cosmetic outcome.

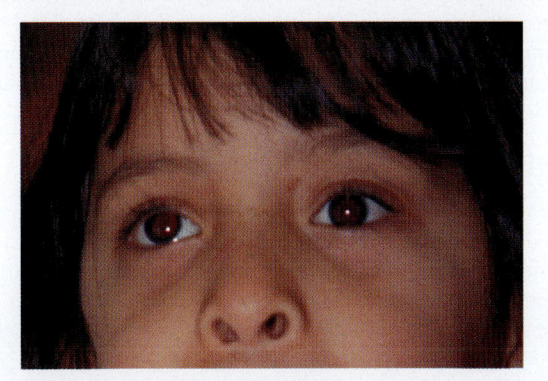

Figure 28.24. Appearance at age 7 years.

ORBITAL CAVERNOUS HEMANGIOMA

General Considerations

Cavernous hemangioma is the most common vascular tumor of the orbit (1–36). In the authors' series of 1,264 orbital masses, the 77 cavernous hemangiomas accounted for 36% of vascular tumors and for 6% of all tumors in the series (1). In a series from Italy, 9% of orbital tumors were cavernous hemangioma (5). In a series specifically on orbital vascular tumors in Turkey, 41% were cavernous hemangioma (4). In a subsequent report by the authors on orbital tumors in the older adult, cavernous hemangioma accounted for 8% of orbital tumors in patients ≥60 years of age (8).

Clinical Features

Orbital cavernous hemangioma is a benign tumor that tends to occur in adulthood as a relatively stationary or slowly progressive lesion that can produce painless proptosis. Because it most often occurs in the muscle cone, it usually produces axial proptosis. It does not generally produce inflammatory signs. Rarely, a cavernous hemangioma can present as an intraosseous lesion in the orbital bones (19–21). Orbital cavernous hemangioma is rarely bilateral (22). Although cavernous hemangioma is generally a solitary lesion, it can sometimes be multiple, particularly when seen in the blue rubber bleb nevus syndrome (23–25). In rare instances, multiple confluent cavernous hemangiomas have involved the orbit and brain simultaneously (30).

Diagnostic Approaches

Modern techniques of neuroimaging have been instrumental in making a more accurate diagnosis of orbital cavernous hemangioma (10). Since the advent of good imaging modalities like CT and MRI, this tumor is often being discovered more often as a coincidental finding when it is small and asymptomatic. As it slowly enlarges, it can produce marked proptosis, compression of the optic nerve, and choroidal folds. Imaging studies demonstrate a well-circumscribed round to ovoid mass, usually in the muscle cone. It shows mild enhancement with contrast agents. The differential diagnosis of a well-circumscribed, round to ovoid, solid orbital mass also includes peripheral nerve sheath tumors (schwannoma and neurofibroma), hemangiopericytoma, fibrous histiocytoma, solitary fibrous tumor, and melanoma. It has been suggested that orbital cavernous hemangioma can be differentiated from schwannoma by contrast-enhancement spread pattern methods on dynamic MRI (31).

Pathology

Histopathologically, orbital cavernous hemangioma is composed of dilated, congested vascular channels separated by connective tissue that contains smooth muscle. The pattern is generally quite typical but on occasion lymphangioma can have similar histopathologic features.

Management

Management of orbital cavernous hemangioma ranges from periodic observation for small, asymptomatic lesions to surgical excision for larger, symptomatic tumors. The surgical approach is determined by the size and location of the tumor. A conjunctival or cutaneous approach may be used for anterior lesions. We have had considerable success removing cavernous hemangiomas that are located in the anterior half of the orbit by a transconjunctival approach. Deep orbital tumors may require a lateral orbitotomy, sometimes with an osteotomy (Kronlein approach). Complete excision is important and meticulous surgery is necessary to avoid incomplete excision and recurrence. Techniques of transcranial approach are used for lesions located at the orbital apex (11). In some cases, an endoscopic approach is used, particularly for tumors deep in the orbit near the apex (14–16).

ORBITAL CAVERNOUS HEMANGIOMA

Selected References

Reviews

1. Shields JA, Shields CL, Scartozzi R. Survey of 1264 patients with orbital tumors and simulating lesions: The 2002 Montgomery Lecture, part 1. *Ophthalmology* 2004;111:997–1008.
2. Shields JA, Bakewell B, Augsburger JJ, et al. Classification and incidence of space-occupying lesions of the orbit. A survey of 645 biopsies. *Arch Ophthalmol* 1984;102:1606–1611.
3. Shields JA, Bakewell B, Augsburger JJ, et al. Space-occupying orbital masses in children: A review of 250 consecutive biopsies. *Ophthalmology* 1986;93:379–384.
4. Gunalp I, Gunduz K. Vascular tumors of the orbit. *Doc Ophthalmol* 1995;89:337–345.
5. Bonavolontà G, Strianese D, Grassi P, et al. An analysis of 2,480 space-occupying lesions of the orbit from 1976 to 2011. *Ophthal Plast Reconstr Surg* 2013;29(2):79–86.
6. Rootman J. Vascular malformations of the orbit: hemodynamic concepts. *Orbit* 2003;22:103–120.
7. Selva D, Strianese D, Bonavolonta G, et al. Orbital venous-lymphatic malformations (lymphangiomas) mimicking cavernous hemangiomas. *Am J Ophthalmol* 2001;131:364–370.
8. Demirci H, Shields CL, Shields JA, et al. Orbital tumors in the older adult population. *Ophthalmology* 2002;109:243–248.

Imaging

9. Thorn-Kany M, Arrue P, Delisle MB, et al. Cavernous hemangiomas of the orbit: MR imaging. *J Neuroradiol* 1999;26:79–86.
10. Ansari SA, Mafee MF. Orbital cavernous hemangioma: role of imaging. *Neuroimaging Clin N Am* 2005;15:137–158.

Management

11. Maus M, Goldman HW. Removal of orbital apex hemangioma using new transorbital craniotomy through suprabrow approach. *Ophthal Plast Reconstr Surg* 1999;15:166–170.
12. Gdal-On M, Gelfand YA. Surgical outcome of transconjunctival cryosurgical extraction of orbital cavernous hemangioma. *Ophthalmic Surg Lasers* 1998;29:969–973.
13. Acciarri N, Giulioni M, Padovani R, et al. Orbital cavernous angiomas: surgical experience on a series of 13 cases. *J Neurosurg Sci* 1995;39:203–209.
14. Muscatello L, Seccia V, Caniglia M, et al. Transnasal endoscopic surgery for selected orbital cavernous hemangiomas: our preliminary experience. *Head Neck* 2013;35:E218–E220.
15. Chen L, White WL, Xu B, et al. Transnasal transsphenoid approach: a minimally invasive approach for removal of cavernous haemangiomas located at inferomedial part of orbital apex. *Clin Experiment Ophthalmol* 2010;38:439–443.
16. Karaki M, Kobayashi R, Mori N. Removal of an orbital apex hemangioma using an endoscopic transethmoidal approach: technical note. *Neurosurgery* 2006;59(1 Suppl 1):ONSE159–ONSE160.
17. Papalkar D, Francis IC, Stoodley M, et al. Cavernous haemangioma in the orbital apex: stereotactic-guided transcranial cryoextraction. *Clin Experiment Ophthalmol* 2005;33:421–423.
18. Rootman DB, Rootman J, Gregory S, et al. Stereotactic fractionated radiotherapy for cavernous venous malformations (hemangioma) of the orbit. *Ophthal Plast Reconstr Surg* 2012;28:96–102.

Case Reports

19. Colombo F, Cursiefen C, Hofmann-Rummelt C, et al. Primary intraosseous cavernous hemangioma of the orbit. *Am J Ophthalmol* 2001;131:151–152.
20. Hwang K. Intraosseous hemangioma of the orbit. *J Craniofac Surg* 2000;11:386–387.
21. Madge SN, Simon S, Abidin Z, et al. Primary orbital intraosseous hemangioma. *Ophthal Plast Reconstr Surg* 2009;25(1):37–41.
22. Shields JA, Hogan RN, Shields CL, et al. Bilateral cavernous haemangiomas of the orbit. *Br J Ophthalmol* 2000;84:928.
23. McCannel CA, Hoenig J, Umlas J, et al. Orbital lesions in the blue rubber bleb nevus syndrome. *Ophthalmology* 1996;103:933–936.
24. Chang EL, Rubin PA. Bilateral multifocal hemangiomas of the orbit in the blue rubber bleb nevus syndrome. *Ophthalmology* 2002;109:537–541.
25. Mojon D, Odel JG, Rios R, et al. Presumed orbital hemangioma associated with the blue rubber bleb nevus syndrome. *Arch Ophthalmol* 1996;114:618–619.
26. Hassler W, Schaller C, Farghaly F, et al. Transconjunctival approach to a large cavernoma of the orbit. *Neurosurgery* 1994;34:859–861.
27. Bajaj MS, Nainiwal SK, Pushker N, et al. Multifocal cavernous hemangioma: a rare presentation. *Orbit* 2003;22:155–159.
28. Kim YH, Baek SH, Choi WC. The transconjunctival approach to a large retrobulbar cavernous hemangioma of the orbit. *Korean J Ophthalmol* 2002;16:37–42.
29. Shields JA, Shields CL, Eagle RC. Cavernous hemangioma of the orbit. *Arch Ophthalmol* 1987;105:853.
30. Puca A, Colosimo C, Tirpakova B, et al. Cavernous hemangioma extending to extracranial, intracranial, and orbital regions. Case report. *J Neurosurg* 2004;101:1057–1060.
31. Tanaka A, Mihara F, Yoshiura T, et al. Differentiation of cavernous hemangioma from schwannoma of the orbit: a dynamic MRI study. *AJR Am J Roentgenol* 2004;183:1799–1804.
32. Yan J, Wu Z. Cavernous hemangioma of the orbit: analysis of 214 cases. *Orbit* 2004;23:33–40.
33. Harris GJ, Perez N. Surgical sectors of the orbit: using the lower fornix approach for large, medial intraconal tumors. *Ophthal Plast Reconstr Surg* 2002;18:349–354.
34. Meena M, Naik M, Honavar S. Acute recurrence of orbital cavernous hemangioma in a young man: a case report. *Ophthal Plast Reconstr Surg* 2012;28:e93–e95.
35. Lee KY, Fong KS, Loh HL, et al. Giant cavernous haemangioma mimicking a fifth nerve neurofibroma involving the orbit and brain. *Br J Ophthalmol* 2008;92:423–425.
36. Paonessa A, Limbucci N, Gallucci M. Are bilateral cavernous hemangiomas of the orbit rare entities? The role of MRI in a retrospective study. *Eur J Radiol* 2008;66:282–286.

Part 3 Tumors of the Orbit

ORBITAL CAVERNOUS HEMANGIOMA

With the advent of CT and MRI, some orbital cavernous hemangiomas are discovered at an early stage, when they are asymptomatic. Such lesions can usually be followed without treatment because they often remain asymptomatic for many years. The patient can be examined once or twice a year with pupil examination, visual acuity, color vision, exophthalmometry, ophthalmoscopy, visual fields, and CT or MRI studies. If the patient begins to develop findings that could cause visual loss, the surgical removal of the tumor is generally appropriate. Like other orbital tumors, they can produce fundus changes like choroidal folds, optic disc edema, and compression of the globe.

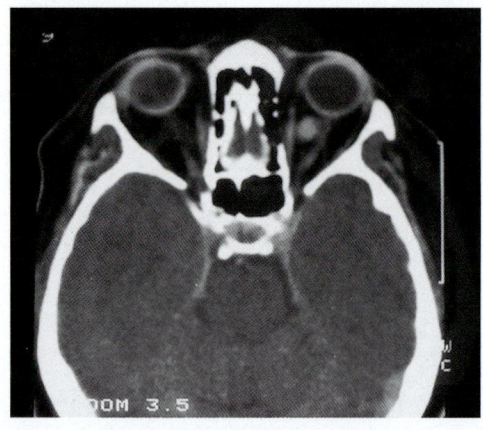

Figure 28.25. Axial computed tomography of small asymptomatic cavernous hemangioma in anterior orbit immediately posterior to the globe and nasal to the optic nerve. Management was periodic observation only.

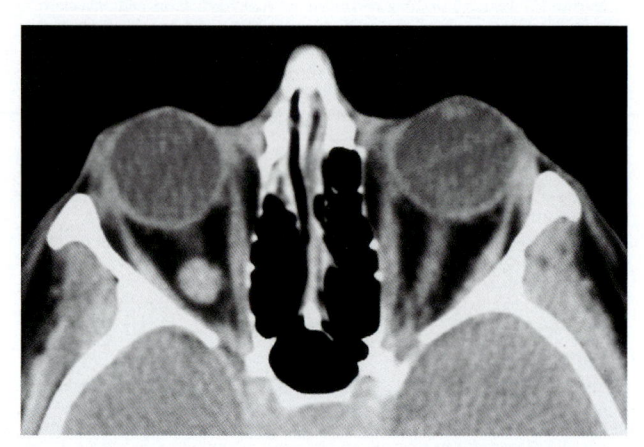

Figure 28.26. Axial computed tomography of small asymptomatic cavernous hemangioma closer to the orbital apex. A lesion like this is difficult to remove surgically. Management was periodic observation only.

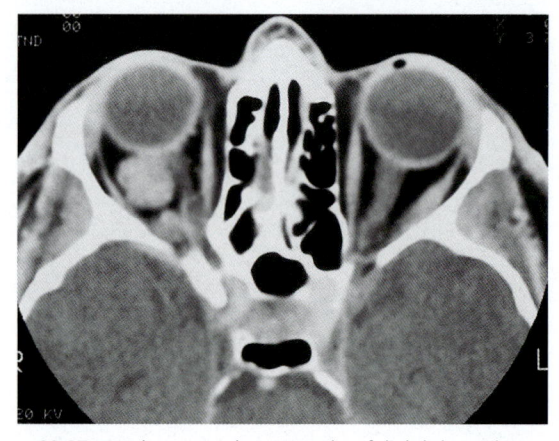

Figure 28.27. Axial computed tomography of slightly larger but asymptomatic cavernous hemangioma in midportion of orbit in muscle cone. Management was periodic observation only.

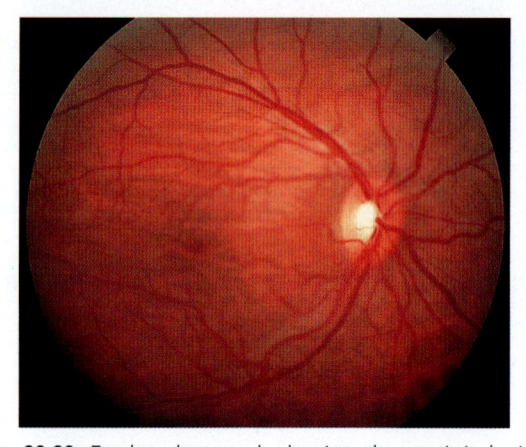

Figure 28.28. Fundus photograph showing characteristic horizontal choroidal folds secondary to another intraconal cavernous hemangioma.

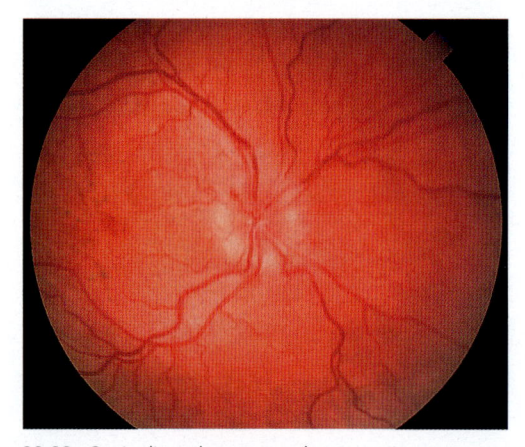

Figure 28.29. Optic disc edema secondary to optic nerve compression by orbital cavernous hemangioma.

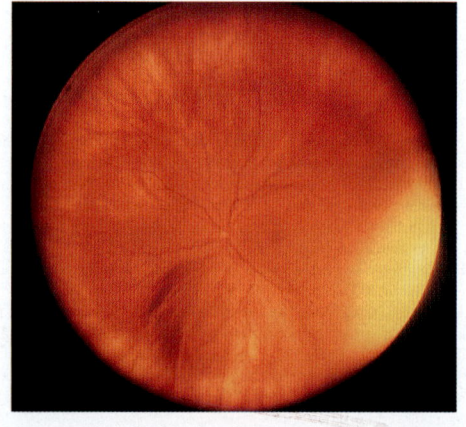

Figure 28.30. Wide-angle fundus photograph showing compression of inferior portion of globe by an orbital cavernous hemangioma. Such an elevation can sometimes be confused with an intraocular neoplasm.

Chapter 28 Orbital Vascular and Hemorrhagic Lesions

ORBITAL CAVERNOUS HEMANGIOMA: SURGICAL REMOVAL BY CONJUNCTIVAL APPROACH

In cases of suspected orbital cavernous hemangioma, one must determine the best approach to surgical removal. If a portion of the tumor is located fairly anteriorly, a conjunctiva approach, rather than cutaneous approach, can be employed in selected cases. An example is shown of a relatively large cavernous hemangioma that was removed by a conjunctival approach. In such instances, a cryoprobe can facilitate removal of the tumor.

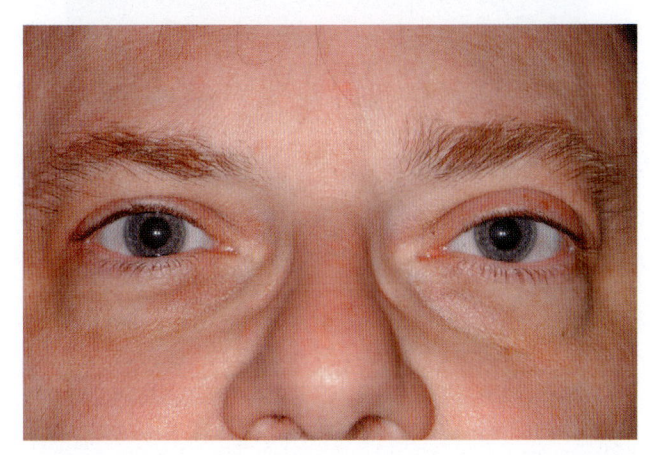

Figure 28.31. Axial proptosis of left eye by orbital cavernous hemangioma.

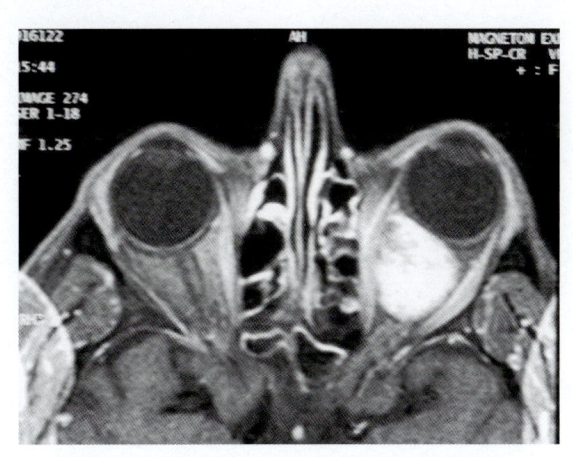

Figure 28.32. Axial magnetic resonance imaging with T1-weighted image and fat suppression, demonstrating large, round, cavernous hemangioma in muscle cone.

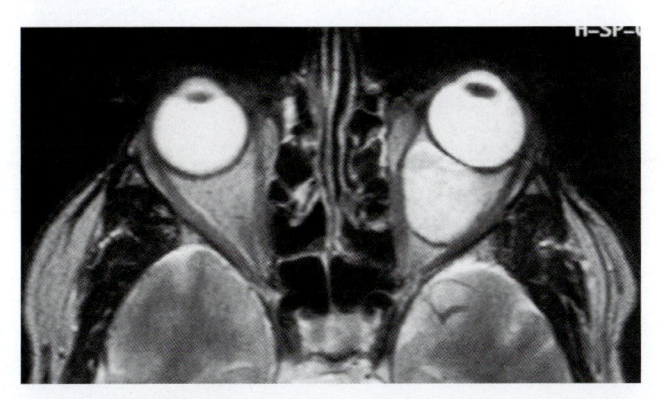

Figure 28.33. Same lesion seen in T1-weighted image. Note that the tumor is causing forward displacement and indentation of the globe. Based on the inferonasal location of the mass, it was elected to remove by a conjunctival approach.

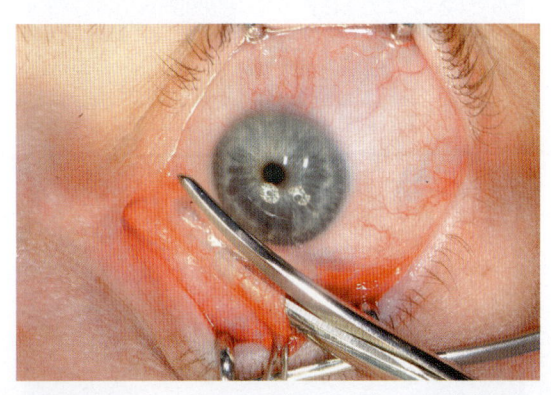

Figure 28.34. Incision with scissors being made in the bulbar conjunctiva inferonasally.

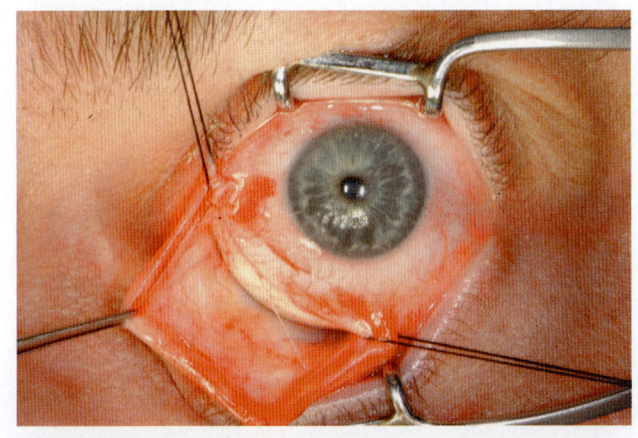

Figure 28.35. The incision has been completed and traction sutures have been placed beneath the insertions of the medial and inferior rectus muscles to assist in rotation of the globe for better exposure.

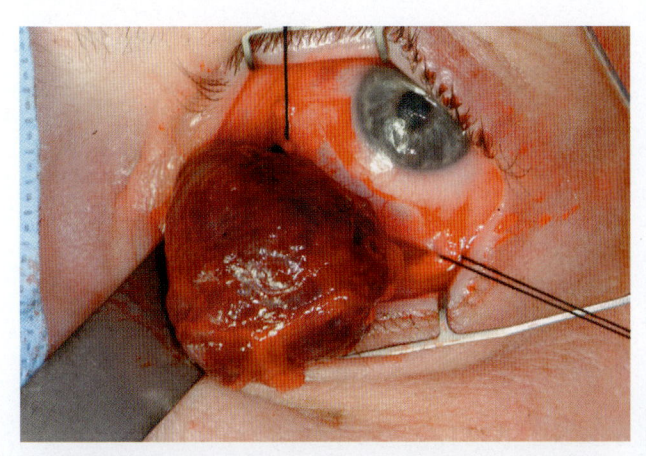

Figure 28.36. Typical orbital cavernous hemangioma being removed. Some sizable cavernous hemangiomas can be removed quickly and successfully by the conjunctival approach.

ORBITAL CAVERNOUS HEMANGIOMA: GLOBE AND OPTIC NERVE COMPRESSION

Depicted is a clinicopathologic correlation of a cavernous hemangioma with globe compression and optic disc edema in which the tumor was removed through a horizontal forniceal conjunctival incision.

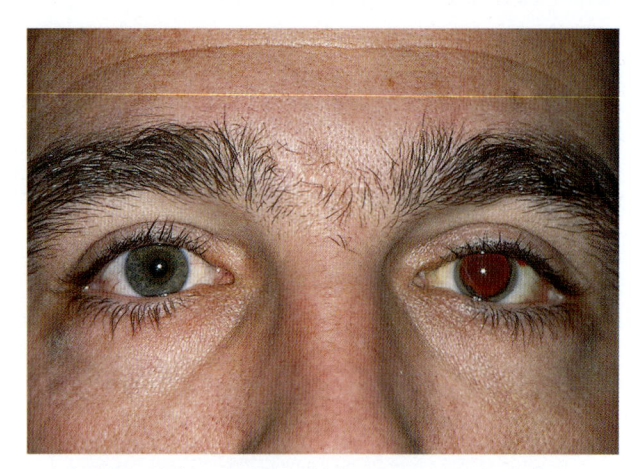

Figure 28.37. Slight proptosis of left eye in a 40-year-old man. The pupil was dilated pharmacologically at the time of the photograph.

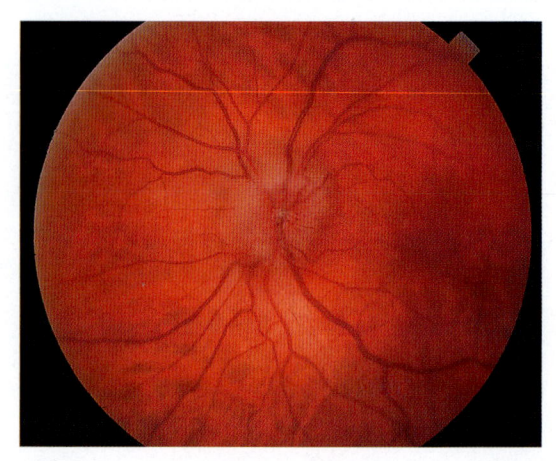

Figure 28.38. Optic disc edema secondary to optic nerve compression by the tumor.

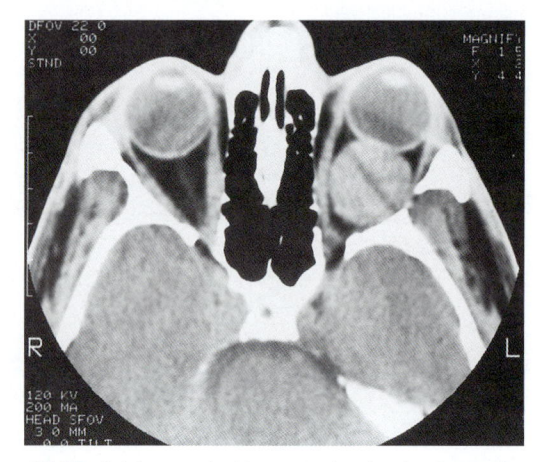

Figure 28.39. Axial computed tomography showing tumor in muscle cone.

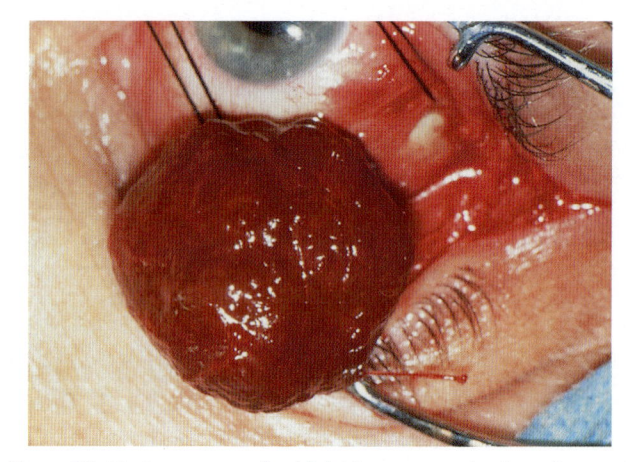

Figure 28.40. Appearance of reddish-blue tumor at the time of removal via an inferotemporal conjunctival incision.

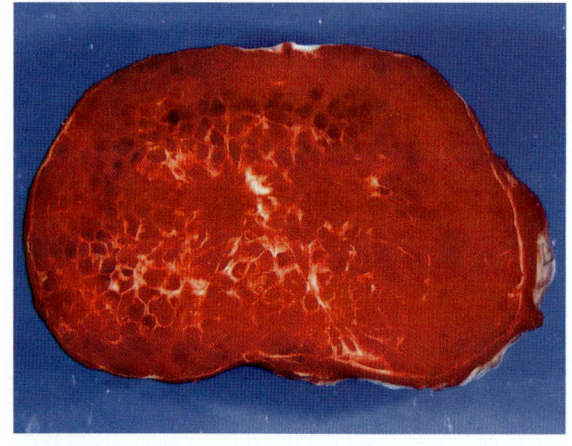

Figure 28.41. Gross appearance after sectioning showing red vascular tumor.

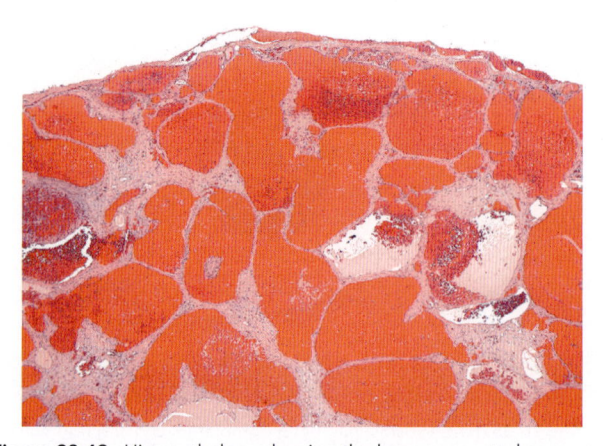

Figure 28.42. Histopathology showing the large congested cavernous vascular channels. (Hematoxylin–eosin ×20.)

Chapter 28 Orbital Vascular and Hemorrhagic Lesions

ORBITAL CAVERNOUS HEMANGIOMA: CLINICOPATHOLOGIC CORRELATION

Larger tumors in the muscle cone or tumors located laterally in the posterior aspect of the orbit can be removed by a superolateral orbitotomy with a skin incision and extraperiosteal approach. An osteotomy (Kronlein approach) is not usually necessary.

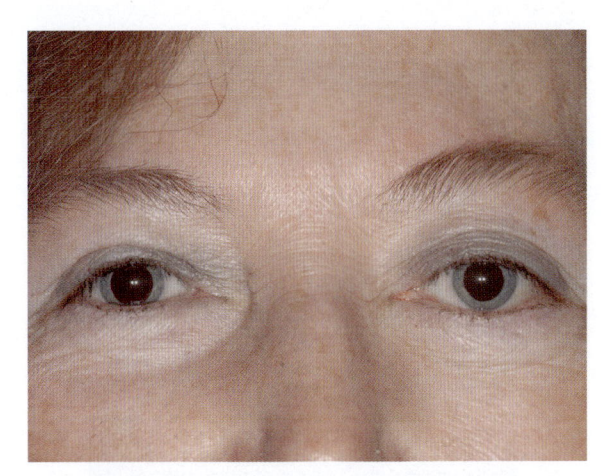

Figure 28.43. Minimal proptosis with mild visual blurring in a middle-aged woman.

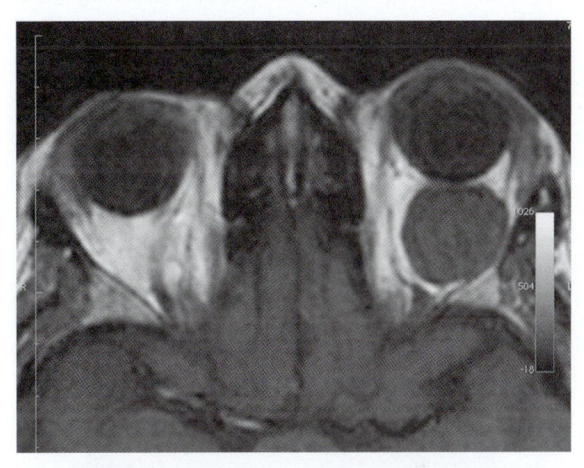

Figure 28.44. Same patient as in Figure 28.43, demonstrating T1-weighted magnetic resonance imaging of large intraconal mass.

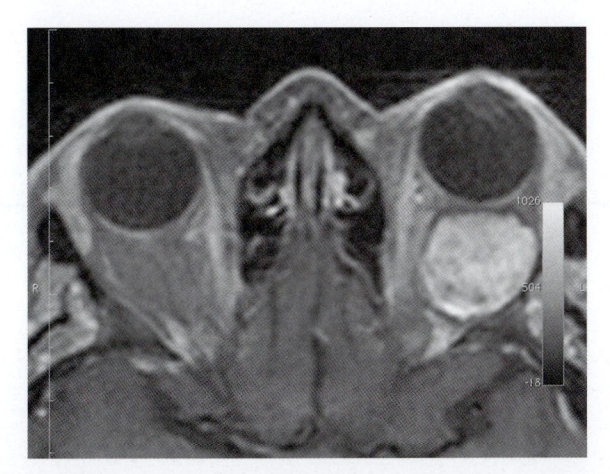

Figure 28.45. On gadolinium-enhanced T1-weighted magnetic resonance imaging, the mass shows bright enhancement.

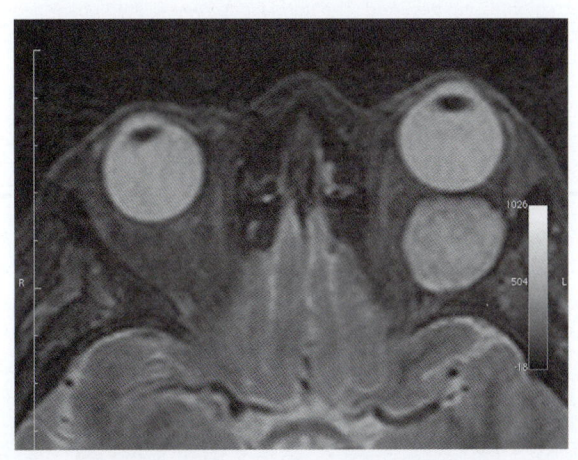

Figure 28.46. On T2-weighted images, the mass shows bright signal compared to vitreous.

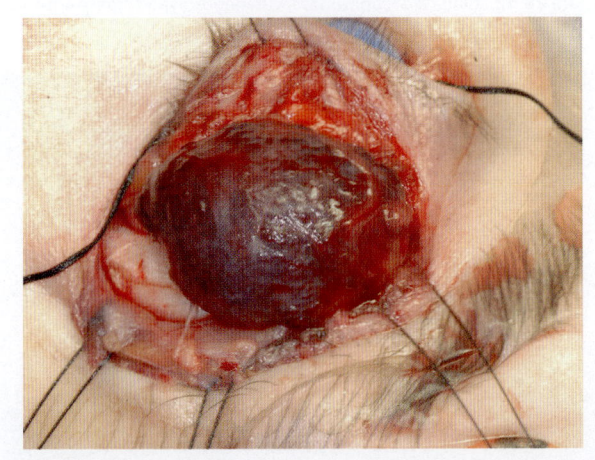

Figure 28.47. Superolateral orbitotomy via eyelid crease incision demonstrating the vascular mass at removal.

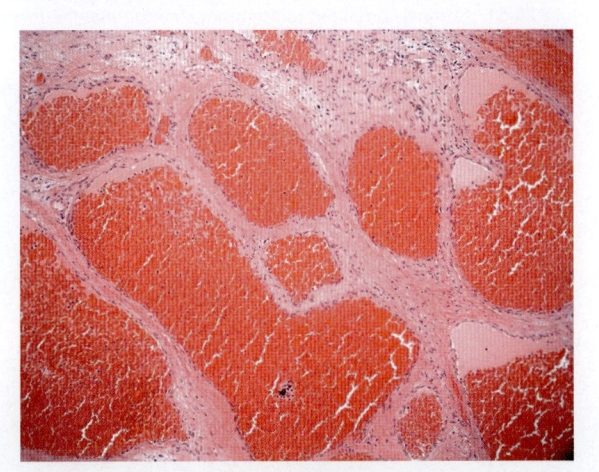

Figure 28.48. Histopathology showing large vascular lakes lined by endothelium and with intervening connective tissue consistent with benign cavernous hemangioma. (Hematoxylin–eosin ×50.)

TUMORS OF THE ORBIT

Part 3 Tumors of the Orbit

ORBITAL CAVERNOUS HEMANGIOMA: SUPERONASAL ORBITOTOMY

In cases where the tumor is nasal to the optic nerve, a superonasal orbitotomy can be employed. Although a conjunctival incision could have been used in the case shown, the skin–extraperiosteal approach offers better surgical exposure. This patient was seen several years ago; today, we may have used a conjunctival approach in such case.

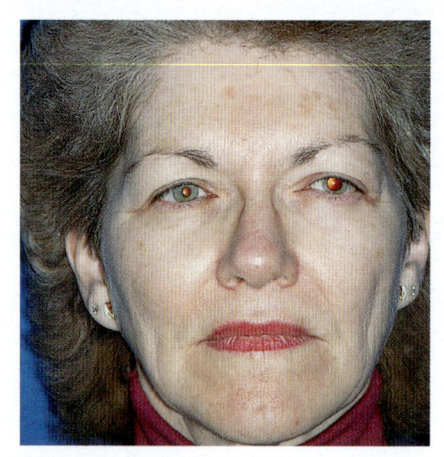

Figure 28.49. Proptosis of left eye in a 52-year-old woman. The patient was followed for 5 years previously and proptosis increased and optic disc compression occurred. The normal pupil was dilated pharmacologically at the time of the photograph.

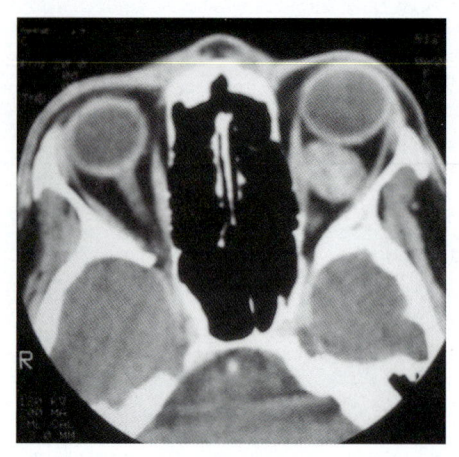

Figure 28.50. Axial computed tomography showing mass in the muscle cone.

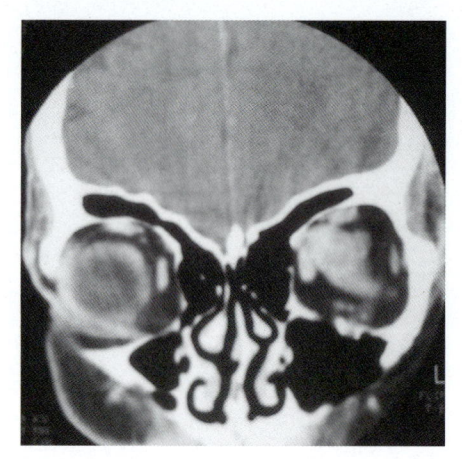

Figure 28.51. Coronal computed tomography showing that the mass is nasal to the optic nerve.

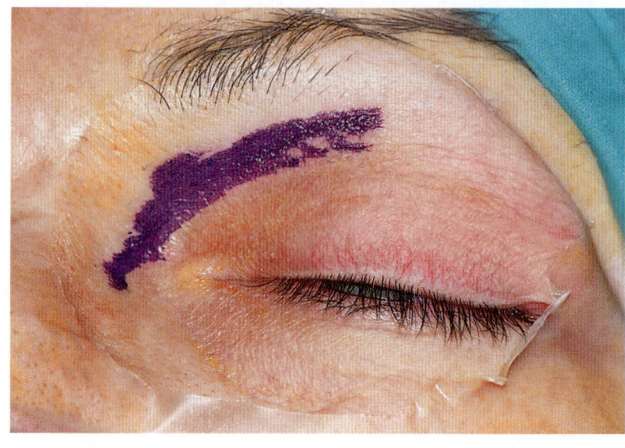

Figure 28.52. Outline of superonasal cutaneous eyelid crease approach.

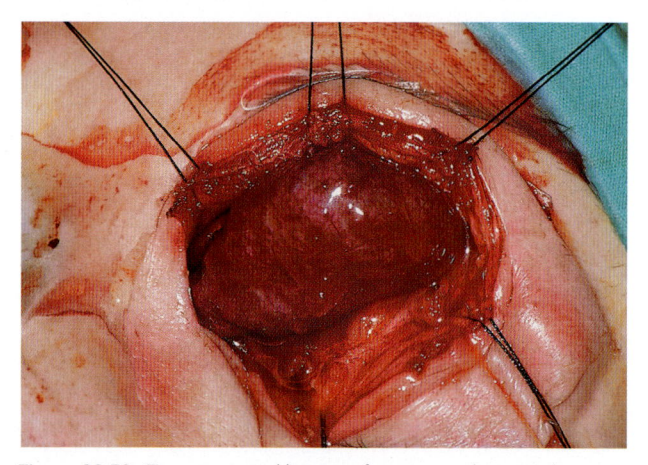

Figure 28.53. Tumor exposed by way of superonasal approach.

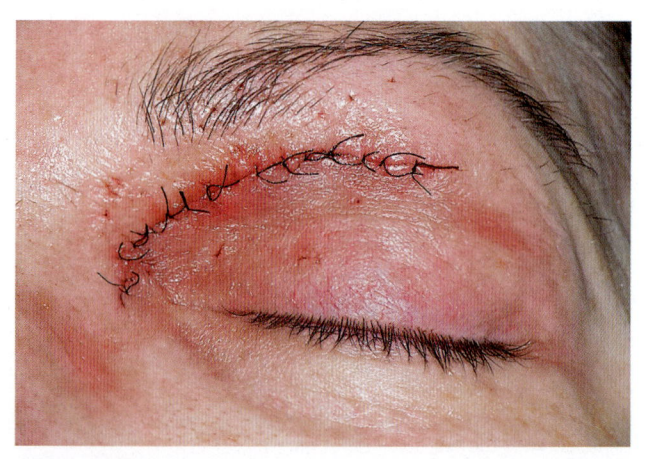

Figure 28.54. Appearance of wound after closure with interrupted 6-0 silk sutures. Today, the authors more often use absorbable 5-0 mild chromic sutures for closure.

Chapter 28 Orbital Vascular and Hemorrhagic Lesions 523

ORBITAL CAVERNOUS HEMANGIOMA: INTRAOSSEOUS TYPE

In rare instances, a cavernous hemangioma can occur in the bone, rather than being confined to the orbital soft tissues.

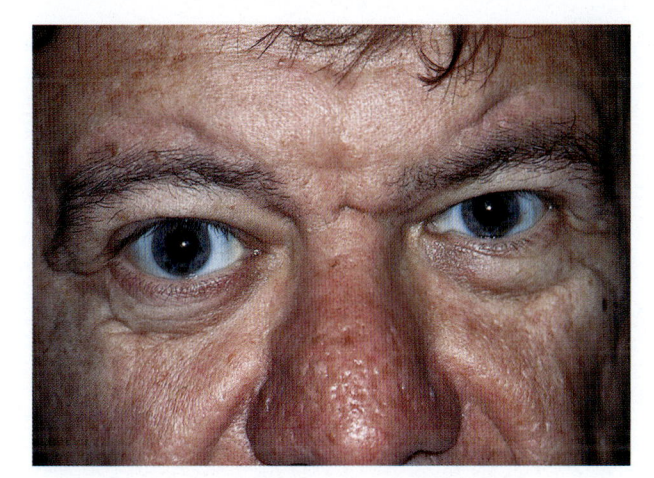

Figure 28.55. Proptosis of right eye in a 57-year-old man.

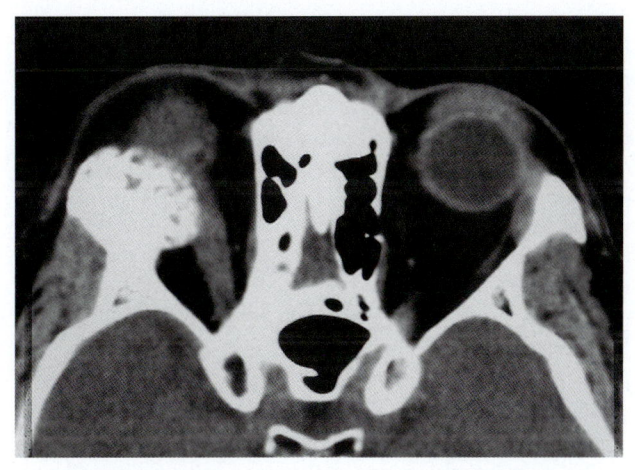

Figure 28.56. Axial computed tomography showing mass within bone on lateral aspect of orbit.

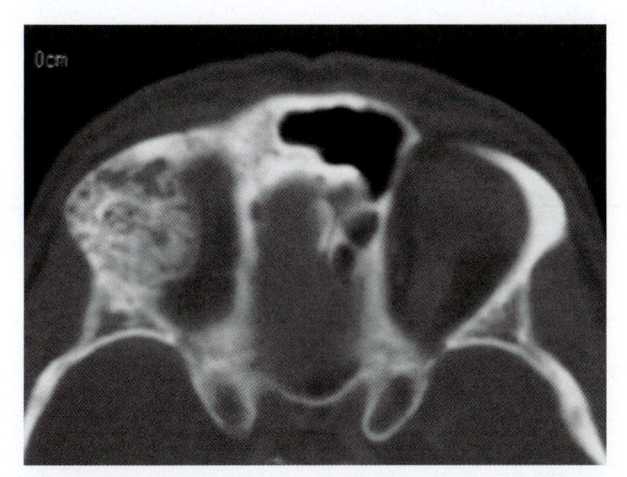

Figure 28.57. Axial computed tomography using bone window technique, showing the lesion.

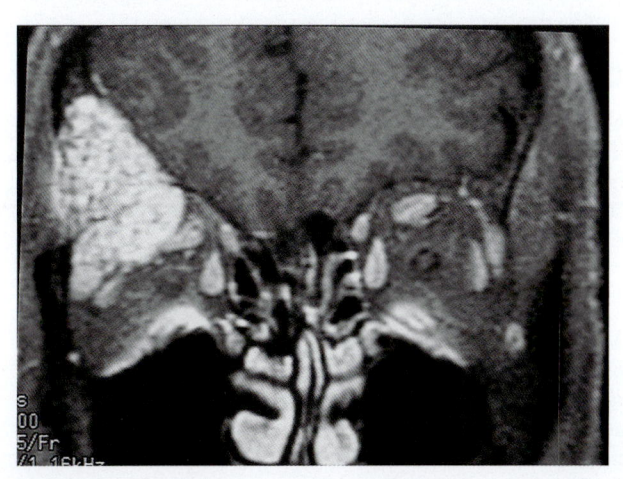

Figure 28.58. Coronal magnetic resonance imaging in T1-weighted image, showing superior extent of the mass.

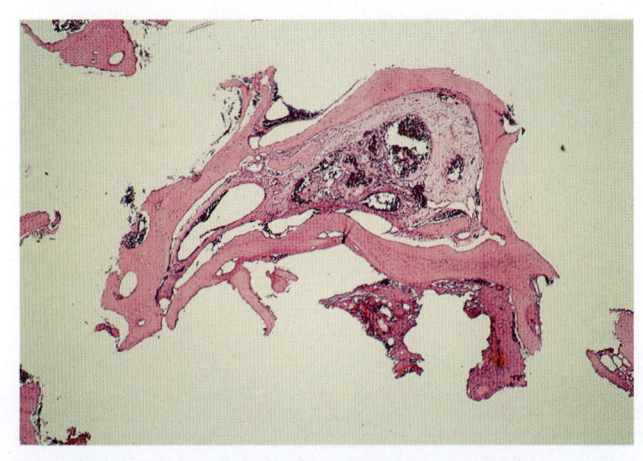

Figure 28.59. Histopathology of intraosseous cavernous hemangioma, showing vascular mass in the bone. (Hematoxylin–eosin ×5.)

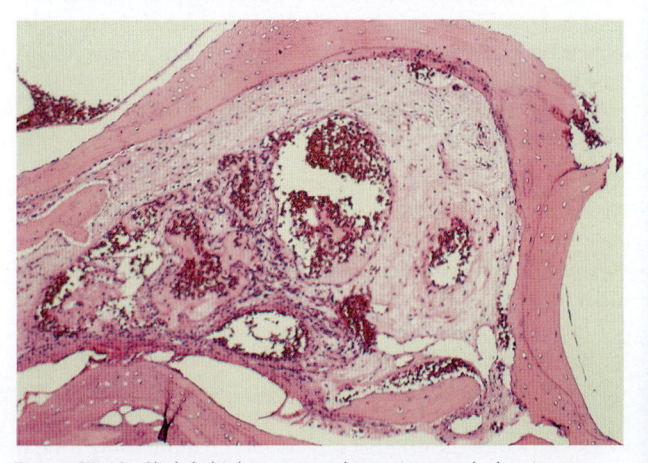

Figure 28.60. Slightly higher-power photomicrograph showing cavernous vascular channels. (Hematoxylin–eosin ×15.)

ORBITAL HEMANGIOPERICYTOMA

General Considerations
There are many published reports on orbital hemangiopericytoma (1–16), but recently there has been controversy about the existence of hemangiopericytoma. Its derivation from vascular pericytes has been questioned and cases have been reclassified as solitary fibrous tumor, based on histopathologic and immunohistochemical observations (7,8). Nevertheless, we have elected to follow tradition for now, and to discuss it under the category of vascular tumors. In the authors' series of 1,264 consecutive space-occupying lesions of the orbit, the 8 hemangiopericytomas accounted for 4% of orbital vascular tumors and for 1% of all lesions (1).

Clinical Features
Orbital hemangiopericytoma occurs mainly in adults and has similar symptoms, signs, and imaging study findings as cavernous hemangioma. With time, however, hemangiopericytoma can be more aggressive, extend throughout the orbit, and even invade the cranial cavity (10,12). About 30% of orbital hemangiopericytomas have histopathologic criteria compatible with malignancy, but distant metastasis is uncommon (5).

Diagnostic Approaches
Clinical features and results of MRI and CT are very similar to other circumscribed orbital tumors such as cavernous hemangioma, solitary fibrous tumor, fibrous histiocytoma, and schwannoma. The diagnosis is generally made histopathologically after surgical removal.

Pathology
Microscopically, hemangiopericytoma consists of spindle to ovoid cells surrounding thin-walled blood vessels lined by flattened endothelial cells (5). The vascular channels often assume a branching or "staghorn" configuration. The tumor is classified into sinusoidal, solid, or mixed patterns depending on the degree of vascularity between the tumor cells. Hemangiopericytoma may be very similar microscopically to solitary fibrous tumor, fibrous histiocytoma, malignant hemangioendothelioma, or angioblastic meningioma. As mentioned, immunohistochemistry and electron microscopy have not clearly established the nature of this neoplasm.

Management
The diagnosis of hemangiopericytoma cannot be made with certainty on clinical evaluation and depends on histopathologic confirmation. Management is the same as for other circumscribed primary tumors. If at all possible, complete excision of the tumor within its capsule should be performed. A tumor that cannot be completely removed has a tendency for late recurrence and more aggressive behavior. The selected approach to surgery should depend on the results of axial and coronal imaging studies. Orbital recurrence, which can develop many years after the original surgery, may require wider orbital exenteration, irradiation, or chemotherapy (6,11).

Selected References

Reviews
1. Shields JA, Shields CL, Scartozzi R. Survey of 1264 patients with orbital tumors and simulating lesions: The 2002 Montgomery Lecture, part 1. *Ophthalmology* 2004;111:997–1008.
2. Shields JA, Bakewell B, Augsburger JJ, et al. Classification and incidence of space-occupying lesions of the orbit. A survey of 645 biopsies. *Arch Ophthalmol* 1984;102:1606–1611.
3. Shields JA, Bakewell B, Augsburger JJ, et al. Space-occupying orbital masses in children: A review of 250 consecutive biopsies. *Ophthalmology* 1986;93:379–384.
4. Gunalp I, Gunduz K. Vascular tumors of the orbit. *Doc Ophthalmol* 1995;89:337–345.
5. Croxatto JO, Font RL. Hemangiopericytoma of the orbit: a clinicopathologic study of 30 cases. *Hum Pathol* 1982;13:210–218.

Management
6. Tijl JW, Koornneef L, Blank LE. Recurrent hemangiopericytoma and brachytherapy. *Doc Ophthalmol* 1992;82:103–107.

Histopathology
7. Goldsmith JD, van de Rijn M, Syed N. Orbital hemangiopericytoma and solitary fibrous tumor: a morphologic continuum. *Int J Surg Pathol* 2001;9:295–302.
8. Furusato E, Valenzuela IA, Fanburg-Smith JC, et al. Orbital solitary fibrous tumor: encompassing terminology for hemangiopericytoma, giant cell angiofibroma, and fibrous histiocytoma of the orbit: reappraisal of 41 cases. *Hum Pathol* 2011;42(1):120–128.

Case Reports
9. Rice CD, Kersten RC, Mrak RE. An orbital hemangiopericytoma recurrent after 33 years. *Arch Ophthalmol* 1989;107:552–556.
10. Kolawole TM, Patel PJ, Boshra Y, et al. Orbital and intracranial haemangiopericytoma. Case report with a short review. *Eur J Radiol* 1988;8:106–108.
11. Setzkorn RK, Lee DJ, Iliff NT, et al. Hemangiopericytoma of the orbit treated with conservative surgery and radiotherapy. *Arch Ophthalmol* 1987;105:1103–1105.
12. Shields JA, Shields CL, Rashid RC. Clinicopathologic correlation of choroidal folds secondary to massive cranio-orbital hemangiopericytoma. *Ophthal Plast Reconstr Surg* 1992;8:62–68.
13. Henderson JW, Farrow GM. Primary orbital hemangiopericytoma. An aggressive and potentially malignant neoplasm. *Arch Ophthalmol* 1978;96:666–673.
14. Jakobiec FA, Howard GM, Jones IS, et al. Hemangiopericytoma of the orbit. *Am J Ophthalmol* 1974;78:816–834.
15. Sullivan TJ, Wright JE, Wulc AE, et al. Haemangiopericytoma of the orbit. *Aust N Z J Ophthalmol* 1992;20:325–332.
16. Karcioglu ZA, Nasr AM, Haik BG. Orbital hemangiopericytoma: clinical and morphologic features. *Am J Ophthalmol* 1997;124:661–672.

Chapter 28 Orbital Vascular and Hemorrhagic Lesions

● ORBITAL HEMANGIOPERICYTOMA: CLINICOPATHOLOGIC CORRELATION

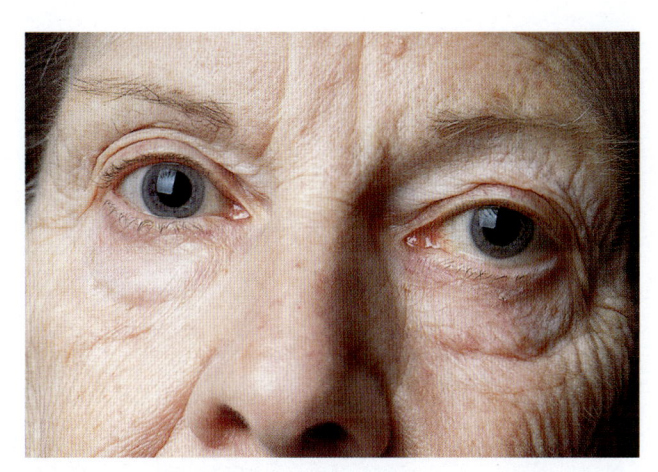

Figure 28.61. Proptosis of the left eye in a 72-year-old woman.

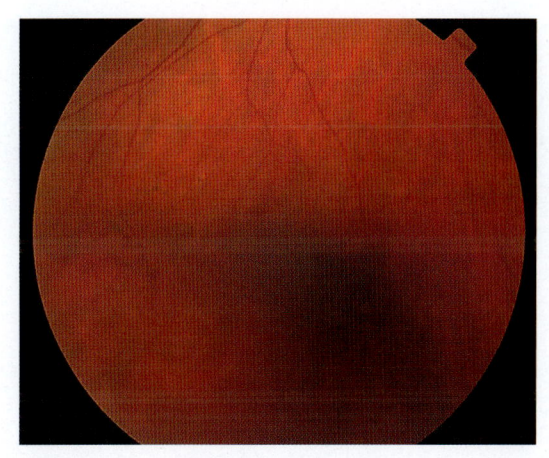

Figure 28.62. Fundus photograph showing compression of the globe inferiorly, simulating a pigmented intraocular tumor.

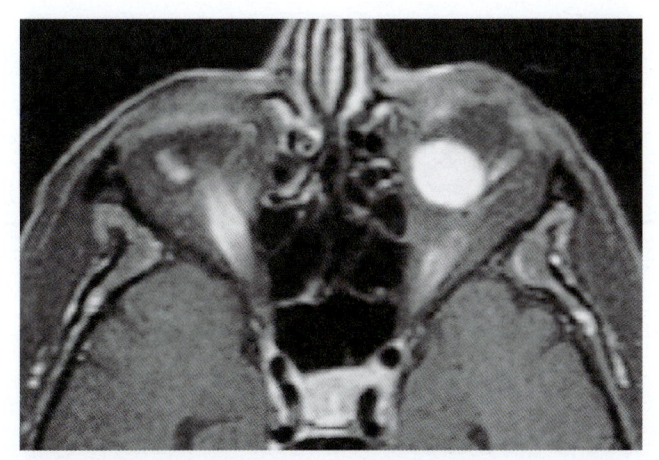

Figure 28.63. Contrast-enhanced axial magnetic resonance imaging in T1-weighted image demonstrating enhancing mass in left orbit.

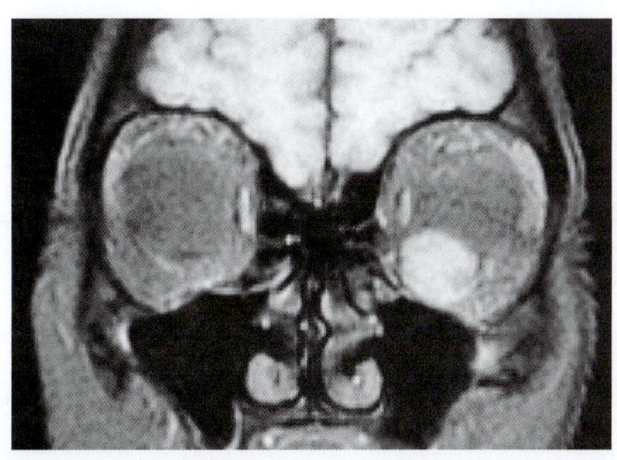

Figure 28.64. Contrast-enhanced coronal magnetic resonance imaging in T1-weighted image showing mass inferior to the globe.

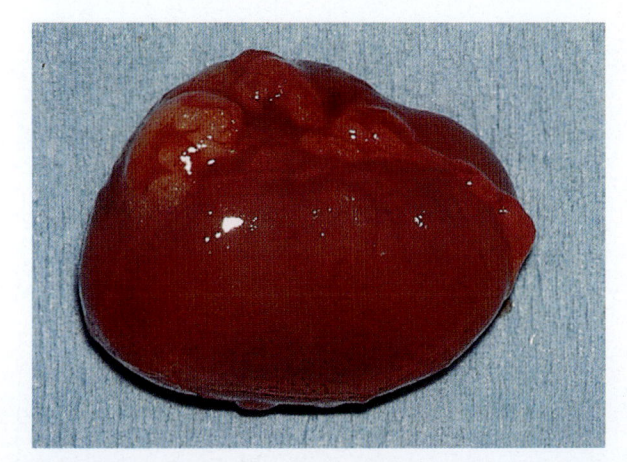

Figure 28.65. Circumscribed red tumor after surgical removal by way of a conjunctival approach.

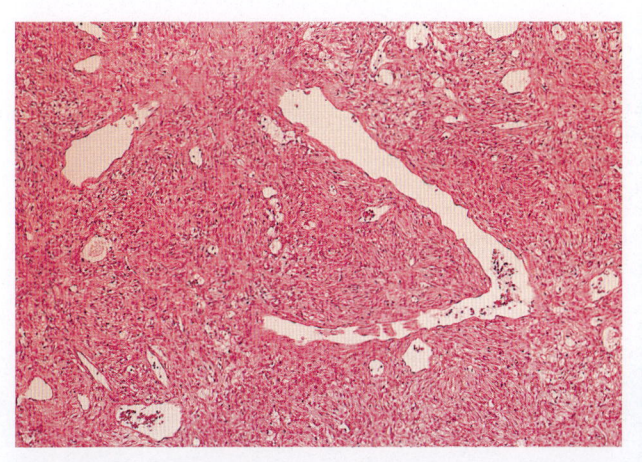

Figure 28.66. Histopathology showing solid vascular lesion with typical "staghorn" branching of the blood vessels. (Hematoxylin–eosin ×50.)

ORBITAL HEMANGIOPERICYTOMA: CLINICOPATHOLOGIC CORRELATION

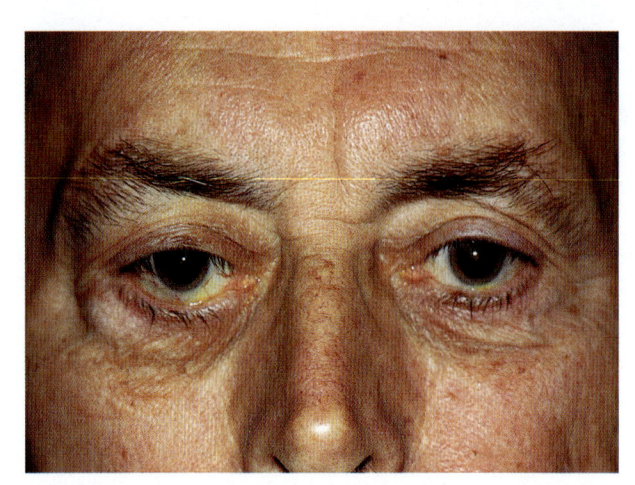

Figure 28.67. Proptosis of the right eye in a 63-year-old man.

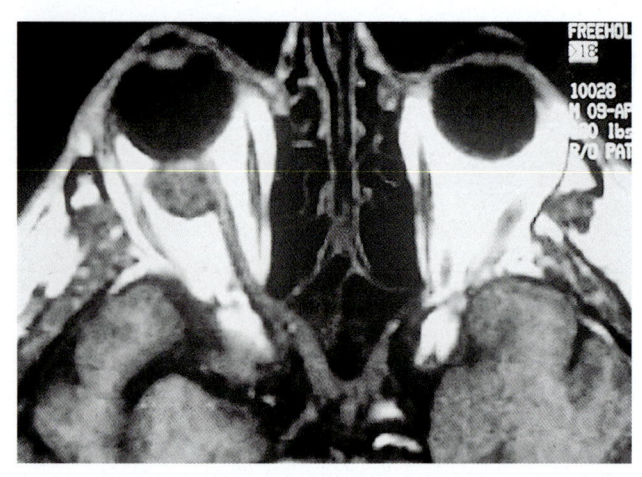

Figure 28.68. Axial MRI in T1-weighted image showing retrobulbar mass compressing the globe.

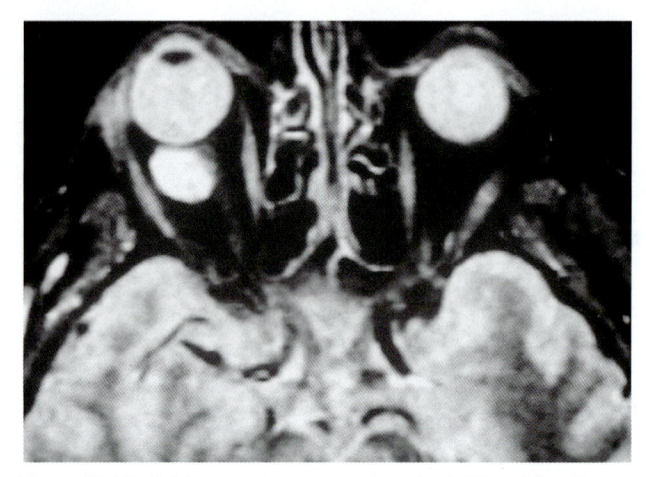

Figure 28.69. Axial magnetic resonance imaging in T2-weighted image showing retrobulbar mass hyperintense to the vitreous.

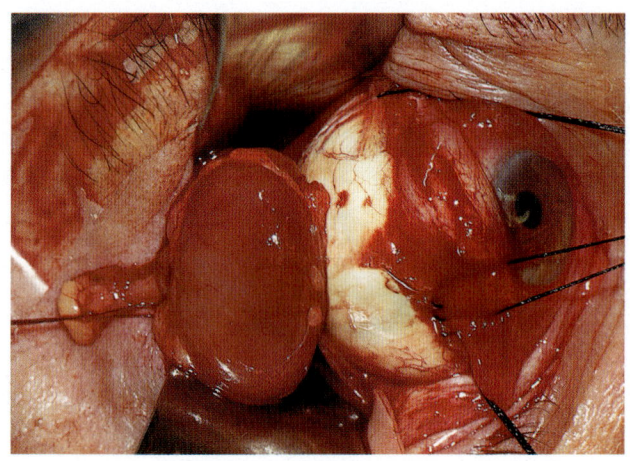

Figure 28.70. Appearance of the red circumscribed mass at the time of surgical removal through a conjunctival approach.

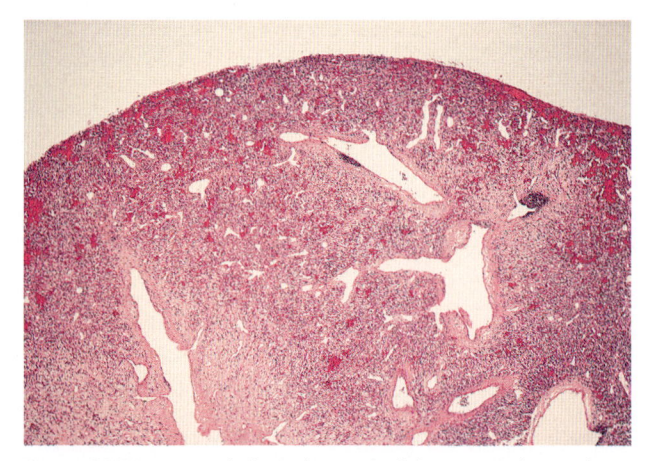

Figure 28.71. Histopathology showing solid tumor with "staghorn" branching pattern to the larger blood vessels. (Hematoxylin–eosin ×25.)

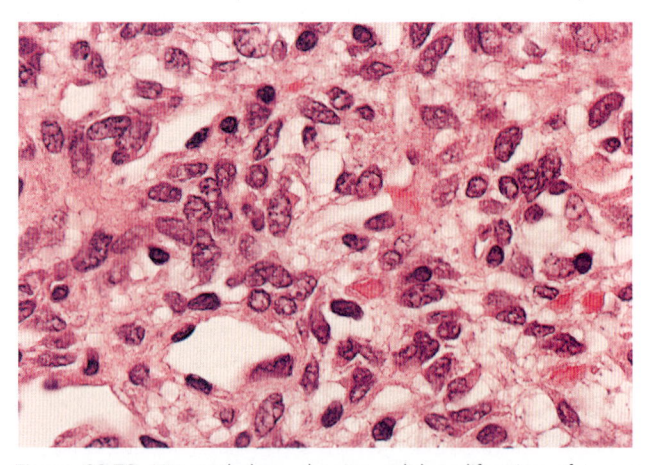

Figure 28.72. Histopathology showing solid proliferation of tumor cells. (Hematoxylin–eosin ×200.)

ORBITAL HEMANGIOPERICYTOMA: AGGRESSIVE TUMOR WITH BRAIN INVASION

In some instances, hemangiopericytoma can undergo malignant transformation and can be locally invasive. Distant metastasis can occasionally develop. A clinicopathologic correlation is shown.

Shields JA, Shields CL, Rashid RC. Clinicopathologic correlation of choroidal folds: secondary to massive cranioorbital hemangiopericytoma. *Ophthal Plast Reconstr Surg* 1992;8:62–68.

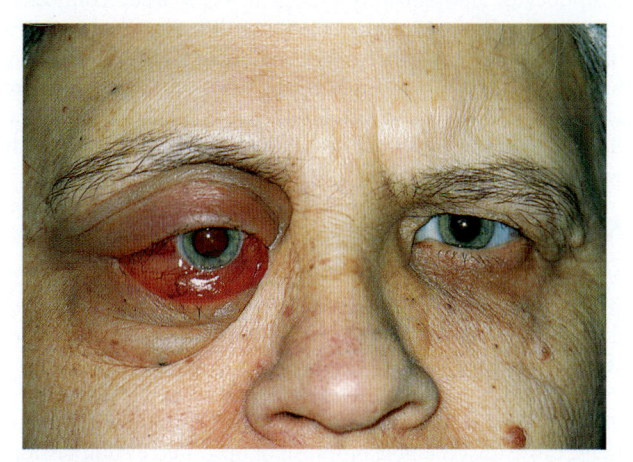

Figure 28.73. Marked proptosis and chemosis of right eye in a 56-year-old woman.

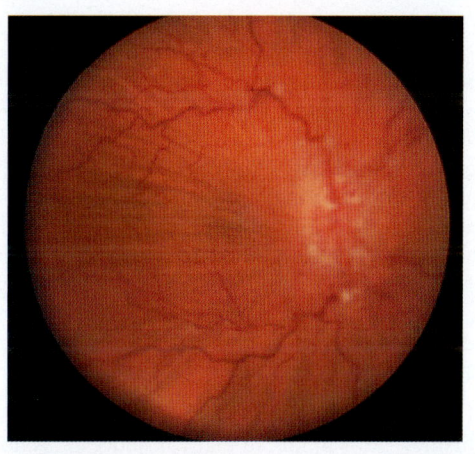

Figure 28.74. Fundus photograph showing optic disc edema and marked choroidal folds secondary to compression of the posterior aspect of the globe by the orbital tumor.

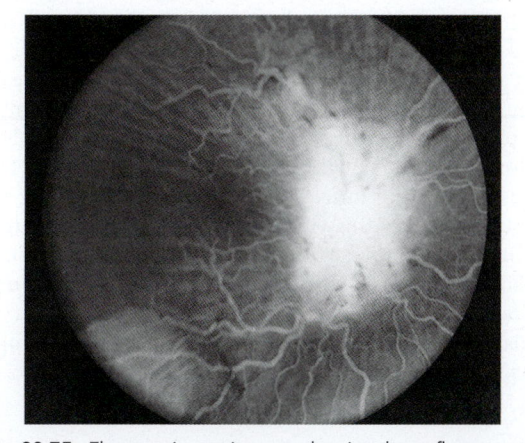

Figure 28.75. Fluorescein angiogram showing hyperfluorescence of the optic disc and radiating choroidal folds.

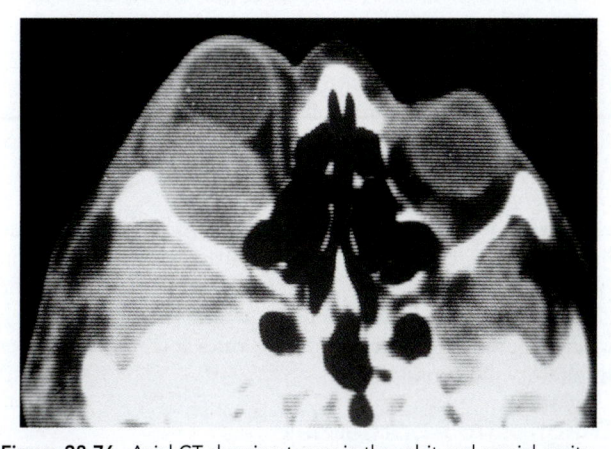

Figure 28.76. Axial CT showing tumor in the orbit and cranial cavity.

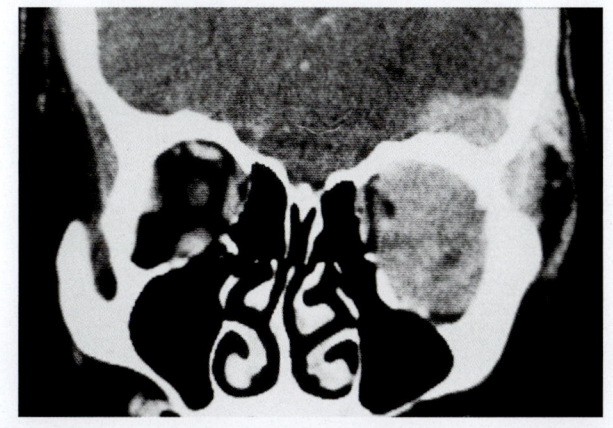

Figure 28.77. Coronal CT further delineating the extent of the tumor. It was removed by orbital exenteration and craniotomy.

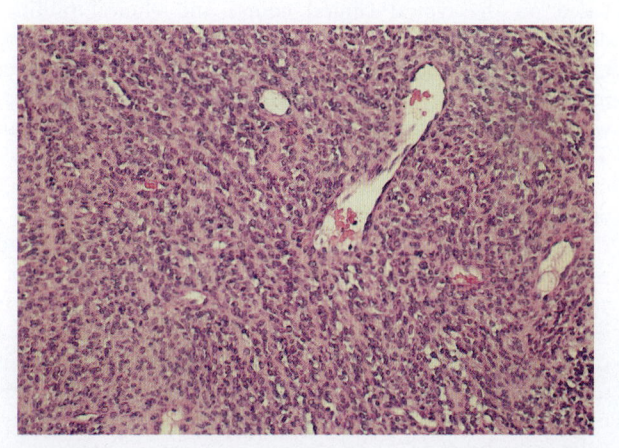

Figure 28.78. Histopathology showing characteristic pattern of hemangiopericytoma. (Hematoxylin–eosin ×50.)

ORBITAL LYMPHANGIOMA

General Considerations

Lymphangioma is a benign vascular lesion that frequently affects the orbit (1–19). In the authors' clinical series of 1,264 consecutive space-occupying orbital lesions, the 54 lymphangiomas accounted for 25% of the 213 vascular lesions and for 4% of all orbital lesions (1). Orbital lymphangioma is probably congenital, but may not become clinically apparent for months or years after birth. In some cases, lymphangioma may be diffuse or multifocal. Such cases may be familial. There has also been controversy with regard to the classification and nomenclature of lymphangioma. Some authorities believe that lymphangioma and varix are very similar or identical lesions (9), whereas others believe they are separate entities (8). We tend to regard them as separate conditions even though there may be some overlap clinically and histopathologically.

Clinical Features

Orbital lymphangioma usually has its clinical onset in children in the first few years of life. In many instances, it is not recognized until the teenage years, when the patient presents with abrupt proptosis, blepharoptosis, and periocular soft tissue swelling or ecchymosis from spontaneous or traumatic hemorrhage. We have also seen several patients whose lymphangioma first became apparent in adulthood and even old age. A conjunctival component, appearing as multiple clear or hemorrhagic cysts, is commonly present and that finding alone should suggest the underlying orbital lesion. These cystic structures filled with blood are seen clinically and/or at the time of surgery and account for the term "chocolate cyst" that is often used to describe this condition. Affected patients may have lymphangiomas elsewhere, particularly on the palate, and such a finding should also suggest the orbital diagnosis. The abrupt hemorrhage in the orbit may gradually resolve and then recur. Proptosis may increase in some cases at the time of upper respiratory infection (10).

Diagnostic Approaches

In most instances, orbital lymphangioma can be suspected based on the typical clinical course and clinical findings described. In addition, MRI and CT show suggestive features that can establish the diagnosis without resorting to an immediate biopsy. The hemorrhagic cystlike spaces, sometimes with a blood–plasma level within the cyst and best seen on T2-weighted MRI, is very suggestive of the diagnosis. However, it should be remembered that hemorrhagic cysts can occur in malignant tumors, such as rhabdomyosarcoma.

Deep orbital lymphangioma can sometimes be round and well defined, simulating cavernous hemangioma. The differentiation is important because dissection of lymphangioma is associated with more complications than surgical excision of a cavernous hemangioma. Orbital lymphangioma has also been seen in association with orbital and intracranial arteriovenous malformation, suggesting an extensive maldevelopment of vascular embryogenesis (6).

Pathology

Histopathologically, lymphangioma consists of dilated ectatic vascular channels filled with clear fluid or blood. Inflammatory lymphocytes are frequently present in the delicate connective tissue septa. The pathogenesis is not well understood and it is difficult to state whether lymphangioma is a true neoplasm, hamartoma, or lymphangiectasia. Some authorities regard lymphangioma as a malformation that arises from sequestration of lymphatic tissue that fails to communicate normally with the lymphatic system.

Management

Management of orbital lymphangioma can be difficult, because complete surgical resection is often not possible owing to poor definition of the lesion and excessive bleeding at the time of surgical manipulation. If visual acuity is not threatened in a young child, a period of observation, allowing the acute hemorrhage to resolve, is warranted. If massive tumor and hemorrhage cause unacceptable proptosis or optic nerve compression, then treatment should be considered. Large hemorrhagic cysts can be aspirated through the eyelid or conjunctiva to provide temporary relief. If malignancy, such as rhabdomyosarcoma, is a diagnostic possibility, exploration with open biopsy is warranted. If surgery is done, the tumor should be debulked as much as possible without damaging the optic nerve or extraocular muscles. The carbon dioxide laser has been used in some cases to control bleeding and facilitate tumor removal (15).

More recently, vascular malformations have been treated with aspiration and intralesional injection of sclerosing agents or tissue glue (16–18). We have found tissue glue a temporary measure but can provide tumor reduction for several months to occasionally a few years. Sclerosing agents are more lasting, but require interventional neuroradiology for localization. Oral sildenafil has been explored to soften and involute lymphangioma (19).

ORBITAL LYMPHANGIOMA

Selected References

Reviews

1. Shields JA, Shields CL, Scartozzi R. Survey of 1264 patients with orbital tumors and simulating lesions: The 2002 Montgomery Lecture, part 1. *Ophthalmology* 2004;111:997–1008.
2. Shields JA, Bakewell B, Augsburger JJ, et al. Classification and incidence of space-occupying lesions of the orbit. A survey of 645 biopsies. *Arch Ophthalmol* 1984;102:1606–1611.
3. Shields JA, Bakewell B, Augsburger JJ, et al. Space-occupying orbital masses in children: A review of 250 consecutive biopsies. *Ophthalmology* 1986;93:379–384.
4. Gunalp I, Gunduz K. Vascular tumors of the orbit. *Doc Ophthalmol* 1995;89:337–345.
5. Rootman J. Orbital venous anomalies. *Ophthalmology* 1998;105:387–388.
6. Katz SE, Rootman J, Vangveeravong S, et al. Combined venous lymphatic malformations of the orbit (so-called lymphangiomas). Association with noncontiguous intracranial vascular anomalies. *Ophthalmology* 1998;105:176–184.
7. Rootman J, Hay E, Graeb D, et al. Orbital-adnexal lymphangiomas. A spectrum of hemodynamically isolated vascular hamartomas. *Ophthalmology* 1986;93:1558–1570.
8. Garrity JA. Orbital venous anomalies. A long-standing dilemma. *Ophthalmology* 1997;104:903–904.
9. Wright JE, Sullivan TJ, Garner A, et al. Orbital venous anomalies. *Ophthalmology* 1997;104:905–913.
10. Iliff WJ, Green WR. Orbital lymphangiomas. *Ophthalmology* 1979;86:914–929.
11. Harris GJ, Sakol PJ, Bonavolonta G, et al. An analysis of thirty cases of orbital lymphangioma. *Ophthalmology* 1990;97:1583–1592.
12. Harris GJ. Orbital vascular malformations: a consensus statement on terminology and its clinical implications. Orbital Society. *Am J Ophthalmol* 1999;127:453–455.
13. Harris GJ. Orbital venous anomalies. *Ophthalmology* 1998;105:388–389.
14. Shields JA, Shields CL. Orbital cysts of childhood. classification, clinical features, and management. *Surv Ophthalmol* 2004;49:281–299.

Management

15. Kennerdell JS, Maroon JC, Garrity JA, et al. Surgical management of orbital lymphangioma with the carbon dioxide laser. *Am J Ophthalmol* 1986;102:308–314.
16. Yue H, Qian J, Elner VM, et al. Treatment of orbital vascular malformations with intralesional injection of pingyangmycin. *Br J Ophthalmol* 2013;97(6):739–745.
17. Boulos PR, Harissi-Dagher M, Kavalec C, et al. Intralesional injection of Tisseel fibrin glue for resection of lymphangiomas and other thin-walled orbital cysts. *Ophthal Plast Reconstr Surg* 2005;21(3):171–176.
18. Hill RH, Shiels WE, Foster JA, et al. Percutaneous drainage and ablation as first line therapy for macrocystic and microcystic orbital lymphatic malformations. *Ophthal Plast Reconstr Surg* 2012;28:119–125.
19. Gandhi NG, Lin LK, O'Hara M. Sildenafil for pediatric orbital lymphangioma. *JAMA Ophthalmol* 2013;131:1228–1230.

ORBITAL LYMPHANGIOMA: CLINICAL AND PATHOLOGIC FEATURES

Patients with lymphangioma can experience intermittent episodes of abrupt proptosis usually owing to spontaneous or traumatic hemorrhage in the tumor and sometimes secondary to inflammation of lymphoid tissue in the tumor at the time of systemic infection.

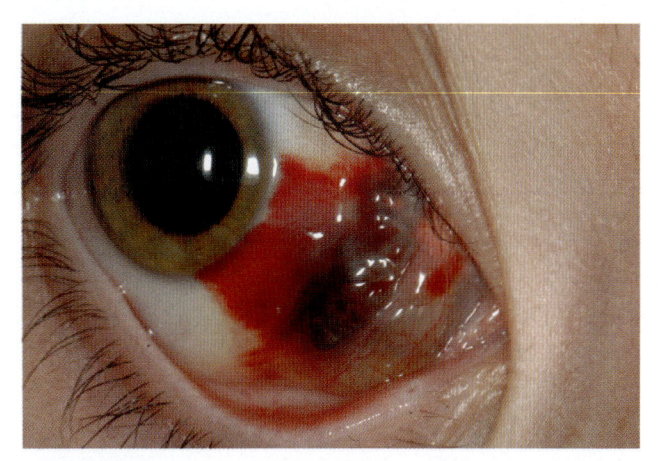

Figure 28.79. Hemorrhagic proptosis from orbital lymphangioma in a 9-year-old girl.

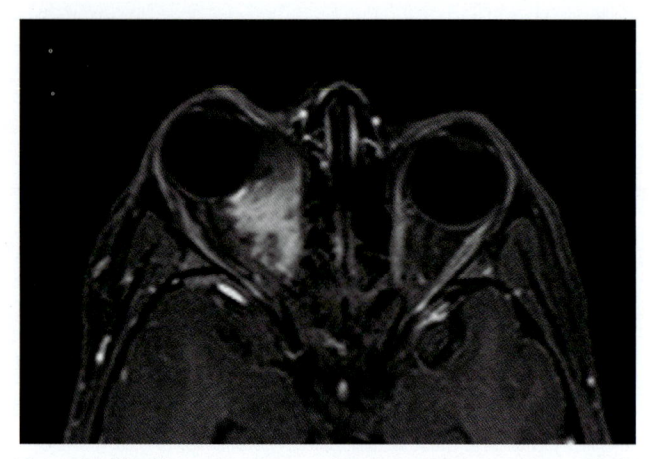

Figure 28.80. Magnetic resonance imaging of patient in Figure 28.79, demonstrating the medial orbital lymphangioma.

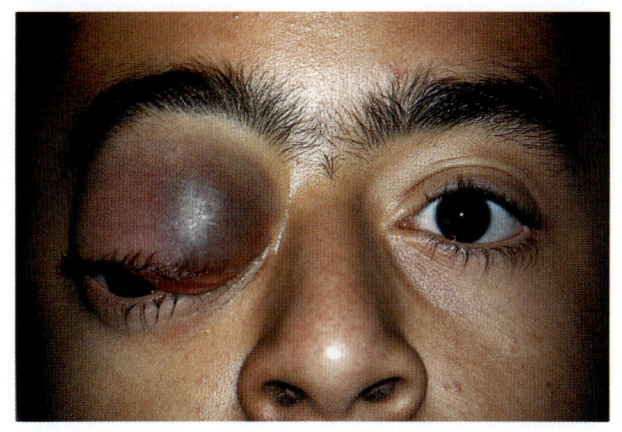

Figure 28.81. Conjunctival involvement by anterior extension of orbital lymphangioma allowing direct visualization of the lesion. Note the diffuse cystic, hemorrhagic nature of the conjunctival component and the blue discoloration to the adjacent lower eyelid.

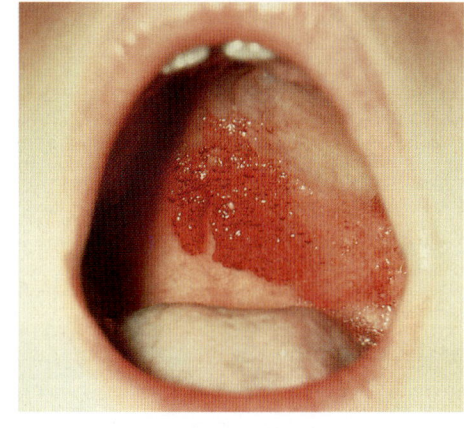

Figure 28.82. Involvement of the hard palate by lymphangioma in a patient with orbital lymphangioma. (Courtesy of Richard Margolies, MD.)

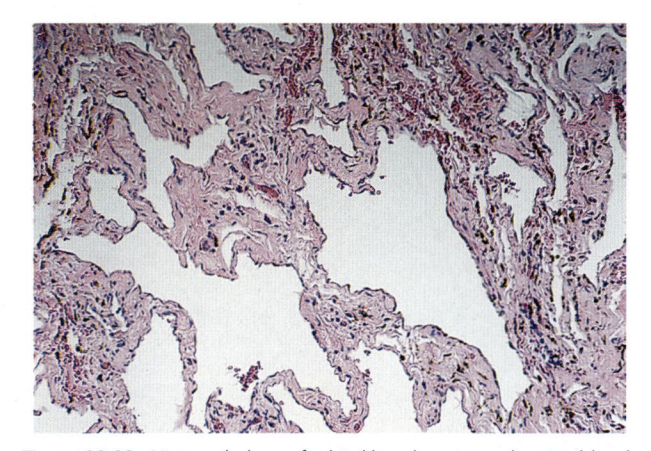

Figure 28.83. Histopathology of orbital lymphangioma showing bloodless, ectatic vascular channels with delicate connective tissue septa. (Hematoxylin–eosin ×40.)

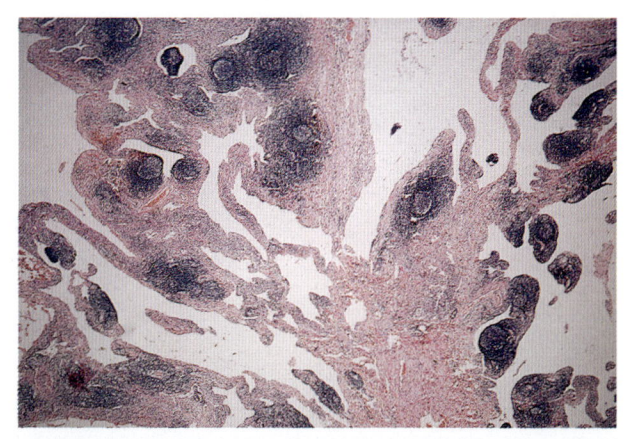

Figure 28.84. Histopathology of another case of orbital lymphangioma showing lymphoid tissue in the connective tissue septae. This lymphoid tissue, like the tonsils, is said to proliferate at the time of upper respiratory infection, making the proptosis worse. (Hematoxylin–eosin ×40.)

Chapter 28 Orbital Vascular and Hemorrhagic Lesions 531

ORBITAL LYMPHANGIOMA: CT AND MRI

CT and MRI studies show very characteristic features in cases of orbital lymphangioma. There is an ill-defined multicystic mass with blood in many of the cysts.

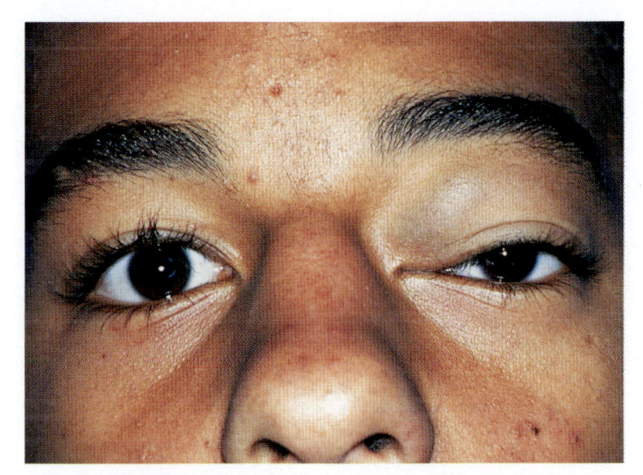

Figure 28.85. Blepharoptosis and fullness of left upper eyelid in a 17-year-old man.

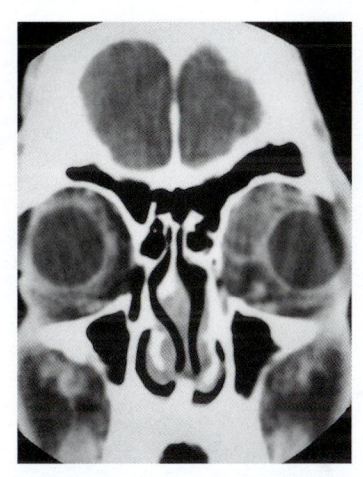

Figure 28.86. Coronal computed tomography of patient shown in Figure 28.85, demonstrating the diffuse, cystic mass superonasal to the globe.

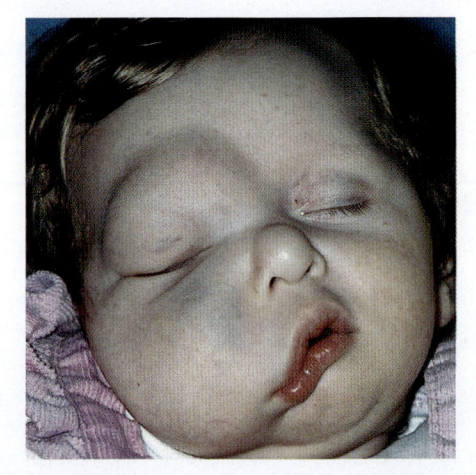

Figure 28.87. Massive orbital and subcutaneous lymphangioma around right eye of a 3-month-old girl.

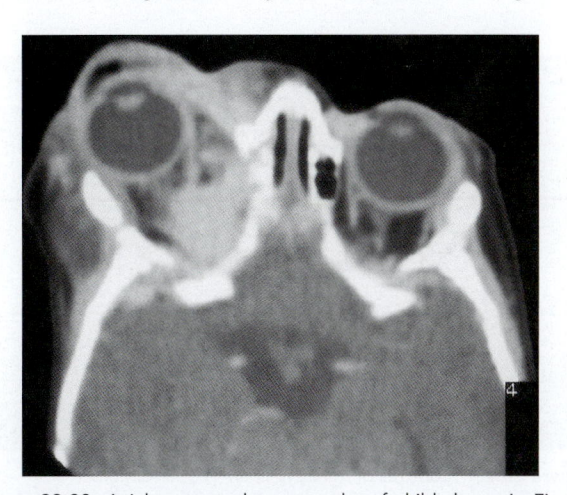

Figure 28.88. Axial computed tomography of child shown in Figure 28.87, revealing diffuse orbital involvement by a multicystic mass.

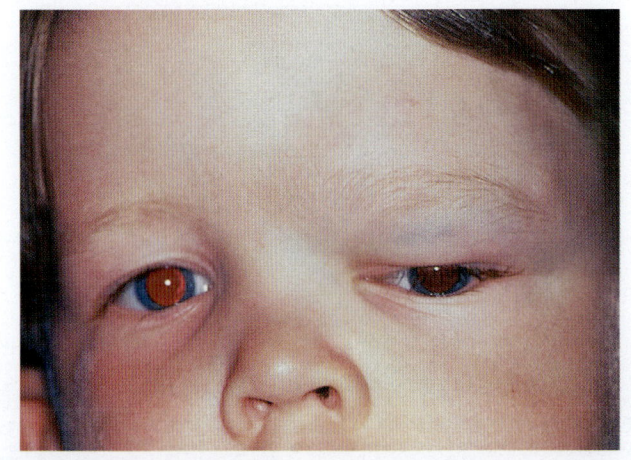

Figure 28.89. Orbital and periocular involvement of left eye in a 3-year-old boy.

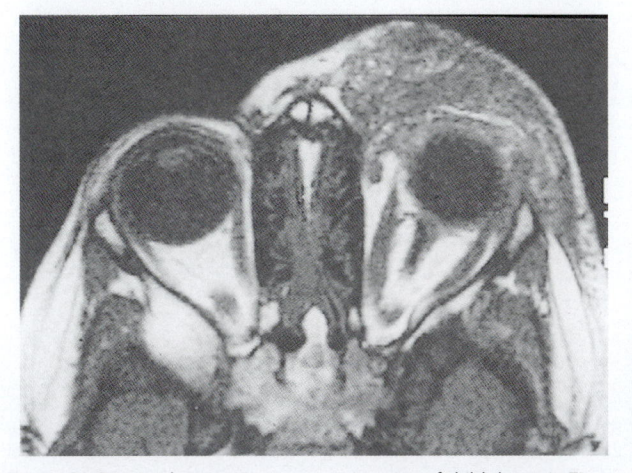

Figure 28.90. Axial magnetic resonance imaging of child shown in Figure 28.89, depicting a diffuse mass anterior and superior to the left eye. The lesion was presumed to be a lymphangioma, but no biopsy was done.

ORBITAL LYMPHANGIOMA: MRI FEATURES AND MANAGEMENT BY ASPIRATION

In some cases, a large hemorrhagic cyst can be identified and aspirated, thus relieving the proptosis without the danger of extensive surgical intervention.

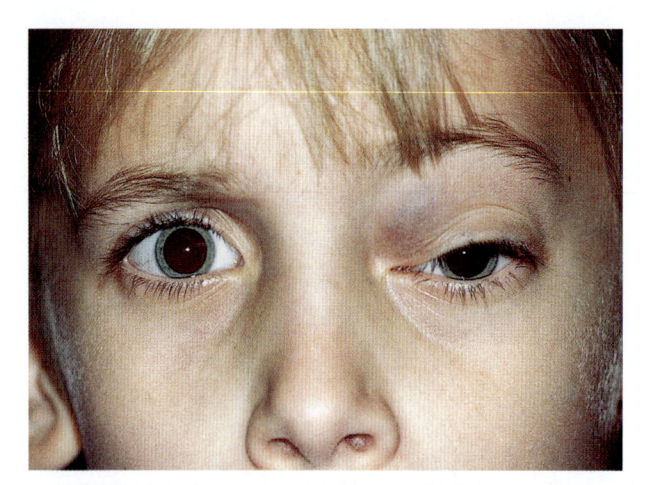

Figure 28.91. Blepharoptosis and fullness of left lower eyelid and downward displacement of the left eye in an 8-year-old boy.

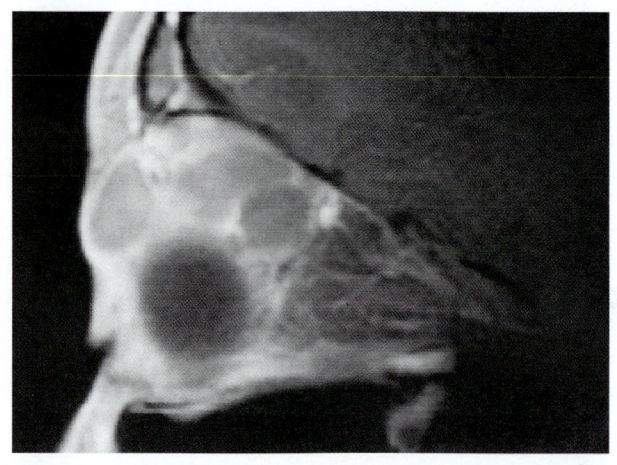

Figure 28.92. Sagittal magnetic resonance imaging in T1-weighted image of child shown in Figure 28.91, revealing extensive multicystic mass involving most of the superior orbit.

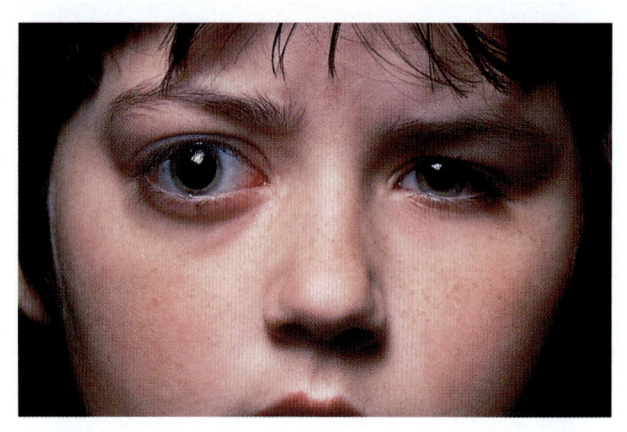

Figure 28.93. Proptosis of right eye in an 11-year-old girl.

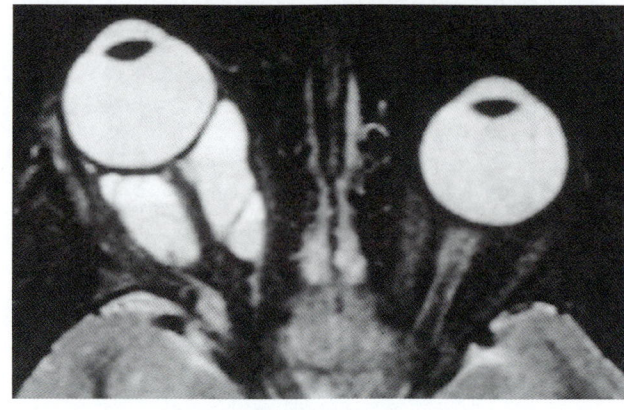

Figure 28.94. Axial magnetic resonance imaging in T2-weighted image of child shown in Figure 28.93, revealing large orbital cysts with a characteristic blood–plasma level.

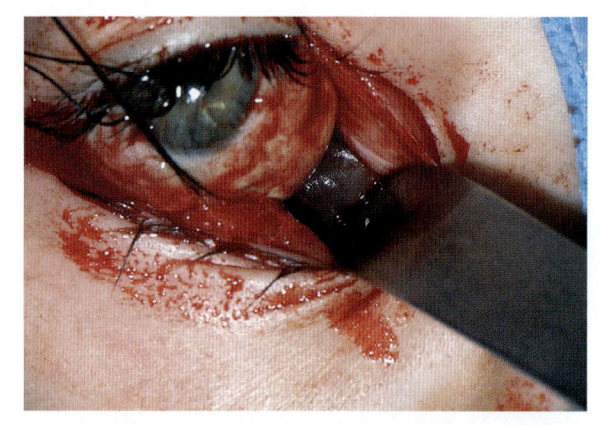

Figure 28.95. Identification of the blood-filled cyst shown in Figure 28.94 after conjunctival forniceal incision and retraction of conjunctival and orbital tissue.

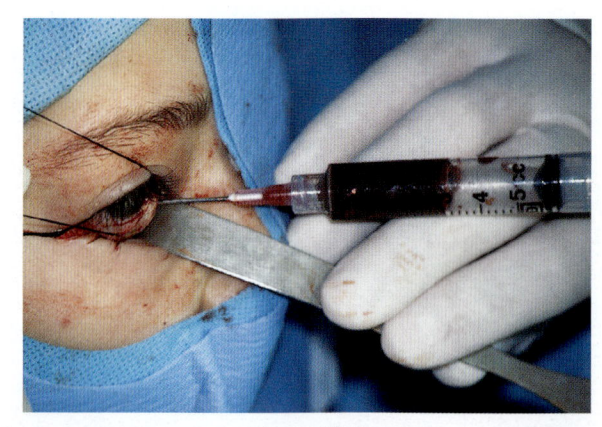

Figure 28.96. Aspiration of blood-filled cyst. This procedure often results in immediate reversal of much of the proptosis. Recurrence after such aspiration may not occur, or may take months or years to develop.

ORBITAL LYMPHANGIOMA: OCCURRENCE IN AN INFANT

Although most orbital lymphangiomas become clinically apparent in slightly older children, this lesion can sometimes be present at birth. A clinicopathologic correlation is illustrated. Although we consider the lesion to be a lymphangioma, some pathologists favored the diagnosis of varix. It may not be possible in many cases to differentiate these two conditions.

Foroozan R, Shields CL, Shields JA, et al. Congenital orbital varices causing extreme neonatal proptosis. *Am J Ophthalmol* 2000;129:693–694.

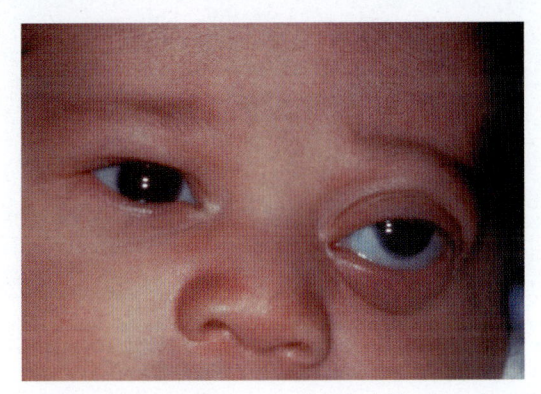

Figure 28.97. Appearance of 1-month-old child with left proptosis owing to orbital lymphangioma.

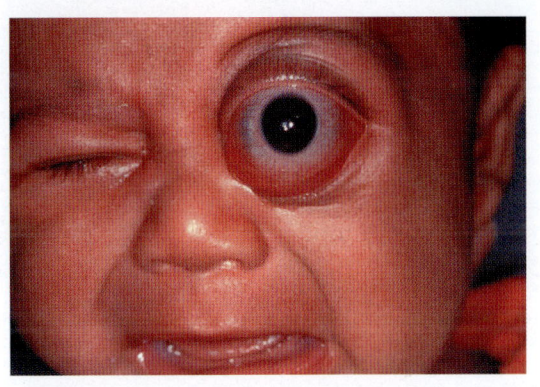

Figure 28.98. Appearance 2 months later showing worsening of proptosis.

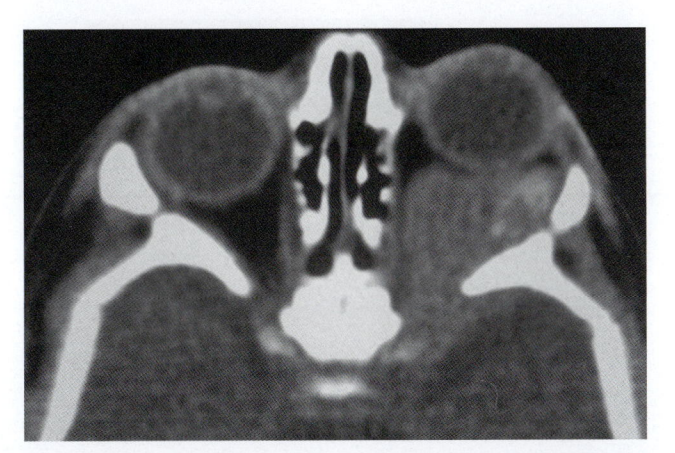

Figure 28.99. Axial magnetic resonance imaging in T1-weighted image demonstrating diffuse mass filling entire orbit with slight extension into the brain.

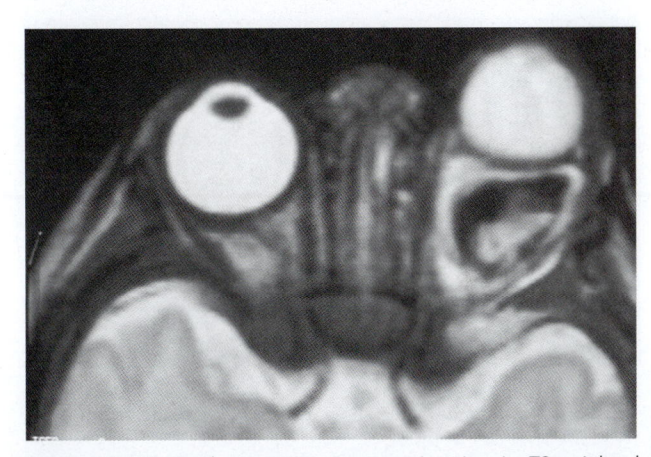

Figure 28.100. Axial magnetic resonance imaging in T2-weighted image better demonstrating the large cysts within the mass. The mass was removed by extensive debulking.

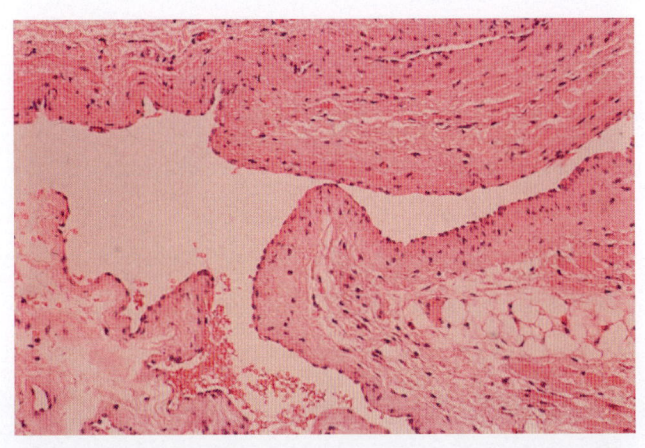

Figure 28.101. Histopathology reveals vascular spaces lined by endothelial cells. Most of the blood that was in the channels was washed out during surgery and processing, but some erythrocytes are present inferiorly. (Hematoxylin–eosin ×20.)

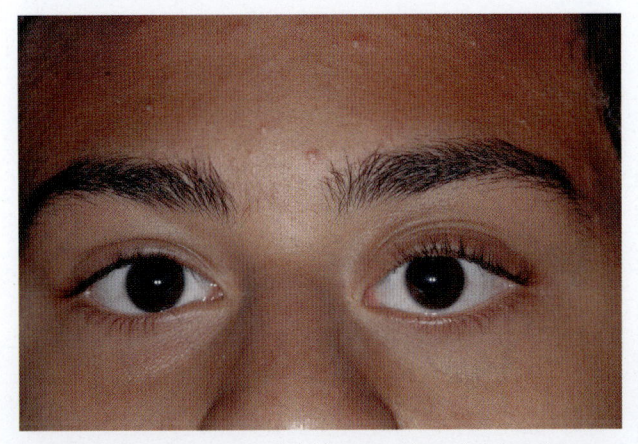

Figure 28.102. Appearance of child 14 years later showing almost stable orbital findings.

ORBITAL LYMPHANGIOMA: OCCURRENCE IN A YOUNG CHILD

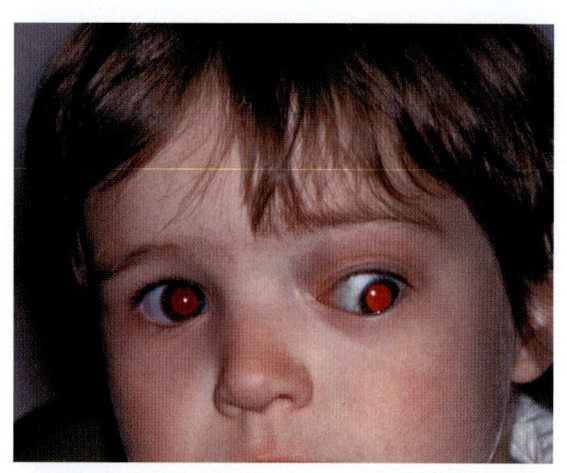

Figure 28.103. Proptosis and inferotemporal displacement of left eye in a 4-year-old girl. The child was normal at birth and the proptosis was of recent onset.

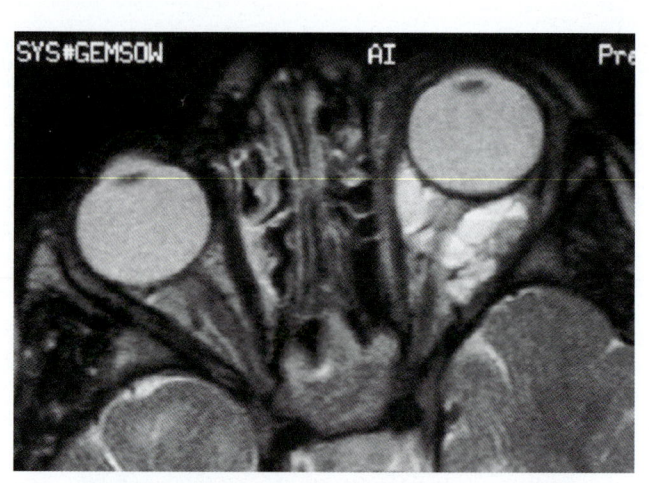

Figure 28.104. Axial magnetic resonance imaging in T2-weighted image showing multicystic mass in left orbit. Some blood–plasma levels can be seen within the hemorrhagic mass.

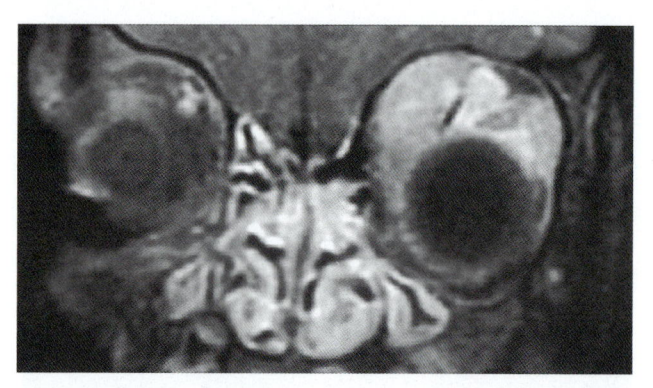

Figure 28.105. Coronal magnetic resonance imaging in T2-weighted image showing that the multicystic mass is located predominantly in the superior portion of the orbit.

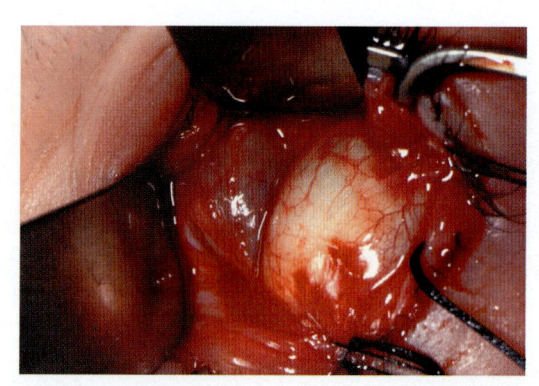

Figure 28.106. Surgical view at time of conjunctival approach. Traction sutures have been placed beneath the insertion of two rectus muscles and retractors are used to expose the superior blood cyst (to the left). It was aspirated and a portion was removed piecemeal.

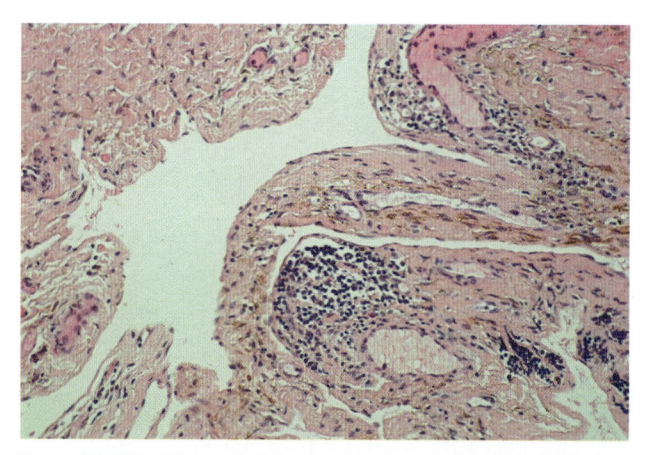

Figure 28.107. Histopathology showing the ectatic channels lined by endothelial cells. Note the diffuse infiltration of lymphocytes in the trabeculae beneath the epithelium. (Hematoxylin–eosin ×40.)

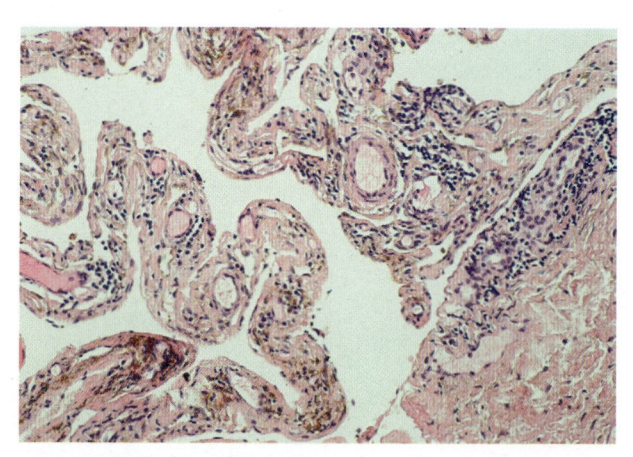

Figure 28.108. Histopathology of another area of the same tumor demonstrating the interconnecting lymph channels and diffuse lymphocytes in the trabeculae. (Hematoxylin–eosin ×40.)

ORBITAL LYMPHANGIOMA: OCCURRENCE IN AN OLDER ADULT

In some instances, orbital lymphangioma is not diagnosed until adulthood. We believe that the tumor in such patients had probably been present since childhood, but had not become apparent.

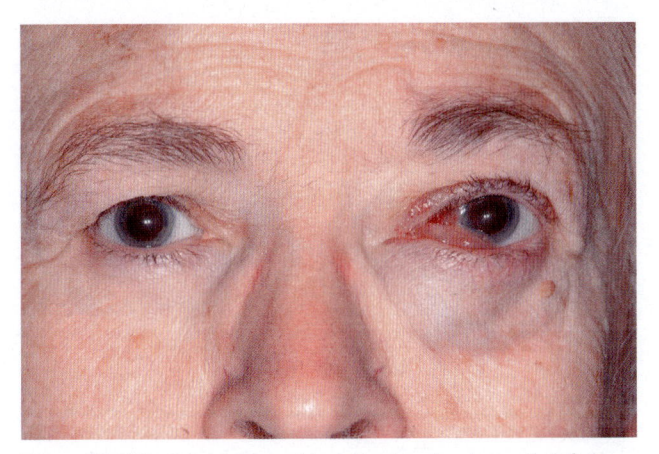

Figure 28.109. Subcutaneous blue discoloration beneath left lower eyelid in a 65-year-old woman. Note also the fleshy mass in the conjunctiva nasally, representing anterior extension of the orbital mass.

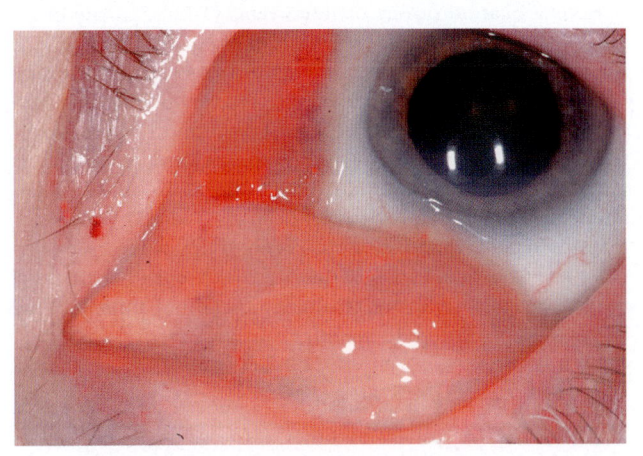

Figure 28.110. Closer view of the conjunctival component of the mass. Note that it is not blue, indicating that the chronic hemorrhage was mainly in the deeper orbital component.

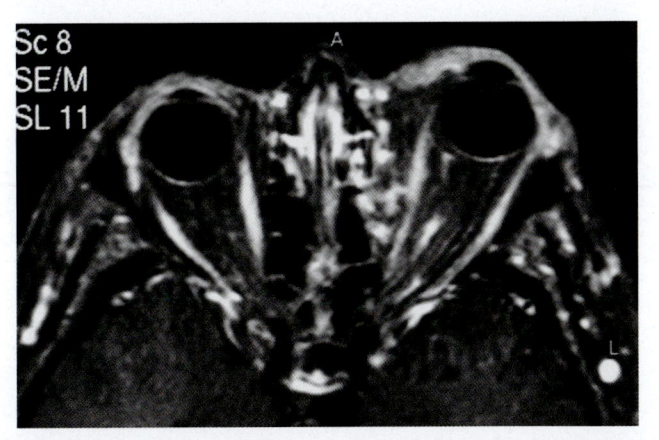

Figure 28.111. Axial magnetic resonance imaging in T1-weighted image, demonstrating proptosis and diffuse, ill-defined left orbital mass.

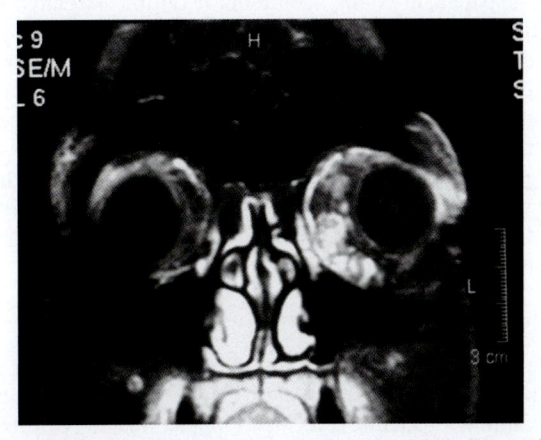

Figure 28.112. Coronal magnetic resonance imaging in T1-weighted image, demonstrating that the multicystic mass is located mostly nasally and inferiorly.

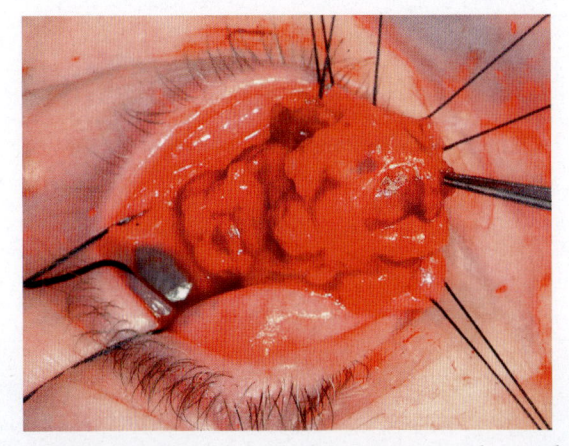

Figure 28.113. Surgical view of multicystic mass as seen after an inferior conjunctival approach.

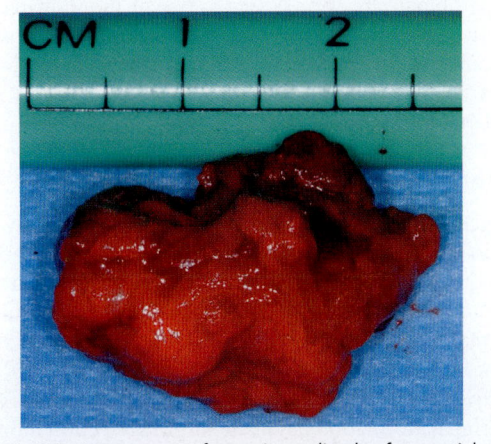

Figure 28.114. Appearance of mass immediately after partial surgical removal. Histopathology showed typical features of lymphangioma.

ORBITAL VARIX

General Considerations

Varix is a dilation of one or more veins (1–26). In the orbit, a varix can become sizable enough to produce a mass effect. There is considerable overlap among orbital venous malformations such as orbital varix, varicocele, and venous angioma, and they probably represent a spectrum. Furthermore, there is controversy as to whether varix and lymphangioma represent the same entity (6,7). The authors believe there are sufficient differences between them with regard to clinical and pathologic features to allow for separate classification. It has been reported that orbital varices can be associated with defects in orbital bone and cephaloceles and that inflammation of a thrombosed varix could predispose to meningitis in such cases (17,18).

Clinical Features

The classic varix usually becomes apparent in young adults and is characterized by positional proptosis, with the proptosis becoming worse with the head bent downward or during Valsalva maneuver. Although orbital varix generally becomes clinically apparent in young adulthood, it can be associated with extreme neonatal proptosis that can be apparent at birth (19). More anteriorly located orbital varix can present as a lacrimal sac mass or subconjunctival mass (13,14). In some instances, chronic inflation and deflation of a varix can lead to enophthalmos.

An unusual variant of orbital varix is the so-called vortex vein varix, which can appear ophthalmoscopically like an intraocular tumor (21). This is discussed in the *Atlas of Intraocular Tumors*.

Diagnostic Approaches

CT and MRI demonstrate a round or irregular mass that may not be apparent until Valsalva maneuver is performed during the scanning procedure (8). Color Doppler imaging can also be used to demonstrate an orbital varix (9).

Pathology

Histopathologically, varix is seen as one or more dilated veins, frequently with thrombosis and hyalinization. A thrombosed varix can lead to a pathologic reaction characterized by intravascular papillary endothelial hyperplasia (IPEH), a subject considered in this book (20).

Management

Management is difficult and controversial. Minimally symptomatic lesions can be observed and more symptomatic ones may require orbitotomy and surgical excision. Exposure of the lesion and embolization with coil has been used to minimize the extent of surgical resection (2). Others have used vascular clips near the orbital apex to manage orbital varix (10). More recently, embolization of orbital varices with cyanoacrylate to "cast" the malformation has made surgical resection more facile (12).

ORBITAL VARIX

Selected References

Reviews

1. Shields JA, Shields CL, Scartozzi R. Survey of 1264 patients with orbital tumors and simulating lesions: The 2002 Montgomery Lecture, part 1. *Ophthalmology* 2004;111:997–1008.
2. Shields JA, Bakewell B, Augsburger JJ, et al. Classification and incidence of space-occupying lesions of the orbit. A survey of 645 biopsies. *Arch Ophthalmol* 1984;102:1606–1611.
3. Shields JA, Bakewell B, Augsburger JJ, et al. Space-occupying orbital masses in children: A review of 250 consecutive biopsies. *Ophthalmology* 1986;93:379–384.
4. Gunalp I, Gunduz K. Vascular tumors of the orbit. *Doc Ophthalmol* 1995;89:337–345.
5. Rootman J, Hay E, Graeb D, et al. Orbital-adnexal lymphangiomas. A spectrum of hemodynamically isolated vascular hamartomas. *Ophthalmology* 1986;93:1558–1570.
6. Garrity JA. Orbital venous anomalies. A long-standing dilemma. *Ophthalmology* 1997;104:903–904.
7. Wright JE, Sullivan TJ, Garner A, et al. Orbital venous anomalies. *Ophthalmology* 1997;104:905–913.

Imaging

8. Shields JA, Dolinskas C, Augsburger JJ, et al. Demonstration of orbital varix with computed tomography and Valsalva maneuver. *Am J Ophthalmol* 1984;97:108–109.
9. Lieb WE, Merton DA, Shields JA, et al. Colour Doppler imaging in the demonstration of an orbital varix. *Br J Ophthalmol* 1990;74:305–308.

Management

10. Beyer R, Levine MR, Sternberg I. Orbital varices: a surgical approach. *Ophthal Plast Reconstr Surg* 1985;1:205–210.
11. Xu D, Liu D, Zhang Z, et al. Gamma knife radiosurgery for primary orbital varices: a preliminary report. *Br J Ophthalmol* 2011;95(9):1264–1267.
12. Couch SM, Garrity JA, Cameron JD, et al. Embolization of orbital varices with N-butyl cyanoacrylate as an aid in surgical excision: results of 4 cases with histopathologic examination. *Am J Ophthalmol* 2009;148(4):614–618.

Case Reports

13. Nasr AM, Huaman AM. Anterior orbital varix presenting as a lacrimal sac mucocele. *Ophthal Plast Reconstr Surg* 1998;14:193–197.
14. Shields JA, Eagle RC Jr, Shields CL, et al. Orbital varix presenting as a subconjunctival mass. *Ophthal Plast Reconstr Surg* 1995;11:37–38.
15. Bullock JD, Goldberg SH, Connelly PJ. Orbital varix thrombosis. *Ophthalmology* 1990;97:251–256.
16. Rosenblum P, Zilkha A. Sudden visual loss secondary to an orbital varix. *Surv Ophthalmol* 1978;23:49–56.
17. Islam N, Mireskandari K, Burton BJ, et al. Orbital varices, cranial defects, and encephaloceles: an unrecognized association. *Ophthalmology* 2004;111:1244–1247.
18. Islam N, Mireskandari K, Rose GE. Orbital varices and orbital wall defects. *Br J Ophthalmol* 2004;88:833–834.
19. Foroozan R, Shields CL, Shields JA, et al. Congenital orbital varices causing extreme neonatal proptosis. *Am J Ophthalmol* 2000;129:693–694.
20. Shields JA, Shields CL, Eagle RC Jr, et al. Intravascular papillary endothelial hyperplasia with presumed bilateral orbital varices. *Arch Ophthalmol* 1999;117:1247–1279.
21. Gunduz K, Shields CL, Shields JA. Varix of the vortex vein ampulla simulating choroidal melanoma: report of four cases. *Retina* 1998;18:343–347.
22. Weill A, Cognard C, Castaings L, et al. Embolization of an orbital varix after surgical exposure. *AJNR Am J Neuroradiol* 1998;19:921–923.
23. Phan IT, Hoyt WF, McCulley TJ, et al. Blindness from orbital varices: case report. *Orbit* 2009;28(5):303–305.
24. McCannel CA, Hoenig J, Umlas J, et al. Orbital lesions in the blue rubber bleb nevus syndrome. *Ophthalmology* 1996;103(6):933–936.
25. Cohen JA, Char DH, Norman D. Bilateral orbital varices associated with habitual bending. *Arch Ophthalmol* 1995;113(11):1360–1362.
26. Kremer I, Nissenkorn I, Feuerman P, et al. Congenital orbital vascular malformation complicated by massive retrobulbar hemorrhage. *J Pediatr Ophthalmol Strabismus* 1987;24(4):190–193.

ORBITAL VARIX: DEMONSTRATION BY INCREASING INTRACRANIAL VENOUS PRESSURE

In some instances, a subtle varix can show marked enlargement and increased proptosis during times of increased venous pressure in the head, induced by bending forward or by Valsalva maneuver. This can be best demonstrated by imaging studies with contrast enhancement.

Shields JA, Dolinskas C, Augsburger JJ, et al. Demonstration of orbital varix with computed tomography and Valsalva maneuver. *Am J Ophthalmol* 1984;97:108–109.

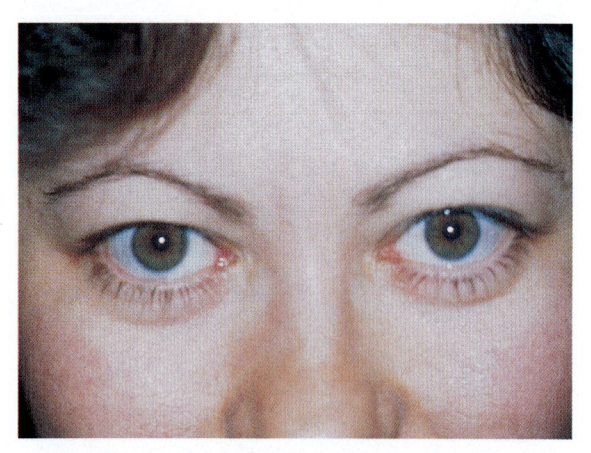

Figure 28.115. Minimal proptosis of the left eye in a 38-year-old woman who complains of a full feeling behind left eye when she bends over.

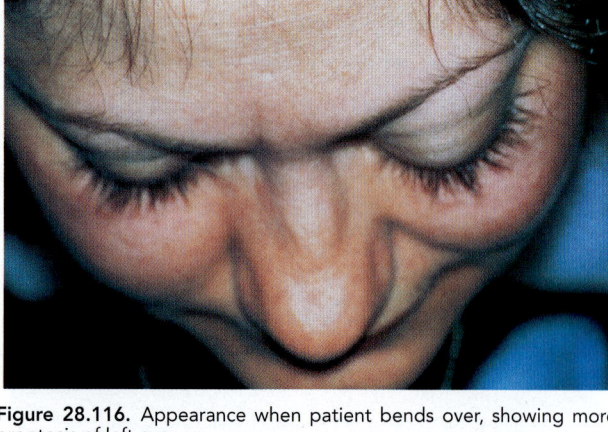

Figure 28.116. Appearance when patient bends over, showing more proptosis of left eye.

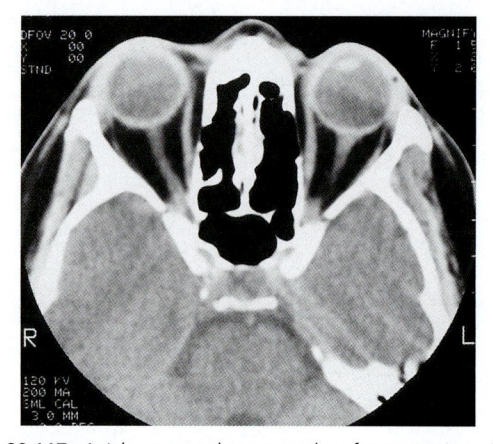

Figure 28.117. Axial computed tomography of same patient showing no apparent orbital mass.

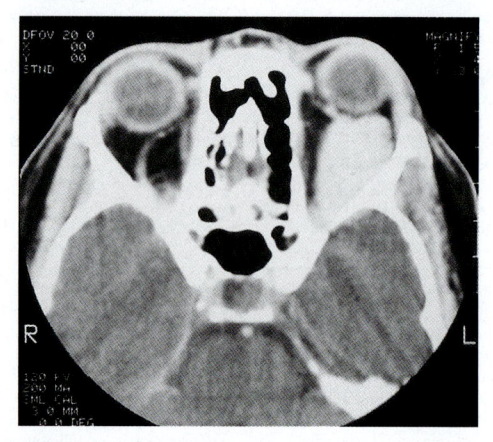

Figure 28.118. Axial computed tomography of same patient with contrast enhancement during Valsalva maneuver. Note that the enhancing orbital mass is now very apparent.

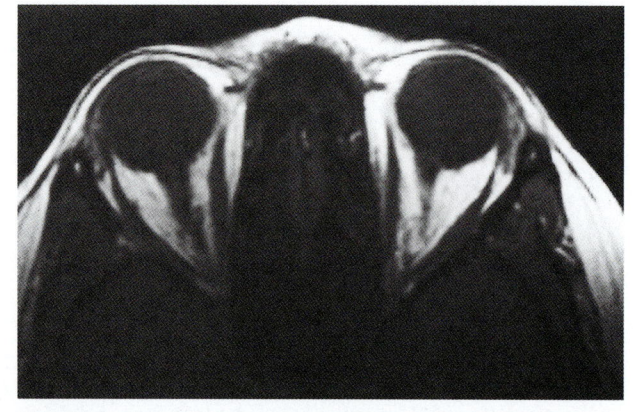

Figure 28.119. Axial magnetic resonance imaging of same patient in T1-weighted image, showing no apparent mass.

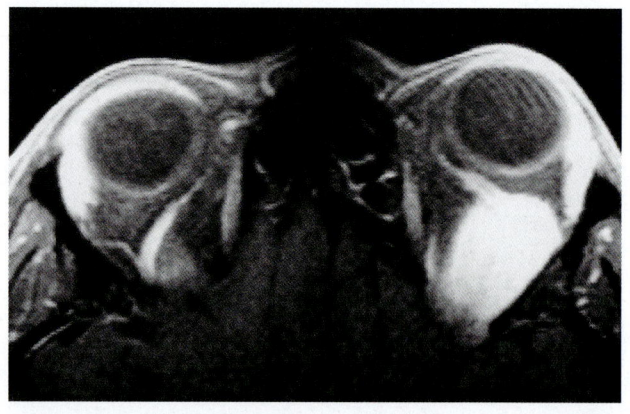

Figure 28.120. Axial magnetic resonance imaging during Valsalva maneuver demonstrated the mass.

Chapter 28 Orbital Vascular and Hemorrhagic Lesions

● ORBITAL VARIX: DEMONSTRATION BY VALSALVA MANEUVER

A patient with unexplained proptosis should be asked to perform a Valsalva maneuver. In most instances, this causes a varix to enlarge, gradually increasing the proptosis after a few seconds. This maneuver should also be performed on a patient who has no proptosis but who experiences a full feeling behind an eye. Two examples are shown.

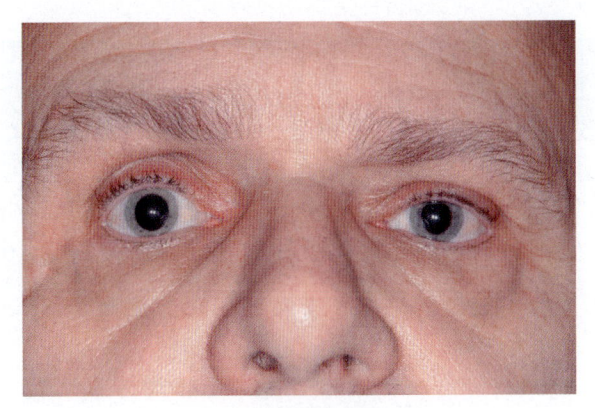

Figure 28.121. Elderly man with proptosis of right eye.

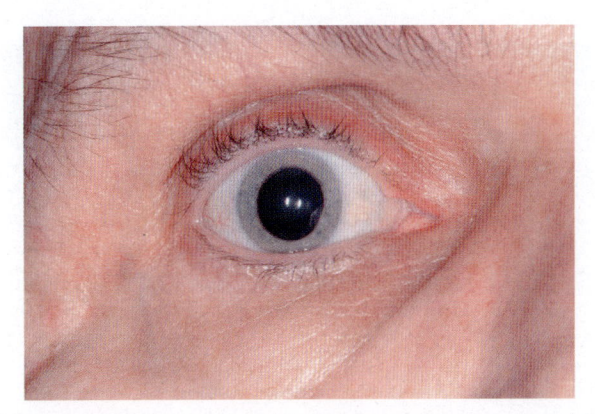

Figure 28.122. Close-up view of right eye revealing proptosis and visible sclera above the corneoscleral limbus, resembling thyroid-associated orbitopathy.

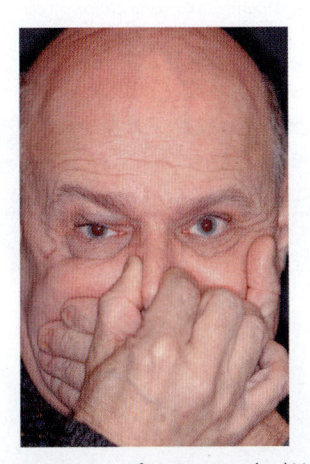

Figure 28.123. Same patient performing standard Valsalva maneuver.

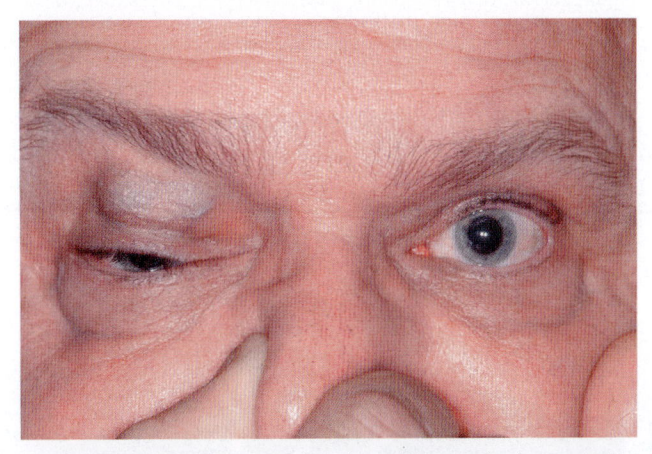

Figure 28.124. Same patient after about 10 seconds, demonstrating blue subcutaneous swelling beneath upper eyelid owing to enlargement of varix, along with proptosis and downward displacement of the globe.

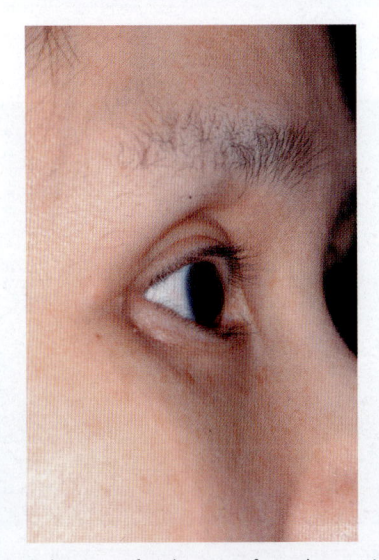

Figure 28.125. Side view of right eye of another patient who complained of a full feeling behind eye when bending over.

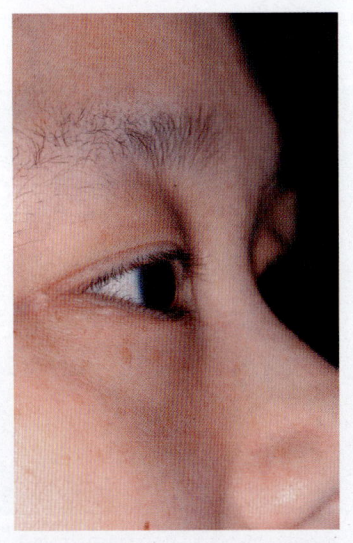

Figure 28.126. Same patient seen in Figure 28.125, demonstrating fullness behind right upper eyelid immediately after Valsalva maneuver.

ORBITAL VARIX: COMPUTED TOMOGRAPHY, MAGNETIC RESONANCE IMAGING, AND COLOR DOPPLER IMAGING

In addition to CT and MRI, color Doppler imaging can also be employed to suggest the diagnosis of orbital varix.

Lieb WE, Merton DA, Shields JA, et al. Color Doppler imaging in the demonstration of an orbital varix. *Br J Ophthalmol* 1990;74:305–308.

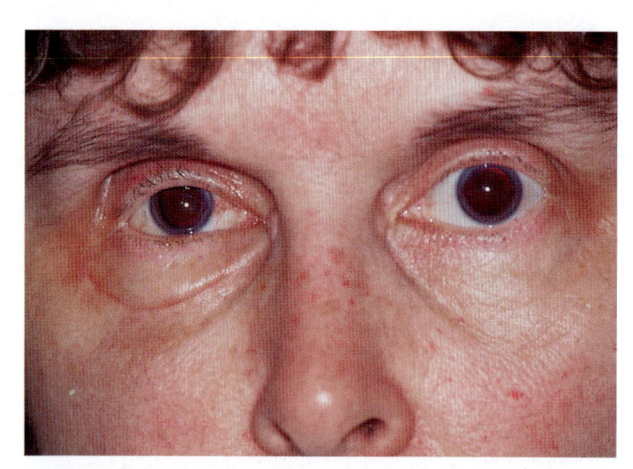

Figure 28.127. Slight enophthalmos of right eye in 59-year-old woman who was referred after she had undergone three right orbitotomies elsewhere to rule out orbital metastasis and no diagnosis had been established.

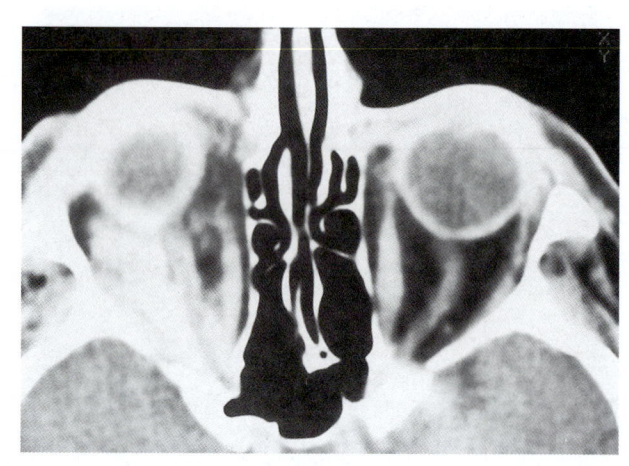

Figure 28.128. Axial computed tomography with contrast agent and Valsalva maneuver demonstrating enhancing mass near floor of the orbit.

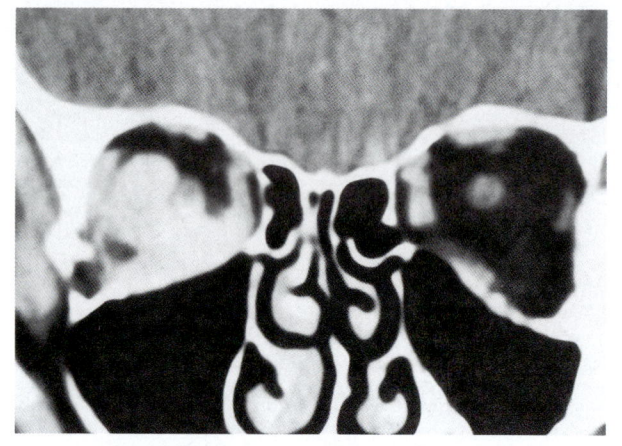

Figure 28.129. Coronal computed tomography with contrast agent and Valsalva maneuver further demonstrating the mass.

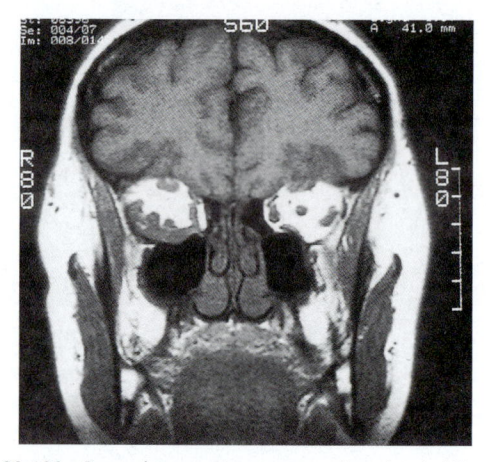

Figure 28.130. Coronal magnetic resonance imaging in T1-weighted image showing irregular mass along floor of right orbit.

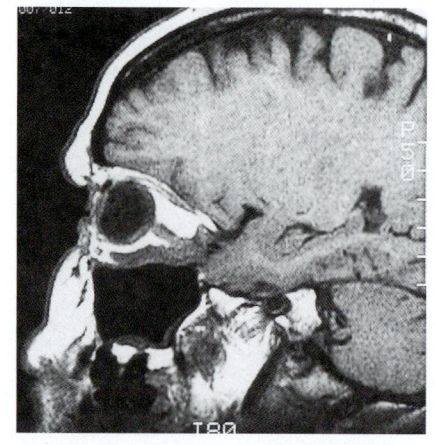

Figure 28.131. Sagittal magnetic resonance imaging in T1-weighted image, further demonstrating the mass near the orbital floor.

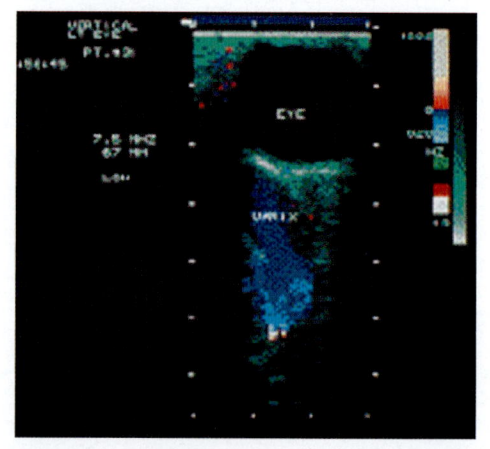

Figure 28.132. Color Doppler imaging of orbital varix showing the dilated retrobulbar vein in blue.

Chapter 28 Orbital Vascular and Hemorrhagic Lesions

● ORBITAL VARIX: ANTERIORLY LOCATED LESION

A varix located in the anterior aspects of the orbit can be clinically apparent through the eyelid or conjunctiva.

Shields JA, Eagle RC Jr, Shields CL, et al. Orbital varix presenting as a subconjunctival mass. *Ophthal Plast Reconstr Surg* 1995;11:37–38.

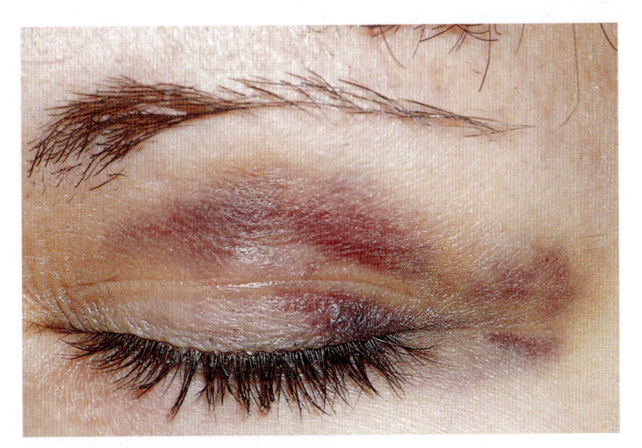

Figure 28.133. Subcutaneous ecchymosis around left eye in a 36-year-old woman with subcutaneous bleeding from an orbital varix that had undergone thrombosis.

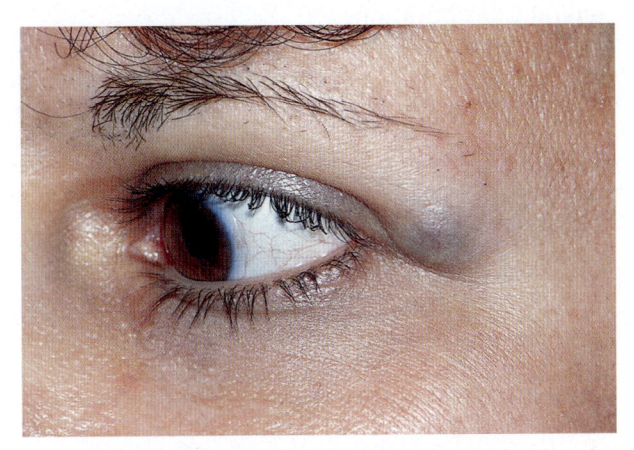

Figure 28.134. Appearance of same patient 6 months after the subcutaneous hemorrhage resolved. Note that the thrombosed varix appears as a blue nodule beneath the skin near the lateral canthus.

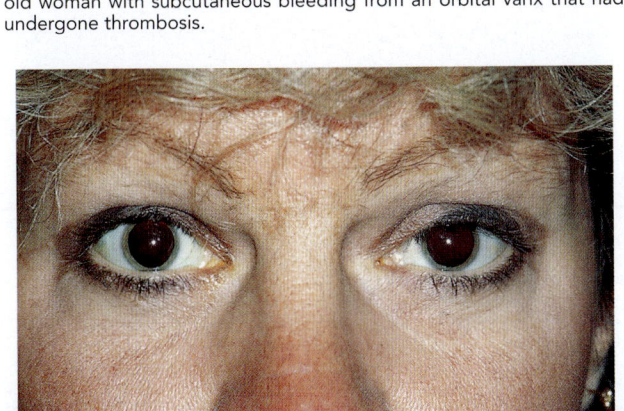

Figure 28.135. Slight blepharoptosis of left eye in a 40-year-old woman.

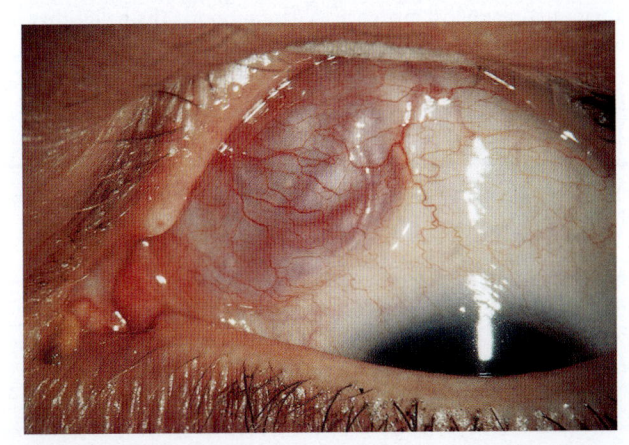

Figure 28.136. Vascular mass in superonasal conjunctival fornix in patient shown in Figure 28.135.

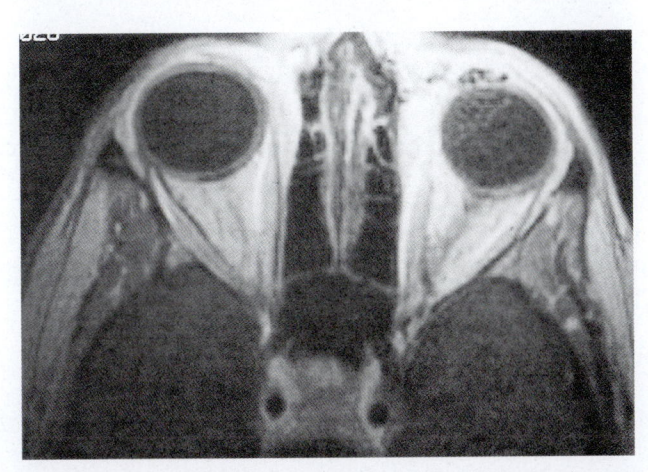

Figure 28.137. Axial magnetic resonance imaging of patient shown in Figure 28.135, demonstrating the irregular vascular mass in anteromedial aspect of orbit.

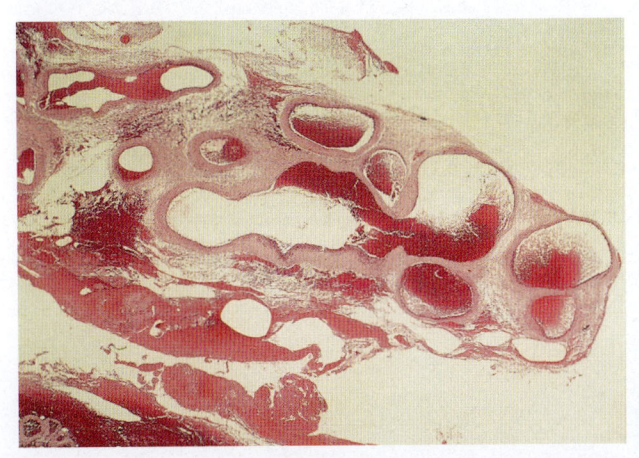

Figure 28.138. Histopathology of same lesion shown in Figure 28.135, demonstrating complex arrangement of dilated veins. (Hematoxylin–eosin ×20.)

ORBITAL MISCELLANEOUS VASCULAR LESIONS: INTRAVASCULAR PAPILLARY ENDOTHELIAL HYPERPLASIA AND GLOMUS TUMOR OF THE ORBIT

Orbital Intravascular Papillary Endothelial Hyperplasia

General Considerations
IPEH is a mass composed of benign endothelial cells that undergo proliferation in a papillary configuration within the lumen of a vascular channel. It may represent an exuberant proliferation of vascular endothelium as a response to the organization of a thrombus, possibly within a varix, cavernous hemangioma or lymphangioma. It can occasionally appear in the orbit as solitary or multiple lesions (1–5).

Clinical Features
Clinically, IPEH is similar to other orbital vascular tumors. There is more likely to be a history of pain if the lesion is preceded by a thrombosed varix. The inflammation caused by the thrombosis can lead to inflammatory edema of the eyelids.

Pathology and Pathogenesis
IPEH is an endothelial cell proliferation into the lumen of blood vessels. In many respects, the benign lesion resembles an angiosarcoma. Most evidence to date supports the belief that it is an unusual type of organizing thrombus.

Diagnostic Approaches
IPEH has similar symptoms and signs like other circumscribed orbital tumors. Pain is a common complaint. On CT and MRI, it appears as a circumscribed mass similar to cavernous hemangioma.

Management
Most cases of IPEH have been managed by excisional biopsy with a preoperative diagnosis of orbital cavernous hemangioma. This seems to be the most appropriate management.

Selected References

Reviews
1. Font RL, Wheeler TM, Boniuk M. Intravascular papillary endothelial hyperplasia of the orbit and ocular adnexa. A report of five cases. *Arch Ophthalmol* 1983;101:1731–1736.
2. Werner MS, Hornblass A, Reifler DM, et al. Intravascular papillary endothelial hyperplasia: collection of four cases and a review of the literature. *Ophthal Plast Reconstr Surg* 1997;13:48–56.

Case Reports
3. Shields JA, Shields CL, Diniz W, et al. Multiple bilateral orbital vascular tumors as a component of intravascular papillary endothelial hyperplasia. *Arch Ophthalmol* 1999;117:1247–1249.
4. Weber FL, Babel J. Intravascular papillary endothelial hyperplasia of the orbit. *Br J Ophthalmol* 1981;65:18–22.
5. Liu D, Shields CL, Lam D. Periocular papillary endothelial hyperplasia (Masson's tumor) in Behçet's disease. *Acta Ophthalmologica* 2012;90:e413–e415.

ORBITAL INTRAVASCULAR PAPILLARY ENDOTHELIAL HYPERPLASIA AND GLOMUS TUMOR

1. Shields JA, Shields CL, Diniz W, et al. Multiple bilateral orbital vascular tumors as a component of intravascular papillary endothelial hyperplasia. *Arch Ophthalmol* 1999;117:1247–1249.
2. Neufeld M, Pe'er J, Rosenman E, et al. Intraorbital glomus cell tumor. *Am J Ophthalmol* 1994;117:539–540.
3. Shields JA, Eagle RC Jr, Shields CL, et al. Orbital-conjunctival glomangiomas involving two ocular rectus muscles. *Am J Ophthalmol* 2006;142:511–513.

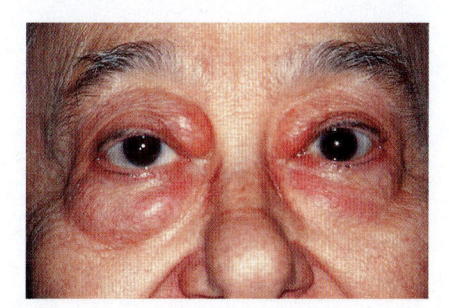

Figure 28.139. Intravascular papillary endothelial hyperplasia causing proptosis and eyelid edema of the right eye in an otherwise healthy 80-year-old woman.

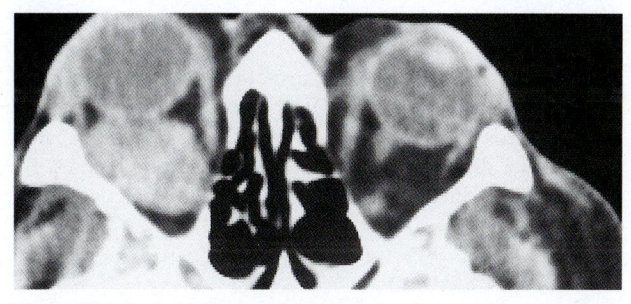

Figure 28.140. Axial computed tomography of patient shown in Figure 28.139, demonstrating a circumscribed retrobulbar tumor resembling a cavernous hemangioma. Additional sections showed similar but smaller masses at the right orbital apex in the soft tissues of the left orbit.

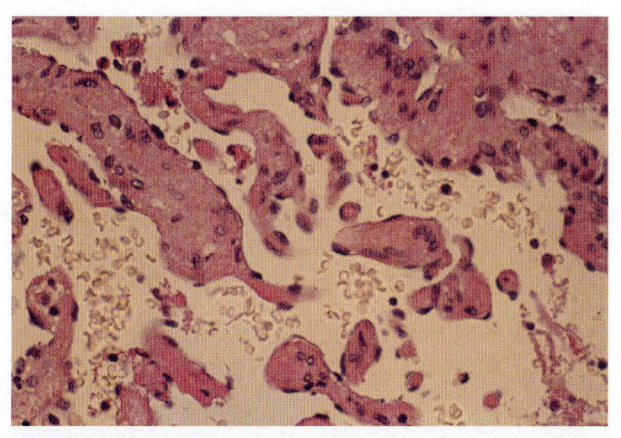

Figure 28.141. Histopathology of lesion shown in Figure 28.139, depicting projections of proliferating endothelial cells into the lumen of a vascular channel. (Hematoxylin–eosin ×100.)

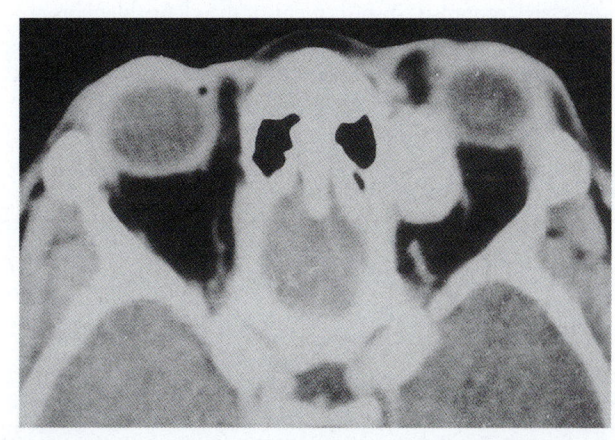

Figure 28.142. Axial computed tomography of an orbital glomus cell tumor in a 35-year-old woman showing a circumscribed mass in superonasal aspect of left orbit. (Courtesy of Jacob Pe'er, MD.)

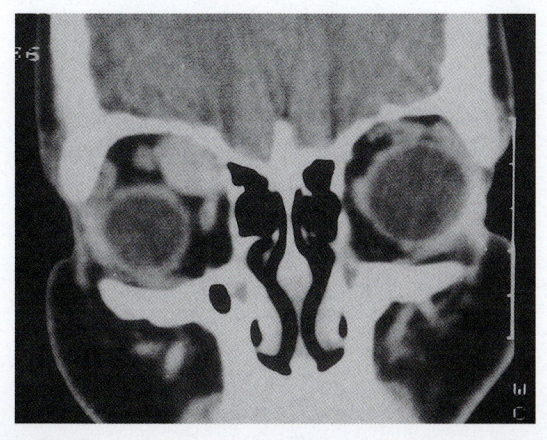

Figure 28.143. Coronal computed tomography of lesion shown in Figure 28.142, showing a superonasal orbital mass. (Courtesy of Jacob Pe'er, MD.)

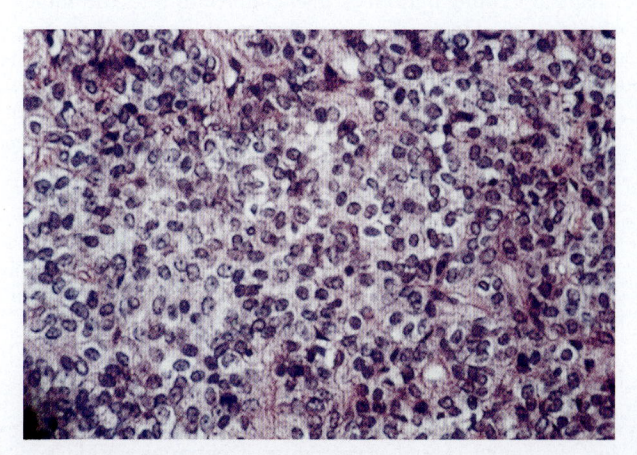

Figure 28.144. Histopathology of lesion shown in Figure 28.142, revealing sheets of polyhedral cells. Immunohistochemical studies supported the diagnosis of glomus tumor. (Hematoxylin–eosin ×125.) (Courtesy of Jacob Pe'er, MD.)

ORBITAL ANGIOSARCOMA

General Considerations

Angiosarcoma (malignant hemangioendothelioma) is a malignant tumor that probably arises from endothelial cells of blood vessels. It can rarely occur in the orbital region (1–9). In a series of 366 cases of angiosarcoma reported from the Armed Forces Institute of Pathology, most involved the skin and soft tissue and only 10 cases (3%) arose in the orbit (2). It has a tendency to occur in young adults and has a predilection for males. Angiosarcoma that arises in the orbit has the capacity to invade locally, with less tendency for distant metastases. No cases were identified in the authors' series of 1,264 consecutive orbital masses (1).

Clinical Features

Orbital angiosarcoma can be localized or diffuse and has no distinct clinical characteristics. The clinical features of an orbital angiosarcoma are similar to those of other malignant and benign orbital tumors. The affected patient may develop progressive proptosis, displacement of the globe, blepharoptosis, and ophthalmoplegia. Tumors in the anterior portion of the orbit can present as a soft subcutaneous mass (5). It can extend from the orbit into the conjunctiva and resemble Kaposi sarcoma of the conjunctiva (2,3).

Diagnostic Approaches

With imaging studies like CT and MRI, orbital angiosarcoma shows findings similar to other orbital tumors. In the early stages, it demonstrates a circumscribed soft tissue mass. When it subsequently infiltrates the surrounding tissues, it becomes diffuse and poorly circumscribed.

Pathology

Histopathologically, angiosarcoma is composed of cords of ovoid pleomorphic endothelial cells separated by fibrous connective tissue. In some cases, large anaplastic cells can assume a papillary configuration or may proliferate into the lumen forming a pseudoglandular appearance. This can lead to diagnostic confusion with intravascular papillary endothelial cell hyperplasia, a benign condition with a similar growth pattern. Immunohistochemical stain for cytoplasmic factor VIII and Ulex europaeus agglutinin I are helpful in identifying the endothelial cell origin of the tumor (2,5). Electron microscopy can assist by detecting Weibel–Palade bodies, which are characteristic ultrastructural features of endothelial cells (2).

The pathogenesis of angiosarcoma is unclear. It possibly develops from the proliferation of endothelial cells of orbital blood vessels.

Management

Orbital angiosarcoma is best managed with wide surgical excision, including orbital exenteration if necessary. Wide excision is crucial because of the tendency of the tumor to infiltrate beyond its clinically visible borders. Although there are insufficient data to support primary irradiation, if there is a question of residual tumor after biopsy or surgical removal, then supplemental radiotherapy, using external beam or plaque brachytherapy techniques (5,000–6,000 cGy) can be considered (10).

Selected References

Reviews

1. Shields JA, Shields CL, Scartozzi R. Survey of 1264 patients with orbital tumors and simulating lesions: The 2002 Montgomery Lecture, part 1. *Ophthalmology* 2004;111:997–1008.
2. Weiss SW, Goldblum JR. Malignant vascular tumors. In: Weiss SW, Goldblum JR, eds. *Enzinger and Weiss's Soft Tissue Tumors.* 4th ed. St. Louis, MO: CV Mosby; 2001:917–954.

Case Reports

3. Carelli PV, Cangelosi JP. Angiosarcoma of the orbit. *Am J Ophthalmol* 1948;31:453–456.
4. Messmer EP, Font RL, McCrary JA, et al. Epithelioid angiosarcoma of the orbit presenting as Tolosa-Hunt Syndrome. *Ophthalmology* 1983;90:1414–1421.
5. Hufnagel T, Ma L, Kuo T. Orbital angiosarcoma with subconjunctival presentation. *Ophthalmology* 1987;94:72–77.
6. Gunduz K, Shields JA, Shields CL, et al. Cutaneous angiosarcoma with eyelid involvement. *Am J Ophthalmol* 1998;125:870–871.
7. Siddens JD, Fishman JR, Jackson IT, et al. Primary orbital angiosarcoma: a case report. *Ophthal Plast Reconstr Surg* 1999;15:454–459.
8. Lopes M, Duffau H, Fleuridas G. Primary spheno-orbital angiosarcoma: case report and review of the literature. *Neurosurgery* 1999;44:405–407.
9. Shuangshoti S, Chayapum P, Suwanwela N, et al. Unilateral proptosis as a clinical presentation in primary angiosarcoma of skull. *Br J Ophthalmol* 1988;72:713–719.
10. De Keizer RJ, de Wolff-Rouendaal D, Nooy MA. Angiosarcoma of the eyelid and periorbital regions. Experience in Leiden with iridium 192 brachytherapy and low-dose doxorubicin chemotherapy. *Orbit* 2008;27:5–12.

ORBITAL ANGIOSARCOMA

1. Gunduz K, Shields JA, Shields CL, et al. Cutaneous angiosarcoma with eyelid involvement. *Am J Ophthalmol* 1998;125:870–871.
2. Messmer EP, Font RL, McCrary JA, et al. Epithelioid angiosarcoma of the orbit presenting as Tolosa–Hunt syndrome. *Ophthalmology* 1983;90:1414–1421.

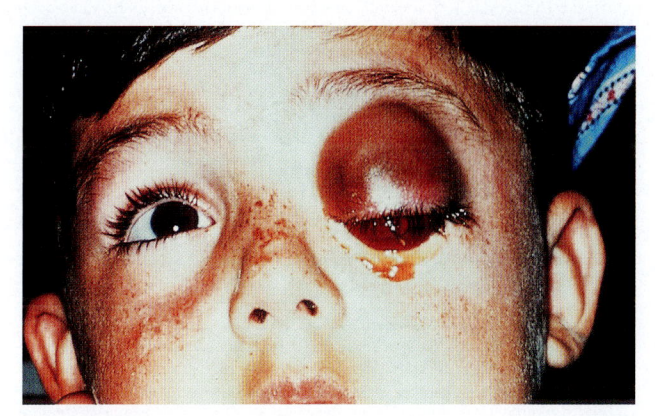

Figure 28.145. Angiosarcoma of left orbit with secondary eyelid and conjunctival involvement in a young boy. (Courtesy of the late Frederick Blodi, MD.)

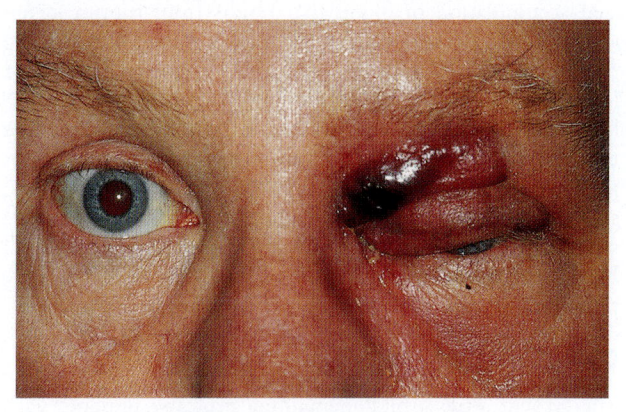

Figure 28.146. Angiosarcoma of the left orbit with secondary extension into the eyelid in a 70-year-old man.

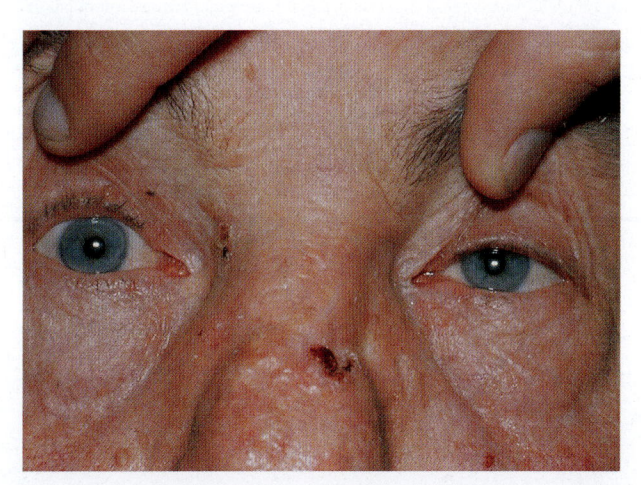

Figure 28.147. Proptosis of the left eye secondary to an epithelioid angiosarcoma of the orbit that produced a Tolosa–Hunt syndrome. (Courtesy of Ramon Font, MD.)

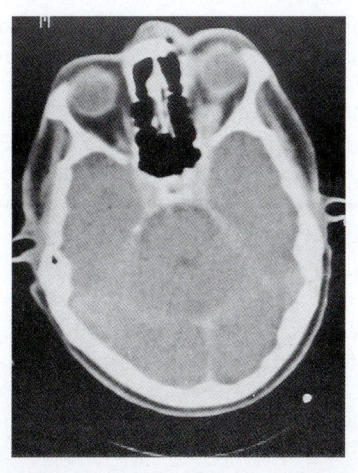

Figure 28.148. Axial computed tomography of patient seen in Figure 28.147, demonstrating an irregular mass near the orbital apex. (Courtesy of Ramon Font, MD.)

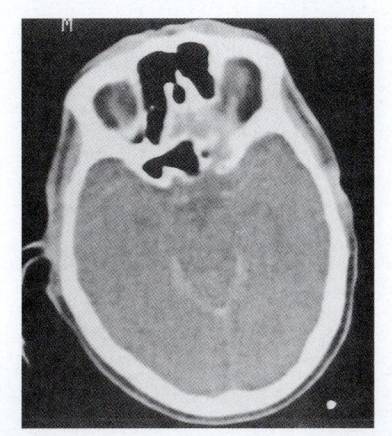

Figure 28.149. Axial computed tomography with a section more inferiorly of lesion seen in Figure 28.148, demonstrating extensive bone destruction near the orbital apex. (Courtesy of Ramon Font, MD.)

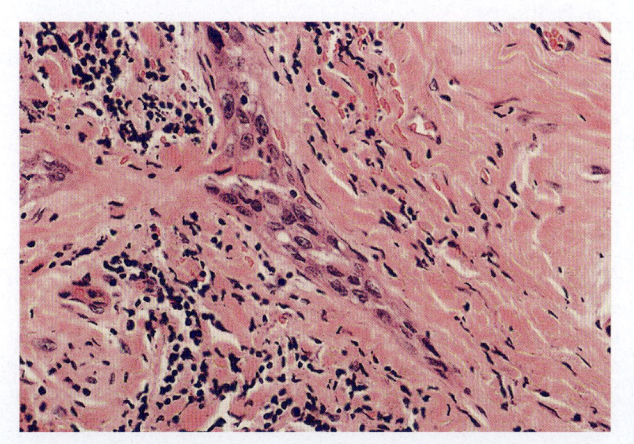

Figure 28.150. Histopathology of lesion shown in Figure 28.148, demonstrating malignant endothelial cells with fibrous tissue stroma. (Hematoxylin–eosin ×200.) After publication of this case, there was debate about the accuracy of the diagnosis and invasive squamous cell carcinoma was considered to be a possibility. (Courtesy of Ramon Font, MD.)

ORBITAL HEMATOMA

General Considerations

Hematoma is not a true vascular neoplasm, but rather a localized accumulation of blood that results from rupture of an artery or vein. It can occur in any part of the body, including the orbit (1–13). The term "hematocele" was previously used for this condition. However, the term "hematoma" is preferable because the lesion lacks an epithelial lining and thus does not meet the criteria for a cyst. Although there are a number of predisposing vascular lesions, including lymphangioma, varix, sudden elevation of cranial venous pressure, underlying bleeding diatheses, and paranasal sinusitis, the majority of orbital hematomas are a result of trauma with or without one of these predisposing conditions (5–12).

Clinical Features

The patient with orbital hematoma typically presents with either an abrupt or gradual onset and progression of unilateral proptosis and displacement of the globe, usually in an inferior direction. Some patients recall a history of prior trauma with eyelid ecchymosis, which may have occurred months or years earlier. Occasionally, the patient recalls no history of trauma. The reason for this occasional delay in the onset of symptoms is unclear. Although some hematomas resolve spontaneously, others become symptomatic and show progressive enlargement, perhaps owing to an osmotic gradient created by the blood products, which allows more absorption of fluid and increase in size.

Diagnostic Approaches

CT and MRI typically show a circumscribed mass in the superior aspect of the orbit with contents compatible with organizing blood on MRI studies. It is usually located between the periorbitum and superior orbital bone, accounting for its well-defined margin. An organizing hematoma in the superior orbit can sometimes gradually erode through the bone and encroach on the brain.

Pathology

Histopathologically, organizing hematoma is characterized by altered blood in various stages of degeneration and organization, with accumulation of cholesterol and a bile pigment called "hematoidin" (9). A fibrous pseudocapsule is often present.

Management

Asymptomatic orbital hematoma that is difficult to approach surgically can be cautiously observed in hopes that it will remain stable or resolve. When treatment is necessary, surgical excision by evacuating the blood and its fibrous tissue capsule is an appropriate choice. When the tumor extends into the cranial cavity, the procedure is often undertaken in conjunction with a neurosurgeon.

Selected References

Reviews
1. Shields JA, Shields CL, Scartozzi R. Survey of 1264 patients with orbital tumors and simulating lesions: The 2002 Montgomery Lecture, part 1. *Ophthalmology* 2004;111: 997–1008.
2. Shields JA, Bakewell B, Augsburger JJ, et al. Classification and incidence of space-occupying lesions of the orbit. A survey of 645 biopsies. *Arch Ophthalmol* 1984;102:1606–1611.
3. Shields JA, Bakewell B, Augsburger JJ, et al. Space-occupying orbital masses in children: A review of 250 consecutive biopsies. *Ophthalmology* 1986;93:379–384.

Case Reports
4. Gunalp I, Gunduz K. Vascular tumors of the orbit. *Doc Ophthalmol* 1995;89: 337–345.
5. Martinez Devesa P. Spontaneous orbital hematoma. *J Laryngol Otol* 2002;116: 960–961.
6. Spence CA, Duong DH, Monsein L, et al. Ophthalmoplegia resulting from an intraorbital hematoma. *Surg Neurol* 2000;54:447–451.
7. Atalla ML, McNab AA, Sullivan TJ, et al. Nontraumatic subperiosteal orbital hemorrhage. *Ophthalmology* 2001;108:183–189.
8. Iwata A, Matsumoto T, Mase M, et al. Chronic, traumatic intraconal hematic cyst of the orbit removed through the fronto-orbital approach—case report. *Neurol Med Chir (Tokyo)* 2000;40:106–109.
9. Lieb WE, Shields JA, Shields CL, et al. Postsurgical hematic cyst simulating a conjunctival malignant melanoma. *Retina* 1990;10:63–67.
10. Kim UR, Arora V, Shah AD, et al. Clinical features and management of posttraumatic subperiosteal hematoma of the orbit. *Indian J Ophthalmol* 2011;59(1):55–8.
11. Yazici B, Gönen T. Posttraumatic subperiosteal hematomas of the orbit in children. *Ophthal Plast Reconstr Surg* 2011;27(1):33–37.
12. Swanenberg IM, Rizzuti AE, Shinder R. Spontaneous subperiosteal hematoma precipitated by anxiety attack. *Orbit* 2013;32(6):402–404.
13. Ali HM, Khairallah AS, Moghazy K. Acute spontaneous extraconal hematic cyst of the orbit. *Saudi J Ophthalmol* 2011;25(1):85–88.

Chapter 28 Orbital Vascular and Hemorrhagic Lesions

● ORBITAL ORGANIZING HEMATOMA

Orbital organizing hematoma is generally a result of orbital trauma and usually occurs in a subperiosteal location in the superior orbit. However, it can occasionally appear in the orbital soft tissue, rather than in a subperiosteal location.

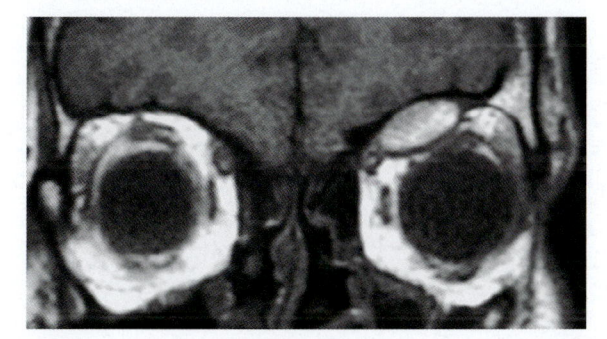

Figure 28.151. Coronal magnetic resonance imaging in T1-weighted image showing typical subperiosteal hematoma in the superior aspect of left orbit in a man who had blunt orbital trauma.

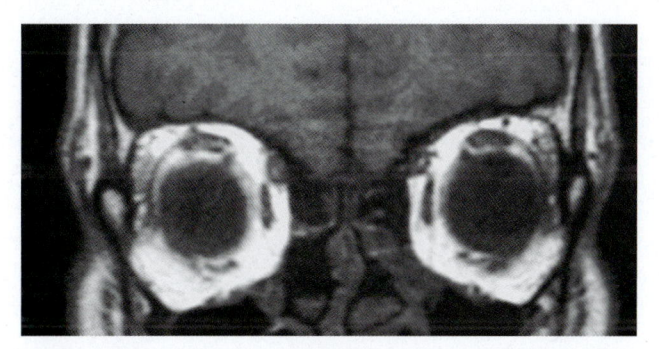

Figure 28.152. Appearance of magnetic resonance imaging in patient shown in Figure 28.151 a few weeks later, demonstrating complete resolution of the blood without treatment.

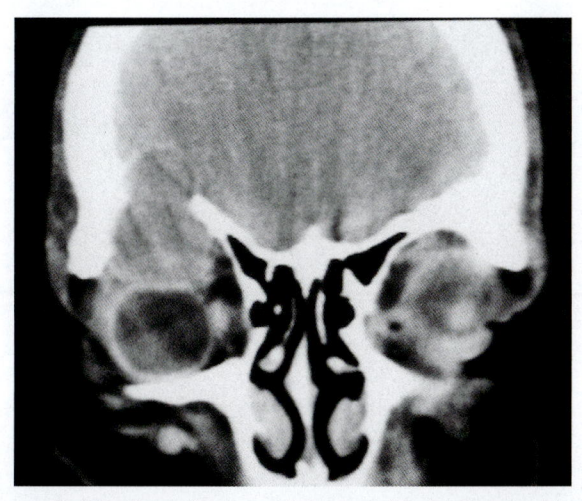

Figure 28.153. Coronal computed tomography of a 32-year-old man with a history of prior ocular trauma. Note the superior orbital mass that displaces the globe downward and extends through the orbital roof into the cranial cavity. This was found surgically and histopathologically to be an organizing hematoma.

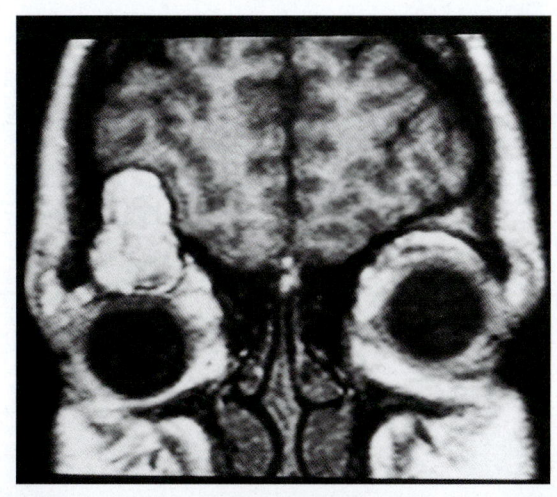

Figure 28.154. Coronal magnetic resonance imaging in T1-weighted image of same patient shown in Figure 28.153 delineating the organizing hematoma.

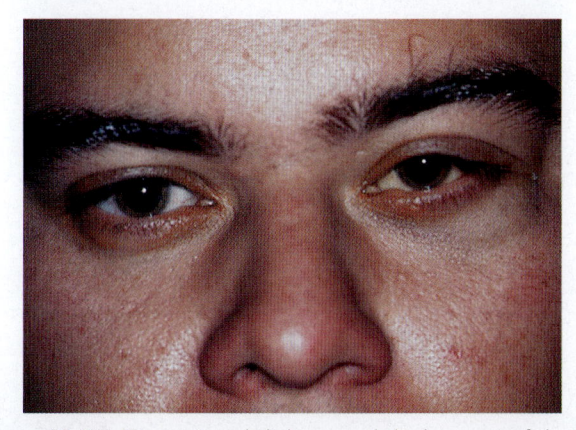

Figure 28.155. Proptosis and slight upward displacement of the left eye in a 26-year-old man.

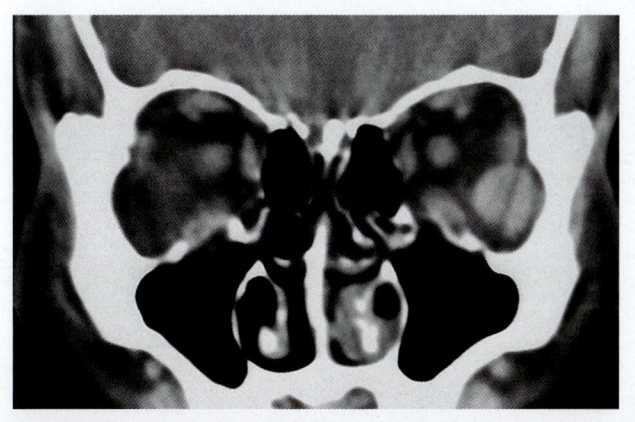

Figure 28.156. Coronal computed tomography of patient shown in Figure 28.155, revealing a circumscribed inferotemporal orbital mass. It proved pathologically to be an organizing hematoma with a dense fibrous pseudocapsule.

CHAPTER 29

ORBITAL PERIPHERAL NERVE TUMORS

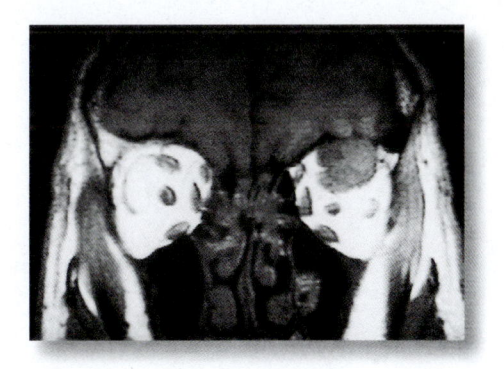

General Considerations

Schwannoma (neurilemoma) is a benign, encapsulated tumor that arises from the Schwann cells that ensheath peripheral nerves. It can arise primarily in the orbit or extend into the orbit from adjacent peripheral nerves (1–22). This tumor accounts for about 1% of all orbital masses (1–4). In the authors' series of 1,264 consecutive space-occupying orbital lesions, the 14 schwannomas accounted for 61% of the 23 peripheral nerve tumors and for 1% of all lesions (1). It was diagnosed at a median age of 37 years with a range from 10 to 84 years.

Clinical Features

Orbital schwannoma usually produces proptosis and displacement of the globe with signs and symptoms similar to those described for orbital cavernous hemangioma. Even though it is a tumor of peripheral nerve sheath origin, it does not usually cause pain. In contrast with neurofibroma, solitary orbital schwannoma is not usually associated with neurofibromatosis.

Diagnostic Approaches

Imaging studies disclose a solid ovoid to elongated mass usually outside the muscle cone along the course of the supraorbital or supratrochlear nerve and occasionally along the infraorbital nerve. Magnetic resonance imaging (MRI) reveals an enhancing mass with signals that vary depending on whether the tumor is solid or cystic. It shows low signal on T1-weighted images and homogeneous postcontrast enhancement (6–10).

Pathology

Histopathologically, schwannoma is a benign proliferation of Schwann cells that can show several variations in one tumor. Some areas are characterized by ribbons or fascicles of spindle cells (Antoni A pattern) and other areas have ovoid clear cells (Antoni B pattern). Large cystoid spaces are sometimes present and can even occupy most of the tumor, suggesting a cystic, rather than a solid lesion.

Ancient schwannoma is a variant of schwannoma that can be confused with a malignant mesenchymal tumor because of increased cellular, nuclear pleomorphism, and hyperchromatism. The variant often shows cyst formation, calcification, hemorrhage, and hyalinization (11).

Although there are no immunohistochemical stains that are specific for Schwann cells, immunohistochemistry can be used to exclude the diagnosis of other spindle cell tumors, like melanoma, leiomyoma, and rhabdomyosarcoma, thus lending support to the diagnosis of schwannoma. Electron microscopy can be used to demonstrate the cytoplasmic wide-spacing collagen that characterizes Schwann cells.

ORBITAL (NEURILEMOMA)

Management

The management of orbital schwannoma is surgical excision. Axial and coronal MRI and/or computed tomography (CT) are essential in determining the best approach to surgical excision. An incisional biopsy should generally not be done for this circumscribed orbital tumor. If the tumor is not completely excised at a fairly early stage, it can show progressive growth, attain a large size, and be more difficult to excise.

ORBITAL (NEURILEMOMA)

Selected References

Reviews

1. Shields JA, Shields CL, Scartozzi R. Survey of 1264 patients with orbital tumors and simulating lesions: the 2002 Montgomery Lecture, part 1. *Ophthalmology* 2004;111:997–1008.
2. Shields JA, Bakewell B, Augsburger DG, et al. Classification and incidence of space-occupying lesions of the orbit. A survey of 645 biopsies. *Arch Ophthalmol* 1984;102:1606–1611.
3. Shields JA, Bakewell B, Augsburger DG, et al. Space-occupying orbital masses in children. A review of 250 consecutive biopsies. *Ophthalmology* 1986;93:379–384.
4. Gunalp I, Gunduz K, Duruk K, et al. Neurogenic tumors of the orbit. *Jpn J Ophthalmol* 1994;38:185–190.
5. Rose GE, Wright JE. Isolated peripheral nerve sheath tumours of the orbit. *Eye* 1991;5:668–673.

Imaging

6. Abe T, Kawamura N, Homma H, et al. MRI of orbital schwannomas. *Neuroradiology* 2000;42:466–468.
7. Carroll GS, Haik BG, Fleming JC, et al. Peripheral nerve tumors of the orbit. *Radiol Clin North Am* 1999;37:195–202.
8. Wang Y, Xiao LH. Orbital schwannomas: findings from magnetic resonance imaging in 62 cases. *Eye (Lond)* 2008;22:1034–1039.
9. Tanaka A, Mihara F, Yoshiura T, et al. Differentiation of cavernous hemangioma from schwannoma of the orbit: a dynamic MRI study. *Am J Roentgenol* 2004;183:1799–1804.

Management

10. Hayashi M, Chernov M, Tamura N, et al. Gamma Knife surgery for abducent nerve schwannoma. Report of 4 cases. *J Neurosurg* 2010;113(Suppl):136–143.

Histopathology

11. Khwarg SI, Lucarelli MJ, Lemke BN, et al. Ancient schwannoma of the orbit. *Arch Ophthalmol* 1999;117:262–264.

Case Reports

12. Rootman J, Goldberg C, Robertson W. Primary orbital schwannomas. *Br J Ophthalmol* 1982;66:194–204.
13. Shields JA, Kapustiak J, Arbizo V, et al. Orbital neurilemoma with extension through the superior orbital fissure. *Arch Ophthalmol* 1986;104:871–873.
14. Tsuzuki N, Katoh H, Ohnuki A, et al. Cystic schwannoma of the orbit: case report. *Surg Neurol* 2000;54:385–387.
15. Lam DS, Ng JS, To KF, et al. Cystic schwannoma of the orbit. *Eye* 1997;11:798–800.
16. Shen WC, Yang DY, Ho WL, et al. Neurilemmoma of the oculomotor nerve presenting as an orbital mass: MR findings. *AJNR Am J Neuroradiol* 1993;14:1253–1254.
17. Faucett DC, Dutton JJ, Bullard DE. Gasserian ganglion schwannoma with orbital extension. *Ophthal Plast Reconstr Surg* 1989;5:235–238.
18. Konrad EA, Thiel HJ. Schwannoma of the orbit. *Ophthalmologica* 1984;188:118–120.
19. Demirci H, Shields CL, Eagle RC Jr, et al. Epibulbar schwannoma in a 17-year-old boy and review of the literature. *Ophthal Plast Reconstr Surg* 2010;26:48–50.
20. de Silva DJ, Tay E, Rose GE. Schwannomas of the lacrimal gland fossa. *Orbit* 2009;28:433–435.
21. Kashyap S, Pushker N, Meel R, et al. Orbital schwannoma with cystic degeneration. *Clin Experiment Ophthalmol* 2009;37:293–298.
22. Sales-Sanz M, Sanz-Lopez A, Romero JA. Bilateral simultaneous ancient schwannomas of the orbit. *Ophthal Plast Reconstr Surg* 2007;23:68–69.

Part 3　Tumors of the Orbit

ORBITAL SCHWANNOMA

Orbital schwannoma most typically occurs in the superior extraconal portion of the orbit and apparently arises from the sheath of the supraorbital nerve. When it is in that location, it is best approached by a superolateral orbitotomy. Most can be successfully removed by a soft tissue approach; osteotomy is only occasionally necessary. A clinicopathologic correlation is presented.

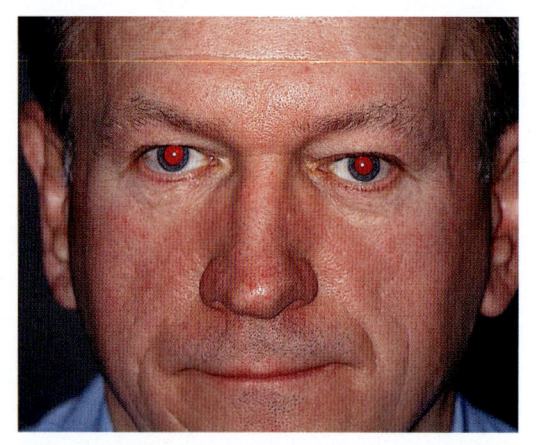

Figure 29.1. Proptosis and downward displacement of the left eye in a 57-year-old man.

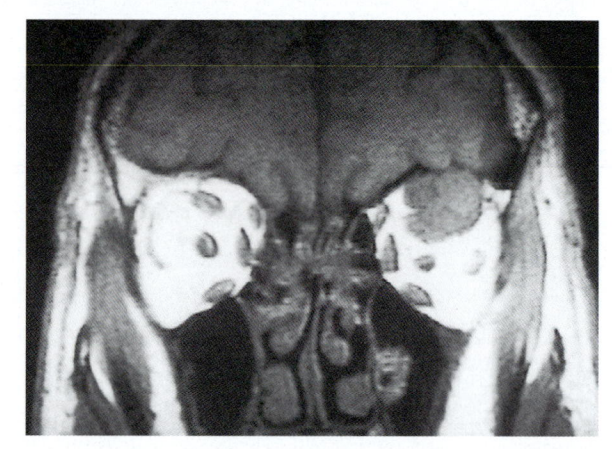

Figure 29.2. Coronal magnetic resonance imaging in T1-weighted image showing circumscribed superior orbital mass. The tumor is hypointense to orbital fat.

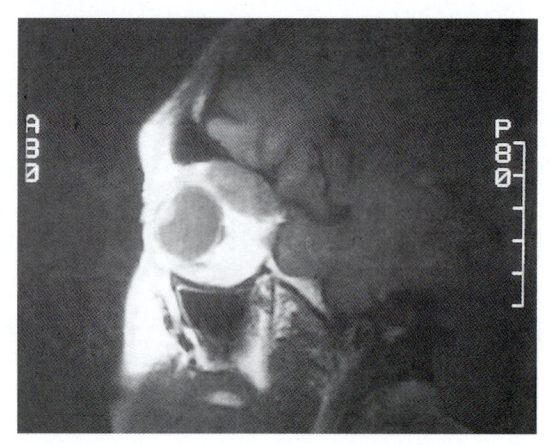

Figure 29.3. Sagittal magnetic resonance imaging in T1-weighted image showing ovoid shape of the superior orbital mass.

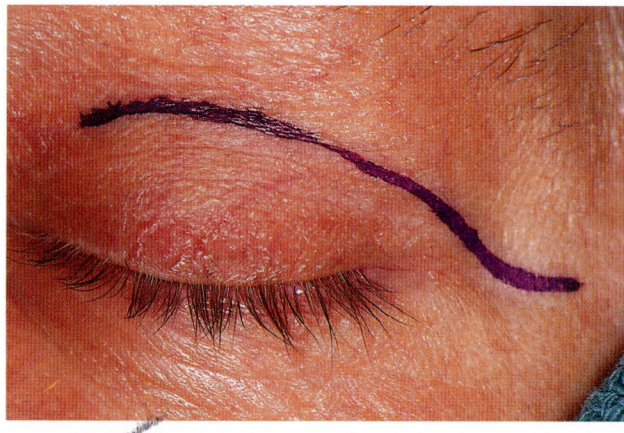

Figure 29.4. Outline of cutaneous incision for removal of the mass. The lesion was removed without complications.

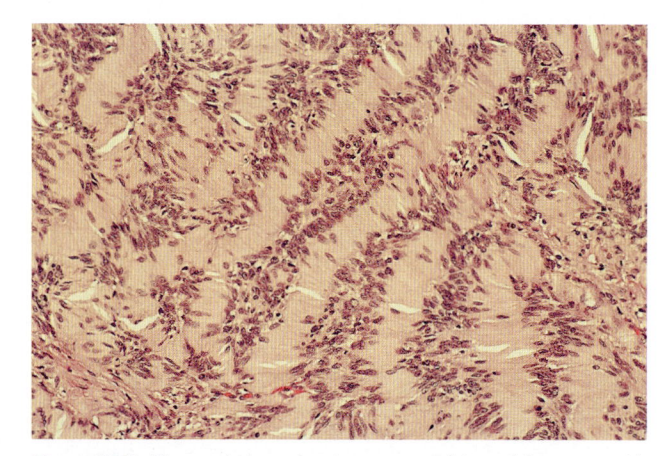

Figure 29.5. Histopathology showing an area of Antoni A pattern with fascicles of nuclei with a ribbon arrangement. (Hematoxylin–eosin ×150.)

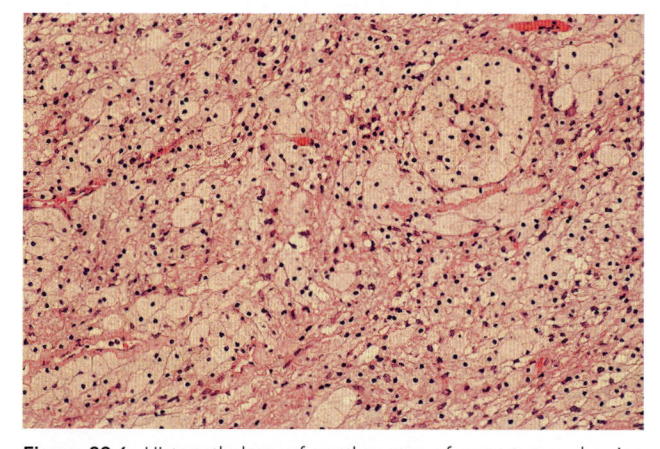

Figure 29.6. Histopathology of another area of same tumor showing Antoni B pattern. (Hematoxylin–eosin ×150.)

ORBITAL SCHWANNOMA

Orbital schwannoma is a benign, slowly growing tumor that can cause compression of the optic nerve and visual impairment. Once the tumor is removed, the optic disc swelling can resolve and the visual acuity can return to normal. However, the choroidal folds tend to remain.

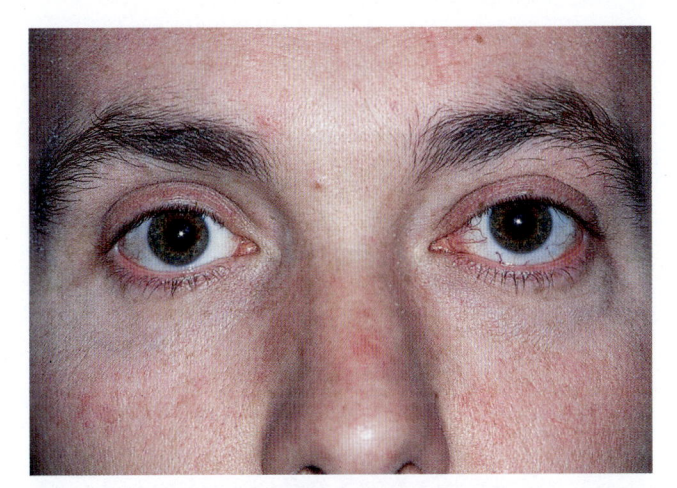

Figure 29.7. Proptosis of the left eye in a 29-year-old man.

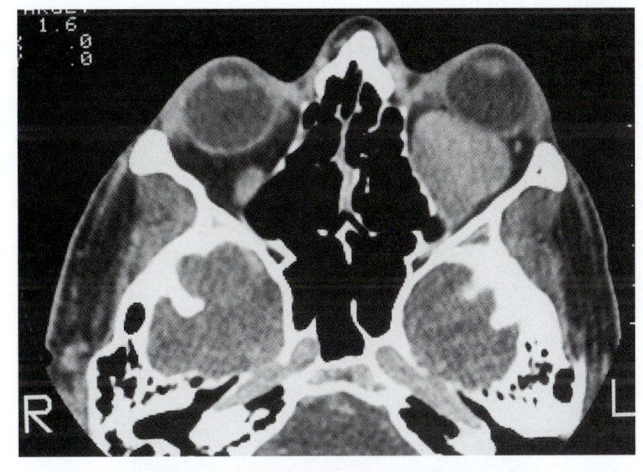

Figure 29.8. Axial computed tomography showing large superior orbital mass. Other sections showed compression of the optic nerve.

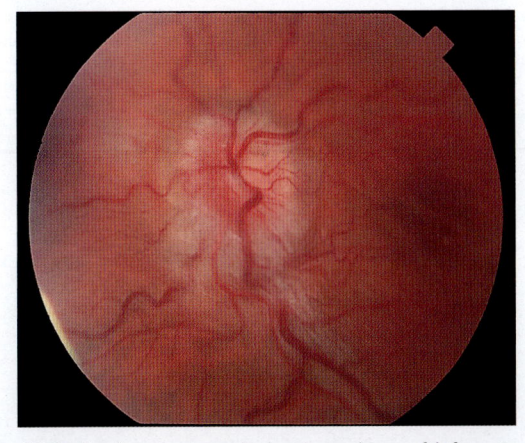

Figure 29.9. Fundus photograph showing edema of left optic nerve, tortuous retinal blood vessels, and choroidal folds. Visual acuity was 6/60.

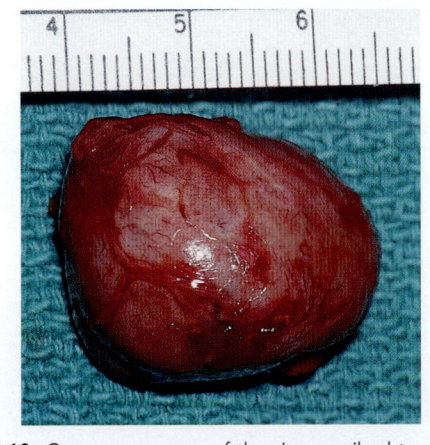

Figure 29.10. Gross appearance of the circumscribed tumor immediately after removal through a superolateral orbitotomy.

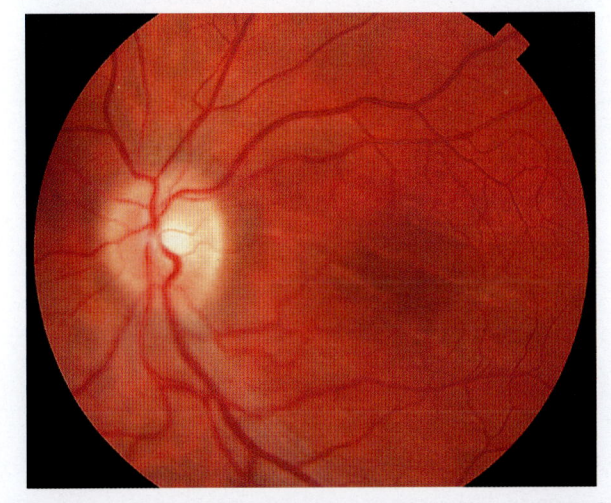

Figure 29.11. Fundus photograph taken 6 months later showing disappearance of the optic disc edema and reversal of the retinal vascular tortuosity. The visual acuity had returned to 6/6. Interestingly, the choroidal folds persisted.

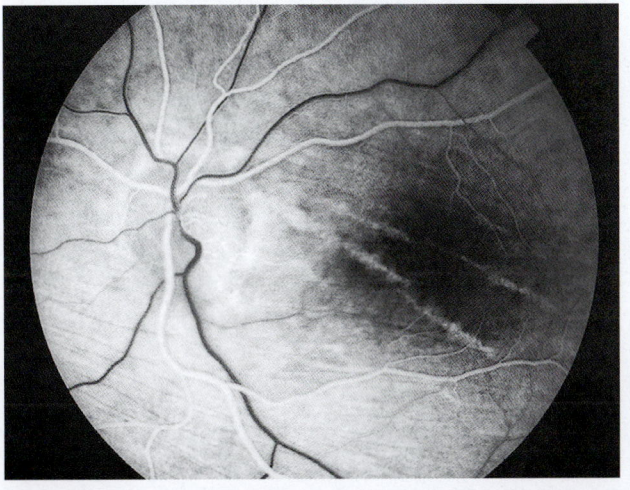

Figure 29.12. Fluorescein angiogram in the arterial phase 6 months after surgery showing transmission hyperfluorescence corresponding to the persistent choroidal folds.

ORBITAL SCHWANNOMA

Because orbital schwannoma is a well-circumscribed, encapsulated tumor, it can sometimes be removed intact by way of lateral orbitotomy despite its large size and posterior location. Illustrated is a clinicopathologic correlation of a large schwannoma in a 33-year-old man who declined a recommended neurosurgical approach and sought another opinion to see if it could be removed without a craniotomy. It was removed intact by way of a superolateral orbitotomy despite the fact that it protruded posteriorly through the superior orbital fissure.

Shields JA, Kapustiak J, Arbizo V, et al. Orbital neurilemoma with extension through the superior orbital fissure. *Arch Ophthalmol* 1986;104:871–873.

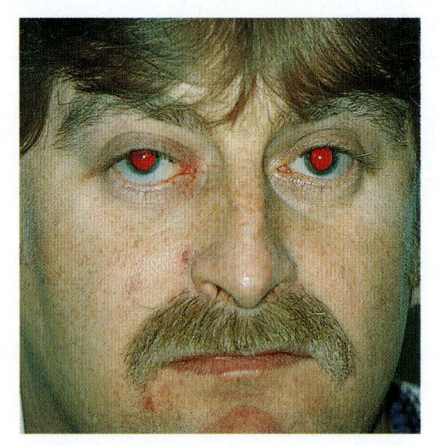

Figure 29.13. Clinical appearance showing proptosis of the right eye.

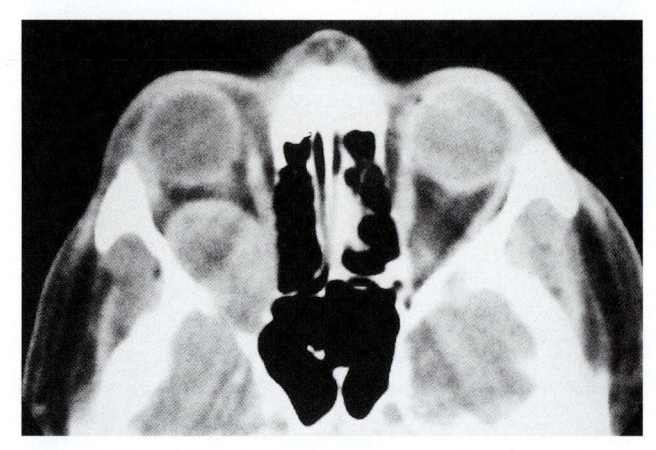

Figure 29.14. Axial CT showing a large, circumscribed mass occupying most of posterior orbit and extending through the superior orbital fissure into the brain.

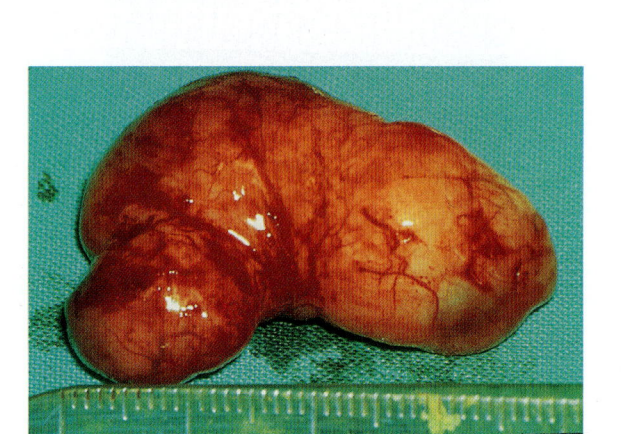

Figure 29.15. Appearance of mass immediately after removal by superotemporal orbitotomy with extraperiosteal approach and osteotomy. The nodular protrusion corresponds to where the tumor protruded posteriorly through the superior orbital fissure.

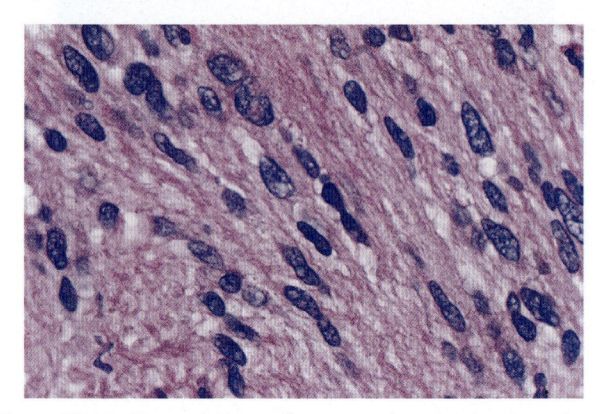

Figure 29.16. Histopathology of an area of tumor showing schwannoma with Antoni A pattern. (Hematoxylin–eosin ×200.)

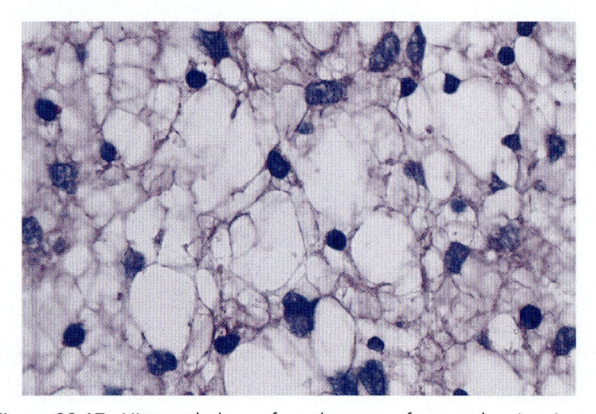

Figure 29.17. Histopathology of another area of tumor showing Antoni B pattern. (Hematoxylin–eosin ×200.)

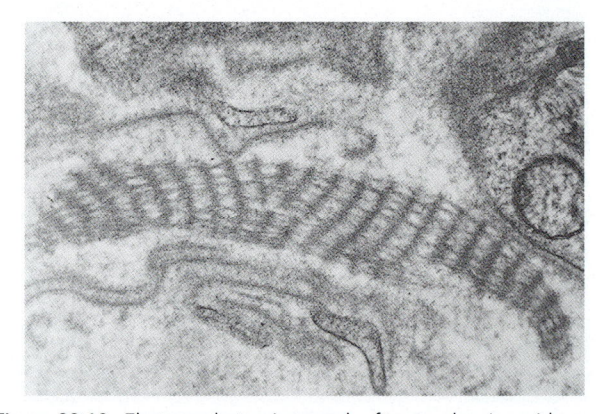

Figure 29.18. Electron photomicrograph of tumor showing wide-spacing collagen in the cytoplasm (Luse body).

Chapter 29 Orbital Peripheral Nerve Tumors 555

ORBITAL SCHWANNOMA: INTRACRANIAL EXTENSION

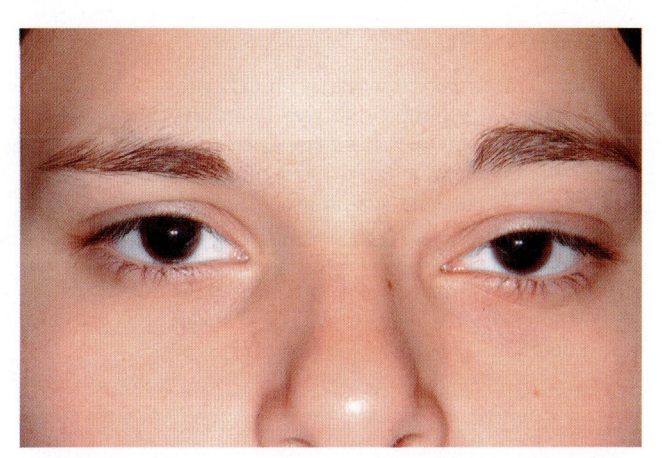

Figure 29.19. Proptosis of left eye in a 16-year-old girl. She had an orbital mass that was found histopathologically after surgical excision to be a schwannoma. It was unclear as to whether the tumor was completely removed.

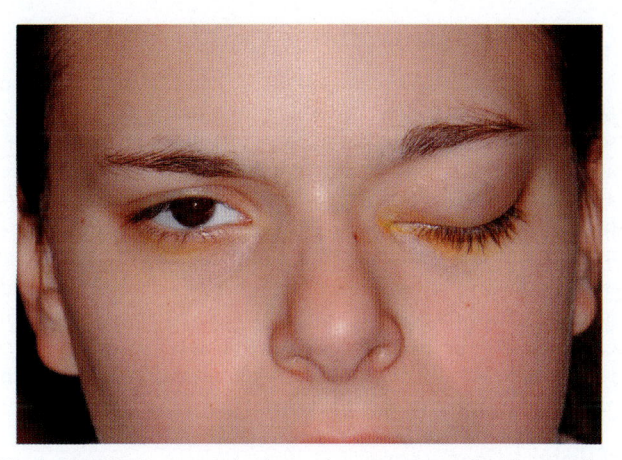

Figure 29.20. Four months later, she was returned with complete blepharoptosis.

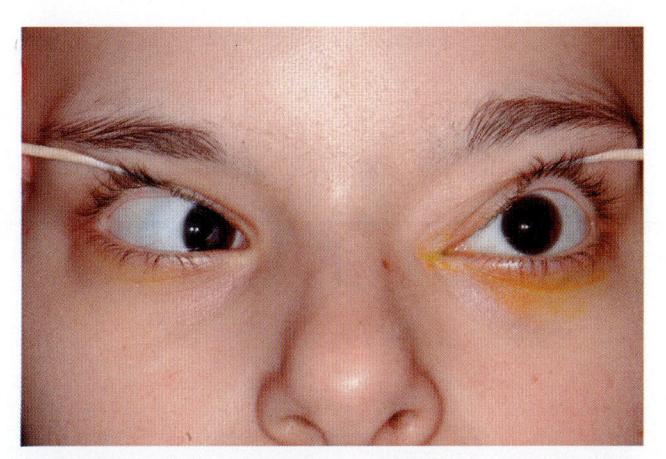

Figure 29.21. On lifting the eyelid, it was found that the left eye had complete absence of ocular motility ("frozen globe").

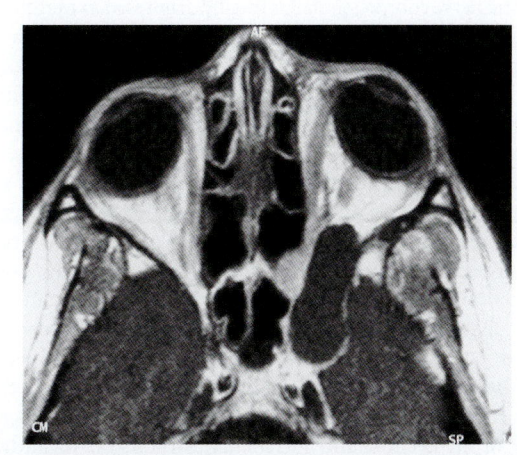

Figure 29.22. Magnetic resonance imaging in T1-weighted image, showing elongated mass extending through the optic foramen. This was apparently not present, or not detected, on the prior imaging studies.

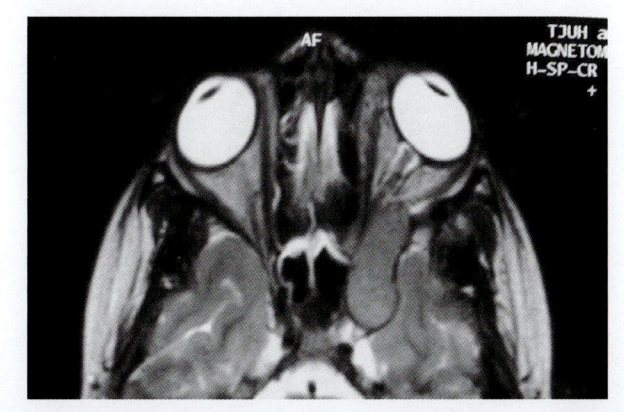

Figure 29.23. Axial magnetic resonance imaging in T2-weighted image, further delineating the well-circumscribed mass.

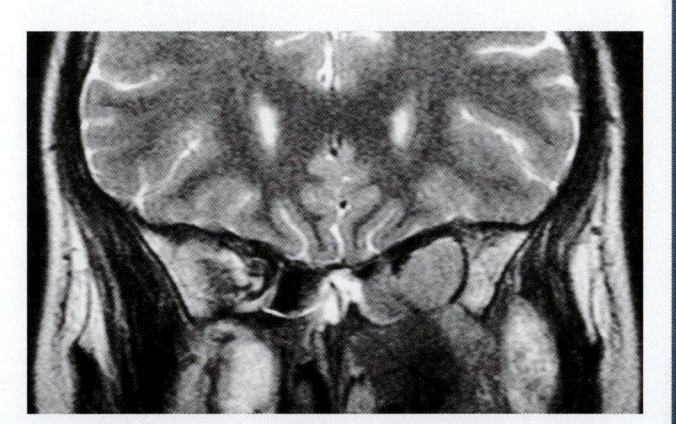

Figure 29.24. Coronal magnetic resonance imaging showing the location of the mass in the region of the optic foramen. The lesion was removed by a neurosurgical approach and there was no recurrence after 4 years of follow-up.

ORBITAL NEUROFIBROMA

General Considerations
Neurofibroma is a benign peripheral nerve tumor that can affect the orbit (1–30). In the authors' series of 1,264 consecutive space-occupying orbital lesions, the 6 neurofibromas accounted for 26% of the 23 peripheral nerve lesions and for <1% of all lesions (1). It can be divided into localized, diffuse, and plexiform types (6). Among our 6 cases, there were 4 plexiform and 2 solitary neurofibromas. The localized type is clinically and radiographically similar to schwannoma and is associated with neurofibromatosis type 1 in about 10% of cases (6). The diffuse type has a variable association with neurofibromatosis and the plexiform type is almost always seen in association with neurofibromatosis.

Clinical Features
Localized neurofibroma produces clinical symptoms and signs similar to schwannoma and other circumscribed orbital tumors and can manifest as proptosis, globe displacement, diplopia, and optic nerve compression. It is usually diagnosed in middle-aged or adult patients and, as mentioned, does not occur in patients with neurofibromatosis type 1. Localized neurofibroma can sometimes occur as multiple orbital tumors in patients without clear evidence of neurofibromatosis. In such cases, pain may be a prominent symptom (19).

Diffuse and plexiform neurofibromas are very similar clinically and radiographically, but are classified separately because of subtle histopathologic differences. They generally become clinically apparent in the first decade of life and show gradual progression, often with involvement of other periocular and ocular tissues, including the uveal tract. The diffuse, poorly defined mass can cause the classic S-shaped curve to the upper eyelid owing to subcutaneous involvement by the tumor. The plexiform form can be very extensive with massive involvement of the orbit, eyelids, and intraocular structures. In addition, patients with neurofibromatosis can have congenital defects in the sphenoid bone that can produce a characteristic pulsating proptosis similar to that seen with encephalocele.

Diagnostic Approaches
With orbital CT and MRI, localized neurofibroma appears as a circumscribed mass that is indistinguishable from schwannoma, described previously. Plexiform and diffuse neurofibromas show an irregular, ill-defined mass, often with extensive periorbital involvement, as mentioned.

Pathology
Localized orbital neurofibroma is circumscribed but lacks a true capsule. The classical case shows interlacing bundles of elongated spindle cells with variable quantities of mucoid material (16). Diffuse and plexiform neurofibromas are composed of a complex intertwining of bundles of enlarged nerves with proliferation of Schwann cells and endoneural fibroblasts in a mucoid matrix. A distinct perineural sheath defines the individual tumor cores.

Management
A patient with suspected localized orbital neurofibroma is usually managed with complete surgical resection of the mass. The diffuse, unresectable plexiform type is typically managed conservatively. However, surgical intervention is often necessary because of bothersome symptoms, threatened vision, or an unacceptable cosmetic appearance. In such instances, debulking surgery is provided, because complete surgical removal may not be possible. Depending on the extent of the disease, a combined approach with neurosurgeons and otolaryngologists may be prudent (11–15).

ORBITAL NEUROFIBROMA

Selected References

Reviews

1. Shields JA, Shields CL, Scartozzi R. Survey of 1264 patients with orbital tumors and simulating lesions: the 2002 Montgomery Lecture, part 1. *Ophthalmology* 2004;111:997–1008.
2. Shields JA, Bakewell B, Augsburger DG, et al. Classification and incidence of space-occupying lesions of the orbit. A survey of 645 biopsies. *Arch Ophthalmol* 1984; 102:1606–1611.
3. Shields JA, Bakewell B, Augsburger DG, et al. Space-occupying orbital masses in children. A review of 250 consecutive biopsies. *Ophthalmology* 1986;93:379–384.
4. Gunalp I, Gunduz K, Duruk K, et al. Neurogenic tumors of the orbit. *Jpn J Ophthalmol* 1994;38:185–190.
5. Rose GE, Wright JE. Isolated peripheral nerve sheath tumours of the orbit. *Eye* 1991;5:668–673.
6. Krohel GB, Rosenberg PN, Wright JE, et al. Localized orbital neurofibromas. *Am J Ophthalmol* 1985;100:458–464.
7. Brownstein S, Little JM. Ocular neurofibromatosis. *Ophthalmology* 1983;91:1595–1599.
8. Avery RA, Dombi E, Hutcheson KA, et al. Visual outcomes in children with neurofibromatosis type 1 and orbitotemporal plexiform neurofibromas. *Am J Ophthalmol* 2013;155:1089–1094.

Imaging

9. De Potter P, Shields CL, Shields JA, et al. The CT and MRI features of an unusual case of isolated orbital neurofibroma. *Ophthal Plast Reconstr Surg* 1992;8:221–227.
10. Reed D, Robertson WD, Rootman J, et al. Plexiform neurofibromatosis of the orbit: CT evaluation. *AJNR Am J Neuroradiol* 1986;7:259–263.

Management

11. Kennerdell JS, Maroon JC. Use of the carbon dioxide laser in the management of orbital plexiform neurofibromas. *Ophthalmic Surg* 1990;2:138–140.
12. Jackson IT, Laws ER Jr, Martin RD. The surgical management of orbital neurofibromatosis. *Plast Reconstr Surg* 1983;71:751–758.
13. Jackson IT. Management of craniofacial neurofibromatosis. *Facial Plast Surg Clin North Am* 2001;9:59–75.
14. Altan-Yaycioglu R, Hintschich C. Clinical features and surgical management of orbitotemporal neurofibromatosis: a retrospective interventional case series. *Orbit* 2010;29:232–238.
15. Snyder BJ, Hanieh A, Trott JA, et al. Transcranial correction of orbital neurofibromatosis. *Plast Reconstr Surg* 1998;102:633–642.

Histopathology

16. Lee LR, Gigantelli JW, Kincaid MC. Localized neurofibroma of the orbit: a radiographic and histopathologic study. *Ophthal Plast Reconstr Surg* 2000;16:241–246.

Case Reports

17. Tada M, Sawamura Y, Ishii N, et al. Massive plexiform neurofibroma in the orbit in a child with von Recklinghausen's disease. *Childs Nerv Syst* 1998;14:210–212.
18. Pittet B, Gumener R, Montandon D. Gigantic neurofibromatosis of the orbit. *J Craniofac Surg* 1997;8:497–500.
19. Shields JA, Shields CL, Lieb WE, et al. Multiple orbital neurofibromas unassociated with von Recklinghausen's disease. *Arch Ophthalmol* 1990;108:80–83.
20. Lyons CJ, McNab AA, Garner A, et al. Orbital malignant peripheral nerve sheath tumours. *Br J Ophthalmol* 1989;73:731–738.
21. Della Rocca RC, Roen J, Labay GR, et al. Isolated neurofibroma of the orbit. *Ophthalmic Surg* 1985;16:634–638.
22. Wiesenfeld D, James PL. Pulsating exophthalmos associated with neurofibromatosis. *J Maxillofac Surg* 1984;12:11–13.
23. Woog JJ, Albert DM, Solt LC, et al. Neurofibromatosis of the eyelid and orbit. *Int Ophthalmol Clin* 1982;22:157–187.
24. Gurland JE, Tenner M, Hornblass A, et al. Orbital neurofibromatosis: involvement of the orbital floor. *Arch Ophthalmol* 1976;94:1723–1725.
25. Kobrin JL, Blodi FC, Weingiest TA, et al. Ocular and orbital manifestations of neurofibromatosis. *Surv Ophthalmol* 1979;24:45–51.
26. Cheng SF, Chen YI, Chang CY, et al. Malignant peripheral nerve sheath tumor of the orbit: malignant transformation from neurofibroma without neurofibromatosis. *Ophthal Plast Reconstr Surg* 2008;24(5):413–415.
27. Pinna A, Demontis S, Maltese G, et al. Absence of the greater sphenoid wing in neurofibromatosis 1. *Arch Ophthalmol* 2005;123:1454.
28. Bajaj MS, Nainiwal SK, Pushker N, et al. Neurofibroma of the lacrimal sac. *Orbit* 2002;21:205–208.
29. Dutton JJ, Tawfik HA, DeBacker CM, et al. Multiple recurrences in malignant peripheral nerve sheath tumor of the orbit: a case report and a review of the literature. *Ophthal Plast Reconstr Surg* 2001;17:293–299.
30. Sadun F, Hinton DR, Sadun AA. Rapid growth of an optic nerve ganglioglioma in a patient with neurofibromatosis 1. *Ophthalmology* 1996;103:794–799.

ORBITAL NEUROFIBROMA: ASSOCIATION WITH NEUROFIBROMATOSIS

Patients with neurofibromatosis can develop a plexiform or a diffuse neurofibroma of the orbit, as well as juvenile pilocytic astrocytoma of the optic nerve. Another orbital manifestation is pulsating proptosis secondary to absence of the greater wing of the sphenoid bone but without an obvious tumor.

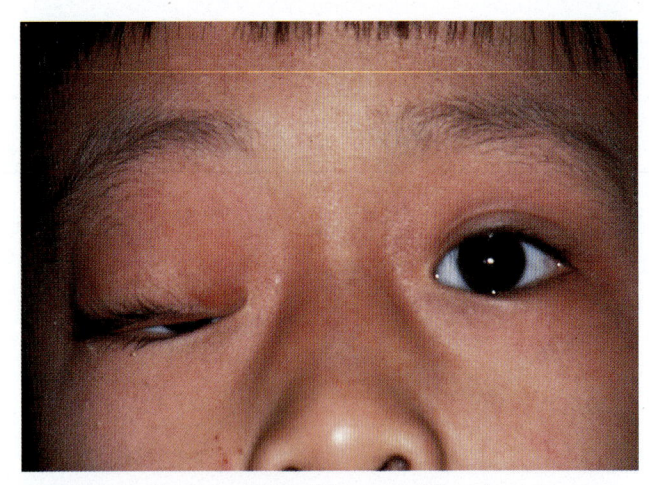

Figure 29.25. Blepharoptosis and proptosis of the right eye in a 6-year-old boy with plexiform neurofibroma of the orbit.

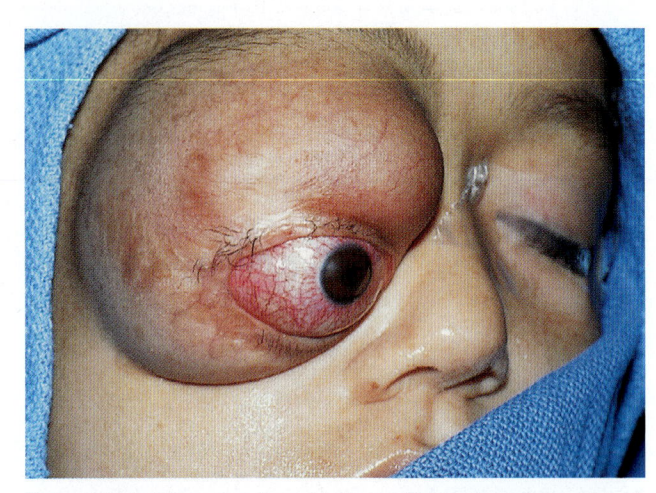

Figure 29.26. More extensive orbital neurofibroma in an 8-year-old girl. (Courtesy of Bruce Johnson, MD.)

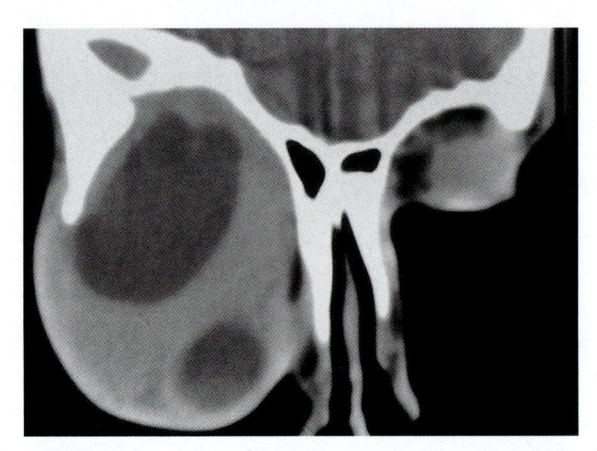

Figure 29.27. Coronal computed tomography of patient shown in Figure 29.26, demonstrating the large orbital mass with clear areas that probably represent mucinous degeneration in the tumor. (Courtesy of Bruce Johnson, MD.)

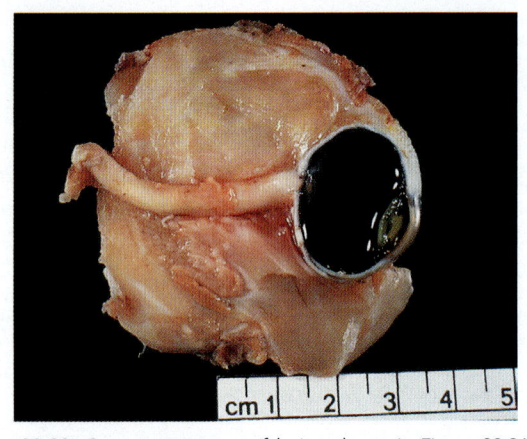

Figure 29.28. Gross appearance of lesion shown in Figure 29.26 after orbital exenteration. Note the advanced diffuse orbital tumor and the long section of grossly normal optic nerve. (Courtesy of Bruce Johnson, MD.)

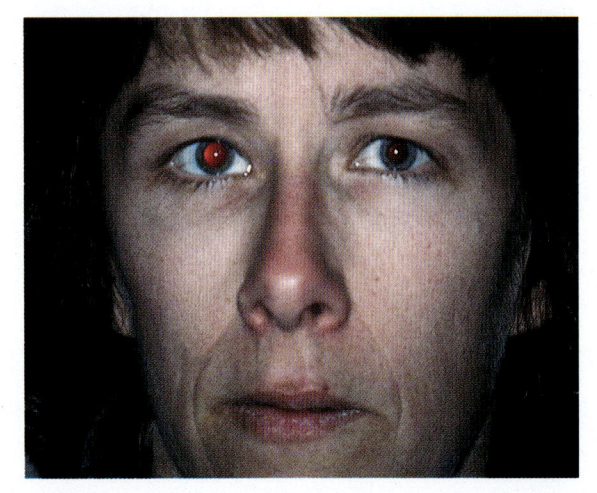

Figure 29.29. Appearance of a 35-year-old woman with neurofibromatosis. She had pulsations of the right eye, but minimal proptosis.

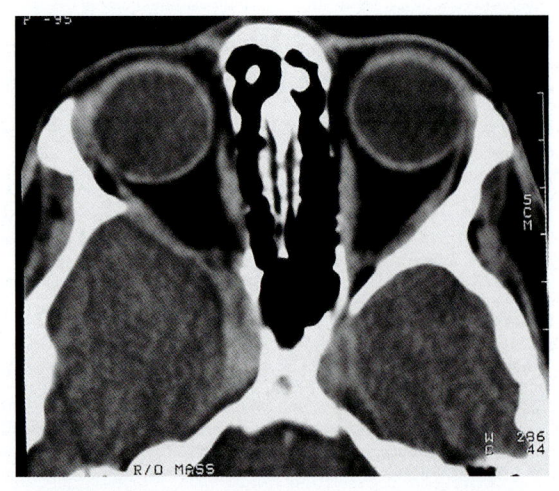

Figure 29.30. Axial computed tomography of patient shown in Figure 29.29. Note the absence of the sphenoid bone that allowed brain pulsations to be transmitted to the orbit.

Chapter 29 Orbital Peripheral Nerve Tumors   559

● ORBITAL NEUROFIBROMA: PROGRESSION OF EYELID, ORBITAL, AND INTRAOCULAR NEUROFIBROMATOSIS

In some instances, neurofibromatosis can involve almost every ocular structure and can demonstrate progressive growth and attain large proportions.

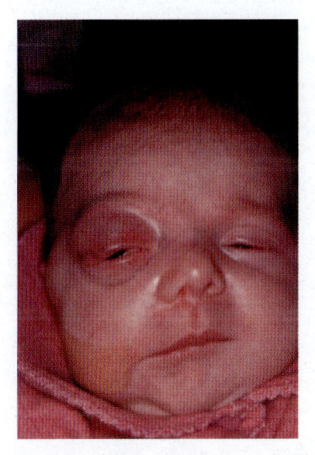

Figure 29.31. One-month-old girl with type 1 neurofibromatosis involving the eyelid, orbit, and globe. There is thickening of upper eyelid, buphthalmos, and proptosis of right eye.

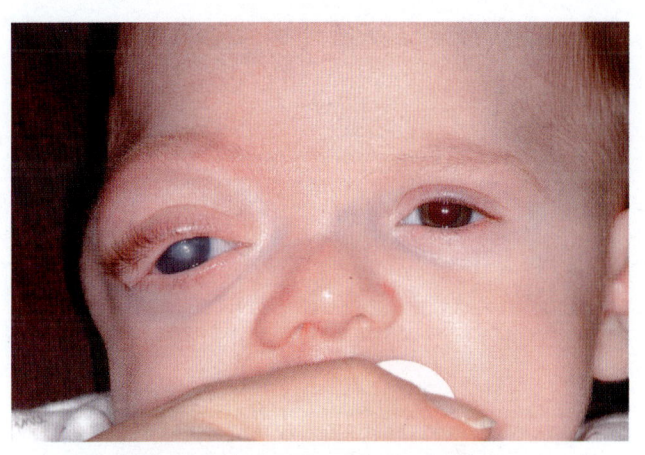

Figure 29.32. Same child at age 4 months showing progression of proptosis and development of a cataract.

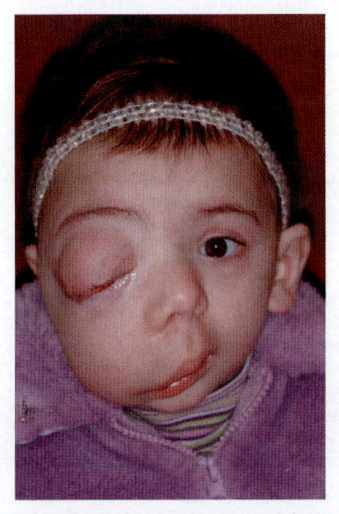

Figure 29.33. Same child at 18 months showing progression of eyelid mass, proptosis, and subcutaneous involvement of right side of face. After much counseling, the parents requested attempted tumor debulking of the tumor and enucleation of the blind right eye, partly for cosmetic reasons.

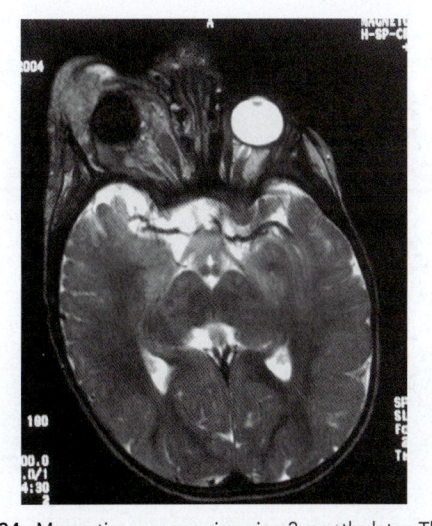

Figure 29.34. Magnetic resonance imaging 2 months later. There is surgical anophthalmos but massive subcutaneous and orbital involvement continues to progress.

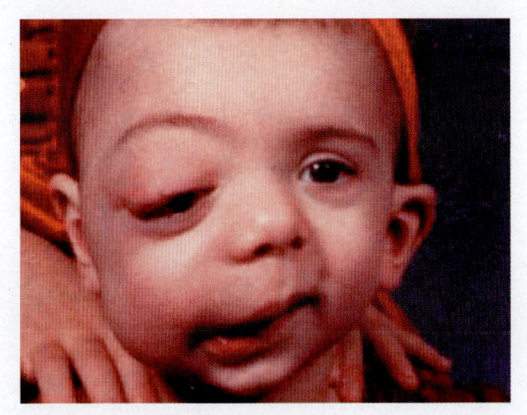

Figure 29.35. Same child at 24 months.

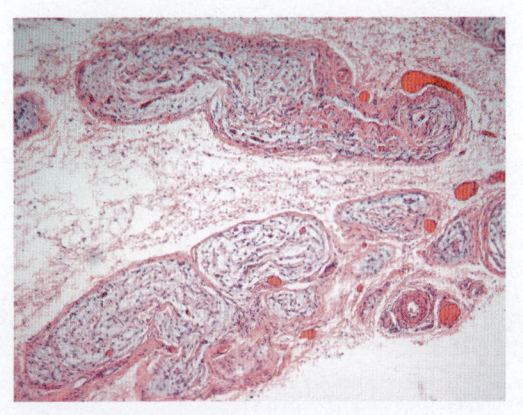

Figure 29.36. Pathology of plexiform neurofibroma of orbit from same child showing enlarged nerve bundles typical of plexiform neurofibroma.

ORBITAL NEUROFIBROMA: SOLITARY TYPE UNASSOCIATED WITH NEUROFIBROMATOSIS

Solitary orbital neurofibroma can occur in the orbit of adults and is often not associated with neurofibromatosis. A clinicopathologic correlation with CT and MRI in a 35-year-old woman is illustrated.

De Potter P, Shields CL, Shields JA, et al. The CT and MRI features of an unusual case of isolated orbital neurofibroma. *Ophthal Plast Reconstr Surg* 1992;8:221–227.

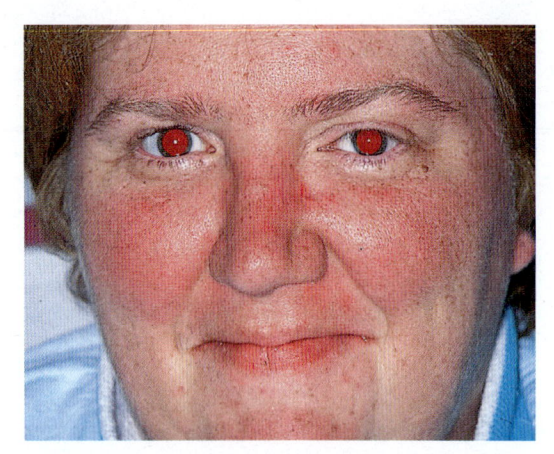

Figure 29.37. Facial appearance showing proptosis of the left eye.

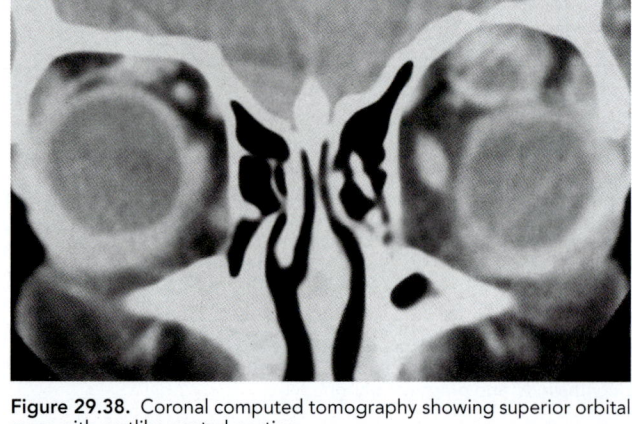

Figure 29.38. Coronal computed tomography showing superior orbital mass with cystlike central portion.

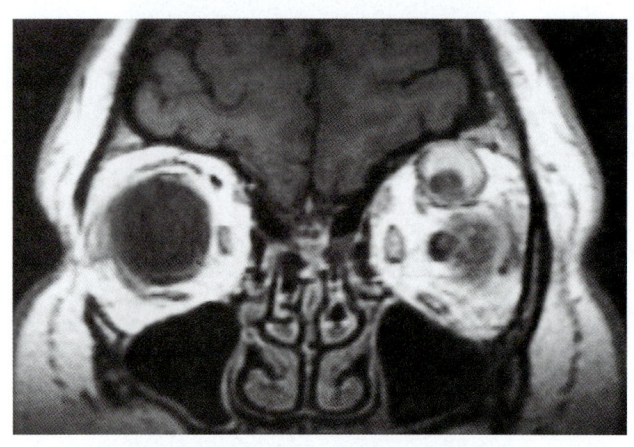

Figure 29.39. Coronal magnetic resonance imaging in T1-weighted image showing the superior orbital mass with low signal component.

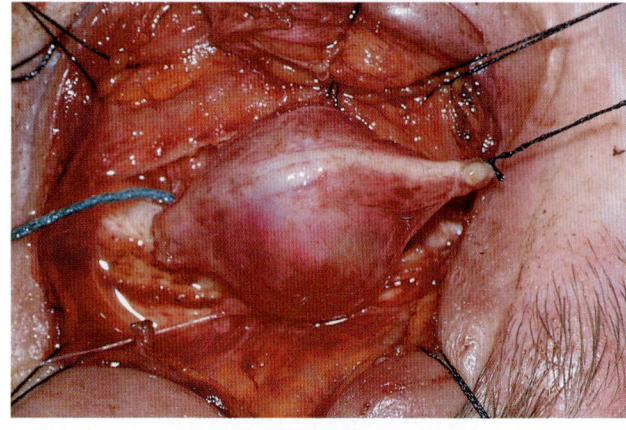

Figure 29.40. Appearance of the mass at the time of surgical exposure. Note the visible nerve coursing along the margin of the mass.

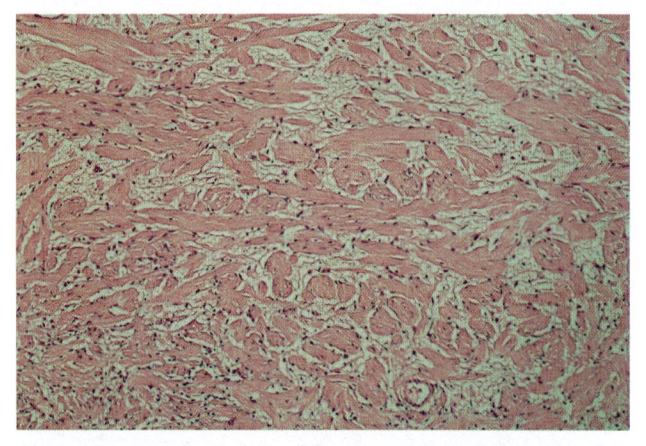

Figure 29.41. Histopathology of the tumor showing large eosinophilic nerve bundles. (Hematoxylin–eosin ×75.)

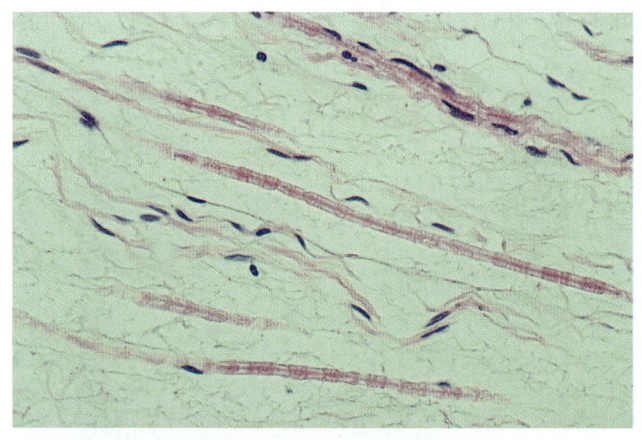

Figure 29.42. Histopathology showing area of extensive mucinous degeneration, corresponding to the low signal component seen on MRI and computed tomography. (Hematoxylin–eosin ×75.)

ORBITAL NEUROFIBROMA: MULTIPLE CIRCUMSCRIBED TYPE UNASSOCIATED WITH NEUROFIBROMATOSIS

Multiple separate neurofibromas can develop in one orbit, apparently unassociated with neurofibromatosis. In the 58-year-old man illustrated here, there was no clinical evidence of neurofibromatosis except for three separate neurofibromas in the right orbit. It is possible that it could represent a forme fruste of von Recklinghausen's neurofibromatosis. The patient's chronic pain completely resolved after surgical removal of the tumors.

Shields JA, Shields CL, Lieb WE, et al. Multiple orbital neurofibromas unassociated with von Recklinghausen's disease. *Arch Ophthalmol* 1990;108:80–83.

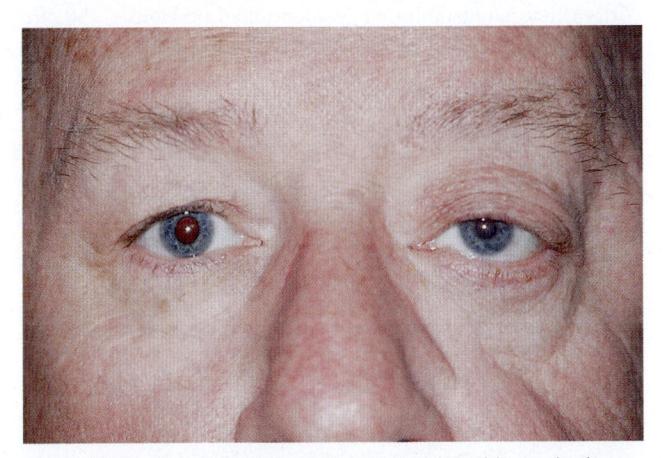

Figure 29.43. Proptosis of the right eye, which had been slowly progressive and painful for several years.

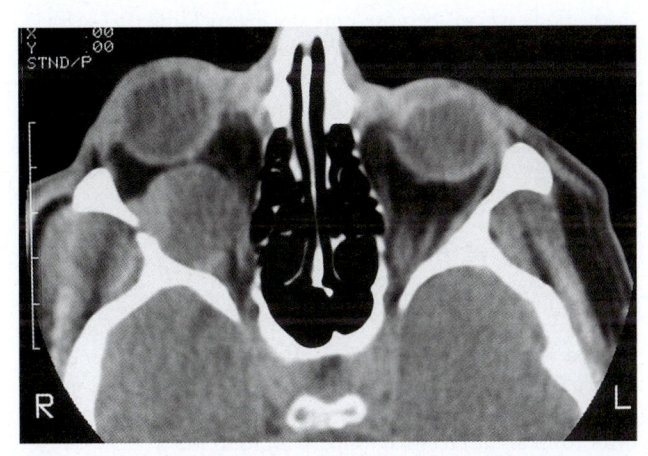

Figure 29.44. Axial computed tomography showing retrobulbar mass and a separate mass in the temporal fossa.

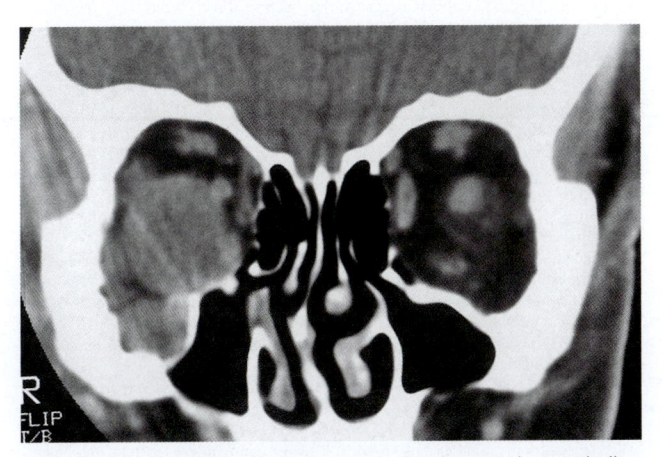

Figure 29.45. Coronal computed tomography showing the retrobulbar mass and a third mass in the inferior aspect of the orbit with displacement of the bony floor of the orbit.

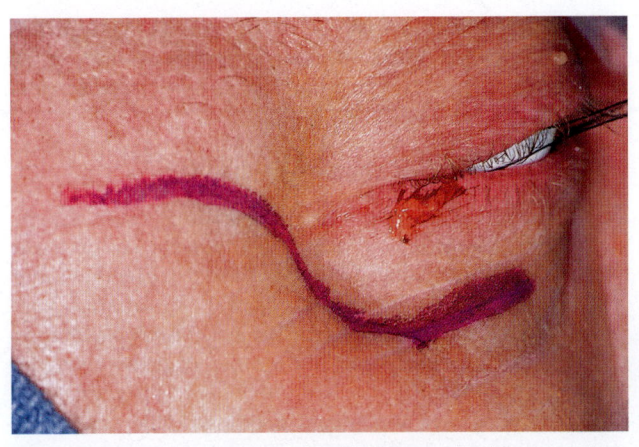

Figure 29.46. Skin incision line for inferotemporal orbitotomy. Three separate masses were removed intact by this approach.

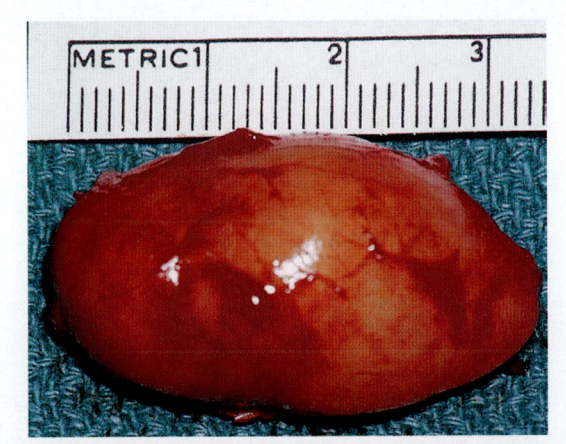

Figure 29.47. Appearance of the retrobulbar mass immediately after surgical removal of all three tumors. Note that the lesion is >30 mm long.

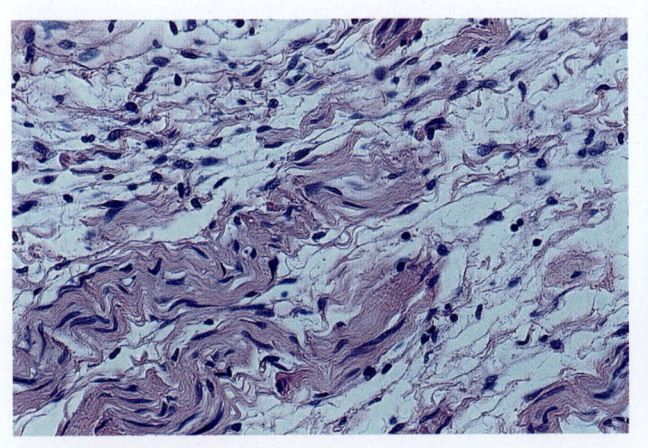

Figure 29.48. Histopathology showing enlarged nerve bundles in a mucoid stroma. (Hematoxylin–eosin ×150.)

ORBITAL PARAGANGLIOMA (CHEMODECTOMA)

General Considerations

Paraganglia are collections of specialized neural crest cells that occur in the adrenal medulla, carotid and aortic bodies, and other similar structures. Paraganglioma (chemodectoma) is a benign neoplasm of paraganglion cells. It can occur anywhere in the body where chemosensory organs are located (1–18).

In the orbit, paraganglioma is believed to arise from the ciliary ganglion. The number of reported orbital cases was drastically reduced when Font et al., after detailed review, reclassified 16 reported cases as alveolar soft part sarcoma (ASPS) (4). Multiple locations can be involved in 10% to 20% of cases, especially if there is a familial predisposition.

Clinical Features

Orbital paraganglioma can become apparent at any age with reported cases having their onset between 4 and 55 years (11). The patient usually develops proptosis, sometimes associated with pain. It has been reported to extend from the orbit into the middle cranial fossa (14) and to secondarily invade the orbit from an intracranial primary location (9).

Diagnostic Approaches

With imaging studies, orbital paraganglioma is usually a well-circumscribed tumor that enhances with contrast agents and is often attached to a rectus muscle. Invasive bone destruction is rare (9,14).

Pathology and Pathogenesis

Paraganglioma is an encapsulated tumor composed of clusters and nests of cells, called "zellballen" that are separated from one another by delicate vascularized septae, and that give the tumor a distinctive pseudoalveolar arrangement. In contrast with ASPS, the nuclei are bland and there is generally no mitotic activity. The histopathologic differential diagnosis includes granular cell tumor (GCT), ASPS, rhabdomyosarcoma, rhabdomyoma, renal cell carcinoma, neuroendocrine carcinoma, melanoma, glomus tumor, and hemangiopericytoma.

True paraganglioma is generally periodic acid-Schiff (PAS) negative and Fontana stain negative. This tumor shows a positive immunohistochemical reaction to neuron-specific enolase, neurofilaments, chromogranin, and synaptophysin. Positive CD 34 outlines the vascular component of the septae. Ultrastructurally, paraganglioma has small, dense core granules measuring 1,000 to 2,000 angstroms in diameter. They represent catecholamine storage in the Golgi apparatus.

The pathogenesis of paraganglioma is unknown, but some cases are familial and multifocal, suggesting a genetic mutation that is still undetermined.

Management

Orbital paraganglioma is almost never diagnosed clinically because it is rare and has no specific features. Like other benign progressive orbital tumors, the recommended management is complete surgical excision. The role of supplemental radiotherapy is not established.

Prognosis

The visual and systemic prognosis is generally good for patients with orbital paraganglioma. As mentioned previously, the rare reported cases of malignant paraganglioma (9,12,14) could represent ASPS.

Selected References

Reviews

1. Shields JA, Shields CL, Scartozzi R. Survey of 1264 patients with orbital tumors and simulating lesions: the 2002 Montgomery Lecture, part 1. *Ophthalmology* 2004; 111:997–1008.
2. Shields JA, Bakewell B, Augsburger DG, et al. Classification and incidence of space-occupying lesions of the orbit. A survey of 645 biopsies. *Arch Ophthalmol* 1984;102:1606–1611.
3. Shields JA, Bakewell B, Augsburger DG, et al. Space-occupying orbital masses in children. A review of 250 consecutive biopsies. *Ophthalmology* 1986;93:379–384.
4. Font RL, Jurco S, Zimmerman LE. Alveolar soft-part sarcoma of the orbit: a clinicopathologic analysis of seventeen cases and a review of the literature. *Hum Pathol* 1982;13:569–579.
5. Lack EE, Cubilla AL, Woodruff JM, et al. Paragangliomas of the head and neck region: a clinical study of 69 patients. *Cancer* 1977;39(2):397–409.

Management

6. Kim CY, Lee SY. Orbital paraganglioma: gamma knife surgery as a therapeutic option. *J Craniofac Surg* 2012;23:1127–1128.

Case Reports

7. Archer KF, Hurwitz JJ, Balogh JM, et al. Orbital nonchromaffin paraganglioma. A case report and review of the literature. *Ophthalmology* 1989;96:1659–1666.
8. Bednar MM, Trainer TD, Aitken PA, et al. Orbital paraganglioma: case report and review of the literature. *Br J Ophthalmol* 1992;76:183–185.
9. Deutsch AR, Duckworth JJ. Nonchromaffin paraganglioma of the orbit. *Am J Ophthalmol* 1969;68:659–663.
10. Laquis SJ, Vick V, Haik BF, et al. Intracranial paraganglioma (glomus tumor) with orbital extension. *Ophthal Plast Reconstr Surg* 2001;17:458–461.
11. Nirankara MS, Greer CH, Chaddah MR. Malignant non-chromaffin paragangliooma in the orbit. *Br J Ophthalmol* 1963;47:357–363.
12. Thacker WC, Duckworth JK. Chemodectoma of the orbit. *Cancer* 1969;23:1233–1238.
13. Tye AA. Nonchromaffin paraganglioma of the orbit. *Ophthalmol Soc Australia* 1961; 21:113–114.
14. Varghese S, Nair B, Joseph TA. Orbital malignant non-chromaffin paraganglioma. Alveolar soft-part sarcoma. *Br J Ophthalmol* 1968;52:713–715.
15. Venkataramana NK, Kolluri VR, Kumar DV, et al. Paraganglioma of the orbit with extension to the middle cranial fossa: case report. *Neurosurgery* 1989;24:762–764.
16. Makhdoomi R, Nayil K, Santosh V, et al. Orbital paraganglioma–a case report and review of the literature. *Clin Neuropathol* 2010;29:100–104.
17. Ahmed A, Dodge OG, Kirk RS. Chemodectoma of the orbit. *J Clin Pathol* 1969; 22:584–588.
18. Mathur SP. Nonchromaffin paraganglioma of the orbit. *Int Surg* 1968;50:336–339.

Chapter 29 Orbital Peripheral Nerve Tumors 563

ORBITAL PARAGANGLIOMA

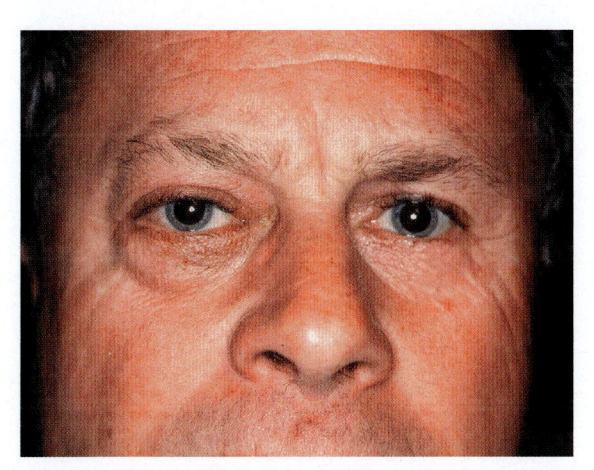

Figure 29.49. Facial appearance of 54-year-old man who has mild proptosis of the right eye. (Courtesy of Phil Aitken, MD.)

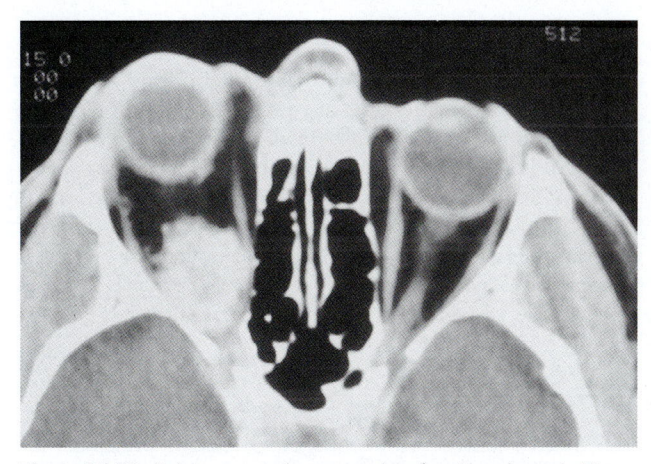

Figure 29.50. Axial computed tomography of patient shown in Figure 29.49, depicting circumscribed mass in posterior orbit with slightly irregular margins. (Courtesy of Phil Aitken, MD.)

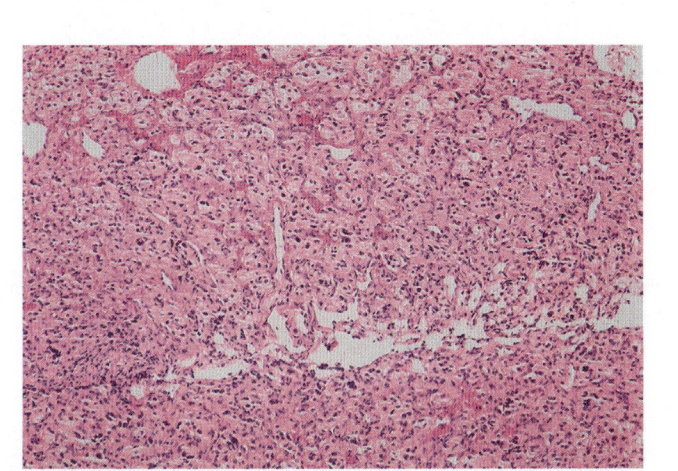

Figure 29.51. Histopathology of lesion shown in Figure 29.49, showing neuroid appearance of cells, forming nests called zellballen, surrounded by a rich capillary network. (Hematoxylin–eosin ×100.) (Courtesy of Phil Aitken, MD.)

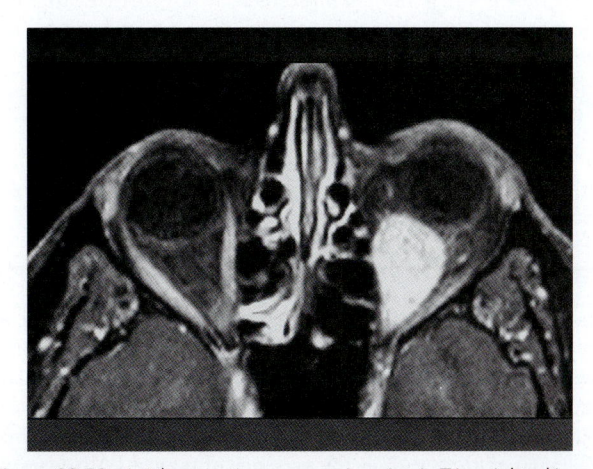

Figure 29.52. Axial magnetic resonance imaging in T1-weighted image in a 53-year-old man who presented with proptosis of left eye showing gadolinium enhancement of circumscribed, elongated mass filling most of the orbit. (Courtesy Janice Safneck, MD.)

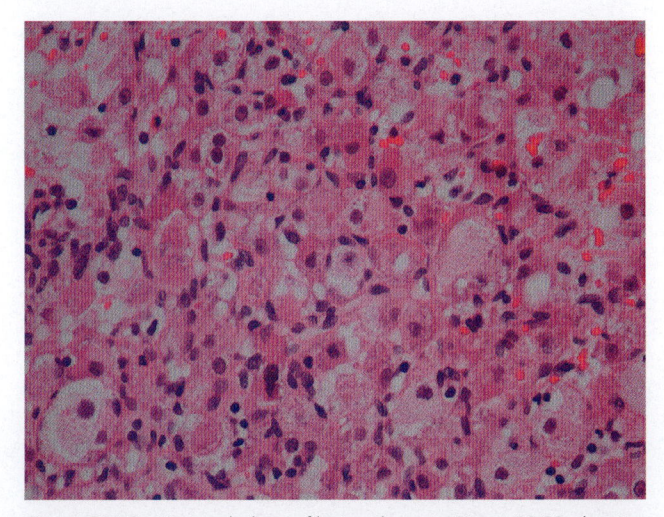

Figure 29.53. Histopathology of lesion shown in Figure 29.52, showing neuroid appearance of cells, small uniform nuclei, and abundant clear cytoplasm, forming nests called zellballen surrounded by a rich capillary network. (Hematoxylin–eosin ×150.) (Courtesy Janice Safneck, MD.)

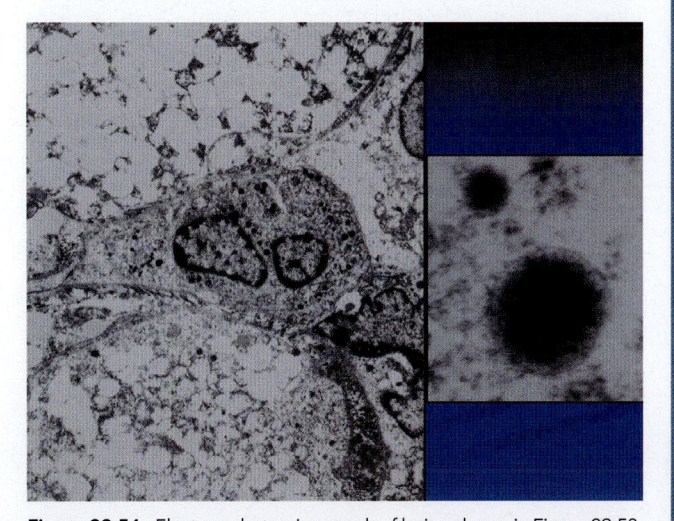

Figure 29.54. Electron photomicrograph of lesion shown in Figure 29.53, depicting cells with osmophilic neurosecretory granules. Inset shows closer view of neurosecretory granule. (Courtesy Janice Safneck, MD.)

TUMORS OF THE ORBIT

ORBITAL ALVEOLAR SOFT PART SARCOMA

General Considerations

ASPS is a soft tissue neoplasm of disputed origin. It is most often found in the extremities of young adults. When it occurs in the head region, it usually involves the tongue or orbit (1–17). It is a rare tumor, with only 1 case (<1%) among 1,264 patients with orbital lesions seen by the authors (1). The largest series of orbital ASPS included 17 cases reported by Font et al. from the Armed Forces Institute of Pathology in 1982 (4). Among the 17 patients, the mean age at diagnosis was 23 years (median age 18 years), with a range of 11 months to 69 years. Most (75%) occurred in females.

Clinical Features

The affected patient with orbital ASPS usually presents with rather rapid onset and progression of proptosis, a course similar to that of other malignant orbital tumors. In the early stages, the tumor is small and circumscribed. If not treated early and effectively, it can become alarmingly aggressive and can fill the orbit and destroy the globe.

Diagnostic Approaches

In the early stages imaging studies of ASPS show a circumscribed mass and in the more advanced stages it is a diffuse, poorly defined mass.

Pathology

Histopathologically, ASPS is characterized by large round to polyhedral cells that assume a pseudoalveolar pattern with the alveolar spaces separated by delicate fibrovascular trabeculae. The loosely cohesive cells sometimes float freely in the alveolar spaces, resembling the alveolar variant of rhabdomyosarcoma. A characteristic feature is the presence of typical PAS-positive, diastase-resistant intracytoplasmic crystalline structures that can be better demonstrated with electron microscopy (4,9). The pathogenesis is still a matter of debate. A leading possibility is that it represents a tumor of neural origin, perhaps a malignant variant of a paraganglioma (chemodectoma) or granule cell tumor.

Management

The best management of orbital ASPS is wide surgical excision followed by irradiation and chemotherapy, similar to the treatment of rhabdomyosarcoma. Local recurrence and metastasis develop in a moderate number of patients (4,5). Metastatic disease can occur, usually to the lungs. In the series of 17 cases, 2 patients died from metastatic disease (4).

ORBITAL ALVEOLAR SOFT PART SARCOMA

Selected References

Reviews

1. Shields JA, Shields CL, Scartozzi R. Survey of 1264 patients with orbital tumors and simulating lesions: the 2002 Montgomery Lecture, part 1. *Ophthalmology* 2004; 111:997–1008.
2. Shields JA, Bakewell B, Augsburger DG, et al. Classification and incidence of space-occupying lesions of the orbit. A survey of 645 biopsies. *Arch Ophthalmol* 1984;102:1606–1611.
3. Shields JA, Bakewell B, Augsburger DG, et al. Space-occupying orbital masses in children. A review of 250 consecutive biopsies. *Ophthalmology* 1986;93:379–384.
4. Font RL, Jurco S, Zimmerman LE. Alveolar soft-part sarcoma of the orbit: a clinicopathologic analysis of seventeen cases and a review of the literature. *Hum Pathol* 1982;13:569–579.
5. Hunter BC, Devaney KO, Ferlito A, et al. Alveolar soft part sarcoma of the head and neck region. *Ann Otol Rhino Laryngol* 1998;107:810–814.

Imaging

6. Grant GD, Shields JA, Flanagan JC, et al. The ultrasonographic and radiologic features of a histologically proven case of alveolar soft-part sarcoma of the orbit. *Am J Ophthalmol* 1979;87:773–777.

Histopathology

7. Alkatan H, Al-Shedoukhy AA, Chaudhry IA, et al. Orbital alveolar soft part sarcoma: Histopathologic report of two cases. *Saudi J Ophthalmol* 2010;24:57–61.
8. Coupland SE, Heimann H, Hoffmeister B, et al. Immunohistochemical examination of an orbital alveolar soft part sarcoma. *Graefes Arch Clin Exp Ophthalmol* 1999;237:266–272.

Case Reports

9. Bunt AH, Bensinger RE. Alveolar soft-part sarcoma of the orbit. *Ophthalmology* 1981;888:1339–1346.
10. Jordan DR, MacDonald H, Noel L, et al. Alveolar soft-part sarcoma of the orbit. *Ophthalmic Surg* 1995;26:269–270.
11. Simmons WB, Haggerty HS, Ngan B, et al. Alveolar soft part sarcoma of the head and neck. A disease of children and young adults. *Int J Pediatr Otorhinolaryngol* 1989;17:139–153.
12. Abrahams IW, Fenton RH, Vidone R. Alveolar soft-part sarcoma of the orbit. *Arch Ophthalmol* 1968;79:185–188.
13. Altamirano-Dimas M, Albores-Saavedra J. Alveolar soft part sarcoma of the orbit. *Arch Ophthalmol* 1966;75:496–499.
14. Khan AO, Burke MJ. Alveolar soft-part sarcoma of the orbit. *J Pediatr Ophthalmol Strabismus* 2004;41:245–246.
15. Mathur SP. Nonchromaffin paraganglioma of the orbit. *Int Surg* 1968;50:336–339.
16. Kim HJ, Wojno T, Grossniklaus HE, et al. Alveolar soft-part sarcoma of the orbit: report of 2 cases with review of the literature. *Ophthal Plast Reconstr Surg* 2013;29:e138–e142.
17. Kashyap S, Sen S, Sharma MC, et al. Alveolar soft-part sarcoma of the orbit: report of three cases. *Can J Ophthalmol* 2004;39:552–556.

ORBITAL ALVEOLAR SOFT PART SARCOMA

Jordan DR, MacDonald H, Noel L, et al. Alveolar soft-part sarcoma of the orbit. *Ophthalmic Surg* 1995;26;269–270.

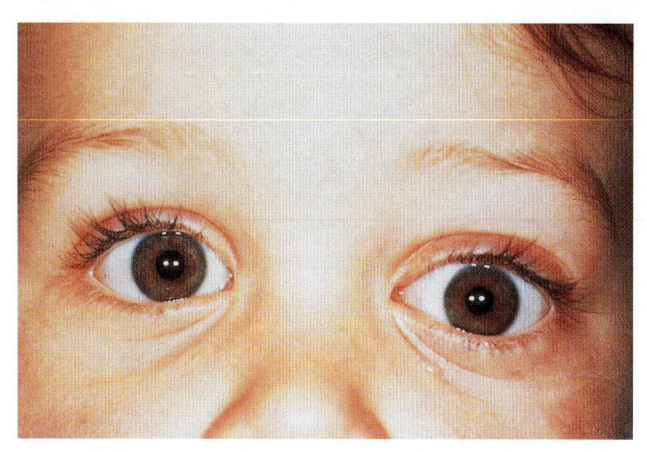

Figure 29.55. Proptosis of the left eye in a 19-month-old boy. (Courtesy of Seymour Brownstein, MD.)

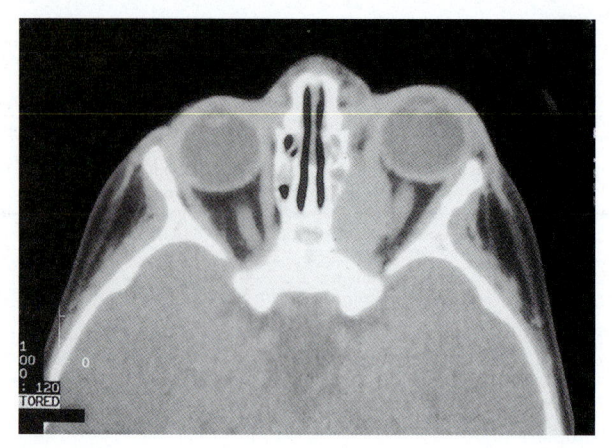

Figure 29.56. Axial computed tomography of patient shown in Figure 29.55, demonstrating solid mass along medial wall of the left orbit. (Courtesy of Seymour Brownstein, MD.)

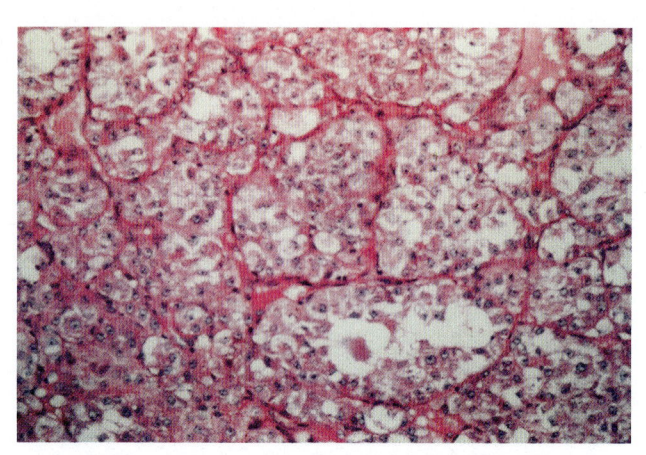

Figure 29.57. Histopathology of orbital alveolar soft part sarcoma demonstrating the alveolar arrangement of the cells and periodic acid–Schiff–positive crystals in cytoplasm. (Periodic acid-Schiff ×100.)

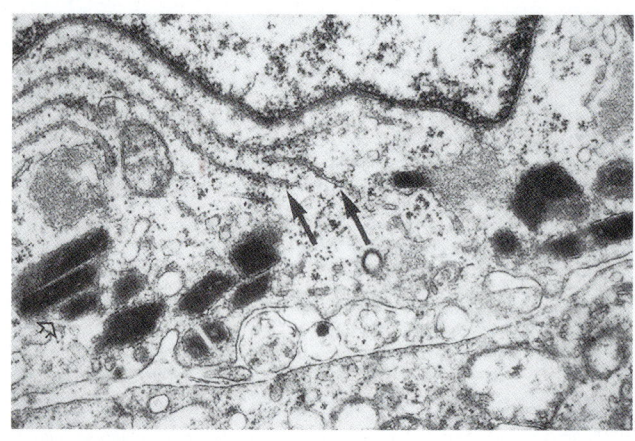

Figure 29.58. Electron microscopy of tumor shown in Figure 29.57, depicting the characteristic crystalline inclusions in the cytoplasm (×10,000). (Courtesy of Seymour Brownstein, MD.)

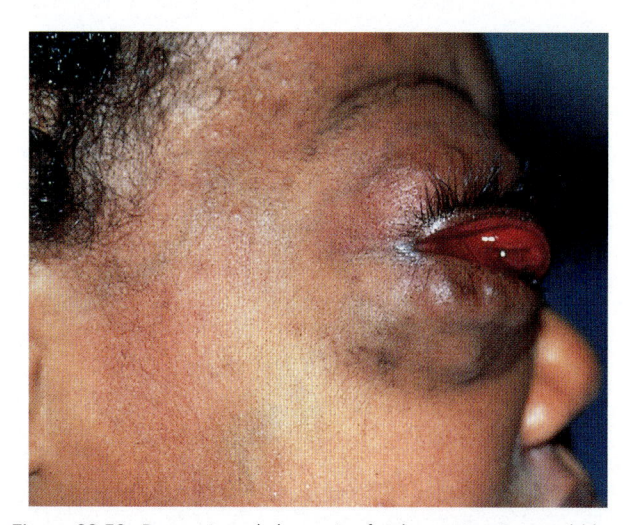

Figure 29.59. Proptosis and chemosis of right eye in a 2-year-old boy with ASPS of the orbit. (Courtesy of Lorenz E. Zimmerman, MD.)

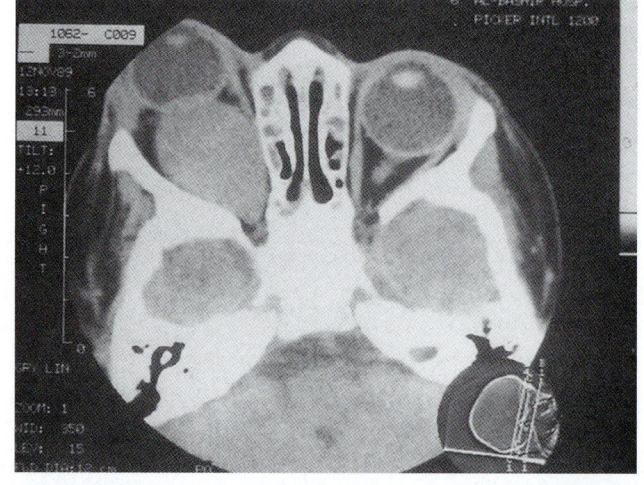

Figure 29.60. Axial computed tomography of the patient shown in Figure 29.59, revealing inferotemporal orbital mass on the left side. The mass was excised and found to be an alveolar soft part sarcoma. (Courtesy of Lorenz E. Zimmerman, MD.)

Chapter 29 Orbital Peripheral Nerve Tumors 567

ORBITAL ALVEOLAR SOFT PART SARCOMA: AGGRESSIVE TUMOR IN A CHILD

In some instances, ASPS can be remarkably aggressive and attain a large size despite treatment efforts. A case example is shown.

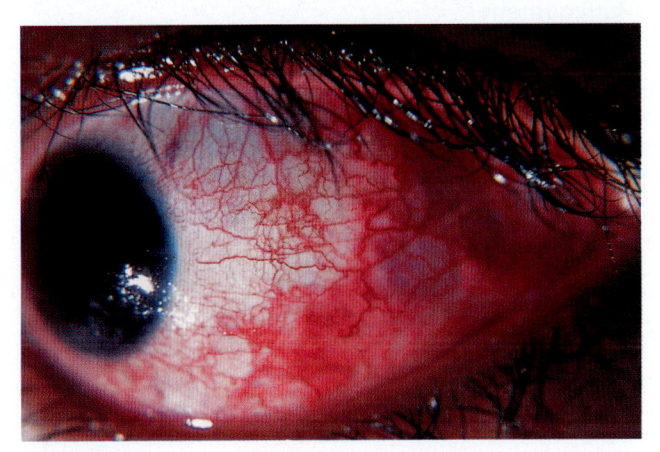

Figure 29.61. Dilated epibulbar blood vessels in the left eye of a 5-year-old child. (Courtesy of John D. Wright, MD.)

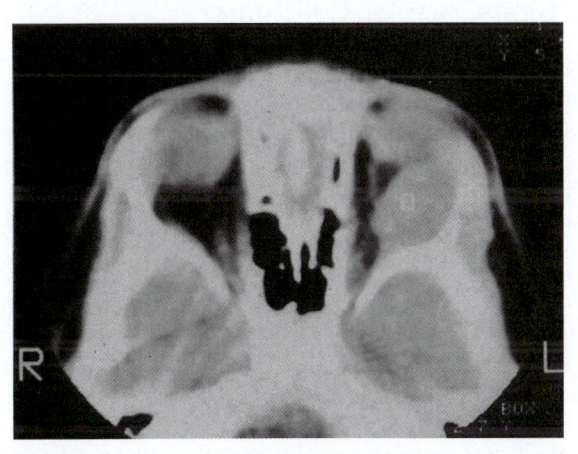

Figure 29.62. Axial computed tomography showing ovoid mass along lateral wall of orbit. The child was treated elsewhere with corticosteroids with a diagnosis of orbital inflammatory pseudotumor, but the lesion continued to progress and biopsy revealed alveolar soft part sarcoma. (Courtesy of John D. Wright, MD.)

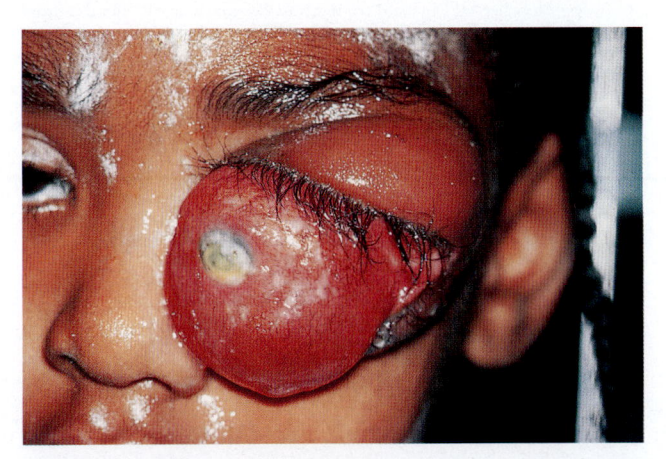

Figure 29.63. Appearance of the patient 3 months later showing marked progression of the lesion. (Courtesy of John D. Wright, MD.)

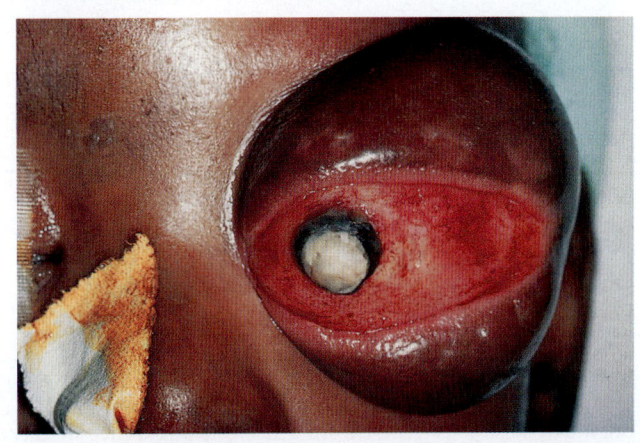

Figure 29.64. Appearance of patient 3 months after Figure 29.63, showing no improvement despite chemotherapy. Orbital exenteration was performed. (Courtesy of John D. Wright, MD.)

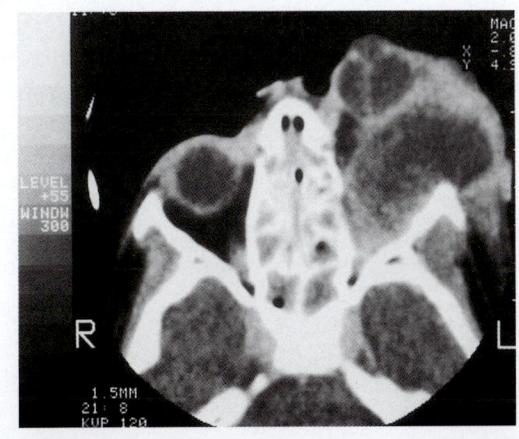

Figure 29.65. Axial computed tomography at time of photograph shown in Figure 29.64 disclosing a massive orbital tumor. (Courtesy of John D. Wright, MD.)

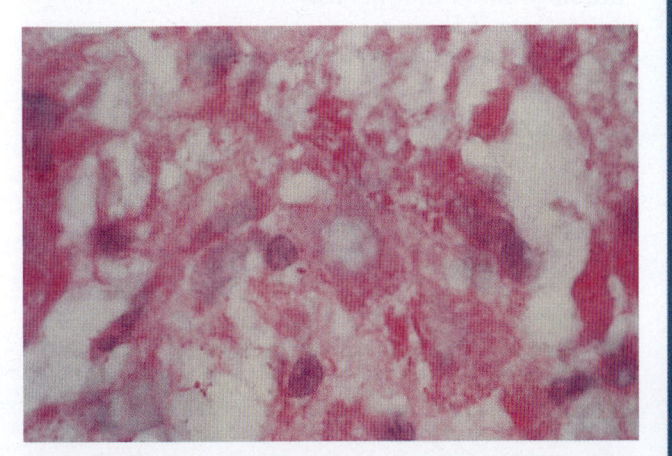

Figure 29.66. Histopathology showing periodic acid-Schiff–positive, diastase-resistant intracytoplasmic structures in the tumor cells. (Periodic acid-Schiff ×300.) (Courtesy of John D. Wright, MD.)

MISCELLANEOUS ORBITAL NEURAL TUMORS: GRANULAR CELL TUMOR, AMPUTATION NEUROMA, AND MALIGNANT PERIPHERAL NERVE SHEATH TUMOR

Orbital Granular Cell Tumor

General Considerations
GCT is a benign neoplasm that can occasionally appear in the orbit (1–22). This tumor generally occurs in dermis, submucosal tissue, and smooth and striated muscle. In the ocular region, it has been known to appear in the conjunctiva, caruncle, lacrimal sac, eyebrow, eyelid, and, rarely, the iris (5). It has rarely been reported to metastasize to the orbit from a primary malignant GCT in the cervical region (7). No convincing cases of GCT were identified in the large series of orbital lesions from Wills Eye Institute (1). Approximately 10% to 15% of reported cases from extraocular areas have been multifocal, but the orbital cases have all been solitary. This tumor can occur in both children and adults (5).

GCT was previously called "granular cell myoblastoma" because it was believed to arise from skeletal muscle. This concept was supported by the fact that the tumor frequently occurred in the oral cavity, particularly the tongue. Most recently, a Schwann cell origin for this tumor has been considered (5).

Clinical Features
GCT is well circumscribed and has clinical and imaging features similar to other well-defined orbital tumors. The clinical features are nonspecific and most cases are not suspected clinically, but are diagnosed histopathologically after surgical excision.

Diagnostic Approaches
Orbital CT and MRI of GCT generally show a round soft tissue mass that has marked contrast enhancement. It is often near an extraocular muscle (6). The close relationship to muscle in some cases does not negate the possibility of a neural origin, because it can arise from a nerve in proximity to the muscle.

Pathology and Pathogenesis
GCT is composed of benign spindle cells with a pronounced granular eosinophilic cytoplasm (8–10). It may resemble oncocytoma, rhabdomyosarcoma, neurofibroma, or schwannoma. Special stains and immunohistochemistry can assist in the differential diagnosis. The cytoplasm is intensely PAS-positive and diastase resistant, suggesting that the granules are not glycogen and thereby excluding the likelihood of a muscle tumor. They are desmin positive and S-100 protein positive, supporting a neural crest origin.

Ultrastructural studies show abundant intercellular basement membrane and spindle cells that may contain characteristic cytoplasmic inclusions called angulated or Bangle bodies (8–10). A malignant variation of this tumor, similar to ASPS, has been reported to occur in about 2% of all GCT.

Management
GCT is rarely diagnosed clinically. Like other slowly progressive, circumscribed, benign tumors, the best management is complete surgical excision if possible. Recurrence appears to be rare after surgical removal. The tumor may be relatively radioresistant (17).

Selected References

Reviews
1. Shields JA, Shields CL, Scartozzi R. Survey of 1264 patients with orbital tumors and simulating lesions: the 2002 Montgomery Lecture, part 1. *Ophthalmology* 2004; 111:997–1008.
2. Shields JA, Bakewell B, Augsburger DG, et al. Classification and incidence of space-occupying lesions of the orbit. A survey of 645 biopsies. *Arch Ophthalmol* 1984;102:1606–1611.
3. Shields JA, Bakewell B, Augsburger DG, et al. Space-occupying orbital masses in children. A review of 250 consecutive biopsies. *Ophthalmology* 1986;93:379–384.
4. McNab AA, Daniel SE. Granular cell tumours of the orbit. *Aust N Z J Ophthalmol* 1991;19:21–27.
5. Jaeger MJ, Green WR, Miller NR, et al. Granular cell tumor of the orbit and ocular adnexae. *Surv Ophthalmol* 1987;3:417–423.

Imaging
6. Ahdoot M, Rodgers IR. Granular cell tumor of the orbit: magnetic resonance imaging characteristics. *Ophthal Plast Reconstr Surg* 2005;21:395–397.

Management
7. Golio DI, Prabhu S, Hauck EF, et al. Surgical resection of locally advanced granular cell tumor of the orbit. *J Craniofac Surg* 2006;17:594–598.

Histopathology
8. Capeans-Tome C, Urdiales-Viedma M. Granular cell tumor of the eye (myoblastoma): ultrastructural and immunohistochemical studies. *Eur J Ophthalmol* 1993; 3:47–52.
9. Goldstein BG, Font RL, Alper MG. Granular cell tumor of the orbit: a case report including electron microscopic observation. *Ann Ophthalmol* 1982;14:231–238.
10. Rodriguez-Ares T, Varela-Duran J, Sanchez-Salorio M, et al. Granular cell tumor of the eye (myoblastoma): ultrastructural and immunohistochemical studies. *Eur J Ophthalmol* 1993;3:47–52.

Case Reports
11. Chaves E, Oliveria AM, Arnaud AC. Retrobulbar granular cell myoblastoma. *Br J Ophthalmol* 1972;56:854–856.
12. Dolman PJ, Rootman J, Dolman CL. Infiltrating orbital granular cell tumor: a case report and literature review. *Br J Ophthalmol* 1987;71:47–53.
13. Drummond JW, Hall DL, Steen WH Jr, et al. Granular cell tumor (myoblastoma) of the orbit. *Arch Ophthalmol* 1979;97:1492–1507.
14. Dunnington JH. Granular cell myoblastoma of the orbit. *Arch Ophthalmol* 1948; 40:14–22.
15. Gonzales-Almaraz G, de Buen S, Tsutsumi V. Granular cell tumor (myoblastoma) of the orbit. *Am J Ophthalmol* 1985;79:606–612.
16. Hashimoto M, Ohtsuka K, Suzuki T, et al. Orbital granular cell tumor developing in the inferior oblique muscle. *Am J Ophthalmol* 1997;124:404–406.
17. Karcioglu ZA, Hemphill GL, Wool BM. Granular cell tumor of the orbit: case report and review of the literature. *Ophthalmic Surg* 1983;14:125–129.
18. Morgan G. Granular cell myoblastoma of the orbit. *Arch Ophthalmol* 1976;94: 2135–2142.
19. Allaire GS, Laflamme P, Bourgouin P. Granular cell tumour of the orbit. *Can J Ophthalmol* 1995;30:151–153.
20. Moriarity P, Garner A, Wright JE. Case report of granular cell myoblastoma arising within the medial rectus muscle. *Br J Ophthalmol* 1983;67:17–22.
21. Singleton EM, Nettleship MB. Granular cell tumor of the orbit: a case report. *Ann Ophthalmol* 1983;15:881–883.
22. Callejo SA, Kronish JW, Decker SJ, et al. Malignant granular cell tumor metastatic to the orbit. *Ophthalmology* 2000;107:550–554.

MISCELLANEOUS ORBITAL NEURAL TUMORS: GRANULAR CELL TUMOR, AMPUTATION NEUROMA, AND MALIGNANT PERIPHERAL NERVE SHEATH TUMOR

Orbital Amputation Neuroma

General Considerations
Amputation neuroma occurs at the stump of severed peripheral nerves and can produce "phantom limb" symptoms. It has developed in the orbit following enucleation, other surgical procedures, and trauma (1–11). The incidence of orbital amputation neuroma is not known. There were no cases in the Wills Eye Hospital clinical series of 1,274 patients (1). In a study of 16 neurogenic orbital tumors from Turkey, there was 1 case of amputation neuroma (4). It may be more common than realized because some are probably small and minimally symptomatic. This is substantiated by a report on patients with orbital pain following enucleation in which four of five biopsies revealed microscopic evidence of amputation neuroma (5).

Clinical Features
Most reported patients with orbital amputation neuroma have had orbital surgical procedures, usually enucleation. Months or years after surgery, the affected patient develops symptoms of a painful mass in the anophthalmic orbit. If enucleation was performed for a malignant intraocular tumor, the possibility of orbital recurrence of the neoplasm is usually the first diagnostic consideration and must be excluded (7). Amputation neuroma has been reported to cause progressive proptosis after orbital trauma, in which case no enucleation had been performed (9).

Diagnostic Approaches
Orbital CT reveals a distinct soft tissue tumor, usually behind the orbital implant (5). Associated conjunctival implantation cysts have also been seen on CT (8). There are probably no specific CT or MRI features of amputation neuroma, but the diagnosis should be suspected in the clinical setting described.

Pathology and Pathogenesis
Amputation neuroma is composed of tangles and whorls of proliferated axons, Schwann cells, and connective tissue. The absence of a distinct perineurium can help to differentiate amputation neuroma from plexiform neurofibroma. However, the typical clinical history and the absence of neurofibromatosis should also be of diagnostic help. The cysts seen on CT in two cases were found to be adjacent conjunctival implantation cysts that were possibly coincidental (8).

Management and Prognosis
The recommended management of an orbital amputation neuroma is surgical excision and orbital reconstruction if necessary. A dermis fat graft or mucous membrane graft may be required for cases that occur in an anophthalmic orbit (8). The systemic prognosis is excellent, because it is benign with no known malignant potential.

Selected References

Reviews
1. Shields JA, Shields CL, Scartozzi R. Survey of 1264 patients with orbital tumors and simulating lesions: the 2002 Montgomery Lecture, part 1. *Ophthalmology* 2004;111:997–1008.
2. Shields JA, Bakewell B, Augsburger DG, et al. Classification and incidence of space-occupying lesions of the orbit. A survey of 645 biopsies. *Arch Ophthalmol* 1984;102:1606–1611.
3. Shields JA, Bakewell B, Augsburger DG, et al. Space-occupying orbital masses in children. A review of 250 consecutive biopsies. *Ophthalmology* 1986;93:379–384.
4. Gunalp I, Gunduz K, Duruk K, et al. Neurogenic tumors of the orbit. *Jpn J Ophthalmol* 1994;38:185–190.

Imaging
5. Abramoff MD, Ramos LP, Jansen GH, et al. Patients with persistent pain after enucleation studied by MRI dynamic color mapping and histopathology. *Invest Ophthalmol Vis Sci* 2001;42:2188–2192.

Case Reports
6. Blodi FC. Amputation neuroma in the orbit. *Am J Ophthalmol* 1949;32:929–932.
7. Folberg R, Bernardino VB Jr, Aguilar GL, et al. Amputation neuroma mistaken for recurrent melanoma in the orbit. *Ophthalmic Surg* 1981;12:275–278.
8. Messmer EP, Camara J, Boniuk M, et al. Amputation neuroma of the orbit. Report of two cases and review of the literature. *Ophthalmology* 1984;91:1420–1423.
9. Sharma K, Kanaujia V, Jain A, et al. Metastasis to optic nerve presenting as ill-fitting prosthesis. *Orbit* 2011;30:118–119.
10. Baldeschi L, Saeed P, Regensburg NI, et al. Traumatic neuroma of the infraorbital nerve subsequent to inferomedial orbital decompression for Graves' orbitopathy. *Eur J Ophthalmol* 2010;20:481–484.
11. Ng DT, Francis IC, Whitehouse SA, et al. Orbital amputation neuroma causing failure of prosthesis wear. *Orbit* 2001;20:57–62.

Orbital Malignant Peripheral Nerve Sheath Tumor

General Considerations
Malignant peripheral nerve sheath tumor (MPNST) accounts for about 5% to 10% of soft tissue sarcomas; between 25% and 50% of them occur in patients with neurofibromatosis type 1 where it may represent malignant degeneration of a benign peripheral nerve sheath tumor (4,5). MPNST can also develop in the orbit spontaneously as a very aggressive malignancy (1–14). Several terms have been applied to malignant tumors that appear to arise from the sheaths of the peripheral nerves, including neurogenic sarcoma, neurofibrosarcoma, and malignant schwannoma (4). Some authors prefer the designation MPNST because it is not clear whether all of these tumors arise purely from the Schwann cell (4,5).

Clinical Features
Most patients are between 20 and 50 years of age at presentation, but there is a tendency for patients with neurofibromatosis to develop the tumor at an earlier age (4,14). In a review of eight cases, two had evidence of neurofibromatosis (4). It has occurred in a 15-month-old child without apparent neurofibromatosis (10). MPNST typically develops in the superonasal aspect of the orbit and produces proptosis and downward displacement of the eye. Unlike benign schwannoma and neurofibroma, it is more likely to produce pain and periocular hypesthesia (4). This tumor most often arises from the supraorbital branch of the trigeminal nerve (5). However, it can occasionally arise from the infraorbital nerve and in the muscle cone. It has a tendency to progress relentlessly along the affected nerves, invade the middle cranial fossa, and even metastasize to distant sites, particularly regional lymph nodes and lung (5). It can secondarily invade the orbit from adjacent structures, including the parotid gland.

Diagnostic Approaches
Little information is available on the CT and MRI findings for MPNST, but the findings appear to be nonspecific and it is not usually possible to make the diagnosis clinically. The mass can be either well circumscribed or more infiltrative and less well defined. There is often bone destruction (4).

Pathology and Pathogenesis
MPNST is composed of poorly differentiated spindle cells with occasional epithelioid cells and multinucleated giant cells. The cytoplasm generally shows variably positive immunoreactivity to S-100 protein. In some children, MPNST shows rhabdomyoblastic differentiation and resembles rhabdomyosarcoma. Such a neoplasm is called a "triton tumor."

Management and Prognosis
Once the diagnosis of MPNST is established histopathologically, the best hope for cure appears to be wide excision of the tumor. This may necessitate exenteration of the orbital contents and removal of adjacent bone. MPNST is generally radioresistant, but radiotherapy and chemotherapy can be employed as supplementary therapy when the lesion cannot be entirely removed surgically. The prognosis for survival in patients with MPNST of the orbit is poor. Many cases prove fatal within 5 years of diagnosis, either owing to direct intracranial extension, regional lymph node metastasis, or distant metastasis (4). In the review of 13 reported cases by Lyons et al., 9 died of their disease within 5 years (5).

Selected References

Reviews
1. Shields JA, Shields CL, Scartozzi R. Survey of 1264 patients with orbital tumors and simulating lesions: the 2002 Montgomery Lecture, part 1. *Ophthalmology* 2004;111:997–1008.
2. Shields JA, Bakewell B, Augsburger DG, et al. Classification and incidence of space-occupying lesions of the orbit. A survey of 645 biopsies. *Arch Ophthalmol* 1984;102:1606–1611.
3. Shields JA, Bakewell B, Augsburger DG, et al. Space-occupying orbital masses in children. A review of 250 consecutive biopsies. *Ophthalmology* 1986;93:379–384.
4. Jakobiec FA, Font RL, Zimmerman LE. Malignant peripheral nerve sheath tumors of the orbit. A clinicopathologic study of eight cases. *Trans Am Ophthalmol Soc* 1985;83:332–336.
5. Lyons CJ, McNab AA, Garner A, et al. Orbital malignant peripheral nerve sheath tumours. *Br J Ophthalmol* 1989;73:731–738.

Case Reports
6. Morton AD, Elner VM, Frueh B. Recurrent orbital malignant peripheral nerve sheath tumor 18 years after initial resection. *Ophthal Plast Reconstr Surg* 1997;13:239–243.
7. Fezza JP, Wolfley DE, Flynn SD. Malignant peripheral nerve sheath tumor of the orbit in a newborn: a case report and review. *J Pediatr Ophthalmol Strabismus* 1997;34:128–131.
8. Briscoe D, Mahmood S, O'Donovan DG, et al. Malignant peripheral nerve sheath tumor in the orbit of a child with acute proptosis. *Arch Ophthalmol* 2002;120:653–655.
9. Dutton JJ, Tawfik HA, DeBacker CM, et al. Multiple recurrences in malignant peripheral nerve sheath tumor of the orbit: a case report and a review of the literature. *Ophthal Plast Reconstr Surg* 2001;17:293–299.
10. Eviatar JA, Hornblass A, Herschorn B, et al. Malignant peripheral nerve sheath tumor of the orbit in a 15-month-old child. Nine-year survival after local excision. *Ophthalmology* 1992;99:1595–1599.
11. Grinberg MA, Levy NS. Malignant neurilemoma of the supraorbital nerve. *Am J Ophthalmol* 1974;78:489–492.
12. Mortada A. Solitary orbital malignant neurilemoma. *Br J Ophthalmol* 1968;52:188–190.
13. Cheng SF, Chen YI, Chang CY, et al. Malignant peripheral nerve sheath tumor of the orbit: malignant transformation from neurofibroma without neurofibromatosis. *Ophthal Plast Reconstr Surg* 2008;24:413–415.
14. Prescott DK, Racz MM, Ng JD. Epithelioid malignant peripheral nerve sheath tumor in the infraorbital nerve. *Ophthal Plast Reconstr Surg* 2006;22:150–151.

ORBITAL MISCELLANEOUS NEURAL TUMORS: GRANULAR CELL TUMOR, AMPUTATION NEUROMA, AND MALIGNANT PERIPHERAL NERVE SHEATH TUMOR

Messmer EP, Camara J, Boniuk M, et al. Amputation neuroma of the orbit. Report of two cases and review of the literature. *Ophthalmology* 1984;91:1420–1423.

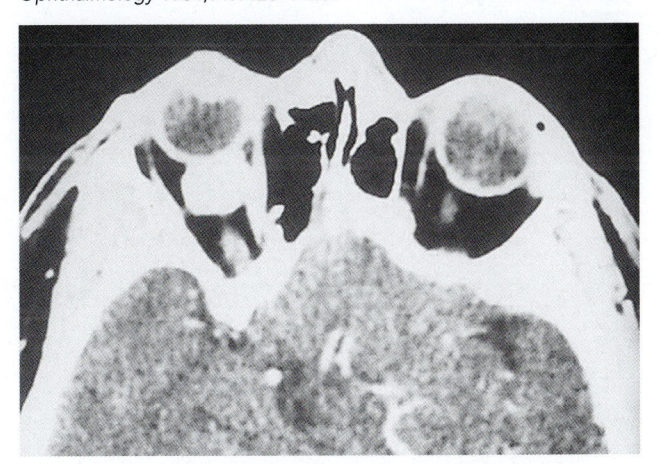

Figure 29.67. Granular cell tumor. Axial computed tomography of a 42-year-old woman who presented with slight pain and diplopia without proptosis. The circumscribed orbital mass located inferior to the optic nerve proved to be a GCT. (Courtesy of Alan Friedman, MD.)

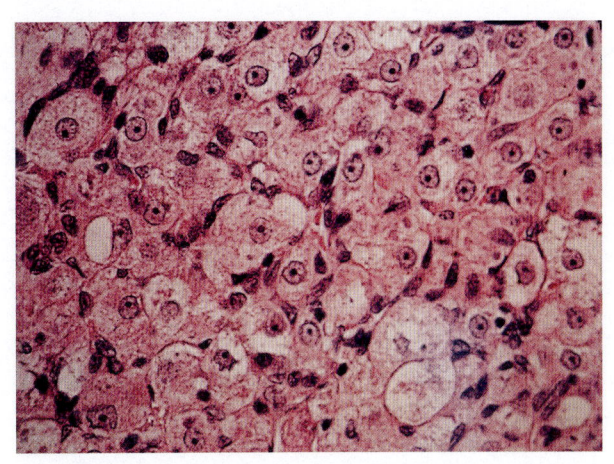

Figure 29.68. Histopathology of granular cell tumor showing large round cells with granular cytoplasm. (Hematoxylin–eosin ×200.)

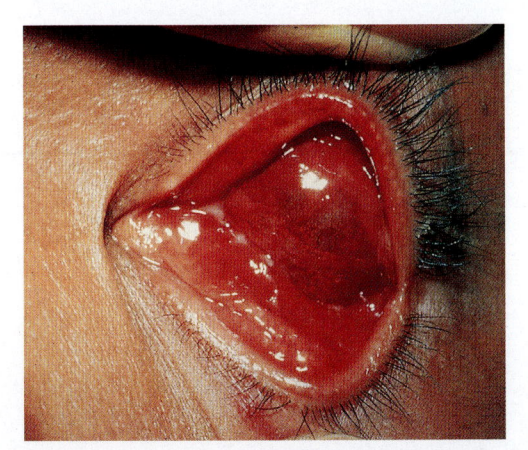

Figure 29.69. Amputation neuroma. Orbital mass in the anophthalmic socket of a 32-year-old man who underwent enucleation at age 7 years for a blind, phthisical eye of uncertain etiology. (Courtesy of Ramon L. Font, MD.)

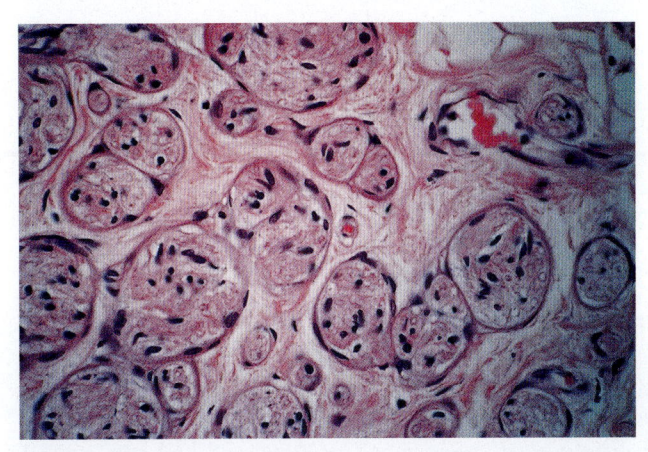

Figure 29.70. Histopathology of case shown in Figure 29.69. Note the proliferating nerve bundles surrounded by a perineural sheath and embedded in dense connective tissue, consistent with amputation neuroma. (Hematoxylin–eosin ×200.) (Courtesy of Ramon L. Font, MD.)

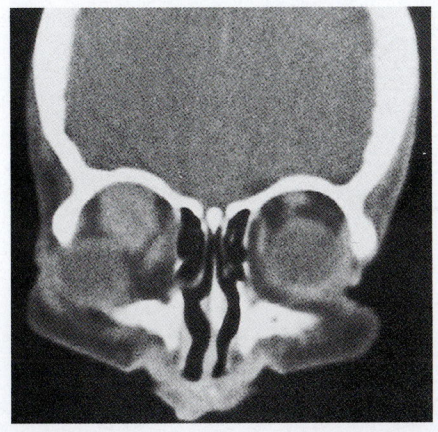

Figure 29.71. Malignant peripheral nerve sheath tumor. Coronal computed tomography showing superior orbital mass in right orbit of a 79-year-old woman. She had three recurrences and eventually died from brain invasion through the orbital roof. (Courtesy of Jurij Bilyk, MD.)

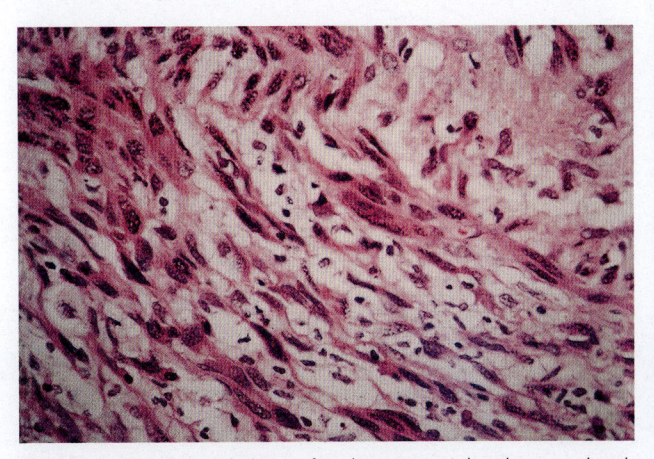

Figure 29.72. Histopathology of malignant peripheral nerve sheath tumor of the orbit showing malignant spindle and epithelioid cells. (Hematoxylin–eosin ×200.) (Courtesy of Jurij Bilyk, MD.)

CHAPTER 30

OPTIC NERVE, MENINGEAL, AND OTHER NEURAL TUMORS

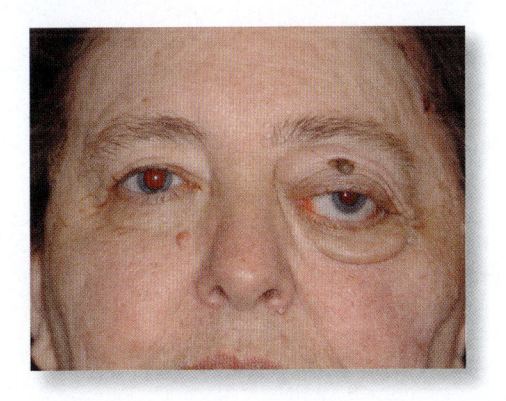

General Considerations

Juvenile pilocytic astrocytoma (JPA; optic nerve glioma) is a well-known and important optic nerve and brain tumor of childhood (1–25). This tumor represents 2% to 5% of brain tumors in children and accounts for about 1% to 2% of all orbital tumors (1–3,15). In the authors' series of biopsy-proven cases, there were 4 cases among 645 biopsied orbital lesions (2). In the authors' subsequent review of biopsy-proven childhood orbital tumors, it accounted for 5 of 250 biopsies (2%) (3). In the authors' most recent clinical series of 1,264 consecutive space-occupying orbital lesions, the 48 JPAs accounted for 46% of the 105 optic nerve lesions and for 4% of all orbital lesions (1).

JPA has an important association with neurofibromatosis type 1 (NF1) (4–16). Although figures vary from series to series, we believe that >50% of patients with JPA of the optic nerve have evidence of NF1. It is generally believed that JPA associated with NF1 is less aggressive and can show spontaneous regression (6,7). In contrast, sporadic JPA has an earlier onset and more severe clinical course than the nonsporadic type associated with NF1 (15). JPA of the optic nerve has also been seen in association with von Hippel–Lindau syndrome, but may be coincidental (21). There is a definite predilection for females (8). On rare occasions, JPA has been seen in association with the morning glory optic disc anomaly, but there is speculation that the dysmorphology of the optic disc extends into the nerve and could represent a pseudoglioma (24). Although it has been usually classified as a hamartoma, recent authors have suggested that this tumor should be classified as a true neoplasm (11).

Clinical Features

Some JPAs of the optic nerve are asymptomatic and are discovered on routine orbital magnetic resonance imaging (MRI) screening in a patient with NF1. Usually, however, JPA is diagnosed in the first or second decade of life when the child presents with progressive visual loss and axial proptosis. This tumor occasionally becomes clinically apparent in adulthood (21). Because there is a high incidence of NF1 associated with this tumor, the affected patient should be evaluated for cutaneous pigmented macules (café-au-lait spots), iris Lisch nodules, and other stigmata of NF1 (12–16). In the early stages, fundus examination might reveal a swollen optic disc and later the disc might become atrophic with a pale appearance and retinochoroidal shunt vessels at the margin. Chronic disc edema can rarely induce a choroidal neovascular membrane in the posterior pole of the eye (18).

OPTIC NERVE JUVENILE PILOCYTIC ASTROCYTOMA (OPTIC NERVE GLIOMA)

JPA located more posteriorly in the intracranial portion of optic nerve, chiasm, or hypothalamus often produces visual loss, strabismus, or nystagmus. Proptosis is not generally present unless the lesion extends anteriorly into the orbit. JPA of the optic nerve can occasionally undergo spontaneous regression, in both sporadic cases and those associated with NF1 (6,7).

Diagnostic Approaches

Computed tomography (CT) and MRI of optic nerve JPA typically shows an ovoid mass corresponding to an enlarged optic nerve. A characteristic kink in the midportion of the tumor is often present. Extension into the optic foramen to the chiasm and brain is common and is best seen with gadolinium-enhanced MRI. The extent of the tumor, as determined by MRI findings, can help to predict visual loss, with postchiasmal lesions causing greatest visual impairment.

Pathology

Gross pathology shows an optic nerve mass that is typically surrounded by the dura mater. Histopathologically, JPA is composed of a benign proliferation of pilocytic (hairlike) astrocytes, sometimes with areas of mucinous degeneration and hemorrhage. More round cells are often present. The astrocytic cell processes sometimes have eosinophilic, cylindrical swellings, called Rosenthal fibers.

Management and Prognosis

The management of JPA of the optic nerve is complex and controversial. Because the lesion is benign, we generally prefer to be as conservative as possible. Biopsy is rarely necessary today, because the diagnosis can usually be established on the basis of the characteristic radiographic findings. On occasion, however, neurosarcoidosis can occasionally show similar imaging features (24). Asymptomatic lesions are often followed initially without treatment and many remain stable for long periods of time (4). Serial examinations should be done for pupillary reaction, visual acuity, visual fields, and color vision of both eyes. Most tumors confined to the orbit remain relatively stable, but slow growth can occasionally occur. If there is progressive enlargement, then chemotherapy is preferred.

There is evidence that subependymal astrocytoma is associated with mTOR mutations and mTOR inhibitors like everolimus and sirolimus can show efficacy. In an analysis of 111 patients with subependymal giant cell astrocytoma of the brain, everolimus induces 50% or greater tumor volume reduction and this was maintained in 38% by 6 months (20). The application of this therapy for orbital astrocytoma has not yet been explored in a large series.

If the patient is blind and has unacceptable proptosis of the affected eye, then complete removal of the mass by lateral orbitotomy is warranted. For those that extend to the orbital apex or more posteriorly, a neurosurgical approach is necessary. It is usually not necessary to remove the blind eye in such cases.

Progressive lesions that involve the chiasm and brain are sometimes fatal and may require chemotherapy and/or radiotherapy. When the tumor is initially confined to the optic nerve, the mortality is <5%. When the hypothalamus is involved, mortality rises to >50% (4).

OPTIC NERVE JUVENILE PILOCYTIC ASTROCYTOMA (OPTIC NERVE GLIOMA)

Selected References

Reviews
1. Shields JA, Shields CL, Scartozzi R. Survey of 1264 patients with orbital tumors and simulating lesions: The 2002 Montgomery Lecture, part 1. *Ophthalmology* 2004;111:997–1008.
2. Shields JA, Bakewell B, Augsburger JJ, et al. Classification and incidence of space-occupying lesions of the orbit. A survey of 645 biopsies. *Arch Ophthalmol* 1984;102:1606–1611.
3. Shields JA, Bakewell B, Augsburger JJ, et al. Space-occupying orbital masses in children: A review of 250 consecutive biopsies. *Ophthalmology* 1986;93:379–384.

General
4. Dutton JJ. Gliomas of the anterior visual pathway. *Surv Ophthalmol* 1994;38:427–452.
5. Khafaga Y, Hassounah M, Kandil A, et al. Optic gliomas: a retrospective analysis of 50 cases. *Int J Radiat Oncol Biol Phys* 2003;13:807–812.
6. Parsa CF, Hoyt CS, Lesser RL, et al. Spontaneous regression of optic gliomas: thirteen cases documented by serial neuroimaging. *Arch Ophthalmol* 2001;119:516–529.
7. Schmandt SM, Packer RJ, Vezina LG, et al. Spontaneous regression of low-grade astrocytomas in childhood. *Pediatr Neurosurg* 2000;32:132–136.
8. Gayre GS, Scott IU, Feuer W, et al. Long-term visual outcome in patients with anterior visual pathway gliomas. *J Neuroophthalmol* 2001;21:1–7.
9. Binning MJ, Liu JK, Kestle JR, et al. Optic pathway gliomas: a review. *Neurosurg Focus* 2007;23(5):E2.
10. McDonnell P, Miller NR. Chiasmatic and hypothalamic extension of optic nerve glioma. *Arch Ophthalmol* 1983;101:1412–1415.
11. Liu GT, Katowitz JA, Rorke-Adams LB, et al. Optic pathway gliomas: neoplasms, not hamartomas. *JAMA Ophthalmol* 2013;131:646–650.

Neurofibromatosis-related
12. Balcer LJ, Liu GT, Heller G, et al. Visual loss in children with neurofibromatosis type 1 and optic pathway gliomas: relation to tumor location by magnetic resonance imaging. *Am J Ophthalmol* 2001;131:442–445.
13. Stern J, Jakobiec FA, Housepian EM. The architecture of optic nerve gliomas with and without neurofibromatosis. *Arch Ophthalmol* 1980;98:505–511.
14. King A, Listernick R, Charrow J, et al. Optic pathway gliomas in neurofibromatosis type 1: the effect of presenting symptoms on outcome. *Am J Med Genet* 2003;122:95–99.
15. Czyzyk E, Jozwiak S, Roszkowski M, et al. Optic pathway gliomas in children with and without neurofibromatosis. *J Child Neurol* 2003;18:471–478.
16. Thiagalingam S, Flaherty M, Billson F, et al. Neurofibromatosis type 1 and optic pathway gliomas: follow-up of 54 patients. *Ophthalmology* 2004;111:568–577.

Imaging
17. Jakobiec FA, Depot MJ, Kennerdell JS, et al. Combined clinical and computed tomographic diagnosis of orbital glioma and meningioma. *Ophthalmology* 1984;91:137–155.

Management
18. Hoyt WF, Baghdassarian SA. Optic glioma of childhood, natural history and rationale for conservative management. *Br J Ophthalmol* 1969;53:793–798.
19. Shriver EM, Ragheb J, Tse DT. Combined transcranial-orbital approach for resection of optic nerve gliomas: a clinical and anatomical study. *Ophthal Plast Reconstr Surg* 2012;28:184–191.
20. Franz DN, Belousova E, Sparangana S, et al. Everolimus for subependymal giant cell astrocytoma in patients with tuberous sclerosis complex: 2-year opern-lable extension of the randomised EXIST-1 study. *Lancet Oncol* 2014;15:1513–1520.

Case Reports
21. Wulc AE, Bergin DJ, Barnes D, et al. Orbital optic nerve glioma in adult life. *Arch Ophthalmol* 1989;107:1013–1016.
22. Nau JA, Shields CL, Shields JA, et al. Optic nerve glioma in a patient with von Hippel-Lindau syndrome. *J Pediatr Ophthalmol Strabismus* 2003;40:57–58.
23. Shields JA, Shields CL, De Potter P, et al. Choroidal neovascular membrane as a feature of optic nerve glioma. *Retina* 1997;17:349–350.
24. Pollock JM, Greiner FG, Crowder JB, et al. Neurosarcoidosis mimicking a malignant optic glioma. *J Neuroophthalmol* 2008;28:214–216.
25. Bandopadhayay P, Dagi L, Robison N, et al. Morning glory disc anomaly in association with ipsilateral optic nerve glioma. *Arch Ophthalmol* 2012;130:1082–1083.

OPTIC NERVE JUVENILE PILOCYTIC ASTROCYTOMA (GLIOMA)

JPA of the optic nerve has typical clinical and CT features. When it is confined to the orbit and produces a blind eye with progressive irreversible proptosis, the tumor can be removed by a lateral orbitotomy. A clinicopathologic correlation is shown.

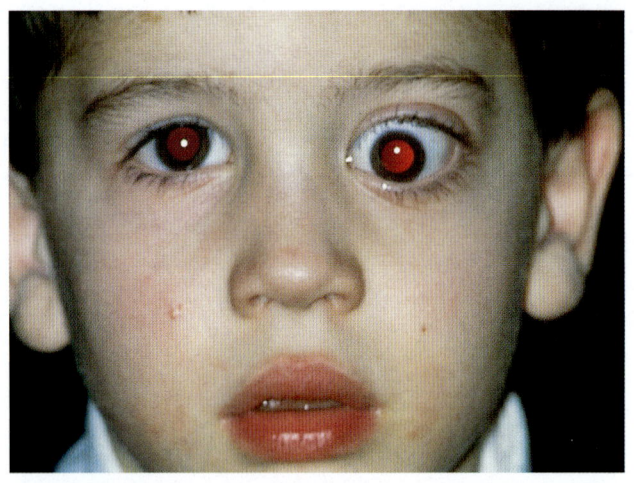

Figure 30.1. Axial proptosis of the left eye in a 4-year-old boy. The proptosis had been progressive for more than a year.

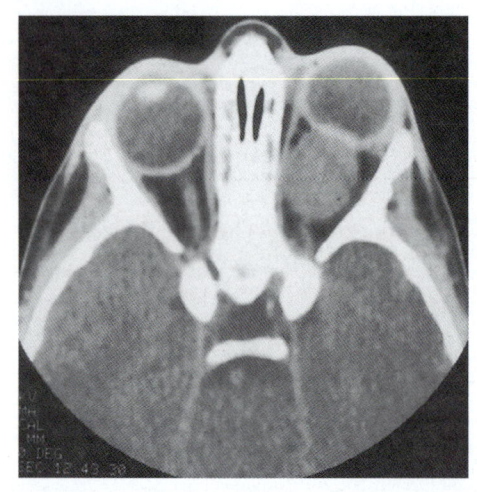

Figure 30.2. Axial computed tomography of patient shown in Figure 30.1, revealing a characteristic, well-defined, ovoid mass affecting the optic nerve. The lesion had shown considerable enlargement compared to a CT done 1 year earlier.

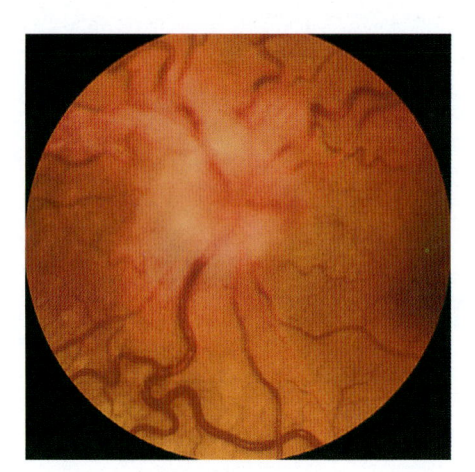

Figure 30.3. Marked swelling of the optic disc of the left eye.

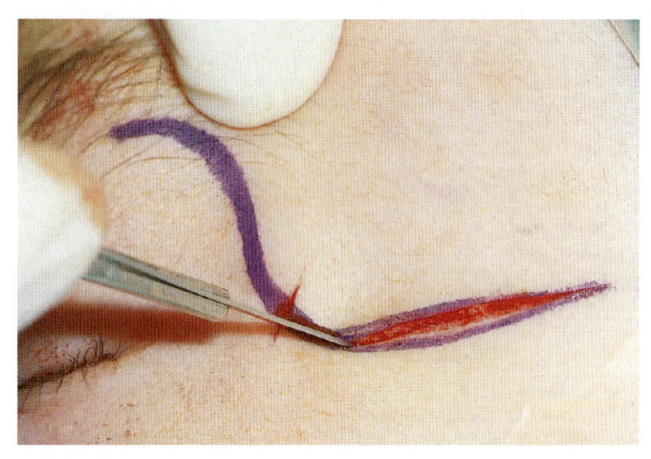

Figure 30.4. The proptosis continued to increase to an unacceptable degree, and surgical excision was elected. Shown is the planned skin incision for a superolateral orbitotomy.

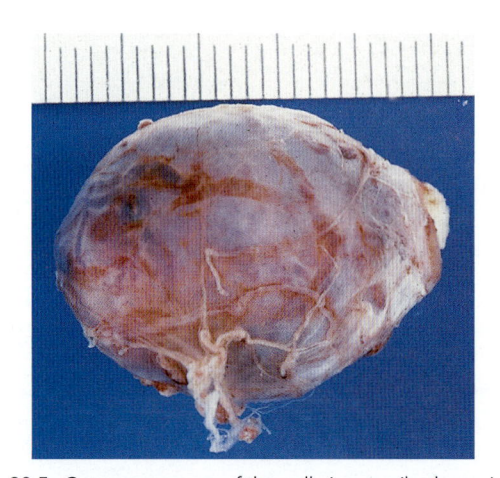

Figure 30.5. Gross appearance of the well-circumscribed mass immediately after surgical removal.

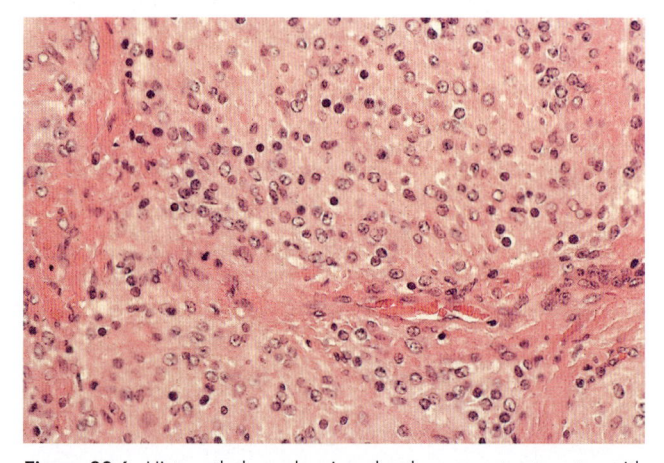

Figure 30.6. Histopathology showing closely compact astrocytes with some round nuclei comprising the tumor. (Hematoxylin–eosin ×100.)

OPTIC NERVE JUVENILE PILOCYTIC ASTROCYTOMA (GLIOMA): MAGNETIC RESONANCE IMAGING

JPA of optic nerve can be diagnosed with either CT or MRI because of its typical imaging features. However, MRI with gadolinium enhancement and fat suppression is the best method for determining whether there is subtle extension of the tumor into the optic canal and chiasmal area. Two examples of MRI are shown.

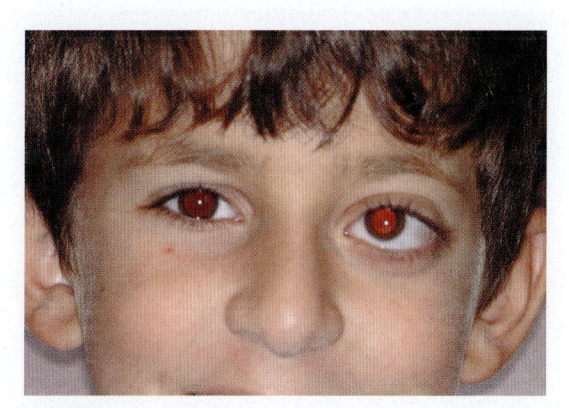

Figure 30.7. Proptosis and upward displacement of right globe in a 12-year-old boy.

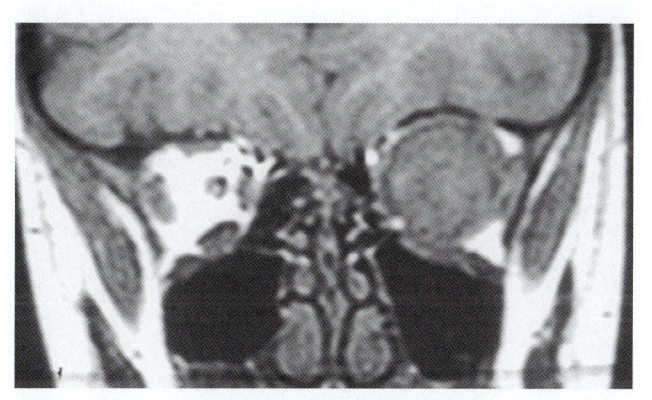

Figure 30.8. Coronal magnetic resonance imaging in T1-weighted image of patient shown in Figure 30.7. Note the large round tumor with its center in the location of the optic nerve.

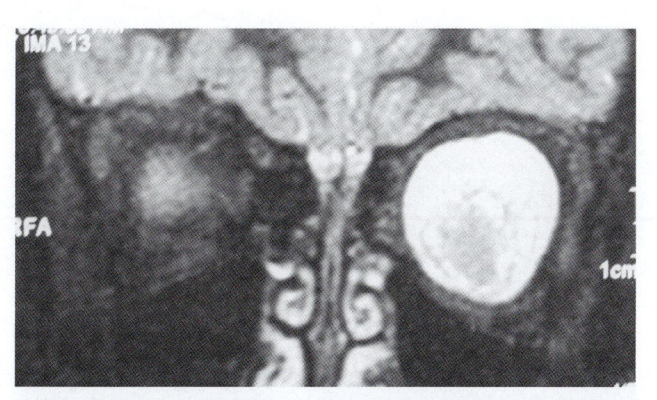

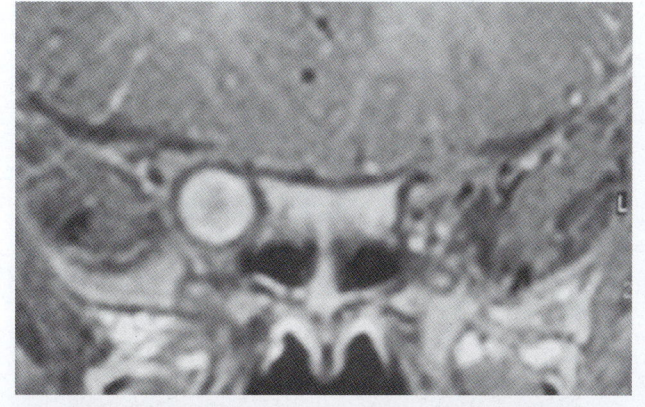

Figure 30.9. Coronal magnetic resonance imaging in T1-weighted image with gadolinium enhancement and fat suppression of patient shown in Figure 30.7. The geographic central area could represent the tumor and the surrounding hyperintense area could represent arachnoidal proliferation around the central tumor.

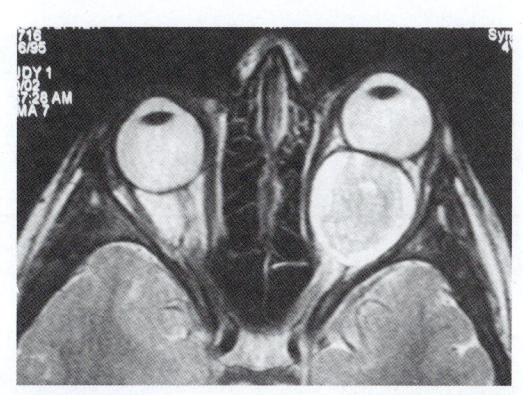

Figure 30.10. Axial magnetic resonance imaging in T2-weighted image of same patient, showing similar findings.

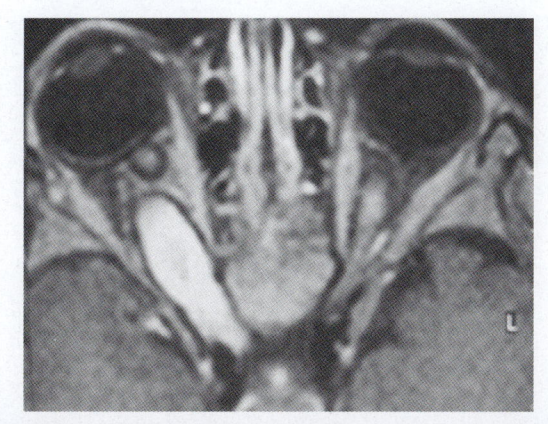

Figure 30.11. Another patient shown with axial magnetic resonance imaging in T1-weighted image with gadolinium enhancement and fat suppression of a posterior orbital juvenile pilocytic astrocytoma with extension into the right optic canal and optic tract. Note the hyperintense fusiform mass and dark rim around the mass that represents cerebrospinal fluid.

Figure 30.12. Coronal magnetic resonance imaging in T1-weighted image with gadolinium enhancement and fat suppression in same patient. This shows extension of the juvenile pilocytic astrocytoma almost to the chiasm.

OPTIC NERVE JUVENILE PILOCYTIC ASTROCYTOMA (GLIOMA)

JPA of the optic nerve has characteristic features with MRI. When the proptosis is more advanced, the proptosis converts from an axial direction to a down-and-out direction, conforming to the contour of the bony orbit. Two related cases are illustrated.

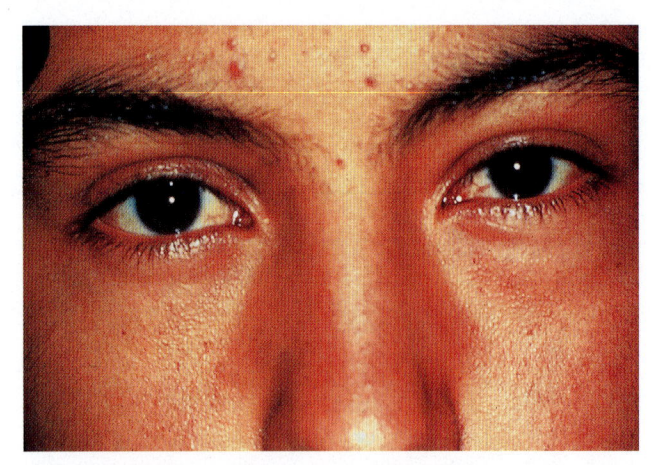

Figure 30.13. Proptosis of left eye in a 15-year-old boy.

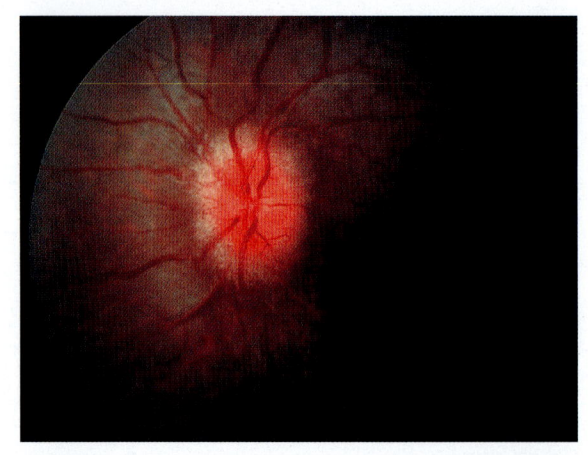

Figure 30.14. Hyperemia and edema of optic disc in patient shown in Figure 30.13.

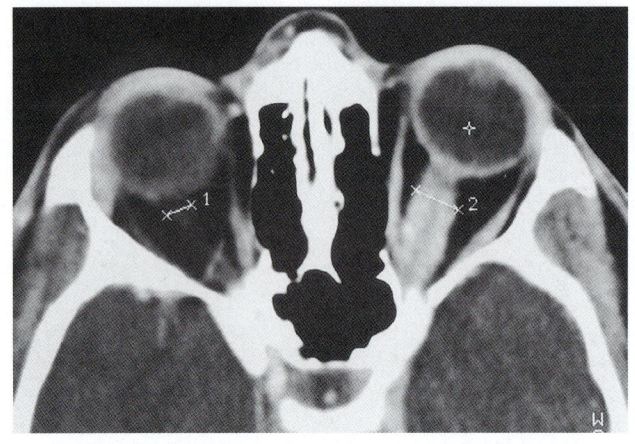

Figure 30.15. Axial computed tomography of patient shown in Figure 30.13. Note the fusiform lesion of the optic nerve.

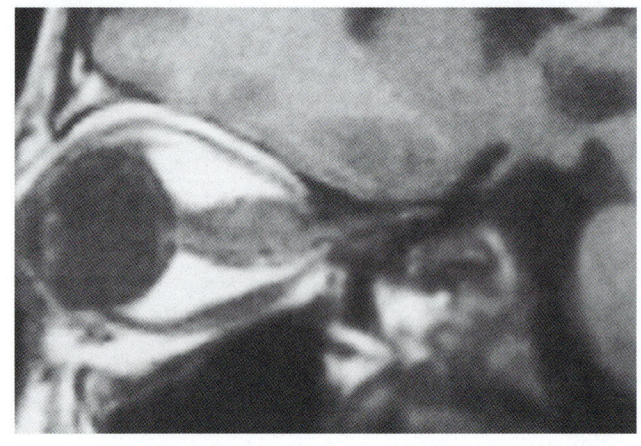

Figure 30.16. Sagittal magnetic resonance imaging in T1-weighted image showing same lesion depicted in Figure 30.15.

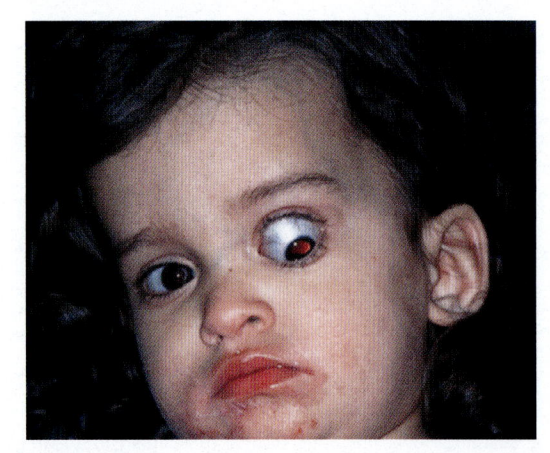

Figure 30.17. Proptosis and downward displacement of the left eye secondary to a juvenile pilocytic astrocytoma in a 2-year-old girl. The eye was blind and the progressive proptosis prompted surgical removal of the tumor.

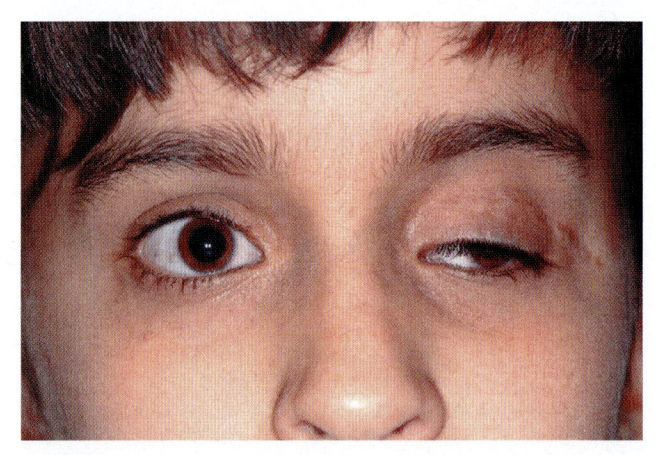

Figure 30.18. Appearance of child shown in Figure 30.17 after removal of the tumor. There is no more proptosis and the blepharoptosis and exotropia are to be corrected in the future.

OPTIC NERVE JUVENILE PILOCYTIC ASTROCYTOMA (GLIOMA): FUNDUS CHANGES

The most common fundus changes with JPA of the optic nerve are a swollen optic disc followed by a retinochoroidal shunt vessel and pallor of the optic disc. The venous stasis secondary to optic disc involvement can prompt development of a juxtapapillary choroidal neovascular membrane.

Shields JA, Shields CL, De Potter, et al. Choroidal neovascular membrane as a presenting feature of optic nerve glioma. *Retina* 1997;17:349–350.

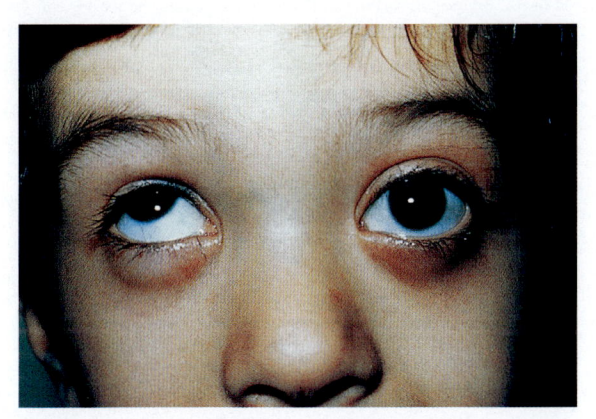

Figure 30.19. Proptosis of left eye and inability of upgaze secondary to a juvenile pilocytic astrocytoma of the optic nerve in a 6-year-old boy.

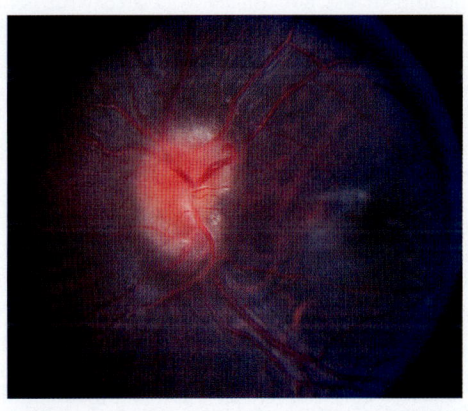

Figure 30.20. Swelling and hyperemia of the optic disc in the child shown in Figure 30.19. Note the retinochoroidal shunt vessel on superotemporal margin of optic disc.

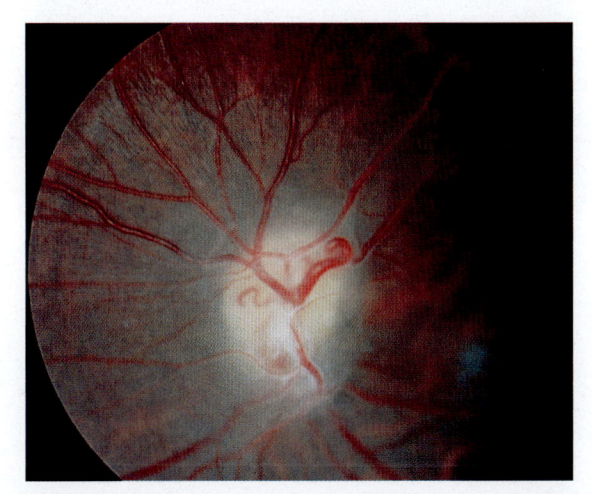

Figure 30.21. Appearance of same optic disc 4 years later. Note the optic disc pallor and distinct retinochoroidal shunt vessel.

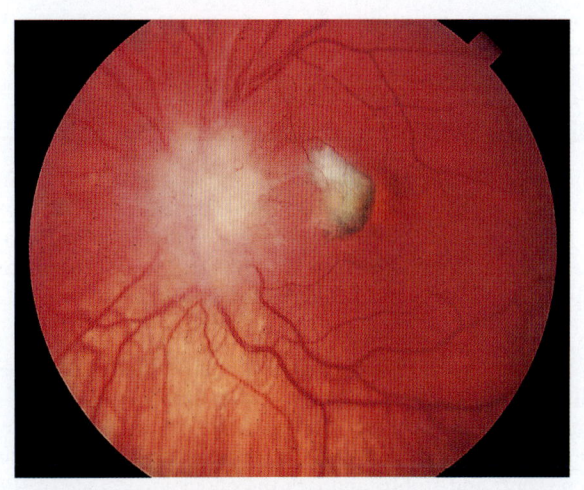

Figure 30.22. Choroidal neovascular membrane temporal to chronically swollen optic disc in a 16-year-old girl. The cause of the optic disc changes and neovascular membrane was not initially determined.

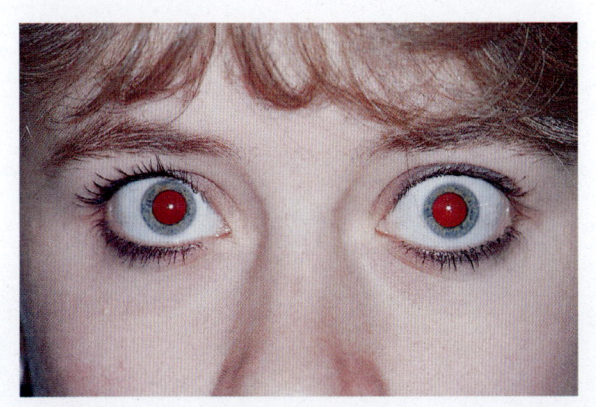

Figure 30.23. A few weeks later the patient shown in Figure 30.22 was realized to have proptosis of the left eye, which prompted an orbital computed tomography and referral.

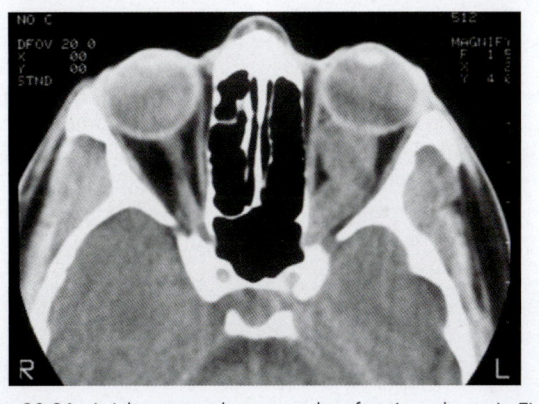

Figure 30.24. Axial computed tomography of patient shown in Figure 30.23, demonstrating the characteristic findings of a juvenile pilocytic astrocytoma of the optic nerve. Note the characteristic kink in the midportion of the nerve nasally.

OPTIC NERVE MALIGNANT ASTROCYTOMA

General Considerations

The benign pilocytic astrocytoma usually has its clinical onset in childhood, under 10 years of age (1–16). There is also a rare malignant form of optic nerve astrocytoma that occurs in adulthood and that is not usually associated with neurofibromatosis. Its clinical features, histopathology, and clinical course are very different from the JPA. Fewer than 50 cases have been published (15). Although it is generally considered to be rare, it is possible that many such cases have gone unreported because the patients usually die rapidly with a "brain tumor" and the precise diagnosis may not always be established.

Clinical Features

The patient characteristically experiences an acute onset of progressive visual impairment in one eye with pain and an afferent pupillary defect. As the tumor rapidly extends to involve the chiasm, there is initially a temporal field defect in the opposite eye followed by rapid loss of vision and bilateral blindness within 5 to 6 weeks of the initial symptoms. Occasionally, only one eye is affected up until the time of death (15). Funduscopic examination discloses optic disc edema with venous congestion. Proptosis is usually mild. Most patients develop hemiparesis and hypothalamic dysfunction and die within 1 year of onset of symptoms (4–16).

Diagnostic Approaches

The diagnosis is seldom made before craniotomy. Imaging studies may show a diffuse mass involving the visual pathways or sometimes a circumscribed round to ovoid orbital mass that can become less well defined as it progresses. The tumor can rapidly invade the central nervous system and cause death.

Pathology

Histopathologically, malignant optic nerve astrocytoma is composed of areas of well-differentiated astrocytes with interspersed areas of anaplastic fibrillary astrocytes. The cells tend to be short and stubby and lack the piloid appearance of JPA. They show pleomorphism and numerous mitotic figures, and tend to aggregate around blood vessels. Tumor giant cells are frequently present.

Management

The best treatment appears to be prompt and wide surgical excision by a transcranial route. Systemic chemotherapy could be useful. Supplemental radiotherapy and orbital exenteration are reserved for extensive, nonresectable disease. The prognosis is poor and most patients die within 6 to 12 months owing to complications of intracranial neoplasm.

Selected References

Reviews

1. Shields JA, Shields CL, Scartozzi R. Survey of 1264 patients with orbital tumors and simulating lesions: The 2002 Montgomery Lecture, part 1. *Ophthalmology* 2004;111: 997–1008.
2. Shields JA, Bakewell B, Augsburger JJ, et al. Classification and incidence of space-occupying lesions of the orbit. A survey of 645 biopsies. *Arch Ophthalmol* 1984;102: 1606–1611.
3. Shields JA, Bakewell B, Augsburger JJ, et al. Space-occupying orbital masses in children: A review of 250 consecutive biopsies. *Ophthalmology* 1986;93:379–384.

Case Reports

4. Hoyt WF, Meshel LG, Lessell S, et al. Malignant optic nerve glioma of adulthood. *Brain* 1974;96:121–132.
5. Wilson WB, Feinsod M, Hoyt WF, et al. Malignant evolution of childhood chiasmal pilocytic astrocytoma. *Neurology* 1976;26:322–325.
6. Mullaney J, Walsh J, Lee WR, et al. Recurrence of astrocytoma of optic nerve after 48 years. *Br J Ophthalmol* 1976;60:539–543.
7. Hamilton AM, Garner A, Tripathi RC, et al. Malignant optic nerve glioma. *Br J Ophthalmol* 1973;57:253–264.
8. Harper CG, Stewart-Wynn EG. Malignant optic gliomas in adults. *Arch Neurol* 1978; 35:731–735.
9. Mattson RH, Peterson EW. Glioblastoma multiforme of the optic nerve. *JAMA* 1966;196:799–800.
10. Rudd A, Rees JE, Kennedy P, et al. Malignant optic nerve gliomas in adults. *J Clin Neuro-Ophthalmol* 1985;5:238–243.
11. Saeb J. Primary tumor of the optic nerve (glioblastoma multiforme). *Br J Ophthalmol* 1949;33:701–708.
12. Spoor TC, Kennerdell JS, Martinez AJ, et al. Malignant gliomas of the optic nerve pathways. *Am J Ophthalmol* 1980;89:284–292.
13. Dario A, Iadini A, Cerati M, et al. Malignant optic glioma of adulthood. Case report and review of the literature. *Acta Neurol Scand* 1999;100:350–353.
14. Matloob S, Fan JC, Danesh-Meeyr HV. Multifocal malignant optic glioma of adulthood presenting as acute anterior optic neuropathy. *J Clin Neurosci* 2011;18: 974–977.
15. Wabbels B, Demmler A, Seitz J, et al. Unilateral adult malignant optic nerve glioma. *Graefes Arch Clin Exp Ophthalmol* 2004;242:741–748.
16. Simao LM, Dine Sultan EN, Hall JK, et al. Knee deep in the nerve. *Surv Ophthalmol* 2011;56:362–370.

Chapter 30 Optic Nerve, Meningeal, and Other Neural Tumors

OPTIC NERVE MALIGNANT ASTROCYTOMA

Malignant optic nerve astrocytoma (glioma) of the visual pathways can cause rapid visual loss, oculomotor palsies, and retinal vascular obstruction.

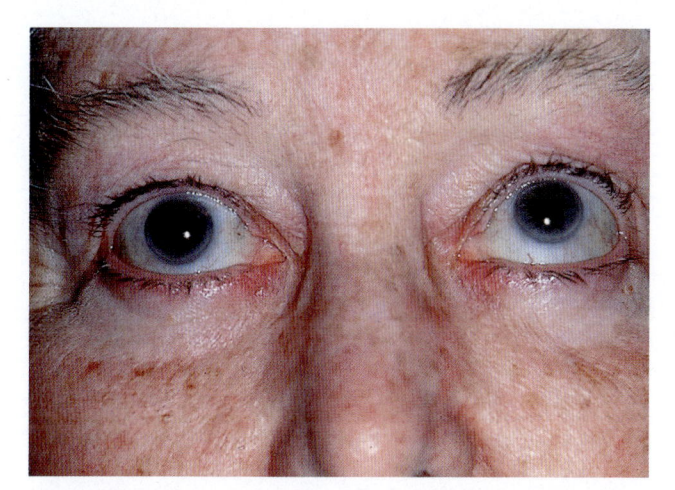

Figure 30.25. Paresis of upgaze of right eye in a 78-year-old woman. (Courtesy of Jurij Bilyk, MD, and Peter Savino, MD.)

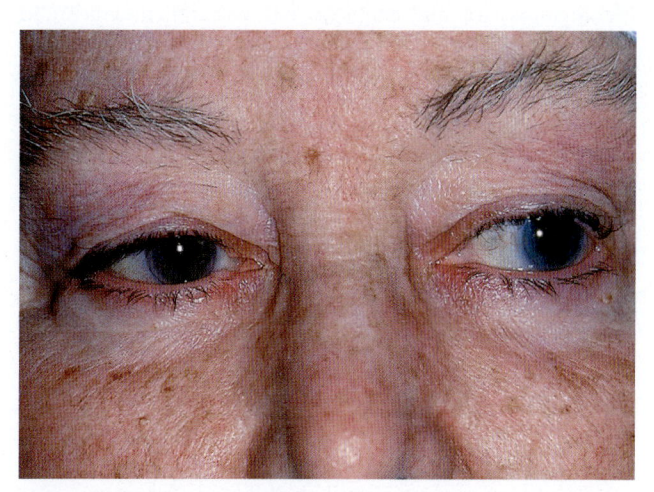

Figure 30.26. Paresis of adduction of right eye in same patient. (Courtesy of Jurij Bilyk, MD, and Peter Savino, MD.)

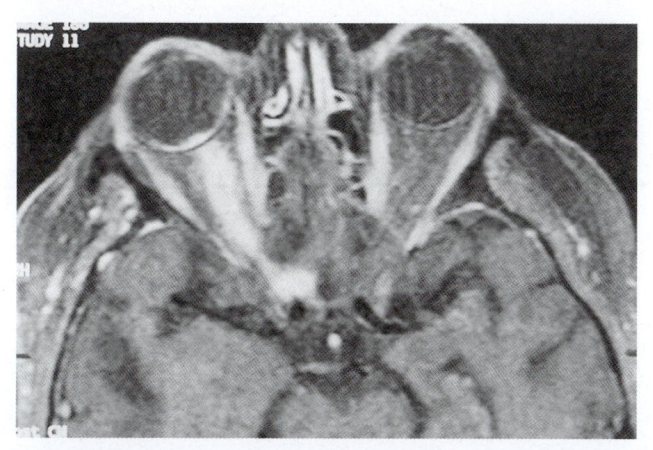

Figure 30.27. Axial magnetic resonance imaging, T1-weighted image, of patient shown in Figures 30.25 and 30.26 demonstrating a diffuse enhancing mass involving the optic nerve to the optic chiasm. (Courtesy of Jurij Bilyk, MD, and Peter Savino, MD.)

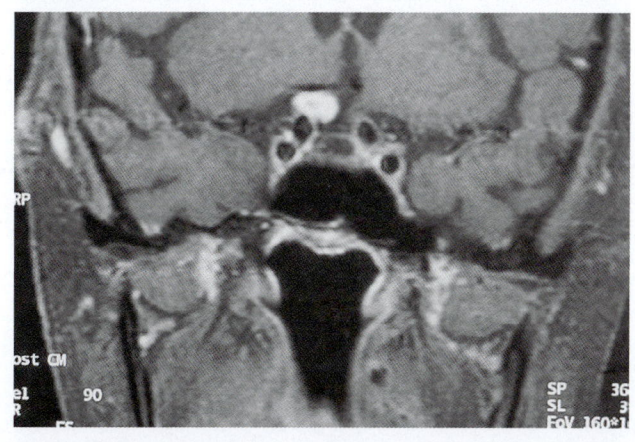

Figure 30.28. Axial magnetic resonance imaging in same patient demonstrating enhancing mass in the optic chiasm. (Courtesy of Jurij Bilyk, MD, and Peter Savino, MD.)

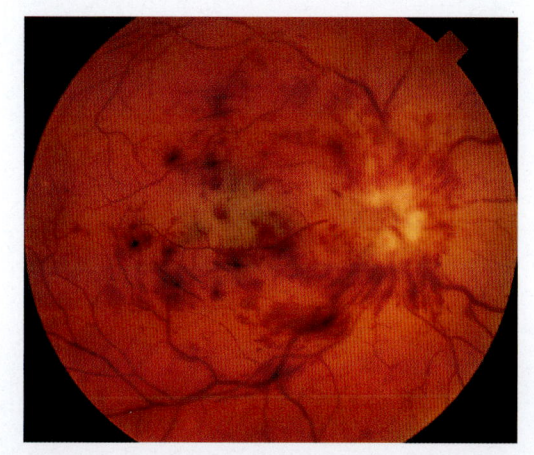

Figure 30.29. Fundus photograph showing optic disc edema, vascular congestion, and hemorrhage in a 52-year-old man with malignant optic nerve glioma. (Courtesy of Lee Jampol, MD.)

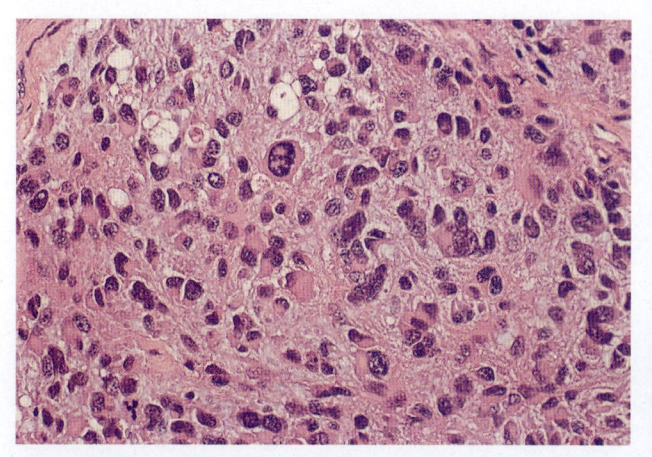

Figure 30.30. Histopathology of malignant optic nerve astrocytoma showing malignant glial cells. (Hematoxylin–eosin ×150.) (Courtesy of Ralph C. Eagle, Jr, MD.)

OPTIC NERVE SHEATH MENINGIOMA

General Considerations

Meningioma is a benign neoplasm that arises from the arachnoid layer of the meninges and frequently affects the orbit. Although there are several types and locations, the most important with regard to the orbit are primary optic nerve sheath meningioma (ONSM) (1–23) and sphenoid wing meningioma (SWM). Like meningiomas elsewhere, these orbital meningiomas are more common in middle-aged women, with most occurring in females. In the authors' clinical series of 1,264 orbital lesions, the 29 ONSMs accounted for 28% of optic nerve and meningeal tumors and for 2% of all orbital masses (1).

Clinical Features

The patient with ONSM generally presents with visual loss and a swollen or atrophic optic disc, often with a characteristic retinochoroidal shunt vessel at the optic disc margin. As the tumor enlarges, there is slowly progressive proptosis of the affected eye. The lesion can occasionally be bilateral. When it is confined to the optic canal (intracanalicular meningioma), it can produce signs of optic neuritis and glaucoma and the diagnosis may be more challenging.

In a 23-year analysis of ONSM of 88 patients, mean age at symptom onset was 40 years and 80% were female (8). Presenting symptoms included decreased visual acuity (80%), transient visual obscurations (15%), pain (7%), and diplopia (4%). Over mean 7-year follow-up, 27% of eyes developed no light perception vision. There were no patient deaths from ONSM.

Diagnostic Approaches

Imaging studies of ONSM show a fusiform or round enlargement in the arachnoid with a relatively normal optic nerve in its center. The normal optic nerve is seen as a negative shadow passing through the center of the lesion (13). Occasionally, ONSM appears as a nodular growth from the optic nerve sheath and may simulate other round, circumscribed orbital tumors. Areas of calcification are often seen in the tumors. In most cases, the findings are so typical that the diagnosis is easily made radiographically, and diagnostic biopsy is rarely necessary. Needle biopsy has been employed to make the diagnosis of ONSM in selected cases (13).

Pathology

The histopathology is similar for ONSM and SWM. Several subtypes are discussed in the literature (5) and are beyond the scope of this text. The most common type is characterized by lobules of tumor cells that resemble the normal meningothelial cells of the arachnoid. Psammoma bodies are often present.

OPTIC NERVE SHEATH MENINGIOMA

Management

Observation only is the preferred treatment for asymptomatic ONSM. The patient should be examined every 6 to 12 months and have testing of visual acuity, color vision, pupillary reaction, visual fields, and orbital MRI. If progression is demonstrated and vision is compromised, then active treatment should be considered. Surgical excision generally involves cutting the optic nerve with resultant absolute blindness. Hence, surgical removal is reserved for advanced tumors with a blind eye and cosmetically unacceptable proptosis. If the tumor is in the anterior two-thirds of the orbit in such instances, removal can usually be accomplished by a lateral orbitotomy approach. More posteriorly located tumors that involve the deep orbit, optic canal, and intracranial optic nerve should be removed by a transcranial route in conjunction with a neurosurgeon. Although surgical removal of the tumor with an attempt to spare the optic nerve has been performed (12,18), patients treated in that manner are at further risk for severe optic atrophy and blindness (18).

The most preferred intervention for progressive ONSM is radiotherapy (14–17,19). Our group has observed that fractionated stereotactic radiotherapy (50–54 Gy) can preserve existing vision in >90% of cases and achieve improved vision in 42%, but longer follow-up is necessary to determine the validity of those observations (16). Radiation retinopathy has been recognized 22 months after stereotactic radiotherapy for ONSM (21). Stereotactic radiosurgery has also been observed to bring about resolution of the retinochoroidal shunt vessels seen with ONSM.

Selected References

Reviews

1. Shields JA, Shields CL, Scartozzi R. Survey of 1264 patients with orbital tumors and simulating lesions: The 2002 Montgomery Lecture, part 1. *Ophthalmology* 2004;111:997–1008.
2. Shields JA, Bakewell B, Augsburger JJ, et al. Classification and incidence of space-occupying lesions of the orbit. A survey of 645 biopsies. *Arch Ophthalmol* 1984;102:1606–1611.
3. Shields JA, Bakewell B, Augsburger JJ, et al. Space-occupying orbital masses in children: A review of 250 consecutive biopsies. *Ophthalmology* 1986;93:379–384.
4. Sibony PA, Krauss HR, Kennerdell JS, et al. Optic nerve sheath meningiomas. Clinical manifestations. *Ophthalmology* 1984;91:1313–1226.
5. Dutton JJ. Optic nerve sheath meningiomas. *Surv Ophthalmol* 1992;37:167–183.
6. Karp LA, Zimmerman LE, Borit A, et al. Primary intraorbital meningiomas. *Arch Ophthalmol* 1974;91:24–28.
7. Wright JE, Call NB, Liaricos S. Primary optic nerve meningioma. *Br J Ophthalmol* 1980;64:553–558.
8. Saeed P, Rootman J, Nugent RA, et al. Optic nerve sheath meningiomas. *Ophthalmology* 2003;11:2019–2030.
9. Margalit NS, Lesser JB, Moche J, et al. Meningiomas involving the optic nerve: technical aspects and outcomes for a series of 50 patients. *Neurosurgery* 2003;53:523–532.

Imaging

10. Jakobiec FA, Depot MJ, Kennerdell JS, et al. Combined clinical and computed tomographic diagnosis of orbital glioma and meningioma. *Ophthalmology* 1984;91:137–155.
11. Stroman GA, Stewart WC, Golnik KC, et al. Magnetic resonance imaging in patients with low-tension glaucoma. *Arch Ophthalmol* 1995;113:168–172.

Management

12. Mark LE, Kennerdell JS, Maroon JC, et al. Microsurgical removal of a primary intraorbital meningioma. *Am J Ophthalmol* 1978;86:704–709.
13. Kennerdell JS, Dubois PJ, Dekker A, et al. CT-guided fine needle aspiration biopsy of orbital optic nerve tumors. *Ophthalmology* 1980;87:491–496.
14. Becker G, Jeremic B, Pitz S, et al. Stereotactic fractionated radiotherapy in patients with optic nerve sheath meningioma. *Int J Radiat Oncol Biol Phys* 2002;54:1422–1429.
15. Pitz S, Becker G, Schiefer U, et al. Stereotactic fractionated irradiation of optic nerve sheath meningioma: a new treatment alternative. *Br J Ophthalmol* 2002;86:1265–1268.
16. Andrews DW, Foroozan R, Yang BP, et al. Fractionated sterotactic radiotherapy for the treatment of optic nerve sheath meningiomas: preliminary observations of 33 optic nerves in 30 patients. *Neurosurgery* 2002;51:890–903.
17. Turbin RE, Thompson CR, Kennerdell JS, et al. A long-term visual outcome comparison in patients with optic nerve sheath meningioma managed with observation, surgery, radiotherapy, or surgery and radiotherapy. *Ophthalmology* 2002;109:890–899.
18. Kennerdell JS, Maroon JC, Malton M, et al. The management of optic nerve sheath meningiomas. *Am J Ophthalmol* 1988;106:450–457.
19. Bloch O, Sun M, Kaur G, et al. Fractionated radiotherapy for optic nerve sheath meningiomas. *J Clin Neurosci* 2012;19:1210–1215.
20. Mark LE, Kennerdell JS, Maroon JC, et al. Microsurgical removal of a primary intraorbital meningioma. *Am J Ophthalmol* 1978;86:704–709.
21. Subramanian PS, Bressler NM, Miller NR. Radiation retinopathy after fractionated stereotactic radiotherapy for optic nerve sheath meningioma. *Ophthalmology* 2004;111:565–567.
22. Carvounis PE, Katz B. Gamma knife radiosurgery in neuro-ophthalmology. *Curr Opin Ophthalmol* 2003;14:317–324.

Histopathology

23. Marquardt MD, Zimmerman LE. Histology of meningiomas and gliomas of the optic nerve. *Human Pathol* 1982;13:226–234.

Chapter 30 Optic Nerve, Meningeal, and Other Neural Tumors

● OPTIC NERVE SHEATH MENINGIOMA

Primary ONSM can take several forms with imaging studies. It is usually an elongated or fusiform lesion but on occasion it can apparently breach the dura mater and assume a globular configuration.

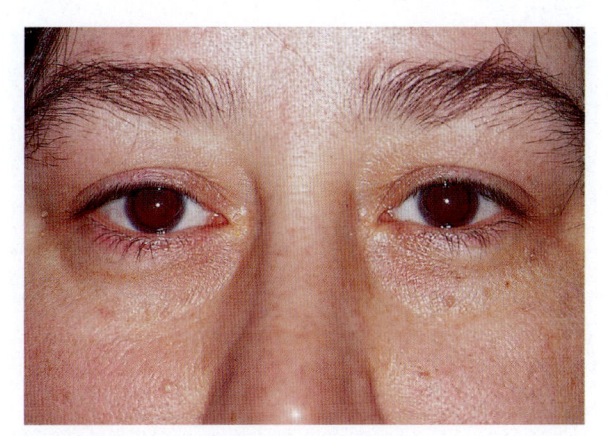

Figure 30.31. Minimal prominence of the right eye in a 38-year-old woman with mild visual loss.

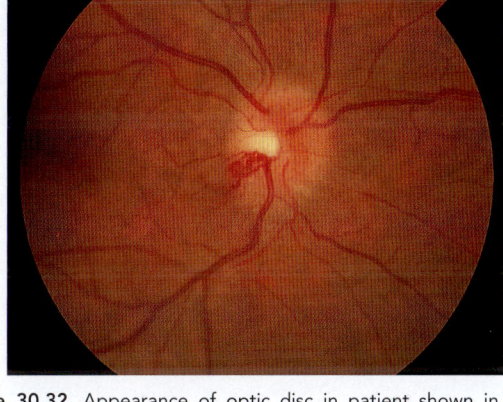

Figure 30.32. Appearance of optic disc in patient shown in Figure 30.31, demonstrating retinochoroidal shunt vessel on inferotemporal margin of optic disc. Photographs 2 years early showed no shunt vessel and it was observed to gradually develop.

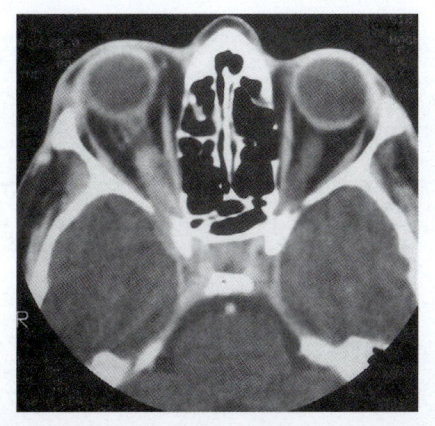

Figure 30.33. Axial computed tomography showing meningioma of right optic nerve sheath.

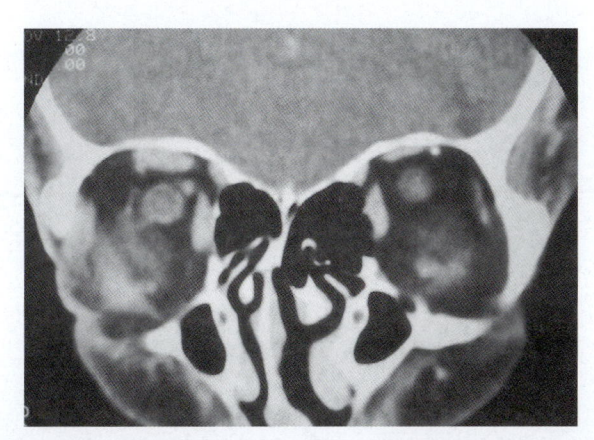

Figure 30.34. Coronal computed tomography showing same lesion depicted in Figure 30.33. Note the enhancement of the arachnoid around right optic nerve.

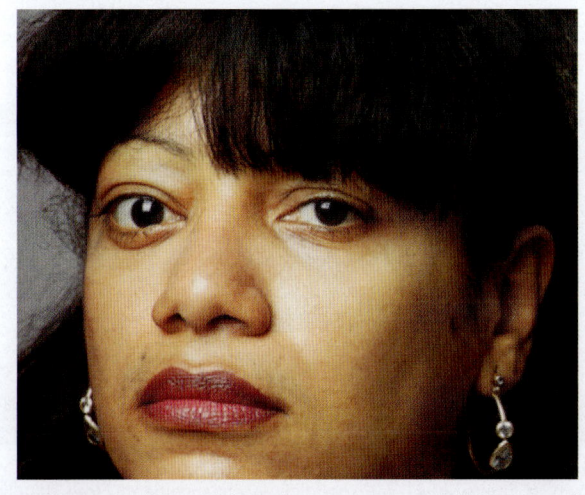

Figure 30.35. Proptosis of the right eye in a 39-year-old woman with an optic nerve sheath meningioma.

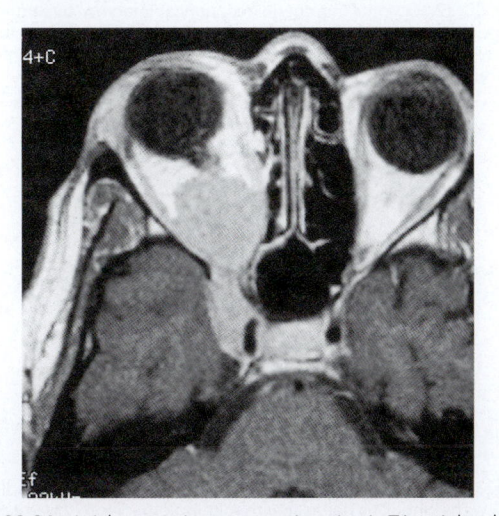

Figure 30.36. Axial magnetic resonance imaging in T1-weighted image of patient shown in Figure 30.35 revealing round mass arising from posterior aspect of optic nerve with extension through the optic canal into the chiasm. The tumor was resected by a transcranial route and histopathologic examination confirmed meningioma.

OPTIC NERVE SHEATH MENINGIOMA: MAGNETIC RESONANCE IMAGING

MRI has become the most useful imaging study to diagnose and determine the extent of ONSM. Gadolinium enhancement and fat suppression afford the best results.

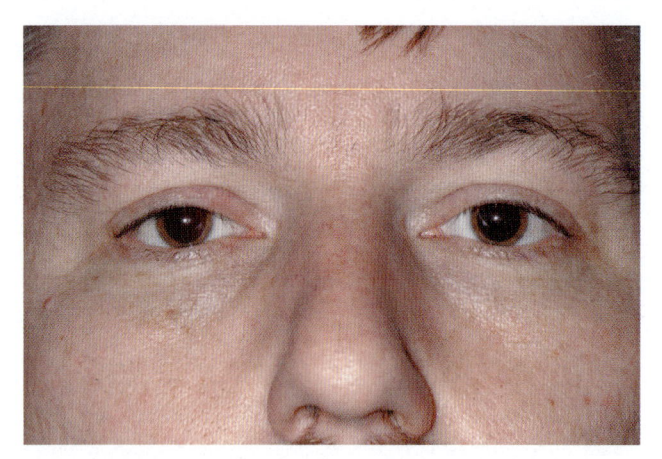

Figure 30.37. Appearance of middle-aged man with painless progressive visual loss in right eye. The eyes externally appear essentially normal.

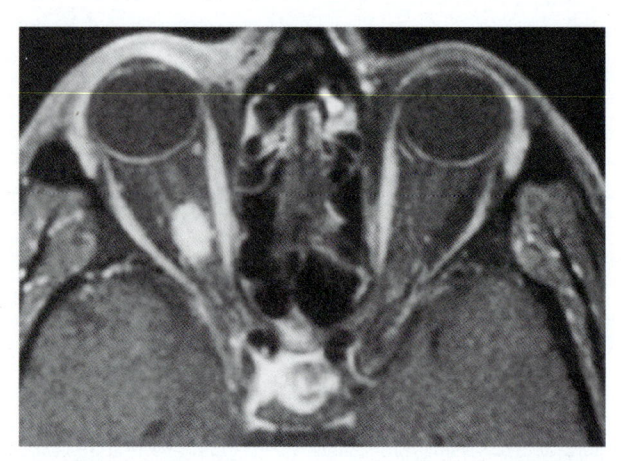

Figure 30.38. Axial magnetic resonance imaging of patient shown in Figure 30.37 with gadolinium enhancement and fat suppression. The enhancing lesion appears to be located in the posterior third of the right optic nerve within the orbit.

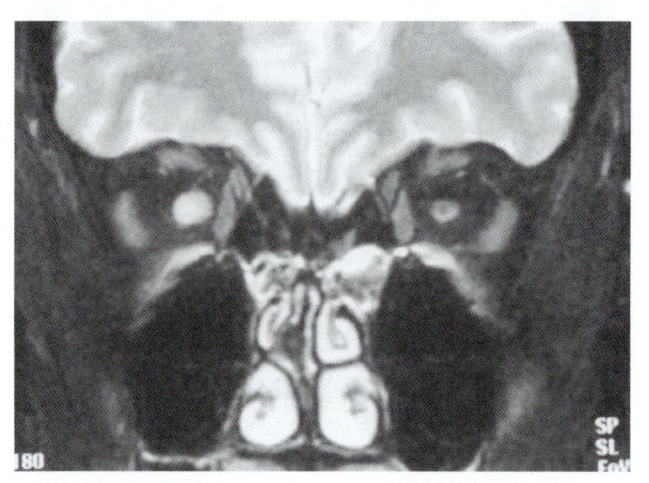

Figure 30.39. Coronal magnetic resonance imaging through posterior aspect of orbits of patient shown in Figure 30.37 with gadolinium enhancement and fat suppression. The lesion appears as an enhancing mass around the optic nerve.

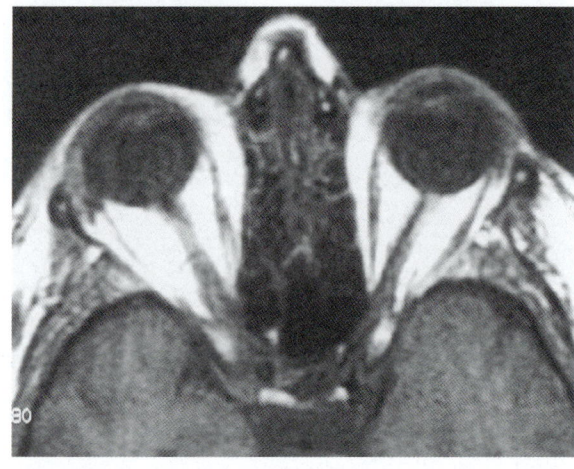

Figure 30.40. Axial magnetic resonance imaging through same region as shown in Figure 30.38 but without fat suppression. The lesion is more difficult to visualize, stressing the importance of fat suppression technique in evaluating such cases.

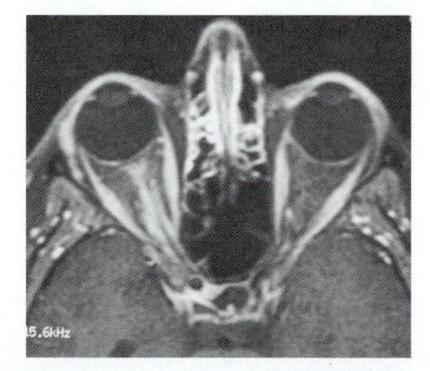

Figure 30.41. Axial magnetic resonance imaging in a middle-aged woman with right optic nerve sheath meningioma. Note the irregular silhouette of the optic nerve with enhancement around the nonenhancing nerve. This "railroad sign" is quite typical of ONSM.

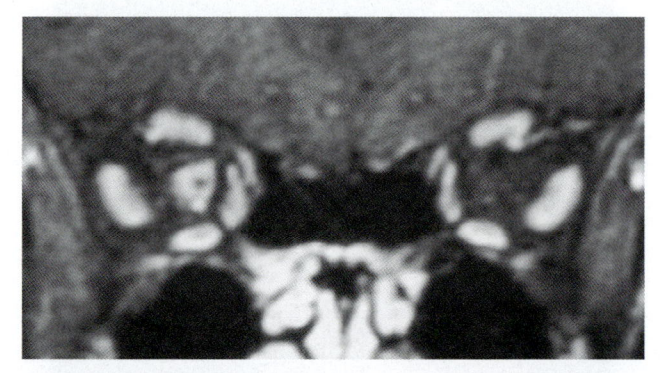

Figure 30.42. Coronal magnetic resonance imaging through lesion shown in Figure 30.41 with gadolinium enhancement. Note that the enhancing lesion around the optic nerve and the dark silhouette of the optic nerve are seen even better. The optic nerve behind the normal contralateral left eye is hardly visible.

Chapter 30 Optic Nerve, Meningeal, and Other Neural Tumors

● OPTIC NERVE SHEATH MENINGIOMA: AGGRESSIVE VARIANT

Incompletely removed meningioma can grow more floridly and be difficult to control. The patient depicted here was seen many years ago and had not received irradiation for the initial tumor after incomplete removal. Recurrence was initially managed elsewhere by enucleation and, ultimately, orbital exenteration and removal of brain meningiomas were necessary.

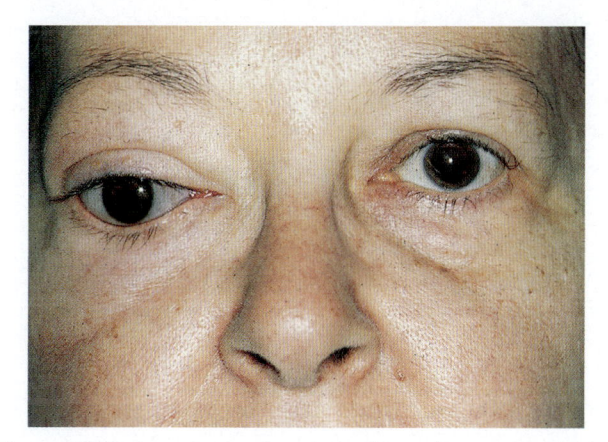

Figure 30.43. Appearance of patient who underwent enucleation elsewhere several years earlier for a blind, uncomfortable eye. She was referred because of recent inability to retain the prosthesis. Results of histopathology could not be obtained and orbital recurrence of uveal melanoma was considered.

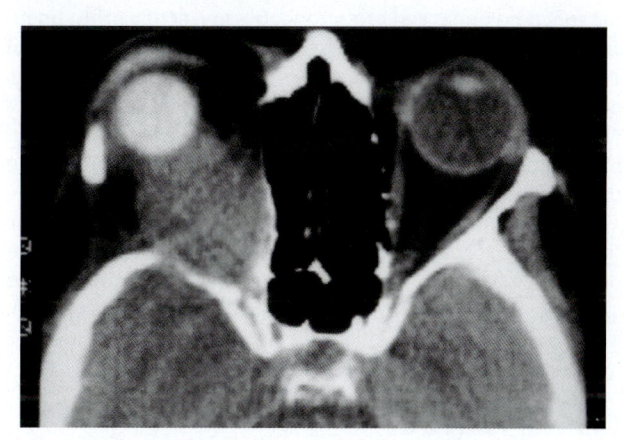

Figure 30.44. Axial computed tomography of patient shown in Figure 40.43, demonstrating orbital mass posterior to the ball implant. Such a patient would be a good candidate for diagnostic orbital fine-needle aspiration biopsy.

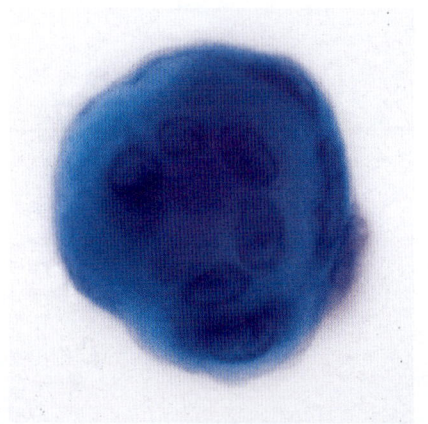

Figure 30.45. Cytology of fine-needle aspiration biopsy of optic nerve sheath meningioma showing a whorl of meningothelial cells. (Papanicolaou ×250.)

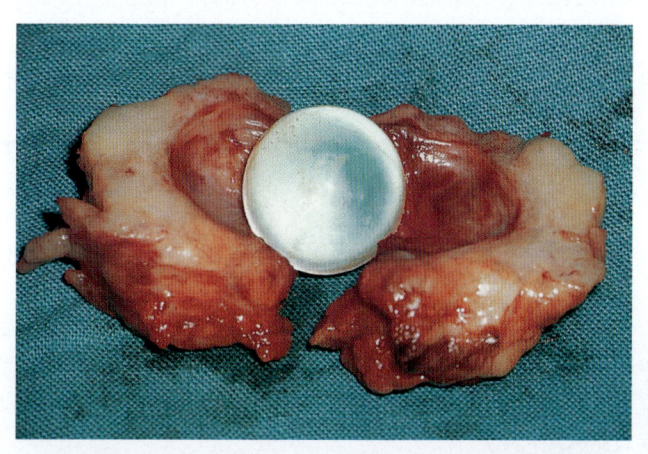

Figure 30.46. Surgical specimen showing ball implant surrounded by dense fleshy tumor tissue. Histopathology confirmed the diagnosis of meningioma and the tumor was believed to be removed completely.

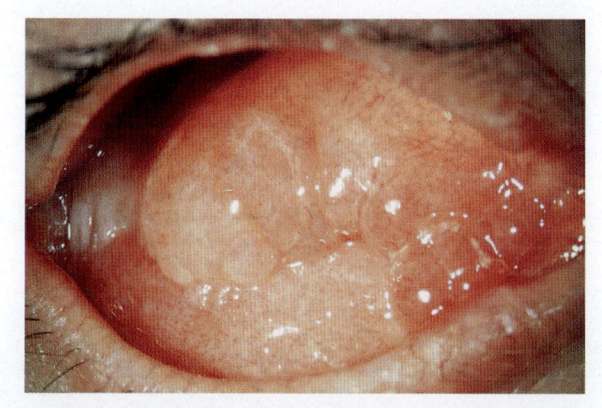

Figure 30.47. Appearance of socket 3 years later showing recurrence of fleshy tumor tissue filling the palpebral fissure.

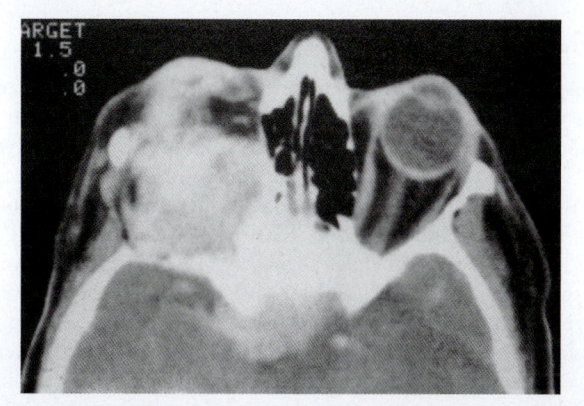

Figure 30.48. Axial computed tomography taken at time of Figure 30.47, demonstrating massive recurrence of the meningioma involving the orbit and intracranial tissues. The tumor was treated successfully by a combined intracranial approach and orbital exenteration. The initial diagnosis was optic nerve sheath meningioma; the hyperostosis was a later development. (Figure 30.44 shows no hyperostosis).

ORBITAL SPHENOID WING MENINGIOMA

General Considerations

SWM is a benign tumor that begins in the arachnoid that lines the sphenoid bones and can secondarily invade the orbit, brain, and temporal fossa (1–20). In the authors' clinical series of 1,264 orbital lesions, the 24 SWMs accounted for 23% of optic nerve and meningeal tumors and for 2% of all orbital masses (1). Hence, the incidence of ONSM and SWM is about equal in a practice of ocular oncology. It was relatively less common in the series of orbital tumors in patients >60 years old (4).

Although most orbital meningiomas are either optic nerve sheath of or sphenoid wing in location, there is a rare variant of ectopic (extradural) orbital meningioma that can be located along the medial, superior, or lateral walls of the orbit (19,20). This ectopic lesion is usually well circumscribed and can have intralesional calcification.

Clinical Features

SWM can produce somewhat different symptoms and signs than the ONSM. The patient is generally a middle-aged woman who initially develops slowly progressive proptosis and fullness of the temporal fossa followed later by visual impairment as the neoplasm encroaches upon the optic canal. Patients with ectopic meningioma typically show painless proptosis with mild or no visual loss (20).

Diagnostic Approaches

The classic clinical manifestations described should strongly suggest the diagnosis of sphenoid wing orbital meningioma. Orbital CT or MRI can further substantiate the diagnosis and determine the extent of the tumor. These studies characteristically show hyperostosis of the involved sphenoid bone and a soft tissue mass that can extend into the orbit, temporal fossa, cranial cavity, and encroach on the optic canal accounting for the visual loss in some patients.

Pathology

The histopathology of SWM is similar to that already described for ONSM. Tumor invasion can be seen within the sphenoid bone.

Management

Surgical excision can be considered with collaboration between an ocular oncologist/oculoplastic surgeon and neurosurgeon if vision is threatened or if there is progressive disease. In an analysis of 39 surgically managed patients with SWM, mean patient age was 48 years and tumor remove appeared total in 39%, near total in 51%, and subtotal in 10%. Recurrence was later detected in 18% over mean follow-up of 41 months (12). Preoperative severe visual field defect was a risk for poor visual outcome whereas hypertrophied sphenoid bone was a favorable factor for good visual outcome. Others have described similar results with extensive intradural and extradural tumor removal as well as drilling of the optic canal (8). Chemotherapy and radiotherapy are also options for SWM if recurrent following surgical resection.

ORBITAL SPHENOID WING MENINGIOMA

Selected References

Reviews

1. Shields JA, Shields CL, Scartozzi R. Survey of 1264 patients with orbital tumors and simulating lesions: The 2002 Montgomery Lecture, part 1. *Ophthalmology* 2004;111:997–1008.
2. Shields JA, Bakewell B, Augsburger JJ, et al. Classification and incidence of space-occupying lesions of the orbit. A survey of 645 biopsies. *Arch Ophthalmol* 1984;102:1606–1611.
3. Shields JA, Bakewell B, Augsburger JJ, et al. Space-occupying orbital masses in children: A review of 250 consecutive biopsies. *Ophthalmology* 1986;93:379–384.
4. Demirci H, Shields CL, Shields JA, et al. Orbital tumors in the older adult population. *Ophthalmology* 2002;109:243–248.
5. Bleeker GM. Orbital meningioma. *Orbit* 1984;3:3–17.
6. Rogers L, Barani I, Chamberlain M, et al. Meningiomas: knowledge base, treatment outcomes, and uncertainties. A RANO review. *J Neurosurg* 2014;24:1–20.

Imaging

7. Smith AB, Horkanyne-Szakaly I, Schroeder JW, et al. From the radiologic pathology archives: mass lesions of the dura: beyond meningioma-radiologic-pathologic correlation. *Radiographics* 2014;34:295–312.

Management

8. Shrivastava RK, Sen C, Constantino PD, et al. Sphenoorbital meningiomas: Surgical limitations and lessons learned in their long-term management. *J Neurosurg* 2005;103:491–497.
9. Verheggen R, Markakis E, Muhlendyck H, et al. Symptomatology, surgical therapy and postoperative results of sphenoorbital, intraorbital-intracanalicular and optic sheath meningiomas. *Acta Neurochir Suppl* 1996;65:95–98.
10. Hakuba A, Liu S, Nishimura S. The orbitozygomatic infratemporal approach: a new surgical technique. *Surg Neurol* 1986;26:271–276.
11. McDermott MW, Durity FA, Rootman J, et al. Combined frontotemporal-orbitozygomatic approach for tumors of the sphenoid wing and orbit. *Neurosurgery* 1990;26:107–116.
12. Oya S, Sade B, Lee JH. Sphenoorbital meningioma: surgical technique and outcome. *J Neurosurg* 2011;114:1241–1249.
13. Forster MT, Daneshvar K, Senft C, et al. Sphenoorbital meningiomas; surgical management and outcome. *Neurol Res* 2014;36:695–700.

Histopathology

14. Marquardt MD, Zimmerman LE. Histopathology of meningiomas and gliomas of the optic nerve. *Human Pathol* 1982;13:226–234.

Case Reports

15. Rodrigues MM, Savino PJ, Schatz NJ. Spheno-orbital meningioma with optociliary veins. *Am J Ophthalmol* 1976;81:666–670.
16. Saul RF, King AB. Spontaneous reduction of growth rate of a large intracranial meningioma. Case Report. *J Clin Neuroophthalmol* 1984;4:133–136.
17. Leipzig B, English J. Sphenoid wing meningioma occurring as a lateral orbital mass. *Laryngoscope* 1984;94:1091–1093.
18. Reale F, Delfini R, Cintorino M. An intradiploic meningioma of the orbital roof: case report. *Ophthalmologica* 1978;177:82–87.
19. Pushker N, Shrey D, Kashyap S, et al. Ectopic meningioma of the orbit. *Int Ophthalmol* 2013;33:707–710.
20. Gunduz K, Kurt RA, Erden E. Ectopic orbital meningioma: report of two cases and literature review. *Surv Ophthalmol* 2014;59:643–648.

SPHENOID WING MENINGIOMA: ORBITAL INVOLVEMENT

If untreated, SWM generally shows slow progression. When the growth causes extreme proptosis or extends toward the optic canal, chiasm, and cavernous sinus, then surgical excision should usually be undertaken, regardless of the risk. If deemed unresectable, then stereotactic irradiation can be considered.

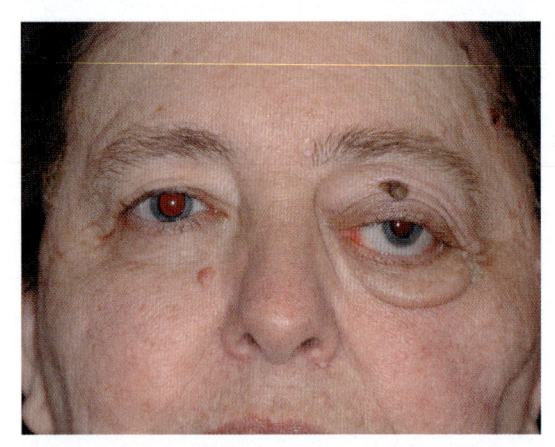

Figure 30.49. Proptosis, blepharoptosis, and downward displacement of left eye in a 56-year-old woman. There is a coincidental papilloma on left upper eyelid.

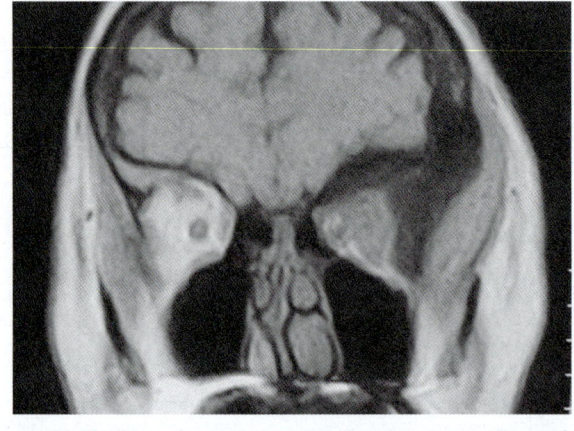

Figure 30.50. Coronal magnetic resonance imaging in T1-weighted image showing the extent of low signal hyperostosis in the left zygomatic, frontal, and temporal bones as well as the bright signal of soft tissue mass.

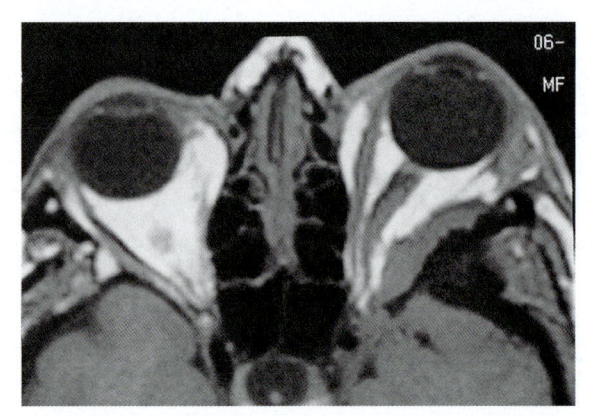

Figure 30.51. Axial magnetic resonance imaging in T1-weighted image of patient shown in Figure 30.49. Note the low signal hyperostosis of the greater wing of the sphenoid bone and the soft tissue component of the tumor in the orbit.

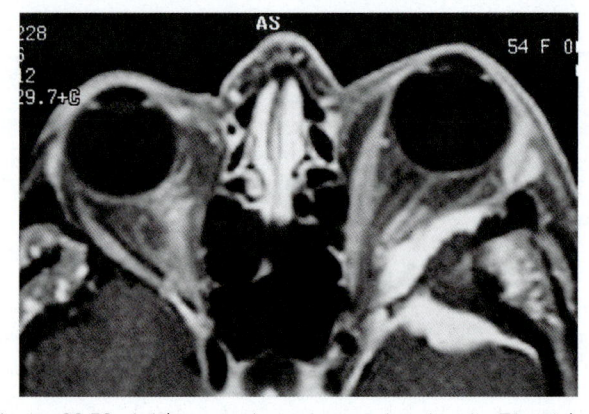

Figure 30.52. Axial magnetic resonance imaging in T1-weighted image with gadolinium enhancement of same patient, showing marked enhancement of the soft tissue component of the placoid tumor in the orbit, brain, and temporal fossa. MRI is superior to computed tomography for defining the extent of the soft tissue involvement.

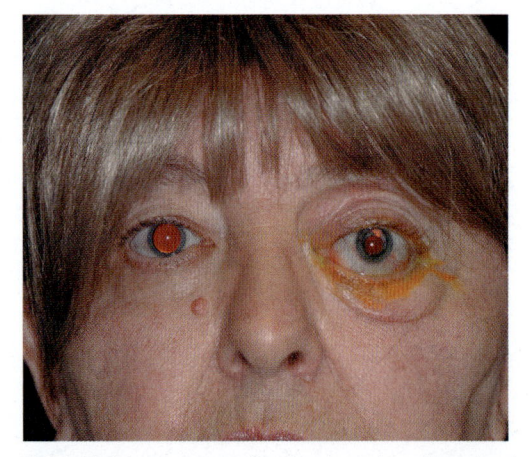

Figure 30.53. Facial appearance of patient 1 year later. Note that the proptosis is worse. Because of progression, the patient agreed to be referred to neurosurgeon for removal, assisted by an ophthalmic oncologist.

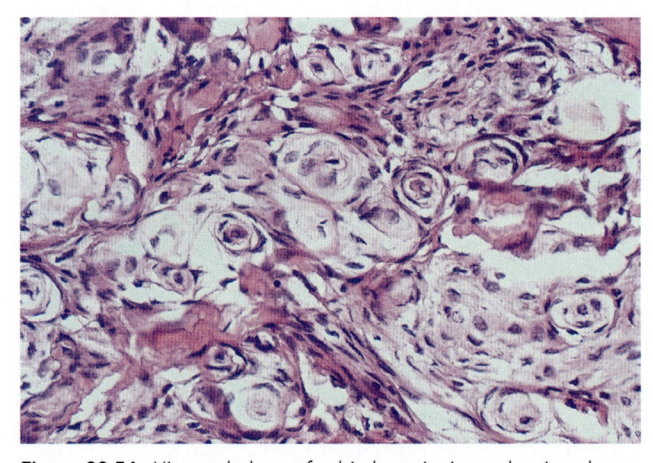

Figure 30.54. Histopathology of orbital meningioma showing characteristic whorls of benign meningothelial cells. (Hematoxylin–eosin ×100.)

Chapter 30 Optic Nerve, Meningeal, and Other Neural Tumors

● SPHENOID WING MENINGIOMA: ORBITAL INVOLVEMENT

Secondary (sphenoid wing) meningioma is a cytologically benign neoplasm that originates in the meninges of the greater or lesser wing of the sphenoid bone and extends secondarily into the orbit soft tissue, meninges of optic nerve, and cranial cavity.

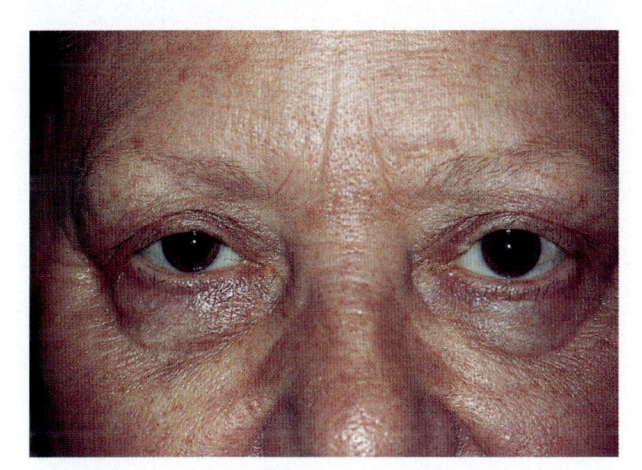

Figure 30.55. Proptosis of the left eye in a 63-year-old woman.

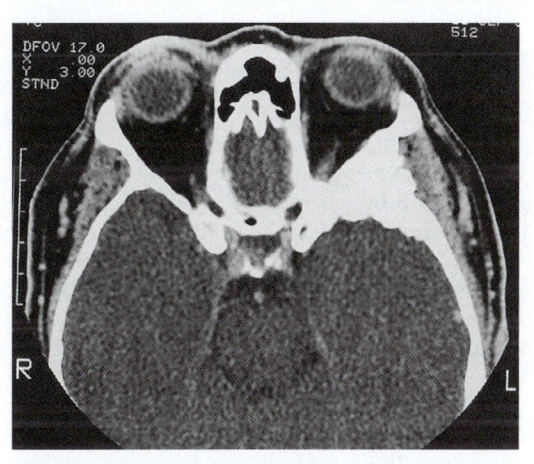

Figure 30.56. Axial computed tomography of patient shown in Figure 30.55, demonstrating hyperostosis of greater wing of sphenoid on left side, a finding characteristic of meningioma.

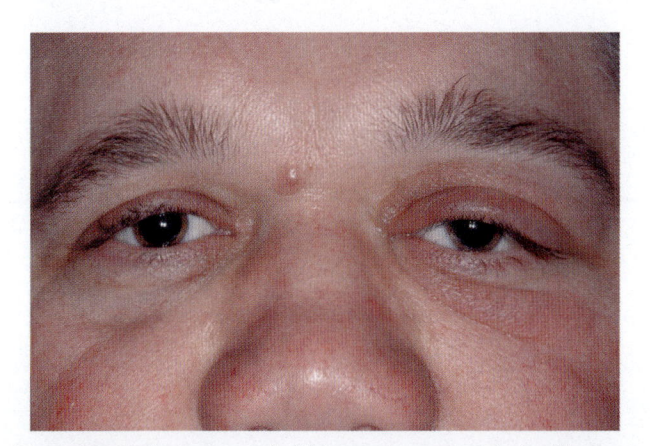

Figure 30.57. Appearance of middle-aged woman with visual loss and pain in region of left eye. There was edema of left upper eyelid and only slight proptosis.

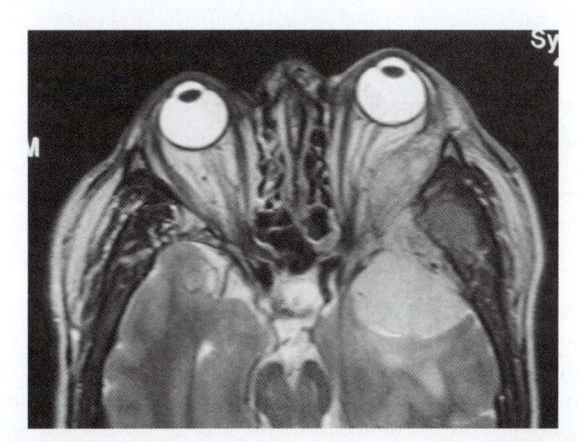

Figure 30.58. Axial magnetic resonance imaging in T2-weighted image, showing proptosis, hyperostosis of sphenoid bone, and soft tissue involvement of orbit and brain.

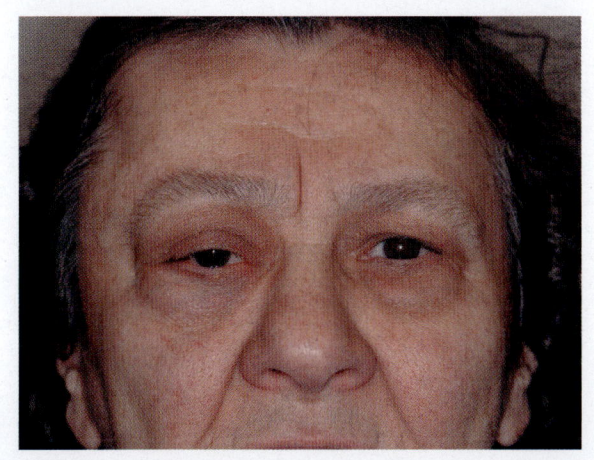

Figure 30.59. Elderly woman with slight right proptosis and blepharoptosis.

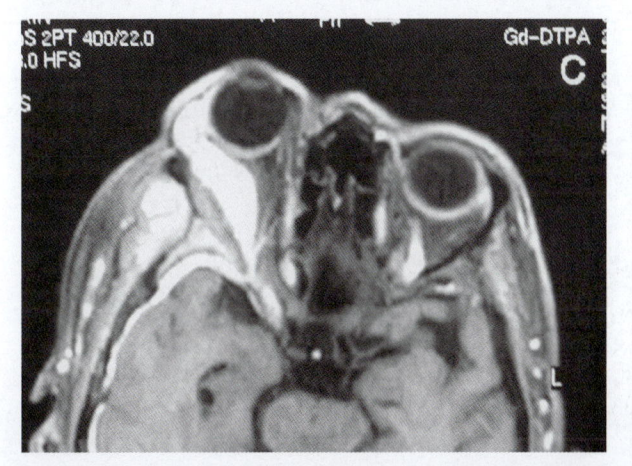

Figure 30.60. Axial computed tomography in T1-weighted image of patient shown in Figure 30.59 with gadolinium enhancement and fat suppression showing the extent of hyperostosis and soft tissue involvement of orbit and temporal fossa. Note the nasal displacement of the optic nerve.

ORBITAL PRIMITIVE NEUROECTODERMAL TUMOR AND PRIMARY ORBITAL NEUROBLASTOMA

Orbital Primitive Neuroectodermal Tumor

General Considerations
Primitive neuroectodermal tumor (PNET) is a neoplasm of childhood that has been diagnosed more frequently in recent years (1–10). Its classification is controversial and some cases of extraskeletal Ewing tumor and other primitive neuroblastic tumors are now being reclassified as PNET based on sophisticated immunohistochemical and genetic studies. PNET arises from the neural crest cells and typically occurs in children with only relatively poor survival (1). This complex subject is discussed elsewhere (1) and this section covers only some of the information on PNETs that have been recognized in the orbit (2–10).

Clinical Features
Orbital primary PNET has been seen primarily in children and young adults. It usually causes rapid unilateral proptosis and displacement of the globe. It has been recognized in the muscle cone and in the extraconal space (2–10). The findings are similar to those seen with rhabdomyosarcoma.

Diagnostic Approaches
Imaging studies may show the lesion anywhere in the orbit. It is circumscribed in the early stages but soon becomes invasive, often with bone destruction. CT and MRI may show features similar to metastatic neuroblastoma to the orbit, discussed later.

Pathology
Microscopically, PNET has several variations (1). The classic tumor is composed of sheets or lobules of small round cells containing darkly staining round to oval nuclei. Variable degrees of fibrous connective tissue may be present. Homer–Wright rosettes are often present and Flexner–Wintersteiner rosettes are occasionally observed. As mentioned, appropriate immunohistochemistry should be done and reviewed by an experienced pathologist to establish the diagnosis.

Management
A biopsy should be done, removing as much tumor tissue as possible, followed by chemotherapy and possibly irradiation, in conjunction with pediatric and radiation oncologists.

Selected References

Reviews
1. Smoll NR. Relative survival of childhood and adult medulloblastomas and primitive neuroectodermal tumors (PNETs). *Cancer* 2012;118:1313–1322.

Case Reports
2. Sen S, Kashyap S, Thanikachalam S, et al. Primary primitive neuroectodermal tumor of the orbit. *J Pediatr Ophthalmol Strabismus* 2002;39:242–244.
3. Alyahya GA, Heegaard S, Fledelius HC, et al. Primitive neuroectodermal tumor of the orbit in a 5-year-old girl with microphthalmia. *Graefes Arch Clin Exp Ophthalmol* 2000;238:801–806.
4. Kiratli H, Bilgic S, Gedikoglu G, et al. Primitive neuroectodermal tumor of the orbit in an adult. A case report and literature review. *Ophthalmology* 1999;106:98–102.
5. Bansal RK, Gupta A. Primitive neuroectodermal tumour of the orbit: a case report. *Indian J Ophthalmol* 1995;43:29–31.
6. Singh AD, Husson M, Shields CL, et al. Primitive neuroectodermal tumor of the orbit. *Arch Ophthalmol* 1994;112:217–221.
7. Wilson WB, Roloff J, Wilson HL. Primary peripheral neuroepithelioma of the orbit with intracranial extension. *Cancer* 1988;62:2595–2601.
8. Chokthaweesak W, Annunziata CC, Alsheikh O, et al. Primitive neuroectodermal tumor of the orbit in adults: a case series. *Ophthal Plast Reconstr Surg* 2011;27:173–179.
9. Romero R, Castano A, Abelairas J, et al. Peripheral primitive neuroectodermal tumour of the orbit. *Br J Ophthalmol* 2011;95:915–920.
10. Shuangshoti S, Menakanit W, Changwaivit W, et al. Primary intraorbital extraocular primitive neuroectodermal (neuroepithelial) tumour. *Br J Ophthalmol* 1986;70:543–538.

ORBITAL PRIMITIVE NEUROECTODERMAL TUMOR AND PRIMARY ORBITAL NEUROBLASTOMA

Orbital Neuroblastoma: Primary Type

General Considerations
The best known neuroblastoma of the orbit is metastatic neuroblastoma from the adrenal gland (1–4). Esthesioneuroblastoma can also secondarily invade the orbit from the adjacent nasal cavity. However, primary orbital neuroblastoma has been reported rarely in the orbit (3,4).

Clinical Features
In contrast to PNET, primary orbital neuroblastoma seems to be more common in adults. It has no unique clinical features and the patient presents with symptoms and signs similar to other orbital tumors.

Diagnostic Approaches
Primary orbital neuroblastoma can begin as a circumscribed tumor that later becomes more invasive. Radiologic features are probably similar to that of PNET and many other orbital neoplasms.

Pathology
Histopathologically, primary orbital neuroblastoma has features that are similar to PNET. This tumor is composed of small round neuroblastic cells arranged in nests, cords, and neuroblastic rosettes. The cytoplasm contains argyrophilic neurosecretory granules. It must be differentiated from neuroendocrine tumors, such as carcinoid (3,4).

Management
Management of primary orbital neuroblastoma is complete surgical resection often combined with chemotherapy and irradiation. The tumor can be aggressive with recurrences and orbital exenteration may eventually be necessary.

For pediatric neuroblastoma, there is new literature regarding therapeutic targeted medication for mutated genes and proteins within the tumor (1,2). Antibodies targeted to GD2, a surface antigen on neuroblastoma cells, can be beneficial for aggressive tumors. These anti-GD2 antibodies stimulate an immune-mediated cytotoxicity directed toward neuroblastoma and are most efficacious for minimal residual disease following standard chemotherapy (2).

Selected References

Management
1. Brodeur GM, Iyer R, Croucher JL, et al. Therapeutic targets for neuroblastomas. *Exper Opin Ther Targets* 2014;18:277–292.
2. Parsons K, Bernhardt B, Strickland B. Targeted immunotherapy for high-risk neuroblastoma – the role of monoclonal antibodies. *Ann Pharmacother* 2013;47:210–218.

Case Reports
3. Jakobiec FA, Klepach GL, Crissman JD, et al. Primary differentiated neuroblastoma of the orbit. *Ophthalmology* 1987;94:255–266.
4. Bullock JD, Goldberg SH, Rakes SM, et al. Primary orbital neuroblastoma. *Arch Ophthalmol* 1989;107:1031–1033.

ORBITAL PRIMITIVE NEUROECTODERMAL TUMOR AND PRIMARY ORBITAL NEUROBLASTOMA

1. Singh AD, Husson M, Shields CL, et al. Primitive neuroectodermal tumor of the orbit. *Arch Ophthalmol* 1994;112:217–221.
2. Jakobiec FA, Klepach GL, Crissman JD, et al. Primary differentiated neuroblastoma of the orbit. *Ophthalmology* 1987;94:255–266.

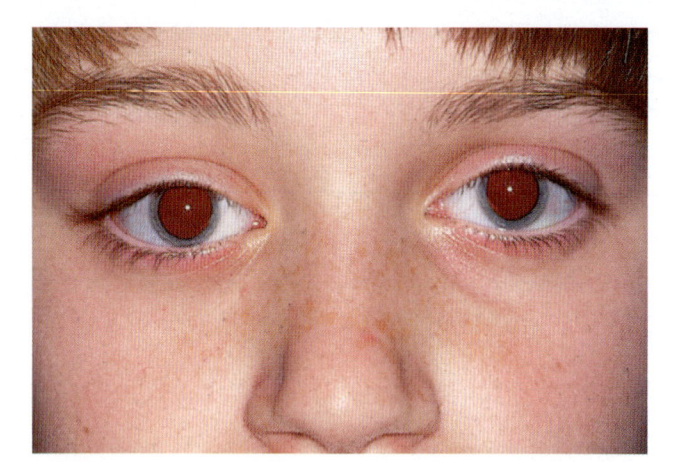

Figure 30.61. Primitive neuroectodermal tumor. Proptosis of the right eye in a 10-year-old girl.

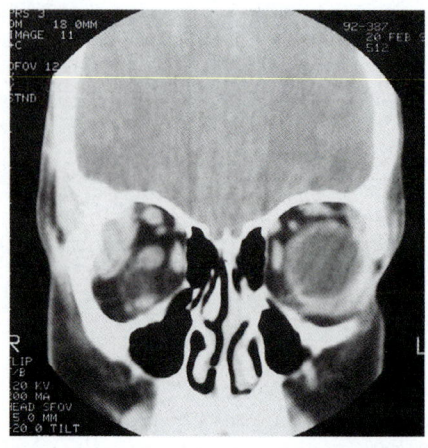

Figure 30.62. Coronal computed tomography of the patient shown in Figure 30.61, demonstrating a superotemporal orbital tumor with bone erosion and hyperostosis.

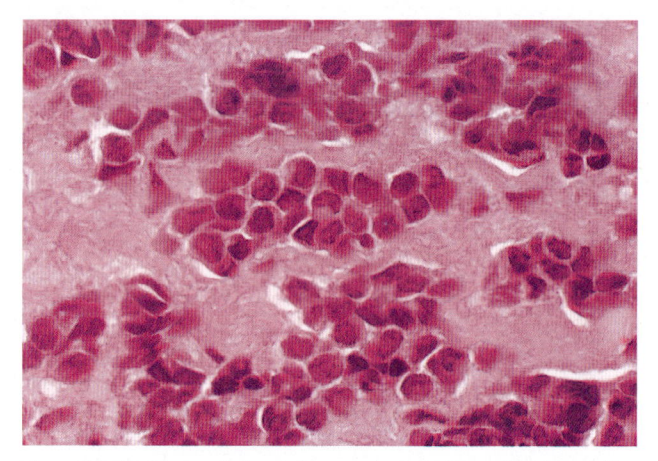

Figure 30.63. Histopathology of tumor shown in Figure 30.61, revealing nests of small cells in a fibrous tissue stroma. (Hematoxylin–eosin ×250.)

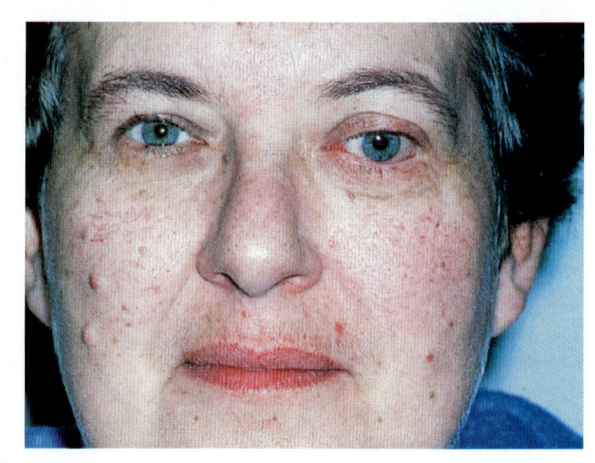

Figure 30.64. Primary orbital neuroblastoma. Proptosis of the left eye in a middle-aged woman. (Courtesy of Frederick Jakobiec, MD.)

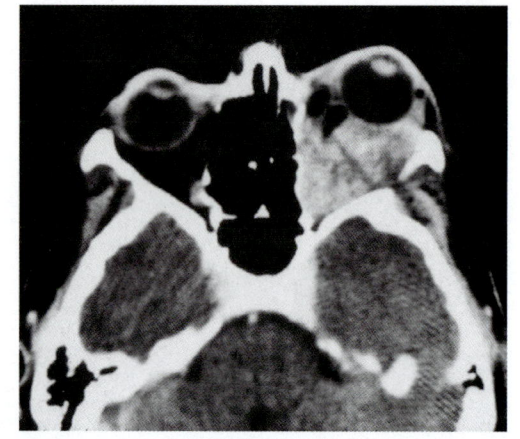

Figure 30.65. Axial computed tomography of woman shown in Figure 30.64, demonstrating large irregular mass filling most of the orbit. (Courtesy of Frederick Jakobiec, MD.)

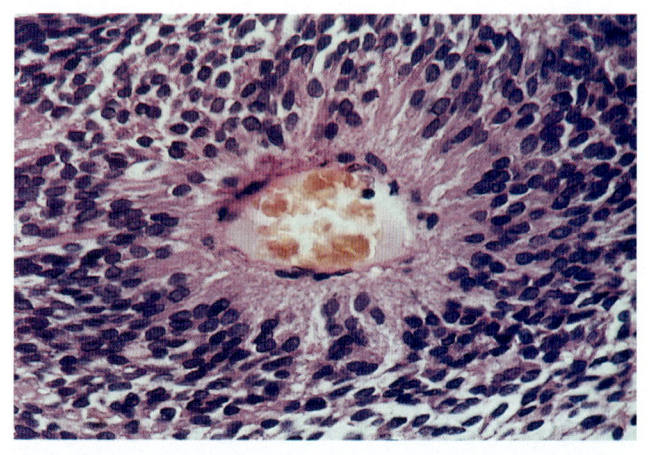

Figure 30.66. Histopathology of lesion shown in Figure 30.64, demonstrating neuroblastic cells with a neuroblastic rosette. (Hematoxylin–eosin ×200.) (Courtesy of Frederick Jakobiec, MD.)

ORBITAL MYOGENIC TUMORS

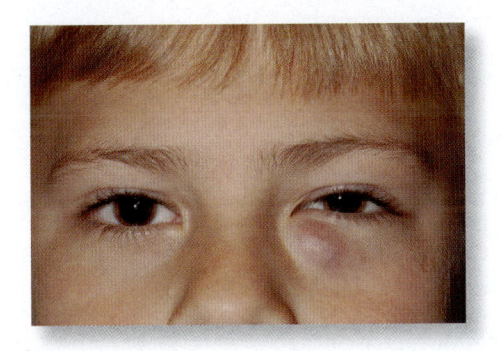

General Considerations

Tumors of skeletal muscle derivation that can develop in the orbit include rhabdomyoma, rhabdomyosarcoma (RMS), and malignant rhabdoid tumor (1–27). Tumors of smooth muscle derivation include leiomyoma and leiomyosarcoma. Orbital rhabdomyoma is extremely rare with only a few cases reported in the literature (25–27). It is generally a circumscribed soft tissue tumor of infancy that is composed of well-differentiated striated muscle cells with a mixture of collagen fibers. We have no examples of orbital rhabdomyoma to illustrate. RMS is the most important myogenic tumor of the orbit.

RMS is the most common primary orbital malignancy of childhood (1–24). In the author's clinicopathologic series, it accounted for only 1% of all biopsied orbital masses (2) and for 4% of all biopsied orbital masses in children (3). In the clinical series of 1,264 patients, 35 cases of orbital RMS accounted for 97% of myogenic tumors and for 3% of all orbital lesions (1). There have been many series (4–6,8–11) and case reports (15–27) on orbital RMS. Orbital RMS generally occurs in the first two decades of life with a mean age at diagnosis of 8 years (4,5). The tumor can originate primarily in the orbit or it can develop in the sinuses or nasal cavity and secondarily extend to involve the orbit. Orbital RMS has been observed many years after orbital irradiation for retinoblastoma (15).

There is a classification of RMS based on the extent and surgical results, called the Intergroup Rhabdomyosarcoma Study Group Staging Classification (Table 31.1).

Clinical Features

The clinical features of orbital RMS can vary considerably from case to case. The patient generally presents with proptosis (80% to 100%), globe displacement (80%), blepharoptosis

Table 31.1 Intergroup Rhabdomyosarcoma Study Group Staging Classification

Group	Description
I	Completely resected localized disease with gross and microscopic confirmation of complete resection and absence of regional lymph node involvement
Ia	Confirmed to muscle or organ of origin
Ib	Contiguous involvement outside the muscle or organ of origin
II	Residual disease and/or regional lymph node involvement
IIa	Grossly resected localized tumor with microscopic residual disease and no evidence of gross residual tumor or regional lymph node involvement
IIb	Completely resected regional lymph node and no microscopic residual tumor
IIc	Grossly resected regional lymph nodes with microscopic residual tumor
III	Incomplete resection with gross residual disease
IV	Distant metastatic disease present at onset

Shields JA, Shields CL. Rhabdomyosarcoma: review for the ophthalmologist. The 2001 Henry Dubins Lecture. *Surv Ophthalmol* 2003;48:39–57.

ORBITAL RHABDOMYOSARCOMA

(30% to 50%), conjunctival and eyelid swelling (60%), palpable mass (25%), and pain (10%). Most patients have proptosis and downward and lateral displacement of the globe owing to the superior or superonasal location of the mass in 70% (4,5). It can occasionally occur as an epibulbar mass without deep orbital involvement (4,5,23).

Diagnostic Approaches

The differential diagnosis of orbital RMS includes orbital cellulitis, nonspecific orbital inflammation ("pseudotumor"), ruptured dermoid cyst, capillary hemangioma, lymphangioma, Langerhans cell histiocytosis, myeloid sarcoma, lymphoma, and most other childhood orbital tumors. The clinical features that serve to differentiate them are described elsewhere in this book and in the literature (7).

Imaging studies are usually helpful in the differentiation. Computed tomography (CT) demonstrates a moderately well circumscribed but irregular orbital mass that is generally confined to soft tissue and usually spares extraocular muscles. Less often it can extend to involve the adjacent orbital bones or sinuses. The tumor shows enhancement with contrast material. It usually has a hypointense signal with respect to orbital fat, but is isointense with respect to extraocular muscles. It generally shows moderate to marked enhancement with gadolinium and is best delineated with fat suppression techniques. On T2-weighted images, the lesion is hyperintense to extraocular muscles and orbital fat. The mass is usually solid but can occasionally show cavitary changes, suggesting the diagnosis of lymphangioma (4,5,21,22).

Pathology

Orbital RMS probably arises from primitive pluripotent mesenchymal cells with a propensity to differentiate toward skeletal muscle (6). Several histologic variations of RMS occur in the orbit. The embryonal type is most common, whereas the alveolar type appears to be the most malignant (4–6). Embryonal RMS is characterized histopathologically by spindle to round cells that show features characteristic of skeletal muscle in various stages of embryogenesis. The predominant cell is an elongated spindle cell that can assume a variety of arrangements and degrees of differentiation. The cytoplasm is generally highly eosinophilic and cross-striations can sometimes be identified on routine histopathologic sections or with special histochemical stains. The alveolar type appears as loosely arranged, malignant cells with septae that are reminiscent of the pulmonary alveoli. The botryoid type may be a variant of the embryonal type that assumes a papillary configuration.

ORBITAL RHABDOMYOSARCOMA

Management
Current management of orbital RMS is reviewed in considerable detail in the recent literature (1–12). Suspected orbital RMS should be managed by a systemic evaluation to exclude metastatic disease including lung, lymph nodes, and other sites. This should be followed by prompt biopsy with histopathologic confirmation of the diagnosis. When possible, the entire tumor should be removed intact. When that cannot be easily accomplished without damage to extraocular muscles or optic nerve, a generous incisional biopsy is sufficient. Once the diagnosis is established histopathologically, most patients are treated with irradiation and chemotherapy, according to guidelines established by the Intergroup Rhabdomyosarcoma Study (7–11).

Prognosis
Orbital RMS can be highly aggressive locally and can invade the brain and adjacent tissues and metastasize to lung, lymph nodes, and other distant sites. Using the modern therapeutic regimen, however, the survival has improved dramatically in recent years. Reports from the 1970s indicated that only 30% were alive after 5 years (13). Today, the survival is >95% for orbital RMS (4,5). Factors that appear responsible for the better prognosis for RMS in the orbital region include the more favorable anatomic location, the earlier stage of the disease at the time of diagnosis, more favorable tumor morphology, and perhaps patient age.

Selected References

Reviews

1. Shields JA, Shields CL, Scartozzi R. Survey of 1264 patients with orbital tumors and simulating lesions: The 2002 Montgomery Lecture, part 1. *Ophthalmology* 2004;111: 997–1008.
2. Shields JA, Bakewell B, Augsburger JJ, et al. Classification and incidence of space-occupying lesions of the orbit. A survey of 645 biopsies. *Arch Ophthalmol* 1984;102: 1606–1611.
3. Shields JA, Bakewell B, Augsburger JJ, et al. Space-occupying orbital masses in children: A review of 250 consecutive biopsies. *Ophthalmology* 1986;93:379–384.
4. Shields CL, Shields JA, Honavar SG, et al. Clinical spectrum of primary ophthalmic rhabdomyosarcoma. *Ophthalmology* 2001;108:2284–2292.
5. Shields CL, Shields JA, Honavar SG, et al. Primary ophthalmic rhabdomyosarcoma in 33 patients. *Trans Am Ophthalmol Soc* 2001;99:133–142.
6. Knowles DM II, Jakobiec FA, Potter GD, et al. Ophthalmic striated muscle neoplasms. *Surv Ophthalmol* 1976;21:219–261.
7. Shields JA, Shields CL. Rhabdomyosarcoma: review for the ophthalmologist. The 2001 Henry Dubins Lecture. *Surv Ophthalmol* 2003;48:39–57.

Management

8. Wharam M, Beltangady M, Hays D, et al. Localized orbital rhabdomyosarcoma. An interim report of the intergroup rhabdomyosarcoma study committee. *Ophthalmology* 1987;94:251–254.
9. Raney RB, Anderson JR, Kollath J, et al. Late effects of therapy in 94 patients with localized rhabdomyosarcoma of the orbit: report from the Intergroup Rhabdomyosarcoma Study (IRS)-III, 1984–1991. *Med Pediatr Oncol* 2000;34:413–420.
10. Raney B, Stoner J, Anderson J, et al., Soft-Tissue Sarcoma Committee of the Children's Oncology Group. Impact of tumor viability at second-look procedures performed before completing treatment on the Intergroup Rhabdomyosarcoma Study Group protocol IRS-IV, 1991–1997: a report from the children's oncology group. *J Pediatr Surg* 2010;45:2160–2168.
11. Cecchetto G, Carretto E, Bisogno G, et al. Complete second look operation and radiotherapy in locally advanced non-alveolar rhabdomyosarcoma in children: A report from the AIEOP soft tissue sarcoma committee. *Pediatr Blood Cancer* 2008;51: 593–597.
12. Seregard S. Management of alveolar rhabdomyosarcoma of the orbit. *Acta Ophthalmol Scand* 2002;80:660–664.
13. Abramson DH, Ellsworth RM, Tretter P, et al. The treatment of orbital rhabdomyosarcoma with irradiation and chemotherapy. *Ophthalmology* 1979;86;1330–1335.

Histopathology

14. Spahn B, Nenadov-Beck M. Orbital rhabdomyosarcoma: clinicopathologic correlation, management and follow-up in two newborns. A preliminary report. *Orbit* 2001; 20:149–156.

Case Reports

15. Wilson MC, Shields JA, Shields CL, et al. Orbital rhabdomyosarcoma fifty seven years after radiotherapy for retinoblastoma. *Orbit* 1996;15:97–100.
16. Cescon M, Grazi GL, Assietti R, et al. Embryonal rhabdomyosarcoma of the orbit in a liver transplant recipient. *Transpl Int* 2003;16:437–440.
17. Jung A, Bechthold S, Pfluger T, et al. Orbital rhabdomyosarcoma in Noonan syndrome. *J Pediatr Hematol Oncol* 2003;25:330–332.
18. Lumbroso L, Sigal-Zafrani B, Jouffroy T, et al. Late malignant melanoma after treatment of rhabdomyosarcoma of the orbit during childhood. *Arch Ophthalmol* 2002; 120:1087–1090.
19. Othmane IS, Shields CL, Shields JA, et al. Primary orbital rhabdomyosarcoma in an adult. *Orbit* 1999;18:183–189.
20. Amato MM, Esmaeli B, Shore JW. Orbital rhabdomyosarcoma metastatic to the contralateral orbit: a case report. *Ophthalmology* 2002;109:753–756.
21. Fetkenhour DR, Shields CL, Chao AN, et al. Orbital cavitary rhabdomyosarcoma masquerading as lymphangioma. *Arch Ophthalmol* 2001;119:1208–1210.
22. Silvana G, Roberto de B, Domenico P, et al. Orbital cavitary rhabdomyosarcoma: a diagnostic dilemma. *Orbit* 2010;29:45–7.
23. Joffe L, Shields JA, Pearah D. Epibulbar rhabdomyosarcoma without proptosis. *J Pediatr Ophthalmol* 1977;14:364–367.
24. Shields JA, Shields CL, Eagle RC, et al. Orbital rhabdomyosarcoma. *Arch Ophthalmol* 1987;105:700–701.
25. Myung J, Kim IO, Chun JE, et al. Rhabdomyoma of the orbit: a case report. *Pediatr Radiol* 2002;32:589–592.
26. Hatsukawa Y, Furukawa A, Kawamura H, et al. Rhabdomyoma of the orbit in a child. *Am J Ophthalmol* 1997;123:142–144.
27. Knowles DM 2nd, Jakobiec FA. Rhabdomyoma of the orbit. *Am J Ophthalmol* 1975; 80:1011–1018.

Chapter 31 Orbital Myogenic Tumors

ORBITAL RHABDOMYOSARCOMA

Orbital RMS usually has characteristic clinical features, imaging studies and histopathology. A typical case is shown with clinico-pathologic correlation and long-term follow-up.

Shields JA, Shields CL, Eagle RC Jr, et al. Orbital rhabdomyosarcoma. *Arch Ophthalmol* 1987;105:700–701.

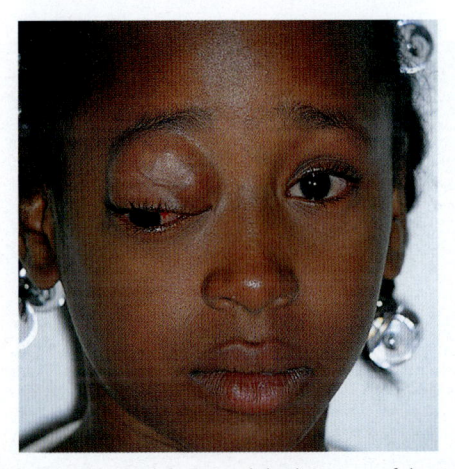

Figure 31.1. Proptosis and downward displacement of the right eye by a superior orbital mass in a 12-year-old girl.

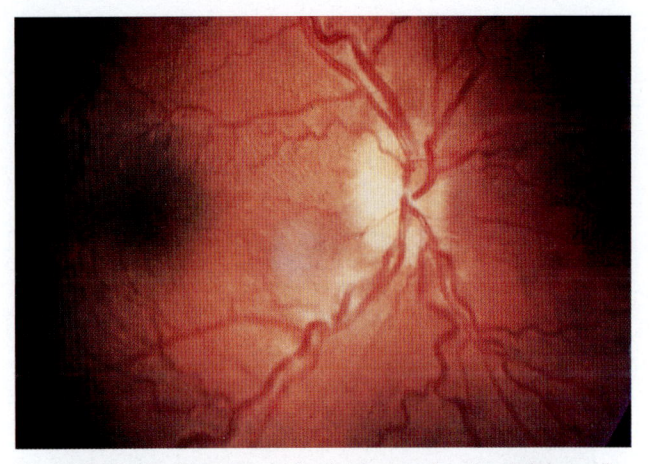

Figure 31.2. Fundus photograph of right eye showing slightly swollen optic disc and tortuous retinal veins secondary to compression of the globe by an orbital mass.

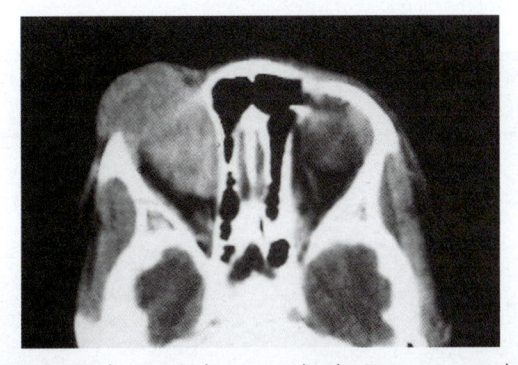

Figure 31.3. Axial computed tomography showing superonasal orbital mass.

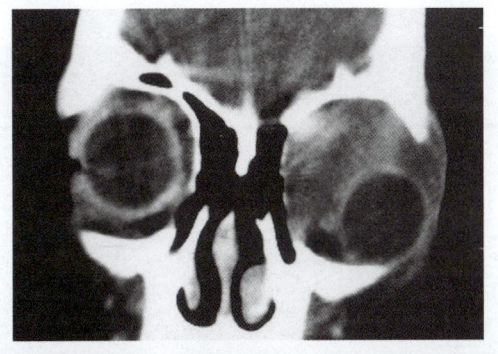

Figure 31.4. Coronal computed tomography showing extent of lesion. Coronal CT or magnetic resonance imaging is important in planning the best approach to either excisional or incisional biopsy. A generous biopsy was done through a superonasal skin incision.

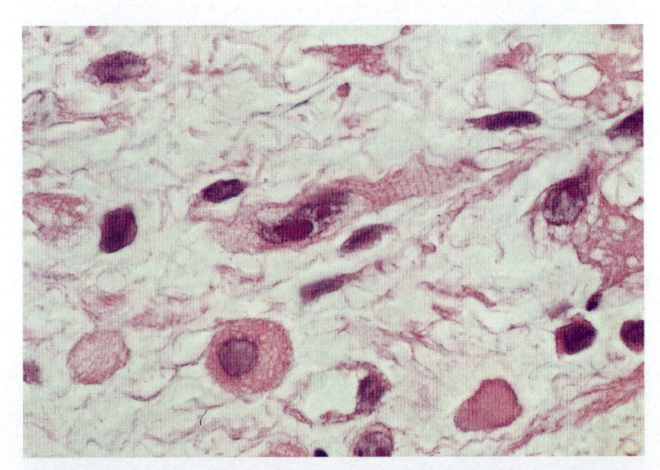

Figure 31.5. Histopathology showing malignant strap cells with cross-striations and some larger round cells with abundant extracellular matrix. (Hematoxylin–eosin ×200.)

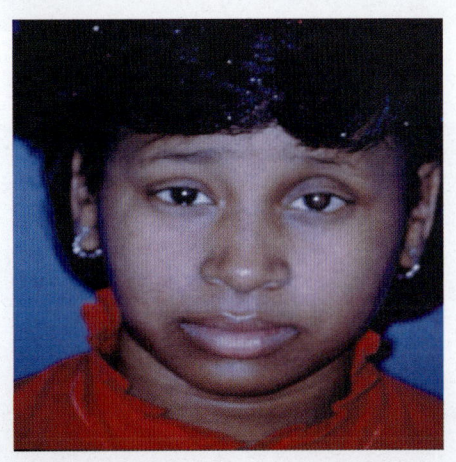

Figure 31.6. Appearance of patient at 22 years old. She had 20/20 vision in the affected right eye.

ORBITAL RHABDOMYOSARCOMA SIMULATING A LYMPHANGIOMA

If not treated promptly, orbital RMS can show rapid progression. An example is illustrated of a cavitary RMS that initially simulated a lymphangioma.

Fetkenhour DR, Shields CL, Chao AN, et al. Orbital cavitary rhabdomyosarcoma masquerading as lymphangioma. *Arch Ophthalmol* 2001;119:1208–1210.

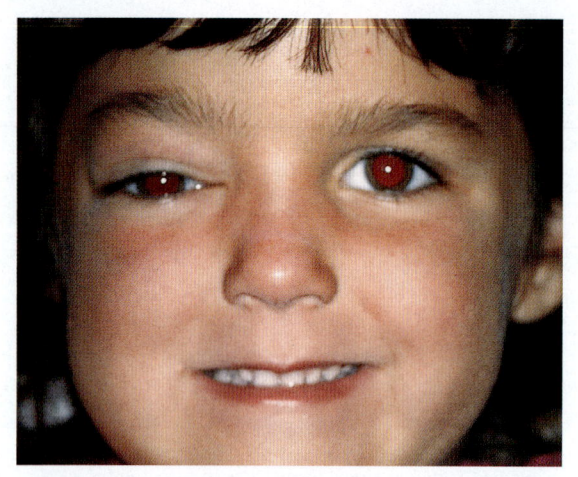

Figure 31.7. Blepharoptosis, proptosis, and downward displacement of right eye in a 4-year-old girl.

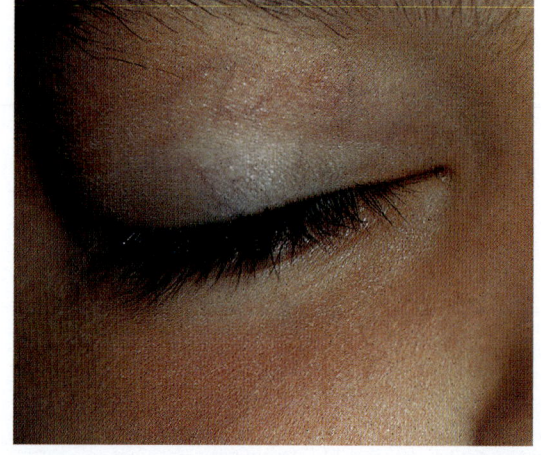

Figure 31.8. Closer view of right eye. A biopsy was not done because the clinical findings and magnetic resonance imaging (shown below) suggested the diagnosis of lymphangioma.

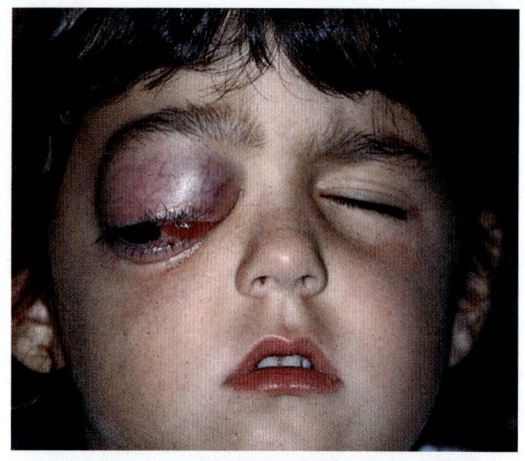

Figure 31.9. Appearance of patient 10 days later, showing rapid progression of proptosis and conjunctival chemosis.

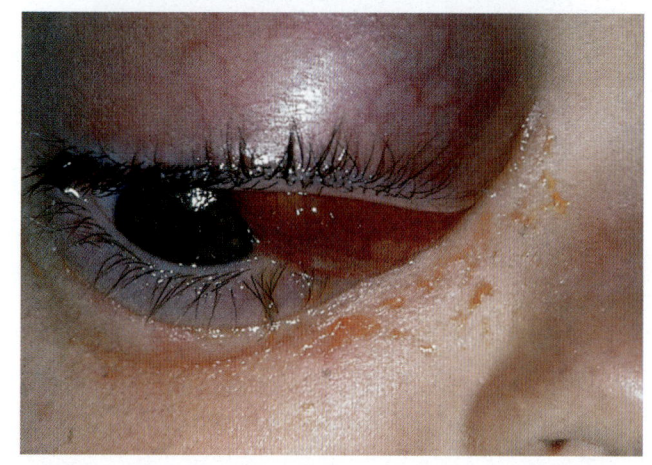

Figure 31.10. Closer view of right eye shown in Figure 31.9.

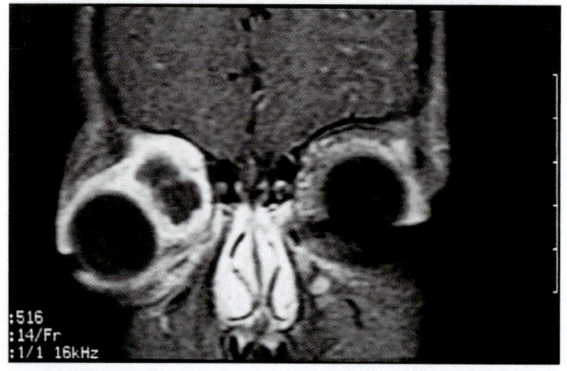

Figure 31.11. Coronal magnetic resonance imaging in T1-weighted image with gadolinium enhancement. Note the nonenhancing central area compatible with blood. This accounted for the original diagnosis of lymphangioma with hemorrhage.

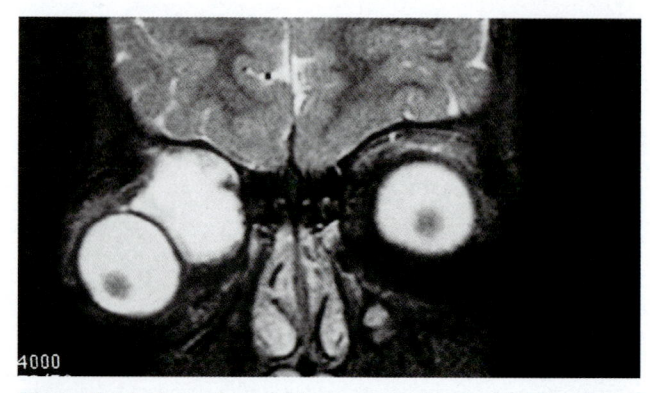

Figure 31.12. Coronal magnetic resonance imaging in T2-weighted image showing extent of the lesion with central cavity suggestive of blood or proteinaceous material.

Chapter 31 Orbital Myogenic Tumors 601

ORBITAL RHABDOMYOSARCOMA: TYPICAL CASE—CLINICAL FEATURES, MRI, AND PATHOLOGY

Orbital RMS typically presents at a mean age of 8 years as an anterior superonasal orbital mass that shows enhancement on typical, but not pathognomonic, radiographic findings. The histopathologic diagnosis can usually be made on the basis of light microscopy, although immunohistochemistry may be necessary for further confirmation.

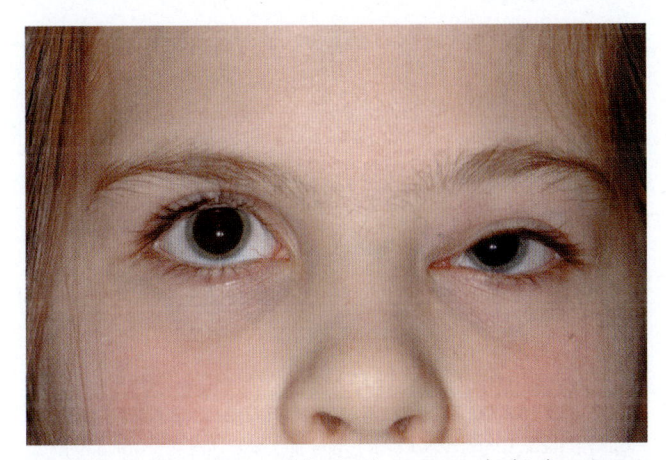

Figure 31.13. Face of 8-year-old girl with superonasal orbital mass causing slight proptosis and downward and lateral displacement of left eye.

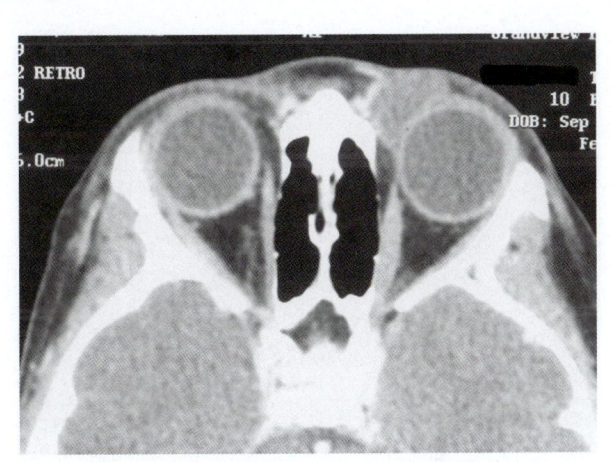

Figure 31.14. Axial computed tomography showing ovoid, circumscribed superonasal anterior orbital mass above the left eye.

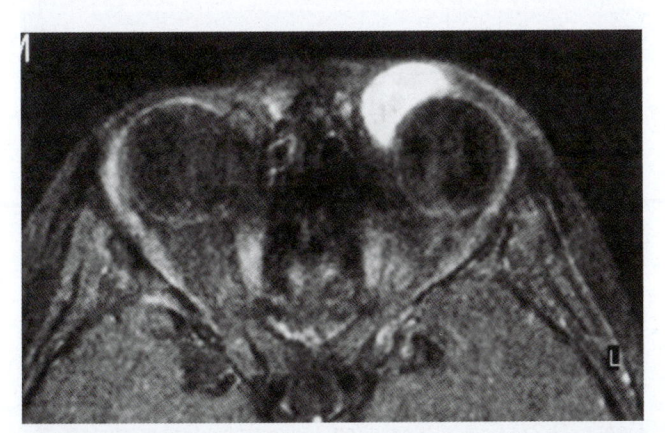

Figure 31.15. Axial magnetic resonance imaging in T1-weighted image with fat suppression and gadolinium enhancement demonstrating the enhancing superonasal mass. Note how the mass conforms to the curvature of the globe.

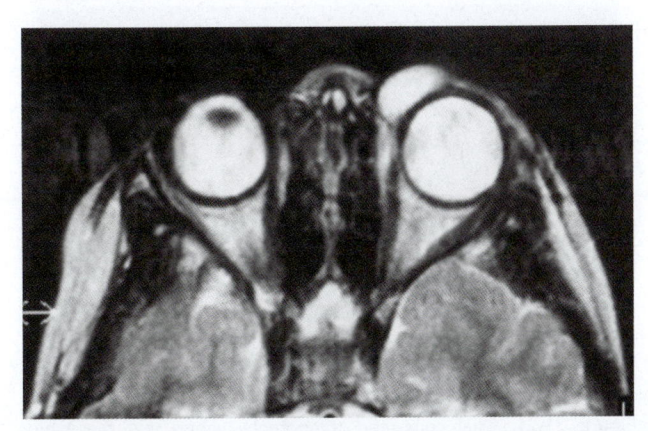

Figure 31.16. Axial magnetic resonance imaging in T2-weighted image demonstrating the extent of the hyperintense mass.

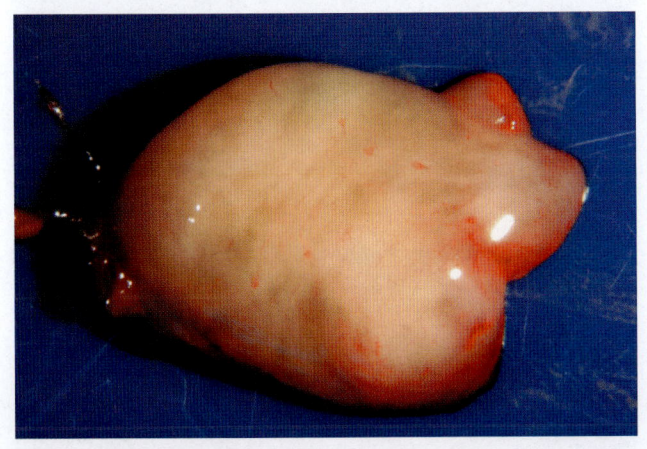

Figure 31.17. Appearance of the mass immediately after complete removal by way of superonasal cutaneous eyelid crease approach. Despite apparent complete removal, the child was treated with irradiation and chemotherapy by standard protocol.

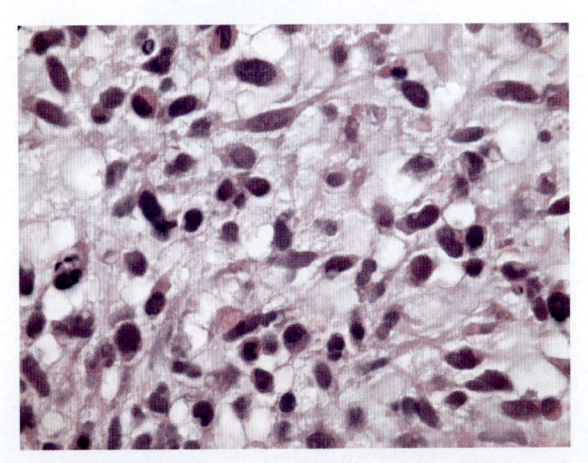

Figure 31.18. Histopathology showing typical malignant strap cells of rhabdomyosarcoma. (Hematoxylin–eosin ×150.)

● ORBITAL RHABDOMYOSARCOMA: PRESENTATION AS A CONJUNCTIVAL MASS

In some instances, a more posteriorly located orbital RMS can present initially in the conjunctival tissues, simulating a primary conjunctival neoplasm. Very large orbital RMS cannot usually be removed intact because the thin pseudocapsule usually ruptures at the time of attempted surgical removal.

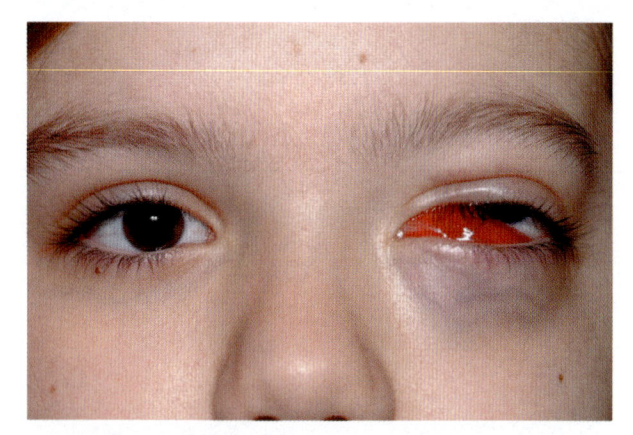

Figure 31.19. Appearance of child who presented with a red subconjunctival mass in the left eye.

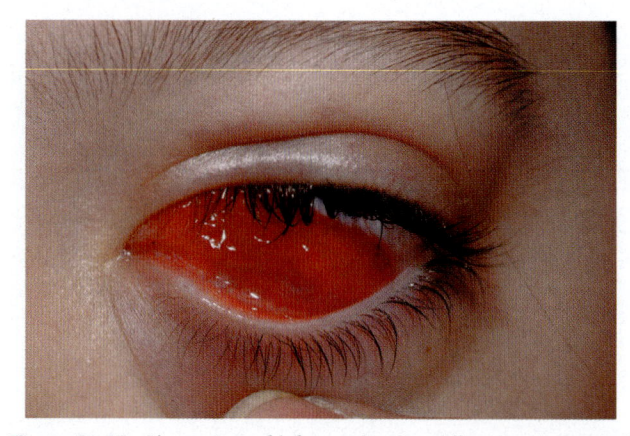

Figure 31.20. Closer view of left eye showing diffuse involvement of the inferior bulbar conjunctiva by a red mass.

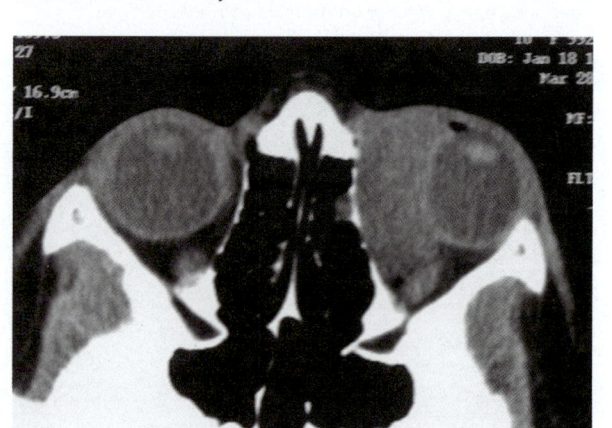

Figure 31.21. Axial computed tomography shows that the tumor extends far posterior into the orbit and is displacing the globe temporally.

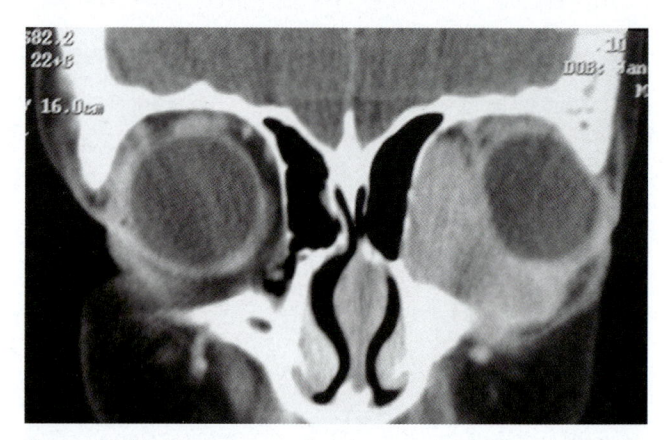

Figure 31.22. Coronal computed tomography further depicts the extent of the neoplasm that occupies most of the inferior and nasal aspects of the orbit.

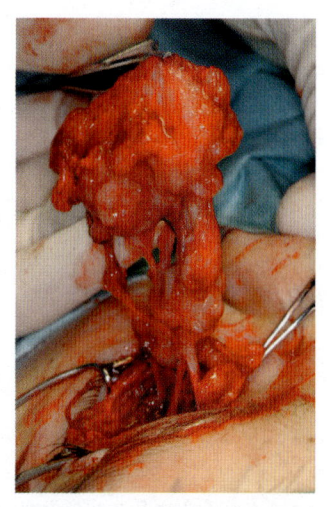

Figure 31.23. Appearance at the time of surgical removal. Despite meticulous surgery, it was not possible to keep the pseudocapsule of the large tumor intact and the tumor leaked into the orbit and had to be removed piecemeal. Microscopic residual tumor was treated by irradiation and chemotherapy by standard protocol.

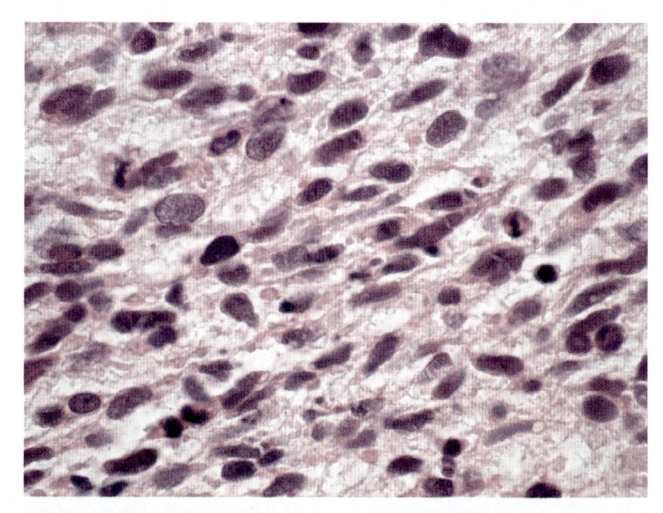

Figure 31.24. Histopathology showing malignant strap cells compatible with rhabdomyosarcoma. (Hematoxylin–eosin ×250.)

Chapter 31 Orbital Myogenic Tumors

ORBITAL RHABDOMYOSARCOMA: BIOPSY APPROACH

As mentioned, the planning of a biopsy of suspected orbital RMS necessitates good axial and coronal imaging studies with computed tomography or magnetic resonance imaging. The goal of surgery is to remove as much of the lesion as possible without damaging vital structures like the optic nerve and extraocular muscles. Another typical case is illustrated in which a smaller tumor was removed intact.

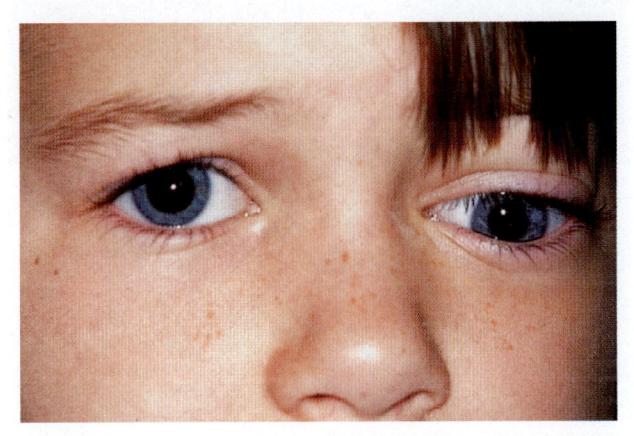

Figure 31.25. Proptosis and downward displacement of the left eye in a 4-year-old girl.

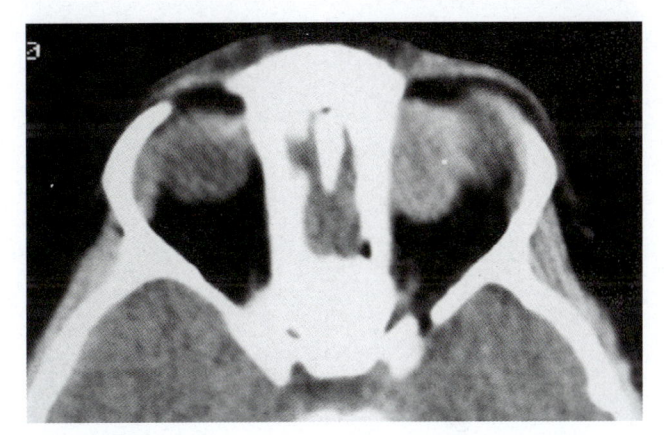

Figure 31.26. Axial computed tomography showing superonasal ovoid orbital mass.

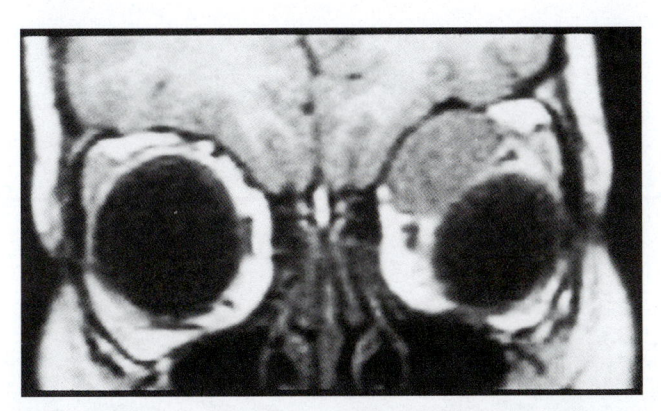

Figure 31.27. Coronal magnetic resonance imaging in T1-weighted image, showing superonasal mass with downward displacement of the globe.

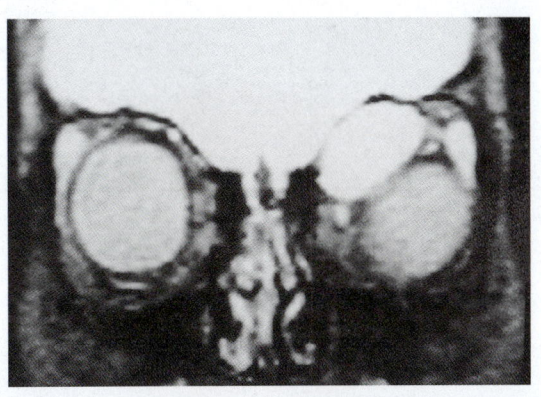

Figure 31.28. Coronal magnetic resonance imaging in T2-weighted image.

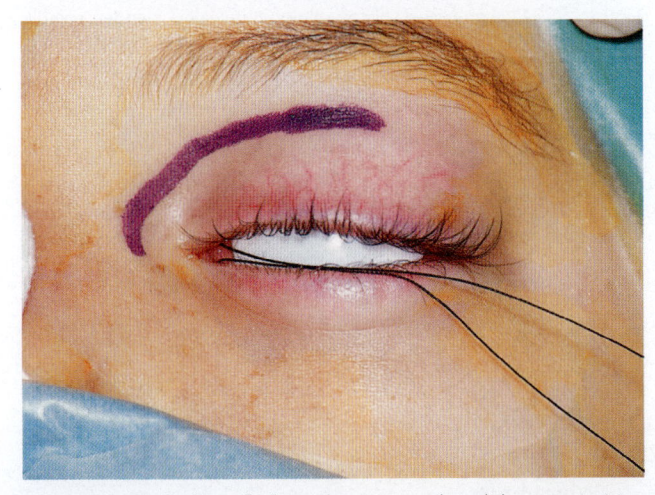

Figure 31.29. Outline of planned superonasal eyelid crease incision based on review of the imaging studies.

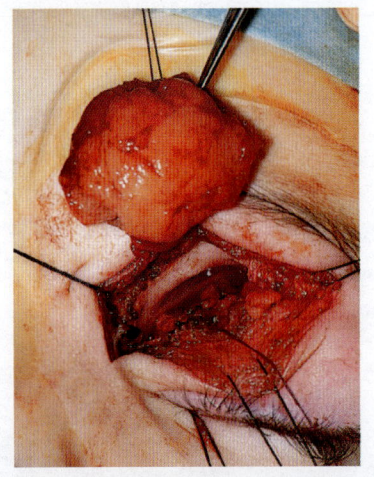

Figure 31.30. View after surgical excision, showing intact tumor. There was no apparent residual tumor in the orbit, either grossly or microscopically. However, the child was treated with irradiation and chemotherapy by standard protocol and is alive and well with no apparent recurrence after several years.

ORBITAL RHABDOMYOSARCOMA: SIMULATING ORBITAL HEMATOMA IN A CHILD

In some instances, RMS can be confined to the anterior orbit, conjunctiva, or eyelid. A case is illustrated that highlights the challenge in differentiation of RMS from orbital hemorrhage post-trauma. In this example, a child sustained an accidental injury to the eye and subsequently developed a hematoma near the site of injury. However, it was later biopsy-proven to represent RMS.

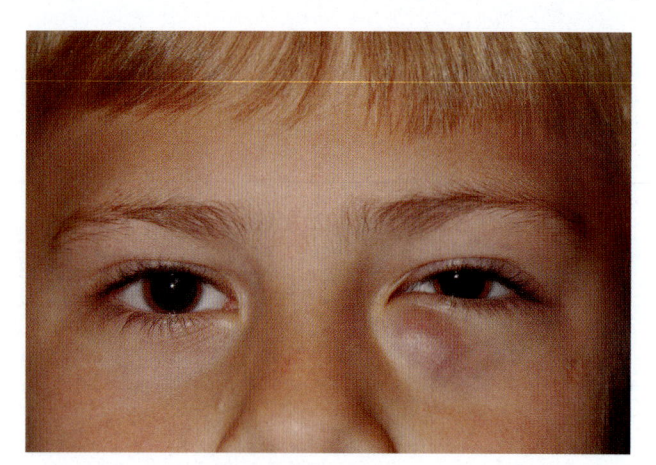

Figure 31.31. Left lower eyelid "hematoma" in an 8-year-old boy following accidental trauma.

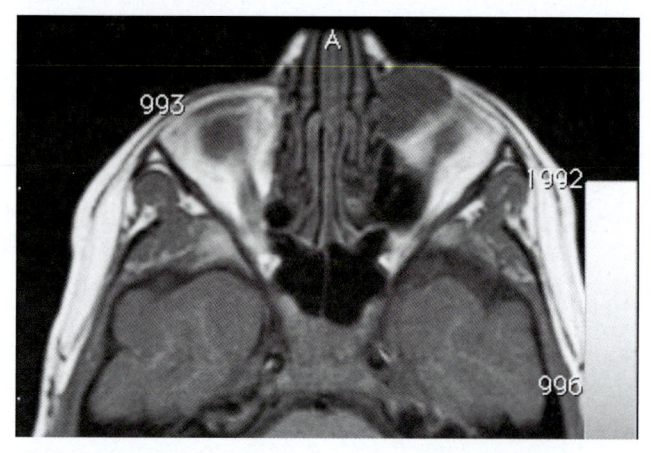

Figure 31.32. Magnetic resonance imaging disclosing a low signal solid mass in the anterior, inferonasal orbit on T1-weighted image.

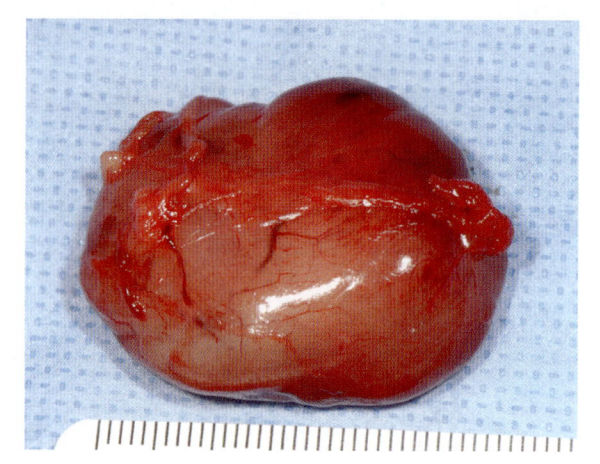

Figure 31.33. Surgical exploration revealing a solid, vascular mass.

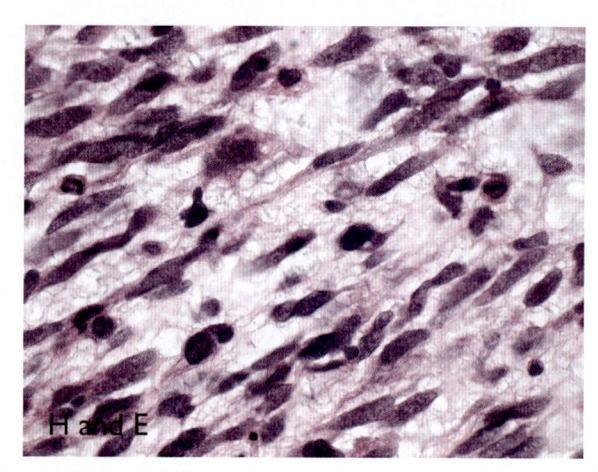

Figure 31.34. High-power histopathology revealed slender spindle cells (strap cells) in loose extracellular matrix, suggestive of rhabdomyosarcoma. (Hematoxylin–eosin ×200.)

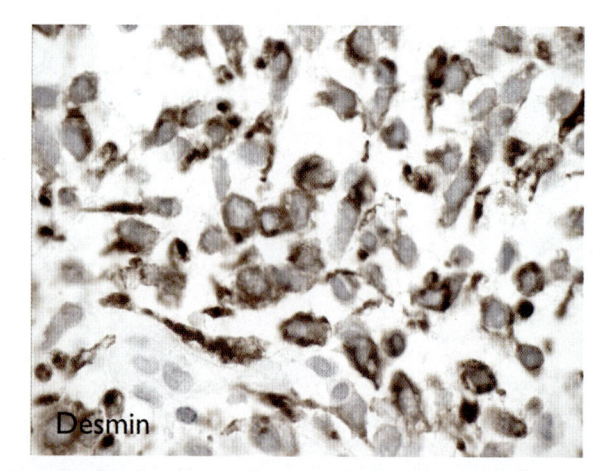

Figure 31.35. Desmin cytoplasmic stain showing positivity, consistent with a tumor of muscle origin such as rhabdomyosarcoma. (Desmin ×200.)

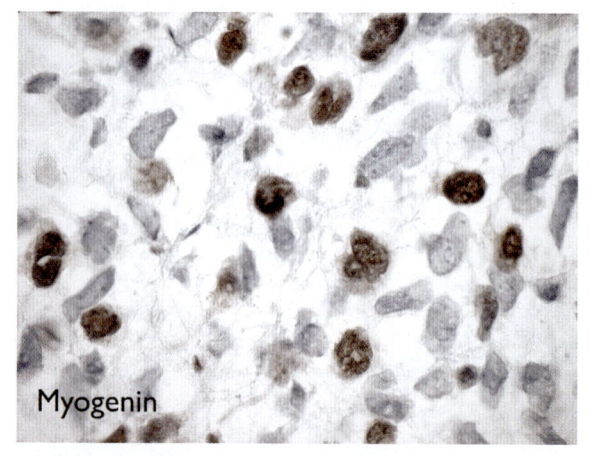

Figure 31.36. Myogenin nuclear stain showing positivity, consistent with a tumor of skeletal muscle differentiation, suggestive of rhabdomyosarcoma. (Myogenin ×200.)

ORBITAL RHABDOMYOSARCOMA: ADVANCED AGGRESSIVE CASES

If not treated soon after its clinical onset, orbital RMS can rapidly progress to an advanced stage. Such advanced cases are not rare in countries with substandard medical care. They often require orbital exenteration as well as chemotherapy and irradiation.

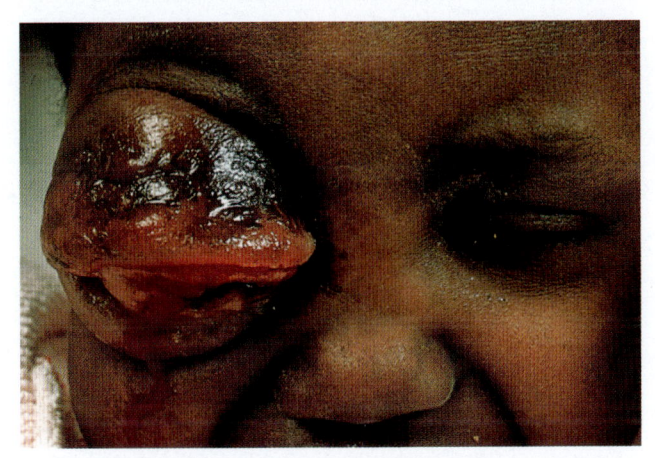

Figure 31.37. Advanced orbital rhabdomyosarcoma in a child from South Africa. (Courtesy of Ellen Ankor, MD.)

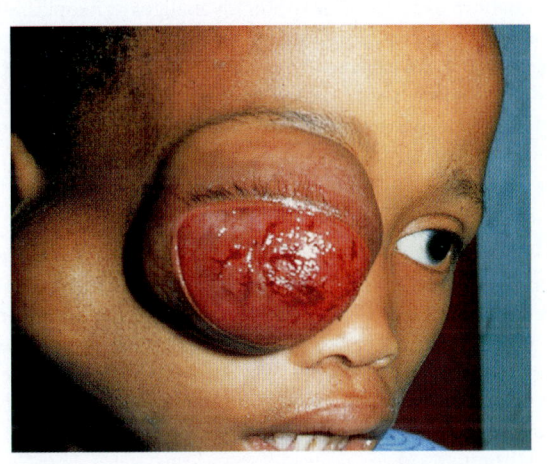

Figure 31.38. Advanced orbital rhabdomyosarcoma with metastasis to preauricular lymph nodes in a child from South Africa. (Courtesy of Ellen Ankor, MD.)

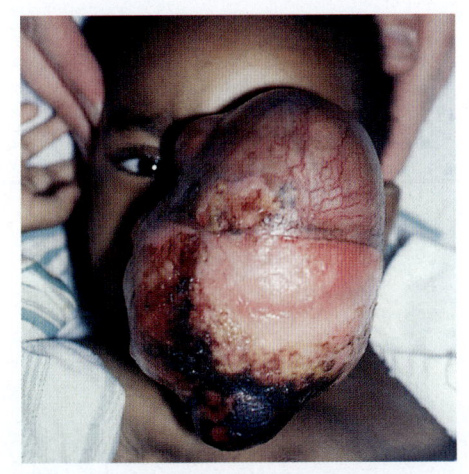

Figure 31.39. Far advanced orbital rhabdomyosarcoma in a child from South Africa. (Courtesy of Eugene Meyer, MD.)

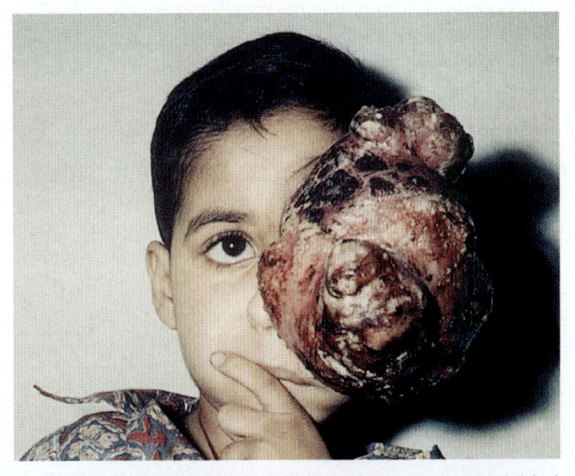

Figure 31.40. Far advanced orbital rhabdomyosarcoma in a child whose parents refused treatment. (Courtesy of Lorenz E. Zimmerman, MD.)

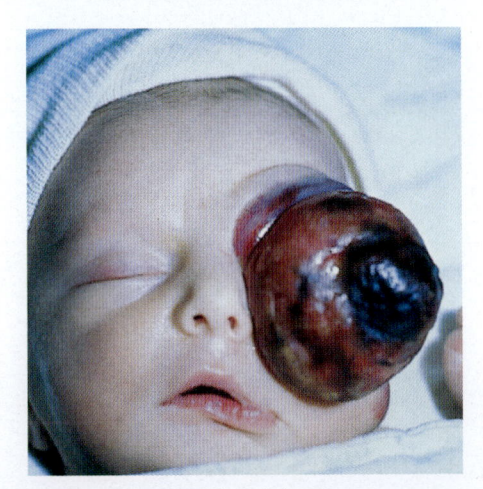

Figure 31.41. Congenital orbital rhabdomyosarcoma present at birth. The child had widespread metastasis at birth and died shortly thereafter. (Courtesy of Nongnard Chan, MD.)

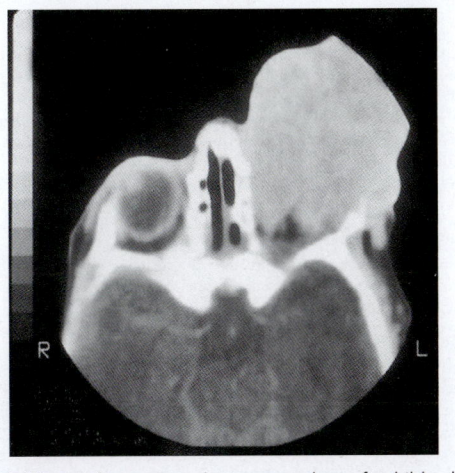

Figure 31.42. Axial computed tomography of child shown in Figure 31.41 demonstrating the extent of the orbital tumor. (Courtesy of Nongnard Chan, MD.)

ORBITAL MALIGNANT RHABDOID TUMOR

General Considerations

Malignant rhabdoid tumor is a highly malignant neoplasm that occurs in the kidney of infants and young children. Although it was originally described as a "rhabdomyosarcomatoid" variant of Wilm tumor, it was subsequently recognized as a distinct entity that can sometimes occur in extrarenal sites including the orbit. Hence the term "extrarenal rhabdoid tumor" has often been used to define this neoplasm (1–11).

Clinical Features

In the orbit, rhabdoid tumors have been diagnosed in both infants and adults (1–11). It generally presents as proptosis and globe displacement. It has been known to produce massive proptosis at birth. The tumor can recur after surgical excision and can invade the sinuses and cranial cavity. It has been described in the orbit after enucleation and irradiation for retinoblastoma (8).

Diagnostic Approaches

Orbital rhabdoid tumor has no specific radiographic features. It is initially a circumscribed neoplasm, but it can become rapidly infiltrative and invade bone (9).

Pathology

Histopathology reveals a poorly differentiated tumor that superficially resembles RMS. It is composed of pleomorphic epithelial cells with prominent nucleoli and many filamentous cytoplasmic inclusions. The cells usually show positive immunoreactivity for vimentin, cytokeratin, and epithelial membrane antigen and negative immunoreactivity for myoglobin, muscle-specific antigen, desmin, and HMB-45.

Management

The treatment is surgical excision, chemotherapy, and radiotherapy, similar to treatment for RMS (4). The prognosis is generally considered very poor.

Selected References

1. Shields JA, Shields CL, Scartozzi R. Survey of 1264 patients with orbital tumors and simulating lesions: The 2002 Montgomery Lecture, part 1. *Ophthalmology* 2004;111:997–1008.
2. Shields JA, Bakewell B, Augsburger JJ, et al. Classification and incidence of space-occupying lesions of the orbit. A survey of 645 biopsies. *Arch Ophthalmol* 1984;102:1606–1611.
3. Shields JA, Bakewell B, Augsburger JJ, et al. Space-occupying orbital masses in children: A review of 250 consecutive biopsies. *Ophthalmology* 1986;93:379–384.

Management

4. Watanabe H, Watanabe T, Kaneko M, et al. Treatment of unresectable malignant rhabdoid tumor of the orbit with tandem high-dose chemotherapy and gamma-knife radiosurgery. *Pediatr Blood Cancer* 2006;47:846–850.

Case Reports

5. Rootman J, Damji KF, Dimmick JE. Malignant rhabdoid tumor of the orbit. *Ophthalmology* 1989;96:1650–1654.
6. Johnson LN, Sexton FM, Goldberg SH. Poorly differentiated primary orbital sarcoma (presumed malignant rhabdoid tumor). *Arch Ophthalmol* 1991;105:1275–1278.
7. Niffenegger JH, Jakobiec FA, Shore JW, et al. Adult extrarenal rhabdoid tumor of the lacrimal gland. *Ophthalmology* 1992;99:567–574.
8. Walford N, Defarrai R, Slater RM, et al. Intraorbital rhabdoid tumour following bilateral retinoblastoma. *Histopathology* 1992;20:170–173.
9. Gunduz K, Shields JA, Eagle RC Jr, et al. Malignant rhabdoid tumor of the orbit. *Arch Ophthalmol* 1998;116:243–246.
10. Stidham DB, Burgett RA, Davis MM, et al. Congenital malignant rhabdoid tumor of the orbit. *J AAPOS* 1999;3:318–320.
11. Gottlieb C, Nijhawan N, Chorneyko K, et al. Congenital orbital and disseminated extrarenal malignant rhabdoid tumor. *Ophthal Plast Reconstr Surg* 2005;21:76–79.

ORBITAL MALIGNANT RHABDOID TUMOR

In young children, malignant rhabdoid tumor can be highly aggressive with recurrence and extension into the central nervous system. A clinicopathologic correlation is shown.

Gunduz K, Shields JA, Eagle RC Jr, et al. Malignant rhabdoid tumor of the orbit. *Arch Ophthalmol* 1998;116:243–246.

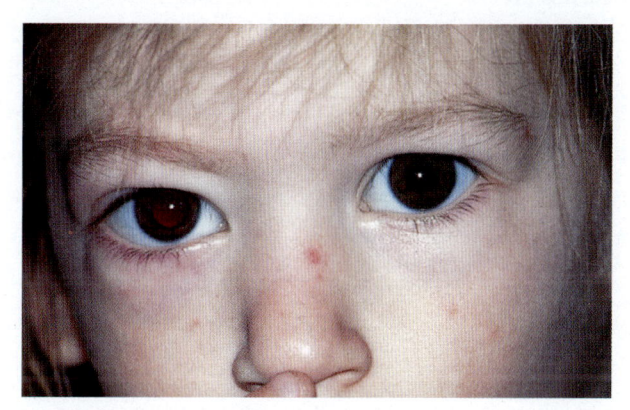

Figure 31.43. Proptosis of the right eye in a 36-month-old girl. The dilated, fixed pupil did not react to light.

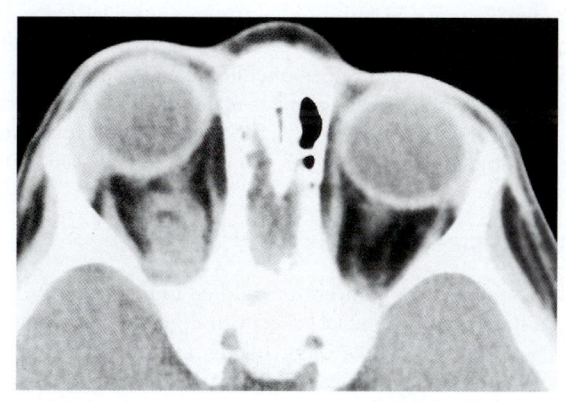

Figure 31.44. Axial computed tomography showing ovoid mass in muscle cone extending to the orbital apex. Piecemeal excisional biopsy revealed features of rhabdoid tumor and the child was treated with chemotherapy (vincristine and actinomycin D) and radiotherapy (5,000 cGy).

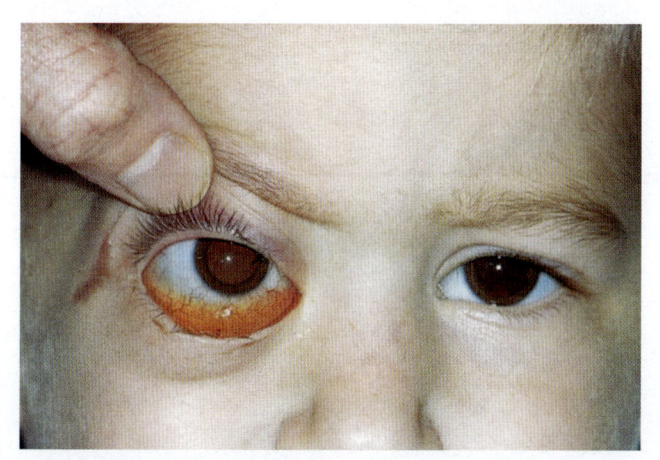

Figure 31.45. About 8 months later the child presented with recurrent proptosis and conjunctival chemosis.

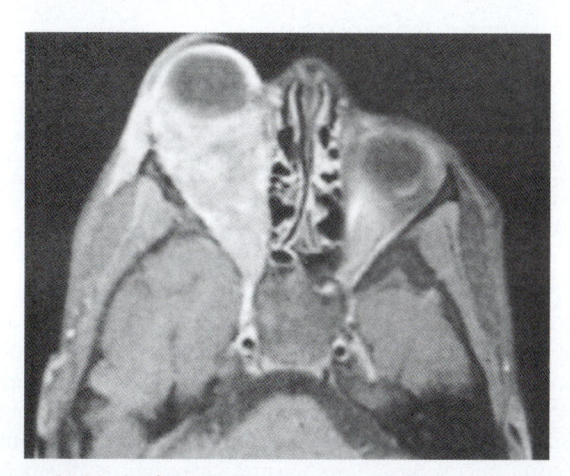

Figure 31.46. Axial magnetic resonance imaging in T1-weighted image, showing massive orbital recurrence. Orbital exenteration was performed followed by irradiation and chemotherapy. A few months later, the tumor recurred in the orbit maxillary sinus and brain and the child died shortly thereafter.

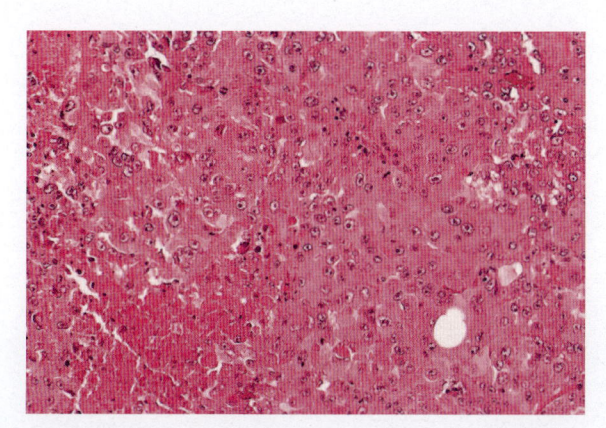

Figure 31.47. Photomicrograph showing sheets of malignant tumor cells. (Hematoxylin–eosin ×50.)

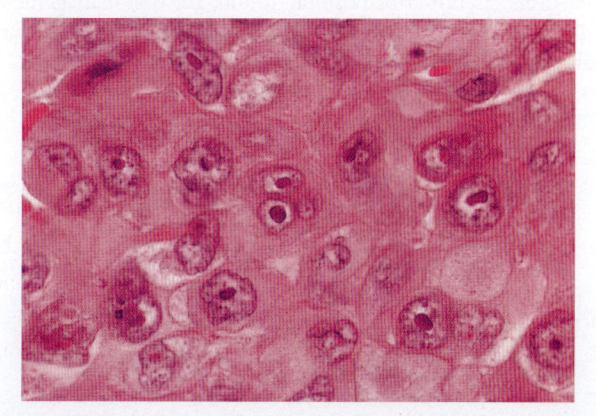

Figure 31.48. Histopathology showing large anaplastic epithelioid cells. (Hematoxylin–eosin ×250.) Immunohistochemistry and electron microscopy supported the diagnosis of extrarenal rhabdoid tumor. The child eventually developed metastasis that proved to be fatal.

ORBITAL LEIOMYOMA

General Considerations

Smooth muscle tumors in the orbit can be benign (leiomyoma) or malignant (leiomyosarcoma) (1–19). They are most common in the genitourinary and gastrointestinal tract, less frequent in the skin, and relatively rare in deep soft tissue. Leiomyoma appears to be a tumor of children and young adults. It occasionally develops in the ocular region, including the orbit (1–19) and even in the uveal tract (5). No orbital leiomyomas were identified in the series of 1,264 orbital lesions seen by the authors (1).

Clinical Features

Orbital leiomyoma can occur in children in the first decade of life, or it can have its clinical onset in adulthood. It can produce symptoms and signs like other benign circumscribed orbital tumors, with slowly progressive proptosis, globe displacement, diplopia, and sometimes blurred vision. It is generally located in the extraconal space and has been seen at the orbital apex. Intracranial extension can occur in advanced or recurrent cases.

Diagnostic Approaches

The diagnosis of orbital leiomyoma is usually made histopathologically after biopsy or surgical excision. Imaging studies generally show a well-circumscribed round to ovoid mass. It usually occurs in the extraconal space, although it can develop anywhere in the orbit. More advanced tumors can breach the capsule and assume a more diffuse pattern.

Pathology

Leiomyoma is composed of well-differentiated spindle cells and may be difficult to differentiate from other spindle cell tumors like schwannoma and solitary fibrous tumor (4). The diagnosis can be confirmed with immunohistochemistry, which shows positivity for smooth muscle antigen, vimentin, and desmin. Electron microscopy shows features characteristic of smooth muscle cells (7).

Management

Like other circumscribed orbital tumors, the best management is complete surgical excision of the mass when possible. Recurrence is well known after incomplete excision.

Selected References

Reviews

1. Shields JA, Shields CL, Scartozzi R. Survey of 1264 patients with orbital tumors and simulating lesions: The 2002 Montgomery Lecture, part 1. *Ophthalmology* 2004;111:997–1008.
2. Shields JA, Bakewell B, Augsburger JJ, et al. Classification and incidence of space-occupying lesions of the orbit. A survey of 645 biopsies. *Arch Ophthalmol* 1984;102:1606–1611.
3. Shields JA, Bakewell B, Augsburger JJ, et al. Space-occupying orbital masses in children: A review of 250 consecutive biopsies. *Ophthalmology* 1986;93:379–384.
4. Jakobiec FA, Howard GM, Rosen M, et al. Leiomyoma and leiomyosarcoma of the orbit. *Am J Ophthalmol* 1975;80:1028–1042.
5. Shields JA, Shields CL, Eagle RC Jr, et al. Observations on seven cases of intraocular leiomyoma. The 1993 Byron Demorest Lecture. *Arch Ophthalmol* 1994;112:521–528.

Histopathology

6. Arat YO, Font RL, Chaudhry IA, et al. Leiomyoma of the orbit and periocular region: a clinicopathologic study of four cases. *Ophthal Plast Reconstr Surg* 2005;21:16–22.

Case Reports

7. Sanborn GE, Valenzuela RE, Green WR. Leiomyoma of the orbit. *Am J Ophthalmol* 1979;87:371–375.
8. Wojno T, Tenzel RR, Nadju M. Orbital leiomyosarcoma. *Arch Ophthalmol* 1983;101:1566–1568.
9. Betharia SM, Arora R, Kishore K, et al. Leiomyoma of the orbit. *Indian J Ophthalmol* 1991;39:35–37.
10. Jolly SS, Brownstein S, Jordan DR. Leiomyoma of the anterior orbit and eyelid. *Can J Ophthalmol* 1995;30:366–370.
11. Vigstrup J, Glenthoj A. Leiomyoma of the orbit. *Acta Ophthalmol (Copenh)* 1982;60:992–997.
12. Saga T, Takeuchi T, Tagawa Y. Orbital leiomyoma accompanied by orbital pseudotumor. *Jpn J Ophthalmol* 1982;26:175–182.
13. Sanborn GE, Valenzuela RE, Green WR. Leiomyoma of the orbit. *Am J Ophthalmol* 1979;87:371–375.
14. Jakobiec FA, Jones IS, Tannenbaum M. Leiomyoma. An unusual tumour of the orbit. *Br J Ophthalmol* 1973;57:825–831.
15. Henderson JW, Harrison EG Jr. Vascular leiomyoma of the orbit: report of a case. *Trans Am Acad Ophthalmol Otolaryngol* 1970;74:970–974.
16. Gunduz K, Gunalp I, Erden E, et al. Orbital leiomyoma: report of a case and review of the literature. *Surv Ophthalmol* 2004;49:237–242.
17. Kulkarni V, Rajshekhar V, Chandi SM. Orbital apex leiomyoma with intracranial extension. *Surg Neurol* 2000;54:327–330.
18. Badoza D, Weil D, Zarate J. Orbital leiomyoma: a case report. *Ophthal Plast Reconstr Surg* 1999;15:460–462.
19. Kaltreider SA, Destro M, Lemke BN. Leiomyosarcoma of the orbit. A case report and review of the literature. *Ophthal Plast Reconstr Surg* 1987;3:35–41.

ORBITAL LEIOMYOSARCOMA

General Considerations

Leiomyosarcoma is a malignant smooth muscle tumor that accounts for 5% to 10% of soft tissue sarcomas. This malignancy has a tendency to occur in middle-aged or older women, particularly those that develop in the uterus. Leiomyosarcoma usually has a more rapid onset and progression than leiomyoma. Orbital leiomyosarcoma is uncommon but several cases have been reported (1–17). A second variant of orbital leiomyosarcoma occurs after irradiation for retinoblastoma, in which cases it is usually diagnosed in older children or young adults (6–9). It has also been reported to metastasize to the orbit from distant primary leiomyosarcoma (14,15). No orbital leiomyosarcomas were identified in the series of 1,264 orbital lesions seen by the authors (1).

Clinical Features

Orbital leiomyosarcoma can produce symptoms and signs like other benign or malignant circumscribed orbital tumors, with progressive proptosis, globe displacement, diplopia, and sometimes blurred vision. It is generally located in the extraconal space. In children with prior irradiation for retinoblastoma, it can appear in the anterior orbit and subcutaneous tissues. Intracranial extension can develop in advanced or recurrent cases.

Diagnostic Approaches

Orbital imaging studies show no features specific to leiomyosarcoma. It may have similar features to leiomyoma and other well-circumscribed orbital tumors. It usually occurs as a well-defined round to ovoid mass anywhere in the orbit. Fine-needle biopsy has been used to diagnose recurrent orbital leiomyosarcoma (5).

Pathology

Histopathology of leiomyosarcoma reveals spindle-shaped cells woven together with abundant cytoplasm, varying sized nuclei, and obvious atypia (4,7–17). There can be storiform pattern and cell necrosis. The anaplastic spindle cells show positive immunoreactivity to smooth muscle antigen, desmin, and vimentin. The cells of leiomyosarcoma differ from leiomyoma in that they have more nuclear pleomorphism, hyperchromatism, giant cells, and mitotic figures.

Management

The best management of orbital leiomyosarcoma is wide excision with capsule intact if possible. This tumor is relatively insensitive to chemotherapy or radiotherapy, but often these must be employed for tumor control. Orbital exenteration may be required in extensive cases.

Selected References

Reviews

1. Shields JA, Shields CL, Scartozzi R. Survey of 1264 patients with orbital tumors and simulating lesions: The 2002 Montgomery Lecture, part 1. *Ophthalmology* 2004;111:997–1008.
2. Shields JA, Bakewell B, Augsburger JJ, et al. Classification and incidence of space-occupying lesions of the orbit. A survey of 645 biopsies. *Arch Ophthalmol* 1984;102:1606–1611.
3. Shields JA, Bakewell B, Augsburger JJ, et al. Space-occupying orbital masses in children: A review of 250 consecutive biopsies. *Ophthalmology* 1986;93:379–384.
4. Jakobiec FA, Howard GM, Rosen M, et al. Leiomyoma and leiomyosarcoma of the orbit. *Am J Ophthalmol* 1975;80:1028–1042.

Imaging

5. Voros GM, Birchall D, Ressiniotis T, et al. Imaging of metastatic orbital leiomyosarcoma. *Ophthal Plast Reconstr Surg* 2005;21:453–456.

Management

6. Padron-Perez N, Mascaro Zamora F, Gutierrez-Miguelez C. Adjuvant pulse dose rate brachytherapy in a secondary leiomyosarcoma of the orbit. *Can J Ophthalmol* 2013;48:e65–e67.

Histopathology/Cytopathology

7. Das DK, Das J, Kumar D, et al. Leiomyosarcoma of the orbit: diagnosis of its recurrence by fine-needle aspiration cytology. *Diagn Cytopathol* 1992;8:609–613.

Case Reports

8. Klippenstein KA, Wesley RE, Glick AD. Orbital leiomyosarcoma after retinoblastoma. *Ophthalmic Surg Lasers* 1999;30:579–583.
9. Folberg R, Cleasby G, Flanagan JA, et al. Orbital leiomyosarcoma after radiation therapy for bilateral retinoblastoma. *Arch Ophthalmol* 1983;101:1562–1565.
10. Font RL, Jurco S 3rd, Brechner RJ. Postradiation leiomyosarcoma of the orbit complicating bilateral retinoblastoma. *Arch Ophthalmol* 1983;101:1557–1561.
11. Mihara F, Gupta KL, Kartchner ZA, et al. Leiomyosarcoma after retinoblastoma radiotherapy. *Radiat Med* 1991;9:183–184.
12. Meekins BB, Dutton JJ, Proia AD. Primary orbital leiomyosarcoma. A case report and review of the literature. *Arch Ophthalmol* 1988;106:82–86.
13. Wojno T, Tenzel RR, Nadji M. Orbital leiomyosarcoma. *Arch Ophthalmol* 1983;101:1566–1568.
14. Hou LC, Murphy MA, Tung GA. Primary orbital leiomyosarcoma: a case report with MRI findings. *Am J Ophthalmol* 2003;135:408–410.
15. Jakobiec FA, Mitchell JP, Chauhan PM, et al. Mesectodermal leiomyosarcoma of the antrum and orbit. *Am J Ophthalmol* 1978;85:51–57.
16. Kaltreider SA, Destro M, Lemke BN. Leiomyoma of the orbit. A case report and review of the literature. *Ophthal Plast Reconstr Surg* 1987;3:35–41.
17. Bakri SJ, Krohel GB, Peters GB, et al. Spermatic cord leiomyosarcoma metastatic to the orbit. *Am J Ophthalmol* 2003;136:213–215.

ORBITAL LEIOMYOMA AND LEIOMYOSARCOMA

1. Gunduz K, Gunalp I, Erden E, et al. Orbital leiomyoma: report of a case and review of the literature. *Surv Ophthalmol* 2004;49:237–242.
2. Meekins BB, Dutton JJ, Proia AD. Primary orbital leiomyosarcoma. A case report and review of the literature. *Arch Ophthalmol* 1988;106:82–86.

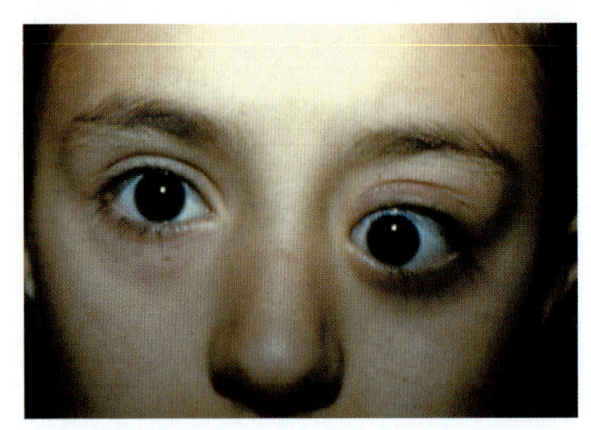

Figure 31.49. Orbital leiomyoma. Proptosis and downward and nasal displacement of the left eye in a 10-year-old girl. It had been slowly progressive for 1 year. (Courtesy of Kaan Gunduz, MD.)

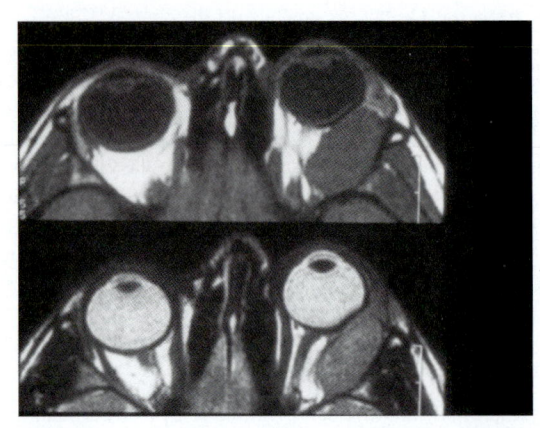

Figure 31.50. Axial magnetic resonance imaging in T1-weighted (*above*) and T2-weighted (*below*) image. The tumor was isointense to the extraocular muscle and cerebral gray matter on T1-weighted images and minimally hyperintense on T2-weighted images. The tumor was totally excised in piecemeal fashion. (Courtesy of Kaan Gunduz, MD.)

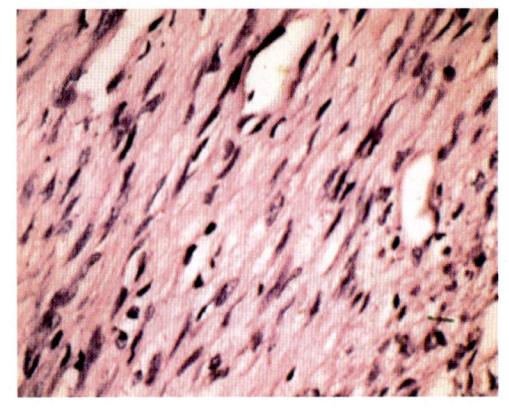

Figure 31.51. Histopathology of lesion shown in Figures 31.49 and 31.50 demonstrating benign spindle cells in a fibrous stroma and dilated sinusoidal capillaries. (Hematoxylin–eosin ×150.) Immunohistochemically, the tumor stained positive with smooth muscle actin, desmin, and vimentin. (Courtesy of Kaan Gunduz, MD.)

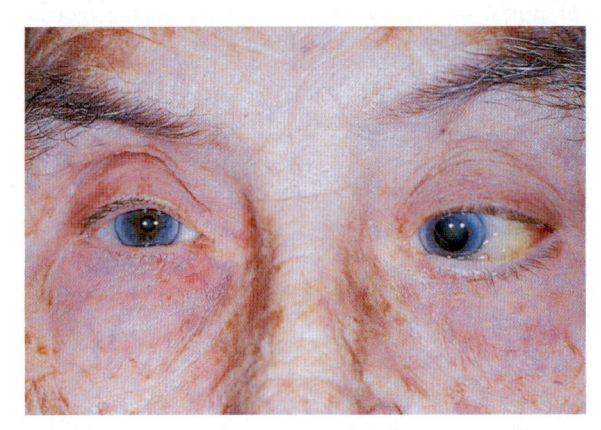

Figure 31.52. Leiomyosarcoma. Proptosis and adduction of the left eye in an 82-year-old woman. (Courtesy of Alan Proia, MD.)

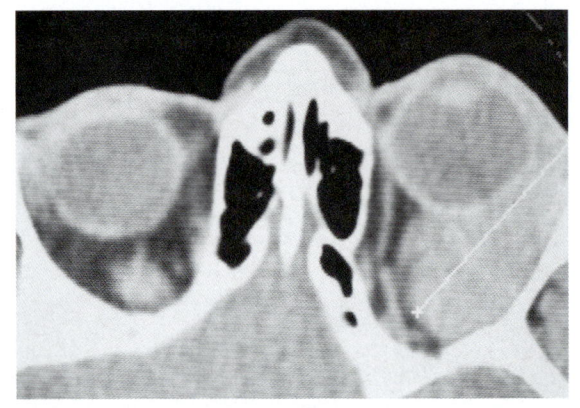

Figure 31.53. Axial computed tomography of patient shown in Figure 31.52, revealing a large mass in retrobulbar space and temporal aspect of orbit. (Courtesy of Alan Proia, MD.)

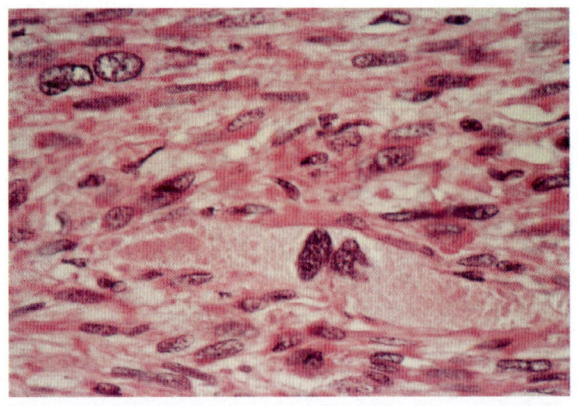

Figure 31.54. Histopathology of lesion shown in Figure 31.53, demonstrating malignant spindle cells. Electron microscopy confirmed the smooth muscle origin of the cells. (Hematoxylin–eosin ×150.) (Courtesy of Alan Proia, MD.)

ORBITAL FIBROUS CONNECTIVE TISSUE TUMORS

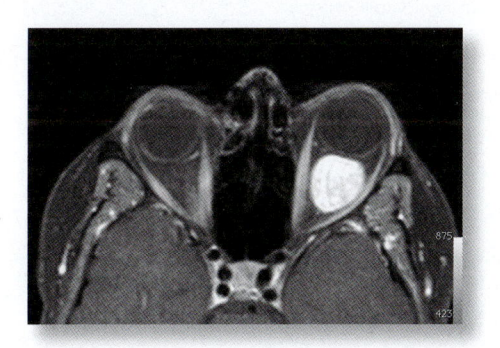

Orbital Nodular Fasciitis

General Considerations
Nodular fasciitis is a benign nodular proliferation of connective tissue that usually involves superficial fascia (1–20). Konwaler et al. originally called it "subcutaneous pseudosarcomatous fibromatosis" (8). It is now recognized to be more common. Its occurrence in the orbital area was elucidated by Font and Zimmerman in 1966 (3) and subsequent reports have expanded on its ophthalmic manifestations (4–20). In the authors' series of 1,264 orbital lesions, there were two cases, accounting for 15% of all fibrocytic lesions and for <1% of all orbital masses (1). It may be more common than indicated in that report because some cases can be misdiagnosed histopathologically as other spindle cell lesions.

Clinical Features
Nodular fasciitis usually occurs in children and has a rather rapid onset and progression. It tends to occur in anterior periocular structures where it is visible or palpable and has rarely been observed in the deep orbit. This tumor can simulate a dermoid cyst clinically (10). In an analysis of 15 children with nodular fasciitis of the head and neck region, the median age at diagnosis was 9 years, all developed an enlarging soft tissue mass, with occasional pain ($n = 2$) (4). Surgical excision was curative in all cases, with no recurrence.

Diagnostic Approaches
The diagnosis of nodular fasciitis can be suspected on the basis of clinical findings and the rapidity of onset, but the diagnosis is confirmed on histopathology after surgical excision. With imaging studies, this tumor shows features typical of other solid masses and has no distinctive findings.

Pathology
The histopathologic diagnosis of nodular fasciitis can be challenging, because it can simulate rhabdomyosarcoma or other soft tissue sarcomas (3,4,6,7). However, pathologists experienced with soft tissue tumors usually can make the diagnosis based on characteristic light microscopic features. Mitotically active stellate or spindle-shaped fibroblasts are often arranged in parallel bundles and extend in all directions, resembling cells in a tissue culture. Numerous newly formed parallel capillaries often ramify through the lesion, forming slitlike spaces reminiscent of those seen in Kaposi sarcoma. With immunohistochemistry, nodular fasciitis shows positive reactions against smooth muscle actin (SMA) and vimentin. With electron microscopy, one sees parallel bundles of actinlike filaments with fusiform densities (6).

Management
Nodular fasciitis is usually well circumscribed and located in the anterior adnexal structures, thus we recommend complete surgical removal when possible. Local recurrence is rare after complete excision (4).

ORBITAL NODULAR FASCIITIS AND FIBROMA

Selected References

Reviews

1. Shields JA, Shields CL, Scartozzi R. Survey of 1264 patients with orbital tumors and simulating lesions: the 2002 Montgomery Lecture, part 1. *Ophthalmology* 2004;111: 997–1008.
2. Shields JA, Bakewell B, Augsburger JJ, et al. Classification and incidence of space-occupying lesions of the orbit. A survey of 645 biopsies. *Arch Ophthalmol* 1984;102: 1606–1611.
3. Font RL, Zimmerman LE. Nodular fasciitis of the eye and adnexa. A report of ten cases. *Arch Ophthalmol* 1966;75:475–481.
4. Hseu A, Watters K, Perez-Atayde A, et al. Pediatric nodular fasciitis in the head and neck: Evaluation and management. *JAMA Otolaryngol Hean Neck Surg* 2015;141(1): 54–59.

Management

5. Graham BS, Barrett TL, Goltz RW. Nodular fasciitis: response to intralesional corticosteroids. *J Am Acad Dermatol* 1999;40:490–492.

Histopathology/Cytopathology

6. Sakamoto T, Ishibashi T, Ohnishi Y, et al. Immunohistologic and electron microscopical study of nodular fasciitis of the orbit. *Br J Ophthalmol* 1991;75:636–638.
7. Kew YT, Cuesta RA. Nodular fasciitis of the orbit diagnosed by fine needle aspiration cytology. A case report. *Acta Cytologica* 1993;37:957–960.

Case Reports

8. Konwaler BE, Keasbey L, Kaplan L. Subcutaneous pseudosarcomatous fibromatosis (fasciitis). *Am J Clin Pathol* 1955;25:241–252.
9. Perry RH, Ramani PS, McAllister SR, et al. Nodular fasciitis causing unilateral proptosis. *Br J Ophthalmol* 1975;59:404–408.
10. Shields JA, Shields CL, Christian C, et al. Orbital nodular fasciitis simulating a dermoid cyst in an 8-month-old child. Case report and review of the literature. *Ophthal Plast Reconstr Surg* 2001;17:144–148.
11. Levitt JM, deVeer A, Oguzhan C. Orbital nodular fasciitis. *Arch Ophthalmol* 1969;81:235–237.
12. Reccia FM, Buckley EG, Townshend LM, et al. Nodular fasciitis of the orbital rim in a pediatric patient. *J Pediatr Ophthalmol Strabismus* 1997;34:316–318.
13. Hymas D, Mamalis N, Pratt DV, et al. Nodular fasciitis of the lower eyelid in a pediatric patient. *Ophthal Plast Reconstr Surg* 1999;15:139–142.
14. Tolls RE, Mohr S, Spencer WH. Benign nodular fasciitis originating in Tenon's capsule. *Arch Ophthalmol* 1966;75:482–483.
15. Meacham CT. Pseudosarcomatous fasciitis. *Am J Ophthalmol* 1974;77:747–749.
16. Ferry AP, Sherman SE. Nodular fasciitis of the conjunctiva apparently originating in the fascia bulbi (Tenon's capsule). *Am J Ophthalmol* 1974;78:514–517.
17. Holds FB, Mamalis N, Anderson RL. Nodular fasciitis presenting as rapidly enlarging episcleral mass in a 3-year-old. *J Pediatr Ophthalmol Strabismus* 1990;27:157–160.
18. Vestal KP, Bauer TW, Berlin AJ. Nodular fasciitis presenting as an eyelid mass. *Ophthalmol Plast Reconstr Surg* 1990;6:130–132.
19. Gupta D, Tailor TD, Keene CD, et al. A case of nodular fasciitis causing compressive optic neuropathy. *Ophthal Plast Reconstr Surg* 2014;30(2):e47–e49.
20. Riffle JE, Prosser AH, Lee JR, et al. Nodular fasciitis of the orbit: a case report and brief review of the literature. *Case Rep Ophthalmol Med* 2011;2011:235956.

ID## ORBITAL NODULAR FASCIITIS AND FIBROMA

Orbital Fibroma

General Considerations
Among the benign fibrous proliferations, fibroma is a difficult lesion to categorize (1–17). In the literature, it appears that some reported cases of orbital fibroma, as well as fibrous histiocytoma, would be reclassified today as solitary fibrous tumor (SFT), based on more recent use of immunohistochemistry. Nevertheless, we have chosen for now to discuss fibroma and SFT separately because they are sometimes difficult to precisely classify.

Clinical Features
Orbital fibroma is a benign neoplasm or possibly a reactive process that can arise from Tenon's fascia or its precursors (3–12). Fibroma in the orbital area usually appears as a palpable firm mass in the anterior orbit that produces proptosis or globe displacement. It can extend anteriorly into the conjunctiva and appear as an irregular, yellow-white mass.

Diagnostic Approaches
There is little specific information on the diagnosis of orbital fibroma. Clinically and with imaging studies, it appears as a solid, anterior, yellow-white mass with irregular borders (5). The diagnosis is rarely suspected clinically and is generally made on histopathology following biopsy or complete removal.

Pathology
Fibroma is composed of a paucicellular population of fibroblasts that are widely separated by abundant collagen. The long, graceful fascicles typical of fibroma and other pure fibroblastic tumors appear different on light microscopy from the twisting storiform pattern of the cells of fibrous histiocytoma. The absence of foci of inflammation is helpful in differentiating fibroma from sclerosing idiopathic orbital inflammation, in which inflammatory cells are detected despite large areas of fibrosis.

Management
The diagnosis of orbital fibroma is not usually made clinically, similar to most primary circumscribed orbital soft tissue tumors. The best management is complete surgical removal. Incomplete surgical removal can lead to recurrence. The approach to surgery is determined by the size and location of the tumor on orbital computed tomography (CT) or magnetic resonance imaging (MRI). Orbital fibromas are probably not radiosensitive, although it might be reasonable to consider radiotherapy in recurrent or unresectable cases with documented progression and complications.

Selected References

Reviews
1. Shields JA, Shields CL, Scartozzi R. Survey of 1264 patients with orbital tumors and simulating lesions: The 2002 Montgomery Lecture, part 1. *Ophthalmology* 2004;111:997–1008.
2. Shields JA, Bakewell B, Augsburger JJ, et al. Classification and incidence of space-occupying lesions of the orbit. A survey of 645 biopsies. *Arch Ophthalmol* 1984;102: 1606–1611.
3. Shields JA, Bakewell B, Augsburger JJ, et al. Space-occupying orbital masses in children: A review of 250 consecutive biopsies. *Ophthalmology* 1986;93:379–384.
4. Prabhu S, Sharanya S, Naik PM, et al. Fibro-osseous lesions of the oral and maxillofacial region: Retrospective analysis for 20 years. *J Oral Maxillofac Pathol* 2013;17: 36–40.

Imaging
5. Hourani R, Taslakian B, Shabb NS, et al. Fibroblastic and myofibroblastic tumors of the head and neck: Comprehensive imaging-based review with pathologic correlation. *Eur J Radiol* 2015;84(2):250–260.

Case Reports
6. Fowler JG, Terplan KL. Fibroma of the orbit. *Arch Ophthalmol* 1942;28:263–271.
7. Case TD, La Piana FG. Benign fibrous tumor of the orbit. *Ann Ophthalmol* 1975;7:813–815.
8. Mortada AK. Fibroma of the orbit. *Br J Ophthalmol* 1971;55:350–352.
9. Stokes WH, Bowers WF. Pure fibroma of the orbit. Report of a case and review of the literature. *Arch Ophthalmol* 1934;11:279–282.
10. Howcroft MJ, Hurwitz JJ. Lacrimal sac fibroma. *Can J Ophthalmol* 1980;15: 196–197.
11. Herschorn BJ, Jakobiec FA, Hornblass A, et al. Epibulbar subconjunctival fibroma. A tumor possibly arising from Tenon's capsule. *Ophthalmology* 1983;90:1490–1494.
12. Ditta LC, Qayyum S, O'Brien TF, et al. Chondromyxoid fibroma of the orbit. *Ophthal Plast Reconstr Surg* 2012;28(5):e105–e106.
13. Ahn M, Osipov V, Harris GJ. Collagenous fibroma (desmoplastic fibroblastoma) of the lacrimal gland. *Ophthal Plast Reconstr Surg* 2009;25(3):250–252.
14. Hartstein ME, Thomas SM, Ellis LS. Orbital desmoid tumor in a pediatric patient. *Ophthal Plast Reconstr Surg* 2006;22(2):139–141.
15. Sigler SC, Wobig JL, Dierks EJ, et al. Cementifying fibroma presenting as proptosis. *Ophthal Plast Reconstr Surg* 1997;13(4):277–280.
16. Schutz JS, Rabkin MD, Schutz S. Fibromatous tumor (desmoid type) of the orbit. *Arch Ophthalmol* 1979;97(4):703–704.
17. Stacy RC, Jakobiec FA, Fay A. Collagenous fibroma (desmoplastic fibroblastoma) of the orbital rim. *Ophthal Plast Reconstr Surg* 2013;29(4):e101–e104.

ORBITAL NODULAR FASCIITIS

Orbital nodular fasciitis usually occurs in young children as a subcutaneous mass. It can sometimes simulate a dermoid cyst.

Shields JA, Shields CL, Christian C, et al. Orbital nodular fasciitis simulating a dermoid cyst in an 8-month-old child. Case report and review of the literature. *Ophthal Plast Reconstr Surg* 2001;17:144–148.

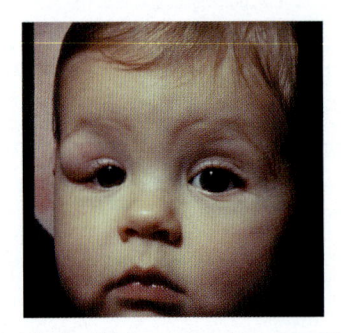

Figure 32.1. Nodular fasciitis in a young boy presenting as a subcutaneous mass beneath lateral aspect of right upper eyelid, resembling a dermoid cyst.

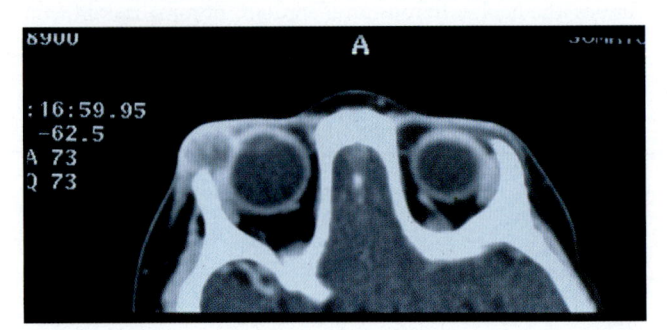

Figure 32.2. Axial computed tomography showing a round mass near superotemporal orbital rim.

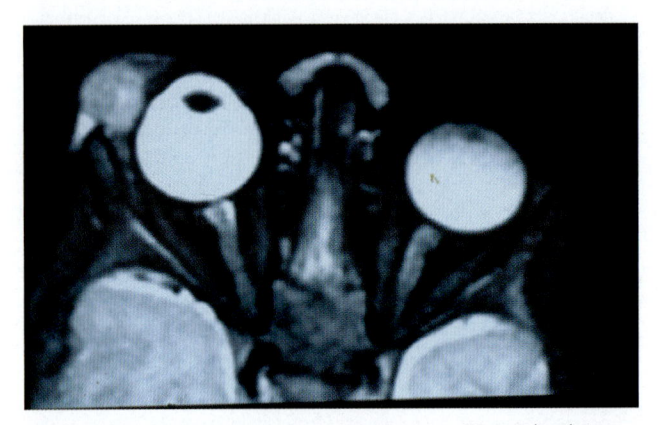

Figure 32.3. Magnetic resonance imaging on T2-weighted image showing the mass with solid internal appearance. It is slightly hyperintense to vitreous on T2.

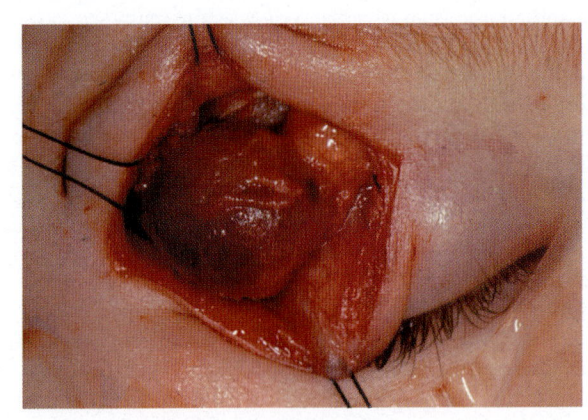

Figure 32.4. Appearance of reddish firm mass exposed at time of surgery by a superotemporal eyelid crease approach.

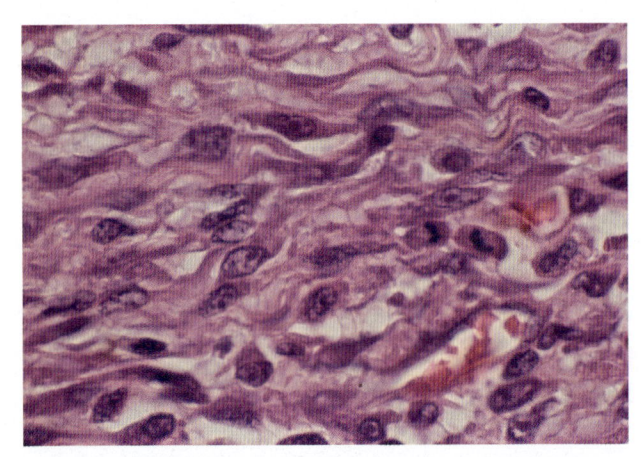

Figure 32.5. Photomicrograph of same lesion showing spindle cells with prominent nucleoli. A mitotic figure is present to the right. On initial diagnostic frozen sections, rhabdomyosarcoma or other malignant spindle cell tumor could not be excluded. However, permanent sections were interpreted as nodular fasciitis by expert soft tissue pathologists. (Hematoxylin–eosin ×200.)

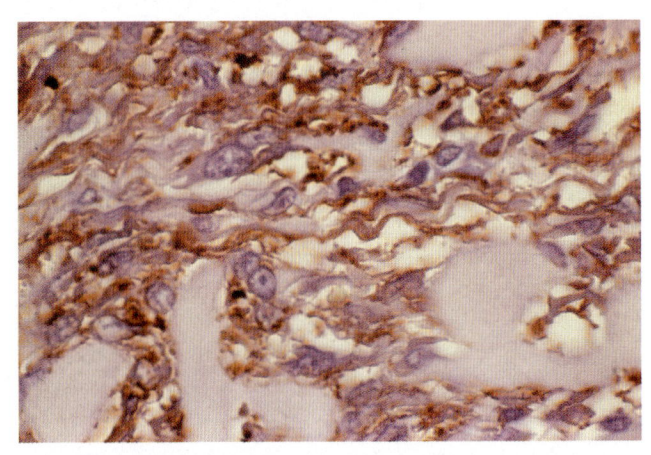

Figure 32.6. Immunohistochemistry shows positive reaction to vimentin. Immunohistochemistry also showed positive reaction for smooth muscle actin. These results supported the diagnosis of nodular fasciitis. (×200.)

Chapter 32 Orbital Fibrous Connective Tissue Tumors

● ORBITAL NODULAR FASCIITIS AND FIBROMA

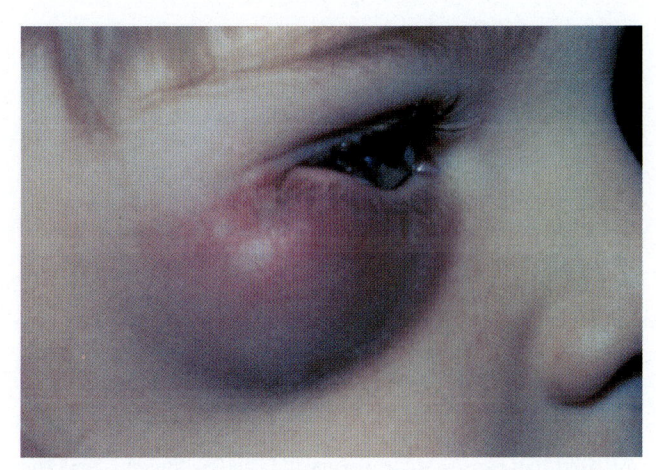

Figure 32.7. Orbital nodular fasciitis presenting as a subcutaneous mass behind lower eyelid in a 2-year-old girl. (Courtesy of Mark Ost, MD.)

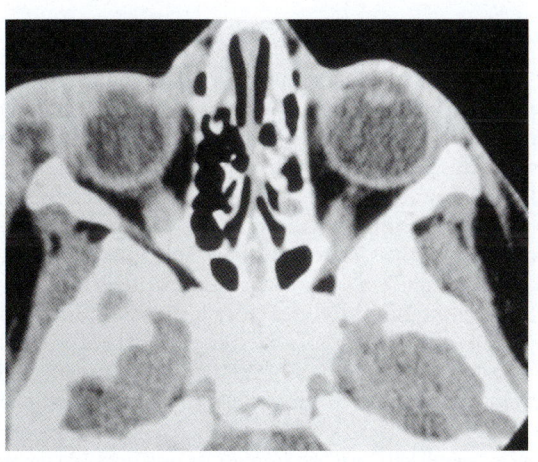

Figure 32.8. Axial computed tomography of the patient shown in Figure 32.7, demonstrating the tumor in the inferotemporal aspect of the orbit and subcutaneous tissue. (Courtesy of Mark Ost, MD.)

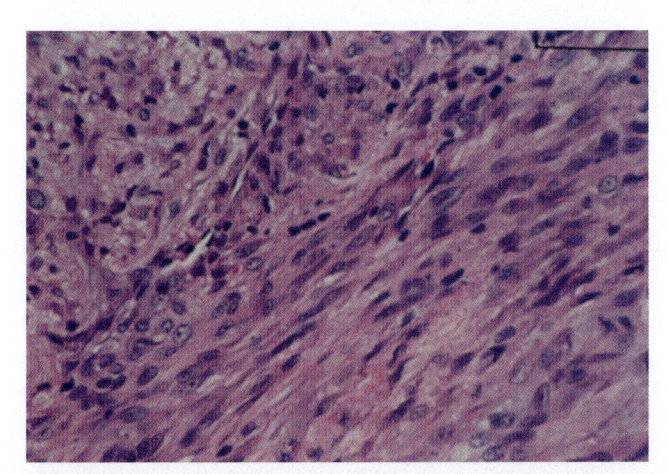

Figure 32.9. Histopathology of nodular fasciitis demonstrating sheets of proliferating fibroblasts and chronic inflammatory cells. (Hematoxylin–eosin ×150.)

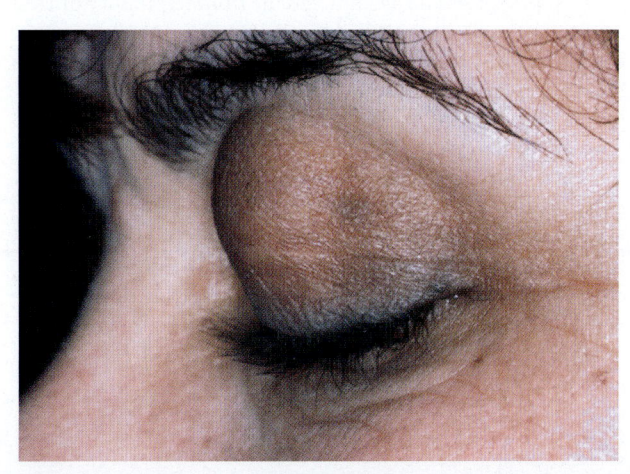

Figure 32.10. Fibroma of superior orbit and subcutaneous tissue in a 49-year-old woman. It was noticed 1 year earlier and had not shown appreciable change. (Courtesy of Mourad Khalil, MD.)

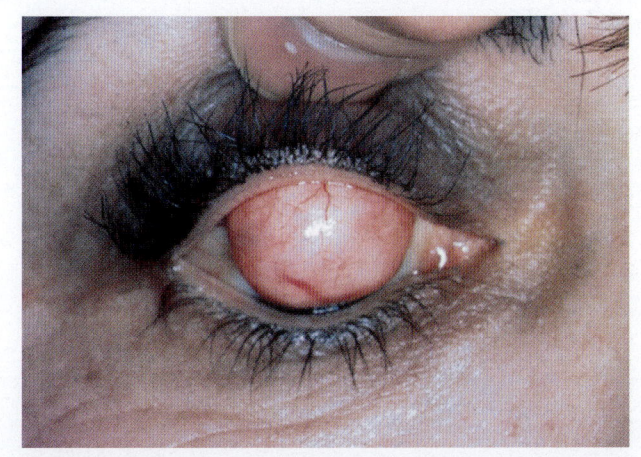

Figure 32.11. Same lesion shown in Figure 32.10 with eyelid elevated. Note the smooth, circumscribed appearance of the lesion. (Courtesy of Mourad Khalil, MD.)

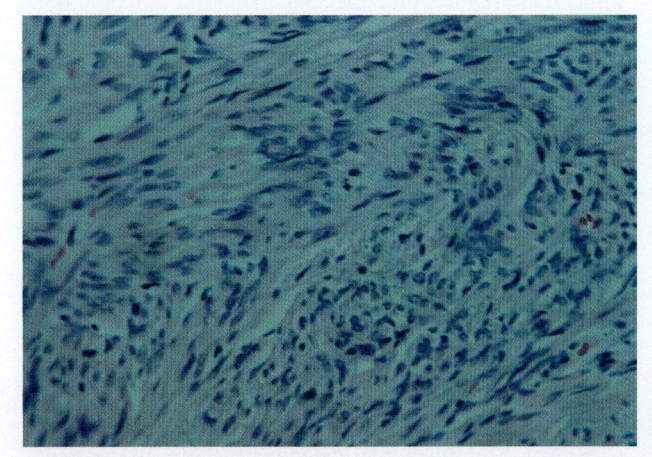

Figure 32.12. Histopathology of lesion shown in Figure 32.11, demonstrating closely packed fibrocytes consistent with fibroma. (Hematoxylin–eosin ×150.) (Courtesy of Mourad Khalil, MD.)

ORBITAL FIBROMATOSIS, MYOFIBROMATOSIS, AND MYOFIBROMA

General Considerations

The fibromatoses (myofibromatoses) are nonencapsulated, nonmetastasizing fibrous tumors that have several clinical variations (1–18). The terminology regarding these entities is confusing because they overlap clinically and histopathologically. Evidence of smooth muscle elements in some lesions is justification for the term "myofibromatosis," and we use the terms interchangeably herein because they are closely related. The fibromatoses appear to represent intermediate lesions between the localized fibromas and the more malignant fibrosarcomas. They can occur at any age and can be a part of generalized fibromatosis or they can be solitary (myofibroma). Orbital involvement has received increasing attention in the literature (6,8–18).

The generalized form (fibromatosis and myofibromatosis) is often present at or shortly after birth as multiple nodules in the dermis, muscle, viscera, and bone. Affected children have a guarded prognosis and as some can die from respiratory distress or diarrhea soon after birth. However, some of the lesions can regress spontaneously. Orbital involvement is uncommon. In the authors' series of 1,264 orbital lesions, only 2 were myofibroma, representing <1% of all lesions and 15% of those 13 cases in the fibrocytic category (1).

The solitary form (myofibroma) appears to be more common in the orbit. The term "infantile myofibroma" is being used more often. There are increasing numbers of such lesions being recognized in the orbital and eyelid region of infants, either in soft tissue or in orbital bones or periosteum (8–18). Myofibroma appears to have an excellent prognosis with a tendency to be self-limited and to remain stable or even regress after incisional biopsy.

Clinical Features

The clinical features of orbital fibromatosis vary with whether the lesion is generalized or localized (6). The most common presentation is a solitary orbital or subcutaneous mass (myofibroma) that produces proptosis and other symptoms and signs of a solitary orbital tumor.

In an analysis of 24 reports in the English literature on orbital myofibroma (1960 to 2011), the mean age at presentation was 35 months with 14 males and 10 females (6). Findings were presented for a mean of 3 months before clinical presentation. The mass involved bone ($n = 17$) or soft tissues ($n = 7$) and reached a mean size of 3 cm. All tumors were well circumscribed.

Diagnostic Approaches

This uncommon diagnosis is rarely suspected clinically. With orbital CTCT and MRI, the lesion appears as a round or irregular soft tissue mass or intraosseous mass with adjacent soft tissue involvement. This tumor can be well circumscribed or irregular. The differential diagnosis includes fibro-osseous lesions, Langerhan's cell histiocytosis, metastatic neuroblastoma, and other bone destructive orbital lesions in children.

Pathology

Microscopically, myofibroblastic tumors are composed of spindle shaped to plump fibroblasts arranged in interlacing fascicles and embedded in a collagenous background matrix (desmoid appearance). There is generally no nuclear atypism or mitotic figures. In one review of 24 published reports, the histopathology features included biphasic, whorled nodular areas of fusiform cells with extracellular collagen (6). That analysis revealed no cases of necrosis but mitoses were seen. Those with immunohistochemistry demonstrated positive reactivity with SMA and vimentin and negative reactivity with muscle specific actin, desmin, myogenin, S100, GFAP, and others (6).

Myofibroma is quite similar to other spindle cell tumors, including infantile hemangiopericytoma, SFT, leiomyoma, and nodular fasciitis. Ultrastructural studies suggest that the predominant cells are fibroblasts and myofibroblasts (1). Difficult cases should be diagnosed by experienced soft tissue pathologists.

Management

The best management of suspected orbital myofibromatosis is surgical excision or generous incisional biopsy. After histopathologic confirmation, the patient should be monitored periodically, but recurrence is uncommon. Little is known about the response to corticosteroids, chemotherapy, or irradiation, but these methods should be withheld until absolutely necessary. As mentioned, the solitary orbital form generally has a favorable prognosis, based on published reports (5–18).

ORBITAL FIBROMATOSIS, MYOFIBROMATOSIS, AND MYOFIBROMA

Selected References

Reviews

1. Shields JA, Shields CL, Scartozzi R. Survey of 1264 patients with orbital tumors and simulating lesions: the 2002 Montgomery Lecture, part 1. *Ophthalmology* 2004;111:997–1008.
2. Shields JA, Bakewell B, Augsburger JJ, et al. Classification and incidence of space-occupying lesions of the orbit. A survey of 645 biopsies. *Arch Ophthalmol* 1984;102:1606–1611.
3. Shields JA, Bakewell B, Augsburger JJ, et al. Space-occupying orbital masses in children: A review of 250 consecutive biopsies. *Ophthalmology* 1986;93:379–384.
4. Prabhu S, Sharanya S, Naik PM, et al. Fibro-osseous lesions of the oral and maxillofacial region: Retrospective analysis for 20 years. *J Oral Maxillofac Pathol* 2013;17:36–40.
5. Hidayat AA, Font RL. Juvenile fibromatosis of the periorbital region and eyelid. A clinicopathologic study of six cases. *Arch Ophthalmol* 1980;98:280–285.
6. Mynatt CJ, Feldman KA, Thompson LD. Orbital infantile myofibroma: a case report and clinicopathologic review of 24 cases from the literature. *Head Neck Pathol* 2011;5:205–215.

Imaging

7. Hourani R, Taslakian B, Shabb NS, et al. Fibroblastic and myofibroblastic tumors of the head and neck: comprehensive imaging-based review with pathologic correlation. *Eur J Radiol* 2015;84(2):250–260.

Case Reports

8. el-Sayed Y. Fibromatosis of the head and neck. *J Laryngol Otol* 1992;106:459–462.
9. Inwards CY, Unni KK, Beabout JW, et al. Solitary congenital fibromatosis (infantile myofibromatosis) of bone. *Am J Surg Pathol* 1991;15:935–941.
10. Shields CL, Husson M, Shields JA, et al. Solitary intraosseous infantile myofibroma of the orbital roof. *Arch Ophthalmol* 1998;116:1528–1530.
11. Westfall AC, Mansoor A, Sullivan SA, et al. Orbital and periorbital myofibromas in childhood: two case reports. *Ophthalmology* 2003;110:2000–2005.
12. Nasr AM, Blodi FC, Lindahl S, et al. Congenital generalized multicentric myofibromatosis with orbital involvement. *Am J Ophthalmol* 1986;102:779–787.
13. Waltermann JM, Huntrakoon M, Beatty EC Jr, et al. Congenital fibromatosis (myofibromatosis). A rare cause of proptosis at birth. *Ann Ophthalmol* 1988;20:394–399.
14. Fornelli A, Salvi F, Mascalchi M, et al. Orbital (desmoid type) fibromatosis. *Orbit* 1999;18:203–210.
15. Weiner JM, Hidayat AA. Juvenile fibrosarcoma of the orbit and eyelid. A study of five cases. *Arch Ophthalmol* 1983;101:253–259.
16. Campbell RJ, Garrity JA. Juvenile fibromatosis of the orbit: a case report with review of the literature. *Br J Ophthalmol* 1991;75:313–316.
17. Schutz JS, Rabkin MD, Schutz S. Fibromatous tumor (desmoid type) of the orbit. *Arch Ophthalmol* 1979;97:703–704.
18. Rodrigues EB, Shields CL, Marr BP, et al. Solitary intraosseous orbital myofibroma in two cases. *Ophthal Plast Reconstr Surg* 2006;22:292–295.

ORBITAL INFANTILE FIBROMATOSIS

1. Waltermann JM, Huntrakoon M, Beatty EC Jr, et al. Congenital fibromatosis (myofibromatosis). A rare cause of proptosis at birth. *Ann Ophthalmol* 1988;20:394–399.
2. Shields CL, Husson M, Shields JA, et al. Solitary intraosseous infantile myofibroma of the orbital roof. *Arch Ophthalmol* 1998; 116:1528–1530.
3. Rodrigues EB, Shields CL, Marr BP, et al. Solitary intraosseous orbital myofibroma in 4 cases. *Ophthal Plast Reconstr Surg* 2006; 22:292–295.

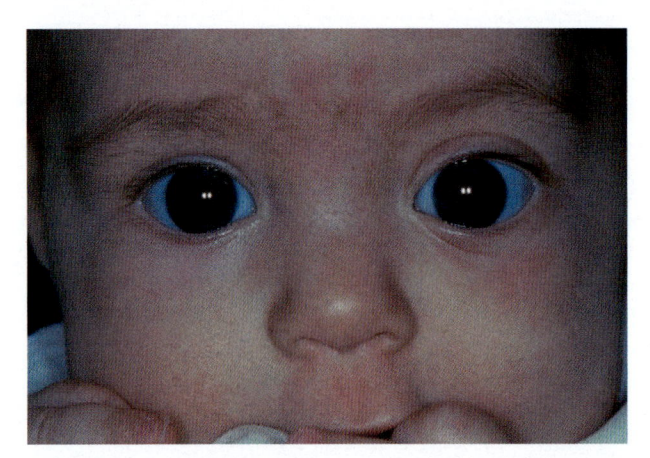

Figure 32.13. Infantile fibromatosis in a 1-month-old girl. Slight proptosis of the left eye that was noted shortly after birth.

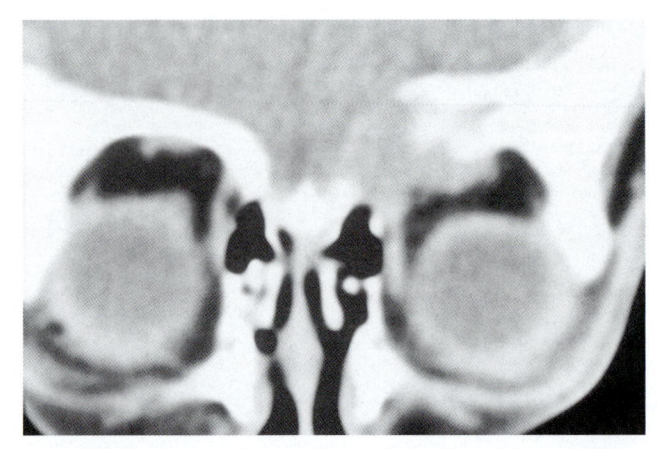

Figure 32.14. Coronal computed tomography of child shown in Figure 32.13, demonstrating a superonasal bone destructive lesion involving the sphenoid bone.

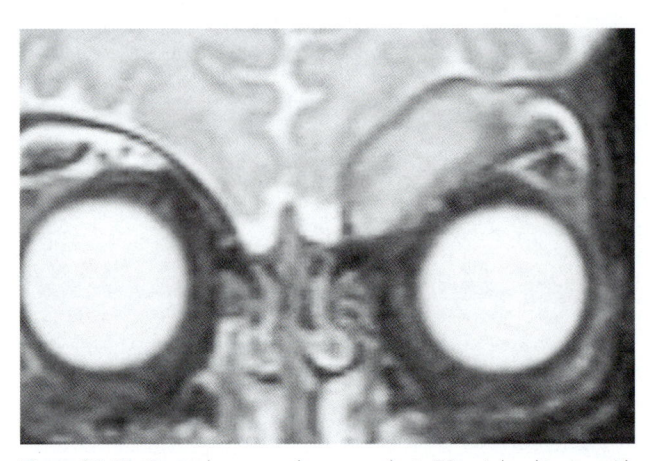

Figure 32.15. Coronal computed tomography in T2-weighted image with gadolinium enhancement, showing the mildly enhancing superonasal mass.

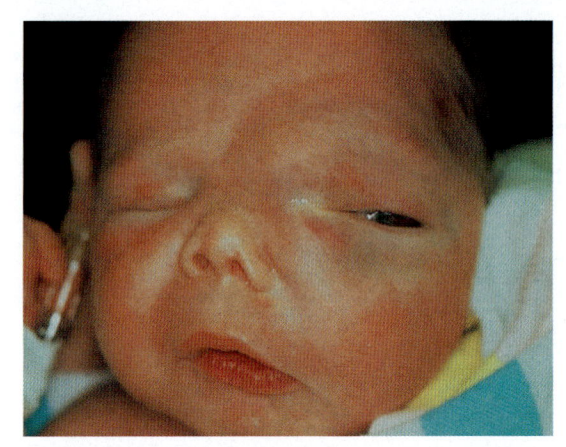

Figure 32.16. Extensive orbital and periorbital fibromatosis in a newborn boy. (Courtesy of Gerhard Cibis, MD.)

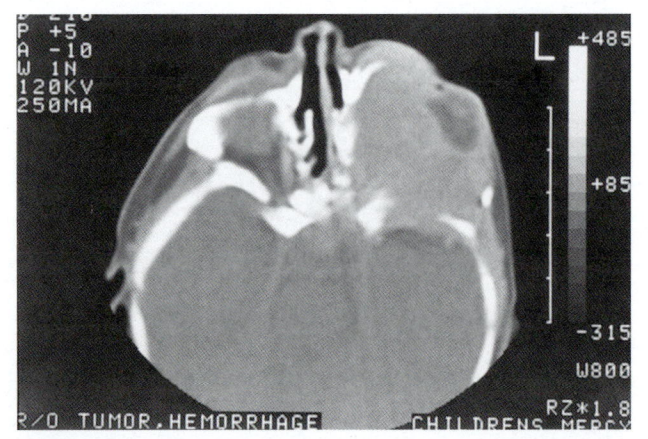

Figure 32.17. Axial computed tomography of child shown in Figure 32.16. The tumor filled the tentire orbit and ethmoid and extended into the cranial cavity of other sections. (Courtesy of Gerhard Cibis, MD.)

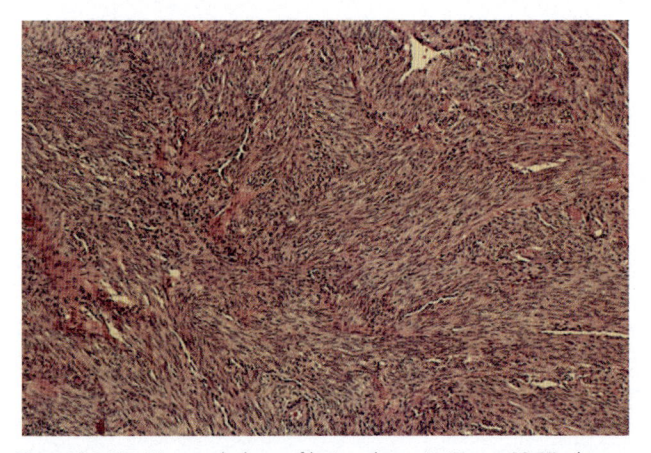

Figure 32.18. Histopathology of lesion shown in Figure 32.17, demonstrating benign spindle cells compatible with fibromatosis. (Hematoxylin–eosin ×80.) (Courtesy of Gerhard Cibis, MD.)

ORBITAL INFANTILE MYOFIBROMATOSIS

1. Waltermann JM, Huntrakoon M, Beatty EC Jr, et al. Congenital fibromatosis (myofibromatosis). A rare cause of proptosis at birth. *Ann Ophthalmol* 1988;20:394–399.
2. Shields CL, Husson M, Shields JA, et al. Solitary intraosseous infantile myofibroma of the orbital roof. *Arch Ophthalmol* 1998; 116:1528–1530.
3. Rodrigues EB, Shields CL, Marr BP, et al. Solitary intraosseous orbital myofibroma in 4 cases. *Ophthal Plast Reconstr Surg* 2006; 22:292–295.

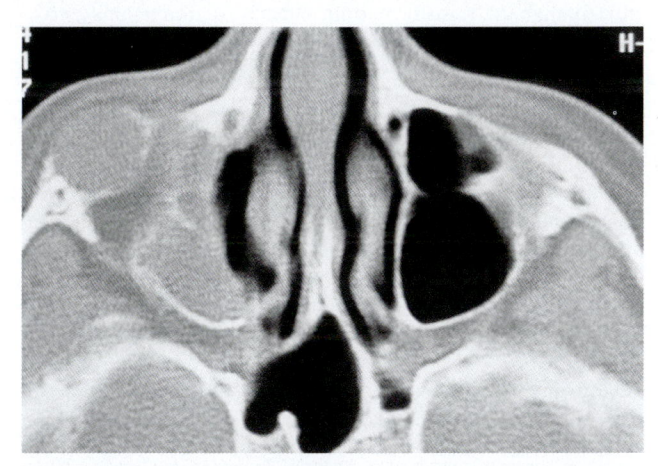

Figure 32.19. Axial computed tomography showing a round mass near floor of orbit in a 6-year-old boy.

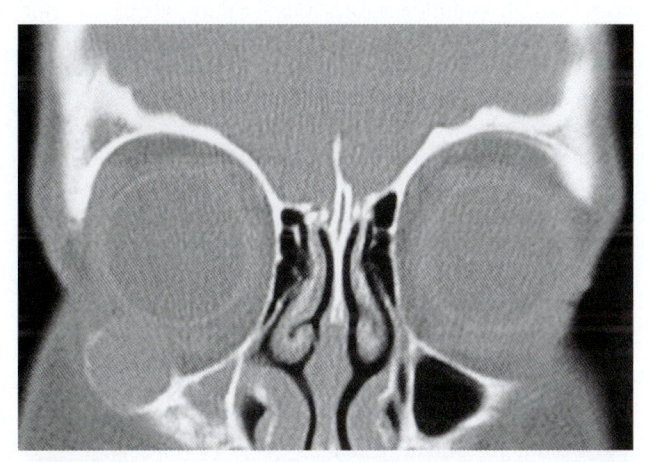

Figure 32.20. Coronal computed tomography with bone window setting of patient shown in Figure 32.19 depicting the round mass surrounded by thin lamella of compressed bone.

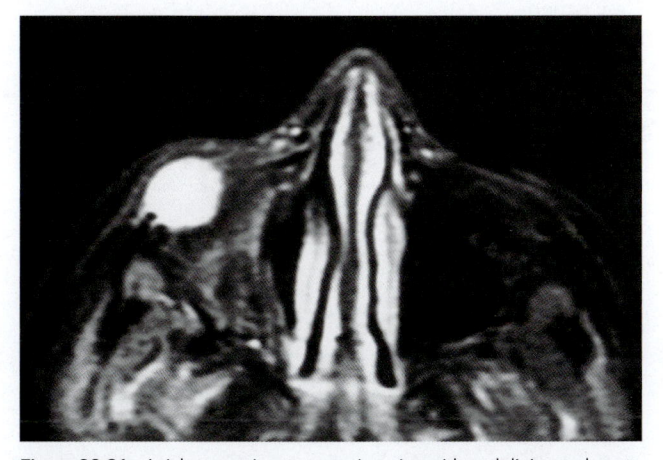

Figure 32.21. Axial magnetic resonance imaging with gadolinium enhancement of same patient showing marked enhancement of round mass.

Figure 32.22. Coronal magnetic resonance imaging with gadolinium showing bright homogeneous enhancement of the mass.

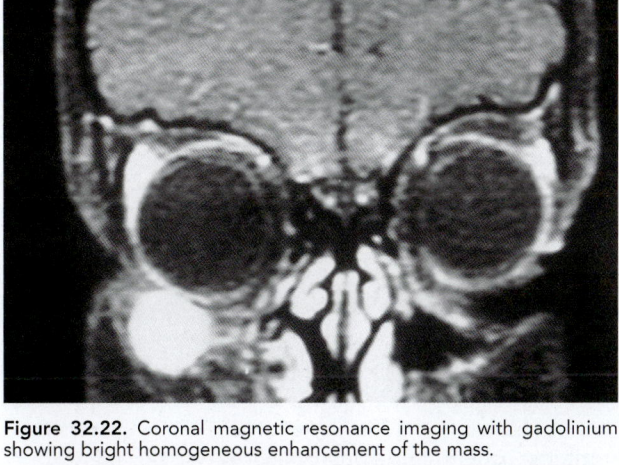

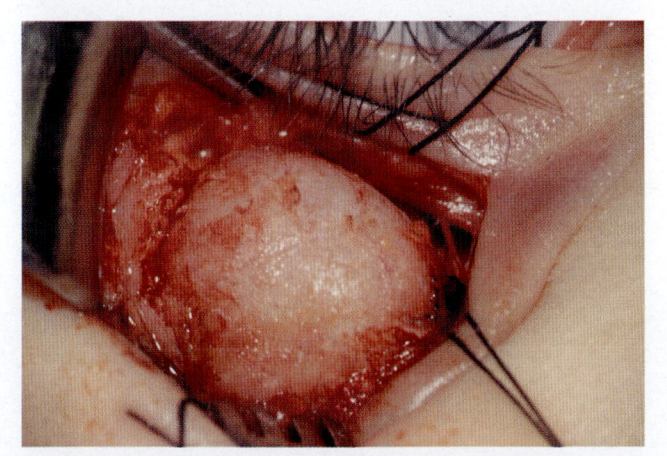

Figure 32.23. The mass was isolated by inferior orbitotomy by an eyelid crease approach and removed intact. Immunohistochemistry (to the right) shows positive reaction to smooth muscle actin (SMA).

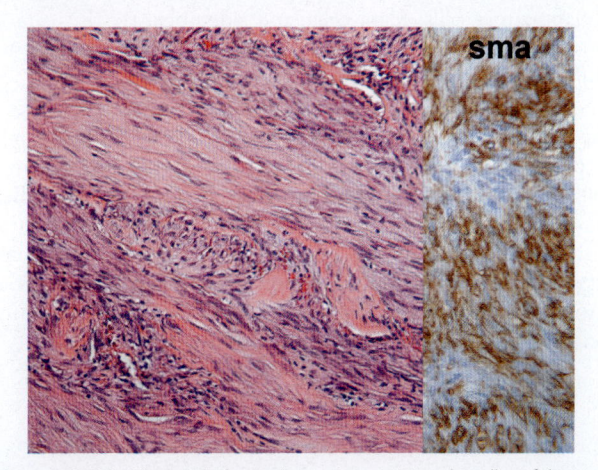

Figure 32.24. Histopathology shows intertwining bundle of benign spindle cells, the small uniform nuclei, and extracellular hyalinization. (Hematoxylin–eosin ×100.) *Inset* (to the right) shows positive immunoreactivity to smooth muscle actin.

ORBITAL FIBROUS HISTIOCYTOMA

General Considerations

Fibrous histiocytoma is a neoplasm composed of fibroblasts and histiocytes (4). This tumor usually occurs in subcutaneous tissue of the extremities. Several years ago, it was recognized to be a relatively common mesenchymal tumor of the orbit and several cases have been identified (1–21). In 1982, Font and Hidayat reported 150 orbital fibrous histiocytomas that had been referred to the Armed Forces Institute of Pathology (4). In the authors' clinical series of 1,264 cases, the 6 fibrous histiocytomas accounted for almost 46% of fibrocytic tumors of the orbit and <1% of all orbital tumors (1). Most fibrous histiocytomas are benign but some are locally aggressive or malignant (15–21). Malignant fibrous histiocytoma can develop after ocular irradiation for heritable retinoblastoma (2). According to newer nomenclature, it is believed that many fibrous histiocytomas are actually SFTs. In a review from the Armed Forces Institute of Pathology of fibroblastic tumors evaluated between 1970 and 2009, there were 23 that were previously diagnosed as fibrous histiocytoma, but according to more recent standards and immunohistochemistry, all 23 were reclassified as SFT (5).

Clinical Features

Orbital fibrous histiocytoma usually presents as a solitary orbital mass with slow onset painless proptosis or dysmotility, symptoms similar to other benign orbital tumors. This tumor can occur anywhere in the orbit, usually is confined to the orbital soft tissue, and has rarely invaded the globe (19).

Diagnostic Approaches

Orbital CT and MRI usually demonstrate a well-circumscribed soft tissue mass that may be similar to schwannoma or cavernous hemangioma. It can rarely erode bone and extend into the cranial cavity.

Pathology

Fibrous histiocytoma has several variations that have been the source of diagnostic difficulty. It is composed of a proliferation of fibroblasts and histiocytes arranged in a characteristic storiform pattern and accompanied by varying numbers of inflammatory cells, foam cells, and siderophages. This tumor possibly arises from a pluripotential cell that has the capacity to differentiate into either fibroblasts or histiocytes.

Based on pathologic criteria, orbital fibrous histiocytoma has been divided into benign (63%), locally aggressive (26%), and malignant categories (11%) (4). In general, histochemical, immunohistochemical, and electron microscopic studies have contributed little to the diagnosis of fibrous histiocytoma, although they can help to exclude other spindle cell tumors like SFT, melanoma, and leiomyoma. Fibrous histiocytoma is usually negative for CD34, whereas SFT is generally uniformly positive (5).

Management

As with other circumscribed orbital tumors, the preferred management is complete surgical resection of the mass within its capsule. Incomplete excision can lead to recurrence and possible malignant transformation. Advanced unresectable cases may require orbital exenteration and/or irradiation.

Selected References

Reviews

1. Shields JA, Shields CL, Scartozzi R. Survey of 1264 patients with orbital tumors and simulating lesions: the 2002 Montgomery Lecture, part 1. *Ophthalmology* 2004;111:997–1008.
2. Shields JA, Bakewell B, Augsburger JJ, et al. Classification and incidence of space-occupying lesions of the orbit. A survey of 645 biopsies. *Arch Ophthalmol* 1984;102:1606–1611.
3. Shields JA, Bakewell B, Augsburger JJ, et al. Space-occupying orbital masses in children: A review of 250 consecutive biopsies. *Ophthalmology* 1986;93:379–384.
4. Font RL, Hidayat AA. Fibrous histiocytoma of the orbit. A clinicopathologic study of 150 cases. *Hum Pathol* 1982;13:199–209.

Histopathology

5. Furusato E, Valenzuela IA, Fanburg-Smith JC, et al. Orbital solitary fibrous tumor: encompassing terminology for hemangiopericytoma, giant cell angiofibroma, and fibrous histiocytoma of the orbit: reappraisal of 41 cases. *Hum Pathol* 2011;42:120–128.
6. Goldsmith JD, van de Rijn M, Syed N. Orbital hemangiopericytoma and solitary fibrous tumor: a morphologic continuum. *Int J Surg Pathol* 2001;9:295–302.

Case Reports

7. Bernardini FP, de Conciliis C, Schneider S, et al. Solitary fibrous tumor of the orbit: is it rare? Report of a case series and review of the literature. *Ophthalmology* 2003;110:1442–1448.
8. Milman T, Finger PT, Iacob C, et al. Fibrous histiocytoma. *Ophthalmology* 2007;114:2369–2370.
9. Bajaj MS, Pushker N, Kashyap S, et al. Fibrous histiocytoma of the lacrimal gland. *Ophthal Plast Reconstr Surg* 2007;23:145–147.
10. Biedner B, Rothkoff L. Orbital fibrous histiocytoma in an infant. *Am J Ophthalmol* 1978;85:548–550.
11. Larkin DF, O'Donoghue HN, Mullaney J, et al. Orbital fibrous histiocytoma in an infant. *Acta Ophthalmol (Copenh)* 1988;66:585–588.
12. Krohel GB, Gregor D. Fibrous histiocytoma. *J Pediatr Ophthalmol* 1980;17:37–39.
13. Verity MA, Elbert JT, Hepler RS. Atypical fibrous histiocytoma of the orbit: an electron-microscopic study. *Ophthalmologica* 1977;175:73–79.
14. al-Hazzaa SA, Specht CS, McLean IW, et al. Benign orbital fibrous histiocytoma simulating a lacrimal gland tumor. *Ophthalmic Surg Lasers* 1996;27:140–142.
15. Liu D, McCann P, Kini RK, et al. Malignant fibrous histiocytoma of the orbit in a 3-year-old girl. Case report. *Arch Ophthalmol* 1987;105:895–896.
16. Ros PR, Kursunoglu S, Batlle JF, et al. Malignant fibrous histiocytoma of the orbit. *J Clin Neuro-Ophthalmol* 1985;5:116–119.
17. Boynton JR, Markowitch W Jr, Searl SS, et al. Periocular malignant fibrous histiocytoma. *Ophthal Plast Reconstr Surg* 1989;5:239–246.
18. Marback EF, Marback PMF, Sento Se DC, et al. Intraocular invasion by malignant orbital fibrous histiocytoma: a case report. *Eur J Ophthalmol* 2001;11:306–308.
19. Shields JA, Husson M, Shields CL, et al. Orbital malignant fibrous histiocytoma following irradiation for retinoblastoma. *Ophthal Plast Reconstr Surg* 2001;17:58–61.
20. Caballero LR, Rodriguez AC, Sopelana AB. Angiomatoid malignant fibrous histiocytoma of the orbit. *Am J Ophthalmol* 1981;92:13–15.
21. Rodrigues MM, Furgiuele FP, Weinreb S. Malignant fibrous histiocytoma of the orbit. *Arch Ophthalmol* 1977;95:2025–2028.

Chapter 32 Orbital Fibrous Connective Tissue Tumors

ORBITAL FIBROUS HISTIOCYTOMA: BENIGN TYPE

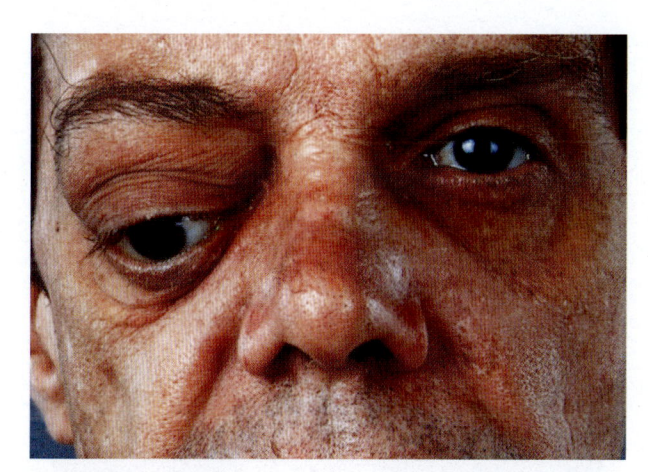

Figure 32.25. Benign fibrous histiocytoma. Proptosis and downward displacement of the left eye in a 49-year-old man. (Courtesy of Norman Charles, MD.)

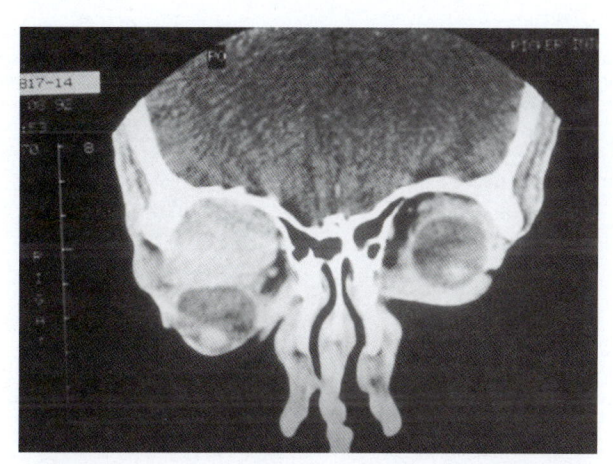

Figure 32.26. Coronal computed tomography of patient seen in Figure 32.25, showing well-circumscribed superior, soft tissue orbital mass with compression of the frontal bone. (Courtesy of Norman Charles, MD.)

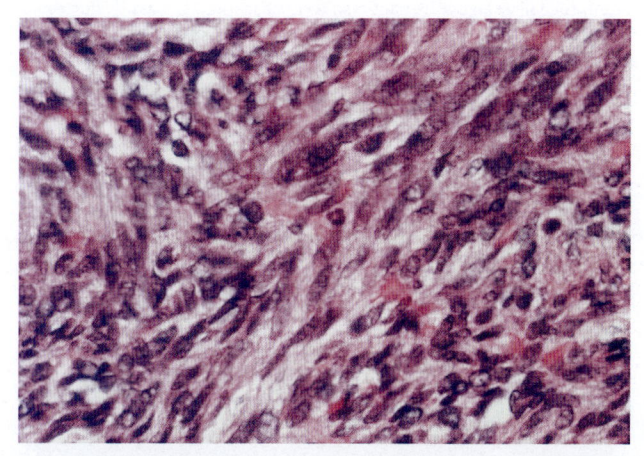

Figure 32.27. Histopathology of lesion shown in Figure 32.26. There are fascicles of spindle cells with interspersed histiocytes. (Hematoxylin–eosin ×200.) (Courtesy of Norman Charles, MD.)

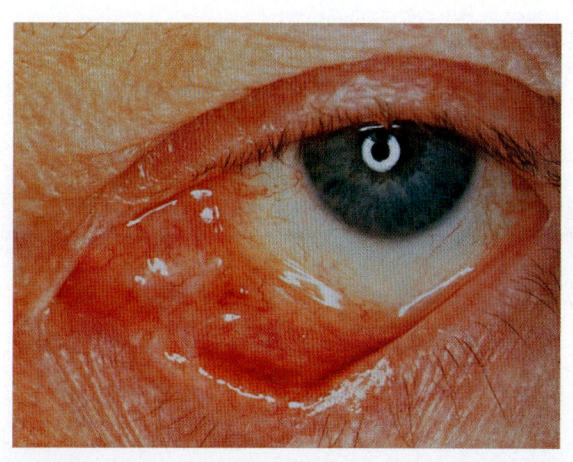

Figure 32.28. Conjunctival mass and ectropion of right lower eyelid in a 62-year-old man. (Courtesy of Douglas Cameron, MD.)

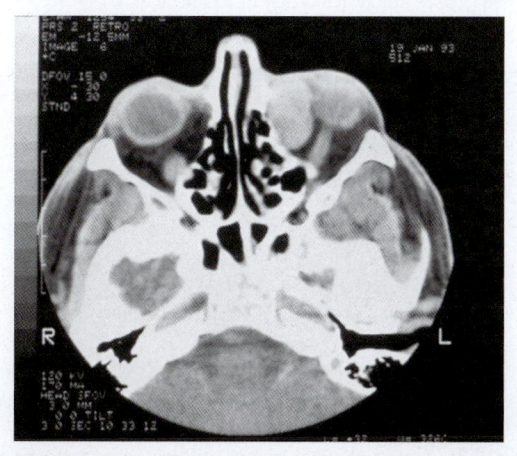

Figure 32.29. Axial computed tomography of patient shown in Figure 32.28, depicting a characteristic well-circumscribed nasal orbital mass. (Courtesy of Douglas Cameron, MD.)

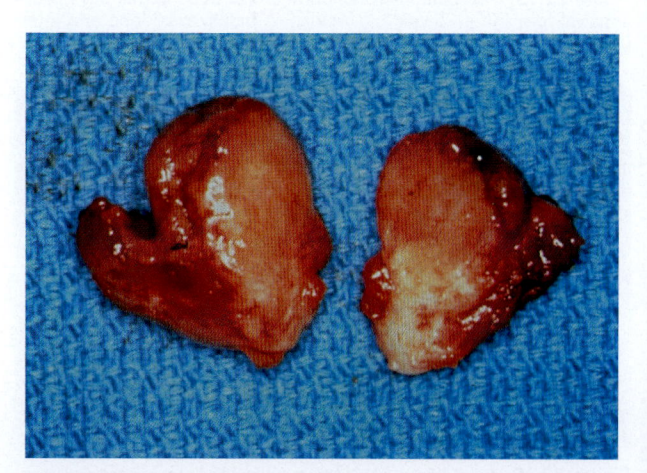

Figure 32.30. Gross appearance of sectioned lesion after surgical excision. Note the yellow appearance of the mass, a feature that is characteristic of fibrous histiocytoma. (Courtesy of Douglas Cameron, MD.)

ORBITAL FIBROUS HISTIOCYTOMA: MALIGNANT TYPE

Locally invasive and malignant fibrous histiocytoma are grouped together because both can exhibit malignant behavior. The former tends to grow locally and the latter has the additional capacity to metastasize. The benign, locally aggressive, and malignant types are usually impossible to differentiate clinically and the diagnosis and classification is made based on histopathologic examination.

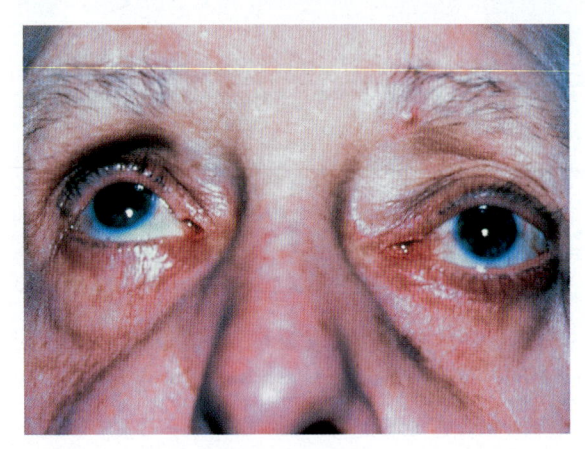

Figure 32.31. Malignant fibrous histiocytoma. Proptosis and restriction of upgaze in left eye of an 85-year-old woman. (Courtesy of Martha Farber, MD.)

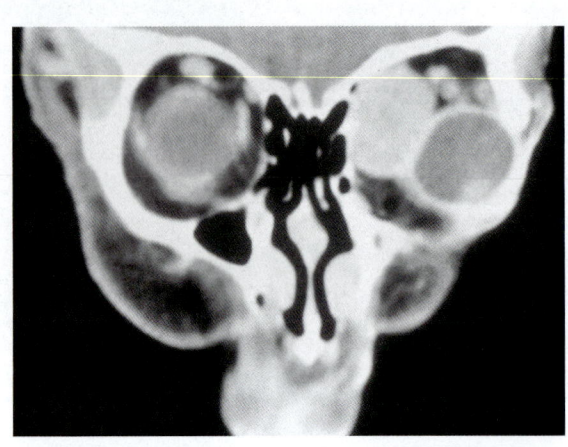

Figure 32.32. Axial computed tomography of patient shown in Figure 32.31, revealing an ovoid, circumscribed nasal orbital mass. (Courtesy of Martha Farber, MD.)

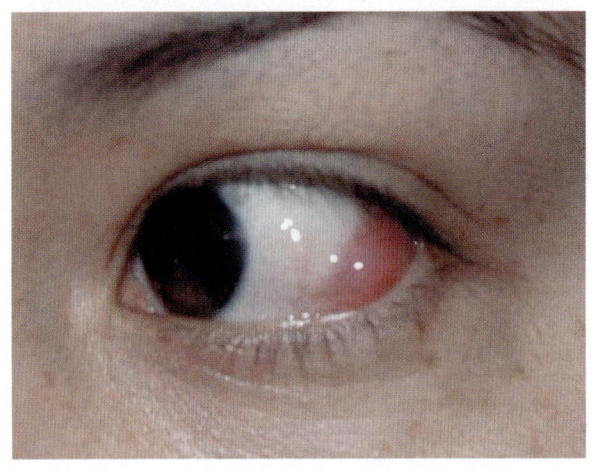

Figure 32.33. Red-pink inferotemporal orbital mass appearing in conjunctival fornix in a 25-year-old woman. A biopsy was done and interpreted elsewhere as a pterygium. (Courtesy of Victor Elner, MD.)

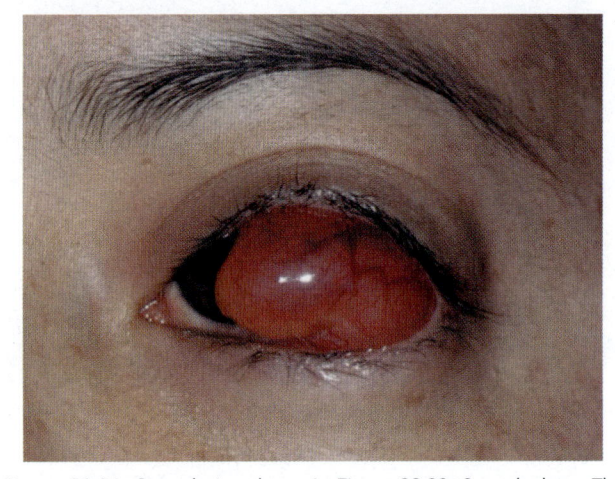

Figure 32.34. Same lesion shown in Figure 32.33, 2 weeks later. The lesion had grown rapidly. (Courtesy of Victor Elner, MD.)

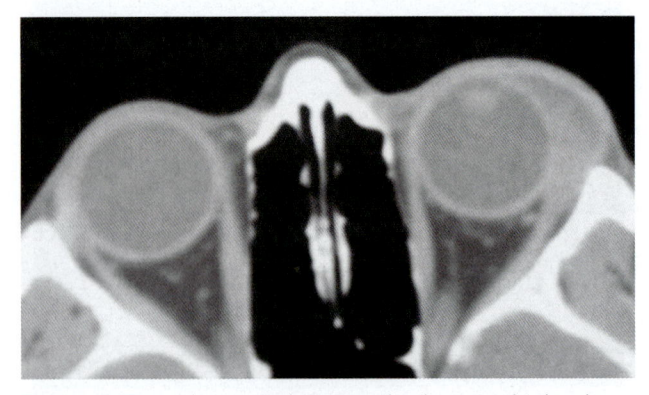

Figure 32.35. Axial computed tomography showing orbital and conjunctival mass. The lesion was removed. (Courtesy of Victor Elner, MD.)

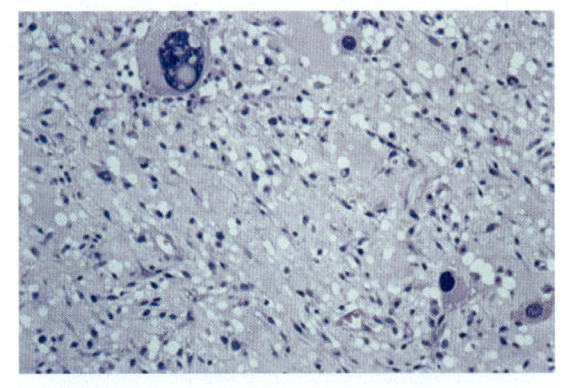

Figure 32.36. Histopathology shows pleomorphic and vacuolated malignant cells in a myxoid matrix. (Hematoxylin–eosin ×250.) The final diagnosis was myxoid malignant fibrous histiocytoma. (Courtesy of Victor Elner, MD.)

ORBITAL FIBROUS HISTIOCYTOMA: MANAGEMENT

The goal of treatment of orbital fibrous histiocytoma is complete excision of the mass within its capsule or pseudocapsule to prevent recurrence and malignant transformation. A benign fibrous histiocytoma that is completely removed may require no further active treatment. A malignant fibrous histiocytoma may require wider surgery or irradiation, depending on the overall clinical circumstances. A case example is shown of a patient referred for excision of a recurrent benign fibrous histiocytoma.

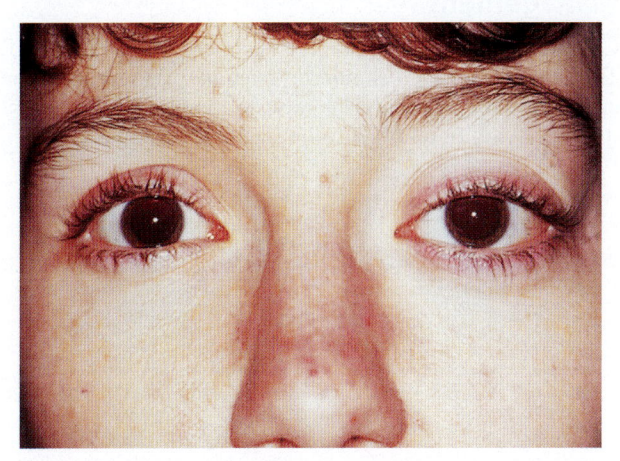

Figure 32.37. Proptosis of the left eye secondary to orbital fibrous histiocytoma in a 24-year-old woman.

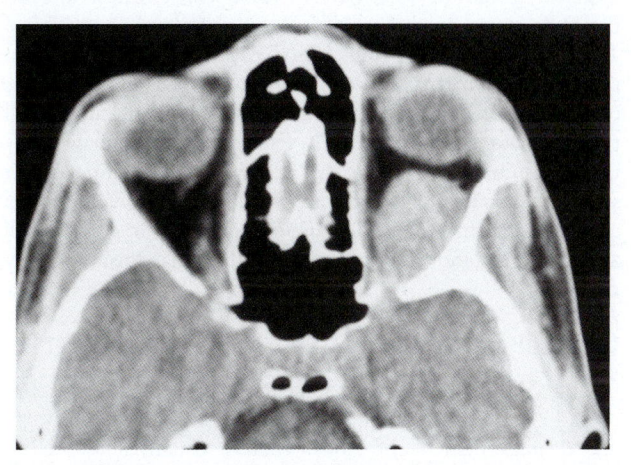

Figure 32.38. Axial computed tomography showing circumscribed orbital mass.

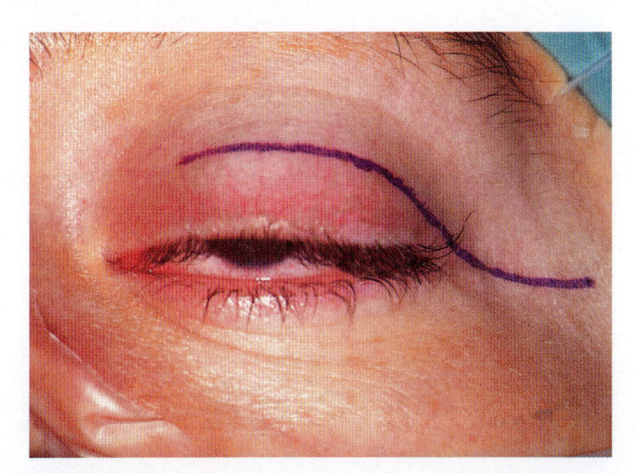

Figure 32.39. Planned superotemporal eyelid crease incision to remove the tumor.

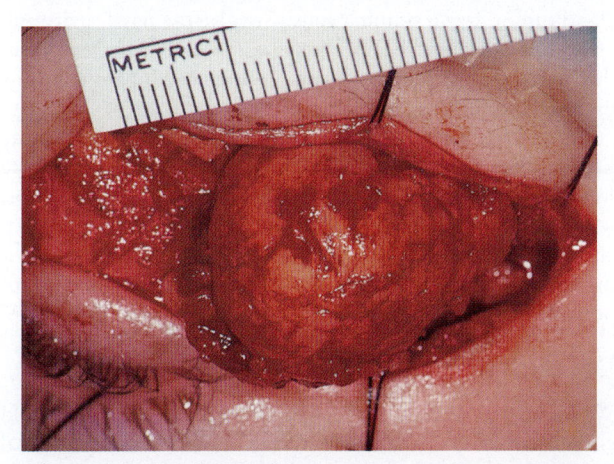

Figure 32.40. Tumor exposed at the time of superolateral orbitotomy.

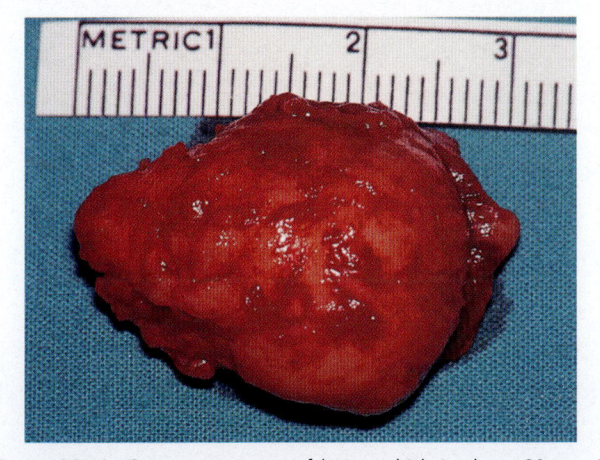

Figure 32.41. Gross appearance of lesion which is about 30 mm in greatest diameter.

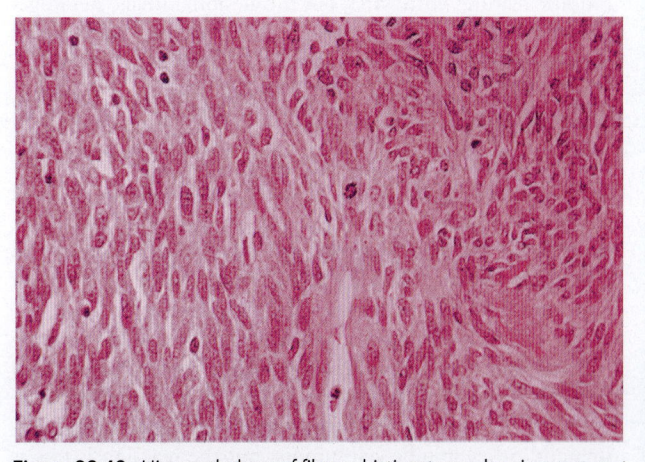

Figure 32.42. Histopathology of fibrous histiocytoma showing compact benign spindle cells. (Hematoxylin–eosin ×150.)

ORBITAL SOLITARY FIBROUS TUMOR

General Considerations

SFT is a neoplasm originally recognized in the pleura and subsequently found in other parts of the body. It is now increasingly diagnosed in the orbit (1–24). In the authors' series of 1,264 orbital tumors, only 1 SFT was identified. Based on the numerous recent reports, however, we speculate that some of the cases in our series were diagnosed as other spindle cell tumors, before SFT was widely recognized. In fact, with the use of immunohistochemistry, not available in some earlier studies, Furusato et al. evaluated 41 cases previously diagnosed as fibrous histiocytoma, hemangiopericytoma, and giant cell angiofibroma, and found that all met the reclassification criteria as SFT (7).

Clinical Features

Orbital SFT is unilateral and occurs in both adults and children (4–24). The patient generally presents with proptosis and displacement of the globe. There is usually a slow clinical course without significant pain or visual loss. This tumor can occur superotemporally and simulate an epithelial lacrimal gland tumor. It can simultaneously involve the nasal cavity and orbit. On occasion, SFT can be aggressive and can extend from the orbit into the central nervous system. Malignant transformation and metastasis are rare.

In one analysis of personal cases and published cases in the English literature on SFT of the head and neck region, there were 153 cases (5). The mean age at presentation was 50 years, with a female:male ratio of 5:4. The tumor size was mean 2.6 cm. All cases expressed cytoplasmic CD34 positivity. Following surgical removal, recurrence was found only in 4 (of 9) with positive margins and 1 (of 10) classified as malignant (5).

Diagnostic Approaches

With imaging studies, orbital SFT appears as a round to ovoid circumscribed mass that is more often located in the extraconal tissues. Smooth remodeling of the adjacent bone is common and suggests the benign behavior of SFT. There are no pathognomonic features with MRI, but intralesional image heterogeneity and a predominantly low T2 signal intensity are believed by some to be distinctive features (6).

Pathology

The histopathology and immunohistochemistry of SFT have been discussed extensively in recent years. Many cases of hemangiopericytoma and other spindle cell neoplasms have been reevaluated and diagnosed as SFT (7–9). In contrast to these other tumors, SFT has a "patternless pattern," without storiform or stag horn features that characterize fibrous histiocytoma and hemangiopericytoma, respectively. The strongly positive immunoreactivity to CD34 supports the diagnosis of SFT and helps exclude other spindle cell tumors (5). Some degree of CD34 positivity can be seen with hemangiopericytoma and other spindle cell tumors, but the reaction is not as profound as with SFT. SFT typically shows positive reaction to vimentin but negative reaction to S-100 protein and muscle and epithelial markers.

Management

Complete surgical resection is the treatment of choice for SFT. The surgical approach should be carefully planned, based on imaging studies. Incomplete excision can lead to recurrent tumor that infiltrates the surrounding tissues and bone (16).

ORBITAL SOLITARY FIBROUS TUMOR

Selected References

Reviews

1. Shields JA, Shields CL, Scartozzi R. Survey of 1264 patients with orbital tumors and simulating lesions: the 2002 Montgomery Lecture, part 1. *Ophthalmology* 2004;111:997–1008.
2. Shields JA, Bakewell B, Augsburger JJ, et al. Classification and incidence of space-occupying lesions of the orbit. A survey of 645 biopsies. *Arch Ophthalmol* 1984;102:1606–1611.
3. Shields JA, Bakewell B, Augsburger JJ, et al. Space-occupying orbital masses in children: A review of 250 consecutive biopsies. *Ophthalmology* 1986;93:379–384.
4. Bowe SN, Wakely PE, Ozer E. Head and neck solitary fibrous tumors: diagnostic and therapeutic challenges. *Laryngoscope* 2012;122:1748–1755.
5. Cox DP, Daniels T, Jordan RC. Solitary fibrous tumor of the head and neck. *Oral Surg Oral Med Oral Pathol Oral Radiol Endod* 2010;110:79–84.

Management

6. Gigantelli JW, Kincaid MC, Soparkar CN, et al. Orbital solitary fibrous tumor: radiographic and histopathologic correlations. *Ophthal Plast Reconstr Surg* 2001;17:207–214.

Histopathology

7. Furusato E, Valenzuela IA, Fanburg-Smith JC, et al. Orbital solitary fibrous tumor: encompassing terminology for hemangiopericytoma, giant cell angiofibroma, and fibrous histiocytoma of the orbit: reappraisal of 41 cases. *Hum Pathol* 2011;42:120–128.
8. Goldsmith JD, van de Rijn M, Syed N. Orbital hemangiopericytoma and solitary fibrous tumor: a morphologic continuum. *Int J Surg Pathol* 2001;9:295–302.
9. Heathcote JG. Pathology update: solitary fibrous tumour of the orbit. *Can J Ophthalmol* 1997;32:432–435.

Case Reports

10. Krishnakumar S, Subramanian N, Mohan ER, et al. Solitary fibrous tumor of the orbit: a clinicopathologic study of six cases with review of the literature. *Surv Ophthalmol* 2003;48:544–554.
11. Bernardini FP, de Conciliis C, Schneider S, et al. Solitary fibrous tumor of the orbit: is it rare? Report of a case series and review of the literature. *Ophthalmology* 2003;110:1442–1448.
12. Polito E, Tosi M, Toti P, et al. Orbital solitary fibrous tumor with aggressive behavior. Three cases and review of the literature. *Graefes Arch Clin Exp Ophthalmol* 2002;240:570–574.
13. Hayashi S, Kurihara H, Hirato J, et al. Solitary fibrous tumor of the orbit with extraorbital extension: case report. *Neurosurgery* 2001;49:1241–1245.
14. Lucci LM, Anderson RL, Harrie RP, et al. Solitary fibrous tumor of the orbit in a child. *Ophthal Plast Reconstr Surg* 2001;17:369–373.
15. Alexandrakis G, Johnson TE. Recurrent orbital solitary fibrous tumor in a 14-year old girl. *Am J Ophthalmol* 2000;130:373–376.
16. DeBacker CM, Bodker F, Putterman AM, et al. Solitary fibrous tumor of the orbit. *Am J Ophthalmol* 1996;121:447–449.
17. Ing EB, Kennerdell JS, Olson PR, et al. Solitary fibrous tumor of the orbit. *Ophthal Plast Reconstr Surg* 1998;14:57–61.
18. Le CP, Jones S, Valenzuela AA. Orbital solitary fibrous tumor: a case series with review of the literature. *Orbit* 2014;33:145–151.
19. Ali MJ, Honavar SG, Naik MN, et al. Orbital solitary fibrous tumor: a rare clinicopathologic correlation and review of literature. *J Res Med Sci* 2013;18:529–531.
20. Polomsky M, Sines DT, Dutton JJ. Solitary fibrous tumor of the orbit with multiple cavities. *Ophthal Plast Reconstr Surg* 2013;29:e117–e119.
21. Patel MM, Jakobiec FA, Zakka FR, et al. Intraorbital metastasis from solitary fibrous tumor. *Ophthal Plast Reconstr Surg* 2013;29:e76–e79.
22. Young TK, Hardy TG. Solitary fibrous tumor of the orbit with intracranial involvement. *Ophthal Plast Reconstr Surg* 2011;27:e74–e76.
23. Feuerman JM, Flint A, Elner VM. Cystic solitary fibrous tumor of the orbit. *Arch Ophthalmol* 2010;128:385–387.
24. Demirci H, Shields CL, Eagle RC Jr, et al. Giant cell angiofibroma, a variant of solitary fibrous tumor, of the orbit in a 16-year-old girl. *Ophthal Plast Reconstr Surg* 2009;25:402–404.

ORBITAL SOLITARY FIBROUS TUMOR

SFT has clinical features similar to other circumscribed orbital tumors. A clinicopathologic correlation is shown.

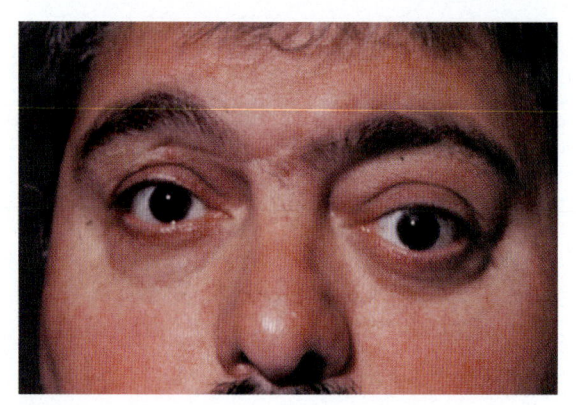

Figure 32.43. Facial appearance of a middle-aged man with proptosis of left eye.

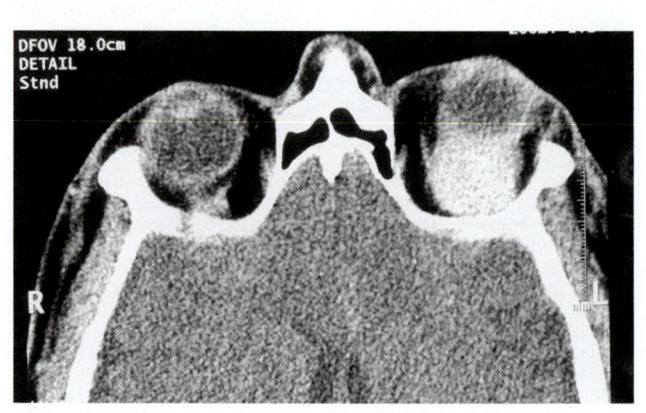

Figure 32.44. Axial computed tomography showing round mass superior to globe.

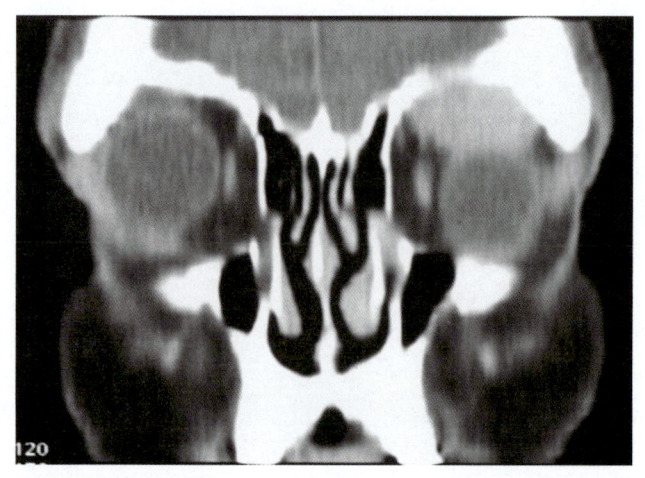

Figure 32.45. Coronal computed tomography showing ovoid circumscribed mass in superior aspect of left orbit.

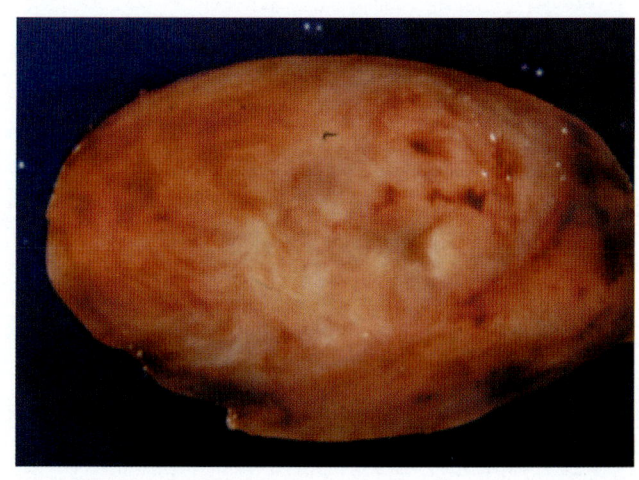

Figure 32.46. Photograph of specimen removed completely by superolateral orbitotomy.

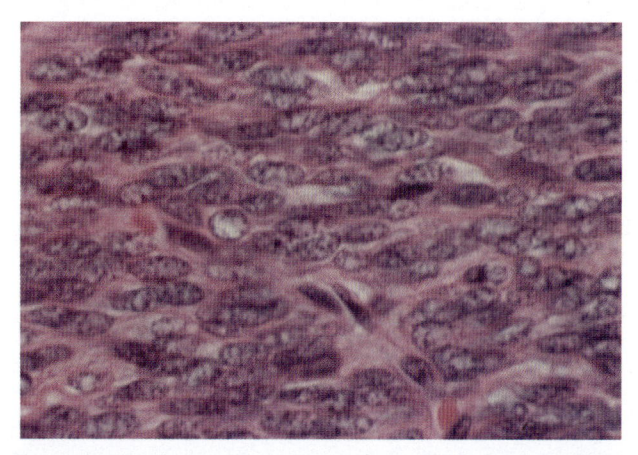

Figure 32.47. Photomicrograph showing uniform closely compact, spindle-shaped cells with features typical of solitary fibrous tumor. (Hematoxylin–eosin ×200.)

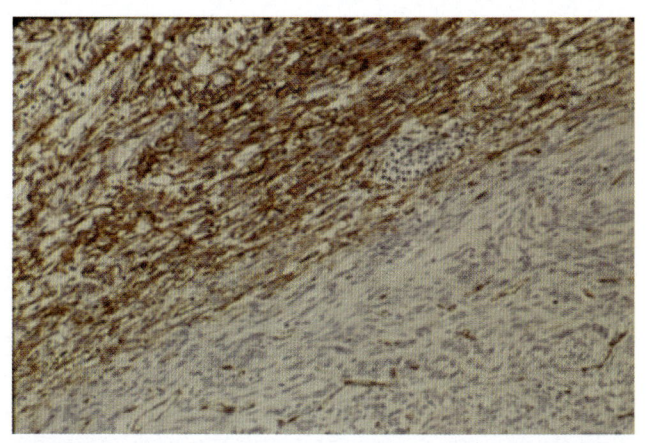

Figure 32.48. Immunohistochemical reaction to CD 34 antigen showing strongly positive area of tumor (above). The area of the tumor below shows less reaction. (×100.)

Chapter 32 Orbital Fibrous Connective Tissue Tumors

ORBITAL SOLITARY FIBROUS TUMOR WITH SLOW-ONSET RECURRENCE

SFT is a low-grade neoplasm. Complete surgical resection is advised. Both cases below had nearly complete surgical resection and both showed slow-onset recurrence several years later.

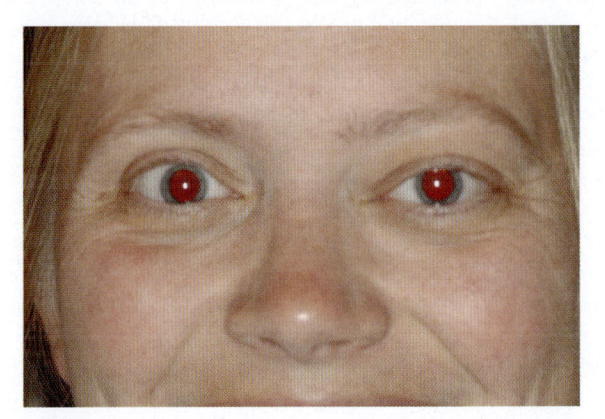

Figure 32.49. Facial appearance of a middle-aged woman with proptosis of left eye.

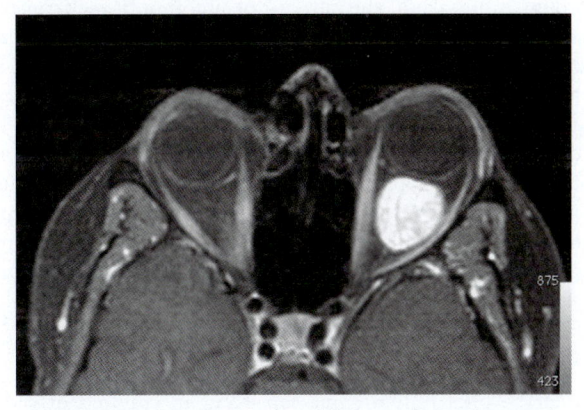

Figure 32.50. Axial T1-weighted, gadolinium-enhanced magnetic resonance imaging of patient in Figure 32.43 revealing well-circumscribed, intraconal soft tissue mass.

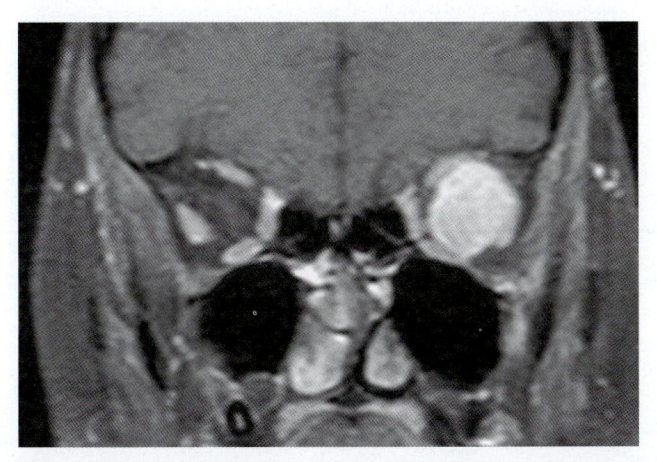

Figure 32.51. Coronal magnetic resonance imaging showing round, enhancing circumscribed mass in muscle cone.

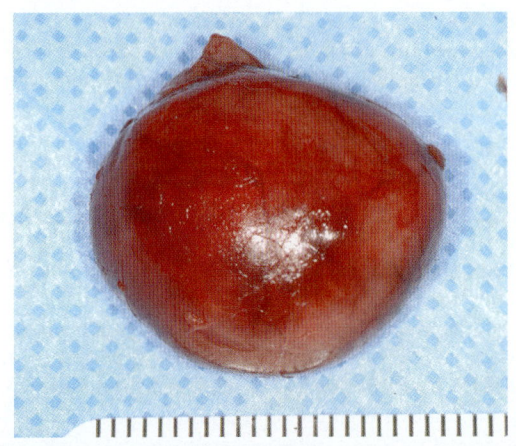

Figure 32.52. Following surgical resection, the specimen appeared to be removed completely and the diagnosis of SFT was confirmed. However, histopathology revealed that tumor extended to the posterior margin. Three years later, this patient required a second surgery to remove orbital tumor recurrence.

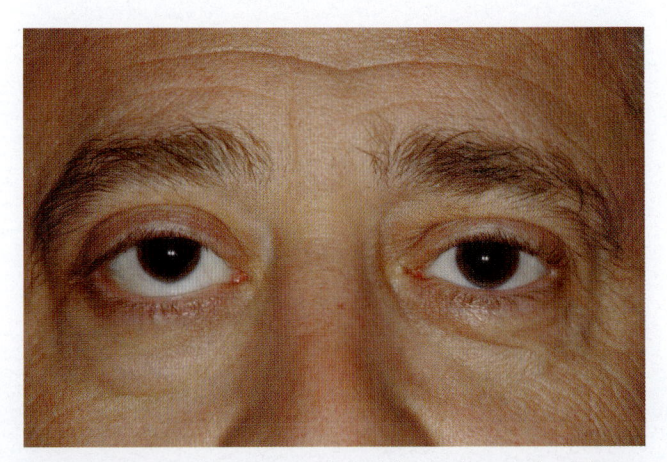

Figure 32.53. Facial appearance of a middle-aged man with subtle proptosis of right eye.

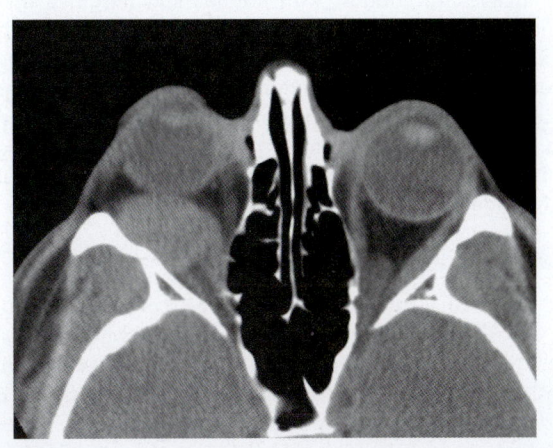

Figure 32.54. Axial computed tomography of patient in Figure 32.47, revealing well-circumscribed, intraconal soft tissue mass. This tumor was removed completely, clinically, but histopathology showed posterior margin involvement. A second surgery to remove slow-onset recurrence was necessary 6 years later.

ORBITAL FIBROSARCOMA

Several years ago, fibrosarcoma was not a rare diagnosis in soft tissue, including the orbit. With the description of other fibrous tumors and the advent of immunohistochemistry, many tumors that would have been called fibrosarcomas are being diagnosed as malignant fibrous histiocytoma, SFT, or other spindle-cell tumors. Hence, fibrosarcoma has become a diagnosis of exclusion, resulting in an apparent decline in its incidence (5). This tumor can occur as a primary orbital tumor in children and adults, a secondary orbital tumor invading from the nasal cavity or sinuses, or after ocular radiotherapy, the heritable retinoblastoma (1–12). Radiation-induced fibrosarcoma, although rare, has become more common than primary orbital fibrosarcoma (8,9).

Clinical Features

Primary orbital fibrosarcoma can occur in children or older adults as a progressive mass, usually in the extraconal space. Children with primary congenital fibrosarcoma may have massive proptosis at birth. The patient with secondary orbital fibrosarcoma tends to develop signs of sinus and orbital disease in middle age. Those with radiation-induced orbital fibrosarcomas develop proptosis and fullness of the temporal fossa from 5 to 35 years after radiotherapy, usually for retinoblastoma.

Diagnostic Approaches

Primary orbital fibrosarcoma is more likely to appear as an irregular but fairly well-circumscribed soft tissue mass in any portion of the orbit. Radiation-induced fibrosarcoma shows a soft tissue mass, usually in the anterior portion of the orbit, often with involvement of the orbit and temporal fossa. The secondary orbital fibrosarcoma would be expected to appear as a poorly circumscribed mass with sinus and nasal cavity involvement along with the orbital tumor.

Pathology and Pathogenesis

Orbital fibrosarcoma is comprised of immature spindle-shaped fibroblasts in a so-called herringbone pattern with interlacing fascicles. In contrast with fibroma and fibromatosis, the tumor is relatively hypercellular and the nuclei have prominent nucleoli and mitotic activity with less intercellular collagen. Electron microscopy and immunohistochemistry can be used to confirm the fibroblastic nature of the tumor by the criteria described earlier and it can help to differentiate fibrosarcoma from other spindle-cell tumors such as rhabdomyosarcoma, schwannoma, and fibrous histiocytoma (5).

Management

The best management of orbital fibrosarcoma is wide surgical excision, including orbital exenteration when necessary. Radiotherapy, chemotherapy, and other modalities are usually considered to be palliative and should be employed when complete surgical excision cannot be accomplished. The systemic prognosis is likewise variable. Patients with secondary and radiation-induced tumors are generally prone to recurrence or to develop other cancers, and have a more guarded prognosis. Primary fibrosarcomas, when confined to the soft tissues of the orbit, could potentially carry a favorable prognosis if completely excised.

Selected References

Reviews

1. Shields JA, Shields CL, Scartozzi R. Survey of 1264 patients with orbital tumors and simulating lesions: the 2002 Montgomery Lecture, part 1. *Ophthalmology* 2004;111: 997–1008.
2. Shields JA, Bakewell B, Augsburger JJ, et al. Classification and incidence of space-occupying lesions of the orbit. A survey of 645 biopsies. *Arch Ophthalmol* 1984;102: 1606–1611.
3. Shields JA, Bakewell B, Augsburger JJ, et al. Space-occupying orbital masses in children: a review of 250 consecutive biopsies. *Ophthalmology* 1986;93:379–384.

Histopathology

4. Jakobiec FA, Tannenbaum M. The ultrastructure of orbital fibrosarcoma. *Am J Ophthalmol* 1974;77:899–917.
5. Folpe AL. Fibrosarcoma: a review and update. *Histopathology* 2014;64:12–25.

Case Reports

6. Weiner JM, Hidayat AA. Juvenile fibrosarcoma of the orbit and eyelid. A study of five cases. *Arch Ophthalmol* 1983;101:253–259.
7. Eifrig DE, Foos RY. Fibrosarcoma of the orbit. *Am J Ophthalmol* 1969;67:244–248.
8. Abramson DH, Ronner H, Ellsworth RM. Second tumors in non-irradiated bilateral retinoblastoma. *Am J Ophthalmol* 1979;84:624–627.
9. Strickland P. Fibromyosarcoma of the orbit. Radiation-induced tumour 33 years after treatment of "bilateral ocular glioma." *Br J Ophthalmol* 1966;50:50–53.
10. Yanoff M, Scheie HG. Fibrosarcoma of the orbit. Report of two patients. *Cancer* 1966;19:1711–1716.
11. Schittkowski MP, Wrede A. Dermatofibrosarcoma protuberans with primary orbital manifestation. *Orbit* 2013;32:117–119.
12. Gosh JM, Lewis CK, Meine JG, et al. Primary dermatofibrosarcoma protuberans invading the orbit. *Ophthalm Plast Reconstr Surg* 2012;28:e65–e67.

Chapter 32 Orbital Fibrous Connective Tissue Tumors

ORBITAL FIBROSARCOMA

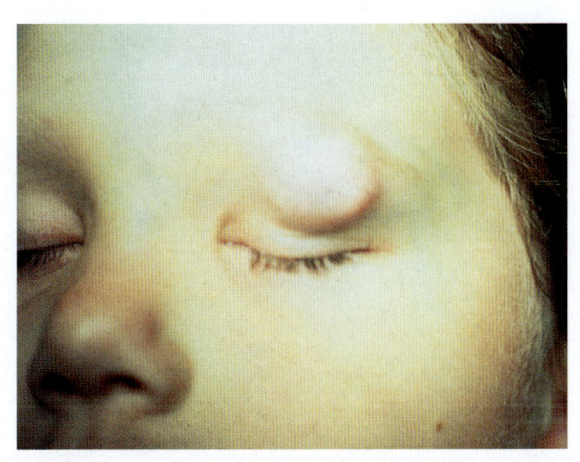

Figure 32.55. Localized primary fibrosarcoma of the superior orbit presenting as a subcutaneous mass in the eyebrow area in a 6-year-old girl.

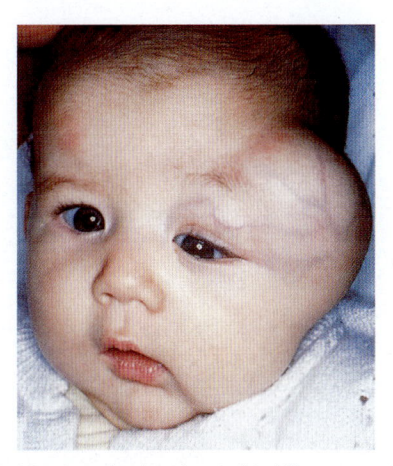

Figure 32.56. Massive orbital and periorbital fibrosarcoma in an infant. (Courtesy of Eduardo Arenas, MD.)

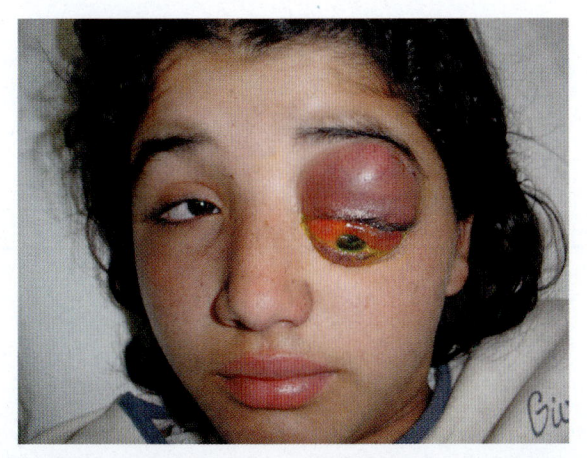

Figure 32.57. Marked proptosis and chemosis in a child with orbital fibrosarcoma. (Courtesy of Marta Chernikoff, MD.)

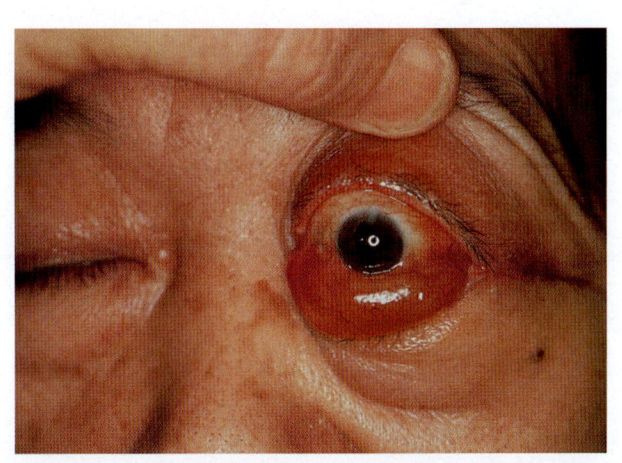

Figure 32.58. Proptosis and chemosis of the left eye in an elderly man secondary to orbital fibrosarcoma. (Courtesy of Charles Lee, MD.)

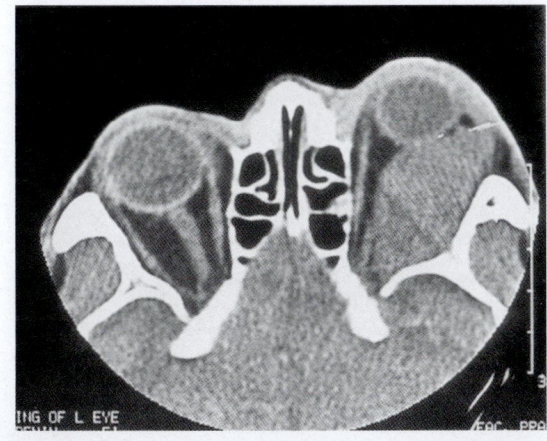

Figure 32.59. Axial computed tomography of patient shown in Figure 32.52, demonstrating the large orbital tumor in soft tissue. (Courtesy of Charles Lee, MD.)

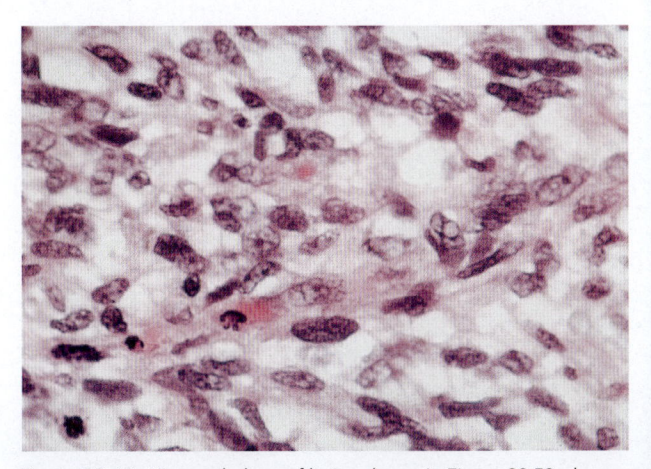

Figure 32.60. Histopathology of lesion shown in Figure 32.53, demonstrating malignant spindle cells. There was some debate as to the exact diagnosis, but most authorities favored the diagnosis of fibrosarcoma. (Hematoxylin–eosin ×150.) (Courtesy of Charles Lee, MD.)

CHAPTER 33

ORBITAL OSSEOUS, FIBRO-OSSEOUS, AND CARTILAGINOUS TUMORS

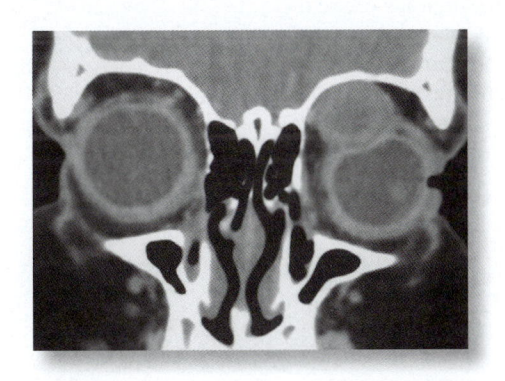

General Considerations

The main tumors of bone are the benign osteoma and the malignant osteosarcoma (1–22). Osteoma is the most common tumor of the nose and paranasal sinuses and the most common neoplasm of the frontal sinus (10). Osteoma that arises from the bones of the frontal sinus, ethmoid sinus, and other periorbital bones can extend into orbit. Osteoma in an ocular oncology practice is relatively uncommon (1–3). In the authors' series of 1,264 orbital lesions, the 4 osteomas accounted for 19% of osseous and fibro-osseous tumors and for <1% of all orbital tumors (1). The true incidence is actually greater, because most lesions originate in the sinuses, have minimal orbital involvement, and are more likely to be managed by otorhinolaryngologists.

Orbital osteoma can sometimes occur with Gardner's syndrome, an autosomal-dominant condition characterized by adenomatous polyposis of the bowel, secondary bowel cancer, typical congenital hyperplastic lesions of the retinal pigment epithelium (RPE), desmoid tumors, and other lesions (12,13). The RPE lesions are discussed in the *Textbook and Atlas of Intraocular Tumors*. A patient with a suspected orbital osteoma should undergo ophthalmoscopy and possible referral to a gastroenterologist.

Clinical Features

Orbital osteoma can occur at any age and there is no predilection for gender. In an analysis of 45 surgically documented cases, men outnumbered women 3:2 and the median age was 37 years (10). Depending on the size and location of the osteoma, this tumor can be asymptomatic or can produce orbital symptoms and signs such as proptosis and displacement of the globe. Osteoma can cause pain, described by the patient as a headache. A hard mass may be visible and palpable at the superior or nasal orbital rim. The bony mass may obstruct the ostia of the sinus and lead to chronic sinusitis or secondary mucocele.

Diagnostic Approaches

Computed tomography of orbital osteoma shows a sessile or pedunculated mass with bone density arising from otherwise normal bone, usually the frontal or ethmoid bones. The ivory type may be identical to bone; the fibrous type is less dense and may resemble fibrous dysplasia.

Pathology

Histopathologically, osteoma has been divided into three types: compact (ivory), cancellous, and fibrous (4–6). It is believed

ORBITAL OSTEOMA

that the compact type is most mature and the fibrous the least mature and that the fibrous type may be part of a continuum incorporating ossifying fibroma and fibrous dysplasia.

Management

Asymptomatic orbital osteoma can sometimes be followed conservatively. The only exception is an osteoma of the sphenoid bone that shows encroachment on the optic canal, in which case earlier surgical excision may be justified. A larger or symptomatic osteoma can be managed by surgical excision. A superonasal lynch incision can be used for the more common superonasal lesion. Another approach is to surgically excise the mass through endoscopic transnasal route to minimize cosmetic defect (7,8). For a more posterior osteoma that involves the orbital roof or cribriform plate, a combined orbitocranial approach or endoscopic approach can be employed. Incomplete removal does not usually lead to recurrence.

ORBITAL OSTEOMA

Selected References

Reviews

1. Shields JA, Shields CL, Scartozzi R. Survey of 1264 patients with orbital tumors and simulating lesions: The 2002 Montgomery Lecture, part 1. *Ophthalmology* 2004;111: 997–1008.
2. Shields JA, Bakewell B, Augsburger JJ, et al. Classification and incidence of space-occupying lesions of the orbit. A survey of 645 biopsies. *Arch Ophthalmol* 1984;102: 1606–1611.
3. Shields JA, Bakewell B, Augsburger JJ, et al. Space-occupying orbital masses in children: A review of 250 consecutive biopsies. *Ophthalmology* 1986;93:379–384.
4. Fu YS, Perzin KH. Non-epithelial tumors of the nasal cavity, paranasal sinuses, and nasopharynx: a clinicopathologic study. II. Osseous and fibro-osseous lesions, including osteoma, fibrous dysplasia, ossifying fibroma, osteoblastoma, giant cell tumor, and osteosarcoma. *Cancer* 1974;33: 1289–1305.
5. Grove AS. Osteomas of the orbit. *Ophthalmic Surg* 1978;9:23–39.
6. Selva D, White VA, O'Connell JX, et al. Primary bone tumors of the orbit. *Surv Ophthalmol* 2004;49:328–342.

Management

7. Selva D, Chen C, Wormald PJ. Frontoethmoidal osteoma: a stereotactic-assisted sino-orbital approach. *Ophthal Plast Reconstr Surg* 2003;19:237–238.
8. Naraghi M, Kashfi A. Endonasal endoscopic resection of ethmoido-orbital osteoma compressing the optic nerve. *Am J Otolaryngol* 2003;24:408–412.

Histopathology

9. Blodi FC. Pathology of orbital bones. The XXXII Edward Jackson Memorial Lecture. *Am J Ophthalmol* 1976;81:1–26.
10. McHugh JB, Mukherji SK, Lucas DR. Sino-orbital osteoma: a clinicopathologic study of 45 surgically treated cases with emphasis on tumors with osteoblastoma-like features. *Arch Pathol* 2009;133:1587–1593.

Case Reports

11. Ataman M, Ayas K, Gursel B. Giant osteoma of the frontal sinus. *Rhinology* 1993; 31:185–187.
12. Whitson WE, Orcutt JC, Walkinshaw MD. Orbital osteoma in Gardner's syndrome. *Am J Ophthalmol* 1986;101:236–241.
13. Van Gehuchten D, Lemagne JM, Weber S, et al. A case of exophthalmos-an early symptom of Gardner's syndrome. *Orbit* 1982;1:61–69.
14. Appalanarsayya K, Murthy AS, Viswanath CK, et al. Osteoma involving the orbit. Case report and review of the literature. *Int Surg* 1970;54:449–453.
15. Borello ED, Argentina R, Sedano HO. Giant osteoid osteoma of the maxilla. *Oral Surg* 1967;23:563–566.
16. Kim AW, Foster JA, Papay FA, et al. Orbital extension of a frontal sinus osteoma in a thirteen-year-old girl. *JAAPOS* 2000;4:122–124.
17. Ma'luf RN, Ghazi NG, Zein WM, et al. Orbital osteoma arising adjacent to a foreign body. *Ophthal Plast Reconstr Surg* 2000;19:327–330.
18. McNab AA. Orbital osteoma in Gardner's syndrome. *Aust N Z J Ophthalmol* 1998; 26:169–170.
19. Miller NR, Gray J, Snip R. Giant mushroom-shaped osteoma of the orbit originating from the maxillary sinus. *Am J Ophthalmol* 1977;83:587–591.
20. Newell FW. Osteoma involving the orbit. *Am J Ophthalmol* 1948;31:1281–1289.
21. Sternberg I, Levine MR. Ethmoidal sinus osteoma: a primary cause of nasolacrimal obstruction and dacryocystorhinostomy failure. *Ophthalmic Surg* 1984;15:295–297.
22. Tarkkanen JV, Mets LP. A case of orbital osteoma. *Acta Ophthalmologica* 1964;42: 1074–1078.

634   Part 3 Tumors of the Orbit

ORBITAL OSTEOMA

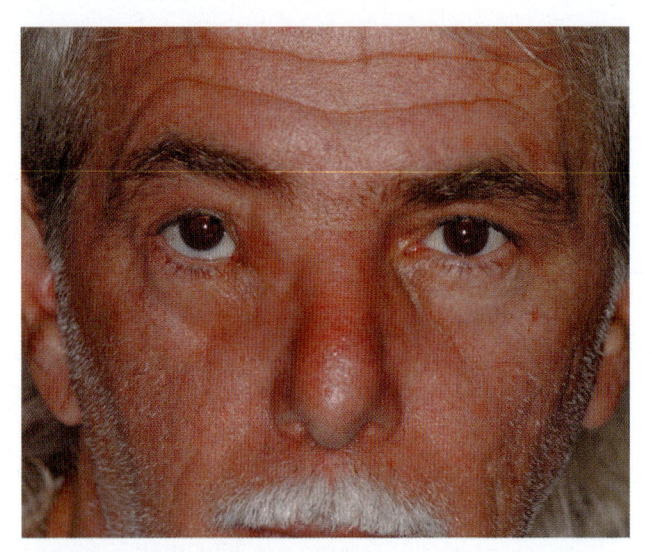

Figure 33.1. Photograph of a 60-year-old man with slowly progressive hard mass in region of right medial canthus.

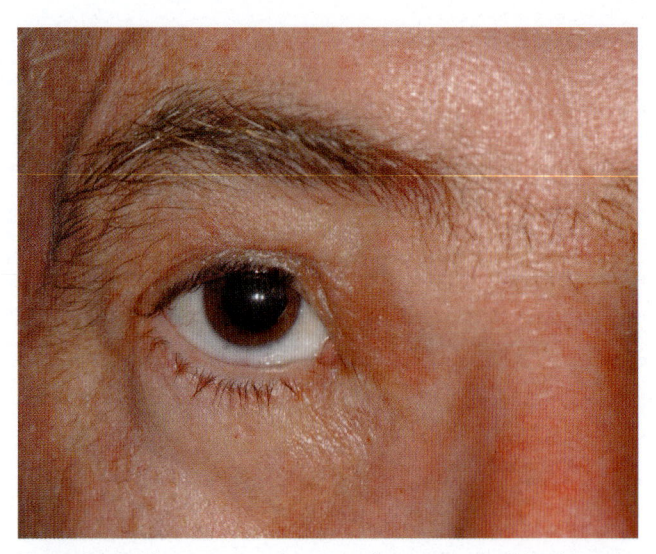

Figure 33.2. Close-up view showing subcutaneous nodule above the medial canthus.

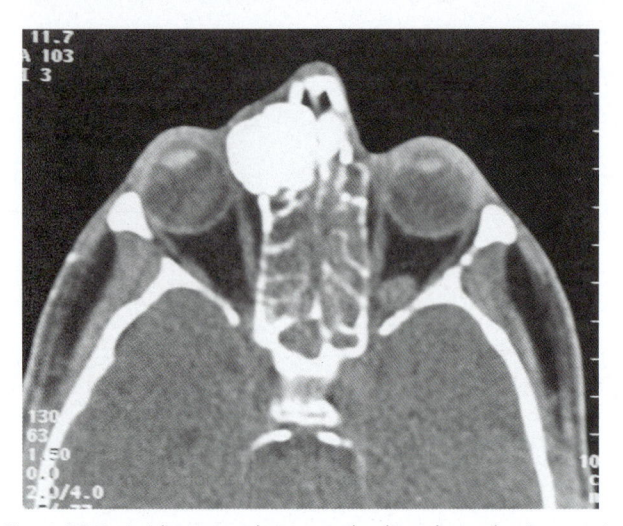

Figure 33.3. Axial computed tomography shows bone density mass in medial aspect of anterior orbit, nasal cavity, and ethmoid sinus.

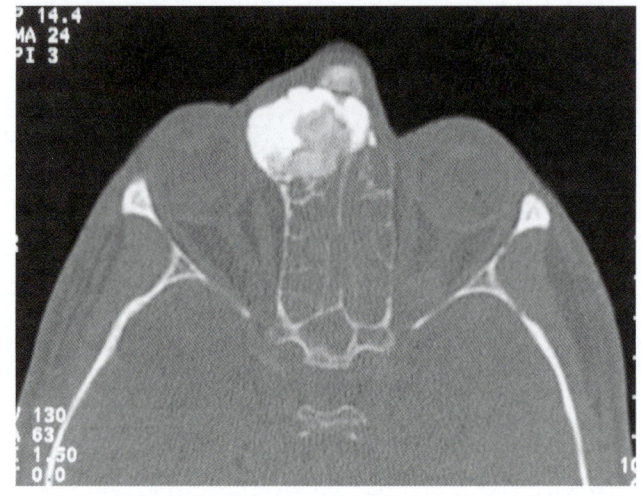

Figure 33.4. Axial computed tomography in bone window setting, showing heterogeneous mass with bone density.

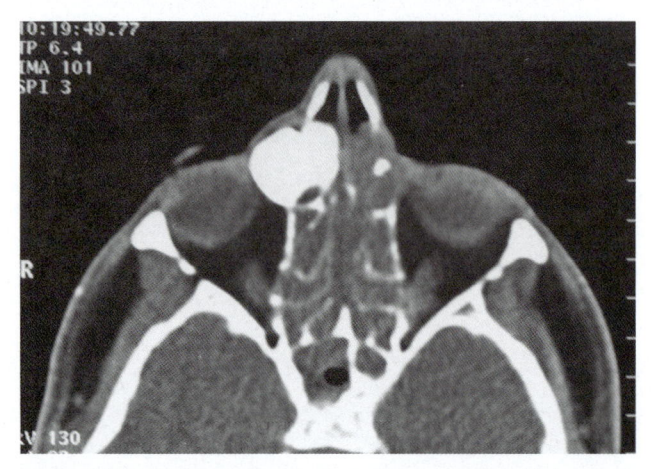

Figure 33.5. Axial computed tomography at a slightly higher level. Note opacity in the contralateral ethmoid sinus. It is uncertain whether the sinusitis is primary or secondary to the osteoma.

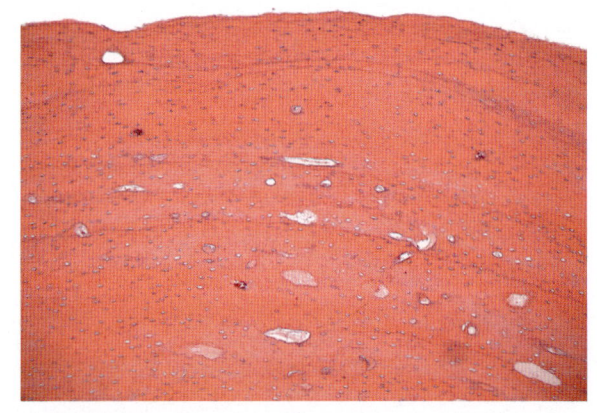

Figure 33.6. Histopathology of orbital osteoma, showing mature bone. (Hematoxylin–eosin ×25.)

ORBITAL OSTEOMA: CLINICOPATHOLOGIC AND IMAGING CORRELATION AND OCCURRENCE IN GARDNER'S SYNDROME

Whitson WE, Orcutt JC, Walkinshaw MD. Orbital osteoma in Gardner's syndrome. *Am J Ophthalmol* 1986;101:236–241.

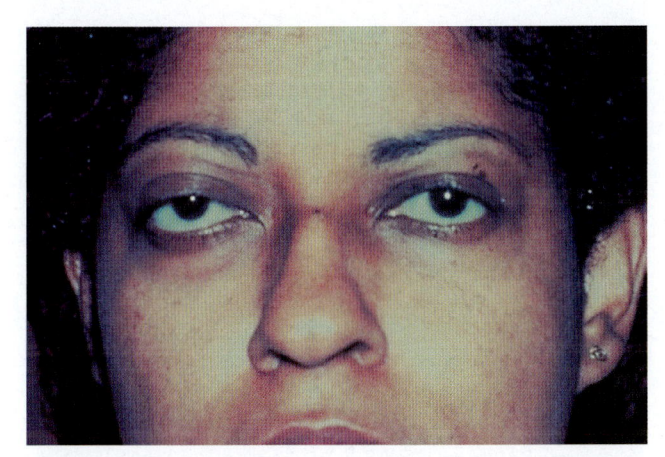

Figure 33.7. Orbital osteoma. Proptosis of the right eye in a 26-year-old woman. (Courtesy of Pearl Rosenbaum, MD and Thomas Slamovitz, MD.)

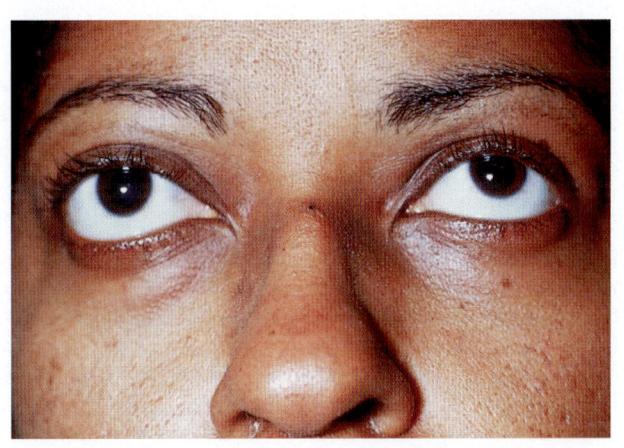

Figure 33.8. Patient shown in Figure 33.7 demonstrating limitation of supraduction of right eye. (Courtesy of Pearl Rosenbaum, MD and Thomas Slamovitz, MD.)

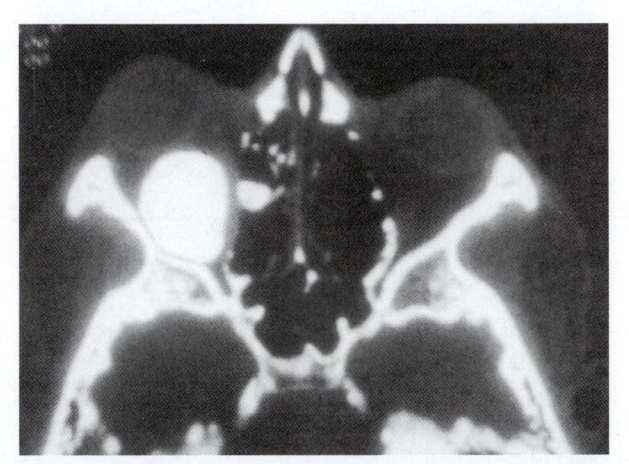

Figure 33.9. Axial computed tomography of patient shown in Figure 33.7, demonstrating a dense mass involving the orbital roof and part of the ethmoid sinus. (Courtesy of Pearl Rosenbaum, MD and Thomas Slamovitz, MD.)

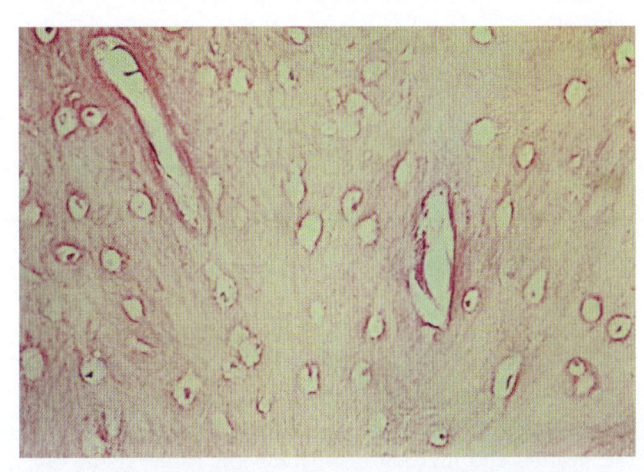

Figure 33.10. Histopathology of lesion shown in Figure 33.9, demonstrating compact bone and minimal fibrous stroma. (Hematoxylin–eosin ×50.) (Courtesy of Pearl Rosenbaum, MD and Thomas Slamovitz, MD.)

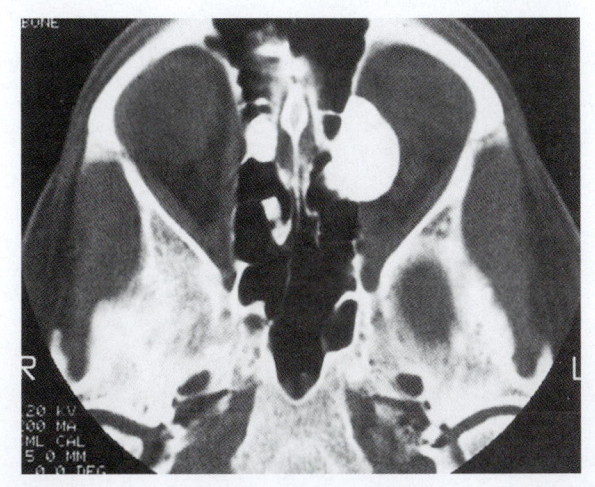

Figure 33.11. Orbital osteoma in Gardner's syndrome. Axial computed tomography showing large bone density mass originating from the medial orbital wall. (Courtesy of James Orcutt, MD.)

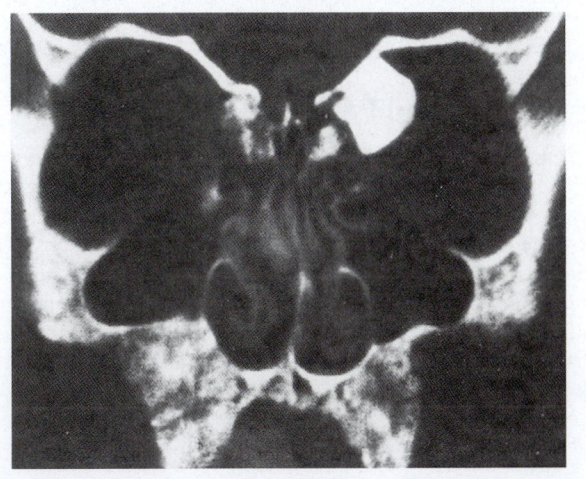

Figure 33.12. Coronal computed tomography of lesion shown in Figure 33.11. (Courtesy of James Orcutt, MD.)

ORBIT OSTEOSARCOMA

General Considerations

Osteosarcoma (osteogenic sarcoma) is the most common primary malignant neoplasm of bone. It occurs twice as frequently as chondrosarcoma and three times more often than Ewing's sarcoma (1). It is a neoplasm of children or young adults that usually originates in long bones and rarely from flat skull bones.

Osteosarcoma can affect the orbital bones as a primary lesion or as a secondary tumor after irradiation for familial retinoblastoma (1–15). It has an increased incidence in patients with Paget's disease and fibrous dysplasia (11,12). There is a close genetic relationship between osteosarcoma and retinoblastoma, with both being linked to a deletion in the long arm of chromosome 13 (7). In the authors' series of 1,264 orbital lesions, the 5 osteosarcomas accounted for 24% of osseous and fibro-osseous tumors and 1% of all orbital tumors (1). All 5 osteosarcomas in our series occurred in patients who had undergone ipsilateral orbital irradiation for hereditary retinoblastoma (1,14). We had no case of primary orbital osteosarcoma (1).

Clinical Features

Primary orbital osteosarcoma characteristically causes a rapid onset and progression of unilateral proptosis, pain, globe displacement, periorbital numbness, eyelid edema, and conjunctival chemosis. When the tumor arises from the ethmoid or frontal bones, there is downward or lateral displacement secondary to a firm, palpable, mass, whereas one arising from the sphenoid wing causes proptosis without a palpable mass (4–6).

Diagnostic Approaches

Orbital CT and magnetic resonance imaging (MRI) generally show an irregular, invasive, destructive bone mass with foci of calcification and invasion of adjacent soft tissue. If the osteoid content is low and the fibrovascular content high, then the lesion appears less dense than bone. In some cases, linear shadows radiate from the main mass because tumor cells grow in fingerlike projections from the main mass. CT shows the bony extent of the lesion; MRI can better delineate the soft tissue component.

Pathology and Pathogenesis

Orbital osteosarcoma is composed of malignant spindle cells with hyperchromatic nuclei and numerous mitotic figures. Osteoid and neoplastic bone formation are readily evident. If there are no bone elements, the lesion is more likely to be diagnosed as a fibrosarcoma. In many cases, the matrix of the tumor contains chondroid and fibromatoid elements and numerous blood vessels (6–8). Thin-walled sinusoidal spaces may contain neoplastic cells, perhaps accounting for the blood-borne metastasis.

Management

Osteosarcoma involving the orbital bones poses a difficult therapeutic challenge. Some authorities advocate preoperative chemotherapy, followed by wide surgical excision, and subsequent chemotherapy or irradiation depending on the clinical and histopathologic findings. The prognosis for patients with osteosarcoma of the orbital bones is generally poor and, historically, most patients have died despite treatment (6). In an analysis of 27 patients with head and neck osteosarcoma, the overall 5-year survival was 55% (6).

Selected References

Reviews

1. Shields JA, Shields CL, Scartozzi R. Survey of 1264 patients with orbital tumors and simulating lesions: the 2002 Montgomery Lecture, part 1. *Ophthalmology* 2004;111: 997–1008.
2. Shields JA, Bakewell B, Augsburger JJ, et al. Classification and incidence of space-occupying lesions of the orbit. A survey of 645 biopsies. *Arch Ophthalmol* 1984;102: 1606–1611.
3. Shields JA, Bakewell B, Augsburger JJ, et al. Space-occupying orbital masses in children: A review of 250 consecutive biopsies. *Ophthalmology* 1986;93:379–384.
4. Fu YS, Perzin KH. Non-epithelial tumors of the nasal cavity, paranasal sinuses, and nasopharynx: a clinicopathologic study. II. Osseous and fibro-osseous lesions, including osteoma, fibrous dysplasia, ossifying fibroma, osteoblastoma, giant cell tumor, and osteosarcoma. *Cancer* 1974;33:1289–1305.
5. Selva D, White VA, O'Connell JX, et al. Primary bone tumors of the orbit. *Surv Ophthalmol* 2004;49:328–342.
6. Ha PK, Eisele DW, Frassica FJ, et al. Osteosarcoma of the head and neck: A review of the Johns Hopkins experience. *Layngoscope* 1999;109:964–969.

Histopathology/Genetics

7. Benedict WF, Fung YK, Murphree AL. The gene responsible for the development of retinoblastoma and osteosarcoma. *Cancer* 1988;62:1691–1694.
8. Blodi FC. Pathology of orbital bones. The XXXII Edward Jackson Memorial Lecture. *Am J Ophthalmol* 1976;81:1–26.

Case Reports

9. de Maeyer VM, Kestelyn PA, Shah AD, et al. Extraskeletal osteosarcoma of the orbit: a clinicopathologic case report and review of the literature. *Indian J Ophthalmol* 2013.
10. Mandel MR, Stewart WB. Periorbital osteosarcoma: an unusual case report and review of the clinical and histopathological features. *Ophthal Plast Reconstr Surg* 1985; 1:129–136.
11. Epley KD, Lasky JB, Karesh JW. Osteosarcoma of the orbit associated with Paget disease. *Ophthal Plast Reconstr Surg* 1998;14:62–66.
12. Goldberg S, Slamovits TL, Dorfman HD, et al. Sarcomatous transformation of the orbit in a patient with Paget's disease. *Ophthalmology* 2000;107:1464–1467.
13. Dhir SP, Munjal VP, Jain IS, et al. Osteosarcoma of the orbit. *J Pediatr Ophthalmol Strabismus* 1980;17:312–314.
14. Abramson DH, Ronner HJ, Ellsworth RM. Second tumors in irradiated bilateral retinoblastoma. *Am J Ophthalmol* 1979;87:624–628.
15. Parmar DN, Luthert PJ, Cree IA, et al. Two unusual osteogenic orbital tumors: presumed parosteal osteosarcomas of the orbit. *Ophthalmology* 2001;108:1452–1456.

Chapter 33 Orbital Osseous, Fibro-osseous, and Cartilaginous Tumors 637

● ORBITAL OSTEOSARCOMA

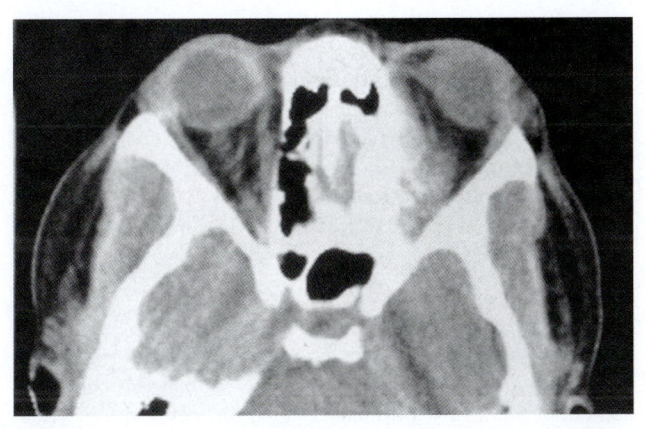

Figure 33.13. Axial computed tomography of a 19-year-old woman with no prior history of retinoblastoma who presented with proptosis of the left eye. Note the diffuse mass in the medial aspect of orbit with involvement of the ethmoid sinus. (Courtesy of Elise Torczynski, MD.)

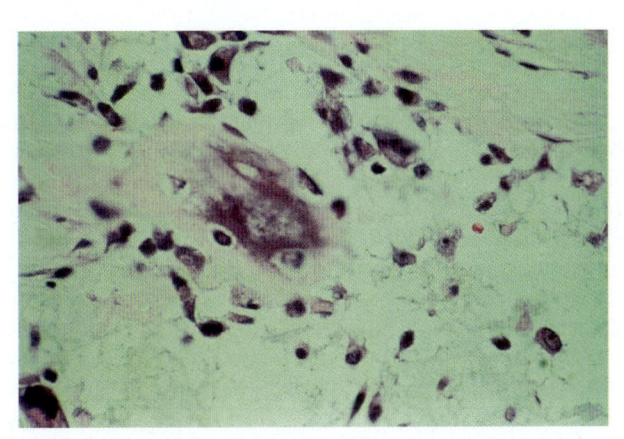

Figure 33.14. Histopathology of lesion shown in Figure 33.13, showing neoplastic cells in a myxomatous matrix. (Hematoxylin–eosin ×200.) (Courtesy of Elise Torczynski, MD.)

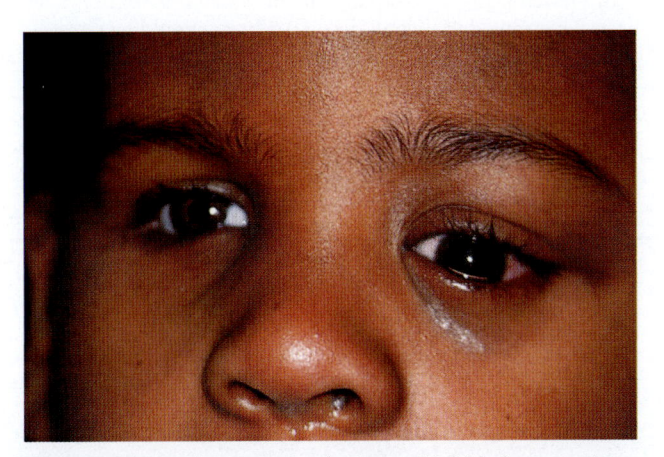

Figure 33.15. Facial appearance of a 5-year-old child who at age 1 year underwent enucleation of the right eye and irradiation of the left eye for retinoblastoma.

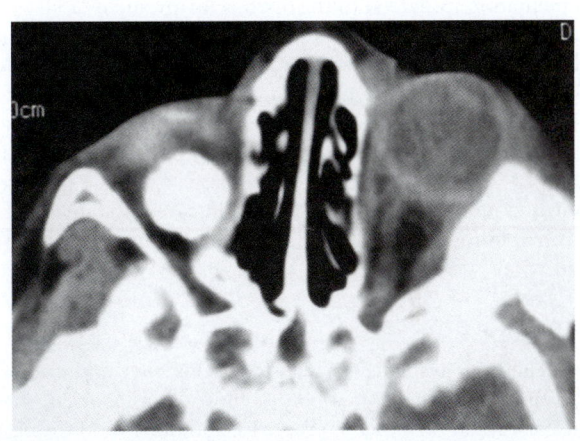

Figure 33.16. Axial computed tomography of child shown in Figure 33.15. Note the orbital implant in the right orbit and the extensive bony mass superotemporally in the left orbit.

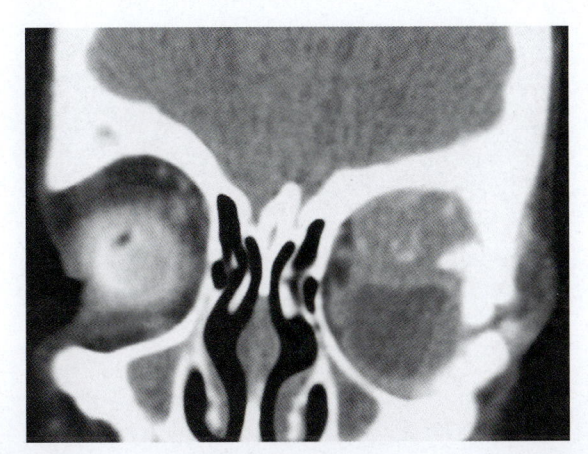

Figure 33.17. Coronal computed tomography of child shown in Figure 33.15. Note the soft tissue component in the superior portion of the left orbit.

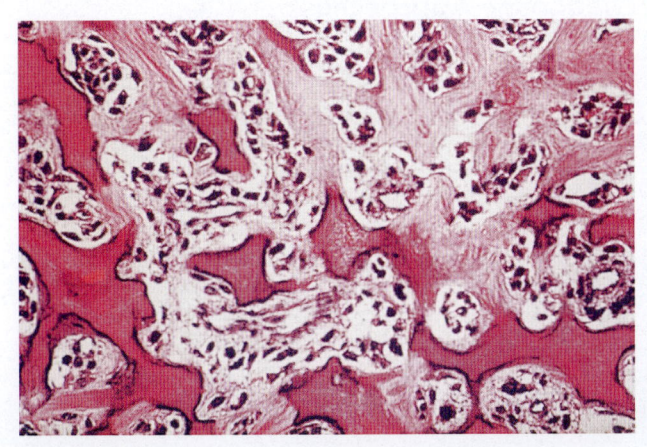

Figure 33.18. Histopathology of another case of osteosarcoma showing bone and malignant spindle cells. (Hematoxylin–eosin ×100.)

ORBITAL FIBROUS DYSPLASIA

General Considerations

Several fibro-osseous lesions can occur in the orbital bones, including fibrous dysplasia, ossifying fibroma, aneurysmal bone cyst, giant cell tumor (osteoclastoma), giant cell reparative granuloma (GCRG), and brown tumor of hyperparathyroidism. Most of these are discussed in more detail elsewhere (1–22) and are not covered in detail here.

Fibrous dysplasia, a fibro-osseous malformation that presumably results from an idiopathic arrest in the maturation of bone at the woven bone stage, can sometimes involve the orbital bones (4–9). It can be monostotic or polyostotic. The monostotic form accounts for 80% of cases, of which 20% affect the craniofacial bones. The frontal bone is most often involved, followed by the sphenoid and ethmoid bones. Orbital fibrous dysplasia is generally of the monostotic form, although it usually involves contiguous bones. The polyostotic form occasionally is found as a part of Albright's syndrome, characterized by precocious puberty in girls and mottled skin pigmentation ipsilateral to the osseous involvement (21).

In the authors' series of 1,264 consecutive space-occupying orbital lesions, the 7 cases of fibrous dysplasia accounted for 33% of fibro-osseous tumors and for 1% of all orbital tumors (1). It was also found to be the most common fibro-osseous lesion among the large series of primary bone tumors of the orbit reported by Selva et al. (5). Fibrous dysplasia has been known to rarely undergo malignant transformation into osteosarcoma, fibrosarcoma, and other neoplasms, particularly after irradiation (5–9).

Clinical Features

Orbital fibrous dysplasia generally has its onset in the first decade (6,8,9). Because the frontal bone is most often involved, there is usually facial asymmetry, proptosis, and downward displacement of the globe. The disease is slowly progressive, although it may slow down or cease in middle life. A secondary aneurysmal bone cyst can develop within fibrous dysplasia (14,18).

Diagnostic Approaches

On computed tomography and MRI, changes in the involved bones range from small translucent zones to large diffuse areas of sclerosis. The lesion can have a "ground glass" appearance and tends to expand the bone with thinning of the overlying cortex (10,11). In the case of sphenoid bone involvement, lateral views best depict the lesion and special optic canal views can detect early compression of the optic foramen. Fibrous dysplasia may have imaging features similar to meningioma, but the latter tends to occur among middle-aged women and may have a homogeneous thickening of bone without the discernible cortical rim (10,11). When necessary, the diagnosis can be confirmed by biopsy.

Pathology

Histopathologically, fibrous dysplasia is composed of benign spindle cells in a fibrous tissue stroma and trabeculae of immature woven bone without osteoblasts. This feature helps to differentiate fibrous dysplasia from ossifying fibroma, in which osteoblasts are usually evident.

Management

Management of fibrous dysplasia of the orbital bones has generally been conservative because the lesion may remain relatively stable for many years. However, in recent years, there has been a tendency by some clinicians to treat this condition earlier. Visual acuity, pupillary evaluation, color vision, visual fields, and coronal CT studies of the optic canals should be done periodically. If the process encroaches on the optic canal or becomes cosmetically unacceptable, then surgical resection and craniofacial reconstruction can be undertaken, usually in conjunction with a neurosurgeon or otolaryngologist. It has been recommended that all dysplastic bone should be removed because progression can continue after incomplete resection (17). Some authors have postulated that visual loss is more likely owing to secondary mucocele or hemorrhage in the lesion.

ORBITAL FIBROUS DYSPLASIA

Selected References

Reviews

1. Shields JA, Shields CL, Scartozzi R. Survey of 1264 patients with orbital tumors and simulating lesions: the 2002 Montgomery Lecture, part 1. *Ophthalmology* 2004;111: 997–1008.
2. Shields JA, Bakewell B, Augsburger JJ, et al. Classification and incidence of space-occupying lesions of the orbit. A survey of 645 biopsies. *Arch Ophthalmol* 1984;102: 1606–1611.
3. Shields JA, Bakewell B, Augsburger JJ, et al. Space-occupying orbital masses in children: a review of 250 consecutive biopsies. *Ophthalmology* 1986;93:379–384.
4. Fu YS, Perzin KH. Non-epithelial tumors of the nasal cavity, paranasal sinuses, and nasopharynx: a clinicopathologic study. II. Osseous and fibro-osseous lesions, including osteoma, fibrous dysplasia, ossifying fibroma, osteoblastoma, giant cell tumor, and osteosarcoma. *Cancer* 1974;33:1289–1305.
5. Selva D, White VA, O'Connell JX, et al. Primary bone tumors of the orbit. *Surv Ophthalmol* 2004;49:328–342.
6. Moore RT. Fibrous dysplasia of the orbit. Review. *Surv Ophthalmol* 1969;13: 321–334.
7. Hullar TE, Lustig LR. Paget's disease and fibrous dysplasia. *Otolaryngol Clin North Am* 2003;36:707–732.
8. Liakos GM, Walder CB, Carruth JA. Ocular complications in craniofacial fibrous dysplasia. *Br J Ophthalmol* 1979;63:611–616.
9. Osguthorpe JD, Gudeman SK. Orbital complications of fibrous dysplasia. *Otolaryngol Head Neck Surg* 1987;97:403–405.

Imaging

10. Faul S, Link J, Behrendt S, et al. MRI features of craniofacial fibrous dysplasia. *Orbit* 1998;17:125–132.
11. Wenig BM, Mafee MF, Ghosh L. Fibro-osseous, osseous, and cartilaginous lesions of the orbit and paraorbital region. Correlative clinicopathologic and radiographic features, including the diagnostic role of CT and MR imaging. *Radiol Clin North Am* 1998;36:1241–1259.

Case Reports

12. Ronner HJ, Trokel SL, Hilal SK. Acute blindness in a patient with fibrous dysplasia. *Orbit* 1982;1:231–234.
13. Moore AT, Buncic JR, Munro IR. Fibrous dysplasia of the orbit in childhood. Clinical features and management. *Ophthalmology* 1985;92:12–20.
14. Yuen VH, Jordan DR, Jabi M, et al. Aneurysmal bone cyst associated with fibrous dysplasia. *Ophthal Plast Reconstr Surg* 2002;18:471–474.
15. Joseph E, Kachhara R, Bhattacharya RN, et al. Fibrous dysplasia of the orbit in an infant. *Pediatr Neurosurg* 2000;32:205–208.
16. Michael CB, Lee AG, Patrinely JR, et al. Visual loss associated with fibrous dysplasia of the anterior skull base. Case report and review of the literature. *J Neurosurg* 2000;92:350–354.
17. Jan M, Dweik A, Destrieux C, et al. Fronto-orbital sphenoidal fibrous dysplasia. *Neurosurgery* 1994;34:544–547.
18. Lucarelli MJ, Bilyk JR, Shore JW, et al. Aneurysmal bone cyst of the orbit associated with fibrous dysplasia. *Plast Reconstr Surg* 1995;96:440–445.
19. Bibby K, McFadzean R. Fibrous dysplasia of the orbit. *Br J Ophthalmol* 1994;78: 266–270.
20. Donoso, LA, Magargal LE, Eiferman RA. Fibrous dysplasia of the orbit with optic nerve decompression. *Ann Ophthalmol* 1982;14:80–83.
21. Sevel D, James HE, Burns R, et al. McCune-Albright syndrome (fibrous dysplasia) associated with an orbital tumor. *Ann Ophthalmol* 1984;16:283–289.
22. Cruz AA, Constanzi M, de Castro FA, et al. Apical involvement with fibrous dysplasia: implications for vision. *Ophthal Plast Reconstr Surg* 2007;23:450–454.

ORBITAL FIBROUS DYSPLASIA

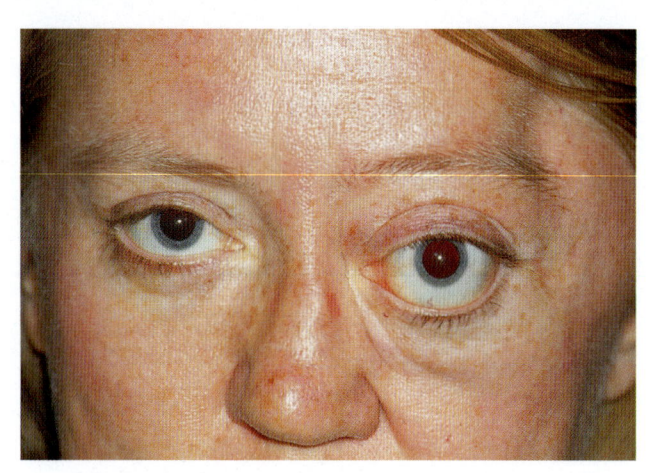

Figure 33.19. Massive proptosis and swelling of the temporal fossa in a 38-year-old woman with fibrous dysplasia.

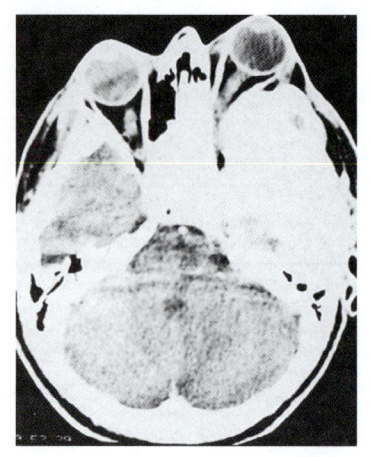

Figure 33.20. Axial computed tomography of patient shown in Figure 33.19, demonstrating the extensive mass involving the orbit, temporal fossa, and cranial cavity.

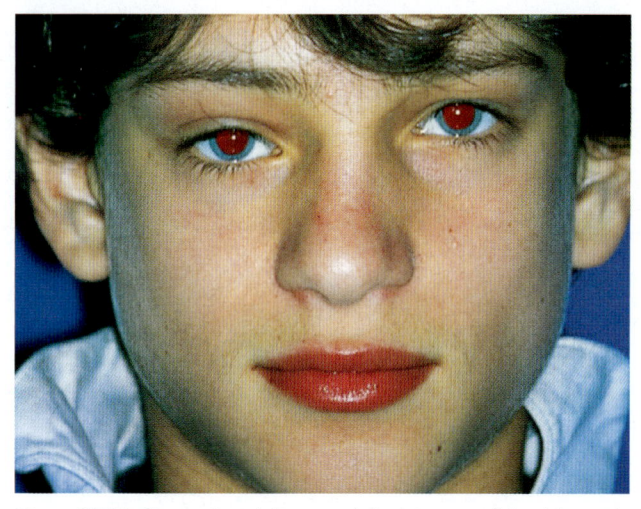

Figure 33.21. Proptosis and downward displacement of the right eye in a 13-year-old boy with fibrous dysplasia.

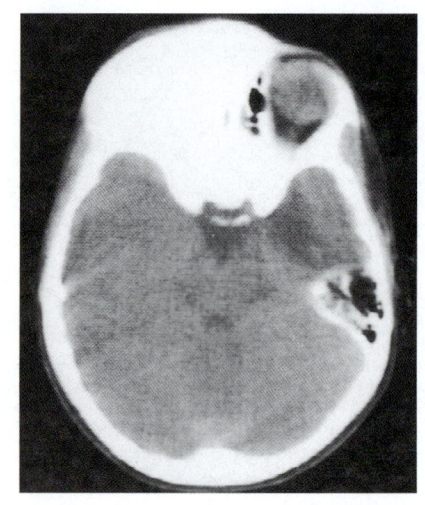

Figure 33.22. Axial computed tomography through superior aspect of the orbit of patient shown in Figure 33.21 demonstrating the extent of the bony lesion.

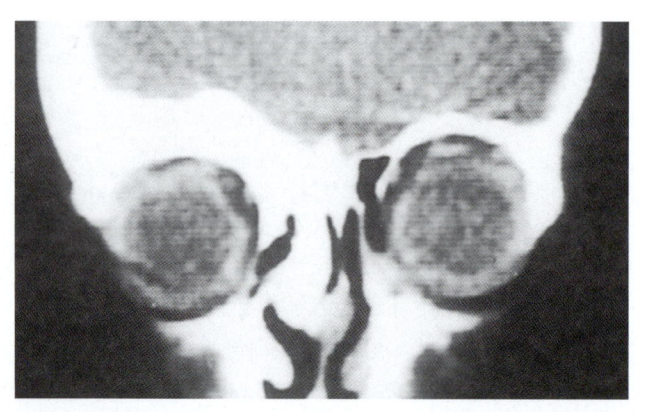

Figure 33.23. Coronal computed tomography of patient shown in Figure 33.21, demonstrating diffuse thickening of the frontal bone.

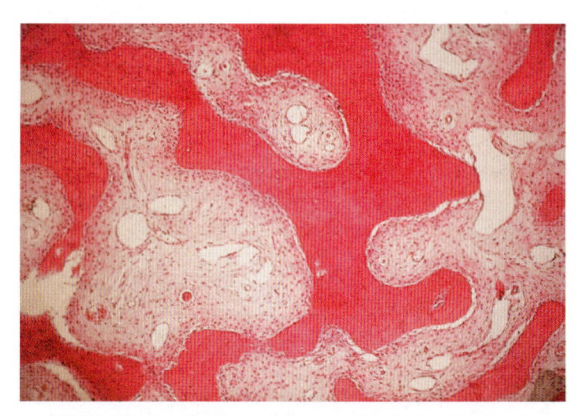

Figure 33.24. Histopathology of fibrous dysplasia showing immature woven bone. (Hematoxylin–eosin ×50.)

Chapter 33 Orbital Osseous, Fibro-osseous, and Cartilaginous Tumors 641

ORBITAL FIBROUS DYSPLASIA

In many cases, fibrous dysplasia may be difficult to differentiate clinically from meningioma.

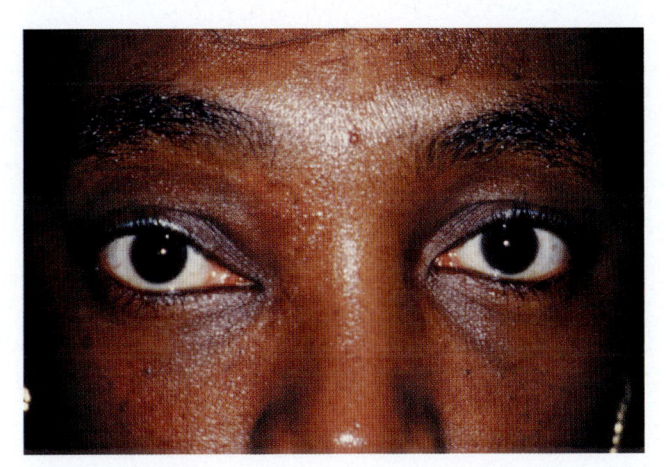

Figure 33.25. Slight proptosis and lateral displacement of right eye in a middle-aged woman.

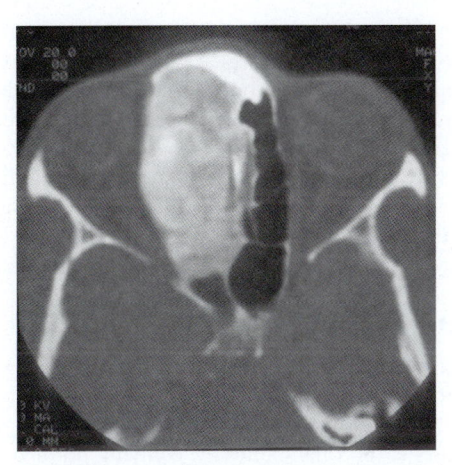

Figure 33.26. Axial computed tomography with bone window setting of patient shown in Figure 33.25 demonstrating extensive fibrous dysplasia in right ethmoid sinus and medial portion of the right orbit.

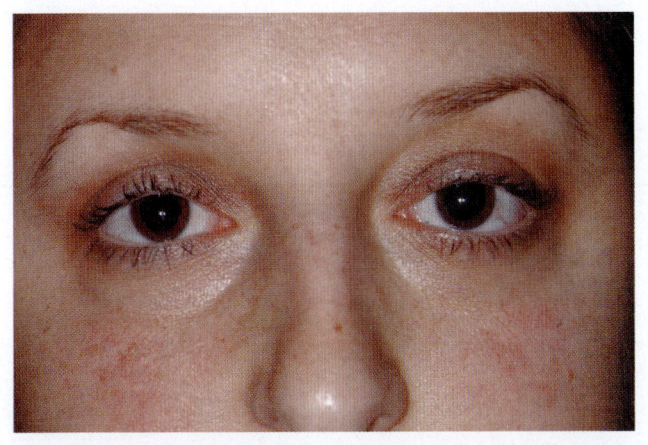

Figure 33.27. Young adult woman with slight upward displacement of left eye and mild left proptosis.

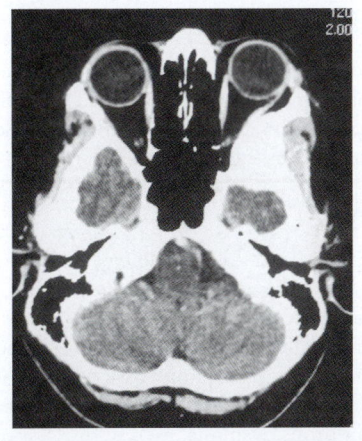

Figure 33.28. Axial computed tomography of patient shown in Figure 33.27, showing fibrous dysplasia involving the sphenoid bone. Note the similarity to the sphenoid wing meningioma discussed earlier.

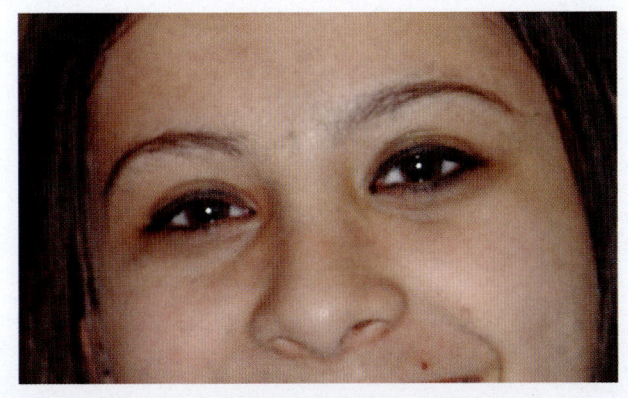

Figure 33.29. Young woman with slight proptosis of left eye.

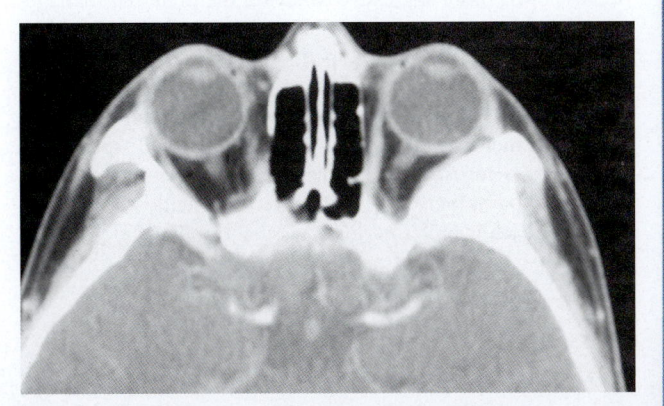

Figure 33.30. Axial computed tomography of patient shown in Figure 33.29, demonstrating extensive involvement of left sphenoid bone. This patient had cutaneous features of Albright's syndrome and orbital fibrous dysplasia.

ORBITAL OSSIFYING FIBROMA

General Considerations

Ossifying fibroma is an acquired benign tumor of bone, in contrast with fibrous dysplasia, which is believed to be an arrest in the normal development of bone (1–20). The lesion has a predilection for the mandible, but, when the orbit is affected, the frontal, ethmoid, and maxillary bones are primarily involved (4–10). This tumor tends to manifest in young adults. In the authors' series of 1,264 consecutive space-occupying orbital lesions, the 3 ossifying fibromas accounted for 14% of the fibro-osseous tumors and for <1% of all orbital tumors (1).

Clinical Features

Ossifying fibroma that involves the orbit produces gradual proptosis and displacement of the globe, the direction depending on which orbital bones are affected. Involvement of the adjacent sinuses is the rule. Clinically, ossifying fibroma seems to be more aggressive than fibrous dysplasia. It begins as a monostotic lesion, but can gradually extend to involve adjacent bones and even extend to the opposite orbit (4–7).

Diagnostic Approaches

Computed tomography of ossifying fibroma demonstrates a round to ovoid expansion of the involved bone that may have a nonhomogeneous matrix and a thin rim of sclerotic bone around the margins of the lesion (8–10).

Pathology

On low magnification histopathology, ossifying fibroma is characteristically composed of benign spindle cells in a vascular fibrous stroma, with scattered bony ossicles that closely resemble psammoma bodies seen in meningioma. Hence, the tumor has been called "psammomatoid ossifying fibroma" (10,13–20). A thin rim of osteoblasts can help to differentiate ossifying fibroma from fibrous dysplasia.

Management

Because of its more aggressive behavior, the preferred management of orbital ossifying fibroma is early surgical removal. Most affected patients have developed progressive symptoms that justify surgical removal combined with craniofacial reconstruction (11–20). In extensive cases, a multidisciplinary approach to management is advisable, including orbital specialists, radiologists, neurosurgeons, otolaryngologists, craniofacial surgeons, and pathologists (11). More recently, endoscopic transnasal approach is preferred for accessible tumors (12).

ORBITAL OSSIFYING FIBROMA

Selected References

Reviews

1. Shields JA, Shields CL, Scartozzi R. Survey of 1264 patients with orbital tumors and simulating lesions: the 2002 Montgomery Lecture, part 1. *Ophthalmology* 2004;111:997–1008.
2. Shields JA, Bakewell B, Augsburger JJ, et al. Classification and incidence of space-occupying lesions of the orbit. A survey of 645 biopsies. *Arch Ophthalmol* 1984;102:1606–1611.
3. Shields JA, Bakewell B, Augsburger JJ, et al. Space-occupying orbital masses in children: A review of 250 consecutive biopsies. *Ophthalmology* 1986;93:379–384.
4. Fu YS, Perzin KH. Non-epithelial tumors of the nasal cavity, paranasal sinuses, and nasopharynx: a clinicopathologic study. II. Osseous and fibro-osseous lesions, including osteoma, fibrous dysplasia, ossifying fibroma, osteoblastoma, giant cell tumor, and osteosarcoma. *Cancer* 1974;33:1289–1305.
5. Selva D, White VA, O'Connell JX, et al. Primary bone tumors of the orbit. *Surv Ophthalmol* 2004;49:328–342.
6. Sarode SC, Sarode GS, Waknis P, et al. Juvenile psammomatoid ossifying fibroma: A review. *Oral Oncol* 2011;47:1110–1116.
7. Wakefield MJ, Ross AH, Damato EM, et al. Review of lateral wall ossifying fibroma. *Orbit* 2010;29:317–320.

Imaging

8. Shields JA, Nelson LB, Brown JF, et al. Clinical, computed tomographic, and histopathologic characteristics of juvenile ossifying fibroma with orbital involvement. *Am J Ophthalmol* 1983;96:650–653.
9. Shields JA, Peyster RG, Augsburger JJ, et al. Massive juvenile ossifying fibroma of maxillary sinus with orbital involvement. *Br J Ophthalmol* 1985;69:392–395.
10. Chung EM, Murphey MD, Specht CS, et al. From the archives of the AFIP. Pediatric orbital tumors and tumorlike lesions: osseous lesions of the orbit. *Radiographics* 2008;28:1193–1214.

Management

11. Hartstein ME, Grove AS Jr, Woog JJ, et al. The multidisciplinary management of psammomatoid ossifying fibroma of the orbit. *Ophthalmology* 1998;105:591–595.

Case Reports

12. Berhouma M, Jacquesson T, Abouaf L, et al. Endoscopic endonasal optic nerve and orbital apex decompression for nontraumatic optic neuropathy: surgical nuances and review of the literature. *Neurosurg Focus* 2014;37:E19.
13. Margo CE, Ragsdale BD, Perman KI, et al. Psammomatoid (juvenile) ossifying fibroma of the orbit. *Ophthalmology* 1985;92:150–159.
14. Jordan DR, Farmer J, DaSilva V. Psammomatoid ossifying fibroma of the orbit. *Can J Ophthalmol* 1992;27:194–196.
15. Tunc M, Char DH. Ossifying fibroma of the lateral orbital wall in an adult. *Orbit* 1999;18:291–293.
16. Fakadej A, Boynton JR. Juvenile ossifying fibroma of the orbit. *Ophthal Plast Reconstr Surg* 1996;12:174–177.
17. Nakagawa K, Takasato Y, Ito Y, et al. Ossifying fibroma involving the paranasal sinuses, orbit, and anterior cranial fossa: case report. *Neurosurgery* 1995;36:1192–1195.
18. Khalil MK, Leib ML. Cemento-ossifying fibroma of the orbit. *Can J Ophthalmol* 1979;14:195–200.
19. Lehrer HZ. Ossifying fibroma of the orbital roof. Its distinction from "blistering" or "intra-osseous" meningioma. *Arch Neurol* 1969;20:536–541.
20. Margo CE, Weiss A, Habal MB. Psammomatoid ossifying fibroma. *Arch Ophthalmol* 1986;104:1347–1351.

ORBITAL OSSIFYING FIBROMA

1. Shields JA, Nelson LB, Brown JF, et al. Clinical, computed tomographic, and histopathologic characteristics of juvenile ossifying fibroma with orbital involvement. *Am J Ophthalmol* 1983;96:650–653.
2. Shields JA, Peyster RG, Augsburger JJ, et al. Massive juvenile ossifying fibroma of maxillary sinus with orbital involvement. *Br J Ophthalmol* 1985;69:392–395.

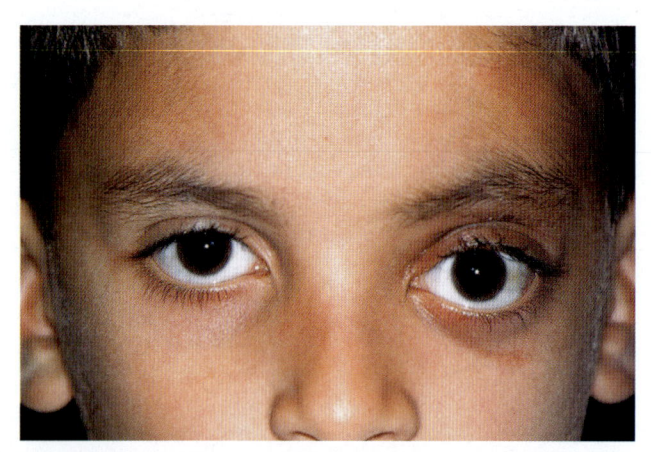

Figure 33.31. Proptosis and downward displacement of the left eye in an 8-year-old boy.

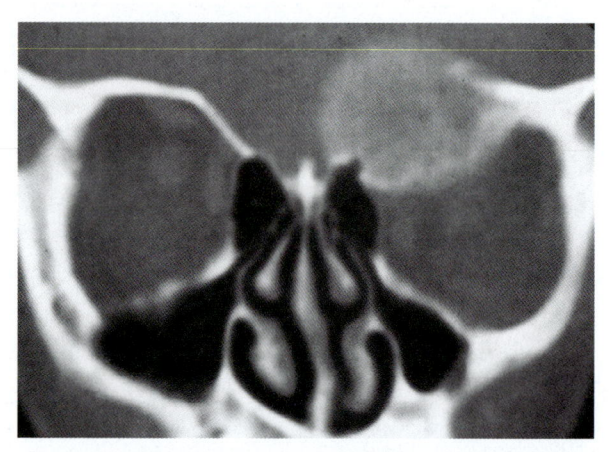

Figure 33.32. Coronal computed tomography of patient shown in Figure 33.31, demonstrating the ovoid heterogeneous mass of the frontal bone and the orbital roof.

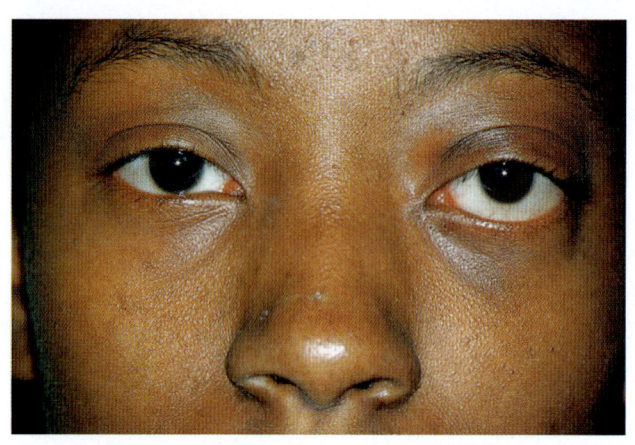

Figure 33.33. Proptosis and upward displacement of the left eye in a 14-year-old girl.

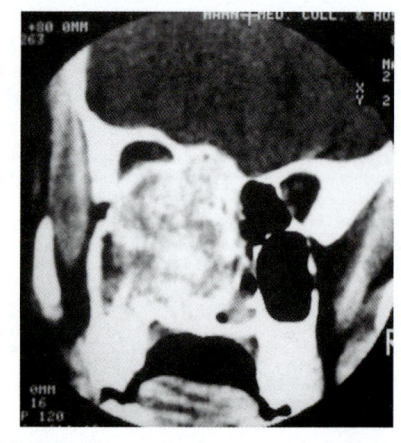

Figure 33.34. Coronal computed tomography of patient shown in Figure 33.33, demonstrating the large mass in maxillary sinus invading through the floor of the orbit.

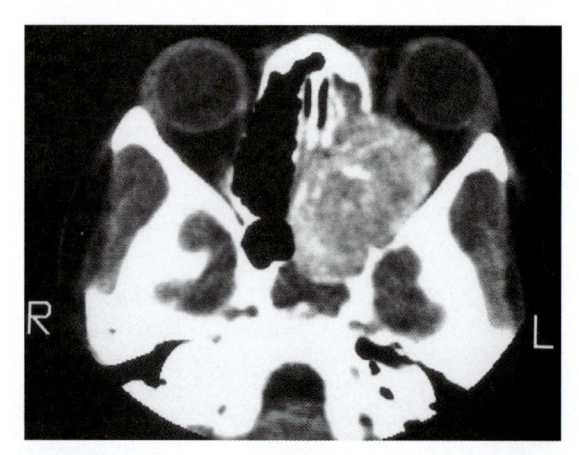

Figure 33.35. Axial computed tomography of patient shown in Figure 33.33, demonstrating the involvement of the posterior aspect of the orbit by the lesion.

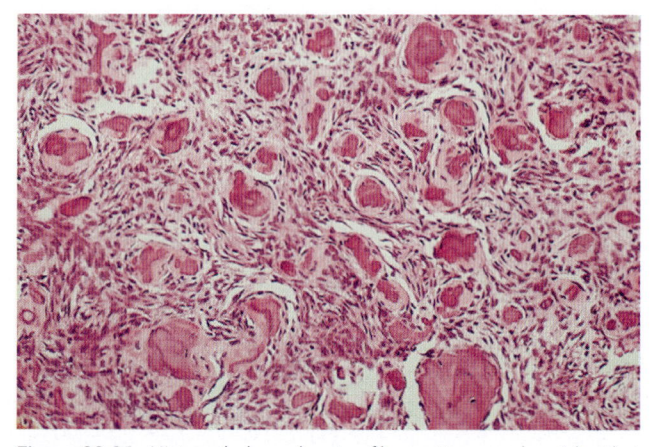

Figure 33.36. Histopathology showing fibrous tissue and ossicles that resemble psammoma bodies. (Hematoxylin–eosin ×100.)

ORBITAL OSSIFYING FIBROMA

Orbital involvement by ossifying fibroma usually has its clinical onset in the first or second decade and has typical radiographic features and histopathologic characteristics.

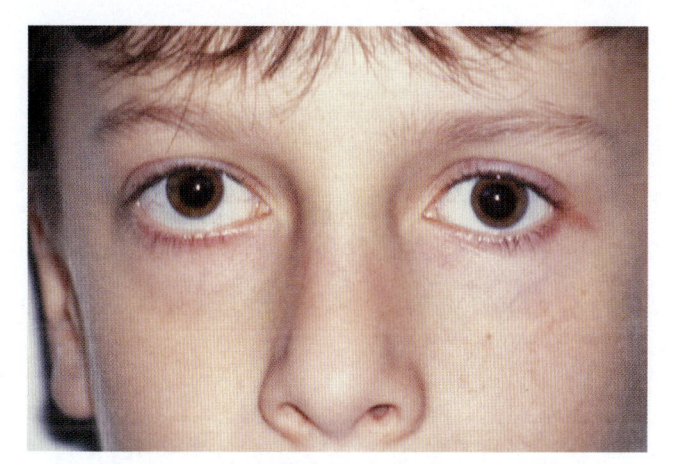

Figure 33.37. Proptosis and upward displacement of right eye in an 11-year-old boy.

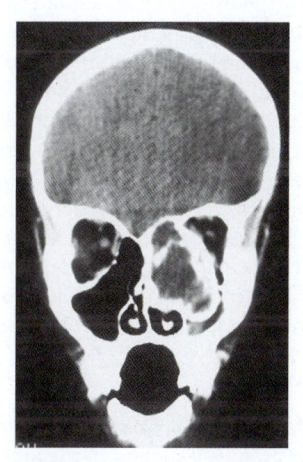

Figure 33.38. Coronal computed tomography of patient shown in Figure 33.37, depicting the bone ossicles that characterize some of these lesions.

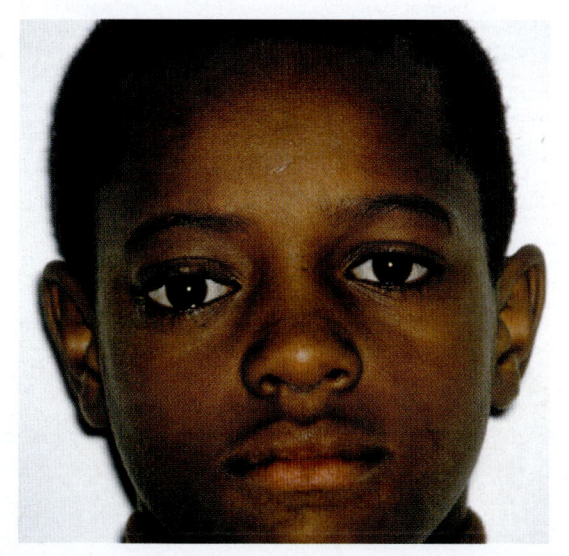

Figure 33.39. Proptosis and downward displacement of right eye in a 10-year-old boy.

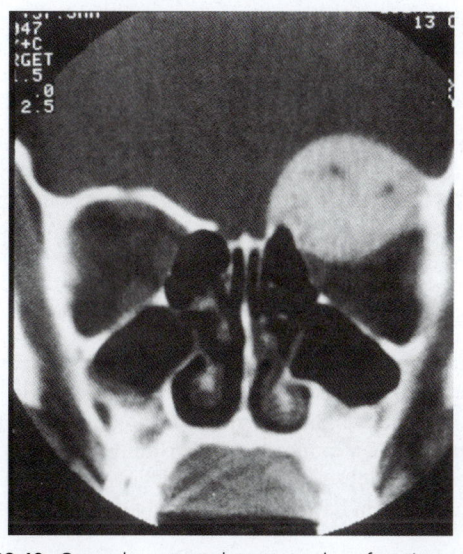

Figure 33.40. Coronal computed tomography of patient shown in Figure 33.39, demonstrating heterogeneous ovoid mass of frontal bone. In this case the right eye is shown on the right, because of rotation.

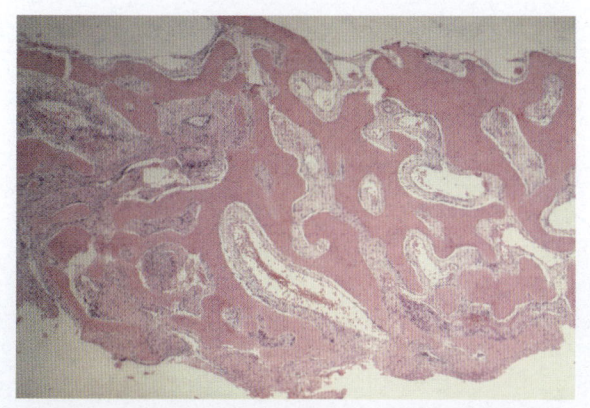

Figure 33.41. Photomicrograph of same patient, showing immature bone with vascularized fibrous connective tissue septae. (Hematoxylin–eosin ×20.)

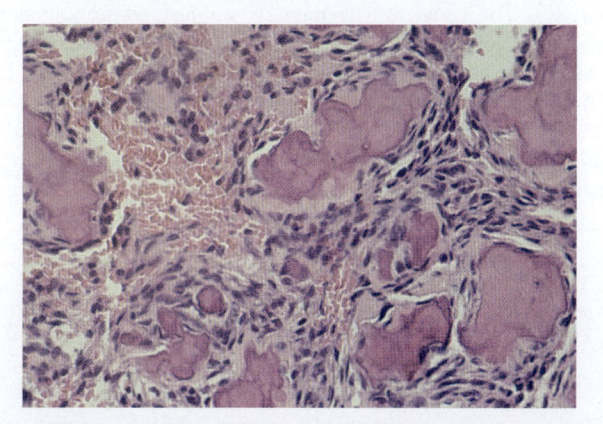

Figure 33.42. Higher-magnification histopathology of same case showing the psammomatoid ossicles that superficially resemble the psammoma bodies often seen in meningiomas. (Hematoxylin–eosin ×100.)

ORBITAL GIANT CELL REPARATIVE GRANULOMA

General Considerations

GCRG is a benign granulomatous lesion that is theorized to be a reparative response to hemorrhage secondary to trauma (1–15). It has been suggested that the word "reparative" be dropped. This would leave the term "giant cell granuloma" to describe this entity. However, there are many different granulomas that contain giant cells and hence that term is not specific enough. Therefore, we retain the term "GCRG" for this discussion, with the realization that a better term may eventually be adopted. GCRG usually occurs in the mandible, maxilla, or phalanges. It can occasionally involve the bones of the skull and orbit (4,5). It is considered rare, with only 1 case recognized in the authors' series of 1,264 orbital lesions (1).

Clinical Features

In the orbit, GCRG generally occurs in children and young adults as a slowly progressive lesion in the orbital roof that can cause proptosis and, less often, downward displacement of the globe, diplopia, pain, and visual loss. Bilateral GCRG has been seen in a patient with cherubism, but the relationship between the two is vague and it may be a coincidental occurrence (15).

Diagnostic Approaches

With imaging studies it appears as a fibro-osseous mass with features similar to ossifying fibroma or aneurysmal bone cyst, often with blood cysts, lysis, and expansion of bone. Clinically and radiographically, it may closely resemble an organizing subperiosteal abscess in the superior orbit.

Pathology

Histopathologically, GCRG consists of a fibrous stroma with giant cells, spindle cells, and organizing blood. It may be difficult to differentiate from organizing hematoma, giant cell tumor, brown tumor of hyperparathyroidism, or other fibro-osseous lesions. The histopathologic details that help in this differentiation have been published (4–13).

Management

There are no established guidelines for management of orbital GCRG. The usual management is surgical excision, generally by curettage (6). Supplemental systemic corticosteroids may hasten resolution of residual mass. Radiotherapy can be attempted for difficult cases, but it is generally not advisable. Some aggressive cases have required orbital exenteration. In other instances, residual tumor has been known to resolve after partial excision (9).

Selected References

Reviews

1. Shields JA, Shields CL, Scartozzi R. Survey of 1264 patients with orbital tumors and simulating lesions: the 2002 Montgomery Lecture, part 1. *Ophthalmology* 2004;111:997–1008.
2. Shields JA, Bakewell B, Augsburger JJ, et al. Classification and incidence of space-occupying lesions of the orbit. A survey of 645 biopsies. *Arch Ophthalmol* 1984;102:1606–1611.
3. Shields JA, Bakewell B, Augsburger JJ, et al. Space-occupying orbital masses in children: A review of 250 consecutive biopsies. *Ophthalmology* 1986;93:379–384.
4. Fu YS, Perzin KH. Non-epithelial tumors of the nasal cavity, paranasal sinuses, and nasopharynx: a clinicopathologic study. II. Osseous and fibro-osseous lesions, including osteoma, fibrous dysplasia, ossifying fibroma, osteoblastoma, giant cell tumor, and osteosarcoma. *Cancer* 1974;33:1289–1305.
5. Selva D, White VA, O'Connell JX, et al. Primary bone tumors of the orbit. *Surv Ophthalmol* 2004;49:328–342.

Histopathology

6. D'Ambrosio AL, Williams SC, Lignelli A, et al. Clinicopathologic review: giant cell reparative egranuloma of the orbit. *Neurosurgery* 2005;57:773–778.

Case Reports

7. Sood GC, Malik SR, Gupta DK, et al. Reparative granuloma of the orbit causing unilateral proptosis. *Am J Ophthalmol* 1967;63:524–527.
8. Sebag J, Chapman P, Truman J, et al. Giant cell granuloma of the orbit with intracranial extension. *Neurosurgery* 1985;16:75–78.
9. Hoopes PC, Anderson RI, Blodi FC. Giant cell (reparative) granuloma of the orbit. *Ophthalmology* 1981;88:1361–1366.
10. Mercado GV, Shields CL, Gunduz K, et al. Giant cell reparative granuloma of the orbit. *Am J Ophthalmol* 1999;127:485–487.
11. Font RL, Blanco G, Soparkar CN, et al. Giant cell reparative granuloma of the orbit associated with Cherubism. *Ophthalmology* 2003;110:1846–1849.
12. Chawla B, Khurana S, Kashyap S. Giant cell reparative granuloma of the orbit. *Ophthal Plast Reconstr Surg* 2013;29:e94–e95.
13. Cecchetti DF, Paula SA, Cruz AA, et al. Orbital involvement in craniofacial brown tumors. *Ophthal Plast Reconstr Surg* 2010;26:106–111.
14. Pherwani AA, Brooker D, Lacey B. Giant cell reparative granuloma of the orbit. *Ophthal Plast Reconstr Surg* 2005;21:463–465.
15. Schultze-Mosgau S, Holbach LM, Wiltfang J. Cherubism: clinical evidence and therapy. *J Craniofac Surg* 2003;14:201–206.

ORBITAL GIANT CELL REPARATIVE GRANULOMA

A clinicopathologic correlation of a lesion diagnosed as a GCRG is shown. The initial diagnosis was aneurysmal bone cyst, but several ophthalmic pathology consultants favored the diagnosis of GCRG.

Mercado GV, Shields CL, Gunduz K, et al. Giant cell reparative granuloma of the orbit. *Am J Ophthalmol* 1999;127:485–487.

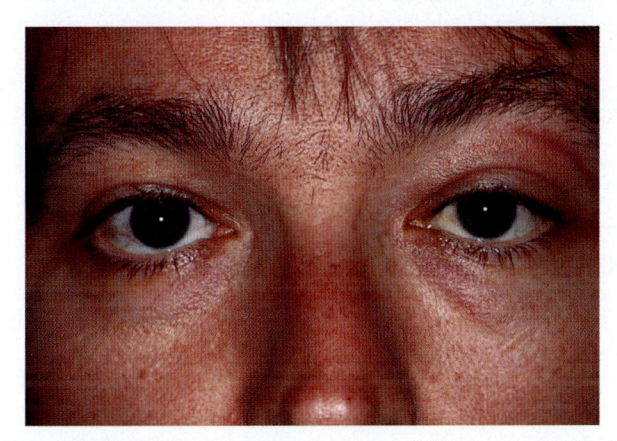

Figure 33.43. Proptosis of the left eye in a 38-year-old man. He is shown here after an incisional biopsy was done. A healed eyelid crease incision is evident.

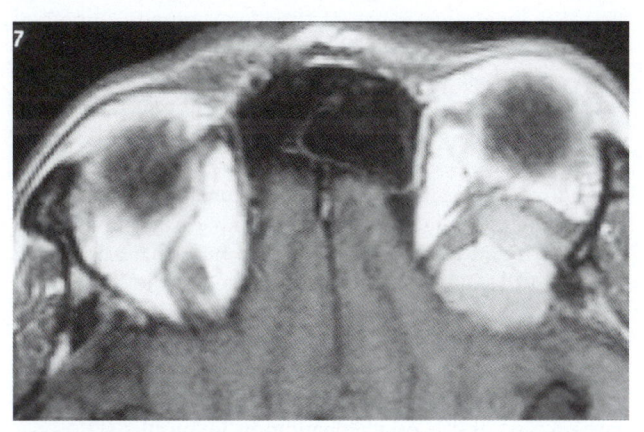

Figure 33.44. Axial magnetic resonance imaging in T1-weighted image demonstrating the cystic character of the lesion with a blood-fluid layer within a cyst.

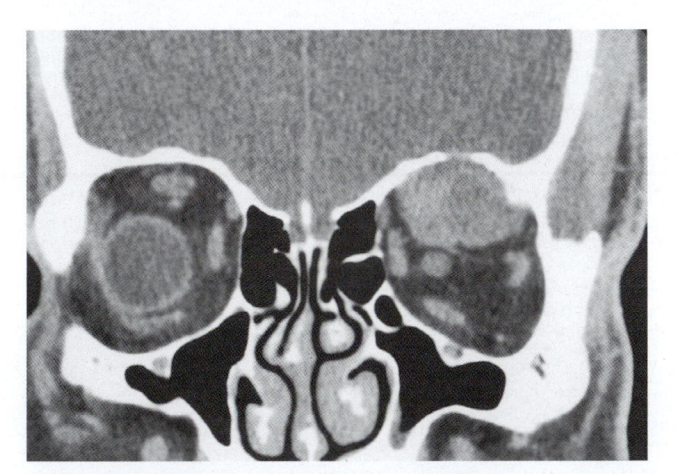

Figure 33.45. Coronal computed tomography showing same mass in orbit superiorly with erosion of the bony roof of the orbit.

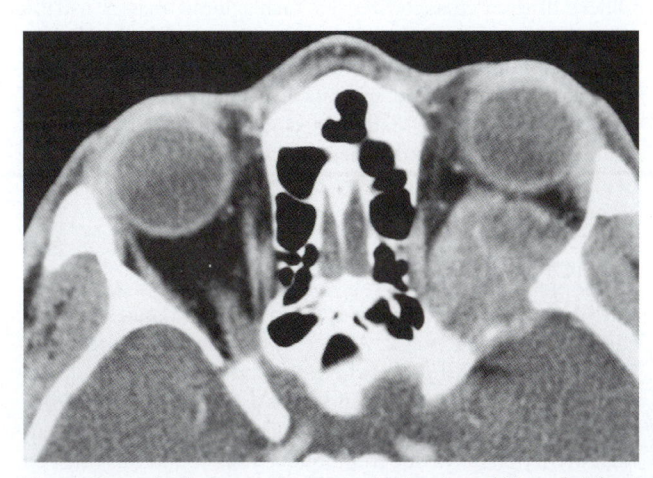

Figure 33.46. Axial computed tomography showing a fairly well-defined mass near the orbital apex. Note the erosion of the lateral wall of the orbit.

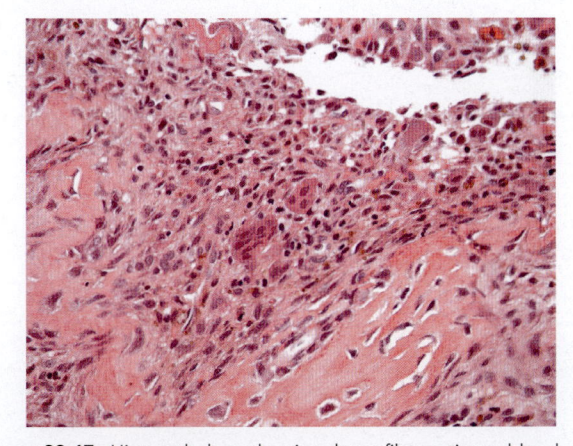

Figure 33.47. Histopathology showing dense fibrous tissue, blood, and giant cells. (Hematoxylin–eosin ×100.)

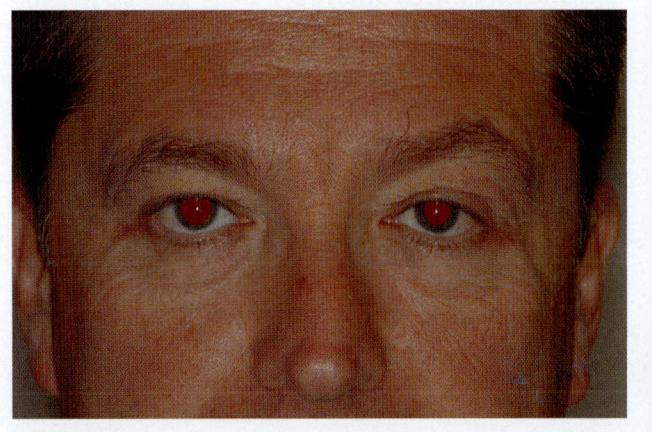

Figure 33.48. At 15-year follow-up, the patient remains healthy without recurrence.

ORBITAL CARTILAGINOUS CHONDROMA

General Considerations

Cartilaginous hamartoma and chondroma are terms that define benign tumors composed almost exclusively of cartilage (1–13). Chondroma is one of the most common tumors of bone (6). Enchondroma is a benign variant of chondroma that arises within bone (13). It can develop in any bone that develops from cartilage. It is often small and asymptomatic, but can occasionally be large enough to produce symptoms.

Acquired cartilaginous tumors of the orbit can be benign (chondroma) or malignant (chondrosarcoma) (5). The trochlea of the superior oblique muscle is the only cartilaginous tissue normally found in the orbit. A benign mass that arises from mature cartilaginous trochlea is designated a true chondroma of the orbit. A tumor that develops from primitive mesenchyme destined to form mature cartilage is better designated as cartilaginous hamartoma. Both true chondroma and cartilaginous hamartoma are rare in the orbit. To our knowledge, we have no cases of true orbital chondroma in our files (1).

Multiple enchondromas (enchondromatoses) can affect the orbit bones in certain syndromes. It has been reported in Ollier's disease, characterized by cartilaginous masses usually located in long bones (11). It has been seen in Maffucci's syndrome, an idiopathic congenital disease characterized by multiple enchondromas and soft tissue hemangiomas (12). One reported patient with Maffucci's syndrome also had multiple bilateral orbital cavernous hemangiomas (12). It is possible that a chondroma can undergo malignant transformation into chondrosarcoma (11).

Clinical Features

Cartilaginous hamartoma can appear in childhood as a circumscribed orbital mass. A true chondroma is more likely to develop in adulthood and is expected to occur as a slowly enlarging hard mass in the upper nasal quadrant of the orbit, corresponding to the area of the trochlea (9). It can compromise the action of the superior oblique muscle and this must be taken into account if surgical removal is considered.

Diagnostic Approaches

There are too few cases to have meaningful information regarding imaging studies of orbital chondroma. It would be expected to appear as a circumscribed orbital mass with bony consistency.

Pathology

Microscopically, chondroma is composed of well-differentiated hyaline cartilage. It can show a mild degree of nuclear atypia that should not be confused with chondrosarcoma (4–6). Enchondroma appears as hypocellular lobules of cartilage enclosed by lamellar bone (13).

Management

Because primary orbital chondroma appears to be slowly progressive, circumscribed lesions, it can be managed by observation or excisional biopsy depending on patient symptoms. The surgical route can vary with the location of the lesion but the typical superonasal anterior tumor arising from the trochlea should be approached by a superonasal orbitotomy using a transconjunctival, cutaneous, or endoscopic transnasal route depending on the clinical and radiographic findings.

Selected References

Reviews

1. Shields JA, Shields CL, Scartozzi R. Survey of 1264 patients with orbital tumors and simulating lesions: the 2002 Montgomery Lecture, part 1. *Ophthalmology* 2004;111:997–1008.
2. Shields JA, Bakewell B, Augsburger JJ, et al. Classification and incidence of space-occupying lesions of the orbit. A survey of 645 biopsies. *Arch Ophthalmol* 1984;102:1606–1611.
3. Shields JA, Bakewell B, Augsburger JJ, et al. Space-occupying orbital masses in children: A review of 250 consecutive biopsies. *Ophthalmology* 1986;93:379–384.
4. Fu YS, Perzin KH. Non-epithelial tumors of the nasal cavity, paranasal sinuses, and nasopharynx: a clinicopathologic study. II. Osseous and fibro-osseous lesions, including osteoma, fibrous dysplasia, ossifying fibroma, osteoblastoma, giant cell tumor, and osteosarcoma. *Cancer* 1974;33:1289–1305.
5. Selva D, White VA, O'Connell JX, et al. Primary bone tumors of the orbit. *Surv Ophthalmol* 2004;49:328–342.
6. Steffner R. Benign bone tumors. *Cancer Treat Res* 2014;162:31–63.

Histopathology

7. Blodi FC. Pathology of orbital bones. The XXXII Edward Jackson Memorial Lecture. *Am J Ophthalmol* 1976;81:1–26.

Case Reports

8. Bowen JH, Christensen FH, Klintworth GK, et al. A clinicopathologic study of a cartilaginous hamartoma of the orbit. A rare cause of proptosis. *Ophthalmology* 1981;88:1356–1360.
9. Jepson CN, Wetzig PC. Pure chondroma of the trochlea. *Surv Ophthalmol* 1966;11:656–659.
10. Pasternak S, O'Connell JX, Verchere C, et al. Enchondroma of the orbit. *Am J Ophthalmol* 1996;122:444–445.
11. DeLaey JJ, DeSchryver A, Kluyskens P, et al. Orbital involvement in Ollier's disease (multiple enchondromatosis). *Int Ophthalmol* 1982;5:149–154.
12. Johnson TE, Nasr AM, Nalbandian RM, et al. Enchondromatosis and hemangioma (Maffucci's syndrome) with orbital involvement. *Am J Ophthalmol* 1990;110:153–159.
13. Harrison A, Loftus S, Pambuccian S. Orbital chondroma. *Ophthal Plast Reconstr Surg* 2006;22:484–485.

Chapter 33 Orbital Osseous, Fibro-osseous, and Cartilaginous Tumors 649

ORBITAL CHONDROMA

Orbital chondroma is extremely rare and we have no recorded cases in the files of the Ocular Oncology Service. A reported case is illustrated.

Harrison A, Loftus S, Pambuccian S. Orbital Chondroma. *Ophthal Plast Reconstr Surg* 2006;22:484–485.

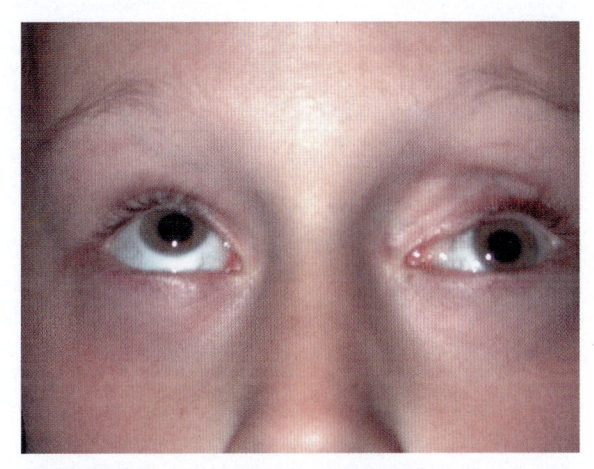

Figure 33.49. Appearance of 9-year-old boy with painless, nontender subcutaneous mass in the left orbit. The left eye has restricted up-gaze.

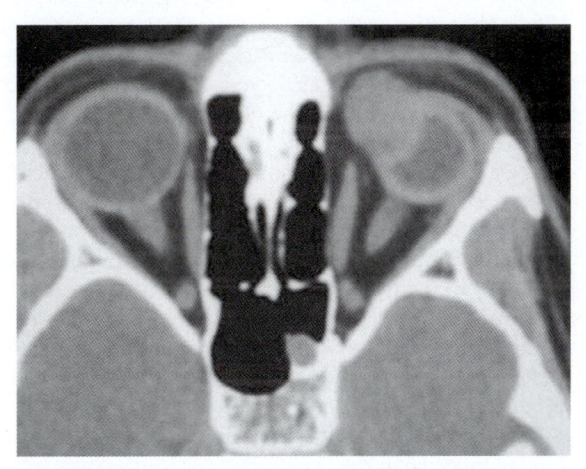

Figure 33.50. Axial computed tomography shows well-circumscribed superonasal left orbital mass displacing the globe.

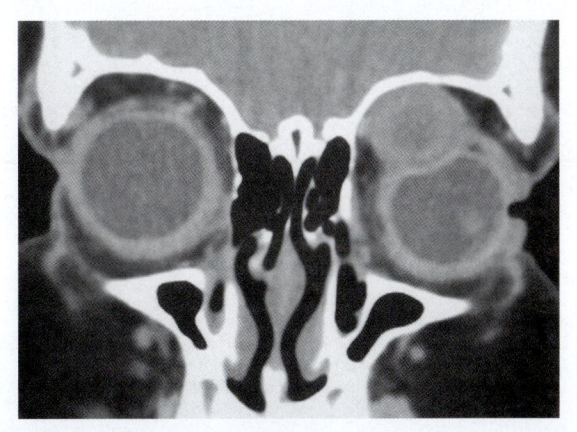

Figure 33.51. Coronal computed tomography showing same lesion.

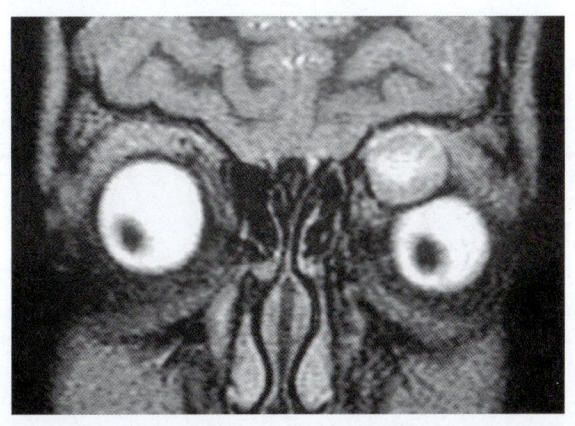

Figure 33.52. Coronal magnetic resonance imaging in T2-weighted image showing that the mass appears cystic and has a hypointense center. The lesion was removed intact.

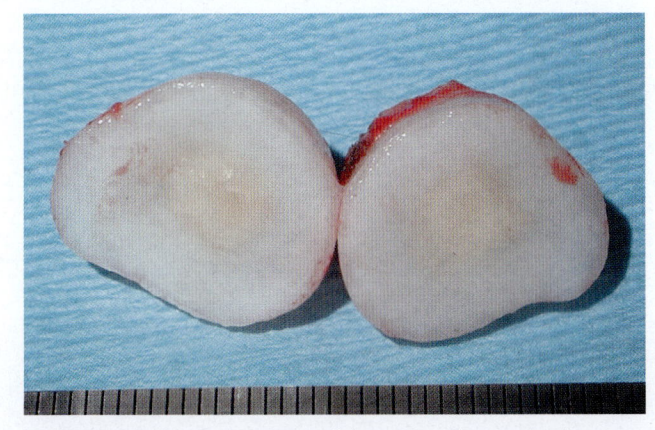

Figure 33.53. Gross appearance of the sectioned mass showing outer white layer and a central yellow avascular core.

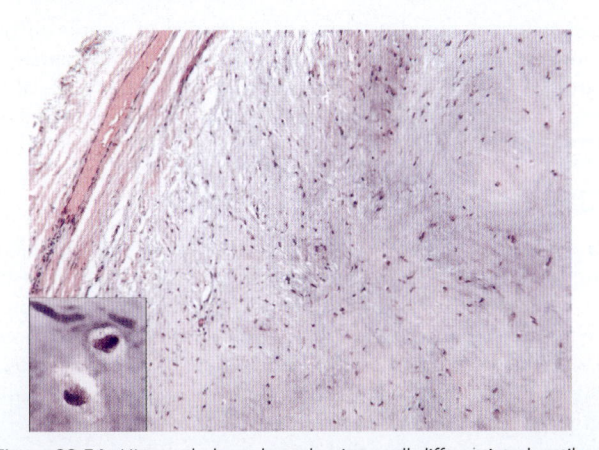

Figure 33.54. Histopathology shows benign, well-differentiated cartilage surrounded by a capsule of mature connective tissue (up and to the left). (Hematoxylin–eosin ×100.) The *inset* shows mononuclear chondrocytes that were scattered sparsely in the lesion. (Hematoxylin–eosin ×100.)

ORBITAL CHONDROSARCOMA

General Considerations

Chondrosarcoma is a neoplasm composed of anaplastic chondrocytes. It usually occurs in long bones, but can occasionally develop in the orbital region (1–23). The three general types of chondrosarcoma that can involve the orbit include the standard type, extraskeletal mesenchymal type, and radiation-induced type (6). All generally invade the orbit from a primary site in the paranasal sinuses and nasal cavity. Low-grade chondrosarcoma can also arise in periorbital areas from multiple enchondromatosis (Ollier's disease). The radiation-induced type can develop after radiotherapy for heritable retinoblastoma (13).

The most common variant of primary chondrosarcoma in the orbit is mesenchymal chondrosarcoma. It can arise from bone or from extraskeletal soft tissue, where it probably develops from primitive mesenchyme that exhibits cartilaginous differentiation. There appears to be a predilection for young adult females. Most comments on chondrosarcoma pertain to extraskeletal mesenchymal chondrosarcoma, which is the type most often reported in the orbit.

Clinical Features

Orbital chondrosarcoma generally occurs in young adults and produces proptosis and displacement of the globe. It can also occur in children as an aggressive, congenital lesion, presenting in the inferior conjunctiva (11). Extraskeletal mesenchymal chondrosarcoma of the orbit can be highly aggressive and invade the cranial cavity.

Diagnostic Approaches

Orbital computed tomography of mesenchymal chondrosarcoma shows a well-defined mass with multiple areas of fine and coarse calcification and moderate contrast enhancement (7). With MRI, the noncalcified portions demonstrate signal intensity lower than or equal to gray matter on T1 images and are isointense to gray matter on T2 images (8).

Pathology

Mesenchymal chondrosarcoma is composed of poorly differentiated mesenchymal tissue with islands of well-differentiated cartilage (4–6,9). Immunohistochemistry has shown variable findings, but most tumors have a positive reaction with vimentin and S-100 protein.

Management

The best management of orbital chondrosarcoma is complete surgical excision. This may necessitate orbital exenteration in advanced cases. Some authors have advocated aggressive chemotherapy and irradiation and have avoided orbital exenteration. The prognosis is generally poor, but a more favorable prognosis has been observed for chondrosarcoma that arises in the pediatric age group (6). It is also believed that extraskeletal mesenchymal chondrosarcoma that occurs in the orbit seems to have a better prognosis than those that arise in other parts of the body.

Selected References

Reviews

1. Shields JA, Shields CL, Scartozzi R. Survey of 1264 patients with orbital tumors and simulating lesions: the 2002 Montgomery Lecture, part 1. *Ophthalmology* 2004;111: 997–1008.
2. Shields JA, Bakewell B, Augsburger JJ, et al. Classification and incidence of space-occupying lesions of the orbit. A survey of 645 biopsies. *Arch Ophthalmol* 1984;102: 1606–1611.
3. Shields JA, Bakewell B, Augsburger JJ, et al. Space-occupying orbital masses in children: A review of 250 consecutive biopsies. *Ophthalmology* 1986;93:379–384.
4. Fu YS, Perzin KH. Non-epithelial tumors of the nasal cavity, paranasal sinuses, and nasopharynx: a clinicopathologic study. II. Osseous and fibro-osseous lesions, including osteoma, fibrous dysplasia, ossifying fibroma, osteoblastoma, giant cell tumor, and osteosarcoma. *Cancer* 1974;33:1289–1305.
5. Selva D, White VA, O'Connell JX, et al. Primary bone tumors of the orbit. *Surv Ophthalmol* 2004;49:328–342.
6. Gadwal SR, Fanburg-Smith JC, Gannon FH, et al. Primary chondrosarcoma of the head and neck in pediatric patients: a clinicopathologic study of 14 cases with a review of the literature. *Cancer* 2000;88:2181–2188.

Imaging

7. Font RL, Ray R, Mazow ML, et al. Mesenchymal chondrosarcoma of the orbit: a unique radiologic-pathologic correlation. *Ophthal Plast Reconstr Surg* 2009;25: 219–222.
8. Shinaver CN, Mafee MF, Choi KH. MRI of mesenchymal chondrosarcoma of the orbit: case report and review of the literature. *Neuroradiology* 1997;39:296–301.

Histopathology

9. Guccion JG, Font RL, Enzinger FM, et al. Extraskeletal mesenchymal chondrosarcoma. *Arch Pathol* 1973;95:336–340.

Case Reports

10. Jacobs JL, Merriam JC, Chadburn A, et al. Mesenchymal chondrosarcoma of the orbit. Report of three new cases and review of the literature. *Cancer* 1994;73: 399–405.
11. Tuncer S, Kebudi R, Peksayar G, et al. Congenital mesenchymal chondrosarcoma of the orbit: case report and review of the literature. *Ophthalmology* 2004;111: 1016–1022.
12. Kashyap S, Sen S, Betharia SM, et al. Mesenchymal chondrosarcoma of the orbit: a clinicopathological study. *Orbit* 2001;20:63–67.
13. Abramson DH, Ronner H, Ellsworth RM. Second tumors in non-irradiated bilateral retinoblastoma. *Am J Ophthalmol* 1979;84:624–627.
14. Bagchi M, Husain N, Goel MM, et al. Extraskeletal mesenchymal chondrosarcoma of the orbit. *Cancer* 1993;72:2224–2226.
15. Lauer SA, Friedland S, Goodrich JT, et al. Mesenchymal chondrosarcoma with secondary orbital invasion. *Ophthal Plast Reconstr Surg* 1995;11:182–186.
16. De Laey JJ, De Schryver A, Kluyskens P, et al. Orbital involvement in Ollier's disease (multiple enchondromatosis). *Int Ophthalmol* 1982;5:149–154.
17. Kiratli H, Dikmetaş O, Tarlan B, et al. Orbital chondrosarcoma arising from paranasal sinuses. *Int Ophthalmol* 2013;33:403–407.
18. Herrera A, Ortega C, Reyes G, et al. Primary orbital mesenchymal chondrosarcoma: case report and review of the literature. *Case Rep Med* 2012;2012:292147.
19. Patel R, Mukherjee B. Mesenchymal chondrosarcoma of the orbit. *Orbit* 2012;31: 126–128.
20. Kaur A, Kishore P, Agrawal A, et al. Mesenchymal chondrosarcoma of the orbit: a report of two cases and review of the literature. *Orbit* 2008;27:63–67.
21. Odashiro AN, Leite LV, Oliveira RS, et al. Primary orbital mesenchymal chondrosarcoma: a case report and literature review. *Int Ophthalmol* 2009;29:173–177.
22. Angotti-Neto H, Cunha LP, Oliveira AV, et al. Mesenchymal chondrosarcoma of the orbit. *Ophthal Plast Reconstr Surg* 2006;22:378–382.
23. Bagchi M, Husain N, Goel MM, et al. Extraskeletal mesenchymal chondrosarcoma of the orbit. *Cancer* 1993;72:2224–2226.

ORBITAL CHONDROSARCOMA

De Laey JJ, De Schryver A, Kluyskens P, et al. Orbital involvement in Ollier's disease (multiple enchondromatosis). *Int Ophthalmol* 1982;5:149–154.

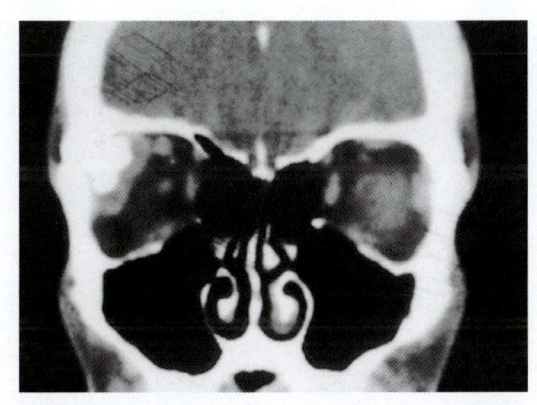

Figure 33.55. Coronal computed tomography of a 21-year-old man with superotemporal orbital mass. Note the bone and soft tissue component of the mass.

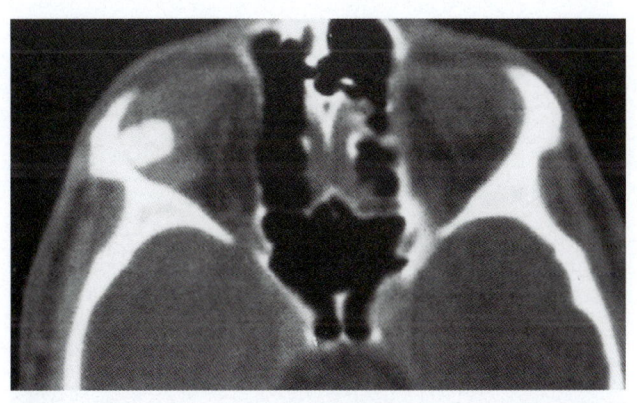

Figure 33.56. Axial computed tomography with bone windows of lesion shown in Figure 33.55 better depicting the bone density in the mass.

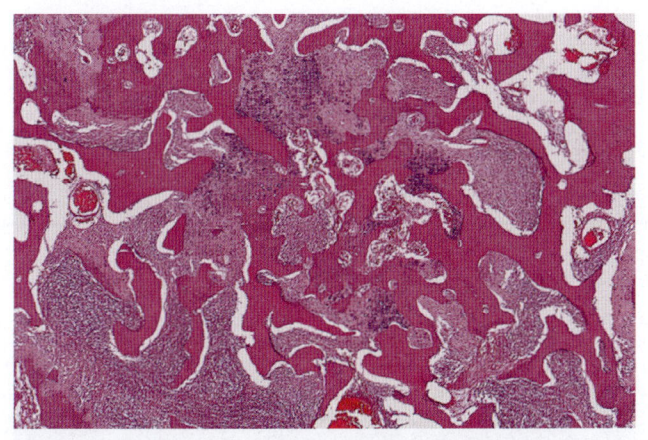

Figure 33.57. Histopathology showing bone spicules and connective tissue. Other areas showed more definitive cartilage. (Hematoxylin–eosin ×80.)

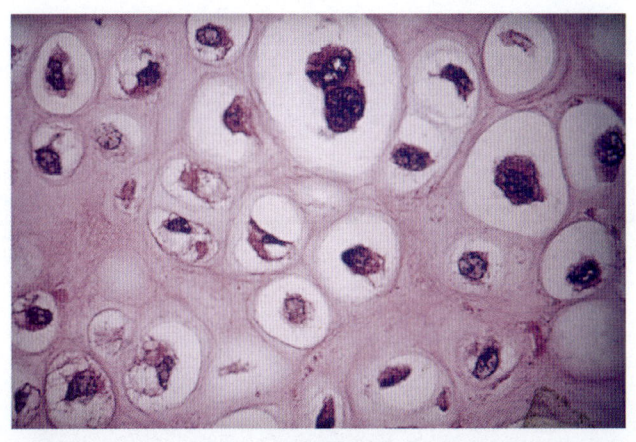

Figure 33.58. Photomicrograph of orbital chondrosarcoma from a child who had undergone irradiation for familial retinoblastoma, showing malignant chondroblasts. (Hematoxylin–eosin ×250.)

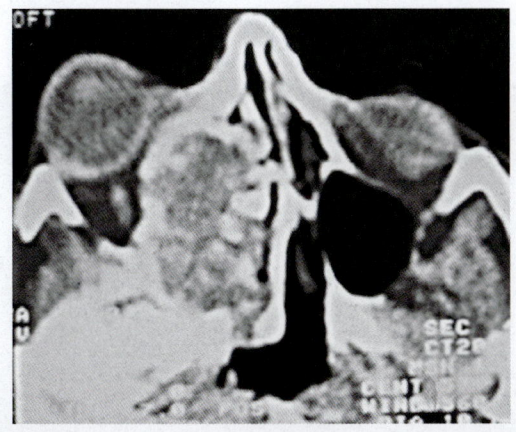

Figure 33.59. Chondrosarcoma associated with Ollier's disease. Axial computed tomography of a 52-year-old woman with Ollier's disease showing mass involving the nose and nasal aspect of the orbit. (Courtesy of J.J De Laey, MD.)

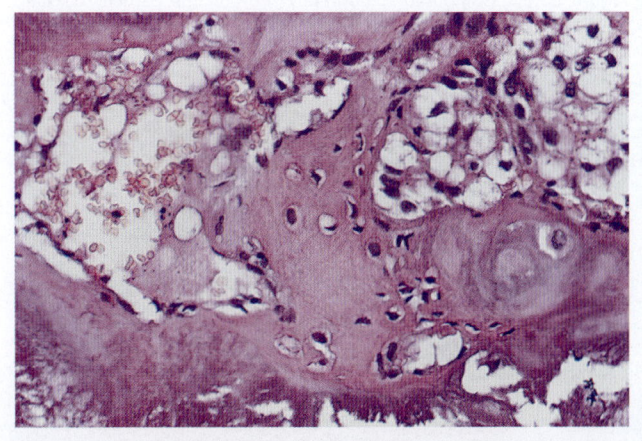

Figure 33.60. Histopathology of lesion shown in Figure 33.59, demonstrating well-differentiated chondrosarcoma. (Hematoxylin–eosin ×75.) (Courtesy of J.J De Laey, MD.)

ORBITAL CHONDROSARCOMA IN A YOUNG WOMAN

Orbital chondrosarcoma generally develops in young patients, especially young woman. Below we illustrated a case that presented with only mild proptosis but was managed with exenteration for complete control.

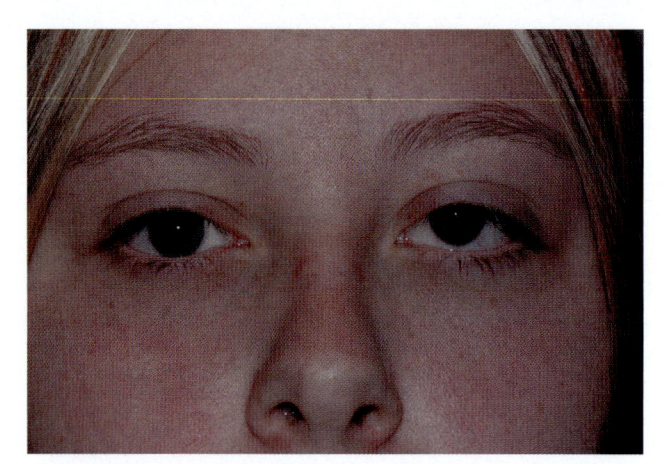

Figure 33.61. Facial appearance of young woman showing mild left proptosis.

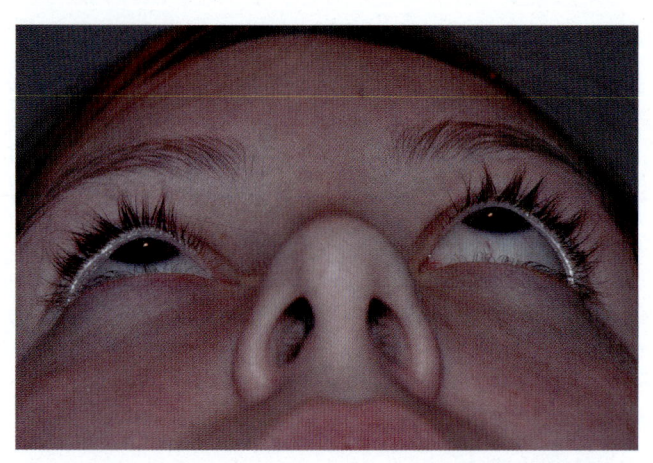

Figure 33.62. Proptosis is more noticeable with this upward view.

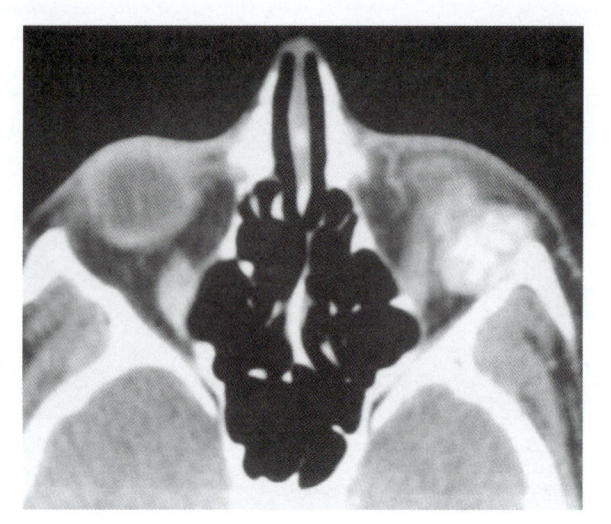

Figure 33.63. Computed tomography showing the partially calcified mass abutting the inferolateral orbital wall.

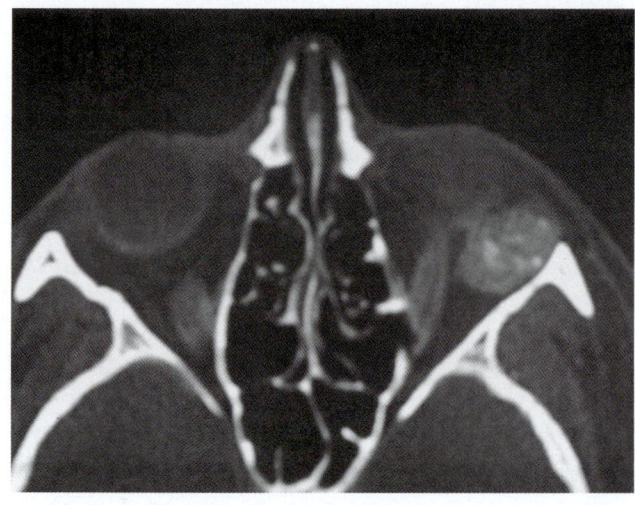

Figure 33.64. Computed tomography (bone windows) demonstrating the "popcorn" calcific flecks within the mass. This "popcorn" calcification is noted in about 75% of chondrosarcomas.

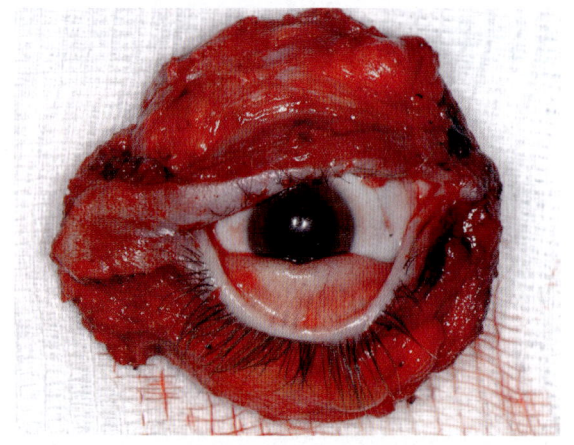

Figure 33.65. Following initial biopsy and establishment of the diagnosis of chondrosarcoma, exenteration was performed.

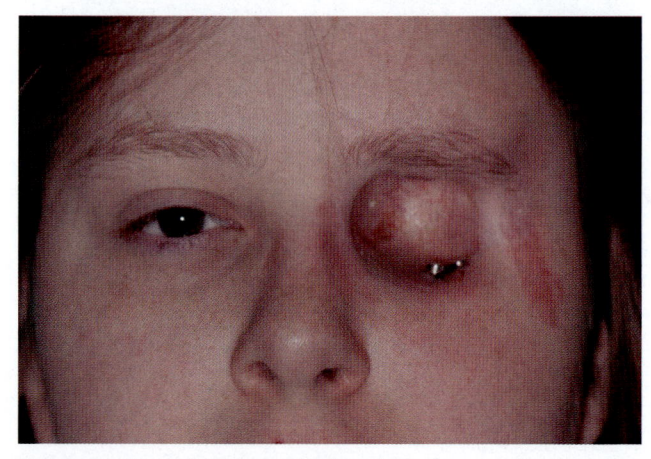

Figure 33.66. Well-healed orbital socket after exenteration. This patient had a magnetic prosthesis and the transcutaneous magnetic hardware is visible in the inferior socket wall.

CHAPTER 34

ORBITAL LIPOMATOUS AND MYXOMATOUS TUMORS

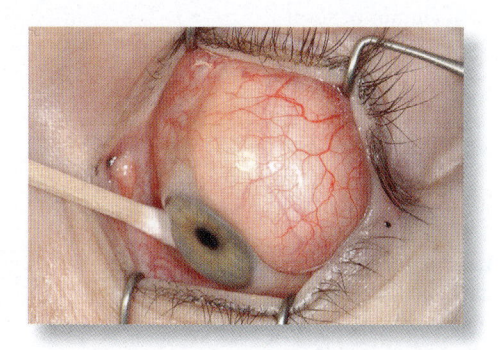

General Considerations

Weakening of the orbital septum with anterior displacement of orbital fat ("baggy eyelids") is common in older individuals. This condition is rarely considered in the differential diagnosis of orbital tumors and is not considered further here. We do discuss, however, a variant that often simulates an orbital or conjunctival neoplasm. This is called orbital fat prolapse.

Orbital fat prolapse is not a true neoplasm, but rather a protrusion of orbital fat through a defect in Tenon's capsule into the conjunctival fornix (1–9). It is included here because affected patients are commonly referred with the diagnosis of dermolipoma, lymphoma, or lacrimal gland epithelial tumor. In the authors' series of 1,264 consecutive space-occupying orbital lesions, the 30 cases of orbital fat prolapse accounted for 47% of lipocytic and myxoid lesions and for 2% of all orbital masses referred to the Oncology Service (1). In the authors' series of 1,643 consecutive conjunctival tumors, orbital fat prolapse presented as a conjunctival mass in 20 cases (1%) and of the 23 lipomatous tumors, this represented 87% (4). However, orbital fat prolapse into the conjunctival fornix is certainly much more common than reflected in both series, which included only more advanced cases that were referred because of suspected tumor. Surprisingly, very little has been published about the specific diagnosis and management of orbital fat prolapse (5–9).

Clinical Features

Orbital fat prolapse can occur in either gender, but has a predilection for obese elderly men (5). Clinically, orbital fat prolapse is characterized by a soft yellow mass, almost always in the superotemporal conjunctival fornix and less commonly in the inferotemporal quadrant. Slit-lamp biomicroscopy demonstrates that the lesion is covered by normal conjunctiva and thin Tenon's fascia and has glistening yellow spherules of fat within the mass. Orbital fat prolapse is often confused clinically with dermolipoma, so it is important to emphasize their differences. Herniated fat occurs in older individuals, is more often bilateral, more compressible, more elevated, has visible lipid globules without hair, and the anterior border is usually convex. In contrast, dermolipoma is generally diagnosed in childhood, is more often unilateral, not compressible, sessile in shape, has a gray-pink color, and frequently has fine white hairs on slit-lamp examination; the anterior border is often concave, being more parallel to the corneoscleral limbus. Dermolipoma can be associated with Goldenhar syndrome. Conjunctival or orbital lymphoma is also included in the differential diagnosis (1,4). If orbital fat prolapse is suspected, it is important to examine the opposite eye because the lesion is often bilateral, although possibly asymmetric.

ORBITAL FAT PROLAPSE

Diagnostic Approaches
Computed tomography (CT) and magnetic resonance imaging (MRI) show the lesion to be consistent with fat and to be directly continuous with the orbital fat posteriorly (7). With imaging studies, the prolapsed fat appears hypointense and is continuous with the orbital fat posteriorly.

Pathology
Histopathologically, orbital fat prolapse is composed of normal orbital lipocytes. On occasion, pathologists who are unfamiliar with this entity may make the diagnosis of simple lipoma or pleomorphic lipoma based on the presence of clumps of suspicious cells called florets.

Management
In most instances, orbital fat prolapse can be managed conservatively by periodic observation only. If it attains a large size and produces ocular irritation, dry eye, or is cosmetically unacceptable, then surgical excision is justified. The prolapsed anterior component can be excised by performing a conjunctival/Tenon's fascia incision, exposing the fat lobules, clamping the posterior aspect of the exposed fat with a hemostat, cutting through the clamped fat with cautery, and allowing the remainder of the lesion to fall back into the orbit (1,2). Then Tenon's fascia is closed separately from the conjunctiva with running or interrupted absorbable sutures to secure the fat and produce a fibrous band to prevent recurrence. Recurrence is uncommon if the initial closure is secure.

Selected References

Reviews
1. Shields JA, Shields CL, Scartozzi R. Survey of 1264 patients with orbital tumors and simulating lesions: the 2002 Montgomery Lecture, part 1. *Ophthalmology* 2004;111: 997–1008.
2. Shields JA, Bakewell B, Augsburger DG, et al. Classification and incidence of space-occupying lesions of the orbit. A survey of 645 biopsies. *Arch Ophthalmol* 1984;102: 1606–1611.
3. Shields JA, Bakewell B, Augsburger DG, et al. Space-occupying orbital masses in children. A review of 250 consecutive biopsies. *Ophthalmology* 1986;93:379–384.
4. Shields CL, Demirci H, Karatza E, et al. Clinical survey of 1643 melanocytic and nonmelanocytic tumors of the conjunctiva. *Ophthalmology* 2004;111:1747–1754.
5. McNab AA. Subconjunctival fat prolapse. *Aust N Z J Ophthalmol* 1999;27:33–36.
6. Kim YD, Goldberg RA. Orbital fat prolapse and dermolipoma: two distinct entities. *Korean J Ophthalmol* 1994;8:42–43.

Imaging
7. Kim E, Kim HJ, Kim YD, et al. Subconjunctival fat prolapse and dermolipoma of the orbit: differentiation on CT and MR imaging. *AJNR Am J Neuroradiol* 2011;32: 465–467.

Management
8. Schwarz F, Randall P. Conjunctival incision for herniated orbital fat. *Ophthalmic Surg* 1980;11:276–279.

Case Reports
9. Jordan DR, Tse DT. Herniated orbital fat. *Can J Ophthalmol* 1987;22:173–177.

Chapter 34 Orbital Lipomatous and Myxomatous Tumors

ORBITAL FAT PROLAPSE

In most instances, orbital fat prolapse is bilateral and fairly symmetric. This bilaterality helps to differentiate it from most neoplasms, which are generally unilateral. Orbitoconjunctival lymphoma can also be bilateral, but it is rarely symmetric and it has a pink, rather than yellow, color.

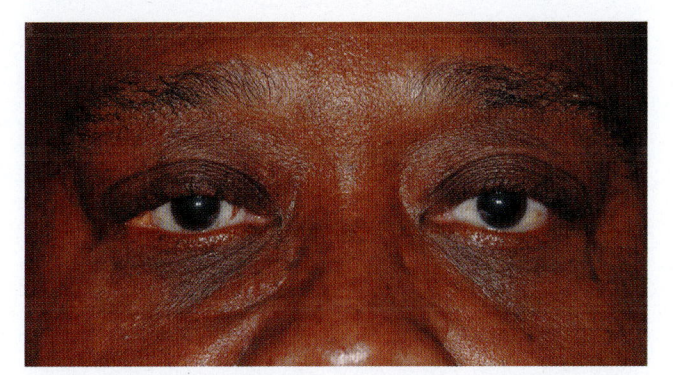

Figure 34.1. Facial appearance of elderly African-American man. A yellow-pink conjunctival lesion can be seen in the lateral canthal region.

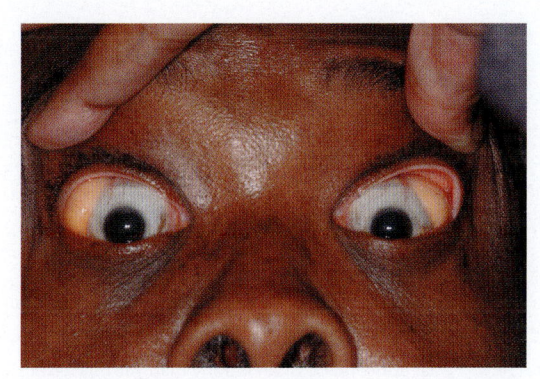

Figure 34.2. Same patient with elevation of both eyelids. The fluctuant, yellow-pink masses can be seen bilaterally.

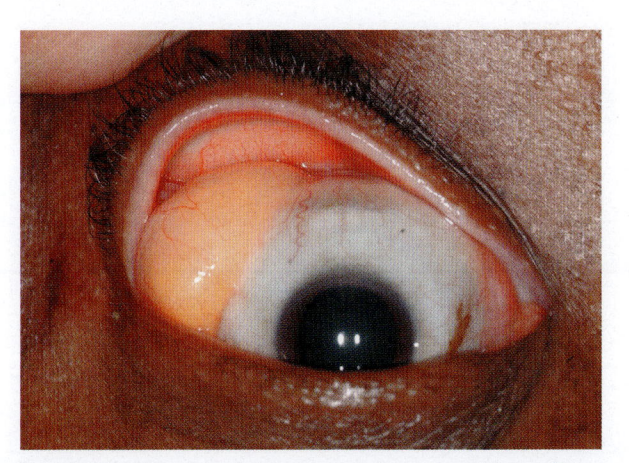

Figure 34.3. Closer view of superotemporal mass in right eye of patient seen in Figure 34.2. The brilliant yellow material within the lesion represents lipid, sometimes forming glistening cholesterol crystals.

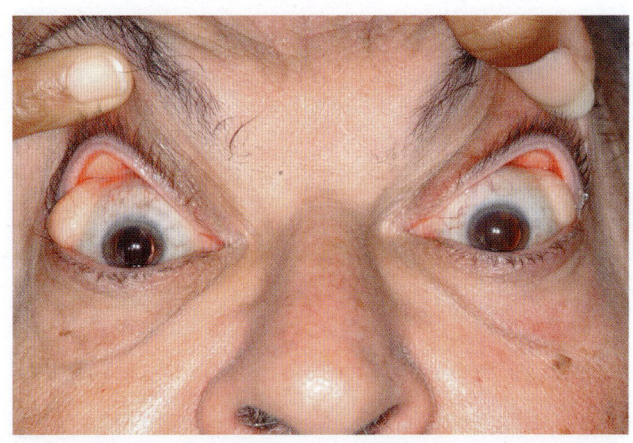

Figure 34.4. Similar bilateral superotemporal masses in an elderly Caucasian man. The upper eyelids are being elevated to afford a better view.

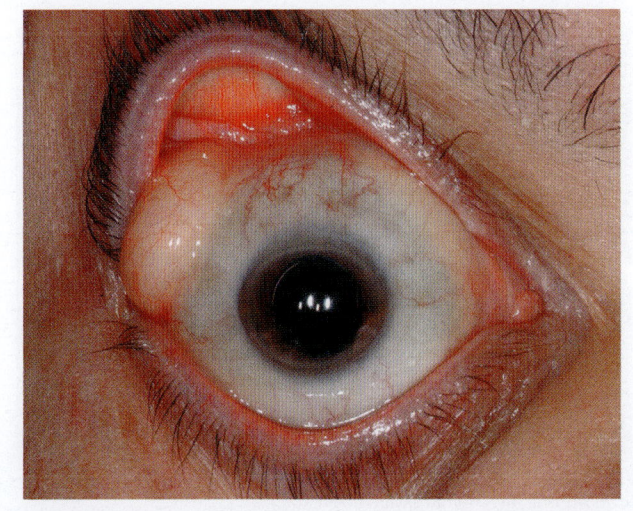

Figure 34.5. Closer view of mass on right eye of patient shown in Figure 34.4.

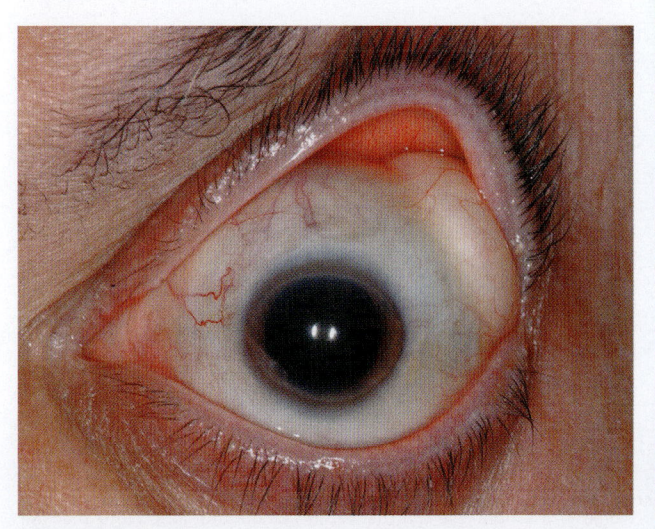

Figure 34.6. Similar but less prominent mass on left side of patient shown in Figure 34.4.

ORBITAL FAT PROLAPSE

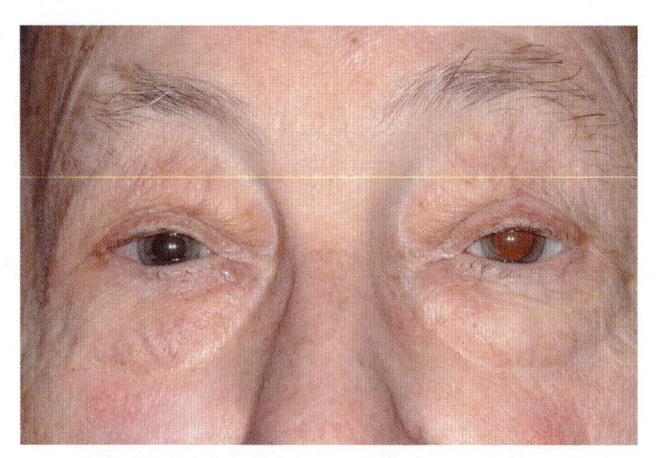

Figure 34.7. Facial appearance of an elderly man with bilateral subcutaneous fluctuant masses owing to herniated orbital fat.

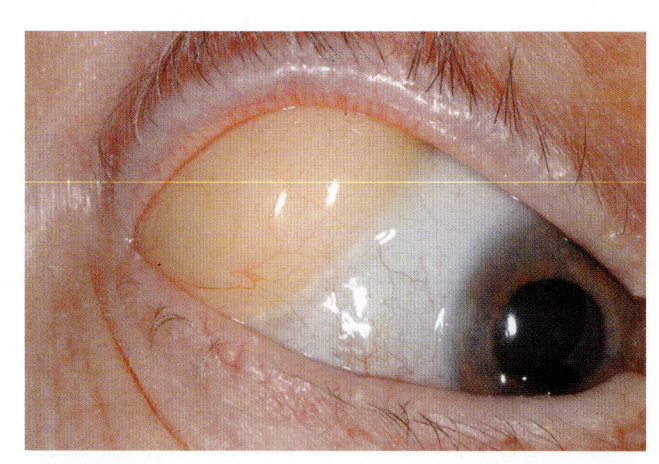

Figure 34.8. Closer view of yellow mass seen in right eye of patient shown in Figure 34.7.

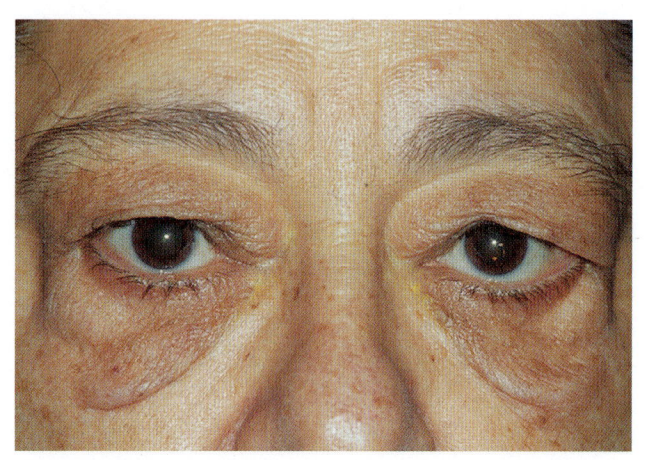

Figure 34.9. Elderly man with bilateral subcutaneous fat similar to patient shown in Figure 34.7. Note the protrusion of the lower eyelids, also owing to fat prolapse.

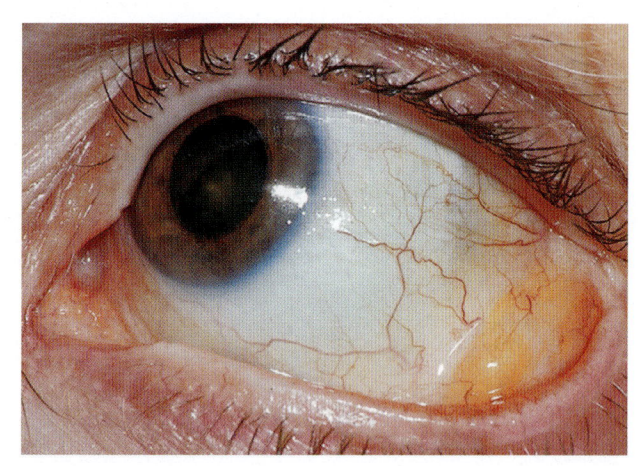

Figure 34.10. Inferotemporal orbital fat prolapse in a 71-year-old woman. Inferotemporal location is less common than superotemporal location.

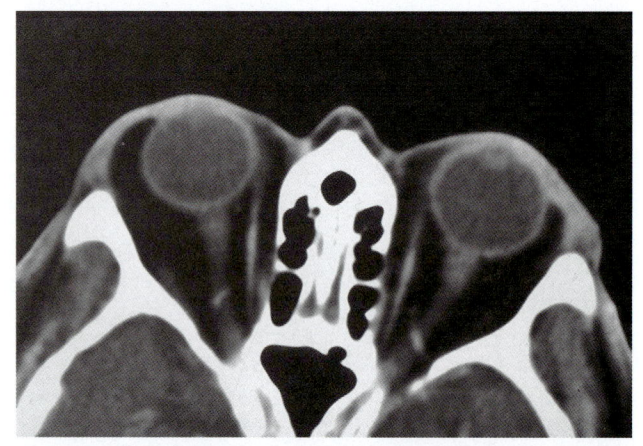

Figure 34.11. Computed tomography of bilateral herniated orbital fat worse in the right eye (on the left in the photograph). Note that the black area represents fat, which extends from the conjunctival fornix into the orbit and is indistinguishable from the orbital fat.

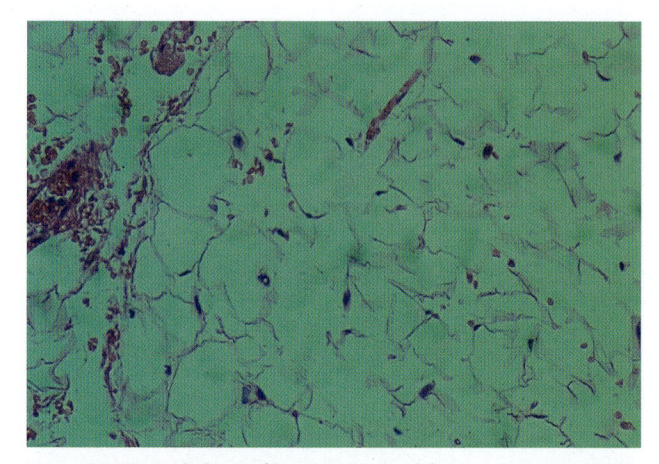

Figure 34.12. Pathology of herniated orbital fat. It is indistinguishable from normal fat. (Hematoxylin–eosin ×50.)

Chapter 34 Orbital Lipomatous and Myxomatous Tumors   657

● ORBITAL FAT PROLAPSE: CLINICAL AND COMPUTED TOMOGRAPHY FEATURES AND SURGICAL APPROACH

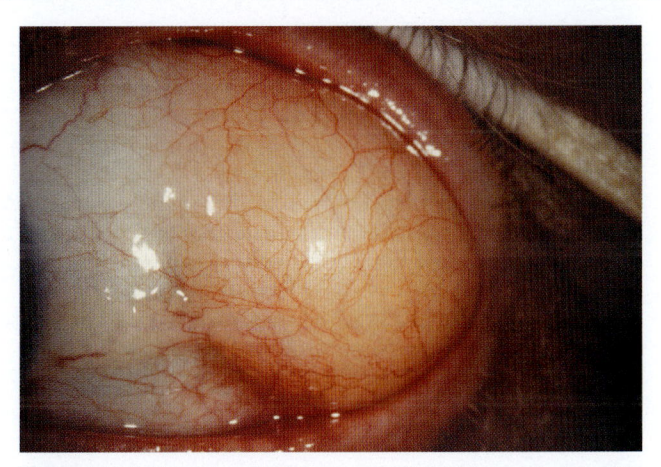

Figure 34.13. Superotemporal herniated orbital fat on left side. This became progressively more prominent and the patient requested surgical excision.

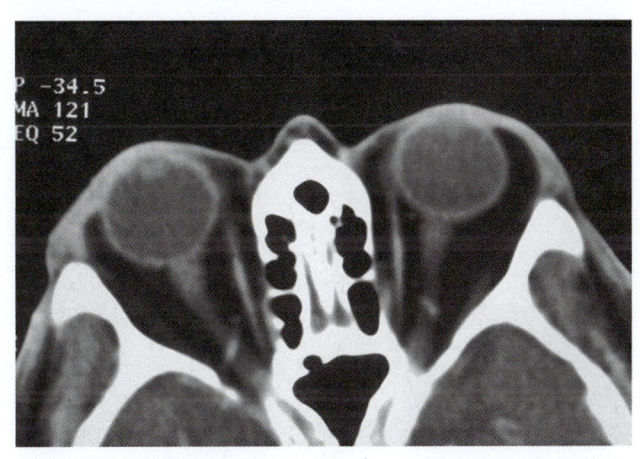

Figure 34.14. Axial computed tomography of lesion shown in Figure 34.13, demonstrating more advanced herniated orbital fat in left orbit.

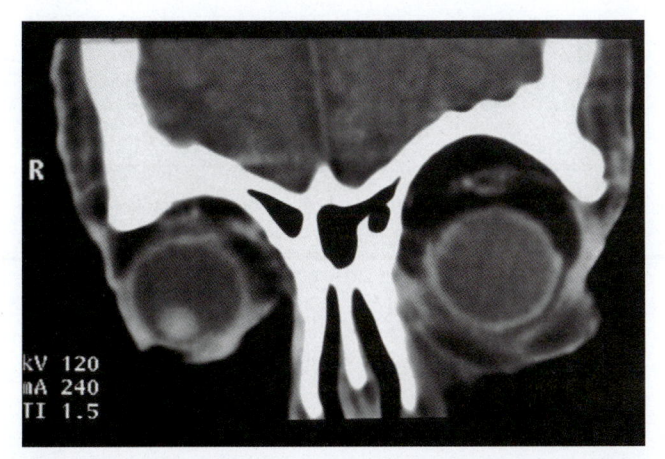

Figure 34.15. Coronal computed tomography through the anterior aspect of the eyes of lesion shown in Figure 34.13. Note the excess orbital fat in left orbit.

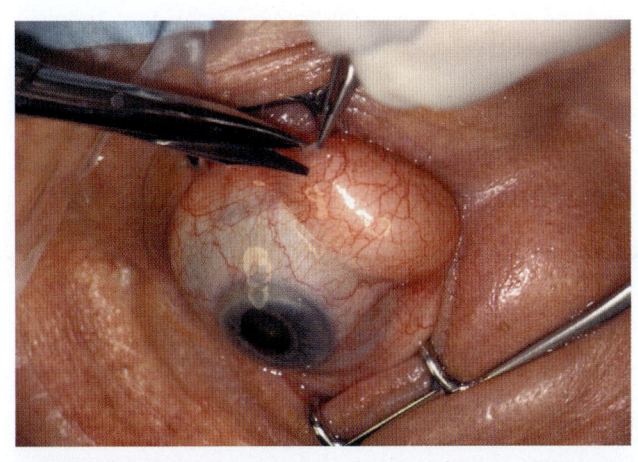

Figure 34.16. Orbital fat exposed at the time of surgery. Scissors are being used to start a conjunctival incision over the mass.

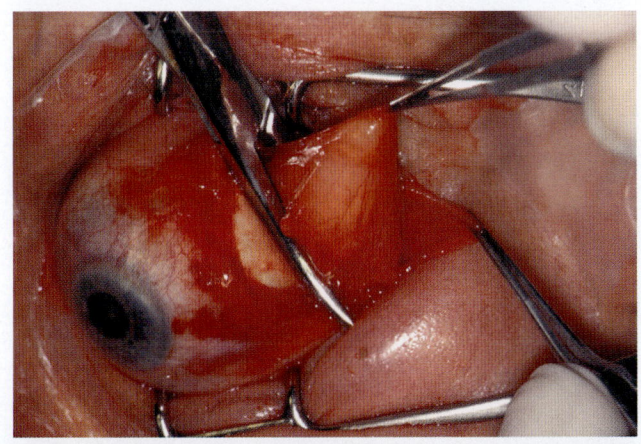

Figure 34.17. The conjunctival incision has been done exposing the fat, which is being lifted with blunt-tipped forceps. A hemostat is being used to clamp the lesion in the anterior aspect of the orbit. Scissors are then used to cut the fat anterior to the hemostat, the hemostat is removed, and the fat allowed to recede into the orbit.

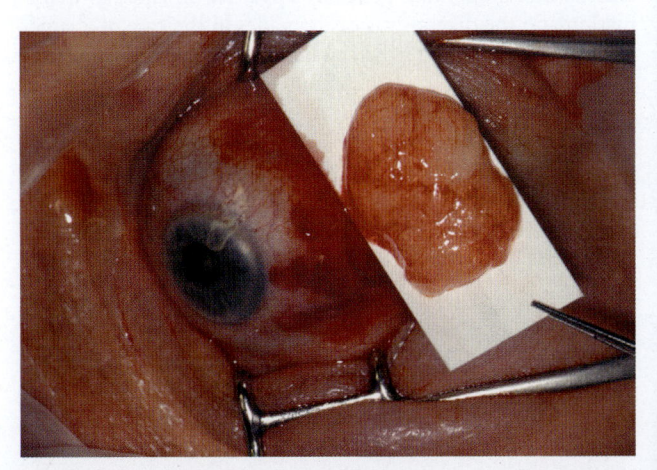

Figure 34.18. The excised tissue is placed on a piece of paper and then sent for histopathologic study. The conjunctival wound is then closed with a running 7-0 absorbable suture. A pressure patch is applied. The residual hemorrhage resolved in a few days.

ORBITAL/CONJUNCTIVAL DERMOLIPOMA

General Considerations

Dermolipoma (lipodermoid) is a choristoma that often affects the orbit and conjunctiva (1–17). It is also discussed in the section on conjunctival tumors. Dermolipoma is a congenital lesion that is often not detected until young adulthood. This tumor might even remain undetected throughout life. In the authors' series of 1,264 consecutive space occupying orbital lesions, the 31 dermolipomas accounted for 3% of all orbital lesions (1). In the authors' series of 1,643 consecutive conjunctival tumors, dermolipoma represented 23 (1%) of all tumors and 58% of conjunctival choristomas (4).

Clinical Features

Orbital/conjunctival dermolipoma is a light pink to yellow, firm, sessile to moderately elevated lesion, the anterior portion of which is usually visible in the conjunctival fornix superotemporally. Fine hairs often protrude from the surface of the mass and are best seen with slit-lamp biomicroscopy. Although yellow lipid globules can be seen, the lipid is not so strikingly apparent as in orbital fat herniation. The lesion can extend anteriorly almost to the limbus and some patients complain of a visual field defect owing to the elevated lesion. It is occasionally bilateral, but often asymmetric. It is usually asymptomatic and is either noticed by the patient or by the physician on routine examination. This lesion can cause mild ocular irritation or a foreign-body sensation. It is generally stationary and mild enlargement can be found over many years, but usually nonsubstantial. There is no predisposition for gender or race. Dermolipoma, like dermoid tumor, can occasionally be associated with certain systemic syndromes, such as Goldenhar syndrome, organoid nevus syndrome, mandibulofacial dysostosis, and others (8–10).

Diagnostic Approaches

Orbital dermolipoma is generally apparent on external examination and the diagnosis is easily made. In the case of a larger lesion, orbital CT and MRI can help to delineate the posterior extent of the lesion (11). These studies disclose a circumscribed oval or elongated mass extending into the orbit superotemporally in close association with the lacrimal gland and orbital fat. It appears solid, rather than cystic, and has attenuation similar to orbital fat.

Pathology and Pathogenesis

Histopathologically, dermolipoma is lined by stratified squamous epithelium, which may be partially keratinized. Underneath the epithelium is a layer of collagen bundles. The deeper portions of the tumor usually contain mature fat, but the fat is not the main component of the lesion. Pilosebaceous elements are occasionally identified. Dermolipomas that contain cartilage and glandular acini are sometimes called complex choristomas and may be a component of the organoid nevus syndrome (9).

Management

Dermolipoma is generally best managed by observation. The patient should be reassured that the lesion has no malignant potential. Large, cosmetically unacceptable dermolipomas can be excised by a conjunctival approach, similar to that described in the section on herniated orbital fat. It may be prudent in some cases to only excise the anterior, subconjunctival portion of the tumor and avoid the orbital portion so as to prevent surgical damage to the lacrimal gland, levator muscle of the eyelid, lateral rectus muscle, and other orbital structures (12–15). The prognosis for life and vision is excellent. The lesion is benign and has no known malignant potential.

Selected References

Reviews

1. Shields JA, Shields CL, Scartozzi R. Survey of 1264 patients with orbital tumors and simulating lesions: the 2002 Montgomery Lecture, part 1. *Ophthalmology* 2004;111: 997–1008.
2. Shields JA, Bakewell B, Augsburger DG, et al. Classification and incidence of space-occupying lesions of the orbit. A survey of 645 biopsies. *Arch Ophthalmol* 1984;102: 1606–1611.
3. Shields JA, Bakewell B, Augsburger DG, et al. Space-occupying orbital masses in children. A review of 250 consecutive biopsies. *Ophthalmology* 1986;93:379–384.
4. Shields CL, Demirci H, Karatza E, et al. Clinical survey of 1643 melanocytic and nonmelanocytic tumors of the conjunctiva. *Ophthalmology* 2004;111:1747–1754.
5. Shields CL, Shields JA. Tumors of the conjunctiva and cornea. *Surv Ophthalmol* 2004; 49:3–24.
6. McNab AA. Subconjunctival fat prolapse. *Aust N Z J Ophthalmol* 1999;27:33–36.
7. Kim YD, Goldberg RA. Orbital fat prolapse and dermolipoma: two distinct entities. *Korean J Ophthalmol* 1994;8:42–43.
8. Khong JJ, Hardy TG, McNab AA. Prevalence of oculo-auriculo-vertebral spectrum in dermolipoma. *Ophthalmology* 2013;120:1529–1532.
9. Shields JA, Shields CL, Eagle RC Jr, et al. Ocular manifestations of the organoid nevus syndrome. *Ophthalmology* 1997;104:549–557.
10. Tranos L. Mandibulofacial dysostosis associated with dermolipoma of the conjunctiva. *Am J Ophthalmol* 1954;37:354–359.

Imaging

11. Kim E, Kim HJ, Kim YD, et al. Subconjunctival fat prolapse and dermolipoma of the orbit: differentiation on CT and MR imaging. *AJNR Am J Neuroradiol* 2011;32: 465–467.

Management

12. McNab AA, Wright JE, Caswell AG. Clinical features and surgical management of dermolipoma. *Aust N Z J Ophthalmol* 1990;18:159–162.
13. Fry CL, Leone CR Jr. Safe management of dermolipomas. *Arch Ophthalmol* 1994; 112:1114–1116.
14. Sa HS, Kim HK, Shin JH, et al. Dermolipoma surgery with rotational conjunctival flaps. *Acta Ophthalmol* 2012;90:86–90.
15. Paris GL, Beard C. Blepharoptosis following dermolipoma surgery. *Ann Ophthalmol* 1973;5:697–699.

Case Reports

16. Ziavras E, Farber MG, Diamond GR. A pedunculated lipodermoid in oculoauriculovertebral dysplasia. *Arch Ophthalmol* 1990;108:1032–1033.
17. Maeng HS, Lee LK, Woo KI, et al. A unique case of dermolipoma located in the lower eyelid. *Ophthal Plast Reconstr Surg* 2010;26:288–289.

Chapter 34 Orbital Lipomatous and Myxomatous Tumors

ORBITAL/CONJUNCTIVAL DERMOLIPOMA: CLINICAL SPECTRUM AND AGE RANGE

Dermolipomas are most likely congenital but, because some are in an occult location, they may not be detected for a few years. Examples are shown of patients who did not have evidence of Goldenhar syndrome.

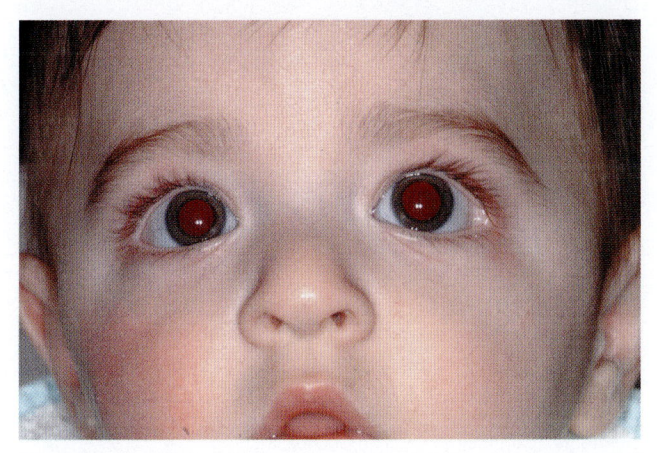

Figure 34.19. Infant with dermolipoma appearing in the lateral canthal area of the left eye.

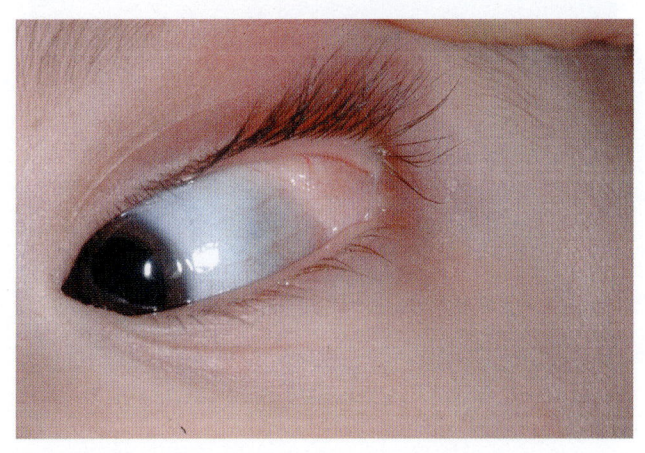

Figure 34.20. Closer view of child shown in Figure 34.19 showing typical dermolipoma appearing beneath conjunctiva superotemporally.

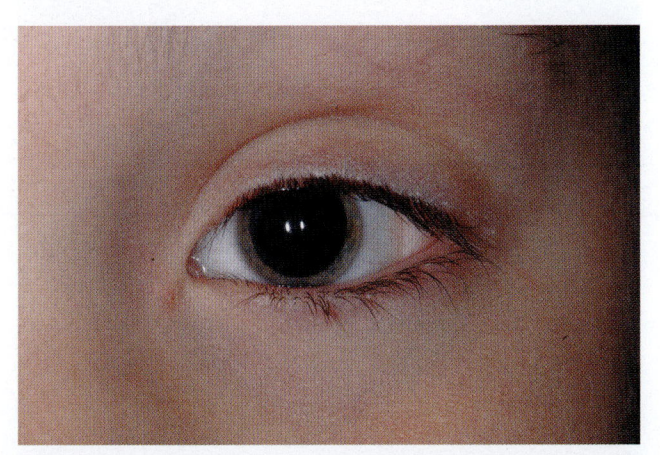

Figure 34.21. Left eye of a 6-year-old child with superotemporal dermolipoma. Although the lesion was probably present since birth, it was first noticed at age 6 years.

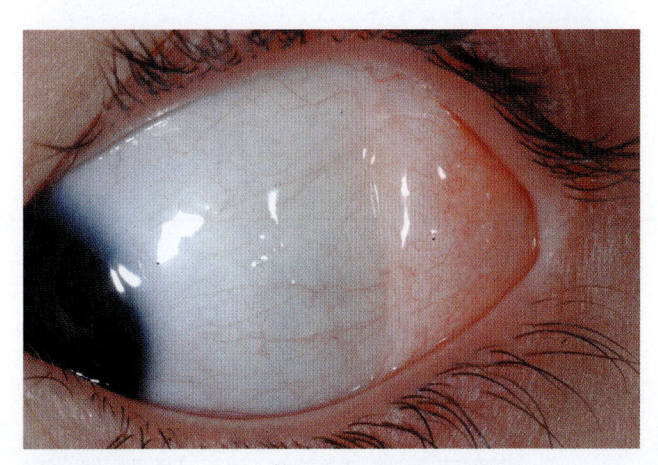

Figure 34.22. Closer view of lesion shown in Figure 34.21.

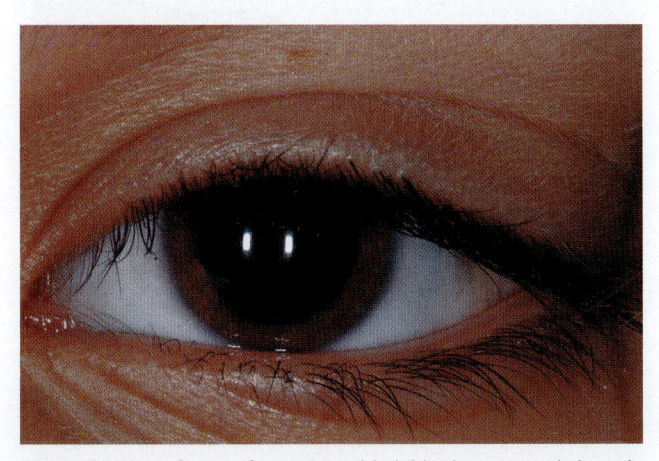

Figure 34.23. Left eye of a 15-year-old child. The temporal dermolipoma is barely visible in primary gaze.

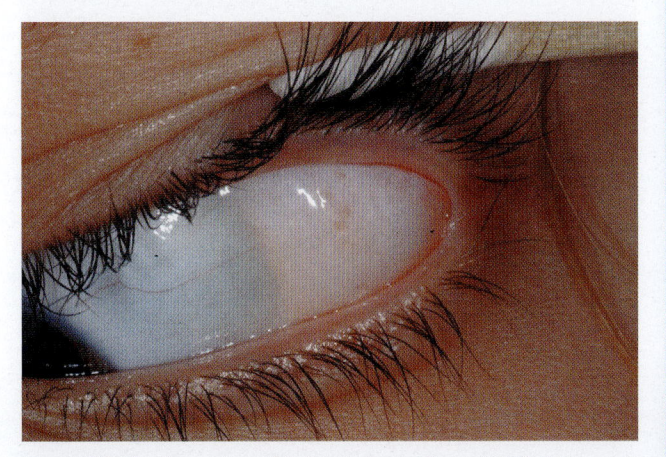

Figure 34.24. Closer view of lesion shown in Figure 34.23. Although it was probably present since birth, the child and parents were unaware of the lesion until the child was 15 years old.

Part 3 Tumors of the Orbit

ORBITAL/CONJUNCTIVAL DERMOLIPOMA: CLINICAL, COMPUTED TOMOGRAPHY, AND HISTOPATHOLOGIC FEATURES

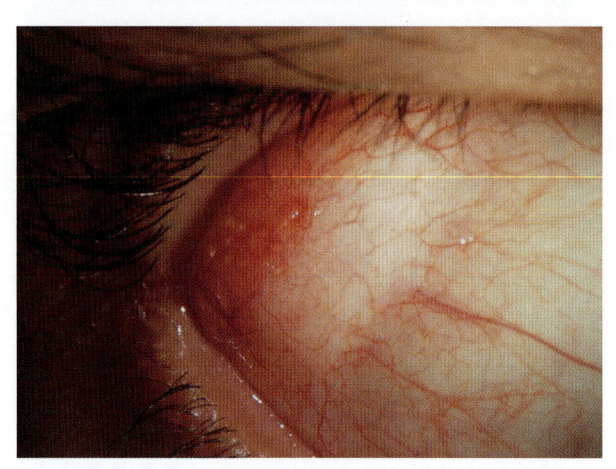

Figure 34.25. Orbitoconjunctival dermolipoma presenting in the superotemporal fornix of a 19-year-old man.

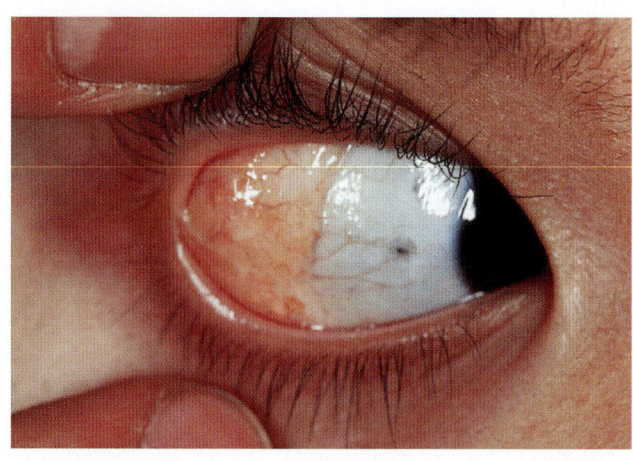

Figure 34.26. Dermolipoma presenting as a superotemporal orbitoconjunctival mass in a 6-year-old girl who had no evidence of Goldenhar syndrome. (Courtesy of Norman Charles, MD.)

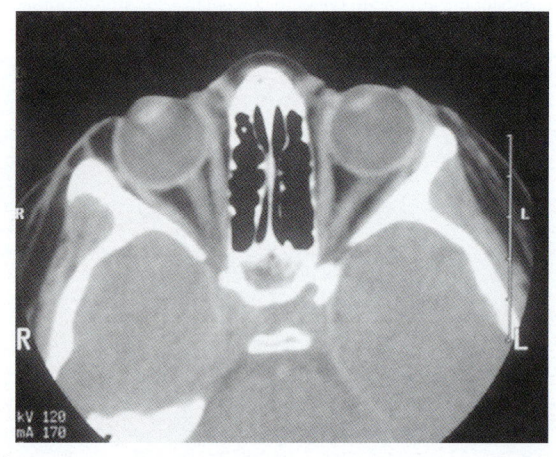

Figure 34.27. Axial computed tomography of patient shown in Figure 34.26 demonstrating triangular lesion temporal to right eye that has a density identical to orbital fat. (Courtesy of Norman Charles, MD.)

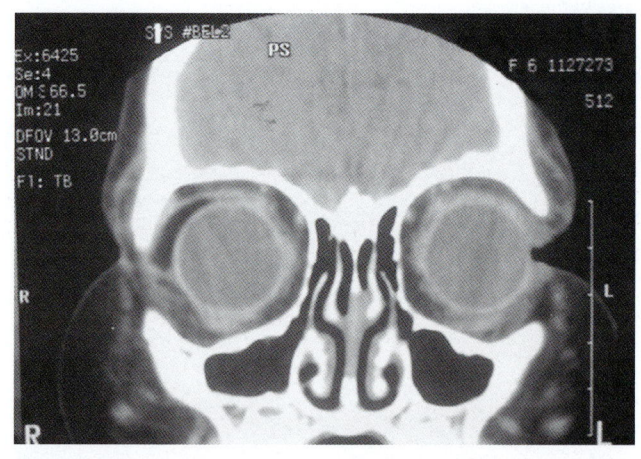

Figure 34.28. Coronal computed tomography of patient shown in Figure 34.26 depicting the same lesion superotemporal to the globe. (Courtesy of Norman Charles, MD.)

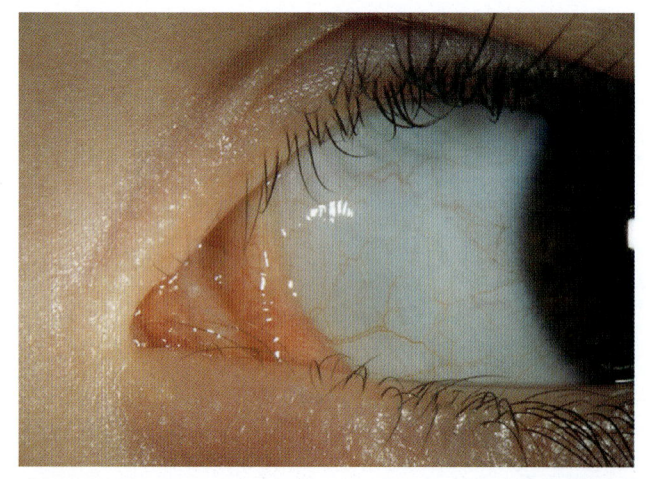

Figure 34.29. Dermolipoma presenting in the medial canthal region of a 2-year-old child with Goldenhar syndrome.

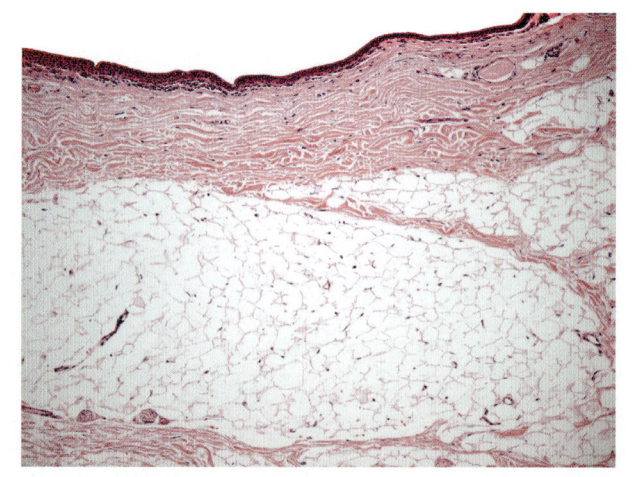

Figure 34.30. Histopathology of orbitoconjunctival dermolipoma showing epithelium, collagenous tissue, and deeper fat. (Hematoxylin–eosin ×50.)

Chapter 34 Orbital Lipomatous and Myxomatous Tumors

ORBITAL/CONJUNCTIVAL DERMOLIPOMA: ASSOCIATION WITH GOLDENHAR SYNDROME

The relationship between conjunctival/corneal dermoid with Goldenhar syndrome is widely recognized. It is less well known that orbital/conjunctival dermolipoma is also a very common finding in patients with Goldenhar syndrome.

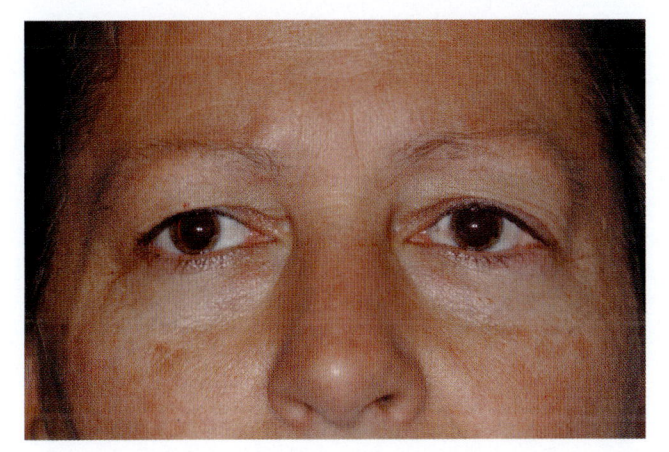

Figure 34.31. Middle-aged woman with subtle dermolipoma in lateral canthus of left eye.

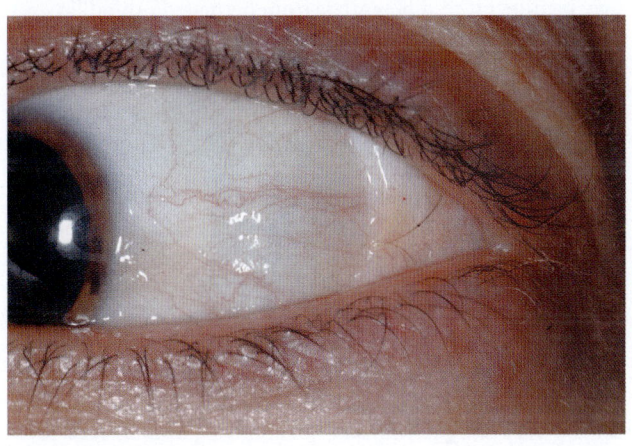

Figure 34.32. Closer view of patient shown in Figure 34.31 on right gaze. Note the dull yellow color to the lesion and the prominent hairs arising from the lesion.

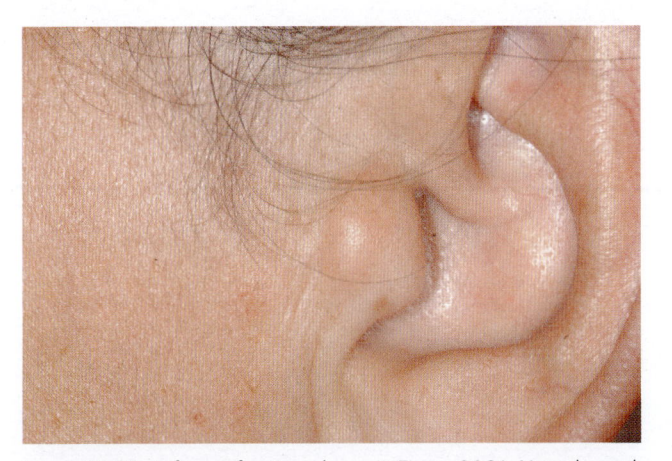

Figure 34.33. Left ear of patient shown in Figure 34.31. Note the nodular appendage in the tragus.

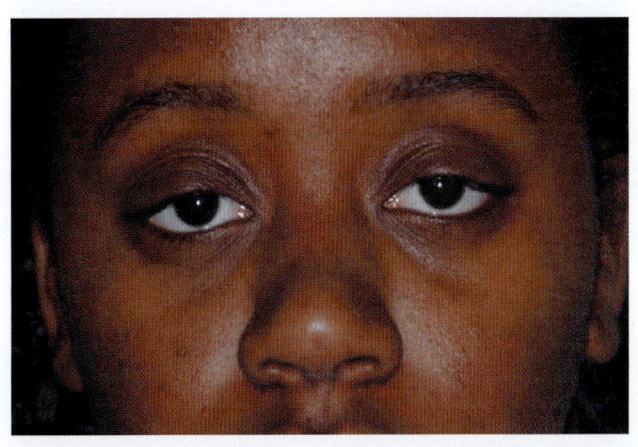

Figure 34.34. Face view of young African-American woman. There is minimal prominence of right lower eyelid temporally.

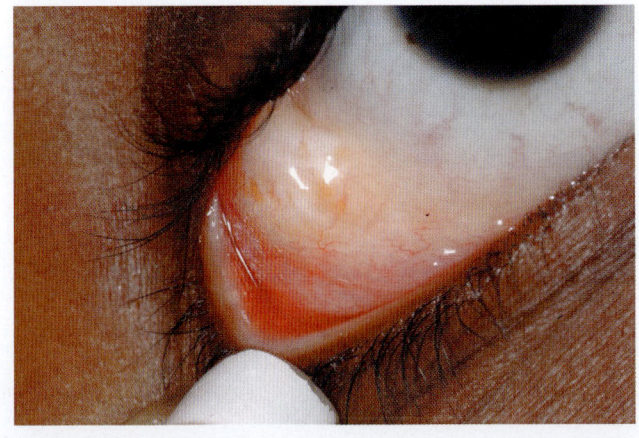

Figure 34.35. Patient shown in Figure 34.34 with right lower eyelid pulled downward. Note the dermolipoma in this atypical location. Most are located superotemporally.

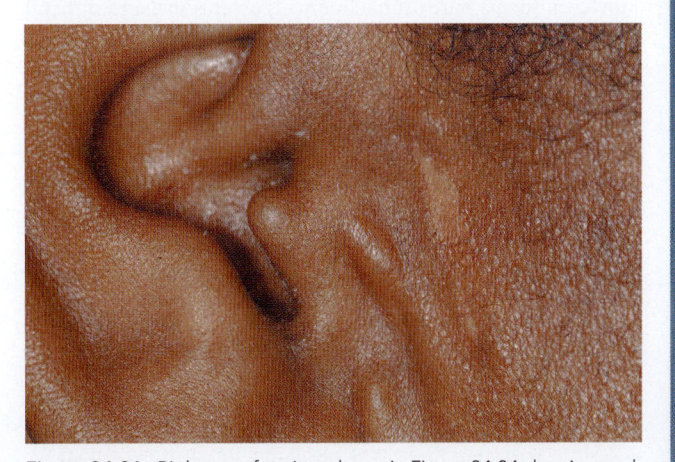

Figure 34.36. Right ear of patient shown in Figure 34.34 showing nodular appendage of tragus.

ORBITAL LIPOMA AND MYXOMA

Orbital lipoma may be difficult to diagnose clinically and radiographically because it blends with normal orbital fat and may be difficult to differentiate from herniated orbital fat.

General Considerations

Lipoma, a benign tumor composed of adipose tissue, is the most common mesenchymal neoplasm (1). It is quite common in subcutaneous tissue in many parts of the body, but is rare in the orbit (1–21). In the orbital region, it is quite likely that some cases diagnosed as orbital lipoma may actually represent herniated orbital fat or normal orbital fat removed as suspected tumor at the time of orbital biopsy. By strict definition, a true orbital lipoma should appear as a distinct mass within orbital fat. Variations of lipoma such as spindle cell lipoma (8,21), angiolipoma (9), pleomorphic lipoma (10), and myolipoma (16) have been recognized in the orbit. Pleomorphic lipoma can be very similar clinically to herniated orbital fat. There were 2 cases (<1%) diagnosed as orbital lipoma among the 1,264 orbital lesions in the authors' series.

Clinical Features

Orbital lipoma usually presents as a circumscribed orbital mass that has similar symptoms and signs to other circumscribed orbital tumors.

Diagnostic Approaches

CT and MRI disclose a mass that may have heterogeneity or may have consistency similar to orbital fat. Lipoma is hyperintense on T1-weighted images. The more vascular lipomas may show contrast enhancement more so than normal fat. The diagnosis is not usually made clinically and the lipoma is recognized histopathologically after surgical excision.

Pathology

Histopathologically, orbital lipoma is a tumor composed of mature lipocytes, and may be quite similar to normal fat cells. However, such a pure orbital lipoma is exceptional and difficult to diagnose microscopically. Some of the variations of lipoma are easier to recognize. Spindle cell lipoma shows mature lipocytes interspersed in a bed of benign spindle cells (4–7,8,21). The pleomorphic lipoma is believed to represent an extremely pleomorphic variant of spindle cell lipoma. It is characterized by the presence of scattered, bizarre giant cells that frequently have a floret-like arrangement of multiple hyperchromatic nuclei around an eosinophilic cytoplasm (10).

Management

Management of orbital lipoma is usually complete surgical excision. The diagnosis is rarely suspected clinically and the tumor is usually managed like any other circumscribed soft tissue mass. The rare case that involves orbital bone requires removal of affected bone. The prognosis is usually excellent.

ORBITAL LIPOMA AND MYXOMA

Selected References

Reviews
1. Shields JA, Shields CL, Scartozzi R. Survey of 1264 patients with orbital tumors and simulating lesions: the 2002 Montgomery Lecture, part 1. *Ophthalmology* 2004;111:997–1008.
2. Shields JA, Bakewell B, Augsburger DG, et al. Classification and incidence of space-occupying lesions of the orbit. A survey of 645 biopsies. *Arch Ophthalmol* 1984;102:1606–1611.
3. Shields JA, Bakewell B, Augsburger DG, et al. Space-occupying orbital masses in children. A review of 250 consecutive biopsies. *Ophthalmology* 1986;93:379–384.

Histopathology
4. Johnson BL, Linn JG Jr. Spindle cell lipoma of the orbit. *Arch Ophthalmol* 1979;97:133–134.
5. Stiglmayer N, Jandrokovicc S, Miklicc P, et al. Atypical lipoma: well differentiated liposarcoma of the orbit with dedifferentiated areas. *Orbit* 2003;22:311–316.
6. Nagayama A, Miyamura N, Lu Z, et al. Light and electron microscopic findings in a patient with orbital myolipoma. *Graefes Arch Clin Exp Ophthalmol* 2003;241:773–776.
7. Jakobiec FA, Nguyen J, Bhat P, et al. MDM2-positive atypical lipomatous neoplasm/well-differentiated liposarcoma versus spindle cell lipoma of the orbit. *Ophthal Plast Reconstr Surg* 2010;26:413–415.

Case Reports
8. Bartley GB, Yeatts RP, Garrity JA, et al. Spindle cell lipoma of the orbit. *Am J Ophthalmol* 1985;100:605–609.
9. Feinfield RE, Hesse RJ, Scharfenberg JC. Orbital angiolipoma. *Arch Ophthalmol* 1988;106:1093–1095.
10. Daniel CS, Beaconsfield M, Rose GE, et al. Pleomorphic lipoma of the orbit: a case series and review of literature. *Ophthalmology* 2003;110:101–105.
11. Brown HH, Kersten RC, Kulwin DR. Lipomatous hamartoma of the orbit. *Arch Ophthalmol* 1991;109:240–243.
12. Miller MH, Yokoyama C, Wright JE, et al. An aggressive lipoblastic tumour in the orbit of a child. *Histopathology* 1990;17:141–145.
13. Ali SF, Farber M, Meyer DR. Fibrolipoma of the orbit. *Ophthal Plast Reconstr Surg* 2013;29:e79–e81.
14. Toledano Fernández N, Stoica BT, Genol Saavedra I, et al. Diplopia from pleomorphic lipoma of the orbit with lateral rectus muscle involvement. *Ophthal Plast Reconstr Surg* 2013;29:e53–e55.
15. Dutton JJ, Escaravage GK Jr, Fowler AM, et al. Lipoblastomatosis: case report and review of the literature. *Ophthal Plast Reconstr Surg* 2011;27:417–421.
16. Borrelli M, Buhlbuck D, Strehl A, et al. Leiomyolipoma of the orbit. *Ophthal Plast Reconstr Surg* 2012;28:e21–e23.
17. Nuruddin M, Osmani M, Mudhar HS, et al. Orbital lipofibromatosis in a child: a case report. *Orbit* 2010;29:360–362.
18. Kim MH, Sa HS, Woo K, et al. Fibrolipoma of the orbit. *Ophthal Plast Reconstr Surg* 2011;27:e16–e18.
19. Shah NB, Chang WY, White VA, et al. Orbital lipoma: 2 cases and review of literature. *Ophthal Plast Reconstr Surg* 2007;23:202–205.
20. Dutton JJ, Wright JD Jr. Intramuscular lipoma of the superior oblique muscle. *Orbit* 2006;25:227–233.
21. Mawn LA, Jordan DR, Olberg B. Spindle-cell lipoma of the preseptal eyelid. *Ophthal Plast Reconstr Surg* 1998;14:174–177.

ORBITAL PLEOMORPHIC LIPOMA: CLINICAL, MAGNETIC RESONANCE IMAGING, AND HISTOPATHOLOGIC FINDINGS

With MRI, orbital pleomorphic lipoma has features almost identical to normal orbital fat. Illustrated is a case of orbital pleomorphic lipoma that presented as a soft mass under the lower eyelid. A typical case is shown.

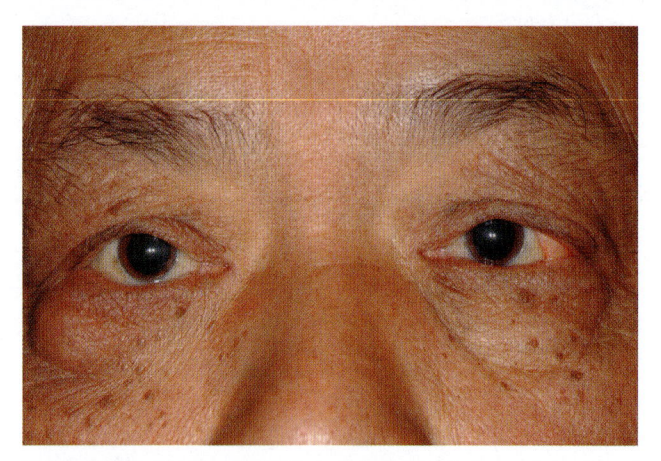

Figure 34.37. Elderly man with conjunctival/orbital mass in region of lateral canthus.

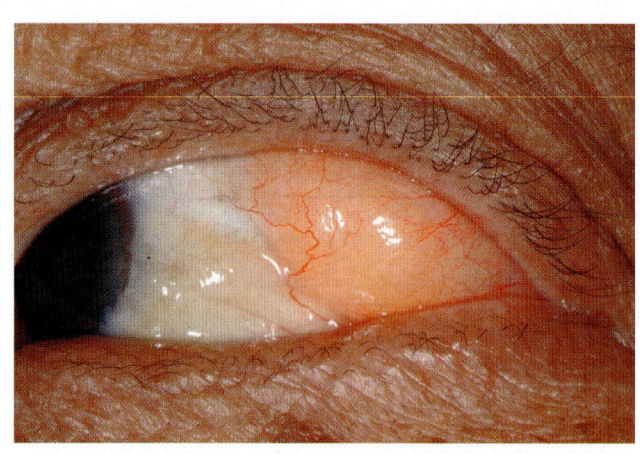

Figure 34.38. Closer view of lesion shown in Figure 34.37.

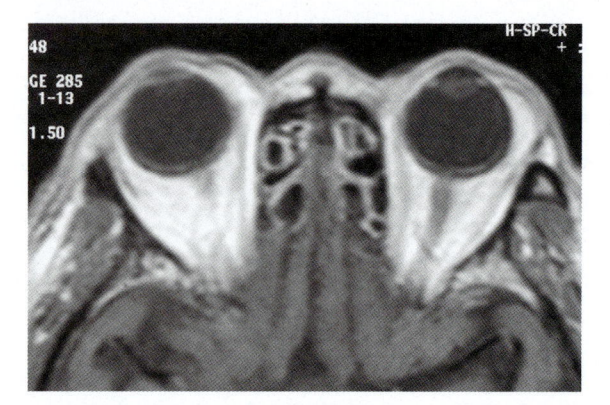

Figure 34.39. Axial magnetic resonance imaging with gadolinium enhancement but without fat suppression. Note that the lesion can be barely seen temporal to left eye (to right in the image).

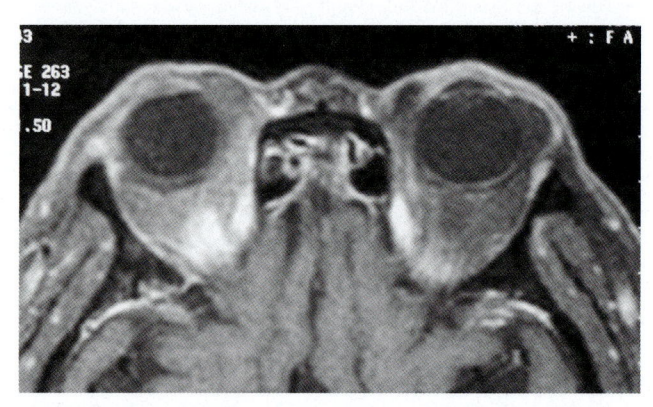

Figure 34.40. Axial MRI with gadolinium enhancement and with fat suppression. The lesion is better seen as a low-signal intensity. The lesion was excised intact.

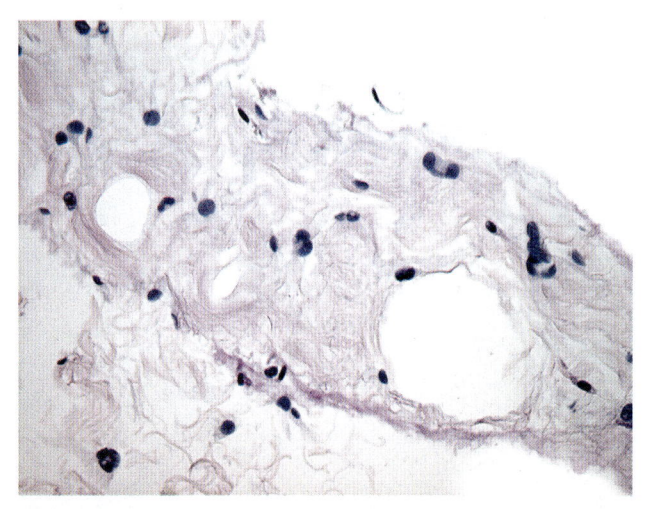

Figure 34.41. Photomicrograph showing mature lipocytes with myxoid change and scattered basophilic nuclei. (Hematoxylin–eosin ×100.)

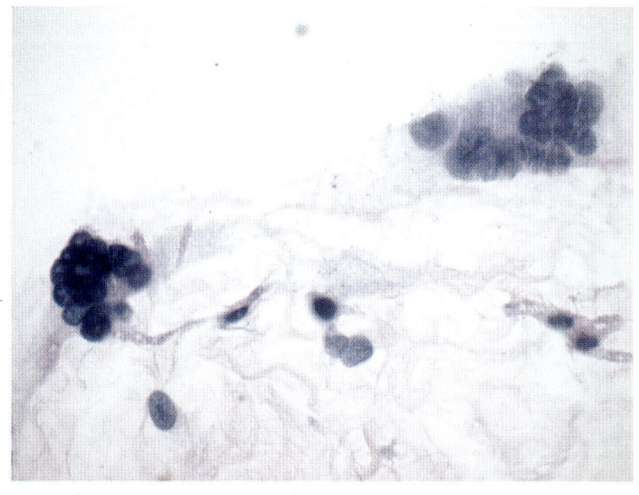

Figure 34.42. Another view of same tumor, showing atypical floret-like giant cells that characterize pleomorphic lipoma. (Hematoxylin–eosin ×250.)

Chapter 34 Orbital Lipomatous and Myxomatous Tumors

ORBITAL LIPOMA: CLINICOPATHOLOGIC VARIATIONS

Orbital lipoma can assume any of several variations. Examples are shown of a spindle cell lipoma, angiolipoma, and pleomorphic lipoma. Another case of pleomorphic lipoma is shown in the *Atlas of Eyelid and Conjunctival Tumors*.

Bartley GB, Yeatts RP, Garrity JA, et al. Spindle cell lipoma of the orbit. *Am J Ophthalmol* 1985;100:605–609.

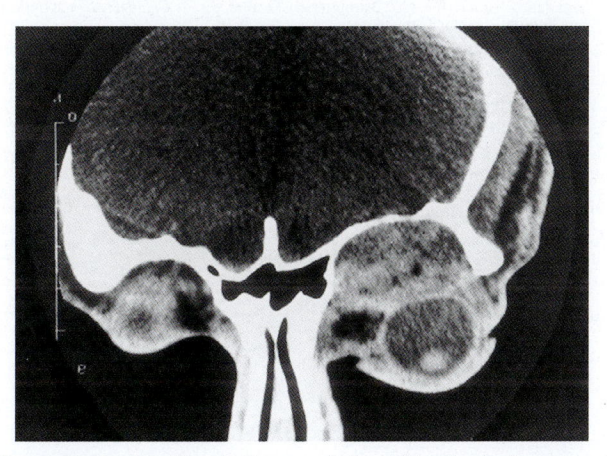

Figure 34.43. Spindle cell lipoma of the orbit. Coronal computed tomography of a 27-year-old man with a 7-year history of progressive fullness of the left upper eyelid. (Courtesy of R. Jean Campbell, MD.)

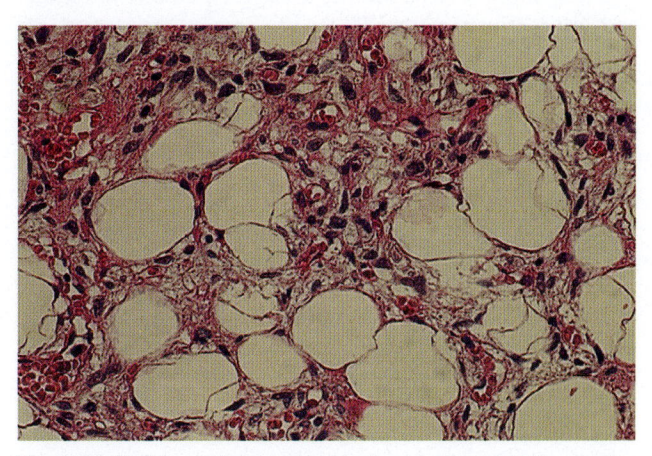

Figure 34.44. Histopathology of lesion shown in Figure 34.43, revealing mature lipocytes and uniform spindle cells. (Hematoxylin–eosin ×160.) (Courtesy of R. Jean Campbell, MD.)

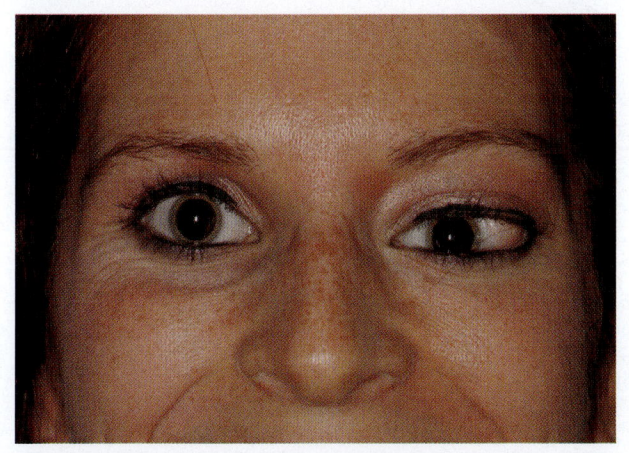

Figure 34.45. Young woman with large, epibulbar mass of the left eye with extension into the orbit causing downward and inward displacement of the globe.

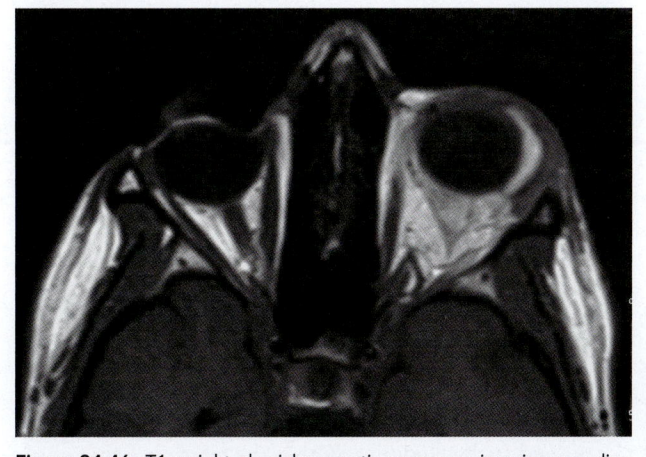

Figure 34.46. T1-weighted axial magnetic resonance imaging revealing an ill-defined bright signal mass filling the entire orbit, overriding the muscles and optic nerve and extending into the temporal epibulbar region.

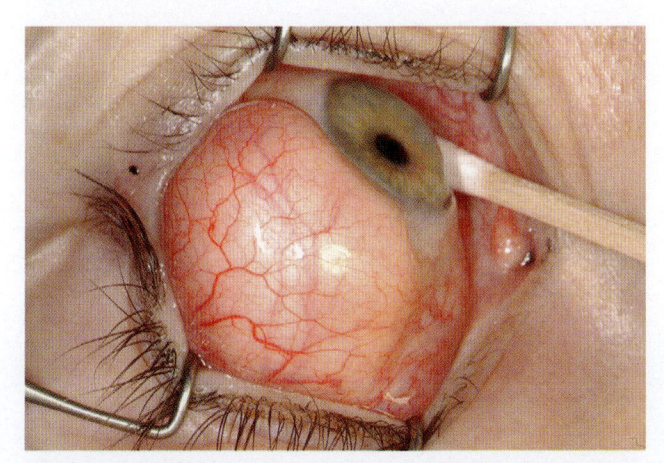

Figure 34.47. Transconjunctival approach was made to remove the large orbital mass.

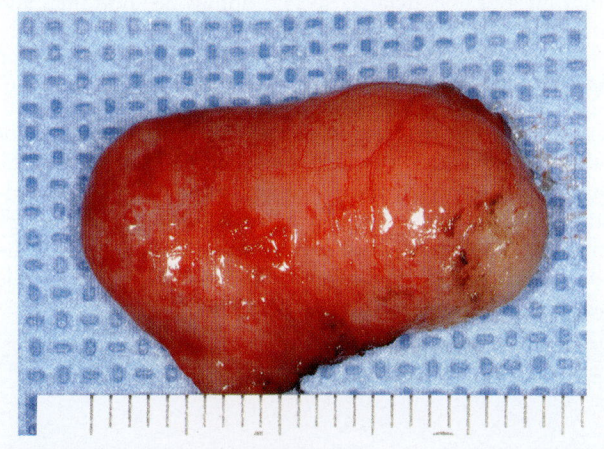

Figure 34.48. At surgery, a lobulated, fatty mass was removed and histopathology confirmed orbital lipoma.

ORBITAL MYXOMA

General Considerations

Myxoma is an uncommon, benign, mesenchymal tumor that generally affects skeletal muscles in the extremities, skin, heart, and genitourinary system (1,2). This tumor rarely occurs in the orbit. In the authors' review of 1,264 orbital tumors, there were no cases of myxoma (1). Myxoma can be a feature of the Carney complex, Mazabraud syndrome, and McCune–Albright syndrome.

Systemic myxoma is classified into five types including intramuscular (typical), cutaneous (superficial angiomyxoma), juxta-articular, nerve sheath (neurothekeoma), and aggressive angiomyxoma (2). These categories are less applicable for orbital tumors (2). Myxoma can produce excessive glycosaminoglycans with prominent hyaluronic acid, but minimal collagen (2). Myxoma and angiomyxoma derive from cells similar to fibroblasts and display low mitotic activity.

Clinical Features

Orbital myxoma usually manifests with painless proptosis. In the few reported cases, this tumor involved mid and posterior aspects of the orbit (2–6). The mass can be a circumscribed and round soft tissue mass to ill defined in appearance.

Diagnostic Approaches

With imaging studies, orbital myxoma demonstrates orbital fat infiltration with enhancement (2,6). There are few published cases in the orbit and the features are not well described.

Pathology

Histopathology of myxoma shows a hypocellular lesion consisting of sparse stellate and spindle cells with small intranuclear and intracytoplasmic vacuolization (2–6). Macrophages and mast cells are sometimes present. Blood vessels are sparse. The cells are surrounded by a basophilic myxoid matrix of hyaluronic acid and chondroitin sulfate. This matrix appears viscous and sticky clinically. Within the matrix are fine fibrillary reticulin fibers. The tumor cells stain positive for vimentin, CD34, and factor XIIIa. Myxoma should be differentiated from myxoid liposarcoma, myxoid fibrous histiocytoma, and myxoid embryonal rhabdomyosarcoma.

Management

Complete surgical resection is the treatment of choice for orbital myxoma. Most excised lesions do not recur (2). If the diagnosis is suspected and the lesion is small and asymptomatic, periodic observation may be appropriate, as is done for small asymptomatic cavernous hemangiomas. Due to the low mitotic cycling, these tumors are expected to show little response to radiotherapy or chemotherapy.

Selected References

Reviews

1. Shields JA, Shields CL, Scartozzi R. Survey of 1264 patients with orbital tumors and simulating lesions: The 2002 Montgomery Lecture, part 1. *Ophthalmology* 2004;111:997–1008.
2. Hidayat AA, Flint A, Marentette L, et al. Myxomas and angiomyxomas of the orbit: a clinicopathologic study of 6 cases. *Ophthalmology* 2007;114:1012–1019.

Case Reports

3. Tawfik HA, Elraey HZ. Orbital myxoma: a case report. *Orbit* 2013;32:200–202.
4. Sánchez-Orgaz M, Grabowska A, Arbizu-Duralde A, et al. Orbital nerve sheath myxoma: a case report. *Ophthal Plast Reconstr Surg* 2011;27:e106–e108.
5. Candy EJ, Miller NR, Carson BS. Myxoma of bone involving the orbit. *Arch Ophthalmol* 1991;109:919–920.
6. Lieb WE, Goebel HH, Wallenfang T. Myxoma of the orbit: A clinicopathologic report. *Graefes Arch Clin Exp Ophthalmol* 1990;228:28–32.

Chapter 34 Orbital Lipomatous and Myxomatous Tumors

ORBITAL MYXOMA

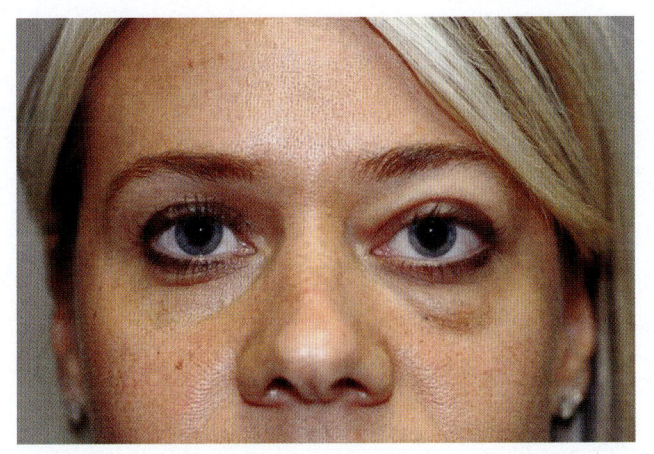

Figure 34.49. Middle-aged woman with mild left proptosis. (Courtesy of Roger Turbin, MD.)

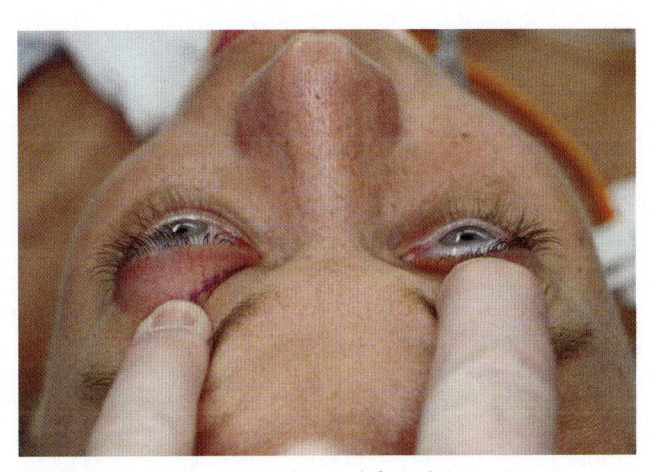

Figure 34.50. Bird's-eye view showing left axial proptosis.

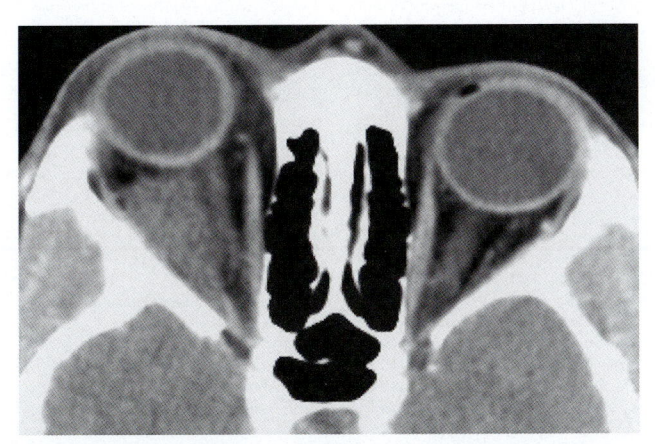

Figure 34.51. Computed tomography showing left orbital mass along lateral wall within muscle cone.

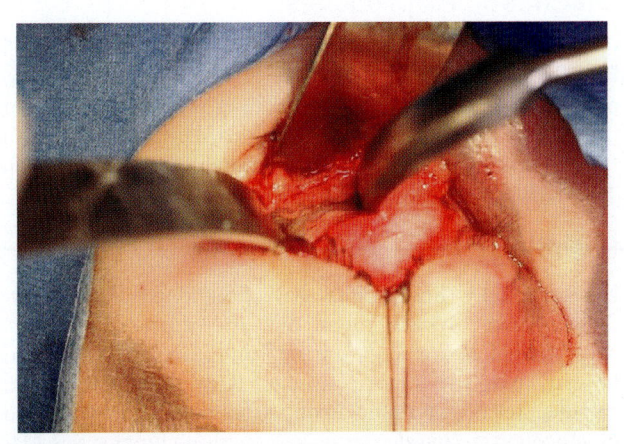

Figure 34.52. At surgery, the mass was ill defined within the orbital tissue.

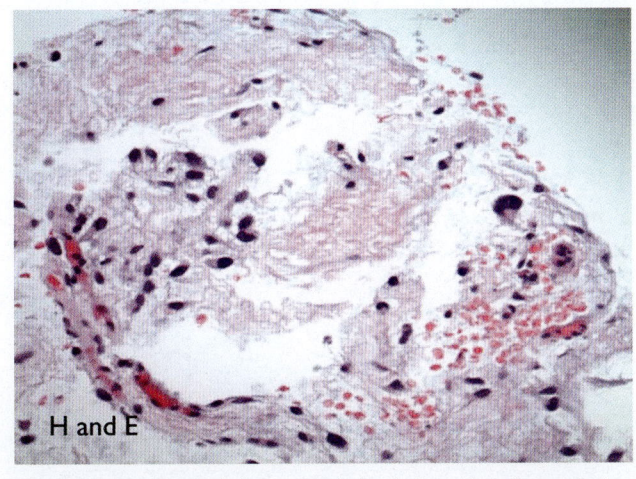

Figure 34.53. Histopathology revealed spindle and stellate cells in a loose matrix. (Hematoxylin–eosin ×200.)

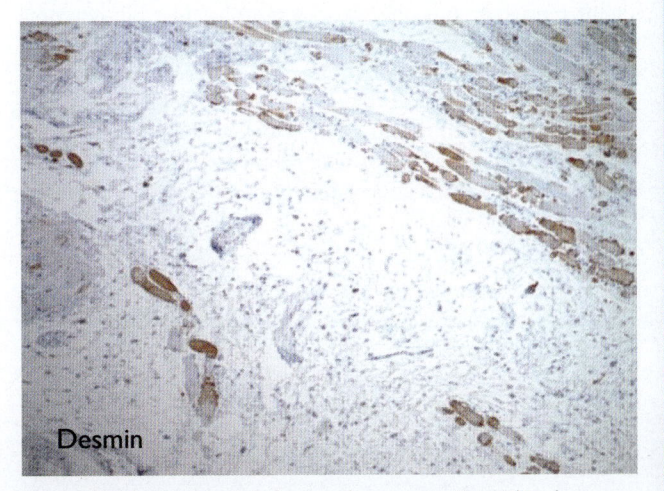

Figure 34.54. Desmin stain for muscle was negative within the tumor, consistent with myxoma. Note the normal muscle strands stain positive as an internal control. (Desmin ×150.)

ORBITAL LIPOSARCOMA

General Considerations

Liposarcoma is a malignant tumor of adipose tissue. It is the most common soft tissue sarcoma of adults (1–18). It occurs most often in the thigh, retroperitoneum, and inguinal region, but has a widespread distribution. It rarely takes origin in the orbital region, where it begins as a slow-growing, circumscribed tumor that may be indistinguishable from other discrete orbital tumors (1–5). There seems to be a slight tendency for orbital liposarcoma to originate in the medial or lateral rectus muscles (4–18). Orbital liposarcoma can occur at any age and reported cases have ranged from 5 to 70 years.

Clinical Features

Orbital liposarcoma generally presents as proptosis or displacement of the globe and cannot be distinguished clinically from most benign or low-grade malignant tumors.

Diagnostic Approaches

Orbital CT and MRI have no specific findings for orbital liposarcoma. The images are expected to vary with the histopathologic findings, which vary by case. With CT, the tumor often has a cystic appearance owing to the large amount of fat and mucin (6). With MRI, the tumor is hyperintense on T1-weighted images.

Pathology

Microscopically, liposarcomas have been divided into well-differentiated, myxoid, round cell, and pleomorphic types. Most orbital liposarcoma are well-differentiated or myxoid liposarcomas. The tumor consists of fairly well-differentiated spindle, stellate, or round lipoblasts suspended in a myxoid or mucopolysaccharide-rich matrix, with a complex vascular system. This is in contrast to a pure myxoma, which shows a sparsity of vessels. In the largest series of primary orbital liposarcoma (seven cases), five were purely differentiated, one was dedifferentiated, and one was pleomorphic (4). Liposarcoma usually does not arise from a pre-existing lipoma, but probably develops from pluripotent mesenchymal cells that have the capacity toward lipocytic differentiation. However, lipoma can rarely undergo dedifferentiation into low-grade liposarcoma. This suggests that the majority of orbital liposarcomas are relatively low grade and a good prognosis is suspected.

Management

The best management of orbital liposarcoma is complete surgical excision. In advanced cases, orbital exenteration may be necessary. However, there seems to be an increasing tendency to avoid exenteration and to employ irradiation (7).

Selected References

Reviews

1. Shields JA, Shields CL, Scartozzi R. Survey of 1264 patients with orbital tumors and simulating lesions: the 2002 Montgomery Lecture, part 1. *Ophthalmology* 2004;111: 997–1008.
2. Shields JA, Bakewell B, Augsburger DG, et al. Classification and incidence of space-occupying lesions of the orbit. A survey of 645 biopsies. *Arch Ophthalmol* 1984;102: 1606–1611.
3. Shields JA, Bakewell B, Augsburger DG, et al. Space-occupying orbital masses in children. A review of 250 consecutive biopsies. *Ophthalmology* 1986;93:379–384.
4. Cai YC, McMenamin ME, Rose G, et al. Primary liposarcoma of the orbit: a clinicopathologic study of seven cases. *Ann Diagn Pathol* 2001;5:255–266.

Imaging

5. Jakobiec FA, Rini F, Char D, et al. Primary liposarcoma of the orbit. Problems in the diagnosis and management of five cases. *Ophthalmology* 1989;96:180–191.
6. McNab AA, Moseley I. Primary orbital liposarcoma: clinical and computed tomographic features. *Br J Ophthalmol* 1990;74:437–439.

Management

7. Cockerham KP, Kennerdell JS, Celin SE, et al. Liposarcoma of the orbit: a management challenge. *Ophthal Plast Reconstr Surg* 1998;14:370–374.

Histopathology

8. Stiglmayer N, Jandrokovicc S, Miklicc P, et al. Atypical lipoma: well-differentiated liposarcoma of the orbit with dedifferentiated areas. *Orbit* 2003;22:311–316.
9. Wagle AM, Biswas J, Subramaniam N, et al. Primary liposarcoma of the orbit: a clinicopathological study. *Orbit* 1999;18:33–36.
10. Naeser P, Mostrom U. Liposarcoma of the orbit: a clinicopathological case report. *Br J Ophthalmol* 1982;66:190–193.

Case Reports

11. Monteiro ML. Liposarcoma of the orbit presenting as an enlarged medial rectus muscle on CT scan. *Br J Ophthalmol* 2002;86:1450.
12. Sabb PC, Syed NA, Sires BS, et al. Primary orbital myxoid liposarcoma presenting as orbital pain. *Arch Ophthalmol* 1996;114:353–354.
13. Lane CM, Wright JE, Garner A. Primary myxoid liposarcoma of the orbit. *Br J Ophthalmol* 1988;72:912–917.
14. Shinder R, Mostafavi D, Nasser QJ, et al. Primary orbital liposarcoma misdiagnosed as thyroid associated orbitopathy. *Orbit* 2012;31:264–266.
15. Doyle M, Odashiro AN, Pereira PR, et al. Primary pleomorphic liposarcoma of the orbit: a case report. *Orbit* 2012;31:168–170.
16. Gire J, Weinbreck N, Labrousse F, et al. Myxofibrosarcoma of the orbit: case report and review of literature. *Ophthal Plast Reconstr Surg* 2012;28:e9–e11.
17. Saeed MU, Chang BY, Atherley C, et al. A rare diagnosis of dedifferentiated liposarcoma of the orbit. *Orbit* 2007;26:43–45.
18. Parmar DN, Luthert PJ, Cree IA, et al. Two unusual osteogenic orbital tumors: presumed parosteal osteosarcomas of the orbit. *Ophthalmology* 2001;108:1452–1456.

Chapter 34 Orbital Lipomatous and Myxomatous Tumors 669

ORBITAL LIPOSARCOMA

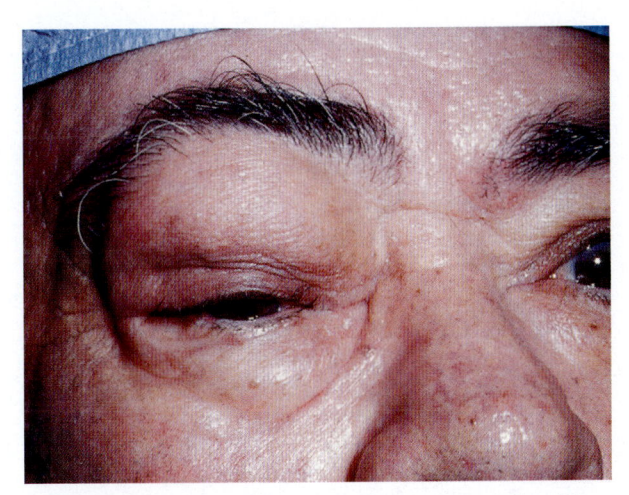

Figure 34.55. Extensive swelling of the right upper eyelid in a 78-year-old man. (Courtesy of Charles Lee, MD.)

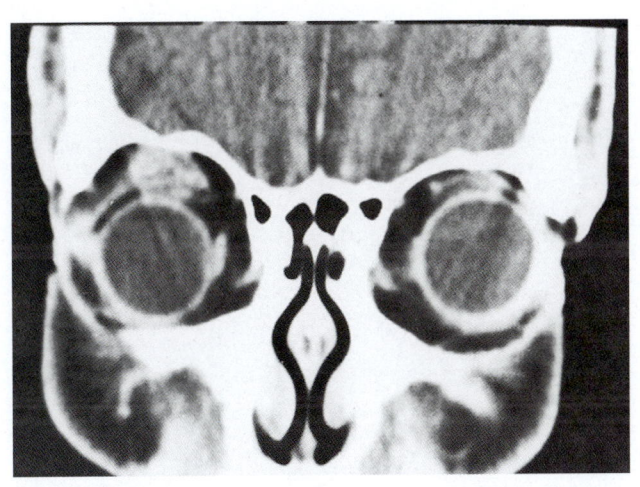

Figure 34.56. Coronal computed tomography of patient shown in Figure 34.49, demonstrating ovoid mass superior to the globe. (Courtesy of Charles Lee, MD.)

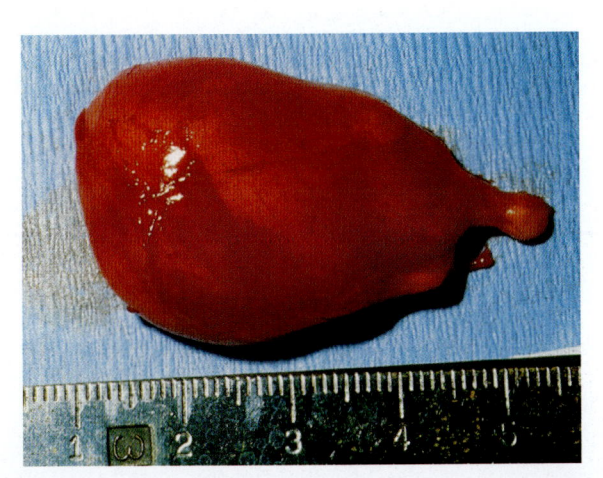

Figure 34.57. Gross appearance of mass shown in Figure 34.49 after excision. (Courtesy of Charles Lee, MD.)

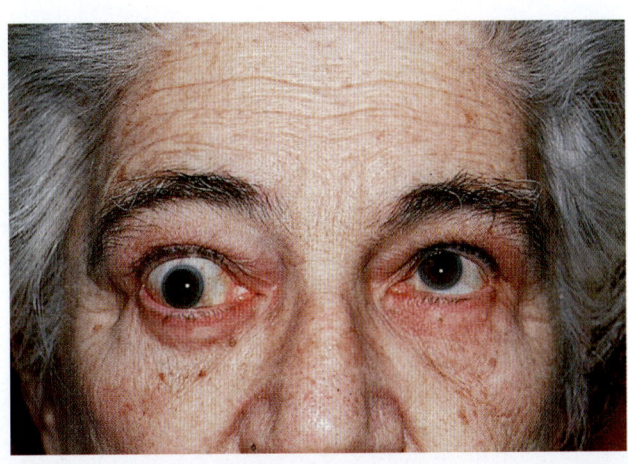

Figure 34.58. Proptosis of the right eye in an elderly woman. (Courtesy of Ralph C. Eagle, Jr, MD.)

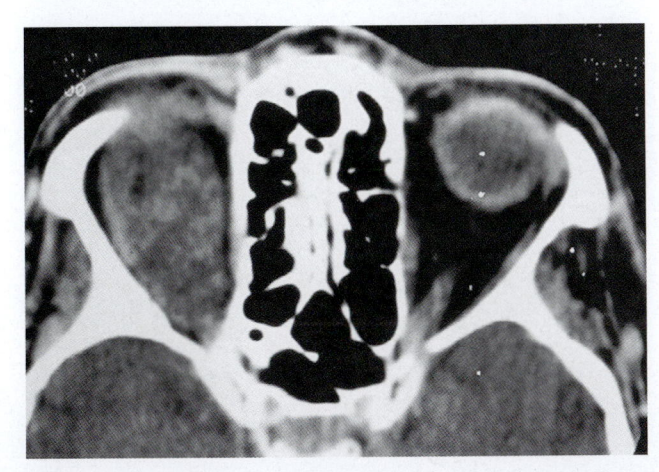

Figure 34.59. Axial computed tomography of patient shown in Figure 34.52, revealing an ovoid mass filling most of posterior orbit. (Courtesy of Ralph C. Eagle, Jr, MD.)

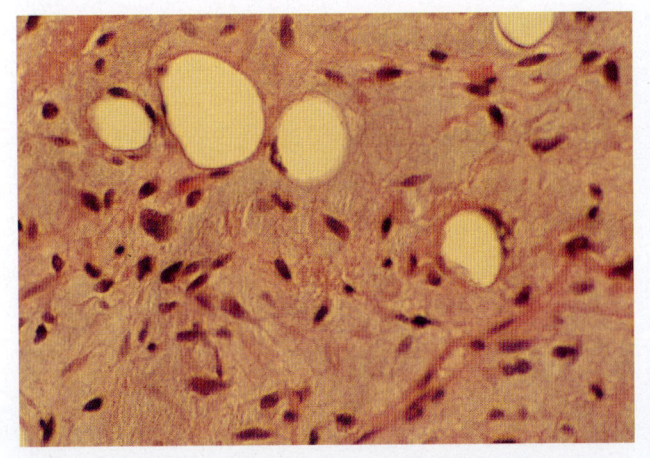

Figure 34.60. Histopathology of lesion shown in Figure 34.52, demonstrating malignant spindle cells in a myxomatous matrix. (Hematoxylin–eosin ×100.) (Courtesy of Ralph C. Eagle, Jr, MD.)

CHAPTER 35

ORBITAL HISTIOCYTIC TUMORS

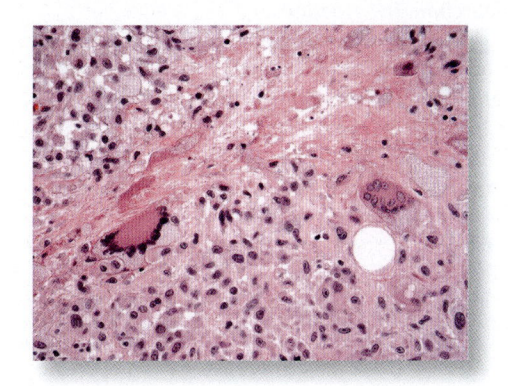

General Considerations

Proliferative disorders of histiocytes comprise a spectrum, ranging from solitary benign inflammatory processes to widely disseminated lesions that exhibit malignant behavior (1–17). Conditions to be considered here include juvenile xanthogranuloma (JXG), adult-onset xanthogranuloma with asthma (AXG), Langerhans' cell histiocytosis (LCH), Erdheim–Chester disease (ECD), sinus histiocytosis with massive lymphadenopathy (SHML), and multinucleate cell angiohistiocytoma. Necrobiotic xanthogranuloma (NXG), a related condition, is discussed in the section on eyelid tumors.

Clinical Features

The general clinical features and other ocular findings in JXG are discussed in the sections on eyelid, conjunctival, and intraocular tumors. Orbital involvement with JXG seems to be more common in the anterior extraconal spaces and presents as eyelid swelling and a palpable mass. Most JXG in the orbit has been solitary, without a history of cutaneous lesions (5,10–15).

Orbital JXG has usually been diagnosed in the first year of life in contrast to lesions in the conjunctiva and eyelid, which can appear in older children or adults (13). Inflammatory signs are usually minimal. Orbital JXG can occasionally be more aggressive and invade orbital bone and the intracranial cavity (7,11,12).

In some cases, xanthogranuloma can affect adults (AXG) and patients often have related asthma (6). The majority of AXG patients is in the fourth or fifth decade of life and simultaneously describe asthma symptoms and an orbital inflammatory picture. Many have periorbital swelling and xanthelasma cutaneous plaques (6,7). The diagnosis is established on biopsy.

Diagnostic Approaches

Imaging studies show an irregular, solid mass that is usually located in the anterior orbital structures. It shows mild to moderate enhancement with contrast agents. The diagnosis is not often made clinically, but is recognized histopathologically after incisional or excisional biopsy.

ORBIT JUVENILE XANTHOGRANULOMA

Pathology

JXG is characterized histopathologically by a proliferation of histiocytes, along with lymphocytes, plasma cells, eosinophils, and typical Touton giant cells that stain positive for lipid. Immunohistochemical markers for histiocytes are positive and S-100 protein is negative. Electron microscopy does not generally show cytoplasmic Birbeck granules, structures that characterize LCH.

Management

If it were possible to diagnosis orbital JXG clinically, a period of observation or oral or perilesional corticosteroids would seem to be appropriate management. However, the diagnosis is rarely made clinically and most cases are removed surgically because of suspicion of neoplasm. If possible, the mass should be removed entirely. If that is not possible and partial biopsy establishes the diagnosis, then corticosteroids are the preferred treatment. More advanced cases with bone involvement may require wide surgical excision and supplemental corticosteroids. Irradiation is generally not warranted.

ORBIT JUVENILE XANTHOGRANULOMA

Selected References

Reviews

1. Shields JA, Shields CL, Scartozzi R. Survey of 1264 patients with orbital tumors and simulating lesions: The 2002 Montgomery Lecture, part 1. *Ophthalmology* 2004;111: 997–1008.
2. Shields JA, Bakewell B, Augsburger JJ, et al. Classification and incidence of space-occupying lesions of the orbit. A survey of 645 biopsies. *Arch Ophthalmol* 1984;102: 1606–1611.
3. Shields JA, Bakewell B, Augsburger JJ, et al. Space-occupying orbital masses in children: A review of 250 consecutive biopsies. *Ophthalmology* 1986;93:379–384.
4. Shields JA, Shields CL. Clinical spectrum of histiocytic tumors of the orbit. *Trans Pa Acad Ophthalmol Otolaryngol* 1990;42:931–937.
5. Vick VL, Wilson MW, Fleming JC, et al. Orbital and eyelid manifestations of xanthogranulomatous diseases. *Orbit* 2006;25:221–225.
6. Jakobiec FA, Mills MD, Hidayat AA, et al. Periocular xanthogranulomas associated with severe adult-onset asthma. *Trans Am Ophthalmol Soc* 1993;91:99–125.
7. Cavallazzi R, Hirani A, Vasu TS, et al. Clinical manifestations and treatment of adult-onset asthma and periocular xanthogranuloma. *Can Respir J* 2009;16:159–162.

Imaging

8. Miszkiel KA, Sohaib SA, Rose GE, et al. Radiological and clinicopathological features of orbital xanthogranuloma. *Br J Ophthalmol* 2000;84:251–258.

Histopathology

9. Hidayat AA, Mafee MF, Laver NV, et al. Langerhans' cell histiocytosis and juvenile xanthogranuloma of the orbit. Clinicopathologic, CT, and MR imaging features. *Radiol Clin North Am* 1998;36:1229–1240.

Case Reports

10. Shields CL, Shields JA, Buchanon H. Solitary orbital involvement with juvenile xanthogranuloma. *Arch Ophthalmol* 1990;108:1587–1589.
11. Sanders TE. Infantile xanthogranuloma of the orbit. A report of three cases. *Am J Ophthalmol* 1966;61:1299–1306.
12. Gaynes PM, Cohen GS. Juvenile xanthogranuloma of the orbit. *Am J Ophthalmol* 1967;63:755–757.
13. Mencia-Gutierrez E, Gutierrez-Diaz E, Madero-Garcia S. Juvenile xanthogranuloma of the orbit in an adult. *Ophthalmologica* 2000;214:437–440.
14. Daien V, Malrieu eliaou C, Rodiere M, et al. Juvenile xanthogranuloma with bilateral optic neuritis. *Br J Ophthalmol* 2011;95:1331–1332.
15. Johnson TE, Alabiad C, Wei L, et al. Extensive juvenile xanthogranuloma involving the orbit, sinuses, brain, and subtemporal fossa in a newborn. *Ophthal Plast Reconstr Surg* 2010;26:133–134.
16. Hammond MD, Niemi EW, Ward TP, et al. Adult orbital xanthogranuloma with associated adult-onset asthma. *Ophthal Plast Reconstr Surg* 2004;20:329–332.
17. Shields CL, Thaler AS, Lally SE, et al. Massive macronodular juvenile xanthogranuloma of the eyelid in a newborn. *J AAPOS* 2014;18:195–197.

ORBITAL JUVENILE XANTHOGRANULOMA

JXG can occur as a solitary orbital mass in infants. A clinicopathologic correlation is illustrated.

Shields CL, Shields JA, Buchanon H. Solitary orbital involvement with juvenile xanthogranuloma. *Arch Ophthalmol* 1990;108:1587–1589.

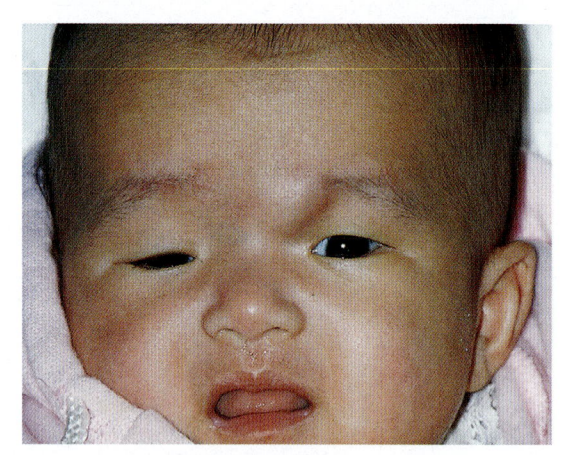

Figure 35.1. Subcutaneous mass superonasal to left eye secondary to juvenile xanthogranuloma in a 3-month-old girl. The mass was noted at birth and had shown gradual enlargement.

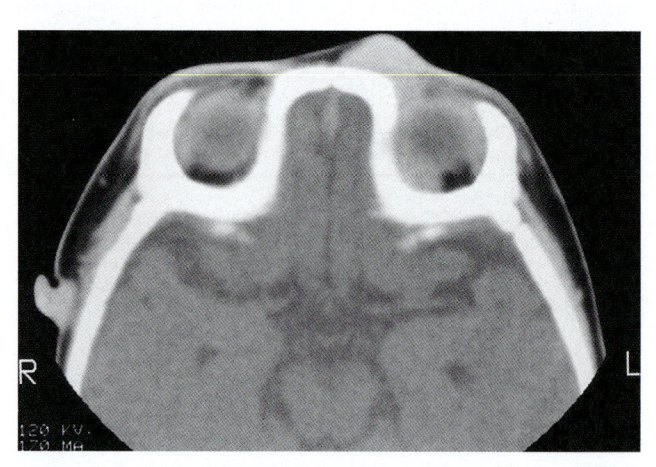

Figure 35.2. Axial computed tomography showing solid mass extending posteriorly along the superonasal wall of the orbit.

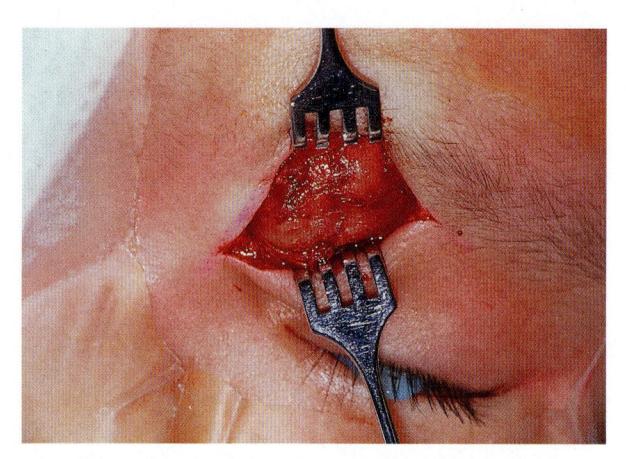

Figure 35.3. A biopsy of the subcutaneous portion of the mass was taken through a superonasal skin incision.

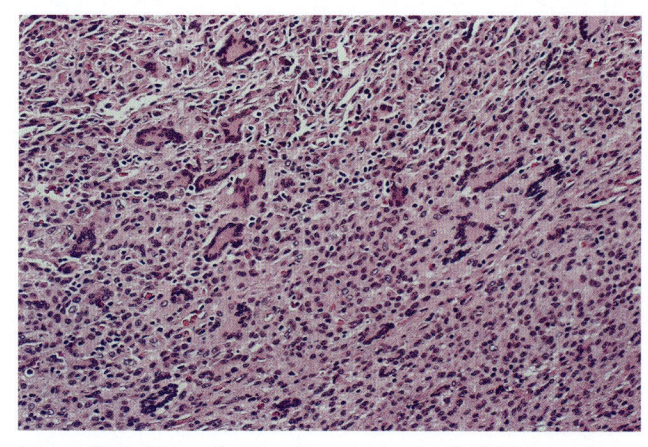

Figure 35.4. Histopathology showing sheets of histiocytes, chronic inflammatory cells, and giant cells. (Hematoxylin–eosin ×50.)

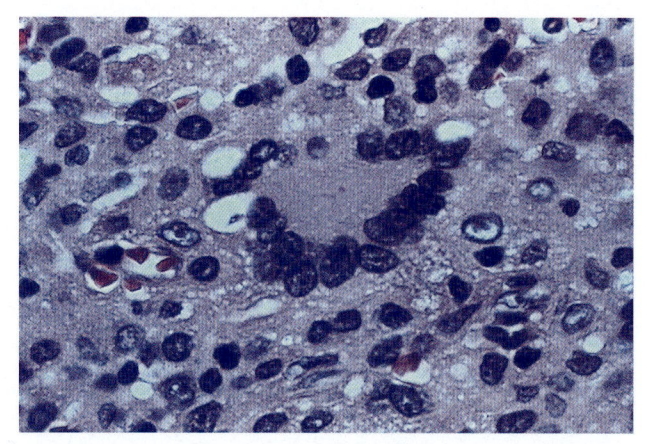

Figure 35.5. Histopathology showing giant cell with some lipid. It was classified as an atypical Touton giant cell. (Hematoxylin–eosin ×250.)

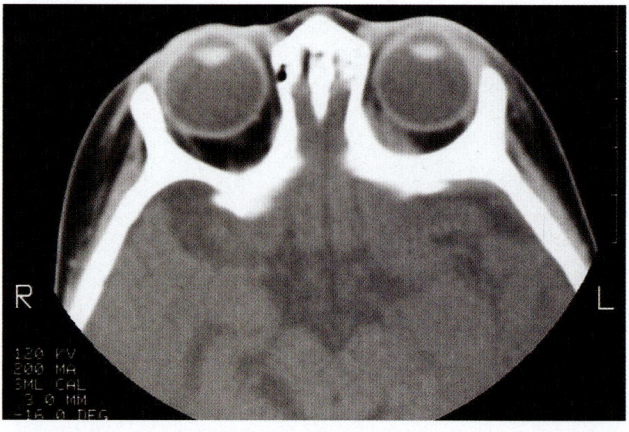

Figure 35.6. Axial computed tomography showing resolution of orbital mass after a course of systemic corticosteroids.

Chapter 35 Orbital Histiocytic Tumors

ORBITAL ADULT-ONSET XANTHOGRANULOMA WITH ASTHMA

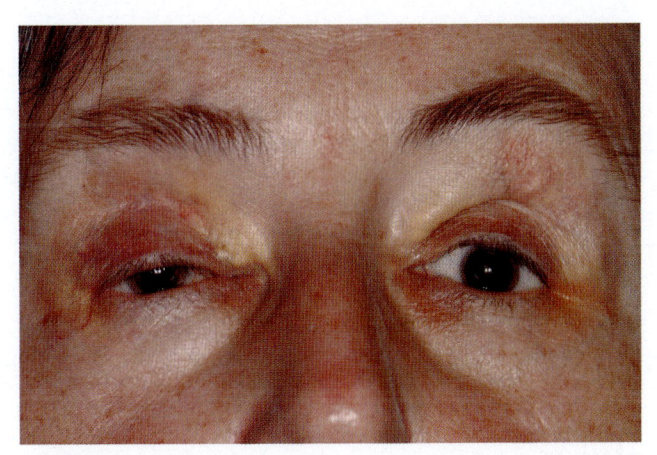

Figure 35.7. Elderly woman with recent onset xanthelasma and asthma, found to have biopsy proven adult-onset xanthogranuloma with asthma.

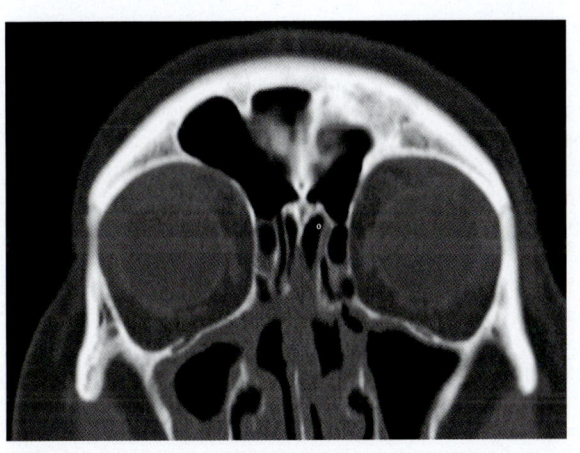

Figure 35.8. Computed tomography of patient in Figure 35.7, demonstrating soft tissue mass in superotemporal right orbit and slightly seen in the lateral left orbit.

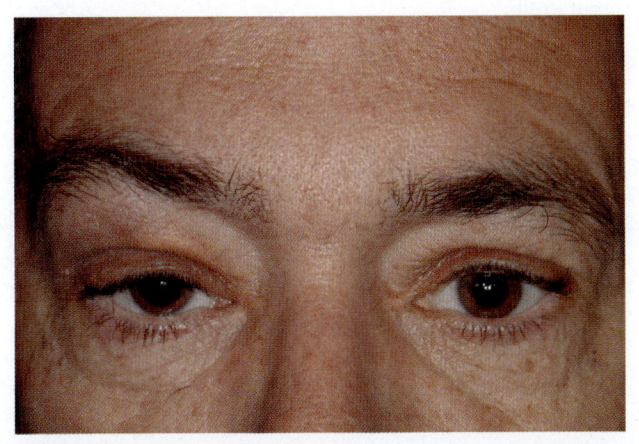

Figure 35.9. Middle-aged man with fullness of right orbit and minimal xanthelasma within the eyelid crease region.

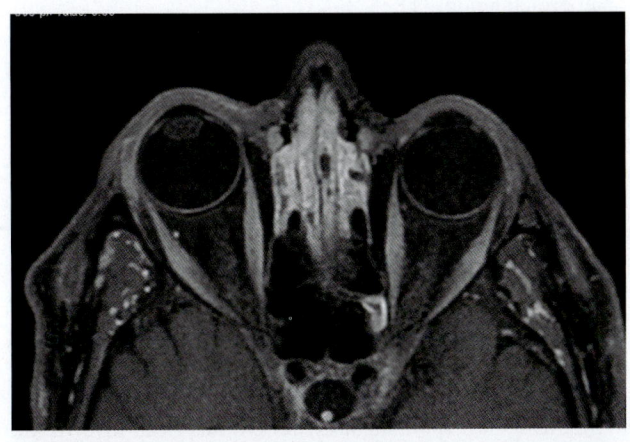

Figure 35.10. Magnetic resonance imaging of patient in Figure 35.9, showing only mild infiltration in right lacrimal gland region. Orbital biopsy confirmed adult-onset xanthogranuloma.

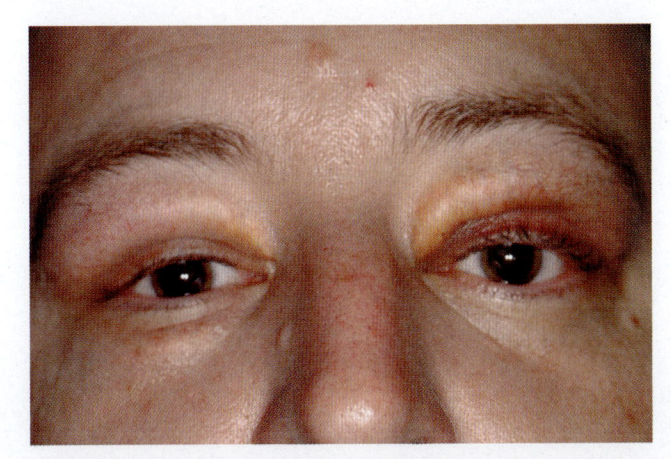

Figure 35.11. Middle-aged woman with bilateral upper eyelid fullness and relatively new onset xanthelasma and mild asthma.

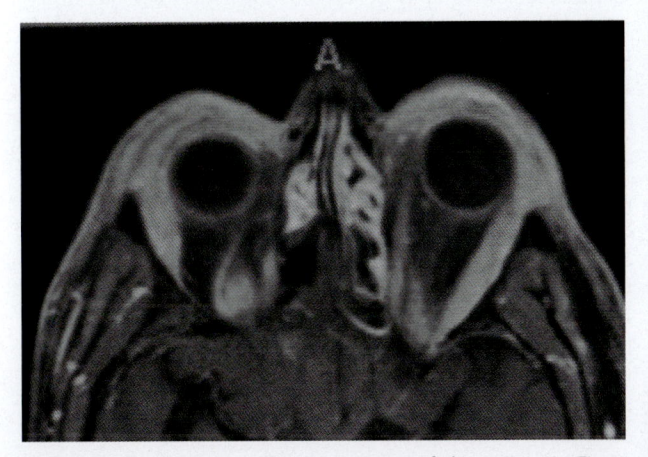

Figure 35.12. Magnetic resonance imaging of the patient in Figure 35.11, showing obvious, ill-defined infiltration laterally in both orbits. Orbital biopsy confirmed adult-onset xanthogranuloma.

ORBITAL LANGERHANS' CELL HISTIOCYTOSIS (EOSINOPHILIC GRANULOMA)

General Considerations

LCH is the currently accepted name for a group of diseases previously included under the term "histiocytosis X," namely eosinophilic granuloma (EG), Hand–Schuller–Christian disease, and Letterer–Siwe disease. The ultrastructural finding of typical rod–shaped or tennis racquet–shaped structures, called Birbeck bodies, suggest that the Langerhans' cell is involved in the disease process (1–24). The Langerhans' cell is a specific variant of dendritic histiocyte that ordinarily resides in the epidermis. The clinical manifestations of LCH vary widely, from a benign, self-limited process to an aggressive systemic condition that can cause death. Some of the more malignant histiocytoses have been reclassified as true histiocytic lymphomas. The most important of these with regard to the orbit is EG, which can occur in the orbital region in children as a solitary lesion of bone. Orbital EG is more common than orbital JXG. In the authors' series of 1,264 orbital lesions, there were 9 EGs and these accounted for 53% of all histiocytic lesions and for 1% of all orbital lesions (1).

Clinical Features

EG usually has typical clinical features, although the clinical findings can vary somewhat from case to case. It generally occurs in the first decade of life as a subacute swelling in the superotemporal aspect of the orbit, often with pain, redness, and tenderness over the affected bone superotemporally (4–23). It can resemble a ruptured dermoid cyst, dacryoadenitis, or idiopathic orbital inflammation ("inflammatory pseudotumor"). EG can occasionally develop in other quadrants and in the deeper orbital tissues, and can sometimes be multifocal. It can rarely be bilateral, with the opposite orbit becoming involved months after the first tumor (15). The lesion tends to gradually heal spontaneously. Rarely LCH can involve the intraocular structures (24).

Diagnostic Approaches

Computed tomography (CT) and magnetic resonance imaging (MRI) have fairly typical features in cases of EG (5,6). In the early stages, the lesion appears as an irregular, enhancing, radiolucent area of expanding bone, often with distinct fragments of bone within the mass. It usually affects the zygomatic and/or frontal bones, but other orbital bones can be affected. With time, the intraosseous lesion breaks through the cortical bone producing a moth-eaten appearance. The soft tissue component usually shows some enhancement with CT and MRI (2). Radiographically, it can resemble metastatic neuroblastoma, which occurs in somewhat younger children. Some degree of intracranial extension is not rare. Multiple osseous lesions are occasionally seen in other orbital and cranial bones (20). Although we generally prefer an open biopsy, fine-needle aspiration biopsy has been used to make the diagnosis in some cases (19).

Pathology

EG is characterized histopathologically as a proliferation of large mononuclear histiocytes with multinucleated giant cells of the Touton type, and scattered eosinophils, lymphocytes, and sometimes bone fragments. Positive immunohistochemistry reaction to S-100 protein is helpful in making the diagnosis. The diagnostic ultrastructural features finding are the Birbeck granules, distinctive rod-shaped or tennis racquet–shaped structures that are characteristic of Langerhans' cells.

Concerning pathogenesis, it is believed that transient immune dysfunction may provoke the cytokine-mediated proliferation of pathologic Langerhans' cells within the bone marrow of the anterolateral frontal bone. These cells cause osteolysis through elaboration of interleukin-1 and prostaglandin E2 (7). New information reveals that patients with LCH and ECD show high frequency of BRAFV600E mutations, detectable in the serum and urine (9). Patients with this mutation can respond to medications targeted against BRAF such as vemurafinib.

Management

Management includes biopsy with possible frozen sections to make a provisional diagnosis, followed by prompt surgical curettage. Systemic or local corticosteroids can be employed (4,8). Cytotoxic agents or low-dose radiotherapy are occasionally used, particularly if there is massive destructive lesions or multifocal lesions. Those with mutation in BRAF can respond to targeted anti-BRAF medications. Occasionally, EG can show spontaneous resolution without treatment (4,18).

ORBITAL LANGERHANS' CELL HISTIOCYTOSIS (EOSINOPHILIC GRANULOMA)

Selected References

Reviews
1. Shields JA, Shields CL, Scartozzi R. Survey of 1264 patients with orbital tumors and simulating lesions: The 2002 Montgomery Lecture, part 1. *Ophthalmology* 2004;111: 997–1008.
2. Shields JA, Bakewell B, Augsburger JJ, et al. Classification and incidence of space-occupying lesions of the orbit. A survey of 645 biopsies. *Arch Ophthalmol* 1984;102: 1606–1611.
3. Shields JA, Bakewell B, Augsburger JJ, et al. Space-occupying orbital masses in children: A review of 250 consecutive biopsies. *Ophthalmology* 1986;93:379–384.
4. Shields JA, Shields CL. Clinical spectrum of histiocytic tumors of the orbit. *Trans Pa Acad Ophthalmol Otolaryngol* 1990;42:931–937.

Imaging
5. Hidayat AA, Mafee MF, Laver NV, et al. Langerhans' cell histiocytosis and juvenile xanthogranuloma of the orbit. Clinicopathologic, CT, and MR imaging features. *Radiol Clin North Am* 1998;36:1229–1240.
6. Goli RS, Cockerham K, Smirniotopoulos JG, et al. The "dural tail sign": not always a meningioma. *Ophthal Plast Reconstr Surg* 1998:126–129.

Management
7. Woo KI, Harris GJ. Eosinophilic granuloma of the orbit: understanding the paradox of aggressive destruction responsive to minimal intervention. *Ophthal Plast Reconstr Surg* 2003;19(6):429–39.
8. Wirtschafter JD, Nesbit M, Anderson P, et al. Intralesional methylprednisolone for Langerhan's cell histiocytosis of the orbit and cranium. *J Pediatr Ophthalmol Strabismus* 1987;14:195–197.

Histopathology/Genetics
9. Hyman DM, Diamond EL, Vibat CR, et al. Prospective blinded study of BRAFV600E mutation detection cell-free DNA of patients with systemic histiocytic disorders. *Cancer Discov* 2015;5(1):64–71.

Case Reports
10. Feldman RB, Moore DM, Hood CI, et al. Solitary eosinophilic granuloma of the lateral orbital wall. *Am J Ophthalmol* 1985;100:318–323.
11. Jordan DR, McDonald H, Noel L, et al. Eosinophilic granuloma. *Arch Ophthalmol* 1993;111:134–135.
12. Glover AT, Grove AS Jr. Eosinophilic granuloma of the orbit with spontaneous healing. *Ophthalmology* 1987;94:1008–1012.
13. Lasso JM, de Erenchun RR, Bazan A. Eosinophilic granuloma of the orbit producing extensive bony destruction in a 32-month-old male infant. *Ann Plast Surg* 2000;44:109–110.
14. Amemiya T. Eosinophilic granuloma of the soft tissue in the orbit. *Ophthalmologica* 1981;182:42–48.
15. Demirci H, Shields CL, Shields JA, et al. Bilateral sequential orbital involvement in eosinophilic granuloma. *Arch Ophthalmol* 2002;120:978–979.
16. Gündüz K, Palamar M, Parmak N, et al. Eosinophilic granuloma of the orbit: report of two cases. *J AAPOS* 2007;11(5):506–508.
17. Gross FJ, Waxman JS, Rosenblatt MA, et al. Eosinophilic granuloma of the cavernous sinus and orbital apex in an HIV-positive patient. *Ophthalmology* 1989;96(4): 462–467.
18. Shetty SB, Mehta C. Langerhans cell histiocytosis of the orbit. *Indian J Ophthalmol* 2001;49:267–268.
19. Smith JH, Fulton L, O'Brien JM. Spontaneous regression of orbital Langerhans cell granulomatosis in a three-year-old girl. *Am J Ophthalmol* 1999;128:119–121.
20. LaBorwit SE, Karesh JW, Hirschbein MJ, et al. Multifocal Langerhans' cell histiocytosis involving the orbit. *J Pediatr Ophthalmol Strabismus* 1998;35:234–236.
21. Kramer TR, Noecker RJ, Miller JM, et al. Langerhans cell histiocytosis with orbital involvement. *Am J Ophthalmol* 1997;124:814–824.
22. Moshegov C, Martin P, Myers P, et al. Langerhans' cell histiocytosis of the frontal bone. *Aust N Z J Ophthalmol* 1994;22:133–138.
23. MacCumber MW, Hoffman PN, Wand GS, et al. Ophthalmic involvement in aggressive histiocytosis X. *Ophthalmology* 1990;97:22–27.
24. Shields CL, Hogarty MD, Kligman BE, et al. Langerhans cell histiocytosis of the uvea with neovascular glaucoma. Diagnosis by needle biopsy and management with intraocular bevacizumab and brachytherapy. *J Am Assoc Ped Ophthalm Strab* 2010;14: 534–5347.

ORBITAL LANGERHANS' CELL HISTIOCYTOSIS (EOSINOPHILIC GRANULOMA): CLINICAL, COMPUTED TOMOGRAPHY, AND PATHOLOGIC FEATURES

Jordan DR, McDonald H, Noel L, et al. Eosinophilic granuloma. *Arch Ophthalmol* 1993;111:134–135.

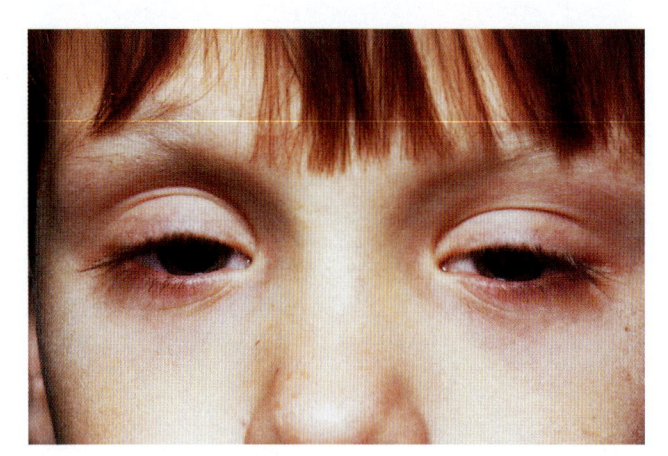

Figure 35.13. Eosinophilic granuloma. Swelling and blepharoptosis of left upper eyelid in a 6-year-old boy.

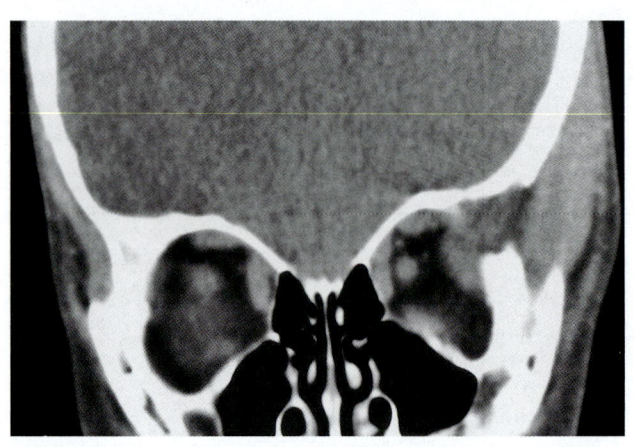

Figure 35.14. Coronal computed tomography of patient shown in Figure 35.7, demonstrating superotemporal bone destructive lesion with extension into the temporal fossa.

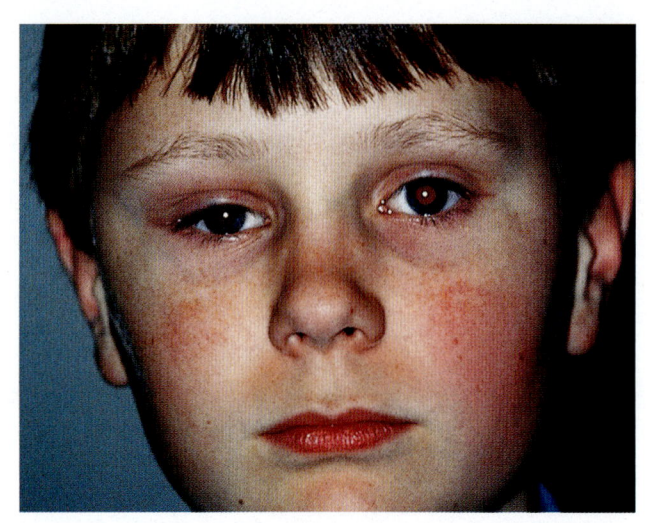

Figure 35.15. Eosinophilic granuloma. Swelling of the temporal fossa and slight blepharoptosis of right upper eyelid in an 8-year-old boy.

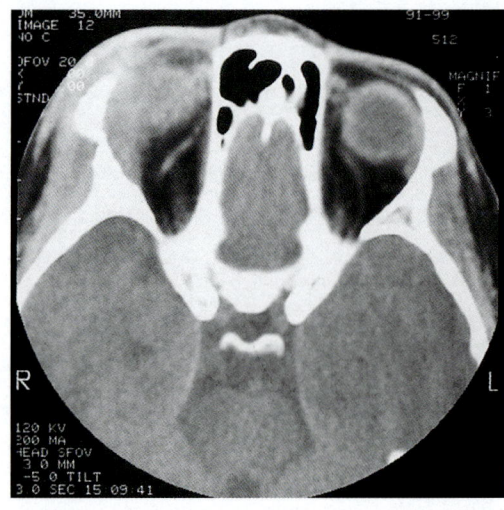

Figure 35.16. Axial computed tomography of patient shown in Figure 35.9, depicting mass in lateral aspect of the orbit and temporal with minor bone destruction.

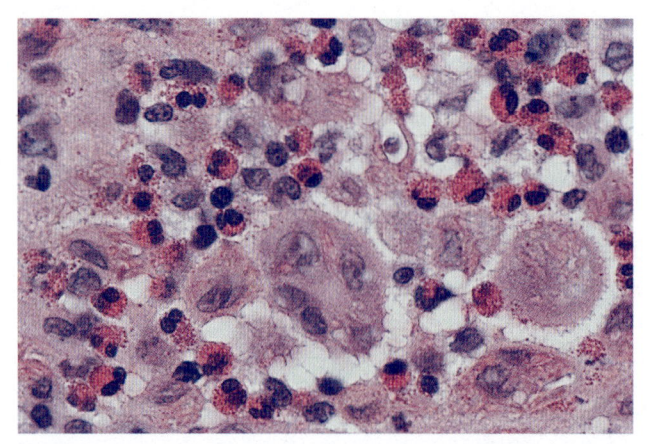

Figure 35.17. Histopathology of eosinophilic granuloma showing admixture of eosinophils, histiocytes and giant cells. (Hematoxylin–eosin ×200.)

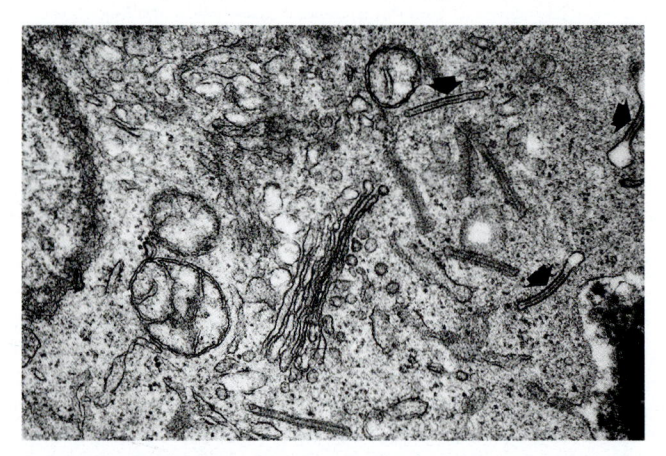

Figure 35.18. Electron photomicrograph showing characteristic Birbeck granules (*arrows*) in the cytoplasm of a histiocyte, a characteristic feature of Langerhans' cell. (×55,000.) (Courtesy of David Jordan, MD.)

Chapter 35 Orbital Histiocytic Tumors

● ORBITAL LANGERHANS' CELL HISTIOCYTOSIS (EOSINOPHILIC GRANULOMA): BILATERAL SEQUENTIAL ORBITAL INVOLVEMENT

In rare instances, bilateral sequential orbital involvement can occur. A case is illustrated of bilateral orbital involvement with spontaneous healing.

Demirci H, Shields CL, Shields JA, et al. Bilateral sequential orbital involvement in eosinophilic granuloma. *Arch Ophthalmol* 2002;120:978–979.

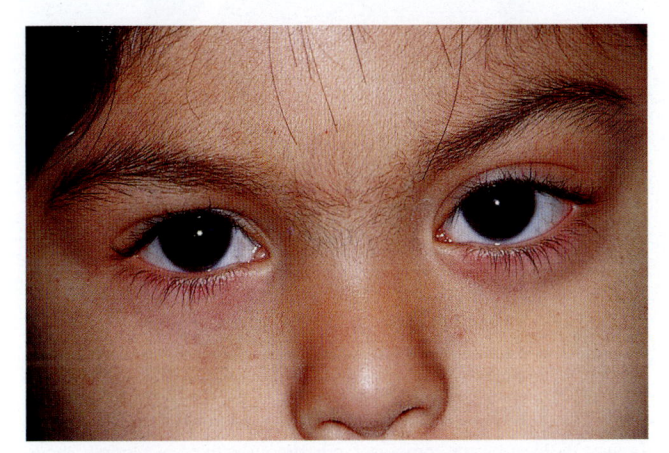

Figure 35.19. Anterior orbital mass causing superotemporal fullness above left eye in a 5-year-old boy.

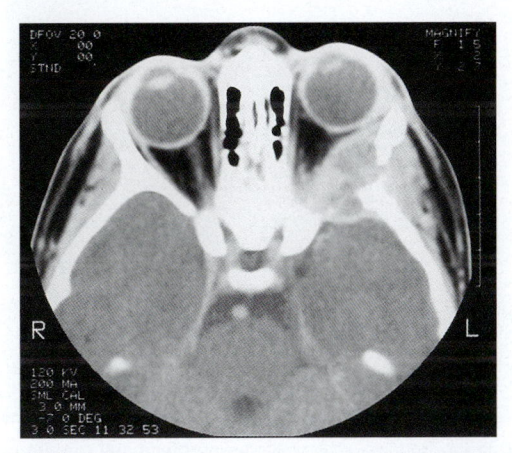

Figure 35.20. Axial computed tomography showing bone destructive mass involving orbit and temporal fossa. A biopsy and curettage was done.

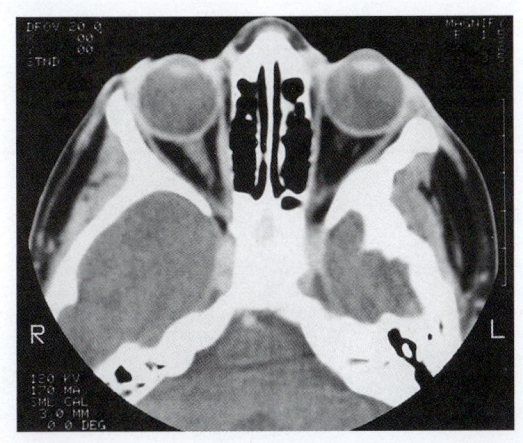

Figure 35.21. Axial computed tomography done 6 months later showing almost complete resolution of mass and remodeling of the bone.

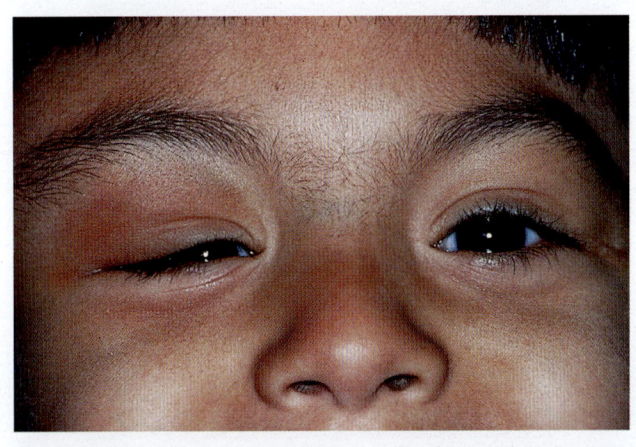

Figure 35.22. Appearance of child 18 months after initial presentation showing acute involvement superotemporally in the right orbit.

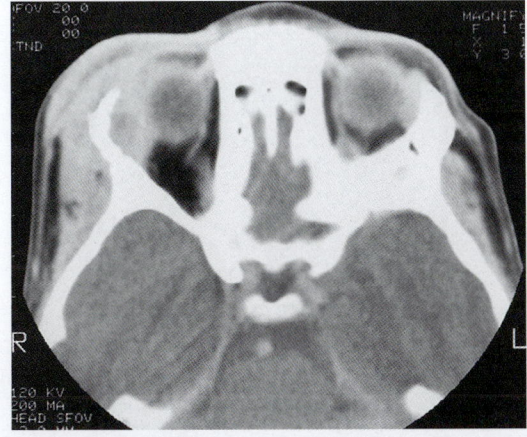

Figure 35.23. Axial computed tomography done at time of Figure 35.16, demonstrating soft tissue and bone involvement in the right orbit. The left orbit has mostly healed, but there is hyperostosis.

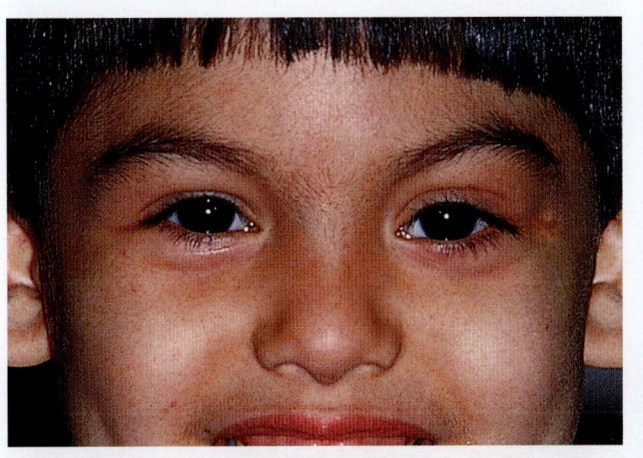

Figure 35.24. Appearance of child 6 months later after both orbits healed spontaneously, demonstrating marked improvement in facial appearance.

ORBITAL LANGERHANS' CELL HISTIOCYTOSIS (EOSINOPHILIC GRANULOMA): MANAGEMENT

In some cases, spontaneous healing can occur. Depicted is a patient who underwent a biopsy for EG and subsequently healed spontaneously without additional treatment.

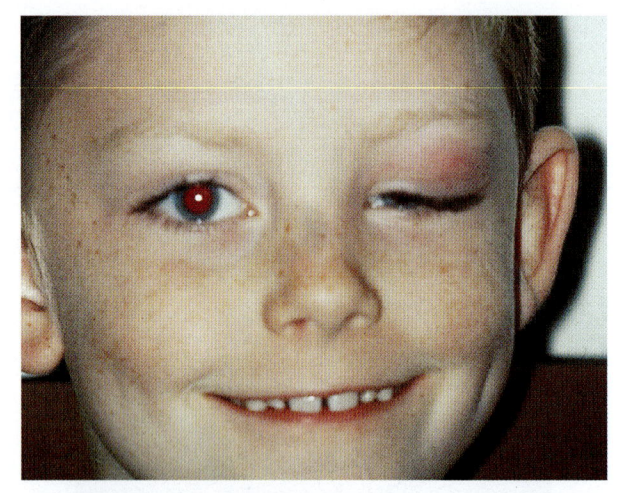

Figure 35.25. Redness and swelling superotemporal to right eye in a 7-year-old boy.

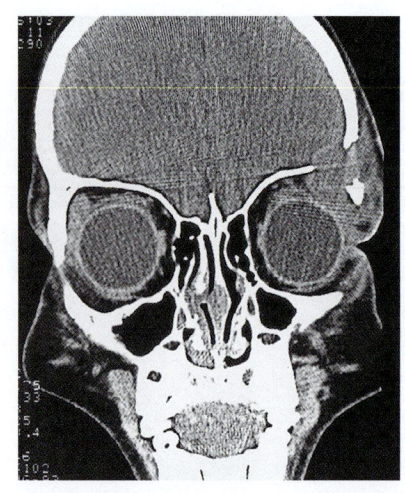

Figure 35.26. Coronal computed tomography with bone window, showing large superotemporal bone destructive lesion involving the left orbit.

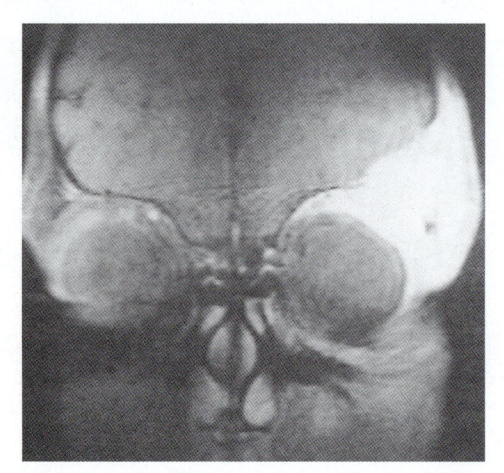

Figure 35.27. Coronal magnetic resonance imaging with gadolinium enhancement and fat suppression demonstrating enhancement of the mass.

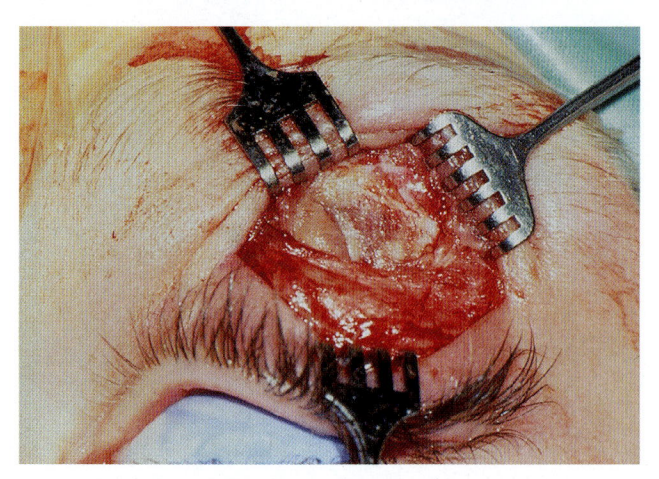

Figure 35.28. Approach to biopsy through a superotemporal cutaneous incision.

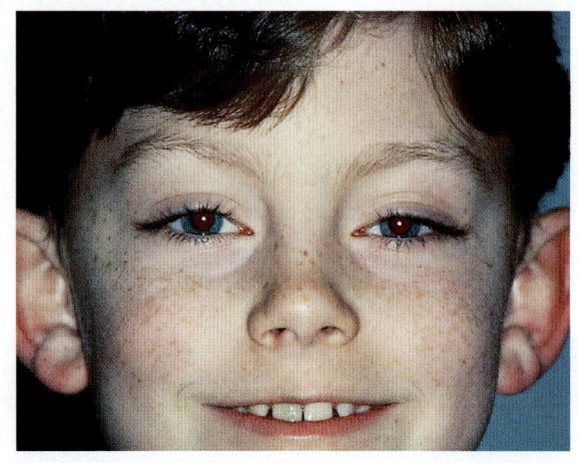

Figure 35.29. Appearance of patient 1 year later showing marked improvement in appearance.

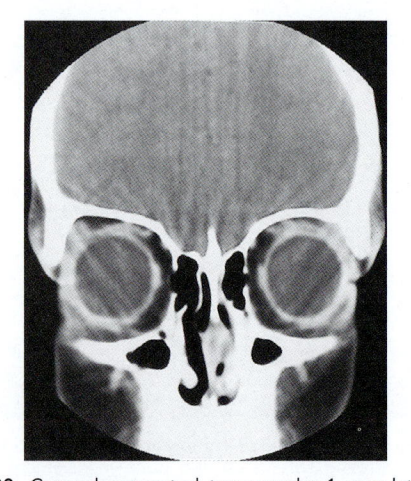

Figure 35.30. Coronal computed tomography 1 year later, showing almost complete healing of the previously destroyed bone.

Chapter 35 Orbital Histiocytic Tumors 681

ORBITAL LANGERHANS' CELL HISTIOCYTOSIS (EOSINOPHILIC GRANULOMA): PRESENTATION AS A HEMORRHAGIC, CYSTIC LESION

On occasion, EG can present as a hemorrhagic, cystic mass. Depicted is such a case that the authors believed at the time of surgical exposure to be an aneurysmal bone cyst.

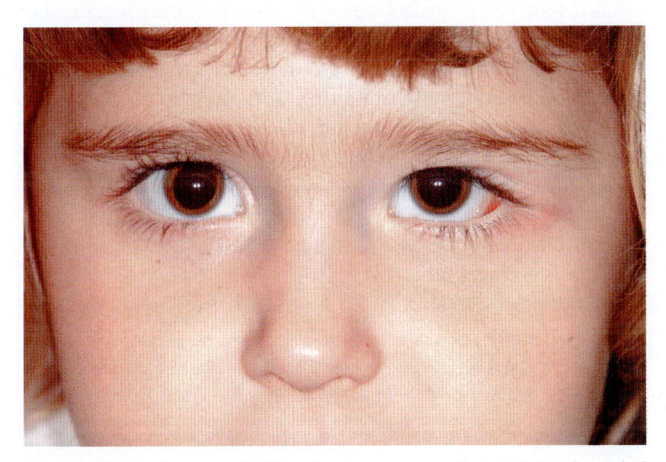

Figure 35.31. Young girl with subcutaneous swelling in lateral canthal area of left eye.

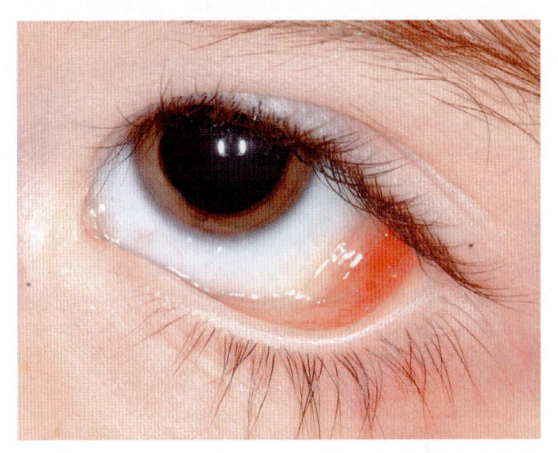

Figure 35.32. Closer view of lateral canthal area showing reddish mass in temporal conjunctiva.

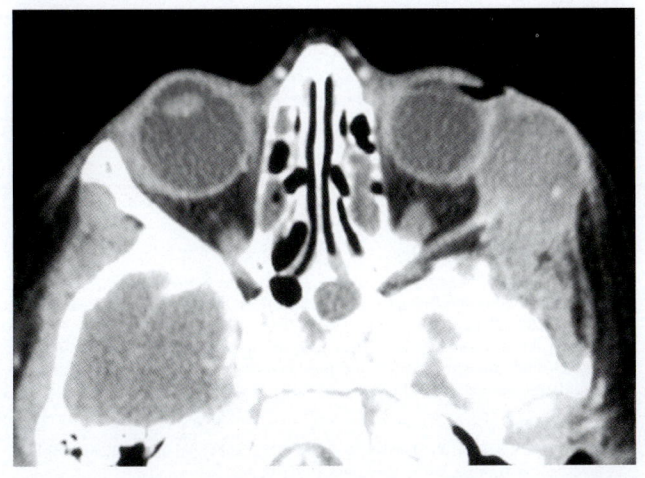

Figure 35.33. Axial computed tomography reveals large, cystic mass replacing lateral orbital bones.

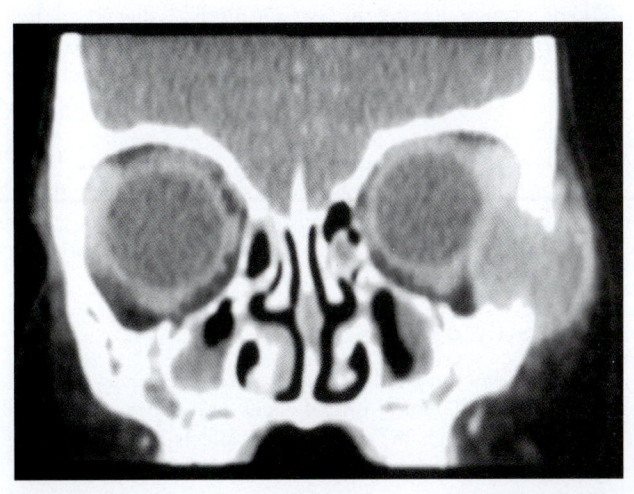

Figure 35.34. Coronal computed tomography shows round cystic mass replacing zygomatic arch.

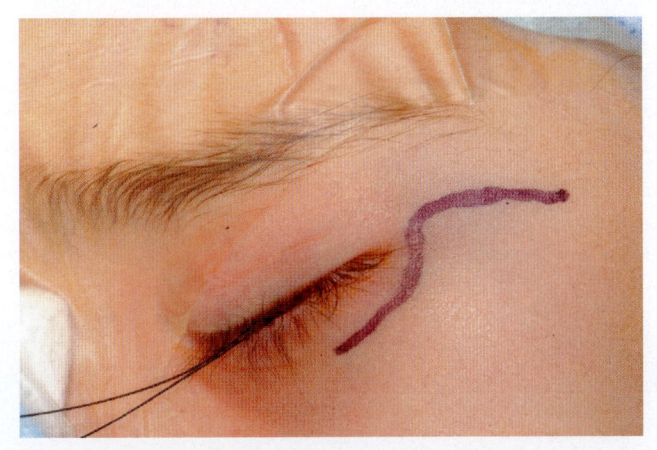

Figure 35.35. Planned surgical excision line for removal of mass.

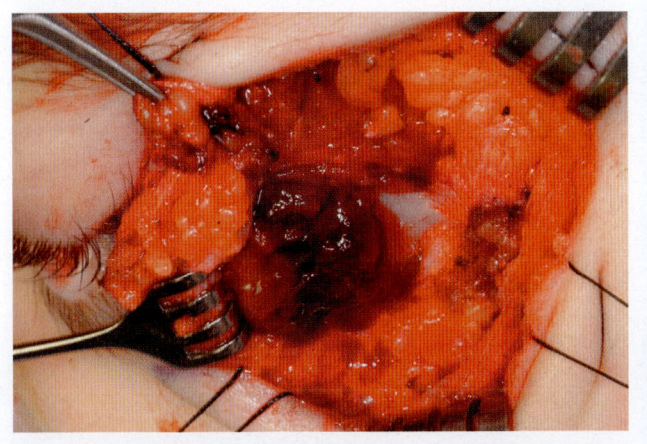

Figure 35.36. Appearance of hemorrhagic, nonencapsulated mass at time of surgical exposure. Histopathology revealed findings compatible with eosinophilic granuloma with hemorrhage.

TUMORS OF THE ORBIT

ORBITAL ERDHEIM–CHESTER DISEASE

General Considerations

LCH is generally a disease of childhood. There are also several important xanthogranulomatous diseases that occur primarily in adulthood and can show orbital involvement. They are generally idiopathic, but can occur as part of specific syndromes, including ECD, adult-onset–associated xanthogranuloma, and NXG with paraproteinemia. NXG with paraproteinemia is also discussed in the sections on *Eyelid and Conjunctival Tumors*.

ECD is an uncommon form of histiocytosis of uncertain etiology characterized by xanthogranulomatous infiltration of many organs including lung, kidney, heart, bones, retroperitoneal tissue, and occasionally the orbit (1–13). Systemic involvement can be severe and lead to death owing to renal or cardiac failure. In the authors' series of 1,264 orbital lesions, the 4 cases of orbital ECD accounted for 25% of histiocytic lesions and for 1% of all orbital tumors (1).

Clinical Features

Orbital involvement can be the initial site of involvement by ECD or it can occur after the systemic disease is diagnosed. It is characterized by proptosis, usually bilateral, and displacement of the globe. The proptosis can be alarmingly severe and cause exposure keratopathy and compressive optic neuropathy with severe visual loss.

A characteristic feature is bilateral atypical xanthelasma (planar xanthomas) of the periocular skin (10). The combination of bilateral xanthelasma and proptosis should arouse suspicion for ECD and the patient should undergo evaluation to detect the associated systemic findings.

Diagnostic Approaches

Imaging studies show diffuse orbital soft tissue masses that can sometimes fill the entire orbital cavity and cause severe proptosis (8). Although the disease often affects long bones, the orbital involvement is usually in soft tissue, without significant bone involvement.

Pathology

Histopathologically ECD is characterized by sheets of xanthoma cells intermixed with lymphocytes and plasma cells, usually with extensive fibrosis. The xanthoma cells are actually histiocytes that have phagocytosed lipid, mainly cholesterol. Scattered Touton giant cells are usually found. Unlike the LCH disorders, ECD does not stain for S-100 protein and ultrastructural studies do not show Birbeck granules.

Newer evidence has revealed BRAFV600E mutation in some ECD patients. In one study of seven cases, this mutation was verified in three (50%) of six tested patients (6). These findings support the belief that ECD is a multi-system clonal entity with neoplastic and inflammatory elements and dependent on impaired BRAF signaling as well as other key sites (6).

Management

In the past most treatments were not particularly effective and severe orbital complications with blindness often ensued. Interferon-alpha is sometimes useful. Currently, all patients are tested for BRAFV600E mutation and if positive, treatment with vemurafenib and other anti-BRAF medications can yield disease control (6,7,9). In one study of eight patients with ECD and BRAFV600E mutation, all of whom failed other therapies, vemurafenib lead to a response in 6 months in all cases and the response was sustained at median 10 months (7).

Selected References

Reviews
1. Shields JA, Shields CL, Scartozzi R. Survey of 1264 patients with orbital tumors and simulating lesions: The 2002 Montgomery Lecture, part 1. *Ophthalmology* 2004;111:997–1008.
2. Shields JA, Bakewell B, Augsburger JJ, et al. Classification and incidence of space-occupying lesions of the orbit. A survey of 645 biopsies. *Arch Ophthalmol* 1984;102:1606–1611.
3. Shields JA, Bakewell B, Augsburger JJ, et al. Space-occupying orbital masses in children: A review of 250 consecutive biopsies. *Ophthalmology* 1986;93:379–384.
4. Shields JA, Shields CL. Clinical spectrum of histiocytic tumors of the orbit. *Trans Pa Acad Ophthalmol Otolaryngol* 1990;42:931–937.
5. Alper MG, Zimmerman LE, LaPiana FG. Orbital manifestations of Erdheim-Chester disease. *Trans Am Ophthalmol Soc* 1983;891:64–85.
6. Mazor RD, Manevich-Mazor M, Kesler A, et al. Clinical considerations and key issues in the management of patients with Erdheim-Chester disease: a seven case series. *BMC Med* 2014;12:221.

Management
7. Haroche J, Cohen-Aubart F, Emile JF, et al. Reproducible and sustained efficacy of targeted therapy with vemurafenib in patients with BRAFV600E-mutated Erheim-Chester disease. *J Clin Oncol* 2015;33(5):411–418.

Histopathology/Genetics
8. De Abreu MR, Chung CB, Biswal S, et al. Erdheim-Chester disease: MR imaging, anatomic, and histopathologic correlation of orbital involvement. *AJNR Am J Neuroradiol* 2004;25:627–630.
9. Hyman DM, Diamond EL, Vibat CR, et al. Prospective blinded study of BRAFV600E mutation detection cell-free DNA of patients with systemic histiocytic disorders. *Cancer Discov* 2014;33(5):411–418.

Case Reports
10. Shields JA, Karcioglu Z, Shields CL, et al. Orbital and eyelid involvement with Erdheim-Chester disease. *Arch Ophthalmol* 1991;109:850–854.
11. Rozenberg I, Wechsler J, Koenig F, et al. Erdheim-Chester disease presenting as malignant exophthalmos. *Br J Radiol* 1986;59:173–177.
12. Karcioglu ZA, Sharara N, Boles TL, et al. Orbital xanthogranuloma: clinical and morphologic features in eight patients. *Ophthal Plast Reconstr Surg* 2003;19:372–381.
13. Valmaggia C, Neuweiler J, Fretz C, et al. A case of Erdheim-Chester disease with orbital involvement. *Arch Ophthalmol* 1997;115:1467–1468.

Chapter 35 Orbital Histiocytic Tumors

● ORBITAL ERDHEIM–CHESTER DISEASE

ECD is characterized by bilateral xanthelasmas and bilateral proptosis. These findings should arouse suspicion of the diagnosis. The orbital involvement is often massive. Two brief cases are illustrated.

Shields JA, Karcioglu Z, Shields CL, et al. Orbital and eyelid involvement with Erdheim-Chester disease. *Arch Ophthalmol* 1991; 109:850–854.

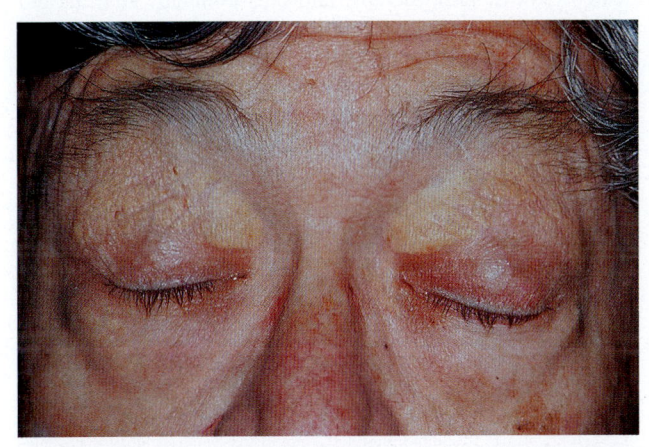

Figure 35.37. Xanthelasma on both upper eyelids in a 78-year-old man with bilateral proptosis and systemic findings of Erdheim–Chester disease, including pulmonary and retroperitoneal fibroses.

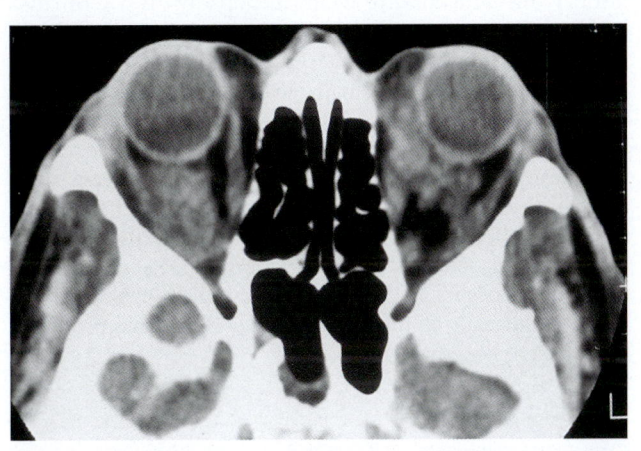

Figure 35.38. Axial computed tomography of patient shown in Figure 35.31, demonstrating patchy involvement of both orbits by soft tissue infiltration.

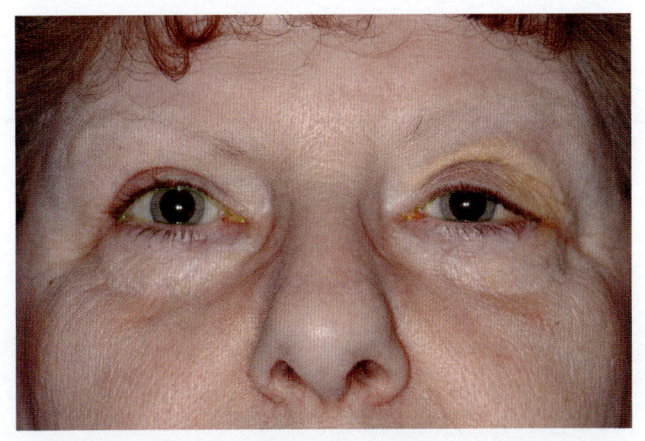

Figure 35.39. Xanthelasma on left upper eyelid in an older woman with atypical unilateral orbital infiltration from Erdheim–Chester disease.

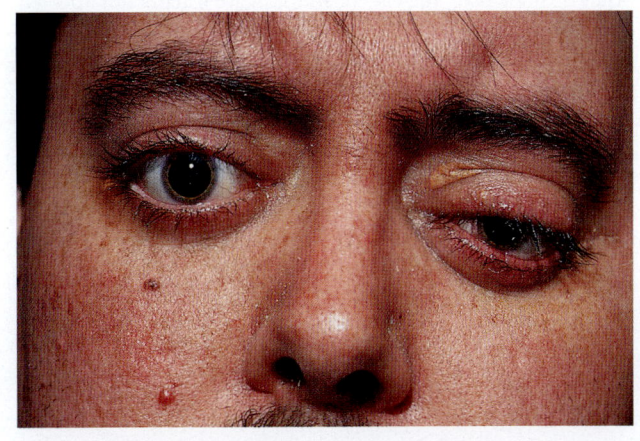

Figure 35.40. Bilateral proptosis and atypical xanthelasmas in a 28-year-old man. The patient had severe visual loss in both eyes secondary to massive orbital involvement and optic nerve compression.

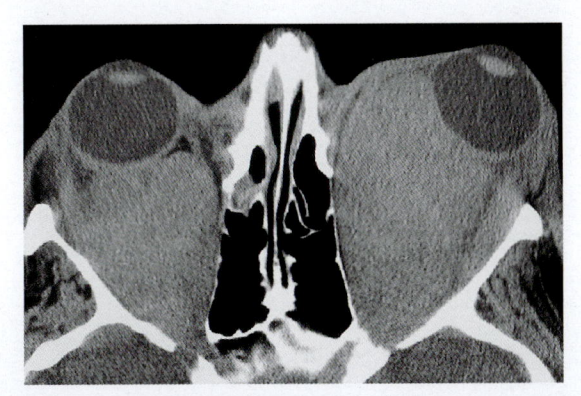

Figure 35.41. Axial computed tomography of patient shown in Figure 35.34, demonstrating massive infiltration of both orbits.

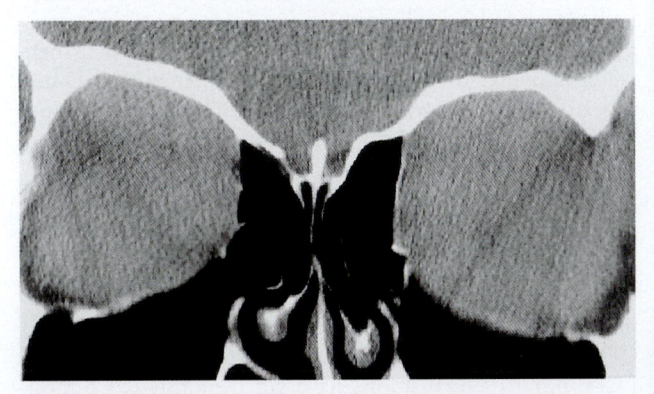

Figure 35.42. Coronal computed tomography through mid-orbit of patient shown in Figure 35.34 further demonstrating the extent of the orbital involvement.

ORBITAL ROSAI–DORFMAN DISEASE (SINUS HISTIOCYTOSIS WITH MASSIVE LYMPHADENOPATHY)

General Considerations

Of these various histiocytic proliferations, sinus histiocytosis is perhaps the best known to involve the orbit (1–15). "Sinus histiocytosis with massive lymphadenopathy" is a term that has been perpetuated in the literature. It is not universally realized that the word "sinus" in the name refers to the sinus of lymph nodes and not the paranasal sinuses. Furthermore, many patients do not have "massive" lymphadenopathy. To circumvent this potential confusion, we have elected to use the common eponym, Rosai–Dorfman (RD) disease until the nature of this entity is better understood. RD disease is a benign, idiopathic, pseudolymphomatous entity with distinctive clinical and histopathologic features (11). Extranodal involvement occurs in 25% of cases and orbital involvement in 10%. Intraocular infiltration by this RD disease has produced clinical signs of uveitis (12,15).

Clinical Features

Orbital RD disease usually occurs during the first or second decades, but it has been diagnosed in adults (6,14). It is somewhat more common in African Americans and males. Unlike other histiocytoses, the viscera and skin are usually not affected (3).

When the orbit is affected, the patient classically presents with a rapid onset of severe cervical lymphadenopathy, mild fever, and unilateral or bilateral proptosis and eyelid edema. A firm, rubbery, nontender mass may be palpable in the superior portion of the orbit, often in the lacrimal gland region. Bilateral lacrimal gland involvement can occur, with or without cervical lymphadenopathy (13).

The differential diagnosis of RD disease from a clinical as well as histopathologic standpoint includes idiopathic orbital inflammation (pseudotumor), rhabdomyosarcoma, lymphoma, leukemia, and LCH.

Diagnostic Approaches

Patients with RD disease may have abnormally elevated total serum proteins and immunoglobulin G. The white blood count is usually normal, but the erythrocyte sedimentation rate may be elevated. Orbital CT and MRI usually show a diffuse irregular soft tissue mass in the superior portion of the orbit. There are no specific radiographic features that differentiate RD disease from these other conditions like lymphoma and nonspecific orbital inflammation (inflammatory pseudotumor).

Pathology

In the lymph nodes and orbital soft tissues, there is a distinctive polymorphous infiltrate of histiocytes that have often phagocytosed erythrocytes, lymphocytes, or plasma cells, a phenomenon called "emperipolesis." The cells are positive for S-100 and CD68 and negative for CD1a and OKT6 (11). In contrast to LCH, ultrastructural studies have not demonstrated Birbeck granules in cases of RD disease (11).

Management

The clinical course of RD disease is variable, making therapeutic decisions more difficult. The disease is often self-limited and corticosteroids, radiotherapy, and chemotherapy may hasten resolution of the lesion. Combinations of chemotherapy and corticosteroids have been known to reverse associated compressive optic neuropathy and airway obstruction associated with RD disease (14). Overall, the prognosis is generally good, but systemic involvement has rarely led to death.

Selected References

Reviews

1. Shields JA, Shields CL, Scartozzi R. Survey of 1264 patients with orbital tumors and simulating lesions: The 2002 Montgomery Lecture, part 1. *Ophthalmology* 2004;111: 997–1008.
2. Shields JA, Bakewell B, Augsburger JJ, et al. Classification and incidence of space-occupying lesions of the orbit. A survey of 645 biopsies. *Arch Ophthalmol* 1984;102: 1606–1611.
3. Shields JA, Bakewell B, Augsburger JJ, et al. Space-occupying orbital masses in children: A review of 250 consecutive biopsies. *Ophthalmology* 1986;93:379–384.
4. Rosai J, Dorfman RF. Sinus histiocytosis with massive lymphadenopathy: a pseudolymphomatous benign disorder. Analysis of 34 cases. *Cancer* 1972;30:1174–1188.
5. Shields JA, Shields CL. Clinical spectrum of histiocytic tumors of the orbit. *Trans Pa Acad Ophthalmol Otolaryngol* 1990;42:931–937.
6. Mohadjer Y, Holds JB, Rootman J, et al. The spectrum of orbital Rosai-Dorfman disease. *Ophthal Plast Reconstr Surg* 2006;22:163–168.
7. Friendly DS, Font RL, Rao NA. Orbital involvement in "sinus" histiocytosis. A report of four cases. *Arch Ophthalmol* 1977;95:2006–2011.
8. Foucar E, Rosai J, Dorfman RF. The ophthalmologic manifestations of sinus histiocytosis with massive lymphadenopathy. *Am J Ophthalmol* 1979;87: 354–357.
9. Zimmerman LE, Hidayat AA, Grantham RL, et al. Atypical cases of sinus histiocytosis (Rosai-Dorfman disease) with ophthalmological manifestations. *Trans Am Ophthalmol Soc* 1988;86:113–135.
10. Vemuganti GK, Naik MN, Honavar SG. Rosai Dorfman disease of the orbit. *J Hematol Oncol* 2008;1:7.
11. Dalia S, Sagatys E, Sokol L, et al. Rosai-Dorfman disease: tumor biology, clinical features, pathology, and treatment. *Cancer Control* 2014;21:322–327.

Case Reports

12. Sartoris DJ, Resnick D. Osseous involvement in sinus histiocytosis with massive lymphadenopathy (Rosai-Dorfman disease). *Eur J Pediatr* 1986;145:238–240.
13. Lee-Wing M, Oryschak A, Attariwala G, et al. Rosai-Dorfman disease presenting as bilateral lacrimal gland enlargement. *Am J Ophthalmol* 2001;131:677–678.
14. Goldberg S, Mahadevia P, Lipton M, et al. Sinus histiocytosis with massive lymphadenopathy involving the orbit: reversal of compressive optic neuropathy after chemotherapy. *J Neuro-Ophthalmol* 1998;18:270–275.
15. Pivetti-Pezzi P, Torce C, Colabelli-Gisoldi RA, et al. Relapsing bilateral uveitis and papilledema in sinus histiocytosis with massive lymphadenopathy (Rosai-Dorfman disease). *Eur J Ophthalmol* 1995;5:59–62.

Chapter 35 Orbital Histiocytic Tumors

● ORBITAL ROSAI–DORFMAN DISEASE (SINUS HISTIOCYTOSIS WITH MASSIVE LYMPHADENOPATHY)

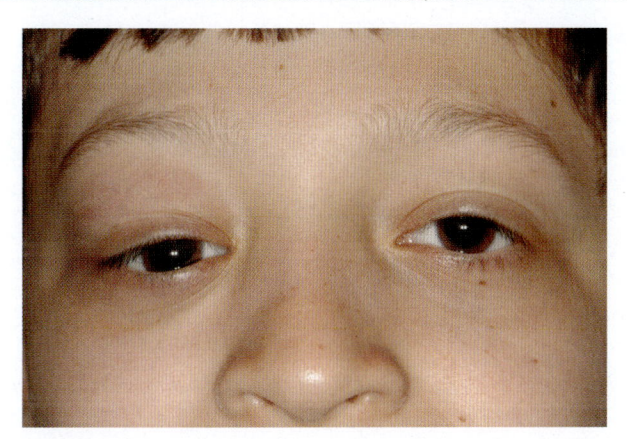

Figure 35.43. Young boy with mass in right anterior orbit.

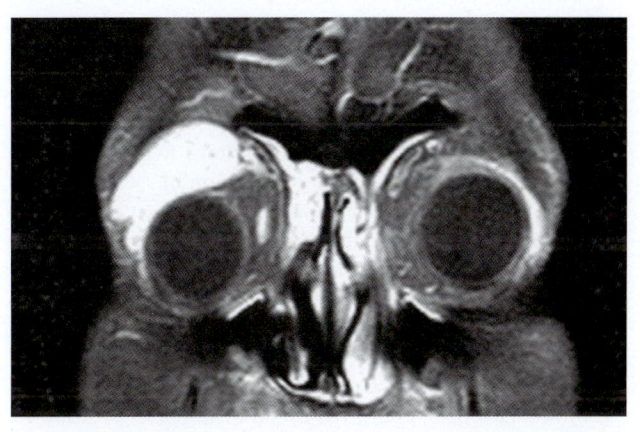

Figure 35.44. Magnetic resonance imaging revealed enhancing soft tissue mass that proved on biopsy to be orbital Rosai–Dorfman disease.

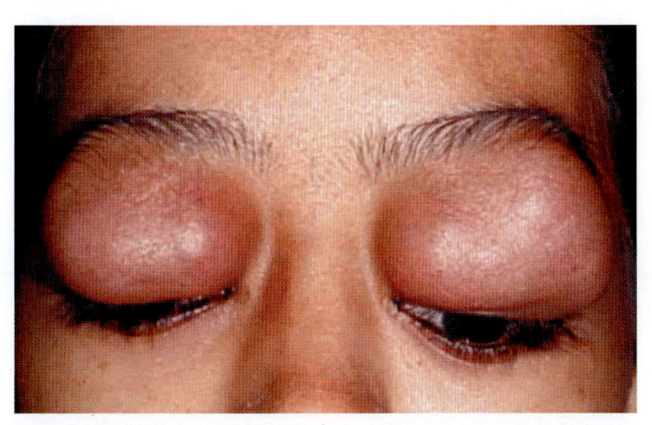

Figure 35.45. Bilateral proptosis and eyelid swelling in a young adult. (Courtesy of Santosh Honavar, MD, and Geeta Vemuganti, MD.)

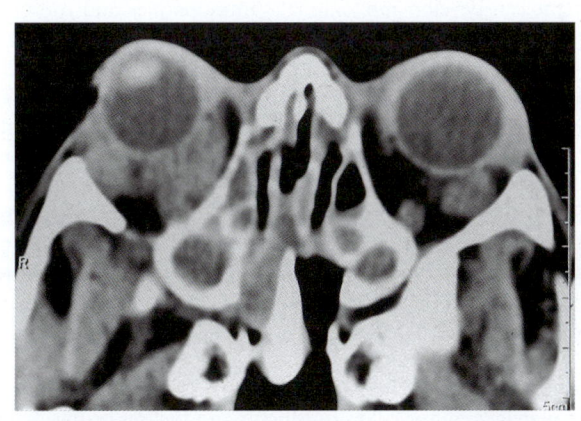

Figure 35.46. Computed tomography of patient in Figure 35.37, showing bilateral diffuse orbital masses, worse in right orbit. The patient was treated with surgical debulking and systemic corticosteroids. (Courtesy of Santosh Honavar, MD and Geeta Vemuganti, MD.)

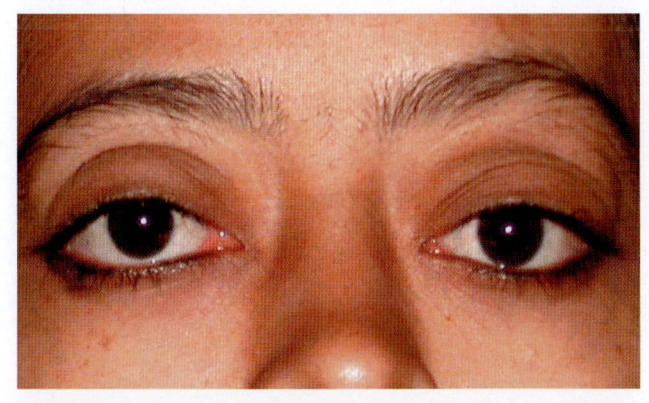

Figure 35.47. Posttreatment appearance of patient shown in Figure 35.37 a few weeks after oral corticosteroids, demonstrating an excellent response. (Courtesy of Santosh Honavar, MD and Geeta Vemuganti, MD.)

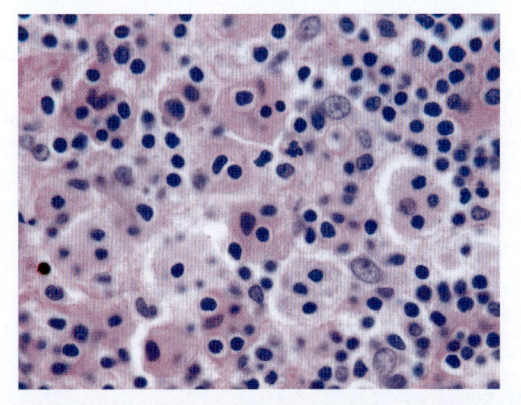

Figure 35.48. Histopathology of orbital sinus histiocytosis with massive lymphadenopathy shows polymorphous infiltrate composed predominately of histiocytes that have often phagocytosed lymphocytes, plasma cells, and erythrocytes (emperipolesis). (Hematoxylin–eosin ×150.)

NECROBIOTIC XANTHOGRANULOMA AND MULTINUCLEATE CELL ANGIOHISTIOCYTOMA

Orbital Necrobiotic Xanthogranuloma

General Considerations
NXG with paraproteinemia is a histiocytic disorder characterized by multiple xanthomatous skin lesions in patients with dysproteinemias (1–14). It is more common in the eyelid area and is also discussed in the *Atlas of Eyelid and Conjunctival Tumors*. However, it occasionally appears in the anterior orbit. This lesion tends occurs in middle-aged to older adults and has a peculiar predilection for the periorbital area.

Clinical Features
The affected patient with anterior orbital involvement typically has the characteristic eyelid yellow xanthelasma in addition to an anterior orbital mass. In some cases the xanthelasma occurs before the mass and in other cases it follows the mass. This condition usually has a progressive clinical course and the patient can develop monoclonal gammopathies and multiple myeloma.

Pathology
NXG is composed of a diffuse polymorphic infiltrate of foamy histiocytes, Touton giant cells, and lymphocytes. The most striking feature is widespread areas of necrobiosis of collagen, a finding that is absent in JXG and ECD. The lipid-containing cells show a positive reaction for monocyte and macrophage markers, but are negative for S-100 protein, which differentiates it from LCH and Rosai–Dorfman disease (sinus histiocytosis).

Management
The management of NXG is difficult and focuses primarily on the treatment of the paraproteinemia (9–12). Corticosteroids and chemotherapy have been employed with some success (9). Radiotherapy may sometimes be effective (10). Newer treatments focus on intravenous immunoglobulin and immunomodulatory medications (11,12).

Selected References

Reviews
1. Shields JA, Shields CL, Scartozzi R. Survey of 1264 patients with orbital tumors and simulating lesions: The 2002 Montgomery Lecture, part 1. *Ophthalmology* 2004;111: 997–1008.
2. Shields JA, Bakewell B, Augsburger JJ, et al. Classification and incidence of space-occupying lesions of the orbit. A survey of 645 biopsies. *Arch Ophthalmol* 1984;102: 1606–1611.
3. Shields JA, Bakewell B, Augsburger JJ, et al. Space-occupying orbital masses in children: A review of 250 consecutive biopsies. *Ophthalmology* 1986;93:379–384.
4. Shields JA, Shields CL. Clinical spectrum of histiocytic tumors of the orbit. *Trans Pa Acad Ophthalmol Otolaryngol* 1990;42:931–937.
5. Robertson DM, Winkelmann RK. Ophthalmic features of necrobiotic xanthogranuloma with paraproteinemia. *Am J Ophthalmol* 1984;97:173–183.
6. Kossard S, Winkelmann RK. Necrobiotic xanthogranuloma with paraproteinemia. *J Am Acad Dermatol* 1980;3:257–270.
7. Cornblath WT, Dotan SA, Trobe JD, et al. Varied clinical spectrum of necrobiotic xanthogranuloma. *Ophthalmology* 1992;99:103–107.
8. Vick VL, Wilson MW, Fleming JC, et al. Orbital and eyelid manifestations of xanthogranulomatous diseases. *Orbit* 2006;25(3):221–225.

Management
9. Plotnick H, Taniguchi Y, Hashimoto K, et al. Periorbital necrobiotic xanthogranuloma and stage I multiple myeloma. Ultrastructure and response to pulsed dexamethasone documented by magnetic resonance imaging. *J Am Acad Dermatol* 1991;25: 373–377.
10. Char DH, LeBoit PE, Ljung BE, et al. Radiation therapy for ocular necrobiotic xanthogranuloma. *Arch Ophthalmol* 1987;105:174–175.
11. Rubinstein A, Wolf DJ, Granstein RD. Successful treatment of necrobiotic xanthogranuloma with intravenous immunoglobulin. *J Cutan Med Surg* 2013;17: 347–350.
12. Abdul-Hay M. Immunomodulatory drugs for the treatment of periorbital necrobiotic xanthogranuloma. *Clin Adv Hematol Oncol* 2013;11:680–681.

Case Reports
13. Codere F, Lee RD, Anderson RL. Necrobiotic xanthogranuloma of the eyelid. *Arch Ophthalmol* 1983;101:60–63.
14. Bullock JD, Bartley GB, Campbell RJ, et al. Necrobiotic xanthogranuloma with paraproteinemia. Case report and a pathogenetic theory. *Ophthalmology* 1986;93:1233.

NECROBIOTIC XANTHOGRANULOMA AND MULTINUCLEATE CELL ANGIOHISTIOCYTOMA

Orbital Multinucleate Cell Angiohistiocytoma

General Considerations
Multinucleate cell angiohistiocytoma is an idiopathic, benign vascular/histiocytic condition (1) that has been recognized mostly in the skin (2,4) and rarely in the anterior orbit (3).

Clinical Features
Multinucleate cell angiohistiocytoma is characterized clinically by multiple, grouped, violaceous, nonpainful, cutaneous papules that generally occur in the extremities of women over 40 years old. The condition has recently been diagnosed in the orbit as a circumscribed anterior orbital mass (2). In one series of 142 cases, the mean age of onset was 50 years and 79% were female. The most commonly affected sites are the hands (30%) and face (29%).

Pathology
Histopathologically, multinucleate cell angiohistiocytoma is characterized by increased numbers of small blood vessels in the dermis, a sparse lymphocytic infiltration, histiocytes, and prominent multinucleated giant cells. Other features include mild dermal fibrosis. Immunohistochemical studies have indicated that the dermal cells are compatible with histiocytes. The pathogenesis is uncertain, but it is believed that this lesion is inflammatory and vascular in origin, but fibrosis and atrophy also play a role (2).

Diagnostic Approaches
The diagnosis depends on the classic clinical features as well as histopathologic confirmation.

Selected References

Reviews
1. Shapiro PE, Nova MP, Rosmarin LA, et al. Multinucleate cell angiohistiocytoma: a distinct entity diagnosable by clinical and histologic features. *J Am Acad Dermatol* 1994;30:417–422.
2. Frew JW. Multinucleate angiohistiocytoma. Clinicopathological correlation of 142 cases with insights into etiology and pathogenesis. *Am J Dermatopathol* 2015;37(3):222–228.

Case Reports
3. Shields JA, Eagle RC Jr, Shields CL, et al. Multinucleate cell angiohistiocytoma of the orbit. *Am J Ophthalmol* 1995;120:402–403.
4. Doane JA, Purdy K, Pasternak S. Generalized multinucleate cell angiohistiocytoma. *J Cutan Med Surg* 2014;18:1–3.

ORBITAL NECROBIOTIC XANTHOGRANULOMA AND MULTINUCLEATE CELL ANGIOHISTIOCYTOMA

Shields JA, Eagle RC Jr, Shields CL, et al. Multinucleate cell angiohistiocytoma of the orbit. *Am J Ophthalmol* 1995;120:402–403.

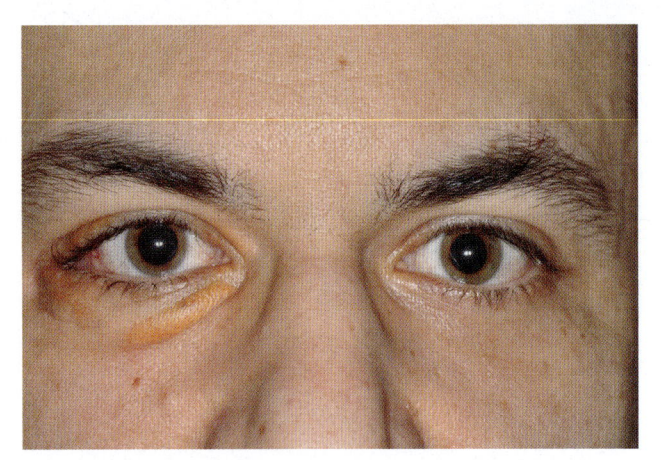

Figure 35.49. Characteristic cutaneous xanthelasma of necrobiotic xanthogranuloma affecting right lower eyelid.

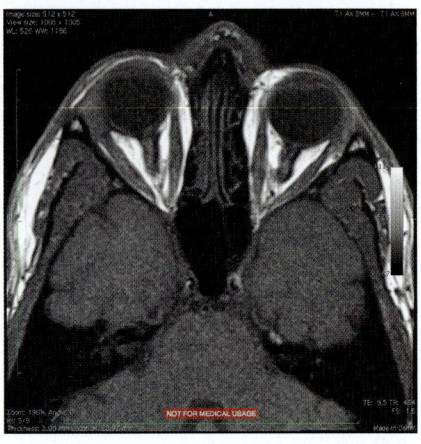

Figure 35.50. T1-weighted axial magnetic resonance imaging showing low signal mass in lacrimal gland fossa of right orbit.

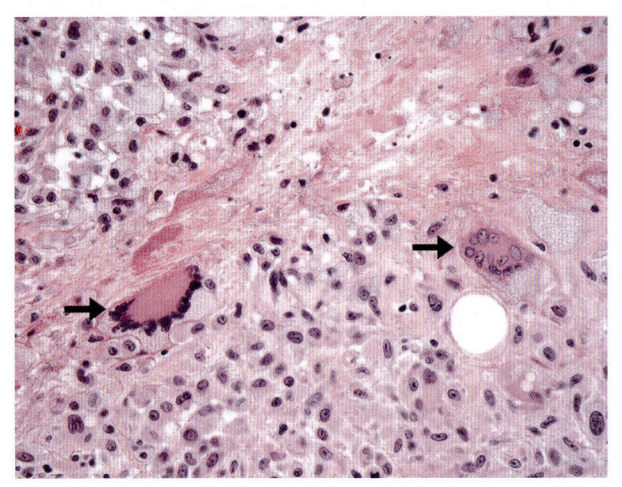

Figure 35.51. Histopathology showing granulomatous inflammation with area of necrosis centrally. *Arrows* point to Touton giant cells. (Hematoxylin–eosin ×150.)

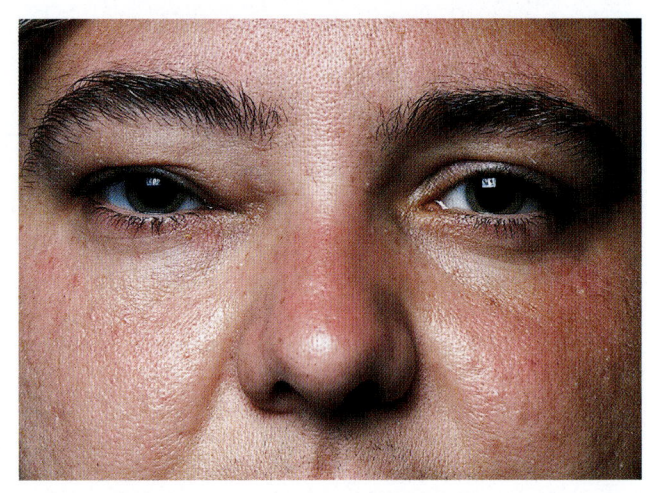

Figure 35.52. Multinucleate cell angiohistiocytoma. Superonasal orbital subcutaneous mass in a 38-year-old woman. She had no cutaneous lesions elsewhere.

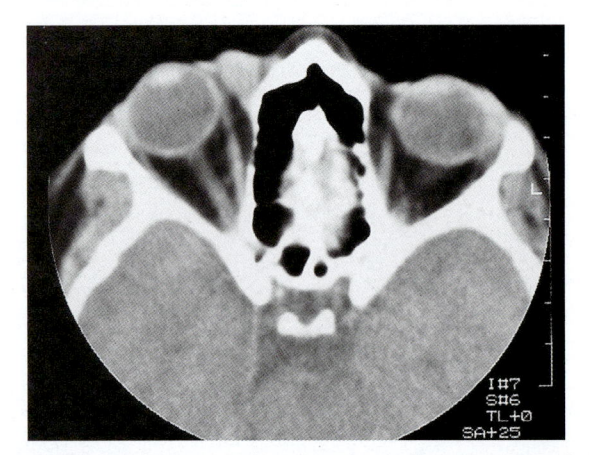

Figure 35.53. Axial computed tomography showing anterior nasal circumscribed orbital mass.

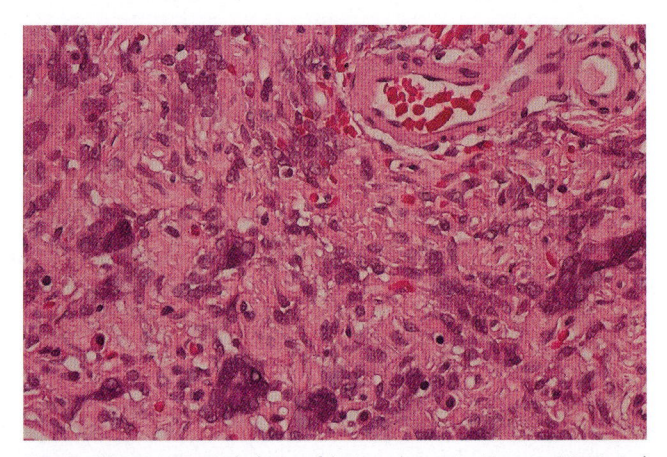

Figure 35.54. Histopathology of lesion shown in Figures 35.46 and 35.47 demonstrating blood vessels, histiocytes, and characteristic multinucleated giant cells. (Hematoxylin–eosin ×200.)

0# ORBITAL PRIMARY MELANOCYTIC TUMORS

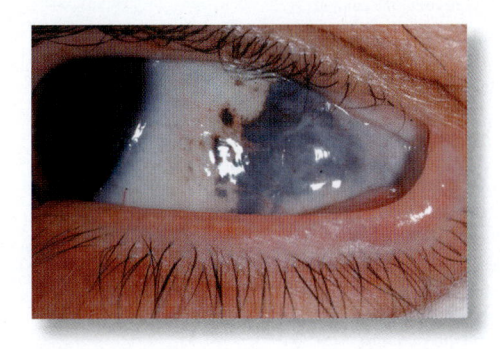

General Considerations

Primary melanocytic orbital tumors include melanoma, melanocytic hamartoma, and melanotic neuroectodermal tumor (MNET) of infancy (retinal anlage tumor). Primary orbital melanoma usually originates from congenital ocular melanocytosis or hypercellular blue nevus that affects the orbital tissue (1–23). Rarely, it can arise from the optic nerve (14) or after orbital irradiation for rhabdomyosarcoma (15). Melanomas from melanocytosis and from blue nevus are similar and are grouped together here. In the authors' review of personal cases, the 10 primary orbital melanomas accounted for 1% of all orbital tumors (1).

Clinical Features

The underlying congenital melanocytic lesion may be evident anteriorly as ocular melanocytosis or blue nevus, but it is often subclinical in the orbit more posteriorly, until it spawns a melanoma later in life. The melanoma that arises from blue nevus or congenital melanocytosis is generally circumscribed, even though the underlying congenital pigmentation is diffuse or patchy. Proptosis in a patient with either congenital ocular melanocytosis or episcleral blue nevus should arouse suspicion for a primary orbital melanoma or orbital extension of uveal melanoma.

Diagnostic Approaches

Computed tomography (CT) and magnetic resonance imaging (MRI) show a circumscribed, enhancing mass in orbital soft tissue, usually in the extraconal space, sometimes in an extraocular muscle. MRI may help to detect the melanin content in the lesion. With time, the tumor can breach its pseudocapsule and diffusely invade the orbit. As part of a diagnostic workup for proptosis, the clinician should inspect the eyelid skin and episclera to look for a blue nevus and perform ophthalmoscopy to rule out uveal melanoma.

Pathology

Grossly and at surgery, orbital melanoma is generally a brown or black circumscribed mass. Microscopically, it is composed of spindle or epithelioid melanoma cells. In many cases, residual areas of cellular blue nevus can be identified. Extensive tumor necrosis is common. Immunohistochemistry demonstrates a positive reaction to melanoma-specific antigens.

Management

Because orbital melanoma is usually well circumscribed, an attempt should be made to remove the entire tumor intact. An incisional biopsy of a circumscribed orbital mass in the setting of congenital ocular melanocytosis is contraindicated if there is a chance of removing the tumor intact. We believe that orbital melanoma is more likely to recur locally or metastasize to distant organs if it is not removed intact. The surrounding flat congenital pigment should be examined at surgery, biopsied, and treated with heavy cryotherapy. Residual or recurrent orbital melanoma should usually be managed by eyelid-sparing orbital exenteration.

ORBITAL MELANOMA ARISING FROM OCULAR MELANOCYTOSIS AND BLUE NEVUS

Selected References

Reviews

1. Shields JA, Shields CL, Scartozzi R. Survey of 1264 patients with orbital tumors and simulating lesions: The 2002 Montgomery Lecture, part 1. *Ophthalmology* 2004;111: 997–1008.
2. Shields JA, Bakewell B, Augsburger JJ, et al. Classification and incidence of space-occupying lesions of the orbit. A survey of 645 biopsies. *Arch Ophthalmol* 1984;102: 1606–1611.
3. Shields JA, Bakewell B, Augsburger JJ, et al. Space-occupying orbital masses in children: A review of 250 consecutive biopsies. *Ophthalmology* 1986;93:379–384.
4. Shields, JA, Shields CL. Orbital malignant melanoma. The 2002 Sean B. Murphy Lecture. *Ophthalmic Plast Reconstr Surg* 2003;19:262–269.
5. Shields CL, Kaliki S, Livesey M, et al. Association of ocular and oculodermal melanocytosis with rate of uveal melanoma metastasis. Analysis of 7872 consecutive eyes. *JAMA Ophthalmology* 2013;131:993–1003.
6. Berman EL, Shields CL, Sagoo MS, et al. Multifocal blue nevus of the conjunctiva. *Survey Ophthalmol* 2008;53:41–49.

Management

7. Shields JA, Shields CL, Demirci H, et al. Experience with eyelid-sparing orbital exenteration: the 2000 Tullos O. Coston Lecture. *Ophthal Plast Reconstr Surg* 2001;17: 355–361.

Case Reports

8. Gunduz K, Shields JA, Shields CL, et al. Periorbital cellular blue nevus leading to orbitopalpebral and intracranial melanoma. *Ophthalmology* 1998;105:2046–2050.
9. Demirci H, Shields CL, Shields JA, et al. Malignant melanoma arising from unusual conjunctival blue nevus. *Arch Ophthalmol* 2000;118:1581–1584.
10. Tellado M, Specht CS, McLean IW, et al. Primary orbital melanoma. *Ophthalmology* 1996;103:929–932.
11. Dutton JJ, Anderson RL, Schleper RL, et al. Orbital malignant melanoma and oculodermal melanocytosis. Report of two cases and review of the literature. *Ophthalmology* 1984;91:497–507.
12. Wilkes SR, Uthman EO, Thornton CN, et al. Malignant melanoma of the orbit in a black patient with ocular melanocytosis. *Arch Ophthalmol* 1984;102:904–906.
13. Mandeville JT, Grove AS Jr, Dadras SS, et al. Primary orbital melanoma associated with an occult episcleral nevus. *Arch Ophthalmol* 2004;122:287–290.
14. DePotter P, Shields CL, Eagle RC Jr, et al. Malignant melanoma of the optic nerve. *Arch Ophthalmol* 1996;114:608–612.
15. Lumbroso L, Sigal-Zafrani B, Jouffroy T, et al. Late malignant melanoma after treatment of rhabdomyosarcoma of the orbit during childhood. *Arch Ophthalmol* 2002; 120:1087–1090.
16. Odashiro AN, Arthurs B, Pereira PR, et al. Primary orbital melanoma associated with a blue nevus. *Ophthal Plast Reconstr Surg* 2005;21:247–248.
17. Rice CD, Brown HH. Primary orbital melanoma associated with orbital melanocytosis. *Arch Ophthalmol* 1990;108:1130–1134.
18. Mahoney NR, Engleman T, Morgenstern KE. Primary malignant melanoma of the orbit in an African-American man. *Ophthal Plast Reconstr Surg* 2008;24:475–477.
19. Mathai AM, Naik R, Pai MR, et al. Orbital melanocytoma. *Orbit* 2008;27:383–387.
20. Lee V, Sandy C, Rose GE, et al. Primary orbital melanoma masquerading as vascular anomalies. *Eye (Lond)* 2002;16:16–20.
21. Polito E, Leccisotti A. Primary and secondary orbital melanomas: a clinical and prognostic study. *Ophthal Plast Reconstr Surg* 1995;11:169–181.
22. Löffler KU, Witschel H. Primary malignant melanoma of the orbit arising in a cellular blue naevus. *Br J Ophthalmol* 1989;73:388–393.
23. Leff SR, Henkind P. Rhabdomyosarcoma and late malignant melanoma of the orbit. *Ophthalmology* 1983;90:1258–1260.

ORBITAL MELANOMA ARISING FROM BLUE NEVUS

Wilkes SR, Uthman EO, Thornton CN, et al. Malignant melanoma of the orbit in a black patient with ocular melanocytosis. *Arch Ophthalmol* 1984;102:904–906.

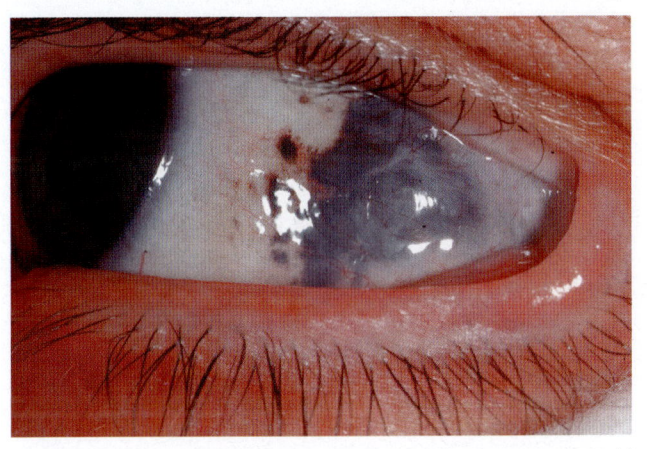

Figure 36.1. Congenital episcleral pigment on left eye in a 59-year-old man with left proptosis. The proptosis was of rather rapid onset and associated with epibulbar hyperemia, signs suggestive of an inflammatory process. It is of interest that the patient also had retinal astrocytomas and other signs of tuberous sclerosis complex, findings that may be unrelated to the orbital lesion.

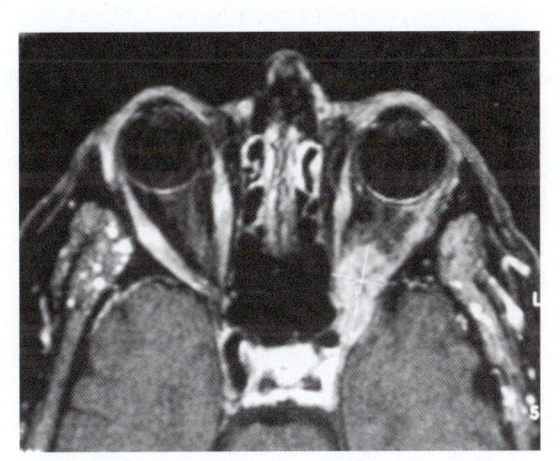

Figure 36.2. Axial orbital magnetic resonance imaging with gadolinium enhancement in T1-weighted image of patient shown in Figure 36.1. Note the deep orbital mass at the apex. At the time of surgery, marked pigmentation was found throughout the temporal portion of the orbit, including the sheath of the lateral rectus muscle.

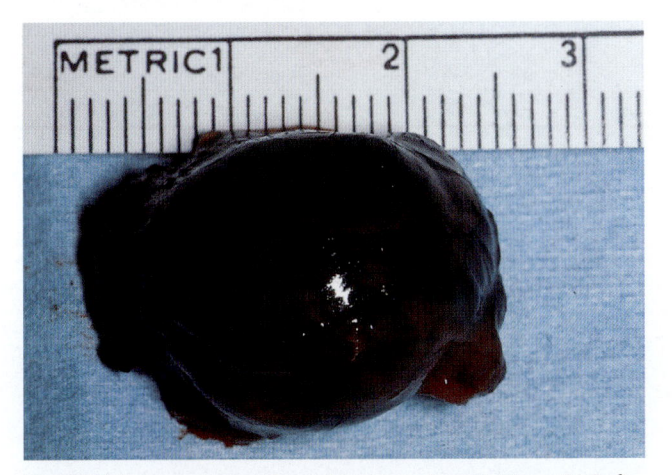

Figure 36.3. Appearance of the orbital mass shown in Figure 36.2 after surgical removal. Care was taken to remove the mass intact.

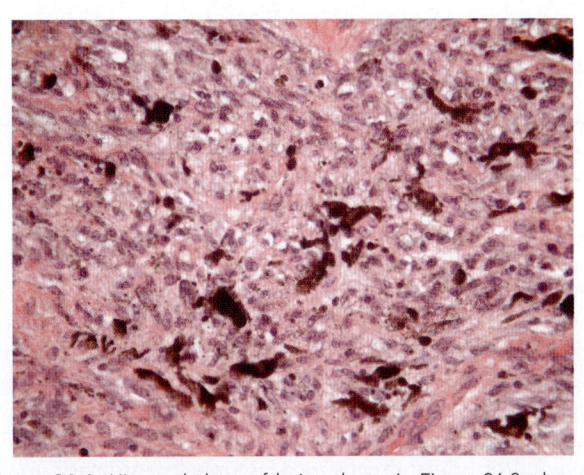

Figure 36.4. Histopathology of lesion shown in Figure 36.3, demonstrating pigmented blue nevus and amelanotic spindle and epithelioid melanoma cells. (Hematoxylin–eosin ×50.)

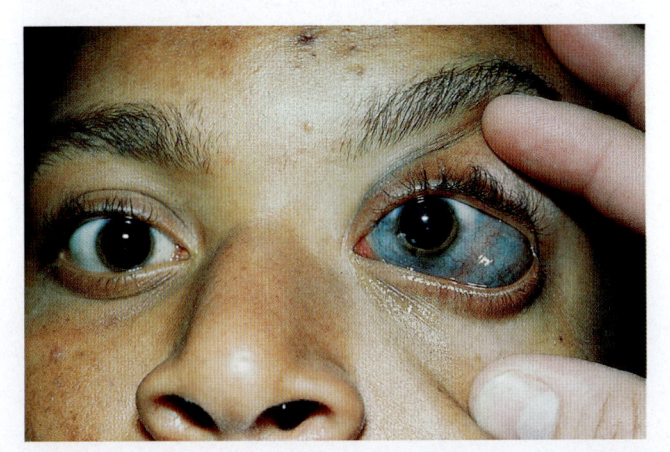

Figure 36.5. African-American patient with ocular melanocytosis with an orbitoconjunctival nodule of recent onset. (Courtesy of Shelby Wilkes, MD.)

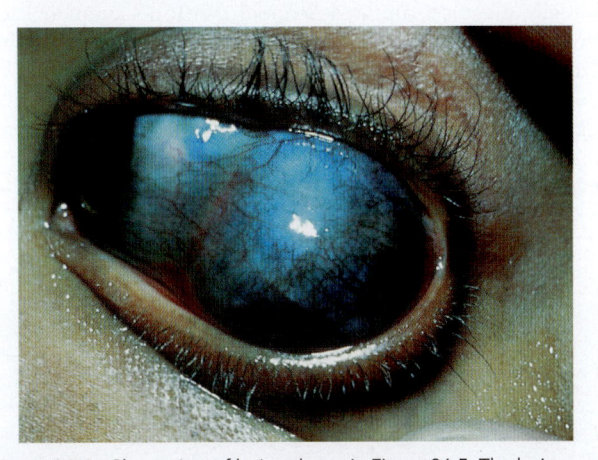

Figure 36.6. Closer view of lesion shown in Figure 36.5. The lesion was excised and proved to be a malignant melanoma arising from ocular melanocytosis. (Courtesy of Shelby Wilkes, MD.)

ORBITAL MELANOMAS ARISING DE NOVO

General Considerations

Orbital melanoma can sometimes arise spontaneously, without an apparent predisposing melanocytic process (1–7). It is possible that such a primary orbital melanoma could arise from subclinical areas of congenital melanocytosis or that it could represent a metastasis from an occult primary melanoma. If there is no evidence of ocular melanocytosis and no demonstrable primary melanoma elsewhere, the lesion can be classified as a presumed de novo primary orbital melanoma.

Clinical Features

The patient with primary orbital soft tissue melanoma generally presents with proptosis or displacement of the eye, findings similar to many other orbital tumors. The diagnosis is not often made clinically, but it can be suspected at surgery when a circumscribed, solid black tumor is detected.

Diagnostic Approaches

Imaging studies like CT or MRI usually reveal a circumscribed orbital mass without bone involvement. Less often, orbital melanoma can be diffuse or poorly circumscribed. It generally shows enhancement with contrast agents.

Management and Prognosis

Concerning management, the presence of an orbital mass in a patient with ocular melanocytosis should prompt suspicion for orbital melanoma. An orbitotomy should generally be performed with an attempt to meticulously remove the mass intact. Incisional biopsy of an orbital melanoma invariably liberates malignant tumor cells into the surrounding tissues, increasing the chance of orbital recurrence and metastasis. At the time of surgery, after the main mass is removed intact, it is advisable to perform small biopsies of adjacent ocular melanocytosis or blue nevus and to do heavy double freeze thaw cryotherapy to the visible areas of melanocytosis. More advanced tumors that cannot be removed entirely may require irradiation and/or orbital exenteration. Retrobulbar primary orbital melanoma has been known to undergo extensive spontaneous necrosis and the yellow, necrotic material seen at surgery can initially suggest a ruptured dermoid cyst (5). Complete excision may be difficult in such cases and eyelid-sparing orbital exenteration may be necessary.

The prognosis for primary orbital melanoma is similar to that of uveal melanoma (5). The 5-year incidence of metastasis is reported to be 38%, with 90% of metastases affecting the liver (4).

Selected References

Reviews

1. Shields JA, Shields CL, Scartozzi R. Survey of 1264 patients with orbital tumors and simulating lesions: The 2002 Montgomery Lecture, part 1. *Ophthalmology* 2004;111: 997–1008.
2. Shields JA, Bakewell B, Augsburger JJ, et al. Classification and incidence of space-occupying lesions of the orbit. A survey of 645 biopsies. *Arch Ophthalmol* 1984;102: 1606–1611.
3. Shields JA, Bakewell B, Augsburger JJ, et al. Space-occupying orbital masses in children: A review of 250 consecutive biopsies. *Ophthalmology* 1986;93:379–384.
4. Shields, JA, Shields CL. Orbital malignant melanoma. The 2002 Sean B. Murphy Lecture. *Ophthalmic Plast Reconstr Surg* 2003;19:262–269.
5. Shields CL, Furuta M, Thangappan A, et al. Metastasis of uveal melanoma millimeter-by-millimeter in 8033 consecutive eyes. *Arch Ophthalmol* 2009;127:989–998.

Case Reports

6. Shields JA, Shields CL, Eagle RC Jr, et al. Necrotic orbital melanoma arising de novo. *Br J Ophthalmol* 1993;77:187–189.
7. DePotter P, Shields CL, Eagle RC Jr, et al. Malignant melanoma of the optic nerve. *Arch Ophthalmol* 1996;114:608–612.

Chapter 36 Orbital Primary Melanocytic Tumors 693

● ORBITAL MELANOMA: DE NOVO PRIMARY TUMORS

In rare instances, melanoma can originate in the orbit as a primary lesion with no history or clinical findings of predisposing congenital melanocytosis or blue nevus. It can occur in the extraneural orbital soft tissue, or in the optic nerve itself. Depicted is a case of presumed primary orbital melanoma arising in soft tissue and another case of melanoma arising primarily in the optic nerve.

1. Shields JA, Shields CL, Eagle RC Jr, et al. Necrotic orbital melanoma arising de novo. *Br J Ophthalmol* 1993;77:187–189.
2. DePotter P, Shields CL, Eagle RC Jr, et al. Malignant melanoma of the optic nerve. *Arch Ophthalmol* 1996;114:608–612.
3. DePotter P, Shields JA, Shields CL, et al. Modified enucleation via lateral orbitotomy for choroidal melanomas with massive orbital extension. *Ophthal Plast Reconstr Surg* 1992;8:109–113.

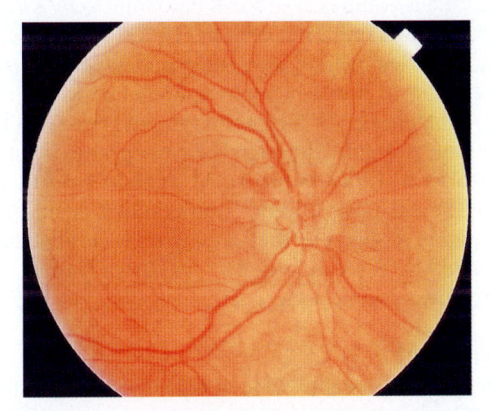

Figure 36.7. Fundus photograph of right eye showing optic disc edema in a 76-year-old man who complained of blurred vision.

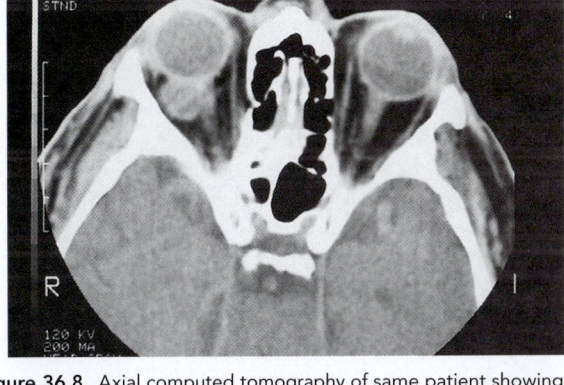

Figure 36.8. Axial computed tomography of same patient showing circumscribed intraconal right retrobulbar mass. The mass was removed via a conjunctival approach.

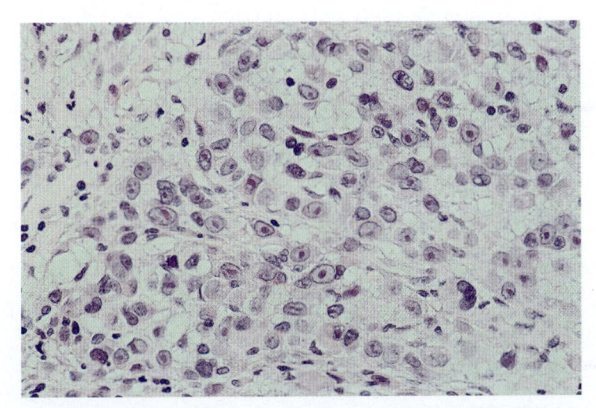

Figure 36.9. Section through a peripheral portion of the mass showing spindle and epithelioid melanoma cells. (Hematoxylin–eosin ×150.)

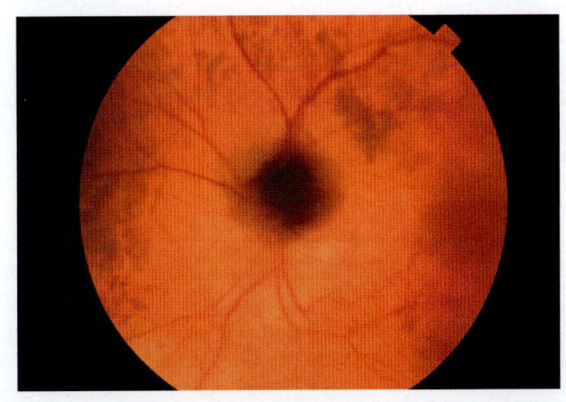

Figure 36.10. Primary melanoma of optic nerve. Fundus photograph of left optic disc showing deeply pigmented mass that was diagnosed clinically as a melanocytoma. It had been followed for years, without change, but the patient then experienced profound visual loss.

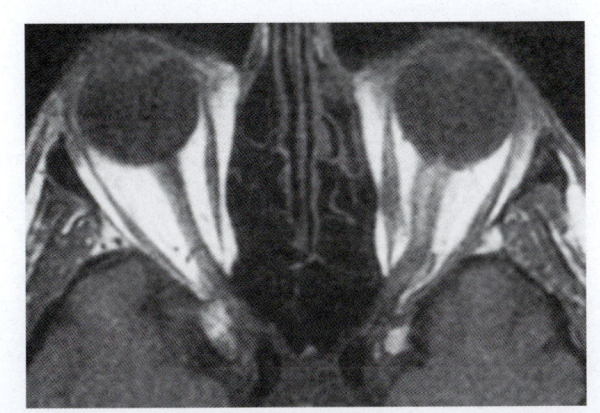

Figure 36.11. Axial magnetic resonance imaging in T1-weighted image and gadolinium enhancement of patient shown in Figure 36.10. Note that a long portion of the larger left optic nerve is showing marked enhancement. The eye was successfully enucleated by a lateral orbitotomy approach and a long section of optic nerve was obtained.

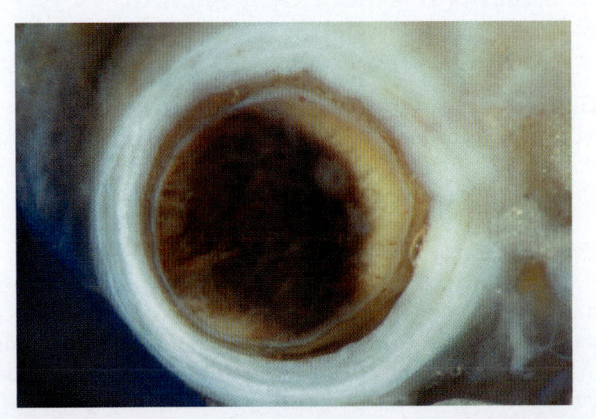

Figure 36.12. Cross-section of optic nerve in mid-orbit, showing pigmented tumor cells in axis of the nerve. The surrounding meninges are not involved by tumor. Histopathologically, the tumor proved to be a highly necrotic mixed cell type melanoma that appeared confined to the optic nerve.

ORBITAL MELANOCYTIC HAMARTOMA AND MELANOTIC NEUROECTODERMAL TUMOR

Rare melanocytic tumors of the orbit include melanocytic hamartoma and MNET, both of which occur in young children (1–11).

Orbital Melanocytic Hamartoma

General Considerations
Melanocytic hamartoma is a rare congenital melanocytic tumor of the orbit (5).

Clinical Features
The lesion reported was a giant melanocytic hamartoma in the orbit of a newborn. It was noted at birth as a black mass that entirely covered the anterior aspect of the orbit, filling the palpebral aperture and obscuring the globe.

Diagnostic Approaches
Little is known about findings on imaging studies of this rare lesion. We speculate that it can occur as a circumscribed or diffuse, poorly circumscribed mass.

Pathology
Pathologically, the lesion seemed to encase the globe as a solid pigmented mass that also diffusely involved the uveal tract (5). Histopathologically, the tumor cells in the orbit were spindle shaped and dendritic, and those in the uvea were round, similar to a melanocytoma. This poorly understood tumor may represent an unusual variant of congenital blue nevus or melanocytoma (5).

Management
Little is known about the management of congenital orbital melanocytic hamartoma. We believe that management should be geared toward the clinical findings and should be similar to treatment of circumscribed blue nevus or other circumscribed tumors. It may require partial excision, enucleation, or orbital exenteration, depending on the extent of the lesion. Malignant potential and prognosis are uncertain because the condition is so rare.

Orbital Involvement by Melanotic Neuroectodermal Tumor

General Considerations
MNET is a congenital, benign, but locally aggressive tumor that begins in the maxillary or zygomatic bones and occasionally affects the orbital soft tissue (6–11).

Clinical Features
Because of the location of MNET, the affected child develops fullness on the side of the face with medial displacement of the eye. The mass is usually hard and immobile to palpation. There is no pain or eyelid ecchymosis, features that help to differentiate it from a metastatic neuroblastoma, which also has a predilection for the zygomatic bone.

Diagnostic Approaches
Imaging studies show a lytic lesion of the affected bones with secondary soft tissue involvement in the orbit.

Pathology
Histopathologically, MNET is composed of two populations of cells. One is composed of small basophilic cells with scanty cytoplasm that resemble neuroblasts. The other consists of large cuboidal cells that contain pigment granules with morphologic characteristics of retinal pigment epithelium (RPE). Rosettes similar to the Flexner–Wintersteiner rosettes of retinoblastoma are commonly found. Although the pathogenesis is uncertain, the similarity to RPE has prompted some investigators to use the term "retinal anlage tumor." Immunohistochemical studies show variable results, but they are generally positive for cytokeratin and HMB-45 and negative for chromogranin, desmin, and carcinoembryonic antigen (7).

Management
Management is generally wide complete excision if possible. Because the lesion usually involves periorbital bone, surgical excision should generally be done in conjunction with an otolaryngologist or a neurosurgeon. Wide surgical margins are necessary to prevent bony recurrence.

Selected References

Reviews
1. Shields JA, Shields CL, Scartozzi R. Survey of 1264 patients with orbital tumors and simulating lesions: The 2002 Montgomery Lecture, part 1. *Ophthalmology* 2004; 111:997–1008.
2. Shields JA, Bakewell B, Augsburger JJ, et al. Classification and incidence of space-occupying lesions of the orbit. A survey of 645 biopsies. *Arch Ophthalmol* 1984;102:1606–1611.
3. Shields JA, Bakewell B, Augsburger JJ, et al. Space-occupying orbital masses in children: A review of 250 consecutive biopsies. *Ophthalmology* 1986;93:379–384.
4. Shields, JA, Shields CL. Orbital malignant melanoma. The 2002 Sean B. Murphy Lecture. *Ophthalmic Plast Reconstr Surg* 2003;19:262–269.

Case Reports
5. Char DH, Crawford JB, Ablin AR, et al. Orbital melanocytic hamartoma. *Am J Ophthalmol* 1981;91:357–361.
6. Hall WC, O'Day DM, Glick AD. Melanotic neuroectodermal tumor of infancy. An ophthalmic appearance. *Arch Ophthalmol* 1979;97:922–925.
7. Franchi G, Sleilati F, Soupre V, et al. Melanotic neuroectodermal tumour of infancy involving the orbit and maxilla: surgical management and follow-up strategy. *Br J Plast Surg* 2002;55:526–529.
8. Kapadia SB, Frisman DM, Hitchcock CL, et al. Melanotic neuroectodermal tumor of infancy. Clinicopathological, immunohistochemical, and flow cytometric study. *Am J Surg Pathol* 1993;17:566–573.
9. Lamping KA, Albert DM, Lack E, et al. Melanotic neuroectodermal tumor of infancy. *Ophthalmology* 1985;92:143–149.
10. Cutler LS, Chaudhry AP, Topazian R. Melanotic neuroectodermal tumor of infancy: an ultrastructural study, literature review and reevaluation. *Cancer* 1981;48:247–270.
11. Nakanishi K, Hori H, Matsubara T, et al. Recurrent melanotic neuroectodermal tumor in the orbit successfully treated with resection followed by pediculated periosteal flaps. *Pediatr Blood Cancer* 2008;51:430–432.

ORBITAL MELANOCYTIC HAMARTOMA AND MELANOTIC NEUROECTODERMAL TUMOR

1. Char DH, Crawford JB, Ablin AR, et al. Orbital melanocytic hamartoma. *Am J Ophthalmol* 981;91:357–361.
2. Hall WC, O'Day DM, Glick AD. Melanotic neuroectodermal tumor of infancy. An ophthalmic appearance. *Arch Ophthalmol* 1979;97:922–925.

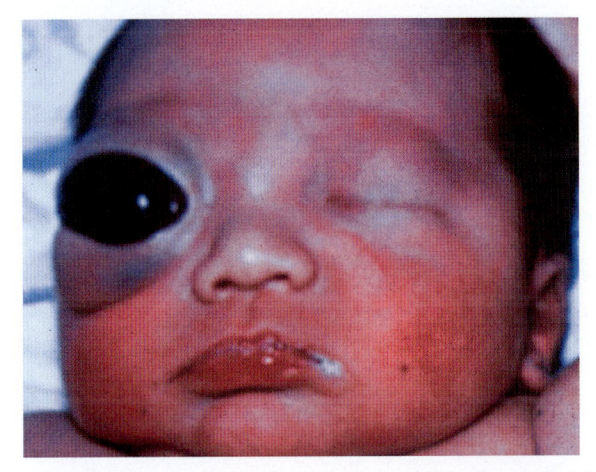

Figure 36.13. Giant melanocytic hamartoma of the orbit in an Asian infant. Note the extensive pigmented mass filling the palpebral aperture. (Courtesy of Devron Char, MD, and Brooks Crawford, MD.)

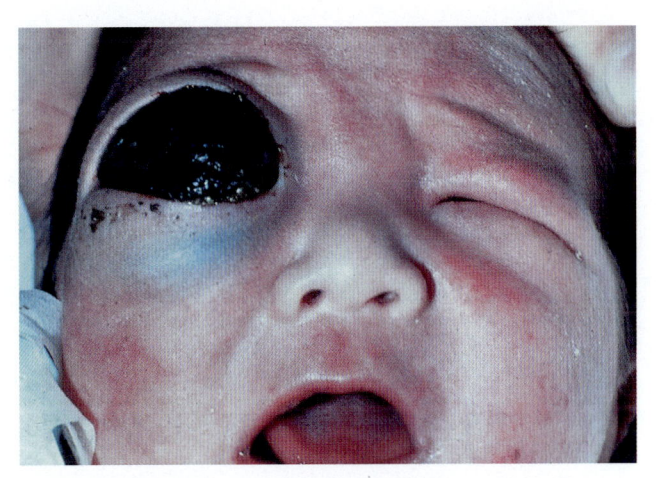

Figure 36.14. Another view of lesion shown in Figure 36.13. (Courtesy of Devron Char, MD, and Brooks Crawford, MD.)

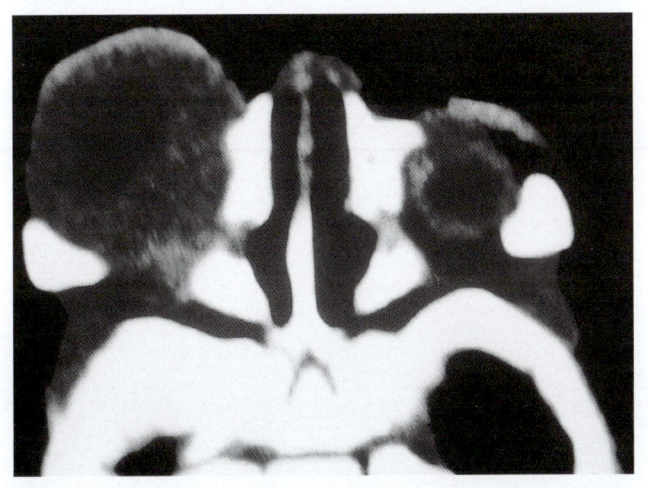

Figure 36.15. Axial computed tomography of lesion shown in Figure 36.13, showing larger right orbit secondary to orbital mass. (Courtesy of Devron Char, MD, and Brooks Crawford, MD.)

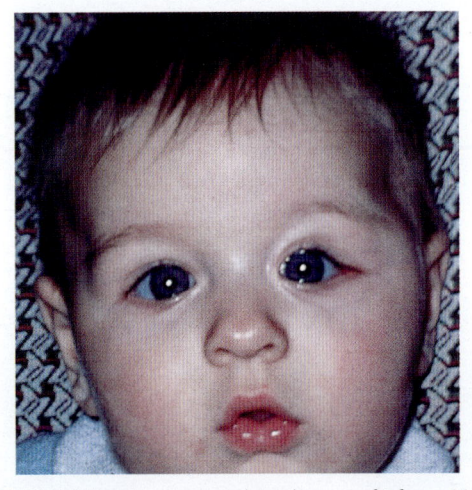

Figure 36.16. Melanotic neuroectodermal tumor of infancy. Medial displacement of the globe in an infant secondary to a lateral orbital mass. (Courtesy of Dennis O'Day, MD.)

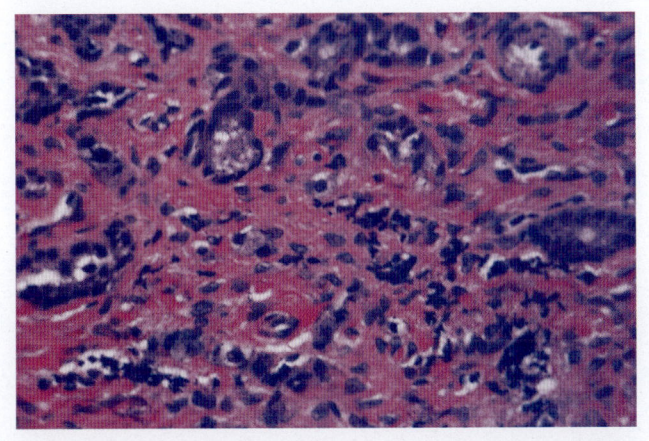

Figure 36.17. Histopathology of lesion shown in Figure 36.16, showing tubules and acini of pigment epithelial cells separated by a connective tissue stroma. (Hematoxylin–eosin ×100.) (Courtesy of Dennis O'Day, MD.)

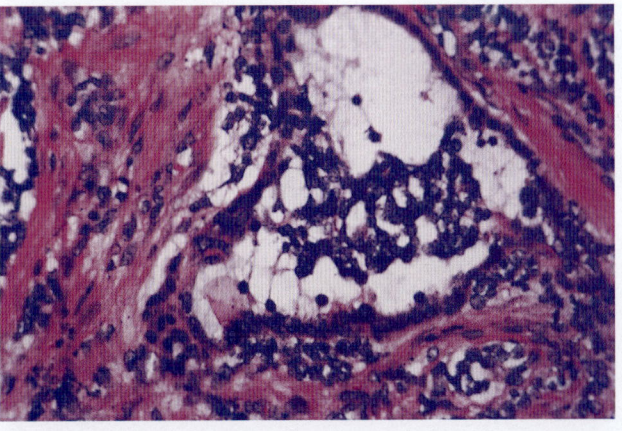

Figure 36.18. Higher magnification photomicrograph of lesion shown in Figure 36.17. (Hematoxylin–eosin ×100.) (Courtesy of Dennis O'Day, MD.)

CHAPTER 37

LACRIMAL GLAND PRIMARY EPITHELIAL TUMORS

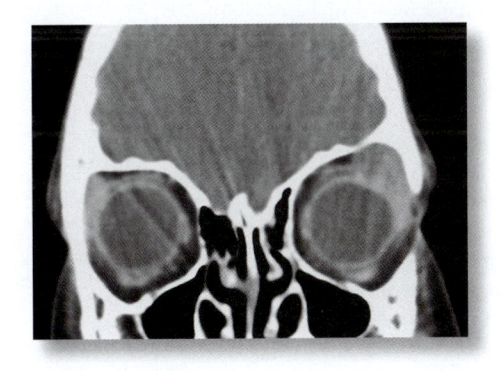

A variety of neoplasms and related lesions can arise in the lacrimal gland (1–15). Lacrimal gland lesions have many similarities to those that occur in the major salivary glands. Lesions of the lacrimal gland can be broadly divided into epithelial and nonepithelial lesions. Nonepithelial lesions such as the lymphoid tumors, inflammations, and other neoplasms that affect the lacrimal gland are covered in other chapters. This chapter covers primary benign and malignant lesions derived from the epithelial structures of the lacrimal gland.

In an analysis of 142 cases of lacrimal gland tumors from the pathology laboratory at Wills Eye Hospital in the USA, the breakdown of lesions included nonepithelial (78%) and epithelial (22%) (6). The nonepithelial lesions included inflammatory dacryoadenitis (64%) and lymphoid tumors (14%), whereas the epithelial tumors included dacryops (6%), pleomorphic adenoma (12%), and malignant epithelial tumors (4%). These findings disprove the old quoted dictum from the 1950s stating that lacrimal gland tumors are 50% epithelial and 50% nonepithelial with 50% benign and 50% malignant (6). A more recent analysis on 268 lacrimal gland biopsies from Australia, findings revealed inflammatory dacryoadenitis (50%), lymphoid tumors (32%), dacryops (3%), pleomorphic adenoma (8%), and malignant epithelial tumors (4%) (9).

A special subset of lacrimal gland tumors includes those with bilateral disease. Recent analysis of 97 cases of bilateral lacrimal gland lesions revealed diagnoses of idiopathic orbital inflammation (pseudotumor) (30%), sarcoidosis (20%), lymphoid tumor (19%), prolapsed lacrimal gland (15%), and dacryops (5%) (12). The authors emphasize that chronic underlying disease was present in 71% of cases (12).

It is important to recall that the lacrimal gland is the only tissue in the orbit that normally contains epithelium and any primary epithelial tumor in the orbit has most likely originated in the lacrimal gland. However, metastatic epithelial neoplasms can reach the orbit by hematogenous spread from distant organs and secondary epithelial neoplasms can invade the orbit from adjacent structures, such as eyelid, conjunctiva, intraocular tissues, paranasal sinuses, and nasopharynx. On rare occasions, congenital ectopic lacrimal gland tissue in the orbit can give rise to cysts and neoplasms (14,15).

True primary epithelial lesions of the lacrimal gland can be divided further into benign and malignant categories. Benign epithelial lesions include ductal epithelial cyst (dacryops) and pleomorphic adenoma (benign mixed tumor). The latter is the only important primary benign epithelial neoplasm of the lacrimal gland. There are several malignant epithelial neoplasms of the lacrimal gland, the most important of which is adenoid cystic carcinoma (ACC). Other less common malignancies include pleomorphic adenocarcinoma (malignant mixed tumor), primary adenocarcinoma, mucoepidermoid carcinoma, primary squamous cell carcinoma, sebaceous carcinoma, acinic cell adenocarcinoma, ductal carcinoma, lymphoepithelial carcinoma, myoepithelial carcinoma, and cystadenocarcinoma. Most of these uncommon neoplasms

INTRODUCTION: LACRIMAL GLAND LESIONS

were discussed in a recent comprehensive review of the subject (7).

Primary epithelial malignancies of the lacrimal gland (PEMLG) occur mostly in middle-aged adults (7). They are less common in the very young and the elderly. However, the important ACC seems to have a biphasic age distribution with some occurring in children in the first or second decade and another group occurring in young to middle-aged adults. There is no known predilection for race or gender.

Estimates regarding the incidence of lacrimal gland lesions vary from series to series depending on the source of the material and specifically which lesions were included in the survey. The following represents fairly accurate estimates regarding lacrimal gland lesions (1,2,6,7).

1. About 10% of orbital space-occupying lesions occur in the lacrimal gland.
2. About 20% of solid lacrimal gland masses are of epithelial origin and 80% are of nonepithelial origin.
3. About 55% of reported epithelial tumors are benign and 45% are malignant.
4. Of PEMLG, specific diagnoses include ACC (60%), pleomorphic adenocarcinoma (20%), primary (de novo) adenocarcinoma (10%), mucoepidermoid carcinoma (5%), and miscellaneous malignant epithelial neoplasms (5%).

In the authors' recent clinical series of 1,264 consecutive patients with orbital tumors from the Wills Eye Hospital Oncology Service, there were 114 (9%) lacrimal gland lesions (1). When dacryops (a cystic lesion) and other nonepithelial tumors were excluded, there were 30 solid primary epithelial tumors, of which 11 were pleomorphic adenoma and 19 were PEMLG. The 19 PEMLGs included 14 ACC (74%), 4 pleomorphic adenocarcinomas (21%), and 1 mucoepidermoid carcinoma (5%). That series, like most other studies, is biased in the sense that more difficult cases or malignant cases are likely to be referred to the Oncology Service. For example, several patients with ACC were referred for further management after incisional biopsy elsewhere disclosed the diagnosis. A completely excised pleomorphic adenoma would be less likely to prompt a referral to the Oncology Service.

Clinically, mass lesions in the lacrimal gland have consistent, but somewhat variable, features. Sizable solid lesions in the lacrimal gland fossa typically cause proptosis and inferior and nasal displacement of the globe. Benign epithelial tumors and lymphomas generally are painless, whereas malignant epithelial tumors and inflammations are more likely to cause pain. With imaging studies, benign tumors are more likely to show normal adjacent bone or smooth fossa formation. In general, malignant epithelial tumors are more likely to exhibit bone destruction as they progress. Clinical symptoms and signs and radiographic features are discussed in greater detail in the following sections.

Concerning prognosis, pleomorphic adenoma carries an excellent prognosis if the tumor can be completely removed within its capsule. Incomplete removal can lead to recurrence and eventual malignant transformation. Primary malignant epithelial tumors of the lacrimal gland are generally much more aggressive neoplasms with a relatively high incidence of local recurrence and distant metastasis despite aggressive treatment, often including orbital exenteration, irradiation, or chemotherapy. However, there is considerable variation in the degree of malignancy among the various malignant epithelial tumors (7).

General References

Reviews

1. Shields JA, Shields CL, Scartozzi R. Survey of 1264 patients with orbital tumors and simulating lesions: the 2002 Montgomery Lecture, part 1. *Ophthalmology* 2004; 111:997–1008.
2. Shields JA, Bakewell B, Augsburger JJ, et al. Classification and incidence of space-occupying lesions of the orbit. A survey of 645 biopsies. *Arch Ophthalmol* 1984; 102:1606–1611.
3. Shields JA, Bakewell B, Augsburger JJ, et al. Space-occupying orbital masses in children: a review of 250 consecutive biopsies. *Ophthalmology* 1986;93:379–384.
4. Reese AB. Expanding lesions of the orbit (Bowman Lecture). *Trans Ophthalmol Soc UK* 1971;91:85–104.
5. Reese AB. The treatment of lesions of the lacrimal gland. *Trans Am Acad Ophthalmol Otolaryngol* 1958;62:679–683.
6. Shields CL, Shields JA, Eagle RC, et al. Clinicopathologic review of 142 cases of lacrimal gland lesions. *Ophthalmology* 1989;96:431–435.
7. Shields, JA, Shields CL, Epstein J, et al. Primary epithelial malignancies of the lacrimal gland. The 2003 Ramon L. Font Lecture. *Ophthalmic Plast Reconstr Surg* 2004;20: 10–21.
8. Andreoli MT, Aakalu V, Setabutr P. Epidemiological trends in malignant lacrimal gland tumors. *Otolaryngol Head Neck Surg* 2015;152(2):279–283.
9. Andrew NH, McNab AA, Selva D. Review of 268 lacrimal gland biopsies in an Australian cohort. *Clin Experiment Ophthalmol* 2015;43(1):5–11.
10. White VA. Update on lacrimal gland neoplasms: Molecular pathology of interest. *Saudi J Ophthalmol* 2012;26:133–135.
11. Ahmad SM, Esmaeli B, Williams M, et al. American Joint Committee on Cancer classification predicts outcome of patients with lacrimal gland adenoid cystic carcinoma. *Ophthalmology* 2009;116:1210–1215.
12. Tang SX, Lim RP, Al-Dahmash S, et al. Bilateral lacrimal gland disease. Clinical features of 97 cases. *Ophthalmology* 2014;121:2040–2046.
13. Demirci H, Shields CL, Shields JA, et al. Orbital tumors in the older adult population. *Ophthalmology* 2002;109:243–248.

Case Reports

14. Rush A, Leone CR Jr. Ectopic lacrimal gland cyst of the orbit. *Am J Ophthalmol* 1981;92:198–201.
15. Green WR, Zimmerman LE. Ectopic lacrimal gland tissue. Report of eight cases with orbital involvement. *Arch Ophthalmol* 1967;78:318–327.

LACRIMAL GLAND DUCTAL EPITHELIAL CYST (DACRYOPS)

General Considerations

Ductal epithelial cyst, often called dacryops, is an inclusion cyst secondary to occlusion of one or more of the ducts that drain tears from the lacrimal gland into the conjunctival fornix (1–24). In a clinical/pathological survey of 1,264 orbital biopsies, dacryops accounted for 19 cases (2%) and represented 17% of all lacrimal gland lesions (1). In a review of 142 lacrimal gland biopsies, dacryops accounted for 6% of cases (4). The frequency is probably higher as most lesions are relatively small and many do not come to clinical recognition or surgical excision. Only 4 of the 19 cases required surgical excision. In rare instances, an epithelial cyst can arise from ectopic lacrimal gland tissue in the orbit (7,17).

Clinical Features

Ductal epithelial cyst usually arises from the palpebral lobe of the lacrimal gland in adults and presents as a unilateral or bilateral, painless, nontender, fluctuant mass in the forniceal conjunctiva superotemporally (8,9). It can occur spontaneously or it can follow dacryoadenitis (8). The lesion is often slowly progressive, but it can remain stable for long periods of time. Dacryops can intermittently discharge tears and then gradually reform. There are reports of dacryops associated with benign mixed tumor as well as mucoepidermoid carcinoma of the lacrimal gland (15,21). In rare cases, dacryops can develop from accessory lacrimal tissue in the conjunctival fornix or caruncle (25). The differential diagnosis includes many of the other conjunctival and orbital cysts discussed elsewhere in these atlases.

Diagnostic Approaches

Ductal epithelial cyst can usually be visualized clinically in the lateral conjunctival fornix, generally surrounding by conjunctival injection. Imaging studies demonstrate a cystic mass corresponding to the anterior part of the lacrimal gland. These studies can help to delineate the posterior extent of the lesion and rule out a solid tumor with an anterior cystic component (15,21). In contrast to dermoid cyst and malignant lacrimal gland tumor, the adjacent bone is normal.

Pathology

Histopathologically, ductal epithelial cyst has a clear lumen and an epithelial lining that consists of one or two layers of somewhat flattened epithelium, similar to a lacrimal gland duct. The inner layer of epithelium is cuboidal and the outer layer is composed of myoepithelial cells. A few mucin-secreting goblet cells can be present. The pathogenesis is multifactorial and related to inflammation and scar tissue that obstructs the duct, followed by secretion and ductal ectasia (8).

An analysis of 15 cases of dacryops histopathologically disclosed origin from the major lacrimal gland in 13 and accessory gland of Krause in 2 (13). The mean patient age was 51 years. All specimens showed goblet cells and luminal pseudoapocrine apical cytoplasmic projections. The dacryops epithelium showed no myoepithelial cells.

Management

As implied, smaller, asymptomatic lesions can be observed and large ones can be resected locally by a superotemporal conjunctival forniceal approach, taking care not to disrupt the ducts that drain the palpebral lobe if possible. Marsupialization of the cyst is another surgical option, particularly in patients who have decreased tear production (12). To avoid standard surgery, some authors have described success using blue-green argon laser to collapse the cyst (11).

Selected References

Reviews

1. Shields JA, Shields CL, Scartozzi R. Survey of 1264 patients with orbital tumors and simulating lesions: the 2002 Montgomery Lecture, part 1. *Ophthalmology* 2004;111: 997–1008.
2. Reese AB. Expanding lesions of the orbit (Bowman Lecture). *Trans Ophthalmol Soc UK* 1971;91:85–104.
3. Reese AB. The treatment of lesions of the lacrimal gland. *Trans Am Acad Ophthalmol Otolaryngol* 1958;62:679–683.
4. Shields CL, Shields JA, Eagle RC, et al. Clinicopathologic review of 142 cases of lacrimal gland lesions. *Ophthalmology* 1989;96:431–435.
5. Andrew NH, McNab AA, Selva D. Review of 268 lacrimal gland biopsies in an Australian cohort. *Clin Experiment Ophthalmol* 2015;43(1):5–11.
6. Shields, JA, Shields CL, Epstein J, et al. Primary epithelial malignancies of the lacrimal gland. The 2003 Ramon L. Font Lecture. *Ophthalmic Plast Reconstr Surg* 2004;20:10–21.
7. Green WR, Zimmerman LE. Ectopic lacrimal gland tissue. Report of eight cases with orbital involvement. *Arch Ophthalmol* 1967;78:318–327.
8. Lam K, Brownstein S, Jordan DR, et al. Dacryops: a series of 5 cases and a proposed pathogenesis. *JAMA Ophthalmol* 2013;131(7):929–932.
9. Smith S, Rootman J. Lacrimal ductal cysts. Presentation and management. *Surv Ophthalmol* 1986;30:245–250.
10. Tang SX, Lim RP, Al-Dahmash S, et al. Bilateral lacrimal gland disease. Clinical features of 97 cases. *Ophthalmology* 2014;121:2040–2046.

Management

11. Pantaleoni FB, Spagnolo S, Martini A, et al. Argon laser photocoagulation in the treatment of the palpebral lobe cysts of the lacrimal gland (dacryops). *Ophthalmic Surg Lasers* 1997;28:690–692.
12. Salam A, Barrett AW, Malhotra R, et al. Marsupialization for lacrimal ductular cysts (dacryops): a case series. *Ophthal Plast Reconstr Surg* 2012;28:57–62.

Histopathology

13. Jakobiec FA, Zakka FR, Perry LP. The cytologic composition of dacryops: an immunohistochemical investigation of 15 lesions compared to the normal lacrimal gland. *Am J Ophthalmol* 2013;155:380–396.

Case Reports

14. Bullock JD, Fleishman JA, Rosset JS. Lacrimal ductal cysts. *Ophthalmology* 1986;93: 1355–1360.
15. Christie DB, Woog JJ, Lahav M. Combined dacryops with underlying benign mixed cell tumor of the lacrimal gland. *Am J Ophthalmol* 1995;11:97–99.
16. Bartley GB. Orbital lobe lacrimal ductal cysts. *Surg Neurol* 1995;43:521.
17. von Domarus H. A lacrimal gland cyst in the orbit. *J Craniomaxillofac Surg* 1987;15:106–109.
18. Sen DK, Thomas A. Simple dacryops. *Am J Ophthalmol* 1967;63:161.
19. Bradey N, Hayward JM. Case report: bilateral lacrimal gland enlargement: an unusual manifestation of dacryops. *Clin Radiol* 1991;43:280–281.
20. Rush A, Leone CR Jr. Ectopic lacrimal gland cyst of the orbit. *Am J Ophthalmol* 1981;92:198–201.
21. Levin LA, Popham J, To K, et al. Mucoepidermoid carcinoma of the lacrimal gland. Report of a case with oncocytic features arising in a patient with chronic dacryops. *Ophthalmology* 1991;98:1551–1555.
22. Brownstein S, Belin MW, Krohel GB, et al. Orbital dacryops. *Ophthalmology* 1984; 91:1424–1428.
23. Morgan-Warren PJ, Madge SN. Lacrimal duct cyst (dacryops) following ocular chemical injury. *Orbit* 2012;31:335–337.
24. Su GW, Patipa M, Font RL. Primary squamous cell carcinoma arising from an epithelium-lined cyst of the lacrimal gland. *Ophthal Plast Reconstr Surg* 2005;21:383–385.
25. Jakobiec FA, Roh M, Stagner AM, et al. Caruncular dacryops. *Cornea* 2015;34: 107–109.

LACRIMAL GLAND DUCTAL EPITHELIAL CYST (DACRYOPS)

In most instances a dacryops is small, asymptomatic, does not prompt a medical consultation, and is detected on routine ocular examination. Occasionally, a dacryops can cause irritation or foreign body sensation and may require symptomatic treatment or surgical removal. Examples of relatively small, asymptomatic dacryops are depicted.

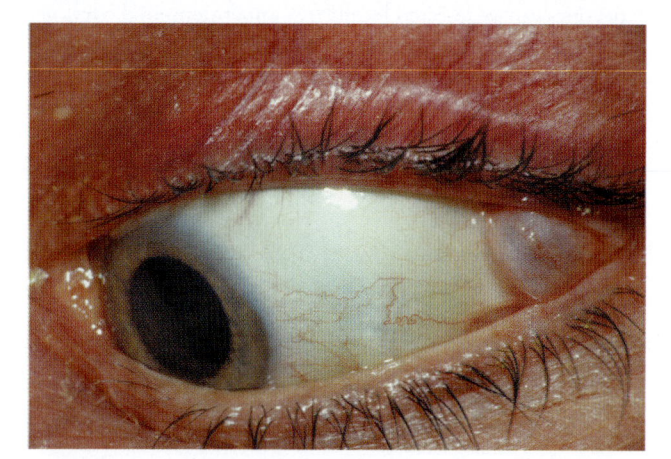

Figure 37.1. Dacryops of left lacrimal gland.

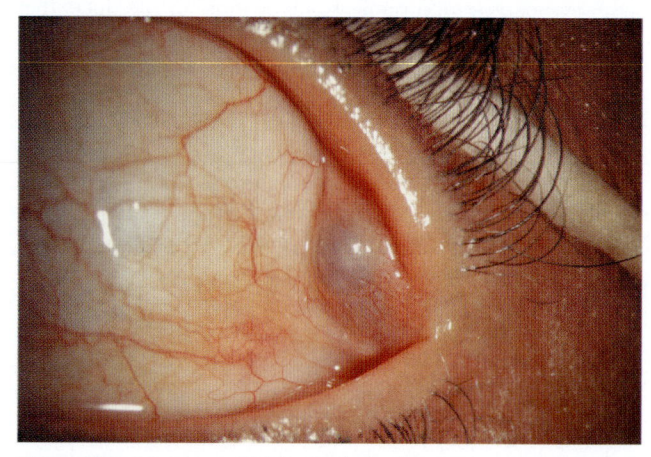

Figure 37.2. Dacryops of left lacrimal gland.

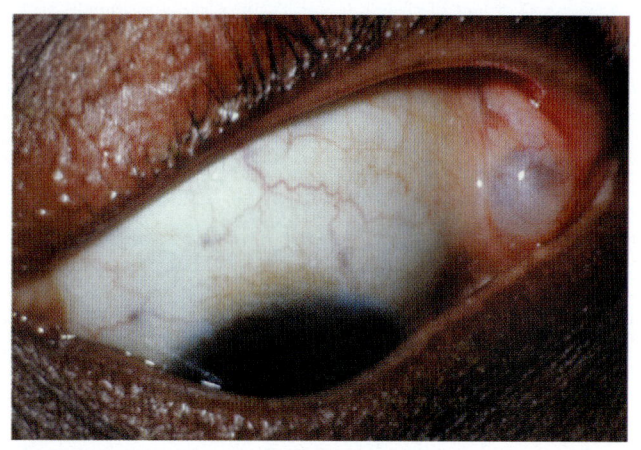

Figure 37.3. Dacryops in African-American patient.

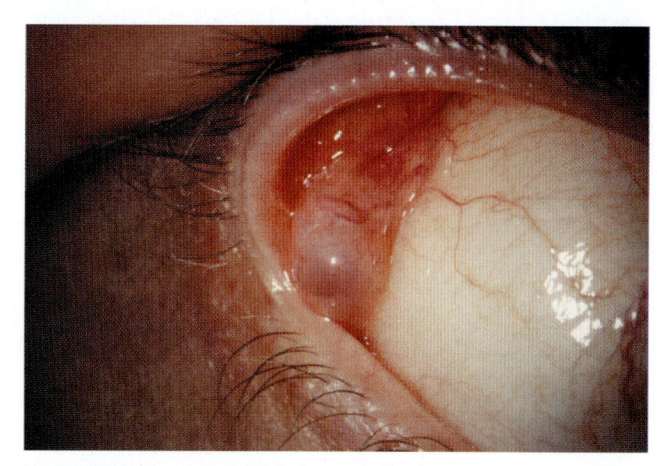

Figure 37.4. Dacryops of right lacrimal gland.

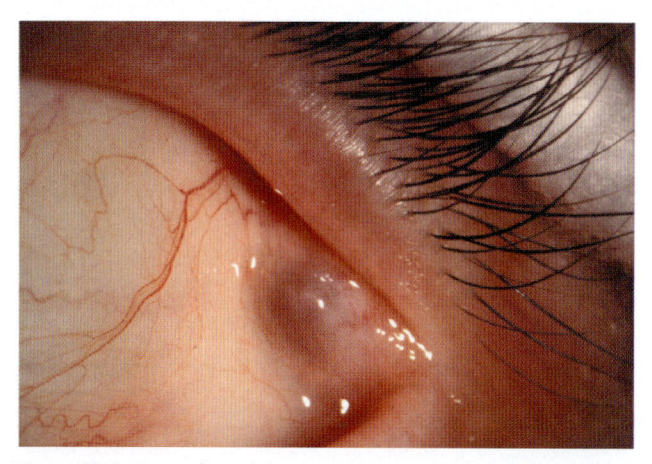

Figure 37.5. Somewhat solid-appearing dacryops of left lacrimal gland.

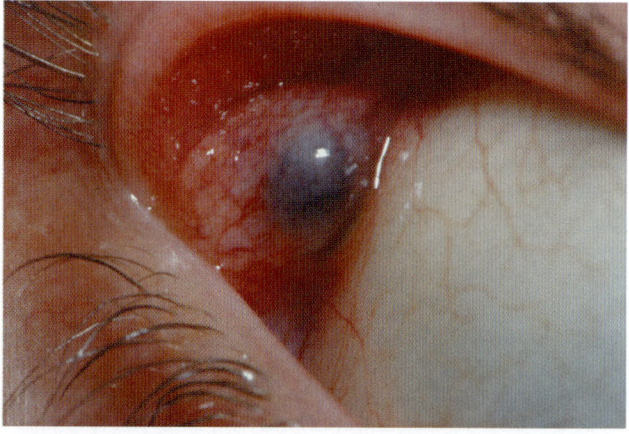

Figure 37.6. Dacryops of right lacrimal gland with a dark blue color.

LACRIMAL GLAND DUCTAL EPITHELIAL CYST (DACRYOPS)

In some instances, dacryops can be larger and cause bothersome symptoms. A case that was studied by computed tomography (CT) and managed by surgical excision is shown.

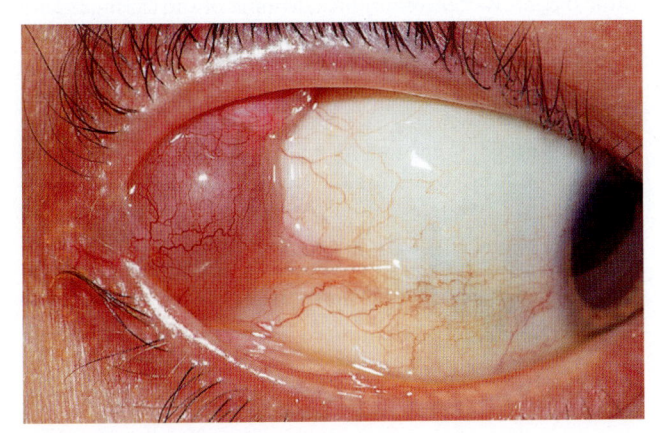

Figure 37.7. Dacryops superotemporally in a 55-year-old man. The lesion was producing persistent discomfort.

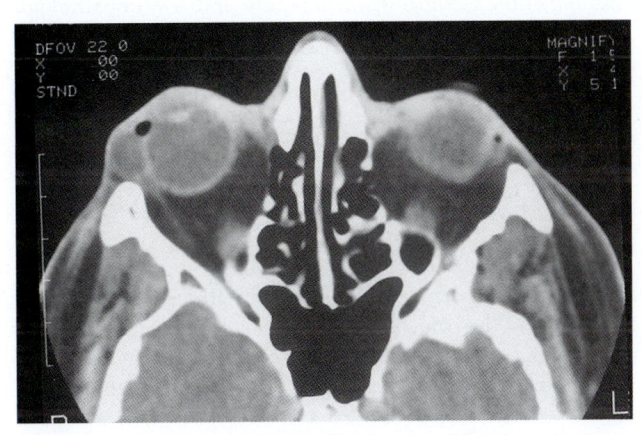

Figure 37.8. Axial computed tomography of patient shown in Figure 37.7, demonstrating cystic lesion near anterior orbital rim.

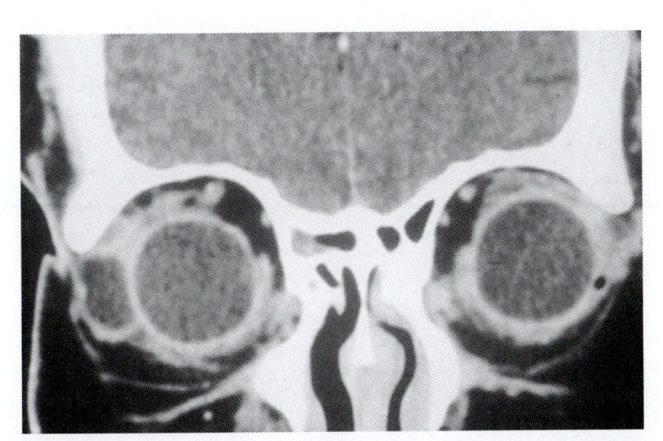

Figure 37.9. Coronal computed tomography showing cystic lesion temporal to the globe.

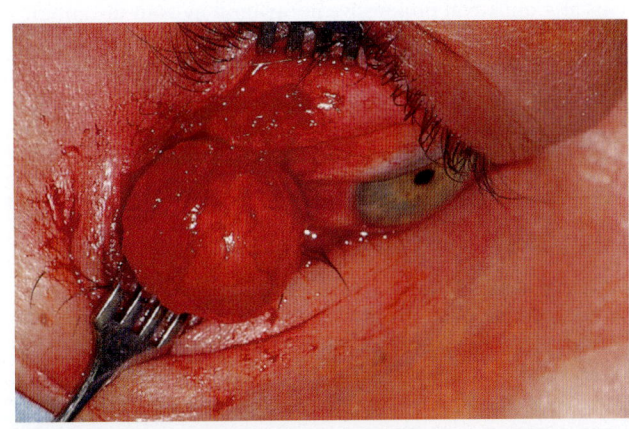

Figure 37.10. Appearance of intact lesion at time of surgical removal by a superotemporal conjunctival approach.

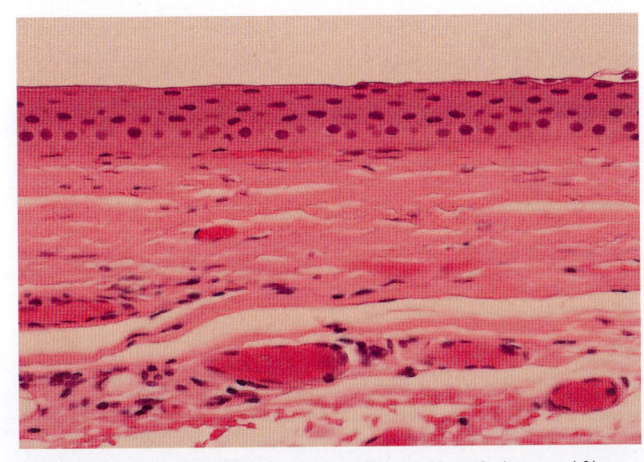

Figure 37.11. Histopathology showing flattened epithelium and fibrous tissue wall of the cyst. (Hematoxylin–eosin ×25.)

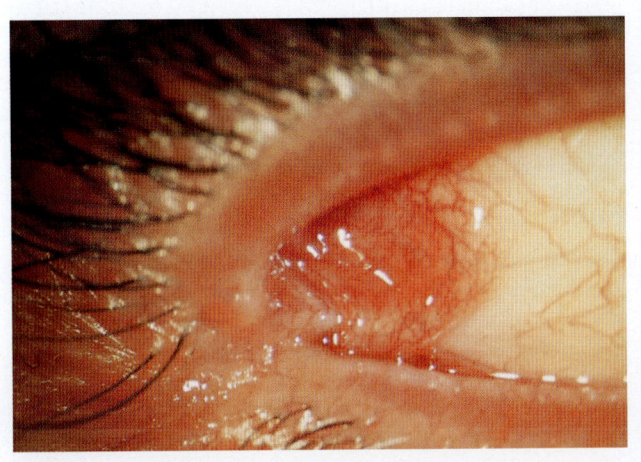

Figure 37.12. Appearance 5 months later showing no recurrence. The patient's symptoms resolved.

LACRIMAL GLAND PLEOMORPHIC ADENOMA (BENIGN MIXED TUMOR)

General Considerations

Tumors of the lacrimal gland are quite similar histopathologically to tumors that arise in the major salivary glands and other minor salivary glands.

Pleomorphic adenoma (benign mixed tumor) is the most important benign epithelial tumor of the lacrimal gland (1–30). In the authors' clinical series of 1,264 orbital tumors, there were 11 pleomorphic adenomas, accounting for 10% of all lacrimal gland lesions and for 1% of all orbital lesions (1). Among 142 lacrimal gland biopsies, pleomorphic adenoma accounted for 12% of cases (4). This tumor usually arises from the orbital lobe of the lacrimal gland, although it has rarely developed in the palpebral lobe or from ectopic lacrimal gland tissue in the orbit (1,6). This tumor is generally found in young to middle-aged adults (mean age, 39 years), but it can occur in children (20,21,25).

Clinical Features

Pleomorphic adenoma of the lacrimal gland generally presents as a unilateral progressive nonpainful mass in the anterior aspect of the orbit superotemporally. As the lesion enlarges, it produces proptosis and downward and nasal displacement of the globe. The relative absence of pain is important in differentiating a pleomorphic adenoma from other malignant lacrimal gland tumors, which characteristically produce more pain (1,14,16).

Diagnostic Approaches

Imaging studies disclose a round to ovoid circumscribed mass in the lacrimal gland fossa with a smooth to slightly irregular surface (10–12). There may be fossa formation in the adjacent bone, but frank bone destruction, as seen with some malignant tumors, is usually not evident. CT is the best method to assess bone involvement, while magnetic resonance imaging with fat suppression and gadolinium enhancement portrays the tumor best (10–12). The anterior portion of the mass seems to stop at or posterior to the orbital rim, suggesting that the lesion affects the orbital lobe but spares the palpebral lobe of the lacrimal gland. There may be an adjacent bony fossa, but true bone erosion is very rare (24). Like malignant epithelial tumors, pleomorphic adenoma shows low to isointense signal on T1-weighted and hyperintense signal on T2-weighted images, and with gadolinium enhancement (12).

Pathology

The histopathology of pleomorphic adenoma of the lacrimal gland varies from case to case. It typically shows a combination of benign epithelial elements and mesenchymal elements, accounting for the name benign mixed tumor (14,15). The epithelial elements can take the form of ducts, cords, and squamous pearls. The mesenchymal elements usually are myxoid material and cartilaginous tissue.

Management

If the diagnosis of pleomorphic adenoma of the lacrimal gland is suspected on the basis of clinical findings and imaging studies, the tumor is generally removed by a superolateral orbitotomy through an eyelid crease incision with an extraperiosteal approach. An osteotomy (Kronlein approach) is rarely necessary. It is generally mandatory to completely excise the mass within its capsule without rupture or incisional biopsy. Incisional biopsy can hinder complete tumor removal and allow for recurrence and possible malignant transformation. With time, pleomorphic adenoma can evolve into pleomorphic adenocarcinoma (malignant mixed tumor) (16).

LACRIMAL GLAND PLEOMORPHIC ADENOMA (BENIGN MIXED TUMOR)

Selected References

Reviews

1. Shields JA, Shields CL, Scartozzi R. Survey of 1264 patients with orbital tumors and simulating lesions: the 2002 Montgomery Lecture, part 1. *Ophthalmology* 2004;111:997–1008.
2. Shields JA, Bakewell B, Augsburger DG, et al. Classification and incidence of space-occupying lesions of the orbit. A survey of 645 biopsies. *Arch Ophthalmol* 1984;102:1606–1611.
3. Reese AB. Expanding lesions of the orbit (Bowman Lecture). *Trans Ophthalmol Soc UK* 1971;91:85–104.
4. Shields CL, Shields JA, Eagle RC, et al. Clinicopathologic review of 142 cases of lacrimal gland lesions. *Ophthalmology* 1989;96:431–435.
5. Andrew NH, McNab AA, Selva D. Review of 268 lacrimal gland biopsies in an Australian cohort. *Clin Experiment Ophthalmol* 2015;43(1):5–11.
6. Wright JE, Stewart WB, Krohel GB. Clinical presentation and management of lacrimal gland tumours. *Br J Ophthalmol* 1979;63:600–606.
7. Wright JE. Factors affecting the survival of patients with lacrimal gland tumours. *Can J Ophthalmol* 1982;17:3–9.
8. White VA. Update on lacrimal gland neoplasms: Molecular pathology of interest. *Saudi J Ophthalmol* 2012;26:133–135
9. Von Holstein SL. Tumours of the lacrimal gland. Epidemiolocial, clinical and genetic characteristics. *Acta Ophthalmol* 2013;6:1–28.

Imaging

10. Jakobiec FA, Trokel SL, Abbott GF, et al. Combined clinical and computed tomographic diagnosis of primary lacrimal fossa lesions. *Am J Ophthalmol* 1982;94:785–807.
11. Font RL, Patipa M, Rosenbaum PS, et al. Correlation of computed tomographic and histopathologic features in malignant transformation of benign mixed tumor of lacrimal gland. *Surv Ophthalmol* 1990;34:449–452.
12. Gunduz K, Shields CL, Gunalp I, et al. Magnetic resonance imaging of unilateral lacrimal gland lesions. *Graefes Arch Clin Exp Ophthalmol* 2003;241:907–913.

Management

13. Tse DT, Folberg R. Technique for incisional biopsy of a lacrimal gland mass when the diagnosis of benign mixed tumor cannot be excluded clinically. *Ophthalmic Surg* 1988;19:321–324.

Histopathology

14. Font RL, Gamel JW. Epithelial tumors of the lacrimal gland: An analysis of 265 cases. In: Jakobiec FA, ed. *Ocular and Adnexal Tumors*. Birmingham, AL: Auscula-pius; 1978:787–805.
15. Chawla B, Kashyap S, Sen S, et al. Clinicopathologic review of epithelial tumors of the lacrimal gland. *Ophthal Plast Reconstr Surg* 2013;29:440–445.

Case Reports

16. Shields JA, Shields CL. Malignant transformation of presumed pleomorphic adenoma of lacrimal gland after 60 years. *Arch Ophthalmol* 1987;105:1403–1405.
17. Hsu HC. Posttraumatic benign pleomorphic adenoma of the lacrimal gland. *Ophthalmologica* 2001;215:235–237.
18. Wharton JA, O'Donnell BA. Unusual presentations of pleomorphic adenoma and adenoid cystic carcinoma of the lacrimal gland. *Aust N Z J Ophthalmol* 1999;27:145–148.
19. Christie DB, Woog JJ, Lahav M. Combined dacryops with underlying benign mixed cell tumor of the lacrimal gland. *Am J Ophthalmol* 1995;119:97–99.
20. Mercado G, Gunduz K, Shields CL, et al. Pleomorphic adenoma of the lacrimal gland in a young patient. *Arch Ophthalmol* 1998;116:962–963.
21. Faktorovich EG, Crawford JB, Char DH, et al. Benign mixed tumor (pleomorphic adenoma) of the lacrimal gland in a 6-year-old boy. *Am J Ophthalmol* 1996;122:446–447.
22. Auran J, Jakobiec FA, Krebs W. Benign mixed tumor of the palpebral lobe of the lacrimal gland. Clinical diagnosis and appropriate surgical management. *Ophthalmology* 1988;95:90–99.
23. Ostrowski ML, Font RL, Halpern J, et al. Clear cell epithelial-myoepithelial carcinoma arising in pleomorphic adenoma of the lacrimal gland. *Ophthalmology* 1994;101:925–930.
24. Hornblass A, Friedman AH, Yagoda A. Erosion of the orbital plate (frontal bone) by a benign tumor of the lacrimal gland. *Ophthalmic Surg* 1981;12:737–742.
25. Stupp T, Pavlidis M, Buchner TF, et al. Pleomorphic adenoma of the lacrimal gland in a child after treatment of acute lymphoblastic leukemia. *Arch Ophthalmol* 2004;122:1538–1540.
26. Shields JA, Shields CL, Eagle RC, et al. Pleomorphic adenoma ("Benign mixed tumor") of the lacrimal gland. *Arch Ophthalmol* 1987;105:560–561.
27. Prabhakaran VC, Cannon PS, McNab A, et al. Lesions mimicking lacrimal gland pleomorphic adenoma. *Br J Ophthalmol* 2010;94:1509–1512.
28. Ramlee N, Ramli N, Tajudin LS. Pleomorphic adenoma in the palpebral lobe of the lacrimal gland misdiagnosed as chalazion. *Orbit* 2007;26:137–139.
29. Currie ZI, Rose GE. Long-term risk of recurrence after intact excision of pleomorphic adenomas of the lacrimal gland. *Arch Ophthalmol* 2007;125:1643–1646.
30. Tong JT, Flanagan JC, Eagle RC Jr, et al. Benign mixed tumor arising from an accessory lacrimal gland of Wolfring. *Ophthal Plast Reconstr Surg* 1995;11:136–138.

LACRIMAL GLAND PLEOMORPHIC ADENOMA: CLINICOPATHOLOGIC CORRELATION

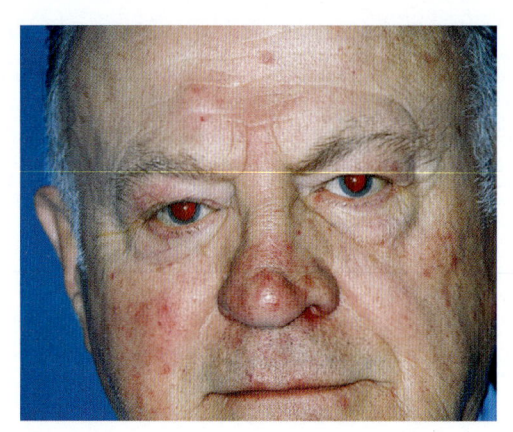

Figure 37.13. Downward displacement of the right eye in a 73-year-old man.

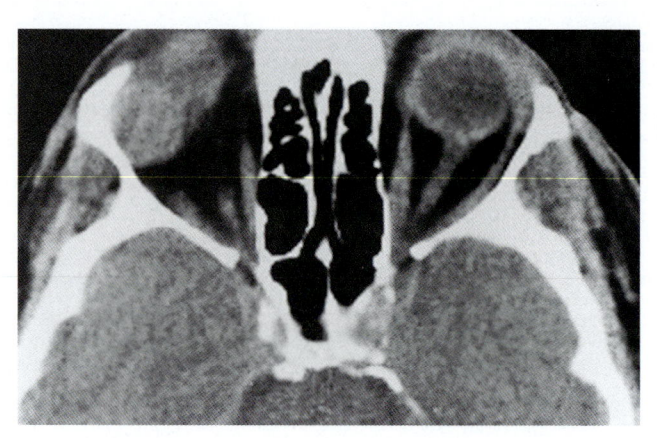

Figure 37.14. Axial computed tomography showing ovoid mass in lacrimal gland fossa.

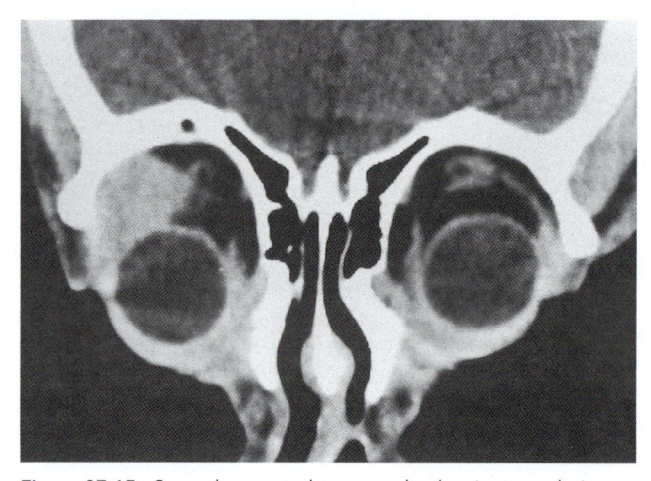

Figure 37.15. Coronal computed tomography showing same lesion.

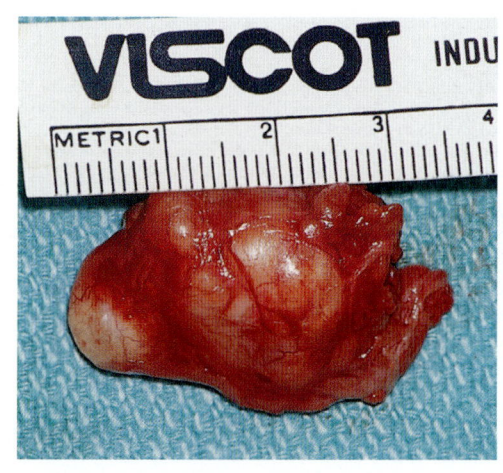

Figure 37.16. Gross appearance of mass after successful surgical removal by superotemporal eyelid crease incision and extraperiosteal approach. Note the lobular surface of the encapsulated mass.

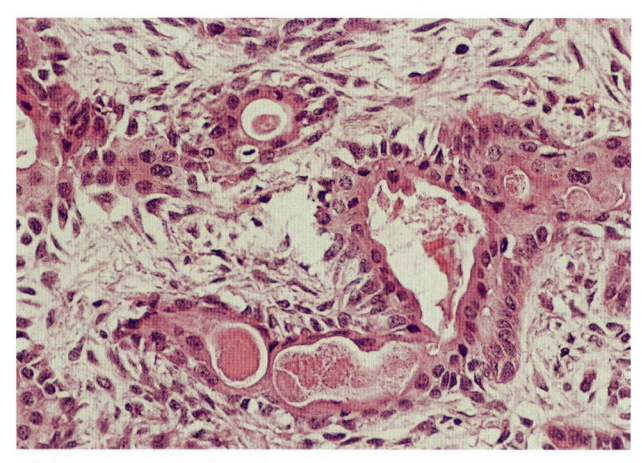

Figure 37.17. Histopathology showing epithelial tubules within myxomatous stroma. (Hematoxylin–eosin ×100.)

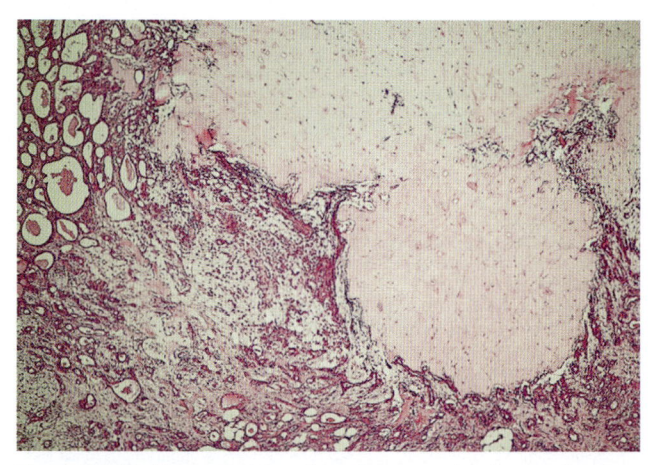

Figure 37.18. Histopathology of another area, showing cartilaginous differentiation. (Hematoxylin–eosin ×50.)

Chapter 37 Lacrimal Gland Primary Epithelial Tumors

● LACRIMAL GLAND PLEOMORPHIC ADENOMA: SURGICAL MANAGEMENT

The goal of treatment is to remove the tumor intact through a superolateral orbitotomy, usually without an osteotomy.

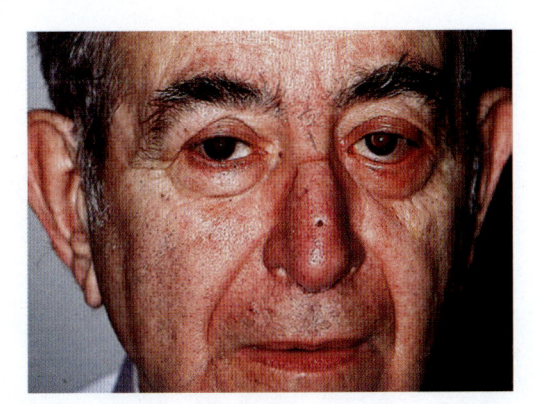

Figure 37.19. Proptosis of the left eye in a 71-year-old man.

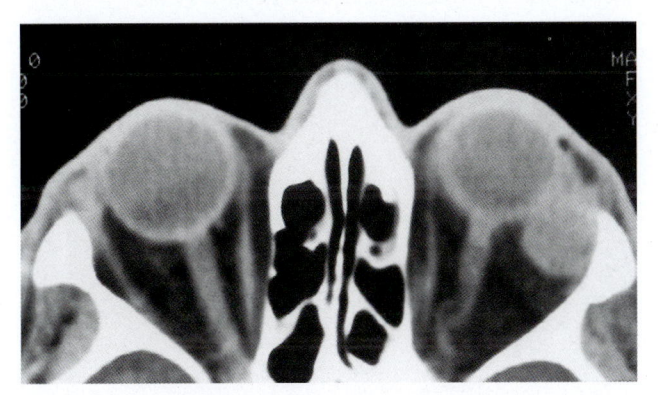

Figure 37.20. Axial computed tomography showing solid, round mass in superotemporal aspect of orbit anteriorly.

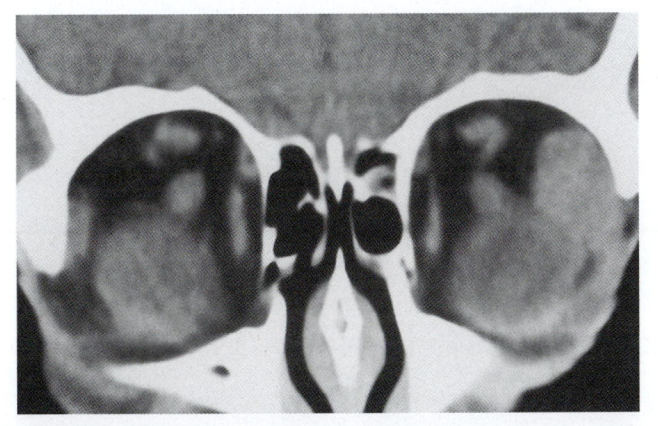

Figure 37.21. Coronal computed tomography showing ovoid mass superotemporal to the globe.

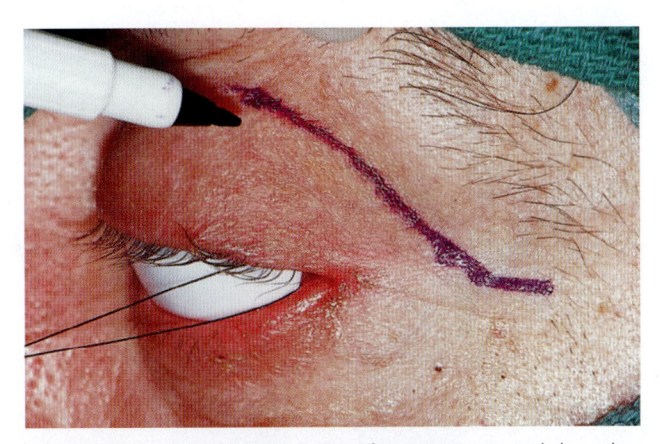

Figure 37.22. Outlined incision to perform tumor removal through a superotemporal cutaneous eyelid crease approach.

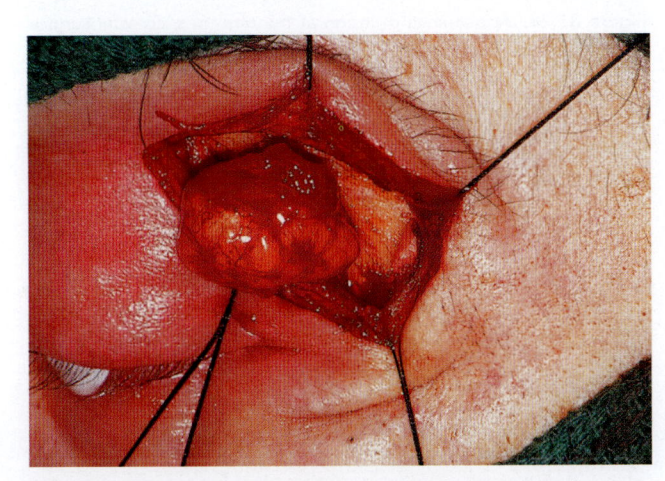

Figure 37.23. Appearance of the tumor as it is being removed.

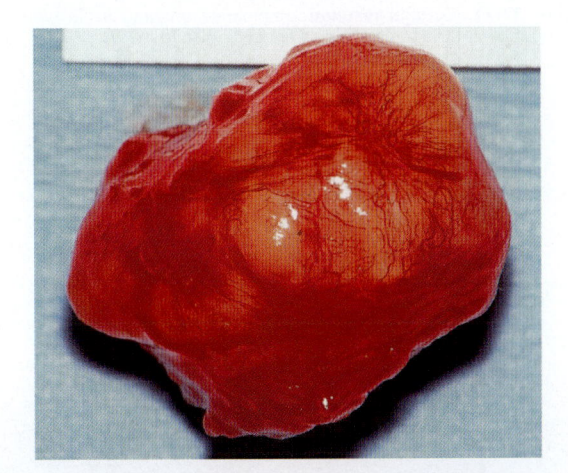

Figure 37.24. Gross appearance of encapsulated mass. Note the characteristic light yellow color and the nodularity of the margin of the lesion. Histopathology revealed typical features of pleomorphic adenoma.

LACRIMAL GLAND PLEOMORPHIC ADENOMA IN A TEENAGER

Pleomorphic adenoma of the lacrimal gland generally appears in middle-aged or older patients. Occasionally, it develops in a younger patient. A clinicopathologic correlation is shown.

Mercado G, Gunduz K, Shields JA, et al. Pleomorphic adenoma of the lacrimal gland in a young patient. *Arch Ophthalmol* 1998;116:962–963.

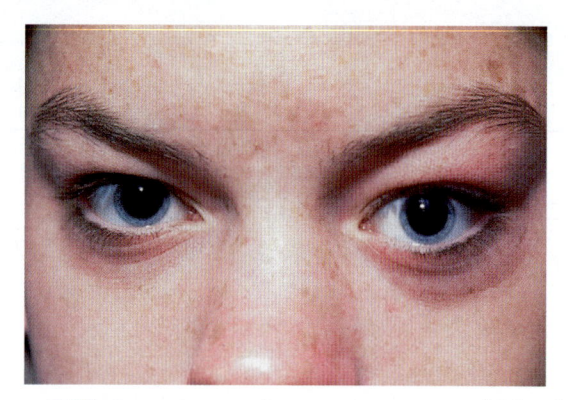

Figure 37.25. Proptosis secondary to a superotemporal left orbital mass in a 15-year-old girl.

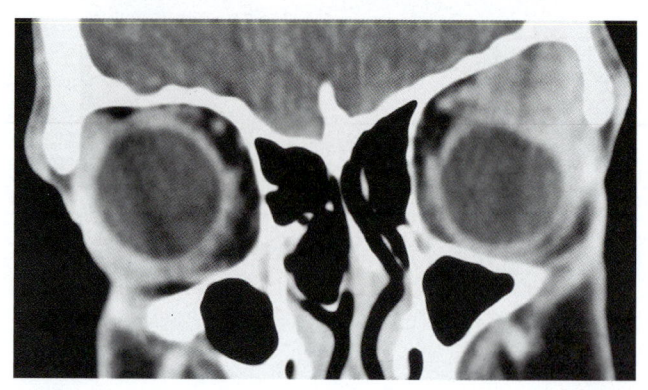

Figure 37.26. Coronal computed tomography showing mass in lacrimal gland fossa. Note that the slow-growing lesion has produced marked fossa in the frontal and zygomatic bones.

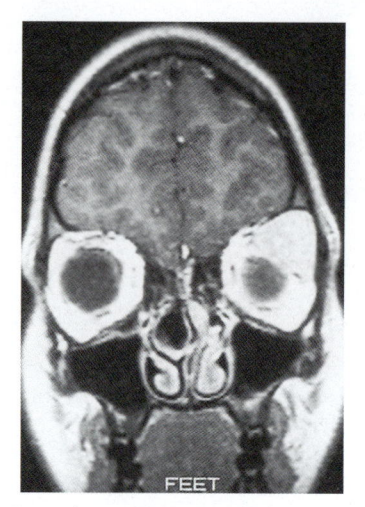

Figure 37.27. Coronal magnetic resonance imaging in T1-weighted image, showing triangular-shaped enhancing solid mass.

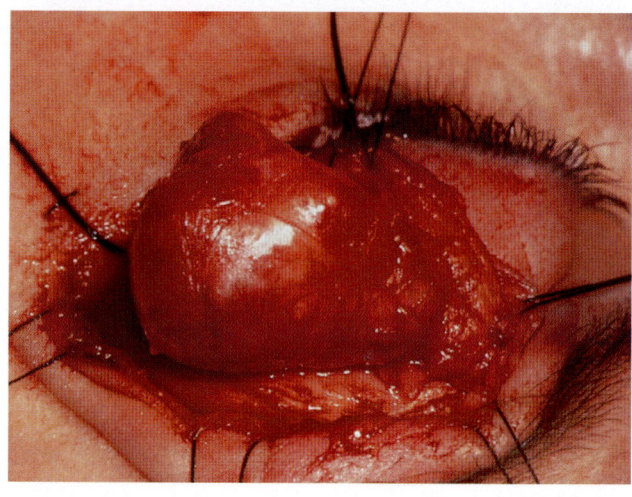

Figure 37.28. Appearance of lesion at the time of successful surgical removal.

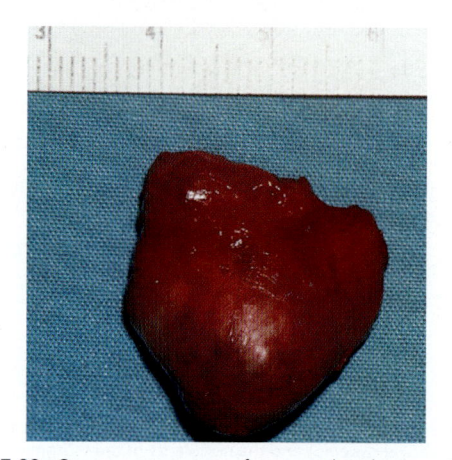

Figure 37.29. Gross appearance of encapsulated mass. Note the characteristic bosselated surface nodularity of the lesion.

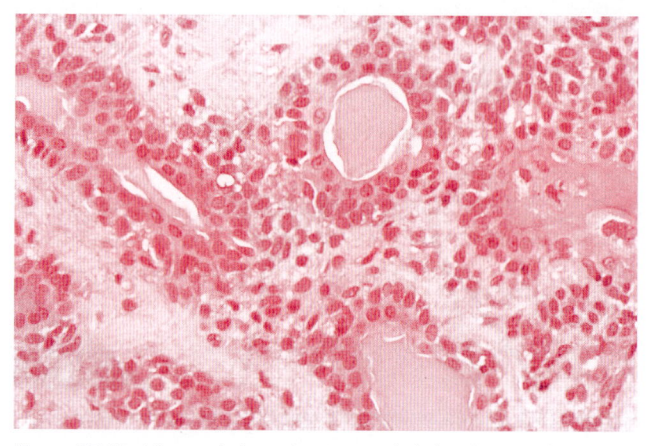

Figure 37.30. Histopathology showing epithelial and mesenchymal elements characteristic of pleomorphic adenoma.

Chapter 37 Lacrimal Gland Primary Epithelial Tumors

● LACRIMAL GLAND PLEOMORPHIC ADENOMA: MAGNETIC RESONANCE IMAGING

The clinical diagnosis of pleomorphic adenoma of lacrimal gland can be supported by orbital magnetic resonance imaging, which shows fairly characteristic features. The MRI characteristics of a typical case are illustrated.

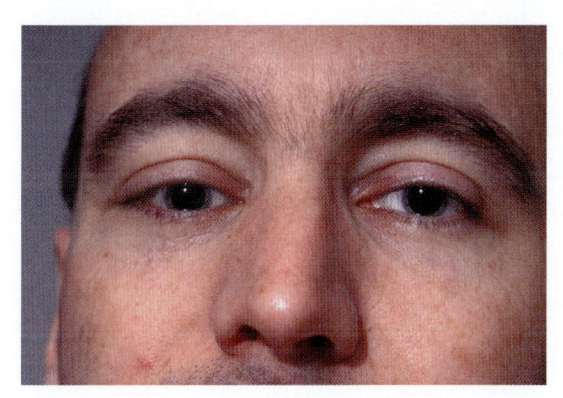

Figure 37.31. Slight downward displacement of right eye in a 40-year-old man.

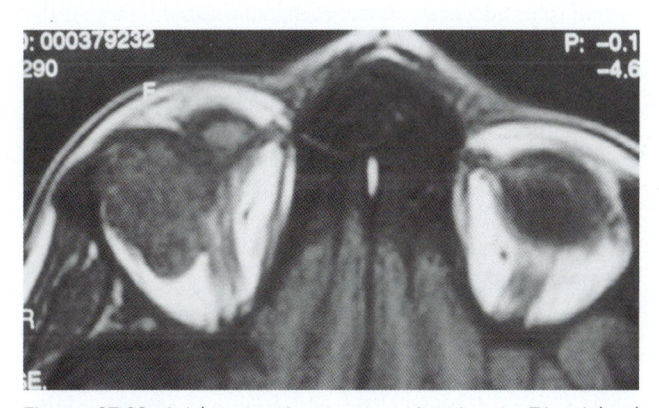

Figure 37.32. Axial magnetic resonance imaging in T1-weighted image, showing hypointense, solid superotemporal orbital mass with characteristic bosselated margins.

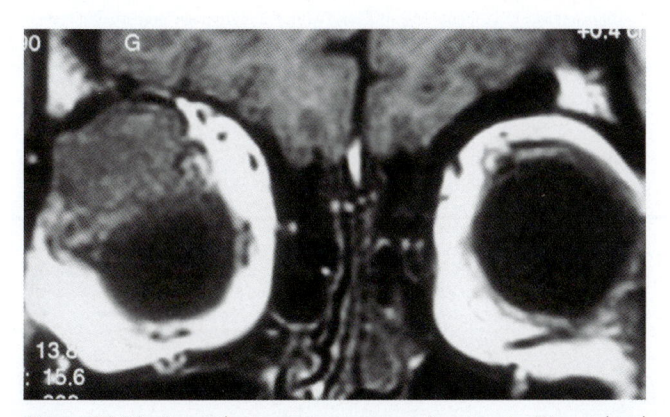

Figure 37.33. Coronal magnetic resonance imaging in T1-weighted image demonstrating superotemporal mass with downward and medial displacement of the globe.

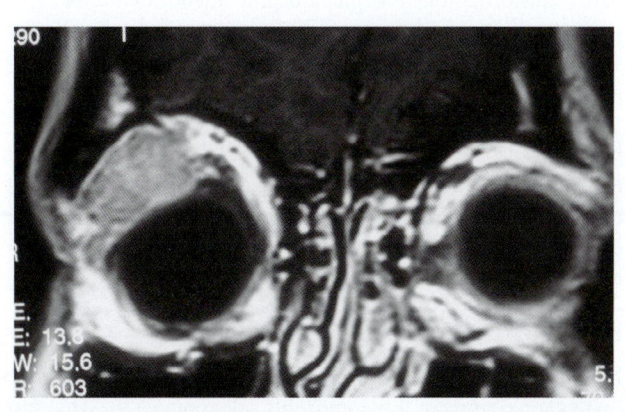

Figure 37.34. Coronal magnetic resonance imaging in T1-weighted image with gadolinium, showing moderate enhancement of the mass.

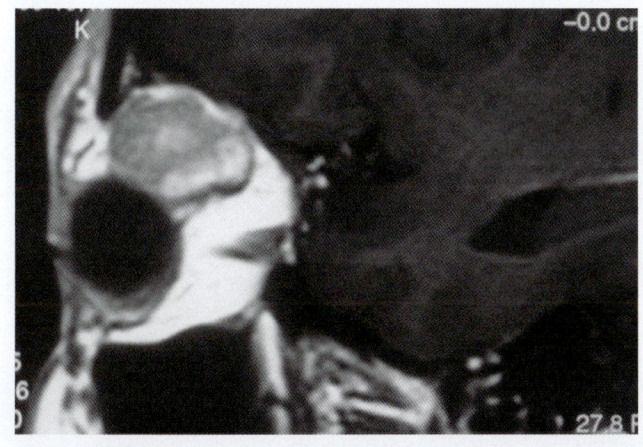

Figure 37.35. Sagittal magnetic resonance imaging in T1-weighted image with gadolinium showing mass superior to globe.

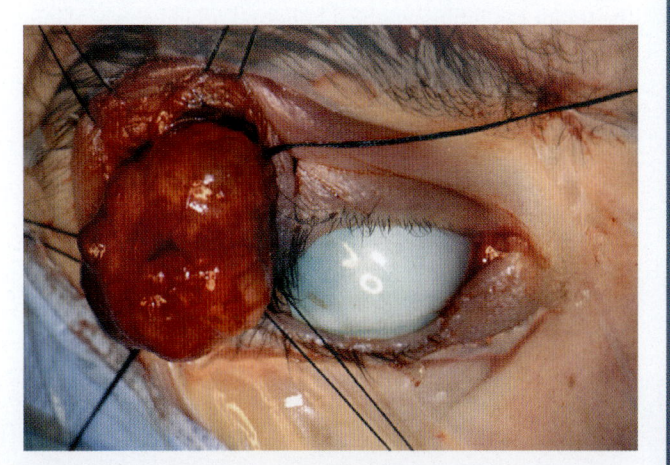

Figure 37.36. Same tumor at time of surgical removal showing circumscribed, encapsulated mass. A plastic protective shield covers the cornea. Histopathology revealed typical features of pleomorphic adenoma.

LACRIMAL GLAND PLEOMORPHIC ADENOCARCINOMA

General Considerations

Pleomorphic adenocarcinoma (malignant mixed tumor) is the second most important PEMLG (1–15). It can occur from spontaneous malignant transformation of a pleomorphic adenoma or from an incompletely excised pleomorphic adenoma. In the authors' clinical series, the 4 pleomorphic adenocarcinomas accounted for 4% of all lacrimal gland fossa lesions and for <1% of 1,264 orbital masses (1). In a recent analysis from data from the Surveillance, Epidemiology, and End Results database regarding 702 malignant tumors of the lacrimal gland, adenocarcinoma represented 4% (10).

Clinical Features

The clinical symptoms and signs are similar to those described for ACC of the lacrimal gland, with proptosis, inferonasal displacement of the globe, motility disturbance, and sometimes pain. One patient with a small asymptomatic lacrimal gland mass for 60 years developed rapid proptosis owing to malignant transformation into pleomorphic adenocarcinoma (13). Local recurrence and distant metastasis are well known. It has been known to cause distant metastasis to bone long before the primary lacrimal gland tumor was discovered (14).

Diagnostic Approaches

CT and magnetic resonance imaging show findings similar to those of ACC. Initially, it is a circumscribed lesion with early bone erosion. As it enlarges, the capsule ruptures and the mass can readily extend diffusely throughout the orbit.

Pathology

Pleomorphic adenocarcinoma is characterized by areas of malignant change in a pleomorphic adenoma (5,9). This can range from small foci of malignant change to massive replacement of the benign tumor by malignant cells. Pleomorphic adenocarcinoma contains fewer glandular structures and the cells have more anaplastic features than pleomorphic adenoma. The tumor can infiltrate orbital bone and orbital nerves. More details of the histopathology are discussed in the literature (11,12).

Management

The management is the same as for ACC. If the lesion is small and circumscribed, it can be removed completely. In more advanced cases that cannot be completely removed, orbital exenteration with possible bone removal may be necessary. Although good follow-up information is lacking on this uncommon malignant tumor, the prognosis appears to be somewhat better than for ACC.

Selected References

Reviews

1. Shields JA, Shields CL, Scartozzi R. Survey of 1264 patients with orbital tumors and simulating lesions: the 2002 Montgomery Lecture, part 1. *Ophthalmology* 2004;111: 997–1008.
2. Shields JA, Bakewell B, Augsburger JJ, et al. Space-occupying orbital masses in children: a review of 250 consecutive biopsies. *Ophthalmology* 1986;93:379–384.
3. Reese AB. Expanding lesions of the orbit (Bowman Lecture). *Trans Ophthalmol Soc UK* 1971;91:85–104.
4. Shields CL, Shields JA, Eagle RC, et al. Clinicopathologic review of 142 cases of lacrimal gland lesions. *Ophthalmology* 1989;96:431–435.
5. Shields, JA, Shields CL, Epstein J, et al. Primary epithelial malignancies of the lacrimal gland. The 2003 Ramon L. Font Lecture. *Ophthalmic Plast Reconstr Surg* 2004; 20:10–21.
6. Andrew NH, McNab AA, Selva D. Review of 268 lacrimal gland biopsies in an Australian cohort. *Clin Experiment Ophthalmol* 2015;43(1):5–11.
7. Wright JE, Stewart WB, Krohel GB. Clinical presentation and management of lacrimal gland tumours. *Br J Ophthalmol* 1979;63:600–606.
8. Wright JE. Factors affecting the survival of patients with lacrimal gland tumours. *Can J Ophthalmol* 1982;17:3–9.
9. Henderson JW, Farrow GM. Primary malignant mixed tumors of the lacrimal gland. Report of 10 cases. *Ophthalmology* 1980;17:466–475.
10. Andreoli MT, Aakalu V, Betabutr P. Epidemiological trends in malignant lacrimal gland tumors. *Otolaryngol Head Neck Surg* 2015;152(2):279–283.

Histopathology

11. Grossniklaus HE, Abbuhl MF, McLean IW. Immunohistologic properties of benign and malignant mixed tumor of the lacrimal gland. *Am J Ophthalmol* 1990;110: 540–549.
12. Perzin KH, Jakobiec FA, Livolsi VA, et al. Lacrimal gland malignant mixed tumors (carcinomas arising in benign mixed tumors): a clinico-pathologic study. *Cancer* 1980; 45:2593–2606.

Case Reports

13. Shields JA, Shields CL. Malignant transformation of presumed pleomorphic adenoma of lacrimal gland after 60 years. *Arch Ophthalmol* 1987;105:1403–1405.
14. Waller RR, Riley FC, Henderson JW. Malignant mixed tumor of the lacrimal gland. Occult source of metastatic carcinoma. *Arch Ophthalmol* 1973;90:297–299.
15. Giliberti FM, Shinder R, Bell D, et al. Malignant mixed tumor of the lacrimal gland in a teenager. *J Pediatr Ophthalmol Strabismus* 2010;26:1–3.

Chapter 37 Lacrimal Gland Primary Epithelial Tumors

LACRIMAL GLAND PLEOMORPHIC ADENOCARCINOMA (MALIGNANT MIXED TUMOR)

Pleomorphic adenocarcinoma can evolve from a pre-existing pleomorphic adenoma of the lacrimal gland after many years. A clinicopathologic correlation is shown.

Shields JA, Shields CL. Malignant transformation of presumed pleomorphic adenoma of lacrimal gland after 60 years. *Arch Ophthalmol* 1987;105:1403–1405.

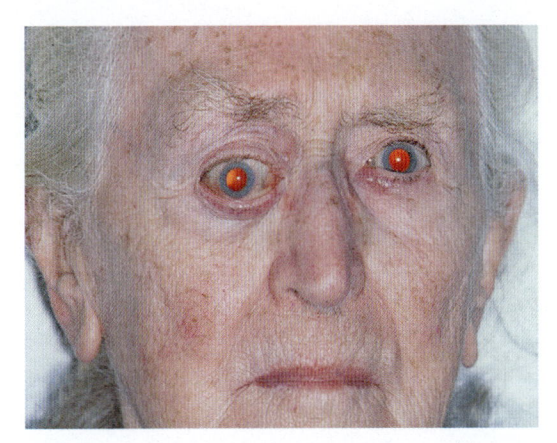

Figure 37.37. Proptosis of the right eye in an 81-year-old woman. Mild proptosis had been noted 60 years earlier and the diagnosis of a benign lacrimal gland tumor was made but no treatment was given. The previously stable proptosis had progressively increased for 18 months.

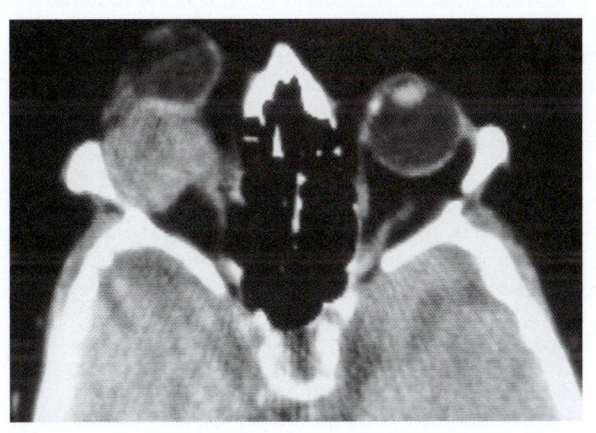

Figure 37.38. Axial computed tomography showing large mass in the lacrimal gland fossa causing severe proptosis. A generous biopsy that was performed under local anesthesia revealed pleomorphic adenocarcinoma, but the patient declined further surgery because of her advanced age and poor cardiovascular status. Orbital radiation was given.

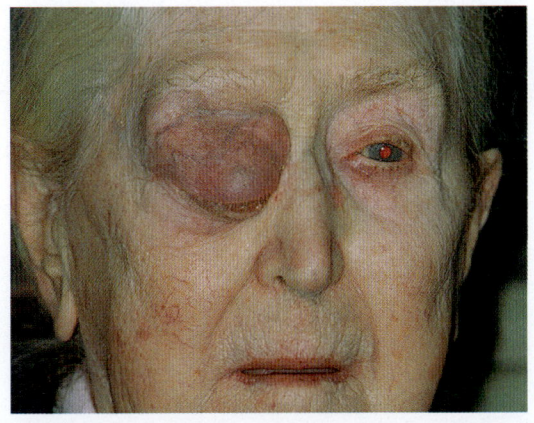

Figure 37.39. Appearance 3 years later when patient developed tumor recurrence with worsening of the proptosis. A protective tarsorrhaphy had been performed to protect the exposed cornea.

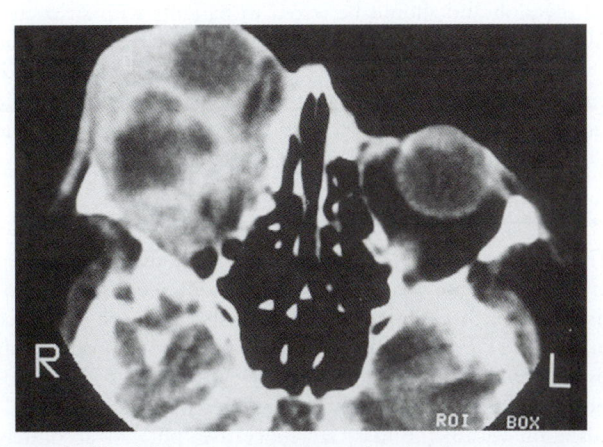

Figure 37.40. Axial computed tomography showing massive tumor recurrence. At this time, the patient agreed to orbital exenteration.

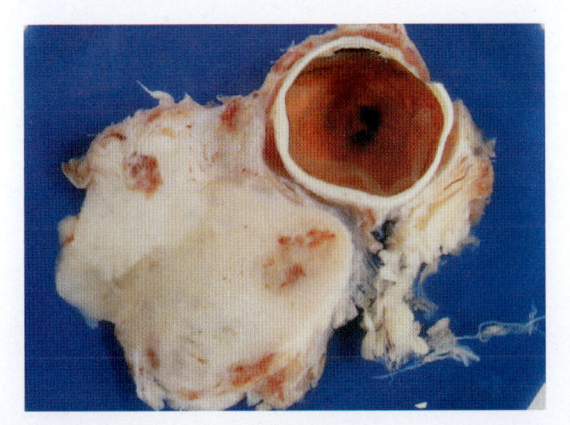

Figure 37.41. Gross section of orbital exenteration specimen showing globe (*above, right*) and massive orbital tumor.

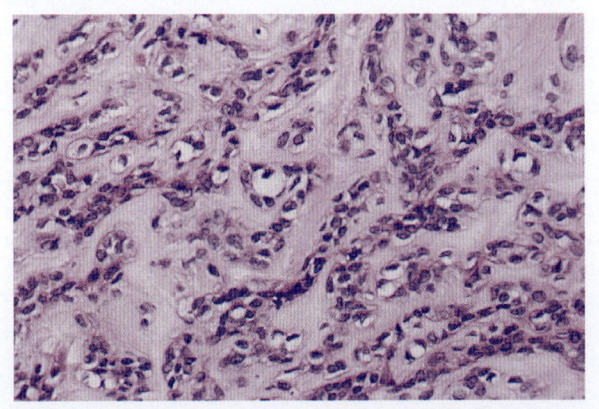

Figure 37.42. Histopathology showing cords of malignant epithelial cells in a myxoid stroma, compatible with pleomorphic adenocarcinoma. (Hematoxylin–eosin ×100.)

LACRIMAL GLAND ADENOID CYSTIC CARCINOMA

General Considerations

Several malignant neoplasms arise from the epithelium of the lacrimal gland. ACC accounts for >60% of malignant epithelial tumors of the lacrimal gland (1–41). In the authors' series of 1,264 consecutive space-occupying orbital lesions, the 14 ACC accounted for 12% of the 114 lacrimal gland lesions and for 1% of all orbital lesions (1). Although it is uncommon, this neoplasm has received considerable attention in the literature mainly because of its highly malignant nature. The mean age at presentation is 40 years, but there is a peculiar bimodal occurrence in the second and fourth decades, with some occurring in the first decade (4–10). It has been suggested that young patients with this tumor may have a more favorable prognosis (9).

Clinical Features

Like other lacrimal gland tumors, ACC causes progressive proptosis and downward and medial displacement of the eye. Unlike benign lacrimal gland tumors, it has a more rapid onset and progression. It is painful in almost half of the cases because of its tendency to invade nerves. Hypesthesia on the ipsilateral cheek and periocular area suggests posterior neural invasion and should be tested in patients with suspected ACC. Exceptionally, ACC has been known to arise in the nasal aspect of the orbit, distant from the main lacrimal gland. Such a tumor could arise from a focus of congenital ectopic lacrimal gland or from accessory lacrimal gland tissue in the conjunctival fornix (32,34).

Diagnostic Approaches

The diagnosis of ACC of lacrimal gland should be suspected on the basis of the symptoms and signs mentioned. The diagnosis can be further substantiated by CT and magnetic resonance imaging. CT generally demonstrates a round or elongated soft tissue mass that sometimes shows irregular outlines. Bone erosion is seen with larger, more aggressive lesions. Foci of calcification within the mass are suggestive, but not absolutely diagnostic, of malignant lacrimal gland tumors. This can sometimes be observed with epibulbar choristomas and dermoid cysts (35). MRI typically shows low to isointense signal on T1-weighted images, hyperintense signal on T2-weighted images, and moderate contrast enhancement.

Pathology

Histopathologically, ACC of the lacrimal gland can assume several patterns (21–24,29). The best known is the typical cystic spaces lined by malignant cells, the so-called "Swiss cheese" pattern. The basaloid pattern is said to impart the worst prognosis (23). More details of the histopathology of ACC are published in broad reviews (21–29).

LACRIMAL GLAND ADENOID CYSTIC CARCINOMA

Management

If ACC of the lacrimal gland is small and circumscribed, it can be removed intact. If it is larger and has breached its capsule, a generous biopsy should be done and if the diagnosis is confirmed on permanent histopathologic sections, then orbital exenteration with removal of affected bone should generally be done. Supplemental radiotherapy and chemotherapy should be considered in advanced cases. In one series, neoadjuvant chemotherapy was employed to shrink the tumor to a smaller size with apparent reduced risk for recurrence and metastatic disease (14,15). In another series, supplemental brachytherapy using a reverse radioactive plaque has been useful for minimal gross or microscopic residual tumor (16).

The prognosis of this malignancy is relatively poor (10,36,37). It is possible that earlier detection with CT or MRI may allow more efficient treatment and a better prognosis in the future.

Selected References

Reviews

1. Shields JA, Shields CL, Scartozzi R. Survey of 1264 patients with orbital tumors and simulating lesions: the 2002 Montgomery Lecture, part 1. *Ophthalmology* 2004;111: 997–1008.
2. Shields JA, Bakewell B, Augsburger JJ, et al. Space-occupying orbital masses in children: a review of 250 consecutive biopsies. *Ophthalmology* 1986;93:379–384.
3. Reese AB. Expanding lesions of the orbit (Bowman Lecture). *Trans Ophthalmol Soc UK* 1971;91:85–104.
4. Shields CL, Shields JA, Eagle RC, et al. Clinicopathologic review of 142 cases of lacrimal gland lesions. *Ophthalmology* 1989;96:431–435.
5. Shields, JA, Shields CL, Epstein J, et al. Primary epithelial malignancies of the lacrimal gland. The 2003 Ramon L. Font Lecture. *Ophthalmic Plast Reconstr Surg* 2004; 20:10–21.
6. Andrew NH, McNab AA, Selva D. Review of 268 lacrimal gland biopsies in an Australian cohort. *Clin Experiment Ophthalmol* 2015;43(1):5–11.
7. Wright JE, Stewart WB, Krohel GB. Clinical presentation and management of lacrimal gland tumours. *Br J Ophthalmol* 1979;63:600–606.
8. Wright JE. Factors affecting the survival of patients with lacrimal gland tumours. *Can J Ophthalmol* 1982;17:3–9.
9. Tellado MV, McLean IW, Specht CS, et al. Adenoid cystic carcinomas of the lacrimal gland in childhood and adolescence. *Ophthalmology* 1997;104:1622–1625.
10. Esmaeli B, Ahmadi MA, Youssef A, et al. Outcomes in patients with adenoid cystic carcinoma of the lacrimal gland. *Ophthal Plast Reconstr Surg* 2004;20:22–26.

Imaging

11. Jakobiec FA, Trokel SL, Abbott GF, et al. Combined clinical and computed tomographic diagnosis of primary lacrimal fossa lesions. *Am J Ophthalmol* 1982;94:785–807.
12. Font RL, Patipa M, Rosenbaum PS, et al. Correlation of computed tomographic and histopathologic features in malignant transformation of benign mixed tumor of lacrimal gland. *Surv Ophthalmol* 1990;34:449–452.
13. Gunduz K, Shields CL, Gunalp I, et al. Magnetic resonance imaging of unilateral lacrimal gland lesions. *Graefes Arch Clin Exp Ophthalmol* 2003;241:907–913.

Management

14. Tse DT, Benedetto P, Dubovy S, et al. Clinical analysis of the effect of intraarterial cytoreductive chemotherapy in the treatment of lacrimal gland adenoid cystic carcinoma. *Am J Ophthalmol* 2006;141(1):44–53.
15. Tse DT, Kossler AL, Feuer WJ, et al. Long-term outcomes of neoadjuvant intraarterial cytoreductive chemotherapy for lacrimal gland adenoid cystic carcinoma. *Ophthalmology* 2013;120(7):1313–1323.
16. Shields JA, Shields CL, Freire JE, et al. Plaque radiotherapy for selected orbital malignancies: preliminary observations: the 2002 Montgomery Lecture, part 2. *Ophthal Plast Reconstr Surg* 2003;19:91–95.
17. Gensheimer MF, Rainey D, Douglas JG, et al. Neutron radiotherapy for adenoid cystic carcinoma of the lacrimal gland. *Ophthal Plast Reconstr Surg* 2013;29(4):256–260.
18. Lewis KT, Kim D, Chan WF, et al. Conservative treatment of adenoid cystic carcinoma with plaque radiotherapy: a case report. *Ophthal Plast Reconstr Surg* 2010;26(2):131–133.
19. Esmaeli B, Golio D, Kies M, et al. Surgical management of locally advanced adenoid cystic carcinoma of the lacrimal gland. *Ophthal Plast Reconstr Surg* 2006;22(5):366–370.
20. Shields JA, Shields CL, Demirci H, et al. Experience with eyelid-sparing orbital exenteration. The 2000 Tullos O. Coston Lecture. *Ophthal Plast Reconstr Surg* 2001;17:355–361.

Histopathology/Genetics

21. Font RL, Gamel JW. Epithelial tumors of the lacrimal gland: an analysis of 265 cases. In: Jakobiec FA, ed. *Ocular and Adnexal Tumors*. Birmingham, AL: Ausculapius; 1978:787–805.
22. Font RL, Gamel JW. Adenoid cystic carcinoma of the lacrimal gland. A clinicopathologic study of 79 cases. In: Nicholson DH, ed. *Ocular Pathology Update*. New York: Masson; 1980:277–283.
23. Lee DA, Campbell RJ, Waller RR, et al. A clinicopathologic study of primary adenoid cystic carcinoma of the lacrimal gland. *Ophthalmology* 1985;92:128–134.
24. Gamel JW, Font RL. Adenoid cystic carcinoma of the lacrimal gland. The clinical significance of a basaloid histologic pattern. *Hum Pathol* 1982;13:219–225.
25. Mendoza PR, Jakobiec FA, Krane JF. Immunohistochemical features of lacrimal gland epithelial tumors. *Am J Ophthalmol* 2013;156(6):1147–1158.
26. White VA. Update on lacrimal gland neoplasms: Molecular pathology of interest. *Saudi J Ophthalmol* 2012;26:133–135.
27. Von Holstein SL. Tumours of the lacrimal gland. Epidemiolocial, clinical and genetic characteristics. *Acta Ophthalmol* 2013;6:1–28.
28. Von Holstein SL, Fehr A, Persson M, et al. Adenoid cystic carcinoma of the lacrimal gland: MYB gene activation, genomic imbalances, and clinical characteristics. *Ophthalmology* 2013;120(10):2130–2138.
29. Chawla B, Kashyap S, Sen S, et al. Clinicopathologic review of epithelial tumors of the lacrimal gland. *Ophthal Plast Reconstr Surg* 2013;29:440–445.

Case Reports

30. Dagher G, Anderson RL, Ossoinig KC, et al. Adenoid cystic carcinoma of the lacrimal gland in a child. *Arch Ophthalmol* 1980;98:1098–1100.
31. Shields JA, Shields CL, Eagle RC Jr, et al. Adenoid cystic carcinoma of the lacrimal gland simulating a dermoid cyst in a 9-year-old child. *Arch Ophthalmol* 1998;116: 1673–1676.
32. Shields JA, Shields CL, Eagle RC Jr, et al. Adenoid cystic carcinoma arising in the nasal orbit. *Am J Ophthalmol* 1997;123:398–399.
33. Kiratli H, Bilgic S. An unusual clinical course of adenoid cystic carcinoma of the lacrimal gland. *Orbit* 1999;18:197–201.
34. Duke TG, Fahy GT, Brown LJ. Adenoid cystic carcinoma of the superonasal conjunctival fornix. *Orbit* 2000;19:31–35.
35. Karatza E, Shields CL, Shields JA, et al. Calcified orbital cyst in an adult simulating a malignant lacrimal gland tumor. *Ophthal Plast Reconstr Surg* 2004;20:397–399.
36. Henderson JW. Adenoid cystic carcinoma of the lacrimal gland, is there a cure? *Trans Am Ophthalmol Soc* 1987;85:312–319.
37. Bartley GB, Harris GJ. Adenoid cystic carcinoma of the lacrimal gland: is there a cure…yet? *Ophthal Plast Reconstr Surg* 2002;18:315–318.
38. Friedrich RE, Bleckmann V. Adenoid cystic carcinoma of salivary and lacrimal gland origin: localization, classification, clinical pathological correlation, treatment results and long-term follow-up control in 84 patients. *Anticancer Res* 2003;23:931–940.
39. Meldrum ML, Tse DT, Benedetto P. Neoadjuvant intracarotid chemotherapy for treatment of advanced adenocystic carcinoma of the lacrimal gland. *Arch Ophthalmol* 1998;116:315–321.
40. Walsh RD, Vagefi MR, McClelland CM, et al. Primary adenoid cystic carcinoma of the orbital apex. *Ophthal Plast reconstr Surg* 2013;29(1):e33–e35.
41. Ali MJ, Honavar SG, Naik MN, et al. Primary adenoid cystic carcinoma: an extremely rare eyelid tumor. *Ophthal Plast Reconstr Surg* 2012;28(2):e35–e36.

Chapter 37 Lacrimal Gland Primary Epithelial Tumors

LACRIMAL GLAND ADENOID CYSTIC CARCINOMA

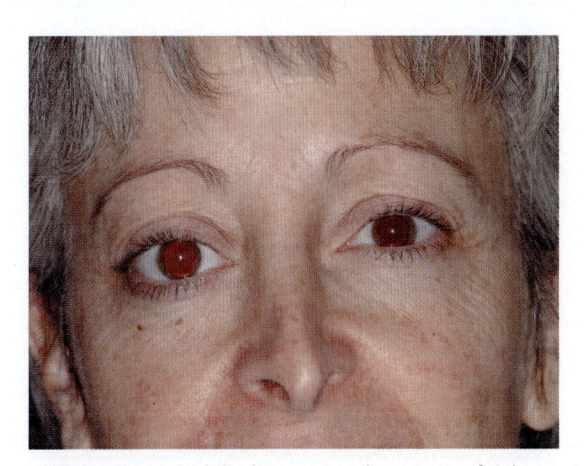

Figure 37.43. Downward displacement and proptosis of right eye in a 50-year-old woman.

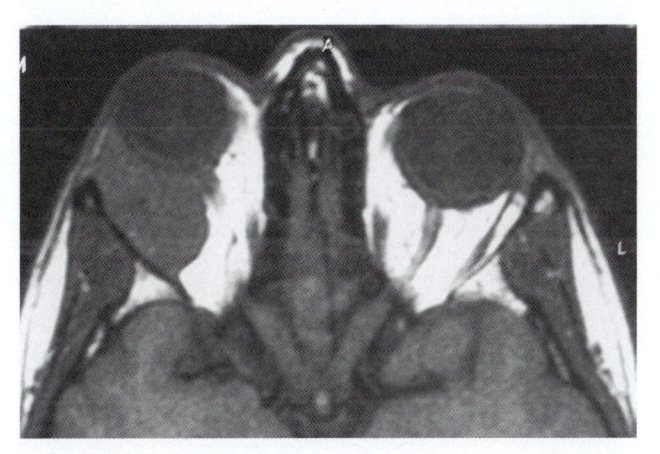

Figure 37.44. Axial magnetic resonance imaging in T1-weighted image showing large ovoid mass in lateral aspect of orbit.

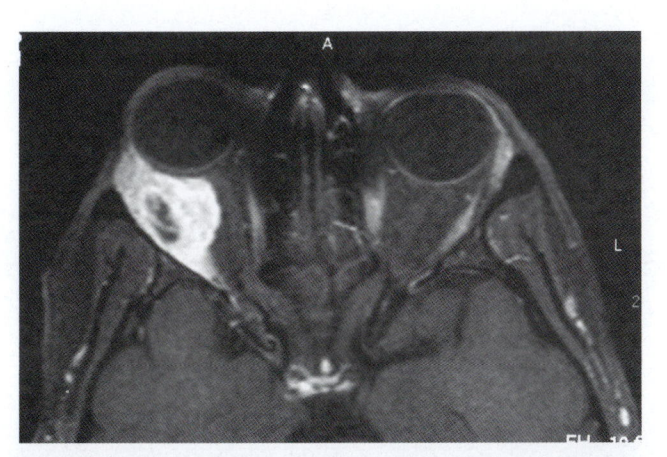

Figure 37.45. Axial magnetic resonance imaging in T1-weighted image with fat suppression and gadolinium enhancement showing enhancement of the mass.

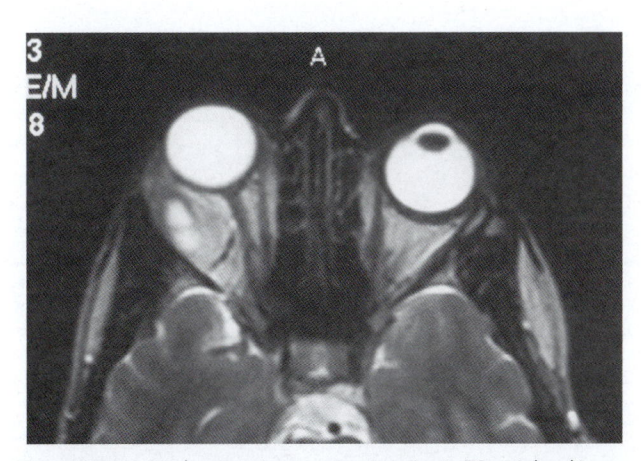

Figure 37.46. Axial magnetic resonance imaging in T2-weighted image demonstrating heterogeneity in the mass.

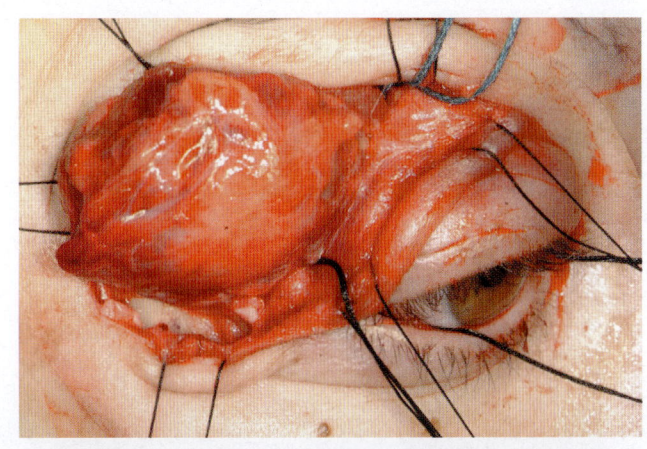

Figure 37.47. Tumor exposed at the time of biopsy. In this case it was removed grossly intact, although the tumor extended to the margin microscopically. The patient was treated with orbital exenteration, irradiation, and chemotherapy.

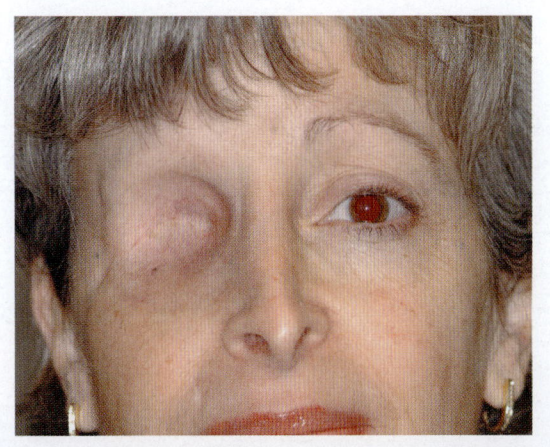

Figure 37.48. Face appearance after eyelid-sparing orbital exenteration. After 2 years, the patient still chose not to have a prosthesis.

Part 3 Tumors of the Orbit

LACRIMAL GLAND ADENOID CYSTIC CARCINOMA: CLINICOPATHOLOGIC CORRELATION OF AN AGGRESSIVE CASE

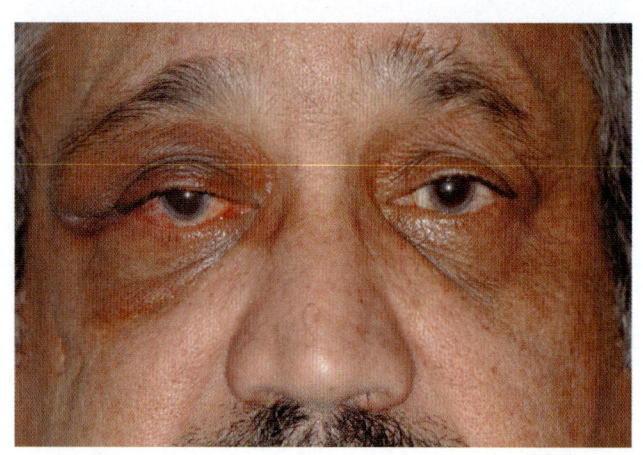

Figure 37.49. Downward displacement and proptosis of right eye in a 61-year-old man.

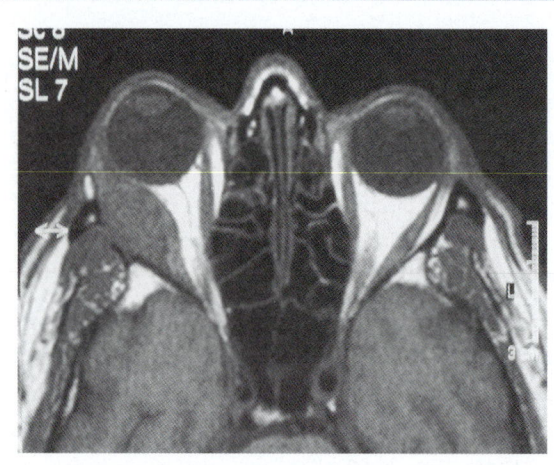

Figure 37.50. Axial magnetic resonance imaging in T1-weighted image showing large fusiform mass in the temporal aspect of the orbit.

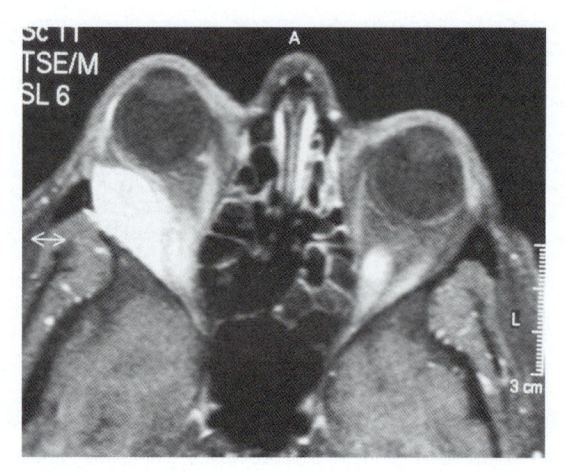

Figure 37.51. Axial magnetic resonance imaging in T1-weighted image with fat suppression and gadolinium enhancement showing large mass and proptosis. There is a suggestion of bone erosion on lateral orbital wall.

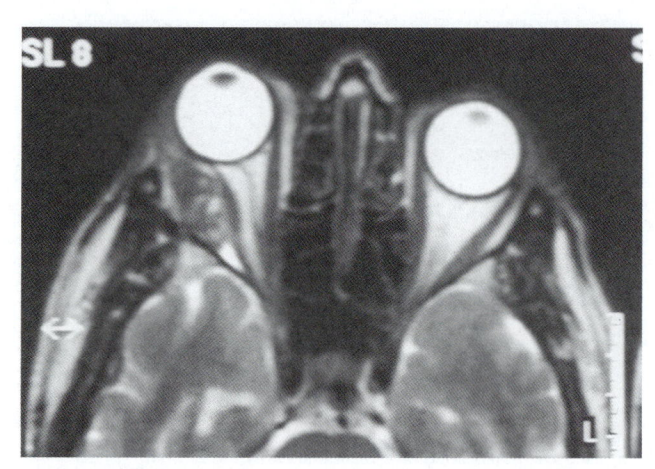

Figure 37.52. Axial magnetic resonance imaging in T2-weighted image showing heterogeneity in the mass. An attempt at excisional biopsy was done, but the entire lesion could not be removed and orbital exenteration was subsequently performed.

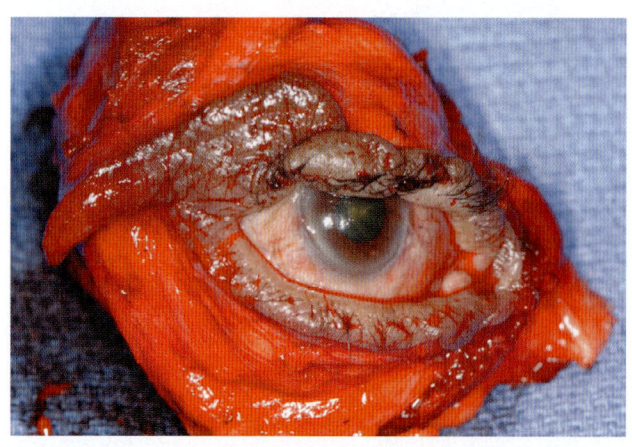

Figure 37.53. Appearance of exenteration specimen.

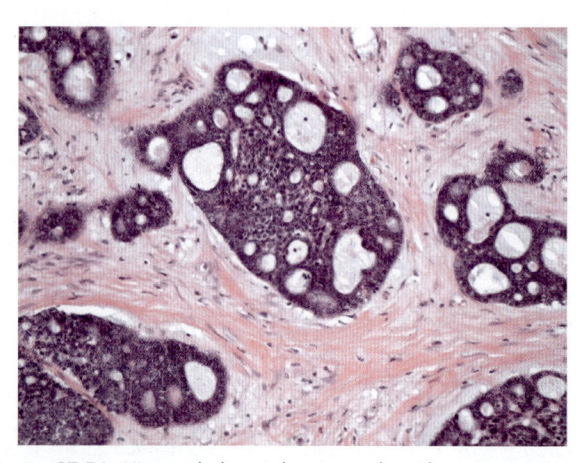

Figure 37.54. Histopathology showing adenoid cystic carcinoma. (Hematoxylin–eosin ×150.)

LACRIMAL GLAND ADENOID CYSTIC CARCINOMA: EARLY DETECTION BY IMAGING STUDIES AND TREATMENT WITH BRACHYTHERAPY

Shields JA, Shields CL, Freire JE, et al. Plaque radiotherapy for selected orbital malignancies: preliminary observations: the 2002 Montgomery Lecture, part 2. *Ophthal Plast Reconstr Surg* 2003;19:91–95.

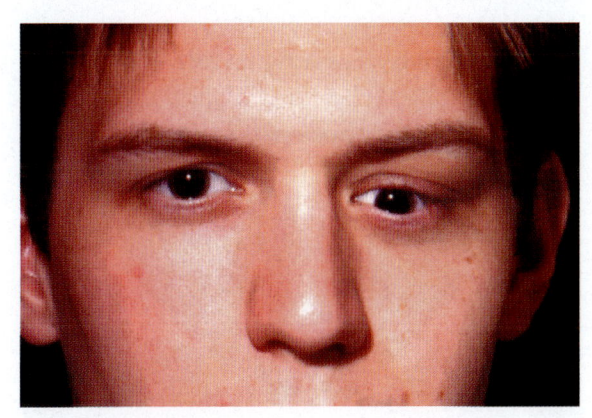

Figure 37.55. Proptosis and downward and nasal displacement of left eye in a young man.

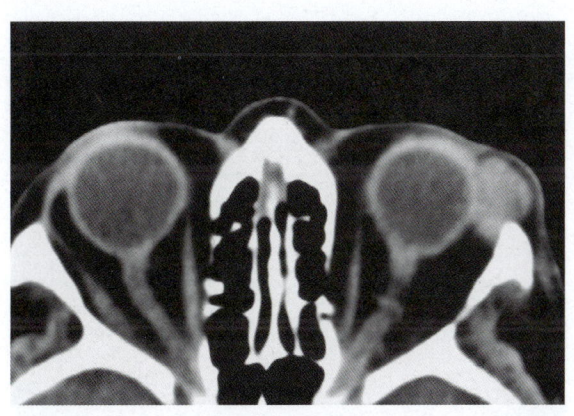

Figure 37.56. Axial computed tomography of patient in Figure 37.49, showing relatively small, well-circumscribed mass arising in left lacrimal gland. The encapsulated lesion was removed intact with no gross or microscopic evidence of residual tumor.

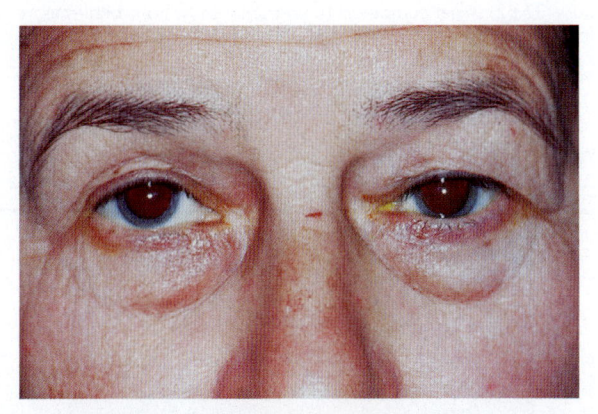

Figure 37.57. Minimal downward displacement of left eye in a 57-year-old woman.

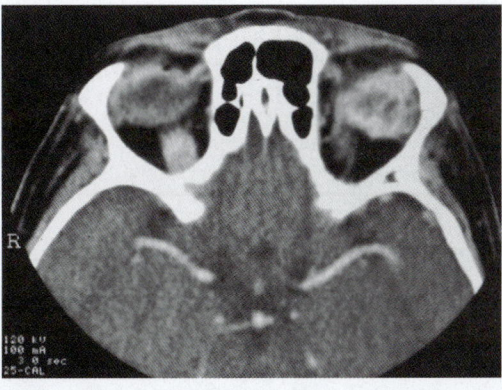

Figure 37.58. Axial computed tomography of patient seen in Figure 37.51, showing orbital mass arising in the lacrimal gland fossa. Note that there are characteristic densities that suggest calcium, a finding seen in many adenoid cystic carcinomas.

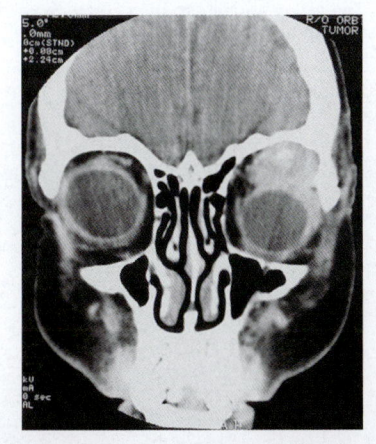

Figure 37.59. Coronal computed tomography showing similar features of the tumor of patient shown in Figure 37.51.

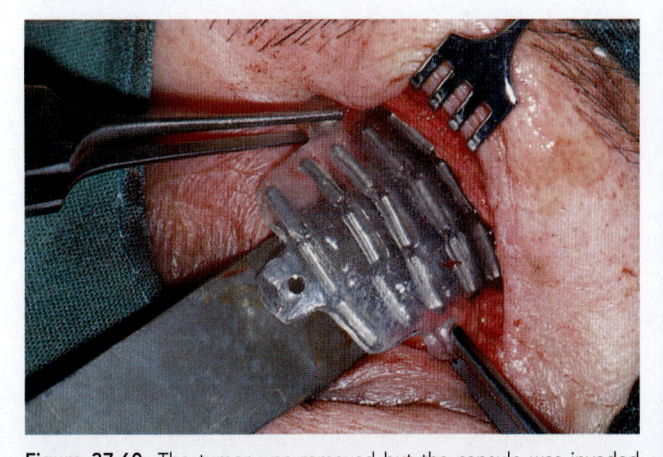

Figure 37.60. The tumor was removed but the capsule was invaded by adenoid cystic carcinoma. Therefore, brachytherapy was employed using a custom-designed radioactive iodine-125 plaque, which is being placed in the superotemporal aspect of the orbit. After 6 years, there was a recurrence in the roof of the orbit and frontal sinus. A combined orbital exenteration and removal of frontal sinus was done. The patient is alive and well after 10 years.

LACRIMAL GLAND ADENOID CYSTIC CARCINOMA: OCCURRENCE IN A CHILD

ACC of the lacrimal gland has a tendency to occur in young children as well as in adults. Depicted is a clinicopathologic correlation and management of such a case in a 9-year-old boy. Treatment included tumor resection followed by brachytherapy.

1. Shields JA, Shields CL, Eagle RC Jr, et al. Adenoid cystic carcinoma of the lacrimal gland in a nine-year-old child. *Arch Ophthalmol* 1998;116:1673–1676.
2. Shields JA, Shields CL, Freire JE, et al. Plaque radiotherapy for selected orbital malignancies: preliminary observations: the 2002 Montgomery Lecture, part 2. *Ophthal Plast Reconstr Surg* 2003;19:91–95.

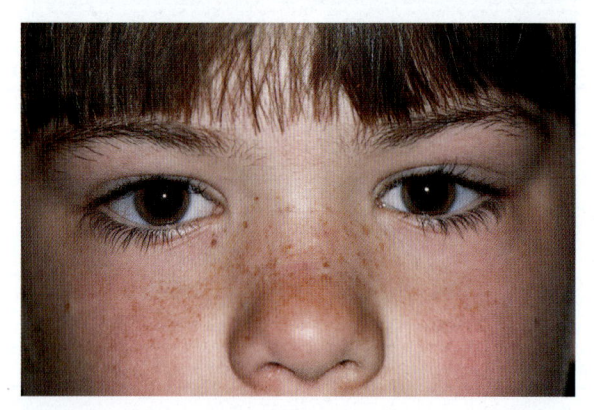

Figure 37.61. Minimal downward displacement of the left eye in a 9-year-old boy who complained of headaches.

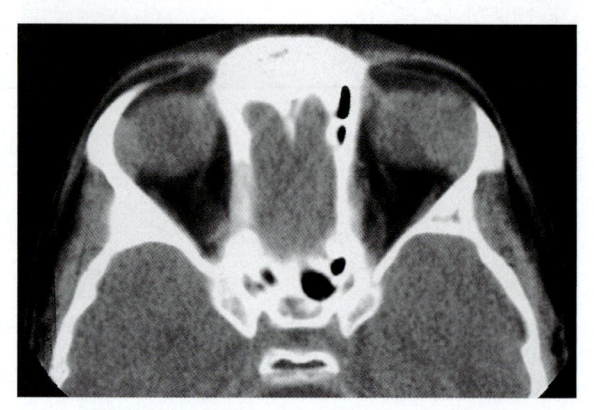

Figure 37.62. Axial computed tomography showing orbital mass arising in the lacrimal gland fossa.

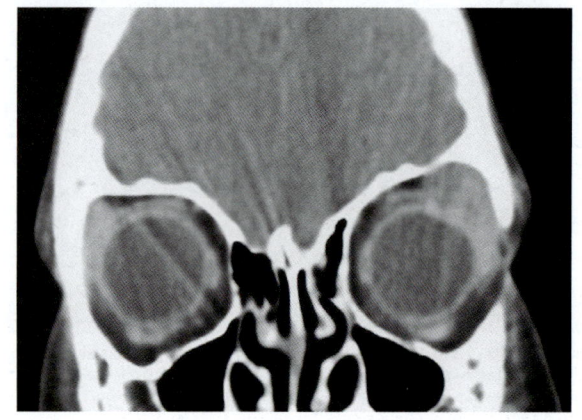

Figure 37.63. Coronal computed tomography showing bony fossa formation from the mass. This pattern raised suspicion for a benign lesion such as a dermoid cyst.

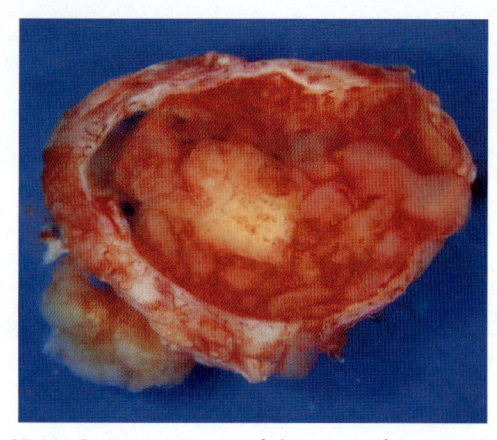

Figure 37.64. Gross appearance of the tumor after surgical removal and sectioning. The lesion appears to be a cyst with yellow material in the center as seen with dermoid cysts.

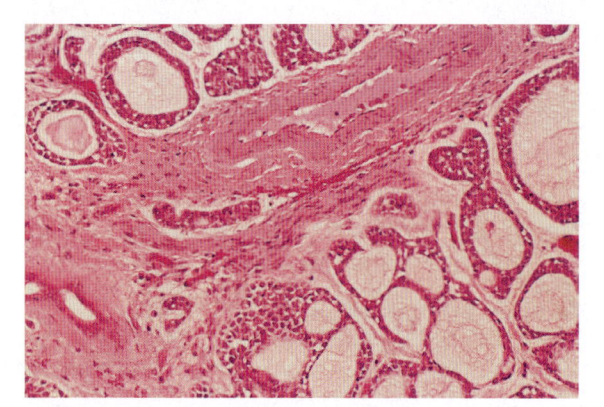

Figure 37.65. Histopathology showing Swiss cheese pattern of adenoid cystic carcinoma. (Hematoxylin–eosin ×100.)

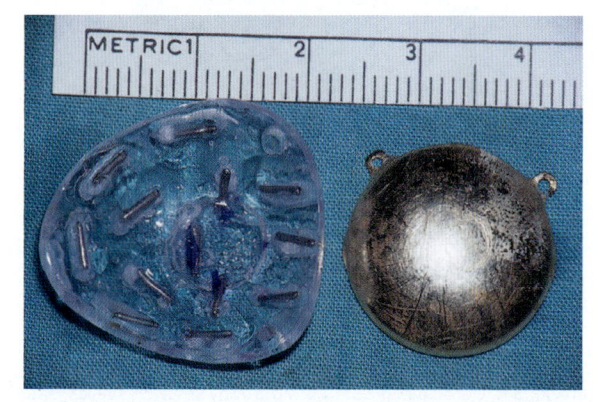

Figure 37.66. Additional frozen sections showed no residual orbital tumor and the visual acuity was perfect, so the patient was treated with brachytherapy using a radioactive plaque rather than orbital exenteration. Shown is the active plaque with I-125 seeds and the gold shield that was placed over the sclera to protect the globe from the irradiation. The lacrimal gland tumor was controlled but he died about 12 years later from disseminated Wilms' tumor, which was believed by oncologists to be unrelated to the lacrimal gland tumor.

LACRIMAL GLAND ADENOID CYSTIC CARCINOMA: ATYPICAL NASAL ORBITAL LOCATION

In rare instances, ACC can occur in an orbital location away from the lacrimal gland. The etiology of such a tumor is uncertain, but it is possible that it could develop from ectopic lacrimal gland. A case is illustrated.

Shields JA, Shields CL, Eagle RC Jr, et al. Adenoid cystic carcinoma arising in the nasal orbit. *Am J Ophthalmol* 1997;123:398–399.

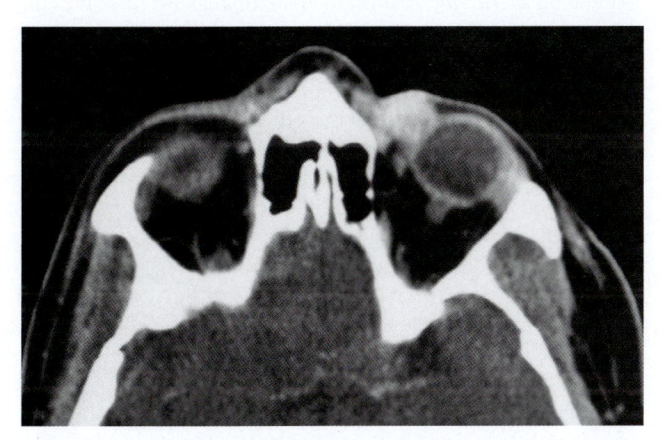

Figure 37.67. Axial computed tomography of a 27-year-old man showing a round mass in the nasal portion of the orbit anteriorly. The patient was managed elsewhere at this time by an incomplete biopsy and the diagnosis of adenoid cystic carcinoma was made.

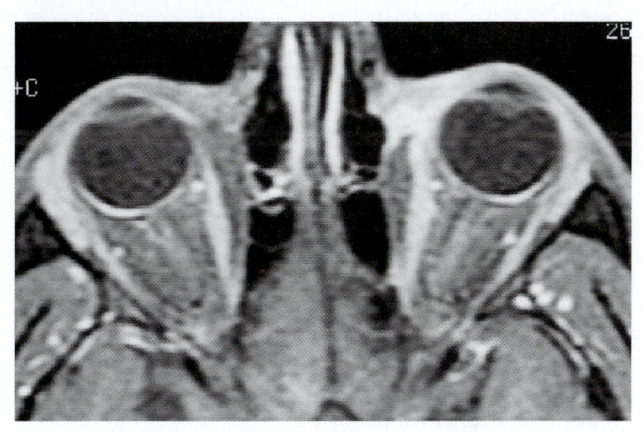

Figure 37.68. Axial magnetic resonance imaging shown 2 weeks later demonstrating enhancing tissue nasally consistent with persistent tumor. Frozen sections revealed diffuse tumor in orbit separate from the circumscribed mass, and an eyelid-sparing orbital exenteration was performed.

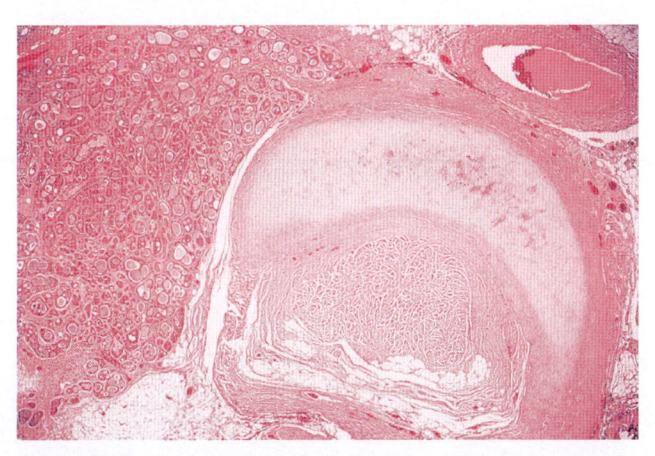

Figure 37.69. Histopathology of exenteration specimen, showing adenoid cystic carcinoma adjacent to the cartilaginous trochlea. (Hematoxylin–eosin ×100.)

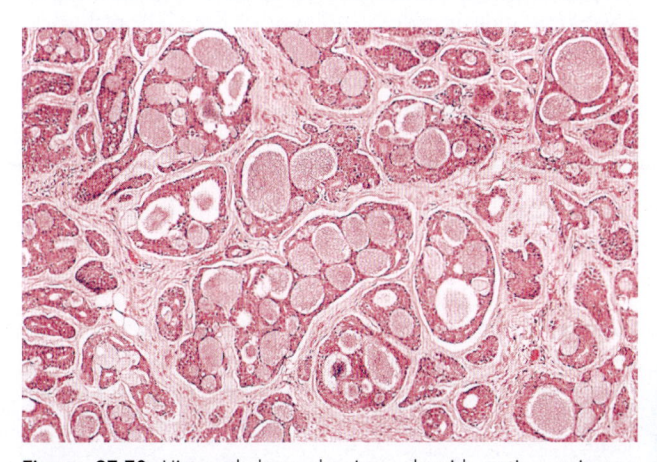

Figure 37.70. Histopathology showing adenoid cystic carcinoma. (Hematoxylin–eosin ×150.)

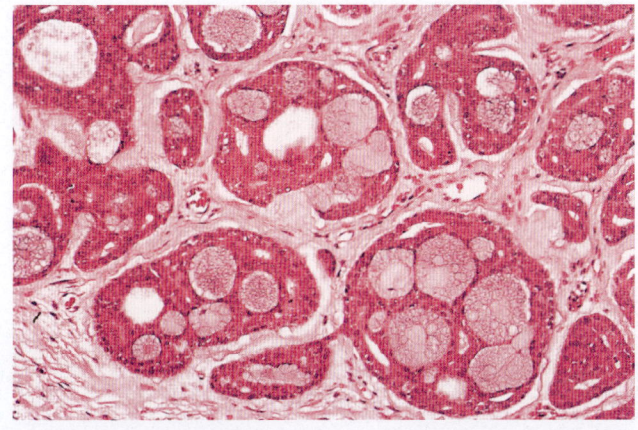

Figure 37.71. Histopathology showing adenoid cystic carcinoma. (Hematoxylin–eosin ×200.)

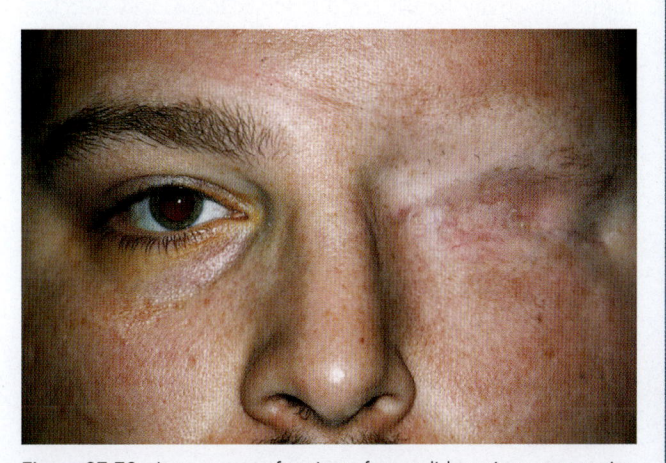

Figure 37.72. Appearance of patient after eyelid-sparing exenteration showing good healing. The patient elected not to have a prosthesis.

LACRIMAL GLAND PRIMARY DUCTAL CARCINOMA

General Considerations

Primary ductal carcinoma is histologically and immunohistochemically similar to salivary duct carcinoma. It is a rare, but highly aggressive salivary gland tumor that histopathologically resembles ductal carcinoma of the breast (1–10). Recognition of primary ductal carcinoma of the lacrimal gland as a separate entity may aid in further delineation of its biologic behavior, management, and prognosis.

Clinical Features

To our knowledge, there are no clinical features that are specific to this neoplasm. It is known to present as a painless, palpable mass under the eyelid superotemporally and to show slow enlargement. It eventually causes progressive blepharoptosis, proptosis, and downward and medial displacement of the eye in keeping with its lacrimal gland location. More advanced tumors can cause pain and diplopia.

Diagnostic Approaches

CT and magnetic resonance imaging show a circumscribed mass that is indistinguishable from other benign or malignant lacrimal gland neoplasms. The lesion shows enhancement with contrast agents. With time, the tumor can develop an ill-defined border secondary to extension outside its capsule.

Pathology

Primary ductal adenocarcinoma of the lacrimal gland is composed of large polygonal cells with vesicular nuclei, prominent nucleoli, and amphophilic cytoplasm. In some areas, the epithelium is vacuolated or shows foci of apocrine-like differentiation. There may be expanded duct-type structures with papillary, cribriform, comedo, and solid patterns, surrounded by prominent basement membrane. Mitotic figures are readily identified. As with ACC, perineural and vascular invasion can occur.

In the case that our group studied, mucicarmine stain disclosed prominent mucin production (10). The tumor showed immunoreactivity for AE1, CK7, CEA, EMA, and BRST-2. Weak focal staining was seen with CK20. Stains for TTF1, PSA, HER-2/neu, ER, P53, and S100 were negative (10). An analysis of five cases revealed uniform positivity for androgen receptor in all cases and three of five overexpressed the HER-2/neu protein (6). Four of five developed metastasis and three died over 5-year follow-up.

Management

The diagnosis is not usually made clinically, but management is the same as for all circumscribed lacrimal gland tumors. The tumor should be removed intact when possible. If excisional biopsy is not possible, then a generous incisional biopsy should be done. If histopathologic studies reveal primary ductal carcinoma that is incompletely excised, then wider local surgery or even orbital exenteration is prudent. Subsequent chemotherapy or radiotherapy should be considered in conjunction with medical oncologists and radiation oncologists. The prognosis is not well known, but the lesion can metastasize to regional lymph nodes and distant sites.

LACRIMAL GLAND PRIMARY DUCTAL CARCINOMA

Selected References

Reviews
1. Shields JA, Shields CL, Scartozzi R. Survey of 1264 patients with orbital tumors and simulating lesions: the 2002 Montgomery Lecture, part 1. *Ophthalmology* 2004;111:997–1008.
2. Shields CL, Shields JA, Eagle RC, et al. Clinicopathologic review of 142 cases of lacrimal gland lesions. *Ophthalmology* 1989;96:431–435.
3. Shields JA, Shields CL, Epstein J, et al. Primary epithelial malignancies of the lacrimal gland. The 2003 Ramon L. Font Lecture. *Ophthalmic Plast Reconstr Surg* 2004;20:10–21.
4. Andrew NH, McNab AA, Selva D. Review of 268 lacrimal gland biopsies in an Australian cohort. *Clin Experiment Ophthalmol* 2015;43(1):5–11.
5. Andreoli MT, Aakalu V, Betabutr P. Epidemiological trends in malignant lacrimal gland tumors. *Otolaryngol Head Neck Surg* 2015;152(2):279–283.

Histopathology
6. Kubota T, Moritani S, Ichihara S. Clinicopathlogic and immunohistochemical features of primary ductal adenocarcinoma of lacrimal gland: five new cases and review of literature. *Graefes Arch Clin Exp Ophthalmol* 2013;251:2071–2076.

Case Reports
7. Katz SE, Rootman J, Dolman PJ, et al. Primary ductal adenocarcinoma of the lacrimal gland. *Ophthalmology* 1996;103:157–162.
8. Nasu M, Haisa T, Kondo T, et al. Primary ductal adenocarcinoma of the lacrimal gland. *Pathol Int* 1998;48:981–984.
9. Krishnakumar S, Subramanian N, Mahesh L, et al. Primary ductal adenocarcinoma of the lacrimal gland in a patient with neurofibromatosis. *Eye* 2003;7:843–845.
10. Milman T, Shields JA, Husson M, et al. Primary ductal adenocarcinoma of the lacrimal gland. *Ophthalmology* 2005;112:2048–2051.

LACRIMAL GLAND PRIMARY DUCTAL CARCINOMA

Primary ductal adenocarcinoma is a well-known neoplasm of the mammary glands. In rare instances, a similar tumor can occur in the lacrimal gland and major salivary glands. A case is shown of a primary ductal carcinoma of the lacrimal gland in an elderly man with no history or findings of cancer elsewhere. Orbital exenteration was performed but the patient subsequently developed regional lymph node metastasis.

Milman T, Shields JA, Husson M, et al. Primary ductal adenocarcinoma of the lacrimal gland. *Ophthalmology* 2005;112:2048–2051.

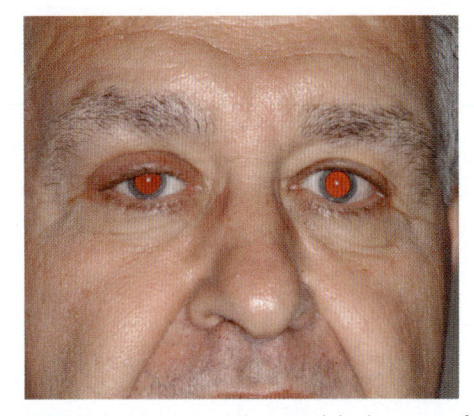

Figure 37.73. Blepharoptosis and downward displacement of right eye in an elderly man. A biopsy of a lacrimal gland lesion had been done elsewhere before referral; histopathologic studies were inconclusive.

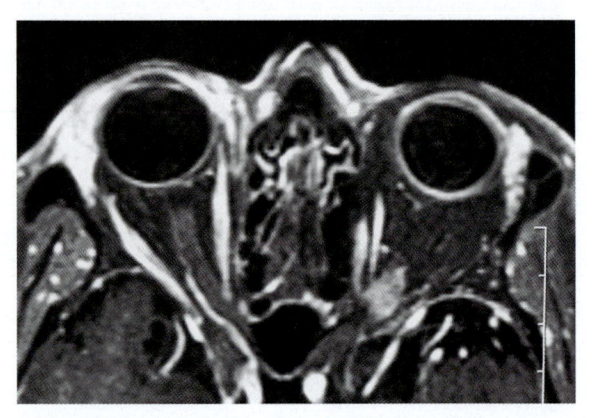

Figure 37.74. Axial magnetic resonance imaging with fat suppression and gadolinium enhancement showing residual enhancing tumor in right lacrimal gland fossa. It was elected to attempt an excisional biopsy for both diagnostic and therapeutic reasons.

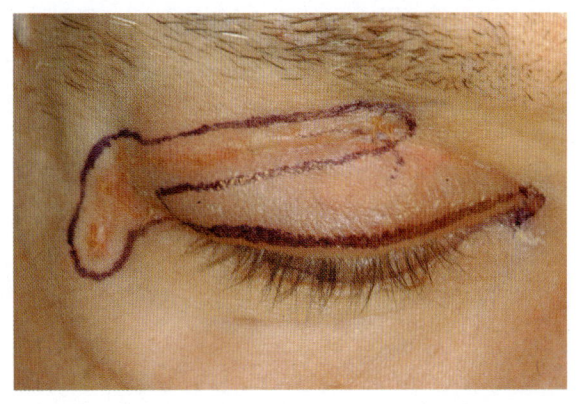

Figure 37.75. Outline of the surgical approach showing plan to remove prior scar and the tumor. Histopathologic studies showed invasive ductal carcinoma with tumor extension to the surgical margins and orbital exenteration was elected.

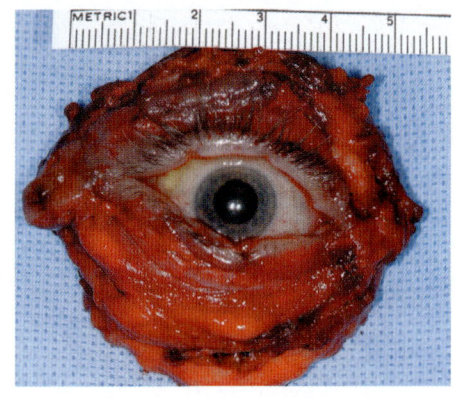

Figure 37.76. Exenteration specimen following eyelid-sparing exenteration technique.

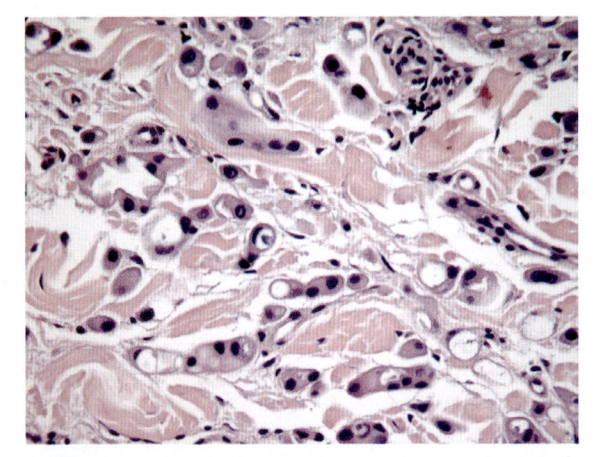

Figure 37.77. Histopathology showing cords of malignant tumor cells in a fibrous stroma, similar to ductal carcinoma of the breast. (Hematoxylin–eosin ×100.)

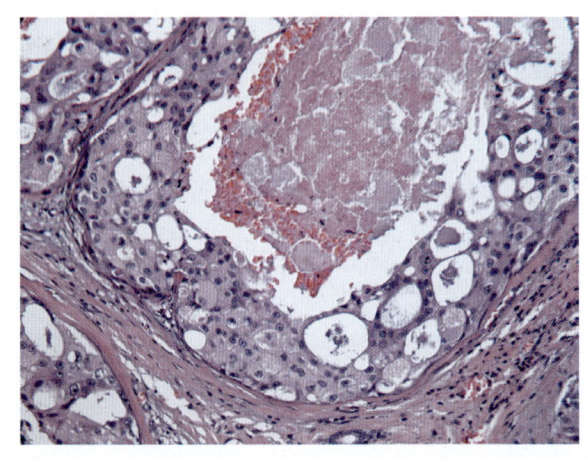

Figure 37.78. Another area showing wall of a ductule with viable malignant tumor cells and areas of necrotic tumor cells in the lumen. (Hematoxylin–eosin ×150.)

Chapter 37 Lacrimal Gland Primary Epithelial Tumors

LACRIMAL GLAND MUCOEPIDERMOID CARCINOMA

Lacrimal gland mucoepidermoid carcinoma is a relatively rare variant of lacrimal gland epithelial malignancies. Below is a well-documented case.

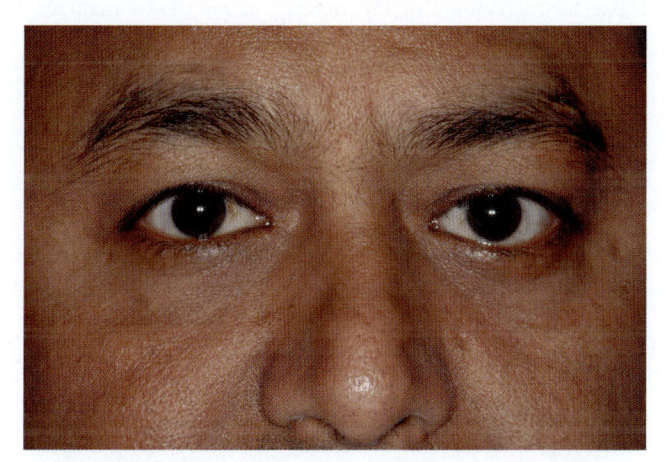

Figure 37.79. Middle-aged man with swelling of left upper eyelid.

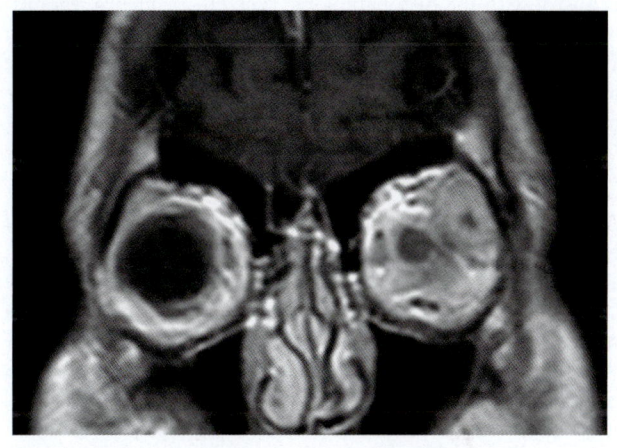

Figure 37.80. Coronal magnetic resonance imaging showing a moderate signal round mass in the left orbit behind the globe.

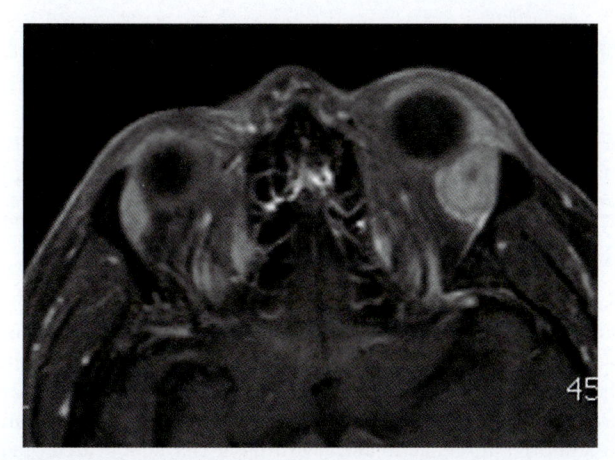

Figure 37.81. Axial magnetic resonance imaging showing circumscribed, enhancing mass in the lacrimal gland region.

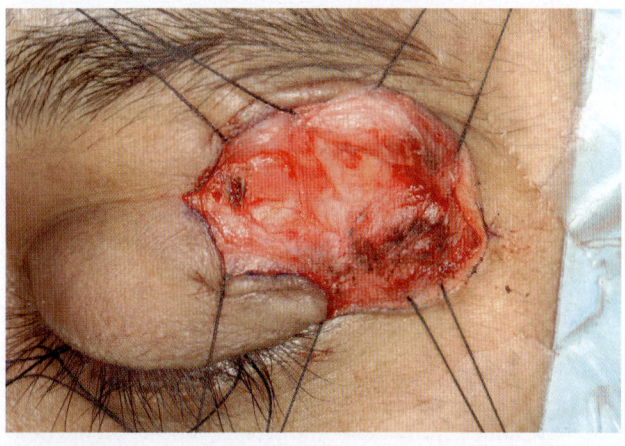

Figure 37.82. Surgical exploration with tumor removal was performed through an eyelid crease incision, extraperiosteal approach.

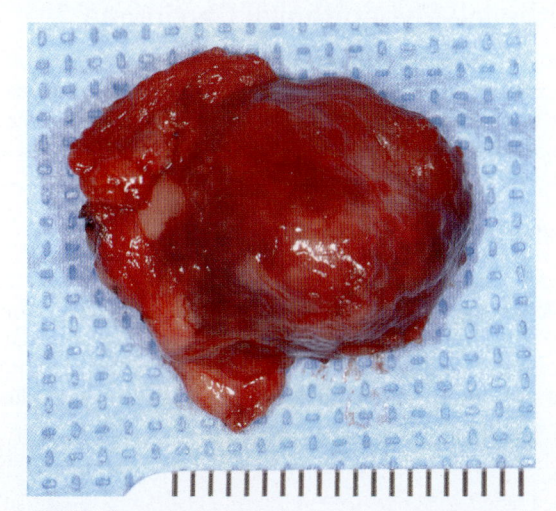

Figure 37.83. The entire lacrimal gland and mass was removed.

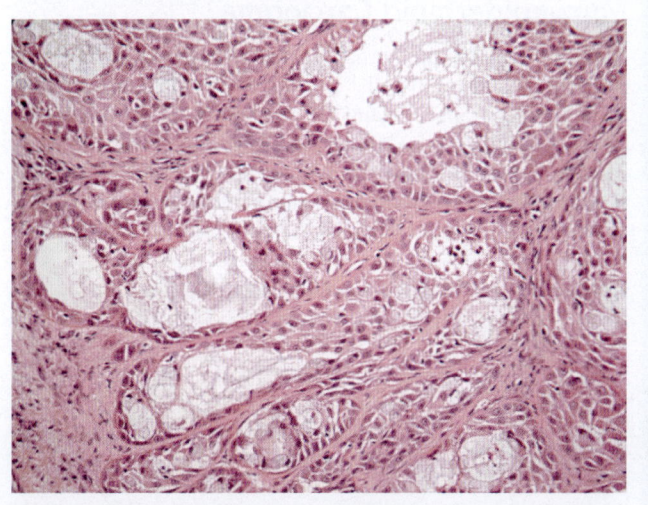

Figure 37.84. Mucoepidermoid carcinoma of the lacrimal gland was found showing characteristic epithelial cells with pools of mucin. (Hematoxylin–eosin ×150.)

HISTOPATHOLOGY OF PRIMARY EPITHELIAL MALIGNANCIES OF LACRIMAL GLAND

Each type of PEMLG has similar clinical and radiographic features, which were previously discussed. However, the prognosis can vary with the histopathologic type (1–3). Hence, the histopathologic differentiation of these neoplasms is important. Presented here is a special section that briefly summarizes the histopathology of most of the PEMLG and illustrates the histopathology of some of them.

Adenoid Cystic Carcinoma

ACC of the lacrimal gland has been subdivided into several histopathologic subtypes, namely cribriform (Swiss cheese), sclerosing, basaloid, comedocarcinoma, and tubular types. The cribriform variant is composed of lobules that contain pools of mucin that give it a Swiss cheese-like appearance. The sclerosing variant consists of epithelial cords, surrounded by a dense hyalinized stroma. The basaloid variant shows solid epithelial lobules with large basophilic nuclei and scanty cytoplasm that superficially resemble basal cell carcinoma; however, it lacks the peripheral palisading that typifies basal cell carcinoma. Although controversial, a poorer prognosis has been ascribed to this variant (1). The comedocarcinoma variant is composed of epithelial lobules with foci of central necrosis. The tubular (ductal) variant is composed of elongated and comma-shaped epithelial tubules lined by two or three layers of cells.

Pleomorphic Adenocarcinoma

Pleomorphic adenocarcinoma shows areas of malignant change in a pleomorphic adenoma. There are variable proportions of myxoid and chondroid elements and malignant epithelial cells.

Primary Adenocarcinoma

Primary adenocarcinoma displays cells that are pleomorphic, mitotically active, arranged in sheets and cords, and frequently manifest lumen formation and some mucin production. Mesenchymal elements are generally absent.

Mucoepidermoid Carcinoma

Mucoepidermoid carcinoma is composed of varying proportions of malignant epithelial cells, often with a prominent cystic component. Special stains are positive for mucin within the cytoplasm and in areas of extracellular pooling. Mucoepidermoid carcinoma demonstrates a spectrum of differentiation; the more differentiated type contains more abundant mucin and carries a better prognosis.

Primary Squamous Cell Carcinoma

Primary squamous cell carcinoma of the lacrimal gland is characterized by a pure proliferation of keratinizing, fairly well-differentiated malignant squamous cells. In contrast to pleomorphic adenocarcinoma, there are no glandular elements. Special stains fail to reveal mucin.

Sebaceous Carcinoma

Sebaceous carcinoma of the lacrimal gland shows anaplastic cells with mitotic activity and cytoplasmic vacuoles that stain for lipid, similar to sebaceous carcinoma of the eyelids.

Acinic Cell Adenocarcinoma

Acinic cell adenocarcinoma shows a microcystic pattern, consisting of vacuolated cells with round nuclei and prominent nucleoli. The zymogen granules in the cytoplasm stain with periodic acid-Schiff, Alcian blue, and colloidal iron. Intracranial extension from acinic cell adenocarcinoma of the lacrimal gland has been observed (1).

Ductal Carcinoma

Ductal carcinoma reveals atypical epithelial cells with a tendency to proliferate in the lumina of the ducts, leading to cystic distension. The cells often form lobules surrounded by basement membrane, similar to ductal carcinoma of the breast.

Lymphoepithelial Carcinoma

Lymphoepithelial carcinoma consists of islands of undifferentiated carcinoma cells permeated and enveloped by an admixture of lymphocytes and macrophages. It is possible that some cases may arise primarily, rather than from a pre-existing benign lymphoepithelial lesion.

Basal Cell Adenocarcinoma

Basal cell adenocarcinoma shows uniform basaloid cells without the myxoid, chondroid, and mesenchymal components of pleomorphic adenoma. It is important to differentiate it from the basaloid type of ACC, because it generally has a better prognosis. The negative Alcian blue stain and negative reaction to smooth muscle actin seen with basal cell adenocarcinoma are helpful in differentiating it from ACC.

Epithelial–Myoepithelial Carcinoma

Epithelial–myoepithelial carcinoma arises from the myoepithelial cells in the lacrimal gland and can show benign or malignant (carcinoma) features. As the name implies, the tumor is composed of a biphasic population of myoepithelial cells and ductal cells.

Cystadenocarcinoma

Cystadenocarcinoma is characterized by malignant cells with numerous cysts, often with a predominant papillary component. The diagnosis is supported by the absence of acinar or mucoepidermoid differentiation and lack of evidence of origin from a pleomorphic adenoma. Cystadenocarcinoma appears to have a better prognosis than most other PEMLG.

HISTOPATHOLOGY OF PRIMARY EPITHELIAL MALIGNANCIES OF LACRIMAL GLAND

Selected References

Reviews

1. Shields JA, Shields CL, Epstein J, et al. Primary epithelial malignancies of the lacrimal gland. The 2003 Ramon L. Font Lecture. *Ophthalmic Plast Reconstr Surg* 2004;20:10–21.
2. Andrew NH, McNab AA, Selva D. Review of 268 lacrimal gland biopsies in an Australian cohort. *Clin Experiment Ophthalmol* 2015;43(1):5–11.
3. Andreoli MT, Aakalu V, Betabutr P. Epidemiological trends in malignant lacrimal gland tumors. *Otolaryngol Head Neck Surg* 2015;152(2):279–283.

LACRIMAL GLAND: HISTOPATHOLOGY OF SELECTED PRIMARY EPITHELIAL MALIGNANCIES

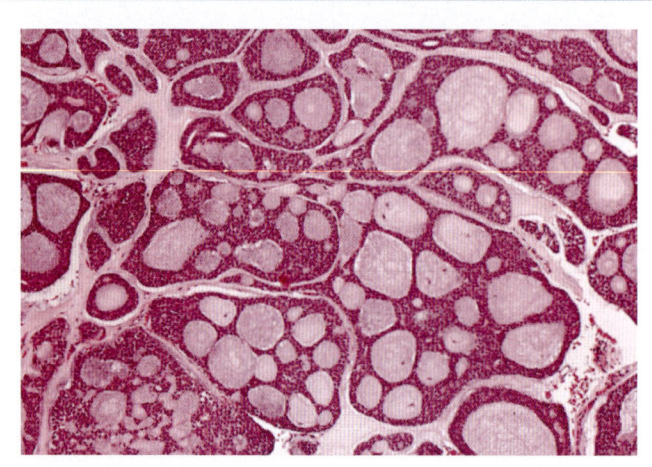

Figure 37.85. Histopathology of cribriform or Swiss cheese variant of adenoid cystic carcinoma of the lacrimal gland showing pools of mucin within lobules of malignant epithelial cells. (Hematoxylin–eosin ×75.)

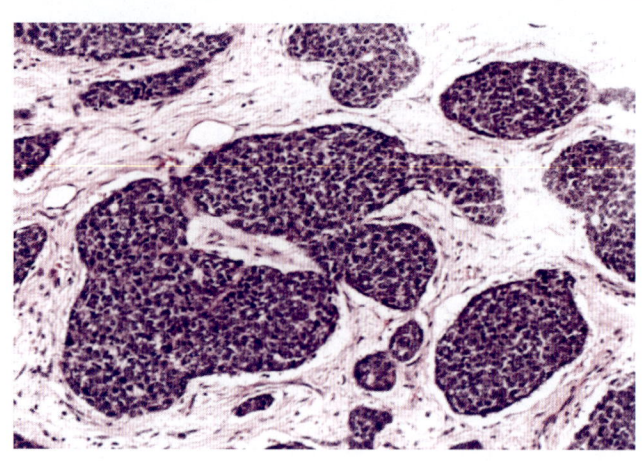

Figure 37.86. Histopathology of basaloid variant of adenoid cystic carcinoma of the lacrimal gland showing the solid lobules of malignant epithelial cells. (Hematoxylin–eosin ×75.)

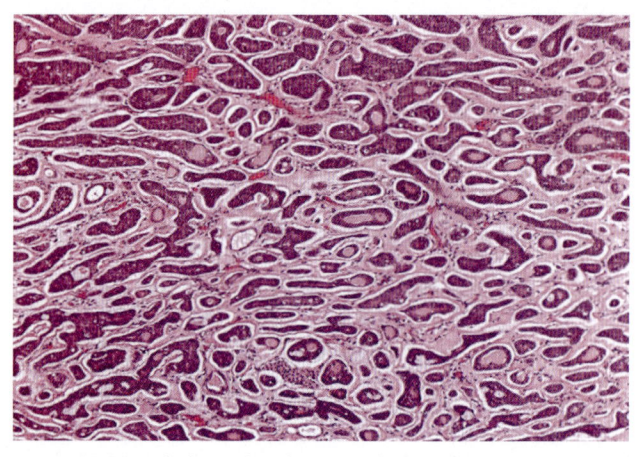

Figure 37.87. Tubular or ductal variant of adenoid cystic carcinoma of the lacrimal gland showing elongated tubules lined by malignant epithelial cells. (Hematoxylin–eosin ×75.)

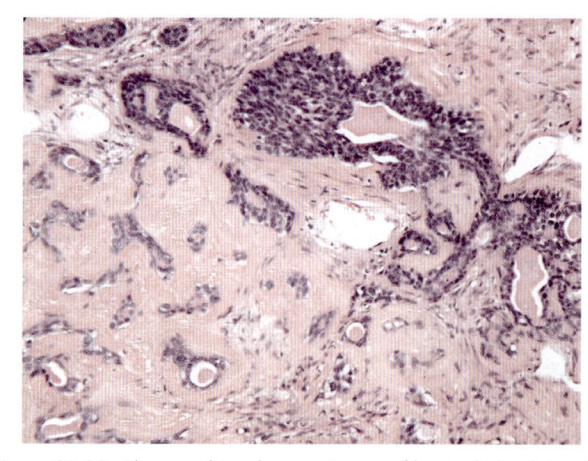

Figure 37.88. Pleomorphic adenocarcinoma of lacrimal gland showing mesenchymal and malignant epithelial cells. (Hematoxylin–eosin ×150.)

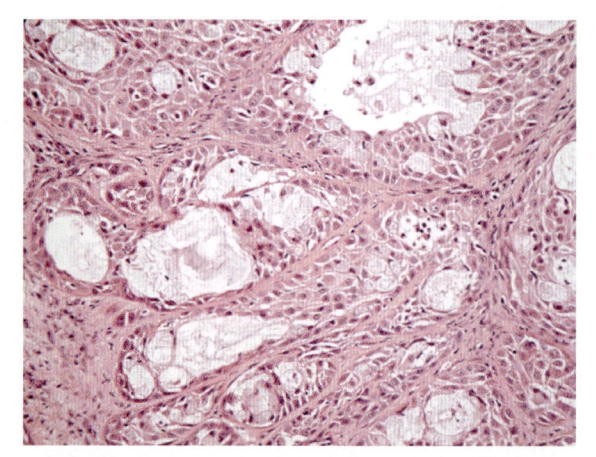

Figure 37.89. Mucoepidermoid carcinoma of lacrimal gland showing malignant epithelial cells with pools of mucin. (Hematoxylin–eosin ×150.) Mucin stains were positive.

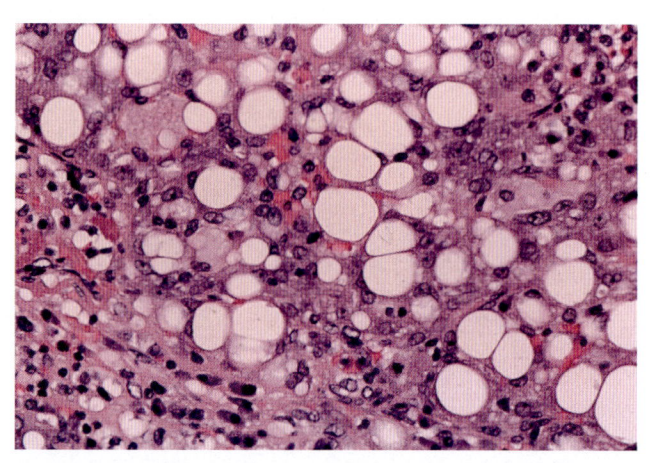

Figure 37.90. Acinic cell carcinoma of the lacrimal gland showing microcystic spaces. (Hematoxylin–eosin ×150.)

CHAPTER 38

ORBITAL METASTATIC CANCER

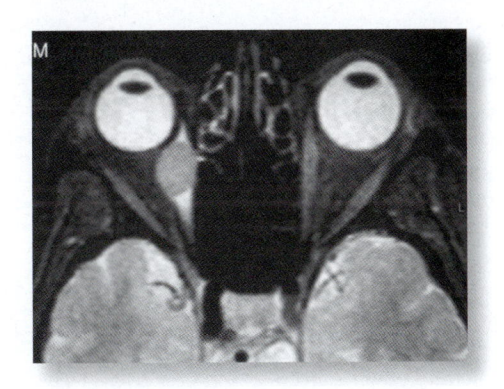

General Considerations

Several types of metastatic cancer can reach the orbital soft tissues or bones by hematogenous routes (1–74). Orbital metastasis can occur in adults and children with different primary tumors in each group. This chapter covers only cancers metastatic to the orbit. Lymphomas and secondary cancers that reach the orbit by direct continuity are covered elsewhere.

In adults, most tumors that metastasize to the orbit are carcinomas that arise in breast, prostate gland, lung, kidney, gastrointestinal tract, and other organs. Carcinoid tumors of the small intestine and appendix have a tendency to metastasize to the orbit, whereas bronchial carcinoid tumors tend to metastasize to the uveal tract (35–40). Cutaneous and uveal melanoma and soft tissue sarcomas can occasionally metastasize to the orbit (41–47). In children, orbital metastases are uncommon and come mainly from adrenal neuroblastoma and less often from Wilms' tumor, and Ewing's tumor (48–53).

Most patients with breast cancer metastasis to the orbit have a history of breast cancer. Many patients with metastasis from lung cancer or carcinoid tumor have no history of cancer and the orbital mass is often the first sign of malignancy. Overall, about 20% of patients who present with orbital metastasis have no history of a primary cancer and the orbital tumor is the first sign of an undiagnosed primary malignancy (5).

Clinical Features

The clinical features of orbital metastasis vary depending on the type of primary neoplasm. Although there are a range of symptoms and signs, the classic presentation is a rather rapid onset of pain, blepharoptosis, proptosis, displacement of the globe, diplopia, and conjunctival and eyelid edema. Some scirrhous tumors, particularly from breast and stomach cancers, can produce a paradoxical enophthalmos because of fibrosis and shrinkage of such tumors (12,17,21,22).

Diagnostic Approaches

Each patient with suspected orbital metastasis should have a history taken and systemic evaluation to rule out a primary cancer. In cases of orbital metastasis, computed tomography (CT) and magnetic resonance imaging (MRI) findings vary with the primary tumor. Metastatic breast cancer to the orbit tends to be confined to soft tissue, is more diffuse in configuration, and grows along fascial planes and muscle (4,5,15–22). Prostate metastasis tends to affect orbital bone (4,5,25–28). Metastatic melanoma, carcinoid tumor, and renal cell carcinoma may be round to ovoid and circumscribed, resembling a benign orbital tumor (29–53). The diagnosis should generally be confirmed by orbital biopsy. If no primary tumor is known, an orbitotomy with open excisional or incisional biopsy is appropriate. If the patient has a known history of cancer and the orbital lesion is anterior, a fine-needle aspiration biopsy (FNAB) can be done to confirm the diagnosis.

ORBITAL METASTATIC CANCER

Pathology

The histopathology of orbital metastasis is generally similar to the primary neoplasm and a discussion of it is beyond the scope of this atlas. Most pathologists who are accustomed to diagnosing metastatic cancer can readily recognize metastasis from breast, lung, gastrointestinal carcinoid tumor, thyroid, kidney, and melanoma on standard hematoxylin and eosin stains. However, some are so poorly differentiated that the diagnosis cannot be readily made and immunohistochemical stains and electron microscopy may be necessary.

An occasional major problem is the diagnosis of a poorly differentiated epithelial malignancy in a patient who has no history of systemic cancer. The onus is on the pathologist to determine if the lesion arose from lacrimal gland, sweat gland tumor of the eyelid, or other similar neoplasms. We have seen cases where it was almost impossible to make this differentiation. The surgeon should always send an adequate history to the pathologist to facilitate diagnosis.

Management

If there is no known primary neoplasm or if a known cancer has no other known metastasis, then an open biopsy should be done by the most accessible route as determined by imaging studies. If the patient has a known primary cancer and possible metastasis elsewhere, then FNAB may be warranted. Subsequent treatment with irradiation, hormone therapy, or chemotherapy is generally employed.

Selected References

Reviews

1. Shields JA, Shields CL, Scartozzi R. Survey of 1264 patients with orbital tumors and simulating lesions: the 2002 Montgomery Lecture, part 1. *Ophthalmology* 2004;111: 997–1008.
2. Shields JA, Bakewell B, Augsburger JJ, et al. Classification and incidence of space-occupying lesions of the orbit. A survey of 645 biopsies. *Arch Ophthalmol* 1984;102: 1606–1611.
3. Shields JA, Bakewell B, Augsburger JJ, et al. Space-occupying orbital masses in children: A review of 250 consecutive biopsies. *Ophthalmology* 1986;93:379–384.
4. Goldberg RA, Rootman J, Cline RA. Tumors metastatic to the orbit: a changing picture. *Surv Ophthalmol* 1990;35:1–24.
5. Shields JA, Shields CL, Brotman HK, et al. Cancer metastatic to the orbit. The 2000 Robert M. Curts Lecture. *Ophthal Plast Reconstr Surg* 2001;17:346–354.
6. Shields CL, Shields JA, Peggs M. Tumors metastatic to the orbit. *Ophthal Plast Reconstr Surg* 1988;4:73–80.
7. Gunalp I, Gunduz K. Metastatic orbital tumors. *Jpn J Ophthalmol* 1995;39:65–70.
8. Amemiya T, Hayashida H, Dake Y. Metastatic orbital tumors in Japan: a review of the literature. *Ophthalmic Epidemiol* 2002;9:35–47.
9. Demirci H, Shields CL, Shields JA, et al. Orbital tumors in the older adult population. *Ophthalmology* 2002;109:243–248.
10. Capone A Jr, Slamovits TL. Discrete metastasis of solid tumors to extraocular muscles. *Arch Ophthalmol* 1990;108:237–243.
11. Ferry AP, Font RL. Carcinoma metastatic to the eye and orbit. I. A clinicopathologic study of 227 cases. *Arch Ophthalmol* 1974;92:276–286.
12. Cline RA, Rootman J. Enophthalmos: a clinical review. *Ophthalmology* 1984;91: 229–237.

Management

13. Tijl J, Koornneef L, Eijpe A, et al. Metastatic tumors to the orbit—management and prognosis. *Graefes Arch Clin Exp Ophthalmol* 1992;230:527–530.

Case Reports

Breast Carcinoma

14. Glassburn JR, Klionsky M, Brady LW. Radiation therapy for metastatic disease involving the orbit. *Am J Clin Oncol* 1984;7:145–148.
15. Demirci H, Shields CL, Chao A, et al. Uveal metastasis from breast cancer in 264 patients. *Am J Ophthalmol* 2003;136:264–271.
16. Huda N, Venable HP. Metastasis of carcinoma of the breast to both orbits. *Am J Ophthalmol* 1967;64:779–780.
17. Shields CL, Shields JA, Mruczek AW. Enophthalmos as the initial manifestation of metastasis from scirrhous carcinoma of the breast. *Ophthalmic Practice* 1989;7:159–160.
18. Reeves D, Levine MR, Lash R. Nonpalpable breast carcinoma presenting as orbital infiltration: case presentation and literature review. *Ophthal Plast Reconstr Surg* 2002; 18:84–88.
19. Saitoh A, Amemiya T, Tsuda N. Metastasis of breast carcinoma to eyelid and orbit of a postmenopausal woman: good response to tamoxifen therapy. *Ophthalmologica* 1997; 211:362–366.
20. Jacobs M, Benger R. Metastatic breast carcinoma of the orbit. *Aust N Z J Ophthalmol* 1989;17:357–361.
21. Manor RS. Enophthalmos caused by orbital metastatic breast carcinoma. *Acta Ophthalmologica* 1974;52:881–884.
22. Shields CL, Stopyra GA, Marr BP, et al. Enophthalmos as initial manifestation of occult mammogram-negative breast carcinoma. *Ophthal Surg Lasers Imaging* 2004; 35:56–57.

Lung Cancer

23. Kulvin MM, Sawchak WG. Tumor of the orbit. Metastatic from malignant bronchial adenoma. *Am J Ophthalmol* 1960;49:833.
24. Shields JA, Shields CL, Eagle RC Jr, et al. Diffuse ocular metastases as an initial sign of metastatic lung cancer. *Ophthalmic Surg Lasers* 1998;29:598–601.

Prostate Cancer

25. Hesse RJ. Orbital metastasis from prostatic carcinoma. *Arch Ophthalmol* 1982;100:64.
26. Winkler CF, Goodman GK, Eiferman RA, et al. Orbital metastases from prostatic carcinoma: identification by an immunoperoxidase technique. *Arch Ophthalmol* 1981;99:1406–1408.
27. Carriere VM, Karcioglu ZA, Apple DJ, et al. A case of prostate carcinoma with bilateral orbital metastasis and the review of the literature. *Ophthalmology* 1982;89:202–206.
28. Baltogiannis D, Kalogeropoulos C, Ioachim E, et al. Orbital metastasis from prostatic carcinoma. *Urol Int* 2003;70:219–222.

Renal Cancer

29. Shields JA, Shields CL, Brucker WK, et al. Metastatic renal cell carcinoma to the orbit. *Ophthalmic Practice* 1989;7:239–242.
30. Mezer E, Gdal-On M, Miller B. Orbital metastasis of renal cell carcinoma masquerading as Amaurosis fugax. *Eur J Ophthalmol* 1997;7:301–304.
31. Bersani TA, Costello JJ Jr, Mango CA, et al. Benign approach to a malignant orbital tumor: metastatic renal cell carcinoma. *Ophthal Plast Reconstr Surg* 1994;10:42–44.
32. Denby P, Harvey L, English MG. Solitary metastasis from an occult renal cell carcinoma presenting as a primary lacrimal gland tumour. *Orbit* 1986;5:21–24.
33. Kindermann WR, Shields JA, Eiferman RA, et al. Metastatic renal cell carcinoma to the eye and adnexae. A report of 3 cases and review of the literature. *Ophthalmology* 1981;88:1347–1350.
34. Shields JA, Shields CL, Eagle RC Jr, et al. Metastatic renal cell carcinoma to the palpebral lobe of lacrimal gland. *Ophthal Plast Reconstr Surg* 2001;17:191–194.

Carcinoid Tumor

35. Couch DA, O'Halloran HS, Hainsworth KM, et al. Carcinoid metastasis to extraocular muscles: case reports and review of the literature. *Orbit* 2000;19:263–269.
36. Honrubia FM, Davis WH, Moore MK, et al. Carcinoid syndrome with bilateral orbital metastases. *Am J Ophthalmol* 1972;72:1118–1121.
37. Divine RD, Anderson RL, Ossoinig KC. Metastatic carcinoid unresponsive to radiation therapy presenting as a lacrimal fossa mass. *Ophthalmology* 1982;89:516–520.
38. Riddle PJ, Font RL, Zimmerman LE. Carcinoid tumors of the eye and orbit: a clinicopathologic study of 15 cases, with histochemical and electron microscopic observations. *Hum Pathol* 1982;13:459–469.
39. Shields CL, Shields JA, Eagle RC, et al. Orbital metastasis from a gastrointestinal carcinoid tumor. *Arch Ophthalmol* 1987;105:968–971.
40. Rush JA, Waller RR, Campbell RJ. Orbital carcinoid tumor metastatic from the colon. *Am J Ophthalmol* 1980;89:636–640.

Skin Melanoma

41. Font RL, Naumann G, Zimmerman LE. Primary malignant melanoma of the skin metastatic to the eye and orbit. *Am J Ophthalmol* 1967;63:738–754.
42. Zografos L, Ducrey N, Beati D, et al. Metastatic melanoma in the eye and orbit. *Ophthalmology* 2003;110:2245–2256.

ORBITAL METASTATIC CANCER

Uveal Melanoma

43. Shields JA, Perez N, Shields CL, et al. Orbital melanoma metastatic from contralateral choroid: management by complete surgical resection. *Ophthalmic Surg Lasers* 2002;33:416–420.
44. Abramson DH, Servodidio CA. Metastatic choroidal melanoma to the contralateral orbit 40 years after enucleation. *Arch Ophthalmol* 1997;115:134.
45. Coupland SE, Sidiki S, Clark BJ, et al. Metastatic choroidal melanoma to the contralateral orbit 40 years after enucleation. *Arch Ophthalmol* 1996;114:751–756.
46. Shields JA, Perez N, Shields CL, et al. Orbital melanoma metastatic from contralateral choroid. Management by complete surgical resection. *Ophthal Surg Lasers* 2002;33:416–420.
47. Shields JA, Shields CL, Shakin EP, et al. Metastasis of choroidal melanoma to the contralateral choroid, orbit, and eyelid. *Br J Ophthalmol* 1988;72:456–460.

Neuroblastoma, Wilms' Tumor, Ewing's Sarcoma

48. Musarella M, Chan HS, DeBoer G, et al. Ocular involvement in neuroblastoma. Prognostic implications. *Ophthalmology* 1984;91:936–940.
49. Lau JJ, Trobe JD, Ruiz RE, et al. Metastatic neuroblastoma presenting with binocular blindness from intracranial compression of the optic nerves. *J Neuroophthalmol* 2004;24:119–124.
50. Apple DJ. Metastatic orbital neuroblastoma originating in the cervical sympathetic ganglionic chain. *Am J Ophthalmol* 1969;68:1093–1095.
51. Fratkin D, Purcell JJ, Krachmer JH, et al. Wilm's tumor metastasis to the orbit. *JAMA* 1977;238:1841–1842.
52. Apple DJ. Wilms' tumor metastatic to the orbit. *Arch Ophthalmol* 1968;80:480–483.
53. Kawachi E, Nunobiki K, Shimada S, et al. A case of Ewing's sarcoma with orbital metastasis. *Folia Ophthalmol Jpn* 1984;35:1840–1845.

Rhabdomyosarcoma

54. Fekrat S, Miller NR, Loury MC. Alveolar rhabdomyosarcoma that metastasized to the orbit. *Arch Ophthalmol* 1993;111:1662–1664.
55. Amato MM, Esmaeli B, Shore JW. Orbital rhabdomyosarcoma metastatic to the contralateral orbit: a case report. *Ophthalmology* 2002;109:753–756.
56. Walton RC, Ellis GS Jr, Haik BG. Rhabdomyosarcoma presumed metastatic to the orbit. *Ophthalmology* 1996;103:1512–1516.

Other Cancers

57. Friedman J, Karesh J, Rodrigues M, et al. Thyroid carcinoma metastatic to the medial rectus muscle. *Ophthal Plast Reconstr Surg* 1990;6:122–125.
58. McCulley TJ, Yip CC, Bullock JD, et al. Cervical carcinoma metastatic to the orbit. *Ophthal Plast Reconstr Surg* 2002;18:385–387.
59. Bartley GB, Campbell RJ, Salomao DR, et al. Adrenocortical carcinoma metastatic to the orbit. *Ophthal Plast Reconstr Surg* 2001;17:215–220.
60. Logrono R, Inhorn SL, Dortzbach RK, et al. Leiomyosarcoma metastatic to the orbit: diagnosis of fine-needle aspiration. *Diagn Cytopathol* 1997;17:369–373.
61. Kaltreider SA, Destro M, Lemke BN. Leiomyosarcoma of the orbit. *Ophthal Plast Reconstr Surg* 1987;3:35–41.
62. Burnstine MA, Frueh BR, Elner VM. Angiosarcoma metastatic to the orbit. *Arch Ophthalmol* 1996;114:93–96.
63. Ballinger WH, Wesley RE. Seminoma metastatic to the orbit. *Ophthal Surg* 1984;15:120–122.
64. Krauss HR, Slamovits TL, Siboney PA, et al. Orbital metastasis of bladder carcinoma (Letter to the Editor). *Am J Ophthalmol* 1982;94:265–266.
65. Lubin JR, Grove AS Jr, Zakov ZN, et al. Hepatoma metastatic to the orbit. *Am J Ophthalmol* 1980;89:268–273.
66. Margo CE, Folberg RF, Zimmerman LE, et al. Endodermal sinus tumor (yolk sac tumor) of the orbit. *Ophthalmology* 1983;90:1426–1432.
67. Rush JA, Older JJ, Ruchman AV. Testicular seminoma metastatic to the orbit. *Am J Ophthalmol* 1981;91:258–260.
68. Scharf Y, Scharf Y, Arieh YB, et al. Orbital metastasis from extra-adrenal pheochromocytoma. *Am J Ophthalmol* 1970;69:638–640.
69. Snyderman HR. Orbital metastasis from tumor of the pancreas. Report of two cases with necropsy findings. *Am J Ophthalmol* 1942;25:1215–1221.
70. Seretan EL. Metastatic adenocarcinoma from the stomach to the orbit. *Arch Ophthalmol* 1981;99:1469.
71. Eldesouky MA, Elbakary MA, Shalaby OE, et al. Orbital metastasis from hepatocellular carcinoma: report of 6 cases. *Ophthal Plast Reconstr Surg* 2014;30:e78–e82.
72. Dhrami-Gavazi E, Lo C, Patel P, et al. Gestational choriocarcinoma metastasis to the extraocular muscle: a case report. *Ophthal Plast Reconstr Surg* 2013;30:e75–e77.
73. Johnson D, Warder D, Plourde ME, et al. Orbital metastasis secondary to Merkel cell carcinoma: case report and literature review. *Orbit* 2013;32:263–265.

Pseudometastasis

74. Foley MR, Moshfeghi DM, Wilson MW, et al. Orbital inflammatory syndromes with systemic involvement may mimic metastatic disease. *Ophthal Plast Reconstr Surg* 2003;19:324–327.

ORBITAL METASTASIS FROM BREAST CANCER

Breast cancer accounts for the majority of orbital metastasis. It usually produces proptosis, with the exception of scirrhous breast cancer, which can contract, causing a paradoxical enophthalmos. CT and MRI show typical, but not pathognomonic, features.

Shields JA, Shields CL, Brotman HK, et al. Cancer metastatic to the orbit. The 2000 Robertt M. Curts Lecture. *Ophthal Plast Reconstr Surg* 2001;17:346–354.

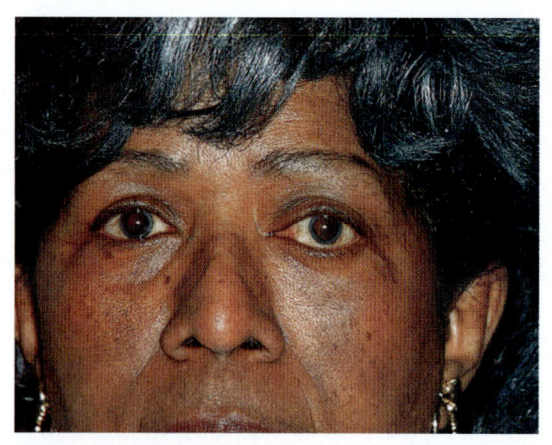

Figure 38.1. Proptosis of left eye secondary to orbital metastasis from breast cancer in a 68-year-old woman.

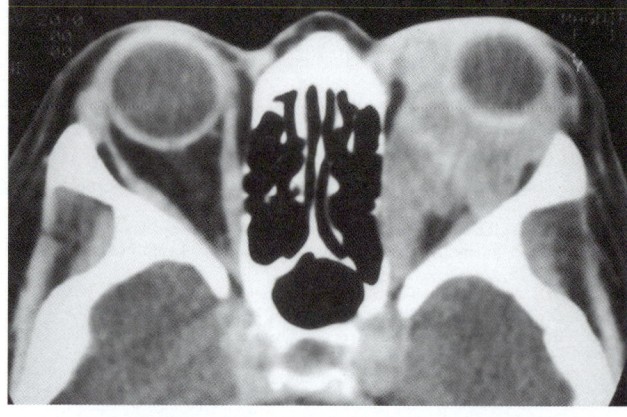

Figure 38.2. Axial computed tomography of patient shown in Figure 38.1 demonstrated a diffuse tumor filling most of the orbit and infiltrating the medial rectus muscle.

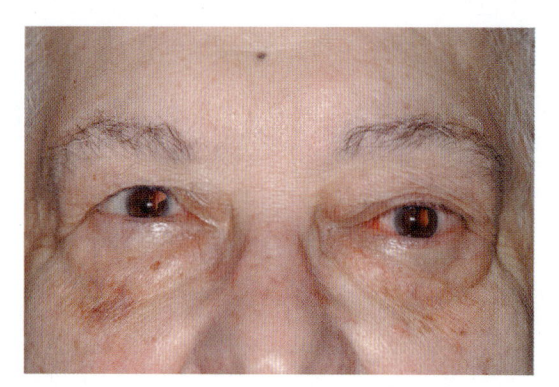

Figure 38.3. Elderly woman with breast cancer metastasis to left orbit showing proptosis, downward displacement of globe, and conjunctival hyperemia.

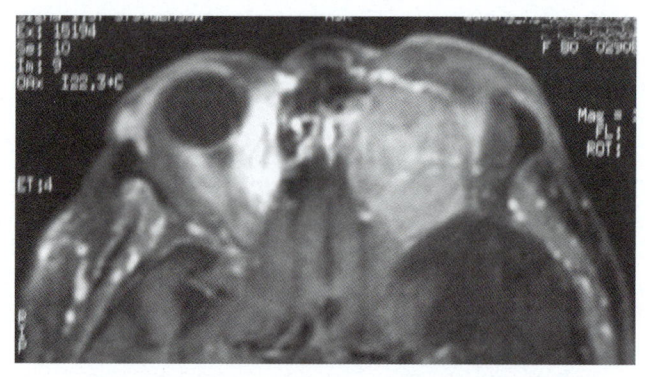

Figure 38.4. Axial magnetic resonance imaging of patient shown in Figure 38.3, T1-weighted image, with fat suppression and gadolinium enhancement, demonstrating large enhancing orbital mass.

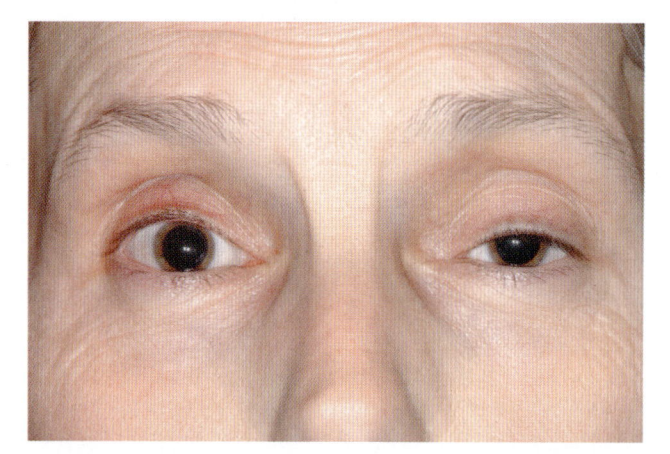

Figure 38.5. Middle-aged woman with breast cancer metastasis to left orbit showing blepharoptosis of left upper eyelid and minimal proptosis.

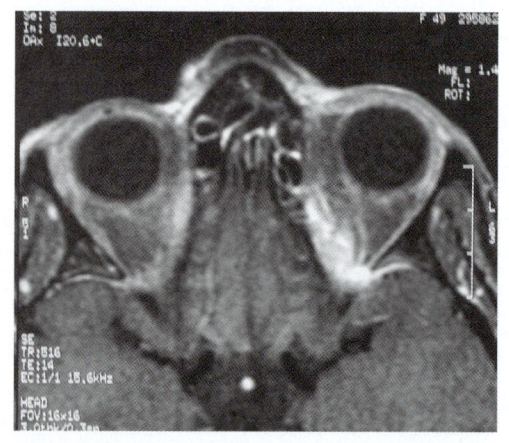

Figure 38.6. Axial magnetic resonance imaging of patient shown in Figure 38.5, T1-weighted image, with fat suppression and gadolinium enhancement, demonstrating minimal enhancement of orbital mass.

ORBITAL METASTASIS FROM BREAST CANCER: CLINICAL VARIATIONS

Orbital metastasis from breast cancer can assume any of several clinical variations. Like orbital metastasis from other primary cancers, and unlike most benign tumors, it tends to have more profound symptoms and signs, with more rapid proptosis, globe displacement, pain, motility disturbance, and conjunctival chemosis.

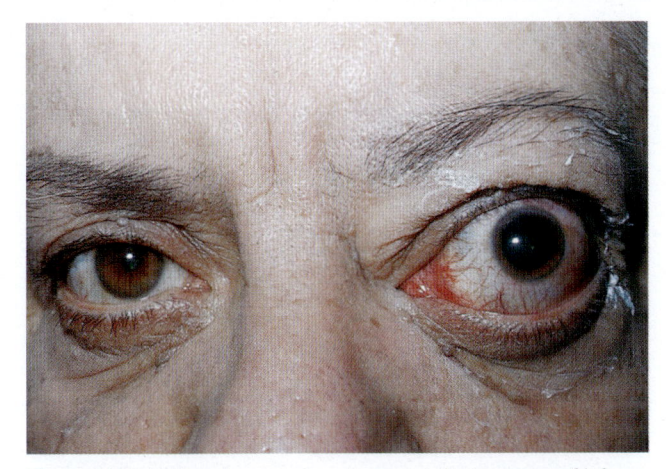

Figure 38.7. Unilateral proptosis and upward displacement of left eye secondary to metastatic breast cancer in a 65-year-old woman.

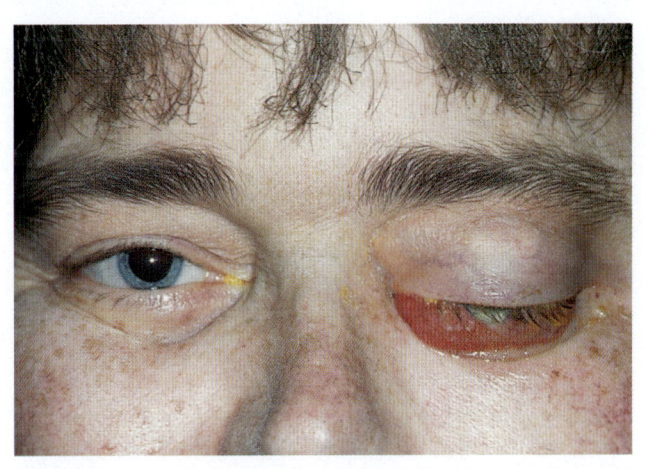

Figure 38.8. Blepharoptosis and conjunctival chemosis in a 47-year-old woman with metastatic breast cancer to the left orbit.

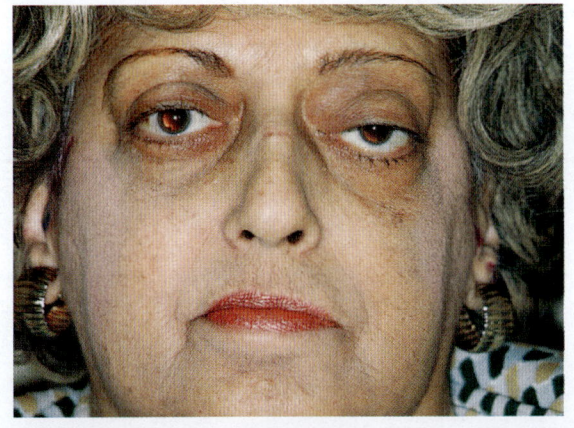

Figure 38.9. Bilateral proptosis and blepharoptosis secondary to bilateral orbital metastasis in a 64-year-old woman.

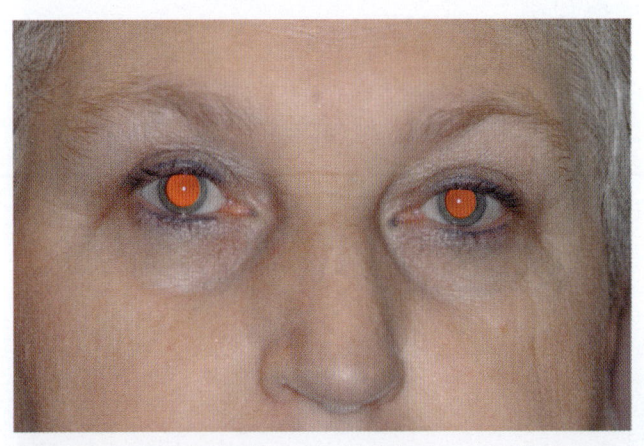

Figure 38.10. Middle-aged woman with slight proptosis of left eye and a history of breast cancer.

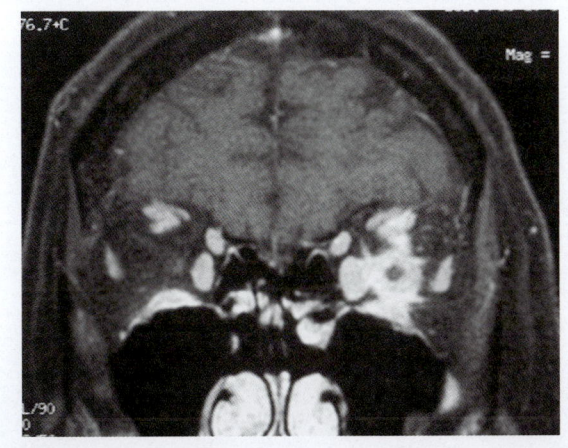

Figure 38.11. Coronal magnetic resonance imaging in T1-weighted image with gadolinium enhancement and fat suppression of patient seen in Figure 38.10 revealing an enhancing infiltrative tumor surrounding optic nerve.

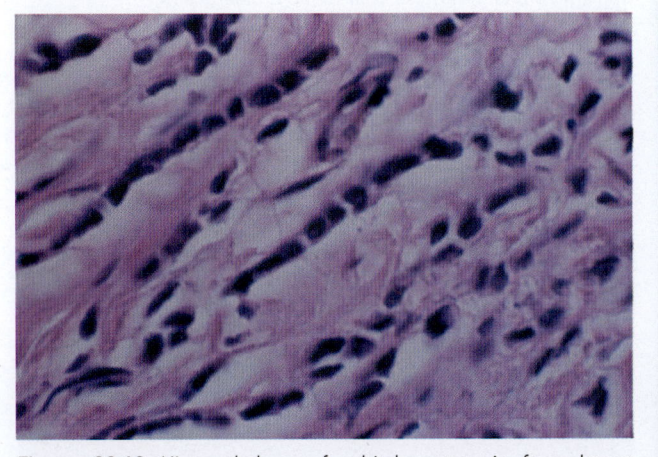

Figure 38.12. Histopathology of orbital metastasis from breast cancer showing cords of malignant tumor cells and fibrous stroma. (Hematoxylin–eosin ×200.)

ORBITAL METASTASIS FROM BREAST CANCER: PARADOXICAL ENOPHTHALMOS

Scirrhous or sclerosing breast cancer metastasis to the orbit can sometimes undergo fibrosis, causing the globe to retract and to produce paradoxical enophthalmos.

1. Shields CL, Shields JA, Mruczek AW. Enophthalmos as the initial manifestation of metastasis from scirrhous carcinoma of the breast. *Ophthalmic Practice* 1989;7:159–160.
2. Shields CL, Stopyra GA, Marr BP, et al. Enophthalmos as initial manifestation of occult mammogram-negative breast carcinoma. *Ophthal Surg Lasers Imaging* 2004;35:56–57.

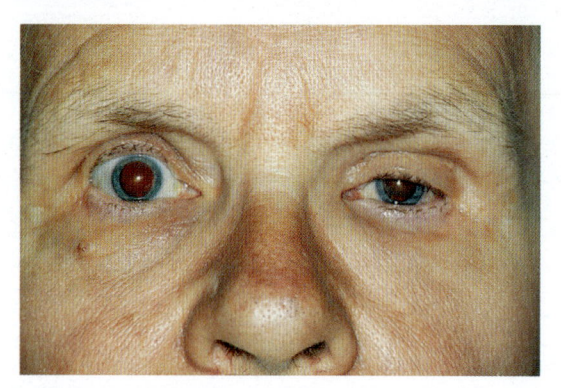

Figure 38.13. Enophthalmos of the left eye secondary to metastatic scirrhous breast cancer to the orbit in a 75-year-old woman. She was referred because of suspected proptosis of the right eye, which proved to be normal.

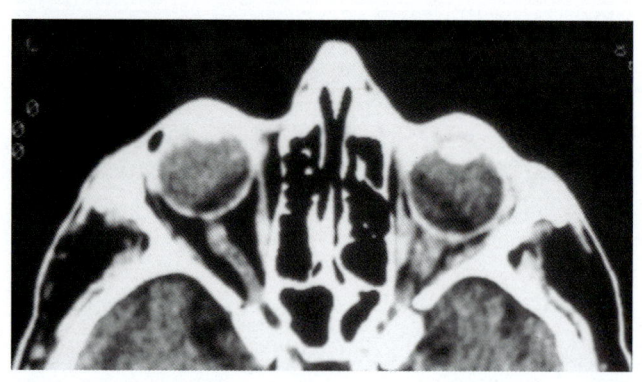

Figure 38.14. Axial computed tomography of patient shown in Figure 38.13. There is diffuse contracting tumor tissue in the medial and posterior orbit, producing the enophthalmos.

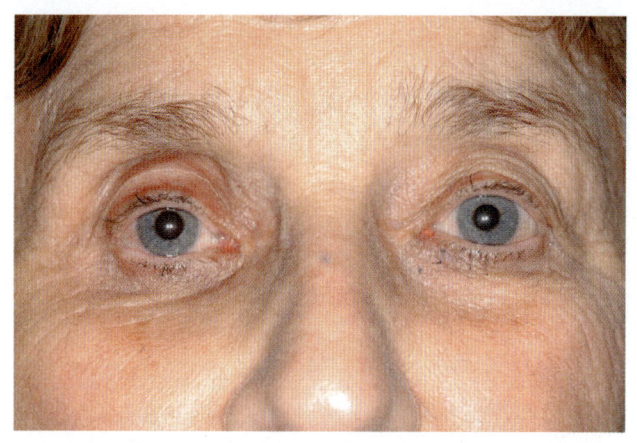

Figure 38.15. Apparent enophthalmos of right eye in elderly woman with right orbital metastasis from scirrhous breast cancer.

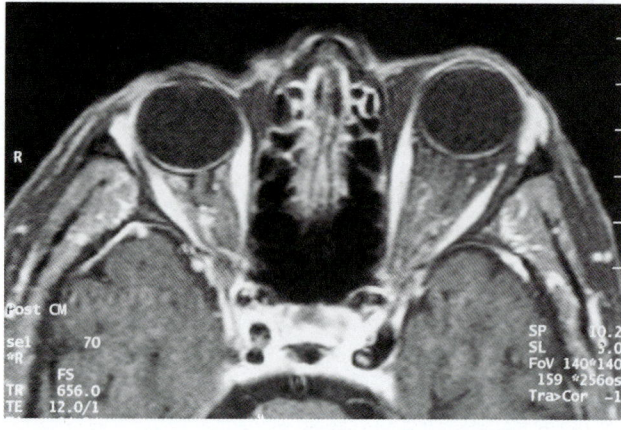

Figure 38.16. Axial magnetic resonance imaging in T1-weighted image showing diffuse mass causing retraction of right eye.

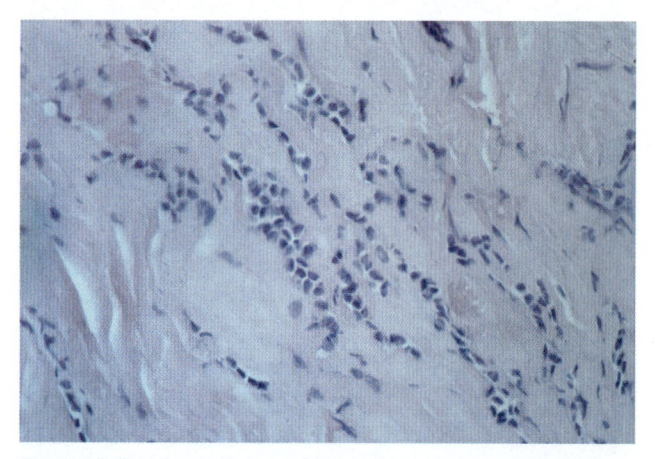

Figure 38.17. Histopathology of lesion shown in Figure 38.16 demonstrating paucicellular mass with extensive fibrosis. (Hematoxylin–eosin ×50.)

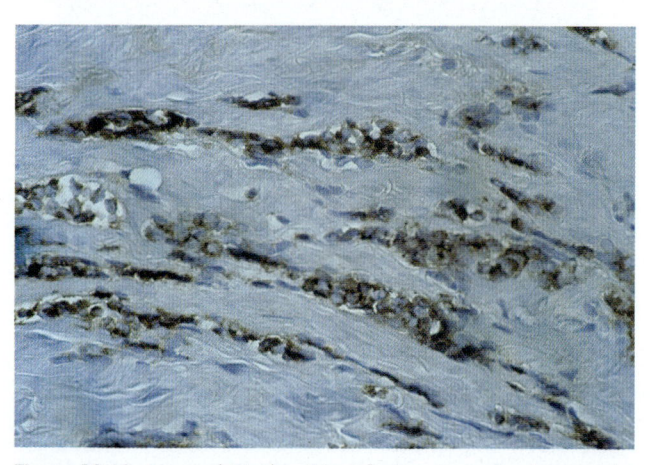

Figure 38.18. Immunohistochemistry of same case, showing positive reaction to breast cancer markers. (BRST ×500.)

ORBITAL METASTASIS FROM BREAST CANCER: BIOPSY TECHNIQUES

Depending on the clinical findings and the size and location of the tumor, either excisional biopsy, incisional biopsy, or FNAB can be performed in cases of suspected orbital metastasis. In many cases, the tumor is diffuse and adherent to adjacent structures and an incisional biopsy is done. When possible, however, excisional biopsy is often advisable.

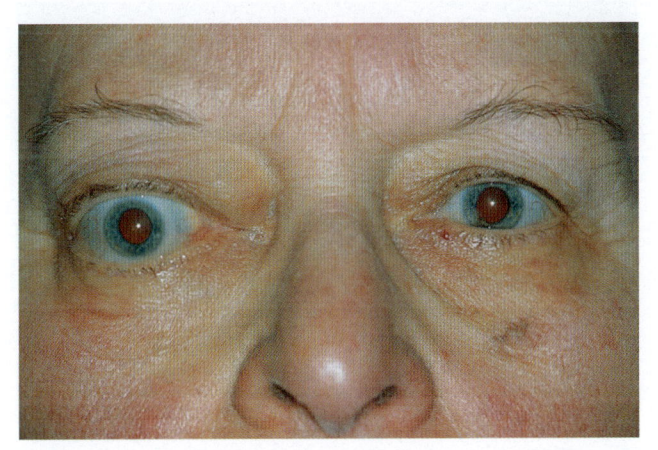

Figure 38.19. Proptosis of the right eye in a 76-year-old woman with breast cancer but no prior history of metastasis.

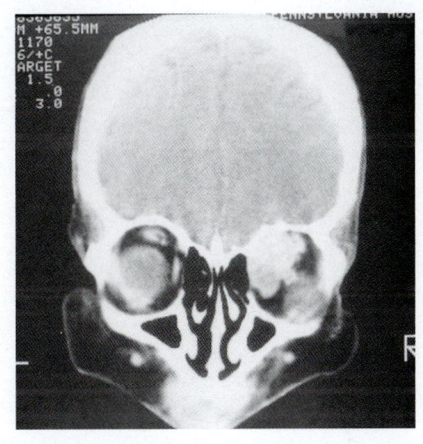

Figure 38.20. Coronal computed tomography of patient seen in Figure 38.19, showing a mass in the superonasal aspect of the right orbit. In such a case, a superonasal cutaneous eyelid crease incision is the best approach to excisional or incisional biopsy.

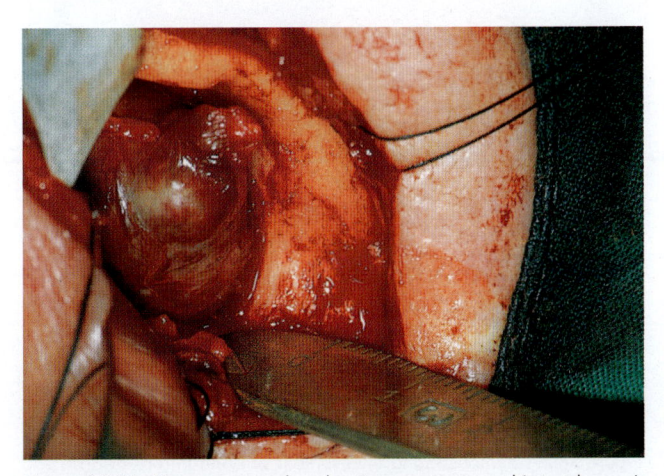

Figure 38.21. Tumor exposed at the time was removed intact by excisional biopsy.

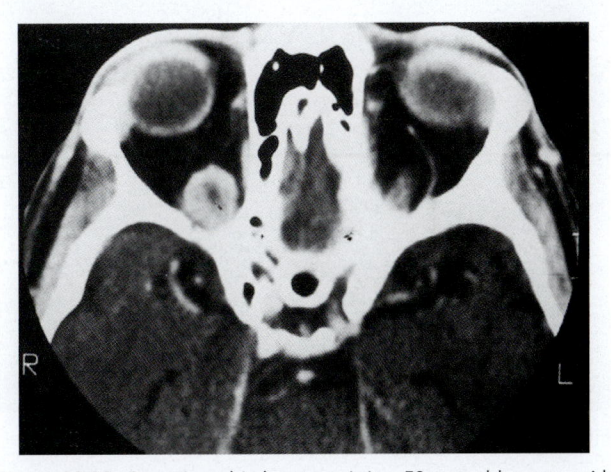

Figure 38.22. Posterior orbital metastasis in a 58-year-old woman with known breast cancer. Axial computed tomography showing small tumor in posterior aspect of orbit.

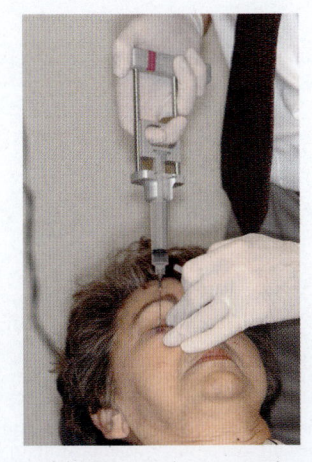

Figure 38.23. A careful, computed tomography-guided fine-needle aspiration biopsy was performed.

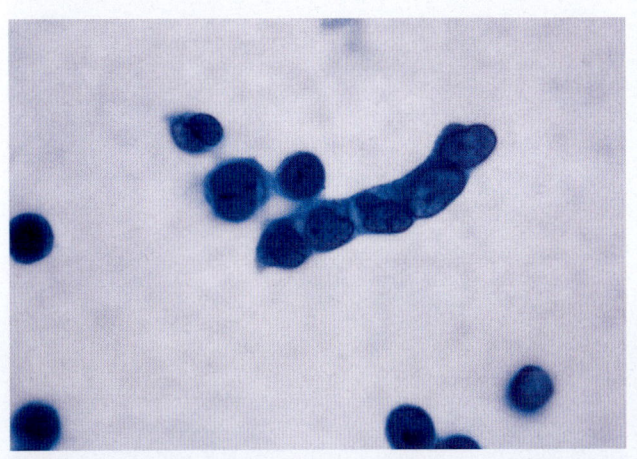

Figure 38.24. Cytopathology of fine-needle aspiration biopsy for orbital metastasis of breast cancer, showing characteristic cells. (Papanicolaou ×250.)

ORBITAL METASTASIS FROM PROSTATE CARCINOMA

Prostate cancer metastatic to the orbital area has a propensity to affect orbital bones as well as soft tissue. Immunohistochemistry for prostate-specific antigen can assist in the histopathologic diagnosis.

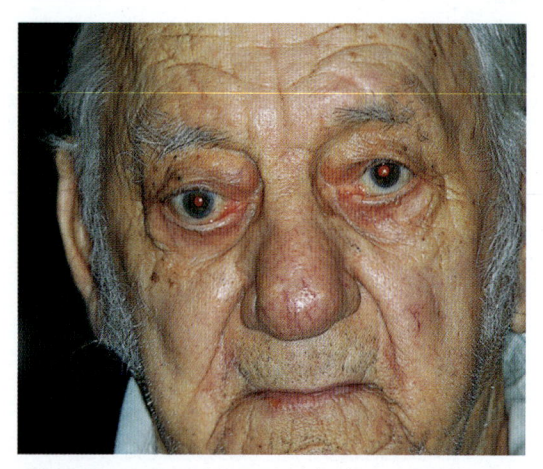

Figure 38.25. Proptosis and downward displacement of the right eye in a 79-year-old man with prostate cancer.

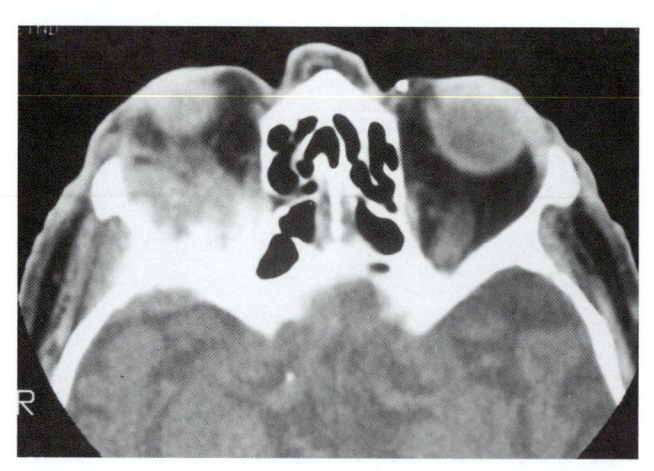

Figure 38.26. Axial computed tomography of patient shown in Figure 38.25, demonstrating extensive bone and soft tissue involvement with metastatic prostate cancer.

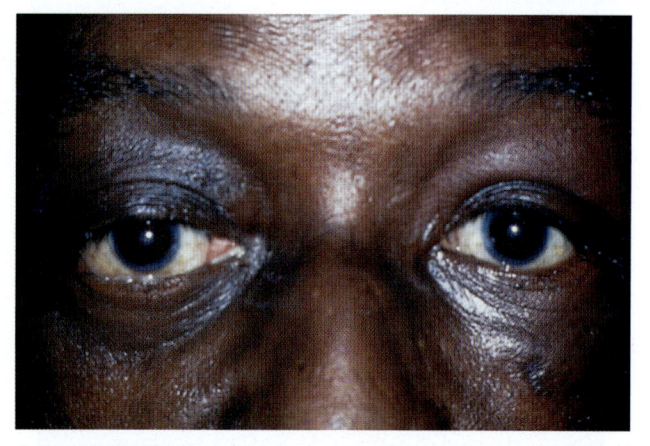

Figure 38.27. Downward displacement of the right eye in a 56-year-old man with prostate cancer.

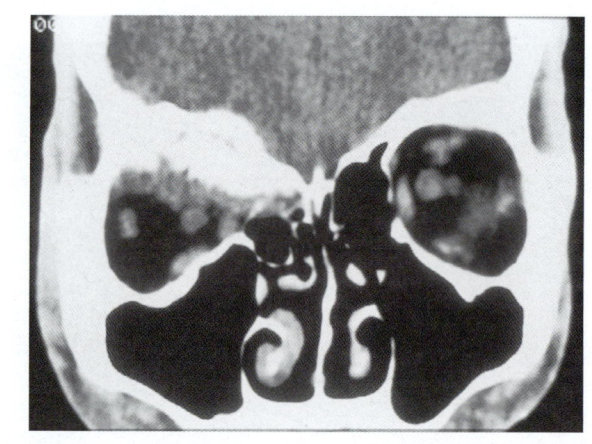

Figure 38.28. Coronal computed tomography of patient shown in Figure 38.27, demonstrating involvement of bone in roof of orbit and mild soft tissue involvement.

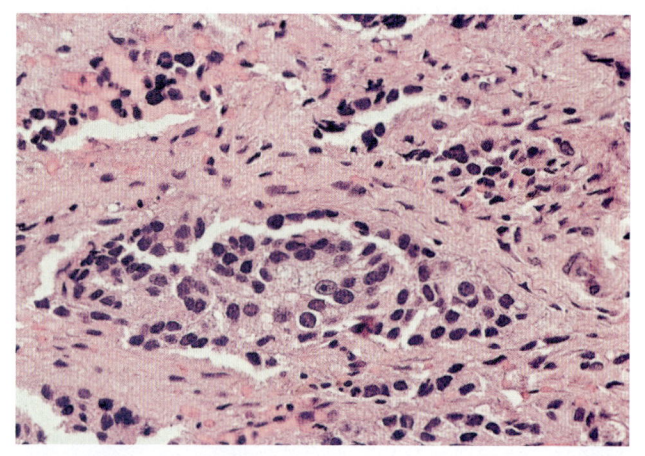

Figure 38.29. Histopathology of orbital biopsy from patient shown in Figure 38.27, demonstrating findings compatible with metastatic prostate cancer. (Hematoxylin–eosin ×150.)

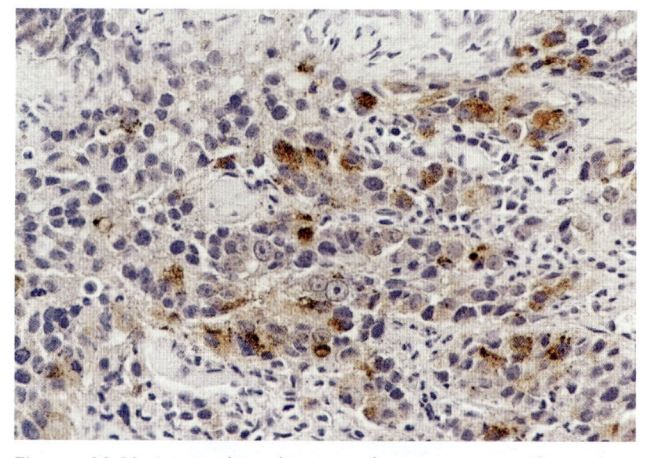

Figure 38.30. Immunohistochemistry for prostate-specific antigen of specimen shown in Figure 38.29, demonstrating immunopositivity. (Hematoxylin–eosin ×150.)

ORBITAL METASTASIS FROM CARCINOID TUMOR

Ocular metastasis from bronchial carcinoid tumor usually involves the uveal tract. In contrast, ocular metastasis from ileal or appendiceal carcinoid tumor tends to affect the orbit. The reason for these metastatic patterns is unknown. A clinicopathologic correlation of a carcinoid tumor of the ileum metastatic to the orbit is shown.

Shields CL, Shields JA, Eagle RC, et al. Orbital metastasis from a carcinoid tumor. Computed tomography, magnetic resonance imaging, and electron microscopic findings. *Arch Ophthalmol* 1987;105:968–971.

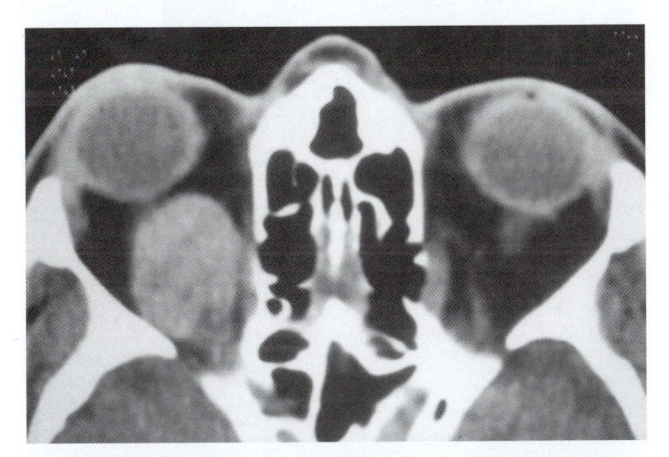

Figure 38.31. Axial computed tomography of a 63-year-old woman with a history of carcinoid tumor of the ileum who developed progressive proptosis of the right eye.

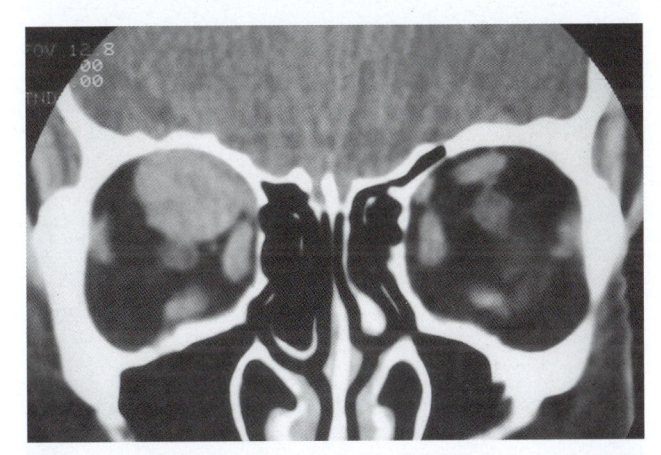

Figure 38.32. Coronal computed tomography showing superior orbital mass.

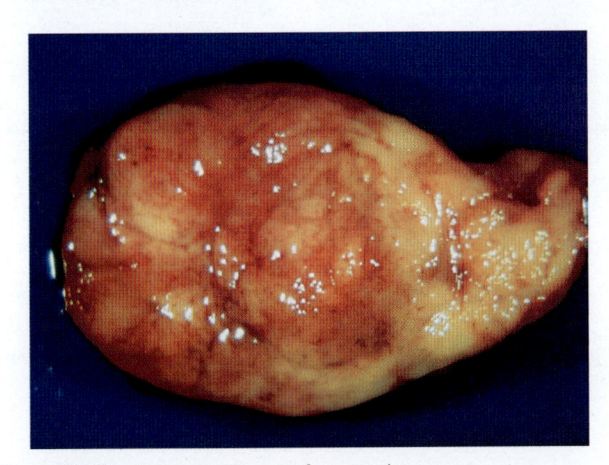

Figure 38.33. Gross appearance of resected tumor.

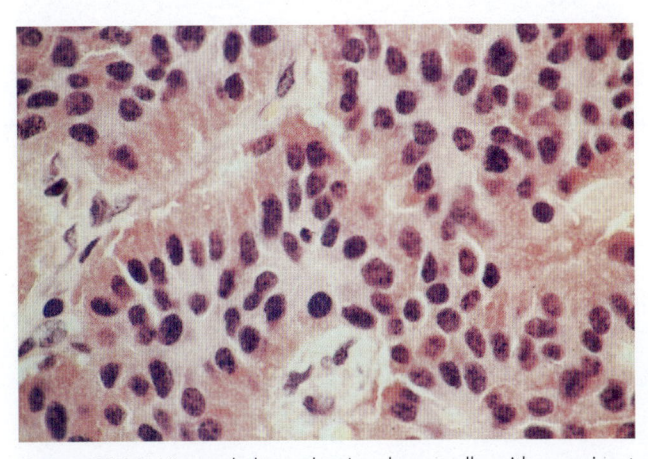

Figure 38.34. Histopathology showing large cells with prominent hyperchromatic eccentric nuclei and granular eosinophilic cytoplasm. (Hematoxylin–eosin ×250.)

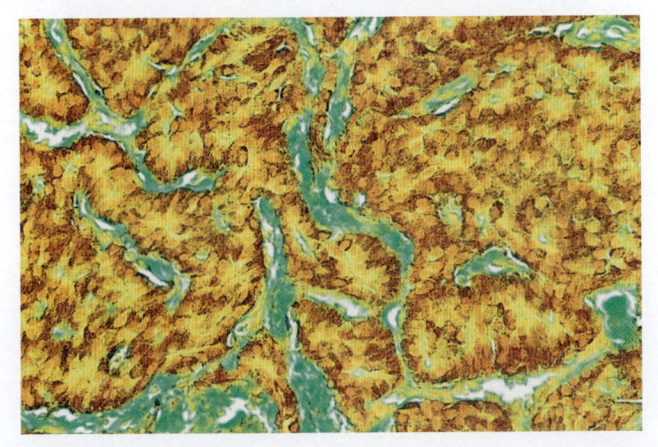

Figure 38.35. Histopathology showing argyrophilic neurosecretory granules. (Grimelius stain ×400.)

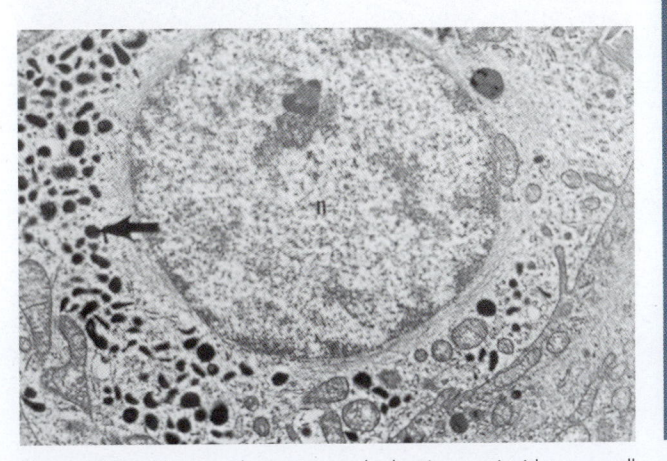

Figure 38.36. Electron photomicrograph showing carcinoid tumor cell with large nucleus and neurosecretory granules in the cytoplasm. (×14,000.)

ORBITAL METASTASIS FROM LUNG CANCER

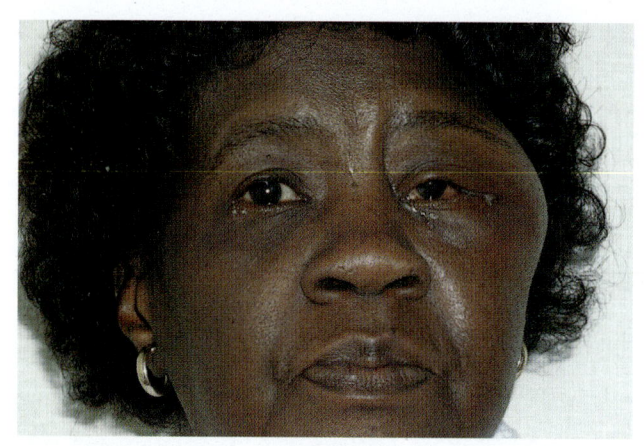

Figure 38.37. Proptosis and swelling of temporal fossa secondary to metastatic lung cancer in a 57-year-old woman.

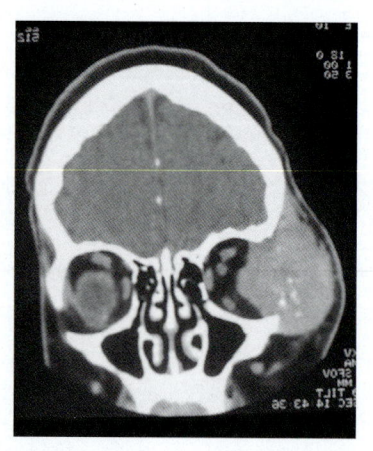

Figure 38.38. Coronal computed tomography of patient shown in Figure 38.37, demonstrating large, bone-destructive tumor.

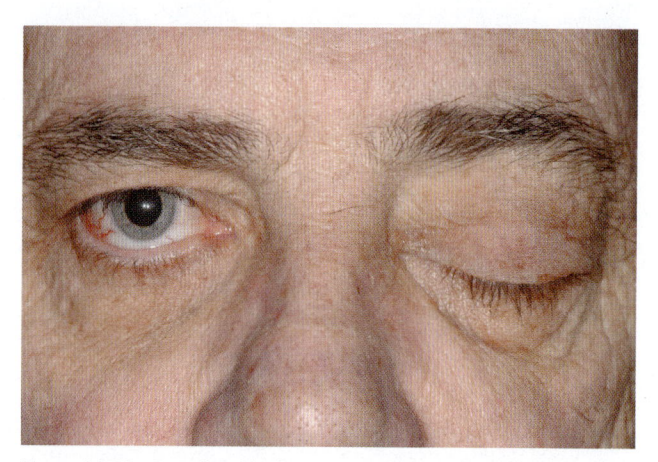

Figure 38.39. Complete blepharoptosis of left upper eyelid as first sign of orbital metastasis from prior lung cancer in a 70-year-old man.

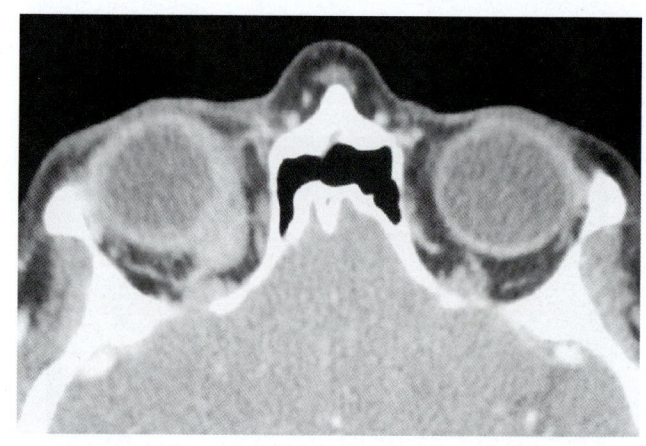

Figure 38.40. Axial computed tomography showing orbital metastasis from lung cancer in midright orbit compressing the globe.

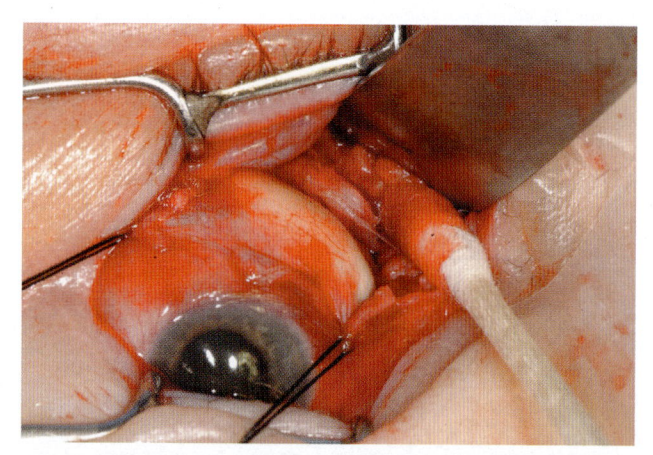

Figure 38.41. Surgical view of patient shown in Figure 38.40 after conjunctival incision. The tumor can barely be visualized. An incisional biopsy was done and metastasis lung cancer was confirmed.

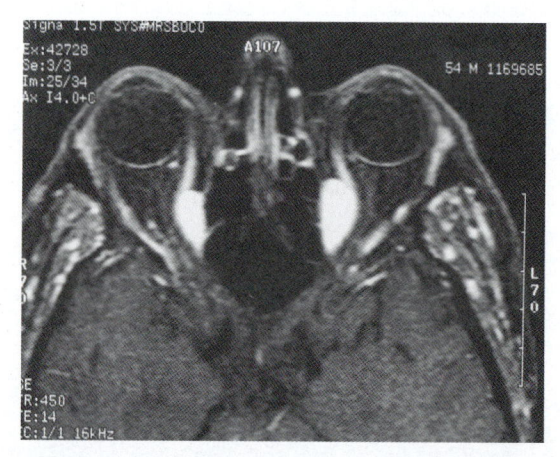

Figure 38.42. T1-weighted magnetic resonance imaging with gadolinium enhancement fat suppression showing bilateral orbital metastasis from lung cancer involving the medial rectus muscle of each eye.

ORBITAL METASTASIS FROM RENAL CELL CARCINOMA

1. Shields JA, Shields CL, Brucker WK, et al. Metastatic renal cell carcinoma to the orbit. *Ophthalmic Practice* 1989;7:239–242.
2. Shields JA, Shields CL, Eagle RC Jr, et al. Metastatic renal cell carcinoma to the palpebral lobe of lacrimal gland. *Ophthal Plast Reconstr Surg* 2001;17:191–194.

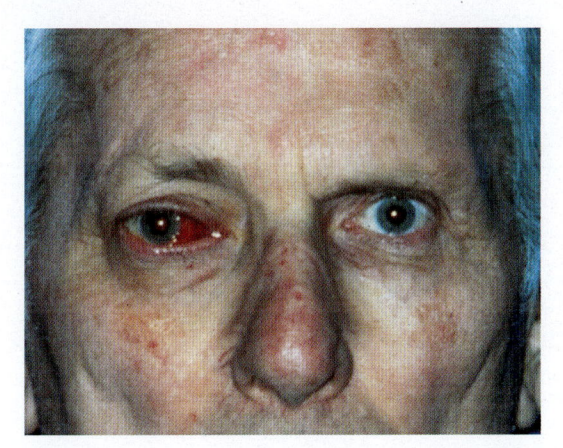

Figure 38.43. Metastatic renal cell carcinoma to the orbit. Proptosis and lateral displacement of the right eye in a 68-year-old man with a history of renal cell carcinoma but no known metastasis. The conjunctival redness is due to a prior biopsy done elsewhere that failed to disclose any tumor cells.

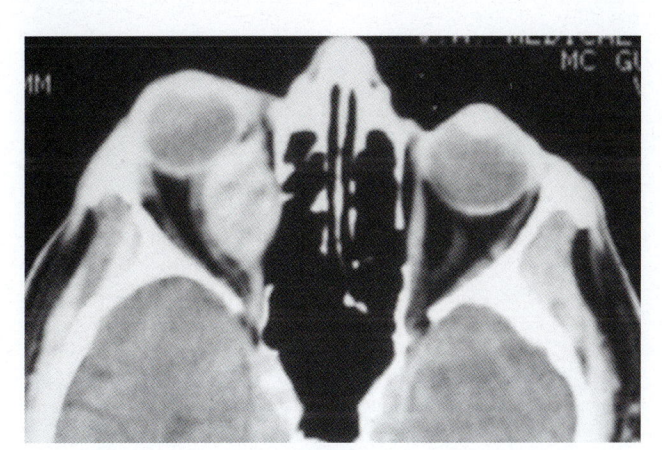

Figure 38.44. Axial computed tomography of patient shown in Figure 38.49, demonstrating ovoid mass in medial aspect of right orbit. The mass was removed.

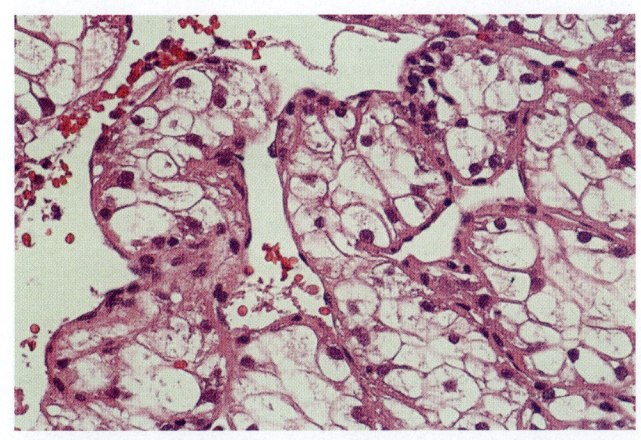

Figure 38.45. Histopathology of lesion shown in Figure 38.43, demonstrating lobules of clear cells compatible with renal cell carcinoma. (Hematoxylin–eosin ×150.)

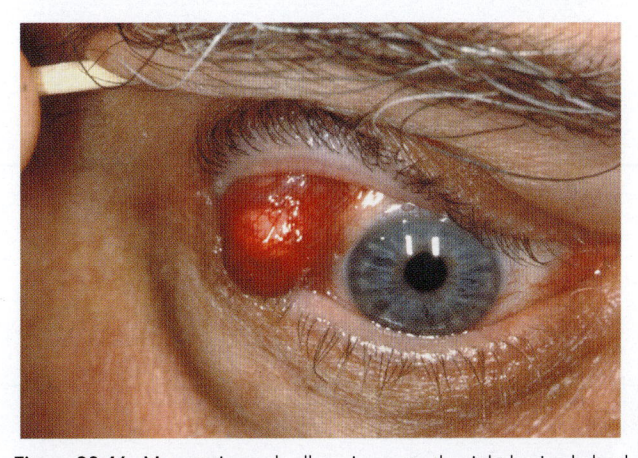

Figure 38.46. Metastatic renal cell carcinoma to the right lacrimal gland in an elderly man. The red color is due to the tendency of metastatic renal cell carcinoma to bleed.

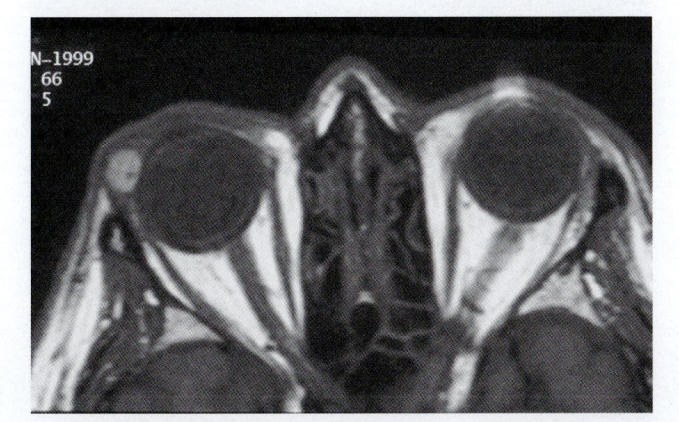

Figure 38.47. Orbital magnetic resonance imaging T1-weighted image with gadolinium enhancement of lesions seen in Figure 38.46, showing enhancing lesion in right lacrimal gland region.

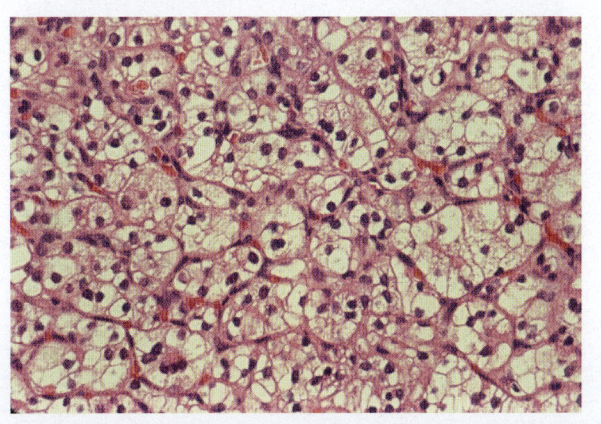

Figure 38.48. Histopathology of lesion shown in Figure 38.53, demonstrating malignant clear cells compatible with renal cell carcinoma. (Hematoxylin–eosin ×150.)

Part 3 Tumors of the Orbit

ORBITAL METASTASIS FROM CUTANEOUS MELANOMA

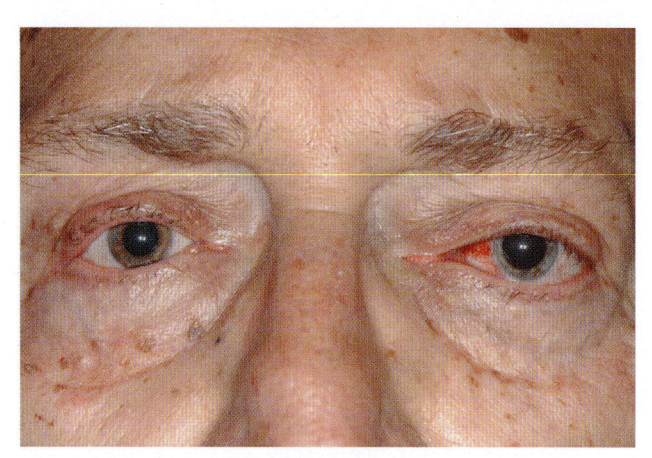

Figure 38.49. Left proptosis and epibulbar hyperemia as first sign of systemic metastasis from cutaneous melanoma in an elderly man.

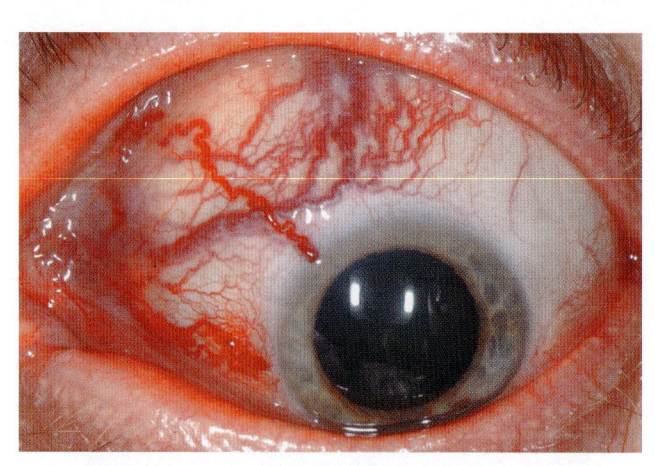

Figure 38.50. Closer view of epibulbar surface showing solid amelanotic mass extending from orbit into the subconjunctival tissues.

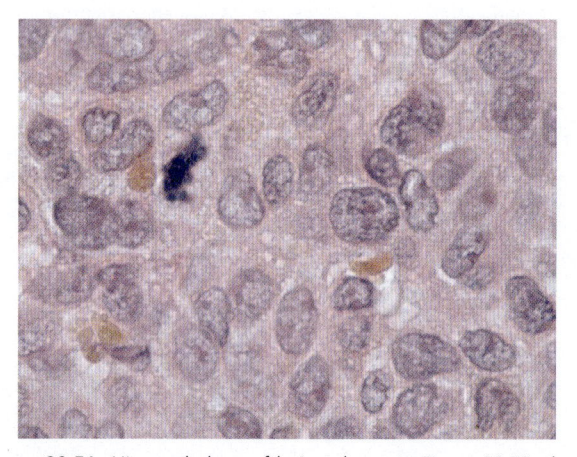

Figure 38.51. Histopathology of lesion shown in Figure 38.50, showing anaplastic epithelioid melanoma cells. Note the mitotic figure. (Hematoxylin–eosin ×250.)

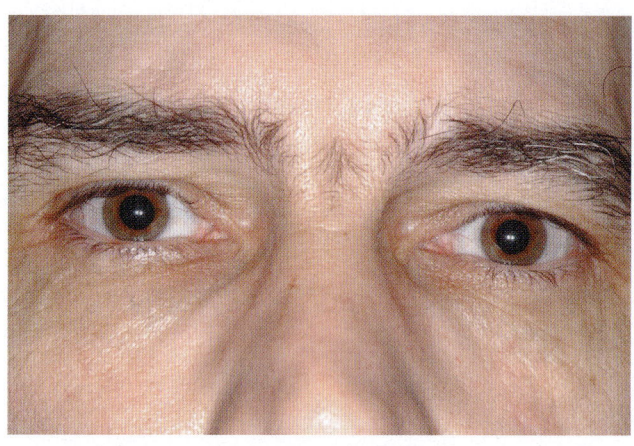

Figure 38.52. Downward displacement of left eye owing to metastatic cutaneous melanoma to the orbit in a middle-aged man.

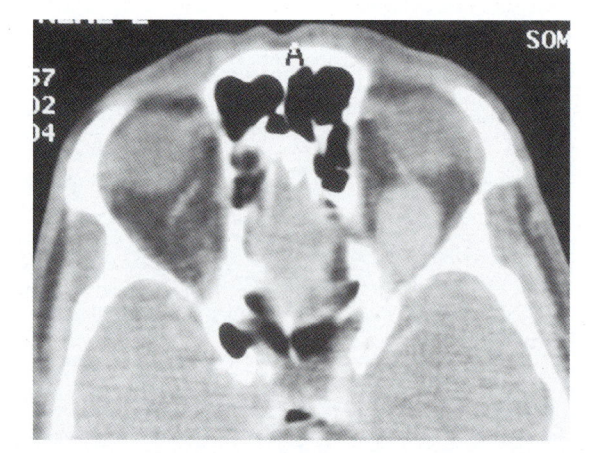

Figure 38.53. Axial computed tomography of patient shown in Figure 38.52. Note the ovoid circumscribed mass in superior aspect of orbit.

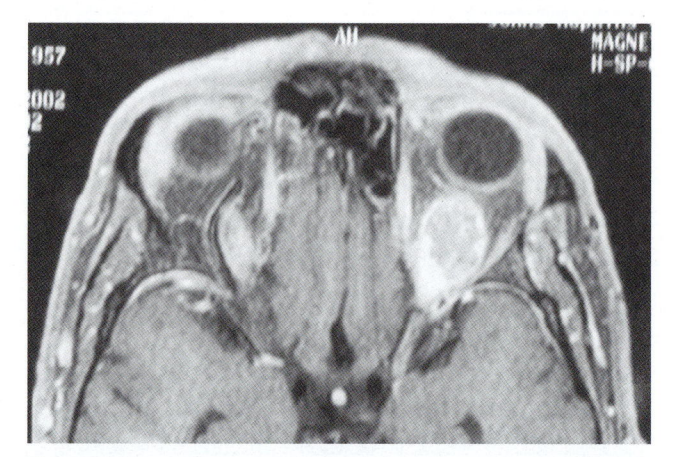

Figure 38.54. Axial magnetic resonance imaging in T1-weighted image with gadolinium enhancement and fat suppression showing enhancement of the mass.

Chapter 38 Orbital Metastatic Cancer   737

● ORBITAL METASTASIS FROM CHOROIDAL MELANOMA

Hematogenous orbital metastasis can occur from uveal melanoma, usually in the setting of systemic metastasis. In such cases, the orbital metastasis is often well circumscribed and affects the extraocular muscles. Two cases are shown of metastasis of choroidal melanoma—one to an ipsilateral rectus muscle and the other to the rectus muscles in the contralateral orbit. Because melanoma metastases are generally well circumscribed, it is often amenable to complete surgical resection as well as irradiation or chemotherapy, depending on the overall circumstances.

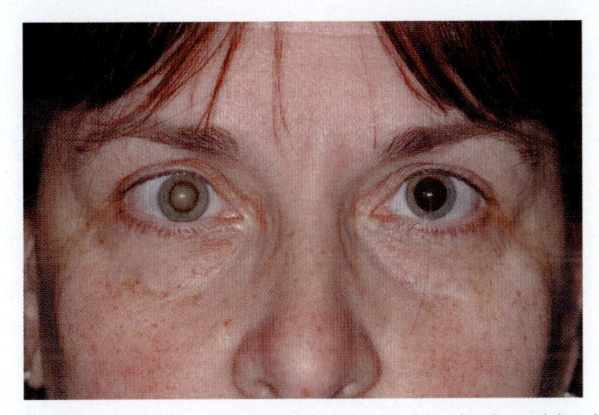

Figure 38.55. In 1989, a 34-year-old woman developed a choroidal melanoma in her right eye and was treated with a radioactive plaque. There was good tumor regression, but she gradually developed radiation retinopathy and cataract. In April 2002, she developed liver metastasis treated with chemoembolization. In August 2003, she developed very subtle swelling of right upper eyelid. Note also the radiation-induced cataract in right eye.

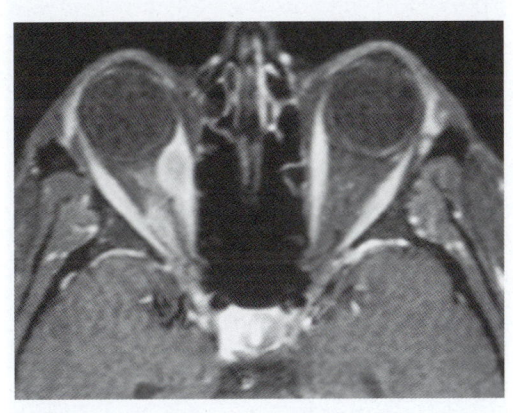

Figure 38.56. Axial magnetic resonance imaging in T1-weighted image shows mass involving right medial rectus muscle.

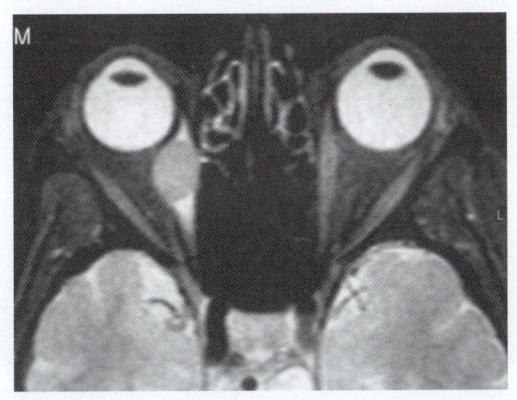

Figure 38.57. Axial magnetic resonance imaging in T2-weighted image showing circumscribed ovoid mass involving medial rectus muscle. On other cuts, a similar mass was detected in the left superior rectus muscle. Widespread metastasis was subsequently detected.

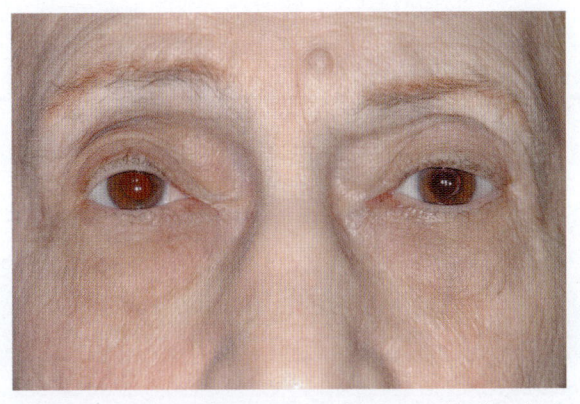

Figure 38.58. In March 1995, a 72-year-old woman developed a large ciliochoroidal melanoma in her right eye and was treated with a radioactive plaque. In April 2002, she developed metastatic melanoma to lung and left orbit. She has mild proptosis of left eye.

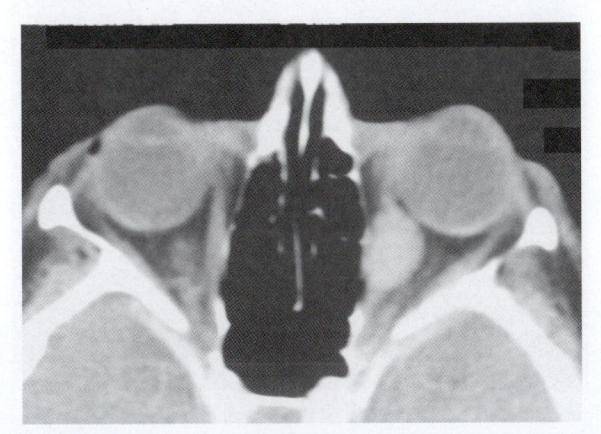

Figure 38.59. Axial computed tomography shows ovoid mass involving the left medial rectus muscle. This was followed and continued to grow; it caused compression of the optic nerve in her only seeing eye, so it was resected by orbitotomy, leaving some tumor tissue in the medial and superior rectus muscles.

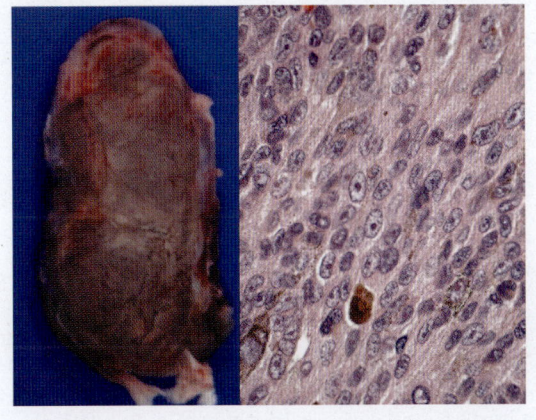

Figure 38.60. Resected tumor appears as a dark ovoid mass that appears to have been removed intact (*left*). Histopathology of metastatic melanoma (*right*). (Hematoxylin–eosin ×250.) The patient retained good visual acuity despite progressive systemic metastasis.

ORBITAL METASTASIS FROM CHOROIDAL MELANOMA TO THE CONTRALATERAL ORBIT

Hematogenous metastasis can occur from choroidal melanoma to the ipsilateral or contralateral orbit. Below is an unusual case in which the contralateral orbit displayed proptosis and metastatic melanoma.

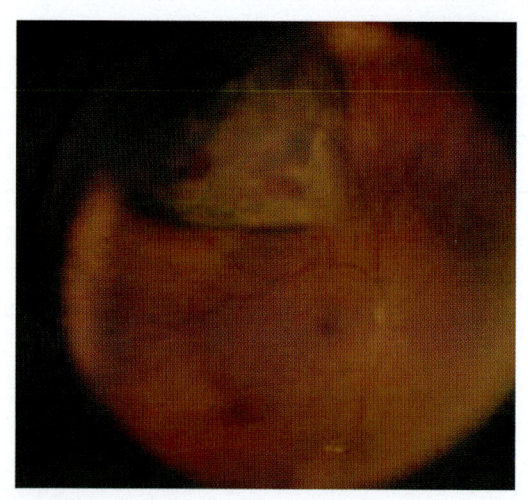

Figure 38.61. Wide-angle image of equatorial melanoma in the right eye of a young woman.

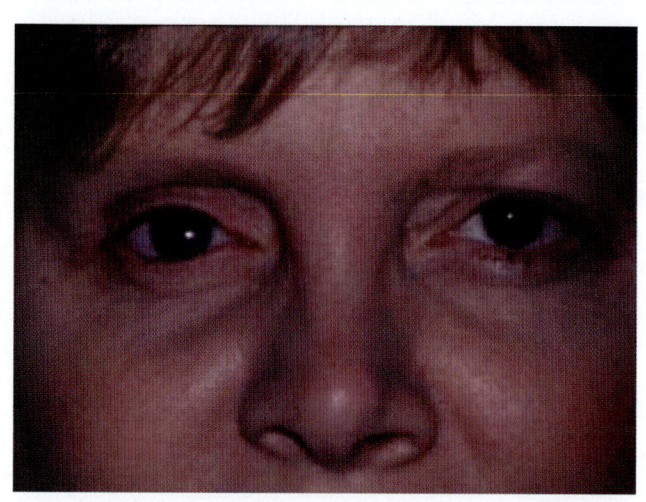

Figure 38.62. Facial photograph of affected patient in Figure 38.61 with new-onset left proptosis.

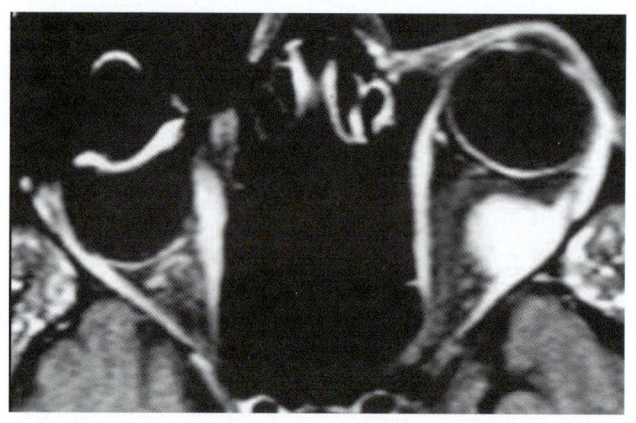

Figure 38.63. Older version magnetic resonance imaging (axial orientation) of orbits showing prosthesis and implant in right orbit and enhancing mass in left orbit.

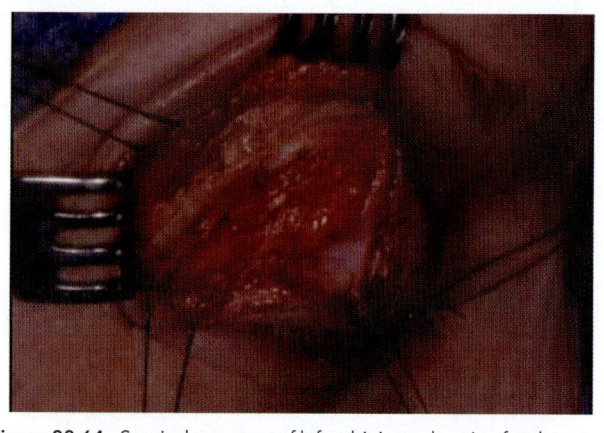

Figure 38.64. Surgical exposure of left orbit in exploration for the mass.

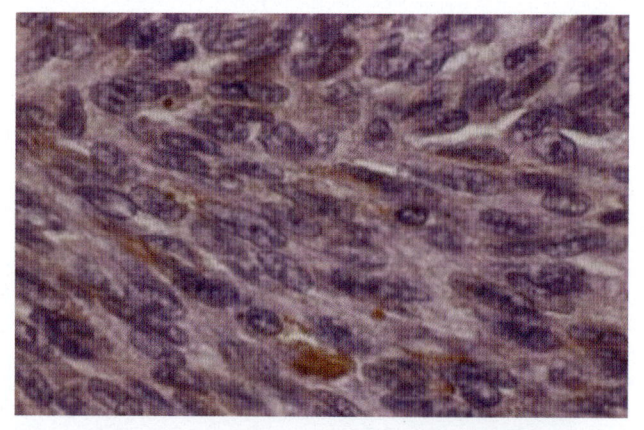

Figure 38.65. Histopathology of the choroidal melanoma was low-grade spindle B melanoma cells. (Hematoxylin–eosin ×200.)

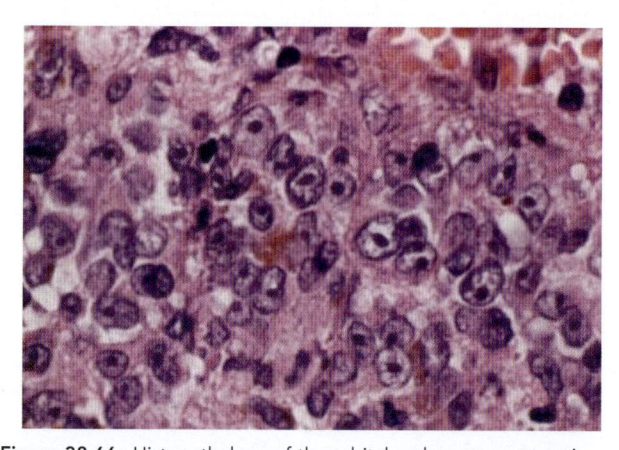

Figure 38.66. Histopathology of the orbital melanoma metastasis was high-grade epithelioid melanoma cells. (Hematoxylin–eosin ×200.)

Chapter 38 Orbital Metastatic Cancer

ORBITAL METASTASIS FROM THYROID CANCER AND ORBITAL METASTASIS FROM AN UNKNOWN PRIMARY SITE

Rare examples are shown of orbital metastasis from thyroid cancer and from an undetermined primary neoplasm.

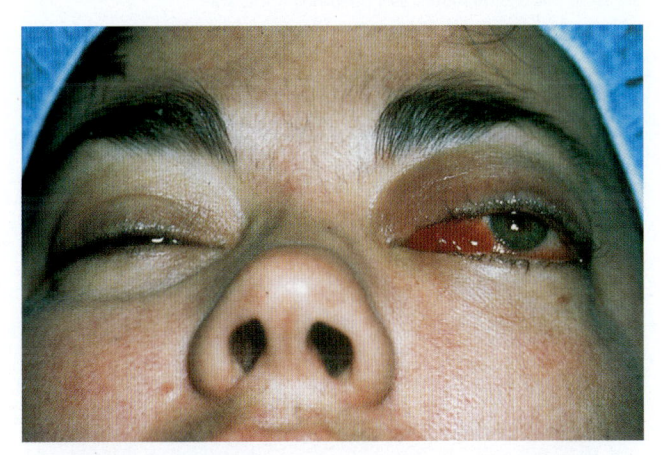

Figure 38.67. Orbital metastasis from Hurthle cell carcinoma of the thyroid gland. Proptosis and chemosis of left eye in a 41-year-old woman. (Courtesy of R. Jean Campbell, MD.)

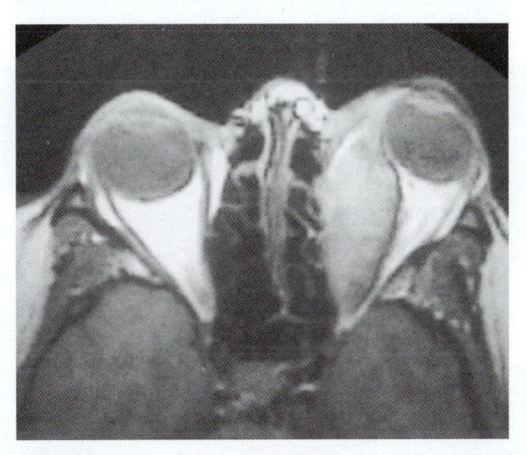

Figure 38.68. Axial magnetic resonance imaging in T1-weighted image of patient seen in Figure 38.61 showing fusiform mass in medial aspect of the orbit, involving the medial rectus muscle. (Courtesy of R. Jean Campbell, MD.)

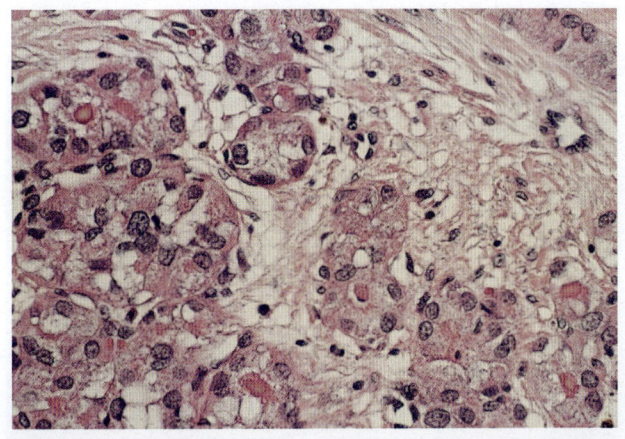

Figure 38.69. Histopathology showing solid lobule and acini of tumor cells. Immunohistochemical stains for thyroglobulin were markedly positive. (Hematoxylin–eosin ×150.) (Courtesy of R. Jean Campbell, MD.)

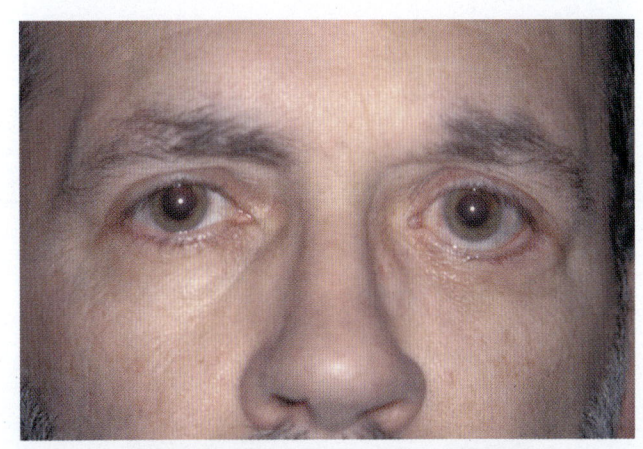

Figure 38.70. Proptosis of left eye in a middle-aged man.

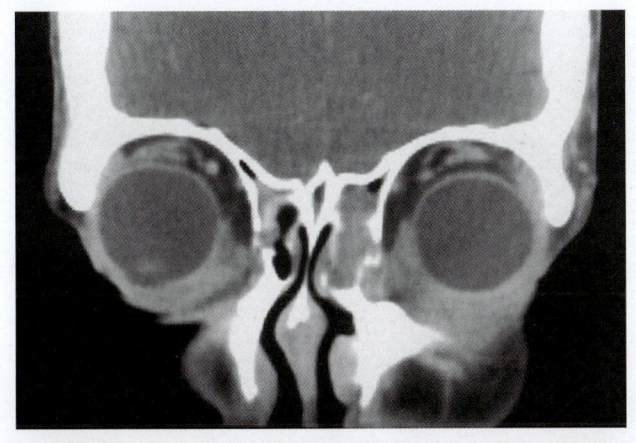

Figure 38.71. Coronal computed tomography shows diffuse, ill-defined mass in inferior aspect of left orbit. Biopsy revealed poorly differentiated adenocarcinoma compatible with metastatic carcinoma. No primary neoplasm was found on extensive systemic evaluation. The lesion was largely removed by a debulking procedure.

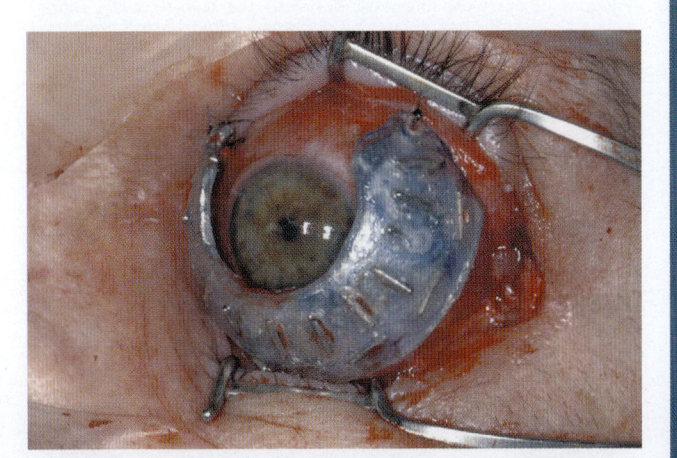

Figure 38.72. Residual orbital tumor in patient shown in Figures 38.64 and 38.65 was treated with plaque brachytherapy after >90% of the tumor was removed surgically. Shown is a custom-designed reversed plaque constructed to protect the globe and to irradiate the residual orbital tumor.

ORBITAL METASTASIS OF ADRENAL NEUROBLASTOMA

Neuroblastoma is the most common neoplasm to exhibit orbital metastasis in children. In most cases of metastatic neuroblastoma, a prior diagnosis of adrenal gland neuroblastoma has been made. In exceptional cases, the orbital metastasis becomes apparent before the primary abdominal mass is found. Two such cases are illustrated.

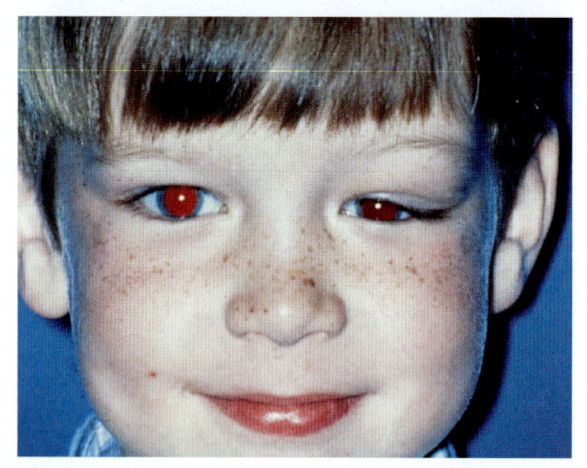

Figure 38.73. Proptosis and blepharoptosis of the left eye in a 6-year-old boy.

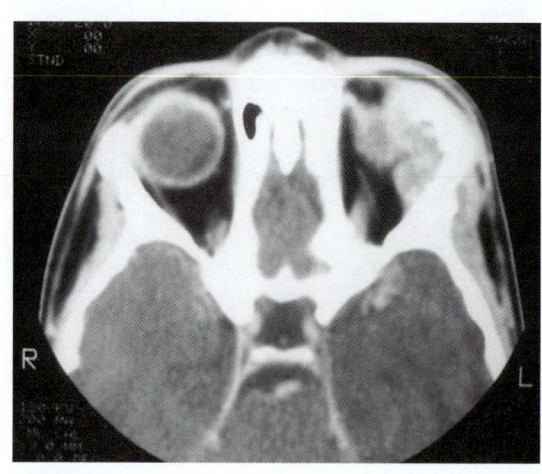

Figure 38.74. Axial computed tomography of patient shown in Figure 38.67, demonstrating irregular mass involving soft tissue and bone in the superotemporal aspect of the orbit.

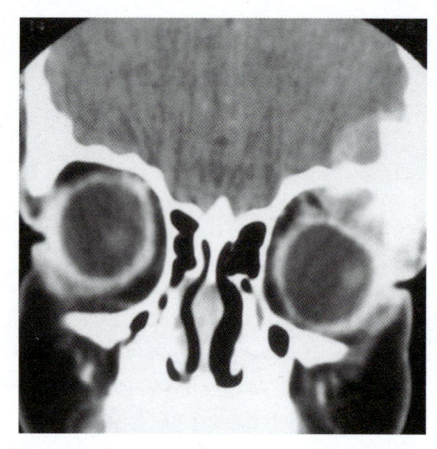

Figure 38.75. Coronal computed tomography showing lesion depicted in Figure 38.68. Note the extension into the cranial cavity. Biopsy revealed metastatic neuroblastoma. A primary adrenal gland tumor was subsequently detected.

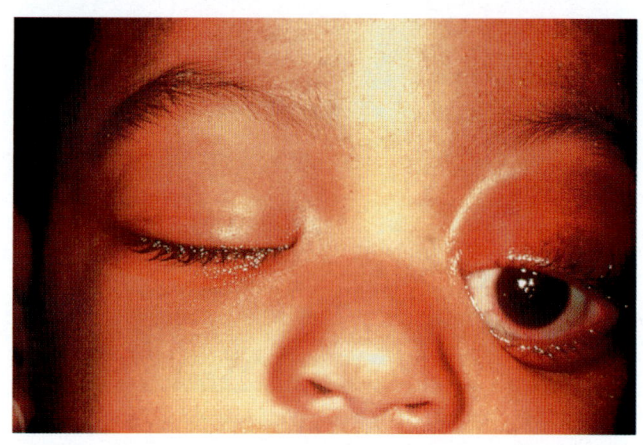

Figure 38.76. Proptosis of the left eye in a 2-year-old girl. (Courtesy of Julia Stevens, MD and Morton Smith, MD.)

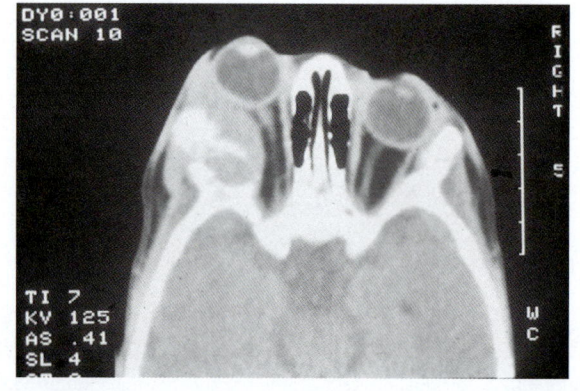

Figure 38.77. Axial computed tomography of patient shown in Figure 38.70, revealing a superotemporal bone-destructive orbital lesion similar to the first patient. (Courtesy of Julia Stevens, MD and Morton Smith, MD.)

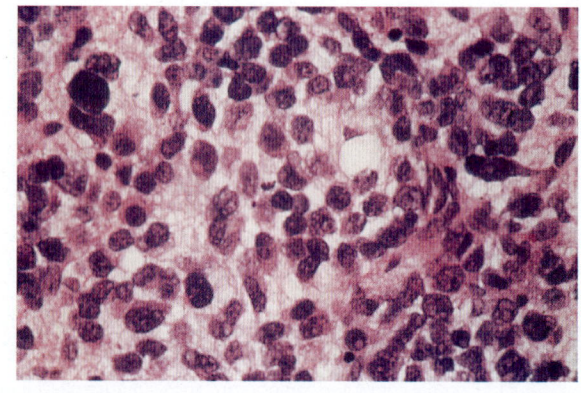

Figure 38.78. Histopathology of lesion shown in Figure 38.71, demonstrating malignant neuroblastic cells. (Hematoxylin–eosin ×250.) (Courtesy of Julia Stevens, MD and Morton Smith, MD.)

ORBITAL METASTASIS: WILMS' TUMOR, EWING'S TUMOR, AND RHABDOMYOSARCOMA

1. Fratkin D, Purcell JJ, Krachmer JH. Wilm's tumor metastasis to the orbit. *JAMA* 1977;238:1841–1842.
2. Kawachi E, Nunobiki K, Shimada S, et al. A case of Ewing's sarcoma with orbital metastasis. *Folia Ophthalmol Jpn* 1984;35:1840–1845.
3. Fekrat S, Miller NR, Loury MC. Alveolar rhabdomyosarcoma that metastasized to the orbit. *Arch Ophthalmol* 1993;111:1662–1664.

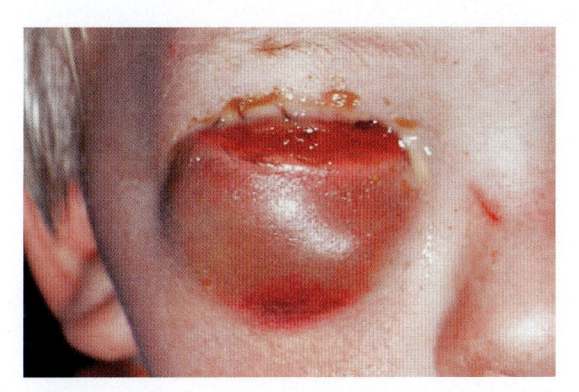

Figure 38.79. Severe proptosis and eyelid hemorrhage secondary to metastatic Wilms' tumor to the right orbit in a young child. (Courtesy of John Purcell, MD.)

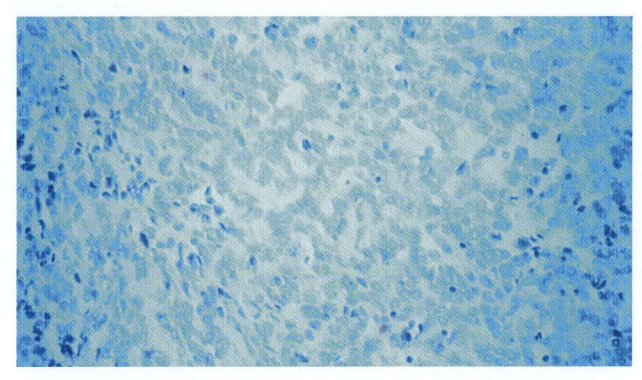

Figure 38.80. Histopathology of lesion shown in Figure 38.73. (Hematoxylin–eosin ×50.) (Courtesy of John Purcell, MD.)

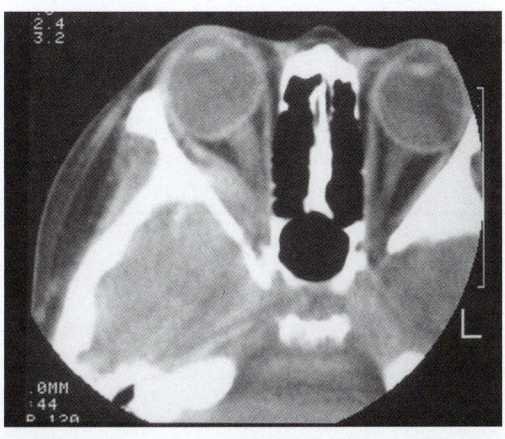

Figure 38.81. Axial computed tomography showing metastatic Ewing's tumor to right orbit along the lateral rectus muscle. (Courtesy of Eiko Kawachi, MD.)

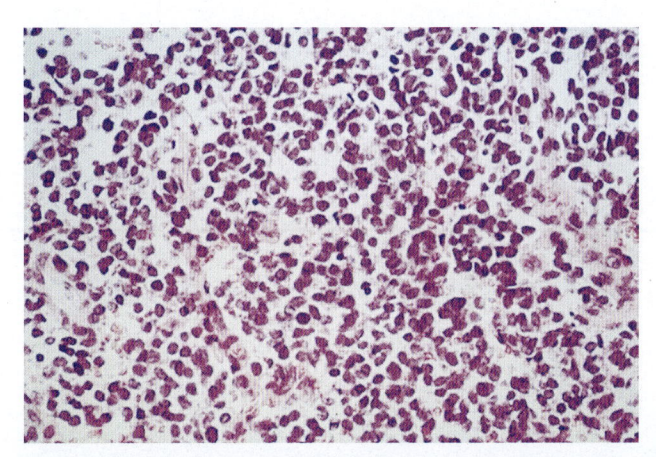

Figure 38.82. Histopathology of lesion shown in Figure 38.75, demonstrating small round cells characteristic of metastatic Ewing's sarcoma to the orbit. (Courtesy of Eiko Kawachi, MD.)

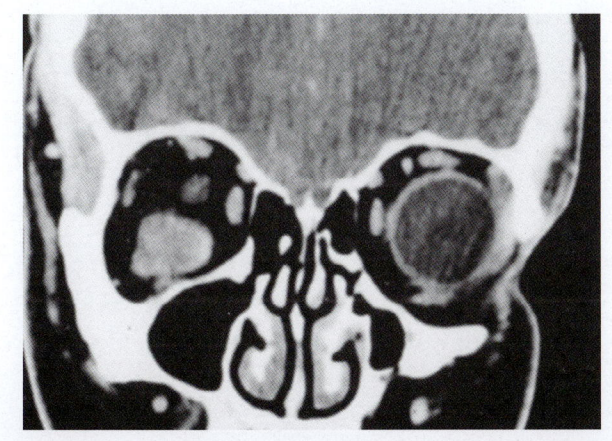

Figure 38.83. Metastatic rhabdomyosarcoma to the orbit in a 22-year-old woman who had a paravaginal alveolar rhabdomyosarcoma. (Courtesy of Neil Miller, MD.)

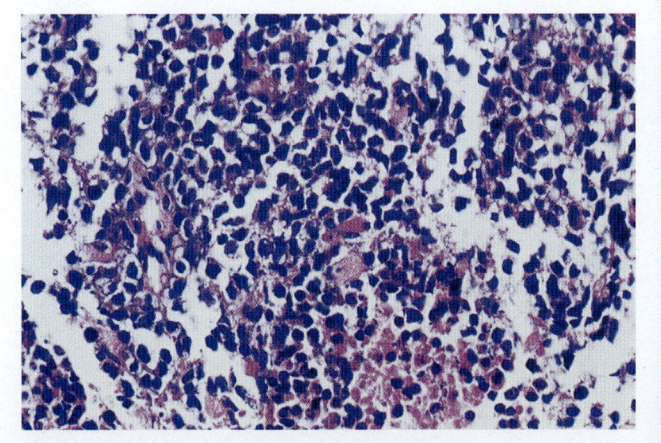

Figure 38.84. Histopathology of lesion shown in Figure 38.77, showing features compatible with metastatic rhabdomyosarcoma. (Hematoxylin–eosin ×100.) (Courtesy of Neil Miller, MD.)

CHAPTER 39

ORBITAL LYMPHOID TUMORS AND LEUKEMIAS

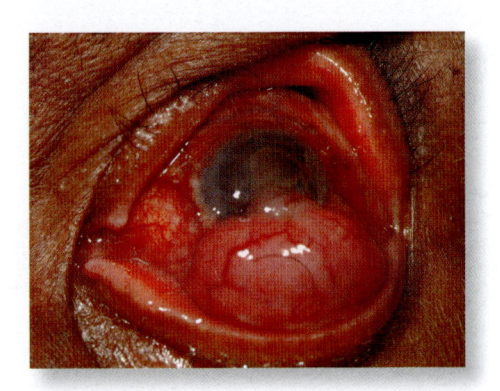

General Considerations

Lymphoma is a malignant neoplasms arising from a clonal proliferation of B- or T-cell lymphocytes (1–3). There are two major groups of lymphoma including Hodgkin lymphoma and non-Hodgkin lymphoma (NHL). The NHLs are categorized on the basis of cell of origin and approximately 80% arise from B lymphocytes, 14% from T lymphocytes, and 6% from natural killer cells (2,3). There are several classifications of ocular adnexal lymphoid tumors including the Revised European American Lymphoma (REAL) classification by the World Health Organization (WHO), the Ann Arbor classification, the American Joint Committee on Cancer (AJCC) classification, and others (3). The REAL classification has been updated by the WHO and below is the WHO 2008 classification of mature B-cell neoplasms (Table 39.1) (3). There is another orbital adnexal lymphoid tumor classification using American Joint Committee on Cancer (AJCC), based on tumor extent and specific location (Table 39.2).

Lymphoma can affect any part of the eye and adnexa. Most are primary tumors of the NHL of B-cell type and the most common primary type in the periocular region is extranodal marginal zone B-cell lymphoma (ENMZL) of mucosa-associated lymphoid tissue (MALT). This low-grade mucosa-associated lymphoid tumor tends to occur in both the orbit and conjunctiva (1–29). Less common orbital lymphoid lesions like Burkitt lymphoma, T-cell lymphoma, plasmacytoma, plasmablastic lymphoma, and leukemias are also discussed. T-cell lymphoma (mycosis fungoides) more typically involves the eyelids.

NHL in the orbit and ocular adnexa region has traditionally been divided into benign (benign reactive lymphoid hyperplasia [BRLH]), intermediate (atypical lymphoid hyperplasia [ALH]), or malignant categories. It is difficult to determine clinically whether a particular lymphoid lesion is benign or malignant and histopathologic evaluation is necessary to categorize these lesions. For reasons of brevity, the term "lymphoma," "lymphoid tumor," or "lymphoproliferative tumor" is used to describe these variations.

In general, orbital lymphoid tumor has characteristic clinical, radiographic, and pathologic features. It usually occurs in older individuals, and is the most common malignant orbital tumor of older patients, accounting for 24% of all orbital malignancies in patients >59 years old (7). Orbital lymphoma can be confined to the orbit or it can be a part of systemic lymphoma. Although estimates vary, the 10-year incidence of systemic lymphoma among patients with orbital lymphoma is approximately 33% for those with unilateral disease and 72% for those with bilateral disease (8).

An unusual form of orbital lymphoma can follow organ transplantation and is believed to result from immunosuppression. This form is termed "post-transplant lymphoproliferative disorder" (PTLD) and is found to be related to Epstein–Barr

ORBITAL NON-HODGKIN LYMPHOMA

Table 39.1 World Health Organization (WHO) 2008 classification of B-cell neoplasms

Non-Hodgkin lymphoma

Chronic lymphocytic leukemia/small lymphocytic lymphoma

B-cell prolymphocytic leukemia

Splenic marginal zone lymphoma

Hairy cell leukemia

Splenic lymphoma/leukemia, unclassifiable
- Splenic diffuse red pulp small B-cell lymphoma
- Hairy cell leukemia—variant

Lymphoplasmacytic lymphoma
- Waldenström macroglobulinemia

Heavy chain diseases
- Alpha heavy chain disease
- Gamma heavy chain disease
- Mu heavy chain disease

Plasma cell myeloma

Solitary plasmacytoma of bone

Extraosseous plasmacytoma

Extranodal marginal zone B-cell lymphoma of mucosa-associated lymphoid tissue (MALT lymphoma)

Nodal marginal zone B-cell lymphoma (MZL)
- Pediatric type nodal MZL

Follicular lymphoma
- Pediatric type follicular lymphoma

Primary cutaneous follicle center lymphoma

Mantle cell lymphoma

Diffuse large B-cell lymphoma (DLBCL), not otherwise specified
- T-cell/histiocyte rich large B-cell lymphoma
- DLBCL associated with chronic inflammation
- Epstein–Barr virus (EBV), DLBCL of the elderly

Lymphomatoid granulomatosis

Primary mediastinal (thymic) large B-cell lymphoma

Intravascular large B-cell lymphoma

Primary cutaneous DLBCL, leg type

ALK+ large B-cell lymphoma

Plasmablastic lymphoma

Primary effusion lymphoma

Large B-cell lymphoma arising in HHV8-associated multicentric Castleman disease

Burkitt lymphoma

B-cell lymphoma, unclassifiable (features between diffuse large B-cell lymphoma and Burkitt lymphoma)

B-cell lymphoma, unclassifiable (features between diffuse large B-cell lymphoma and Hodgkin lymphoma)

Hodgkin Lymphoma

Nodular lymphocyte-predominant Hodgkin lymphoma

Classical Hodgkin lymphoma
- Nodular sclerosis classical Hodgkin lymphoma
- Lymphocyte-rich classical Hodgkin lymphoma
- Mixed cellularity classical Hodgkin lymphoma
- Lymphocyte-depleted classical Hodgkin lymphoma

Jaffe ES. The 2008 WHO classification of lymphomas: implications for clinical practice and translational research. *Hematology* 2009;523–531.

ORBITAL NON-HODGKIN LYMPHOMA

Table 39.2 American Joint Committee on Cancer (AJCC) classification of ocular adnexal lymphoma

Clinical stage	Definition
Primary tumor (T)	
Tx	Tumor extent cannot be assessed
T0	Tumor absent
T1	Tumor in conjunctiva
T1a	Tumor in bulbar conjunctiva
T1b	Tumor in palpebral, forniceal, caruncular conjunctiva
T1c	Tumor extensive in conjunctiva
T2	Tumor in orbit
T2a	Tumor in orbit anteriorly
T2b	Tumor in orbit and lacrimal gland
T2c	Tumor in orbit posteriorly
T2d	Tumor in orbit and nasolacrimal system
T3	Tumor in preseptal eyelid
T4	Tumor in orbit plus additional bone or brain
T4a	Tumor in additional nasopharynx
T4b	Tumor in additional bone
T4c	Tumor in additional sinuses
T4d	Tumor in additional brain
Regional lymph node (N)	
Nx	Regional lymph nodes cannot be assessed
N0	Regional lymph node involvement absent
N1	Regional lymph node ipsilateral involvement present
N2	Regional lymph node contralateral/bilateral involvement present
N3	Regional lymph node remote from ocular region present
N4	Central lymph node involvement present
Distant metastasis (M)	
M0	Distant metastasis cannot be assessed
M1a	Distant involvement in noncontiguous tissue (parotid, lung, liver, spleen, kidney, breast)
M1b	Distant involvement in bone marrow
M1c	Both M1a and M1b present

Edge SB, Byrd DR, Compton CC, et al, eds. Carcinoma of the conjunctiva. In: AJCC Cancer Staging Manual. 7th ed. New York, NY: Springer; 2010:583–589.

virus (EBV)-related lymphoma, best managed with reduction in immune suppression to allow the host immune system to control the viral-related condition (29).

Clinical Features

Orbital lymphoma typically presents as a painless, slowly progressive, unilateral or bilateral anterior orbital mass that can often be palpable through the eyelid or conjunctiva as a rubbery mass. It is important in such cases to inspect the conjunctiva for the typical fleshy (salmon patch) infiltration and to check the uveal tract for iris or choroidal infiltration that, if present, strongly suggests that the orbital lesion is lymphoma.

Diagnostic Approaches

The patient with a suspected orbital lymphoma should undergo a thorough systemic evaluation to detect and determine the extent of any associated systemic lymphoma. With regard to the orbital lesion, computed tomography (CT) and magnetic resonance imaging (MRI) disclose an ovoid or elongated mass that tends to mold to adjacent orbital structures and shows moderate enhancement with contrast agents. It is usually confined to soft tissue. Bone involvement is uncommon. Orbital lymphoid tumor can occur anywhere in the orbit and is commonly confined to the lacrimal gland. Lymphoid tumors that arise in the lacrimal gland should be differentiated from primary epithelial tumors of the lacrimal gland. Lymphoid tumors generally have an oblong, ovoid, or pancake contour and mold to the globe and orbital bones, usually without producing a bony fossa or bony erosion. In contrast, epithelial tumors of the lacrimal gland tend to have a more rounded contour and tend to compress the bone, producing a fossa or sometimes true bone destruction.

Pathology

Most benign or malignant orbital lymphomas are of the B-cell type, classified histopathologically as ENMZL of MALT (8,10). There is a spectrum of orbital lymphoma ranging from BRLH to ALH to frank lymphoma. BRLH is characterized by a polymorphous array of small round lymphocytes and plasma cells. Mitotically active germinal centers are frequently present. ALH is an intermediate form between BRLH and frank malignant lymphoma. It is composed of monomorphous sheets of lymphocytes. In contrast with BRLH, the nuclei are somewhat larger, prominent nucleoli can be present, and abortive follicles can be observed. Malignant NHL is characterized by more anaplastic cells with larger cleaved nuclei, more nuclear pleomorphism, and frequent prominent nucleoli. Lymph follicles and endothelial cell proliferation are absent or less evident (9,22,24).

Management

Management of suspected orbital lymphoma is individualized to each case. An excisional or incisional orbital biopsy is generally advisable and the best approach to biopsy is determined by imaging studies. Prior communication with a pathologist is important so that the excised tissue can be appropriately processed for immunohistochemistry and flow cytometry. The surgeon should debulk the entire tumor or as much of the orbital tumor as possible, attempting to avoid damage to vital orbital structures.

Systemic physical examination and imaging studies should be performed to rule out remote lymphoma (8). If the patient has established systemic lymphoma and the orbital lesion is located anteriorly beneath the skin, a fine-needle biopsy can help to establish the orbital diagnosis, thus avoiding an open biopsy. If systemic lymphoma is present and chemotherapy is advised, then the orbital lesion can usually be followed while on chemotherapy with no further treatment. If no systemic lymphoma is found, then the orbital lymphoma can be treated with local orbital radiotherapy using 2,000 to 2,500 cGy for more benign lesions and 3,500 to 4,000 cGy for malignant lesions (1,8,10,14–17). Other alternative therapies include systemic intravenous or local injection of rituximab immunotherapy. In one analysis of 10 patients with orbital lymphoma and no systemic disease who were treated with intravenous rituximab, complete lymphoma control at mean 2.5-year follow-up was found in 36% and additional radiotherapy was necessary in those who had partial response or recurrence (64%) (19). Even if evaluation for systemic lymphoma is negative, the patient should have yearly or biyearly follow-up for the development of systemic lymphoma.

In an analysis of treatment outcome based on AJCC (Table 39.2) versus Ann Arbor classification of lymphoma, it was found that results were more often related to the histopathology (Table 39.1) rather than the tumor size of specific location as in these classifications (4). In another analysis on 130 patients classified by AJCC 7th edition for ocular adnexal lymphoma (Table 39.2), treatment varied depending on histologic type (Table 39.1) and increasing AJCC tumor category was associated with worse 5-year survival (5). Specifically, 5-year survival was 68% for T1, 59% for T2, 29% for T3, and 33% for T4.

Orbital ENMZL requires special mention because of the recent revelations regarding its relationship to gastric MALT lymphoma and *Helicobacter pylori* and *Chlamydia* species. There is currently interest in treating some cases of MALT lymphoma of the conjunctiva and orbit with antibiotics directed toward these organisms.

Selected References

Reviews

1. Shields JA, Shields CL, Scartozzi R. Survey of 1264 patients with orbital tumors and simulating lesions: the 2002 Montgomery Lecture, part 1. *Ophthalmology* 2004;111: 997–1008.
2. Coupland SE, Damato B. Lymphomas involving the eye and ocular adnexa. *Curr Opin Ophthalmol* 2006;17:523–531.
3. Jaffe ES. The 2008 WHO classification of lymphomas: implications for clinical practice and translational research. *Hematology* 2009;523–531.
4. Graue GF, Finger PT, Maher E, et al. Ocular adnexal lymphoma staging and treatment: American Joint Committee on Cancer versus Ann Arbor. *Eur J Ophthalmol* 2013;23:344–355.
5. Sniegowski MC, Roberts D, Bakhoun M, et al. Ocular adnexal lymphoma: validation of American Joint Committee on Cancer seventh edition staging guidelines. *Br J Ophthalmol* 2014;98:1255–1260.
6. Aronow ME, Portell CA, Rybicki LA, et al. Ocular adnexal lymphoma: assessment of a tumor node metastasis staging system. *Ophthalmology* 2013;120:1915–1919.
7. Demirci H, Shields CL, Shields JA, et al. Orbital tumors in the older adult population. *Ophthalmology* 2002;109:243–248.
8. Demirci H, Shields CL, Karatza EC, et al. Orbital lymphoproliferative tumors: Analysis of clinical features and systemic involvement in 160 cases. *Ophthalmology* 2008;115:1626–1631.
9. Cockerham GC, Jakobiec FA. Lymphoproliferative disorders of the ocular adnexa. *Int Ophthalmol Clin* 1997;37:39–59.
10. Coupland SE, Krause L, Delecluse HJ, et al. Lymphoproliferative lesions of the ocular adnexa. Analysis of 112 cases. *Ophthalmology* 1998;105:1430–1441.
11. Lauer SA. Ocular adnexal lymphoid tumors. *Curr Opin Ophthalmol* 2000;11: 361–366.
12. Malek SN, Hatfield AJ, Flinn IW. MALT lymphomas. *Curr Treat Options Oncol* 2003;4:269–279.
13. Tranfa F, Di Matteo G, Strianese D, et al. Primary orbital lymphoma. *Orbit* 2001;20: 119–124.

Management

14. Yeo JH, Jakobiec FA, Abbott GF, et al. Combined clinical and computed tomographic diagnosis of orbital lymphoid tumors. *Am J Ophthalmol* 1982;94:235–245.
15. Kennerdell JS, Flores NE, Hartsock RJ. Low-dose radiotherapy for lymphoid lesions of the orbit and ocular adnexa. *Ophthal Plast Reconstr Surg* 1999;15:129–133.
16. Bolek TW, Moyses HM, Marcus RB Jr, et al. Radiotherapy in the management of orbital lymphoma. *Int J Radiat Oncol Biol Phys* 1999;44:31–36.
17. Lee SW, Suh CO, Kim GE, et al. Role of radiotherapy for primary orbital lymphoma. *Am J Clin Oncol* 2002;25:261–265.
18. Harada K, Murakami N, Kitaguchi M, et al. Localized ocular adnexal mucosa-associated lymphoid tissue lymphoma treated with radiation therapy: a long-term outcome in 86 patients with 104 treated eyes. *Int J Radiat Oncol Biol Phys* 2014;88: 650–654.
19. Tuncer S, Tanyildiz B, Basaran M, et al. Systemic rituximab immunotherapy in the management of primary ocular adnexal lymphoma: single institution experience. *Curr Eye Res* 2014;23:1–6.
20. Rath S, Connors JM, Dolman PJ, et al. Comparison of American Joint Committee on Cancer TNM-based staging system (7th edition) and Ann Arbor classification for predicting outcome in ocular adnexal lymphoma. *Orbit* 2014;33:23–28.
21. Rasmussen PK, Coupland SE, Finger PT, et al. Ocular adnexal follicular lymphoma: a multicenter international study. *JAMA Ophthalmol* 2014;132:851–858.

Histopathology

22. Knowles DM II, Jakobiec FA. Ocular adnexal lymphoid neoplasms: clinical, histopathologic, electron microscopic, and immunologic characteristics. *Hum Pathol* 1982;13:148–162.
23. Nicolo M, Truini M, Sertoli M, et al. Follicular large-cell lymphoma of the orbit: a clinicopathologic, immunohistochemical and molecular genetic description of one case. *Graefes Arch Clin Exp Ophthalmol* 1999;237:606–610.
24. Medeiros LJ, Harris NL. Lymphoid infiltrates of the orbit and conjunctiva. A morphologic and immunophenotypic study of 99 cases. *Am J Surg Pathol* 1989;13:459–471.

Case Reports

25. Adkins JW, Shields JA, Shields CL, et al. Plasmacytoma of the eye and orbit. *Int Ophthalmol* 1996;20:339–343.
26. Park KL, Goins KM. Hodgkin's lymphoma of the orbit associated with acquired immunodeficiency syndrome. *Am J Ophthalmol* 1993;116:111–112.
27. Font RL, Laucirica R, Patrinely JR. Immunoblastic B-cell malignant lymphoma involving the orbit and maxillary sinus in a patient with acquired immune deficiency syndrome. *Ophthalmology* 1993;100:966–970.
28. Font RL, Shields JA. Large cell lymphoma of the orbit with microvillous projections ("porcupine lymphoma"). *Arch Ophthalmol* 1985;103:1715–1719.
29. Douglas RS, Goldstein SM, Katowitz JA, et al. Orbital presentation of posttransplantation lymphoproliferative disorder: a small case series. *Ophthalmology* 2002;109: 2351–2355.

ORBITAL NON-HODGKIN LYMPHOMA: CLINICAL, COMPUTED TOMOGRAPHY, AND MAGNETIC RESONANCE IMAGING FEATURES

Orbital lymphoma has rather characteristic clinical and radiographic features that should strongly suggest the diagnosis.

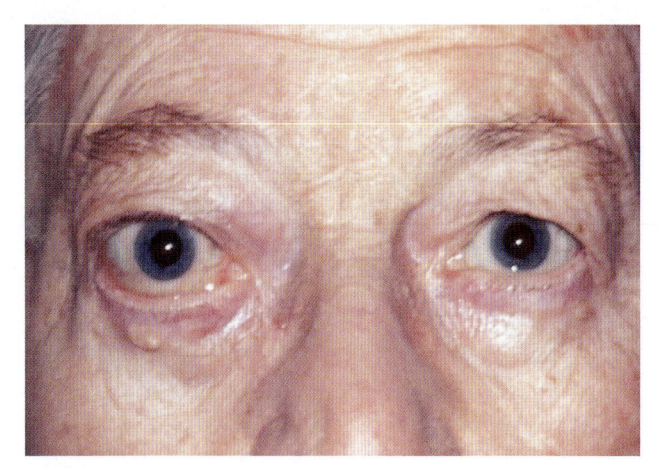

Figure 39.1. Slight proptosis of the right eye in a 90-year-old man with no prior history of lymphoma.

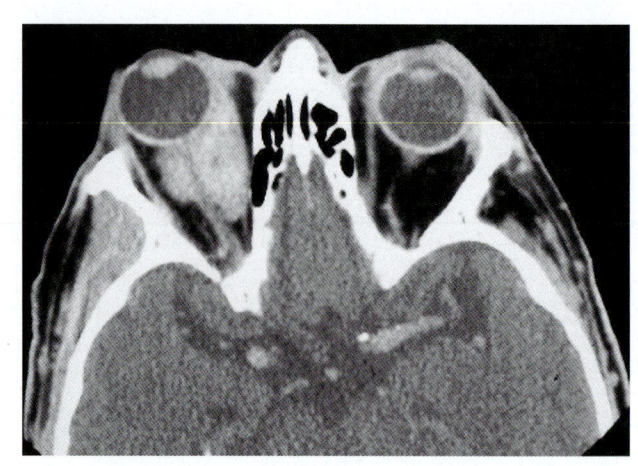

Figure 39.2. Axial computed tomography of patient shown in Figure 39.1. Note the characteristic diffuse orbital mass that molds to the globe and optic nerve. In such a case, incisional biopsy can be done under local anesthesia.

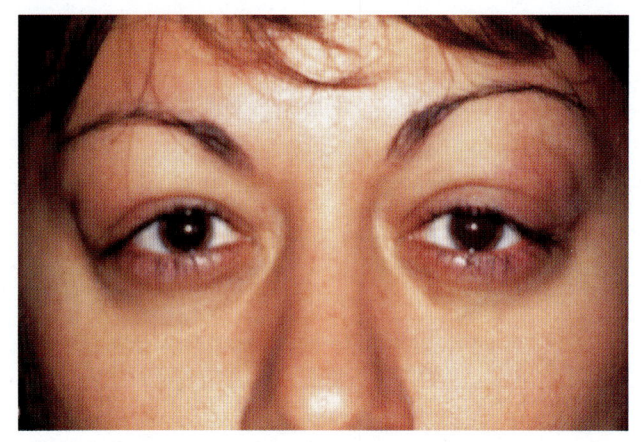

Figure 39.3. Bilateral lacrimal gland involvement by lymphoma. Note the superotemporal orbital fullness bilaterally in this 37-year-old woman.

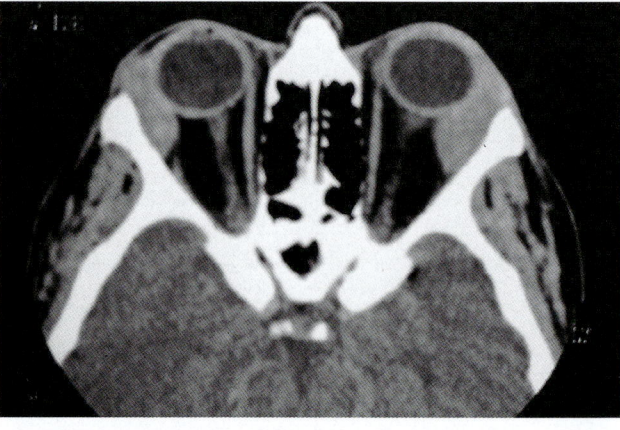

Figure 39.4. Axial computed tomography of patient shown in Figure 39.3, showing the bilateral orbital masses that affect the lacrimal glands and mold to the globe and orbital bone.

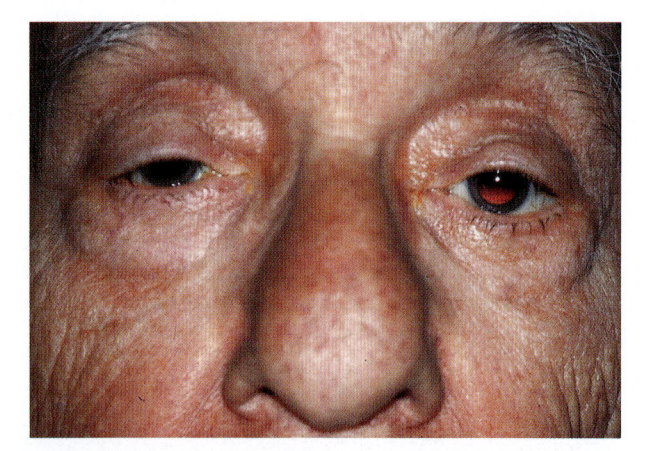

Figure 39.5. Proptosis and blepharoptosis of the right eye in an 86-year-old man.

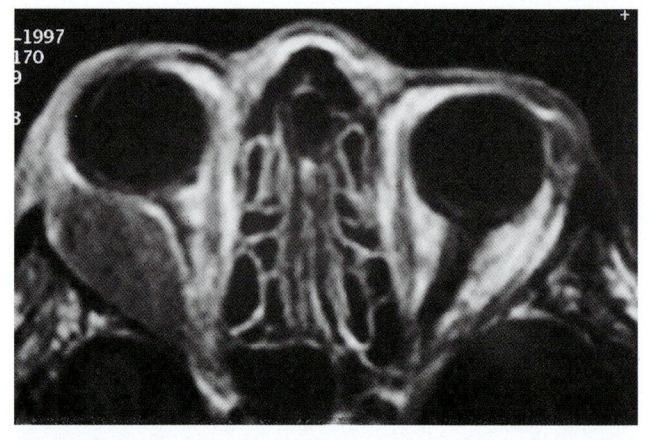

Figure 39.6. Axial magnetic resonance imaging in T1-weighted image of patient shown in Figure 39.5 showing diffuse ovoid mass in temporal aspect of the right orbit.

Chapter 39 Orbital Lymphoid Tumors and Leukemias

ORBITAL NON-HODGKIN LYMPHOMA: CLINICAL VARIATIONS AND PATHOLOGY

In a patient with suspected orbital lymphoma, it is important to perform a complete ocular examination. The finding of typical lymphoma of the conjunctiva or uveal tract should strongly suggest that the orbital lesion is lymphoma.

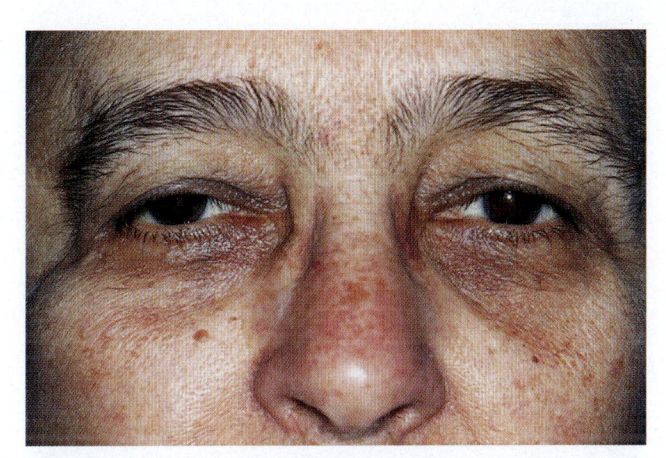

Figure 39.7. Minimal blepharoptosis and proptosis of right eye in a 68-year-old woman.

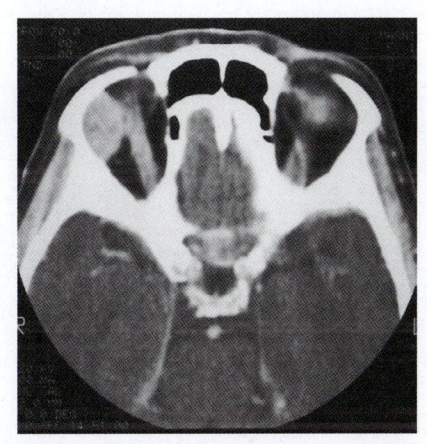

Figure 39.8. Axial computed tomography showing ovoid mass in superotemporal aspect of orbit in patient seen in Figure 39.7.

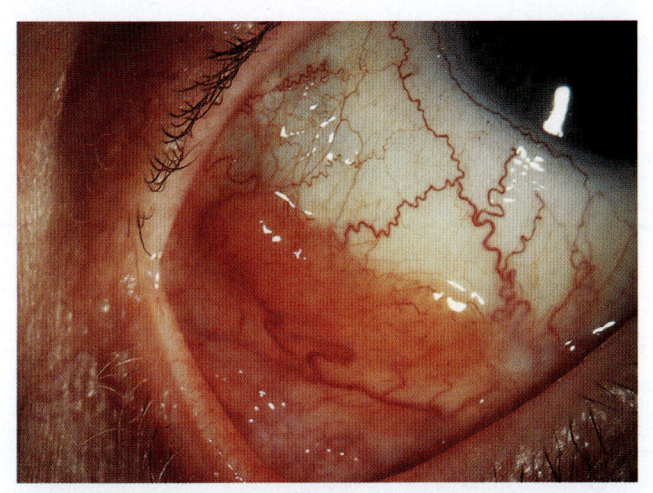

Figure 39.9. Subtle lymphoid infiltration in inferotemporal conjunctival fornix in same patient.

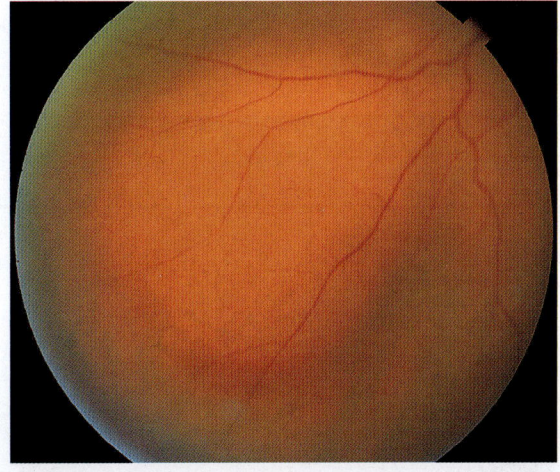

Figure 39.10. Yellow-orange lymphoid infiltrate in choroid inferotemporally in same patient. The patient declined treatment and the orbital, conjunctival, and choroidal lesions enlarged very slowly.

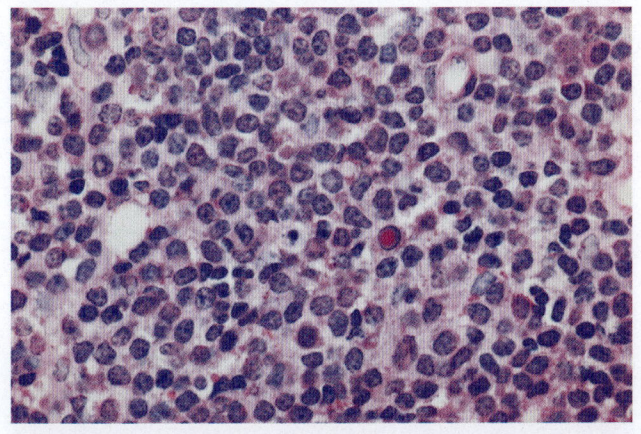

Figure 39.11. Histopathology of another case showing low-grade orbital lymphoma. Note the well-differentiated lymphocytes and the eosinophilic intranuclear inclusion body (Dutcher body) near the center of the field. (Hematoxylin–eosin ×200.)

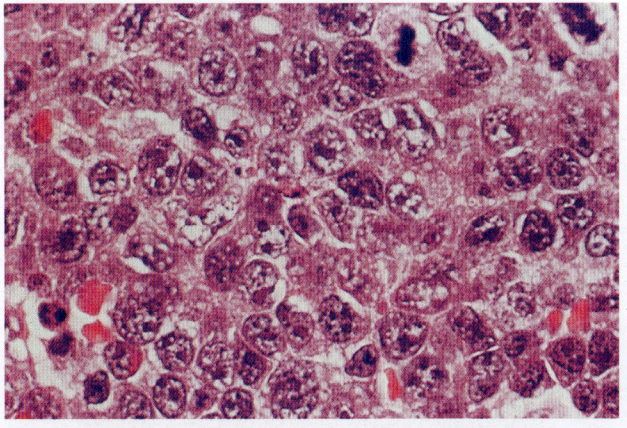

Figure 39.12. Histopathology of malignant orbital lymphoma showing poorly differentiated lymphocytes. (Hematoxylin–eosin ×250.)

ORBITAL LACRIMAL GLAND LYMPHOMA: CLINICAL AND MAGNETIC RESONANCE IMAGING CORRELATIONS

Lymphoma can occur anywhere in the orbit and it seems to have a slight predilection for the lacrimal gland. Like other orbital lymphomas, it can be unilateral or bilateral and isolated or part of systemic lymphoma. It usually presents as a painless, slowly growing, anterior orbital mass that is often visible or palpable through the skin. Imaging studies like computed tomography and magnetic resonance imaging are invaluable in making the diagnosis and determining the approach to biopsy. Cases are shown, each of which was confirmed histopathologically.

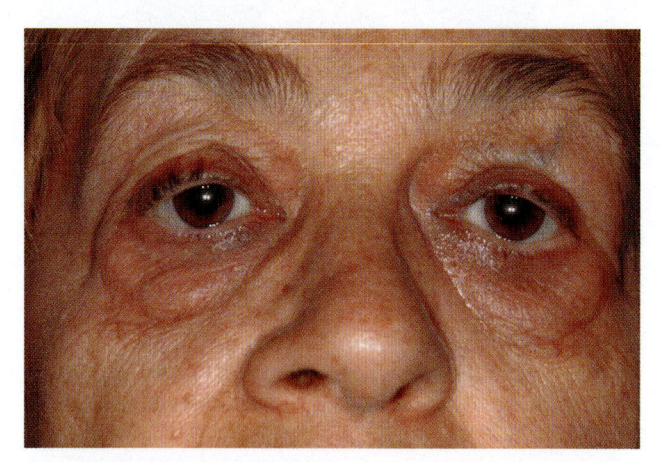

Figure 39.13. Elderly man with bilateral lacrimal gland masses.

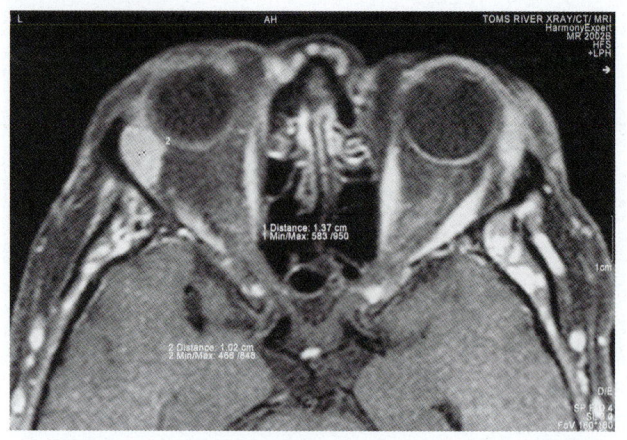

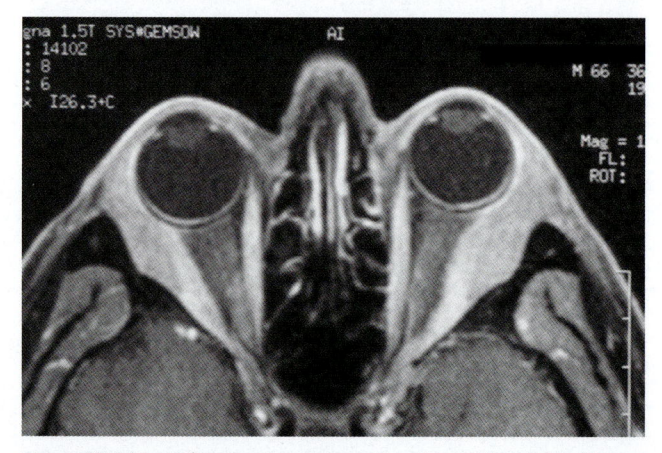

Figure 39.14. Axial magnetic resonance imaging in T1-weighted image and gadolinium enhancement of patient shown in Figure 39.13. Note the moderately enlarged right lacrimal gland and mildly enlarged left lacrimal gland.

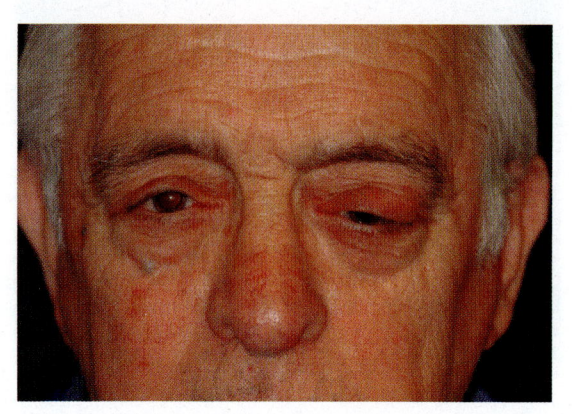

Figure 39.15. Elderly man with clinical evidence of left lacrimal gland mass.

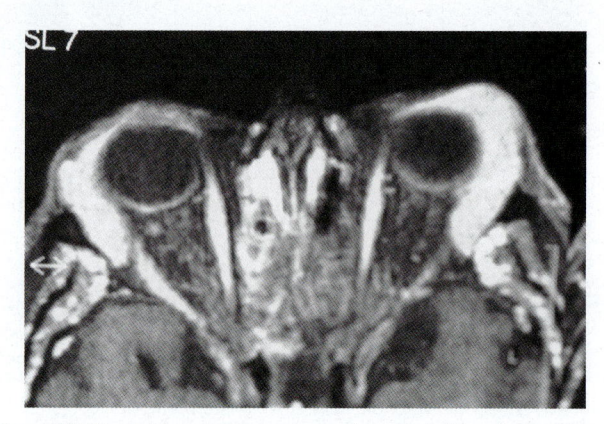

Figure 39.16. Axial magnetic resonance imaging in T1-weighted image and gadolinium enhancement of patient shown in Figure 39.15. Note how the mass molds to the globe and orbital bones.

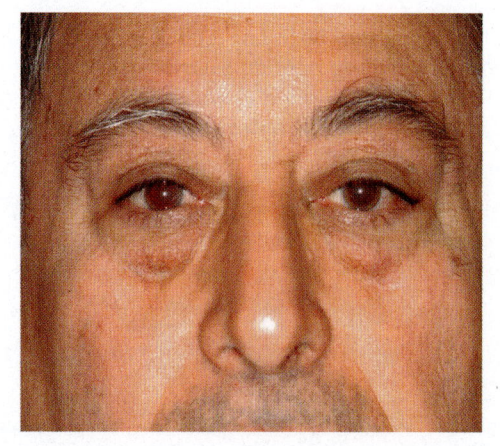

Figure 39.17. Elderly man with bilateral fullness in orbits superotemporally but no pain.

Figure 39.18. Axial magnetic resonance imaging in T1-weighted image and gadolinium enhancement of patient depicted in Figure 39.17 showing bilateral elongated masses extending from the lacrimal glands along the lateral rectus muscles.

ORBITAL NON-HODGKIN LYMPHOMA: DIAGNOSIS AND MANAGEMENT

In most instances, a biopsy is indicated for suspected orbital lymphoma. If there is no known lymphoma, an open biopsy is done using the most accessible approach as determined by axial and coronal computed tomography or magnetic resonance imaging. Small anterior circumscribed tumors should be excised completely if possible. Large nonresectable tumors should have incisional biopsy, still removing as much of the tumor as possible. If the patient has known lymphoma that has already been diagnosed and staged, a fine-needle aspiration biopsy can be performed to confirm the orbital diagnosis. The orbital tumor can respond to either irradiation or chemotherapy.

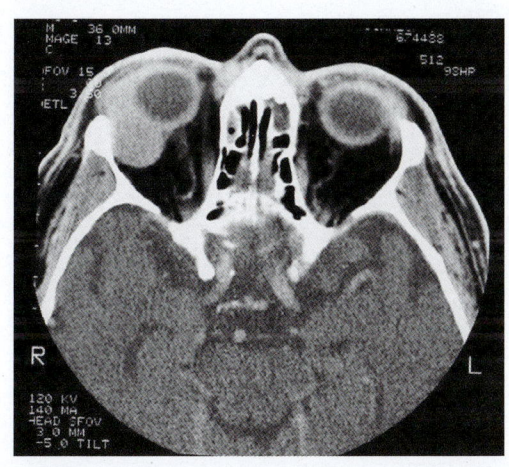

Figure 39.19. Axial computed tomography showing well-circumscribed orbital lymphoma involving the lacrimal gland. Because the tumor requires a biopsy and is surgically accessible, it is advisable to remove the tumor entirely, rather than performing an incisional biopsy.

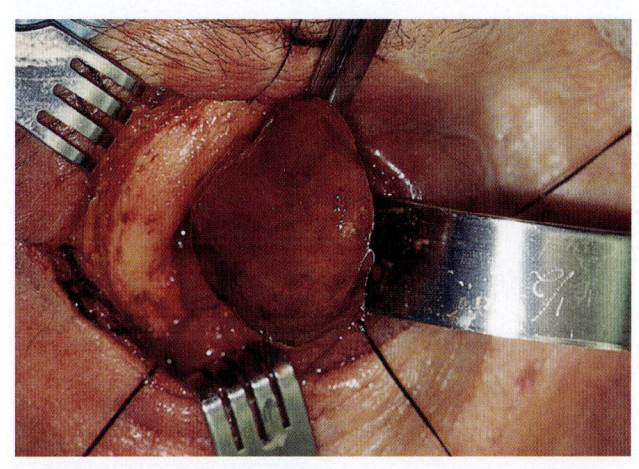

Figure 39.20. Entire tumor being removed through superotemporal orbitotomy without an osteotomy.

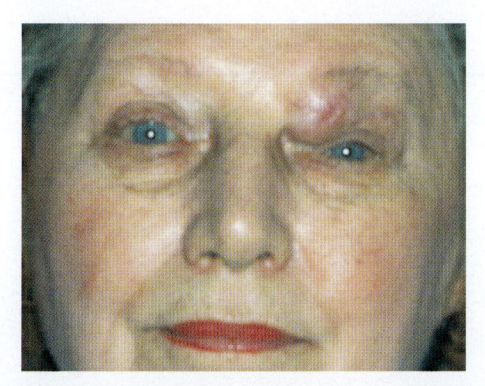

Figure 39.21. Superonasal anterior orbital mass presenting as a subcutaneous lesion in a 71-year-old woman with known lymphoma. In such a case, a fine-needle aspiration biopsy performed in the office is sufficient to confirm the suspected diagnosis.

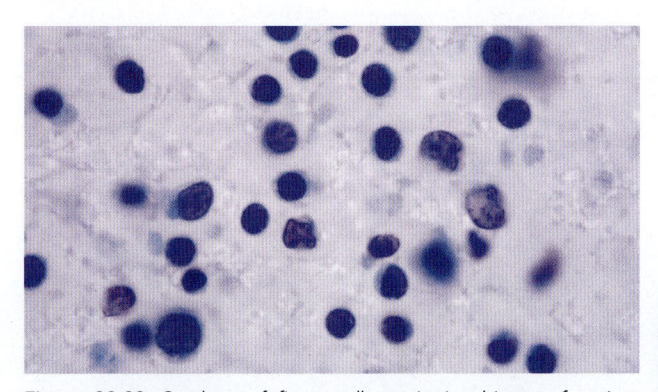

Figure 39.22. Cytology of fine-needle aspiration biopsy of patient shown in Figure 39.21. Note the large and small lymphocytes. Diagnosis was low-grade malignant lymphoma. (Papanicolaou ×300.)

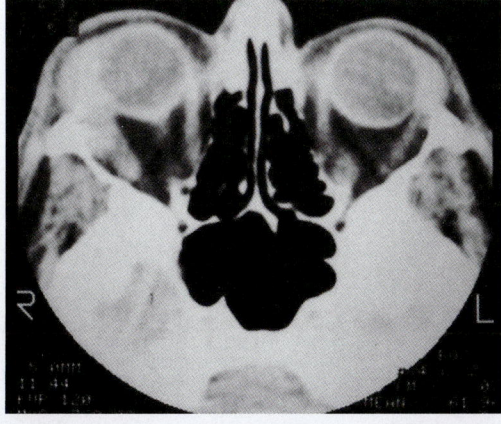

Figure 39.23. Response of orbital lymphoma to irradiation. Axial computed tomography shows a diffuse right temporal orbital mass in a 70-year-old man.

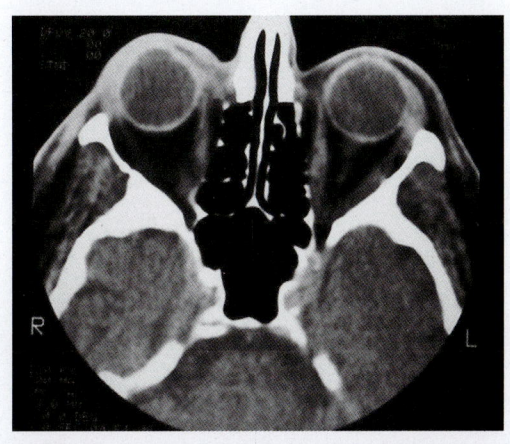

Figure 39.24. Postirradiation axial computed tomography of patient shown in Figure 39.23, demonstrating complete regression of the tumor.

ORBITAL LYMPHOMA: ATYPICAL FORMS

Most orbital lymphomas are typical non-Hodgkin B-cell lymphoma (1–8). However, unusual variants do occur. An example is shown of a large cell lymphoma with microvillous projections. This rare form of lymphoma may be confused with an epithelial tumor with light microscopy and even with electron microscopy (9).

Cutaneous T-cell lymphoma (mycosis fungoides) can also affect the orbit and adnexa (10,11). This type appears to be much more aggressive than B-cell lymphoma and can grow rapidly and destroy the eye. Most patients who develop orbital T-cell lymphoma already have systemic T-cell lymphoma (mycosis fungoides). The treatment is similar to that described for B-cell lymphoma. The prognosis is guarded.

Selected References

Reviews

1. Coupland SE, Damato B. Lymphomas involving the eye and ocular adnexa. *Curr Opin Ophthalmol* 2006;17:523–531.
2. Jaffe ES. The 2008 WHO classification of lymphomas: implications for clinical practice and translational research. *Hematology* 2009;523–531.
3. Graue GF, Finger PT, Maher E, et al. Ocular adnexal lymphoma staging and treatment: American Joint Committee on Cancer versus Ann Arbor. *Eur J Ophthalmol* 2013;23:344–355.
4. Sniegowski MC, Roberts D, Bakhoun M, et al. Ocular adnexal lymphoma: validation of American Joint Committee on Cancer seventh edtion staging guidelines. *Br J Ophthalmol* 2014;98:1255–1260.
5. Aronow ME, Portell CA, Rybicki LA, et al. Ocular adnexal lymphoma: assessment of a tumor node metastasis staging system. *Ophthalmology* 2013;120:1915–1919.
6. Demirci H, Shields CL, Karatza EC, et al. Orbital lymphoproliferative tumors: Analysis of clinical features and systemic involvement in 160 cases. *Ophthalmology* 2008;115:1626–1631.
7. Cockerham GC, Jakobiec FA. Lymphoproliferative disorders of the ocular adnexa. *Int Ophthalmol Clin* 1997;37:39–59.
8. Coupland SE, Krause L, Delecluse HJ, et al. Lymphoproliferative lesions of the ocular adnexa. Analysis of 112 cases. *Ophthalmology* 1998;105:1430–1441.

Case Reports

9. Font RL, Shields JA. Large cell lymphoma of the orbit with microvillous projections ("porcupine lymphoma"). *Arch Ophthalmol* 1985;103:1715–1719.
10. Meekins B, Proia AD, Klintworth GK. Cutaneous T-cell lymphoma presenting as rapidly enlarging ocular adnexal tumor. *Ophthalmology* 1985;91:1288–1293.
11. Shields CL, Shields JA, Eagle RC Jr. Rapidly progressive T-cell lymphoma of conjunctiva. *Arch Ophthalmol* 2002;120:508–589.

ORBITAL LYMPHOMA: ATYPICAL FORMS: LARGE CELL LYMPHOMA WITH MICROVILLOUS PROJECTIONS AND CUTANEOUS T-CELL LYMPHOMA

1. Font RL, Shields JA. Large cell lymphoma of the orbit with microvillous projections ("porcupine lymphoma"). *Arch Ophthalmol* 1985;103:1715–1719.
2. Meekins B, Proia AD, Klintworth GK. Cutaneous T-cell lymphoma presenting as rapidly enlarging ocular adnexal tumor. *Ophthalmology* 1985;91;1288–1293.

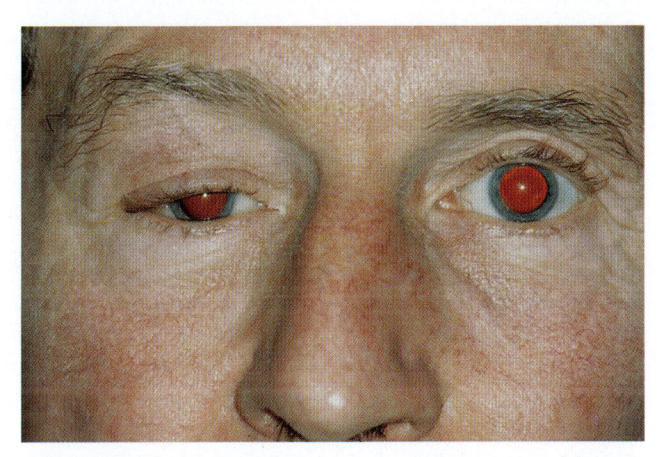

Figure 39.25. Blepharoptosis and downward displacement of the right eye in a 57-year-old man.

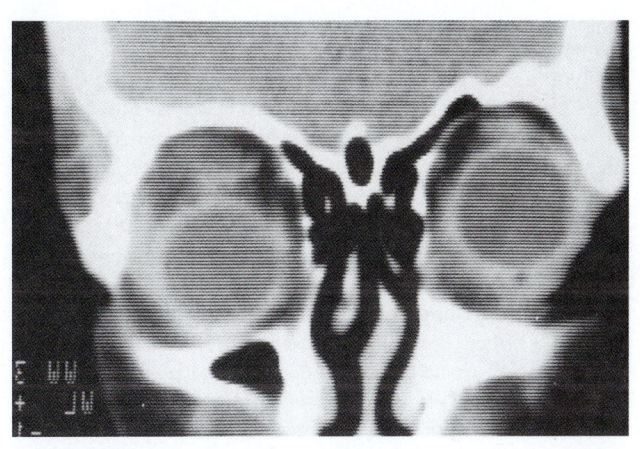

Figure 39.26. Coronal computed tomography showing superotemporal orbital mass in patient seen in Figure 39.25. There was bone erosion evident on many sections.

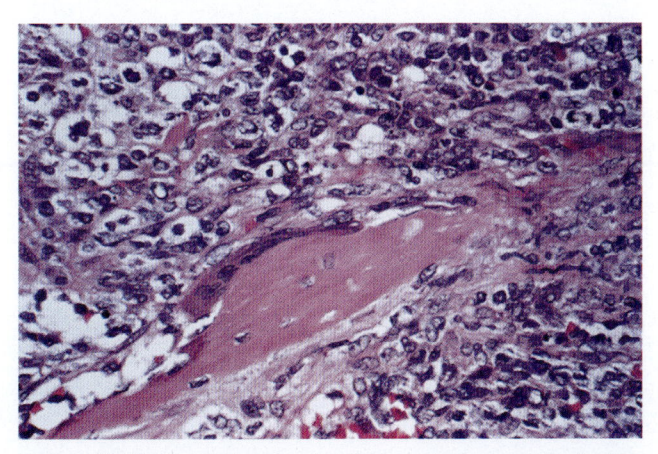

Figure 39.27. Histopathology showing anaplastic tumor cells. The diagnosis could not be determined on the basis of light microscopy. (Hematoxylin–eosin ×100.)

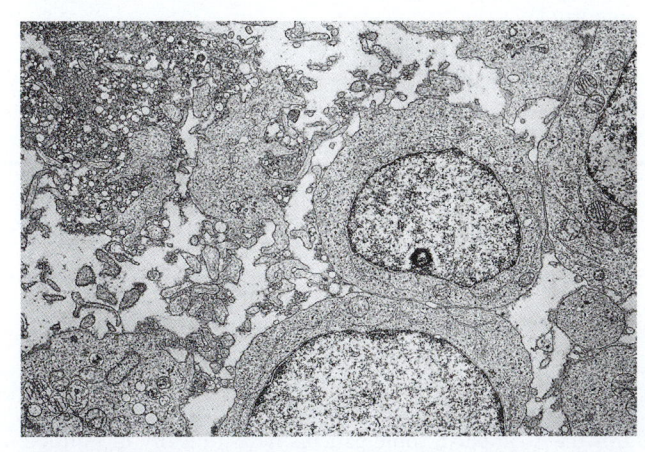

Figure 39.28. Electron photomicrograph showing lymphoid cells with microvillous projections, resembling an epithelial tumor. However, these findings are characteristic of a large cell lymphoma with microvillous projections ("porcupine" lymphoma).

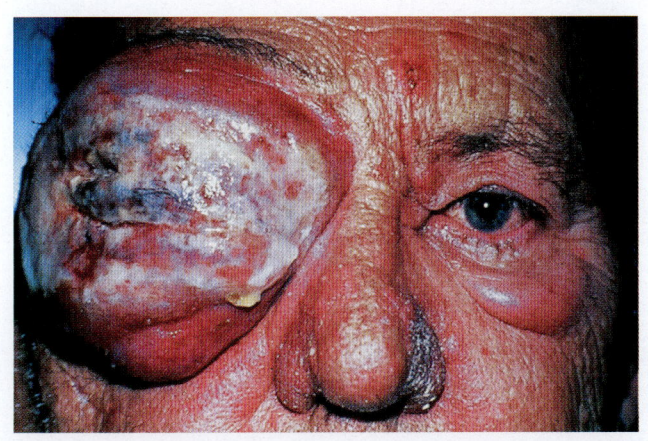

Figure 39.29. Massive orbital involvement and destruction of the eye by aggressive T-cell lymphoma (mycosis fungoides). (Courtesy of Gordon Klintworth, MD.)

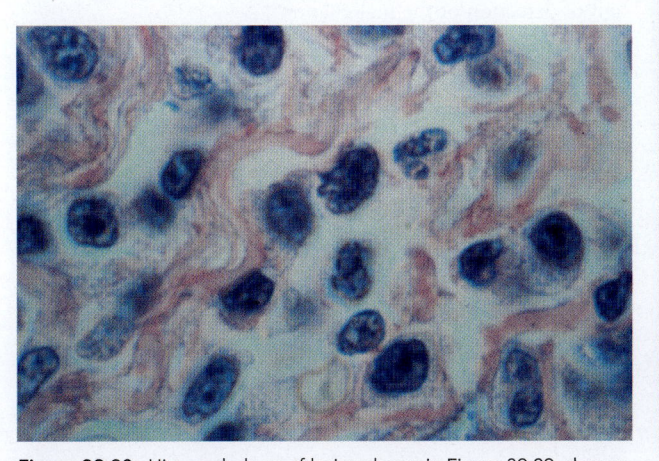

Figure 39.30. Histopathology of lesion shown in Figure 39.29, demonstrating malignant T cells. (Hematoxylin–eosin ×400.) (Courtesy of Gordon Klintworth, MD.)

ORBITAL PLASMACYTOMA AND LYMPHOPLASMACYTOID TUMORS

General Considerations

Tumors composed of pure plasma cells (plasmacytomas) or those composed of B lymphocytes and plasma cells (lymphoplasmacytoid tumors) are closely related to the various lymphomas as discussed above (1–27). The plasma cell is actually a B lymphocyte that produces a large amount of immunoglobulin. Lymphoplasmacytoid tumors are closer in the spectrum to lymphoma. Plasmacytoma is a tumor composed predominantly of plasma cells and is closer in the spectrum to multiple myeloma. Multiple myeloma is a plasma cell neoplasm characterized by plasma cell infiltration of bone marrow and by monoclonal immunoglobulin (Bence–Jones protein) in the serum. A solitary form of extramedullary plasma cell tumor can occur in the upper respiratory tract, gastrointestinal tract, or lymph nodes. It is relatively rare in the orbit, where it can occur as a soft tissue or bony lesion (6,12–15). Plasmacytoma can involve the orbit as a solitary lesion or as part of multiple myeloma. The majority of patients with solitary plasmacytoma will eventually develop multiple myeloma. In the authors' clinical series, the six cases of plasmacytoma accounted for 4% of all orbital lymphoid tumors and for <1% of all orbital tumors (1).

Waldenström macroglobulinemia is a malignancy of lymphoplasmacytoid cells that secrete immunoglobulin M. It has systemic symptoms and signs similar to lymphoma. Affected patients can develop lymphoma and myeloma.

Clinical Features

The clinical features of orbital plasmacytoma are similar to those of NHL. This tumor typically presents in a middle-aged to elderly patient with proptosis and displacement of the eye. This tumor can be seen in children or adults without myeloma (12). The patient might experience pain, especially if there is intralesional hemorrhage or orbital bone involvement. In some instances, orbital plasmacytoma can present as a fungating growth. As implied, some patients have a history of multiple myeloma and others need long-term follow-up with monitoring for myeloma. Orbital plasmacytoma is occasionally initial sign of insufficiently controlled multiple myeloma or the first sign of detection of the malignancy.

Diagnostic Approaches

A patient with suspected or biopsy-proven orbital plasma cell tumor should undergo systemic evaluation to exclude multiple myeloma or other dysproteinemias. Like orbital lymphoma, computed tomography or magnetic resonance imaging of orbital plasmacytoma shows a diffuse or ovoid mass. Bleeding in areas of necrosis of orbital plasmacytoma can simulate orbital cellulitis clinically (11). It is more likely, however, to show erosion of bone, particularly in patients with multiple myeloma. Solitary soft tissue plasmacytoma can also be associated with myeloma. It is possible that some cases actually originate in orbital bone and secondarily affect the orbital soft tissue.

Pathology

Multiple myeloma is a plasma cell neoplasm characterized by plasma cell infiltration of bone marrow and monoclonal immunoglobulin in the serum. Orbital plasmacytoma can range from well-differentiated mature plasma cells to poorly differentiated anaplastic plasma cells.

Management

Management includes incisional or excisional biopsy confirmation followed by radiotherapy if the tumor is not completely removed. Associated multiple myeloma is usually treated with high-dose chemotherapy, with radiation to local lesions. Solitary orbital plasmacytoma without myeloma can be treated with radiotherapy and show a favorable response.

ORBITAL PLASMACYTOMA AND LYMPHOPLASMACYTOID TUMORS

Selected References

Reviews

1. Shields JA, Shields CL, Scartozzi R. Survey of 1264 patients with orbital tumors and simulating lesions: the 2002 Montgomery Lecture, part 1. *Ophthalmology* 2004;111:997–1008.
2. Coupland SE, Damato B. Lymphomas involving the eye and ocular adnexa. *Curr Opin Ophthalmol* 2006;17:523–531.
3. Jaffe ES. The 2008 WHO classification of lymphomas: implications for clinical practice and translational research. *Hematology* 2009;523–531.
4. Coupland SE, Krause L, Delecluse HJ, et al. Lymphoproliferative lesions of the ocular adnexa. Analysis of 112 cases. *Ophthalmology* 1998;105(8):1430–1441.
5. Adkins JW, Shields JA, Shields CL, et al. Plasmacytoma of the eye and orbit. *Int Ophthalmol* 1977;20:339–343.
6. Knapp AJ, Gartner S, Henkind P. Multiple myeloma and its ocular manifestations. *Surv Ophthalmol* 1987;31:343–351.
7. Orellana J, Friedman AH. Ocular manifestations of multiple myeloma, Waldenstrom's macroglobulinemia, and benign monoclonal gammopathy. *Surv Ophthalmol* 1981;26:157–169.
8. de Smet MD, Rootman J. Orbital manifestations of plasmacytic lymphoproliferations. *Ophthalmology* 1987;94:995–1003.

Histopathology

9. Shields JA, Cooper H, Donoso LA, et al. Immunohistochemical and ultrastructural study of unusual IgM lambda lymphoplasmacytic tumor of the lacrimal gland. *Am J Ophthalmol* 1986;101:451–457.
10. Khalil MK, Huang S, Viloria J, et al. Extramedullary plasmacytoma of the orbit: case report with results of immunocytochemical studies. *Can J Ophthalmol* 1981;16:39–42.

Case Reports

11. Rappaport K, Liesegang TJ, Menke DH, et al. Plasmacytoma manifesting as recurrent cellulitis and hematic cyst of the orbit. *Am J Ophthalmol* 1996;122:595–597.
12. Sharma MC, Mahapatra AK, Gaikwad S, et al. Primary extramedullary orbital plasmacytoma in a child. *Childs Nerv Syst* 1996;12:470–472.
13. Gonnering RS. Bilateral primary extramedullary orbital plasmacytomas. *Ophthalmology* 1987;94:267–270.
14. Ezra E, Mannor G, Wright JE, et al. Inadequately irradiated solitary extramedullary plasmacytoma of the orbit requiring exenteration. *Am J Ophthalmol* 1995;120:803–805.
15. Aboud N, Sullivan T, Whitehead K. Primary extramedullary plasmacytoma of the orbit. *Aust N Z J Ophthalmol* 1995;23:235–239.
16. Agrawal PK, Mittal S, Gupta P, et al. Plasmacytoma of orbit. *Indian J Ophthalmol* 1993;41:34–36.
17. Tung G, Finger PT, Klein I, et al. Plasmacytoma of the orbit. *Arch Ophthalmol* 1988;106:1622.
18. Nikoskelainen E, Dellaporta A, Rice T, et al. Orbital involvement by plasmacytoma. Report of two cases. *Acta Ophthalmol (Copenh)* 1976;54:755–761.
19. McFadzean RM. Orbital plasma cell myeloma. *Br J Ophthalmol* 1975;59:164–165.
20. Levin SR, Spaulding AG, Wirman JA. Multiple myeloma. Orbital involvement in a youth. *Arch Ophthalmol* 1977;95:642–644.
21. Jampol LM, Marsh JC, Albert DM, et al. IgA-associated lymphoplasmacytic tumor involving the conjunctiva, eyelid, and orbit. *Am J Ophthalmol* 1975;97:279–284.
22. Kottler UB, Cursiefen C, Holbach LM. Orbital involvement in multiple myeloma: first sign of insufficient chemotherapy. *Ophthalmologica* 2003;217:76–78.
23. Uceda-Montanes A, Blanco G, Saornil MA, et al. Extramedullary plasmacytoma of the orbit. *Acta Ophthalmol Scand* 2000;78:601–603.
24. Fay AM, Leib ML, Fountain KS. Multiple myeloma involving the orbit. *Ophthal Plast Reconstr Surg* 1998;14:67–71.
25. Sen S, Kashyap S, Betharia S. Primary orbital plasmacytoma: A case report. *Orbit* 2003;22:317–319.
26. Hsu VJ, Agarwal MR, Chen CS, et al. IgA orbital plasmacytoma in multiple myeloma. *Ophthal Plast Reconstr Surg* 2010;26(2):126–127.
27. Lazaridou MN, Micallef-Eynaud P, Hanna IT. Soft tissue plasmacytoma of the orbit as part of the spectrum of multiple myeloma. *Orbit* 2007;26(4):315–318.

ORBITAL PLASMACYTOMA AND LYMPHOPLASMACYTOID TUMORS

Lymphoplasmacytoid tumors can occur in the orbit in association with Waldenström macroglobulinemia, myeloma, or as an apparent isolated entity. The tumors are usually low grade.

Shields JA, Cooper H, Donoso LA, et al. Immunohistochemical and ultrastructural study of unusual IgM lambda lymphoplasmacytic tumor of the lacrimal gland. *Am J Ophthalmol* 1986;101:451–457.

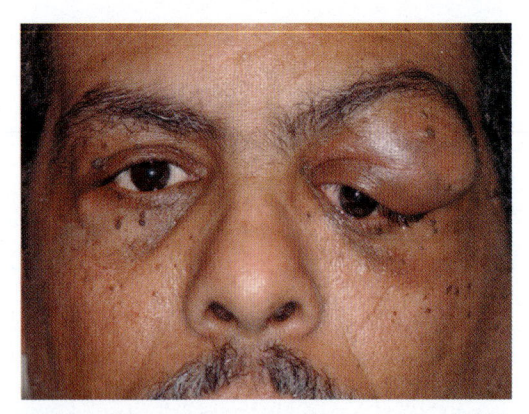

Figure 39.31. A 50-year-old man with a 20-year history of Waldenström macroglobulinemia developed a progressively enlarging, painless mass superotemporal to the left eye.

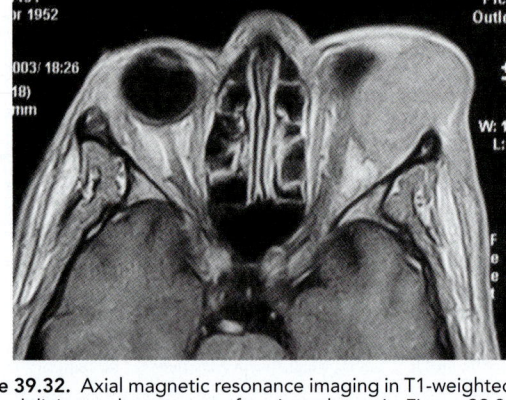

Figure 39.32. Axial magnetic resonance imaging in T1-weighted image and gadolinium enhancement of patient shown in Figure 39.31. Note the large enhancing mass in the region of the left lacrimal gland.

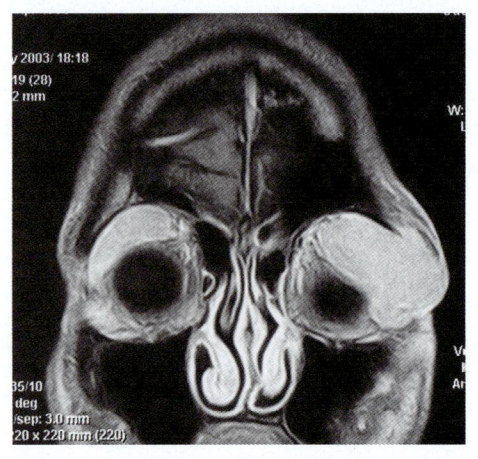

Figure 39.33. Coronal magnetic resonance imaging of same patient reveals bilateral superotemporal orbital masses. Review of a prior small biopsy revealed diffuse non-Hodgkin B-cell lymphoma consistent with marginal zone lymphoma of mucosa-associated lymphoid tissue. The patient showed a dramatic response to 4 weeks of rituxan treatment.

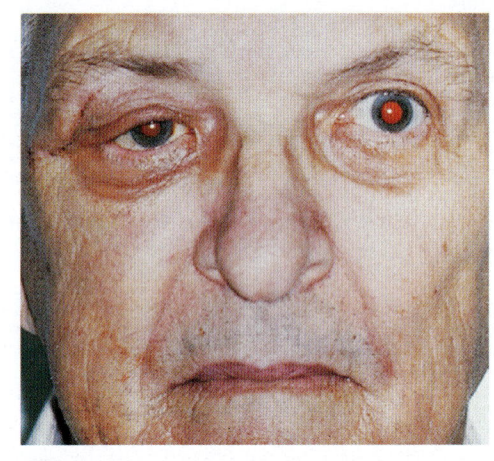

Figure 39.34. Lymphoplasmacytoid tumor. Blepharoptosis and slight proptosis of the right eye of a 72-year-old man.

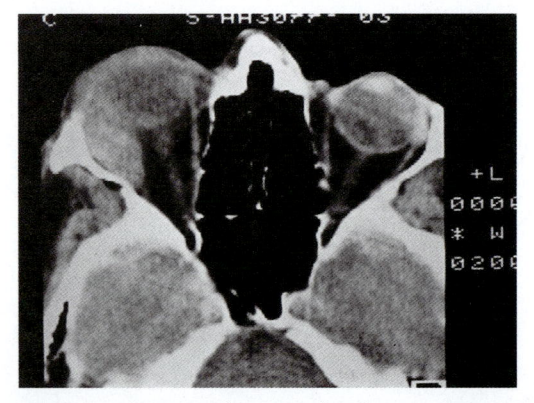

Figure 39.35. Axial computed tomography of patient shown in Figure 39.34, depicting an ovoid tumor in the superotemporal orbit affecting mainly the lacrimal gland. The tumor was completely excised by way of a superotemporal orbitotomy.

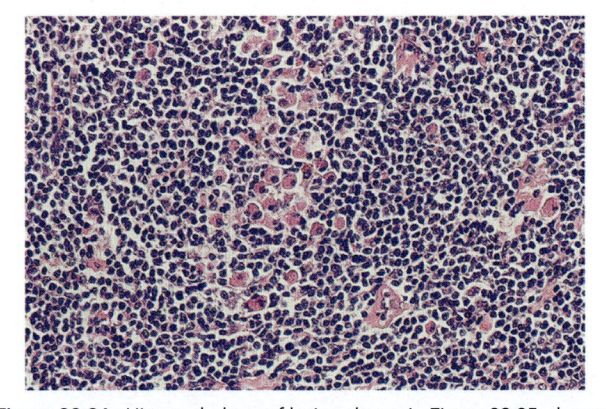

Figure 39.36. Histopathology of lesion shown in Figure 39.35, demonstrating diffuse sheets of small lymphocytes with scattered swollen plasma cells. (Hematoxylin–eosin ×100.)

Chapter 39 Orbital Lymphoid Tumors and Leukemias

ORBITAL PLASMACYTOMA: ASSOCIATION WITH MULTIPLE MYELOMA

Malignant plasmacytoma can occur in the orbit in patients with multiple myeloma. It has a tendency to involve orbital bone but can sometimes be confined to soft tissue.

Adkins JW, Shields JA, Shields CL, et al. Plasmacytoma of the eye and orbit. *Int Ophthalmol* 1977;20:339–343.

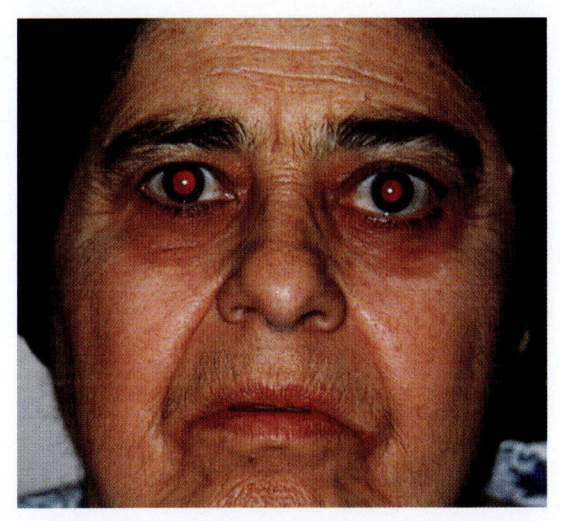

Figure 39.37. Orbital plasmacytoma as part of multiple myeloma. A 76-year-old woman with a 3-year history of immunoglobulin G lambda multiple myeloma treated with chemotherapy developed proptosis of the left eye.

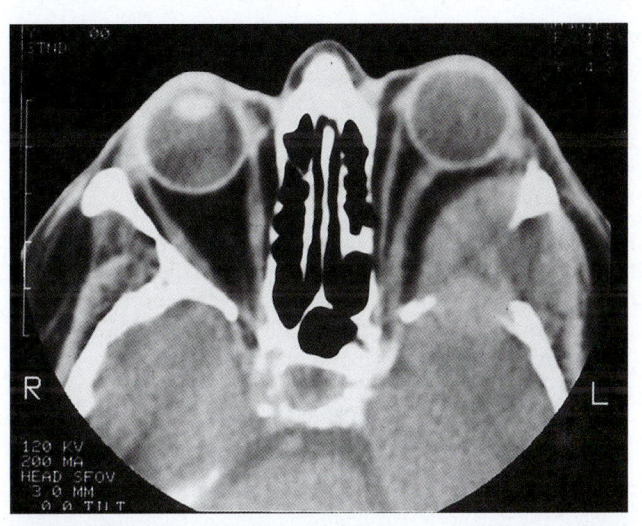

Figure 39.38. Axial computed tomography of patient shown in Figure 39.37, demonstrating diffuse temporal orbital mass with medial displacement of the optic nerve, destruction of the zygomatic bone, and extension into the brain and temporal fossa.

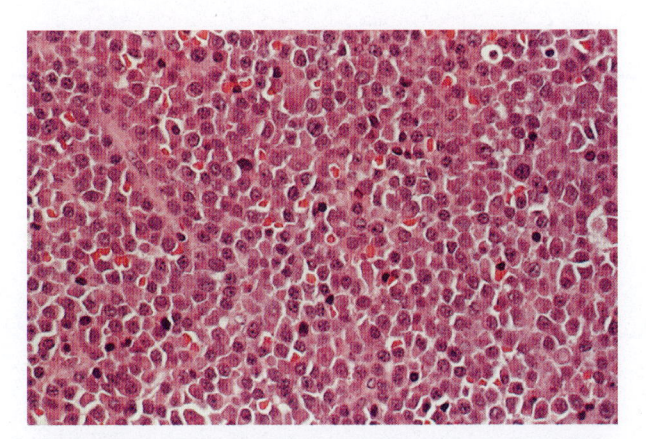

Figure 39.39. Histopathology of lesion shown in Figure 39.38, demonstrating sheets of atypical plasma cells. (Hematoxylin–eosin ×75.)

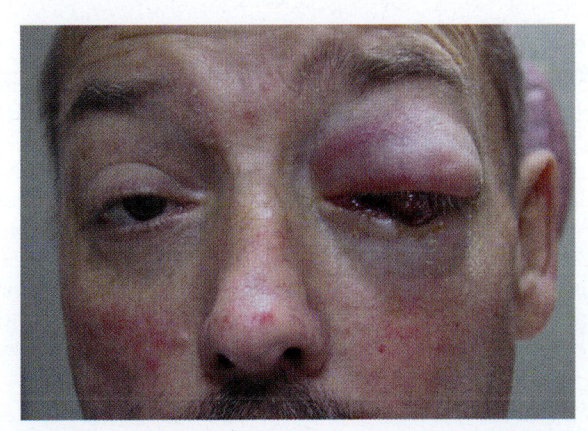

Figure 39.40. Left proptosis and eyelid swelling in a 52-year-old patient with known multiple myeloma.

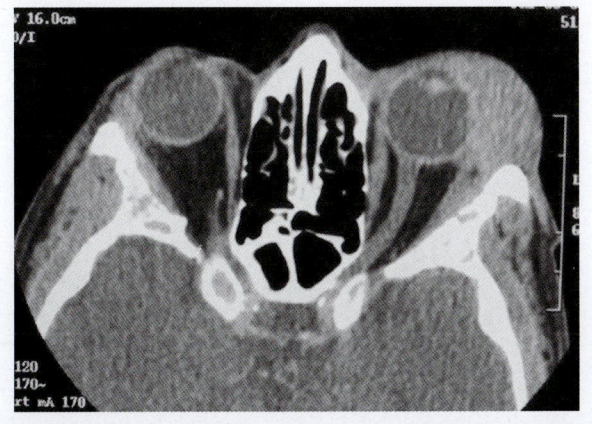

Figure 39.41. Axial magnetic resonance imaging in T1-weighted image with gadolinium enhancement in patient shown in Figure 39.40. Note the large soft tissue orbital mass affecting the lacrimal gland.

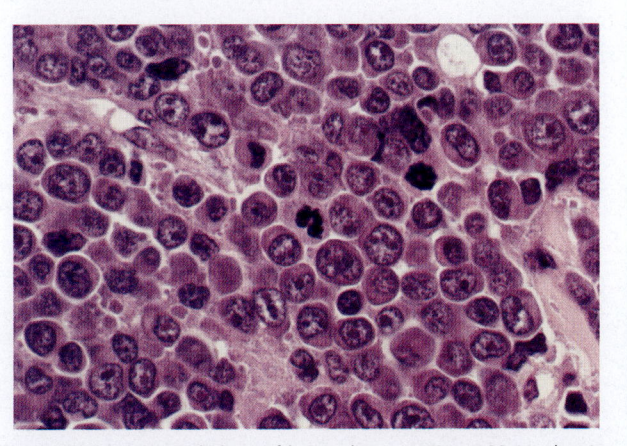

Figure 39.42. Histopathology of lesion shown in Figure 39.41, showing malignant plasma cell tumor with mitotic activity. (Hematoxylin–eosin ×200.)

ORBITAL PLASMABLASTIC LYMPHOMA

General Consideration

Plasmablastic lymphoma, originally described to occur in the oral cavity, is rarely found at other sites (1–4). However, there are isolated reports of orbital involvement (3–4). This rare variant of NHL that has recently been classified under diffuse large B-cell lymphoma (1). This disease can be associated with human immunodeficiency virus (HIV) infection, but also can occur in immunocompetent patients.

Clinical Features

Plasmablastic lymphoma is a rare variant of diffuse large B-cell lymphoma that exhibits a highly aggressive course and is often fatal. It can begin in the orbital soft tissues, but can extend into the brain, sinuses, and even into the globe. About 80% of affected patients are immunosuppressed (1–4).

Diagnostic Approaches

The diagnosis can be suspected in the case of a rapidly expanding orbital mass. Imaging studies including MRI and CT can suggest the diagnosis. An aggressive lymphoma is often a diagnostic consideration but the diagnosis is not usually suspected clinical and biopsy with histopathologic and immunohistochemical studies are necessary to establish the diagnosis.

Pathology

Plasmablastic lymphoma is a variant of diffuse large B-cell lymphoma and can demonstrate a "starry sky" appearance similar to that seen with Burkitt's lymphoma. The cells resemble B immunoblasts, but express the immunophenotype of plasma cells. They lack the immunohistochemical surface markers of B cells, and express IgG, favoring a plasmablastic identity (2–4). The pathogenesis of plasmablastic lymphoma is unclear, but the disorder is thought to be derived from post-germinal center, terminally differentiated, activated B lymphocyte or plasmablasts. There is a strong association with EBV infection.

Management

The management of plasmablastic lymphoma is not well established, and the disease is often rapidly fatal. In cases with symptomatic orbital involvement, palliative radiation or chemotherapy can be employed.

Selected References

1. Jaffe ES. The 2008 WHO classification of lymphomas: implications for clinical practice and translational research. *Hematology* 2009;523–531.
2. Delecluse HJ, Anagnostopoulos I, Dallenbach F, et al. Plasmablastic lymphomas of the oral cavity: a new entity associated with the human immunodeficiency virus infection. *Blood* 1997;89:1413–1420.
3. Morley AM, Verity DH, Meligonis G, et al. Orbital plasmablastic lymphoma–comparison of a newly reported entity with diffuse large B-cell lymphoma of the orbit. *Orbit* 2009;28(6):425–429.
4. Mulay K, Ali MJ, Reddy VA, et al. Orbital plasmablastic lymphoma: a clinicopathological correlation of a rare disease and review of literature. *Clin Ophthalmol* 2012;6:2049–2057.

Chapter 39 Orbital Lymphoid Tumors and Leukemias

ORBITAL PLASMABLASTIC LYMPHOMA

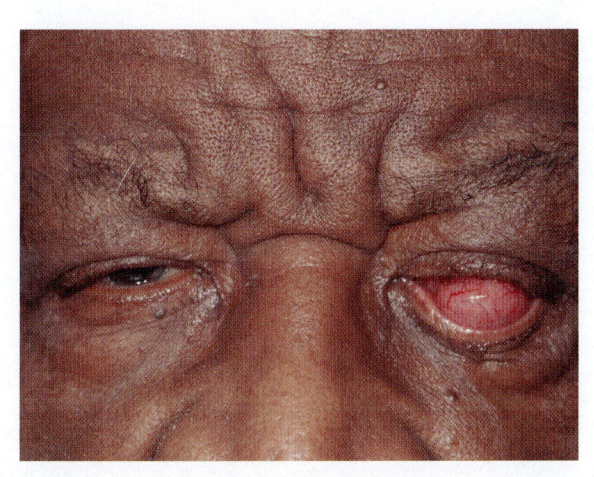

Figure 39.43. A 77-year-old immunocompetent African-American male with rapid onset of visual loss and mass emanating from the inferior fornix.

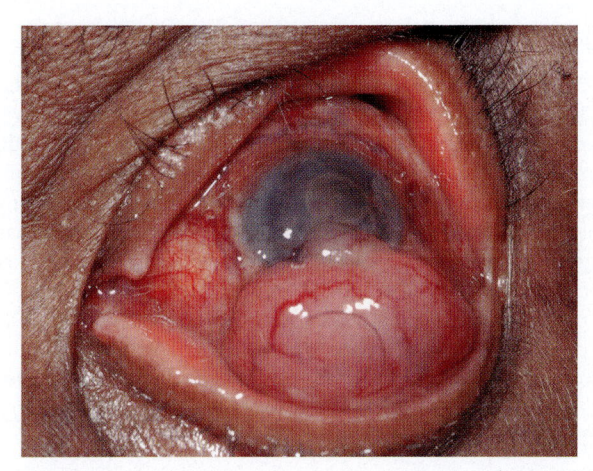

Figure 39.44. The large amelanotic mass of patient in Figure 39.43 appearing in the conjunctival fornix, but also involving the orbit and intraocular structures.

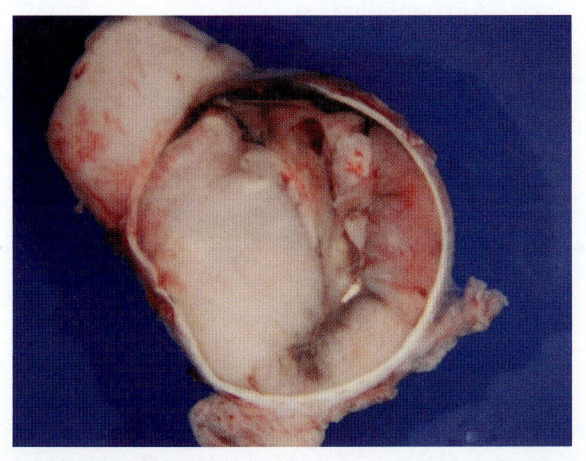

Figure 39.45. Following enucleation of the eye with contiguous orbital tumor the extent of this malignancy is appreciated.

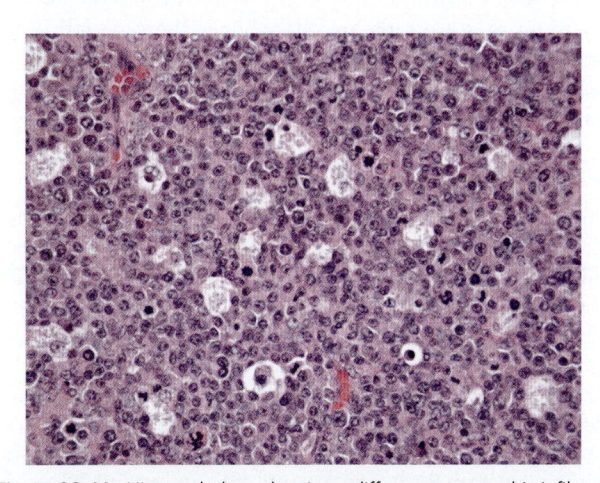

Figure 39.46. Histopathology showing a diffuse monomorphic infiltrate of large plasmacytoid cells and occasional plasmablasts, with admixed tingible-body macrophages. These features, along with immunohistochemistry, were consistent with plasmablastic lymphoma.

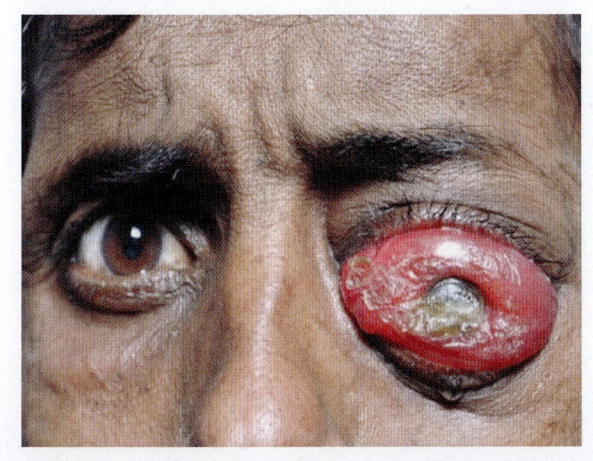

Figure 39.47. A 57-year-old immunocompromised Asian-Indian male with marked periorbital edema and notable corneal dryness.

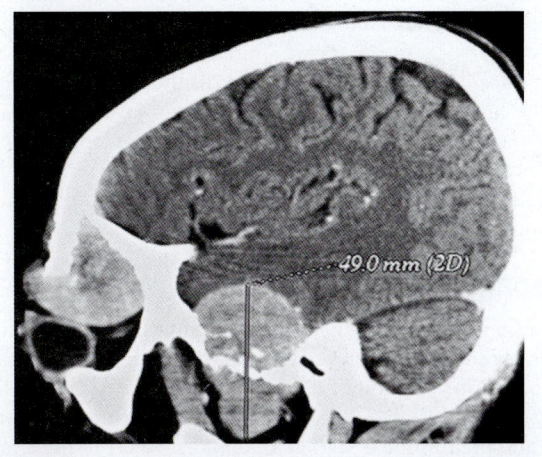

Figure 39.48. Coronal view computed tomography of patient in Figure 39.47, showing diffuse heterogeneous superior orbital as well as brain mass. Biopsy confirmed plasmablastic lymphoma.

ORBITAL BURKITT LYMPHOMA

General Considerations
Burkitt lymphoma is a non-Hodgkin B-cell lymphoma that is being recognized more frequently in the orbit (1–14). Early descriptions of Burkitt lymphoma characterized it as a rapidly progressive, solid lymphoma with a predilection for the jaw and abdomen of certain African children (2). This tumor accounts for approximately 50% of childhood malignant tumors in East Africa (4). Three distinct forms of Burkitt lymphoma have been recognized including the African type, non-African (American) type, and an acquired immunodeficiency syndrome (AIDS) type, each of which can involve the orbital soft tissue or bone and can extend into the globe (2–14). Only one case (American type) was identified in the series of 1,264 orbital lesions reported by the authors (5).

Clinical Features
In the African form, orbital involvement is common secondary to invasion from the maxillary bone. The American form typically involves lymph nodes, bone marrow, and viscera. The AIDS-related form is more aggressive and mainly affects the central nervous system in patients with AIDS (6).

Diagnostic Approaches
An abdominal and orbital mass with proptosis and upward displacement of the globe unilaterally or bilaterally in an African child is highly suggestive of the diagnosis. Orbital computed tomography and magnetic resonance imaging demonstrate a maxillary mass with secondary orbital involvement. Imaging of the American form usually shows an irregular mass in the paranasal sinuses with secondary orbital invasion. The AIDS-related form can involve both orbital soft tissue and bone (12,13). A patient with suspected Burkitt lymphoma should have a systemic evaluation for lymphoma and HIV infection.

Pathology
Burkitt lymphoma is a proliferation of closely packed B lymphocytes. Interspersed histiocytes containing phagocytosed debris cause the classic "starry sky" appearance on low-magnification microscopy. Evidence of the EBV can be found in the majority of cases. Chromosomal abnormalities, particularly a translocation of chromosome 8 to the long arm chromosome 14, occur in many cases. It now seems clear that EBV plays some role in the pathogenesis of Burkitt lymphoma, but the precise role is not clear.

Management
Management parallels that for the systemic disease. In general, a biopsy should be done combined with attempted debulking of the lesion. This tumor is extremely sensitive to chemotherapeutic agents using cyclophosphamide, vincristine, methotrexate, and prednisone. External irradiation (30 Gy to the affected area) can be used in some cases that appear resistant to chemotherapy. The prognosis has improved greatly in recent years.

Selected References

Reviews
1. Jaffe ES. The 2008 WHO classification of lymphomas: implications for clinical practice and translational research. *Hematology* 2009;523–531.
2. Burkitt D. A sarcoma involving the jaws in African children. *Br J Surg* 1958;46:218–223.
3. Burkitt D, O'Conor GT. Malignant lymphoma in African children. I. A clinical syndrome. *Cancer* 1961;14:258–269.
4. Templeton AC. Orbital tumours in African children. *Br J Ophthalmol* 1971;55:254–261.
5. Shields JA, Shields CL, Scartozzi R. Survey of 1264 patients with orbital tumors and simulating lesions: the 2002 Montgomery Lecture, part 1. *Ophthalmology* 2004;111:997–1008.
6. Reifler DM, Warzynski MJ, Blount WR, et al. Orbital lymphoma associated with acquired immune deficiency syndrome (AIDS). *Surv Ophthalmol* 1994;38:371–380.

Case Reports
7. Edelstein C, Shields JA, Shields CL, et al. Non-African Burkitt lymphoma presenting with oral thrush and an orbital mass in a child. *Am J Ophthalmol* 1997;124:859–861.
8. Weisenthal RW, Streeten BW, Dubansky AS, et al. Burkitt lymphoma presenting as a conjunctival mass. *Ophthalmology* 1995;102:129–134.
9. Payne T, Karp LA, Zimmerman LE. Intraocular involvement in Burkitt's lymphoma. *Arch Ophthalmol* 1971;85:295–298.
10. Feman SS, Niwayama G, Hepler RS, et al. "Burkitt tumor" with intraocular involvement. *Surv Ophthalmol* 1969;14:106–111.
11. Zak TA, Fisher JE, Afshani E. Infantile non-African Burkitt's lymphoma presenting as bilateral fulminant exophthalmos. *J Pediatr Ophthalmol Strabismus* 1982;19:294–298.
12. Blakemore WS, Ehrenberg M, Fritz KJ, et al. Rapidly progressive proptosis secondary to Burkitt's lymphoma. Origin in the ethmoidal sinuses. *Arch Ophthalmol* 1983;101:1741–1744.
13. Brooks HL, Downing J, McClure JA, et al. Orbital Burkitt's lymphoma in a homosexual man with acquired immune deficiency. *Arch Ophthalmol* 1984;102:1533–1537.
14. Gupta R, Yadav JS, Yadav S, et al. Orbital involvement in nonendemic Burkitts lymphoma. *Orbit* 2012;31(6):441–445.

Chapter 39 Orbital Lymphoid Tumors and Leukemias

ORBITAL BURKITT LYMPHOMA

1. Edelstein C, Shields JA, Shields CL, et al. Non-African Burkitt's lymphoma presenting with oral thrush and an orbital mass in a child. *Am J Ophthalmol* 1997;124:859–861.
2. Brooks HL, Downing J, McClure JA, et al. Orbital Burkitt's lymphoma in a homosexual man with acquired immune deficiency. *Arch Ophthalmol* 1984;102:1533–1537.

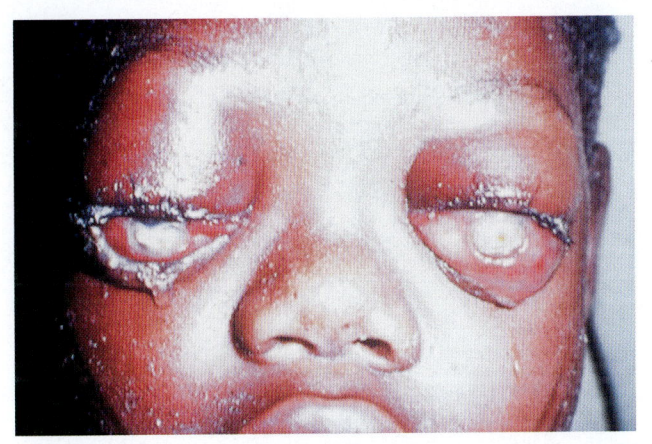

Figure 39.49. African Burkitt lymphoma. Massive bilateral orbital involvement with secondary exposure keratopathy and corneal ulceration in an African child. (Courtesy of Armed Forces Institute of Pathology, Washington, DC.)

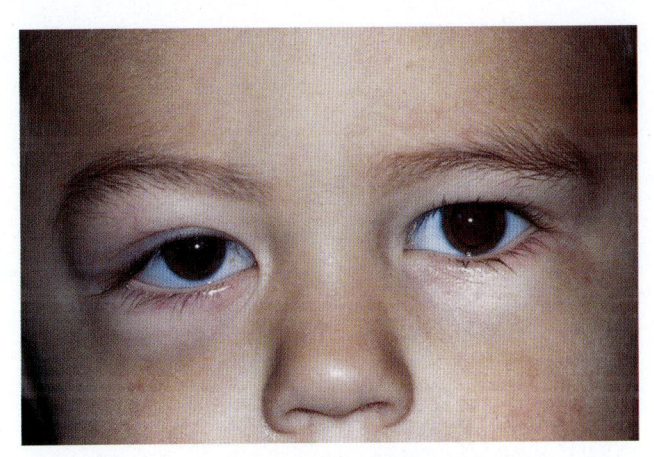

Figure 39.50. Non-African Burkitt lymphoma. Eyelid swelling and proptosis of the right eye in a 26-month-old child.

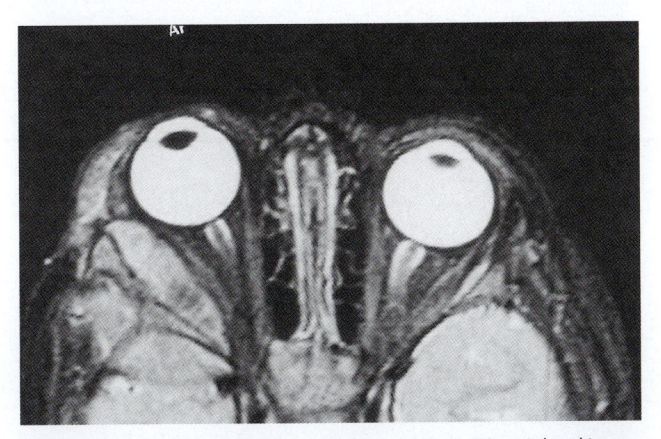

Figure 39.51. Axial magnetic resonance imaging in T2-weighted image of patient shown in Figure 39.44, demonstrating elongated mass along the lateral wall of the orbit.

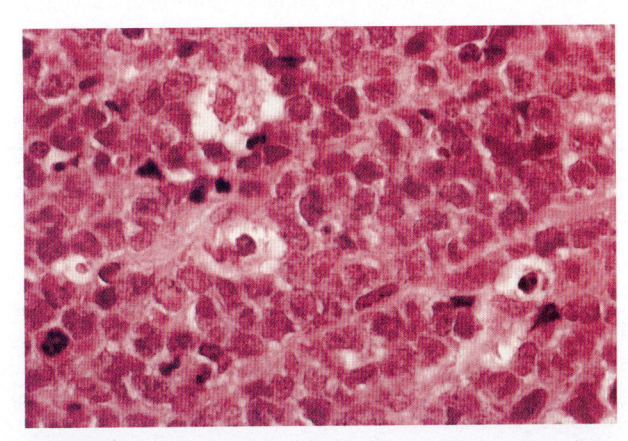

Figure 39.52. Histopathology of lesion shown in Figure 39.45, depicting the sheets of lymphocytes with islands of histiocytes. (Hematoxylin–eosin ×300.)

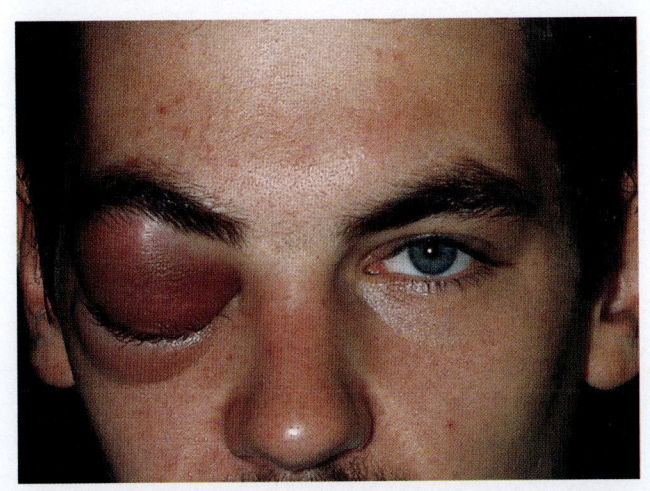

Figure 39.53. AIDS-related Burkitt lymphoma. Acute eyelid swelling and proptosis in a teen-aged man. (Courtesy of H. Logan Brooks, MD.)

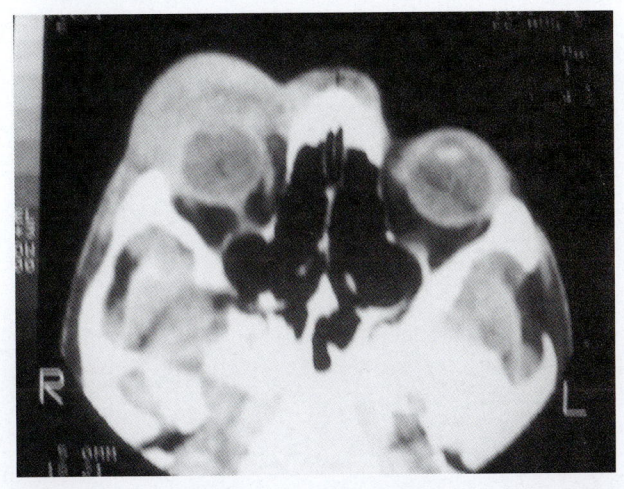

Figure 39.54. Axial computed tomography of patient shown in Figure 39.47 demonstrating diffuse anterior orbital involvement by the tumor. It showed a dramatic response to chemotherapy. (Courtesy of H. Logan Brooks, MD.)

ORBITAL POST-TRANSPLANT LYMPHOPROLIFERATIVE DISORDER

General Considerations

PTLD is a described entity that consists of a polyclonal and/or monoclonal lymphocytic proliferation that follows 2% of organ transplant recipients who are under intensive immunosuppression (1–7). Some affected patients have had prior infection with EBV. It can affect a range of tissues including central nervous system, gastrointestinal tract, cervical lymph nodes, and tonsils. Some cases are being recognized in the ocular region, including the orbit.

Clinical Features

PTLD can occur in the orbit, eyelid, conjunctiva, uveal tract, and retina. It is also discussed elsewhere in this text. Orbital PTLD presents with similar features to classic orbital lymphoma, with the exception that the disease followed organ transplant. This condition should be suspected in any immunosuppressed transplant patient who presents with a lymphoid lesion in the orbital region.

Pathology

Although histopathologic and immunohistochemical characteristics vary, the cells are of lymphocytes of B-cell lineage. A pathology classification of PTLD has been proposed and can be used in predicting prognosis (4).

Management

Treatment of orbital involvement by PTLD depends on the extent of involvement and histopathologic features. An attempt should be made to decrease the immunosuppression and allow the host immune system to recover. Like other orbital lymphoid tumors, small localized lesions can be excised and large lesions can be confirmed by biopsy and treated with radiotherapy. The prognosis varies with the extent of disease. Some patients experience complete recovery and others have a fatal outcome.

ORBITAL POST-TRANSPLANT LYMPHOPROLIFERATIVE DISORDER

Selected References

Reviews
1. Jaffe ES. The 2008 WHO classification of lymphomas: implications for clinical practice and translational research. *Hematology* 2009;523–531.
2. Strazzabosco M, Corneo B, Iemmolo RM, et al. Epstein-Barr virus-associated post transplant lympho-proliferative disease of donor origin in liver transplant recipients. *J Hepatol* 1997;26:926–934.
3. Douglas RS, Goldstein SM, Katowitz JA, et al. Orbital presentation of posttransplantation lymphoproliferative disorder: a small case series. *Ophthalmology* 2002;109:2351–2355.

Histopathology/Genetics
4. Knowles DM, Cesarman E, Chadburn A, et al. Correlative morphologic and molecular genetic analysis demonstrates three distinct categories of posttransplantation lymphoproliferative disorders. *Blood* 1995;85:552–565.

Case Reports
5. Pomeranz HD, McEvoy LT, Lueder GT. Orbital tumor in a child with posttransplantation lymphoproliferative disorder. *Arch Ophthalmol* 1996;114:1422–1423.
6. Clark WL, Scott IU, Murray TG, et al. Primary intraocular posttransplantation lymphoproliferative disorder. *Arch Ophthalmol* 1998;116:1667–1669.
7. Chan SM, Hutnik CM, Heathcote JG, et al. Iris lymphoma in a pediatric cardiac transplant recipient: clinicopathologic findings. *Ophthalmology* 2000;107:1479–1482.

ORBITAL POST-TRANSPLANT LYMPHOPROLIFERATIVE DISORDER

Douglas RS, Goldstein SM, Katowitz JA, et al. Orbital presentation of posttransplantation lymphoproliferative disorder: a small case series. *Ophthalmology* 2002;109:2351–2355. (Courtesy of Roberta Gausas, MD.)

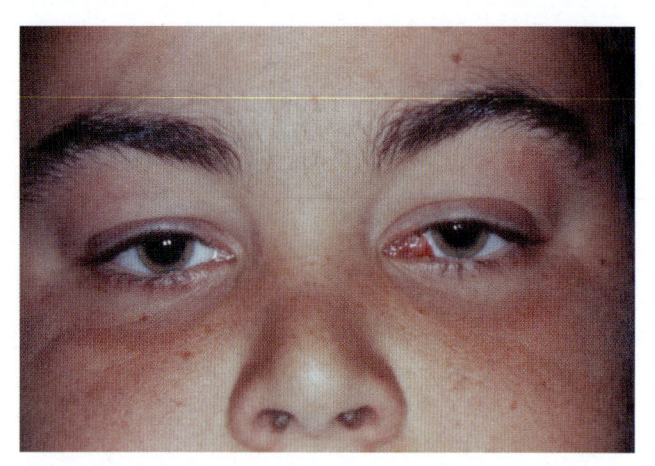

Figure 39.55. Orbital–conjunctival post-transplant lymphoproliferative disorder. Face of an 8-year-old boy showing fleshy mass in medial canthal area of left eye.

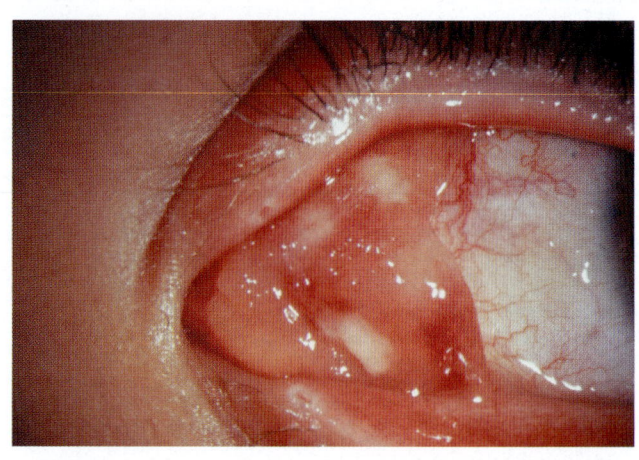

Figure 39.56. Closer view shows multinodular, fleshy mass in medial aspect of conjunctiva and caruncle.

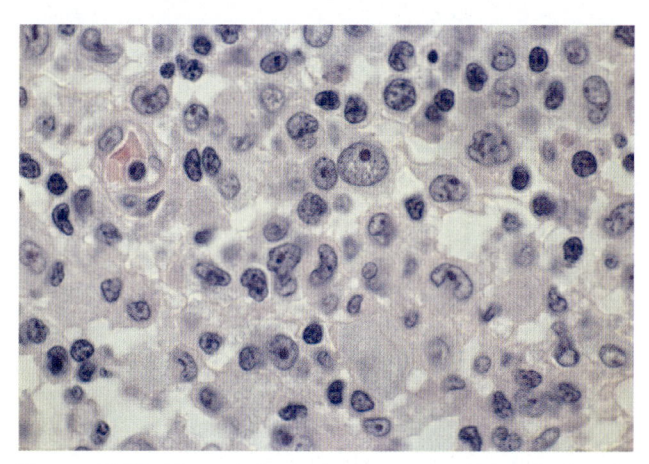

Figure 39.57. Histopathology showing atypical lymphoid cells. (Hematoxylin–eosin ×300.)

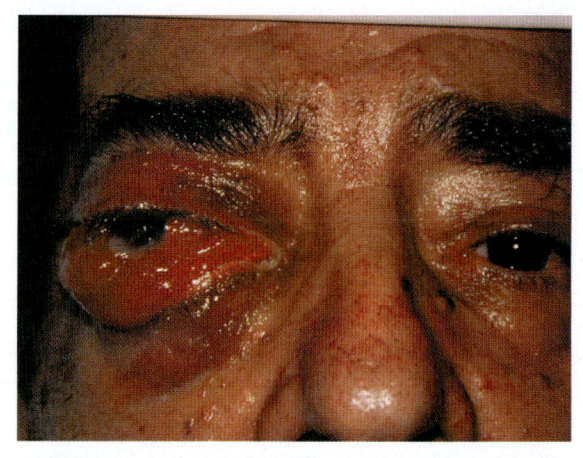

Figure 39.58. Marked proptosis and conjunctival and eyelid edema in a 61-year-old man who underwent heart transplantation 42 months earlier. (Courtesy of Roberta Gausas, MD.)

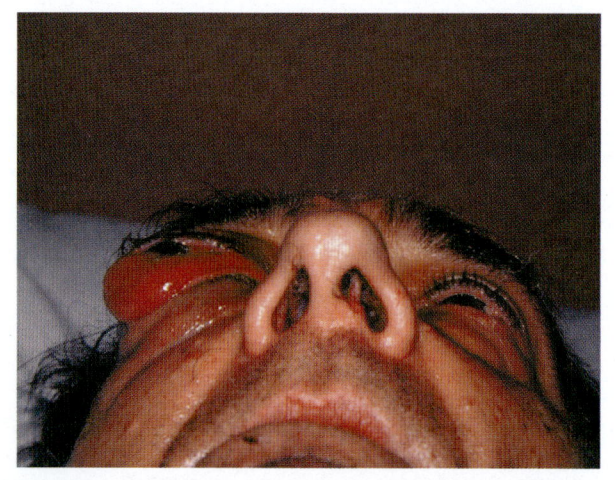

Figure 39.59. Another view of lesion shown in Figure 39.58, showing better the proptosis and eyelid edema. (Courtesy of Roberta Gausas, MD.)

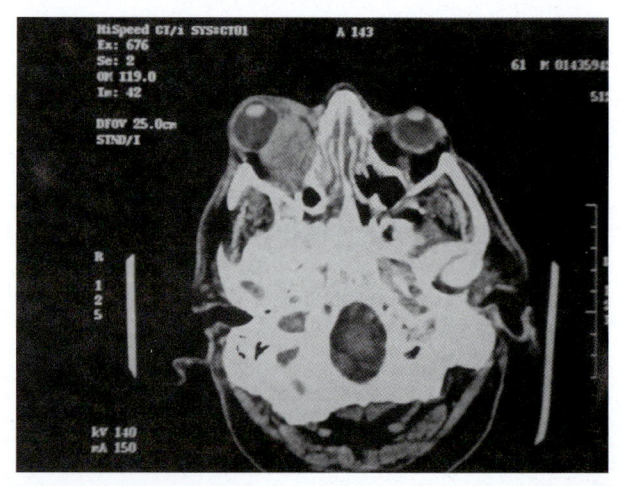

Figure 39.60. Axial computed tomography showing large nasal orbital mass causing proptosis and displacement of the globe. Histopathology showed an infiltrate of large B lymphocytes with immunoblastic and plasmacytic differentiation. (Courtesy of Roberta Gausas, MD.)

ORBITAL POST-TRANSPLANT LYMPHOPROLIFERATIVE DISORDER

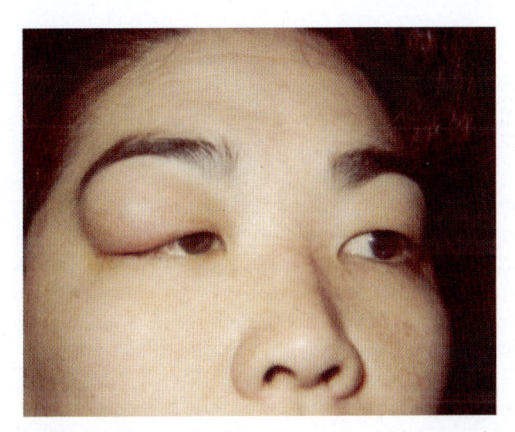

Figure 39.61. A 45-year-old Asian woman noted 2-year history of swollen right upper eyelid with recent worsening. She was immune-suppressed following renal transplant for glomerulonephritis. (Courtesy of Mary Stefanyszyn, MD.)

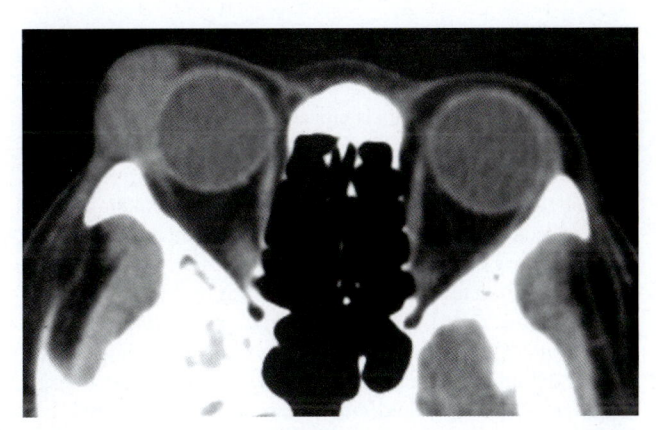

Figure 39.62. Axial computed tomography of patient in Figure 39.61, demonstrating circumscribed soft tissue mass in right orbit anteriorly.

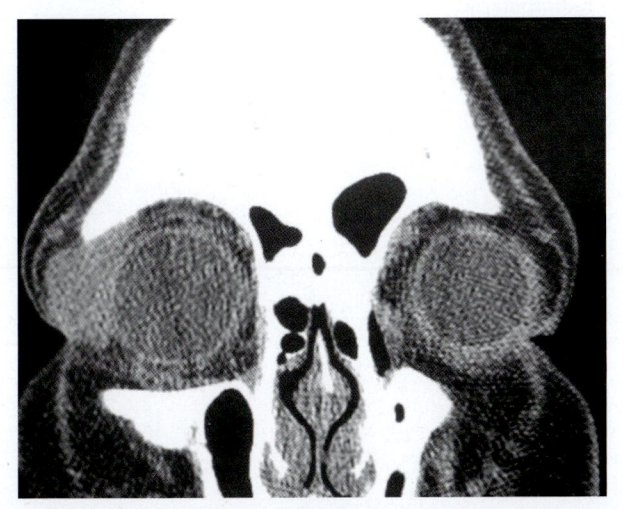

Figure 39.63. Coronal computed tomography showing the mass apparently emanating from lacrimal gland fossa.

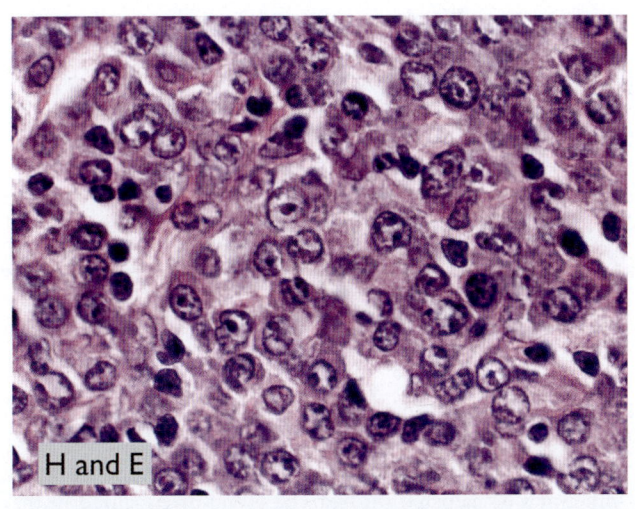

Figure 39.64. Following surgical excision, histopathology show monomorphic lymphocytes with prominent nucleoli. (Hematoxylin–eosin ×150.)

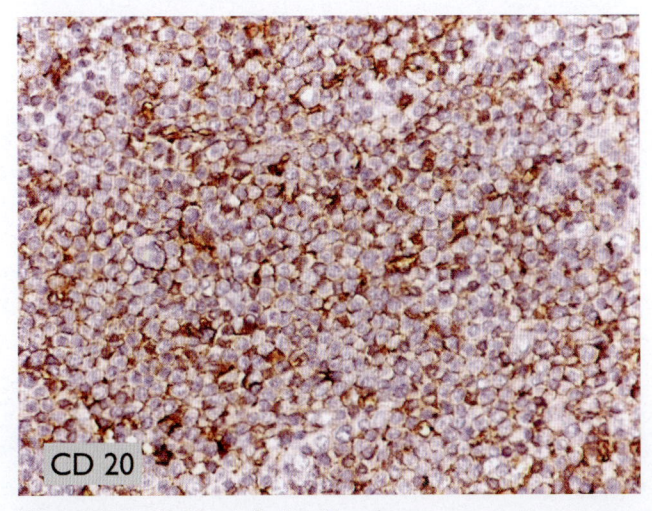

Figure 39.65. CD 20 stain for B-cell lymphocytes was positive, suggesting B-cell lymphoma. (CD 20 ×100.)

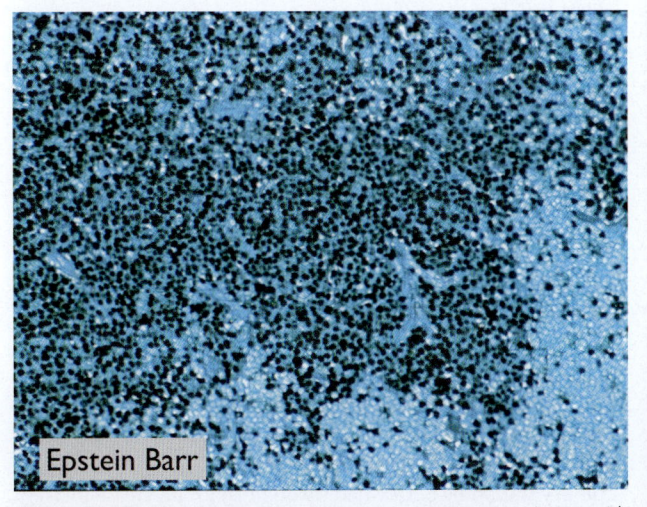

Figure 39.66. Epstein–Barr virus stain was positive, consistent with post-transplant lymphoproliferative disorder. The patient was managed with reduction in immune suppression. (EBV ×100.)

ORBITAL–ORBITAL INVOLVEMENT BY LEUKEMIA (MYELOID SARCOMA)

General Considerations

Leukemia is a well-known neoplastic proliferation of abnormal leukocytes. Although the classification of leukemia is complex and continues to change, the main types are acute lymphoblastic leukemia, chronic lymphocytic leukemia, acute myelogenous myeloid leukemia, and chronic myelogenous leukemia. Any form of leukemia can affect the orbit and orbital involvement can be the first sign of systemic disease (1–24). The best-known form of orbital leukemia is soft tissue invasion by myelogenous leukemia, also called myeloid sarcoma, granulocytic sarcoma, or chloroma (5,11). As several variants of acute myeloid leukemia by definition have few or no cells of granulocytic lineage, the broader term "myeloid sarcoma" is currently preferred. It is important to realize that the orbital myeloid sarcoma can occur before the recognition of blood or bone marrow involvement (2). Therefore, myeloid sarcoma must be included in the differential diagnosis of an otherwise normal child who presents with a unilateral or bilateral orbital tumor.

Orbital myeloid sarcoma is usually considered to be rare. However, it is more prevalent in the Middle East, Asia, and Africa (2). Many large clinical series have come from Turkey (5) and India (11,14,22). In the authors' series of 1,264 orbital lesions, there were 3 cases of chronic lymphocytic leukemia, 3 cases of acute myeloid leukemia, and 2 cases of acute lymphocytic leukemia with orbital involvement (3). In most instances, orbital myeloid sarcoma occurs in young children (4). It is rare among orbital tumors of childhood, accounting for only 1 of 250 cases in a prior report from our department (4).

Clinical Features

The patient is typically a child in the first of decade of life who presents with unilateral or bilateral eyelid edema, proptosis, or displacement of the globe. A firm rubbery mass can sometimes be palpated through the eyelid or visualized in the conjunctiva as a red-pink fleshy mass. The clinical differential includes lymphoma, metastatic neuroblastoma, and idiopathic orbital inflammation ("inflammatory pseudotumor"). Orbital involvement by acute myeloid sarcoma is relatively rare among orbital tumors and pseudotumors. However, in the setting of simultaneous bilateral orbital tumors in children, myeloid sarcoma appears to be one of the most likely diagnoses. Any child with an orbital mass of uncertain origin, particularly if it is bilateral, should be evaluated for acute myeloid leukemia (13).

Diagnostic Approaches

Any child with an orbital mass should have initially a complete blood count or other studies to exclude leukemia. If the blood count is elevated, a bone marrow biopsy is generally performed to establish the diagnosis. Orbital magnetic resonance imaging and computed tomography disclose an orbital soft tissue mass that enhances with contrast agents. This soft tissue mass can occasionally involve bone and extend into the temporal fossa. A biopsy should be performed through an eyelid crease incision or skin incision in the temporal fossa if there is a palpable mass.

Pathology

Histopathologically, myeloid sarcoma is composed of round cells that are similar to cells seen in large cell lymphoma (2,9–11). However, the nuclei are more oval and the cytoplasm is more granular. When the pathologist renders a diagnosis of lymphoma from an orbital biopsy in a child, the alternative diagnosis of leukemia should also be entertained. In such cases, the Leder stain or immunohistochemical stains for lysosome (muramidase) for identification of cytoplasmic esterase can be done to substantiate the diagnosis of leukemia. Electron microscopy can also be helpful in difficult cases (11).

Management

The management involves treatment of the systemic leukemia with appropriate chemotherapeutic agents. The orbital tumor generally responds well to the chemotherapy. It is also sensitive to radiotherapy.

ORBITAL–ORBITAL INVOLVEMENT BY LEUKEMIA (MYELOID SARCOMA)

Selected References

Reviews

1. Jaffe ES. The 2008 WHO classification of lymphomas: implications for clinical practice and translational research. *Hematology* 2009;523–531.
2. Zimmerman L, Font RL. Ophthalmologic manifestations of granulocytic sarcoma (myeloid sarcoma or chloroma). *Am J Ophthalmol* 1975;30:975–990.
3. Shields JA, Shields CL, Scartozzi R. Survey of 1264 patients with orbital tumors and simulating lesions: the 2002 Montgomery Lecture, part 1. *Ophthalmology* 2004;111:997–1008.
4. Shields JA, Bakewell B, Augsburger DG, et al. Space-occupying orbital masses in children. A review of 250 consecutive biopsies. *Ophthalmology* 1986;93:379–384.
5. Cavdar AO, Arcasoy A, Babacan E, et al. Ocular granulocytic sarcoma (chloroma with acute myelomonocytic leukemia in Turkish children. *Cancer* 1978;41:1606–1609.
6. Kincaid MC, Green WR. Ocular and orbital involvement in leukemia. *Surv Ophthalmol* 1983;27:211–232.
7. Rosenthal AR. Ocular manifestations of leukemia. A review. *Ophthalmology* 1983;90:899–905.
8. Brownstein S, Thelmo W, Olivier A. Granulocytic sarcoma of the orbit. *Can J Ophthalmol* 1975;10:174–183.

Histopathology

9. Davis JL, Parke DW II, Font RL. Granulocytic sarcoma of the orbit. A clinicopathologic study. *Ophthalmology* 1985;92:1758–1762.
10. Singh T, Jayaram G, Gupta AK. Cytologic diagnosis of myeloid sarcoma. *Am J Ophthalmol* 1985;99:496–497.
11. Aggarwal E, Mulay K, Honavar SG. Orbital extra-medullary granulocytic sarcoma: Clinicopathologic correlation with immunohistochemical features. *Surv Ophthalmol* 2014;59:232–235.

Case Reports

12. Michelson JB, Shields JA, Leonard BC, et al. Periorbital chloroma and proptosis in a two-year old with acute myelogenous leukemia. *J Pediatr Ophthalmol* 1975;12:255–258.
13. Shields JA, Stopyra GA, Marr BP, et al. Bilateral orbital myeloid sarcoma as initial sign of acute myeloid leukemia. *Arch Ophthalmol* 2003;121:138–142.
14. Shome DK, Gupta NK, Prajapati NC, et al. Orbital granulocytic sarcomas (myeloid sarcomas) in acute nonlymphocytic leukemia. *Cancer* 1992;70:2298–2301.
15. Ohta K, Kondoh T, Yasuo K, et al. Primary granulocytic sarcoma in the sphenoidal bone and orbit. *Childs Nerv Syst* 2003;19:674–679.
16. Consul BN, Kulshrestha OP, Mehrotra AS. Bilateral proptosis in acute myeloid leukemia. *Br J Ophthalmol* 1967;51:65–67.
17. Rajantie J, Tarkkanen A, Rapola J, et al. Orbital granulocytic sarcoma as a presenting sign in acute myelogenous leukemia. *Ophthalmologica* 1984;189:158–161.
18. Jordan DR, Noel LP, Carpenter BF. Chloroma. *Arch Ophthalmol* 1991;109:734–735.
19. Watkins LM, Remulla HD, Rubin PA. Orbital granulocytic sarcoma in an elderly patient. *Am J Ophthalmol* 1997;123:854–856.
20. Stockl FA, Dolmetsch M, Saornil A, et al. Orbital granulocytic sarcoma. *Br J Ophthalmol* 1997;1:1084–1088.
21. Bhattacharjee K, Bhattacharjee H, Das D, et al. Chloroma of the orbit in a non leukemic adult: a case report. *Orbit* 2003;22:293–297.
22. Gujral S, Bhattarai S, Mohan A, et al. Ocular extramedullary myeloid cell tumour in children: an Indian study. *J Trop Pediatr* 1999;45:112–115.
23. Mangla D, Dewan M, Meyer DR. Adult orbital myeloid sarcoma (granulocytic sarcoma): two cases and review of the literature. *Orbit* 2012;31(6):438–440.
24. Esmaeli B, Medeiros LJ, Myers J, et al. Orbital mass secondary to precursor T-cell acute lymphoblastic leukemia: a rare presentation. *Arch Ophthalmol* 2001;119(3):443–446.

ORBITAL MYELOID SARCOMA (LEUKEMIA)

Davis JL, Parke DW II, Font RL. Granulocytic sarcoma of the orbit. A clinicopathologic study. *Ophthalmology* 1985;92:1758–1762.

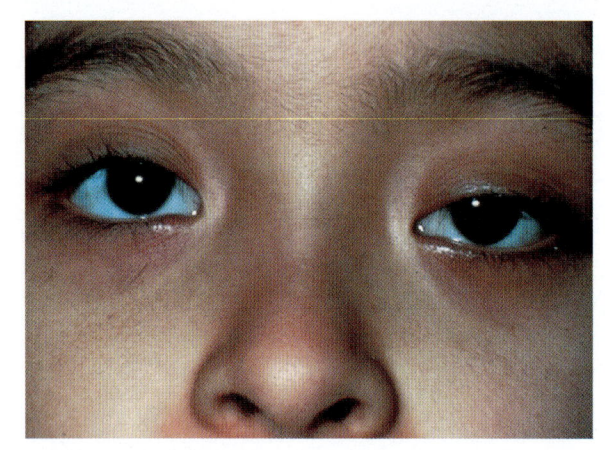

Figure 39.67. Blepharoptosis and proptosis of left eye owing to granulocytic sarcoma in a 9-year-old girl. (Courtesy of Ramon Font, MD.)

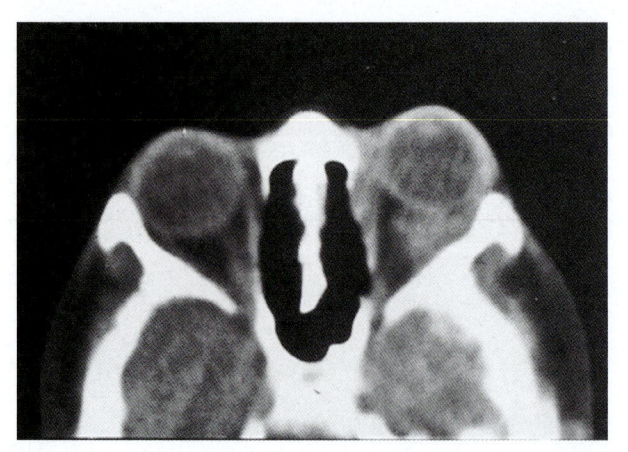

Figure 39.68. Axial computed tomography of patient shown in Figure 39.67, depicting an irregular orbital mass. Biopsy of an associated brain lesion revealed granulocytic sarcoma. It was almost 1 month later that the patient developed positive blood studies for leukemia. (Courtesy of Ramon Font, MD.)

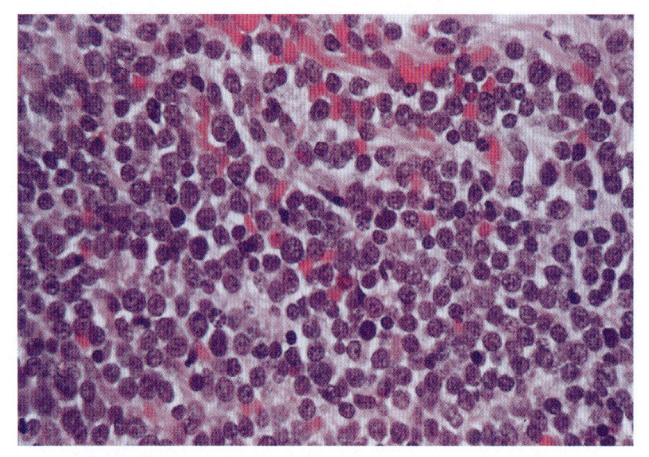

Figure 39.69. Histopathology of tumor seen in Figure 39.67, showing poorly differentiated blast cells. (Hematoxylin–eosin ×150.) (Courtesy of Ramon Font, MD.)

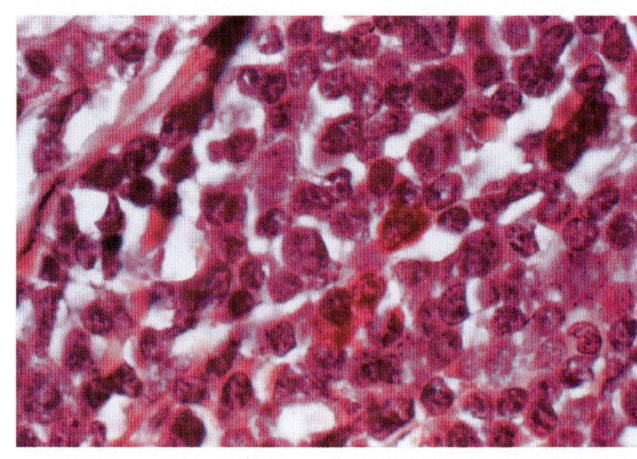

Figure 39.70. Leder stain of tumor shown in Figure 39.67, depicting the cytoplasmic granules. (Leder stain ×250.) (Courtesy of Ramon Font, MD.)

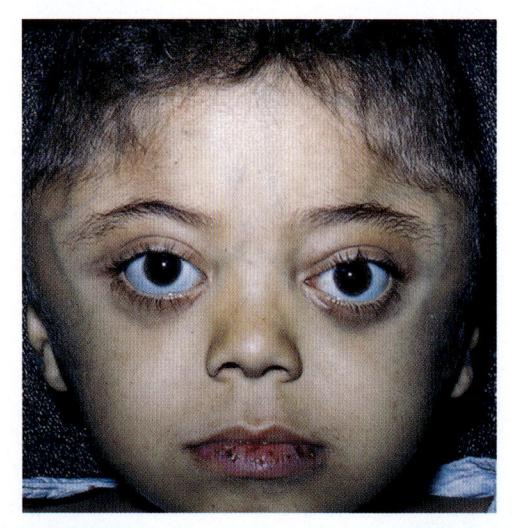

Figure 39.71. Bilateral masses in orbit and temporal fossa in child with leukemia. Note the pallor of the skin.

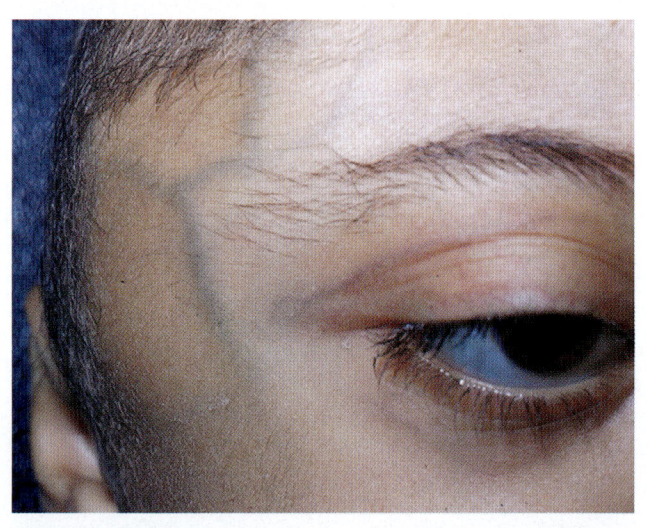

Figure 39.72. Close view of right eye and temporal area in child shown in Figure 39.71. Note the dilated temporal vein.

● ORBITAL MYELOID SARCOMA (LEUKEMIA): BILATERAL ORBITAL INVOLVEMENT

Orbital myeloid sarcoma is an uncommon cause of proptosis in children. However, when one considers bilateral simultaneous orbital tumors of childhood, myeloid sarcoma is one of the most common etiologies.

Shields JA, Stopyra GA, Marr BP, et al. Bilateral orbital myeloid sarcoma as initial sign of acute myeloid leukemia. *Arch Ophthalmol* 2S003;121:138–142.

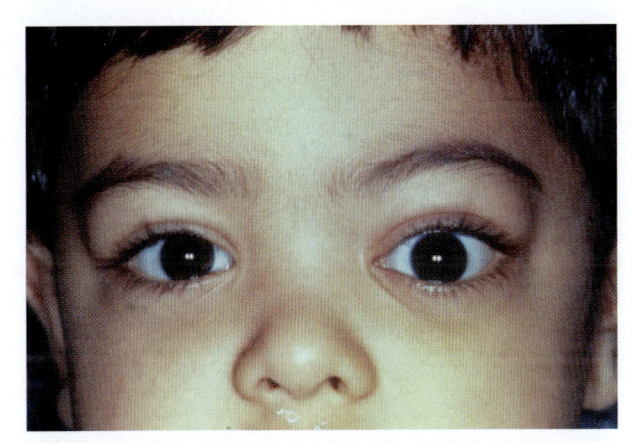

Figure 39.73. A previously healthy, 25-month-old boy developed painless progressive proptosis of his left eye over 2 weeks.

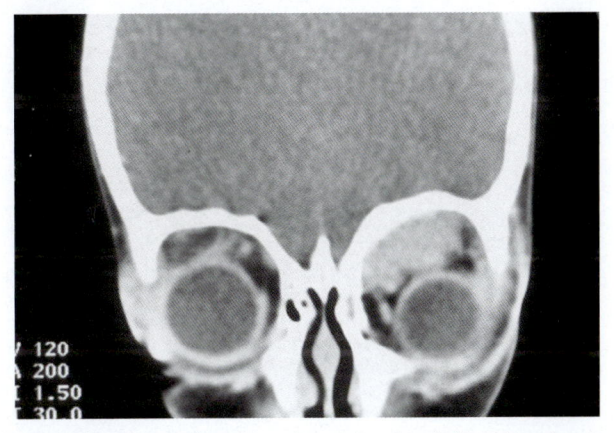

Figure 39.74. Coronal computed tomography of the orbits showing bilateral superior orbital masses. The mass in the left orbit (*to the right*) is larger and more clearly seen.

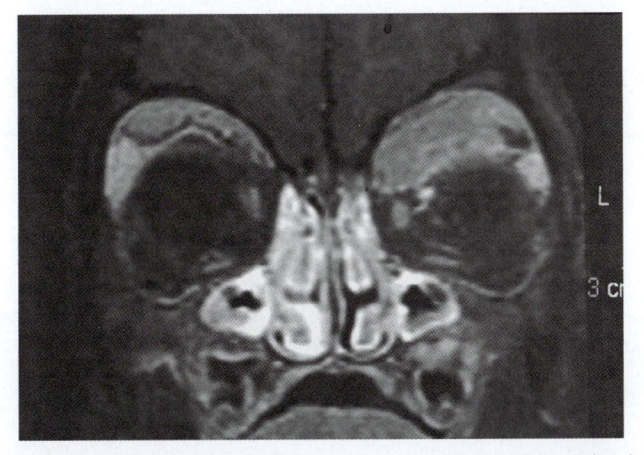

Figure 39.75. Coronal magnetic resonance imaging in T1-weighted image with gadolinium enhancement showing soft tissue masses in the superior aspect of each orbit.

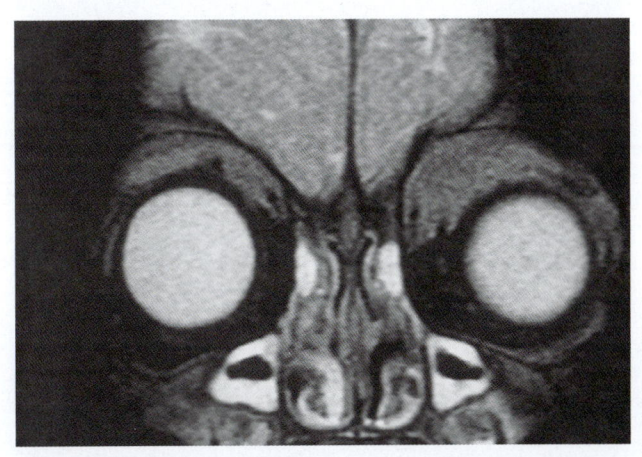

Figure 39.76. Coronal magnetic resonance imaging in T2-weighted image with gadolinium enhancement depicting the extent of the superior orbital tumors.

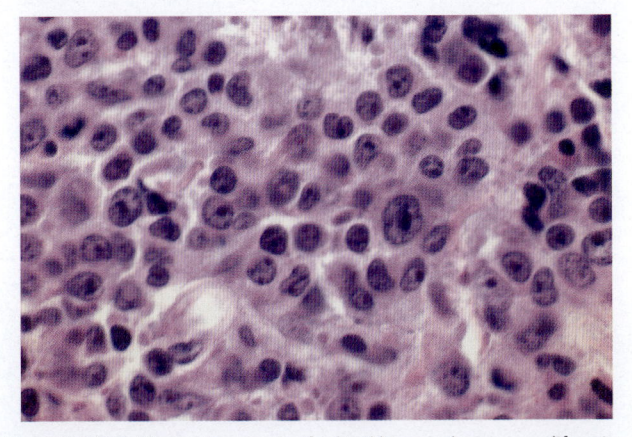

Figure 39.77. Photomicrograph of orbital biopsy showing proliferation of poorly differentiated cells with irregular nuclear contours, typical of monoblasts. (Hematoxylin–eosin ×250.) The Leder stain was positive, supporting the diagnosis.

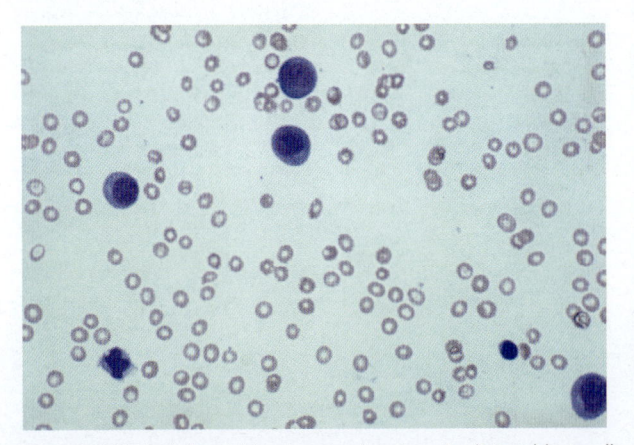

Figure 39.78. Peripheral blood stain showing circulating blast cells compatible with diagnosis of myeloid leukemia. (Hematoxylin–eosin ×400.)

CHAPTER 40

ORBITAL SECONDARY TUMORS

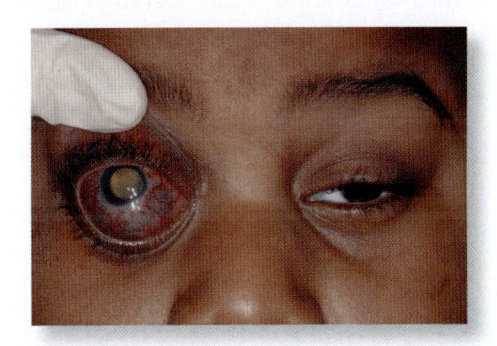

General Considerations

By traditional definition, an orbital secondary tumor is a neoplasm that has invaded the orbital tissues to form a neoplastic site in adjacent structures such as eyelid, conjunctiva, intraocular structures, sinuses, nasopharynx, and brain (1–34). This is to be differentiated from a metastatic orbital tumor in which the lesion reaches the orbit from a distant cancer by hematogenous or neural routes. In this chapter, we provide an overview of the subject, followed by selected examples of specific lesions that invade the orbit.

The main eyelid tumors that can involve the orbit secondarily include basal cell carcinoma, sebaceous gland carcinoma, squamous cell carcinoma, cutaneous melanoma, and Merkel cell carcinoma. Conjunctival tumors include melanoma and squamous cell carcinoma, particularly the mucoepidermoid and spindle cell variants. Intraocular tumors include uveal melanoma and retinoblastoma, and, rarely, medulloepithelioma and acquired epithelial tumors of the ciliary body. Sinus tumors that can secondarily invade the orbit include carcinoma of the ethmoid or maxillary sinus and, rarely, rhabdomyosarcoma. Nasopharyngeal tumors include carcinoma, juvenile angiofibroma, and esthesioneuroblastoma. Intracranial tumors include sphenoid wing meningioma and, rarely, glioblastoma. Most of the tumors that can secondarily invade the orbit have been discussed in other chapters and the other atlases. In the authors' clinical series, the 142 secondary orbital tumors accounted for 11% of the 1,264 orbital lesions. That series was somewhat biased because of the large number of patients with uveal melanoma and retinoblastoma seen by the authors and the fewer cases of primary sinus carcinoma referred to the authors (1).

Clinical Features

The clinical features of a secondary orbital tumor necessarily vary with the type and location of the primary neoplasm. In many instances, there is a prior history of excision or other management of a periorbital lesion. This is particularly true of eyelid, conjunctival, lacrimal sac, and intraocular tumors. In cases of sinus or nasopharyngeal tumors and sphenoid wing meningioma, the orbital manifestations are commonly the initial features of the disease.

Diagnostic Approaches

In cases of suspected secondary orbital tumor, it is important to take a detailed medical history and to perform an ocular and systemic evaluation. External ocular examination, slit-lamp biomicroscopy, and fundus examination can reveal the primary tumor. Imaging studies, particularly computed tomography (CT) and magnetic resonance imaging (MRI), are mandatory to determine the extent of orbital involvement and to assess the status of a primary lesion in the eyelid, conjunctiva, globe, paranasal sinuses, nasopharynx, or brain.

Pathology

The histopathology of a secondary orbital tumor necessarily varies with the type of neoplasm. The pathology of these tumors is covered in textbooks and elsewhere in the current atlases.

ORBITAL SECONDARY TUMORS

Management

The management of orbital extension of the various periorbital tumors can vary greatly from case to case. Each case must be individualized. In general, wide surgical resection often followed by irradiation or chemotherapy are treatment options. Massive orbital extension by primary eyelid and conjunctival tumors (basal cell carcinoma, squamous cell carcinoma, melanoma, etc.) are usually managed initially by wide surgical excision, which includes orbital exenteration (6). Massive orbital extension of uveal melanoma (23) or retinoblastoma (24–27) may also require orbital exenteration, but there are various alternatives for mild degrees of orbital involvement, including techniques of irradiation and chemotherapy. Mild degrees of secondary orbital invasion by lymphoma, metastatic carcinoma, rhabdomyosarcoma, and esthesioneuroblastoma can usually be managed by irradiation. Orbital extension of sphenoid wing meningiomas can be managed by surgical excision, irradiation, or both, depending on the clinical situation. There are many other situations where treatment depends on the entire clinical situation.

These sources cite many other references on specific tumors that secondarily involve the orbit.

Selected References

Reviews

1. Shields JA, Shields CL, Scartozzi R. Survey of 1264 patients with orbital tumors and simulating lesions: The 2002 Montgomery Lecture, part 1. *Ophthalmology* 2004;111:997–1008.
2. Shields JA, Bakewell B, Augsburger JJ, et al. Classification and incidence of space-occupying lesions of the orbit. A survey of 645 biopsies. *Arch Ophthalmol* 1984;102:1606–1611.
3. Shields JA, Bakewell B, Augsburger JJ, et al. Space-occupying orbital masses in children: A review of 250 consecutive biopsies. *Ophthalmology* 1986;93:379–384.
4. Demirci H, Shields CL, Shields JA, et al. Orbital tumors in the older adult population. *Ophthalmology* 2002;109:243–248.
5. Glover AT, Grove AS Jr. Orbital invasion by malignant eyelid tumors. *Ophthal Plast Reconstr Surg* 1989;5:1–12.

Management

6. Shields JA, Shields CL, Suvarnamani C, et al. Orbital exenteration with eyelid sparing: indications, technique and results. *Ophthalmic Surg* 1991;22:292–297.
7. Shields JA, Shields CL, De Potter P. Surgical approach to conjunctival tumors. The 1994 Lynn B. McMahan Lecture. *Arch Ophthalmol* 1997;115:808–815.

Case Reports

Eyelid Basal Cell Carcinoma

8. Madge SN, Khine AA, Thaller VT, et al. Globe-sparing surgery for medial canthal basal cell carcinoma with anterior orbital invasion. *Ophthalmology* 2010;117:2222–2228.

Eyelid Sebaceous Carcinoma

9. Shields JA, Demirci H, Marr BP, et al. Sebaceous carcinoma of the ocular region. *Surv Ophthalmol* 2005;50:103–122.
10. Shields JA, Demirci H, Marr BP, et al. Sebaceous carcinoma of the eyelids. Personal experience with 60 cases. *Ophthalmology* 2004;111:2151–2157.
11. Rao NA, Hidayat AA, McLean IW, et al. Sebaceous gland carcinoma of the ocular adnexa: A clinicopathologic study of 104 cases with five year follow-up data. *Hum Pathol* 1982;13:113–122.
12. Priyadarshini O, Biswas G, Biswas S, et al. Neoadjuvant chemotherapy in recurrent sebaceous carcinoma of eyelid with orbital invasion and regional lymphadenopathy. *Ophthal Plast Reconstr Surg* 2010;26:366–368.

Eyelid Squamous Cell Carcinoma

13. Detorakis ET, Ioannakis K, Giatromanolaki A, et al. Selective removal of sebaceous gland carcinoma of the lower eyelid with orbital infiltration. *Ophthalmic Surg Lasers Imaging* 2007;38:413–416.

Eyelid Melanoma

14. Johnson TE, Tabbara KF, Weatherhead RG, et al. Secondary squamous cell carcinoma of the orbit. *Arch Ophthalmol* 1997;115:75–78.
15. Shields JA, Elder D, Arbizo V, et al. Orbital involvement with desmoplastic melanoma. *Br J Ophthalmol* 1987;71:279–285.
16. Dithmar S, Meldrum ML, Murray DR, et al. Desmoplastic spindle-cell melanoma of the eyelid with orbital invasion. *Ophthal Plast Reconstr Surg* 1999;15:134–136.

Conjunctival Melanoma

17. Polito E, Leccisotti A. Primary and secondary orbital melanomas: a clinical and prognostic study. *Ophthal Plast Reconstr Surg* 1995;11:169–181.
18. Shields CL, Markowitz JS, Belinsky I, et al. Conjunctival melanoma. Outcomes based on tumor origin in 382 consecutive cases. *Ophthalmology* 2011;118:389–395.
19. Shields CL, Shields JA, Gunduz K, et al. Conjunctival melanoma: Risk factors for recurrence, exenteration, metastasis and death in 150 consecutive patients. *Arch Ophthalmol* 2000;118:1497–1507.
20. Crawford JB. Conjunctival melanomas: prognostic factors. A review and analysis of a series. *Trans Am Ophthalmol Soc* 1980;78:467–502.
21. Paridaens AD, McCartney AC, Minassian DC, et al. Orbital exenteration in 95 cases of primary conjunctival malignant melanoma. *Br J Ophthalmol* 1994;78:520–528.

Uveal Melanoma

22. Shields JA, Shields CL, Gunduz K, et al. Clinical features predictive of orbital exenteration for conjunctival melanoma. *Ophthal Plast Reconstr Surg* 2000;16:173–178.
23. Shields JA, Shields C. Massive orbital extension of posterior uveal melanoma. *J Ophthal Plast Reconstr Surg* 1991;7:238–251.

Retinoblastoma

24. Ellsworth RM. Orbital retinoblastoma. *Trans Am Ophthalmol Soc* 1974;72:88.
25. Shields CL, Shields JA, Baez K, et al. Optic nerve invasion of retinoblastoma. Metastatic potential and clinical risk factors. *Cancer* 1994;73:692–698.
26. Hungerford J, Kingston J, Plowman N. Orbital recurrence of retinoblastoma. *Ophthalmic Paediatr Genet* 1987;8:63–68.
27. Kaliki S, Shields CL, Shah SU, et al. Postenucleation adjuvant chemotherapy with vincristine, etoposide, and carboplatin for the treatment of high-risk retinoblastoma. *Arch Ophthalmol* 2011;129:1422–1427.

Sinus Tumors

28. Conley JJ. Sinus tumors invading the orbit. *Trans Am Acad Ophthalmol Otolaryngol* 1966;70:615–619.
29. Johnson LN, Krohel GB, Yeon EB, et al. Sinus tumors invading the orbit. *Ophthalmology* 1984;91:209–217.

Other Tumors

30. Rakes SM, Yeatts RP, Campbell RJ. Ophthalmic manifestations of esthesioneuroblastoma. *Ophthalmology* 1985;92:1749–1753.
31. Elner VM, Burnstine MA, Goodman ML, et al. Inverted papillomas that invade the orbit. *Arch Ophthalmol* 1995;113:1178–1183.
32. Perlman JI, Specht CS, McLean IW, et al. Oncocytic adenocarcinoma of the lacrimal sac: report of a case with paranasal sinus and orbital extension. *Ophthalmic Surg* 1995;26:377–379.
33. Moshari A, Bloom EE, McLean IW, et al. Ectopic chordoma with orbital invasion. *Am J Ophthalmol* 2001;131:400–401.
34. Herwig MC, Fischer HP, Moore CE, et al. Orbital invasion of a maxillary ameloblastoma. *Ophthalmology* 110:251–254.

ORBITAL INVASION FROM EYELID BASAL CELL CARCINOMA

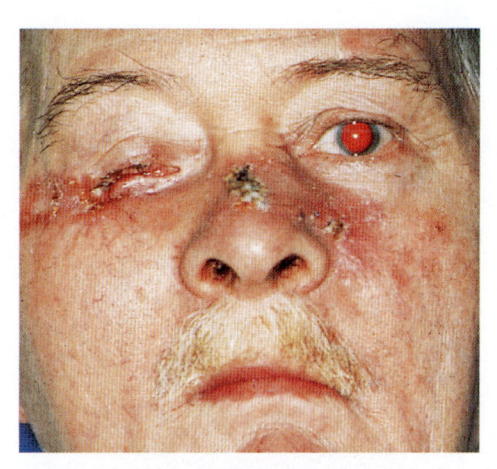

Figure 40.1. Neglected basal cell carcinoma near lateral canthus with secondary orbital invasion in a 63-year-old man. The motility of the eye was markedly restricted owing to diffuse orbital involvement.

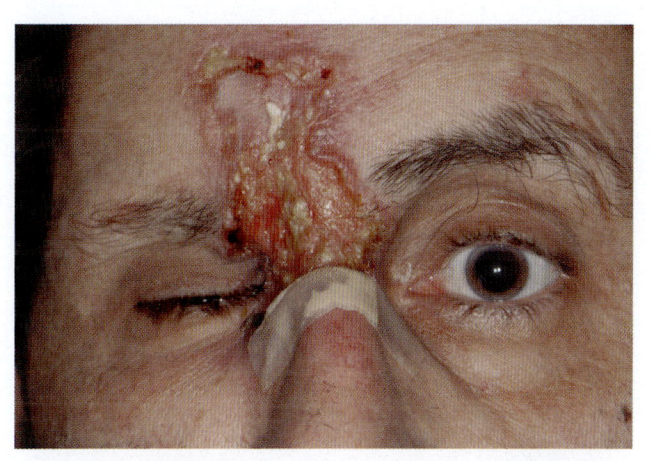

Figure 40.2. Neglected basal cell carcinoma of nasal bridge and forehead with secondary orbital invasion causing right blepharoptosis and dysmotility in a 67-year-old man.

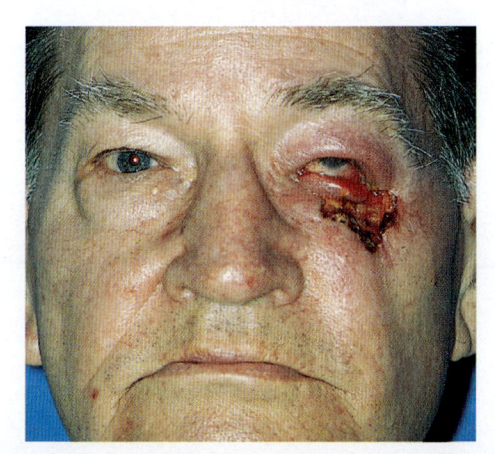

Figure 40.3. Neglected basal cell carcinoma of lower eyelid and lateral canthus with secondary orbital invasion causing upward displacement of the right eye in a 69-year-old man. The motility of the eye was markedly restricted.

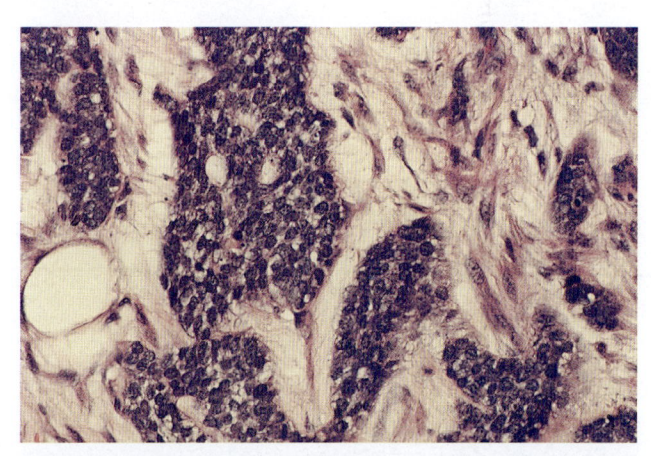

Figure 40.4. Histopathology of lesion shown in Figure 40.3 after orbital exenteration. Note the morpheaform basal cell carcinoma in a fibrous connective tissue stroma. (Hematoxylin–eosin ×200.)

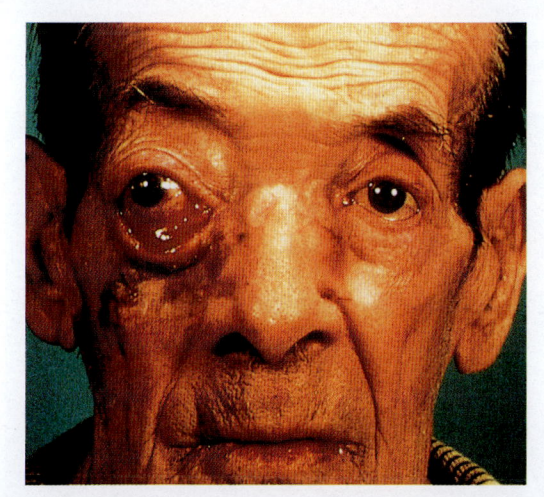

Figure 40.5. Orbital invasion by basal cell carcinoma of the lower eyelid in a 66-year-old man. He had excision of a basal cell carcinoma from right lower eyelid 16 years earlier but he did not return for follow-up. Note that the globe is displaced superiorly and laterally. (Courtesy of Moshe Lahav, MD.)

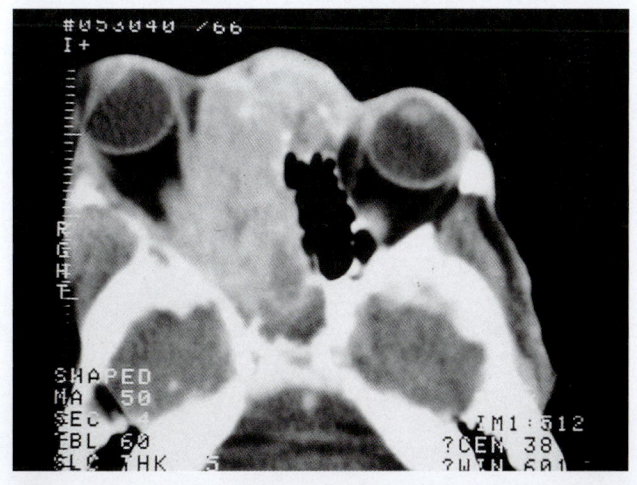

Figure 40.6. Axial computed tomography of patient shown in Figure 40.5. Note the massive tumor replacing the medial aspect of the orbit and ethmoid sinus with extension into the cranial cavity. (Courtesy of Moshe Lahav, MD.)

ORBITAL INVASION FROM EYELID SEBACEOUS CARCINOMA: SIMULATING A PRIMARY LACRIMAL GLAND TUMOR

Sebaceous gland carcinoma can occasionally invade the lacrimal gland and surrounding tissues from a diffuse tumor in the eyelid, simulating a primary neoplasm of the lacrimal gland.

Shields JA, Font RL. Meibomian gland carcinoma presenting as a lacrimal gland tumor. *Arch Ophthalmol* 1974;92:304–308.

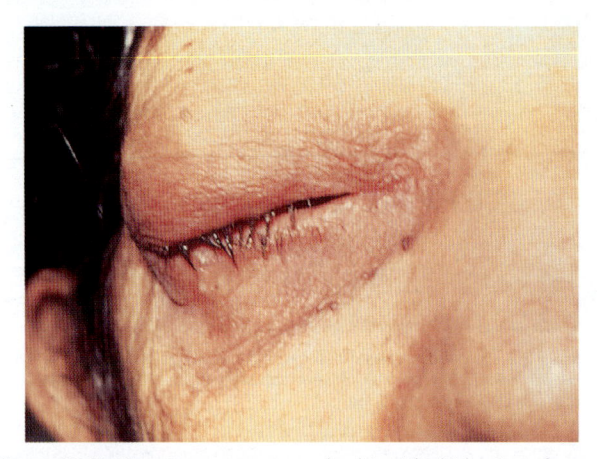

Figure 40.7. Mass in superotemporal orbit with thickening of upper eyelid in a 65-year-old woman. The eyelids were mildly thickened by the eyelid neoplasm. A small lacrimal gland biopsy done elsewhere revealed a malignancy and orbital exenteration was done.

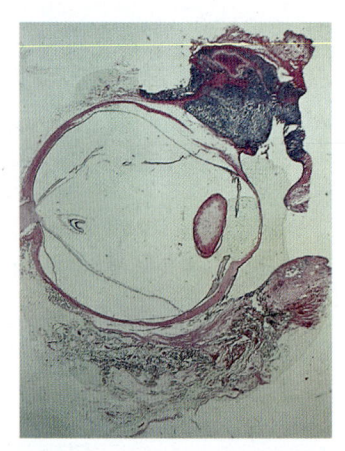

Figure 40.8. Low-magnification photomicrograph showing basophilic mass superior to the globe in the lacrimal gland.

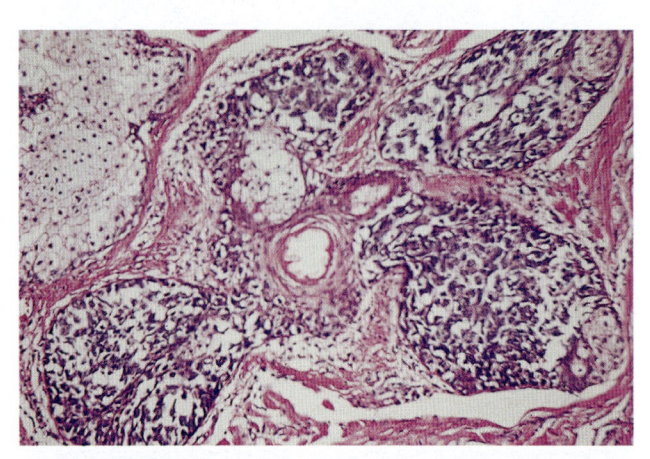

Figure 40.9. Photomicrograph of tarsal region, showing lobules of sebaceous gland carcinoma. (Hematoxylin–eosin ×125.)

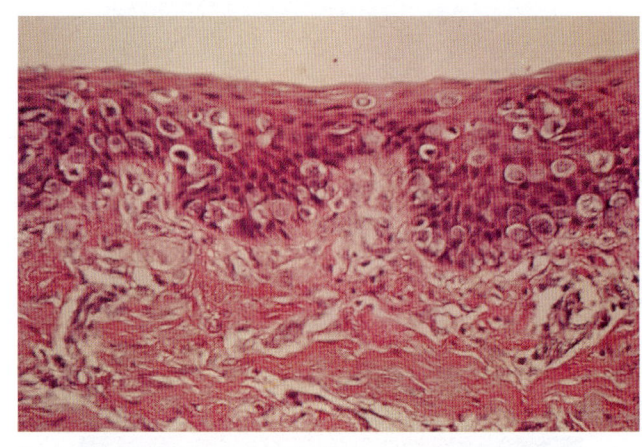

Figure 40.10. Photomicrograph showing Pagetoid invasion of sebaceous gland carcinoma in the epidermis. (Hematoxylin–eosin ×75.)

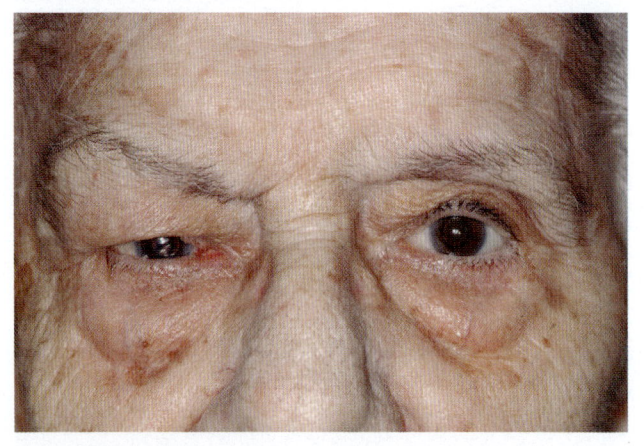

Figure 40.11. Elderly woman presenting with right mass in lacrimal gland area. Although there was a suggestion of primary lacrimal gland neoplasm, the thickened eyelids suggested sebaceous carcinoma. The lesion was removed surgically and residual eyelid/conjunctival tumor was treated with plaque brachytherapy.

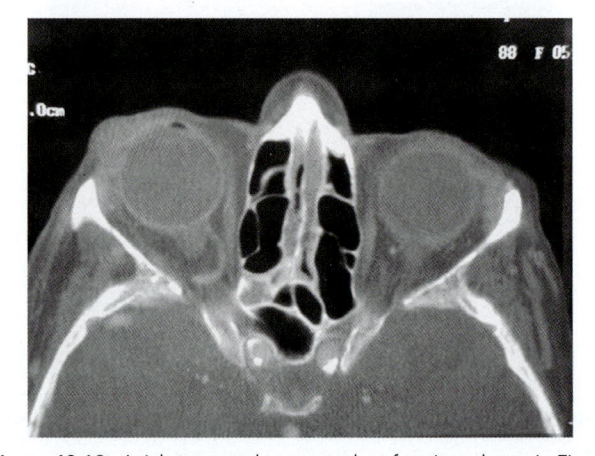

Figure 40.12. Axial computed tomography of patient shown in Figure 40.11, revealing a diffuse mass in lacrimal gland region, suggesting a primary lacrimal gland lymphoma.

ORBITAL INVASION FROM EYELID MELANOMA

Cutaneous melanoma has a tendency in some cases to invade the dermis by neurotropic mechanisms and to recur as a deep nodule. An eyelid melanoma can invade the soft tissues of the orbit by a similar mechanism. This is particularly true of desmoplastic melanoma, which can exhibit deeper invasion along nerves, a process called "neurotropism."

Shields JA, Elder D, Arbizo V, et al. Orbital involvement with desmoplastic melanoma. *Br J Ophthalmol* 1987;71:279–285.

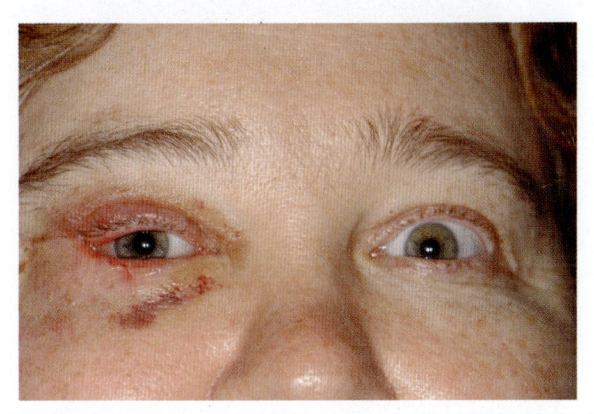

Figure 40.13. Young woman with history of primary melanoma of right lower eyelid. She had biopsy elsewhere and recurrent eyelid melanoma was diagnosed.

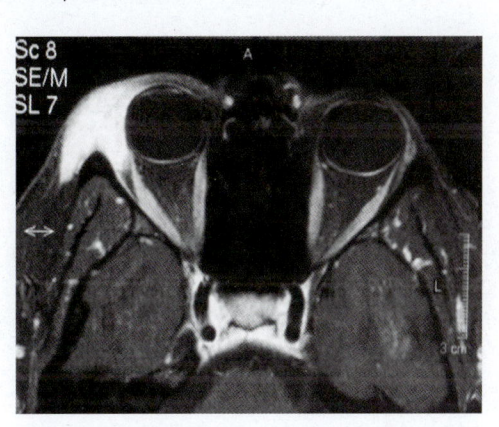

Figure 40.14. Axial magnetic resonance imaging in T1-weighted image with gadolinium enhancement and fat suppression of patient shown in Figure 40.13. Note extension of the eyelid mass into the anterior temporal aspect of the orbit. The patient underwent orbital exenteration but later developed overt systemic metastasis.

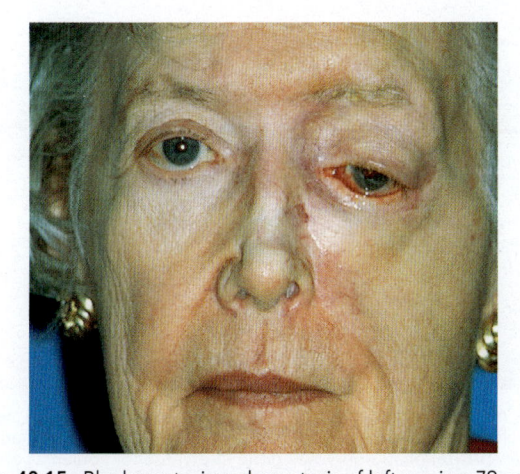

Figure 40.15. Blepharoptosis and proptosis of left eye in a 79-year-old woman who had excision of a cutaneous melanoma from left medial canthal area 5 years earlier.

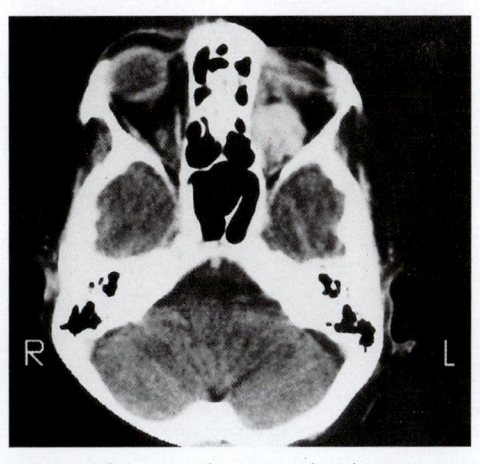

Figure 40.16. Axial computed tomography showing circumscribed tumor in the posterior aspect of the orbit.

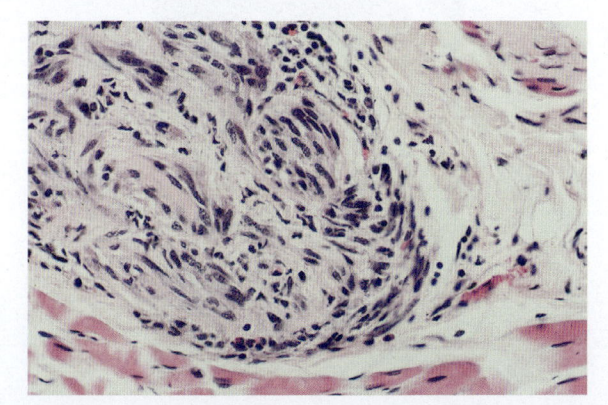

Figure 40.17. Histopathology of reexamined cutaneous lesions showing spindle cells invading a nerve. (Hematoxylin–eosin ×100.)

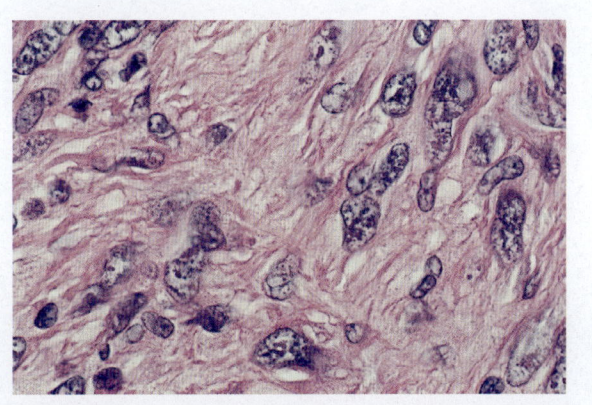

Figure 40.18. Photomicrograph of another area of orbital tumor showing anaplastic spindle and epithelioid cells. Immunohistochemistry of both the original eyelid lesion and the orbital recurrence confirmed the diagnosis of melanoma. (Hematoxylin–eosin ×250.)

ORBITAL INVASION FROM CONJUNCTIVAL SQUAMOUS CELL CARCINOMA

In most instances, conjunctival squamous cell carcinoma can be controlled by carefully performed early surgery. If it is not treated early or if it is incompletely excised, orbital recurrence can develop. This is particularly true in immunosuppressed patients. In such instances, eyelid-sparing orbital exenteration is often required to achieve tumor control.

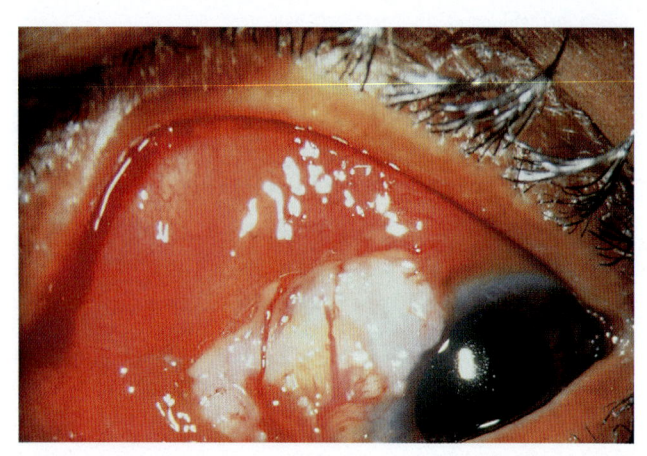

Figure 40.19. Advanced, neglected squamous cell carcinoma on the left eye of a 70-year-old man. Orbital computed tomography showed extension into the orbit with compression of the equator of the globe.

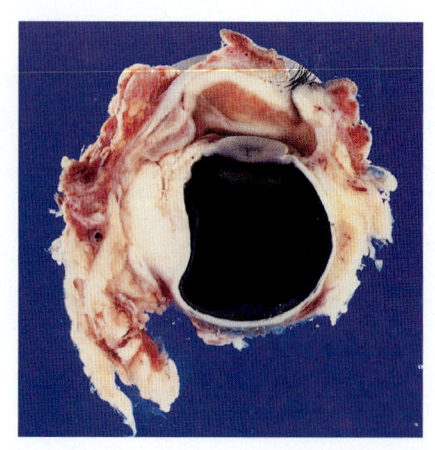

Figure 40.20. Exenteration specimen of patient shown in Figure 40.19, demonstrating white solid tumor extending posteriorly along the surface of the globe (*left*).

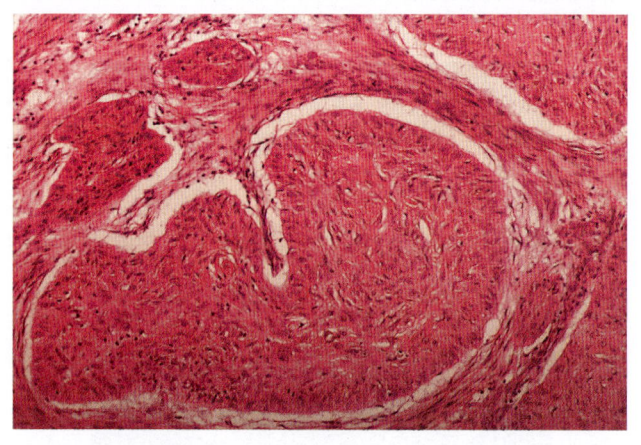

Figure 40.21. Histopathology of lesion shown in Figure 40.20, revealing invasive spindle-shaped cells with keratinization. (Hematoxylin–eosin ×25.)

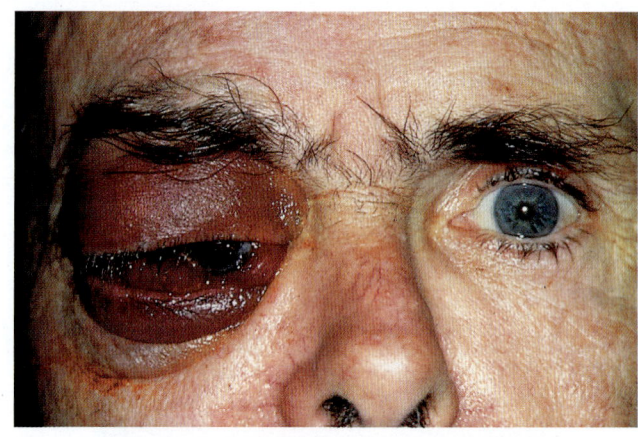

Figure 40.22. Proptosis, eyelid ecchymosis, and conjunctival hemorrhagic chemosis in a 56-year-old man who was immunosuppressed after liver transplantation. Surgery was done elsewhere for conjunctival squamous cell carcinoma and this represented recurrence.

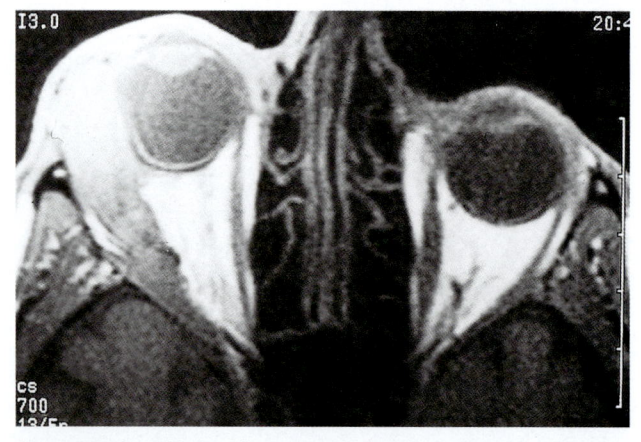

Figure 40.23. Orbital axial magnetic resonance imaging in T1-weighted image of patient shown in Figure 40.22, demonstrating tumor invasion along lateral wall of orbit.

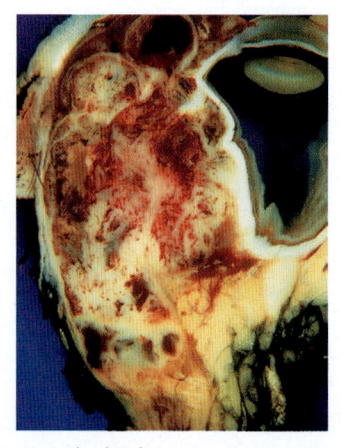

Figure 40.24. Sectioned orbital exenteration specimen demonstrating a large hemorrhagic mass temporal to the globe.

ORBITAL INVASION FROM CONJUNCTIVAL MELANOMA

In rare instances, conjunctival melanoma is far advanced at the time of the initial diagnosis and primary orbital exenteration is necessary. Much more commonly, however, orbital invasion of conjunctival melanoma occurs after a number of prior resections of very aggressive conjunctival melanoma, particularly the type that arises from primary acquired melanosis.

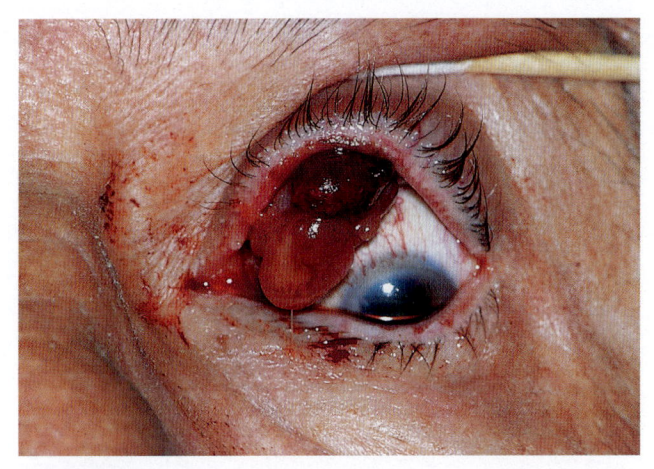

Figure 40.25. Recurrent conjunctival melanoma in superonasal fornix with anterior orbital invasion in a 64-year-old man.

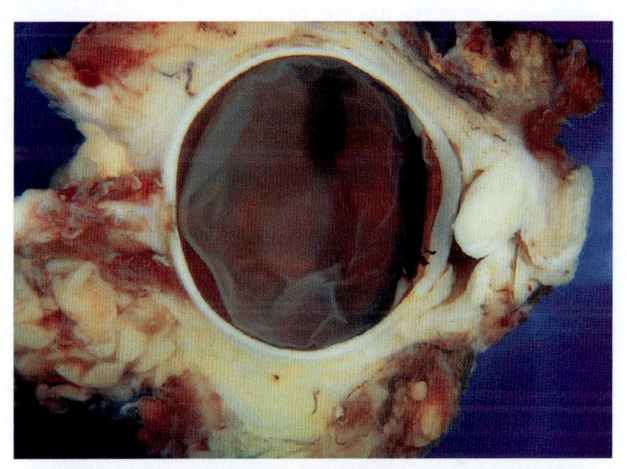

Figure 40.26. Sectioned orbital exenteration specimen from patient shown in Figure 40.25 revealing nodules of amelanotic melanoma anteriorly.

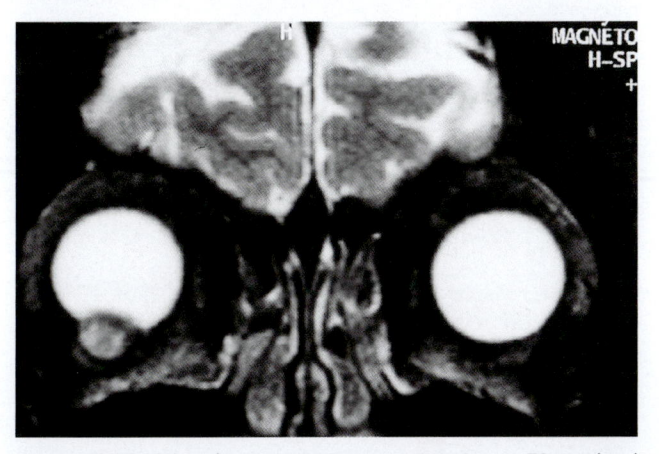

Figure 40.27. Coronal magnetic resonance imaging in T2-weighted image showing inferior orbital melanoma in a 50-year-old woman who had prior excisions of conjunctival melanoma.

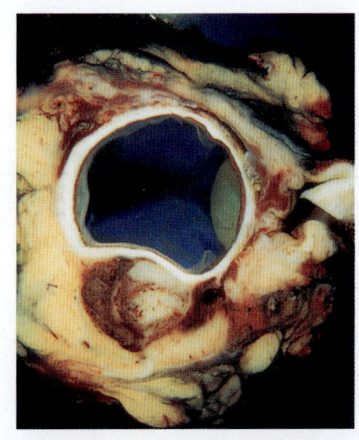

Figure 40.28. Sectioned orbital exenteration specimen from patient shown in Figure 40.27. Note the large tumor nodule indenting the sclera inferiorly.

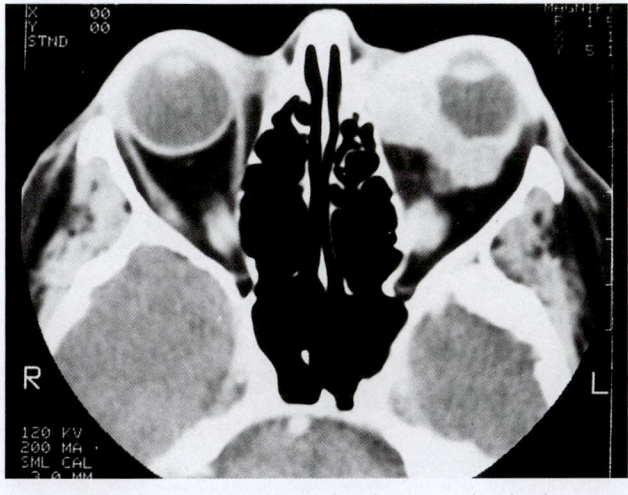

Figure 40.29. Recurrent conjunctival melanoma with orbital invasion surrounding the left globe in a 72-year-old woman.

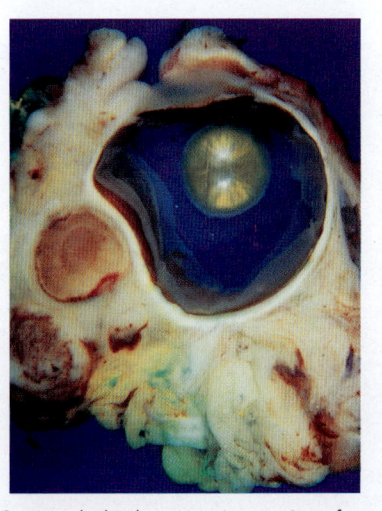

Figure 40.30. Sectioned orbital exenteration specimen from patient shown in Figure 40.29. Note the large tumor nodule indenting the sclera nasally.

ORBITAL INVASION FROM CONJUNCTIVAL MELANOMA IN A YOUNG AFRICAN AMERICAN

Conjunctival melanoma tends to occur in Caucasian patients. In rare instances, this malignancy can arise in non-Caucasians. In our practice of ocular oncology, we have seen several cases of relatively aggressive conjunctival melanoma in young African-American persons.

Shields CL, Markowitz JS, Belinsky I, et al. Conjunctival melanoma. Outcomes based on tumor origin in 382 consecutive cases. *Ophthalmology* 2011;118:389–395.

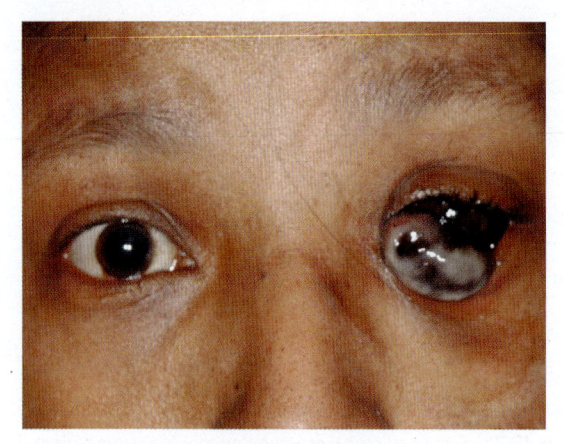

Figure 40.31. Massive conjunctival melanoma in a young African-American woman that grew over a few years.

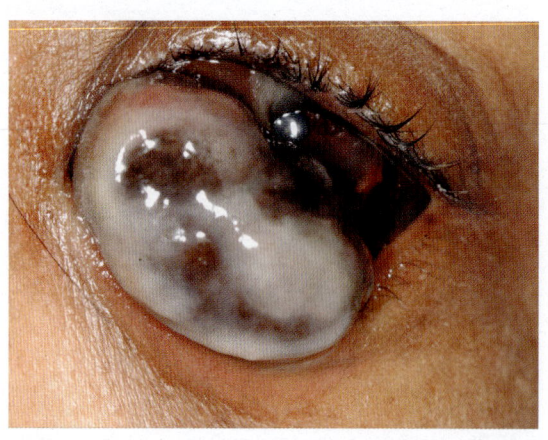

Figure 40.32. Close up view of patient in Figure 20.31 demonstrating the multinodular dark-brown mass completely overhanging the cornea and eyelid.

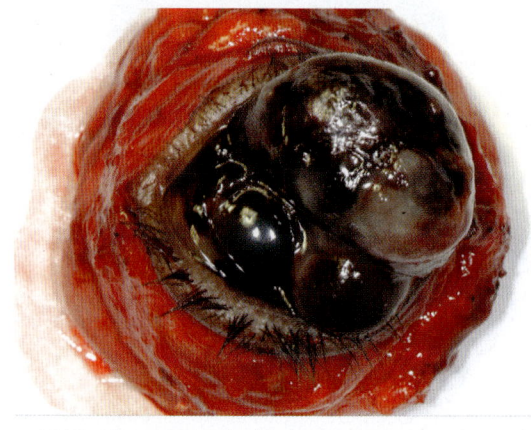

Figure 40.33. Photograph of orbital exenteration specimen showing extensive melanoma.

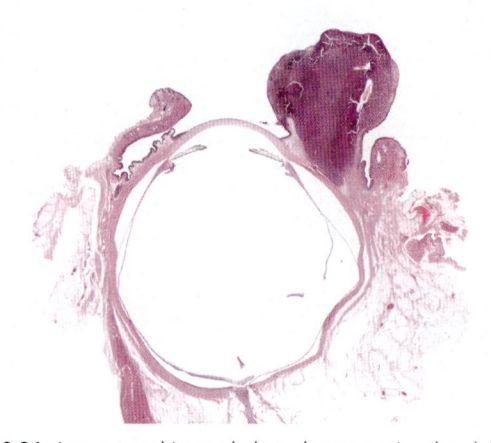

Figure 40.34. Low-power histopathology demonstrating the globe and the pedunculated tumor emanating from the conjunctiva and anterior orbital region. (Hematoxylin–eosin ×2.)

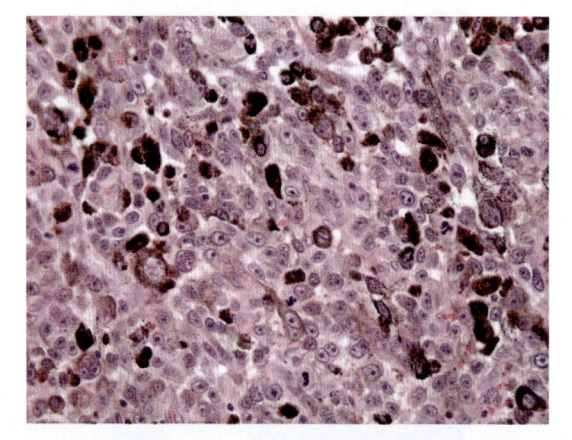

Figure 40.35. High-power histopathology demonstrating tightly packed epithelioid melanoma cells, some with pigment and some without pigment. (Hematoxylin–eosin ×150.)

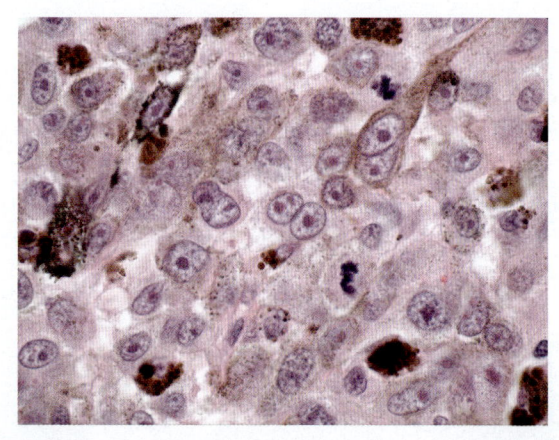

Figure 40.36. High-power histopathology demonstrating anaplastic melanoma cells with prominent nucleoli, binucleate cells, and brisk mitotic activity. (Hematoxylin–eosin ×250.)

ORBITAL INVASION FROM UVEAL MELANOMA: MASSIVE ORBITAL INVOLVEMENT

On occasion uveal melanoma can show extensive orbital invasion. It usually occurs after a long delay in diagnosis. This subject is also discussed in the *Atlas of Intraocular Tumors*.

Shields CL, Shields JA, Yarian DL, et al. Intracranial extension of choroidal melanoma via the optic nerve. *Br J Ophthalmol* 1987;71:172–176.

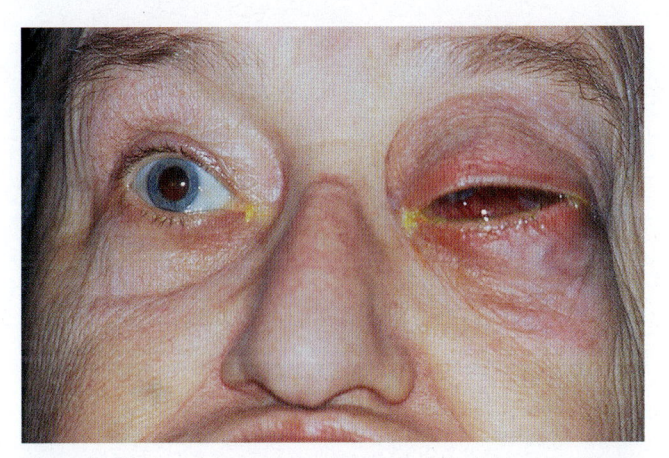

Figure 40.37. Facial view showing proptosis of the right eye in 62-year-old woman who had been treated with medication and cyclocryotherapy for "glaucoma secondary to central retinal vein occlusion" and eventually developed proptosis and pain.

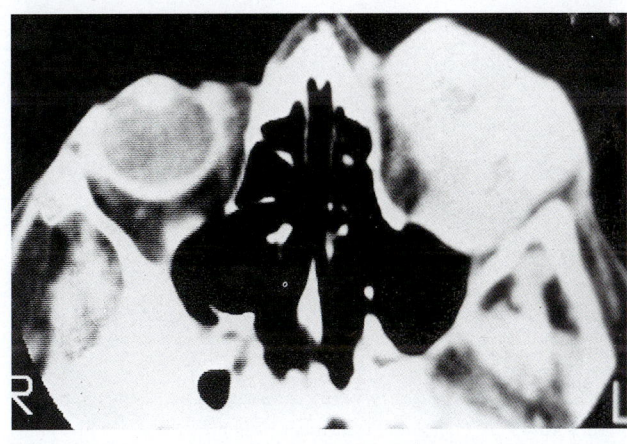

Figure 40.38. Axial computed tomography of patient shown in Figure 40.31 showing that the globe and the entire orbit are filled with solid tumor. A fine-needle aspiration biopsy through the inferior conjunctival fornix disclosed melanoma cells and orbital exenteration was performed.

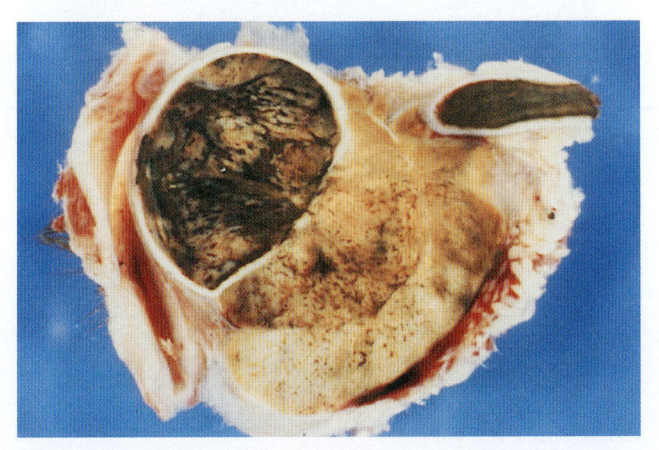

Figure 40.39. Sagittal section through the exenteration specimen of patient shown in Figure 40.31 showing melanoma entirely filling the globe and orbit and replacing the optic nerve. The orbital tumor proved to be melanoma composed almost entirely of large epithelioid melanoma cells.

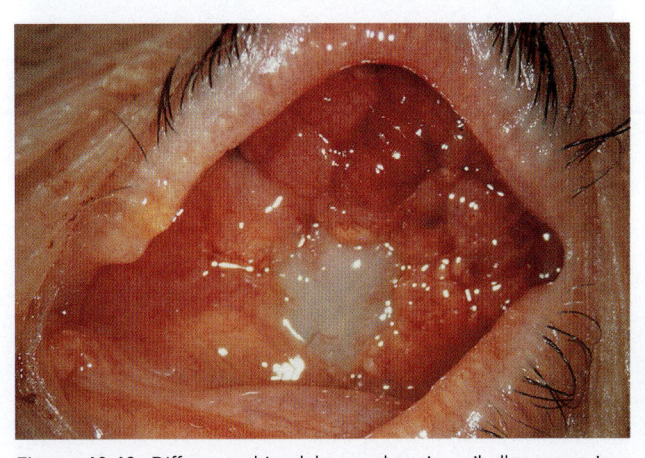

Figure 40.40. Diffuse, multinodular amelanotic epibulbar mass in a woman who underwent cataract surgery about a year earlier because of "phakolytic glaucoma."

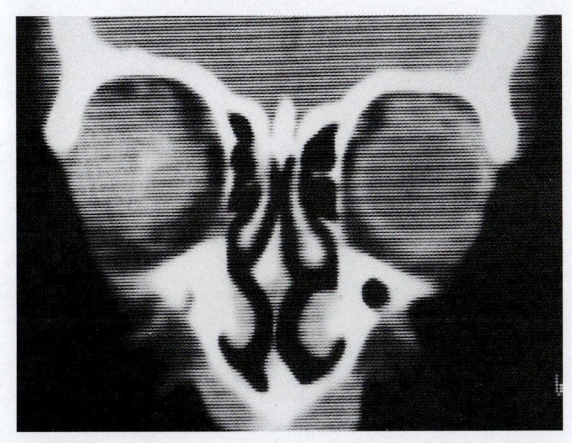

Figure 40.41. Coronal computed tomography of patient shown in Figure 40.40 demonstrating diffuse solid tumor encircling the globe.

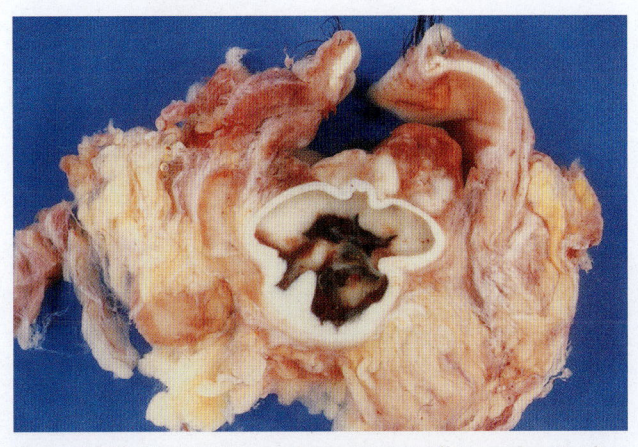

Figure 40.42. Exenteration specimen showing diffuse amelanotic ciliary body melanoma with massive extension outside the globe.

ORBITAL INVASION FROM MASSIVE CHOROIDAL MELANOMA

Ghassemi F, Palamar M, Shields CL, et al. Black tears (melanodacryorrhea) from uveal melanoma. *Arch Ophthalmol* 2008;126(8):1166–1168.

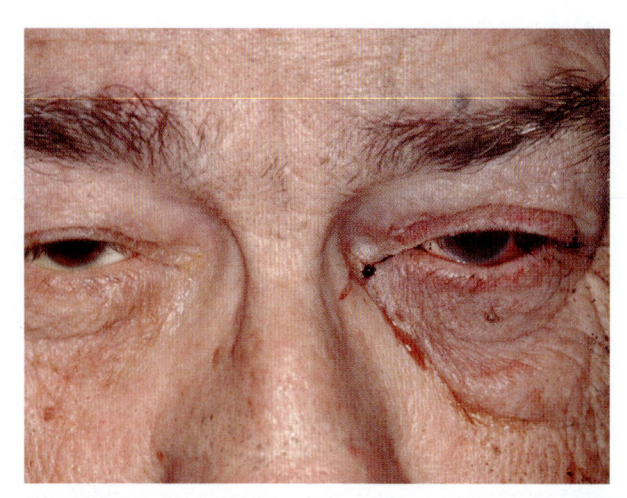

Figure 40.43. A 71-year-old Caucasian male noted black debris in his tears.

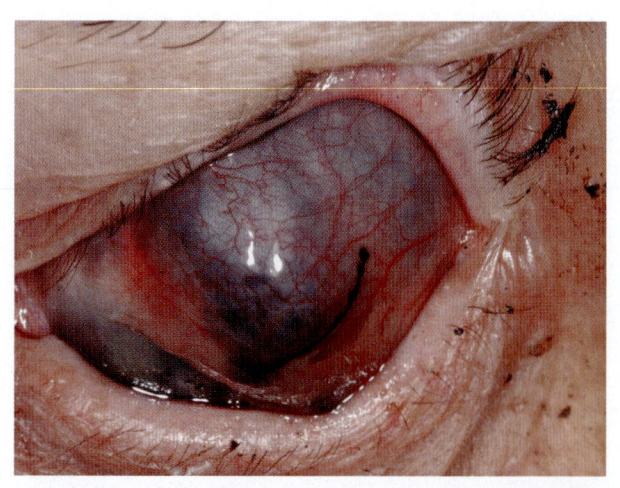

Figure 40.44. On the surface of the globe of the patient in Figure 40.43, a dark mass suspicious for melanoma was noted. Ophthalmoscopy revealed large choroidal melanoma with extrascleral extension.

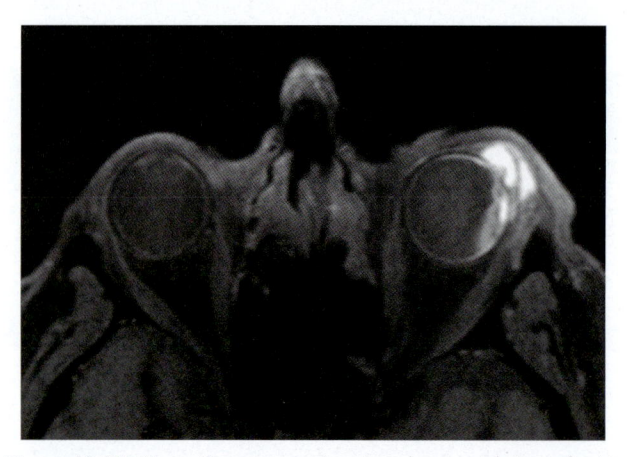

Figure 40.45. Magnetic resonance imaging shows axial view of orbit demonstrating the enhancing intraocular melanoma and secondary orbital invasion.

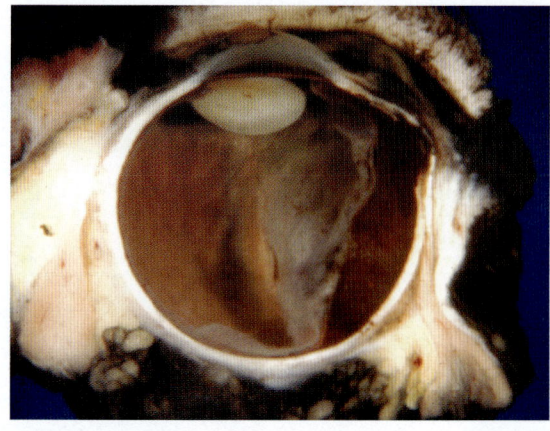

Figure 40.46. Orbital exenteration was performed and the large intraocular melanoma is seen.

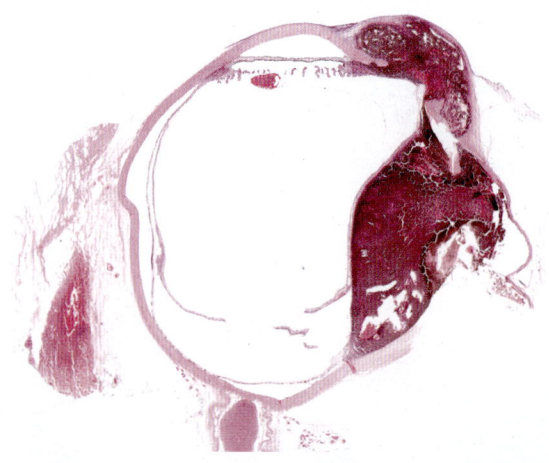

Figure 40.47. Low-power histopathology demonstrating the uveal and secondary orbital portions of the melanoma. (Hematoxylin–eosin ×2.)

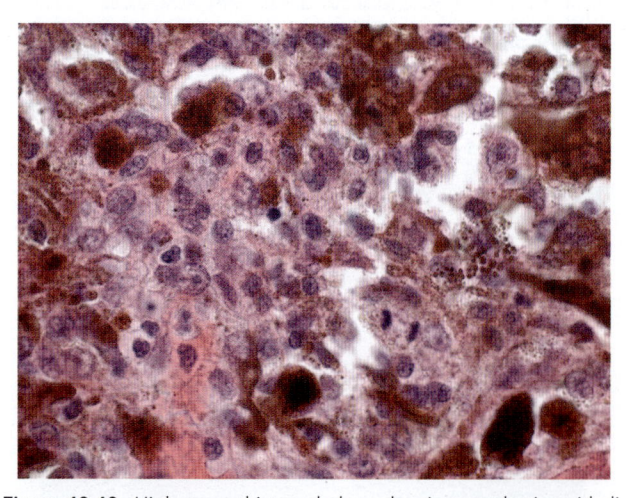

Figure 40.48. High-power histopathology showing anaplastic epithelioid melanoma cells with mitotic activity. (Hematoxylin–eosin ×200.)

ORBITAL INVASION FROM RETINOBLASTOMA

Retinoblastoma can occasionally exhibit extensive orbital invasion. This is rare in medically developed countries but is fairly common in areas of the world where advanced medical care may not be readily available. Orbital extension of retinoblastoma generally is associated with a worse prognosis and is often fatal. This subject is discussed in the *Atlas of Intraocular Tumors*.

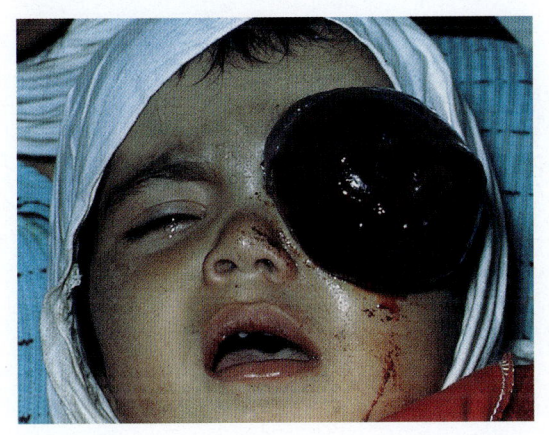

Figure 40.49. Massive extraocular extension of retinoblastoma in a child from the Middle East. (Courtesy of Hormoz Chams, MD.)

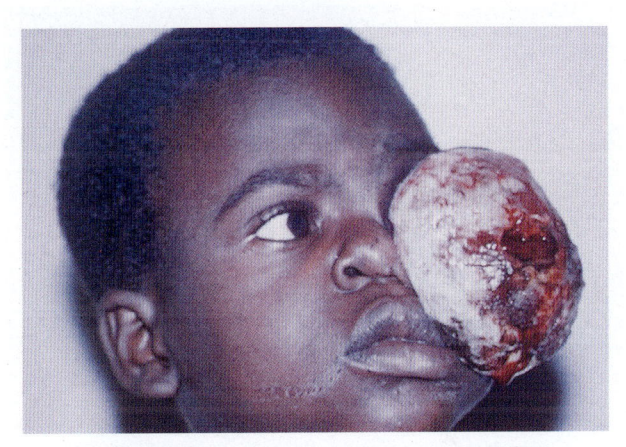

Figure 40.50. Massive extraocular extension of retinoblastoma in a child from Africa. (Courtesy of Armed Forces Institute of Pathology, Washington, DC.)

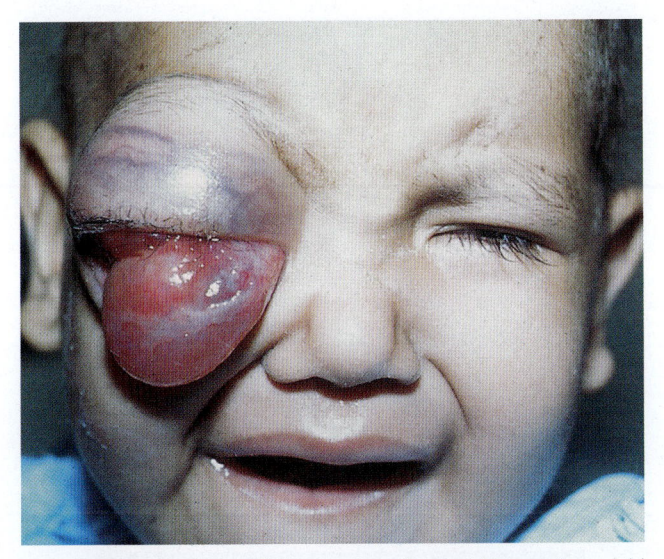

Figure 40.51. Marked orbital extension of retinoblastoma in a child from Latin America. (Courtesy of Imelda Pifano, MD.)

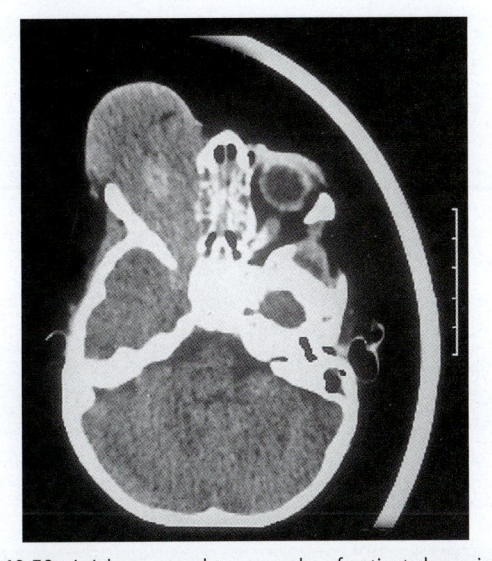

Figure 40.52. Axial computed tomography of patient shown in Figure 40.51 demonstrating massive intraocular and orbital tumor.

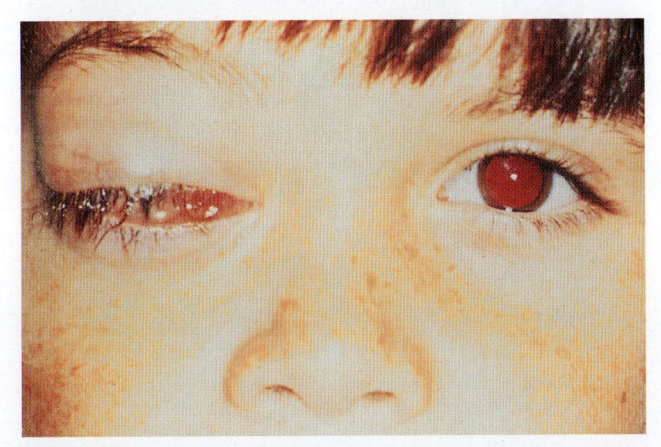

Figure 40.53. Extensive orbital swelling in a 10-year-old boy who had undergone prior enucleation elsewhere for retinoblastoma.

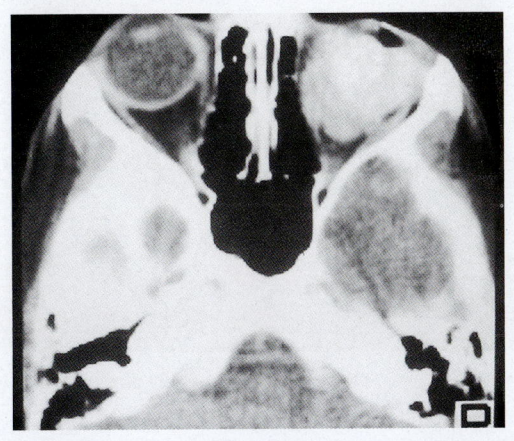

Figure 40.54. Axial computed tomography of patient shown in Figure 40.53 demonstrating massive retinoblastoma surrounding the orbital implant.

ORBITAL INVASION FROM MASSIVE UNRECOGNIZED RETINOBLASTOMA

Shields CL, Schoenfeld E, Kocher K, et al. Lesions simulating retinoblastoma (pseudoretinoblastoma) in 604 cases. *Ophthalmology* 2013;120:311–316.

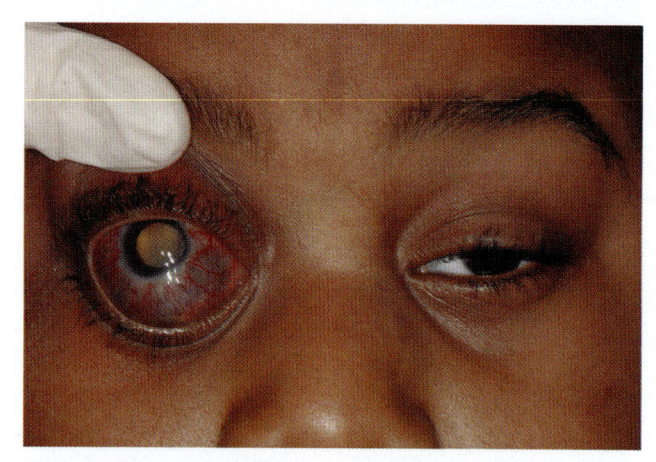

Figure 40.55. Six-year-old boy with unrecognized retinoblastoma, misdiagnosed as Coats disease and followed for nearly 1 year. Suspicion for retinoblastoma eventually prompted referral to our center.

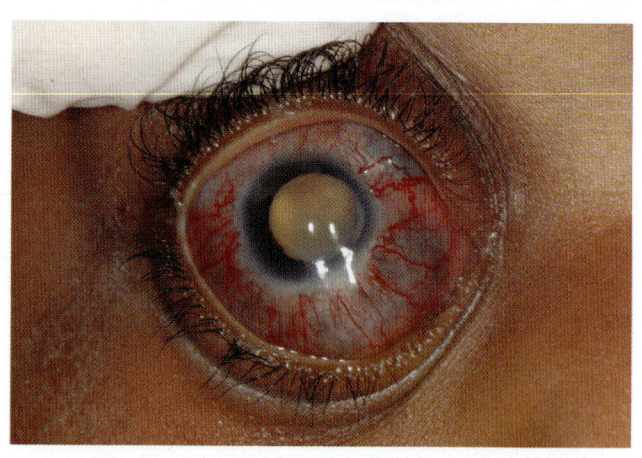

Figure 40.56. Close up view of patient in Figure 40.55, demonstrating the bupthalmic eye, congestion, and leukocoria.

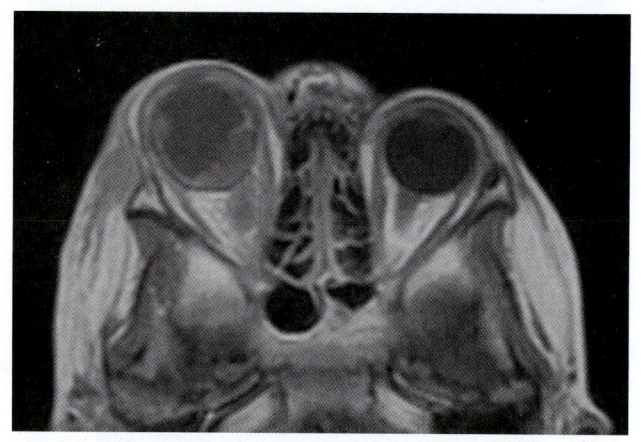

Figure 40.57. Axial magnetic resonance imaging of orbit demonstrating enlarged globe with a mass extending into the orbit consistent with retinoblastoma with massive orbital invasion.

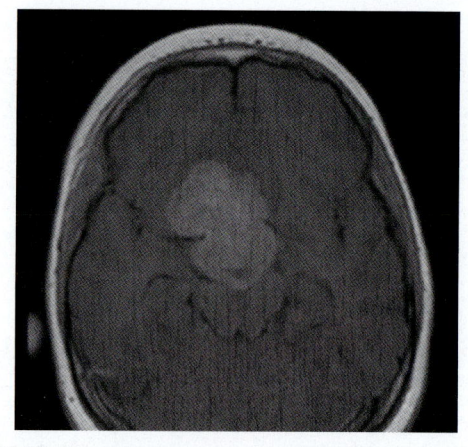

Figure 40.58. Magnetic resonance imaging of brain showing large mass in brain suspicious for retinoblastoma invasion.

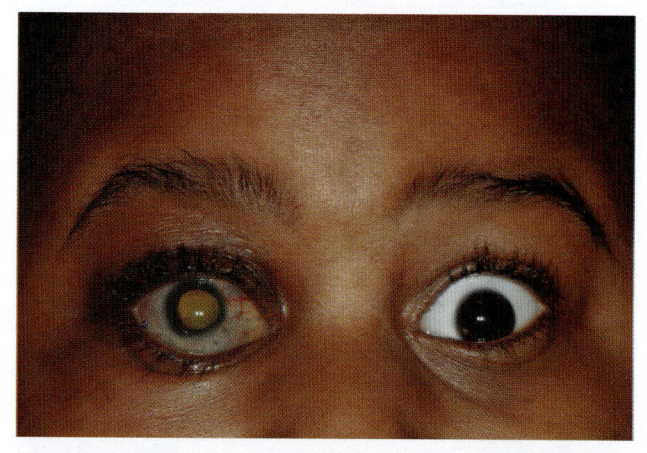

Figure 40.59. Following two cycles of chemotherapy the tumor showed marked regression. This child was treated for 12 months with chemotherapy, followed by radiotherapy and enucleation. He was alive and well after 3 years.

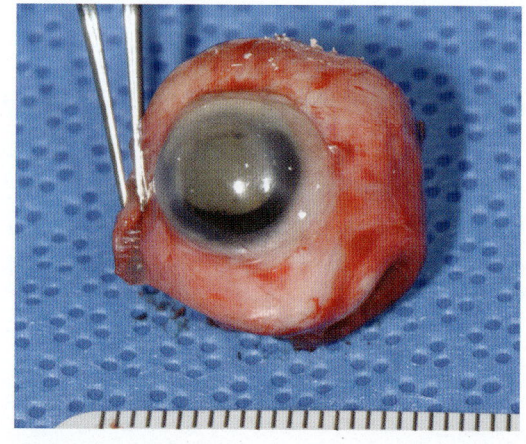

Figure 40.60. The enucleated globe was shrunken and had no residual tumor on histopathology.

ORBITAL INVASION FROM PARANASAL SINUS CANCERS

Paranasal sinus cancers, particularly those originating in the ethmoid and maxillary sinuses, can secondarily invade the orbit. Although the majority is squamous neoplasms, a variety of sarcomas, osseous, and fibro-osseous tumors can originate in the sinuses and secondarily invade the orbit. As expected, ethmoid sinus carcinoma tends to displace the globe laterally and maxillary sinus carcinoma displaces the globe superiorly. Treatment of squamous carcinoma with orbital invasion involves surgical excision in conjunction with an otolaryngologist with appropriate irradiation and chemotherapy.

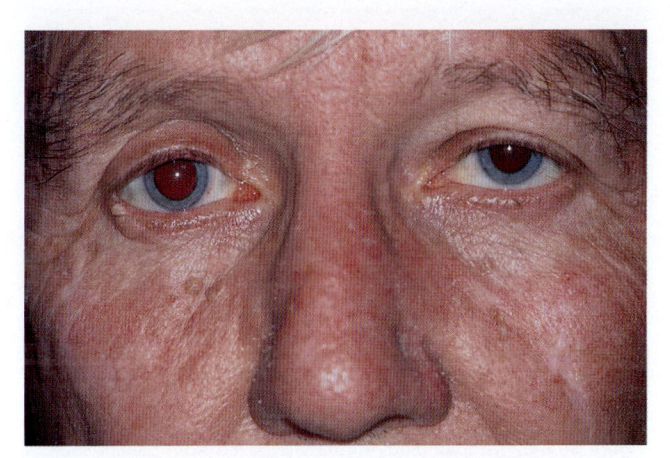

Figure 40.61. Maxillary sinus carcinoma with slight orbital extension. Slight upward displacement of the left eye in a 68-year-old man.

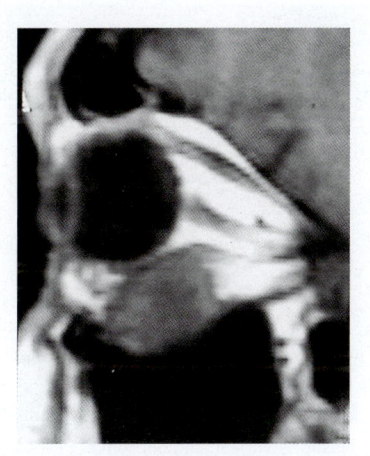

Figure 40.62. Sagittal magnetic resonance imaging in T1-weighted image of patient shown in Figure 40.61, demonstrating a mass arising from roof of maxillary sinus with preferential growth into the orbital soft tissues.

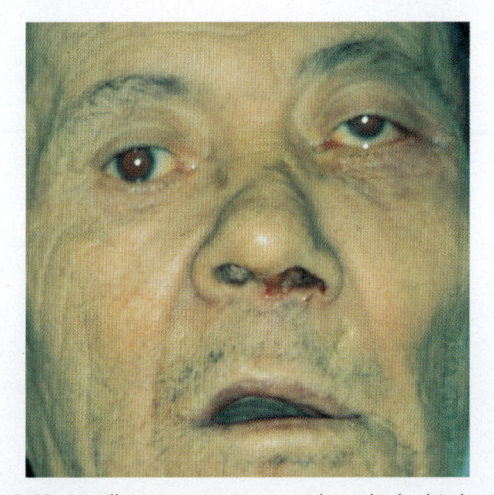

Figure 40.63. Maxillary sinus carcinoma with marked orbital extension. Upward displacement of the left eye in an 80-year-old man.

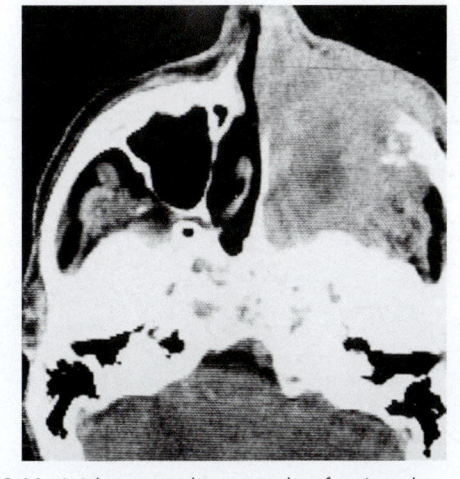

Figure 40.64. Axial computed tomography of patient shown in Figure 40.63 depicting massive neoplasm in the maxillary sinus.

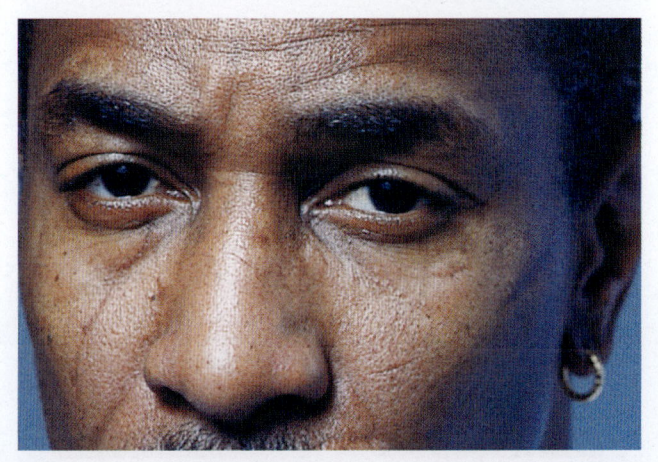

Figure 40.65. Ethmoid sinus carcinoma with orbital extension. Slight lateral displacement of the left eye in a 46-year-old man.

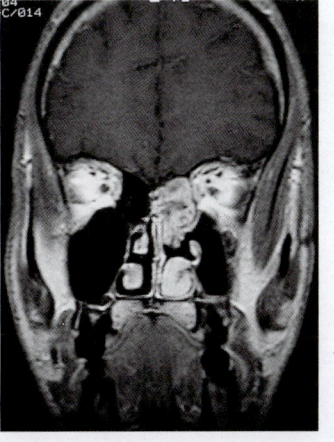

Figure 40.66. Coronal magnetic resonance imaging of patient shown in Figure 40.65. Note the mass in the left ethmoid sinus and nasal cavity with extension into the medial aspect of the orbit.

ORBITAL INVASION FROM NASOPHARYNGEAL CANCERS

Nasopharyngeal neoplasms can also secondarily invade the orbit. Juvenile angiofibroma is an uncommon tumor that affects young males. It is locally invasive, but does not tend to metastasize. Nasopharyngeal carcinoma is most common, but a number of other tumors can exhibit similar behavior. Tumors in this location can produce involvement of multiple cranial nerves. Esthesioneuroblastoma is a neurogenic neoplasm that arises from the olfactory sensory epithelium in the roof of the nasal cavity.

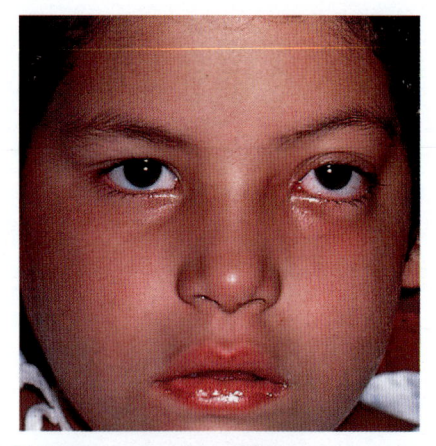

Figure 40.67. Nasopharyngeal angiofibroma. Proptosis and upward displacement of the left eye in a 7-year-old girl. A large vascular mass was subsequently removed. (Courtesy of Dr Robert Levine.)

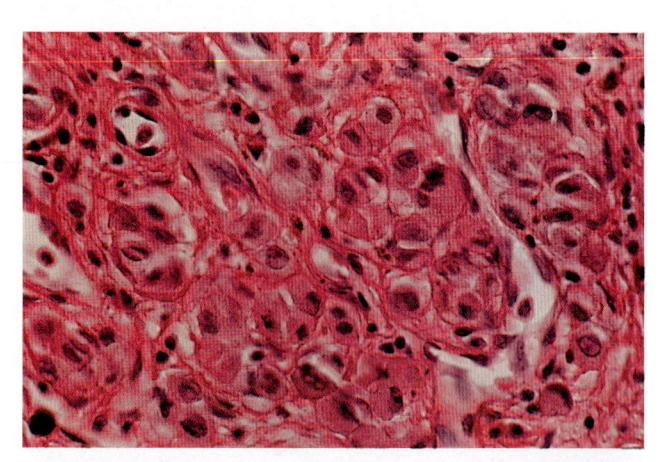

Figure 40.68. Histopathology of mass removed from patient seen in Figure 40.67, demonstrating vascular neoplasm with ovoid and spindle cells. (Hematoxylin–eosin ×200.) (Courtesy of Robert Levine, MD.)

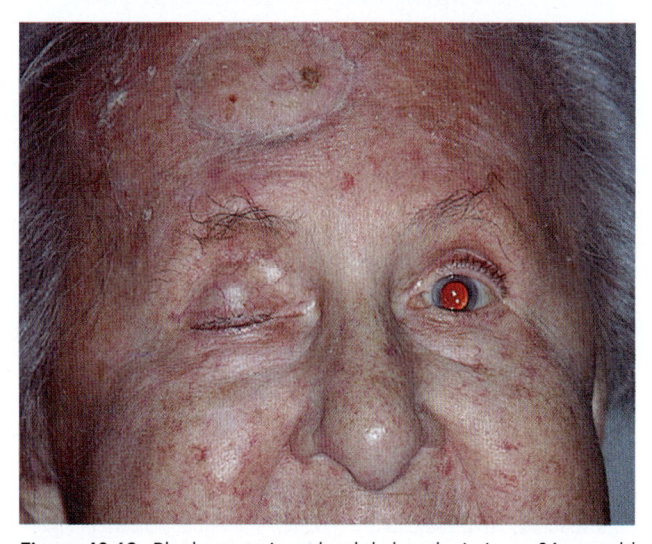

Figure 40.69. Blepharoptosis and ophthalmoplegia in an 84-year-old woman with orbital extension of nasopharyngeal carcinoma.

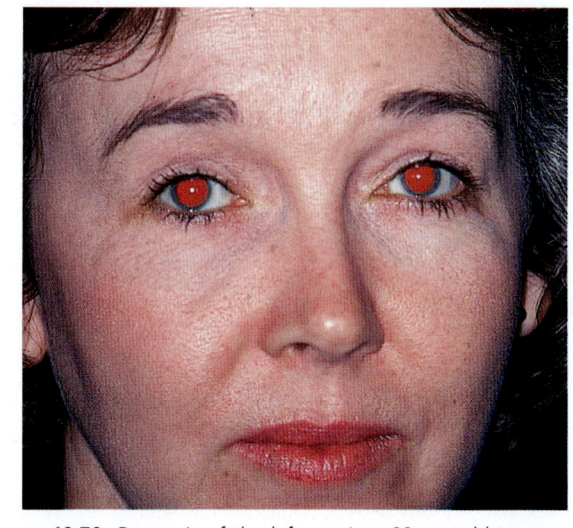

Figure 40.70. Proptosis of the left eye in a 39-year-old woman with esthesioneuroblastoma.

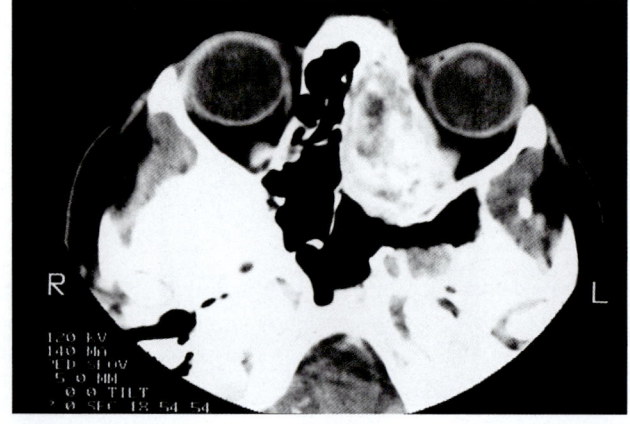

Figure 40.71. Axial computed tomography of patient shown in Figure 40.70, demonstrating a large, irregular mass involving the nasal cavity and medial aspect of the orbit.

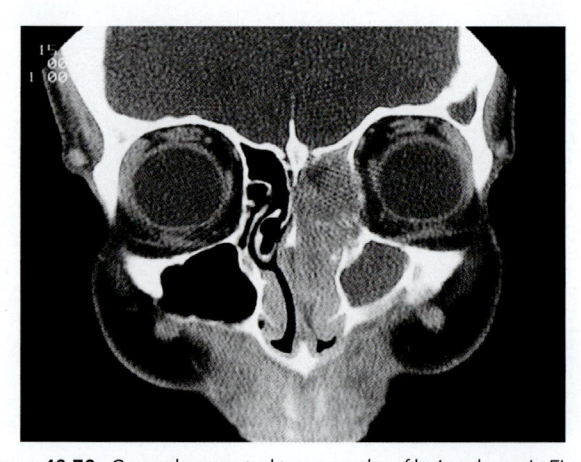

Figure 40.72. Coronal computed tomography of lesion shown in Figure 40.70, showing a diffuse nasopharyngeal mass.

SURGICAL MANAGEMENT OF ORBITAL TUMORS

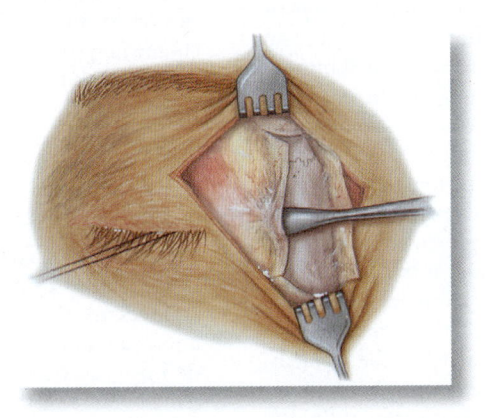

The details of surgical approaches to orbital tumors and pseudotumors are discussed elsewhere (1–5). Enucleation is discussed in the *Atlas of Intraocular Tumors* and is not covered here. Illustrated and briefly described here are the indications and techniques of orbital fine-needle aspiration biopsy (FNAB), conjunctival approach, cutaneous approaches, and orbital exenteration (1–5). In general, well-circumscribed tumors should be managed with excisional biopsy. Poorly circumscribed, diffuse tumors are best managed by incisional biopsy. The diagnostic method chosen depends largely on orbital imaging studies and varies with the size and location of the lesion and the suspected diagnosis. Local anesthesia can be used for most FNAB and for very anterior relative small orbital lesions. For larger lesions in the midportion or posterior portion of the orbit, general anesthesia is preferable.

Fine-Needle Aspiration Biopsy

FNAB is a useful method for obtaining a diagnosis in selected cases (1). It is used most often to confirm the diagnosis of orbital lymphoma or metastasis in a patient who has known systemic lymphoma or a primary neoplasm. If lymphoma or metastases are suspected and there is no known systemic malignancy, incisional or excisional biopsy usually should be done to provide more tissue for histopathologic study. FNAB should generally not be used for circumscribed orbital tumors in which complete excision is anticipated. Cases where FNAB is indicated have been illustrated throughout this atlas.

There are different methods of performing FNAB for orbital tumors. A pistol grip instrument (Asper-gun) can be used with a 25- or 22-gauge needle. If the orbital lesion is palpable through the skin, the needle can be placed directly into the mass and aspiration done to draw tumor cells into the needle bore. Orbital FNAB can also be performed by a similar technique that is used frequently for intraocular tumors. By this method, a similar needle is attached to a plastic connector tubing about 25 mm long, which is in turn attached to a 10-cc syringe. The needle is guided into the lesion and aspiration is performed to draw tumor cells into the needle bore.

Once the tumor cells are in the syringe, there are two methods of placing the cells onto a slide for cytopathologic stains. One is to use a syringe to express the cells immediately onto a slide and spread them with another glass slide to facilitate staining. The second method, which our cytopathologists prefer, is to immediately place the needle into a small bottle of cytological fixative and to aspirate it immediately into a syringe. This flushes the cells in the needle bore into the preservative solution. The syringe is then submitted immediately for preparation for cytopathologic studies. The solution undergoes centrifugation with a millipore filter technique is to allow a higher yield and better distribution of the cells for cytopathologic study.

SURGICAL MANAGEMENT OF ORBITAL TUMORS

Conjunctival Approach

A conjunctival approach is frequently the best method for selected anterior orbital tumors. It usually requires less surgical time and avoids performing a skin incision and suture removal. The authors use it more frequently for circumscribed anterior orbital tumors that are most likely benign, like cavernous hemangioma, schwannoma, and soft tissue dermoid cysts. An incision is made in the retrolimbal conjunctiva or the conjunctival fornix and Tenon's fascia is separated by spreading with scissors. Two or three rectus muscles are isolated with nylon sutures for rotation of the globe. Blunt dissection with scissors-spreading, cotton-tipped applicator sticks, or firm periosteal elevator is performed until the tumor is exposed and an attempt is made to remove the tumor intact (excisional biopsy) when possible. Caution is used when cutting any structure in the orbit to avoid bisecting muscles, nerves, or vascular tissue.

In using the conjunctival approach inferotemporally, the surgeon should identify the inferior oblique muscle and isolate it with a rubber drain. For superotemporal lesions, the superior oblique muscle must be identified and protected from damage. In the case of an anterior nasal lesion, a transcaruncular approach with a vertical incision on the temporal side of the caruncle can provide adequate exposure. The tumor can be removed primarily or with assistance of a cryoprobe to facilitate removal. When the tumor has been removed, the conjunctiva is closed with running 7-0 absorbable sutures, antibiotic or corticosteroid ointment is applied, and a patch is placed on the eye until the next day at which time the patient undergoes an office examination with visual acuity, pupil evaluation, and motility check.

Cutaneous Approach

A cutaneous approach, which provides somewhat better surgical exposure, is generally preferred for larger, more posteriorly located tumors and for tumors that involve the orbital lobe of the lacrimal gland. Depending on the location and size of the lesion as determined by axial and coronal imaging studies, the incision should be made superotemporally, superonasally, inferotemporally, inferonasally, or directly nasally. A subcutaneous injection of local anesthesia combined with epinephrine along the incision line is performed to achieve better hemostasis. Transconjunctival 4-0 silk bridal sutures can be used to isolate rectus muscles in the quadrants of the tumor, so that they can be continuously identified during the procedure.

Once the skin incision is completed, either a transeptal or transperiosteal entry into the orbit can be used, also depending on the imaging and surgical findings. Anterior lesions are reached through transeptal whereas mid or posterior lesions are reached by reansperiosteal approach. Blunt dissection should be employed as much as possible in the orbital soft tissues. With a transeptal approach, the lesion can be approached directly by gently separating the orbital fat and identifying nearby extraocular muscles and retracting them with sutures or rubber drains. The tumor can be removed directly.

With the extraperiosteal approach, the skin incision is carried down to the periosteum about 3 mm outside the orbital rim. A periosteal elevator is used to separate the periosteum from the orbital bone and this separation is carried as far posterior as necessary in the orbit. This approach minimizes bleeding in the extraperiosteal plane and prevents premature exposure of the orbital fat. The periosteum is then separated with scissors and the orbital fat is exposed in the area of the tumor. The tumor is then slowly dissected and carefully removed. When hemostasis is attained, the subcutaneous tissues and skin is closed with absorbable sutures. We generally prefer 5-0 absorbable sutures for periosteal closure and 6-0 absorbable sutures for skin closure. Antibiotic ointment is applied to the cutaneous wound and a patch is placed for 1 to 2 days. For orbits at risk for swelling and hemorrhage, the patient undergoes an office examination the following day. For those with minimal manipulation and relatively minor dissection, we wait 2 to 3 weeks to re-examine the patient.

Regardless of the surgical approach, it is best to remove tumors entirely if that can be achieved without damage to vital structures like the extraocular muscles and optic nerve. In the case of a noncircumscribed or very large tumor, it may be necessary to remove the lesion piecemeal. If the diagnosis is uncertain and there is residual tumor in the orbit, a diagnostic frozen section can be performed to determine whether to remove more of the tumor before terminating the procedure. In the case of radiosensitive malignant tumors like lymphoma and metastasis, it may not be necessary to remove the entire tumor. In the case of nonradiosensitive malignant tumors, an attempt should be made for complete excision if possible.

SURGICAL MANAGEMENT OF ORBITAL TUMORS

Orbital Exenteration

Orbital exenteration is used for massive orbital extension of uveal melanoma, orbital extension of primary eyelid and conjunctival malignancies, and certain primary orbital malignancies. When possible, an eyelid-sparing technique should be employed (4,5). After general anesthesia is administered, an outline of the planned skin incision is made with a sterile marking pencil for 360 degrees. If the eyelids are to be sacrificed because of tumor involvement, the line is drawn outside the eyelids but inside the eyebrow superiorly. If the eyelid skin is to be preserved, the 360-degree line is drawn just outside the cilia.

A subcutaneous injection of local anesthesia combined with epinephrine along the incision line is performed to achieve better hemostasis. The skin incision is made and dissection is carried down to the periosteum. For the eyelid-sparing technique, the skin and orbicularis muscle are separated from the tarsus as the periosteum is approached, to preserve a myocutaneous flap for later closure. For the eyelid-sacrificing approach, separation of the subcutaneous tissue is carried directly to the underlying orbital rim. The periosteum is then incised for 360 degrees and the bone is exposed. A periosteal elevator is used to separate the periosteum from the bone as far posterior as possible toward the orbital apex. Large enucleation scissors are then used to make a "blind" cut through the optic nerve, muscles, and adjacent tissues at the orbital apex and the globe and other orbital contents are pulled forward and removed. The orbit is then immediately packed with gauze and hemostasis is obtained by standard methods.

If the eyelid-sparing technique is used, closure of the subcutaneous tissue is performed with 5-0 absorbable sutures and closure of the skin with and 6-0 absorbable sutures. If the eyelids are sacrificed, the orbit can be packed with gauze and allowed to granulate primarily or a skin graft or rotational myocutaneous flaps can be used to close the defect.

Selected References

1. Shields JA. Basic principles of management. In: Shields JA, ed. *Diagnosis and Management of Orbital Tumors*. Philadelphia, PA: WB Saunders; 1989:47–66.
2. Rootman J, Stewart B, Goldberg RA. *Orbital Surgery. A Conceptual Approach*. Philadelphia, PA: Lippincott Raven; 1995.
3. Dutton J. *Atlas of Oculoplastic and Orbital Surgery*. Philadelphia, PA: Lippincott Williams and Wilkins; 2013.
4. Shields JA, Shields CL, Suvarnamani C, et al. Orbital exenteration with eyelid sparing: indications, technique and results. *Ophthalmic Surg* 1991;22:292–297.
5. Shields JA, Shields CL, Demirci H, et al. Experience with eyelid-sparing orbital exenteration. The 2000 Tullos O. Coston Lecture. *Ophthal Plast Reconstr Surg* 2001;17:355–361.

ORBITAL SURGERY: INSTRUMENTATION AND CONJUNCTIVAL APPROACH

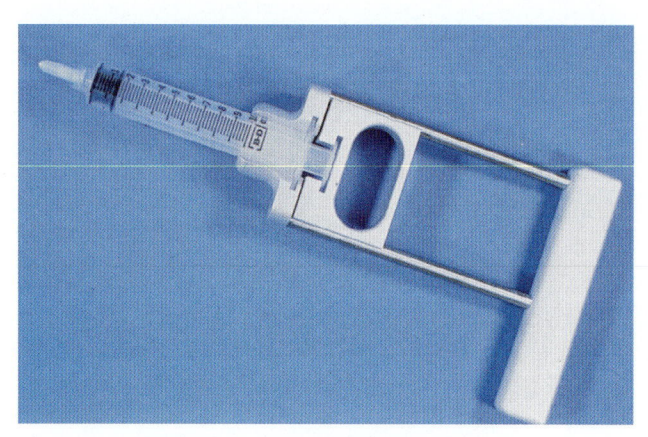

Figure 41.1. Aspiration instrument used for fine-needle aspiration biopsy of orbital tumors.

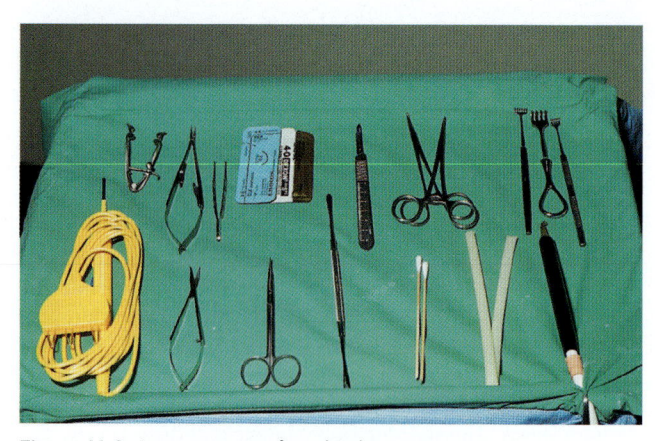

Figure 41.2. Instrument tray for orbital surgery.

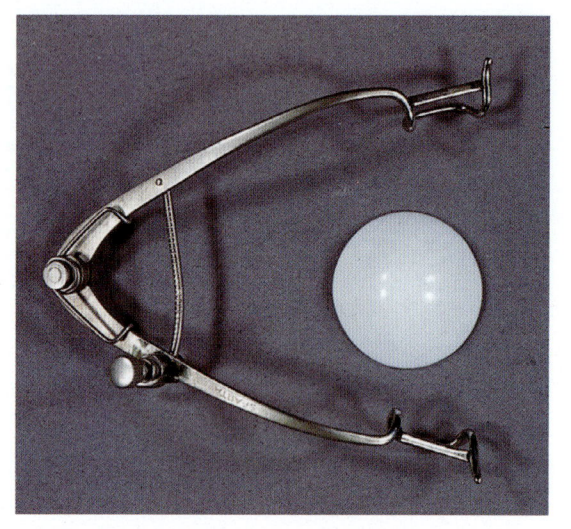

Figure 41.3. Eyelid speculum and corneal shield used for orbital surgery.

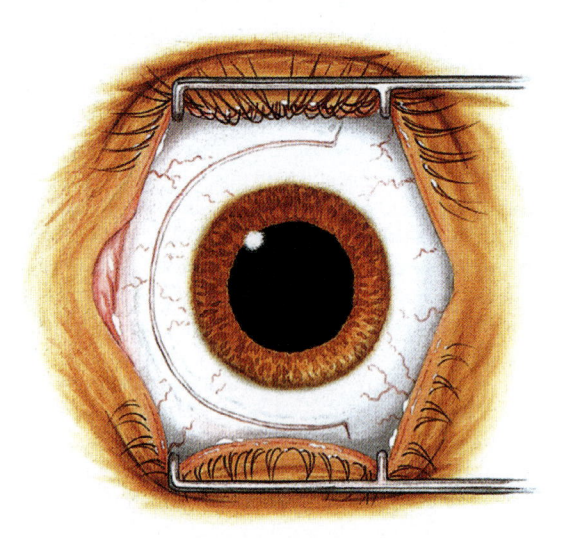

Figure 41.4. Conjunctival incision for removal of medial orbital tumor.

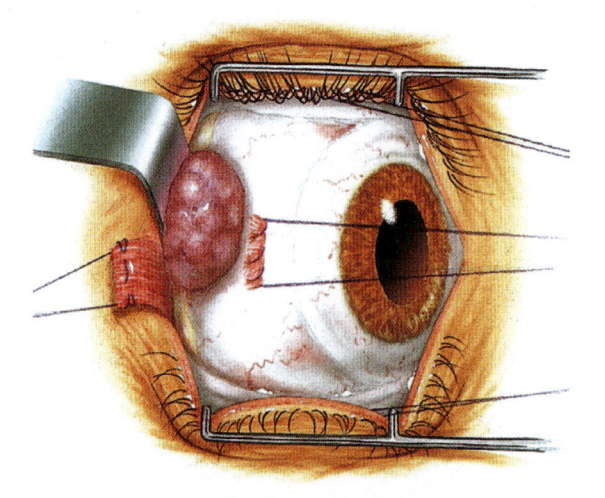

Figure 41.5. Tumor exposed after incision through conjunctiva and Tenon's capsule. Note that in this case the medial rectus muscle was disinserted for better exposure. In most cases, it is not necessary to disinsert the muscle.

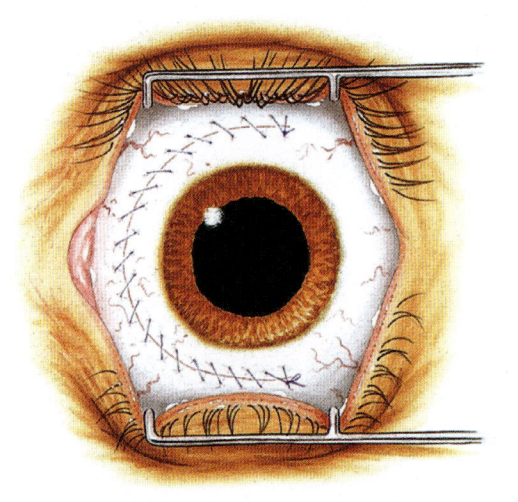

Figure 41.6. Closure with running absorbable suture after tumor removal.

Chapter 41 Surgical Management of Orbital Tumors

ORBITAL SURGERY: CUTANEOUS SUPERONASAL APPROACH

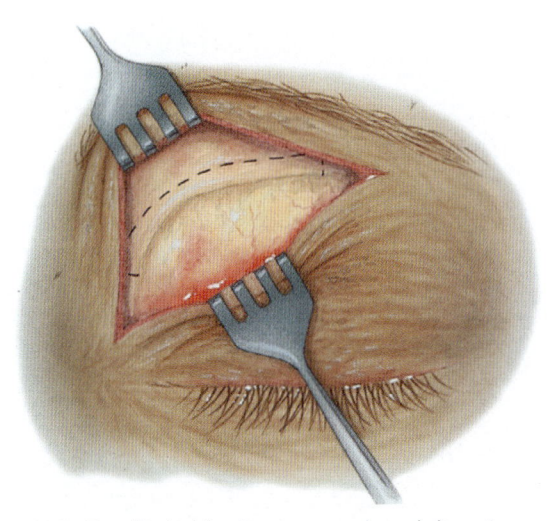

Figure 41.7. The skin incision has been made and dissection carried through the orbicularis muscle to expose the periosteum. *Dotted line* indicates where the periosteum is to be cut.

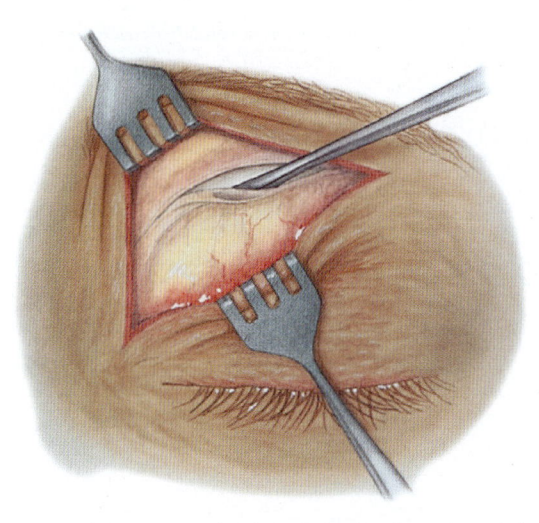

Figure 41.8. The periosteum has been incised and a periosteal elevator is being used to separate the periosteum from the orbital wall exposing the bone.

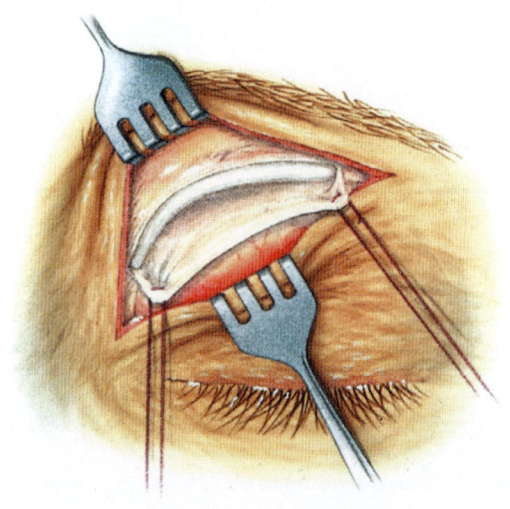

Figure 41.9. The periorbital area is exposed and ready for incision to enter the orbit.

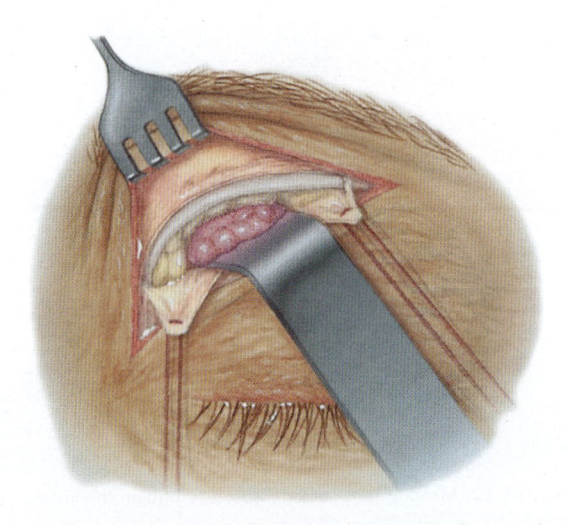

Figure 41.10. The periorbitum has been incised and soft tissue dissection has revealed the tumor to be removed.

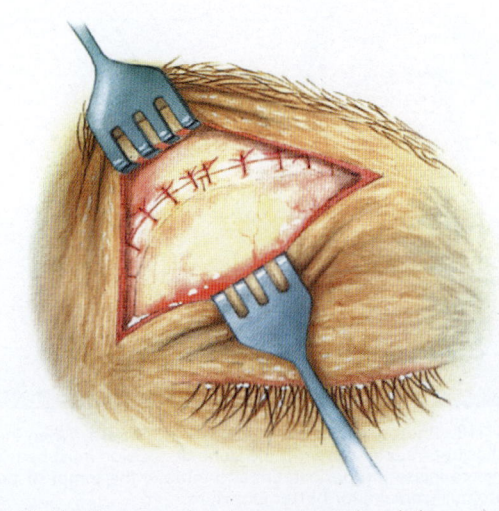

Figure 41.11. The tumor has been removed and the periosteum is closed with interrupted 5-0 absorbable sutures.

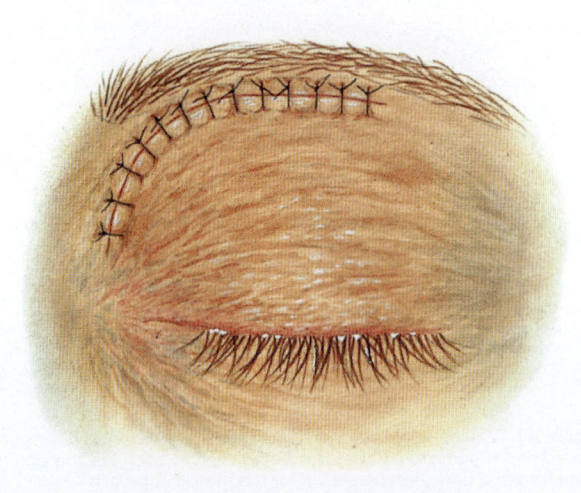

Figure 41.12. The skin has been closed with interrupted 6-0 absorbable sutures.

Part 3 Tumors of the Orbit

ORBITAL SURGERY: CUTANEOUS SUPEROTEMPORAL APPROACH

For more accessible tumors, the tumor can be removed by this approach without performing an osteotomy.

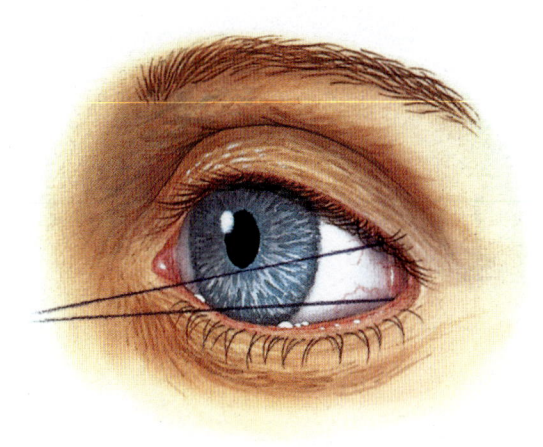

Figure 41.13. A traction suture is first placed beneath the lateral rectus muscle for traction and for identification of the muscle during surgery.

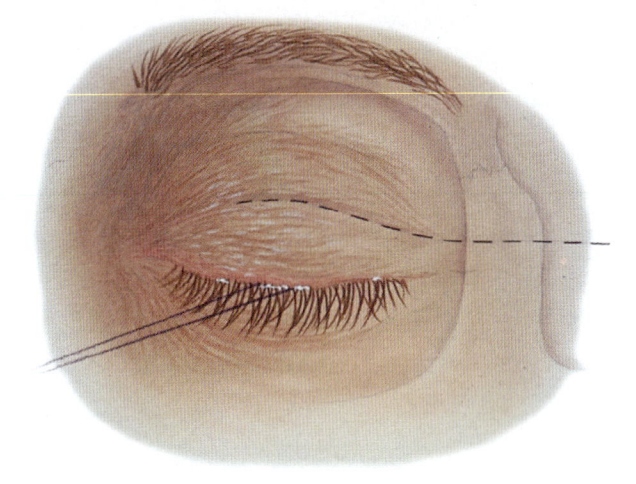

Figure 41.14. *Dotted line* indicating the location of the eyelid crease incision for superolateral orbitotomy.

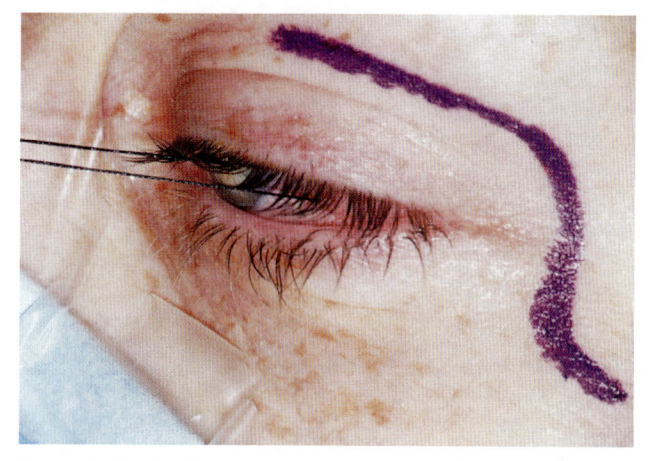

Figure 41.15. Marking pen has been used to outline the incision of a superolateral orbitotomy.

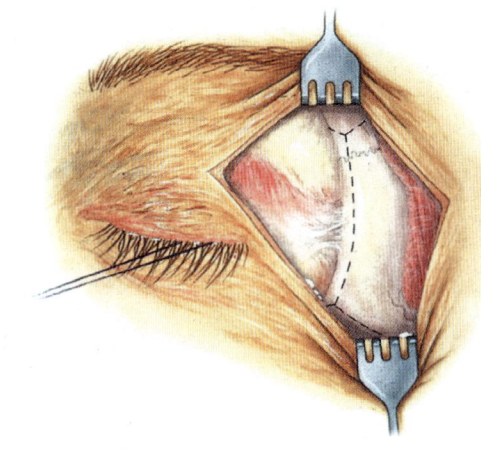

Figure 41.16. Outline of periosteal incisions shown by *dotted lines.*

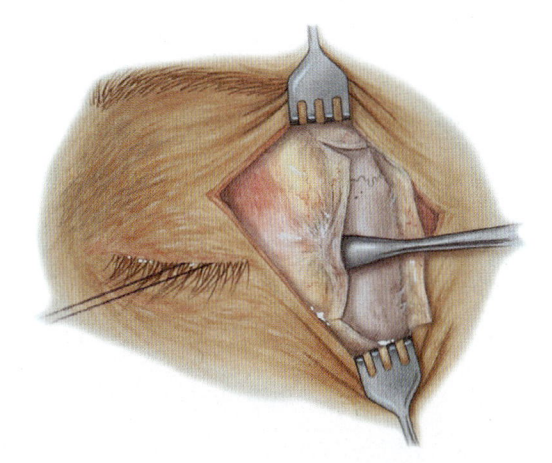

Figure 41.17. The skin, orbicularis muscle, and periosteum have been incised and a periosteal elevator is being used to separate the periosteum from the bone, as was shown for the medial approach.

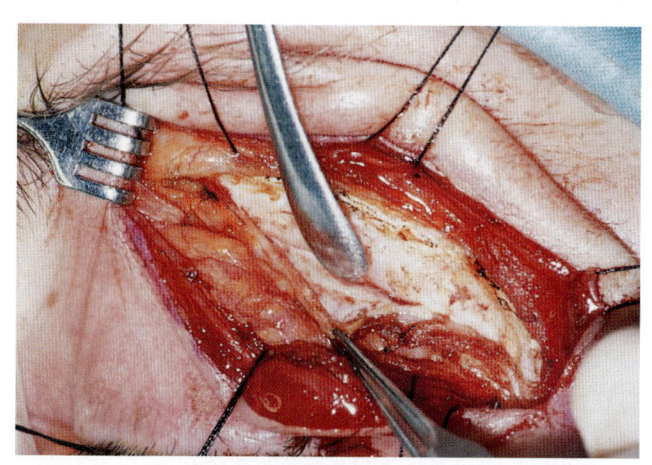

Figure 41.18. Photograph of periosteal elevator in use. When the periorbitum has been separated from the bone, a decision must be made as to whether to incise the periosteum and remove the tumor or perform an osteotomy (Kronlein) for better exposure.

Chapter 41 Surgical Management of Orbital Tumors 791

● ORBITAL SURGERY: CUTANEOUS SUPEROTEMPORAL APPROACH

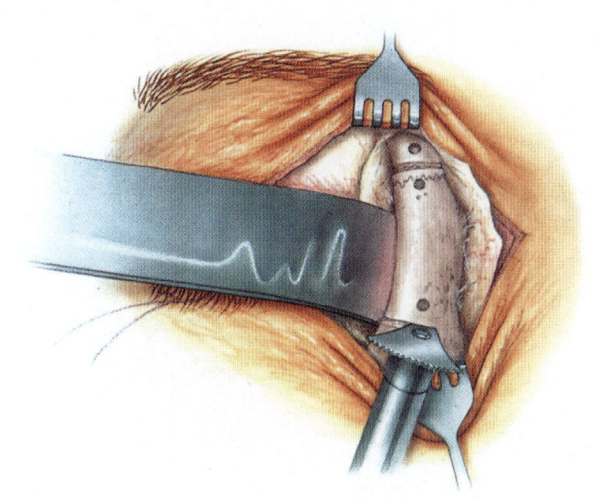

Figure 41.19. A decision has been made to perform an osteotomy. Four holes are drilled through the bone for reconstruction later and two cuts with an electric saw are made through the bone between the holes.

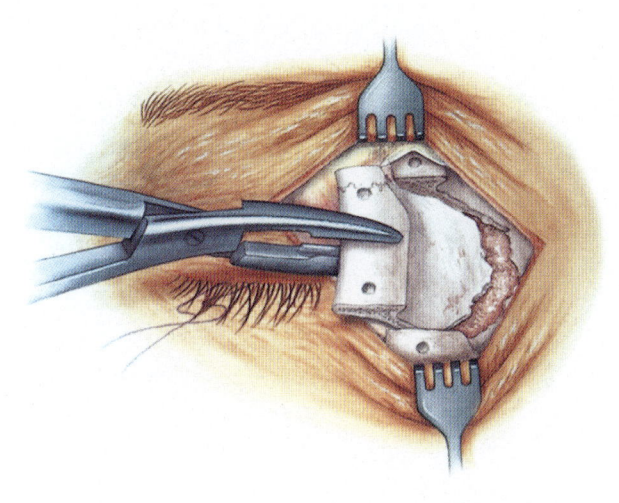

Figure 41.20. The bone flap is broken and reflected with a bone rongeur.

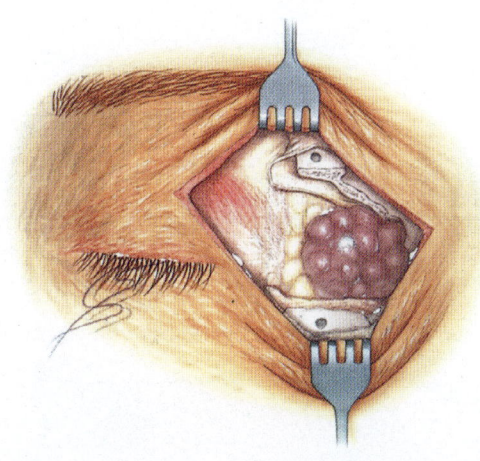

Figure 41.21. The bone flap is reflected, the periosteum incised, and soft tissue dissection has allowed exposure of the tumor.

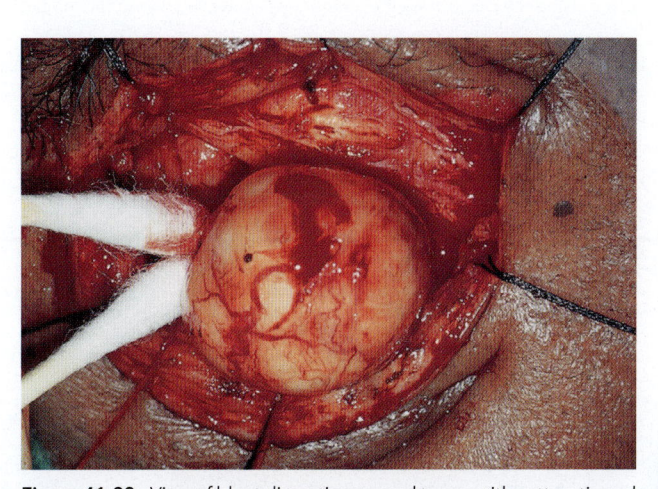

Figure 41.22. View of blunt dissection around tumor with cotton-tipped applicators. The periosteal elevator can also be used to create a separation between the tumor and the adjacent soft tissue.

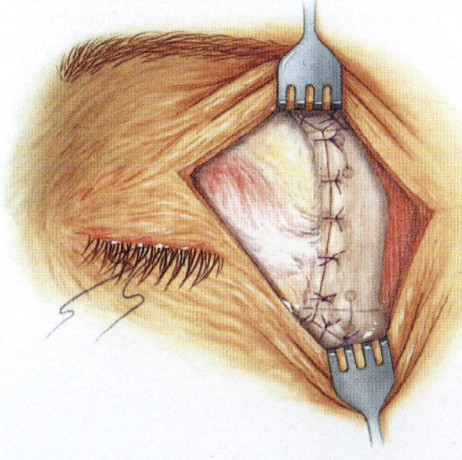

Figure 41.23. The tumor has been removed, the bone flap replaced with sutures through the drill holes, and the periosteum has been sutured.

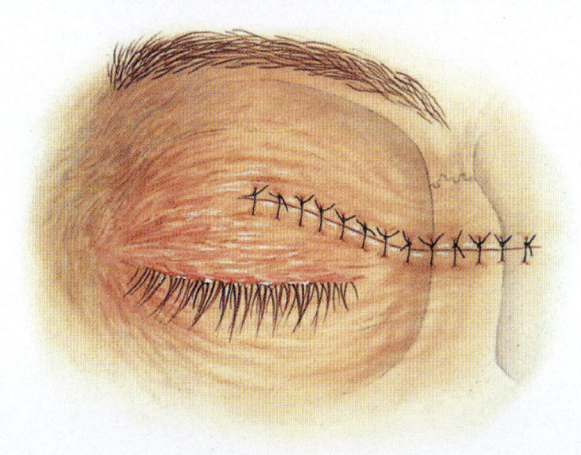

Figure 41.24. The skin has been closed with interrupted 6-0 silk sutures.

TUMORS OF THE ORBIT

ORBITAL SURGERY: EXENTERATION

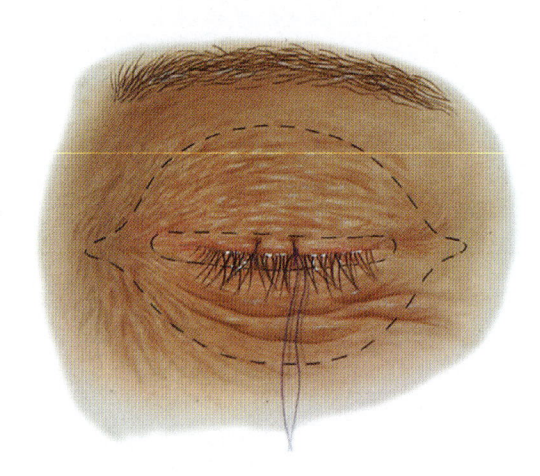

Figure 41.25. It is important to decide whether to remove the eyelids with the specimen or whether to spare the eyelid. The *outer dotted line* shows the incision for removing the eyelids and the *inner dotted line*, just outside the cilia, shows the incision for an eyelid-sparing technique.

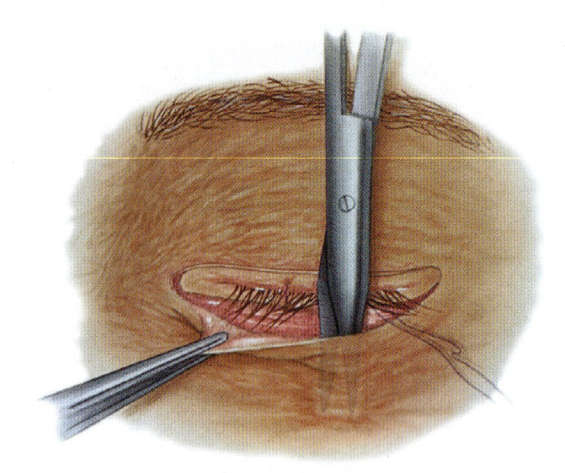

Figure 41.26. The skin incision has been made for an eyelid-sparing exenteration and the skin is separated for 360 degrees to the periosteum around the orbital rim.

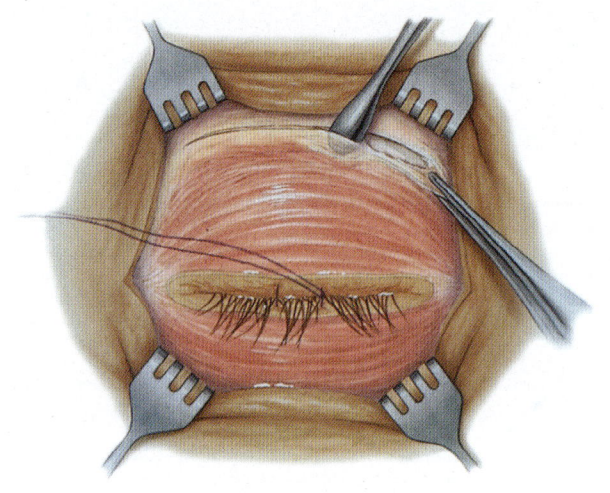

Figure 41.27. The periosteum has been exposed for 360 degrees and is being separated from the bone with a periosteal elevator.

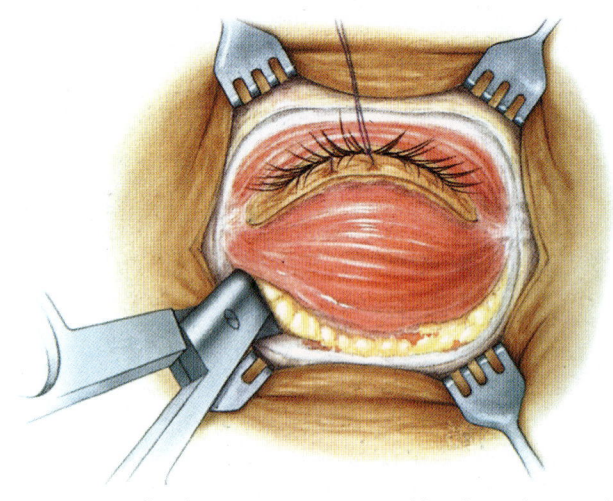

Figure 41.28. After the periosteum is separated from bone almost to the orbital apex, long scissors are inserted between the bone and the periosteum and used to cut the optic nerve, extraocular muscles, and adjacent tissue, allowing removal of the orbital contents mostly within the periosteum.

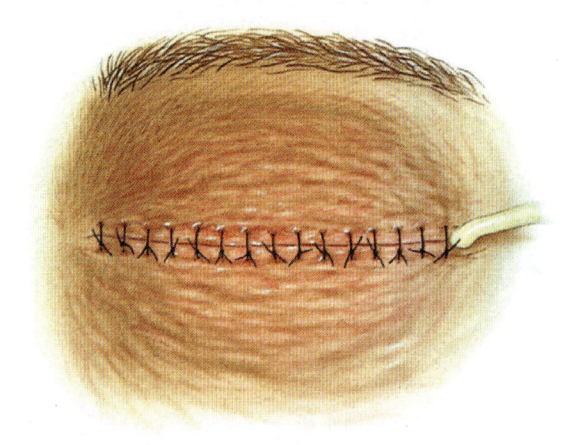

Figure 41.29. After hemostasis is achieved at the orbital apex, the eyelid flaps are sutured together and a drain is inserted.

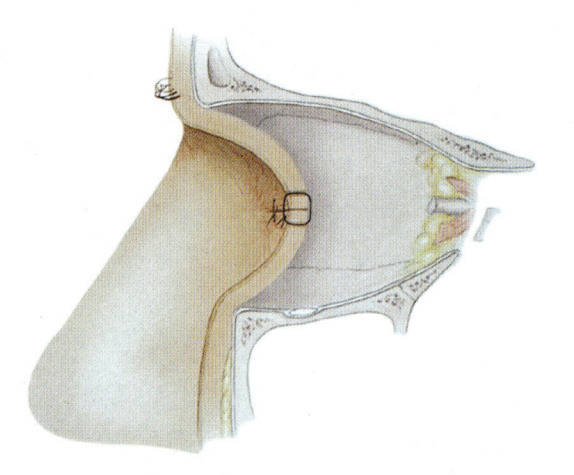

Figure 41.30. Side view showing eyelids sutured together with interrupted 5-0 absorbable sutures.

Chapter 41 Surgical Management of Orbital Tumors

● ORBITAL EXENTERATION PROSTHESES

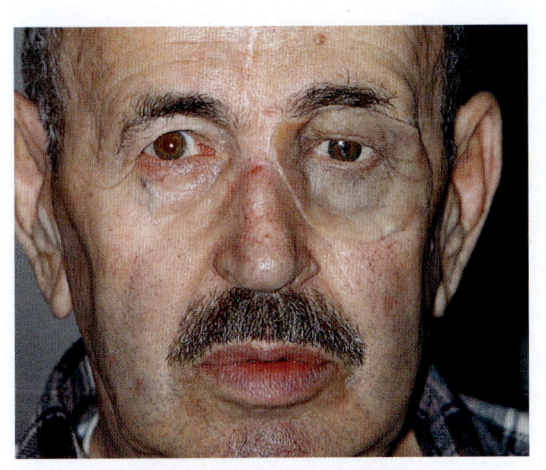

Figure 41.31. Glued on prosthesis for left orbit of elderly man who underwent eyelid-sacrificing orbital exenteration for orbital invasion of eyelid basal cell carcinoma.

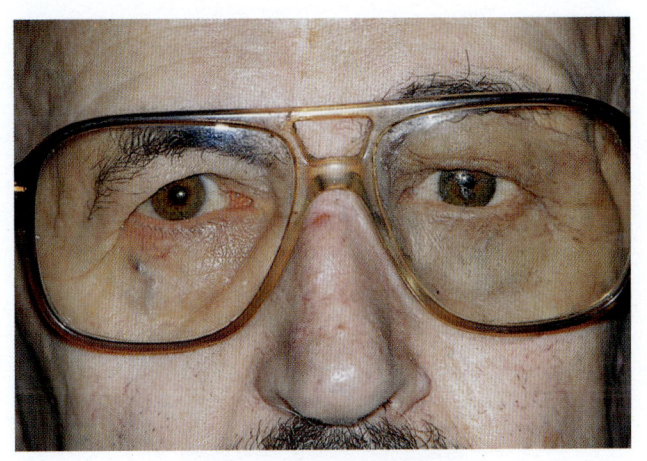

Figure 41.32. Patient shown in Figure 41.31 wearing glasses.

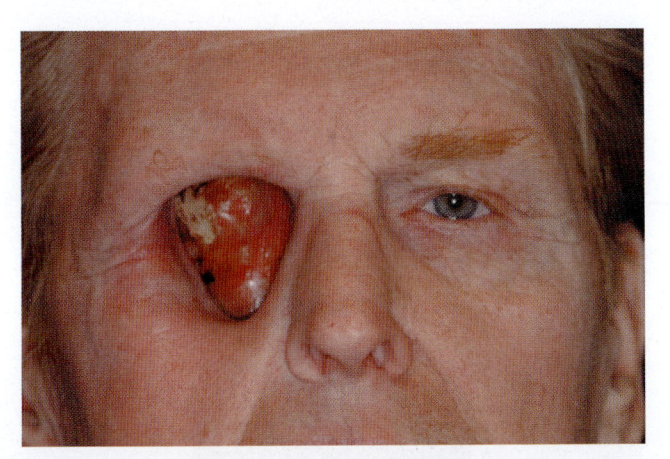

Figure 41.33. Facial appearance of man who underwent orbital exenteration for adenoid cystic carcinoma of lacrimal gland.

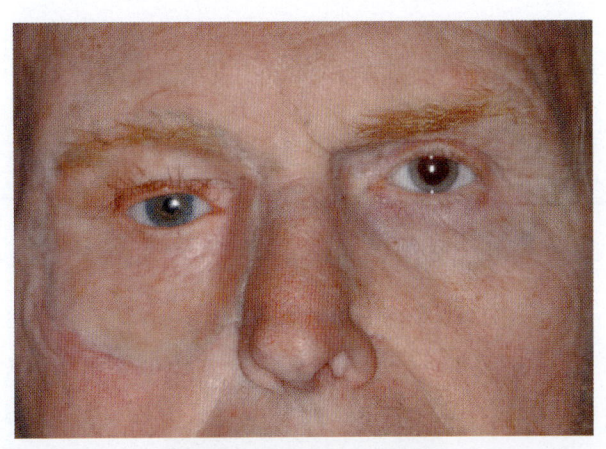

Figure 41.34. Patient shown in Figure 41.33 with glued-on prosthesis.

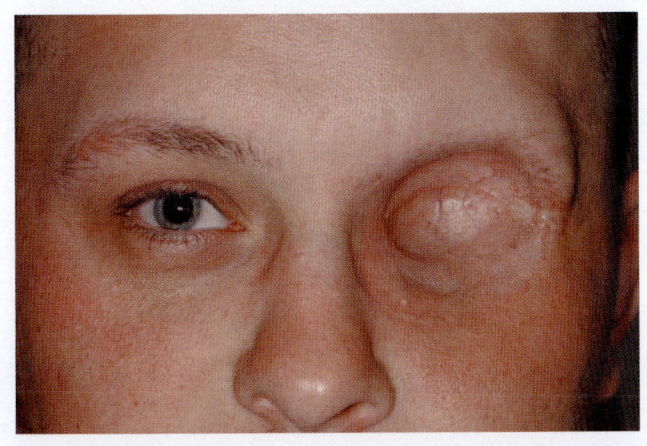

Figure 41.35. Appearance of young man who had undergone eyelid-sparing orbital exenteration.

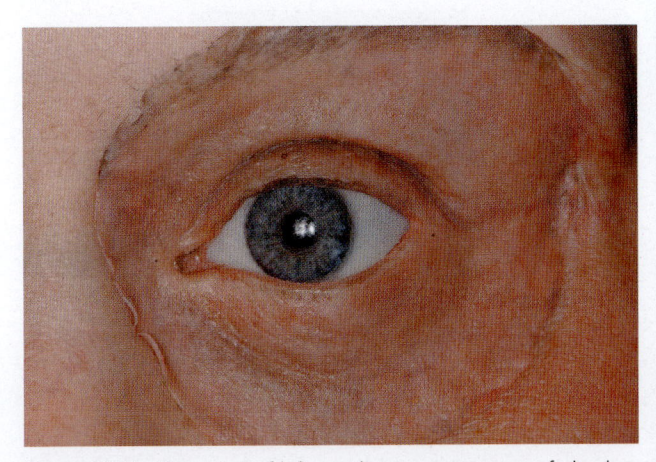

Figure 41.36. Close view of left eye showing appearance of glued-on prosthesis.

ORBITAL EXENTERATION: COSMETIC REHABILITATION

Following exenteration, cosmetic rehabilitation differs among patients. Some patients prefer simply wearing a patch, others wear frosted eyeglasses, and others wear a prosthesis. These various methods are illustrated below.

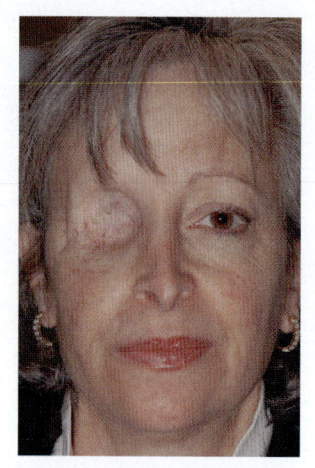

Figure 41.37. Well-healed socket following exenteration for orbital invasion from lacrimal gland adenoid cystic carcinoma.

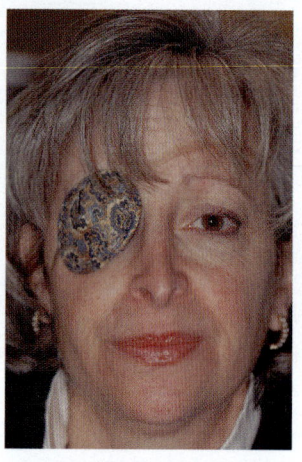

Figure 41.38. Cosmetic rehabilitation with custom made pirate's patch with elastic band matching skin tone.

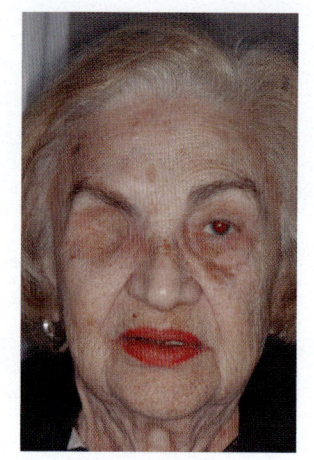

Figure 41.39. Well-healed socket following exenteration for orbital invasion from eyelid sebaceous carcinoma.

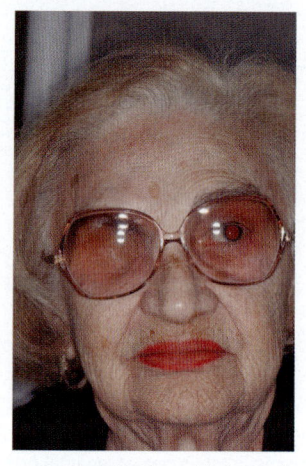

Figure 41.40. Cosmetic rehabilitation with frosted eyeglass.

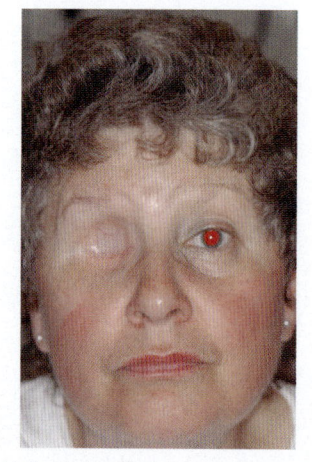

Figure 41.41. Well-healed socket following exenteration for orbital invasion from conjunctival melanoma.

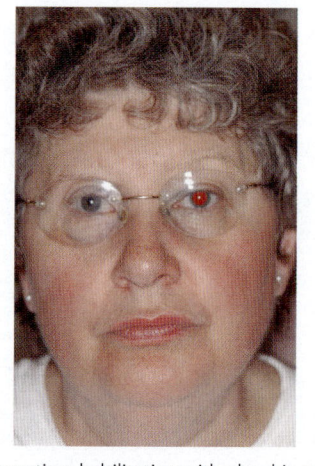

Figure 41.42. Cosmetic rehabilitation with glued-in prosthesis.

INDEX

Note: Figures are noted with a page number first succeeded by the notation for the specific figure in italic numerals: for example, figure 1–27 on page 3 is shown as 3:*1–27*.

A

Abscess
  eyelid, 220, 221:*12.31–12.32*
  Serratia marcescens, conjunctival, 418
  Staphylococcus aureus
    conjunctival, 418, 420:*24.43*
    eyelid, 220
Acanthosis, actinic keratosis and, 20
ACC. *See* Adenoid cystic carcinoma
Acinic cell adenocarcinoma, lacrimal gland, 722
  histopathology, 724:*37.90*
Acquired hemangioma, eyelid (cherry hemangioma)
  CIN and, 286
  molluscum contagiosum infection, eyelid and, 207
  squamous cell carcinoma, invasive and, 286
Acquired immunodeficiency syndrome (AIDS), 286
  conjunctival invasive SCC and, 292
  KS and, 364
Actinic keratosis
  conjunctival, 283, 285:*18.3–18.5*
  cutaneous, eyelid, 20, 23:*2.7–2.12*
  eyelid, 20, 22:*2.1–2.6*
  management, 20
Acute orbital myositis, nonspecific, 455:*26.37–26.42*
Adenocarcinoma. *See also* Acinic cell adenocarcinoma, lacrimal gland; Basal cell adenocarcinoma, lacrimal gland; Pleomorphic adenocarcinoma, lacrimal gland
  primary, lacrimal gland, 697–698, 722
  sweat gland, eyelid, 76, 78:*4.25–4.30*, 79:*4.31–4.36*
    apocrine, 76, 79:*4.33–4.34*
    eccrine, 76, 78:*4.25*
    mucinous, 76, 78:*4.25–4.30*
Adenoid cystic carcinoma (ACC), 722
  lacrimal gland, 697, 698, 708, 710–711, 713:*37.42–37.48*
    atypical orbital location of, 716:*37.67–37.72*
    in children, 716:*37.61–37.66*
    clinicopathologic correlation, 714:*37.49–37.54*
    early detection of, by imaging studies, 715:*37.55–37.60*
Adenoma, eyelid sebaceous, 49, 50. *See also specific adenomas*
Adnexal, orbital capillary hemangioma and involvement of, 509, 514:*28.13–28.18*
Adult-onset-associated xanthogranuloma, orbital, 671, 675:*35.7–35.12*. *See also* Juvenile xanthogranuloma

African-Americans
  CRCP in, 322
  melanoma, conjunctival in, 337:*19.103–19.104*, 337:*19.107–19.108*
AIDS. *See* Acquired immunodeficiency syndrome
Albright's syndrome, fibrous dysplasia and, 638
Alcohol epitheliectomy, conjunctival melanoma, 332–333, 341:*19.127–19.132*
Aldara. *See* Imiquimod
Alveolar soft part sarcoma (ASPS)
  orbital, 564, 566:*29.55–29.60*
    aggressive tumor in child, 567:*29.61–29.66*
  paraganglioma, orbital and, 562
Amelanotic melanoma, conjunctival, 340:*19.121–19.126*
5-aminolevulinic acid, nevoid BCC syndrome, 31
Amphotericin B
  mycotic infections, eyelid, 218
Amputation neuroma, orbital, 569, 571:*29.69–29.70*
Amyloidosis
  conjunctival, 422, 424:*24.55–24.60*, 425:*24.61–24.66*
  eyelid, 223, 225:*13.1–13.6*
  systemic, 422
Aneurysmal bone cyst, orbital, 638
Angiolipoma, orbital, 662
"Angiolymphoid hyperplasia with eosinophilia" (ALHE), 468
Angiosarcoma (malignant hemangioendothelioma)
  orbital, 544, 545:*28.145–28.150*
Apocrine hidrocystoma, eyelid, 198, 199:*11.7–11.12*
Arteriovenous malformation, orbital lymphangioma and, 528
Asian-Indians, conjunctival melanoma in, 337:*19.105–19.106*
Asians
  CRCP in, 322
ASPS. *See* Alveolar soft part sarcoma
Astrocytoma, optic nerve malignant, 580, 581:*30.25–30.30*
Atypical mycobacterium infection, conjunctival, 418, 420:*24.46*

B

Bacterial infections, eyelid, 220, 221:*12.31–12.36*
Baggy eyelids, 653

Balloon cell nevus, 308
Basal cell adenocarcinoma, lacrimal gland, 722
Basal cell carcinoma (BCC). *See also* Nevoid BCC syndrome
  eyelid, 30–31
    advanced cases, 36:*2.49–2.54*
    clinical variations, 30, 35:*2.43–2.48*
    imiquimod, topical for, 31, 40:*2.73–2.78*
    morpheaform type, 30, 34:*2.37–2.42*
    nevoid BCC syndrome (Gorlin–Goltz syndrome), 31, 37:*2.55–2.60*, 38:*2.61–2.66*, 39:*2.67–2.72*
    nodular and noduloulcerative type, 30, 33:*2.31–2.36*
    orbital exenteration for, 42:*2.85–2.90*
    pentagonal full-thickness eyelid resection for, 40:*2.73–2.78*
    surgical management, results of, 41:*2.79–2.84*
  PEH, eyelid and, 12, 13:*1.25*
BCC. *See* Basal cell carcinoma
B-cell lymphoma, 164:*9.1–9.6*, 165:*9.7–9.12*
Benign acquired melanosis, 324
Benign mixed tumor. *See* Pleomorphic adenoma
Benign reactive lymphoid hyperplasia (BRLH), 379
  conjunctival, 383:*22.1–22.6*
Blastomyces dermatitidis, 218
Blastomycosis, eyelid, 218, 219:*12.25–12.26*
Blepharopathy, radiation, 24, 25:*2.13–2.18*
Blepharoptosis, conjunctival amyloidosis and, 422
Blue nevus
  association with orbital and brain melanoma, 112:*6.79–6.84*, 113:*6.85–6.90*
  cavernous hemangioma, conjunctival and, 358
  cellular, 110
    eyelid, 110, 111:*6.73–6.78*, 112:*6.79–6.84*, 113:*6.85–6.90*
    periocular, 110
  common, 10
  conjunctival, 308
  melanoma, orbital arising from, 689, 691:*36.1–36.6*
  orbital melanoma, 111:*6.73–6.78*
Brain
  hemangiopericytoma, orbital invasion in, 527:*28.73–28.78*
  melanoma
    conjunctival metastasis to, 333, 347:*19.163–19.168*
Breast cancer, metastatic
  PEH, eyelid and, 12

795

BRLH. *See* Benign reactive lymphoid hyperplasia
Brooke's tumor, 81
Brown tumor of hyperparathyroidism, orbital, 638

C

Calcified scleral plaque, 430
Cantharidin, eyelid molluscum contagiosum infection, 207
Capillary hemangioma. *See also* Congenital capillary hemangioma, eyelid
   cavernous hemangioma and, 360
   conjunctival, 349, 360, 361:*20.31–20.36*
      infantile, 360
   lymphangioma and, 360
   orbital, 509–510, 512:*28.1–28.6*
      adnexal/eyelid involvement, simultaneous in, 509, 514:*28.13–28.18*
      clinical variations, 509, 513:*28.7–28.12*
      regression, 509, 513:*28.7–28.12*
      surgical resection of, 510, 515:*28.19–28.24*
Carney complex
   melanocytic nevus and, 308
   myxoma and, 376
Cartilaginous hamartoma, orbital, 648, 649:*33.49–33.54*
Cartilaginous tumors
   acquired orbital, 648, 649:*33.49–33.54*
   orbital, 631–652
Caruncle
   cavernous hemangioma, 401:*23.40*
   cysts, 393, 400:*23.31–23.36*
   fibroma, 401:*23.42*
   KS, 401:*23.39*
   lymphoma, 401:*23.41*
   melanoma, 394, 397:*23.13–23.18*
   nevus, 393, 396:*23.7–23.12*
   oncocytoma, 393, 398:*23.19–23.24*
   papilloma, 393, 395:*23.1–23.6*
   pyogenic granuloma, 401:*23.37–23.38*
   sebaceous tumors, 393, 399:*23.25–23.30*
   tumors, 393–401
      conjunctival, 393–401
      miscellaneous, 394, 401:*23.37–23.42*
Cavernous hemangioma
   capillary hemangioma and, 360
   caruncular, 401:*23.40*
   conjunctival, 349, 358, 359:*20.27–20.28*
   hemangiopericytoma, orbital and, 524
   orbital, 516, 518:*28.25–28.30*
      clinicopathologic correlation, 516, 521:*28.43–28.48*
      globe/optic nerve compression, 516, 520:*28.37–28.42*
      intraosseous type, 516, 523:*28.55–28.60*
      schwannoma and, 550
      supertemporal orbitotomy, 516, 521:*28.43–28.48*
      supranasal orbitotomy, 516, 522:*28.49–28.54*
      surgical removal of, by conjunctival approach, 516, 519:*28.31–28.36*
Chalazion, eyelid, 210, 212:*12.7–12.12*
   clinical variations, 210, 213:*12.13–12.18*
Chemodectoma. *See* Paraganglioma
Cherry hemangioma. *See* Acquired hemangioma, eyelid
Cherubism, GCRG and, 646
Childhood conjunctival papilloma, 267–268, 270:*17.1–17.6*

cimetidine management of, 268, 271:*17.7–17.12*
Children. *See also* Infants
   ACC, lacrimal gland in, 716:*37.61–37.66*
   ASPS, orbital aggressive tumor in, 567:*29.61–29.66*
   fibrosarcoma in, 628, 629:*32.55–32.60*
   JPA, optic nerve in, 574
   leiomyoma, orbital in, 608
   lymphangioma, orbital in, 534:*28.103–28.108*
   malignant rhabdoid tumor, orbital in, 606, 607:*31.43–31.48*
   nodular fascitis in, 611, 614:*32.1–32.6*
   osteosarcoma in, 636, 637:*33.15–33.18*
   RMS, orbital in, 595–596
Chondroma
   chondrosarcoma transformation of, 648, 650
   orbital, 648, 649:*33.49–33.54*
Chondroma, syringoma, 74
Chondrosarcoma
   chondroma transformation into, 650
   extraskeletal mesenchymal type, 650
   orbital, 650, 651:*33.55–33.60*
      in young woman, 652:*33.61–33.66*
   radiation-induced type, 650
   standard type, 650
Choristomas
   complex
      conjunctival, 264, 265:*16.43–16.48*
      epibulbar, association with organoid nevus syndrome, 264, 266:*16.49–16.54*
   conjunctival, 251–266
      lacrimal gland, 262, 263:*16.37–16.42*
      respiratory, 262, 263:*16.37–16.42*
   epibulbar, 251–266
Churg–Strauss syndrome, conjuctival neoplasm simulated by, 414, 415:*24.31–24.36*
Cidofovir
   CIN, 286
   conjunctival invasive SCC, 293
Ciliary body melanoma, extraocular extension of, 430
Cimetidine (Tagamet), 268, 271:*17.7–17.12*
CIN. *See* Conjunctival intraepithelial neoplasia
Clark classification, melanoma, 324
Clear cell hydradenoma, 70
Coccidioides immitis, 218
Coccidioidomycosis, eyelid, 218, 219:*12.27*
Complexion-related conjunctival pigmentation (CRCP)
   conjunctival, 323:*19.61–19.66*
Congenital capillary hemangioma, eyelid (strawberry hemangioma)
   orbital, 509
Conjunctiva
   abscess, 418, 420:*24.43*, 420:*24.51–24.54*
   actinic keratosis, 283, 285:*18.3–18.5*
   amyloidosis, 422, 424:*24.55–24.60*, 425:*24.61–24.66*
   benign epithelial tumors, 267–281
   blue nevus, 308
   capillary hemangioma, 349, 360, 361:*20.31–20.36*
      infantile, 360
   caruncular tumors, 393–401
   cavernous hemangioma, 349, 358, 359:*20.27–20.28*

   cavernous hemangioma, orbital and surgical removal through, 516, 519:*28.31–28.36*
   choristomas, 251–266
      complex, 264, 265:*16.43–16.48*
      lacrimal gland, 262, 263:*16.37–16.42*
      respiratory, 262, 263:*16.37–16.42*
   CRCP, 322, 323:*19.61–19.66*
   dacryoadenoma, 280, 281:*17.37–17.42*
   dermoid, 251–252, 253:*16.1–16.6*, 254:*16.7–16.12*
      atypical variations, 255:*16.13–16.18*
   dermolipoma, 256, 258:*16.19–16.24*, 658, 659:*34.19–34.24*
      age range, 659:*34.19–34.24*
      bilobed variants of, 256, 259:*16.25–16.30*
      clinical features of, 658, 660:*34.25–34.30*
      clinical spectrum, 659:*34.19–34.24*
      computed tomography features of, 658, 660:*34.25–34.30*
      Goldenhar syndrome and, 658, 661:*34.31–34.36*
      histopathologic features of, 658, 660:*34.25–34.30*
      pedunculated variants of, 256, 259:*16.25–16.30*
   diffuse neonatal hemangiomatosis, 360
   episcleral sentinel vessels, 358, 359:*20.30*
   epithelial inclusion cyst, 403, 405:*24.1–25.6*
   epithelium, tumors of, 283–305
   FH, 372, 373:*21.13–21.18*
   fibroma, 374, 375:*21.19–21.20*
   foreign bodies, 408, 410:*24.13–24.18*, 411:*24.19–24.24*
   GCT, 370, 371:*21.11–21.12*
   glomus tumor, 362, 363:*20.39–20.42*
   hemangiopericytoma, 362, 363:*20.37–20.38*
   hereditary benign intraepithelial dyskeratosis, 278, 279:*17.31–17.36*
   JXG, 374, 375:*21.23–21.24*
   KA, 276, 277:*17.26–17.30*
   keratotic plaque, 283, 285:*18.1–18.2*, 285:*18.6*
   KS, 349, 364, 365:*20.43–20.48*
   leukemia, 388
   leukemia infiltrate in, 389:*22.25–22.30*
   leukemic tumors, 379–392
   ligneous conjunctivitis, 416, 417:*24.37–24.42*
   lipoma, 376, 377:*21.27–21.28*
   lymphangiectasia, 354, 356:*20.13–20.16*
   lymphangioma, 349, 354, 356:*20.17–20.18*, 357:*20.19–20.24*
   lymphoid tumors, 380–381
   lymphoma
      atypical forms, 385:*22.13–22.17*
      radiotherapy response of, 385:*22.16*, 385:*22.18*
   macrovessels, 358, 359:*20.29*
   malignant melanoma, 332–333
   melanocytic nevus, 308–309
   melanoma
      alcohol epitheliectomy, 332–333, 341:*19.127–19.132*
      amelanotic variations, 340:*19.121–19.126*
      brain metastasis of, 333, 347:*19.163–19.168*
      cryotherapy, 332–333, 341:*19.127–19.132*
      de novo-arising tumors of, 338:*19.109–19.114*, 339:*19.115–19.120*

diffuse tumors or, before/after treatment, 342:*19.133–19.138*
lymph nodes, preauricular metastasis of, 333, 347:*19.163–19.168*
in non-Caucasians, 337:*19.103–19.108*
orbital exenteration, 332–333, 346:*19.157–19.162*
PAM and evolution of, 335:*19.91–19.96*, 336:*19.97–19.102*
plaque radiotherapy for, 345:*19.151–19.156*
sentinel lymph node biopsy and localization of, 333, 344:*19.145–19.150*
surgical resection, 332–333, 341:*19.127–19.132*
tumor with scleral invasion and, 343:*19.139–19.144*
malignancies with topical chemotherapy and interferon, 438:*25.19–25.24*
metastasis, 390, 391:*22.31–22.36*
from cutaneous melanoma, 392:*22.37–22.42*
metastatic tumors, 379–392
myxoma, 376, 377:*21.25–21.26*
neoplasms
Churg–Strauss allergic granulomatosis simulating, 414, 415:*24.31–24.36*
miscellaneous infectious lesions simulating, 418, 420:*24.43–24.48*, 421:*24.49–24.54*
miscellaneous lesions simulating, 403–432
with plaque brachytherapy, 440:*25.31–25.36*
with plaque radiotherapy, 439:*25.25–25.30*
neurofibroma, 367–368, 369:*21.1–21.6*
neuroma, 367–368
nevi in, 308–309
nodular fascitis, 374, 375:*21.21–21.22*
non-Hodgkin lymphoma, 384:*22.7–22.12*
B-cell type, 380
orbital cyst of
associated with Stevens–Johnson syndrome, 485:*27.55–27.60*
secondary type, after enucleation, 483:*27.43–27.48*
secondary type, after retinal detachment surgery, 484:*27.49–27.54*
organizing hematoma, 406
secondary to silicone sponge for retinal detachment repair, 407:*24.7–24.12*
PAM, 324–326
melanoma and, 324, 330:*19.79–19.84*, 331:*19.85–19.90*
mild involvement of, 328:*19.67–19.72*
moderately severe, 329:*19.73–19.78*
papilloma of adulthood in, 272, 274:*17.13–17.18*
atypical variations of, 272, 275:*17.19–17.24*
papilloma of childhood in, 267–268, 270:*17.1–17.6*
cimetidine management of, 268, 271:*17.7–17.12*
PEH, 276, 277:*17.25*
pigmented melanoma simulated by miscellaneous lesions of, 430
plasmacytic tumors, 380–381
PTLD, 386, 387:*22.19–22.24*
pyogenic granuloma, 350

plaque radiotherapy treatment for, 350, 353:*20.7–20.12*
primary type, 352:*20.1–20.6*
reticulohistiocytoma, 376, 377:*21.29–21.30*
RMS, orbital presenting as mass in, 602:*31.19–31.24*
SCC, invasive of, 292–294
advanced, 298:*18.43–18.48*
atypical variations, 301:*18.61–18.66*
early, 297:*18.37–18.42*
en bloc eye wall resection for, 302:*18.67–18.72*
intraocular invasion, 304:*18.79–18.84*
mucoepidermoid, 305:*18.85–18.90*
orbital invasion, 303:*18.73–18.78*
papillomatous corneal involvement, extensive in, 300:*18.55–18.60*
tarsal conjunctiva involvement in, 299:*18.49–18.54*
schwannoma, 370, 371:*21.7–21.10*
surgical management of, 437:*25.13–25.18*
primary acquired melanosis, 436:*25.7–25.12*
primary acquired melanoma, 436:*25.7–25.12*
tumors, 249–440, 367–377
melanocytic, 307–347
secondary, 390
surgical resection of limbal, 435:*25.1–25.6*
vascular, 349–365
varix, 349, 358, 359:*20.25–20.26*
vascular lesions of, miscellaneous, 358
Conjunctival intraepithelial neoplasia (CIN), 286
actinic keratosis and, 283
fleshy configurations, 288:*18.7–18.12*
keratotic plaque and, 283
leukoplakia, 289:*18.13–18.18*
limbus clinical locations of, 290:*18.19–18.24*
papillomatous configurations, 288:*18.7–18.12*
superficial corneal invasion, 291:*18.30–18.30*
Conjunctivitis, ligneous, 416, 417:*24.37–24.42*
Cornea
CIN and superficial invasion in, 291:*18.25–18.30*
dermoid, 254:*16.7–16.12*
atypical variations, 255:*16.13–16.18*
pyogenic granuloma, 350, 353
SCC, conjunctival and involvement of papillomatous, 300:*18.55–18.60*
Cowden's disease, multiple eyelid trichilemmoma and, 86, 87:*5.14*
CRCP. *See* Complexion-related conjunctival pigmentation
Cryotherapy, conjunctival melanoma, 332–333, 341:*19.127–19.132*
Cutaneous malignancies, nevoid BCC syndrome with, 38:*2.61–2.66*
Cyclophosphamide, eyelid Wegener's granulomatosis, 216
Cyclosporine, ligneous conjunctivitis, 416
Cylindromas, multiple, 81
Cystadenocarcinoma, lacrimal gland, 722
Cystic lesions

eyelid, simulating neoplasms, 195–205
orbital, 471

D

Dacryoadenoma, conjunctival, 280, 281:*17.37–17.42*
Dacryocystitis, acute lacrimal sac, 242:*14.23–14.24*
Dacryops. *See* Ductal epithelial cyst, lacrimal gland
De novo arising tumors, melanoma conjunctival, 338:*19.109–19.114*, 339:*19.115–19.120*
metastasis and, 692
orbital, 692
Dermoid
conjunctival, 251–252, 253:*16.1–16.6*, 254:*16.7–16.12*
atypical variations, 255:*16.13–16.18*
corneal, 254:*16.7–16.12*
atypical variations, 255:*16.13–16.18*
Dermoid cyst
eyelid, 204
clinicopathologic correlation, 204, 205:*11.25–11.30*
nodular fascitis simulating, 611
Dermolipoma (lipodermoid), 251
conjunctival, 256, 258:*16.19–16.24*, 658, 659:*34.19–34.24*
age range, 659:*34.19–34.24*
bilobed variants of, 256, 259:*16.25–16.30*
clinical features of, 658, 660:*34.25–34.30*
clinical spectrum, 659:*34.19–34.24*
computed tomography features of, 658, 660:*34.25–34.30*
Goldenhar syndrome and, 658, 661:*34.31–34.36*
histopathologic features of, 658, 660:*34.25–34.30*
pedunculated variants of, 256, 259:*16.25–16.30*
fat prolapse, orbital and, 653–654
orbital, 256, 258:*16.19–16.24*, 658, 659:*34.19–34.24*
age range, 659:*34.19–34.24*
clinical features of, 658, 660:*34.25–34.30*
clinical spectrum, 659:*34.19–34.24*
computed tomography features of, 658, 660:*34.25–34.30*
Goldenhar syndrome and, 658, 661:*34.31–34.36*
histopathologic features of, 658, 660:*34.25–34.30*
Diffuse neonatal hemangiomatosis
cavernous hemangioma, conjunctival and, 358
conjunctival, 360
Dinitrochlorobenzene, childhood conjunctival papilloma, 268
DNS. *See* Dysplastic nevus syndrome
Down's syndrome, multiple syringomas and, 67
Ductal carcinoma, lacrimal gland, 722
Ductal epithelial cyst, lacrimal gland (dacryops), 697, 699, 700:*37.1–37.6*, 701:*37.7–37.12*
Dyskeratosis, 19. *See also* Hereditary benign intraepithelial dyskeratosis, conjunctival

Dysplastic nevus, 307, 308
Dysplastic nevus syndrome (DNS)
  malignant melanoma, conjunctival and, 332
  melanocytic nevus and, 307
  PAM and, 324

E

EBV. See Epstein–Barr virus (EBV)
Ecchymosis, eyelid and orbital hematoma, 546
Eccrine acrospiroma, 70
  eyelid, 71:4.7–4.12
Eccrine hidrocystoma, eyelid, 195, 197:11.1–11.6
  apocrine hidrocystoma v., 195
Eccrine hydradenoma, 70
ECD. See Erdheim–Chester disease
EG. See Eosinophilic granuloma
Ehlers–Danlos syndrome, multiple syringomas and, 67
Elliptical excision, eyelid tumor, 245:15.5, 246:15.7–15.12
En bloc wall resection, conjunctival SCC, 302:18.67–18.72
Enchondromas, multiple, 648
Enucleation
  amputation neuroma and, 568
Eosinophilic granuloma (EG), 676
Epibulbar complex
  choristomas, organoid nevus syndrome associated with, 264, 266:16.49–16.54
  RMS, orbital presenting as mass in, 604:31.31–31.36
Epibulbar osseous choristoma, 260, 261:16.31–16.36
Epidermal inclusion cyst, eyelid (epidermoid cyst), 202, 203:11.19–11.24
Epidermal nevus syndrome. See Sebaceous nevus, eyelid
Epidermoid cyst. See Epidermal inclusion cyst, eyelid
Episclera
  neurofibroma, conjunctival in, 368, 368:21.4–21.6
  ocular melanocytosis pigmentation and, 320
  sentinel vessels, conjunctival, 358, 359:20.30
Episcleritis
  diffuse, 412, 413:24.25
  neoplasms simulating, 412
  nodular, 412, 413:24.26
Epithelial cysts. See also Ductal epithelial cyst, lacrimal gland
  inclusion, conjunctival, 403, 405:24.1–24.6
Epithelial-myoepithelial carcinoma, lacrimal gland, 722
Epithelial tumors. See also Primary epithelial malignancies of lacrimal gland
  conjunctival
    benign, 267–281
    malignant, 283–305
    premalignant, 283–305
  lacrimal gland primary, 697–724
Epithelioid cell nevus, 308, 314:19.21–19.22
Epstein–Barr virus (EBV)
  PTLD and
    conjunctival, 386, 387:22.24
  Erdheim–Chester disease (ECD)
    orbital, 671, 682, 683:35.37–35.42
Esthesioneuroblastoma, 593

Ewing tumor
  extraskeletal, PNET classification and, 592
Eyelid
  abscess, 220, 221:12.31–12.32
  actinic keratosis, 20, 22:2.1–2.6
    cutaneous, 20, 23:2.7–2.12
  acquired capillary hemangioma, 142, 143:8.31–8.36
  amyloidosis, 223, 225:13.1–13.6
  angiosarcoma, 158
    clinical variations, 159:8.91–8.96
  apocrine hidrocystoma, 198, 199:11.7–11.12
  bacterial infections, 220, 221:12.31–12.36
  BCC, 30–31
    advanced cases, 36:2.49–2.54
    clinical variations, 30, 35:2.43–2.48
    imiquimod, topical for, 31, 40:2.73–2.78
    morpheaform type, 30, 34:2.37–2.42
    nevoid BCC syndrome (Gorlin–Goltz syndrome), 31, 37:2.55–2.60, 38:2.61–2.66, 39:2.67–2.72
    nodular and noduloulcerative type, 30, 33:2.31–2.36
    orbital exenteration for, 42:2.85–2.90
    pentagonal full-thickness eyelid resection for, 40:2.73–2.78
    surgical management, results of, 41:2.79–2.84
  blastomycosis, 218, 219:12.25–12.26
  capillary hemangioma, orbital and involvement of, 509, 514:28.13–28.18
  chalazion, 210, 212:12.7–12.12
    clinical variations, 210, 213:12.13–12.18
  coccidioidomycosis, 218, 219:12.27
  congenital capillary hemangioma
    deep type, 138:8.7–8.12
    regression of deep type, 140:8.19–8.24
    regression of superficial type, 139:8.13–8.18
    strawberry hemangioma, 134–135
    superficial type, 137:8.1–8.6
    surgical removal, 141:8.25–8.30
  dermoid cyst, 204
    clinicopathologic correlation, 204, 205:11.25–11.30
  eccrine acrospiroma, 70, 71:4.7–4.12
  eccrine hidrocystoma, 195, 197:11.1–11.6
  epidermal inclusion cyst, 202, 203:11.19–11.24
  epidermis
    benign tumors of, 3–18
    malignant tumors of, 19–48
    premalignant tumors of, 19–48
  facial angiofibroma, 184
    with tuberous sclerosis complex, 185:10.25–10.30
  GCT, 228, 229:13.13–13.14
  glomus tumor, 152, 153:8.67–8.72
  granulomatous diseases, miscellaneous, 214–216
  IFK, 10, 11:1.19–1.24
  inflammatory lesions of, simulating neoplasms, 207–221
  KA, 14, 15:1.31–1.36
    case description, 16:1.37–1.42
    clinicopathologic correlation in, 17:1.43–1.48
    management by excision and skin graft, 16:1.37–1.42

lesions
  cystic, simulating neoplasms, 195–205
lipoid proteinosis, 226, 227:13.7–13.12
lymphangioma, 150, 151:8.61–8.66
lymphoma, 162
malakoplakia, 228, 229:13.15–13.16
melanocytic nevus, 93
  age variations, 93, 96:6.7–6.12
  clinical variations of, 93, 98:6.19–6.24
  congenital, 93, 100:6.31–6.36
  largecongenital periocular type, 93, 101:6.37–6.42
  nonpigmented types, 93, 97:6.13–6.18
  pigmented types, 93, 95:6.1–6.6
  race variations, 93, 96:6.7–6.12
  small lesion excision technique/pathology, 93, 99:6.25–6.30
melanocytic tumors, 92–117
melanoma, primary, 116:6.97–6.102
  surgical excision, 117:6.103–6.108
miscellaneous fibrous, 190
molluscum contagiosum infection, 207, 209:12.1–12.6
mucormycosis, 218, 219:12.28–12.30
mycotic infections, 218, 219:12.25–12.30
myxomatous tumors, 190
necrotizing fasciitis, 220, 221:12.33–12.36
neoplasms simulated by miscellaneous conditions of, 223–231
neurothekeoma, 125:7.13–7.18
nevus flammeus (port wine hemangioma), 144, 145:8.37–8.42
  association with Sturge–Weber syndrome, 147:8.49–8.54
  clinical variations and follow-up, 146:8.43–8.42
nodular fasciitis, 186, 188:10.31–10.36
  clinicopathologic correlation, 189:10.37–10.42
nonspecific keratosis, 14, 18:1.49–1.54
orbital simple primary cyst, 480
PEH, 12, 13:1.25–1.30
phakomatous choristoma, 230, 231:13.19–13.24
pilomatrixoma, 88
  in adults, 89:5.19–5.24
  in children (surgical excision), 90:5.25–5.30
  histopathology, 91:5.31–5.36
  surgical excision, 91:5.31–5.36
plasmacytoma, 168, 169:9.25–9.30
pleomorphic adenoma, 74, 75:4.19–4.24
primary idiopathic type, 482:27.37–27.42
pseudoneoplastic lesions, 228
pseudorheumatoid nodule (granuloma annular), 215, 217:2.21–2.22
reconstruction, 243
sarcoidosis, 214, 217:2.19–2.20
SCC, 43–44, 45:2.91–2.96
  aggressive invasive tumors in, 47:2.103–2.108
  deep cystic recurrent tumors in, 48:2.109–2.114
  diffuse involvement of upper eyelid in, 46:2.97–2.102
Schwannoma, 125:7.13–7.18
sebaceous carcinoma, 51–53
  aggressive clinical course, 61:3.43–3.48
  clinical variations, 58:3.25–3.30

diffuse neoplasm, 60:*3.37–3.42*
diffuse neoplasm masquerading as inflammation, 56:*3.13–3.18*
histopathology, 58:*3.25–3.30*
large tumor and rotational forehead flap, 64:*3.61–3.66*
meibomian gland origin, 54:*3.1–3.6*
MTS associated with, 52, 59:*3.31–3.36*
pedunculated variant of, 57:*3.19–3.24*
pentagonal full-thickness eyelid resection, 62:*3.49–3.54*
pentagonal resection, 63:*3.55–3.60*
posterior lamellar eyelid resection and reconstruction, 65:*3.67–3.72*
semicircular flap reconstruction, 63:*3.55–3.60*
Zeis gland origin, 55:*3.7–3.12*
sebaceous cyst, 200, 201:*11.13–11.18*
sebaceous gland tumors, 49–65
sebaceous nevus, 28, 29:*2.25–2.30*
SK, 6, 8:*1.7–1.12*, 9:*1.13–1.18*
subepidermal calcified nodule, 228, 229:*13.17–13.18*
sweat gland
  adenocarcinoma of, 76, 78:*4.25–4.30*, 79:*4.31–4.36*
  tumors, 67–79
syringocystadenoma papilliferum, 72, 73:*4.13–4.18*
syringoma, 67, 68, 69:*4.1–4.6*
trichilemmoma, 86, 87:*5.13–5.18*
trichoadenoma, 84, 85:*5.7–5.12*
trichoepithelioma, 81, 82, 83:*5.1–5.6*
trichofolliculoma, 84, 85:*5.7–5.12*
tumors, 1–248
  elliptical excision, 246:*15.7–15.12*
  epidermis, benign, 3–18
  hair follicle, 81–91
  lacrimal drainage system, 233–242
  reconstruction of, 243
  surgical management of, 243–248
  sweat gland, 67–79
varix, 148, 149:*8.55–8.60*
Wegener's granulomatosis, 216, 217:*12.23–12.24*
xanthelasma, 178:*10.1–10.6*
xanthoma, 176, 178:*10.1–10.6*
xeroderma pigmentosum, 26, 27:*2.19–2.24*

F
Fat prolapse, orbital, 653–654, 655:*34.1–34.6*, 656:*34.7–34.12*
  clinical features of, 657:*34.13–34.18*
  computed tomography features of, 657:*34.13–34.18*
  surgical approach, 657:*34.13–34.18*
Ferguson–Smith syndrome, eyelid KA and, 14
FH. *See* Fibrous histiocytoma
Fibroma. *See also* Ossifying fibroma
  caruncular, 401:*23.42*
  conjunctival, 374, 375:*21.19–21.20*
  orbital, 613, 615:*32.10–32.12*
Fibromatosis
  infantile, 616, 618:*32.13–32.18*
  orbital, 616, 618:*32.13–32.18*
Fibro-osseous tumors, orbital, 631–652
Fibrosarcoma
  in children, 628, 629:*32.55–32.60*
  orbital, 628, 629:*32.55–32.60*
  radiation-induced, 628

Fibrous connective tissue tumors, orbital, 611–629
Fibrous dysplasia
  malignant transformation, 638
  monostotic, 638
  orbital, 638, 640:*33.19–33.24*, 641:*33.25–33.30*
  polystotic, 638
Fibrous histiocytoma (FH)
  benign, 620, 621:*32.25–32.30*
  conjunctival, 372, 373:*21.13–21.18*
  fibroma, orbital and, 613
  fibrosarcoma diagnosis and, 628
  lacrimal sac, 241:*14.15–14.16*
  locally aggressive, 620
  malignant, 620, 622:*32.31–32.36*
  management of, 620, 623:*32.37–32.42*
  orbital, 620
    benign, 620, 621:*32.25–32.30*
    malignant, 620, 622:*32.31–32.36*
    management of, 620, 623:*32.37–32.42*
Fibrous tumors. *See also* Solitary fibrous tumor
  conjunctival, 367–377
Fine-needle aspiration biopsy (FNAB), 725
5-fluorouracil (5-FU)
  actinic keratosis, eyelid, 22:*2.2*
  KA, eyelid, 14
  trichilemmoma, eyelid and, 86
Focal hyperkeratosis, eyelid actinic keratosis and, 19
Foreign bodies, conjunctival, 408, 410:*24.13–24.18*, 411:*24.19–24.24*
5-FU. *See* 5-fluorouracil

G
Gardner syndrome
  epidermal inclusion cyst, eyelid and, 202
  osteoma, orbital and, 631–632
GCRG. *See* Giant cell reparative granuloma
GCT. *See* Granular cell tumor
Giant cell reparative granuloma (GCRG)
  bilateral, 646
  orbital, 638, 646, 647:*33.43–33.48*
Giant cell tumor, orbital (osteoclastoma), 638
Glaucoma, ocular melanocytosis and secondary, 320
Glomangioma. *See* Glomus tumor
Glomus tumor (glomangioma)
  conjunctival, 362, 363:*20.39–20.42*
  orbital, 542, 543:*28.142–28.144*
Goldenhar's syndrome
  dermoid, conjunctival, 251
  dermolipoma and, 658, 661:*34.31–34.36*
  fat prolapse, orbital and, 653
Goltz syndrome, 31
Gorlin–Goltz syndrome. *See* Nevoid BCC syndrome
Granular cell myoblastoma, 568
Granular cell tumor (GCT)
  ASPS and, 564
  conjunctival, 370, 371:*21.11–21.12*
    PEH and, 370
  eyelid, 228, 229:*13.13–13.14*
  orbital, 568, 571:*29.67–29.68*
Granulocytic sarcoma, 388
Granuloma annulare. *See* Pseudorheumatoid nodule, eyelid
Granulomatosis, allergic simulating conjuctival neoplasm, 414, 415:*24.31–24.36*
Granulomatous diseases, miscellaneous, 214–216

H
Hamartoma. *See* Cartilaginous hamartoma, orbital; Melanocytic hamartoma, orbital
Hand–Schuller–Christian disease, 676
Hemangiopericytoma
  conjunctival, 362, 363:*20.37–20.38*
  orbital, 524
    aggressive tumor with brain invasion, 527:*28.73–28.78*
    clinicopathologic correlation, 525:*28.61–28.66*, 526:*28.67–28.72*
    recurrence, 524
    SFT and, 624
Hematic cyst. *See* Organizing hematoma
Hematocele. *See* Organizing hematoma
Hematoma, orbital, 546. *See also* Organizing hematoma
Hemiparesis, optic nerve malignant astrocytoma and, 580
Hemorrhagic lesions
  LCH, orbital presenting as cystic, 676, 681:*35.31–35.36*
  orbital, 509–547
Hereditary benign intraepithelial dyskeratosis, conjunctival, 278, 279:*17.31–17.36*
Hidrocystoma
  apocrine, 67
    eccrine v., 195
    eyelid, 198, 199:*11.7–11.12*
  clear cell, 70
  eccrine, 67
    eyelid, 195, 197:*11.1–11.6*
Histiocytic tumors, orbital, 671–688
HPV. *See* Human papillomavirus
Human papillomavirus (HPV)
  childhood papilloma and, 267
  CIN and, 286
  conjunctival invasive SCC and, 292
  lacrimal sac neoplasms and, 234
Hyperimmunoglobulinemia E (Job's syndrome), 210
Hyperparathyroidism, brown tumor of, 638
Hyperplasia, 49, 50. *See also* Benign reactive lymphoid hyperplasia; Intravascular papillary endothelial hyperplasia, orbital
  squamous epithelium benign, 3
Hypesthesia, MMPNST and periocular, 570
Hypodontia, apocrine hidrocystoma and, 198
Hypothalamic dysfunction, optic nerve malignant astrocytoma and, 580

I
IFK. *See* Inverted follicular keratosis, eyelid
Imiquimod (Aldara)
  actinic keratosis, eyelid, 20
  BCC, eyelid, 31, 40:*2.73–2.78*
  KA, eyelid, 14
  SCC, eyelid, 43
Incisional biopsy, eyelid tumor, 243
Infants
  capillary hemangioma, conjunctival, 360
  fibromatosis, 616, 618:*32.13–32.18*
  JXG, 674:*35.1–35.6*
  lymphangioma, orbital in, 533:*28.97–28.102*
  MNET of, 689
  myofibroma, 618:*32.13–32.18*, 619:*32.19–32.24*

Inflammatory lesions, neoplasms simulating
    eyelid, 207–221
α-Interferon, childhood conjunctival
    papilloma, 268
Interferon α-2b
    capillary hemangioma, 510
    CIN, 286
    conjunctival invasive SCC, 293
Intravascular papillary endothelial hyperplasia,
    orbital (IPEH), 542, 543:28.142–28.144
Inverted follicular keratosis, eyelid, 10,
    11:1.19–1.24
IPEH. See Intravascular papillary endothelial
    hyperplasia, orbital

J
Job's syndrome. See Hyperimmunoglobulinemia E
JPA. See Juvenile pilocytic astrocytoma
Juvenile pilocytic astrocytoma (JPA),
    optic nerve, 574, 576:30.1–30.6,
    578:30.13–30.18
    fundus changes, 574, 579:30.19–30.24
    magnetic resonance imaging, 574,
    577:30.7–30.12
Juvenile xanthogranuloma (JXG)
    conjunctival, 374, 375:21.23–21.24
    infantile, 674:35.1–35.6
    orbital, 671–672, 674:35.1–35.6
JXG. See Juvenile xanthogranuloma

K
KA. See Keratoacanthoma
Kaposi sarcoma (KS), 154
    AIDS and, 364
    angiosarcoma resembling, 544
    caruncular, 401:23.39
    conjunctival, 349, 364, 365:20.43–20.48
    eyelid
        in immunosuppressed patients,
            156:8.79–8.84
        in nonimmunosuppressed patient,
            155:8.73–8.78
        treatment with radiotherapy,
            157:8.85–8.90
Keratinocytes, eyelid actinic keratosis and
    mildly atypical, 19
Keratoacanthoma (KA)
    conjunctival, 276, 277:17.26–17.30
    eyelid, 14, 15:1.31–1.36
        case description, 16:1.37–1.42
        clinicopathologic correlation in,
            17:1.43–1.48
        management by excision and skin graft,
            16:1.37–1.42
Keratoconjunctivitis sicca, dermolipoma and,
    256
Keratotic plaque, conjunctival, 283,
    285:18.1–18.2, 285:18.6
"Kimura disease," 468
KS. See Kaposi sarcoma

L
Lacrimal drainage system tumors, 233–242
Lacrimal gland primary epithelial tumors,
    697–724. See also Primary epithelial
    malignancies of lacrimal gland
Lacrimal glands. See also Primary epithelial
    malignancies of lacrimal gland
    ACC, 697–698, 710–711, 713:37.42–37.48
        atypical orbital location of,
            716:37.67–37.72
        in children, 716:37.61–37.66
        clinicopathologic correlation,
            714:37.49–37.54
        early detection of, by imaging studies,
            715:37.55–37.60
    acinic cell adenocarcinoma, 722
        histopathology, 724:37.90
    adenocarcinoma, primary, 722
    basal cell adenocarcinoma, 722
    cystadenocarcinoma, 722
    ductal carcinoma, 722
    ductal epithelial cyst, 697, 699,
        700:37.1–37.6, 701:37.7–37.12
    epithelial-myoepithelial carcinoma, 722
    mucoepidermoid carcinoma, 697–698,
        721:37.79–37.84, 722
        histopathology, 724:37.89
    pleomorphic adenocarcinoma, 708,
        709:37.37–37.42, 722
        histopathology, 724:37.88
    pleomorphic adenoma, 697–698, 702,
        709:37.67–37.72
        clinicopathologic correlation,
            704:37.13–37.18
        magnetic resonance imaging,
            707:37.31–37.36
        surgical management, 705:37.19–37.24
        in teenager, 706:37.25–37.30
    primary ductal carcinoma, 718,
        720:37.73–37.78
    SCC, primary, 722
    sebaceous carcinoma, 722
Lacrimal sac
    dacryocystitis, acute, 242:14.23–14.24
    fibrous histiocytoma, 241:14.15–14.16
    infections, 242:14.19–14.24
    inflammations, 242:14.19–14.24
    leiomyoma, 241:14.13–14.14
    MALT lymphoma, 241:14.17–14.18
    melanoma, 233, 238, 239:14.7–14.12
    neoplasms, 233
    pseudotumors, 240
    pyogenic granuloma, 242:14.19–14.20
    squamous carcinoma, 233, 236, 237:14.1–14.4
    squamous cell carcinoma (SCC), 233
    squamous papilloma, 233, 236,
        237:14.5–14.6
    tumors, miscellaneous, 240,
        241:14.13–14.18
Langerhans cell histiocytosis (LCH), orbital,
    671–672, 676
    bilateral sequential orbital involvement in,
        676, 679:35.19–35.24
    features, 676, 678:35.13–35.18
    management of, 676, 680:35.25–35.30
    orbital
        LCH, 680:35.25–35.30
        presentation as hemorrhagic cystic lesion,
            676, 681:35.31–35.36
LCH. See Langerhans cell histiocytosis
Leiomyoma
    in adulthood, 608
    in children, 608
    lacrimal sac, 241:14.13–14.14
    orbital, 608, 610:31.49–31.51
Leiomyosarcoma, orbital, 609,
    610:31.49–31.51
Lentigomaligna (LM), eyelid, 106,
    107:6.55–6.60
    surgical excision, 106, 108:6.61–6.66
Lentigomaligna melanoma (LMM), 106, 114
    eyelid, 109:6.67–6.72
Lesions. See also specific lesions
    conjunctival, miscellaneous, 358
    conjunctival neoplasms simulated by
        miscellaneous, 403–432
    infectious, conjunctival neoplasms
        simulated by, 418, 420:24.43–24.48,
        421:24.49–24.54
    pigmented melanoma simulated by
        miscellaneous, 430
Letterer–Siwe disease, 676
Leukemias
    conjunctiva and infiltrate of,
        389:22.25–22.30
    conjunctival, 388
Leukemic tumors, conjunctival, 379–392
Leukoplakia, CIN, 289:18.13–18.18
Lhermitte–Duclos disease, 86
Ligneous conjunctivitis, conjunctival, 416,
    417:24.37–24.42
Lipodermoid. See Dermolipoma
Lipoid proteinosis, eyelid (Urbach–Wiethe
    disease), 226, 227:13.7–13.12
Lipoma. See also Dermolipoma; Myolipoma,
    orbital; Pleomorphic lipoma, orbital;
    Spindle cell lesions
    conjunctival, 376, 377:21.27–21.28
    orbital, 662
        clinicopathologic variations, 665:34.43–34.48
Lipomatous tumors
    conjunctival, 367–377
    orbital, 653–670
Liposarcoma, orbital, 668, 669:34.55–34.60
Lymphangiectasia, conjunctival, 354,
    356:20.13–20.16
Lymphangioma
    capillary hemangioma and, 360
    conjunctival, 349, 354, 356:20.17–20.18,
        357:20.19–20.24
    diffuse, 528
    multifocal, 528
    orbital, 528
        aspiration management of, 532:28.95–28.96
        in children, 534:28.103–28.108
        clinical features, 530:28.79–28.84
        computed tomography, 531:28.85–28.88
        infantile, 533:28.97–28.102
        magnetic resonance imaging,
            531:28.89–28.90, 532:28.91–28.94
        in older adults, 535:28.109–28.114
        pathologic features, 530:28.79–28.84
    varix and, 528
Lymph nodes. See also Sentinel lymph node
    biopsy
    melanoma, conjunctival metastasis to, 333,
        347:19.163–19.168
    primary ductal carcinoma metastasis to, 720
Lymphoid hyperplasia, conjunctival benign
    reactive, 383:22.1–22.6
Lymphoid tumors
    conjunctival, 380–381
Lymphoma. See also specific lymphomas
    caruncular, 401:23.41
    conjunctival
        atypical forms, 385:22.13–22.17

radiotherapy response of, 385:*22.16*, 385:*22.18*
systemic, conjunctival, 380
eyelid involvement
advanced cases, 166:*9.13–9.18*
B-Cell, 164:*9.1–9.6*, 165:*9.7–9.12*
T-Cell, 167:*9.19–9.24*
systemic, conjunctival, 380

M

Macrovessels, conjunctival, 358, 359:*20.29*
Maffucci's syndrome, orbital cavernous hemangiomas and, 648
Malakoplakia, eyelid, 228, 229:*13.15–13.16*
Malignant hemangioendothelioma. *See* Angiosarcoma
Malignant melanoma
conjunctival, 332–333
epithelial inclusion cyst and, 403
eyelid primary, 114, 115:*6.91–6.96*
nonpigmented varieties, 116, *6.97–6.102*
organizing hematoma and, 406
pigmented varieties, 116, *6.97–6.102*
surgical excision, 117, *6.103–6.108*
Malignant peripheral nerve sheath tumor, orbital (MPNST), 570, 571:*29.71–29.72*
Malignant rhabdoid tumor, orbital, 606, 607:*31.43–31.48*
MALT. *See* Mucosa-associated lymphoid tissue
MALT lymphoma. *See* Mucosa-associated lymphoid tissue lymphoma
Mandibulofacial dysostosis, dermolipoma and, 658
Marfan's syndrome, multiple syringomas and, 67
MCA. *See* Multinucleate cell angiohistiocytoma
Melanocytic hamartoma, orbital, 689, 694, 695:*36.13–36.15*
Melanocytic nevus
conjunctival, 308–309
blue nevus variant of, 317:*19.37–19.42*
clinical variations, 314:*19.19–19.24*
extralimbal location, 315:*19.25–19.30*
giant type, 318:*19.43–19.48*
lesions with prominent cysts, 316:*19.31–19.36*
non-Caucasian, 319:*19.49–19.54*
nonpigmented type, 312:*19.7–19.12*
partially pigmented type, 313:*19.13–19.18*
pigmented type, 311:*19.1–19.6*
Melanocytic tumors
conjunctival, 307–347
primary, orbital, 689–695
Melanocytosis, ocular. *See also* Oculodermal melanocytosis
congenital, scleral involvement with, 321:*19.55–19.60*
episcleral pigment, 320
melanoma, orbital arising from, 689
scleral pigment, 320, 321:*19.55–19.60*
Melanoma. *See also specific melanomas*
caruncular, 394, 397:*23.13–23.18*
Clark classification of, 324
conjunctival
alcohol epitheliectomy, 332–333, 341:*19.127–19.132*
amelanotic variations, 340:*19.121–19.126*
brain metastasis of, 333, 347:*19.163–19.168*
cryotherapy, 332–333, 341:*19.127–19.132*
de novo-arising tumors of, 338:*19.109–19.114*, 339:*19.115–19.120*
diffuse tumors or, before/after treatment, 342:*19.133–19.138*
lymph nodes, preauricular metastasis of, 333, 347:*19.163–19.168*
in non-Caucasians, 337:*19.103–19.108*
orbital exenteration, 332–333, 346:*19.157–19.162*
PAM and evolution of, 335:*19.91–19.96*, 336:*19.97–19.102*
plaque radiotherapy for, 345:*19.151–19.156*
sentinel lymph node biopsy and localization of, 333, 344:*19.145–19.150*
surgical resection, 332–333, 341:*19.127–19.132*
tumor with scleral invasion and, 343:*19.139–19.144*
lacrimal sac, 233, 238, 239:*14.7–14.12*
orbital
arising de novo, 692, 693:*36.7–36.12*
arising from blue nevus, 689, 691:*36.1–36.6*
arising from ocular melanocytosis, 689
PAM and, 324–326, 330:*19.79–19.84*, 331:*19.85–19.90*
pigmented
conjunctival miscellaneous lesions simulating, 430, 432:*24.85–24.90*
scleral miscellaneous lesions simulating, 430
staphyloma simulating, 430, 431:*24.79–24.84*
Melanotic Freckle of Hutchinson, 106, 107:*6.55–6.60*
Melanotic neuroectodermal tumor (MNET)
infantile, 689
orbital, 689, 694, 695:*36.16–36.18*
Meningeal tumors, 573–594
Meningioma, fibrous dysplasia and, 641
Meningitis, orbital varices and, 536
Merkel cell carcinoma, 126, 128:*7.19–7.24*
clinical appearance, 126, 130:*7.31–7.36*
clinical variations, 144, 146:*8.43–8.48*
clinicopathologic correlation, 126, 129:*7.25–7.30*, 186, 189:*10.37–10.42*
follow-up, 142, 146:*8.43–8.48*
management, 126, 129:*7.25–7.30*
metastatic neoplasms to, 170, 171:*9.31–9.36*, 171:*9.37–9.42*
neurofibroma, 120
nevus flammeus, 144, 145:*8.37–8.42*
nodular fasciitis, 186, 188:*10.31–10.36*
oculodermal melanocytosis and clinical features of, 102, 104:*6.43–6.48*
with paraproteinemia, 182, 183:*10.19–10.24*
pathology, 126, 131:*7.37–7.42*
surgical technique, 126, 130:*7.31–7.36*
Metastatic neoplasms to eyelids, 170
Metastatic tumors, 171:*9.31–9.36*, 172:*9.37–9.42*
conjunctival, 379–392, 390, 391:*22.31–22.36*, 392:*22.31–22.36*
from choroidal melanoma, 173:*9.43–9.48*
from cutaneous melanoma, 392:*22.37–22.42*, 393:*22.37–22.42*
Methotrexate, eyelid KA, 14
Mitomycin
childhood conjunctival papilloma, 268
CIN, 268
conjunctival invasive SCC, 293
Mitomycin C (MMC)
CIN, 286
MMC. *See* Mitomycin C
MNET. *See* Melanotic neuroectodermal tumor
Molluscum contagiosum infection
conjunctival, 418, 420:*24.44*
eyelid, 207, 209:*12.1–12.6*
MPNST. *See* Malignant peripheral nerve sheath tumor, orbital
MTS. *See* Muir–Torre syndrome
Mucoepidermoid carcinoma, 722
lacrimal gland, 697–698, 721:*37.79–37.84*
SCC, conjunctival, 305:*18.85–18.90*
Mucormycosis
eyelid, 218, 219:*12.28–12.30*
Mucosa-associated lymphoid tissue (MALT) lymphoma, 379
lacrimal sac, 241:*14.17–14.18*
Muir–Torre syndrome (MTS), 49
epidermal inclusion cyst, eyelid and, 202
KA, eyelid and, 14
sebaceous carcinoma, eyelid and, 52, 59:*3.31–3.36*
sebaceous gland tumors and, 49
Multinucleate cell angiohistiocytoma, orbital (MCA), 671, 687, 688:*35.52–35.54*
Multiple endocrine neoplasia type 2b, neuromas and, 367
Mycotic infections
eyelid, 218, 219:*12.25–12.30*
Myofibroma
infants, 616, 619:*32.19–32.24*
orbital, 616, 619:*32.19–32.24*
Myofibromatosis, orbital, 616
Myogenic tumors, orbital, 595–610
Myolipoma, orbital, 662
Myxoma
conjunctival, 376, 377:*21.25–21.26*
orbital, 666, 667:*34.49–34.54*
Myxomatous tumors
conjunctival, 367–377
orbital, 653–670

N

Necrobiotic xanthogranuloma (NXG)
eyelid, 686
orbital, 686, 688:*35.49–35.51*
with paraproteinemia
orbital, 682, 686
Necrotizing fasciitis, eyelid, 220, 221:*12.33–12.36*
Neomycin, eyelid BCC, 31
Neoplasms
conjunctival
Churg–Strauss allergic granulomatosis simulating, 414, 415:*24.31–24.36*
miscellaneous infectious lesions simulating, 418, 420:*24.43–24.48*, 421:*24.49–24.54*

Neoplasms (*continued*)
  miscellaneous lesions simulating, 403–432
  cystic lesions, eyelid simulating, 195–205
  episcleritis simulating, 412
  eyelid miscellaneous conditions simulating, 223–231
  inflammatory lesions simulating eyelid, 207–221
  lacrimal sac, 233
  malignant, sunlight exposure and eyelid, 24
  scleritis simulating, 412
Nervous system, malignant rhabdoid tumor extension into, 607:*31.43–31.48*
Neural tumors, 573–594
  conjunctival, 367–377
  orbital, miscellaneous, 568–570
Neurilemoma. *See* Schwannoma
Neuritis, optic, 582
Neuroblastoma. *See also specific neuroblastomas*
  orbital primary, 593, 594:*30.64–30.66*
  PNET classification and, 592
Neurofibroma
  eyelid, 120
  conjunctival, 367–368, 369:*21.1–21.6*
  diffuse
    conjunctival, 367–368, 369:*21.1–21.6*
    orbital, 556
  episcleral, conjunctival, 369:*21.4–21.6*
  localized, 122:*7.1–7.6*, 556
  multiple circumscribed, 561:*29.43–29.48*
  neurofibromatosis and, 558:*29.25–29.30*, 559:*29.31–29.36*
  orbital, 556, 560:*29.37–29.42*
    multiple circumscribed type of, 561:*29.43–29.48*
  plexiform, 123:*7.7–7.12*
    amputation neuroma and, 569
    conjunctival, 367–368, 369:*21.3*
    orbital, 556
  solitary
    conjunctival, 368–369
    orbital, 560:*29.37–29.42*
Neurofibromatosis
  JPA and, 574
  malignant melanoma, conjunctival and, 332
  neurofibroma and, 559:*29.31–29.36*
    orbital, 558:*29.25–29.30*
  PAM and, 324
Neuroma
  amputation, orbital, 569
  conjunctival, 368–369
Nevoid BCC syndrome, 30, 31, 37:*2.55–2.60*
  with multiple cutaneous malignancies, 38:*2.61–2.66*
  with odontogenic keratocyst, 39:*2.67–2.72*
Nevus. *See also specific forms of nevus*
  caruncular, 393, 396:*23.12–23.17*
Nodular fasciitis (pseudosarcomatous fasciitis)
  in children, 611, 614:*32.1–32.6*
  conjunctival, 374, 375:*21.21–21.22*
  orbital, 611, 614:*32.1–32.6*, 615:*32.7–32.9*
Non-Hodgkin lymphoma
  B-cell
    conjunctival, 379–380
    conjunctival, 384:*22.7–22.12*
Nonne–Milroy–Meige disease, 354
Nonspecific keratosis, eyelid, 14, 18:*1.49–1.54*
NXG. *See* Necrobiotic xanthogranuloma

O

Ocular melanocytosis
  clinical features, 104:*6.43–6.48*
  congenital spectrum of pigmentation, 105:*6.49–6.54*
Ocular surface squamous neoplasia (OSSN), 286
Oculodermalmelanocytosis (Nevus of Ota), 102
  blue nevus and, 110
  clinical features of, 104:*6.43–6.48*
  congenital, pigmentation spectrum of, 105:*6.49–6.54*
Odontogenic keratocyst, nevoid BCC syndrome with, 39:*2.67–2.72*
Ollier's disease, multiple enchondromas and, 648
Oncocytoma, caruncular, 393, 398:*23.19–23.24*
ONSM. *See* Optic nerve sheath meningioma
Onychodystrophy, apocrine hidrocystoma and, 198
Optic nerves
  astrocytoma, malignant, 516, 581:*30.25–30.30*
  cavernous hemangioma, orbital and compression of, 516, 520:*28.37–28.42*
  glioma, 574, 576:*30.1–30.6*, 578:*30.13–30.18*
    fundus changes, 574, 579:*30.19–30.24*
    magnetic resonance imaging, 577:*30.7–30.12*
  JPA, 574, 576:*30.1–30.6*, 578:*30.13–30.18*
    fundus changes, 574, 579:*30.19–30.24*
    magnetic resonance imaging, 574, 577:*30.7–30.12*
  tumors, 573–594
Optic nerve sheath meningioma (ONSM), 582–583, 585:*30.31–30.36*
  aggressive variant, 587:*30.43–30.48*
  magnetic resonance imaging, 583, 586:*30.37–30.42*
Orbit
  adult-onset-associated xanthogranuloma, 671, 675:*35.7–35.12*
  amputation, orbital, 569, 571:*29.69–29.70*
  aneurysmal bone cyst, 638
  angiolipoma, 662
  angiosarcoma, 544, 545:*28.145–28.150*
  ASPS, 564, 566:*29.55–29.60*
    aggressive tumor in child, 567:*29.61–29.66*
  brown tumor of hyperparathyroidism, 638
  capillary hemangioma, 509–510, 512:*28.1–28.6*
    adnexal/eyelid involvement, simultaneous in, 509, 514:*28.13–28.18*
    clinical variations, 509, 513:*28.7–28.12*
    regression, 509, 513:*28.7–28.12*
    surgical resection of, 510, 515:*28.19–28.24*
  cartilaginous hamartoma, 648, 649:*33.49–33.54*
  cartilaginous tumors, 631–652
  cavernous hemangioma, 516, 518:*28.25–28.30*
    clinicopathologic correlation, 516, 521:*28.43–28.48*
    globe/optic nerve compression, 516, 520:*28.37–28.42*
    intraosseous type, 516, 523:*28.55–28.60*
    supertemporal orbitotomy, 516, 521:*28.43–28.48*
    supranasal orbitotomy, 516, 522:*28.49–28.54*
    surgical removal of, by conjunctival approach, 516, 519:*28.31–28.36*
  chondroma, 648, 649:*33.49–33.54*
  chondrosarcoma, 650, 651:*33.55–33.60*
    in young woman, 652:*33.61–33.66*
  dermolipoma, 658, 659:*34.19–34.24*
    age range, 659:*34.19–34.24*
    clinical features of, 658, 660:*34.25–34.30*
    clinical spectrum, 659:*34.19–34.24*
    computed tomography features of, 658, 660:*34.25–34.30*
    Goldenhar syndrome and, 658, 661:*34.31–34.36*
    histopathologic features of, 658, 660:*34.25–34.30*
  ECD, 671, 682, 683:*35.37–35.42*
  fat prolapse, 653–654, 655:*34.1–34.6*, 656:*34.7–34.12*
    clinical features of, 657:*34.13–34.18*
    computed tomography features of, 657:*34.13–34.18*
    surgical approach, 657:*34.13–34.18*
  FH, 620
    benign, 620, 621:*32.25–32.30*
    malignant, 620, 622:*32.31–32.36*
    management of, 620, 623:*32.37–32.42*
  fibroma, 613, 615:*32.10–32.12*
  fibromatosis, 616, 618:*32.13–32.18*
  fibro-osseous tumors, 631–652
  fibrosarcoma, 628, 629:*32.55–32.60*
  fibrous dysplasia, 638, 640:*33.19–33.24*, 641:*33.25–33.30*
  GCRG, 638, 646, 647:*33.43–33.48*
  GCT, 568, 571:*29.67–29.68*
  giant cell tumor, 638
  glomus tumor, 542, 543:*28.142–28.144*
  hemangiopericytoma, 524
    aggressive tumor with brain invasion, 527:*28.73–28.78*
    clinicopathologic correlation, 525:*28.61–28.66*, 526:*28.67–28.72*
    recurrence, 524
  hematoma, 546
  hemorrhagic lesions, 509–547
  histiocytic tumors, 671–688
  IPEH, 542, 543:*28.142–28.144*
  JXG, 671–672, 674:*35.1–35.6*
  LCH, 671–672, 676
    bilateral sequential orbital involvement in, 676, 679:*35.19–35.24*
    features, 676, 678:*35.13–35.18*
    management of, 676, 680:*35.25–35.30*
    presentation as hemorrhagic cystic lesion, 676, 681:*35.31–35.36*
  leiomyoma, 595, 608, 610:*31.49–31.51*
  leiomyosarcoma, 595, 609, 610:*31.49–31.51*
  lipoma, 662
    clinicopathologic variations, 665:*34.43–34.48*
  lipomatous tumors, 653–670
  liposarcoma, 668, 669:*34.55–34.60*
  lymphangioma, 528
    aspiration management of, 532:*28.95–28.96*

in children, 534:*28.103–28.108*
clinical features, 530:*28.79–28.84*
computed tomography,
  531:*28.85–28.88*
infantile, 533:*28.97–28.102*
magnetic resonance imaging,
  531:*28.89–28.90*, 532:*28.91–28.94*
in older adults, 535:*28.109–28.114*
pathologic features, 530:*28.79–28.84*
malignant rhabdoid tumor, 606,
  607:*31.43–31.48*
MCA, 671, 687, 688:*35.52–35.54*
melanocytic hamartoma, 689, 694,
  695:*36.13–36.15*
melanocytic tumors, primary, 689–695
melanoma
  arising de novo, 692, 693:*36.7–36.12*
  arising from blue nevus, 689,
    691:*36.1–36.6*
  arising from ocular melanocytosis, 689
MNET, 689, 694, 695:*36.16–36.18*
MPNST, 570, 571:*29.71–29.72*
myofibroma, 616, 619:*32.19–32.24*
myofibromatosis, 616
myogenic tumors, 595–610
myolipoma, 662
myxoma, 666, 667:*34.49–34.54*
myxomatous tumors, 653–670
neuroblastoma, primary, 593, 594:*30.64–30.66*
neurofibroma, 556
  multiple circumscribed type of,
    561:*29.43–29.48*
  neurofibromatosis and,
    558:*29.25–29.30*
  solitary, 560:*29.37–29.42*
nodular fasciitis, 611, 614:*32.1–32.6*,
  615:*32.7–32.9*
NXG, 682, 686, 688:*35.49–35.51*
organizing hematoma, 546,
  547:*28.151–28.156*
osseous tumors, 631–652
ossifying fibroma, 638, 642,
  643:*33.31–33.36*, 644:*33.37–33.42*
osteoma, 631–632, 634:*33.1–33.6*
  clinicopathologic correlation,
    635:*33.7–33.12*
  imaging correlation, 635:*33.7–33.12*
osteosarcoma, 636, 637:*33.15–33.18*
paraganglioma, 562, 563:*29.49–29.54*
peripheral nerve tumors, 549–571
pleomorphic lipoma, 662,
  664:*34.37–34.42*
PNET, 592, 594:*30.61–30.63*
pseudotumors, 671–688
RD disease, 684, 685:*35.43–35.48*
rhabdomyoma, 595
RMS, 595–597, 599:*31.1–31.6*,
  600:*31.7–31.12*
  advanced aggressive cases of,
    605:*31.37–31.42*
  biopsy approach, 603:*31.25–31.30*
  clinical features, 601:*31.13–31.18*
  magnetic resonance imaging,
    601:*31.13–31.18*
  pathology, 601:*31.13–31.18*
  presentation as conjunctival mass,
    602:*31.19–31.24*
  presentation as epibulbar mass,
    604:*31.31–31.36*

simulating orbital hematoma in child,
  604:*31.31–31.36*
SCC and invasion of, conjunctival,
  303:*18.73–18.78*
schwannoma, 550, 552:*29.1–29.6*,
  553:*29.7–29.12*, 554:*29.13–29.18*
  intracranial extension, 555:*29.19–29.24*
SFT, 624, 626:*32.43–32.48*
  with slow-onset recurrence,
    627:*32.49–32.54*
SHML, 671, 684, 685:*35.43–35.48*
SWM, 583
SWM and involvement of,
  590:*30.49–30.54*, 591:*30.55–30.60*
tumors
  neural, miscellaneous, 568–570
varix, 536
  anteriorly located lesion of,
    541:*28.133–28.138*
  color Doppler imaging,
    540:*28.131–28.132*
  computed tomography, 540:*28.127–28.128*
  imaging, 540:*28.127–28.132*
  intracranial venous pressure increase
    demonstrating, 538:*28.115–28.120*
  magnetic resonance imaging,
    540:*28.129–28.130*
  Valsalva maneuver demonstrating,
    539:*28.121–28.126*
vascular lesions, 509–547
  miscellaneous, 543
venous malformations, 536
Orbital angiolymphoid hyperplasia with
  eosinophilia and Kimura disease,
  469:*26.67–26.72*
Orbital aspergillosis, 461
Orbital Burkitt lymphoma, 760, 761:*39.49–39.54*
Orbital cephalocele, 496
  anterior (ethmoidal) type, 498:*27.97–27.102*
  posterior (sphenoidal) type, 499:*27.103–27.108*
Orbital colobomatous cyst, 493:*27.79–27.84*
  bilateral occurrence, clinicopathologic
    correlation, 494:*27.85–27.90*
  clinical variations, ultrasonography, and
    pathology, 495:*27.91–27.96*
Orbital congenital cystic eye, 490
  discovered in utero, 491:*27.73–27.78*
Orbital dermoid cyst, 472
  deep orbital type, 479:*27.31–27.36*
  dumbbell type, 477:*27.19–27.24*
  surgical resection, 478:*27.25–27.30*
  lesion of conjunctival origin in an adult,
    476:*27.13–27.18*
  lesion of conjunctival origin in a child,
    475:*27.7–27.12*
  typical case of epidermal origin,
    474:*27.1–27.6*
Orbital exenteration
  melanoma, conjunctival, 332–333,
    346:*19.157–19.162*
  tumor, eyelid, 243
Orbital granulomatosis with polyangiitis
  (Wegener granulomatosis), 466,
  467:*26.61–26.66*
Orbital hydatid cyst, 507:*27.127–27.132*,
  508:*27.133–27.138*
Orbital inflammation, idiopathic
  nongranulomatous
  in adulthood, 452:*26.19–26.24*

clinical and radiologic spectrum,
  453:*26.25–26.30*
childhood, 454:*26.31–26.36*
Orbital invasion from eyelid basal cell
  carcinoma, 773:*40.1–40.6*
  simulating a primary lacrimal gland tumor,
    774:*40.7–40.12*
Orbital invasion from eyelid melanoma,
  775:*40.13–40.18*
  conjunctival squamous cell carcinoma,
    776:*40.19–40.24*
  conjunctival melanoma, 777:*40.25–40.30*
  young African American, 778:*40.31–40.36*
Orbital invasion from uveal melanoma
  massive choroidal melanoma,
    780:*40.43–40.48*
  massive orbital involvement, 779:*40.37–40.42*
  massive unrecognized retinoblastoma,
    782:*40.55–40.60*
  nasopharyngeal cancers, 784:*40.67–40.72*
  paranasal sinus cancers, 783:*40.61–40.66*
  retinoblastoma, 781:*40.49–40.54*
Orbital lacrimal gland lymphoma
  magnetic resonance imaging correlations,
    750:*39.13–39.18*
Orbital lymphoid tumors and leukemias, 743
Orbital lymphoma
  and cutaneous T-cell lymphoma,
    753:*39.25–39.30*
  with microvillous projections,
    753:*39.25–39.30*
Orbital metastatic cancer, 725
  of adrenal neuroblastoma, 740:*38.73–38.78*
  biopsy techniques, 731:*38.19–38.24*
  from breast cancer, 728:*38.1–38.6*
  from carcinoid tumor, 733:*38.31–38.36*
  from choroidal melanoma, 737:*38.55–38.60*
  contralateral orbit, 738:*38.61–38.66*
  clinical variations 729:*38.7–38.12*
  from cutaneous melanoma, 736:*38.49–38.54*
  Ewing's tumor, 741:*38.79–38.84*
  histopathology of, 726
  from lung cancer, 734:*38.37–38.42*
  paradoxical enophthalmos, 730:*38.13–38.18*
  from prostate carcinoma, 732:*38.25–38.30*
  from renal cell carcinoma, 735:*38.43–38.48*
  rhabdomyosarcoma, 741:*38.79–38.84*
  from thyroid cancer, 739:*38.67–38.72*
  unknown primary site, 739:*38.67–38.72*
  Wilms' tumor, 741:*38.79–38.84*
Orbital mucocele, 500, 502:*27.109–27.114*
  clinical, imaging, and histopathologic
    correlations:503:*27.115–27.120*
Orbital mucormycosis, 460
Orbital mycotic infections
  aspergillosis and mucormycosis,
    463:*26.49–26.54*
Orbital myeloid sarcoma (Leukemia), 766,
  768:*39.67–39.72*
  bilateral orbital involvement,
    769:*39.739.78*
Orbital non-Hodgkin lymphoma, 744–746
  clinical variations and pathology,
    749:*39.7–39.12*
  computed tomography, 748:*39.1–39.6*
  diagnosis and management,
    751:*39.19–39.24*
  magnetic resonance imaging features,
    748:*39.1–39.6*

Orbital parasitic cysts, 506
Orbital plasmablastic lymphoma, 759:39.43–39.48
Orbital plasmacytoma
  association with multiple myeloma, 757:39.37–39.42
  lymphoplasmacytoid tumors, 756:39.31–39.36
Orbital post-transplant lymphoproliferative disorder, 762, 764:39.55–39.60, 765:39.61–39.66
Orbital respiratory epithelial cyst, 504, 505:27.121–27.126
Orbital sarcoidosis, 464, 465:26.55–26.60
Orbital secondary tumors, 771–772
Orbital surgery
  cosmetic rehabilitation, 794:41.37–41.42
  cutaneous superonasal approach, 789:41.7–41.12
  cutaneous superotemporal approach, 790:41.13–41.18, 791:41.19–41.24
  exenteration:792:41.25–41.30
    prostheses, 793:41.31–41.36
  instrumentation and conjunctival approach, 788:41.1–41.6
Orbital teratoma (teratomatous cyst), 486, 489:27.67–27.72
  discovered in utero, 488:27.61–27.66
Orbital tuberculosis, 459:26.43–26.48
Orbital tumors, surgical management of, 785–787
Organizing hematoma (hematic cyst, hematocele)
  conjunctival, 406
    secondary to silicone sponge for retinal detachment repair, 407:24.7–24.12
  orbital, 546, 547:28.151–28.156
Organoid nevus syndrome
  dermolipoma and, 658
  epibulbar complex choristomas associated with, 264, 266:16.49–16.54
Orthokeratosis, eyelid actinic keratosis and, 19
Osseous tumors, orbital, 631–652
Ossifying fibroma
  orbital, 638, 642, 643:33.31–33.36, 644:33.37–33.42
  psammomatoid, 642
OSSN. See Ocular surface squamous neoplasia
Osteoclastoma. See Giant cell tumor, orbital
Osteogenic sarcoma. See Osteosarcoma
Osteoma
  cancellous, 631–632
  compact (ivory), 631–632
  fibrous, 631
  orbital, 631–632, 634:33.1–33.6
    clinicopathologic correlation, 635:33.7–33.12
    imaging correlation, 635:33.7–33.12
Osteosarcoma (osteogenic sarcoma)
  in children, 636, 637:33.15–33.18
  orbital, 636, 637:33.15–33.18
  primary, 636
  secondary, 636

P

Palmar-plantar hyperkeratosis, apocrine hidrocystoma and, 198
PAM. See Primary acquired melanosis
Papilloma, caruncular, 393, 395:23.1–23.6

Papilloma, conjunctival
  of adulthood, 272, 274:17.13–17.18
    atypical variations of, 272, 275:17.19–17.24
  of childhood, 267–268, 270:17.1–17.6
    cimetidine management of, 268, 271:17.7–17.12
Paraganglioma (Chemodectoma)
  ASPS and, 562, 564
  orbital, 562, 563:29.49–29.54
PEH. See Pseudoepitheliomatous hyperplasia
PEMLG. See Primary epithelial malignancies of lacrimal gland
Pentagonal full-thickness excision with semicircular flap, eyelid tumor, 247:15.13–15.18
Periorbital dermatitis, eyelid molluscum contagiosum infection and, 207
Peripheral nerve tumors, orbital, 549–571. See also Malignant peripheral nerve sheath tumor, orbital
Phakomatous choristoma, eyelid (Zimmerman's tumor), 230, 231:13.19–13.24
Pilar cyst. See Sebaceous cyst, eyelid
Pilomatrix carcinoma, 88
Pilomatrixoma, eyelid, 88
  in adults, 89:5.19–5.24
  in children (surgical excision), 90:5.25–5.30
  histopathology, 91:5.31–5.36
  surgical excision, 91:5.31–5.36
Pinguecula, 426, 427:24.67–24.72
Plaque radiotherapy
  melanoma, conjunctival, 345:19.151–19.156
  pyogenic granuloma, conjunctival treatment with, 350, 353:20.7–20.12
Plasmacytic tumors
  conjunctiva, 380–381
Plasmin, ligneous conjunctivitis, 416
Pleomorphic adenocarcinoma, lacrimal gland, 722
  histopathology, 724:37.88
Pleomorphic adenoma (benign mixed tumor)
  eyelid, 74, 75:4.19–4.24
  lacrimal glands, 697–698, 702, 709:37.67–37.72
    clinicopathologic correlation, 704:37.13–37.18
    magnetic resonance imaging, 707:37.31–37.36
    surgical management, 705:37.19–37.24
    in teenager, 706:37.25–37.30
Pleomorphic lipoma, orbital, 662, 664:34.37–34.42
PNET. See Primary neuroectodermal tumor, orbital
Porocarcinoma, 76, 79:4.35–4.36
Porosyringoma, 70
Post-transplant lymphoproliferative disorder (PTLD)
  conjunctival, 386, 387:22.19–22.24
  EBV and, 386, 387:22.24
Precancerous melanosis, 324
Primary acquired melanosis (PAM), 233
  conjunctival, 324–325
    melanoma and, 324, 330:19.79–19.84, 331:19.85–19.90
    mild involvement of, 328:19.67–19.72
    moderately severe, 329:19.73–19.78

malignant melanoma, conjunctival and, 332
melanoma, conjunctival evolution from, 335:19.91–19.96, 336:19.97–19.102
with/without atypia, 324–325
Primary ductal carcinoma
  lacrimal glands, 718, 720:37.73–37.78
  lymph node metastasis of, 720
Primary epithelial malignancies of lacrimal gland (PEMLG), 698
  histopathology of, 722
Primary neuroectodermal tumor, orbital (PNET), 592, 594:30.61–30.63
Psammomatoid ossifying fibroma, 642
Pseudoepitheliomatous hyperplasia (PEH)
  conjunctival, 276, 277:17.25
  eyelid, 12, 13:1.25–1.30
  GCT, conjunctival and, 370
Pseudohypopyon, 403
Pseudoneoplastic lesions, eyelid, 228
Pseudorheumatoid nodule, eyelid (granuloma annulare), 215, 217:2.21–2.22
Pseudosarcomatous fasciitis. See Nodular fasciitis
Pseudotumors
  lacrimal sac, 240
  orbital, 671–688
Pterygium, 428, 429:24.73–24.78
PTLD. See Post-transplant lymphoproliferative disorder
Punch biopsy, eyelid tumor, 245:15.1–15.2
Pyogenic granuloma
  caruncular, 403:23.37–23.38
  classification, 350
  conjunctival, 350
    plaque radiotherapy treatment for, 350, 353:20.7–20.12
    primary type, 352:20.1–20.6
  corneal, 350, 353
  lacrimal sac, 242:14.19–14.20
  terminology, 350

R

"Racial melanosis," 322, 323:19.61–19.66
Radiotherapy
  lymphoma, conjunctival response to, 385:22.16, 385:22.18
  plaque, conjunctival melanoma, 345:19.151–19.156
RD disease. See Rosai–Dorfman (RD) disease
Reticulohistiocytoma, conjunctival, 376, 377:21.29–21.30
Retin-A. See Tretinoin
Retinal detachment
  silicone sponge for, organizing hematoma secondary to, 407:24.7–24.12
Retinoblastoma
  leiomyosarcoma and, 609
  malignant rhabdoid tumor and, 606
  osteosarcoma and, 636
Rhabdomyoma, orbital, 595
Rhabdomyosarcoma (RMS)
  alveolar type, 596
  botryoid type, 596
  childhood, 595–596
  embryonal, 596
  metastasis, 596
  MPNST and, 570

orbital, 595–597, 599:*31.1–31.6*, 600:*31.7–31.12*
    advanced aggressive cases of, 605:*31.37–31.42*
    biopsy approach, 603:*31.25–31.30*
    clinical features, 601:*31.13–31.18*
    magnetic resonance imaging, 601:*31.13–31.18*
    pathology, 601:*31.13–31.18*
    presentation as conjunctival mass, 602:*31.19–31.24*
    presentation as epibulbar mass, 604:*31.31–31.36*
    simulating orbital hematoma in child, 604:*31.31–31.36*
Rhinosporidiosis, conjunctival, 418, 420:*24.47–24.48*
Rituximab, conjunctival lymphoma, 381
RMS. *See* Rhabdomyosarcoma
Rosai–Dorfman (RD) disease, orbital, 684, 685:*35.43–35.48*

S

Salicylic acid, eyelid molluscum contagiosum infection, 207
Sarcoidosis
    conjunctival, 218, 421:*24.49–24.50*
    eyelid, 214, 217:*2.19–2.20*
Sarcoma, granulocytic, 388. *See also specific sarcomas*
SCC. *See* Squamous cell carcinoma
Schöpf–Schulz–Passarge syndrome, 198
Schwann cells, 549
Schwannoma (neurilemoma)
    conjunctival, 370, 371:*21.7–21.10*
    epibulbar, conjunctival, 371:*21.7–21.10*
    orbital, 550, 552:*29.1–29.6*, 553:*29.7–29.12*, 554:*29.13–29.18*
    intracranial extension, 555:*29.19–29.24*
Sclera
    melanoma, conjunctival and tumor invasion in, 343:*19.139–19.144*
    ocular melanocytosis pigmentation and, 320, 321:*19.55–19.60*
    pigmented melanoma simulated by miscellaneous lesions of, 430
    staphyloma, melanoma simulated by, 430, 431:*24.79–24.84*
Scleritis, 412, 413:*24.29–24.30*
    neoplasms simulating, 412
    nodular, 412, 413:*24.27–24.28*
Sebaceous carcinoma
    lacrimal gland, 722
Sebaceous carcinoma, eyelid, 51–53
    aggressive clinical course, 61:*3.43–3.48*
    clinical variations, 58:*3.25–3.30*
    comedocarcinoma, 52
    diffuse neoplasm, 60:*3.37–3.42*
    diffuse neoplasm masquerading as inflammation, 56:*3.13–3.18*
    histopathology, 58:*3.25–3.30*
    large tumor and rotational forehead flap, 64:*3.61–3.66*
    lobular, 52
    meibomian gland origin, 54:*3.1–3.6*
    mixed, 52
    MTS associated with, 52, 59:*3.31–3.36*
    papillary, 52
    pedunculated variant of, 57:*3.19–3.24*
    pentagonal full-thickness eyelid resection, 62:*3.49–3.54*
    pentagonal resection, 63:*3.55–3.60*
    periocular gland, classification of, 51:*3.1t*
    posterior lamellar eyelid resection and reconstruction, 65:*3.67–3.72*
    semicircular flap reconstruction, 63:*3.55–3.60*
    Zeis gland origin, 55:*3.7–3.12*
Sebaceous cyst, eyelid (pilar cyst), 200, 201:*11.13–11.18*
Sebaceous nevus, eyelid, 28
    association with periocular, 29:*2.25–2.30*
Sebaceous tumors
    caruncular, 393, 399:*23.25–23.30*
    eyelid and gland, 49–65
    gland, 49–65
Seborrheic keratosis, eyelid (SK), 6, 8:*1.7–1.12*, 9:*1.13–1.18*
    acanthotic type, 6, 8:*1.11*
Sentinel lymph node biopsy, conjunctival melanoma localization and, 333, 344:*19.145–19.150*
Serratia marcescens abscess, conjunctival, 418, 421:*24.51–24.54*
SFT. *See* Solitary fibrous tumor
Shaving biopsy, eyelid tumor, 243, 245:*15.3–15.4*
SHML. *See* Sinus histiocytosis with massive lymphadenopathy
"Sign of Leser-Trelat"
    IFK, eyelid and, 10
    SK, eyelid and, 6
Silicone sponge for retinal detachment, organizing hematoma secondary to, 407:*24.7–24.12*
Sinus histiocytosis with massive lymphadenopathy, orbital (SHML), 671, 684, 685:*35.43–35.48*
SK. *See* Seborrheic keratosis, eyelid
Skin flap, eyelid tumor, 243
Skin graft, eyelid tumor, 243, 245:*15.6*
Solitary fibrous tumor (SFT), 524
    fibroma, orbital and, 613
    fibrosarcoma diagnosis and, 628
    orbital, 624, 626:*32.43–32.48*
        with slow-onset recurrence, 627:*32.49–32.54*
Sphenoid wing meningioma (SWM), 582
    orbital, 583
    orbital involvement, 590:*30.49–30.54*, 591:*30.55–30.60*
Spindle cell lesions
    fibroma, orbital and, 613
    fibrosarcoma diagnosis and, 628
    SFT and, 624
Spindle cell lipoma, 662
Squamous carcinoma, lacrimal sac, 233, 236, 237:*14.1–14.6*
Squamous cell carcinoma (SCC)
    conjunctival
        advanced invasive type of, 298:*18.43–18.48*
        atypical variations, 301:*18.61–18.66*
        early invasive type, 297:*18.37–18.42*
        en bloc eye wall resection for, 302:*18.67–18.72*
        intraocular invasion, 304:*18.79–18.84*
        orbital invasion, 303:*18.73–18.78*
        papillomatous corneal involvement, extensive in, 300:*18.55–18.60*
        sunlight exposure and, 296:*18.31–18.36*
        tarsal conjunctiva involvement in, 299:*18.49–18.54*
    cutaneous actinic keratosis, eyelid associated with, 23:*2.7–2.12*
    eyelid, 43–44, 45:*2.91–2.96*
        aggressive invasive tumors in, 47:*2.103–2.108*
        deep cystic recurrent tumors in, 48:*2.109–2.114*
        diffuse involvement of upper eyelid in, 46:*2.97–2.102*
    invasive, 286
        conjunctival, 292–294
        eyelid, 43, 47:*2.103–2.108*
    lacrimal gland, 722
    lacrimal sac, 233
    mucoepidermoid, 292
        conjunctival, intraocular invasion, 305:*18.85–18.90*
    PEH, eyelid and, 12
    primary, 722
    in situ, eyelid, 43
    spindle cell, 292
Squamous cell neoplasia, epithelial, 286
Squamous papilloma, 3–4
    eyelid, 3–4, 5:*1.1–1.6*
        multiple, 3
        pedunculated, 3, 5:*1.2–1.5*
        sessile, 3, 5:*1.1*
        solitary, 3
    lacrimal sac, 233, 236, 237:*14.5–14.6*
Staphylococcus aureus
    abscess
        conjunctival, 418, 420:*24.43*
        eyelid, 220
Staphyloma, 430
    melanoma simulated by, 430, 431:*24.79–24.84*
Steven–Johnson syndrome
    epithelial inclusion cyst and, 403
Strawberry hemangioma. *See* Congenital capillary hemangioma, eyelid
Strontium-90, CIN, 286
Sturge–Weber syndrome
    cavernous hemangioma, conjunctival and, 358
Subepidermal calcified nodule, eyelid, 228, 229:*13.17–13.18*
Sunlight exposure
    CIN and, 286
    malignant melanoma and conjunctival, 332
    malignant neoplasms, eyelid and, 24
    SCC, conjunctival, 296:*18.31–18.36*
Supertemporal orbitotomy, orbital cavernous hemangioma, 516, 521:*28.43–28.48*
Supranasal orbitotomy, orbital cavernous hemangioma, 516, 522:*28.49–28.54*
Surveillance, Epidemiology, and End Results program, conjunctival melanoma and, 332
Sweat glands
    eccrine, adenocarcinoma of, 76, 78:*4.25*
    eccrine acrospiroma of, 70, 71:*4.7–4.12*
    mucinous, adenocarcinoma of, 76, 78:*4.25–4.30*
    tumors, eyelid, 67–79
SWM. *See* Sphenoid wing meningioma

Syringocystadenoma papilliferum, eyelid, 72, 73:*4.13–4.18*
Syringoma
  chondroid, 74
  eyelid, 67, 68, 69:*4.1–4.6*

T

Tagamet. *See* Cimetidine
TB. *See* Tuberculosis
T-cell lymphoma, 166
  eyelid involvement in, 167:*9.19–9.24*
Thalidomide, eyelid sarcoidosis, 214
Thyroid-related ophthalmopathy, 443, 446:*26.1–26.6*
  clinical and radiologic variations, 447:*26.7–26.12*
  orbital cellulitis and abscess, 449:*26.13–26.18*
Tretinoin (Retin-A), 207
Trichilemmal carcinoma, 87:*5.17*, 87:*5.18*
Trichilemmoma
  eyelid, 86, 87:*5.13–5.18*
  multiple facial, 86
Trichloroacetic acid
  apocrine hidrocystoma, 198
Trichloroacetic acid, eyelid sebaceous gland tumors, 49
Trichoadenoma, eyelid, 84, 85:*5.7–5.12*
Trichoepithelioma
  eyelid, 81, 82, 83:*5.1–5.6*
  multiple, 81
  solitary, 81
  facial, 83:*5.1–5.6*
Trichofolliculoma, eyelid, 84, 85:*5.7–5.12*
Triton tumor, 570
Tuberculosis (TB)
  conjunctival, 418, 420:*24.45*
Tumors. *See also specific tumors*
  caruncular, miscellaneous, 393, 401:*23.37–23.42*
  conjunctiva
    secondary, 390
  conjunctival, 249–440, 367–377
    epithelium, malignant, 283–305
    epithelium, premalignant, 283–305
  eyelid, 1–248
    elliptical excision, 246:*15.7–15.12*
    epidermis, benign, 3–18
    hair follicle, 81–91
    lacrimal drainage system, 233–242
    malignant, 19–48
    premalignant, 19–48
    sebaceous gland, 49–65
    surgical management of, 243–248
    sweat gland, 67–79
  lacrimal drainage system, eyelid, 233–242
  lacrimal sac, miscellaneous, 240, 241:*14.13–14.18*
  meningeal, 573–594
  optic nerve, 573–594
Turner's syndrome, lymphangioma and, 354

U

Urbach-Wiethe disease. *See* Lipoid proteinosis, eyelid
Uveal melanoma
  melanocytosis, ocular and, 320

V

Valsalva maneuver, orbital varix demonstrated by, 539:*28.121–28.126*
Varix
  conjunctival, 350, 358, 359:*20.25–20.26*
  lymphangioma and, 528
  orbital, 536
    anteriorly located lesion of, 541:*28.133–28.138*
    color Doppler imaging, 540:*28.131–28.132*
    computed tomography, 540:*28.127–28.128*
    imaging, 540:*28.127–28.132*
    intracranial venous pressure increase demonstrating, 538:*28.115–28.120*
    magnetic resonance imaging, 540:*28.129–28.130*
    Valsalva maneuver demonstrating, 539:*28.121–28.126*
  vortex vein, 536
Vascular lesions, orbital, 509–547
  miscellaneous, 543
Vascular tumors
  conjunctival, 349–365
Venous malformations, orbital, 536
Vimentin
  chondrosarcoma, orbital, 650
  malignant rhabdoid tumor and, 606
  SFT, 624
Von Hippel–Lindau syndrome, JPA and, 573
Vortex vein varix, 536

W

Wegener granulomatosis
  eyelid, 216, 217:*12.23–12.24*
Weibel–Palade bodies, angiosarcoma and, 544
Wilm's tumor
  malignant rhabdoid tumor and, 606

X

Xanthelasma, 178:*10.1–10.6*
  association with systemic conditions, 179:*10.7–10.12*
Xanthogranuloma
  adult-onset, 374, 671, 675:*35.7–35.12*. *See also* Juvenile xanthogranuloma
  eyelid juvenile, 180, 181:*10.13–10.18*
  eyelid juvenile fibromatosis, fibrous histiocytoma, and fibrosarcoma, 192:*10.43–10.48*
  eyelid myxoma 193:*10.49–10.54*
  eyelid necrobiotic with paraproteinemia, 182, 183:*10.19–10.24*
  multicentric reticulohistiocytosis, 193:*10.49–10.54*
Xanthoma, 176, 178:*10.1–10.6*
Xanthomatous tumors, conjunctival, 367–377
Xeroderma pigmentosum
  eyelid, 26, 27:*2.19–2.24*
  FH, conjunctival and, 372
  malignant melanoma, conjunctival and, 332

Z

Zimmerman's tumor. *See* Phakomatous choristoma, eyelid